ANNALS OF OTOLOGY, RHINOLOGY & LARYNGOLOGY

ANNALS OF HEAD AND NECK MEDICINE AND SURGERY

Founded in 1892

≈

PUBLISHED BIMONTHLY
BY THE
ANNALS PUBLISHING COMPANY

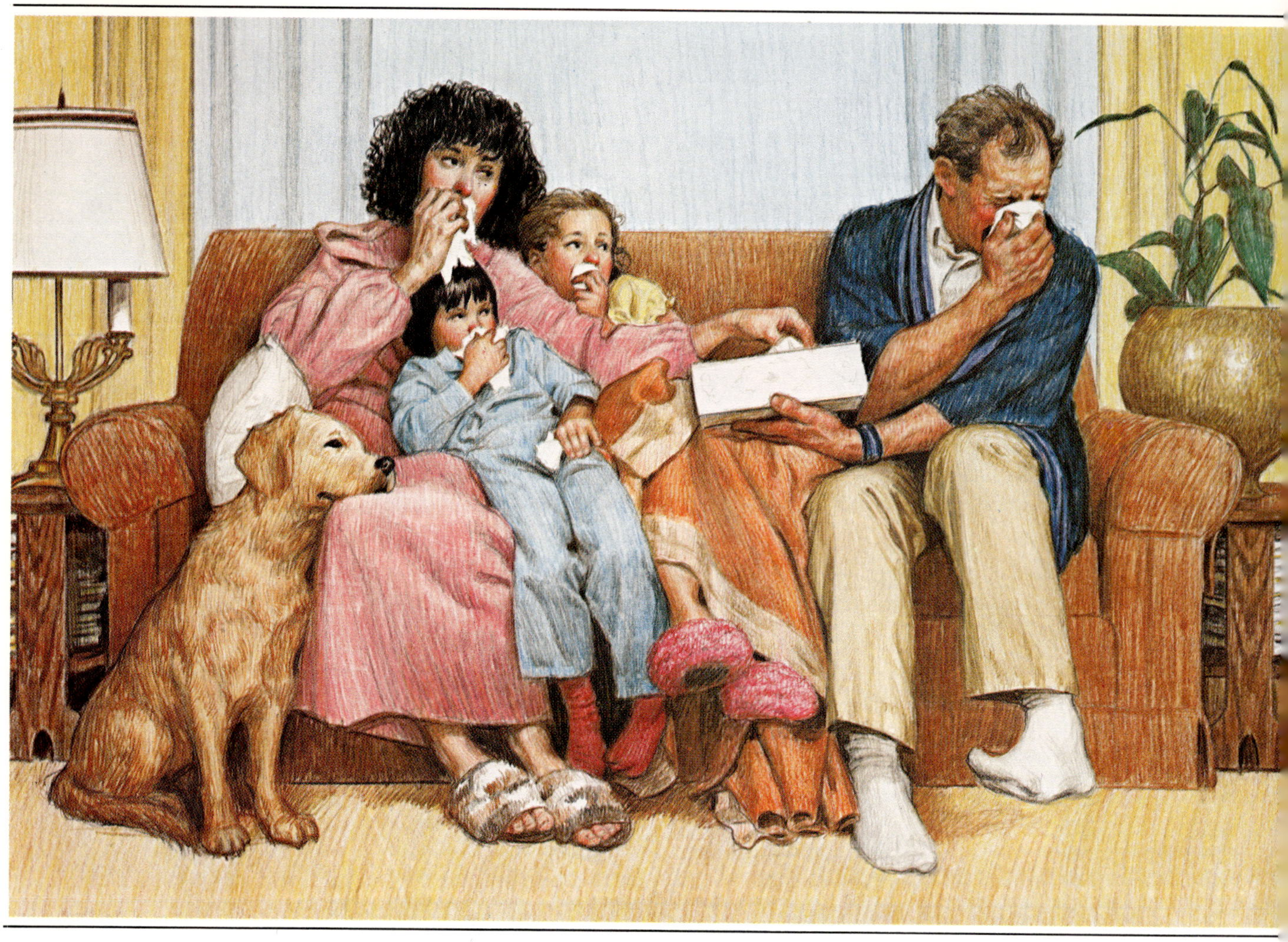

For your family of congested patients

Our family of recommendable cold products

Available without Rx

Sudafed® S.A.

(pseudoephedrine HCl) 120 mg

Sustained action nasal decongestant

Potent 12-hour relief without drowsiness!

Available in 120 mg capsules in packages of 10s and 40s.

Not recommended for children under 12 years of age.

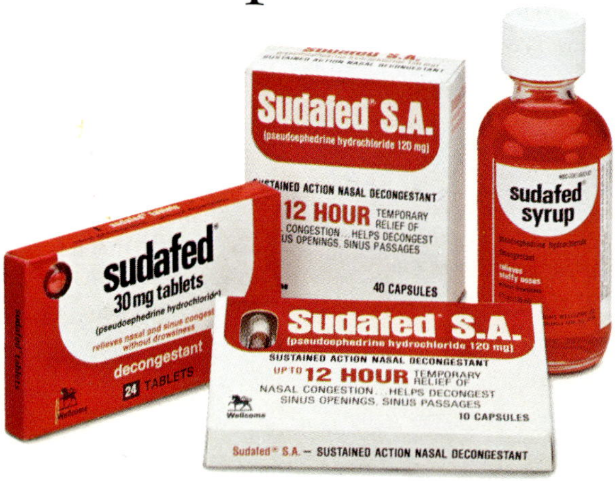

Sudafed®

(pseudoephedrine HCl) 30 mg

Unclogs the stuffy nose without closing the patient's eyes!

Available in 30 mg tablets and a tasty raspberry-flavored syrup containing 30 mg per 5 cc.

Young or old — the decongestant you can recommend with confidence has the name SUDAFED on it.

For reliable and potent decongestion without drowsiness

Wellcome

Burroughs Wellcome Co.
Research Triangle Park
North Carolina 27709

ANNALS OF OTOLOGY, RHINOLOGY AND LARYNGOLOGY

ANNALS OF HEAD AND NECK MEDICINE AND SURGERY

VOL. 91 — JANUARY-FEBRUARY 1982 — NO. 1

CONTENTS

PART I

Dedication. B. F. McCabe, MD 1

A Brief History of the *Annals* 1892-1982. B. H. Senturia, MD 2

Editorial. B. H. Senturia, MD 4

Cochlear Hydrops in Association with Collapsed Saccule and Ductus Reuniens. K. Kitamura, MD; H. F. Schuknecht, MD; R. S. Kimura, PhD 5

Spatial Occupancy of Vessels and Facial Nerve in the Facial Canal. A. Ogawa, MD, DMS; I. Sando, MD, DMS 14

Tympanometric Configurations and Middle Ear Findings in Experimental Otitis Media. G. S. Giebink, MD; K. A. Heller; E. R. Harford, PhD 20

Argon Laser Stapedotomy. B. J. Gantz, MD; H. A. Jenkins, MD; S. Kishimoto, MD; U. Fisch, MD 25

Mucormycosis of the Temporal Bone. R. Gussen, MD; R. F. Canalis, MD 27

Acute Morphological Changes in Guinea Pig Cochlea Following Electrical Stimulation. A Preliminary Scanning Electron Microscope Study. L. G. Duckert, MD, PhD; J. M. Miller, PhD 33

Intracranial Complications of Sinusitis in Children. A Sequela of Periapical Abscess. I. Brook, MS, MD; E. M. Friedman, MD 41

Vestibular Ganglion of the Squirrel Monkey. C. D. Fermin, PhD; M. Igarashi, MD 44

Revascularization of Skin Using a Myovascular Pedicle. An Animal Model for Free and Myocutaneous Flaps. R. Sergeant, FRCS; W. R. Panje, MD 53

Fluorescence Bronchoscopy. A New Technique and Further Results. D. Hürzeler, MD 57

Auditory Brainstem Responses as Indicators of Hearing Aid Performance. P. Kileny, PhD 61

Management of Paranasal Sinus Schwannomas. M. A. Shugar, MD; W. W. Montgomery, MD; E. J. Reardon, MD 65

Humoral and Cell-Mediated Immunity in Peripheral Blood Following Introduction of Antigen into the Middle Ear. A. F. Ryan, PhD; P. H. Cleveland, PhD; M. T. Hartman, BA; A. Catanzaro, MD 70

Granulocyte Proteases in Middle Ear Effusions. B. Carlsson, MD; C. Lundberg, MD; K. Ohlsson, MD 76

Comparative Anatomy of Eustachian Tube and Middle Ear Cavity in Animal Models for Otitis Media. H. J. Daniel III, PhD; R. S. Fulghum, PhD; J. E. Brinn, PhD; K. A. Barrett, MS 82

Experimental Viral Infections of the Inner Ear. III. Viremic Spread of Reovirus to Hamster Eighth Nerve Ganglion Cells. L. E. Davis, MD 90

Carcinoma of the Anterior Tongue. B. Leipzig, MD; C. W. Cummings, MD; C. T. Chung, MD; J. T. Johnson, MD; R. H. Sagerman, MD 94

Combined Pectoralis Major Myocutaneous Flap with Medially Based Deltopectoral Flap for Closure of Large Pharyngocutaneous Fistulas. R. H. Maisel, MD; S. L. Liston, MD 98

Characteristics of Tissue Plasminogen Activator from Paranasal Mucous Membrane in Chronic Sinusitis. T. Kosugi, MD; O. Matsuo, MD; H. Mihara, MD; K. Hirano, MD; M. Hamaya, MD 101

Nasal Decongestant Effect of Propylhexedrine. L. H. Hamilton, PhD 106

Nasal Cycle and Postural Variations in Nasal Resistance. M. Hasegawa, MD 112

Indications of Congenital Palatal Incompetence before Diagnosis. H. L. Morris, PhD; L. J. Krueger, MA; R. M. Bumsted, MD 115

Vocal Symptoms in Parkinson Disease Treated with Levodopa. A Case Report. W. S. Schley, MD; E. Fenton, PhD; S. Niimi, MD 119

A Case of Cysticercosis Cerebri. Neurotologic Implications. S. J. Millen, MD; J. L. Pulec, MD 122

Obituary — Samuel Rosen 126

Programs: Combined Otolaryngological Spring Meetings
- American Broncho-Esophagological Association 127
- American Laryngological Association 128
- American Laryngological, Rhinological and Otological Society, Inc. 128
- American Neurotology Society 129
- American Otological Society, Inc. 129
- American Society for Head and Neck Surgery 130

Index to Advertisers 47a

Part II

Degeneration and Regeneration of Olfactory Epithelium in the Mouse. A Scanning Electron Microscopic Study. D. H. Matulionis, PhD; W. Breipohl, MD; K. P. Bhatnagar, PhD .... Supplement 89

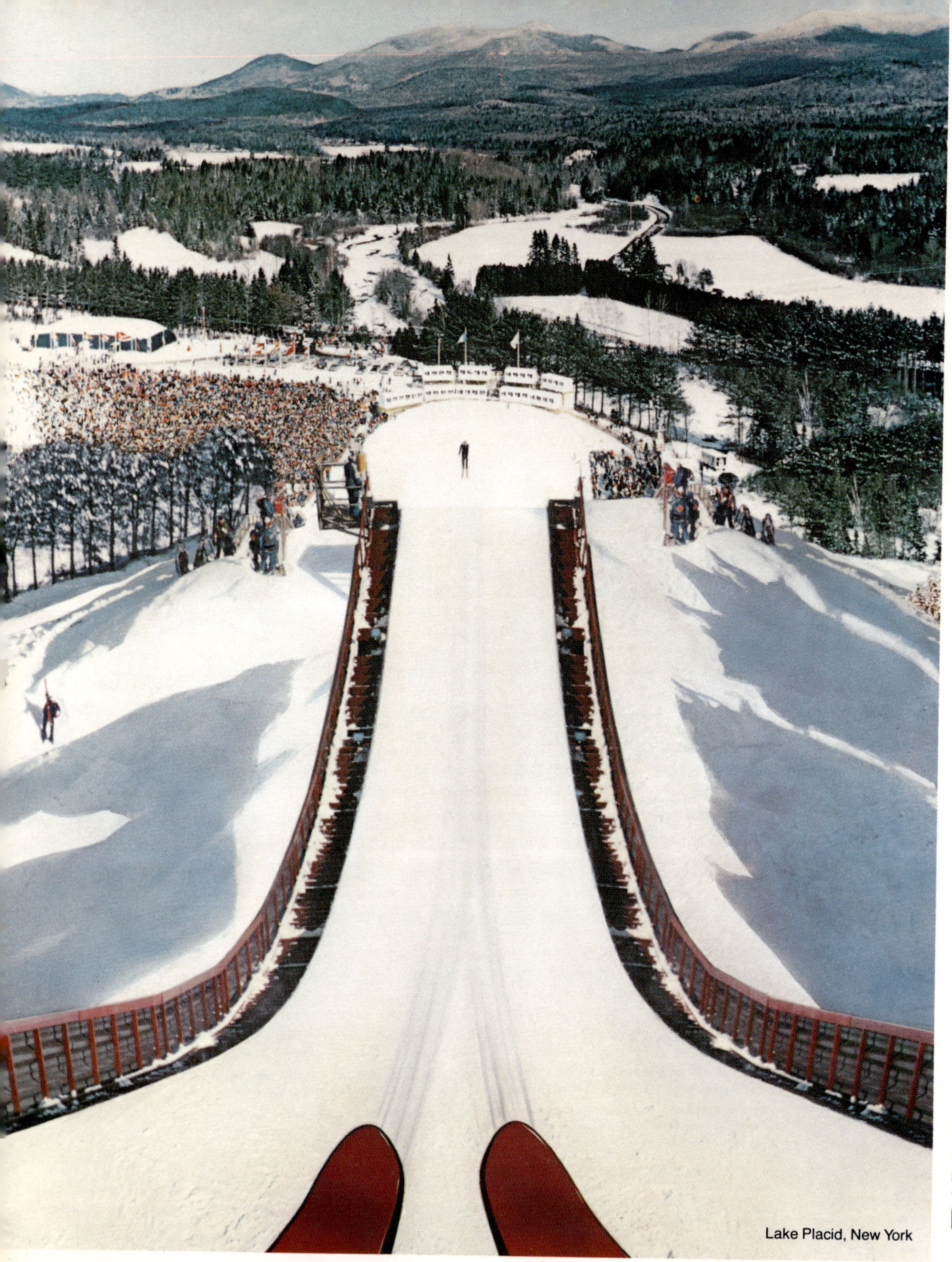

Lake Placid, New York

ANNALS OF OTOLOGY, RHINOLOGY & LARYNGOLOGY

ANNALS OF HEAD & NECK MEDICINE & SURGERY

VOL. 91 MARCH-APRIL 1982 NO. 2

CONTENTS

PART I

Bone Resorption in Human Cholesteatomas. P. Bretlau, MD; C. H. Sørensen, MD; M. B. Jørgensen, MD; E. Dabelsteen, DDS 131

Inner Ear Pathology Following Injury to the Eighth Cranial Nerve and the Labyrinthine Artery. I. Sando, MD, DMS; A. Ogawa, MD, DMS; B. W. Jafek, MD, FACS 136

Benign Mucous Membrane Pemphigoid. R. J. H. Smith, MD; R. B. Sessions, MD; S. F. Bean, MD 142

Basic Principles of Chemotherapy in the Treatment of Metastatic Head and Neck Cancer. S. W. Needleman, MD 145

Bacteriology of the Maxillary Sinus of Rhesus Monkeys. E. D. Shapiro, MD; E. R. Wald, MD; W. Doyle, PhD; D. Rohn, BA 150

Head and Neck Carcinoma in Patients Under 40 Years of Age. P. J. Carniol, MD; M. P. Fried, MD 152

Collagenase Activity in Squamous Cell Carcinoma of the Human Parotid Gland. C-C. Huang, PhD; A. Blitzer, DDS, MD; M. Abramson, MD 156

Tetracycline Bone Labeling: An Improved Technique Using Incident Fluorescence. R. F. Canalis, MD; J. Lechago, MD, PhD 160

Sudden Deafness Due to Infection by *Mycoplasma pneumoniae*. E. Shanon, MD; D. Zikk, MD; C. Redianu, MD; E. Eylan, MD 163

Biofeedback Rehabilitation in Seventh Nerve Paralysis. M. A. Corral-Romero, MD; A. Bustamante-Balcárcel, MD ... 166

Standardization of Acoustic Reflex Latency: A Study in Humans and Nonhuman Primates. C. A. Mangham, Jr, MD, MS; P. A. Burnett, MS; R. C. Lindeman, MD 169

Oxatomide in the Treatment of Chronic Allergic Rhinitis. E. Vannieuwenhuyse, MD; W. De Proost, MD; F. Degreef, MD; J. Callier, MD 175

Comparison of Normal Eustachian Tube Function in the Rhesus Monkey and Man. E. I. Cantekin, PhD; W. J. Doyle, PhD; C. D. Bluestone, MD 179

Semicircular Canal Structure During Postnatal Development in Cat and Guinea Pig. I. S. Curthoys, PhD; R. H. I. Blanks, PhD; C. H. Markham, MD 185

Vaterite Otoconia in Two Cases of Otoconial Membrane Dysplasia. C. G. Wright, PhD; R. C. Rouse, PhD; L-G. Johnsson, MD; A. G. Weinberg, MD; D. G. Hubbard, MD 193

Bony Auditory Tube and Otitis Media with Effusion. R. B. Duncan, FRACS 200

An Inexpensive Effective Cryoprobe for Palliative Care. N. R. T. Pashley, MD, FRCS(C) 204

Latency of Auditory Nerve Response in Neonates One to Eight Hours Old. A. Rubinstein, BA; H. Sohmer, PhD 205

Functional Patency of the Cochlear Aqueduct. B. Carlborg, MD; B. Densert, MD; O. Densert, MD 209

Evidence for Presynaptic Parasympathetic Receptors on Nasal Blood Vessels. R. T. Jackson, PhD 216

Typhoid Fever and Cochleovestibular Lesions. J. R. Escajadillo, MD; G. Alatorre, MD; A. Zárate, MD 220

Binocular Counterrolling During Sustained Body Tilt in Normal Humans and in a Patient with Unilateral Vestibular Nerve Section. S. G. Diamond, BA; C. H. Markham, MD; N. Furuya, MD 225

X-Ray Study of the Month. Rhabdomyosarcoma of the Nasopharynx. R. Eavey, MD; A. L. Weber, MD; G. Healy, MD 230

Obituary — French K. Hansel, MD 232

Book Reviews 233

Letter to the Editor 234

Information for Authors 235

Index to Advertisers 36a

PART II

The American Board of Otolaryngology: 1950-1979. W. P. Work, MD .... Supplement 90

PART III

Cochlear Implants: Progress and Perspectives. W. R. House, MD; K. I. Berliner, PhD; Editors .... Supplement 91

In Allergic Rhinitis..

Inflammation reduced-
nasal passages cleared through safe
topically applied steroid contro

Dramatic Clinical Benefits Demonstrate

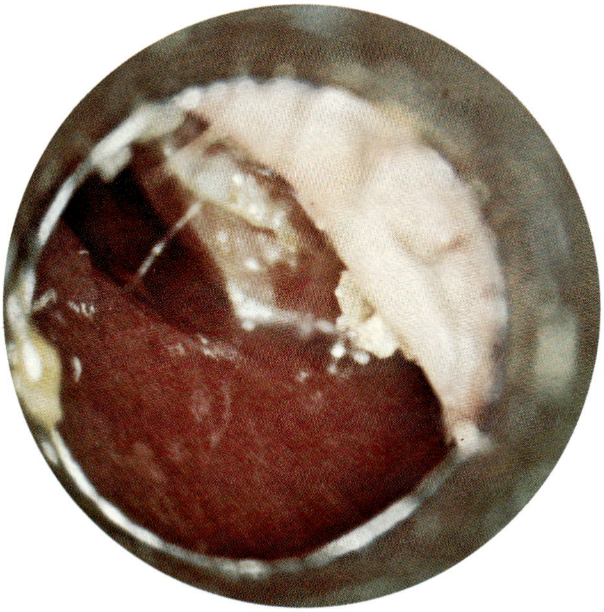

Before Vancenase treatment
Left nostril before VANCENASE Nasal Inhaler treatment:
See marked swelling of turbinate with partially obstructed airway, moderate amount of thin and thickened secretions, red mucosa.

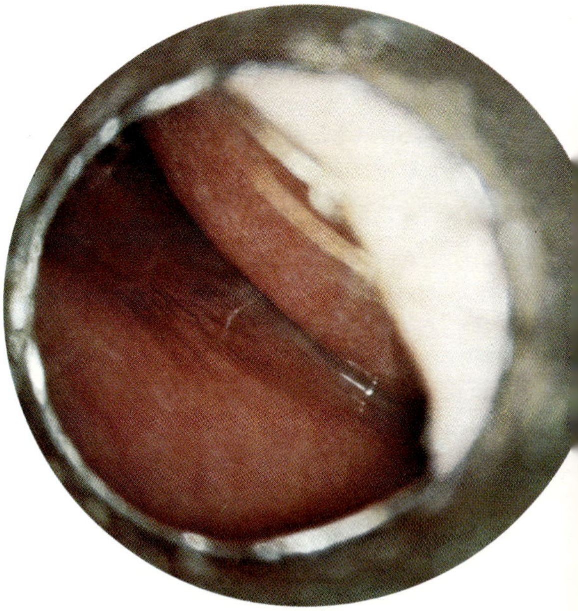

After Vancenase Treatment
Left nostril after using VANCENASE Nasal Inhaler for eight weeks:
Note marked reduction of turbinate size with improvement in nasal patency; minimal secretion, pir (normal) mucosa.

Case history and photograph courtesy of John T. Connell, M.D., Englewood, New Jersey. Dosage was two puffs in each nostril t.i.d. There were no adverse side effects.

ANNALS OF OTOLOGY, RHINOLOGY & LARYNGOLOGY
ANNALS OF HEAD & NECK MEDICINE & SURGERY
VOL. 91 MAY-JUNE 1982 NO. 3

CONTENTS

PART I

The Giant Apical Air Cell Syndrome: A New Entity. E. M. Kraus, MD; B. F. McCabe, MD 237
The Price of Preservation of Hearing in Acoustic Neuroma Surgery. M. Tos, MD; J. Thomsen, MD, PhD 240
Warthin's Tumor, a Multifocal Disease. J. M. A. Shugar, MD; P. M. Som, MD; H. F. Biller, MD 246
Deafness in Cryoglobulinemia. Y. Nomura, MD; M. Tsuchida, MD; S. Mori, MD; T. Sakurai, MD 250
Longitudinal Study of the Efficacy of Ampicillin in the Treatment of Pneumococcal Otitis Media in a Chinchilla Animal Model. J. S. Supance, MD; G. Marshak, MD; W. J. Doyle, PhD; E. I. Cantekin, PhD 256
Occurrence of Additional Primary Neoplasms in Patients with Laryngeal Carcinoma in Israel (1960-1976). E. Deviri, MD; A. Bartal, MD; M. Goldsher, MD, MSc; I. Eliachar, MD; R. Steinitz, MD; E. Robinson, MD 261
Accuracy of Auditory Brainstem Evoked Response with Hearing Level Unknown. L. E. Smith, MD; F. B. Simmons, MD 266
Distribution of Antileukoprotease in Upper Respiratory Mucosa. U. Fryksmark, MD; K. Ohlsson, MD; Å. Polling, BSc; H. Tegner, MD 268
Early- and Middle-AER Components to Clicks as Response Indices for Neonatal Hearing Screening. H. A. Frye-Osier, MS; R. Goldstein, PhD; J. E. Hirsch, PhD; K. Weber, LPN 272
Vocal Quality, Articulation and Audiological Characteristics of Children and Young Adults with Diagnosed Allergies. B. M. Baker, PhD; C. D. Baker, PhD; H. T. Le, MD 277
Malleus Handle Probe: A Middle Ear Diagnostic Procedure. R. B. Duncan, FRCS, FRACS 281
Effectiveness of Middle Ear Electrical Stimulation for Activating Central Auditory Pathways. B. M. Clopton, PhD; M. M. Bosma, BSc 285
Monophasic Extraskeletal Mandibular Fixation in Head and Neck Surgery. S. D. Schaefer, MD; G. A. Wessberg, DDS; S. L. Heaton, MD 292
Hair-Clip Type Piston Artificial Stapes and the Safety Auger. Tung M-S., MD 297
Bilateral Middle Ear Carcinomas Associated with Waldenström's Macroglobulinemia. G. B. Brookes, FRCS 299
Effects of Conductive Hearing Loss on Auditory Brainstem Response. T. J. McGee, PhD; J. D. Clemis, MD 304
Cortical, Subcortical, and Brainstem Dysfunction: A Correlation in Dyslexic Children. L. W. Welsh, MD; J. J. Welsh, MD; M. Healy, MA; B. Cooper, PhD 310
Alexander's Law: A Model and Resulting Study. M. J. Doslak, PhD; L. F. Dell'Osso, PhD; R. B. Daroff, MD 316
Familial Laryngeal Abductor Paralysis with Presumed Autosomal Dominant Inheritance. G. Morelli, MD; C. Mesolella, MD; F. Costa, MD; B. Testa, MD; V. Ventruto, MD; B. Santulli, MD 323
Tracheoesophageal Fistula: A Complication of Foreign Body. M. N. Obiako, MD 325
Otitis Media Secondary to Ampicillin-Resistant *Hemophilus Influenzae:* An Update. R. H. Schwartz, MD; W. J. Rodriguez, MD, PhD; W. N. Khan, MD 328
Conditioned Middle Ear Muscle Tinnitus: A Case Report. M. E. Collard, MA; C. A. Wagner, MS; F. R. Tingwald, MD 330
Simultaneous Round and Oval Window Fistulae in a Child. N. R. T. Pashley, MB, FRCS(C) 332
Intrinsic Malignant Schwannoma of the Larynx: A Case Report. H. L. DeLozier, MD 336
Aneurysmal Bone Cyst of the Sphenoid in a Child. C. P. Kimmelman, MD; W. P. Potsic, MD; L. Schut, MD 339
Pathology Consultation. Malignant Mixed Tumor. J. G. Batsakis, MD 342
X-Ray Study of the Month. Hypertelorism in Nasal and Paranasal Sinus Polyposis. A. L. Weber, MD; W. R. Wilson, MD; W. W. Montgomery, MD 344
Book Reviews 346
Books Received 348
Index to Advertisers 30a
Information for Authors .... March-April 1982; 235

PART II

Fibrous Dysplasia: A Review of the Disease and its Manifestations in the Temporal Bone. G. T. Nager, MD; D. W. Kennedy, MD; E. Kopstein, MD .... Supplement 92

PART III

Experimental Otitis Media in Chinchillas .... Supplement 93
I. Baseline Immunological Investigation. N. Watanabe, MD; B. R. Briggs, BS; D. J. Lim, MD
II. Comparison of the Middle Ear Immune Responses to S *Pneumoniae* Types 3 and 23. N. Watanabe, MD; T. F. DeMaria, PhD; D. M. Lewis, PhD; G. Mogi, MD; D. J. Lim, MD

ANNALS OF OTOLOGY, RHINOLOGY & LARYNGOLOGY

ANNALS OF HEAD & NECK MEDICINE & SURGERY

VOL. 91 JULY-AUGUST 1982 NO. 4

CONTENTS

PART 1

In Memoriam — Ben H. Senturia, MD; 1910-1982 349
Tribute. B. F. McCabe, MD 350
Obituary. Victor Goodhill, MD 351
Eighth Daniel C. Baker, Jr, Memorial Lecture. Subcertification: A Dilemma for Otolaryngology — Head and Neck Surgery. G. F. Reed, MD 352
Office Telescopic Photography of the Larynx. E. Yanagisawa, MD, FACS 354
Laryngeal Sarcoidosis: Report of 13 Patients. H. B. Neel III, MD, PhD; T. J. McDonald, MD 359
Laryngotracheal Invasion by Thyroid Carcinoma. M. Friedman, MD; V. K. Shelton, MD; E. M. Skolnik, MD; F. G. Berlinger, MD; M. Arab, MD 363
Age-Related Changes in the Epithelium of the Monkey Larynx. M. P. Stearns, FRCS; C. W. Cummings, MD, FACS 370
Classification and Approach to Patients with Functional Voice Disorders. J. A. Koufman, MD; P. D. Blalock, MA 372
Pathogenesis of Vocal Cord Polyps. O. Kleinsasser, MD 378
Endoscopic Rehabilitation of the Airway in Laryngeal Paralysis. F. R. Kirchner, MD, FACS 382
Predictive Factors of Success or Failure in the Endoscopic Management of Laryngeal and Tracheal Stenosis. G. T. Simpson, MD, MPH; M. S. Strong, MD; G. B. Healy, MD; S. M. Shapshay, MD; C. W. Vaughan, MD 384
Diagnosis and Conservative Surgical Management of Chondrosarcoma of the Larynx. J. N. Hicks, MD; E. E. Walker, MD; E. E. Moor, MD 389
Chondrosarcoma of the Larynx: Excision of Massive Recurrence. F. E. LeJeune, Jr, MD, FACS; H. W. Van Horn III, MD; G. H. Farr, MD 392
Extended Transantral Approach to Pterygomaxillary Tumors. C. J. Krause, MD; S. R. Baker, MD 395
Primary Management of Laryngeal Trauma. S. D. Schaefer, MD 399
Assessment of Intubation in Croup and Epiglottitis. J. J. Zulliger, MD; D. E. Schuller, MD; T. P. Beach, MD; J. P. Garvin, MD; H. G. Birck, MD; J. E. Frank 403
Treatment of Severe Subglottic Stenosis Without Tracheotomy: A Preliminary Report. L. D. Holinger, MD 407
Infant Tracheotomy. C. R. Gerson, MD; G. F. Tucker, Jr, MD 413
Laryngeal Paralysis in Children: A Long-Term Retrospective Study. S. R. Cohen, MD; K. A. Geller, MD; J. W. Birns, MD; J. W. Thompson, MD 417
Laryngeal Papilloma: Results of Treatment with the CO_2 Laser and Podophyllum. H. H. Dedo, MD; R. K. Jackler, MD 425
Leukocyte Interferon in Patients with Juvenile Laryngeal Papillomatosis. H. Goepfert, MD; R. B. Sessions, MD; J. U. Gutterman, MD; A. Cangir, MD; W. J. Dichtel, MD; M. Sulek, MD 431
Cricothyroidotomy: The Impact of Antecedent Endotracheal Intubation. E. A. Weymuller, Jr, MD; C. W. Cummings, MD 437
Nerve-Muscle Pedicle Reinnervation of the Larynx: Avoiding Pitfalls and Complications. H. M. Tucker, MD 440
Surgery of the Inferior Nasal Turbinates. W. H. Saunders, MD 445
Correction of Posterior Glottic Incompetence Following Horizontal Partial Laryngectomy. H. F. Biller, MD; W. Lawson, MD, DDS; S. Sacks, MD 448
Tracheostomal Stenosis Following Total Laryngectomy. E. N. Myers, MD, FACS; L. J. Gallia, DDS, MD 450
Predicting Esophageal Speech. G. A. Gates, MD; E. M. Hearne III, PhD 454
Primary Vocal Rehabilitation Using the Blom-Singer and Panje Voice Prostheses. M. D. Maves, MD; R. E. Lingeman, MD 458
Chemical Modulation of the Hypoxic Fraction in the Treatment of Head and Neck Cancer. R. R. Weichselbaum, MD; T. J. Ervin, MD; D. Miller, MD 461
Pathology Consultation. Metastatic Patterns of Salivary Gland Neoplasms. J. G. Batsakis, MD 465
Book Reviews 467
Letter to the Editor 467
Information for Authors 468
Books Received 19a
Index to Advertisers 32a

PART 2

Microcrypt Extensions of Tonsillar Crypts. S. Maeda, MD; G. Mogi, MD; M. Oh, MD .... Supplement 94

PART 3

Endotracheal Artificial Larynx. V. S. Dayal, MB, FRCS(C); M. L. G. Joy, PhD, PEng; R. E. Moon, MD, FRCP(C); A. Lo, BASc; A. Jares .... Supplement 95

PART 4

Postnatal Development of the Vestibular Aqueduct and Endolymphatic Sac *and* Dimensional Anatomy of the Vestibular Aqueduct and the Endolymphatic Sac (Rugose Portion) in Human Temporal Bones. Statistical Analysis of 79 Bones. A. Kodama, MD; I. Sando, MD .... Supplement 96

ANNALS OF OTOLOGY, RHINOLOGY & LARYNGOLOGY

ANNALS OF HEAD & NECK MEDICINE & SURGERY

VOL. 91 SEPTEMBER-OCTOBER 1982 NO. 5

CONTENTS

PART 1

Papers Presented at the Meeting of the American Otological Society, Inc. Part 1.

Singular Neurectomy Update. R. R. Gacek, MD ... 469

Infratemporal Fossa Approach for Glomus Tumors of the Temporal Bone. U. Fisch, MD ... 474

Polytomography and Congenital Anomalies of the Ear. J. W. Wright, Jr, MD; J. W. Wright III, MD; G. Hicks, MD ... 480

Normal Neonatal Brainstem Auditory Evoked Potentials. H. H. Zubick, PhD; M. P. Fried, MD; P. Feudo, Jr, MA; M. F. Epstein, MD; M. Strome, MD ... 485

Harmonic Acceleration Tests as a Measure of Vestibular Compensation. W. Rubin, MD ... 489

Comparison of Vestibular Subjective Sensation and Nystagmus Responses During Computerized Harmonic Acceleration Tests. V. Honrubia, MD; H. A. Jenkins, MD; R. W. Baloh, MD; H. R. Konrad, MD; R. D. Yee, MD; P. H. Ward, MD ... 493

CT Air-Contrast Scanning of the Internal Auditory Canal. R. Anderson, MD; J. Olson, Col, USAF, MC; R. Dowart, Maj, USAF, MC; M. Merkle, MD; S. Schaefer, MD ... 501

Hindbrain Circulation and Its Evaluation by Dynamic Computed Tomography. G. E. Valvassori, MD; G. D. Dobben, MD ... 506

Anatomic Specificity of Central Vestibular Signs in Posterior Fossa Lesions. A. Kumar, MD, FRCS(Ed); M. Mafee, MD; N. Torok, MD ... 510

Stapedectomy — A Long-Term Report. J. J. Shea, MD ... 516

What Can Be Done for the Recruiting Ear? M. Schiff, MD; R. E. Sandlin, PhD ... 521

Effect of Mastoid Cavity Modification on Middle Ear Sound Transmission. J. T. McElveen, MD; R. L. Goode, MD; C. Miller, MS; S. A. Falk, MD ... 526

The Homograft Tympanic Membrane After 12 Years. R. E. Wehrs, MD ... 533

Lyophilized Partial Ossicular Replacement Allografts. M. F. W. Smith, MD; J. T. McElveen, MD ... 538

Pathology Consultation. Midfacial Necrotizing Diseases. J. G. Batsakis, MD ... 541

X-Ray Study of the Month. Intracavernous Internal Carotid Artery Aneurysm. A. L. Weber, MD; K. R. Davis, MD; R. G. Ojemann, MD; M. Negri, MD ... 543

Book Reviews ... 546

Books Received ... 549

Information for Authors ... 550

Index to Advertisers ... 26a

PART 2

Papers Presented at the Meeting of the American Otological Society, Inc. Part 2. ... Supplement 97

Cochlear and Otoconial Abnormalities in Capsular Otosclerosis with Hydrops. L-G. Johnsson, MD; J. E. Hawkins, Jr, DSc; R. C. Rouse, PhD; F. H. Linthicum, Jr, MD ... 3

Behavior of the Vestibular Nerve Following Labyrinthectomy. H. F. Schuknecht, MD ... 16

The Facial Canal: Normal Anatomy, Variations and Anomalies. B. Proctor, MD; G. T. Nager, MD ... 33

Speech and Language Development in a Parent-Infant Total Communication Program. A. Dee, MA; I. Rapin, MD; R. J. Ruben, MD ... 62

PART 3

Tissue Impedance and Current Flow in the Implanted Ear: Implications for the Cochlear Prosthesis. F. A. Spelman, PhD; B. M. Clopton, PhD; B. E. Pfingst, PhD

Neural Mechanisms Relevant to the Design of an Auditory Prosthesis: Location and Electrical Characteristics. B. M. Clopton, PhD; F. A. Spelman, PhD ... Supplement 98

ANNALS OF OTOLOGY, RHINOLOGY & LARYNGOLOGY

ANNALS OF HEAD & NECK MEDICINE & SURGERY

VOL. 91 NOVEMBER-DECEMBER 1982 NO. 6

CONTENTS

PART 1

Chevalier Jackson Lecture. Esophagology: An Update. A. M. Olsen, MD 551
Observations on So-Called Idiopathic Vocal Cord Paralysis. P.H. Ward, MD; G. Berci, MD 558
Congenital Hereditary Bilateral Abductor Vocal Cord Paralysis. K. M. Grundfast, MD; G. Milmoe, MD 564
Atlantoaxial Instability Revisited. An Alert for Endoscopists. M. L. Norton, MD, JD; M. A. Ghanma, MD 567
Laryngeal Malignancies and Computerized Tomography. A Correlation of Tomographic and Histopathologic Findings. J. A. Schild, MD; G. E. Valvassori, MD; M. F. Mafee, MD; W. A. Bardawil, MD 571
Tracheostoma Valve for Postlaryngectomy Voice Rehabilitation. E. D. Blom, PhD; M. I. Singer, MD; R. C. Hamaker, MD, FACS 576
Factors in Successful Deglutition Following Supraglottic Laryngeal Surgery. T. C. Flores, MD; B. G. Wood, MD; H. L. Levine, MD; L. K. Koegel, Jr, MD; H. M. Tucker, MD 579
Complications of Intubation. W. M. Keane, MD; J. C. Denneny, MD; L. D. Rowe, MD; J. P. Atkins, Jr, MD 584
Wegener's Granulomatosis of the Subglottis and the Upper Portion of the Trachea. T. J. McDonald, MD; H. B. Neel III, MD; R. A. DeRemee, MD 588
Wegener's Granulomatosis Appearing Initially in the Trachea. J. C. Arauz, MD; R. Fonseca, MD 593
Anatomic Abnormalities in Obstructive Sleep Apnea. D. Wilms, MD; J. Popovich, MD; W. Conway, MD; S. Fujita, MD; F. Zorick, MD 595
Brainstem Evoked Potentials in Adult Sleep Apnea. N. L. Snyderman, MD; J. T. Johnson, MD; M. Møller, MD, PhD; P. B. Thearle, RN 597
Use of Foley Catheter for Removal of Esophageal Foreign Bodies. A Survey. W. F. McGuirt, MD 599
A Simple Endoscopic Intubation Technique in Esophageal Obstruction. E. T. Edens, MD; J. J. van Overbeek, MD 602
Incendiary Characteristics of Endotracheal Tubes with the Carbon Dioxide Laser. Supplemental Report. C. T. Yarington, Jr, MD; G. E. Thompson, MD 605
Heat Sink Protection Against Lasering Endotracheal Cuffs. F. E. LeJeune, Jr, MD, FACS; C. Guice, MD; F. LeTard, MD, DABA; H. Marice, MD 606
Universal Endoscopic Coupler for Carbon Dioxide Laser Surgery. R. H. Ossoff, DMD, MD; M. S. Karlan, MD 608
Anesthetic Gas Scavenger for Use During Open Rigid Bronchoscopy. D. J. Steward, MB, FRCP(C); B. Fearon, MD, FRCS(C) 610
Scanning Electron Microscopic Examination of Nonbeating Cilia. J. P. Dudley, MD; L. Eisner; J. D. Cherry, MD 612
Dynamics of Venturi Jet Ventilation Through the Operating Laryngoscope. P. Woo, MD; S. Eurenius, BS 615
Foregut Cysts in Infants and Children. Diagnosis and Management. S. R. Cohen, MD; K. A. Geller, MD; J. W. Birns, MD; J. W. Thompson, MD; B. W. Meyer, MD; G. G. Lindesmith, MD 622
Pediatric Tracheostomy. Experience During the Past Decade. R. F. Wetmore, MD; S. D. Handler, MD; W. P. Potsic, MD 628
Home Care of the Pediatric Patient with a Tracheotomy. R. J. Ruben, MD; L. Newton, MD; D. Jornsay, RN, PNP; R. Stein, MD; H. Chambers, MD; J. Liquori, CSW; C. Lawrence, MA, RN 633
Bronchoscopic Limited Lavage for Cystic Fibrosis Patients. An Adjunct to Therapy. B. F. Rothmann, MD; L. H. Walker, MD; R. T. Stone, MD; F. W. Seguin, MD 641
Respiratory Rehabilitation with Transtracheal Oxygen System. H. J. Heimlich, MD 643
Tracheobronchial Obstruction from Metastatic Distant Malignancies. S. M. Shapshay, MD; M. S. Strong, MD 648
Hematoporphyrin-Derivative Phototherapy for Local Treatment of Cancer of the Tracheobronchial Tree. D. A. Cortese, MD; J. H. Kinsey, PhD 652
Pediatric Caustic Ingestion. J. S. Adam, MD; H. G. Birck, MD 656
Mediastinoscopy for Extrathoracic Malignancies. L. W. Welsh, MD; J. J. Welsh, MD; J. C. Chinnici, DO, MS; G. F. Huck, Jr, MD 659
X-Ray Study of the Month. Chemodectomas (Nonchromaffin Paragangliomas) of the Glomus Jugulare, Glomus Vagale and Carotid Body. A. L. Weber, MD; K. R. Davis, MD; J. B. Nadol, Jr, MD 666
Letters to the Editor 670
Book Review 670
Index 671
Instructions to Authors 21a
Statement of Ownership 32a
Index to Advertisers 34a

PART 2

Computed Tomography of the Neck. C. R. Martinez, MD; H. Kashima, MD; B. W. Gayler, MD; S. S. Siegelman, MD ..... Supplement 99

PART 3

First National Conference on Research Goals and Methods in Otolaryngology. Recommendations of the Writing Groups. G. A. Gates, MD ..... Supplement 100

DEDICATION

The first act of the new editor of the *Annals* is to join with the entire staff in dedicating this issue of the journal to Ben H. Senturia, MD. His editorship of this organ is the capstone of a brilliant career. Random House defines "annals" as "a history of events; historical records generally." Ben has made the *Annals* just that: a history of otolaryngology. But it is more than that, it is a chronicle of events which is meticulously edited. Ben has such great respect for his readers and such a grasp of concepts and language that he will work with his authors for weeks or months to revise and polish a manuscript to crystalline clarity. Nine of ten manuscripts go back to authors after critical review for revision, and frequently more than once. He guides his copyeditors in polishing the final manuscript with the precision and discipline of a watchmaker. Bringing to birth each issue is a complex event involving not just manuscript selection but choosing and cropping illustrations, cajoling the typesetters to deliver proofs on time, keeping the printer on his deadline, and insisting upon no sacrifice in quality in every step of the operation. It is small wonder then that many authors consider the *Annals* the finest journal of otolaryngology-head and neck medicine and surgery in the world, and will publish only in it. It has been a privilege and a great learning experience to have been his coeditor the past six years. The journal and its readers are fortunate that Ben has agreed not to leave the *Annals*, but simply to turn over more of the decision-making to the new editor.

It is also fitting to dedicate this issue to his wife Nancy, ever supportive and helpful, and a tower of love.

Brian F. McCabe, MD
Editor

A BRIEF HISTORY OF THE *ANNALS* 1892-1982

The year 1982 marks two important milestones in the history of the *Annals of Otology, Rhinology & Laryngology — Annals of Head and Neck Medicine and Surgery:* it is the 90th anniversary of our founding and the occasion of the appointment of our sixth editor, Dr. Brian F. McCabe.

The *Annals of Ophthalmology and Otology* was the title under which the journal was first published in Kansas City, Missouri, by Dr. James P. Parker in January 1892. The first volume consisted of 212 pages and was widely acclaimed. The reputation of the journal spread rapidly and by 1896 the number of published papers had increased so much that the fifth volume contained 1,380 pages. It was evident that the size of the journal had gotten out of hand, and in 1896 it was announced that the journal would be divided into the components of ophthalmology, neurology, otology, and rhinology and laryngology.

The publication devoted to the ear, nose and throat appeared in 1897 as Volume Six, under the title *Annals of Otology, Rhinology & Laryngology*. This volume contained 528 pages including 25 original communications, almost half of which are case reports or descriptions of new instruments. Abstracts constituted a large part of the earlier volumes, as did society proceedings of the American Laryngological Association; the American Laryngological, Rhinological and Otological Association; the French Otological Society and the Section of Laryngology and Otology of the British Medical Association. However, the balance shifted rapidly and original communications soon became the primary feature of the journal. In 1900, 34 papers were published along with the journal's first photomicrographs. Five years later the lead article was illustrated with the first color page which consisted of four drawings of mucous membranes and glands.

The name of Dr. Hanau W. Loeb appeared as a member of the Editorial Board from 1895 to 1899. In 1896 the demand for more rhinology and laryngology articles made it desirable to have a special editor in St. Louis, and Dr. Loeb assumed charge of these areas; later he purchased the journal and became its editor and publisher. A man of great intelligence and energy, Dr. Loeb helped organize the Marion Sims Medical College in St. Louis which later became the Medical Department of St. Louis University, was Head of its Department of Otolaryngology, and became Dean of the School of Medicine. He devoted great energy and fervor to improving the scientific standards of the journal and its reputation throughout the world. The *Annals* remained under Dr. Loeb's direction until 1926.

In 1927, Dr. L. W. Dean, Professor of Otolaryngology at Washington University School of Medicine, was appointed Editor-in-Chief; he immediately asked Dr. Arthur W. Proetz, one of his brilliant colleagues, to become his Associate Editor. After nine years of this arrangement, Dr. Dean named Dr. Proetz Coeditor and transferred to him major responsibility for the journal. Upon Dr. Dean's death in 1943, Dr. Proetz became Editor and continued in this capacity for 23 years.

Dr. Arthur Proetz was a brilliant scientist and an outstanding clinician and administrator; he was also a man of many interests and accomplishments which included photography, art, music and drama. It was no wonder that under his direction, the *Annals* grew progressively in scientific and editorial quality to become one of the outstanding otolaryngologic journals in the world.

It was my privilege to serve as Associate Editor under Dr. Proetz for eight years before assuming the editorship in 1966. As Clinical Professor of Otolaryngology at Washington University School of Medicine and Director of the Department of Otolaryngology at The Jewish Hospital of St. Louis, I was fortunate to know many authors whose research and clinical studies were important contributions to the *Annals*. During these past 15 years, the *Annals* has striven to maintain the highest standards, while aspiring at the same time to creative and thoughtful innovation. The changes to a bimonthly and to the larger journal format as well as the supplement program were enthusiastically received everywhere. In 1980, as part of a national trend to make journal titles reflect the more comprehensive nature of our specialty, the name of the journal was expanded to the *Annals of Otology, Rhinology & Laryngology — Annals of Head and Neck Medicine and Surgery*.

The *Annals* has become a fully international journal, with authors and subscribers in every part of the world. In terms of content, it clearly reflects the evolution and expansion which have characterized science, medicine and otolaryngology in this century. In 1981 the *Annals* published 143 papers and 11 supplements, and the journal is richly illustrated not only with color — 7 full pages — but also with a broad range of figures representing the most sophisticated technology of both medical science and the printer's art.

In 1982, on our 90th anniversary, we are very fortunate to have Dr. Brian F. McCabe, Head of the Department of Otolaryngology at the University of Iowa School of Medicine, assume the editorship of the *Annals*. Dr. McCabe is widely known for his many clinical, research and academic achievements. Under his direction, we look forward to progressive growth and the maintenance of continued high scientific and editorial standards.

Despite the inroads of inflation and high costs, the grandchildren and great-grandchildren of Dr. Loeb, who are the present publishers of the *Annals*, have informed Dr. McCabe that it is their desire that we continue to produce one of the finest possible ear, nose and throat journals in the world. It will be the prime objective of the editors and the editorial staff to fulfill this request.

Ben H. Senturia, MD

EDITORS of the *ANNALS*

JAMES P. PARKER, MD
Founder, Editor and Publisher
1892-1896

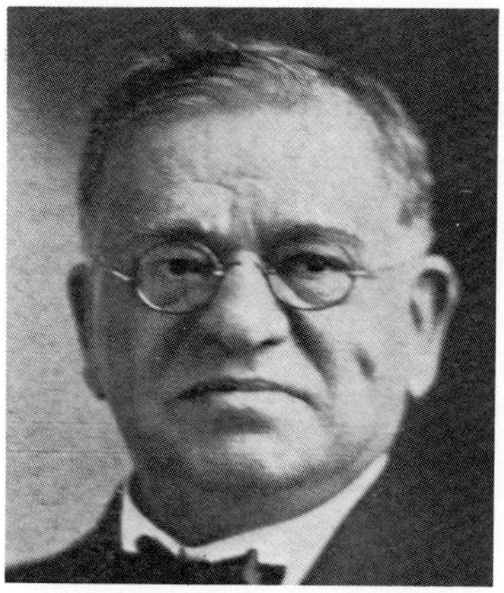

HANAU W. LOEB, MD
Editor 1900-1926

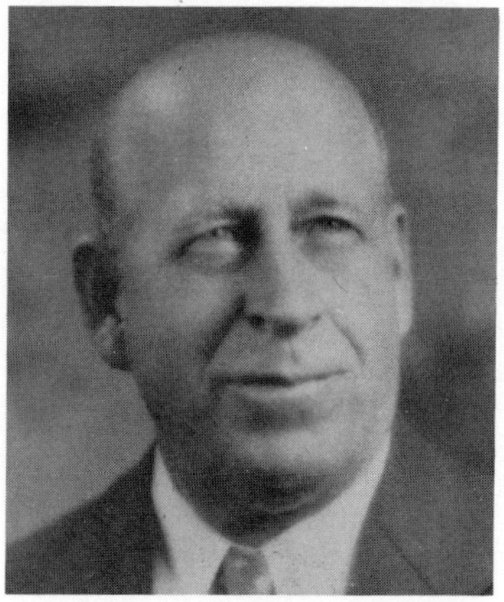

L. W. DEAN, MD
Editor 1927-1935, Coeditor 1936-1943

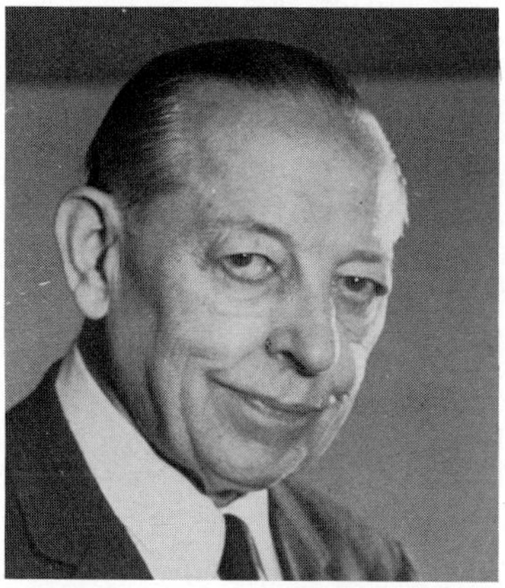

ARTHUR W. PROETZ, MD
Associate Editor 1927-1935, Coeditor 1936-1943,
Editor 1944-1966

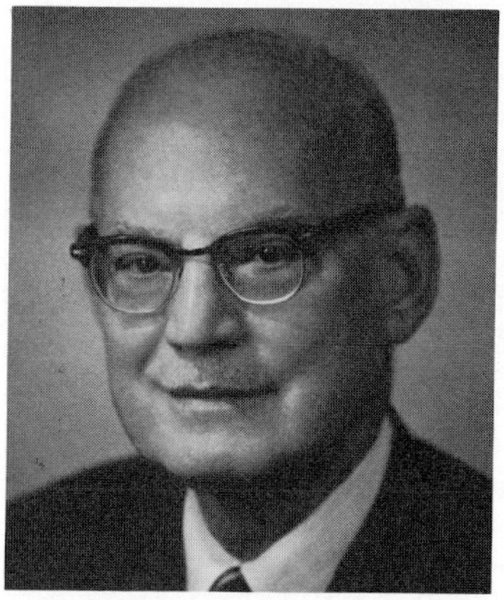

BEN H. SENTURIA, MD
Associate Editor 1958-1966, Editor 1966-1981,
Coeditor 1982-

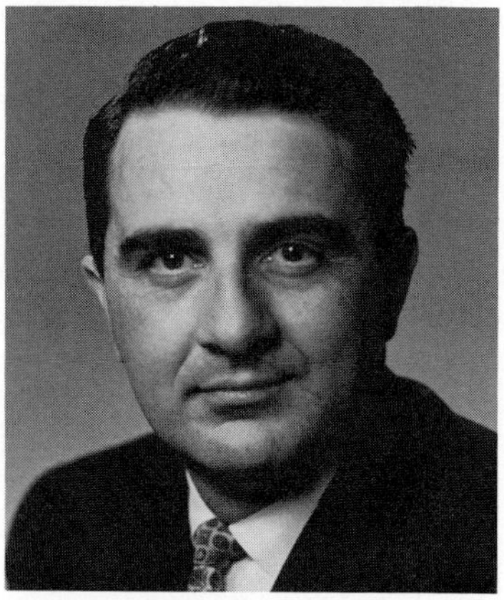

BRIAN F. MCCABE, MD
Associate Editor 1972-1975, Coeditor 1976-1981,
Editor 1982-

EDITORIAL

It is a distinct pleasure and honor for me to announce that the Board of Directors has appointed Dr. Brian F. McCabe Editor of the *Annals of Otology, Rhinology & Laryngology* as of January 1, 1982. Dr. McCabe is widely respected among otolaryngologists and head and neck specialists for his many clinical, research and academic achievements. These include Professor of Otolaryngology and Chairman of the Department of Otolaryngology and Maxillofacial Surgery at the University of Iowa College of Medicine; Director on the American Board of Otolaryngology; numerous administrative positions in our national societies; and the publication of a large number of papers in nationally recognized journals. For the past six years, he has been an active and effective Coeditor of the *Annals* and he has demonstrated a sensitivity to and understanding of the need for a strong, independent, scientific and clinically oriented journal of otolaryngology.

At the request of Dr. McCabe and the Board, I shall remain active as Coeditor to provide such advice and help as I can offer. It is the present plan of the Board to have the Editor's office and a part of the editorial staff in Iowa City under Dr. McCabe's supervision, and to maintain in St. Louis a large segment of the editorial work and the production phases of the *Annals* under the supervision of Dr. McCabe and myself.

In great measure the maintenance of high production standards and efficiency of the *Annals* has been a result of the intelligence and unique and multitalented competence of our Managing Editor, Bess E. Arick. Everyone who has had occasion to interact with her knows of her enthusiasm and dedication to the *Annals*. Early in 1982, Mrs. Arick will retire to the Boston area, where her children and grandchildren live. She has set standards which all of us will strive to maintain.

We are very fortunate to have Sara Jenkins to assume the position of Managing Editor, and Kenneth A. Cooper, Jr., to take on the tasks of Business Manager. They are looking forward to cooperating with Dr. McCabe in providing our readers with the outstanding editorial input and good service to which they have grown accustomed.

With this first issue of the year we welcome to the Board of Editors Jack D. Clemis, MD, Seymour R. Cohen, MD, and Yasuya Nomura, MD. We thank Wesley H. Bradley, MD, and Richard R. Gacek, MD, for their past help and guidance and are happy that both Dr. Bradley and Dr. Gacek have agreed to continue their association with the *Annals* by serving on the Emeritus Board.

I wish to thank the *Annals* staff, associates and contributors who have put up with my publishing idiosyncrasies. It is my sincere feeling that all of us have the potential for accomplishing more than we give ourselves credit; it merely requires that we set our standards and arrange our goals so that they may be intelligently and happily accomplished. With this in mind, I have routinely asked our contributors, especially our younger colleagues, to strive for excellence, and with few exceptions, all of us in the editorial office have been pleased with the results.

I considered it one of the outstanding accomplishments of my medical career to have been chosen, in 1958, by Dr. Arthur Proetz to be his Associate Editor, and to be selected as his successor in 1966. For the past 15 years, the *Annals* has provided me with one of the most gratifying experiences of my life. I have had the opportunity to work intimately and constructively with outstanding members of our profession all over the world and to interact on a personal level with our authors, reviewers and subscribers. I hope and pray that Dr. McCabe will enjoy this same unique and happy experience.

Ben H. Senturia, MD
Coeditor

Ann Otol 91:1982

COCHLEAR HYDROPS IN ASSOCIATION WITH COLLAPSED SACCULE AND DUCTUS REUNIENS

KEN KITAMURA, MD

HAROLD F. SCHUKNECHT, MD ROBERT S. KIMURA, PhD

BOSTON, MASSACHUSETTS

Histopathological evidence from five human temporal bones with endolymphatic hydrops limited to the cochlea shows pathological obliteration of their saccules and/or ductus reunientes. We suggest that this finding supports the theory of longitudinal flow of endolymph. The anatomical distribution of endolymphatic hydrops is related to the location of the blockage which may occur anywhere from the ductus reuniens to the endolymphatic sac. Atrophy of sensorineural structures of the cochlea is severe in these five temporal bones and is presumed to be caused by the original disorders rather than occurring secondary to the endolymphatic hydrops.

Endolymphatic hydrops is found in several disorders including Menière's disease,[1,2] syphilitic labyrinthitis,[3,4] and inflammatory disease.[5,6] It has been proposed that a possible cause for hydrops in Menière's disease is loss of the resorptive function of the endolymphatic sac. This is based on both animal studies in which hydrops followed ablation of the sac[7,8] and human temporal bone studies.[9,10] Kimura et al[11] recently demonstrated in experiments on guinea pigs that obliteration of the ductus reuniens can produce hydrops limited to the cochlea. A logical explanation for isolated cochlear hydrops is interruption of the normal longitudinal flow of endolymph from the cochlea to endolymphatic sac.

We have studied 59 temporal bones in the collection of the Massachusetts Eye and Ear Infirmary which exhibit cochlear hydrops. Five of them showed hydrops limited to the cochlea and all were accompanied by obliteration of the saccules and/or ductus reunientes.

RESULTS

A study was made of the position of the membranous walls in the saccules and ductus reunientes of 59 temporal bones with cochlear hydrops. Some temporal bones were excluded from this study because artifact and postmortem change precluded evaluation of the position of their membranous walls. The clinical diagnoses were Menière's disease in 37; labyrinthitis in association with otitis media, surgical or traumatic fistulization of the bony labyrinth, syphilis, or viral disease in 16; and obliterated vestibular aqueduct in 3. The cause of hydrops in the remaining three ears is unknown.

The most frequent finding is a normal or dilated endolymphatic space in both the saccule and ductus reuniens (49 of 59 temporal bones). In three ears there is saccular collapse following hydrops which is presumably the result of rupture of the saccular walls and patent ductus reunientes. Both ears from one patient showed hydrops of the saccules and collapsed ductus reunientes which could be the result of the severe autolytic change related to antemortem ischemia in association with cerebral anoxia (caused by cardiac arrest). The saccular space is obliterated and ductus reuniens is patent in one ear in which a stapedectomy was performed. The remaining four temporal bones from three patients show obliterated endolymphatic spaces of their saccules and ductus reunientes.

CASE REPORTS

The following cases show cochlear hydrops in association with collapsed saccules and/or ductus reunientes.

Case 1

The patient, an 83-year-old male, stated that he had been totally deaf in his left ear all his life. He had noticed diminished hearing in his right ear since age 27. There was no history of vertiginous attacks. He died at age 83 of a brainstem infarction. No audiogram was available.

Right Ear. An otosclerotic lesion has fixed the anterior margin of the footplate. There is scattered mild loss of hair cells and cochlear neurons. The position of Reissner's membrane is normal. The vestibular organs appear normal. The ductus reuniens is normal and patent.

Left Ear. There is otosclerotic fixation of the footplate at the anterior margin of the oval window. There is cochlear endolymphatic hydrops, most severe at the basal end (Fig. 1). Reissner's membrane is in contact with the walls of the scala vestibuli in part of the cochlea. The organ of Corti is

From the Department of Otolaryngology, Harvard Medical School and Massachusetts Eye and Ear Infirmary, Boston.

REPRINTS — Harold F. Schuknecht, MD, Department of Otolaryngology, Massachusetts Eye and Ear Infirmary, 243 Charles St., Boston, MA 02114.

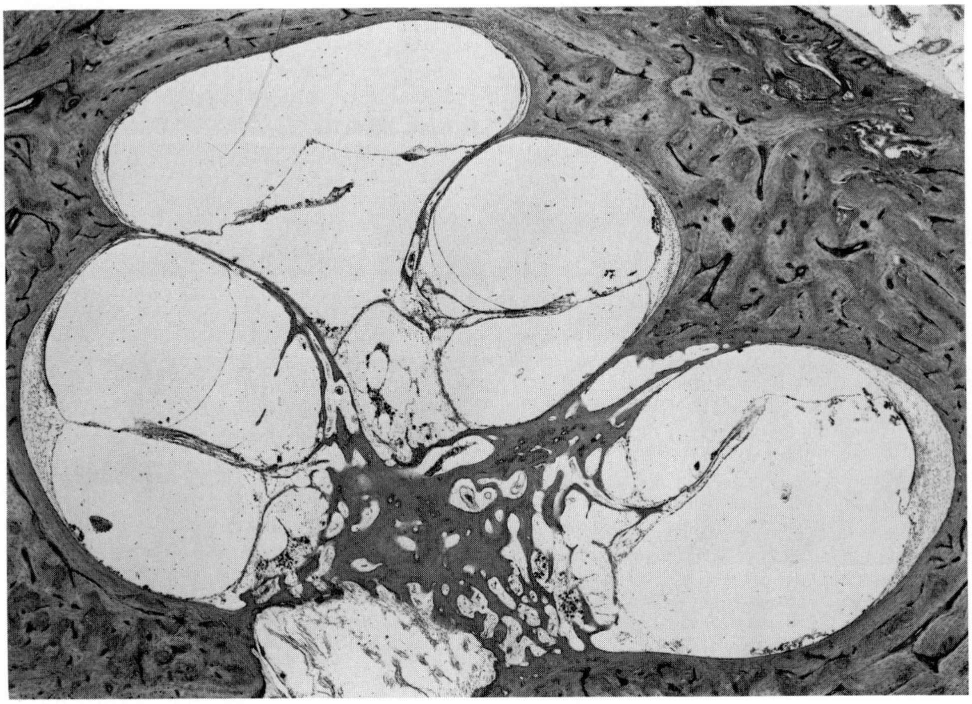

Fig. 1. (Case 1) Left ear. There is severe endolymphatic hydrops and severe loss of cochlear neurons. Rupture of the basilar membrane in the basal turn is probably due to preparation artifact.

severely atrophied throughout the cochlea; it appears as a small mound of undifferentiated tissue and the hair cells are totally missing in all turns. There is 90% loss of cochlear neurons in the basal and apical turns, and moderate loss in the middle turn. The stria vascularis shows total atrophy in the basal 19 mm and 90% loss in the remainder of the cochlea. The tectorial membrane is missing throughout the cochlea.

All of the hair cells of the saccular macula are missing, but patches of supporting cells remain. The saccular wall is collapsed and adherent to a granular amorphous basophilic material presumed to be the degenerated otolithic membrane. The endolymphatic lumen of the saccule is obliterated (Fig. 2). The ductus reuniens is collapsed and its lumen is obliterated. The utricle, (Fig. 3) semicircular canals, endolymphatic duct, and sac appear normal.

Comment. The absence of hydrops of the pars superior (utricle and canals) suggests that a generalized hydropic condition was not present before collapse of the saccule and ductus reuniens.

Case 2

The patient, a 53-year-old female, had normal auditory function and speech development up to age four. Following a severe attack of measles, she became totally deaf and subsequently relied on sign language for communication. At age 53 she died of acute myocardial infarction. No history of vertigo was reported.

Right Ear. Reissner's membrane is moderately distended and in contact with the walls of the scala

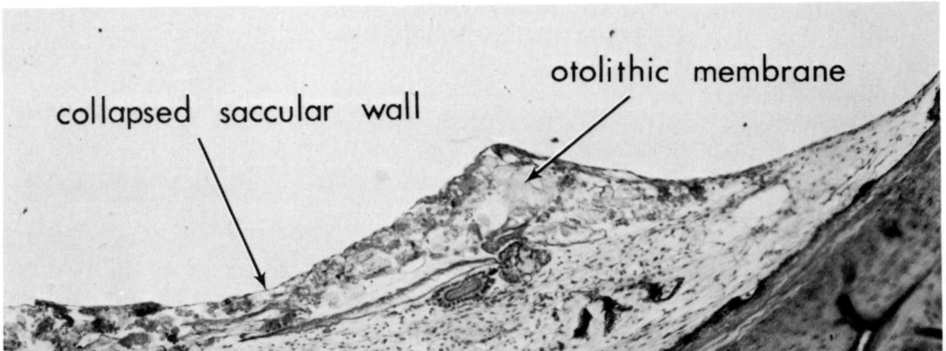

Fig. 2. (Case 1) Left ear. The wall of the saccule is collapsed and adherent to the otolithic membrane. There is severe atrophy of the sensory epithelium.

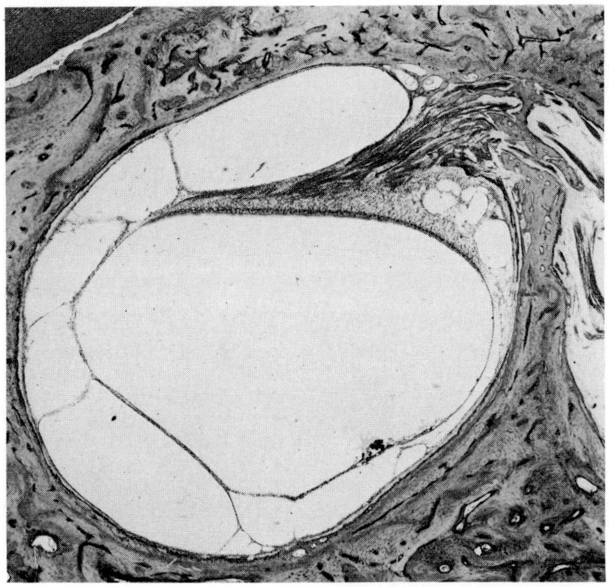

Fig. 3. (Case 1) Left ear. Normal utricle.

vestibuli in some areas (Fig. 4). The hair cells are missing in the basal 18 mm of the cochlea. Some hair cells are preserved in the middle turn and 60% remain in the apical turn. There is loss of about 90% of the cochlear neurons in the basal turn, 50 to 80% in the middle turn, and 20% in the apical turn. The tectorial membrane is partly encapsulated in the basal turn, distorted in the middle turn, and normal in the apical turn. About 20 to 50% of the stria vascularis is atrophied. There is loss of connective cells in the basal 4 to 11 mm of the limbus. Connective tissue and new bone formation are noted in the scala vestibuli in the basal turn.

The saccular macula shows severe atrophy of the sensory epithelium. In some areas the sensory epithelium is missing and in other areas it is disorganized and contains scattered basophilic deposits. Irregular basophilic granular deposits on the macula probably represent the degenerated otolithic membrane. The wall of the saccule is collapsed onto the otolithic membrane. The endolymphatic lumen of the saccule is obliterated (Fig. 5). The ductus reuniens is obliterated in part proximal to the saccule, but patent and dilated in the area close to the basal turn of the cochlea.

The utricular macula and wall are normal. The superior and lateral cristae show areas of cystic atrophy and basophilic deposits; however, hair cell populations appear normal. Bone is seen in the perilymphatic spaces of the anterior third of the lateral semicircular canal and in the midportion of the posterior semicircular canal. The endolymphatic duct and sac appear normal.

Left Ear. Reissner's membrane is atrophied and collapsed onto the organ of Corti; however, it is intact throughout. In the midbasal turn the organ of Corti is completely missing, and in the middle and apical turns it consists of a mound of undifferentiated cells. Ninety percent of the cochlear neurons are missing in the basal turn and 30% in the middle and apical turns. A small remnant of stria vascularis remains in the middle turn. There is bone and fibrous tissue in the scala tympani of the basal turn near the round window membrane. Bone and connective tissue are also shown on the internal wall of the scala vestibuli of the basal turn.

The lumens and walls of the saccule and ductus

Fig. 4. (Case 2) Right ear. Midmodiolar section showing moderately distended Reissner's membrane. There is loss of about 90% of the cochlear neurons in the basal turn, 50 to 80% in the middle turn, and 20% in the apical turn.

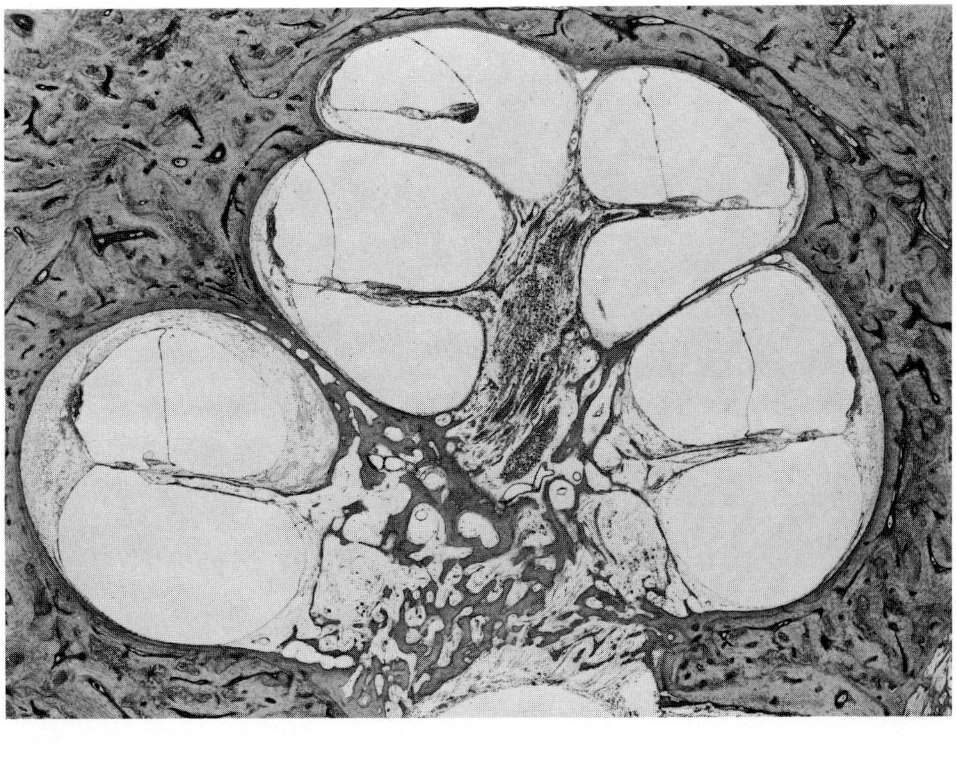

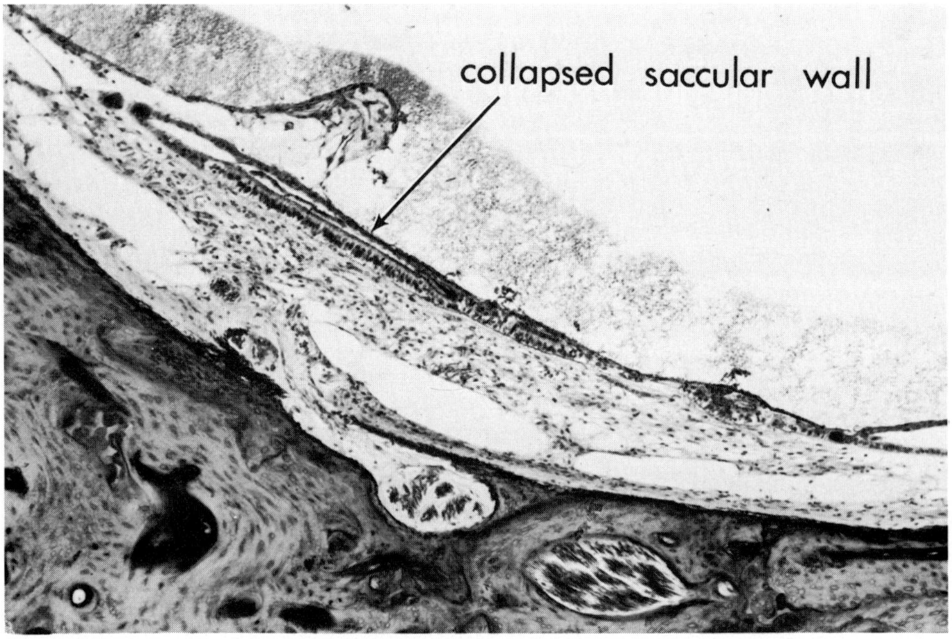

Fig. 5. (Case 2) Right ear. The saccular macula shows severe atrophy of the sensory epithelium. The saccular wall is collapsed and the endolymphatic lumen of the saccule is obliterated.

reuniens are normal. The saccular macula shows patchy atrophy with loss of hair cells and basophilic deposits as well as clear spaces and shrinking of the otolithic membrane. The utricular macula and cristae, as well as their walls, appear normal. There is bone in the perilymphatic spaces of the lateral and posterior semicircular canals. There are basophilic deposits on the rugose portion of the endolymphatic sac; however, the epithelium appears normal.

Comment. Fibrosis and new bone formation in the perilymphatic space has been previously reported in meningogenic measles labyrinthitis.[5] Endolymphatic hydrops was exhibited in the cochleae and the vestibules of both ears. In the present case cochlear hydrops has occurred in the right ear which has the obliterated saccule and ductus reuniens but not in the left where these structures are patent. The evidence suggests that the inflammatory process, which had involved both ears, was probably not the cause of the hydrops in the right ear.

Case 3

The patient, an 84-year-old female, experienced a progressive hearing loss and was profoundly deaf at the time of her terminal admission to the hospital for pneumonia. No episodes of vertigo were described.

Right Ear. There is severe endolymphatic hydrops of the cochlear duct, most severe at the basal end (Fig. 6). The organ of Corti is atrophied throughout with nearly total loss of hair cells. There is 70 to 80% loss of cochlear neurons in the basal and middle turns, and 90% loss in the apical turn. The tectorial membrane is encapsulated and spherically deformed or flattened throughout the cochlea. The stria vascularis is missing in the basal 9 mm, and 50 to 90% atrophied in the remainder of the cochlea.

The saccular macula and saccular nerve are severely degenerated and all of the hair cells are missing. The wall of the saccule is collapsed onto the otolithic membrane and its endolymphatic lumen is obliterated (Fig. 7A). The ductus reuniens is obliterated and contains otolithic membrane crystals (Fig. 6).

The utricular wall and macula and the cristae and walls of the semicircular canals appear normal. The endolymphatic duct and sac appear normal.

Left Ear. The cochlear duct shows moderate endolymphatic hydrops (Fig. 8). There is severe atrophy of the organ of Corti with hair cells totally missing in the basal 12 mm and 70 to 80% loss in the middle and apical turns. Sixty to 90% of the cochlear neurons are missing. The tectorial membrane is flattened and collapsed onto the organ of Corti. The stria vascularis is missing in the basal 4 mm and 70 to 80% atrophied in other areas.

The walls of the saccule and ductus reuniens are collapsed and their lumens are obliterated. The saccular macula shows severe atrophy of its sensory epithelium and only scattered hair cells remain (Fig. 7B).

The utricular macula and wall as well as all walls and cristae of the semicircular canals appear normal. The endolymphatic duct and sac are normal.

Case 4

The patient, a 55-year-old female, had a bilateral progressive hearing loss first noted at the age of 14. Audiometric tests at the age of 41 showed a bilateral combined sensorineural and conductive hearing loss

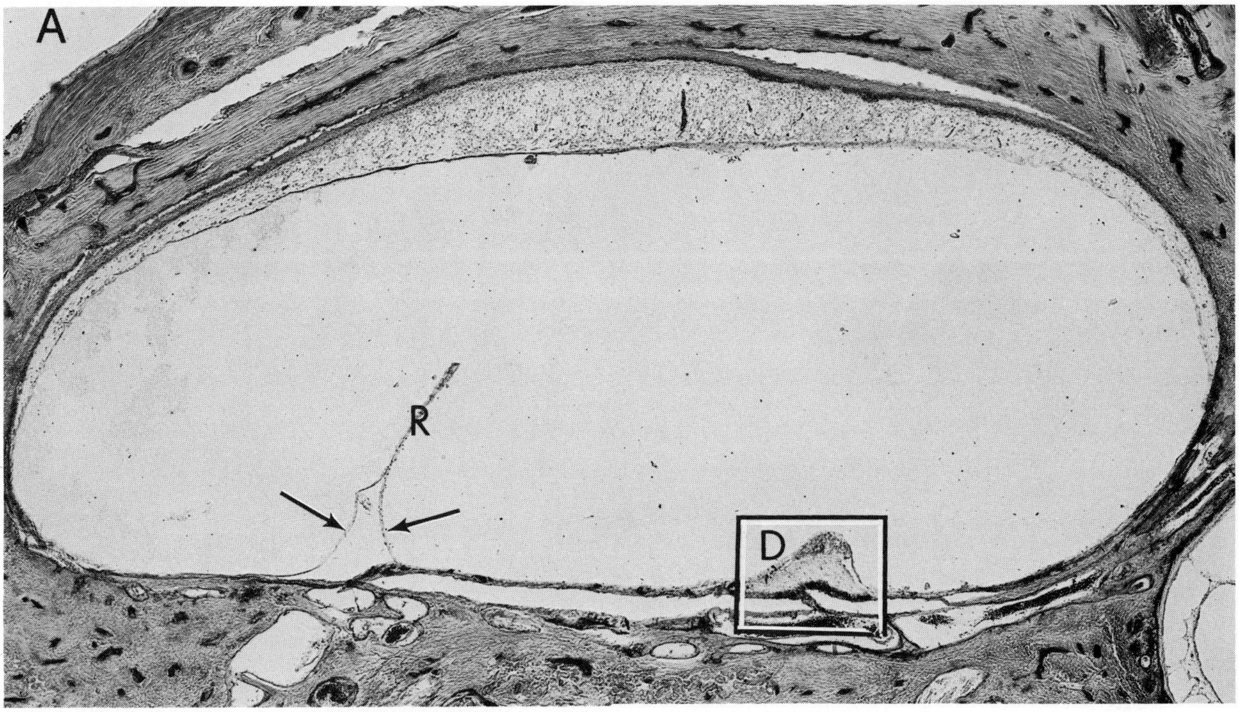

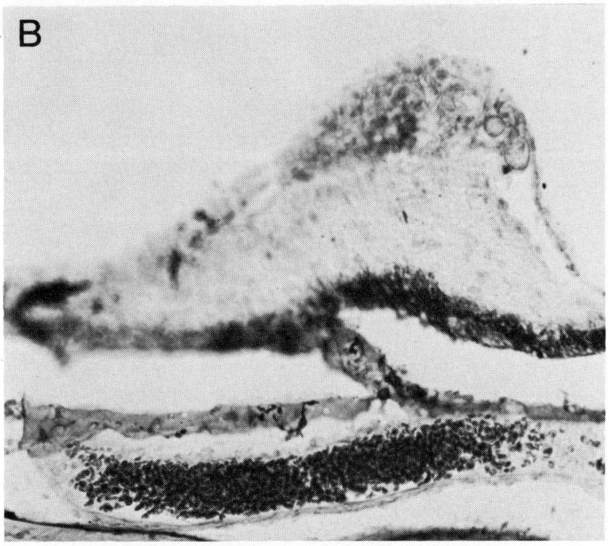

Fig. 6. (Case 3) Right ear. A) Severe endolymphatic hydrops is seen at the basal end of the cochlear duct. Reissner's membrane is severely distended (R) and ductus reuniens (D) is collapsed. B) Higher magnification view of the ductus reuniens.

with discrimination scores of 76% on the right and 86% on the left. A stapedectomy was performed on her right ear. The stapes footplate was partly removed and a Teflon®-wire prosthesis was introduced. She noted no subjective improvement in hearing postoperatively; however, eight months later she had a sudden aggravation of the hearing loss in that ear. A surgical exploration was performed but no cause for the hearing loss was found and hearing was not improved. At the age of 49 she complained of episodic vertigo with nausea. At the age of 55 she died of mammary carcinoma.

Right Ear. The footplate of the stapes is greatly thickened by otosclerotic bone and has a central surgically created opening marking the position of the Teflon-wire piston. The silhouette of the piston extends deeply into the vestibule and is lined by a fibrous membrane containing scattered small foreign body giant cells (Fig. 9).

There is moderately severe hydrops of all turns of the cochlea (Fig. 9). There is a loss of 50% of the hair cells in the basal and middle turns and 20% loss in the apical turn. Cochlear neurons show 30 to 50% loss, most severe in the basal and apical turns. There is loss of 50% of the stria vascularis in the 14 to 29 mm region; however, it appears normal in the basal and apical regions.

The saccular wall is collapsed onto the otolithic membrane and its endolymphatic lumen is obliterated. The saccular macula shows an area of cellular disruption with loss of hair cells. This lesion is in spatial contiguity with the silhouette of the Teflon-

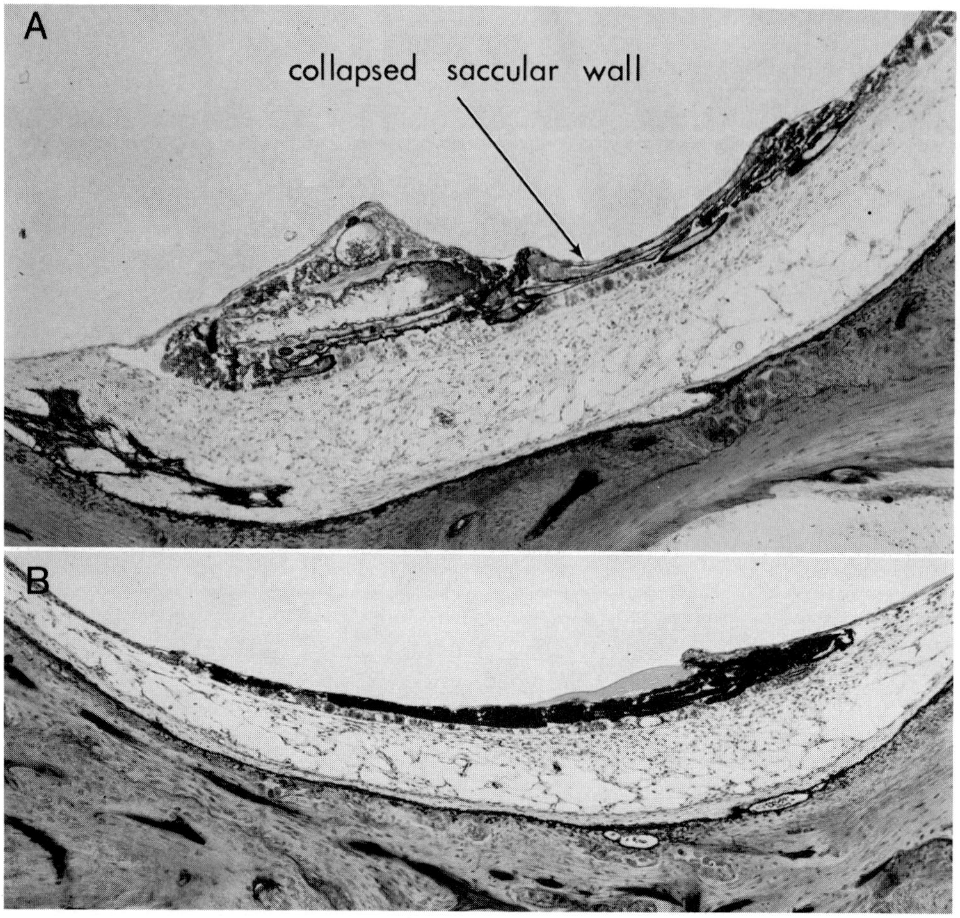

Fig. 7. (Case 3) The saccular walls are collapsed onto the otolithic membranes and their endolymphatic lumens are obliterated in both ears. A) Right saccule. B) Left saccule.

wire piston (Fig. 10). The ductus reuniens is dilated. The utricular macula and cristae and their walls appear normal; the endolymphatic duct and sac are normal.

Left Ear. There is an otosclerotic lesion involving the footplate and bases of the crura which involves the cochlear bony wall anterior to the oval window but does not extend to the endosteum. A separate otosclerotic lesion has blocked the round window niche. The position of Reissner's membrane is normal. Hair cell and neuronal populations of the cochlea are near normal. The stria vascularis shows patchy atrophy. The vestibular sense organs and nerves appear normal. The ductus reuniens is normal and patent.

Comment. It seems probable that the introduction of an excessively long piston-type prosthesis caused direct trauma to the saccule with collapse of its wall and obliteration of its lumen, followed by hydrops of the cochlear duct and ductus reuniens.

DISCUSSION

The pattern of pathological change common to these five ears is: 1) obliteration of the lumen of the saccule, 2) endolymphatic hydrops limited to the cochlear duct, 3) atrophy of the organ of Corti, and 4) preservation of some stria vascularis.

The literature reveals reports of 16 ears with endolymphatic hydrops confined to the cochlea.[12-18] Twelve of the 21 ears (including the 5 reported here) show obliterated saccules and/or ductus reunientes. Two ears have completely obliterated cochlear ducts in the extreme basal ends of the cochleae with partly collapsed saccules. In the remaining seven ears the saccular walls are described to be partly collapsed except in two in which no comments were made as to the condition of the ductus reunientes. Gussen[18] related the cochlear endolymphatic hydrops to mechanical interference of endolymph flow and considered it to be retrograde to the collapsed saccule.

Kimura et al[11] observed hydrops limited to the cochlea after obliteration of the ductus reuniens in 35 of 52 guinea pig ears. In a series of 11 animals in which the endolymphatic duct was blocked two months after surgical obstruction of the ductus reuniens, they observed hydrops in all cochleae and saccules and in ten utricles. These animal studies and the human temporal bone findings reported here support the theory of longitudinal flow of endolymph from cochlea to endolymphatic sac. They also suggest that interruption of the endolymph pathway to the endolymphatic sac at any point leads to hydrops of the isolated segment of endolymphatic system.

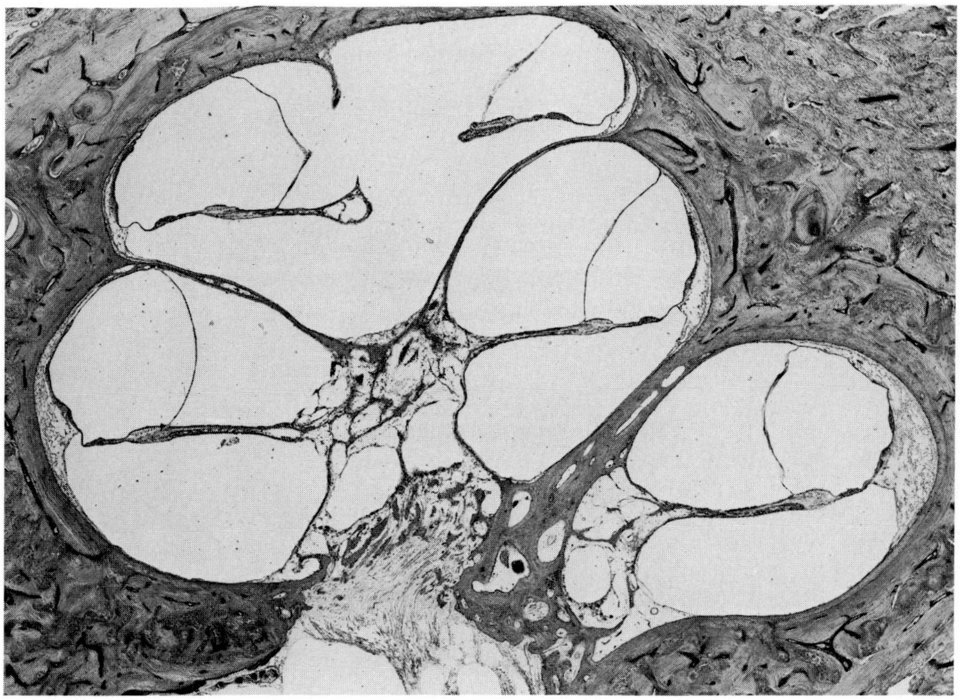

Fig. 8. (Case 3) Left ear. There is moderate cochlear endolymphatic hydrops and severe loss of cochlear neurons.

There are reports in the literature describing collapsed saccular walls without cochlear hydrops. Lindsay and Zajtchuk[19] reported the findings in a 23-year-old female who had deafness caused by head trauma. Although the saccular wall was collapsed and adherent to the degenerated macula, there was no endolymphatic hydrops in the cochlear duct. Alford[20] described four temporal bones showing cochleosaccular degeneration caused by maternal rubella in which the saccular walls were collapsed and the cochlear ducts showed the tendency to be collapsed. One of the temporal bones reported by Sando et al[17] demonstrated an almost completely collapsed ductus reuniens and saccule as well as collapsed cochlear duct.

There are two possible explanations for the absence of cochlear hydrops in the presence of a collapsed saccule. 1) It seems probable that cochlear hydrops would only develop if blockage of the endolymph pathway is complete. Kimura et al[11] found in their guinea pig experiment that complete blockage of the ductus reuniens is essential to produce cochlear hydrops. The saccular walls in the cases reported by Alford[20] and Lindsay and Zajtchuk[19] do not appear to be entirely collapsed. 2) Another pos-

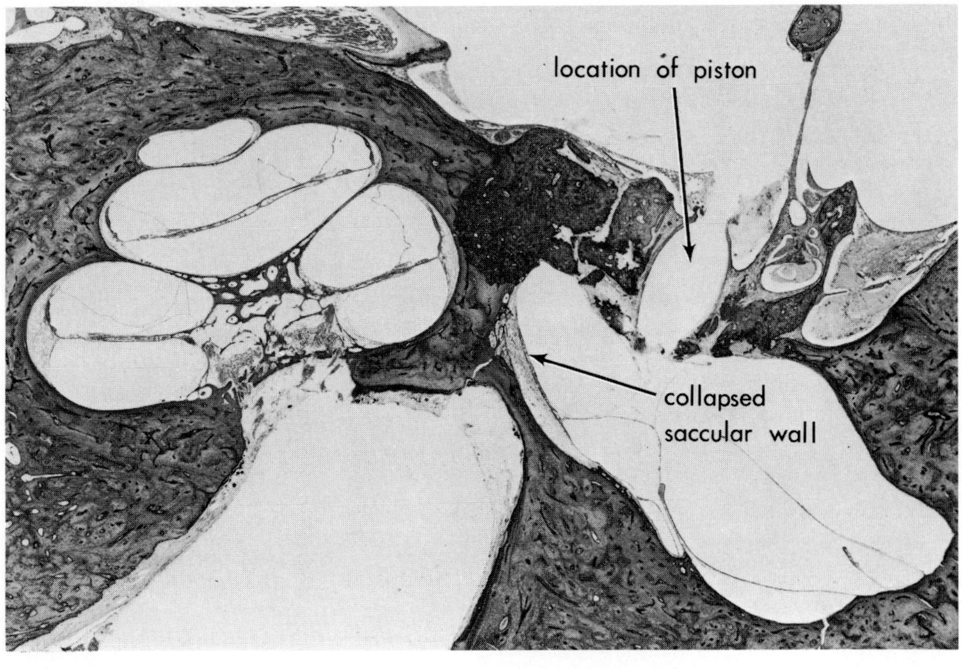

Fig. 9. (Case 4) Right ear. Moderate cochlear hydrops is seen and the silhouette of the piston extends deeply into the vestibule.

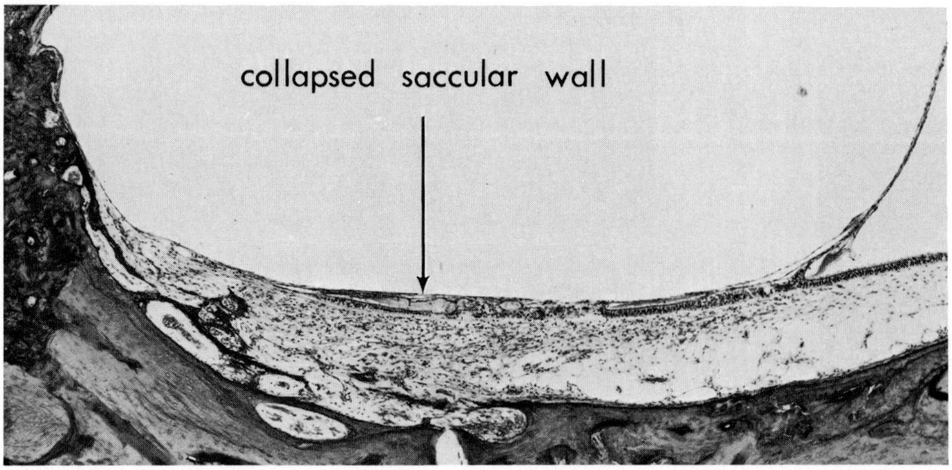

Fig. 10. (Case 4) Right ear. The saccular wall is collapsed and its endolymphatic lumen is obliterated.

sible requirement for the development of cochlear hydrops is the presence of functional stria vascularis. Without it no endolymph would be produced and thus no hydrops would occur. Sando et al[17] reported that the stria vascularis was severely atrophic throughout the cochlea in an ear without hydrops in spite of collapsed saccule and ductus reuniens. Although our five cases show some atrophy of the striae vasculares, each has some remaining stria vascularis. This condition was also true for other cases of cochlear hydrops reported in the literature.[12,14-18]

Atrophy of the organ of Corti, most severe in the basal turn, is a constant feature shown in these ears and is presumed to be the direct result of the disease that caused the blocked saccule and/or ductus reuniens. In our four cases the etiology is unknown in cases 1 and 3, measles labyrinthitis in case 2, and surgical trauma in case 4. In addition, we have found six temporal bones among our collection which show severe atrophy of the organ of Corti without cochlear hydrops and with minimal pathology in the vestibular sensory structures. In these ears the membranous walls of the saccules and ductus reunientes are normal. The etiology for the cochlear pathology is thought to be measles in four ears and whooping cough in two ears.

Only case 4 complained of vertigo. This symptom consisted of recurring episodes of a spinning sensation with nausea of short duration, similar to but less severe than the classic attacks of vertigo occurring in Menière's disease. We suspect that these ears with their collapsed saccules and partially atrophied striae vasculares are incapable of generating and pooling large volumes of endolymph in the vestibular system. This condition would obviate the occurrence of ruptures of the membranous labyrinth with potassium paralysis of the vestibular system, such as is postulated as the cause for episodic vertigo in Menière's disease.[21]

ACKNOWLEDGMENTS — The authors wish to express their appreciation to Ms. Carol Ota for her help in the preparation of this manuscript. They would also like to thank Ms. Diane Jones and Ms. Barbara Burgess for their kind assistance in this study.

REFERENCES

1. Hallpike CS, Cairns H. Observations on the pathology of Meniere's syndrome. Proc Roy Soc Med 1938; 31:1317-36.

2. Schuknecht HF, Benitez JT, Beekhuis J. Further observations on the pathology of Meniere's disease. Ann Otol Rhinol Laryngol 1962; 71:1039-54.

3. Karmody C, Schuknecht HF. Deafness in congenital syphilis. Arch Otolaryngol 1966; 83:18-27.

4. Belal A Jr, Linthicum FH Jr. Pathology of congenital syphilitic labyrinthitis. Am J Otolaryngol 1980; 1:109-18.

5. Nager FR. Beiträge zur Histologie der erworbenen Taubstummheit. Z Ohrenheilkd 1907; 54:217-44.

6. Paparella MM, Sugiura S. The pathology of suppurative labyrinthitis. Ann Otol Rhinol Laryngol 1967; 76:554-86.

7. Kimura RS, Schuknecht HF. Membranous hydrops in the inner ear of the guinea pig after obliteration of the endolymphatic sac. Pract Oto Rhino Laryngol 1965; 27:343-54.

8. Schuknecht HF, Northrop C, Igarashi M. Cochlear pathology after destruction of the endolymphatic sac in the cat. Acta Otolaryngol (Stockh) 1968; 65:479-87.

9. Egami T, Sando I, Black FO. Hypoplasia of the vestibular aqueduct and endolymphatic sac in endolymphatic hydrops. Trans Am Acad Ophthalmol Otolaryngol 1978; ORL 86:327-41.

10. Schuknecht HF. Rationale of surgical procedures for Menière's disease. Presented at the International Symposium on Pathogenesis, Diagnosis and Treatment of Meniere's Disease. Dusseldorf, Germany, May 12-14, 1980.

11. Kimura RS, Schuknecht HF, Ota CY, Jones DD. Obliteration of the ductus reuniens. Acta Otolaryngol (Stockh) 1980; 89: 295-309.

12. Lindsay JR, von Schulthess G. An unusual case of labyrinthine hydrops. Acta Otolaryngol (Stockh) 1958; 49:315-24.

13. Lindsay JR, Matz GJ. The differentiation of acquired congenital from genetically determined inner ear deafness. Ann Otol Rhinol Laryngol 1966; 75:830-43.

14. Cohn AM, Beal DD, Kohut RI. Inner ear pathology in unilateral congenital deafness. Ann Otol Rhinol Laryngol 1968; 77:43-54.

15. Lindsay JR. Profound childhood deafness. Inner ear pa-

thology. Ann Otol Rhinol Laryngol 1973; 82 Suppl 5:1-121.

16. Gussen R, Adkins WY Jr. Saccule degeneration and ductus reuniens obstruction. Arch Otolaryngol 1974; 99:132-5.

17. Sando I, Harada T, Loehr A, Sobel JH. Sudden deafness. Histopathologic correlation in temporal bone. Ann Otol Rhinol Laryngol 1977; 86:269-79.

18. Gussen R. Saccule otoconia displacement into cochlea in cochleosaccular degeneration. Arch Otolaryngol 1980; 106:161-6.

19. Lindsay JR, Zajtchuk J. Concussion of the inner ear. Ann Otol Rhinol Laryngol 1970; 79:699-709.

20. Alford BR. Rubella-la bête noire de la médecine. Laryngoscope 1968; 78:1623-59.

21. Schuknecht HF. Pathology of the ear. Cambridge: Harvard University Press, 1974:453-65.

≈

NINCDS NOTES*

INSTITUTE INVITES TINNITUS RESEARCH APPLICATIONS

The NINCDS Communicative Disorders Program is soliciting research proposals on tinnitus, a common adult hearing problem. The Institute, which recently awarded several research grants in this area, is particularly interested in studies defining the auditory properties of tinnitus and identifying the disorder's causes and physiological correlates. Other high-priority needs are investigations to explore the masking of tinnitus and to develop animal models and improved methods of treatment. Information on application procedures may be obtained from Dr. Earleen Elkins, Communicative Disorders Program, NINCDS, Federal Building, Room 1C08, 7550 Wisconsin Avenue, Bethesda, MD 20205; tel: (301) 496-5061.

POSTDOCS SOUGHT FOR CHEMOSENSORY TRAINING

Applications from clinical investigators interested in postdoctoral research training in the clinical measurement of taste and smell function are being sought by NINCDS's Communicative Disorders Program. The announcement for training appears in the NIH Guide for Grants and Contracts, Vol. 10, No. 10. Additional information on these training opportunities is available from Dr. Jack Pearl, Communicative Disorders Program, NINCDS, Federal Building, Room 1C14, 7550 Wisconsin Avenue, Bethesda, MD 20205; tel: (301) 496-5061.

NINCDS SOLICITS INSTITUTIONAL TRAINING GRANT PROGRAMS IN SPEECH AND LANGUAGE

Nonprofit institutions have been invited by NINCDS to propose grant supported programs for training scientists in methods of investigating speech and language disorders. The Institute's Communicative Disorders Program, under guidelines established for National Research Service Awards, is seeking to encourage research careers in speech and language by providing postdoctoral laboratory and clinical research experience in these disciplines. Of particular interest are proposals providing for study of impaired language or speech development, language problems in infantile autism, stuttering, and voice disorders. Program proposals which include adult aphasia and dysarthrias associated with neurological disorders are also being sought. Domestic private or public institutions may apply for grants. Information on application procedures may be obtained from Dr. Christy L. Ludlow, Communicative Disorders Program, NINCDS, Federal Building, Room 1C13, 7550 Wisconsin Avenue, Bethesda, MD 20205; tel: (301) 496-5061.

----

*This information is prepared monthly by the Office of Scientific and Health Reports, National Institute of Neurological and Communicative Disorders and Stroke, National Institutes of Health, Building 31, Room 8A06, Bethesda, MD 20205; (301) 496-5751.

Ann Otol 91:1982

SPATIAL OCCUPANCY OF VESSELS AND FACIAL NERVE IN THE FACIAL CANAL

AKIRA OGAWA, MD, DMS
TOKYO, JAPAN

ISAMU SANDO, MD, DMS
PITTSBURGH, PENNSYLVANIA

The vascularity and spatial relationships of the contents of the labyrinthine portion of the facial canal were studied by measuring the diameters of arteries, the areas of the arteries, veins, facial nerve, and facial canal; and by expressing these areas as percentages of the areas of the facial canal and facial nerve. These results were compared for each of these segments of the facial canal. Using temporal bone sections which contained transverse or oblique sections of the three representative (labyrinthine, tympanic, and mastoid) portions of the facial canal, the size of the largest artery, and the area of the sectioned vessels, facial nerve, and facial canal were measured. Relative values of measured areas were calculated as an index of spatial occupancy of vessels and facial nerve in the canal. By comparing these results in three portions, we could demonstrate that, in the labyrinthine portion, the internal diameter of the main artery was less than four tenths of the diameter of the arteries in the other portions, and that the ratio of spatial occupancy of the vessels to the canal and to the nerve in the labyrinthine portion was extremely small compared with that in the other two portions. We also found that the labyrinthine and tympanic portions of the canal have less extra space for the nerve than does the mastoid portion. Considering both the vascularity of the three portions of the facial canal, and the spatial relationships of elements in the canal in each of the three segments of the canal, we feel that the facial nerve in the labyrinthine portion of the facial canal is indeed anatomically the most vulnerable portion of the nerve in its course through the temporal bone.

INTRODUCTION

Many authors have discussed the arterial supply to the facial nerve and the spatial relationship that the facial nerve bears to the canal.[1-5] In 1954 and 1956 Blunt[3,4] pointed out that in the labyrinthine portion of the canal there is no anastomosing arterial arcade making this portion the one weak link in an otherwise continuous arterial anastomotic chain throughout the facial canal. Because at that time[6] the lesion of Bell's palsy was believed to occur most commonly in the mastoid portion of the canal, Blunt did not perceive that the unique structure of the blood supply to the labyrinthine portion could possibly be associated with the etiology of this disease.

Recently, as a result of the development of a surgical technique to approach the internal auditory canal and the labyrinthine portion of the facial nerve,[7-9] it has been discovered that this portion of the nerve is most frequently involved in Bell's palsy as well as in traumatic herpetic and neoplastic lesions.[9] Also it has been found that the labyrinthine segment of the facial canal is the narrowest part of this structure in the temporal bone.[10]

Although the arterial supply and spatial relationship of the facial nerve to the facial canal have been discussed previously, no detailed study of these subjects in different portions of the facial canal has yet been reported.

The purpose of this paper is to investigate the vascularity of the facial nerve, as well as the spatial relationship of the facial nerve to the facial canal in its three different portions (labyrinthine, tympanic, and mastoid). These studies may help increase our understanding of the etiology of Bell's palsy.

MATERIALS AND METHOD

From our human temporal bone collection, 18 bones were selected for the present study. They were carefully chosen according to the following criteria: 1) No bones were studied which had been obtained from individuals who suffered from a congenital disease or an acquired disease which could lead to pathologic changes in the structure of the temporal bone. 2) Only specimens which included all labyrinthine, tympanic, and mastoid portions of the facial canal in either cross section or oblique section were studied; those in which the canal was seen in longitudinal section were not included in this study.

These bones had been removed from cadavers in the routine manner, fixed in 10% formalin solution, dehydrated in graded solutions of ethanol, embedded in celloidin, and sectioned horizontally at 20μ. Every tenth section was stained with hematoxylin and eosin (H & E). Additional sections were stained by the Verhoeff-van Gieson method to differentiate the artery from the vein.

The diameter of the largest artery and the sum of the areas of the arteries and veins and the areas of the facial nerve and facial canal in the labyrinthine, tympanic, and mastoid portions of each temporal bone were measured. 1) The measurements in the labyrinthine portion were made just proximal to the geniculate ganglion (Figs. 1 and 2). 2) The tympanic measurements were made in the middle of the tympanic portion (Figs. 3 and 4). 3) The measurements in the mastoid portion were made at the same level as the lowest point of the cochlea (Fig. 5). As described by Lindeman,[5] parts of the tympanic and mastoid portions of the canal were found to be dilated. These were locations where blood vessels entered the surrounding bone tissue. In this study, these parts were not used in determining the diameters and areas mentioned above.

The internal diameter of the largest artery in each of the three representative portions of the facial canal was measured using an eyepiece scale built into the microscope. The internal diameter was measured because it was always possible to detect endotheli-

From the Departments of Otolaryngology and Pathology, University of Pittsburgh School of Medicine, Eye and Ear Hospital of Pittsburgh. This study was supported by Research Grant NS 13787 from the National Institute of Neurological and Communicative Disorders and Stroke.

REPRINTS — Isamu Sando, MD, DMS, Department of Otolaryngology, University of Pittsburgh School of Medicine, Eye and Ear Hospital of Pittsburgh, Pittsburgh, PA 15213.

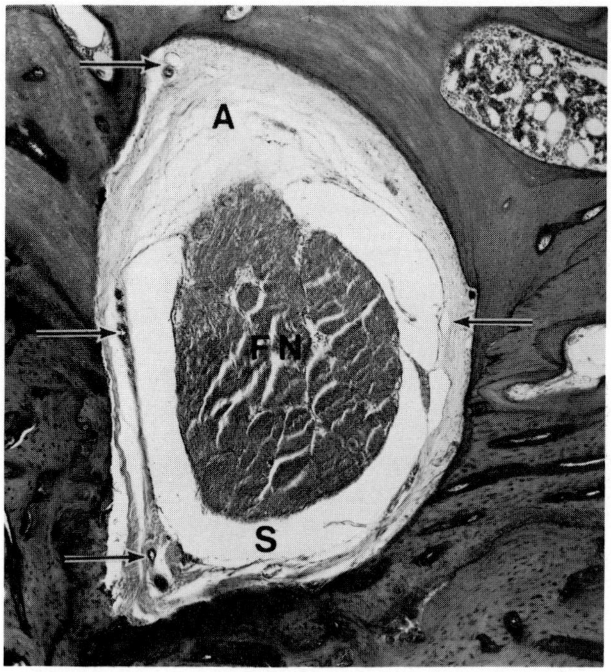

Fig. 1. (Bone 13) Labyrinthine portion of the facial canal. Several small vessels (arrows) are shown in the peripheral connective tissue. A clear space (S) surrounds most of the facial nerve (FN) except for the area (A) close to the geniculate ganglion, which might contain cerebrospinal fluid as described by Fisch.[11] (H & E, x52)

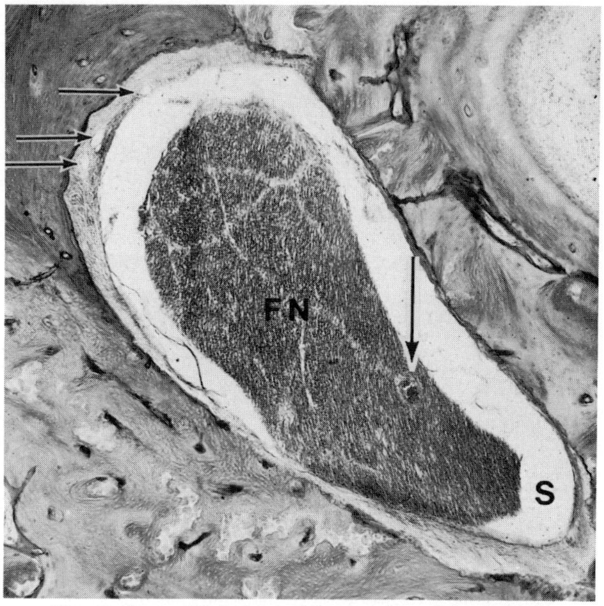

Fig. 2. (Bone 10) Labyrinthine portion of the facial canal. In this portion of the canal a small space surrounds the facial nerve (FN). The ratio of the area of the nerve to that of the canal is almost the same as the mean of this portion. Note that no perineurium surrounding the nerve was observed. An artery (large arrow) which is shown in the nerve bundle is exceptionally large for this portion. A few small veins (small arrows) may be seen in the peripheral connective tissue. S - Cerebrospinal fluid space. (H & E, x52)

um more clearly than to differentiate the tunica adventitia, which was often indistinct in those sections stained with H & E. When an artery had been sectioned obliquely, the minimum width of the lumen was taken as the diameter of this artery.

Enlarged pictures of the vessels, facial nerve, and facial canal in each portion of the facial canal were drawn in a projector apparatus. From these enlargements, the areas of the vascular lumen, facial nerve, and facial canal were measured using a compensating polar planimeter. Then the actual areas of the arteries, veins, nerve, and canal were determined by multiplying the area measured on the enlargement by the inverse of the magnification used. Because many specimens had been sectioned obliquely, the areas of these structures would be greater on oblique sections than these areas measured on more transversely sectioned specimens. However, in general, the proportion of the area of one structure to the area of another would not be affected by the angle of sectioning.

When the sum of the areas of the arteries and veins and the areas of the facial nerve and facial canal in each of the three segments of the canal had been determined, we calculated the following ratios to determine the degree to which each segment of the facial canal was occupied by vessels or the facial nerve. We also calculated an index of vascularity for the facial nerve in each segment. We then compared these indices for each of the portions of the canal: ratio of sum of areas of a) sectioned arterial lumens to area of the facial canal, b) sectioned arterial lumens to area of the facial nerve, c) sectioned venous lumens to area of the facial

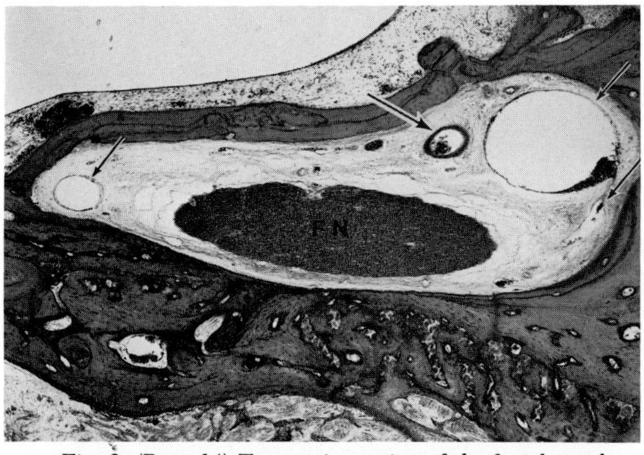

Fig. 3. (Bone 14) Tympanic portion of the facial canal. An artery (large arrow) and veins (small arrows) are notable. Facial nerve (FN) is covered by the perineurium. (H & E, x49)

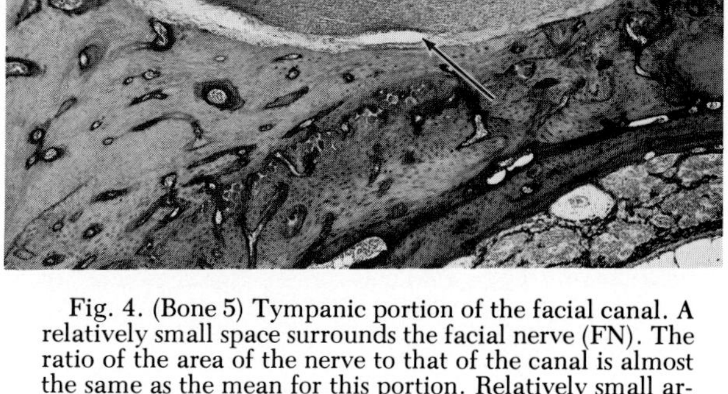

Fig. 4. (Bone 5) Tympanic portion of the facial canal. A relatively small space surrounds the facial nerve (FN). The ratio of the area of the nerve to that of the canal is almost the same as the mean for this portion. Relatively small arteries (large arrows) and a moderate number of venous lumens (small arrows) are visible. (H & E, x45)

TABLE 1. INTERNAL DIAMETER OF LARGEST ARTERY IN EACH PORTION OF FACIAL CANAL

	Portion (μ)		
Bone No.	*Lab*	*Tym*	*Mast*
1	20	20	30
2	20	70	70
3	20	30	70
4	(-)*	70	50
5	20	40	30
6	30	50	150
7	20	100	60
8	20	130	110
9	30	50	90
10	50	60	40
11	20	50	40
12	20	30	60
13	20	70	160
14	30	160	40
15	20	40	90
16	30	110	70
17	30	40	90
18	(-)*	70	120
Mean†	25.0(a)	66.1(b)	76.1(b)
SD	8.2	37.3	38.8

Lab - Labyrinthine portion of the canal; Tym - Tympanic portion of the canal; Mast - Mastoid portion of the canal.

*No artery was detected in this specimen.

†The mean value (a) is significantly different from mean value (b) by Student's t test ($p<0.01$).

canal, d) sectioned venous lumens to area of the facial nerve, and ratio of the area of sectioned facial nerve to the area of the facial canal. In all of these studies, vessels which were smaller than 10 μ in diameter were neglected. Statistical analysis of the means and variances of these values was carried out by the Student's t test and F test, respectively.

RESULTS

Internal Diameter of the Largest Artery. The artery was detected in the labyrinthine portion in 16 out of 18 bones. Its mean diameter was 25.0 ±8.2 μ(M±SD). In the tympanic and mastoid portions two or three arteries were detected in all 18 bones. The largest artery in the tympanic portion had a mean diameter of 66.1±37.3 μ and 76.1±38.8 μ and in the mastoid portion respectively. The results of these measurements are shown in Table 1. The arterial diameter in the labyrinthine portion was significantly smaller than that in both the tympanic and mastoid portions ($p<0.01$).

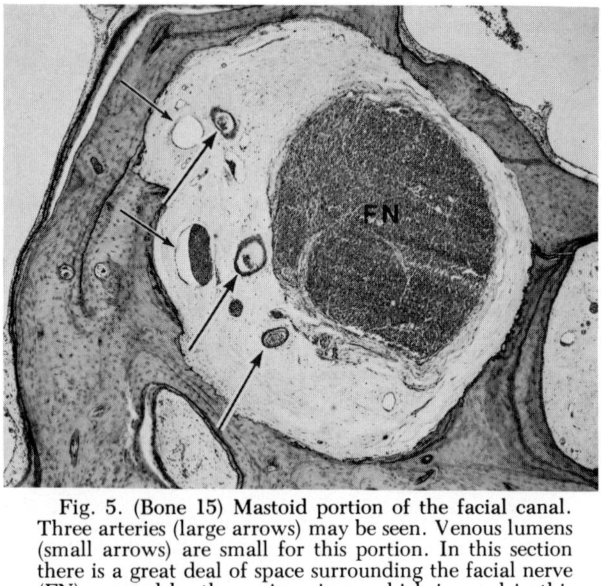

Fig. 5. (Bone 15) Mastoid portion of the facial canal. Three arteries (large arrows) may be seen. Venous lumens (small arrows) are small for this portion. In this section there is a great deal of space surrounding the facial nerve (FN) covered by the perineurium, which is usual in this portion of the canal. (H & E, x45)

TABLE 2. RATIO OF SUM OF AREAS OF SECTIONED ARTERIAL LUMENS TO AREA OF FACIAL CANAL

	Portion (%)		
Bone No.	*Lab*	*Tym*	*Mast*
1	0.0	0.2	0.1
2	0.0	1.2	0.5
3	0.1	0.1	0.3
4	(-)*	0.7	0.3
5	0.1	0.2	0.1
6	0.1	0.3	0.5
7	0.1	0.5	0.4
8	0.6	1.0	0.8
9	0.0	0.3	0.8
10	0.2	1.2	0.3
11	0.1	0.3	1.2
12	0.0	0.2	0.4
13	0.1	0.7	1.3
14	0.2	1.9	0.1
15	0.0	0.2	0.7
16	0.2	1.1	0.5
17	0.1	0.8	0.8
18	(-)*	0.4	0.7
Mean†	0.12(a)	0.63(b)	0.54(b)
SD	0.14	0.49	0.35

Ratio of Sum of Areas of Sectioned Arterial Lumens to Area of the Facial Canal or the Facial Nerve. As shown in Table 2, the ratio of the sum of luminal areas of sectioned arteries to areas of the facial canal was 0.12±0.14% (M±SD) in the labyrinthine portion, 0.63±0.49% in the tympanic portion, and 0.54±0.35% in the mastoid portion.

TABLE 3. RATIO OF SUM OF AREAS OF SECTIONED ARTERIAL LUMENS TO AREA OF FACIAL NERVE

	Portion (%)		
Bone No.	*Lab*	*Tym*	*Mast*
1	0.0	0.3	0.1
2	0.1	3.1	1.9
3	0.4	0.2	10.0
4	(-)*	1.4	0.8
5	0.1	0.3	0.2
6	0.3	1.1	4.7
7	0.1	0.8	1.3
8	0.9	2.3	2.7
9	0.0	0.5	2.3
10	0.4	2.0	0.6
11	0.1	1.6	3.9
12	0.1	0.4	1.0
13	0.2	2.1	6.0
14	0.4	6.8	0.7
15	0.1	0.4	1.9
16	0.4	2.8	2.0
17	0.1	1.4	2.1
18	(-)*	0.9	1.9
Mean†	0.23(a)	1.58(b)	2.45(b)
SD	0.23	1.58	2.44

TABLE 4. RATIO OF SUM OF AREAS OF SECTIONED VENOUS LUMENS TO AREA OF FACIAL NERVE

Bone No.	Lab	Portion (%) Tym	Mast
1	0.9	7.9	0.6
2	0.5	12.8	6.4
3	0.7	3.2	14.9
4	0.5	6.8	5.8
5	1.3	8.6	4.2
6	0.2	13.6	18.0
7	1.0	1.9	7.0
8	0.3	5.9	11.0
9	0.7	3.9	6.8
10	0.3	1.2	1.3
11	0.6	14.2	9.0
12	0.8	5.4	7.9
13	0.4	5.1	3.4
14	0.3	23.1	11.4
15	0.3	1.9	2.5
16	0.4	8.3	8.9
17	0.9	9.4	8.6
18	0.3	14.5	9.7
Mean†	0.58(a)	8.21(b)	7.63(b)
SD	0.31	5.67	4.51

The ratio in the labyrinthine portion was significantly less than that in the other two portions ($p<0.001$). The ratio of the total luminal area of sectioned arteries to the facial nerve area was $0.23\pm0.23\%$ ($M\pm SD$) in the labyrinthine portion, $1.58\pm1.58\%$ in the tympanic portion, and $2.45\pm2.44\%$ in the mastoid portion. These are shown in Table 3. Again, the ratio in the labyrinthine portion was significantly smaller than that in the other two portions ($p<0.001$).

Ratio of Sum of Areas of Sectioned Venous Lumens to Area of the Facial Canal or the Facial Nerve. Table 4 shows the ratio of sum of areas of sectioned veins to the area of the facial canal, which was $0.58\pm0.31\%$ ($M\pm SD$) in the labyrinthine portion, $8.21\pm5.67\%$ in the tympanic portion, and $7.63\pm4.51\%$ in the mastoid portion. The ratio in the labyrinthine portion was significantly less than that observed in the remaining two portions ($p<0.001$). As shown in Table 5, the total area of sectioned veins averaged $1.12\pm0.63\%$ ($M\pm SD$) of that of the area of the facial nerve in the labyrinthine portion, $22.89\pm23.36\%$ of that in the tympanic portion, and $31.43\pm35.84\%$ of the area of the facial nerve in the mastoid portion. Again, the ratio in the labyrinthine portion was significantly smaller than that in the other two portions ($p<0.001$).

TABLE 5. RATIO OF SUM OF AREAS OF SECTIONED VENOUS LUMENS TO AREA OF FACIAL NERVE

Bone No.	Lab	Portion (%) Tym	Mast
1	2.1	13.2	1.7
2	1.1	32.3	24.4
3	2.1	6.6	43.1
4	1.1	13.6	16.1
5	2.0	15.7	8.3
6	0.4	52.6	159.6
7	1.9	2.9	23.3
8	0.6	14.1	36.1
9	0.1	6.7	19.8
10	0.5	2.0	2.5
11	1.3	68.1	30.3
12	1.4	10.0	21.2
13	1.0	15.4	16.0
14	0.7	84.9	69.1
15	0.7	2.8	6.9
16	0.9	21.1	38.2
17	1.7	17.7	23.3
18	0.6	32.4	25.9
Mean†	1.12(a)	22.89(b)	31.43(b)
SD	0.63	23.36	35.84

TABLE 6. RATIO OF AREA OF SECTIONED FACIAL NERVE TO FACIAL CANAL

Bone No.	Lab	Portion (%) Tym	Mast
1	44.4	59.3	36.1
2	45.4	37.4	26.2
3	35.3	49.1	34.6
4	50.1	50.0	35.7
5	62.5	54.9	50.7
6	43.2	25.9	11.3
7	50.7	63.4	30.2
8	62.6	41.8	30.5
9	47.8	59.0	34.1
10	53.6	62.1	51.4
11	46.6	20.8	29.8
12	54.2	53.5	37.2
13	35.1	33.2	21.4
14	38.0	27.2	16.4
15	41.5	66.8	36.2
16	51.3	39.3	23.2
17	56.4	53.1	37.0
18	50.0	44.6	37.4
Mean†	48.26(a)	46.74(a)	32.19(b)
SD	8.06	13.80	10.21

Ratio of the Area of Sectioned Facial Nerve to that of Facial Canal. As shown in Table 6, the facial nerve occupied $48.26\pm8.06\%$ ($M\pm SD$) of the canal in the labyrinthine portion, $46.74\pm13.80\%$ in the tympanic portion, and $32.19\pm10.21\%$ of the canal in the mastoid portion. The former two values were significantly larger than the third ($p<0.001$).

DISCUSSION

Until recently, it was thought that Bell's palsy was most probably caused by primary or secondary ischemia. Recently, however, viral infection has been implicated in the etiology of this disorder.[11-14] Edema and ischemia of the nerve would be expected to occur with this disorder regardless of the cause, and engorgement of the vein due to the edema of the nerve would lead to further increased edema of the nerve.[15] These changes must occur within the facial canal, which as a closed space allows only limited possibility for expansion of soft tissue. Therefore, the condition of the arterial and venous contents of the canal and the spatial relationship that the nerve bears to the canal appear to be important factors in the occurrence of Bell's palsy.

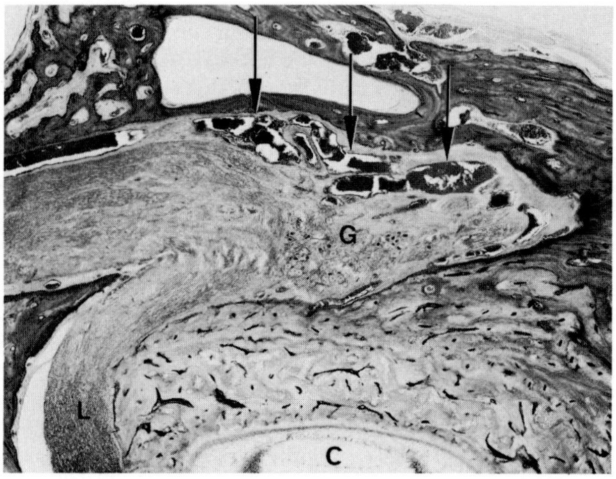

Fig. 6. Rich vascularity (arrows) in the horizontally sectioned geniculate ganglion (G) area is in striking contrast to the poor vascularity in the labyrinthine portion (L). C - Cochlea. (H & E, x27)

Until recently, it had been thought that the most frequent site of the lesion of Bell's palsy was the mastoid portion of the nerve, just above the stylomastoid foramen.[6,16-18] Several investigators examined this portion of the canal for evidence of an anatomical factor predisposing to Bell's palsy, but they found no evidence of compromised blood supply to any part of the facial nerve below the geniculate ganglion which would especially predispose it to ischemia, the result of vascular spasm.[3] They also searched for narrowing in the vertical portion of the facial canal,[5] but found none.

It is now possible to approach the labyrinthine portion of the facial canal and the internal auditory canal through the middle cranial fossa.[7-9] This development has shown clinically that the labyrinthine portion of the nerve is the most frequent site of the lesion of Bell's palsy.[19,20] This seems reasonable, since it has been reported that this particular portion of the canal is the narrowest[10] and that there is no anastomosing arterial arcade in the canal (this latter will be discussed later).

Regarding the vascularity of the facial canal, to our knowledge, there is no clear description of the blood supply in the labyrinthine portion. Blunt[3,4] reported that the arterial blood supply of the facial nerve derives proximally from the anterior inferior cerebellar artery, the nerve in the internal auditory meatus being supplied by the internal auditory artery. He did not describe the particular sources of the blood supply to the labyrinthine portion. Sunderland and Cossar[2] stated that the branches of the petrosal artery proceed centrally along the facial nerve as far as the meatal entrance to the labyrinthine portion of the facial canal. They also found that fine branches from the internal auditory artery, anterior inferior cerebellar artery, and basilar artery supplied the nerve between the brainstem and the geniculate ganglion. Nager and Nager[1] reported that one of the branches of the petrosal artery enters the geniculate ganglion and divides into two vessels, one of which travels centrally to the fundus of the internal auditory meatus.

From the descriptions supplied by these investigators, it appears that the vascular supply to the labyrinthine portion of the facial nerve is derived from the fine branches of the petrosal artery or of the internal auditory artery or both; in addition, it appears that this portion had no anastomosing arterial arcade. Therefore the labyrinthine portion seems to be poorly vascularized compared with the other two portions, which are supplied from an arterial arcade formed by direct anastomosis between the stylomastoid artery and the petrosal artery.[1,3] This anastomosis is of profound functional significance since it ensures adequate vascularization of the intracanalicular segment of the facial nerve, even after obstruction of one or another of its component vessels.[4] Blunt[3] also found that the petrosal artery provides the main arterial supply to the geniculate ganglion and that there is no direct link between the petrosal artery and the branch of the internal auditory artery. The labyrinthine portion, therefore, is the one weak link in an otherwise continuous arterial anastomosing chain.

In the present study, the relatively poor vascularity of the labyrinthine portion was demonstrated, which is in striking contrast to the geniculate ganglion area (Fig. 6). This was determined by the measurement of the largest artery, the arterial area, and the venous area in the canal. The internal diameter of the largest artery in the labyrinthine portion was found to be less than 40% on the average, of that of the main artery measured in the other two portions. The ratio in the labyrinthine portion of the sum of areas of sectioned arterial lumens to the area of both the facial canal and the facial nerve was much smaller than that same ratio in the tympanic and the mastoid portions.

In the labyrinthine portion, the ratio of the sum of areas of sectioned veins to the canal and to the nerve was also much smaller than that observed in the tympanic portion and the mastoid portion. However, there was no significant difference between the above mentioned ratios of the arteries and veins in the tympanic and mastoid portions. From this study it seems clear to us that due to its poor vascularization, the labyrinthine portion of the facial nerve could easily become ischemic.

Edema of the facial nerve may be closely related to the efficiency of venous drainage. Veins in the canal could easily become engorged as a result of swelling of the facial nerve, which in turn would increase the edema. This situation may be more likely to occur in the labyrinthine portion of the canal because this portion, according to our study, was revealed to have a poor venous system compared with the other two portions.

Just as the vascularity of different portions of the

facial canal is significant in the etiology of Bell's palsy, we feel that the spatial condition of the nerve in the canal is also one of the important factors in the etiology of this disorder. Sunderland and Cossar[2] found that the nerve occupied 20-50% of the canal. Lindeman[5] measured only the mastoid portion of the canal, using a method very similar to that used in our study, and stated that the nerve occupied 25-50% of the bony canal and that no particular narrowing within the mastoid portion of the facial canal could be seen. However, Fisch[10] measured diameters of the facial nerve and canal at three different points along the nerve, similar to those which we chose to study. He found that unoccupied space in the facial canal was least in the labyrinthine portion.

The results of the present study demonstrate that the facial nerve area in both the labyrinthine and tympanic portions occupies on an average more than 45% of the canal, while in the mastoid portion the nerve occupies only 32%. This means that the labyrinthine and tympanic portions of the canal have less extra space for the nerve than does the mastoid portion of the canal. Thus it may be seen how the nerve may be damaged so easily.

We feel that the most reasonable finding of our investigation was extremely poor vascularity of the labyrinthine portion of the facial canal. This poor vascularity combined with the unique arterial supply described by Blunt[3] could easily lead to ischemia of the facial nerve. In comparison we feel that the finding of narrowing of the labyrinthine portion is less significant. However, both poor vascularity and narrowing of the canal in relation to the facial nerve in the labyrinthine portion appear to be one of the significant etiologies of Bell's palsy.

Presently Dr. Ogawa is an Assistant Professor, Department of Otolaryngology, Tokyo Medical and Dental University, Tokyo, Japan.

ACKNOWLEDGMENT — The authors express their appreciation to Eugene N. Myers, MD, and Mark May, MD, for giving us good advice and to Julio A. Martinez, MD, for special staining. Appreciation is also expressed to Mrs. Ruth Anderson and Mrs. Ellie Lee for their kind assistance in this study.

REFERENCES

1. Nager GT, Nager M. The arteries of human middle ear with particular regard to the blood supply of the auditory ossicles. Ann Otol Rhinol Laryngol 1953; 62:923-49.

2. Sunderland S, Cossar DF. The structure of the facial nerve. Anat Rec 1953; 116:147-62.

3. Blunt MJ. The blood supply of the facial nerve. J Anat 1954; 88:520-6.

4. Blunt MJ. The possible role of vascular changes in the etiology of Bell's palsy. J Laryngol Otol 1956; 70:701-13.

5. Lindeman H. The fallopian canal, an anatomical study of its distal part. Acta Otolaryngol (Stockh) 1960 Suppl 158:204-11.

6. Cawthorne T. Peripheral facial paralysis. Some aspects of its pathology. Laryngoscope 1946; 56:653-64.

7. House WF. Surgical exposure of the internal auditory canal and its contents through the middle cranial fossa. Laryngoscope 1961; 71:1363-85.

8. Pulec JL. Total decompression of the facial nerve. Laryngoscope 1966; 76:1015-28.

9. Fisch U. Operations of the facial nerve in its labyrinthine and meatal courses. In: Miehlke A, ed. Surgery of the facial nerve. Philadelphia: WB Saunders, 1973:175-205.

10. Fisch U. Total facial nerve decompression and electroneurography. In: Silverstein H. Morrell H, eds. Neurological surgery of ear. Birmingham, Ala: Aesculapius Publishing Company, 1977:21-33.

11. Peiterson E, Caunt AE. The incidence of herpes zoster antibodies in patient with peripheral facial palsy. J Laryngol Otol 1970; 84:65-70.

12. McCormick DP. Herpes simplex virus as a cause of Bell's palsy. Lancet 1972; 1:937-9.

13. Tomita H, Hayakawa W, Hondo R. Varicella-zoster in idiopathic facial palsy. Arch Otolaryngol 1972; 95:364-8.

14. May M. Bell's palsy: progressive ascending paralysis, therapeutic implications. Laryngoscope 1978; 88:61-72.

15. Groves J. Facial nerve. In: Hinchcliffe R, Harrison D, eds. Scientific foundation of otolaryngology. Chicago: Year Book Medical Publishers Inc, 1976:429-59.

16. Sullivan JA. Recent advances in the surgical treatment of facial paralysis and Bell's palsy. Laryngoscope 1952; 63:449-60.

17. Jongkees LBW. Treatment of Bell's palsy. Neurology 1957; 7:697-701.

18. McGovern FH. A review of the experimental aspects of Bell's palsy. Laryngoscope 1969; 78:324-33.

19. Fisch U, Esslen E. Total intratemporal exposure of the facial nerve. Arch Otolaryngol 1972; 95:335-41.

20. May M. Total facial nerve exploration: transmastoid, extralabyrinthine and subtemporal indications and results. Laryngoscope 1979; 89:906-17.

Ann Otol 91:1982

TYMPANOMETRIC CONFIGURATIONS AND MIDDLE EAR FINDINGS IN EXPERIMENTAL OTITIS MEDIA

G. SCOTT GIEBINK, MD

KELLEY A. HELLER

EARL R. HARFORD, PhD

MINNEAPOLIS, MINNESOTA

Relationships between ventilation of the middle ear (ME) system and pathogenic bacteria in the upper respiratory tract were explored in an animal model to better understand the etiopathogenesis of otitis media. Otitis media developed in 12 of 18 chinchillas inoculated intranasally with *Streptococcus pneumoniae* followed by bilateral ME deflation (negative pressure). Otitis media with effusion developed in 19 of 36 ears examined ten days after inoculation. The development of purulent effusion after ten days was highly correlated with persistent negative ME pressure for at least 48 hours after deflation, while most ears that developed serous effusion after ten days had normal ME pressure 48 hours after deflation. Tympanometric validation of the presence or absence of effusion and type of effusion was obtained ten days after inoculation. A low compliance tympanogram detected 90% of the purulent effusions and was 100% specific for this type of effusion. In contrast, three of four serous effusions were associated with normal pressure/normal compliance tracings suggesting that the physical characteristics or volume of ME effusion and/or the histopathology of the ME cleft are reflected in the tympanometric configuration.

Otitis media (OM) is a common childhood illness effecting the majority of children on at least one occasion before entering school. Although the suppurative complications of acute OM, such as mastoiditis and meningitis, have diminished in frequency with the widespread use of antimicrobials, hearing impairment remains a major sequela of this disease effecting children's language and scholastic skills. Acoustic impedance measurement as a means of evaluating middle ear (ME) physiologic function is gaining wide interest among otologists and pediatricians. Tympanometry resolves many of the disadvantages of conventional otologic assessment for otitis media with effusion (OME) and has proven to be a reliable, objective and noninvasive procedure.[1-4]

While the incidence and epidemiology of OM is well-described,[5-7] the pathogenesis of this condition is not understood. Clinical and experimental studies suggest that a triad of factors, including ME ventilation, pathogenic microbes in the upper respiratory tract, and inflammatory and immunologic host responses, are intimately involved in OM pathogenesis.[8] Laboratory examination of middle ear effusion (MEE) from patients with OM reveals distinct effusion types, which have been classified as purulent, serous and mucoid, yet observations in humans and experimental animals show that effusions change their biochemical, microbiologic and cytologic characteristics over time.[8-11] Thus, OM is a spectrum of different clinical entities which appear to have a common etiopathogenesis.

Animal models of OM have been employed to explore the pathogenesis of this condition. Functional or mechanical obstruction of the eustachian tube produces serous of mucoid OM,[10,12-15] and inoculation of the ME with *Streptococcus pneumoniae* produces purulent OM.[11] While intranasal inoculation of chinchillas with pneumococci did not yield a high incidence of OM, middle ear deflation (negative pressure) applied several days after intranasal inoculation greatly increased the incidence of purulent OM, thereby supporting the hypothesis that both compromised ME ventilation and pathogenic respiratory tract bacteria are important in the pathogenesis of purulent OM.[16] Tympanometry has been utilized to further explore the relationships between ventilation of the ME system and pathogenic bacteria in the upper respiratory tract in the production of experimental OM. This report describes ME pressure/tympanic membrane (TM) compliance characteristics which antedate the development of OM in chinchillas, as well as the pressure/compliance characteristics associated with direct observations of the ME cleft and effusion.

METHODS

Otitis media was produced in healthy young adult chinchillas, one to two years of age, following intranasal inoculation with *S pneumoniae* type 7F (American type 51). Virulence of the strain was maintained by monthly passage in mice, and serotype was confirmed throughout the experiments by the quellung reaction using antiserum to type 7 *S pneumoniae* (Statens Seruminstitut, Copenhagen, Denmark). Pneumococci were cultured in nutrient broth and frozen in glycerol-buffered albumin at −70 C for dilution prior to each experiment.[16] The inoculum for each experiment was prepared by thawing an aliquot of the frozen pneumococcal suspension immediately before inoculation and diluting it in sterile phosphate-buffered saline (PBS; pH 7.4) to a concentration of 2×10^5 pneumococci/ml. Chinchillas anesthetized with 15 mg ketamine hydrochloride IM were inoculated intranasally by

From the Departments of Pediatrics and Otolaryngology, University of Minnesota School of Medicine, Minneapolis. Supported by grant number NS14538 from the National Institute of Neurological and Communicative Disorders and Stroke, contract number N01 AI 52533 and grant number AI-17160 from the National Institute of Allergy and Infectious Diseases.

REPRINTS — G. Scott Giebink, MD, Box 483, Mayo Building, University of Minnesota School of Medicine, Minneapolis, MN 55455.

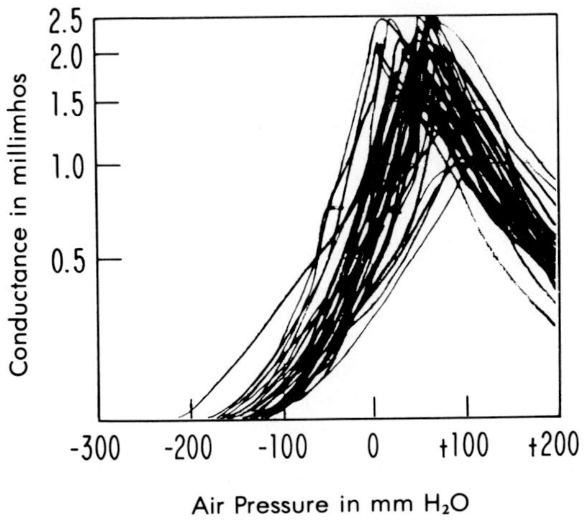

Fig. 1. The range of tympanometric configurations from 43 healthy anesthetized chinchillas (86 ears). All tympanograms showed peak compliance between 15 and 106 mm H_2O (mean = 60 mm H_2O).

dripping 0.5 ml of the bacterial suspension into the nares, maintaining the animals in a supine position for several minutes.

Middle ear deflation was performed bilaterally two days following pneumococcal inoculation. The fur over the ME bulla was plucked and the skin prepared aseptically. Immediately prior to deflation, the nasopharynx of each chinchilla was rinsed with 0.5 ml sterile PBS. Negative pressure was applied to the ME by inserting a 23 gauge needle attached to a mercury manometer into the epitympanic bulla. Negative pressure (−30 mm Hg) was applied to each ear while an observer noted TM retraction. Deflation was maintained in each ear for five minutes.

At regular intervals, the TM of each chinchilla were examined using an operating microscope, and tympanometry was performed using a Grason-Stadler 1722 Middle Ear Analyzer. Bone wax (Lukens Laboratory) was liberally applied to the tympanometer tip to insure an airtight seal. When properly inserted, the tympanometric tracing began between 0.25 and 1.25 millimhos. Duplicate readings were taken of each ear. Tympanic membrane color and opacity were described at each examination, and presence of an air-fluid level, bubbles, or perforation was noted. All chinchillas were sacrificed ten days after pneumococcal inoculation, and the ME cavities were examined for effusion and culture on 5% sheep's blood agar.

RESULTS

Tympanometry was performed on 86 healthy uninfected chinchillas to establish the normal tympanometric configuration of an anesthetized chinchilla. These tympanograms were plotted on the pressure compliance axes to construct the upper and lower range of normal (Fig. 1). Results clustered in a single configuration with peak compliance between 15 and 106 mm H_2O pressure, which was defined as the normal (type A) tympanogram. One chinchilla was studied before and during anesthesia to determine if there was ME hyperinflation during anesthesia which might account for the positive pressure peak observed in anesthetized animals. The peak TM compliance was 47 mm H_2O before anesthesia, 67 mm H_2O during anesthesia and 54 mm H_2O immediately on awakening.

Eighteen chinchillas were inoculated intranasally with *S pneumoniae* followed two days later by bilateral ME deflation. Nasal colonization with pneumococci was established in all 18 animals, and 12 (67%) developed OME. Three animals (17%) developed bilateral purulent effusions which cultured *S pneumoniae*. Seven animals (39%) developed unilateral purulent pneumococcal OM, and three of these seven had sterile serous effusion in the contralateral ear. Two animals (11%) developed bilateral OM with sterile serous effusions. Three animals (17%) showed a unilateral change in TM color and opacity at sacrifice but effusion was not obtained.

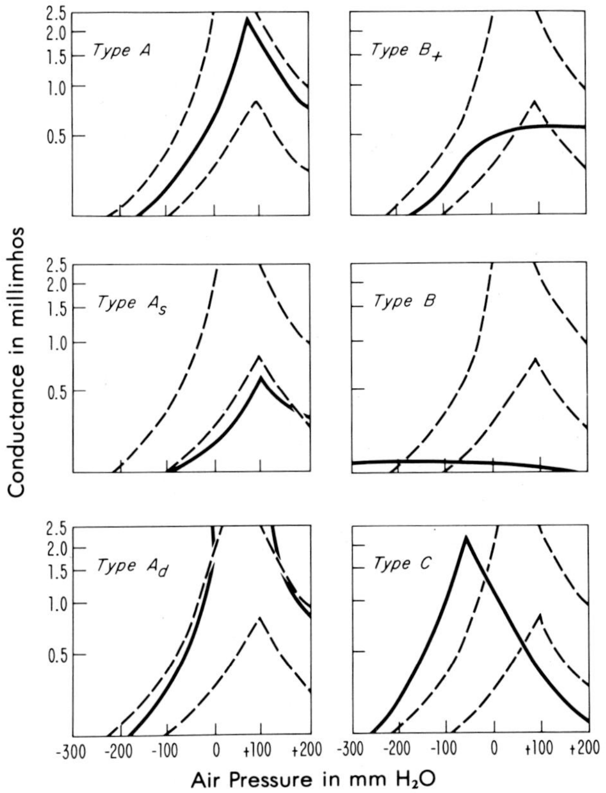

Fig. 2. Tympanogram configurations in chinchillas. Type A tympanogram shows peak TM compliance between 15 and 106 mm H_2O. Type A_s tympanogram has a peaked configuration with normal pressure but reduced compliance. Type A_d tympanogram has an open configuration with no peak but pressure within the normal range. Type B_+ tympanogram shows an initial rise in compliance as pressure is increased but no peak. Type B tympanogram shows no change in compliance as pressure is increased. Type C tympanogram shows nearly normal compliance with negative ME pressures (<6 mm H_2O).

Tympanometry was performed on inoculated chinchillas two days following ME deflation to determine ventilation deficits associated with the subsequent development of OM, and again at sacrifice for tympanometric validation of effusion. The resulting tympanometric configurations clustered into six unique types which were classified using modifications from human tympanometric configurations described by Jerger based on the Madsen impedance bridge[1] (Fig. 2).

TABLE 1. TYMPANOMETRIC CONFIGURATIONS 2 DAYS AFTER ME DEFLATION AND SUBSEQUENT DEVELOPMENT OF OM IN 18 CHINCHILLAS

ME Finding at Sacrifice	*No. Ears*	*No. Ears with Specified Tympanometric Configuration 48 Hours After Deflation*					
		A	A_d	A_s	B_+	B	C
OME							
Purulent, pneumococcal	13	0	0	0	8	0	5
Serous, sterile	6	4	0	0	2	0	0
Red/opaque TM without effusion	3	3	0	0	0	0	0
No OM	13	11	0	1	0	0	1
Total no. ears		18	0	1	10	0	6

Ears that developed effusion during the ten days after inoculation and ME deflation showed persistent negative ME pressure and low compliance tympanograms when measured 48 hours after deflation (Table 1). A type B_+ or C tympanometric configuration 48 hours after deflation was observed in 15 of 19 ears that developed OME during the ensuing eight days but in only 1 of 13 ears that did not develop OM ($X^2 = 15.676$, $p < .001$). All 13 ears that subsequently developed purulent effusions which cultured pneumococci showed a B + or C configuration 48 hours after deflation (Table 1). However, only two ears that developed OM with sterile serous effusion showed a B_+ configuration, and none showed type C configurations 48 hours after deflation. One ear with a sterile serous effusion could not be tested. All three ears showing TM opacity or color changes but without effusion at sacrifice had normal type A configurations 48 hours after deflation. Of the 13 ears which showed no evidence of OM at sacrifice, 12 showed normal ME pressure (11 type A and 1 type A_s), and one showed negative ME pressure (type C) 48 hours after deflation.

Tympanometric validation of effusion was performed on 30 ears available for examination ten days after inoculation when the animals were sacrificed (Table 2). The type B_+ and B configurations were observed in 9 of 14 ears with effusion and in none of 16 ears without effusion ($X^2 = 14.694$, $p < .001$). Nine of ten ears with purulent effusion showed a B_+ or B configuration, while none of the four ears with sterile serous effusion showed this configuration ($p = .005$ by Fisher's exact test). In fact, three of the four ears with sterile serous effusion had normal type A configurations, and one had a negative pressure type C configuration. Effusion volume was not measured. All three ears with TM color or opacity changes without effusion had normal type A tympanograms. Eight of the 13 ears which showed no evidence of OM had normal ME pressure (7 type A, 1 type A_d), and 5 showed negative type C configurations. Thus, negative ME pressure persisted in five ears for eight days after deflation with pneumococci present in the nasopharynx without the development of OM.

DISCUSSION

Middle ear deflation was employed in this animal model because observations in humans have shown that negative ME pressure accompanies and often precedes the development of OM.[17-20] Tympanometry was employed to measure ME pressure since others have demonstrated a close correlation between electroacoustic impedance measurement and actual intratympanic air pressures.[21] Although anesthesia may have accounted for some positive ME pressure in chinchillas, they manifested a static positive pressure by the instrument used in this study.

Previous studies have shown that intranasal inoculation of pneumococci in chinchillas with normal ME pressure yielded a very low incidence (13%) of OM; ME deflation increased the incidence of OM in this animal model by five-fold.[16] A deflation pressure of −30 mm Hg was selected because this pressure caused functional eustachian tube obstruction but did not cause acute histopathologic alteration of the ME mucoperiosteal lining.[22] Because all animals subjected to pneumococcal inoculation and ME deflation did not develop OM, we hypothesized that the duration of negative pressure in the ME was directly related to subsequent development of OM. Tympanometric measurements 48 hours after deflation confirmed this hypothesis: five of six type C configurations were

TABLE 2. TYMPANOMETRIC CONFIGURATIONS AND ME FINDINGS AT SACRIFICE IN 15 CHINCHILLAS 10 DAYS AFTER PNEUMOCOCCAL INOCULATION

ME Finding	*No. Ears*	*No. Ears with Specified Tympanometric Configuration at Sacrifice*					
		A	A_d	A_s	B_+	B	C
OME							
Purulent, pneumococcal	10	1	0	0	8	1	0
Serous, sterile	4	3	0	0	0	0	1
Red/opaque TM without effusion	3	3	0	0	0	0	0
No OM	13	7	1	0	0	0	5
Total no. ears		14	1	0	8	1	6

recorded in ears that subsequently developed purulent OM. Since four of the six ears that developed sterile serous effusion had normal tympanograms 48 hours after deflation, the pathogenesis of this condition seems to be associated with a shorter duration of negative pressure than is required for the development of purulent effusion.

Several clinical reports have correlated tympanometric configuration with presence or absence of MEE in patients with OM.[4,23-26] Jerger proposed a method for classifying tympanometric configurations based on TM compliance and external canal pressure at peak compliance using the Madsen impedance bridge.[1] This schemata was further refined by Paradise et al, who described 15 tympanometric variants each associated with a greater or lesser probability of effusion.[27] Middle ear pressure and compliance are not well correlated and can therefore be used as independent indicators of the state of the ME.[25] Our observations in the experimental model confirm these clinical studies by demonstrating that ears with effusion have a lower compliance, a smaller gradient and lower pressure than dry ears. Our study supports the observation by Beery et al by failing to demonstrate a relationship between ME pressure and presence of effusion.[28]

The B_+ tympanometric configuration showed the greatest sensitivity (57%) and specificity (100%) for OME in chinchillas, whereas the type B configuration was comparably insensitive (10%) but equally specific (100%) for presence of an effusion (Table 2). Although a variant similar to our B_+ configuration was not described in human patients by Paradise et al,[27] the Class III tracing in humans described by Beery et al is similar to the B_+ tracing in chinchillas.[28] Among ears without effusion, the type A configuration was 63% sensitivity and 71% specific for this condition. The type C configuration detected 38% of ears without effusion but was 68% specific for this condition.

Purulent effusions which cultured pneumococci were associated with tympanometric configurations which were distinctly different from ears with sterile serous effusions. Type B_+ configurations were found exclusively in association with a purulent effusion (Table 2) ($p < .001$, Fisher's exact test). Three of four serous effusions showed normal type A configurations, while only one of ten purulent effusions showed a type A configuration ($p = .04$). These results suggest that TM compliance and/or ME pressure is directly related to the physical characteristics of ME fluids and the histopathology of the ME cleft. Histologic examination of the chinchilla ME cleft following intranasal inoculation of pneumococci and ME deflation has shown mucosal edema, hyperemia, hemorrhage and extensive leukocyte infiltration during the first week after deflation followed by epithelial metaplasia, granulation tissue and osteoneogenesis during the second, third and fourth week.[22] The ME cleft of chinchillas with serous MEE showed mucosal edema and widening of the subepithelial space with vascular dilations and proliferation of loose fibrous connective tissue. Leukocyte infiltration was considerably less in serous than purulent OM.[10]

Wiederhold et al has also examined the tympanometric configurations of low and high viscosity effusions in cats after ligation of the eustachian tube.[29] The shape of the tympanogram was not a completely reliable indication of effusion. Effusion volume, however, did correlate with tympanogram configuration. All ears with at least 0.4 ml of fluid had flat (type B) tympanograms, whereas 43% of ears with less than 0.4 ml of fluid had very shallow tympanograms. Cantekin et al have also suggested that the false-negative tympanograms recorded on ears with serous effusion may be due to a small volume of low-viscosity fluid which may have an undetectable contribution in the mass component of the acoustic impedance without changing overall compliance of the ME system.[30] We did not measure effusion volume in the chinchillas but in previous studies have noted that effusion volume varies between 0.05 and 1.4 ml.

Only a single report has correlated type of effusion with tympanometric configuration in human patients.[31] In that report low viscosity (serous) effusions were found in all ears with low compliance/normal pressure tympanograms and in half of the ears low compliance/high negative pressure tympanograms; high viscosity (mucoid) effusions were obtained only on ears with low compliance/high negative pressure tympanograms. To our knowledge, there have been no reports describing the tympanometric characteristics of purulent effusion, nor has the ME cleft been explored in any of these patients to observe pathologic evidence of OM for correlation with the tympanometric configuration.

These results in an animal model suggest that tympanometry might be applied in expanded clinical studies similar to those of Groothuis et al for studying the pathogenesis of OM by describing the physiological function of the ME system during longitudinal observations.[17] This study confirms the utility of tympanometry in detecting MEE and supports the use of this technique for evaluating children with OM for whom an objective measurement of outcome is required.

REFERENCES

1. Jerger J. Clinical experience with impedance audiometry. Arch Otolaryngol 1970; 92:311-24.

2. Brooks DN. Electroacoustic impedance bridge studies in normal ears of children. J Speech Hear Res 1971; 14:247-53.

3. McCandless GA, Thomas GK. Impedance audiometry as a screening procedure for middle ear disease. Trans Am Acad Ophthalmol Otolaryngol 1974; 78:98-102.

4. Bluestone CD, Cantekin EI. Design factors in the characterization and identification of otitis media and certain related conditions. Ann Otol Rhinol Laryngol 1979; 88 Suppl 60:13-28.

5. Howie VM, Ploussard JH, Sloyer JL. The "otitis-prone" condition. Am J Dis Child 1975; 129:676-8.

6. Report of a survey by the Medical Research Council's Working-Party for Research in General Practice: acute otitis media in general practice. Lancet 1957; 2:510-4.

7. Klein JO. Epidemiology of otitis media. In: Harford ER, Bess FH, Bluestone CD, Klein JO, eds. Impedance screening for middle ear disease in children. New York: Grune & Stratton, 1978.

8. Giebink GS, Quie PG. Otitis media: the spectrum of middle ear inflammation. Ann Rev Med 1978; 29:285-306.

9. Paparella MM. Middle ear effusions: definitions and terminology. Ann Otol Rhinol Laryngol 1976; 85 Suppl 25:8-11.

10. Juhn SK, Paparella MM, Kim CS, et al. Pathogenesis of otitis media. Ann Otol Rhinol Laryngol 1977; 86:481-92.

11. Giebink GS, Payne EE, Mills EL, et al. Experimental otitis media due to *Streptococcus pneumoniae*: immunopathogenic response in the chinchilla. J Infect Dis 1976; 134:595-604.

12. Paparella MM, Juhn SK, Hiraide F, et al. Cellular events involved in middle ear fluid production. Ann Otol Rhinol Laryngol 1970; 79:766-80.

13. Miller J, Donaldson J. Primate model for studies of clinical problems of middle ear functions. Ann Otol Rhinol Laryngol 1976; 85 Suppl 25:194-201.

14. Rankin JD, Karmody CS. Serous otitis media: an experimental model. Arch Otolaryngol 1970; 92:14-23.

15. Goycoolea MV, Paparella MM, Carpenter AM, et al. A longitudinal study of cellular changes in experimental otitis media. Otolaryngol Head Neck Surg 1979; 87:685-700.

16. Giebink GS, Berzins IK, Schiffman G, Quie PG. Experimental otitis media in chinchillas following nasal colonization with type 7F *Streptococcus pneumoniae*: prevention after vaccination with pneumococcal capsular polysaccharide. J Infect Dis 1979; 140:716-23.

17. Groothuis JR, Sell SHW, Wright PF, et al. Otitis media in infancy: tympanometric findings. Pediatrics 1979; 63:435-42.

18. Van Dishoeck HAE. Negative pressure and loss of hearing in tubal catarrh. Acta Otolaryngol (Stockh) 1941; 29:303-12.

19. Perlman HB. Quantitative tubal function. Arch Otolaryngol 1943; 38:453-65.

20. Thomsen KA. Investigations on the tubal function and measurement of the middle ear pressure in pressure chamber. Acta Otolaryngol (Stockh) 1958; 140 Suppl: 269-78.

21. Eliachar I, Sando I, Northern JL. Measurement of middle ear pressure in guinea pigs. Arch Otolaryngol 1974; 99:172-6.

22. Meyerhoff WL, Giebink GS, Shea D. Pneumococcal otitis media following middle ear deflation. Ann Otol Rhinol Laryngol 1981; 90:72-6.

23. Brooks DN. An objective method of detecting fluid in the middle ear. Int Audiol 1968; 7:280-6.

24. Grimaldi PMGB. The value of impedance testing in the diagnosis of middle ear effusion. J Laryngol Otol 1976; 90:141-52.

25. Haughton PM. Validity of tympanometry for middle ear effusions. Arch Otolaryngol 1977; 103:505-13.

26. Shurin PA, Pelton SI, Finkelstein J. Tympanometry in the diagnosis of middle ear effusion. N Engl J Med 1977; 296:412-7.

27. Paradise JL, Smith CG, Bluestone CD. Tympanometric detection of middle ear effusion in infants and young children. Pediatrics 1976; 58:198-210.

28. Beery QC, Andrus WS, Bluestone CD, et al. Tympanometric pattern classification in relation to middle ear effusions. Ann Otol Rhinol Laryngol 1975; 84:56-64.

29. Wiederhold ML, Zajtchuk JT, Vap JG, Paggi RE. Hearing loss in relation to physical properties of middle ear effusions. Ann Otol Rhinol laryngol 1980; 89 Suppl 68:185-9.

30. Cantekin EI, Beery QC, Bluestone CD. Tympanometric patterns found in middle ear effusions. Ann Otol Rhinol Laryngol 1977; 86 Suppl 41:16-20.

31. Bluestone CD, Beery QC, Paradise JL. Audiometry and tympanometry in relation to middle ear effusions in children. Laryngoscope 1973; 83:594-604.

Ann Otol 91:1982

ARGON LASER STAPEDOTOMY

BRUCE J. GANTZ, MD
SEIJI KISHIMOTO, MD
HERMAN A. JENKINS, MD
UGO FISCH, MD
ZURICH, SWITZERLAND

The argon laser has been used clinically to perform stapedotomies in patients with otosclerosis. In order to determine if this device induces histologic changes in the inner ear, stapedotomies were performed in cats. Saccular membrane fistulas, in line with the path of the laser beam, were found in 3 of 8 ears. The unpredictable nature of the argon laser in the ear is discussed.

INTRODUCTION

Recently, it has been proposed that the argon laser be employed clinically for fenestration of the stapes footplate in the treatment of otosclerosis.[1,2] A similar argon laser is now commercially available for otologic surgery. This report presents our preliminary findings investigating the light microscopic changes in the middle ear and vestibule following argon laser fenestration of the stapes footplate in cats.

MATERIAL AND METHODS

Seven healthy adult cats with no evidence of ear disease were used in this series of experiments. The animals were anesthetized with intraperitoneal injections of Nembutal and the middle ear exposed through a postauricular approach. Bilateral laser fenestrations of the stapes footplate were performed in four animals using a Spectraphysics model 770 argon laser mounted on a Zeiss Opmi-one operating microscope. Three animals with intact normal ears were used as controls.

Prior to fenestration of the footplate, the stapes crura were removed by vaporization with the laser. Initially, a rosette pattern of small fenestra was created on the footplate and the central portion was vaporized, usually with a single pulse. Care was taken not to pass the laser beam directly through the fenestration. A beam intensity of 1.5 W and an exposure time of 0.1 seconds were used in all experiments.

Immediately following creation of the fenestra, the animals with bilateral lesions were fixed using vital perfusion of Heidenhain-Susa. Temporal bones were removed immediately following perfusion and prepared for light microscopic observation using routine celloidin techniques. Twenty-micron serial sections were stained with hematoxylin and eosin.

RESULTS

The argon laser was successful in creating a stapedial footplate fenestration in all eight experimental ears. A carbon char was present at the margin of the fenestra but did not extend beyond the boundaries of the stapes. In three animals a coagulum was present in the oval window niche. The bone in the area of the fenestration was completely vaporized. There were no fragments of bone debris in the vestibule, but in two ears the vestibule exhibited an amorphous eosinophilic material. The margins of all fenestrae also contained the same amorphous material.

In three ears a perforation of the saccular membrane was present (Fig. 1A). These perforations were in direct line with the laser fenestration of the footplate. The perforations were of variable sizes from 50-150 μ in diameter. The margins of the saccular perforations did not exhibit a marginal char like the bone. The only alteration in the saccular membrane at the light microscopic level was a slight thickening at the margins of the perforation (Fig. 1B). The macula of the saccule appeared intact without evidence of alteration at this magnification. The other five experimental ears exhibited undisturbed saccular membranes (Fig. 2). Control ears had intact stapes footplates and intact saccular anatomy.

DISCUSSION

During the initial experiments with the argon laser it became quickly apparent that the number of laser pulses required to create a stapedial footplate fenestration was quite variable. The factor that influenced this most was pigmentation present in the bone. When slight pigmentation was present, a superficial carbon char was easily achieved and a fenestration accomplished in 2-3 pulses of the laser beam. When the footplate was void of pigmentation, a char was not produced until a small amount of blood was placed over the footplate. Previous authors have discussed the importance of pigmentation when using the argon laser since its concentrating effect depends on absorption by pigmented tissues. Absorption of the beam by pigmented tissues is what makes the argon laser most useful, for example, in retinal surgery.

The absence of pigmentation of the bone partially explains the saccular membrane perforations. Because of the lack of pigmentation, the number of laser pulses required to create a char is increased. Stahle and his coworkers[3] have shown that internal damage can be produced in the cochlea with the argon laser without producing a bony defect. They discuss the fact that internal damage was difficult to predict because of the variability of thickness, density, and mineralization of the bone.

From the ENT-Department, University Hospital, Zurich, Switzerland. This work was supported in part by NIH, Teacher-Investigator Awards KO 7 Ns 00 570-01 CDR and KO 5 Ns 00294.

REPRINTS — Prof. U. Fisch, ENT-Department, University Hospital, Raemistr. 100, 8091 Zurich, Switzerland.

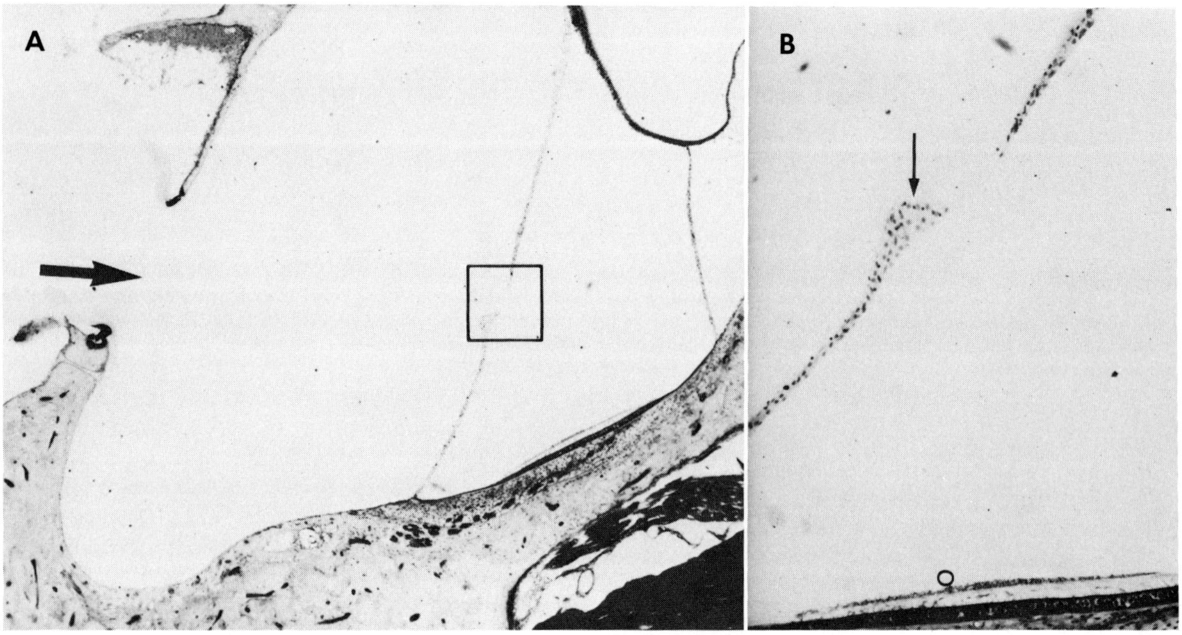

Fig. 1. A) Cat ear following creation of a fenestration (arrow) in the stapes footplate with the argon laser. Saccular membrane exhibits perforation (box) in direct line with the path of the laser beam. B) Magnification of A showing perforation of margin (arrow) due to cellular swelling. Otoconia (O) appear undisturbed at this magnification.

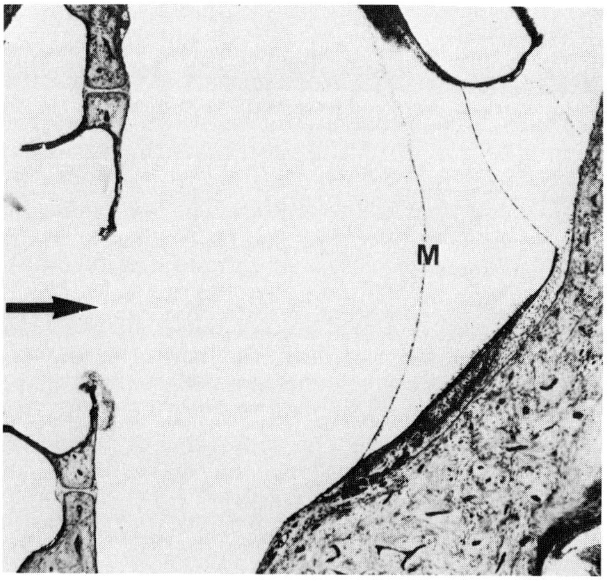

Fig. 2. Cat ear following argon laser stapedotomy. The fenestration of the stapes and path of the laser beam are demonstrated by the arrow. The saccular membrane (M) was intact in this ear.

Other factors influencing inner ear damage by the argon laser include duration of the laser beam pulse and focusing of the laser beam. Even though the pulse duration is quite short, 0.1 seconds, the final bit of bone may be vaporized at the beginning of the pulse allowing the beam to penetrate more distally. The distal progression of the beam is counteracted by using a short focal length beam. Focusing often requires trial and error with the short focal length laser beam and is a problem when dealing with less than a millimeter of tolerance, as encountered in the inner ear.[4,5]

The unpredictable combination of footplate thickness, lack of pigmentation in the bone, transmission of the laser beam through the bone, and degree of mineralization is compounded in the patient with otosclerosis. In view of the fact that saccular membrane fistulas occurred in 37% of the ears following argon laser stapedotomy, the safety of this procedure at the present technical level must be questioned. It is hoped that the questions raised by these initial experiments will stimulate further investigative work before the argon laser is deployed on a more widespread clinical basis in stapes surgery.

ACKNOWLEDGMENT — Bruce J. Gantz, MD, is a clinical fellow from the Department of Otolaryngology, University of Iowa, Iowa City, and Herman A. Jenkins, MD, is a clinical fellow from the Department of Surgery, Division of Head and Neck, UCLA School of Medicine, Los Angeles.

The authors wish to thank Mrs. Eva Knecht for her technical assistance in the preparation of the histologic material.

REFERENCES

1. Perkins, RC. Laser stapedotomy for otosclerosis. Laryngoscope 1980; 90:228-40.

2. Sataloff J. Experimental use of laser in otosclerotic stapes. Arch Otolaryngol 1967; 85:58-60.

3. Stahle J, Hoegberg L, Engstrom B. The laser as a tool in inner ear surgery. Acta Otolaryngol (Stockh) 1972; 73:27-37.

4. Wilpizeski CR. Otological applications of lasers. In: Wolbarsht ML, ed. Laser applications in medicine and biology. Vol. 3. New York: Plenum Publishing Corporation, 1977: 289-328.

5. Wilpizeski CR, Maiorello RP, Reddy JB, et al. Otological applications of lasers: basic background. Trans Pa Acad Ophthalmol Otolaryngol 1977; 30:185-92.

MUCORMYCOSIS OF THE TEMPORAL BONE

RUTH GUSSEN, MD RINALDO F. CANALIS, MD

LOS ANGELES, CALIFORNIA

Mucormycosis of the temporal bone is described in a 60-year-old female with uncontrolled diabetes mellitus whose symptoms related to cranial nerve palsies and hearing loss, following spread of infection from the nasopharynx. The infection spread along the eustachian tube and tensor tympani muscle to the base of the skull, involving the internal carotid artery with mycotic thrombosis and rupture. Subsequent spread occurred from this area predominantly along nerve pathways and as mycotic emboli in blood vessels of the labyrinth and middle ear. Infection also spread from the anterior middle ear wall through the oval window into the vestibule. The temporal bone changes were those of granulomatous inflammation with necrosis and ischemic infarction.

The widespread use of corticosteroids, broad-spectrum antibiotics and chemotherapeutic agents has resulted in better control of many chronic diseases. However, along with the beneficial effects of these drugs, the resulting altered immunologic status of these patients has contributed to a marked increase in the incidence of aggressive fungal infections. Among those involving the head and neck, mucormycosis remains the most rapidly fatal. In this region the disease most commonly involves initially the nose and paranasal sinuses, usually spreading to the eye and eventually intracranially. Otologic manifestations may be present and are occasionally prominent.

The histopathologic changes of mucormycosis involving the facial and intracranial structures are well known. In contrast, those associated with the otologic manifestations of the disease have been described in only two temporal bone reports, one cited by Schuknecht[1] and described in more detail by McGill,[2] and the second by Meyerhoff.[3] Recently, two patients with mucormycosis originating in the nasopharynx and presenting with multiple cranial nerve palsies were reported by Bahna et al.[4] Despite aggressive treatment, one of these patients with a total unilateral hearing loss succumbed to the disease. This patient's temporal bones are the basis of this report and are especially interesting because they show some of the behavioral features of the disease within the ear and demonstrate routes of infection.

CASE REPORT

The patient was a 60-year-old female with adult onset diabetes mellitus diagnosed in 1969. In mid-February 1978 she was admitted to a local hospital in ketoacidosis. During her initial evaluation, she was noted to have paralysis of cranial nerves III, V, VII, IX, XI and XII. Following control of her ketoacidosis, she was transferred to UCLA Medical Center for further study. On admission, the patient was in no acute distress and her vital signs were within normal limits. The cranial nerve deficits were again documented, as well as bilateral hearing loss more pronounced in the right ear. She denied vertigo and there was no nystagmus. The rest of the physical examination was negative except for diffuse muscular weakness and mild intentional tremor on the left side. General laboratory data were within normal limits except for a blood glucose of 265 mg% and urinalysis positive for sugar. A chest radiograph was normal. Sinus x-ray films showed diffuse mucoperiosteal thickening and a nasopharyngeal mass. A computerized axial tomographic (CAT) study showed cloudy sphenoid sinuses.

Nasopharyngeal examination revealed a predominantly right-sided, ulcerated mass covered by greenish exudate. The right tympanic membrane was dull, stiff and lacked normal anatomical landmarks. The left tympanic membrane was hypomobile but otherwise normal. Audiogram revealed a moderate sensorineural hearing loss in the left ear and total sensorineural hearing loss in the right. Biopsy of the nasopharyngeal mass demonstrated acute inflammatory reaction, muscle necrosis and numerous nonseptate hyphae consistent with the diagnosis of mucormycosis.

Treatment was started with amphotericin B, 30 mg twice a day. However, the patient became increasingly lethargic without appreciable change in her blood chemistry. A repeat CAT scan revealed extension of the disease to the right internal carotid artery, the sphenoid sinus and posterior ethmoidal cells. No evidence of intracranial involvement was noted. The patient was placed on intravenous ampicillin, 300 mg every six hours. Three days later she underwent extensive debridement of the nasopharyngeal lesion, sphenotomy, right external ethmoidectomy and a right Caldwell-Luc operation. Following surgery there was slight improvement of her

From the Division of Head and Neck Surgery and the Department of Pathology, School of Medicine, University of California, Los Angeles. Supported by USPHS Grant NS-06606 from the National Institute of Neurological and Communicative Disorders and Stroke.

REPRINTS — Ruth Gussen, MD, Department of Surgery, Division of Head and Neck, 32-34 Rehabilitation Center, University of California, Los Angeles, CA 90024.

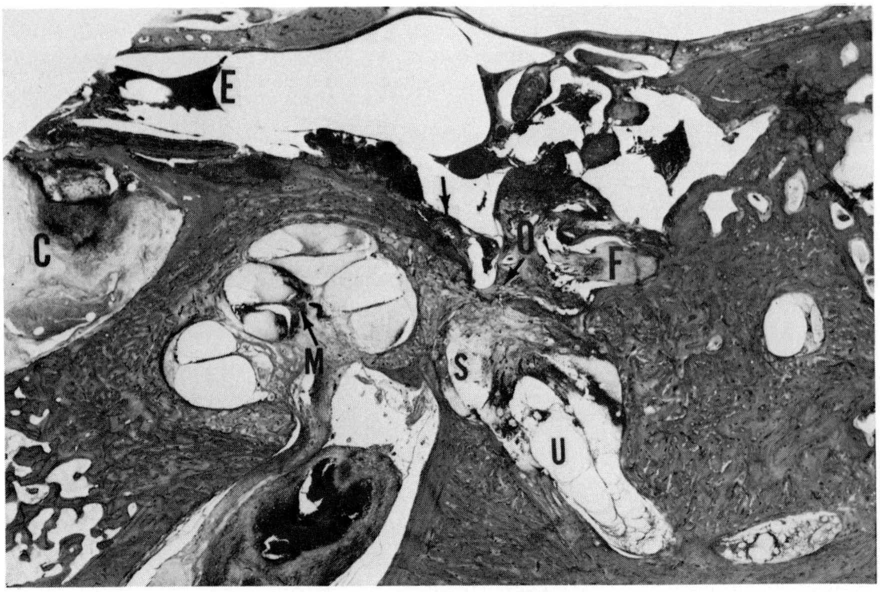

Fig. 1. Right temporal bone. Note inflammation and necrosis involving carotid canal (C) and wall of eustachian tube (E). Facial nerve canal is eroded and facial nerve (F) and tympanic nerve (arrow) are necrotic. Scar tissue is continuous between middle ear and vestibule through annular ligament (O, arrow). Note necrosis of modiolus of middle cochlear turn (M, arrow) and labyrinthitis, with relative sparing of basal turn. Note large necrotic focus in vestibular nerve with compression of cochlear nerve. The saccule (S) and utricle (U) are necrotic. (H&E, x6.5)

mental status, but no change in cranial nerve palsies was noted. Twenty days after the operation she had profuse oral bleeding which subsided spontaneously. Three days later the patient had a massive, uncontrollable hemorrhage and cardiorespiratory arrest.

AUTOPSY FINDINGS

The nasopharyngeal mucosa was ulcerated, hemorrhagic and necrotic and demonstrated numerous large, broad, nonseptate branching hyphae on microscopic examination. The underlying muscular wall was also necrotic and invaded by fungus. The right infratemporal region showed extensive edema, necrosis and congestion. Microscopic examination demonstrated widespread granulomatous inflammation and necrosis, and the presence of fungus. There was no evidence of meningitis. Cranial nerves V, VII and VIII on the right side were markedly edematous. Microscopic examination showed granulomatous lesions and fungus in cranial nerve V. There was a recent infarct in the right parietal lobe of the brain and a thrombosed meningeal artery with no granulomatous reaction or fungi.

TEMPORAL BONE FINDINGS.

Right. There was widespread fungal involvement with large necrotic areas and focal granulomatous lesions with epithelioid cells and multinucleated giant cells. Large, nonseptate hyphae were easily demonstrated in certain locations within the inner and middle ear, as well as in blood vessels and nerve tissue (Figs. 1 and 2).

A large necrotic inflammatory mass was present in the anterior portion of the temporal bone involving the eustachian tube, petrous carotid canal, and adjacent trigeminal nerve (Figs. 1 and 2). The petrous marrow contained irregular foci of granulomatous inflammation. The internal carotid artery wall was necrotic and its lumen was filled with masses of hyphae. The vessel wall was ruptured and appeared collapsed. The pericarotid tissue was necrotic and filled with polymorphonuclear leukocytes and hyphae. Inferiorly, the bony septum between the carotid canal and the eustachian tube was completely resorbed and there was continuity of the necrotic inflammatory mass in the two areas (Fig. 3). Superior to this region, where the bony septum was intact, hyphae were noted within the vascular canals of the bone. Extension of the anterior inflammatory mass proceeded along the greater superficial petrosal nerve and tensor tympani muscle, involving the geniculate ganglion and facial nerve. The latter was necrotic in its entire middle ear course to the origin of the chorda tympani nerve (Figs. 1 and 2). The stapedius muscle was also necrotic with hyphae present in the muscle and facial nerve throughout its course. The stylomastoid artery was thrombosed by hyphae. The facial nerve was also involved into the internal auditory canal, the disease extending to the superior vestibular and a portion of the inferior vestibular nerves (Figs. 1 and 2). The cochlear nerve was compressed by the large inflammatory mass involving these structures, but was not directly involved by the infection. The more cranial portions of the facial and vestibular nerves, within the internal auditory meatus, demonstrated very early, recent lesions (Fig. 1); hyphae were present.

The oval window region demonstrated dense scar tissue, infiltrated by chronic inflammatory cells. The annular ligament, anteriorly, was replaced by this scar tissue which was continuous from the middle ear into the vestibule. No fungus was seen in this region.

The cochlea demonstrated necrosis of the modiolus in the distal descending basal and middle turns, which included the modiolar blood vessels in these areas (Figs. 1 and 4). Hyphae were present in nerve

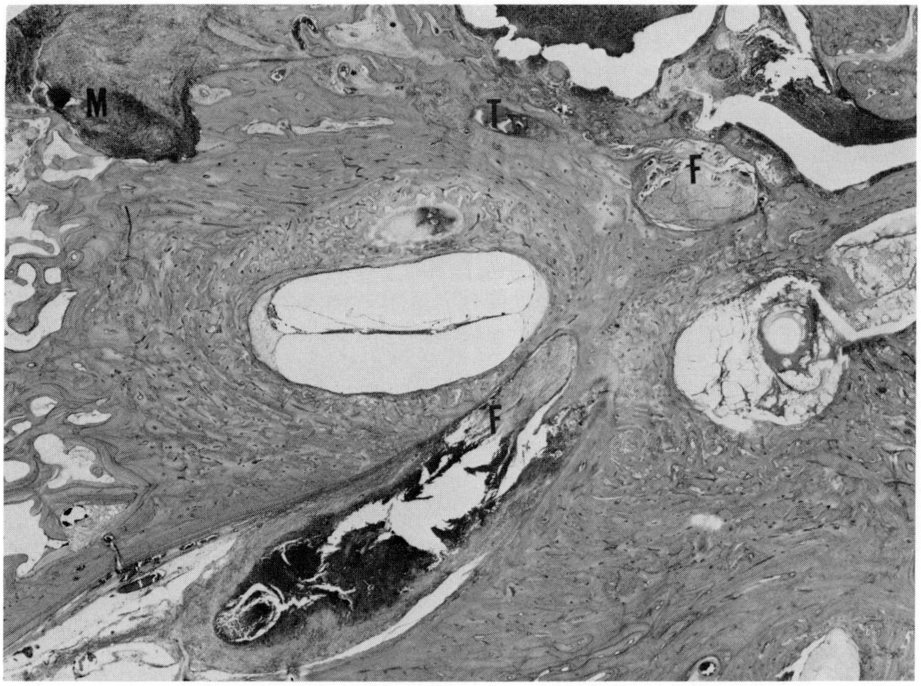

Fig. 2. Inflammatory mass present anteriorly (M) with involvement of tympanic nerve (T) and facial nerve (F) in its course horizontally and into the internal auditory canal with spread to the superior vestibular nerve. Note exudate in middle ear. (H&E, x9.75)

fibers and in the vessels extending into the spiral bony lamina and interscalar bony septa. Hyphae were also present in the perilymph of the scala vestibuli of the middle turn. Marked necrosis and inflammatory response was evident in the cochlear soft tissues of the middle and apical turns, with relative sparing of the ascending basal limb. The larger cochlear veins demonstrated vasculitis with prominent cellular proliferation about the normally thin-walled vessels (Fig. 4).

The vestibular organs were all completely necrotic, with inflammatory cell infiltration. Fungus was seen in one submacular vessel of the saccule and a few hyphae were seen in the perilymph space of the posteroinferior region of the vestibule.

Jacobson's nerve was involved superiorly, and continued necrotic and invaded by fungus all the way to the glossopharyngeal ganglia within the cranial opening of the cochlear aqueduct.

The endolymphatic duct system demonstrated necrosis of its sinus with flat, atrophic epithelium lining the isthmus and rugal portions of the sac. The vein in the paravestibular canaliculus appeared somewhat smaller than usual, but was otherwise unremarkable.

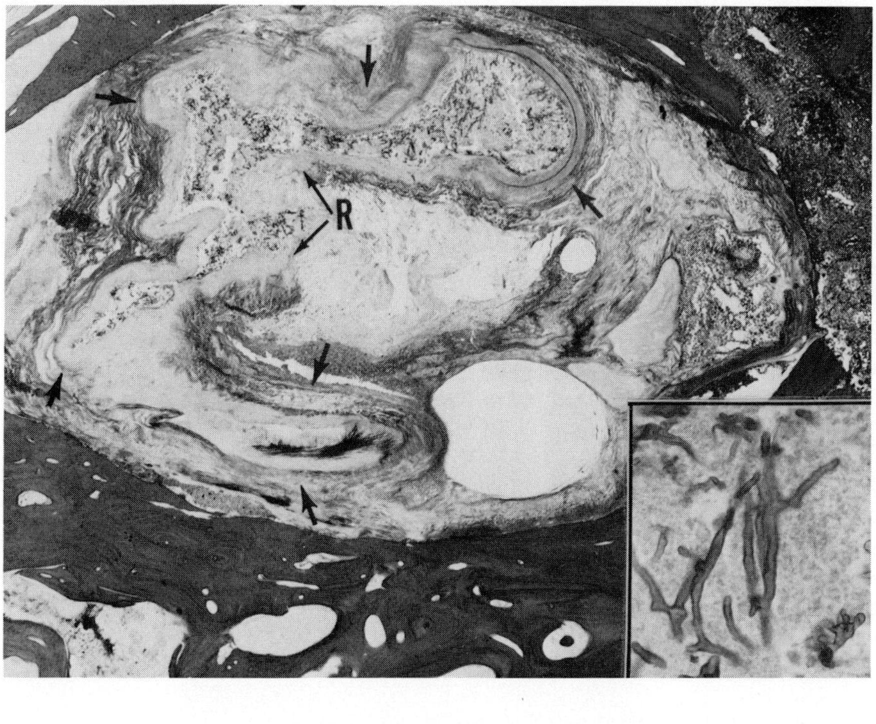

Fig. 3. Petrous carotid canal. Note collapse and rupture of arterial wall (R). Arrows outline collapsed arterial wall. Lumen is filled with masses of hyphae (insert). At right note erosion of bone of carotid canal by inflammatory mass. (H&E, x21)

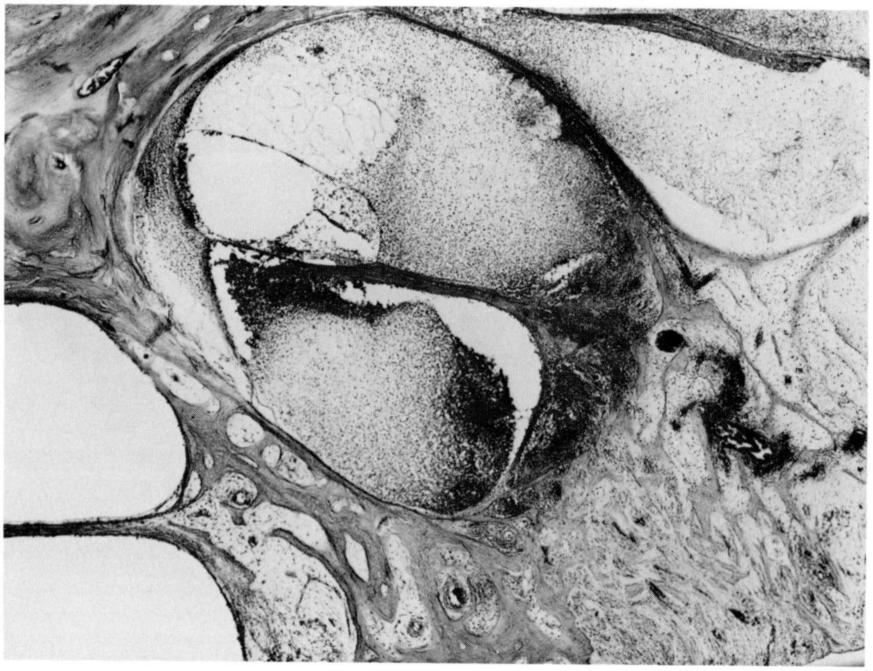

Fig. 4. High power view of middle turn demonstrating severe labyrinthitis associated with vasculitis and necrosis of modiolar elements. (H&E, x45)

The middle ear contained foci of fibrinopurulent exudate with early granulation tissue formation. No fungus could be demonstrated in the middle ear save for those within the muscles and nerves. The tympanic membrane was intact.

Left. Granulomatous inflammation was present in the petrous marrow in the inferiormost portion of the specimen. No fungus could be demonstrated. The cochlea revealed decreased spiral ganglion cells in the proximal basal turn, as well as considerable lipochrome pigment in the stria vascularis of the descending basal, middle and apical turns. There was focal strial atrophy throughout the cochlea.

DISCUSSION

Mucormycosis was first described by Paltauf[5] in 1885 and initially reported in the American literature by Gregory et al[6] in 1943. The disease is caused by fungi of the Rhizopus and Mucor species, which belong to the class Phycomycetes. Absidia has also been implicated.[7] These organisms, characterized by large, branching nonseptate hyphae, are frequently found in soil, dust, manure and decaying organic material. They have also been cultured from the respiratory and digestive tracts of asymptomatic individuals.[8] Under favorable conditions, usually related to debilitating illness, phycomycetes may become pathogenic. Uncontrolled diabetes mellitus remains the most commonly associated entity. In addition to the head and neck, the lungs, skin, heart and gastrointestinal tract may be separately involved. A disseminated form of the disease also exists.[9] Diagnosis is readily made by biopsy, although culture in Sabouraud media is needed for species identification. Treatment is based on control of the underlying metabolic imbalance, debridement or excision of the lesion, and intravenous amphotericin B. Prognosis is guarded.

Mucormycosis involvement of the ear was initially described by Huckel[10] in 1886. In modern times, reports of ear pain, drainage and facial nerve paralysis developing during the course of the disease have periodically appeared in the literature[1-4,9-21] However, confirmation of Mucor infection of the temporal bone has been reported in only four fatal cases[2,3,12,17] and in one survivor.[21] Temporal bones were studied in two of these cases.

Schuknecht[1] briefly cited, and McGill[2] reported on the temporal bone findings in a 38-year-old diabetic male with rhinocerebral mucormycosis who died of rupture of the internal carotid artery. This patient exhibited predominant involvement of the nasopharynx and presented with multiple cranial nerve palsies. Both ears were involved. The tympanic cavities and mastoids were filled with hemorrhagic fluid and desquamated epithelial cells. The tensor tympani muscles and petrous marrow were infiltrated by lymphocytes, plasma cells and multinucleated cells. New bone formation was present in the right carotid canal, while the left carotid canal was partially destroyed. The labyrinth was unaffected.

Meyerhoff et al[3] recently described a case of mucormycosis in a 48-year-old male with acute myelogenous leukemia. Death was attributed to meningoencephalitis, and fungal infection was not identified until autopsy. Temporal bone sections (side unspecified) revealed Mucor hyphae in the middle ear, internal auditory canal, cochlea and vestibule. Hyphae appeared to have invaded the inner ear through the oval window annulus and round window membrane. A serous precipitate was present in the endolymphatic and perilymphatic spaces of the cochlea and semicircular canals.

The present case demonstrated massive, widespread mucormycosis of the temporal bone. Infection originated in the nasopharynx and extended along the wall of the eustachian tube and fibers of the tensor tympani muscle. It also extended along the sphenoid bone into the base of the skull involving the petrous marrow. From the eustachian tube and tensor tympani muscle, the infection progressed into the anterior wall of the middle ear. The internal carotid artery appears to have been invaded at this level following breakdown of the bony wall separating it from the eustachian tube. From this area infection proceeded along the greater superficial petrosal nerve and the geniculate ganglion, with distal spread along the fallopian canal. Infection along the facial nerve also extended into the internal auditory canal. Additional spread through the annular ligament of the oval window into the vestibule was also noted. Extension from the middle ear into the internal auditory canal is most likely because the inflammatory lesions within this canal are progressively more recent in the cranial direction. The scar tissue in the oval window and vestibule, continuous through the annular ligament region, also represents an older process. The rest of the middle ear and mastoid demonstrated the changes of an acute fibrinopurulent otitis media, less severe in the mastoid. No hyphae were seen within these spaces, so that the fungus appeared to be confined to nerve and muscle compartments within the middle ear wall.

Cochlear mucormycosis resulted predominantly from fungal invasion of the modiolar arteries with necrosis of the modiolus in the middle and apical turns, and spread of the fungi into the scala vestibuli of the middle turn. Notably less involvement of the proximal basal turn may be explained by fungus thromboses of the distal, smaller caliber modiolar vessels. The vestibular organs were similarly compromised by fungal invasion of vessels, as well as by spread of infection from the inflammatory mass within the internal auditory canal. The entire labyrinth also suffered ischemic changes due to the widespread vascular involvement.

The internal carotid artery findings are interesting in that the thrombus consisted of fungus with no blood elements evident so that the rupture noted at this level did not result in fatal bleeding, probably because of proximal thrombosis. Postmortem identification of the vessel responsible for the terminal hemorrhage was difficult because of the extensive necrosis in the infratemporal space.

The neural involvement by Mucor in this case is striking, suggesting that the fungus, in addition to its affinity for vessel walls, may also have an affinity for spread along nerve fibers. To our knowledge, this type of neural extension has not been previously described in otitic mucormycosis. Recently, however, McGill[2] reported similar findings in a case of aspergillosis involving the temporal bone.

To conclude, involvement of the temporal bone by mucormycosis may occur via three major routes. In the first, preceding chronic otitis media favors superimposed fungus infection. This represents primary mucormycosis and may remain restricted to the middle ear and mastoid. An example of this type has been described by Bergstrom et al.[21] The second, or meningeal route, follows intracranial extension and invasion through the internal auditory canal. This is exemplified by Meyerhoff et al's case.[3] Finally, the third route of invasion originates from the nasopharynx and extends along the eustachian tube and tensor tympani muscle. This is exemplified by McGill's case[2] and by the present case.

ACKNOWLEDGMENT — The author is indebted to Mrs. Ada Dörr for her invaluable technical assistance, and to Mr. Howard Tribe for photography.

REFERENCES

1. Schuknecht HF. Pathology of the ear. Cambridge: Harvard University Press, 1974; 262-3.

2. McGill TJI. Mycotic infection of the temporal bone. Arch Otolaryngol 1978; 104:140-4.

3. Meyerhoff WL, Paparella MM, Oda M, Shea D. Mycotic infections of the inner ear. Laryngoscope 1979; 89:1725-34.

4. Bahna M, Ward PH, Konrad H. Nasopharyngeal mucormycotic osteitis: a new syndrome characterized by initial presentation of multiple cranial nerve palsies. Otolaryngol Head Neck Surg 1980; 88:146-53.

5. Paltauf A. Mycosis mucorina. Virchows Arch 1885; 102: 543-64.

6. Gregory JE, Golden A, Haymaker W. Mucormycosis of the central nervous system. A report of three cases. Bull Johns Hopkins Hosp 1943; 73:403-19.

7. Dubos RJ, Hirsch JG. Bcterial and mycotic infections of man. Philadelphia: JB Lippincott, 1965; 178.

8. Martinson FD. Rhinophycomycosis. J Laryngol Otol 1963; 77:691-705.

9. Bryan GT, Read CH, Zimmerman GR. Disseminated mucormycosis in a child with diabetes mellitus. J Iowa State Med Soc 1958; 48:193-6.

10. Huckel A. Zur Kenntniss der Biologie des Mucor corymbifer. Beitrage zur Pathologischer Anatomie 1886; 1:117-31.

11. DeWeese DD, Schleuning AJ II, Robinson LB. Mucormycosis of the nose and paranasal sinuses. Laryngoscope 1965; 75:1398-405.

12. Abramson E, Wilson D, Arky RA. Rhinocerebral phycomycosis in association with diabetic ketoacidosis. Ann Intern Med 1967; 66:735-42.

13. Harris JS. Mucormycosis: a report of a case. Pediatrics 1955; 16:857-67.

14. Foushee S, Beck WC. Mucormycosis of the central nervous system. North Car Med J 1956; 17:26-31.

15. Gass JDM. Acute orbital mucormycosis. Arch Otolaryngol 1961; 65:214-20.

16. Bank H, Shibolet S, Gilat T, Altmann G, Heller H. Mucormycosis of the head and neck structures: a case with survival. Br

Med J 1962; 1:766-8.

17. Smith HW, Kirchner AJ. Cerebral mucormycosis. Arch Otolaryngol 1968; 68:715-28.

18. LaTouche CJ, Sutherland TW, Telling M. Rhinocerebral mucormycosis. Lancet 1963; 2:811-3.

19. Hoaglund RJ, Sube J, Bishop RH, Holding BF Jr. Mucormycosis. Am J Med Sci 1961; 242:415-22.

20. Faillo P, Sube HP, Anderson NH. Mucormycosis of the paranasal sinuses and the maxilla. Oral Surg 1959; 12:304-9.

21. Bergstrom L, Hemenway GW, Barnhart RA. Rhinocerebral and otologic mucormycosis. Ann Otol Rhinol Laryngol 1970; 79:70-81.

≈

ACUTE MORPHOLOGICAL CHANGES IN GUINEA PIG COCHLEA FOLLOWING ELECTRICAL STIMULATION

A PRELIMINARY SCANNING ELECTRON MICROSCOPE STUDY

LARRY G. DUCKERT, MD, PhD JOSEF M. MILLER, PhD

SEATTLE, WASHINGTON

A major area of concern in the development of the cochlear prosthesis involves the effects of the implant on inner ear anatomy and function. This study examined one aspect of host-implant interaction — the effects of cochlear implantation with and without electrical stimulation on cochlear morphology in the guinea pig. To accomplish this, a series of normal guinea pigs were acutely implanted bilaterally with a scala tympani multiple electrode prosthesis. One ear was stimulated with continuous 1 kHz sinusoidal current of constant intensity for a period of three hours. The contralateral control ear was not stimulated. Current intensities tested ranged from 0.1 mA to 1 mA rms. After stimulation the animals were sacrificed, perfused with fixative and the temporal bones were microdissected for examination using the scanning electron microscope. Morphological changes observed in the stimulated ear ranged from hair cell and supporting cell degeneration to complete destruction of the basilar membrane and organ of Corti overlying the electrode. These changes occurred at current intensities ranging from 0.4 mA to 1 mA and were conspicuously absent in the implanted but unstimulated control ears. The current intensities employed in this experiment were within operating ranges presently used in long-term behavioral studies in other animal models. To what degree the morphological changes observed in this study may effect the function of the prosthesis or host responses on a long-term basis cannot be determined from this experiment. However, our observations do demonstrate that electrical stimulation of the cochlea is not benign and point out the need for further evaluation to help define safe standards for use of the prosthesis.

The development of a cochlear prosthesis to rehabilitate the patient with sensorineural deafness has stimulated considerable interest within the scientific community and has generated numerous challenging problems. The introduction of an artificial device into the cochlea for the purpose of direct electrical stimulation of the auditory system raises many questions regarding the effects of such implantation on preexisting temporal bone morphology. One major concern must be the development of a prosthetic device that will produce minimal additional damage to cochlear sensory and neural components and thus not further compromise cochlear function and limit the usefulness of the prosthetic device.

Concerns include: mechanical trauma caused at surgery, host reaction to the foreign body, and effects of electrical current. While it is more or less apparent that the traumatic placement of a cochlear prosthesis may produce degenerative changes within the temporal bone, pathology consequent to electrical stimulation is somewhat less obvious and certainly less well understood. The significance of this problem has been discussed in the literature,[1-3] yet published data addressing this problem is scant.

The purpose of this investigation was to assess the effects of acute cochlear implantation and electrical stimulation on the guinea pig cochlea using the scanning electron microscope. The goal has been to help identify factors which could affect development of the prosthesis and standards for its use.

LITERATURE REVIEW

The question of whether the cochlea can survive long-term implantation has been approached by a number of investigators using conventional histological techniques in animal models.

Using light histopathology techniques Schindler and Merzenich[4] demonstrated destructive changes involving the organ of Corti in cats implanted with scala tympani electrodes within weeks. Severe destruction of the organ of Corti and loss of hair cells and supporting elements was observed in the section of the basilar partition overlying the electrode. In a

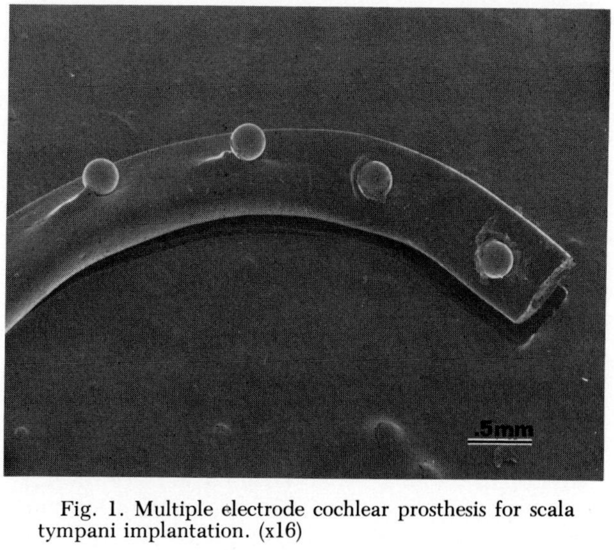

Fig. 1. Multiple electrode cochlear prosthesis for scala tympani implantation. (x16)

From the University of Washington, School of Medicine, Department of Otolaryngology, Seattle. Funded in part by NIH Grant NS 13056-03.

REPRINTS — Larry G. Duckert, MD, PhD, University of Washington, School of Medicine, Department of Otolaryngology, RL-30, Seattle, WA 98199.

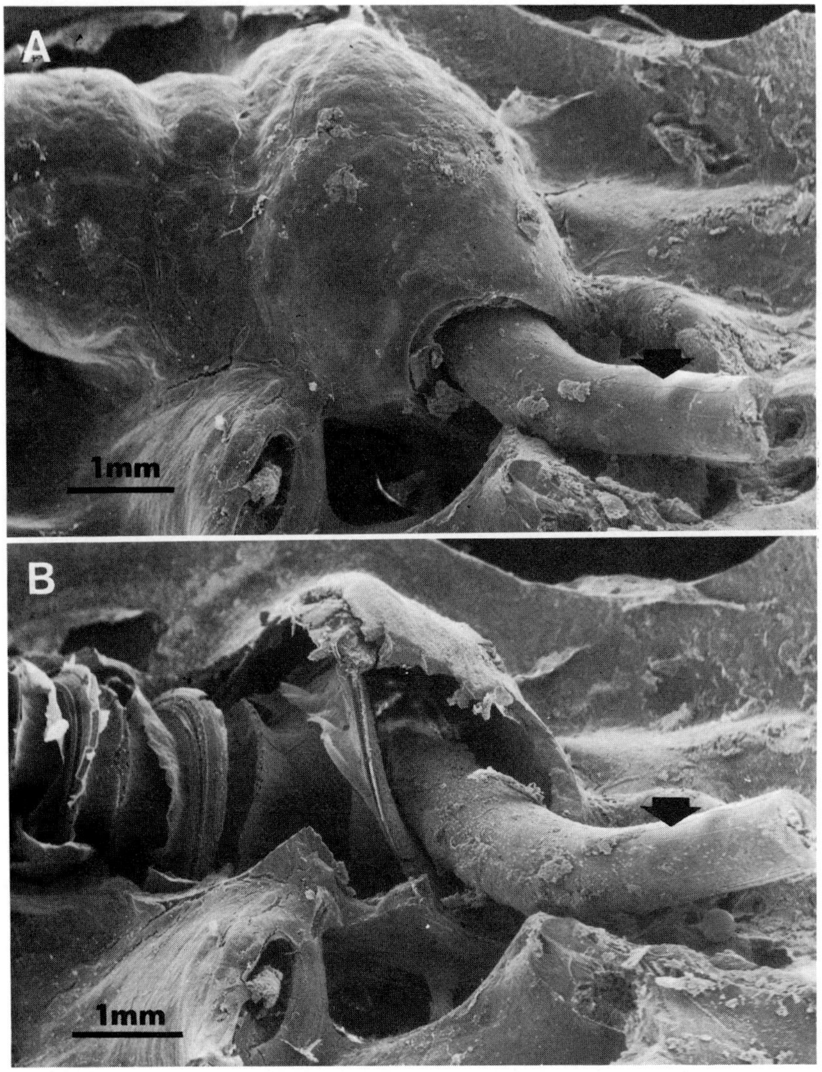

Fig. 2. Guinea pig cochlea. A) With prosthesis (arrow) intact in round window before dissection. B) After dissection. (x15)

later study in cats, Schindler[5] and Schindler et al[6] confirmed these earlier findings and added that neural degeneration was seen only in areas of basilar membrane rupture and loss of supporting elements in the organ of Corti. Significant ganglion cell survival after implantation in cats was also reported by Simmons.[7] Neural degeneration did occur, however, related to surgical trauma, tears in the basilar membrane and infection.

Using monkeys as the experimental model and scala tympani implants, Sutton et al[8] and Miller and Sutton[9] described morphological changes in the cochlea following implantation including ruptures in the basilar membrane, fractures of the osseous spiral lamina, osteoneogenesis and loss of spiral ganglion cells.

Histopathological observations also have recently been reported from one human implanted with chronic scala tympani electrodes.[10] Neural degeneration was the most striking finding as well as bony overgrowth in these specimens. Based on these studies, it has been suggested that the cat may have a robust cochlea which tolerates insults associated with the scala tympani prosthesis better than the primate or human.

In general while some effects of cochlear implantation of cochlear morphology have been reported, the data are limited and in some areas conflicting. Moreover, in these studies it is not possible to separate the morphological effects resulting from electrical stimulation versus the trauma of surgery and foreign body reaction. It is in this area specifically that this study will contribute to our basic knowledge.

METHODS

The animal model for the experiment was the guinea pig. Twelve young (200-250 g body weight) healthy animals were used. Each was evaluated for the presence of a Preyer's reflex. At the time of surgery the external and middle ear was examined for signs of present or past infection. If any indication of nonnormal auditory function was observed, the subject was eliminated from the investigation. The animals were anesthetized with a combination of xylozine and ketamine and the bulla opened via a postauricular incision. The round window was exposed and the round

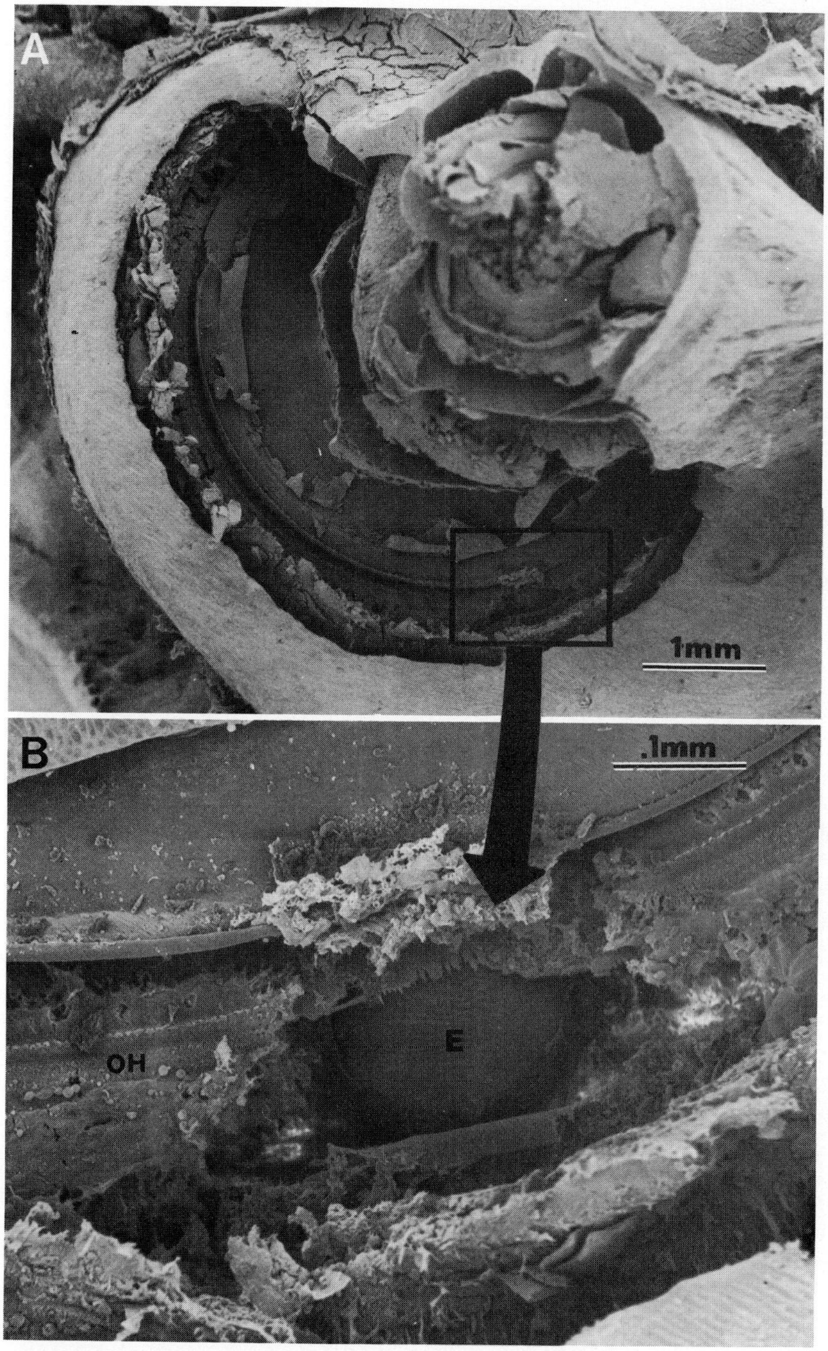

Fig. 3. A) Scanning electron micrograph of guinea pig cochlea stimulated for three hours at 0.500 mA current intensity. The bracketed area demonstrates an area of destruction in organ of Corti and basilar membrane overlying the electrically stimulated electrode. (x16) B) Higher magnification photomicrograph of bracketed area showing the scala tympani electrode (E) through defect in organ of Corti. OH - Outer hair cells. (x160)

window membrane incised. The multiple electrode system designed after Michelson[11] was then implanted into the scala tympani[12] bilaterally in all animals. The electrode consists of three to four platinum-iridium wires terminating in ball tips protruding from a molded silicon rubber matrix. The electrodes are staggered at 1 mm distances along the implant (Fig. 1). Implant diameter occupied approximately 50% of the scala tympani.

The electrodes were held in place with a carboxylate cement until sacrifice. One ear of each animal was stimulated with continuous 1 kHz sinusoidal current of constant intensity for a period of three hours. The contralateral control ear was not stimulated. Current intensities tested ranged from 0.1 mA rms. After stimulation, the animals were sacrificed and the tissue fixed by intracardiac perfusion using 2.5% phosphate-buffered gluteraldehyde followed by postfixation for one hour in 1% osmium tetroxide. The temporal bones were removed with the prosthesis intact and the bone overlying the basal turn in proximity to the implant was removed with a diamond burr (Fig. 2A, B). After microdissection, the tissue was prepared for observation with scanning electron microscope. The specimens were dehydrated in an ethanol series and critical point dried using CO_2.[13] The tissue was mounted on aluminum stubs using carbon suspension and gold coated prior to examination with the scanning electron microscope (ETEC B1).

RESULTS

Morphological changes involving the organ of Corti were found in the ears stimulated at current intensities ranging from 0.4 mA to 1 mA. Morphological alteration was not seen in ears stimulated at current intensities below 0.4 mA. The most dramatic findings were destructive lesions in the basal

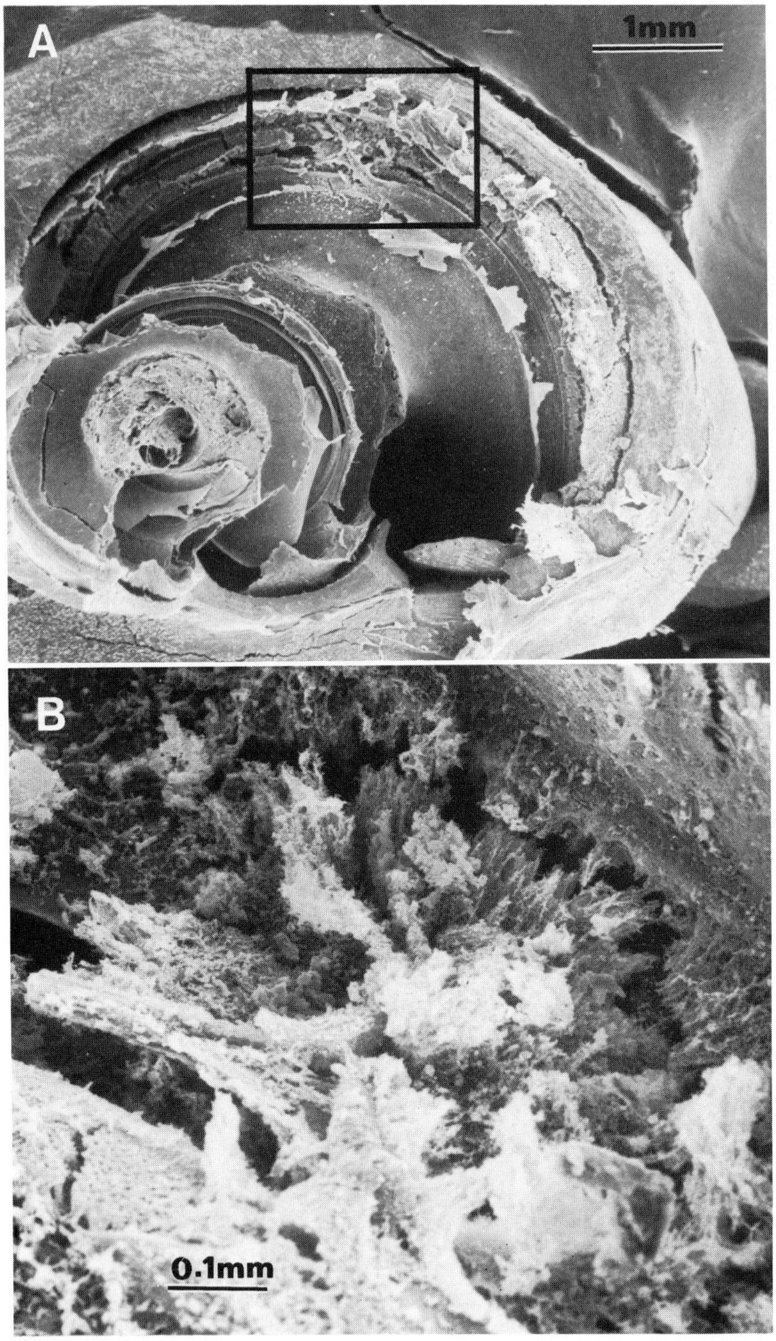

Fig. 4. A) Scanning electron photomicrograph of guinea pig cochlea stimulated for three hours at 1 mA current intensity. The bracketed area demonstrates the region of the organ of Corti destroyed by electrical stimulation. (x16) B) Higher magnification photomicrograph of bracketed area showing destruction of normal cochlear anatomy. (x175)

turn overlying the stimulated scala tympani electrodes. In some specimens the sensory cells, supporting cells and basilar membrane were completely destroyed and the electrodes were visible through the defect (Fig. 3A, B). In other stimulated ears the lesions consisted of a well-defined region of necrosis where hair cell and supporting cells were reduced to an amorphous debris (Fig. 4A, B). Adjacent to the areas of complete destruction, the organ of Corti was frequently collapsed and the outer rows of hair cells were disorganized. Degenerative changes involving both the outer hair and supporting cells were observed. The outer hair cell stereocilia were blunted and fused and bleb formation was present (Fig. 5A). In some areas the apical surfaces of the degenerating hair cells appeared granular and the stereocilia collapsed (Fig. 6A). The Deiter cell phalangeal processes were also distorted and disorganized. "Ballooning" of the cell surface was frequently observed (Fig. 6A). In contrast to the outer hair cells, the inner hair cells appeared to be intact.

The degenerative changes were limited to the basal turn sparing the more apical turns (Fig. 7). Examination of the unstimulated but implanted control ears demonstrated no degenerative lesions and normal anatomy preserved throughout (Figs.

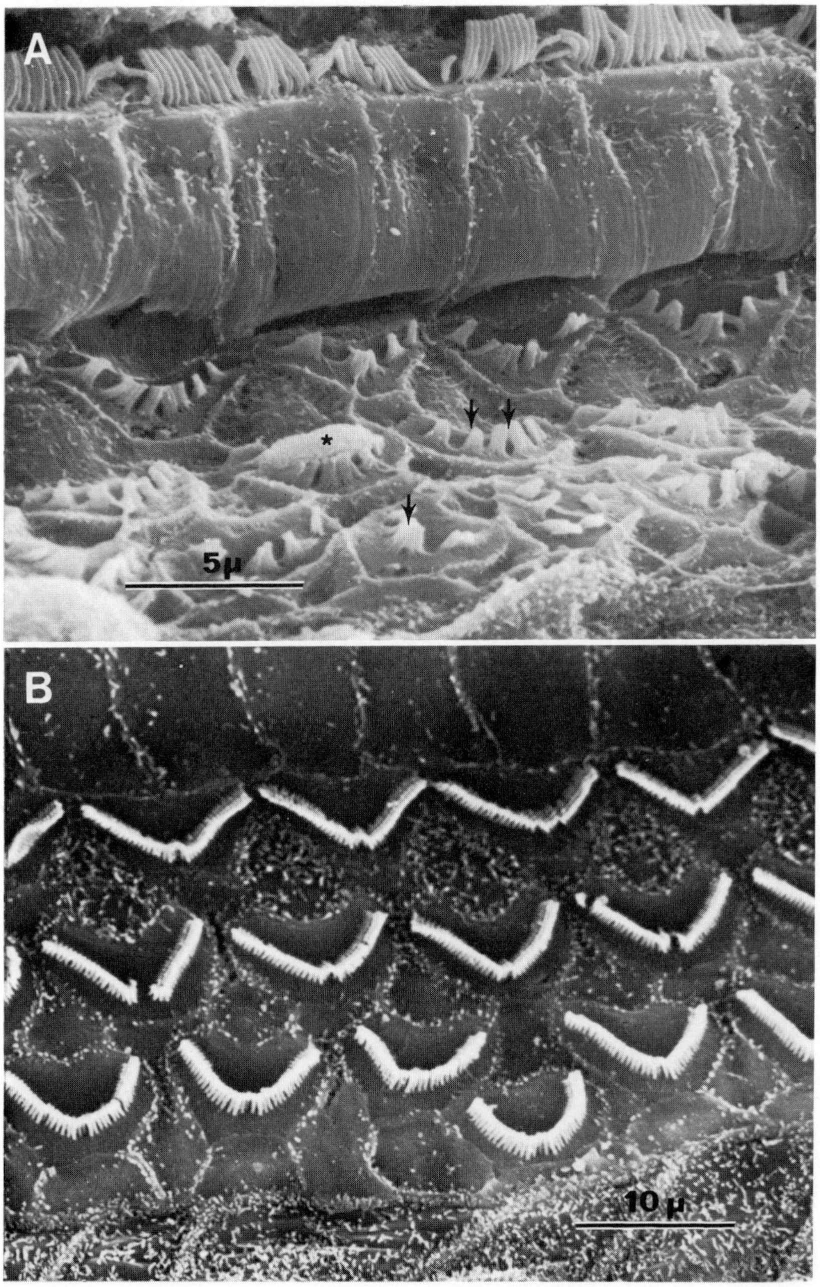

Fig. 5. A) Organ of Corti in close proximity to the destructive lesion. The organ of Corti is collapsed. Degenerating outer hair cells show bleb formation (asterisk) and fusion of stereocilia (arrows). (x4,400) B) Outer hair cells from implanted but unstimulated control ear. Hair cell integrity is preserved. (x1,750)

5B and 6B). Shrinkage artifacts including cracks and fissures within the organ of Corti were frequently present in the basal turns of both the control and stimulated ears and were easily differentiated from premortum changes.

DISCUSSION

Morphological changes observed in the stimulated ears ranged from complete destruction of the organ of Corti and basilar membrane to lesser degenerative changes within the organ of Corti at current intensities ranging from 1.0 mA down to 0.4 mA rms. While it is clear that the lesions resulted from electrical stimulation, the exact mechanism by which the changes occur is unknown. Similar destructive changes in the cochlear sensory cells, including cellular disruption, degeneration of microvilli and nuclear damage, have been observed by other investigators using similar current intensities (0.5 mA).[14]

The charge density at the threshold of damage (0.4 mA rms) based on the geometric surface area of the electrode used in this study is 214.8 $\mu C/cm^2$/phase. Based on calculations from Spelman et al,[15] the threshold for gas production at this experimental electrode is estimated at 0.56 mA rms (300.7 $\mu C/cm^2$/phase). It seems likely therefore that a significant amount of the destructive changes observed at the higher current intensities were a result of gas formation. Certainly the pattern and severity

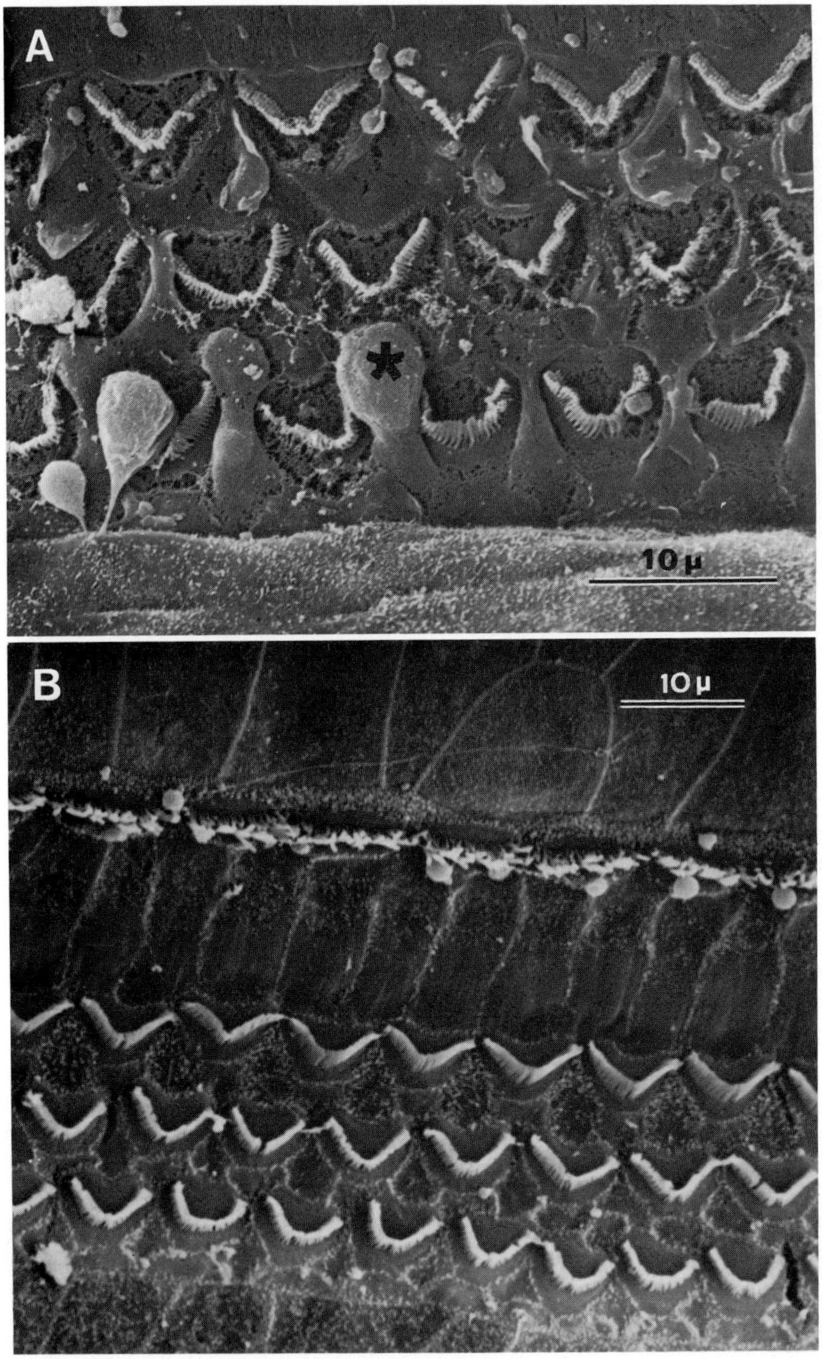

Fig. 6. A) Organ of Corti in close proximity to a destructive lesion overlying stimulated electrode. The phalangeal processes of the Deiter cells appear "ballooned" (asterisk), in other areas collapsed. The apical surface of the degenerating outer hair cells appear granular. (x2,200) B) Organ of Corti from implanted but unstimulated control ear showing normal anatomy. (x855)

of destruction observed in this study suggests that the lytic lesions of the organ of Corti were secondary to direct mechanical insult rather than some subtle chemical or metabolic event. Direct thermal agitation also remains a potential destructive process. It should be emphasized that great care was taken to insure that no direct current component was present during stimulation.

The same destructive event may occur to a lesser degree in the remaining areas of the basal turn resulting in the observed cellular degeneration. Degenerative changes in hair cells including fusion of the stereocilia and bleb formation has been observed as a result of acoustic exposure.[16-18] It has been suggested that these changes may constitute a nonspecific reaction to a variety of noxious influences.[16,19] It is apparent that the degenerative changes were not limited to the sensory cells alone but also involved the adjacent supporting cells including the Deiter and pillar cells. This also suggests that the noxious event was nonspecific.

It must be pointed out that the degenerative changes observed in these cells could be confused with ischemic changes and fixation artifact induced during tissue preparation. This seems unlikely, however, since the changes were distributed in

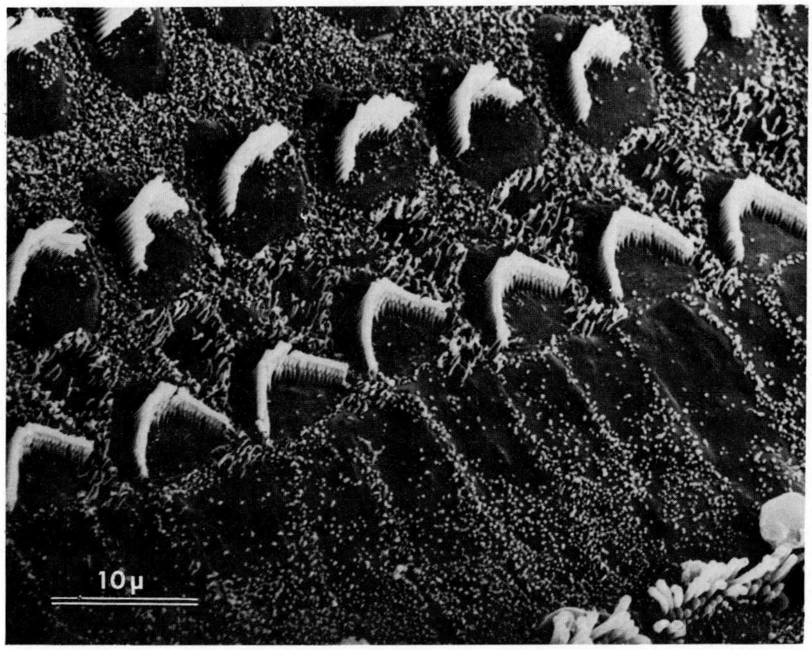

Fig. 7. Outer rows of hair cells from apical turn of pathologically altered, electrically stimulated cochlea showing normal anatomy. (x16,600)

proximity to the electrode while the more apical portions of the cochlea were spared. Good tissue preservation was also evidenced in the control ears, suggesting that the changes observed represent premortum degenerative changes and autolysis. The sparing of the inner hair cells in contrast to the degeneration of the supporting cells which are normally more resistent to ischemic changes also supports this conclusion.

Other potential explanations for the observed degenerative changes include exposure to cytotoxic products of electrolysis, chemical changes in the endolymph or perilymph, or cross-contamination of the inner ear fluids resulting from breakdown of the physiological barriers[20] adjacent to the electrode. It would appear unlikely that vascular compromise or disruption of the normal cochlear microcirculation as a result of implantation alone, at least on the acute basis, is responsible for the observed changes since the implant was small and the implanted but unstimulated control ears were without morphological alteration.

While the lesions were consistently produced after the 0.4 mA threshold was surpassed, poor correlation was found between current intensity above the threshold value and the amount of cochlear damage observed. The expected monotonic relationship between current intensity and cochlear damage certainly was not found. It can be conjectured that such a relationship between current intensity and morphological alteration did not appear to exist due to uncontrolled variations in the tissue to electrode interaction. Although it was endeavored to consistently place the electrode in direct apposition to the basilar membrane, differences in electrode orientation were unavoidable and could have contributed to the inconsistency observed. It is also possible that early degenerative changes produced by lower current intensities occurred in deeper tissue levels not subject to scrutiny with the scanning electron microscope.

For electrode measurements obtained at this laboratory the calculated threshold of damage at 214.8 $\mu C/cm^2$/phase (geometric surface area) can be converted to 70 $\mu C/cm^2$/phase based on actual surface area. This value may be compared to a threshold value of 40 $\mu C/cm^2$/phase for chronic stimulation which produced changes in brainstem evoked responses and subsequent histopathological changes.[21] These changes occurred after "hundreds of hours" of continuous stimulation. The current values determined in this study to produce damage after chronic stimulation overlap those intermittent stimuli applied to behaviorly trained primates.[22] Charge density values based on geometric surface areas of 50 $\mu C/cm^2$/phase have been used in humans.[23] It is to be noted that in these behavioral investigations intermittent stimuli are used. The biological effect of modifying the parameters of duration, intermittency, and intensity of stimulus is not known. Generalization of results from this preliminary study is difficult. The results make it clear that significant harmful effects are possible. With appropriate systematic controlled study, these effects can be better defined and results more readily applied to man obtained.

In summary, the results of this study serve to point out the potentially destructive nature of the electrically stimulated prosthesis. The morphological changes may have serious implications regarding long-term host response and electrode function. The results demonstrate the need for further evaluation of the cochlear prosthesis implanted for chronic periods of time with and without electrical stimulation to more fully assess the feasibility of this rehabilitative device.

REFERENCES

1. Tonndorf J. Cochlear prosthesis. A state-of-the-art review. Ann Otol Rhinol Laryngol 1977; 86:1-19.

2. Hambrecht FT, Reswick HD, eds. Functional electrical stimulation. Application in neural prosthesis. New York: Marcel Dekker, 1977:543.

3. Hambrecht FT. Neural prostheses. Ann Rev Biophys Bioeng 1979; 8:239-67.

4. Schindler RA, Merzenich MM. Chronic intracochlear electrode implantation: Cochlear pathology and acoustic nerve survival. Ann Otol Rhinol Laryngol 1974; 83:202-16.

5. Schindler RA. The cochlear histopathology of chronic intracochlear implantation. J Laryngol Otol 1975; 40:445-57.

6. Schindler RA, Merzenich MM, White MW, et al. Multielectrode intracochlear implants. Arch Otolaryngol 1977; 103:691-9.

7. Simmons FB. Permanent intracochlear electrodes in cats, tissue tolerance and cochlear microphonics. Laryngoscope 1967; 77:171-86.

8. Sutton D, Miller JM, Pfingst BE, et al. Cochlear pathology associated with a silicon rubber implant in monkey and guinea pig scala tympani. Proceedings of Midwinter Research Meeting. Assoc Res Otolaryngol 1978; 24.

9. Miller JF, Sutton D. Cochlear prosthesis: morphological considerations. J Laryngol Otol (in press).

10. Johnsson L-G, House WF. Bilateral cochlear implants, histological findings in a pair of human temporal bones. Laryngoscope 1979; 89:759-62.

11. Michelson RP. Electrical stimulation of the human cochlea. Arch Otolaryngol 1971; 93:317-23.

12. Pfingst BE, Donaldson JA, Miller JM. Behavioral evaluation of the cochlear prosthesis. Proceedings of midwinter meeting. Assoc Res Otolaryngol 1978; 22.

13. Anderson TF. Techniques for the preservation of 3-dimensional structure in preparing specimens for the electron microscope. Trans NY Acad Sci 1951; 13:130-4.

14. Fourcin AN, Rosen SM, Moore BCJ, et al. External electrical stimulation of the cochlea: clinical, psychophysical, speech-perceptual and histological findings. Br J Audiol (in press).

15. Spelman R, Pfingst B, Powers W, et al. Biophysics of the implanted ear: electrical parameters. In: Prosthetic and technical devices for the deaf. McPherson D, ed. New York: National Technical Information Services 1978:312-23.

16. Bredberg G, Ades HY, Engstrom Y. Scanning electron microscopy of the normal and pathologically altered organ of Corti. Acta Otolaryngol (Stockh) 1972; Suppl 301:3-46.

17. Soudijn ER. Scanning electron microscopic study of the organ of Corti in normal and sound-damaged guinea pigs. Ann Otol Rhinol Laryngol 1976; 29:1-46.

18. Hunter-Duvar IM. A technique for preparation of cochlear specimens for assessment with the scanning electron microscope. Acta Otolaryngol (Stockh) 1978; Suppl 351:2-23.

19. Wersall J. Problems and pitfalls in studies of cochlear hair cell pathology. In: Moller AR, ed. Basic mechanisms in hearing. New York: Academic Press 1973:235-56.

20. Bohne BA. Mechanisms of noise damage in the inner ear. In: Henderson D, Hamernik RP, Dosanjh DS, Mills JH, eds. Effects of noise on hearing. New York: Raven Press 1976:14-68.

21. Walsh SM, Leake-Jones PA, Vurek L, et al. Effects of chronic electrical stimulation of auditory nerve in cat. Presented at ARO Midwinter Meeting, St. Petersburg, Fla., 1980.

22. Pfingst BE, Donaldson JA, Miller JM, et al. Psychophysical evaluation of cochlear prostheses in a monkey model. Ann Otol Rhinol Laryngol 1979; 88:613-25.

23. Mathews RG. Sound processing for an auditory prosthesis. Tech. Report No. 5306-3. Integrated Circuits Laboratory, Stanford University, Stanford, Calif., 1978.

INTRACRANIAL COMPLICATIONS OF SINUSITIS IN CHILDREN
A SEQUELA OF PERIAPICAL ABSCESS

ITZHAK BROOK, MS, MD ELLEN M. FRIEDMAN, MD
WASHINGTON, DC

The cases of two children with periapical abscess in the upper incisors, sinusitis, and intracranial abscess are described. The ethmoid and maxillary sinuses were involved in both patients. Subdural empyema occurred in both, and one of the children had also cerebritis and brain abscess. Anaerobic bacteria were isolated from the infected subdural empyemas. *Peptostreptococcus intermedius* and microaerophilic streptococci were recovered in one patient and *Fusobacterium* sp in the other. Surgical drainage and appropriate antimicrobial therapy resulted in complete eradication of the infection in both patients. The role of anaerobic bacteria and the therapy directed against them in periapical abscess and the sinusitis and intracranial abscess which follow are discussed.

INTRODUCTION

An alveolar abscess is the extension of a necrotic or putrescent pulp into the periapical area, causing necrosis of bone and tissue in the affected area with the accumulation of pus. As the abscess progresses, more tissue may be involved, including adjacent teeth, and the pressure of accumulated pus may produce a sinus tract to the exterior or to the oral or nasal cavity.[1]

Serious complications from periapical infections are relatively rare, considering the number of infected teeth that occur in the population. However, in some cases the infection spreads to tissues in other portions of the oral cavity, causing submandibular or superficial sublingual abscesses. Abscesses may be produced also in the submaxillary triangle or in the parapharyngeal or submasseteric space.[2]

In the maxilla, periapical infection may affect only the soft tissues of the face. It may also extend to the infratemporal space including the sinuses and from there to the central nervous system where it can cause serious complications such as subdural empyema, brain abscess or meningitis.[3]

This report describes two children with intracranial complication of periapical abscess in the upper incisors. The infection spread to the central nervous system through the maxillary and frontal sinuses. The purpose of this report is to alert physicians and dentists to the rare occurrence of this complication even in the antibiotic era.

METHODS

Material for culture was obtained aseptically from the infected sites, after the adjacent mucous membrane was swabbed with Betadine®, or through direct aspirate of the involved sinuses or subdural space during surgery. Specimens were transported immediately to the microbiology laboratory using a syringe and corked needle and were plated within 30 minutes of collection. Gram stain preparations were made of all specimens.

Sheep blood, chocolate, and MacConkey's agar plates were inoculated for aerobes. The plates were incubated at 37 C aerobically (MacConkey's) or under 5% CO_2, and examined at 24 and 48 hours. For anaerobes, the material was plated onto prereduced vitamin-K_1-enriched *Brucella* blood agar, an anaerobic blood agar plate containing kanamycin and vancomycin, and anaerobic blood plate containing phenylethyl alcohol and placed into enriched thioglycolate broth (containing hemin, sodium bicarbonate and vitamin K_1).[4] The plates were incubated in GasPak® jars (BBL, Cockeysville, Md) and examined at 48 and 96 hours. The thioglycolate broth was incubated in anaerobic conditions for 14 days. Anaerobes were identified by techniques previously described.[4] Aerobic bacteria were identified using conventional methods.[5]

CASE REPORTS

Case 1. A six-year-old male presented with a frontal headache, fever, nasal congestion, and swelling under his left eye of three days' duration. Two weeks earlier he had broken his left upper incisor. Two days prior to admission, he was seen at the Outpatient Department, where skull and sinus films revealed opacifications of the left ethmoid and left maxillary sinuses. Oral ampicillin therapy was started but this condition did not improve.

Physical examination on admission revealed an enlargement of the left cervical and left submandibular lymph nodes and marked cellulitis, with swelling and purple discoloration of the left maxillary area which extended to the upper lid. The patient had a clear mucoid discharge from his left nostril. An abscess was noted in the root of the left upper incisor.

Laboratory findings were Hgb 12.3 g/dl, Hct 36.7%, WBC 20,000/mm^3 (segments 72, bands 1, lymphocytes 18, mononuclears 9), platelet count normal, ESR 45 mm/first hour, and blood cultures negative. Sinus x-rays showed marked density of the left ethmoid and maxillary sinuses and an abscess in the root of the right upper incisor. Bone scan showed increased uptake in the left ethmoid and

From the Departments of Infectious Diseases and Otolaryngology, and the Clinical Microbiology Laboratories, Children's Hospital National Medical Center; and George Washington University School of Medicine, Washington, DC.

REPRINTS — Itzhak Brook, MD, MS, Naval Medical Research Institute, National Naval Medical Center, Bethesda, MD 20014.

maxillary sinuses, suggesting osteomyelitis. A computerized tomography (CT) scan confirmed these findings and showed evidence of subdural empyema.

A Caldwell-Luc procedure, ethmoid drainage, and frontal craniotomy were performed. Frank pus was obtained from the sinus as well as the subdural space. A direct extension of the inflammation through the cribriform plate was evident during surgery. The dental abscess was drained and the affected incisor was extracted. Gram stain of the left ethmoid sinus and subdural empyema aspirates showed Gram-positive cocci in chains, and the culture of the subdural aspirate yielded *Peptostreptococcus intermedius* and microaerophilic streptococci. The patient was started on an eight-day course of IV therapy with ampicillin (150 mg/kg/day) and oxacillin (150 mg/kg/day). The facial swelling decreased slowly and there was a slow resolution of the sinusitis. The patient was discharged and oral ampicillin therapy was continued for 14 days. One year follow-up in the ENT and dental clinics showed complete resolution of the sinusitis and dental abscess.

Case 2. A seven-year-old male presented with localized pain over the left forehead of two weeks' duration. Three weeks prior to his admission, he began to complain of pain in his right upper incisor, and a temporary filling was done at this tooth. Three days before admission his temperature rose to 38.2 C, and the following day he started to receive oral erythromycin therapy. However, the child became restless, combative, and uncooperative. His headaches continued to be throbbing, he started to vomit, and he developed bilateral periorbital cellulitis.

On admission the patient was found to be irritable, restless, uncooperative, and disoriented. His temperature was 38.1 C, pulse 84, and respiration 28/min. Physical and neurological examination were normal, except for bilateral periorbital cellulitis and periapical abscess in the right upper incisor. Laboratory findings were Hgb 12/g/dl, Hct 35.5%, WBC 21,500/mm^3 (10 bands, 80 segments, 9 mononuclears, 1 lymphocytes) and ESR 59 mm/first hour. Blood cultures were negative and CT scan was normal. Sinus x-rays revealed right maxillary and ethmoid sinusitis. Lumbar puncture showed 15 WBC/cu mm; 8 of the cells were lymphocytes and 7 segments. The protein was 63 mg/dl and glucose 59 mg/dl. The periapical abscess was drained, and the cultures obtained from that sample grew *Bacteroides melaninogenicus*, *Bacteroides bivius*, *Fusobacterium* sp, and *Veillonella parvula*.

The patient was started on parenteral therapy with chloramphenicol and methicillin. During the first four days of his hospitalization his condition gradually deteriorated. His temperature spiked to 39 C and he became more delirious and combative. On the fifth day, bilateral papilledema and a sluggish left pupil developed. He was started on parenteral mannitol for the treatment of brain edema. Repeat CT scan on the seventh day showed a shift of the midline to the right and an increased flow in the left parietal area, consistent with cerebritis. Repeat brain scans showed continued evidence of cerebritis. He remained febrile after seven days of therapy and his condition did not improve. At that time metronidazole was added to the therapy. Repeat CT scan 16 days after admission showed formation of a walled abscess.

Surgical drainage was carried out, and a large purulent subdural effusion over the left frontal area and a smoldering cerebritis were found. About 30 cc of purulent fluid were removed, and cultures of that material grew *Fusobacterium* sp. Following surgery, the patient's condition and mental status slowly improved. The patient was discharged from the hospital after 37 days, which included 30 days of antimicrobial therapy. He was followed in the neurology clinic for one year, and showed complete cure of the infection, and no neurological sequelae.

DISCUSSION

We have described two children with intracranial abscess following periapical abscess of the upper incisor teeth. Both patients presented with frontal headache and maxillary and ethmoid sinusitis. CT scan was instrumental in the early diagnosis of the intracranial infection and the ability of CT scan to detect the transformation of cerebritis into a brain abscess was demonstrated in the second child. The bacteria recovered from the patients' abscesses were only anaerobic. However, since both received antimicrobial therapy prior to sample collection, other organisms, including aerobes, could have been eliminated.

Aerobic bacteria are usually recovered from inflamed pulp and root canal. These include *Streptococcus salivarius*, *Streptococcus faecalis*, and Gram-negative rods.[6,7] A number of studies of the bacteriology of root canals have been done in which anaerobes have been detected.[3] However, the quality of these studies varies considerably and the anaerobic techniques are generally not optimal. A variety of anaerobes have been isolated in these past studies, accounting for 25 to 30% of the root canal isolates. These include anaerobic streptococci, *Bacteroides* sp, *Propionibacterium* sp, *Veillonella* sp, and others.[8]

Anaerobes were isolated from cases of periodontal abscesses. Gilmer and Moody[9] inoculated aspirates from acute and chronic alveolar abscesses and found that aerobic streptococci predominated but fusiform bacilli were found in some abscesses, sometimes in pure culture. In three abscesses, these workers found a slow-growing, black, pigment-producing anaerobic organism. More recent studies[3] reported the isolation of a variety of anaerobes in periodontal abscess. These included anaerobic cocci, anaerobic Gram-negative bacilli, and anaerobic Gram-positive bacilli.

We have also found anaerobic organisms to be the predominant isolate in periodontal abscesses in children, outnumbering aerobes eight to one.[10] The recovery of anaerobes in periapical abscess is of importance because of the association of anaerobes with many serious infections arising from dental foci. These include bacteremia, endocarditis, sinusitis, meningitis, subdural empyema, brain abscess, and pulmonary empyema.[3]

Intracranial suppuration following tooth extraction or dental infection is an uncommon but extremely serious complication.[3,11] Most intracranial infections of buccodental origin result in cavernous sinus thrombosis, at times associated with brain abscess,[3,12] or subdural empyema.[3,13] Isolated brain abscesses occur much less frequently, and subdural empyema of odontogenic origin is rare.

In 1945 Haymaker[14] presented 28 fatal cases of central nervous system infections which occurred following tooth extraction. This series included eight cases of brain abscess and three cases of subdural empyema. He pointed out that infections of the molar teeth are more likely to cause intracranial complications because pus arising in the back of the jaw tends to collect between the muscles of mastication and spread upward in the fascial planes, whereas infection arising in the front of the jaw has free access to the oral cavity. Since Haymaker's publication, additional examples of brain abscess[13] and subdural empyema[15,16] of odontogenic origin have been reported. However, the techniques for cultivation of anaerobic bacteria were usually not strict, and thus the number of anaerobic isolates were small.

Our findings support the role of anaerobes in periapical abscess, the sinusitis, and the intracranial infections that follow. This data warrants the use of appropriate antimicrobial coverage for anaerobic as well as aerobic organisms and early surgical drainage when indicated. As more centers begin to utilize techniques for the detection of anaerobic bacteria, the yield of anaerobes in periapical abscess and its complications will undoubtedly increase.

Most of the anaerobic pathogens isolated from the abscesses are sensitive to penicillin. However, some strains of *B melaninogenicus* and *Bacteroides oralis* are resistant to penicillins.[17,18] Although these organisms were not recovered from our patients, other investigators have isolated them.[8] The recovery of these penicillin-resistant organisms requires antimicrobial agents such as clindamycin, chloramphenicol, carbenicillin, or cefoxitin.[3] Although we wish to emphasize the need for judicious selection of antimicrobial agents, it is essential to note that the treatment of periapical abscess may require surgical intervention and that surgical drainage of these cases is therefore an integral part of the management.

REFERENCES

1. Gorlin RJ, Goman HM, eds. Thoma's oral pathology. 6th ed. St. Louis: CV Mosby, 1970.

2. Rogers AH. The oral cavity as a source of potential pathogens in focal infection. Oral Surg 1976; 42:245-8.

3. Finegold SM. Anaerobic bacteria in human disease. New York: Academic Press, 1977.

4. Sutter VL, Vargo VL, Finegold SM. Wadsworth anaerobic bacteriology manual. 2nd ed. Los Angeles: UCLA Extension Division, 1975.

5. Lennette EH, Spaulding EH, Traunt JR. Manual of clinical microbiology. 2nd ed. Washington: American Society for Microbiology, 1974.

6. Akpata ES. Total viable count of microorganisms in the infected dental pulp. J Dent Res 1974; 53:1330-3.

7. Kalman MI. The microbial status of the root canal during endodontic treatment. NY State Dent J 1964; 30:419-24.

8. Fulghum RS, Wiggins CB, Mullaney TP. Pilot study for detecting obligate anaerobic bacteria in necrotic dental pulps. J Dent Res 1973; 52:637.

9. Gilmer TL, Moody AM. A study of the bacteriology of alveolar abscess and infected root canals. JAMA 1914; 63:2023-4.

10. Brook I, Grimm S, Kielich RB. Bacteriology of acute periapical abscess in children. J Endodontics (in press).

11. Hollin SA, Hayashi H, Gross SW. Intracranial abscesses of odontogenic origin. Oral Surg 1967; 23:277-93.

12. Dixon OJ. Dental infection as a cause of cavernous sinus thrombosis. Dental Cosmos 1929; 71:121-4.

13. Koepf SW, Rosedale RS, Learn GE. Infection of Gasserian ganglion following tooth extraction. J Am Dent Assoc 1937; 24:1843-6.

14. Haymaker W. Fatal infections of the central nervous system and meninges after tooth extraction with an analysis of 28 cases. Am J Ortho Oral Surg 1945; 31:117-88.

15. Kemper JW, Aseltine LF. Intracranial lesions resulting from dental infection. Am J Ortho Oral Surg 1944; 30:701-3.

16. Bacchi JG. Brain abscesses and oral surgery. Dent Items Interest 1946; 68:597-600.

17. Sutter VL, Finegold SM. Susceptibility of anaerobic bacteria to 23 antimicrobial agents. Antimicrob Agents Chemother 1976; 10:736-52.

18. Brook I, Calhoun L, Yocum P. Beta lactamase isolates of *Bacteroides* sp. from children. Antimicrob Agents Chemother 1980; 18:164-6.

VESTIBULAR GANGLION OF THE SQUIRREL MONKEY

CÉSAR D. FERMIN, PhD MAKOTO IGARASHI, MD

HOUSTON, TEXAS

The vestibular ganglia of adult squirrel monkeys (*Saimiri sciureus*) were studied with the aid of light and electron microscopy. The vestibular ganglia are formed by small and large neurons (perikarya). The perikarya's outermost surface is surrounded by 2-20 lamellae of compact myelin. The compact myelin sheath varies its thickness around one perikaryon. The sheath generally thins out in the vicinity of the axon hillock. Occasionally, the compact myelin transforms completely into loose myelin for a length of 2-5 μ. Two to eight lamellae of loose myelin usually face the cytoplasm of the neurons. This myelin arrangement is constant in the majority of the cells examined regardless of shape and/or size. Large myelinated perikarya form the majority of the ganglion cells. There are, however, a few neurons that lack a true compact myelin sheath. Others are surrounded by very few lamellae of loose myelin. The general morphology of the neurons was compared to the available literature on other species. Possible variation on the myelination pattern due to fixation differences, and variation on perikaryal size due to the angle of cut and irregular shape of the cells are also discussed.

INTRODUCTION

The fine structure of the vestibular ganglia has been studied in several species, including man,[1-3] primates,[3,4] cats,[3,5] and guinea pigs.[3] The above studies, coupled with ultrastructural studies of the spiral ganglia[6-12] have given investigators controversial opinions about the shape, size, myelination and distribution patterns of the vestibular ganglion cells. Comparisons between spiral and vestibular ganglion cells have been made.[1,3] Mainly due to the lack of detailed ultrastructural information, particularly in primates, we have initiated this electron microscopic study, in order to ascertain if morphological variation exists among the neurons within one ganglion of the squirrel monkey. Since the variation of the neurons among different species could have a functional significance, this report provides information about this small primate that is extensively used in otological research, and that very well fits between some of the species previously studied.

MATERIALS AND METHODS

The vestibular ganglia of adult squirrel monkeys were fixed overnight by immersion with 2% glutaraldehyde in 0.2 M phosphate buffer, pH 7.2-7.4 at 2-5 C. The tissue was subsequently postfixed in 1% buffered osmium tetroxide for 1-2 hours, embedded in Epon 812® and sectioned on a MT2 Porter-Blum ultramicrotome.

Thick sections (1-2 μ) of Epon-embedded material were stained with 1% toluidine blue and 1% paraphenylenediamine and examined under a light microscope. Material fixed in formaldehyde, embedded in celloidin, and stained with hematoxylin and eosin was also examined for purposes of orientation. Thin sections were doubly stained with uranyl acetate[13] and with lead citrate[14] and examined under a JEM-100 CX electron microscope.

Values relative to size are given for the cut surface area of the neurons instead of their diameter due to the irregularity of cell bodies. Serial (2 μ) sections were chosen, one every 30 μ, in order to avoid repetitious count. The values shown here for the somal surface area were calculated with an Apple II computer through a graphic tablet. Average values are given for more than 100 cells.

For measurement we have chosen axons displaying the very smooth and round shape within a bundle. The values for the axonal diameter were obtained from cross sections in order to eliminate possible variations due to the angle of cutting.

RESULTS

The squirrel monkey vestibular ganglion frequently shows V-shaped cell arrangement with its vertex toward the end-organs and its sides toward the brain (Fig. 1). The ganglion is formed by large (average 706 μ^2) and small (average 537.1 μ^2) neurons (Fig. 2). Capillaries are occasionally seen less than 1 μ from the neurons and their nerve fibers (Fig. 2). The perikarya are generally ovoid and have an irregular contour; that is more obvious under the electron microscope (Fig. 3). Around the perikarya there are many collagen fibers that usually locate close to the extracellular coat (glycocalyx) of the Schwann cells (Figs. 4 and 5).

The compact myelin sheath varies its thickness around one perikaryon (Figs. 3 and 6). The sheath generally thins out in the vicinity of the axon hillock. Occasionally, the compact myelin transforms completely into loose myelin for a length of 2-5 μ (Fig. 7). Two to eight lamellae of loose myelin usually face the cytoplasm of the neuron. The number of lamellae of compact myelin ranges between 2 and 20. This myelin arrangement is found in the majority of the cells examined regardless of shape and/or size (Figs. 3 and 6). Large myelinated perikarya form the majority of the ganglion cells. There are, however, about 5% of neurons lacking a true compact myelin sheath (Figs. 2, 4, and 5). Other neurons are surrounded by a very few lamellae of loose myelin. The alternating pattern of the

From the Department of Otorhinolaryngology and Communicative Sciences, Baylor College of Medicine, Houston. This study was supported by NINCDS grant NS-10940.

REPRINTS — Makoto Igarashi, MD, Department of Otorhinolaryngology and Communicative Sciences, Baylor College of Medicine, 1200 Moursund Ave., Houston, TX 77030.

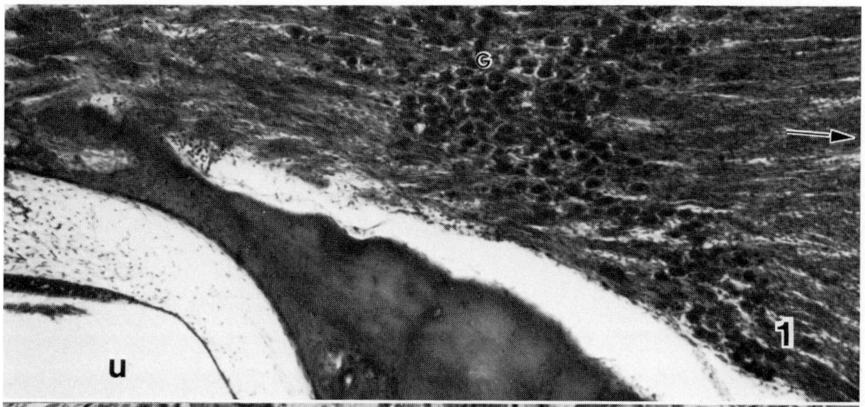

Fig. 1. Light micrograph of the squirrel monkey vestibular ganglion (G). Arrow points toward the brain. U - Utricle. Celloidin section 25 μ thick. (x94)

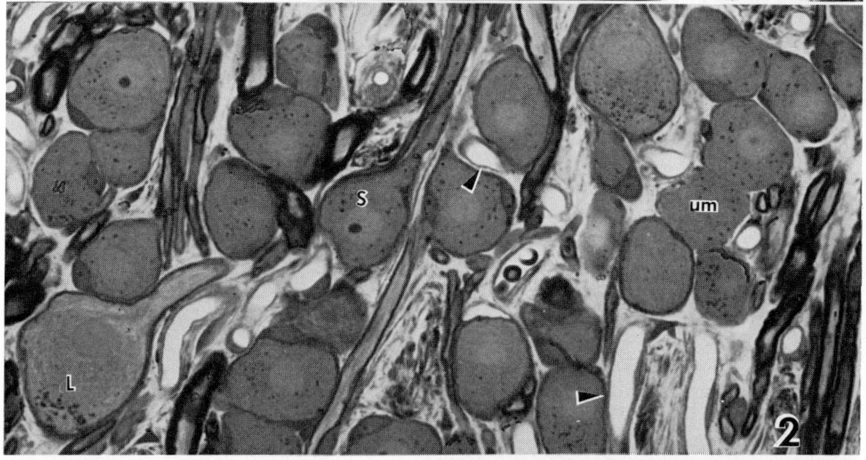

Fig. 2. Light micrograph of 2 μ thick section. Large (L), small (S) and unmyelinated (um) neuron. Arrowheads point to capillary near neurons. (x467)

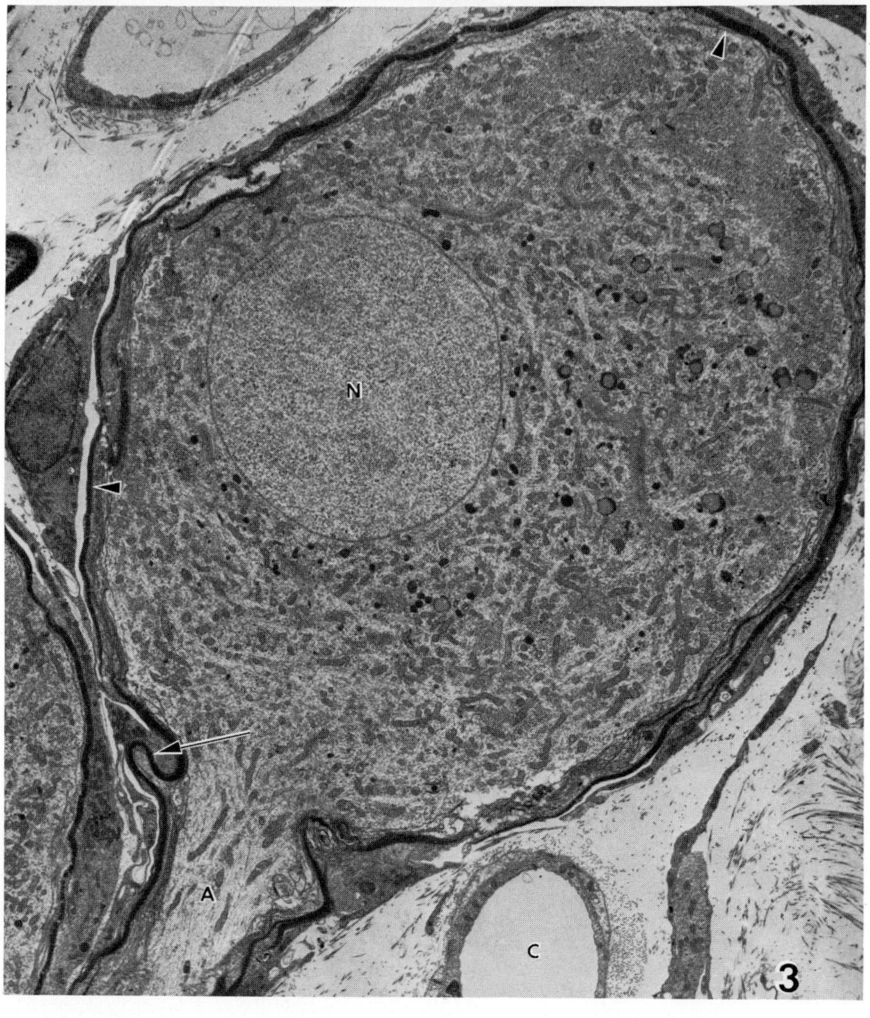

Fig. 3. Large myelinated perikaryon with euchromatic nucleus (N) and axon (A). Arrow points to cytoplasmic finger-like extension and arrowheads indicate the variation of the compact myelin. C - Capillary. (Transmission electron micrograph [TEM], x3,446)

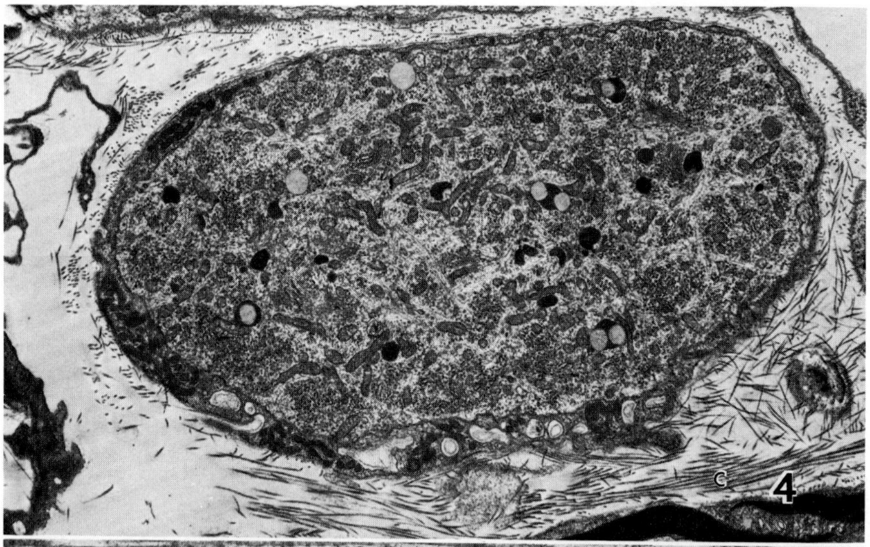

Fig. 4. Section of an unmyelinated neuron proximal to the axon hillock. C - Collagen fibrils. (TEM, x5,600)

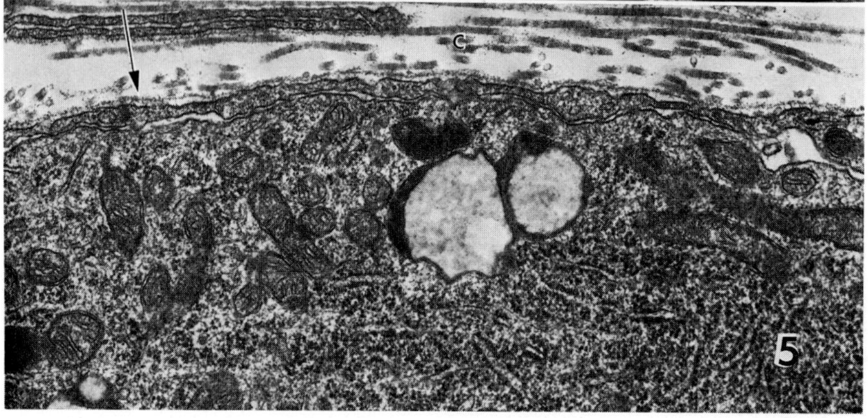

Fig. 5. Higher magnification of unmyelinated neuron showing details of cytoplasm. Schwann cell external coat (arrow) and collagen fibers (C) are located very closely. (TEM, x21,540)

perikaryal myelin, between loose and compact, sometimes proceeds to the axon, where they are recognized as Schmidt-Lanterman clefts (Fig. 8). These clefts are more frequently seen following the first node of Ranvier, which is often preceded by a naked axonal segment that can reach up to 20 μ in length before becoming heavily myelinated with up to 60 layers of compact myelin (Fig. 9).

The perikaryal myelin is formed by Schwann cells that sometimes display two nuclei. Light microscopic examination of 20-25 μ thick sections through different focusing planes shows that there could be up to four Schwann cells contributing to the perikaryal myelin. The Schwann cells have many dark mitochondria and usually elliptical nuclei with dispersed heterochromatin (Fig. 7). Sometimes a nucleolar complex is envisioned. Occasionally, Schwann cells form extensive invaginations in the proximity to the initial axonal segment (Fig. 7). Sometimes small myelinated bodies (1-2 μ diameter) were identified. These bodies are formed by the first Schwann cell lamellae (Fig. 10). Frequently vesiculated structures are wrapped by the myelin of these bodies. Some of these resemble mitochondria (Fig. 11). All perikarya have granular cytoplasm with abundant polysomes that are formed by rosettes of three to six ribosomes (Figs. 10 and 12). The polysomes, together with free ribosomes and also short cisterns of rough endoplasmic reticulum are grouped randomly throughout the cytoplasm (Figs. 3 and 5). Up to five mitochondria per square micron can be counted on any given portion of the cell. They are approximately 0.25 μ in diameter and up to 4 μ in length. The inner cristae of mitochondria are loosely arranged and of a light appearance as compared to those in the mitochondria of the Schwann cells (Fig. 10). Occasionally the neuronal plasmalemma invaginates into the cytoplasm to form coated vesicles (Fig. 13).

There are are several Golgi complexes on each cell and, occasionally, a few multivesicular bodies. There are numerous dense osmiophilic granules, approximately 0.5 μ in diameter, surrounded by a double membrane and very often located close to lipid droplets (Fig. 12). These dense granules, as most other organelles, are not preferentially positioned within the cytoplasm (Fig. 3) although they are occasionally located close to Golgi complexes (Figs. 12 and 14). Very few microtubules are seen. Contrarily, abundant neurofilaments are located proximal to the axon hillock (Fig. 7) where often large amounts of polysomes and rough endoplasmic reticulum are also observed.

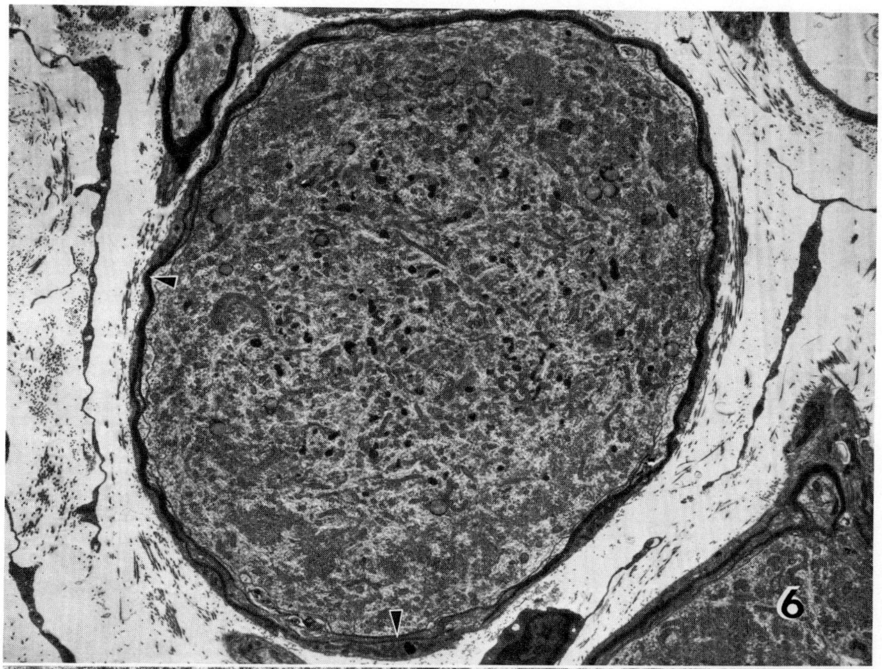

Fig. 6. Section of a neuron in the vicinity of the axon hillock. Arrowheads show a variation in the thickness of compact myelin. (TEM, x3,590)

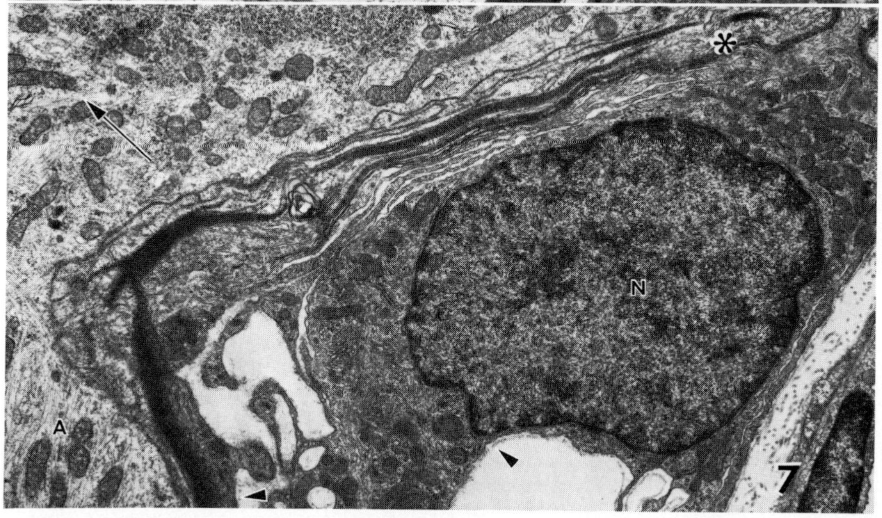

Fig. 7. Section at the level of the initial axonal segment (A) showing extensive cytoplasmic invaginations of the Schwann cell cytoplasm. Asterisk (*) shows the point where the compact myelin has transformed into loose myelin. Note cell coat (arrowhead) and heterochromatin in the nucleus (N). The arrow points to neurofilaments in neuron. (TEM, x9,693)

The perikaryal nuclei, approximately 10 μ in diameter, are void of heterochromatin. They are almost spherical and seldom positioned centrally (Fig. 3). The nucleolar complexes are not seen in all cells. They are approximately 2 μ in diameter and they are generally eccentrically positioned within the nuclei. Although both constituents of the nucleolar complexes can be seen in the same cells, in most cells only the nucleolemma (pars fibrosa) is seen, while in other cells mainly the pars amorpha (granulosa) predominates (Fig. 14).

The nerve fibers are heavily or lightly myelinated. Their diameters range between 2-8 μ. Although the peripheral (toward the vestibule) initial segment of the fiber was occasionally wider than the central (toward the brain) initial segment, the fibers themselves did not show significant variation after the first node of Ranvier. In cross section, a third type constitutes a small number of unmyelinated fibers with a single Schwann cell layer surrounding them. All nerve fibers have varicosities that alternate repeatedly with narrower axonal segments (Fig. 8). These varicosities are more numerous within the limits of the ganglion and they are readily seen in freshly fixed preparations viewed under the phase microscope. At the varicosities, the neurofilaments are less densely packed, and the number of mitochondria usually increases.

The axonal initial segment may or may not be myelinated. When the initial segment is myelinated, the number of myelin sheaths is less than that in the regions after the first node of Ranvier. In those cells where the initial segment is not myelinated, there is a single layer of Schwann cell cytoplasm that extends from the soma and wraps around the axon. Following the first node of Ranvier, there is an increase in the number of myelin lamellae. Characteristic of this region are Schmidt-

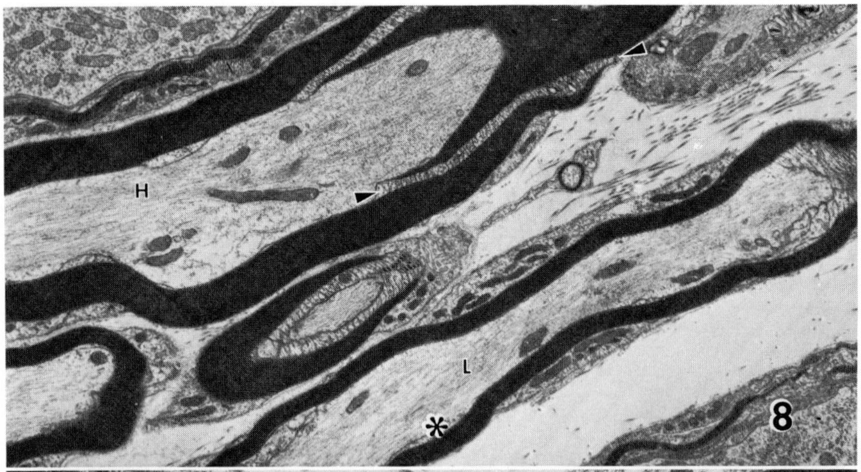

Fig. 8. Longitudinal section through a heavily (H) and a lightly (L) myelinated nerve fiber. Notice Schmidt-Lanterman cleft between arrowheads. Varicosity of the nerve is indicated by (*). (TEM, x5,888)

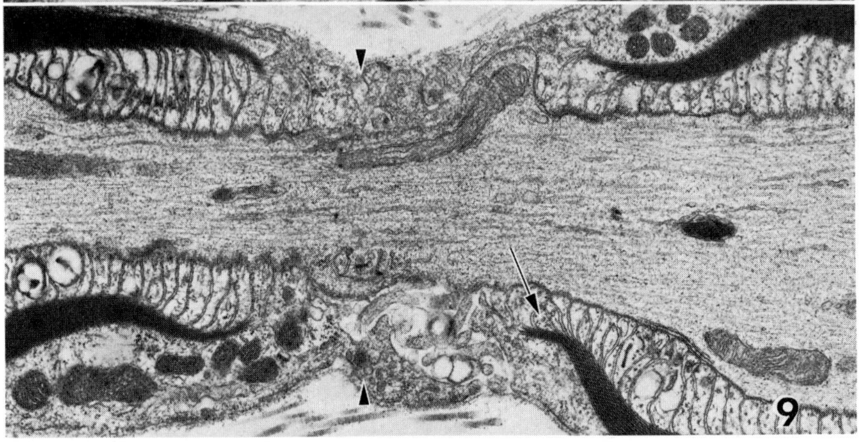

Fig. 9. High magnification of a node of Ranvier. Section across the two arrowheads will result in an unmyelinated nerve fiber. The arrow points to dense particles in the paranodal region as well as the end of the compact myelin. (TEM, x16,586)

Lanterman clefts. Sometimes, up to six Schmidt-Lanterman clefts can be seen per 40 μ of axonal length. Many electron dense particles are always seen between the myelin layers at the clefts (Fig. 15). The same type of particle also exists in the paranodal cytoplasm (Fig. 9).

DISCUSSION

As previously reported,[2,3] in the squirrel monkey vestibular ganglia there are small and large neurons (Fig. 2); however, the majority of the ganglion cells are large neurons (Fig. 3). Although small neurons with nuclei were seen in all sections, the authors consider that classification of these irregularly shaped neurons cannot be elucidated with certainty until scanning electron microscopic investigation is carried out. Through that manner size rather than diameter or surface area will be investigated appropriately. A tangential section through one of the large neurons with a peripherally positioned nucleus may very well be identified as a cell with morphological characteristics similar to that of the neurons of a smaller size. Neuronal size is more homogenous in 25 μ thick sections where the chance to visualize whole cells is greater (Fig. 1). Occasionally, scattered neurons were observed certain distances away from the ganglia proper. Scattered neurons have also been reported in the vestibular ganglia,[3] and in the spiral ganglia of other species,[8] but their functional significance is not known.

Although we were able to identify heavily or lightly myelinated (Fig. 3), and unmyelinated neurons (Figs. 4 and 5), we are presently unable to correlate the myelination pattern with cytoplasmic appearance of these neurons, ie, granular and filamentous with myelinated and nonmyelinated perikarya.

The cytoplasmic organelles of the neurons are randomly distributed. Serial thick (1-2 μ) sections of Epon-embedded materials indicate that cytoplasmic differences among perikarya may result from cutting these irregularly shaped cells through different planes. In these bipolar neurons both nerve fibers do not always exit exactly at opposite sides from the cytoplasm of the perikarya (Fig. 16). This is illustrated by the fact that generally in 1-2 μ serial sections, only one fiber is cut along with the soma (Figs. 2 and 3). In addition, these neurons have nuclei that are not always centrally positioned; this fact eliminates the possibility of using either the nuclei or the nucleolar complexes as a marker for measurement when the cells are cut through their centers. Moreover, there are more neurofilaments in the vicinity of the axon hillock than in the central portion of the cells (Fig. 17). Different sectioning planes could result in sections with cells of the same

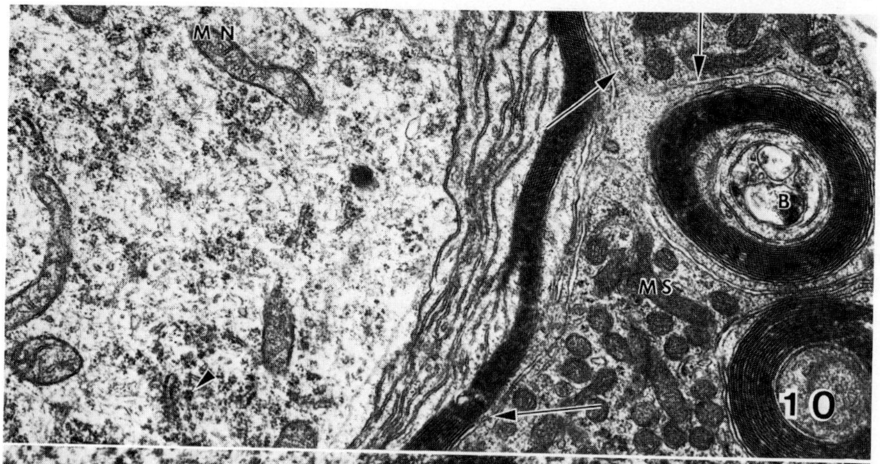

Fig. 10. Myelinated bodies (B) in Schwann cell. Myelin lamella (arrows) detaches from compact myelin and wraps around one of the bodies. Note the difference between neuronal (MN) mitochrondria and Schwann cell (MS) mitochrondria. Polysome at the arrowhead. (TEM, x17,950)

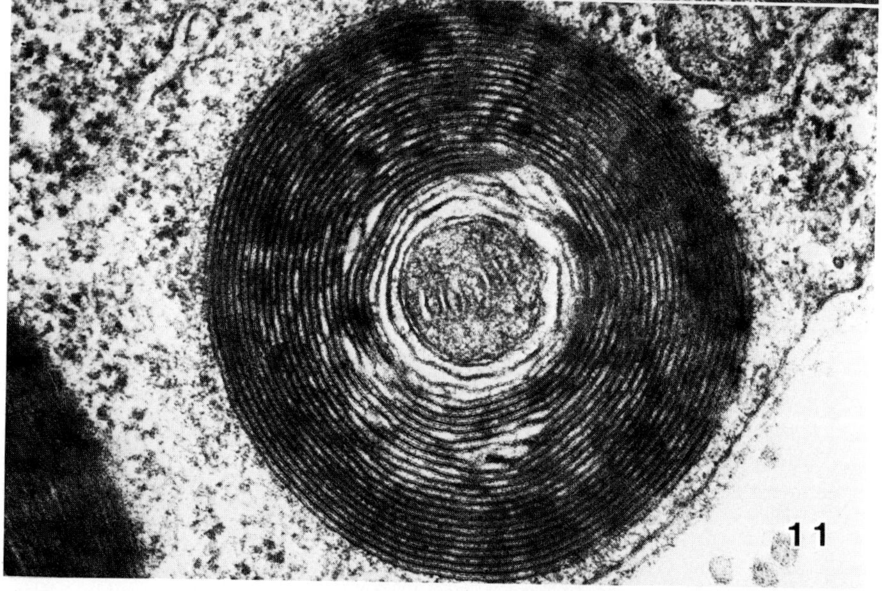

Fig. 11. Higher magnification of a myelinated body within Schwann cell. (TEM, x71,800).

type, but with different cytoplasmic appearance and myelination patterns. However, our observations on the squirrel monkey vestibular ganglia do not necessarily emphasize that correlation between myelination pattern and cytoplasmic appearance exists among the vestibular neurons of other animals. In our preparation approximately 5% of the vestibular neurons did not have a true myelin sheath. They were not preferentially positioned at a particular location, and their cytoplasmic appearance was not different than the other neurons within the ganglion (Figs. 2, 4, and 5). In other species, approximately 10% of the vestibular neurons followed the above pattern.[3] In the same study myelination and cytoplasmic appearance were correlated.

The granular appearance of the vestibular perikarya (Figs. 4, 5, and 12) is the result of large amounts of polysomes, free ribosomes, and short cisterns of endoplasmic reticulum that are randomly distributed throughout the somal cytoplasm. Mitochondria are also distributed throughout the cytoplasm in a random manner. The large number of mitochondria and the ribosomal machinery attest to a high metabolic activity among these neurons. Testimony of the above observation is also the presence of euchromatic nuclei,[15] lightly stained, both under the light and the electron microscope (Figs. 2, 3, and 14). Microtubules were not predominant, and multivesicular bodies were very rarely observed.

There was no significant difference between central and peripheral processes of the neurons. The processes were heavily or lightly myelinated (Fig. 8). The third type of unmyelinated nerve fiber, which was observed in our cross sections and reported by other investigators,[3] could be the result of cutting through the nodes of Ranvier (Fig. 9) where the fibers usually narrow down.

Although longitudinal sections as well as surface preparations show the presence of various nerve fiber diameters, cross sections of nerve fibers have a limitation in indicating actual nerve fiber diameter because the existence of varicosities can alter it. In the chick statoacoustic ganglion, for instance, the nerve varicosities account for some of the diameter difference observed in cross sections.[16]

The Schwann cell cytoplasm is denser and less

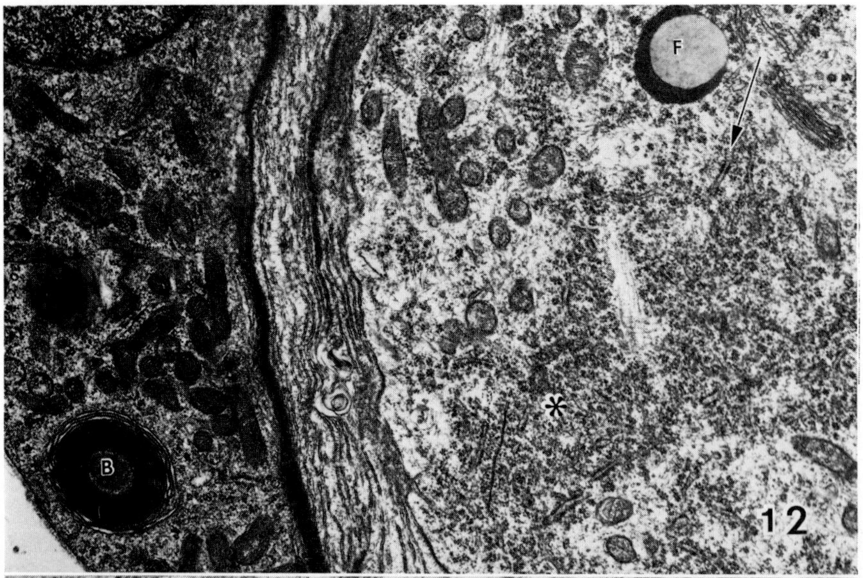

Fig. 12. Cytoplasmic detail of a perikaryon is seen (right). Lipid droplet (F), short cistern of rough endoplasmic reticulum (arrow) and group of polysomes (*). A myelinated body (B) is seen in the Schwann cell (left). (TEM, x14,360)

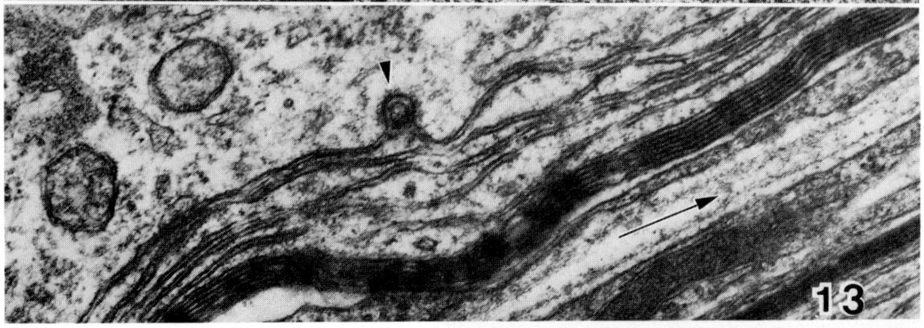

Fig. 13. Coated vesicle is surrounded by perikaryon plasma membrane (arrowhead). Notice that coats of two cells are in close contact with each other (arrow). (TEM, x43,080)

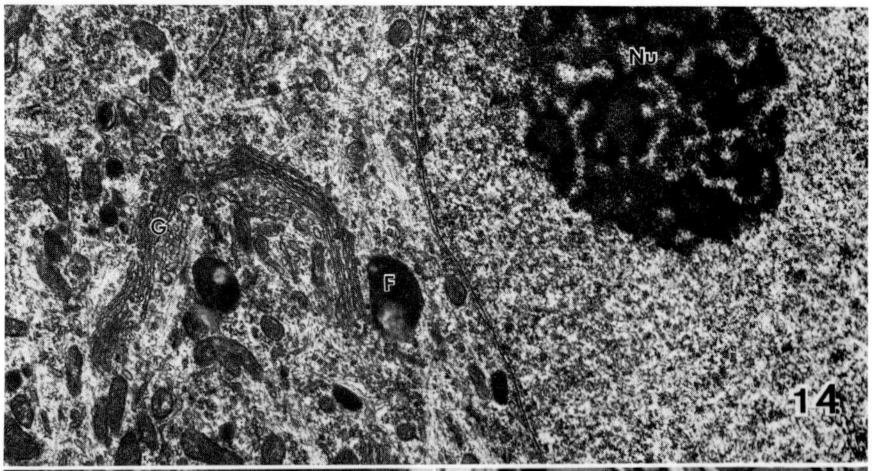

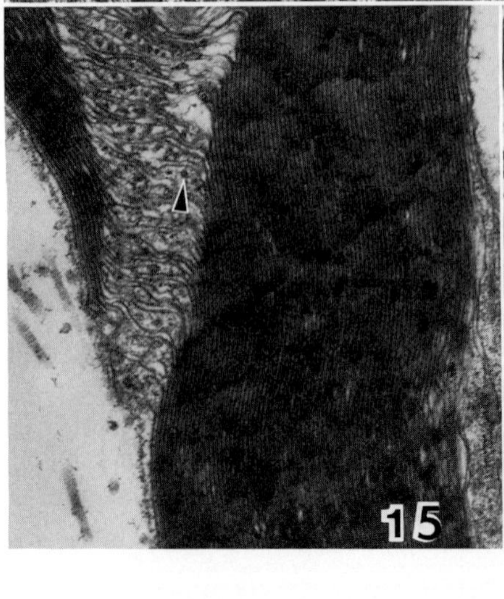

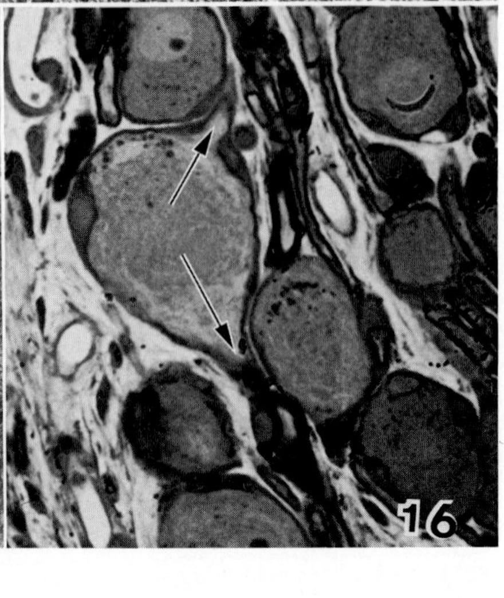

Fig. 14. Golgi complex (G) and lipid droplet (F). Note euchromatic nucleus of perikaryon. Nu -Nucleolus. (TEM, x14,360)

Fig. 15. Dense particles are sandwiched between myelin lamellae of Schmidt-Lanterman cleft (arrowhead). (TEM, x28,720)

Fig. 16. Light micrograph of a 2 μ thick section. Notice that the fibers do not exist at exactly opposite extremes (arrows). (TEM, x539)

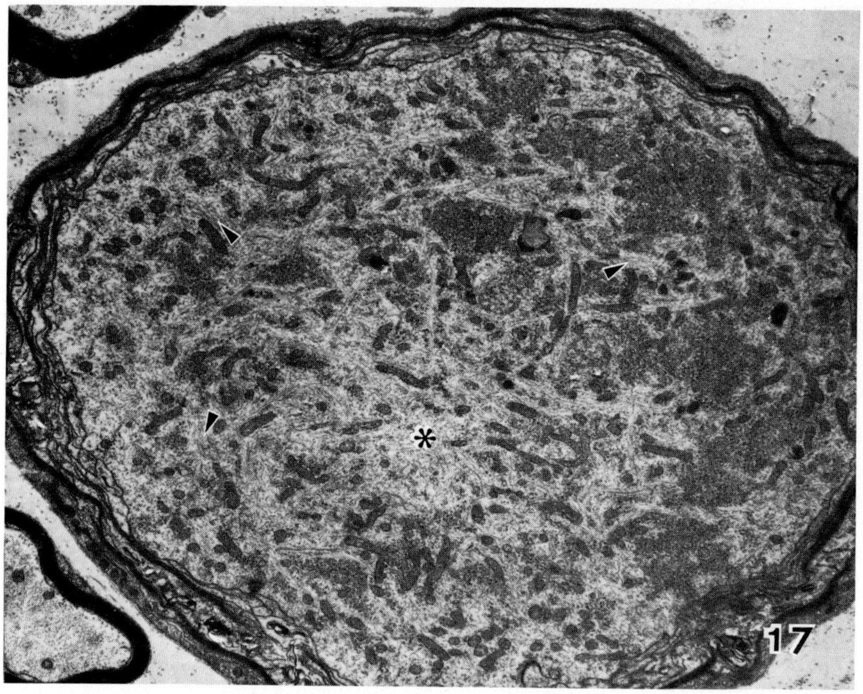

Fig. 17. Cross section near the axon hillock (*) of a myelinated perikaryon. Notice abundance of neurofilaments (arrowheads) in this region. (TEM, x5,600)

granular than that of the soma myelinated by Schwann cells. Mitochondria are smaller, darker, and have more cristae than those of the perikaryal mitochondria. The nuclei are generally heterochromatic instead of euchromatic. Two nuclei in one Schwann cell is not uncommon. This finding can be the result of cutting a single nucleus in two places since the Schwann cells wrap around the soma. While doing so Schwann cell nuclei are usually flattened and deformed; ie, the nuclei lose their spherical appearance. At the site of the extensive invaginations of the Schwann cell cytoplasm (Fig.7), the cell coat is prominent even within closed processes. These processes could have a functional significance especially since the Schwann cells are the ones contacting the interstitial fluid. Cytoplasmic extensions of this type are known to increase surface area. Cell coat is essential for cell-cell interaction and recognition.[15] In chick developing statoacoustic ganglion, for instance, the Schwann cells lose their coat at the site of contact with the nerve fibers once axonal recognition has been made.[16]

Within the Schwann cell cytoplasm we saw myelinated bodies (Figs. 10 and 11). These bodies have been observed in the spiral[4] and in the vestibular[7] ganglia of other species. At least in the squirrel monkey, these bodies seem to be the result of transverse cuts through finger-like projections of the perikarya (Fig. 3). The number of myelin lamellae of these bodies is about the same as those of the soma. The bodies, however, are almost always compactly myelinated whereas the soma displays both loose and compact myelin.

Figure 18 summarizes the main morphological features of the myelinated vestibular neurons in the squirrel monkey. It should be pointed out that slight variation of the myelin arrangement among perikarya and nerve fibers is often observed within a ganglion. In some neurons, the myelin continues on to the initial segment with the same number of lamellae found around the body. In others, however, myelination ends at the axon hillock and restarts after the first node of Ranvier. This diagram

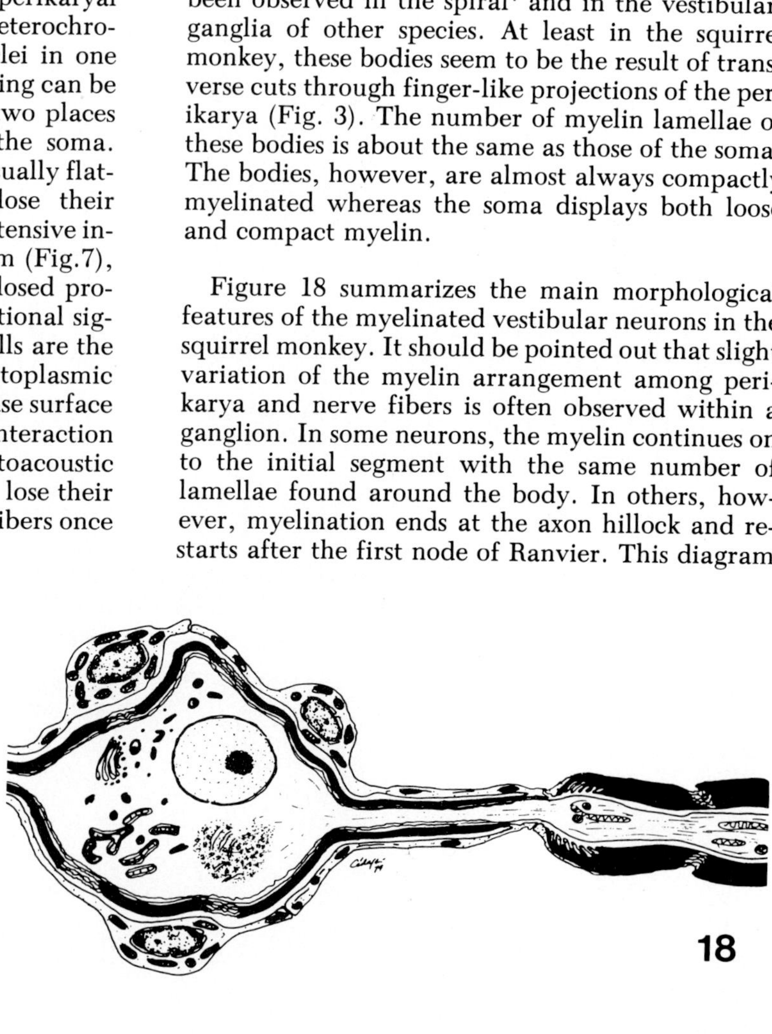

Fig. 18. Diagrammatic drawing of a vestibular neuron, its axon, myelin arrangement and Schwann cell. Some neurons and their nerve fibers are covered with a thinner myelin sheath. In other neurons, myelination ends at the axon hillock and restarts after the first node of Ranvier. The soma of some neurons is unmyelinated whereas the fibers are myelinated both before and after the first node of Ranvier. Nevertheless, this diagram represents the majority of ganglion cells, regardless of size and/or shape.

does not apply to unmyelinated neurons. Analysis of the initial segment of these neurons and myelination pattern after the first node of Ranvier was not possible.

In our preparation, we have observed numerous Schmidt-Lanterman clefts predominantly in heavily myelinated fibers (Fig. 8). On several fibers chosen randomly, and from sections at least 30 μ apart, we were able to count Schmidt-Lanterman clefts every 10-20μ in segments of heavily myelinated fibers and every 20-30 μ in segments of lightly myelinated fibers. Long (up to 100 μ) axonal segments are usually separating the segments where the clefts are frequent. Not all fibers within a ganglion follow this pattern though. Although these interruptions of the compact axonal myelin have been observed in vivo,[17] we wonder whether different tissue fixation could alter their frequency, because Schmidt-Lanterman clefts have not been reported previously with the frequency that we have observed. It is well known that the percentage of glutaraldehyde and the molarity of the vehicle of the fixative are important for the preservation of some structures.[18] The ultrastructural preservation of some tissue types differs between primary osmium fixation and primary glutaraldehyde fixation.[19] Also, a different buffer system yields different results on penetration of the fixative, stainability, and cellular appearance.[20] For instance, when the statoacoustic ganglia of chicks (counterpart of mammalian spiral ganglion) is fixed with glutaraldehyde in either cacodylate buffer or phosphate buffer, the contour of the soma as well as the myelin arrangement differ (Fermin CD. Personal observation).

ACKNOWLEDGMENT — We express our appreciation to Dr. Glenn C. Thompson for providing us with the Apple-II microcomputer and the program for data analysis.

REFERENCES

1. Perre J, Sterkers NM, Ohresser M, Foncin JF. Sur la gaine des cellules ganglionnaires de Scarpa chez l'homme. CR Acad Sci (Paris) 1975; 280:1405-7.

2. Bergström B. Morphological studies of the vestibular nerve. Acta universitatis upsaliensis. Abstracts of Uppsala dissertations from Faculty of Medicine 1973; 159:7-38.

3. Ballantyne J, Engström H. Morphology of the vestibular ganglion cells. J Laryngol Otol 1969; 83:19-42.

4. Perre J, Riche D, Foncin JF. Sur la gaine des cellules ganglionnaires de Scarpa chez le babouin (*Papio papio*). Arch Otolaryngol 1977; 83:279-83.

5. Densert O. A fluorescence and electron microscopic study of the adrenergic innervation in the vestibular ganglion and sensory areas. Acta Otolaryngol (Stockh) 1975; 79: 96-107.

6. Kellerhals B, Engstrom H, Ades HE. Die morphologie des ganglion spirale cochleae. Acta Otolaryngol (Stockh) 1967; Suppl 226: 5-78.

7. Adamo NJ, Daigneault EA. Ultrastructural features of neurons and nerve fibers in the spiral ganglia of cats. J Neurocytol 1973; 2:91-103.

8. Ylikoski J, Collan Y, Palva T. Ultrastructural features of spiral ganglion cells: a study of patients with hearing loss of varying origins. Arch Otolaryngol 1978; 104:84-8.

9. Awataguchi S, Yamamoto N. Fine structure of the eighth nerve ganglion in the toad. Auris Nasus Larynx 1974; 1:77-87.

10. Ross MD, Burkel W. Multipolar neurons in the spiral ganglion of the rat. Acta Otolaryngol (Stockh) 1973; 76:381-94.

11. Tomsen E. The ultrastructure of the spiral ganglion in guinea pigs. Acta Otolaryngol (Stockh) 1967; Suppl 224: 442-8.

12. Rosenbluth J. The fine structure of the acoustic ganglia in the rat. J Cell Biol 1962; 12:329-59.

13. Watson ML. Staining of tissue for electron microscopy with heavy metals. J Biophys Biochem Cytol 1958; 4:475-578.

14. Reynolds ES. The use of lead citrate at high pH as an electron opaque stain in electron microscopy. J Cell Biol 1963; 17:208-12.

15. De Robertis EPD, De Robertis EMF Jr. Cell and molecular biology, 7th ed. Philadelphia: Saunders, 1980.

16. Cohen GM, Fermin CD. Differentiation and myelination of the embryonic chick's statoacoustic ganglion. Abstracts of the Second Midwinter Research Meeting. Association for Research in Otolaryngology, St. Petersburg Beach, Florida, 1978.

17. Truex RC, Carpenter AB. Human neuroanatomy, 6th ed. Baltimore: Williams & Wilkins, 1969.

18. Mathieu O, Claasen H, Weibel ER. Differential effect of glutaraldehyde and buffer osmolarity on cell dimensions: a study on lung tissue. J Ultrastruct Res 1978; 63:20-34.

19. Santos-Sacchi J. Differential effects of primary fixation with glutaraldehyde and osmium upon the membranous system of strial and external sulcus cells. Acta Otolaryngol (Stockh) 1978; 86:56-63.

20. Wood LR, Luft JH. The influence of buffer systems on fixation with osmium tetroxide. J Ultrastruct Res 1965; 12:22-45.

Ann Otol 91:1982

REVASCULARIZATION OF SKIN USING A MYOVASCULAR PEDICLE

AN ANIMAL MODEL FOR FREE AND MYOCUTANEOUS FLAPS

R. SERGEANT, FRCS
ROTTINGDEAN, SUSSEX, ENGLAND

WILLIAM R. PANJE, MD
IOWA CITY, IOWA

Myovascular pedicles developed from the rat hind limb allowed for revascularization of groin skin. This result confirms previous work. The myovascularized skin could be used as a free flap or as an experimental animal model in the study of myocutaneous flaps.

INTRODUCTION

Over the last decade the technique of suturing together blood vessels less than 3 mm in diameter has emerged from the experimental laboratory into clinical practice. Free flap reconstruction of surgical and traumatic defects using these microvascular techniques has now established itself in clinical practice as a useful and consistently successful procedure.[1,2] The most frequently used flap is based on the superficial circumflex iliac vessels in the groin area;[3] less commonly the skin from the dorsum of the foot based on the dorsalis pedis vessels has been utilized.[4] The relative lack of donor free flap sites dependent upon a direct cutaneous vascular supply and the need for vessels at least 1.5 mm in diameter to achieve reliable anastomosis remain as disadvantages to the further development of microsurgical reconstruction.

In 1969 Schechter et al[5] showed that revascularization of canine skin was possible using a myovascular pedicle. The observation that such skin could be transferred as a free flap is of considerable interest now that free flaps have gained clinical acceptance. The ability to selectively revascularize areas of skin or tissue units, ie, bowel, bone, neuromuscular tissue, with a suitably sized vascular pedicle for microvascular anastomosis would widen the scope and possibilities for microvascular tissue transplantation.

Myocutaneous flaps have deservedly received great impetus in the recent clinical literature. These compound flaps have demonstrated a wide range of reliable usefulness in reconstruction of head and neck defects. However, to better understand physiology and biochemistry of the myocutaneous flap, an animal model that represents the human situation would seem appropriate.

Using the rat, a myovascularized skin flap model was developed that confirms previous observations found in the dog. In addition this experimental flap was examined histologically, by perfusion studies, and physiologically as to its applicability to represent an animal model for the human myocutaneous flap.

METHODS

Twenty-two male rats (Biolab) weighing between 250 and 350 g were anesthetized using intraperitoneal Nembutal. A U-shaped thigh skin flap based in the inguinal region was elevated to expose the inguinal fat pad, and the inferior epigastric and femoral vessels. The subcutaneous elevation was continued onto the anterior abdominal wall to divide the myocutaneous vessels in the lower abdominal quadrant adjacent to the thigh. The inguinal fat pad was excised following ligation and division of the inferior epigastric vessels at their origin. The femoral vessels were ligated and divided just distal to the origin of a constant muscular branch that supplies the adductor muscles of the thigh. A 6 x 5 x 2 mm block of gracilis was elevated on the vascular pedicle just described. Elevation proximally of the femoral vessels resulted in a long vascular pedicle such that the muscle block could be sutured using 9 monofilament nylon to the undersurface of the elevated abdominal wall skin. The skin flap was replaced and the wound closed (Fig. 1).

Five rats were used as controls, and in these no myovascular pedicle was elevated although identical elevation of the skin of the thigh and abdomen was performed. Between the 18th and 25th day following flap elevation the animals were divided into groups for subsequent experimentation.

Experiment 1. In the five control rats a 4 cm disc of skin situated centrally in the previously elevated skin flap was dissected free and then sutured back in situ. Six rats with myovascular pedicles had similar discs of skin, centered on the muscle block, elevated. These skin discs, whose only attachment was the myovascular pedicle, were sutured back in situ. In all rats, on return of the skin discs, intravenous fluorescein was given prior to examination under ultraviolet light. The subsequent fate of the skin discs was recorded.

Experiment 2. Flaps measuring 8 x 4 cm were elevated in five rats such that the only point of attachment near the lower end of the flap was the myovascular pedicle, all other sources of blood supply being sacrificed. The flaps after elevation were sutured back in position. Five rats, previously unoperated, were used as controls, and in these, similar size flaps were elevated based only on the inferior epigastric vessels. These flaps were also sutured back in position. In five rats 8 x 4 cm flaps were raised on each side of the animal. On the right side the flap was supplied only by the myovascular pedicle and on the left side by the inferior epigastric vessels. Thus ten neovascularized flaps were available for assessment, together with ten controls. The flaps were examined, following intravenous fluorescein, under ultraviolet light shortly after return and suturing. Final assessment was made at the fifth day.

From the Department of Otolaryngology and Maxillofacial Surgery, Division of Head and Neck Surgery, University of Iowa Hospitals, Iowa City.
REPRINTS — William R. Panje, MD, Department of Otolaryngology and Maxillofacial Surgery, University of Iowa Hospitals, Iowa City, IA 52242.

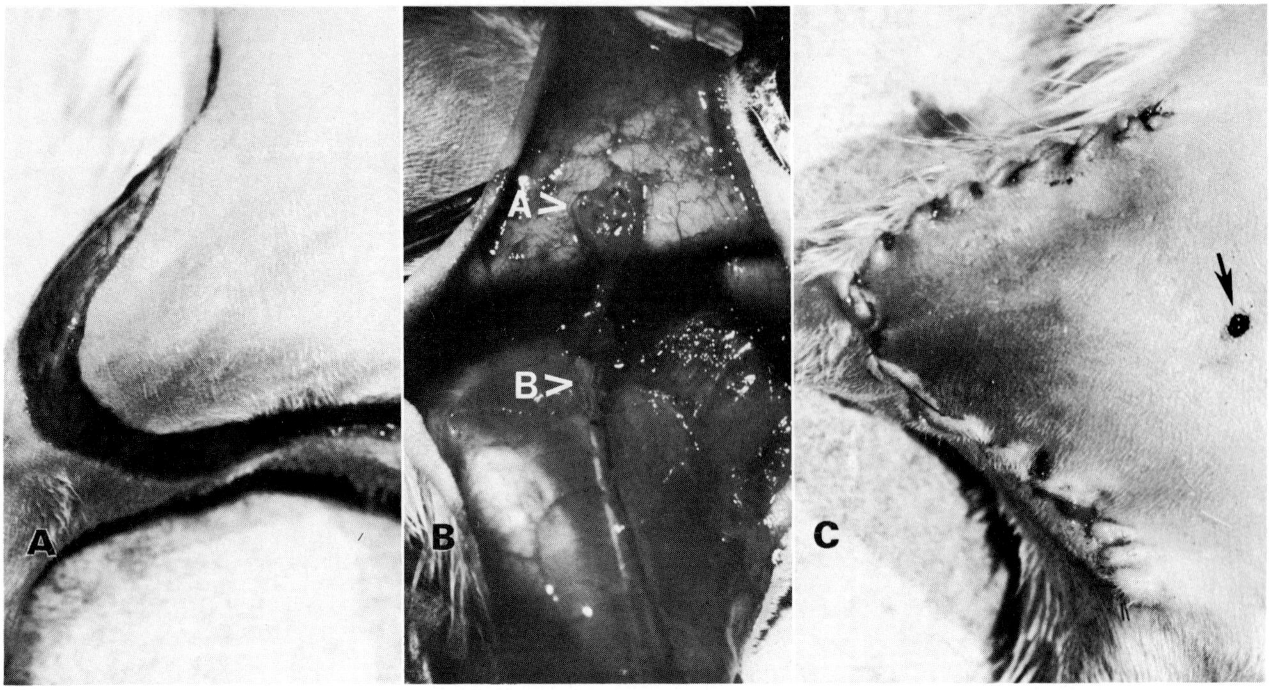

Fig. 1. A) Rat groin and leg with medially pedicled "cutaneous"groin flap. B) Gracilis muscle applied to undersurface of reflected groin flap (arrow A). Vascular pedicle entering femoral vessels (arrow B). C) Cutaneous groin flap sutured in place. Black dot (arrow) marks area to which gracilis myovascular pedicle has been attached.

Rats demonstrate a marked tendency to devour their own skin flaps. In the bilateral group the abdominal wall was protected by means of a cervical collar and all rats were caged individually.

Experiment 3. Three rats with myovascular pedicles were sacrificed at 28 days. The skin and underlying muscle block were serially sectioned.

Experiment 4. In one rat a 4 cm disc of skin based on the myovascular pedicle was raised. An intravenous injection of India ink into the dorsal vein of the penis perfused the flap. The animal was sacrificed and the skin with its underlying myovascular pedicle was serially sectioned.

Experiment 5. Vinylite plastic casts of the vascular tree in the lower half of two rats with myovascular pedicles were made according to E. Rose (personal communication).

RESULTS

The results of experiments 1 and 2 are tabulated in the table. In reference to experiments 3, 4, and 5, serial sections through the myovascular pedicle at 28 days show the presence of neocapillaries between the muscle and subdermal plexus of the skin flap. Carbon particles (India ink) were shown to be present in the subdermal plexus of the flap isolated in its myovascular pedicle prior to injection. Vinylite casts demonstrated the gross anatomical change in the vascular pattern.

DISCUSSION

The blood supply of skin is dependent on the subdermal vascular plexus and its vascular connections. In these experiments the plane of flap elevation is just deep to the subdermal vascular plexus and all vascular connections except at the base of the flap are divided. The muscle block when sutured in situ is adjacent to the subdermal plexus. The acute inflammatory response and organization of the hematoma between skin and muscle results in the formation of neocapillaries which unite the subdermal vascular plexus to vessels in the muscle block. These vessels were demonstrated in the serial sections of the muscle and skin (experiment 3). The vascular continuity at capillary level has been demonstrated histologically with serial sections performed following the injection of India ink (experiment 4). The Vinylite casts, not surprisingly, failed to show vascular continuity between the muscle block and subdermal plexus of the skin flap. The casts, however, did demonstrate a nutrient vessel to the adductor muscle mass of the thigh.

In the first experiment all control skin discs failed to fluoresce and were gangrenous by the fifth day. In the muscle pedicle group complete flap survival was noted in all animals despite the effects of self-inflicted trauma and resuturing required at 24 hours in two rats. This experiment clearly shows that it is possible to revascularize skin and that such may be elevated as a flap on a new and discrete vascular pedicle.

The second experiment attempts to determine the area of viable skin that can be maintained by the standard size muscle block and pedicle. In both the control and experimental groups flap loss occurred distally and extended the full width of the flap. Flap loss has been assessed, therefore, as a single linear measurement. Of the ten neovascularized flaps elevated, one was eaten prior to assessment

FLUORESCENCE AND FLAP VIABILITY IN EXPERIMENTS 1 AND 2

Rats	*Rat No.*	*Area of Fluorescence (cm)*	*Area of Viability at 5th Day (cm)*	*Remarks*
Experiment 1. Skin disc				
Control group (N = 5)		Nil	Nil	
Pedicle group (N = 6)		Complete	Complete	In 2 rats resuturing wound required at 24 hr
Experiment 2.				
Myovascular pedicle group	1	4.0 x 8.0	4.0 x 8.0	
	2	4.0 x 8.0	4.0 x 7.0	
	3	4.0 x 8.0	Nil	Eaten
	4	4.0 x 4.0	4.0 x 4.5	
	5	0.5 x 0.5	4.0 x 3.5	
	6	4.0 x 5.0	4.0 x 7.0	
	7	4.0 x 4.0	4.0 x 6.0	
	8	4.0 x 5.0	4.0 x 6.5	
	9	4.0 x 6.5	4.0 x 8.0	
	10	4.0 x 6.0	4.0 x 6.0	
Control group	1	Nil	Nil	Eaten
	2	Nil	Nil	Eaten
	3	Nil	Nil	Animal death, cause unknown
	4	4.0 x 8.0	4.0 x 6.5	
	5	4.0 x 6.0	4.0 x 6.0	
	6	4.0 x 6.0	4.0 x 8.0	
	7	4.0 x 8.0	4.0 x 7.0	
	8	4.0 x 8.0	4.0 x 8.0	
	9	4.0 x 8.0	4.0 x 8.0	
	10	4.0 x 8.0	4.0 x 8.0	

and in another the vascular pedicle was traumatized at the time of elevation, resulting in poor fluorescence and considerable flap loss by the fifth day. These two animals were excluded from analysis. Of the remaining six some flap loss was noted, the range being 1 to 3.5 cm. The mean linear flap loss was 1.4 cm.

The experimental control was an axial pattern flap based on the inferior epigastric vessels. Again 10 flaps were raised; 2 flaps were eaten and one animal died leaving 7 flaps for analysis. Complete survival was noted in four and in the remaining three, linear flap loss occurred of 1, 1.5, and 2 cm. The mean linear flap loss was 0.6 cm.

In this small group of animals no statistically significant results can be expressed. Nevertheless the standard muscle block and vascular pedicle is able to maintain the viability of a flap on the average 4 x 6.6 cm. If the area of muscle in contact with the flap is related to the total area of viable flap, the

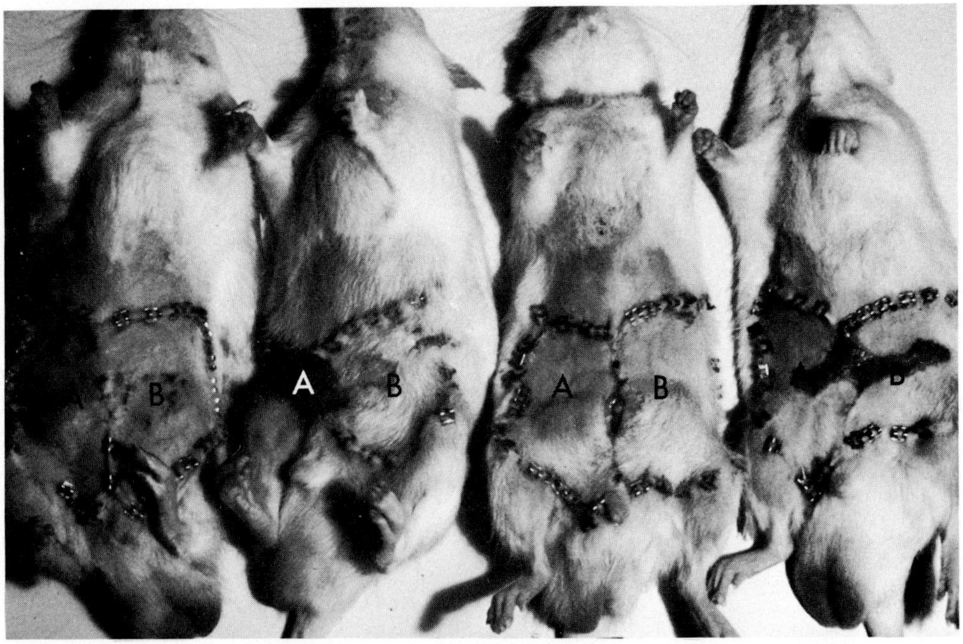

Fig. 2. Rat abdomens from experiment 2 at ten days postoperative. Note similarity of flap survival in each animal. Control group (A); Experimental myovascularized flap group (B).

ratio is 1:66. The result compares favorably with the size of flap (4 x 7.4 cm) maintained by the animal's own inferior epigastric vessels (Fig. 2).

CONCLUSION

These experiments confirm that it is possible to revascularize an area of skin with a discrete myovascular pedicle. Such skin with its newly selected vascular pedicle could be readily transferred as a free flap. In clinical practice the mobilization of a comparatively small muscle block and vascular pedicle would cause minimal morbidity and no functional loss yet ultimately yield a flap, ie, skin and vessel diameter suitable for microvascular reconstructive surgery.

With the recent promulgation of myocutaneous flaps,[6,7] development of a small animal skin-muscle flap model would be important for further explorations into the possible uses of this flap. Previous anatomical studies have demonstrated that animal models, except for the pig and monkey, are unsuitable for definitive cutaneous flap research which can apply to the human.[8] Animal skin is supplied through a dual vascular system separated by a thin muscle layer (panniculus carnosum). In contrast, human integument receives its principal vascular supply through musculocutaneous perforators. By removing the animal's panniculus carnosum and its underlying blood supply and directly applying a vascularized muscle pedicle to the subdermal plexus as done in this experiment, one is essentially creating a myocutaneous unit that duplicates the human situation. The significance of this experiment animal flap model as used herein can be seen in the development of the human myocutaneous "paddle" flap concept. The "paddle" flap is a myocutaneous flap in which there is a cutaneous extension without underlying muscle. The cutaneous extension provides for thinness and suppleness not easily achieved with the pure compound arrangement. The skin-only extension is a random flap and, unlike the axial skin-muscle arrangement, is more subject to failure with greater length-width ratios. From this experiment a comparatively small myovascular pedicle (5 x 6 mm), when attached to skin, was able to maintain viability of a moderately large proportion of a delayed cutaneous-only flap. The relative area of muscle to skin was 1:66. This concept has now been applied to the human situation and will be reported at a later date.

Clearly the need exists for further experimentation to substantiate the validity of the rat myovascularized skin flap concept to duplicate the human situation. The revascularization of bone and composite tissues are planned areas for further free flap experimentation. The use of various drugs will also be investigated as to their effect on how and when to reverse the dying myovascularized skin flap.

REFERENCES

1. Harii K, Ohman K, Torii S, et al. Free groin skin flaps. Br J Plast Surg 1975; 28:225-37.

2. Panje WR, Krause CJ, Bardach J, Baker S. Reconstruction of intraoral defects with the free groin flap. Arch Otolaryngol 1977; 103:78-83.

3. Smith PJ, Foley B, McGregor IA, Jackson IT. The anatomical basis of the groin flap. Plast Reconstr Surg 1972; 49:41-7.

4. McCraw JB, Furlow T Jr. The dorsalis pedis arterialized flap. Plast Reconstr Surg 1975; 55:177-85.

5. Schechter GL, Biller HF, Ogura JH. Revascularized skin flaps. Laryngoscope 1969; 79:1647-65.

6. Panje WR. Myocutaneous trapezius flap. Head Neck Surg 1980; 2:206-12.

7. Panje WR. Myocutaneous flaps vs free flaps. Otolaryngol Clin North Am 1982 (in press).

8. Daniel RK, Williams HB. The free transfer of skin flaps by microvascular anastomosis: an experimental study and a reappraisal. Plast Reconstr Surg 1973; 52:16-31.

Ann Otol 91:1982

FLUORESCENCE BRONCHOSCOPY
A NEW TECHNIQUE AND FURTHER RESULTS

DIETRICH HÜRZELER, MD

ZÜRICH, SWITZERLAND

A new method of fluorescence bronchoscopy is presented which uses a standard light source and a special filter combination to permit the carrying out of fluorescence bronchoscopy with a surface marking method by means of inhaling a fluorescein solution. Normal mucous membrane, or mucous membrane with no histological change other than inflammation, which is cleansed by ciliary activity, does not usually fluoresce for a period longer than about two hours after the inhalation. There were, it is true, 13 false positive fluorescences out of 52 fluorescing areas in the mucous membrane. Correctly recorded were 39 cases of positive, ie, visible tumors, metaplasias, accumulation of mucous glands in the epithelium, and mucous membrane which had undergone a neoplastic change in the sense of a lymphangitis carcinomatosa or a mucous membrane carcinosis; these all caused fluorescence. The false negative results amounted to only two nonfluorescing tumors and one metaplasia. These diagnoses arise from the first 100 patients examined by this method. The fact must be especially emphasized that out of the 58 carcinoma cases, there were 7 where neoplastic changes in the mucous membrane were diagnosed by the fluorescence technique, although they had not been recognized macroscopically either by the naked eye or by the Hopkins optical technique.

INTRODUCTION

Preliminary results with ultraviolet (UV) fluorescence bronchoscopy were reported two years ago at the meeting of the American Broncho-Esophagological Association.[1] Since then, further experience has been accumulated and a new technique adopted.

TECHNIQUE

Requirements. J. Reling, of the firm of J. L. Storz, drew the author's attention to the fact that fluorescence can be excited not only by UV light but also by visible light (Fig. 1). This area ranges from 400 to 770 nm (1 nm = 10^{-9} m). The light required for optimal production of fluorescence lies in the dark blue band, at a wavelength of 495-498 nm. There are also two further exciting frequencies in UV light which have been used hitherto, namely 325 and 280 nm. The fluorescent light generated lies in the green-yellow range. It starts at 480 nm and reaches a maximum at 525 nm.

Apparatus. These requirements can be met by apparatus designed as follows. The UV light source is no longer necessary but is replaced by a conventional endoscope light source of any make equipped to accept a cooled dark blue filter in front. The filter must meet the following specifications: it should transmit light over a narrow waveband only, as close as possible to 495 nm, with a steep drop in the curve beyond this point and practically no more light being transmitted beyond 500 nm. The Zeiss exciter filter 500, an interference filter, has been specially developed for this purpose. On account of its instability to heat, this filter must be air-cooled. Certain chemicals such as formaldehyde

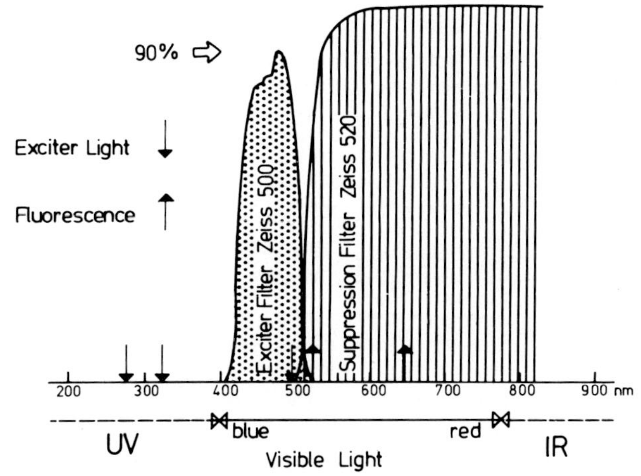

Fig. 1. Areas of fluorescence excited by ultraviolet and visible light sources. UV - Ultraviolet; IR - Infrared.

vapor or Aldosan, a disinfectant, can also bleach the filter. This narrow band of blue light is transmitted through an ordinary glass fiber-bundle light carrier. The special quartz fiber-bundle light carrier is unnecessary, since no UV light is to be transmitted. This light-conducting fiber-bundle is attached to a viewing optical system having any chosen viewing angle, and assures optimal illumination of the field of vision with the exciter light. In theory, a fiber-bronchoscope could also be attached. The author, however, has not yet gained any experience with this, since no suitable light source possessing a filter drawer has so far been available.

In order to exclude the exciter light, which lies in the visible light range and would be reflected within the bronchial tree, so that only the induced fluorescent light can be seen, a yellow suppression filter

From the Department of Oto-Rhino-Laryngology, Triemli Municipal Hospital, Zürich, Switzerland.

Presented at the meeting of the Second World Congress for Bronchology, Düsseldorf, West Germany, June 2-4, 1980.

REPRINTS — PD Dr. med. D. Hürzeler, Klosbachstr. 107, CH-8032 Zürich, Switzerland.

is fitted to the optical eyepiece or the fiber bronchoscope eyepiece. Here too, a special filter combined with the Zeiss 500 exciter filter is available. This is the Zeiss suppression filter 520, an absorption filter with a very steep cutoff at about 500 to 515 nm. Its transmission factor amounts to 90% at 530 nm and as much as 95% at 540 nm, and it thus passes practically all of the fluorescent light generated. The very small amount of overlap between these two filters allows so little light passing through that it can practically not be seen.

With these two filters, therefore, the generated fluorescent light is all that can be seen. If, however, there is a great deal of fluorescing material in the bronchial tree, as is observed especially in cases of chronic bronchitis, the fluorescent light generated illuminates the bronchi to such an extent that their contours can be seen. This disturbing phenomenon can be alleviated by drawing off the overexcessive amount of fluorescing secretion present. It is recommended that this be done under careful, directed control by means of a catheter, the flexible instrument guide according to Maassen and the 0°-optical system, or by means of careful lavage.

From the point of view of the apparatus, therefore, the whole method has been reduced to the use of these two filters, the blue exciter filter Zeiss 500 in the light source and the yellow suppression filter Zeiss 520 on the optical eyepiece. Since the UV light source and the quartz fiber light carrier are dispensed with, one can no longer speak of UV bronchoscopy. The method is one of fluorescence bronchoscopy.

Experiments. The experiments carried out with this equipment have shown that the bronchial tree is excellently illuminated, even with right-angle or retrograde viewing, and that the energy of the inducing light is very great and gives rise to a very considerable degree of fluorescence, even of the smallest particles. After numerous experiments, the author has reached the conclusion that the inhalation of fluorescein in this procedure must be done one or two hours before the bronchoscopy is carried out, since even after four hours nonciliar areas can still fluoresce.

Practical Procedure. The new procedure is carried out as follows. On arrival for ambulant bronchoscopy, or at least one or preferably two hours before the treatment, the patient inhales 5 ml of a sterile aqueous 5% fluorescein solution together with a β_2 stimulator, by means of a pressure inhaler. A nose clip during inhalation prevents a wrong breathing technique, and yellow coloration of the tongue and lips indicates correct absorption of the fluorescein. The patient is encouraged to cough vigorously and to expectorate following the inhalation to support the automatic cleansing of the surfaces. The bronchoscopy is first carried out in accordance with the usual routine. Any yellow stained secretions that may be present do not interfere with the examination in any way.

TABLE 1. FINAL DIAGNOSES OF FIRST 100 CASES

Diagnosis		*No.*
Central carcinoma cases		27
Peripheral carcinoma cases, not visible by endoscope or fiber bronchoscope		24
Operated cases examined by bronchoscope to check area of resection	5	
Lung metastases associated with primary tumors located elsewhere		7
Other diagnoses including lung disorders where bronchoscopy used to clarify diagnosis		42

For the bronchoscope, one of the usual light sources is used, and for the optics, a new modified Storz light source is used, which already has a built-in dark blue exciter filter Zeiss 500. As well as these, the filter revolver contains two further light blue filters (Schott BG 23) of different density, which according to earlier work have been found to make it possible to increase the contrast between yellow tones and red tones (eg, with tubercles).

When the routine examination is finished, the bronchoscope illumination is switched off and the bronchial tree is viewed with the optical system in the blue exciter light. One immediately sees the fluorescing areas as well as the blue image of the bronchial tree. Under some circumstances, it may be difficult to decide whether what one sees is a secretion permanently located on the parietal surfaces, or a true fluorescence of the mucous membrane. Delicate laminated reticular and punctiform fluorescence mostly indicates true parietal fluorescence; where intensive fluorescence occurs in longitudinal strips, it is likely to be a matter of an adherent secretion. Careful, directed withdrawal by suction, which must not initiate any bleeding, or even lavage, will usually permit differentiation. All bleeding must be avoided since the maximum light absorption of hemoglobin lies exactly in the wavelength of the induced fluorescent light, and blood will therefore completely extinguish all fluorescence. For definitive verification of the situation, the yellow suppression filter Zeiss 520 is placed on the eyepiece. If a fluorescent area is seen on the parietal surface, both filters are taken off so that the area can be observed in normal light. In this way, it is easy to decide whether the area concerned appears macroscopically inconspicuous or perhaps does show certain changes. In any case, this area in the mucous membrane can be submitted to a visually directed biopsy by means of the optical system.

TABLE 2. FLUORESCENCE WITH CENTRAL TUMORS (27 CASES WITH 35 BIOPSIES)

Tumor fluorescence		21*	6†(4 due to blood)
Proximal fluorescence		7	20
Biopsies carried out		7	1
Normal mucous membrane	2		1
Metaplasias	3		
Tumor infiltrations	2		

*Positive fluorescence.
†Negative fluorescence.

TABLE 3. FLUORESCENCE WITH PERIPHERAL TUMORS (24 CASES, 19 BIOPSIES)

Fluorescence	14*	10†
Biopsies carried out	14	5
Normal mucous membrane	6	5
Metaplasias	3	
Tumor infiltrations	5	

*Positive fluorescence.
†Negative fluorescence.

CASE STUDIES

The first 100 cases (35 with the UV light source, 65 with the new procedure), examined successively without special selection but excluding the test experiments, are illustrated in Table 1. Of these cases, 15 were contributed by the ENT Clinic of the Cantonal Hospital of St. Gallen, and the remaining 85 by the City Hospital of Triemli.

RESULTS

The following have shown positive fluorescence: neoplasms, metasplastic changes in the mucous membrane or massive accumulations of mucous cells in the mucous membrane. Unchanged epithelium, or epithelium which is histologically changed only by inflammation, does not usually show fluorescence. Tables 2-5 give a numerical breakdown of the results.

FLUORESCENCE

With Visible Tumors. Of the 27 visible tumors, 21 showed a positive fluorescence (Table 2). Two showed no fluorescence in spite of having appeared strongly and unmistakably to be malignant changes in macroscopic examination. With four of the tumors, spitting of blood had been evident even at the first examination, so that the tumor was covered by blood. For this reason, any fluorescence was extinguished and could not be registered. Proximal to these tumors, in the macroscopically unchanged epithelium, there were seven additional fluorescing areas. These indicated three metaplastically changed areas and two tumor infiltrations. In the whole of this group, there were thus 26 correct positive and 2 false positive results as well as 2 (+ 4) false negative results.

With Peripheral Tumors. In the 24 cases with peripheral tumors which could not be seen even with the fiber bronchoscope, there were 14 fluorescing areas in the mucous membrane which were macroscopically inconspicuous. Of these, 8 were correct positives (3 metaplasias and 5 tumor infiltrations). This group contained the largest number of false positive results (6), ie, in six cases, a layer of fluorescing secretion was incorrectly interpreted as true parietal fluorescence. For the patients, however, this was no negative conclusion, inasmuch as by means of the directed biopsy of these areas of mucous membrane it was possible to rule out serious disease.

TABLE 4. FLUORESCENCE WITH METASTASES (7 CASES, 5 BIOPSIES)

Fluorescence	3*	4†
Biopsies carried out	3	2
Normal mucous membrane	1	2
Metaplasias	1	
Tumor infiltration	1§	

*Positive fluorescence.
†Negative fluorescence.
§Breakthrough.

TABLE 5. FLUORESCENCE WITH REMAINING BRONCHOPULMONARY DISORDERS (42 CASES, 35 BIOPSIES)

Fluorescence	7*	35†
Biopsies carried out	7	28
Normal mucous membrane	4	27
Metaplasias	3	1
Tumor infiltrations	0	

*Positive fluorescence.
†Negative fluorescence.

With Metastases. In the seven cases with lung metastases associated with foreign tumors, only three fluorescing areas were found. One of these had already been recognized macroscopically as malignant, being a tumor breakthrough of a lymph node metastasis in the central bronchial tree. Together with the fluorescing metaplasia, there were therefore two results which were correct positives and one which was false positive.

With Remaining Bronchopulmonary Disorders. Among the 42 noncarcinomatous cases examined, 7 mucous membrane areas showed fluorescence; 3 metaplasias are to be assessed as correct positive results and 4 normal mucous membrane areas as false positives. Of the 35 nonfluorescing areas, the mucous membrane was found in 27 of 28 routine biopsies to be normal or only affected by inflammation, and only once did the biopsy show a metaplasia. This last case must be added to the false negative cases of the carcinomatous group.

SUMMARY

In the 100 examinations, there were altogether 52 fluorescing mucous membrane areas of tumors (Table 6). In 28 cases, a tumor was already macro-

TABLE 6. RESULTS OF FLUORESCENCE STUDIES (N = 100)

	No. of Cases	*No. of Areas*
Diagnoses		
Tumor cases	58	
Other bronchopulmonary disorders	42	
Fluorescence		
Positive	52*	
Negative	75*	
Verification of biopsy		
Correct positive		39
Correct negative		35
False positive		13
False negative		3 (+ 4)
Neoplastic infiltration discovered by fluorescence only	7	

*Visible tumors counted twice.

scopically visible (27 central tumors and one central lymph node breakthrough in a lung metastasis). There were 22 tumors which fluoresced. Together with the 10 fluorescing metaplasias or accumulation of mucous glands and 7 tumor infiltrations which were not macroscopically recognizable, 39 correct positive fluorescences were therefore observed. Thirty-six routine biopsies were taken from the 69 nonfluorescing, macroscopically unchanged mucous membrane areas central to a tumor and areas where no tumor could be seen. In 35 of these biopsies, the mucous membrane proved to be histologically normal or affected only in inflammation, and only once was a metaplasia found which had not fluoresced. In this series of examinations, therefore, 35 gave correct negative results. Altogether, 13 mucous membrane areas which were normal or only affected by inflammation showed fluorescence, ie, a deposited fluorescing mucus layer was interpreted as true parietal fluorescence. These are the false positive results. The two nonfluorescing tumors, the nonfluorescing metaplasia and the four tumors covered by blood are to be counted with the false negative results. They are in the minority. On the other hand, it is to be noted that a tumor infiltration of a macroscopically unchanged mucous membrane was on seven occasions only discovered by the fluorescence.

ACKNOWLEDGMENT — We offer our sincere thanks to Dr. med. H. H. Wespi, Superintendent of the Ear, Nose and Throat Clinic and Facial Surgery Section of the Cantonal Hospital of St. Gallen, for his cooperation.

REFERENCES

1. Hürzeler D. Ultraviolet-fluorescence bronchoscopy in early detection of bronchogenic carcinoma. Ann Otol Rhinol Laryngol 1978; 87:1-5.

≈

CASSELBERRY AWARD

AUDITORY BRAINSTEM RESPONSES AS INDICATORS OF HEARING AID PERFORMANCE

PAUL KILENY, PhD

EDMONTON, ALBERTA, CANADA

A procedure involving the utilization of auditory brainstem responses (ABR) to indicate effective amplification is reported. The procedure involves eliciting ABRs by clicks presented in sound field to the aided ear and the estimation of an aided ABR threshold. The method allows for the selection of the ear responding best to amplification in very young or uncooperative hearing-impaired patients. Case studies including electroacoustical analyses of the amplified click stimuli and aided ABRs are presented.

One of the important factors in the successful management of the hearing-impaired infant is the provision of effective amplification.[1] Due to increasingly widespread utilization of electrophysiological diagnostic methods, an accurate diagnosis of hearing loss is now possible at a very young age.[2-4] However, the initial selection of a suitable hearing aid for the severely and especially the profoundly hearing-impaired infant is still a fairly arbitrary procedure.[1] This report deals with the utilization of auditory brainstem responses (ABR) as indicators of effectiveness of amplification. While this procedure cannot replace ongoing evaluation and long-term behavioral observations it has the potential to provide a better starting point. Its applications would be mainly in hearing-impaired infants or developmentally delayed youngsters.

METHODS

Brainstem responses were recorded by a vertex to ipsilateral earlobe surface electrode configuration. The contralateral earlobe or the forehead served as ground. The impedance between any two electrodes was below 3,000Ω. The responses were preamplified (10^4), filtered with a bandpass of 150-3,000 Hz and averaged following 2,048 stimulus presentation by a Nicolet Ca-1000 averager or a Nicolet Med-80 minicomputer (Nicolet Instrument Corp., Madison, Wis.). The averaged time period was 20 ms. The responses obtained were displayed on the built-in oscilloscope for inspection and peak latency measurements, and plotted on paper with an X-Y recorder.

Clicks were obtained by delivering 100 μs duration rectangular pulses alternated in polarity to a TDH-39 earphone at a rate of 17/s. In some cases 500 Hz tone pips were also utilized to elicit unaided auditory brainstem responses. These originated from 500 Hz sine waves gated with rise and fall times of 4 ms (2 cycles) and no plateau. The tone pips were delivered at a constant polarity and were embedded in continuous high pass filtered white noise with a cutoff of 1,500 Hz as described elsewhere.[5] Stimulus intensities are expressed in dB HL and are based on averaged normal adult thresholds. Because of the characteristics of the specific hearing aids, the click signals were modified both in spectral frequency and temporal characteristics as illustrated in Figures 1 and 2. Figure 1 shows the click waveform generated by a TDH-39 earphone as measured in a 6 cm^3 coupler, as modified by a Phonic Ear® (H. C. Electronics, Inc., Mill Valley, Calif.) HC 880 aid and by a Maico-P311 postauricular aid. Figure 2 illustrates changes in the frequency spectrum of clicks when amplified by the above-mentioned hearing aids. Hearing aid output was measured in a 2 cm^3 coupler. The click stimuli were delivered to the respective hearing aids by the TDH-39 earphone positioned 5 cm from its input.

The infants and children presented in this report were tested asleep in a crib. When necessary, they were sedated with an intramuscular injection (0.05 cm^3/0.45 kg) consisting of 16.7 mg meperidine, 8.3 mg chlorpromazine and 8.3 mg promethazine per 1 cm^3 of solution.

After establishing unaided ABR thresholds, a hearing aid was placed in the patient's ear. In most cases custom-made earmolds were available at the time of testing. Click stimuli were delivered to the aided ear by a TDH-39 earphone suspended from an adjustable arm at a distance of 5 cm from the microphone of the hearing aid. Depending upon the necessity to mask, the contralateral ear was either left open or covered by an earphone. Whenever possible, aided thresholds were established, however the presence of aided responses elicited by 45 or 55 dB HL clicks in cases of severe or profound hearing loss were considered to be indicative of effective amplification.

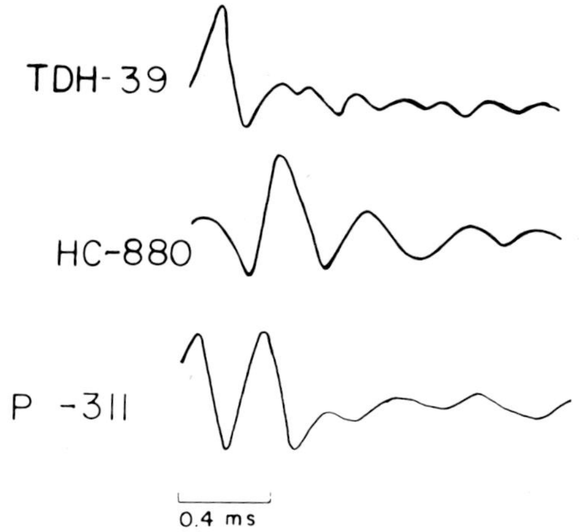

Fig. 1. Modifications of temporal characteristics of condensation clicks when delivered in sound field by a TDH-39 earphone to two different hearing aids. Top trace (TDH-39): 80 dB HL clicks measured in a 6 cm^3 coupler; middle and bottom traces (HC-880, P-311): 40 dB HL clicks delivered to the respective hearing aids measured in a 2 cm^3 coupler.

From the Department of Audiology, Glenrose Hospital, Edmonton, Alberta, Canada. This project was funded by a Glenrose Hospital Special Education and Research Grant.

REPRINTS — Paul Kileny, PhD, Department of Audiology, Glenrose Hospital, 10230-111 Avenue, Edmonton, Alberta T5G OB7, Canada.

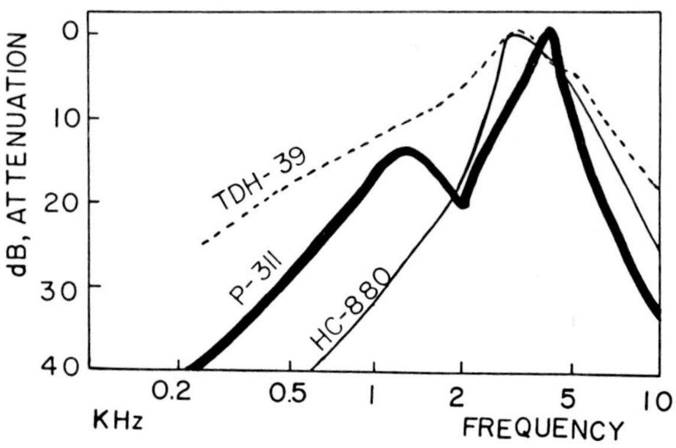

Fig. 2. Frequency spectrum envelopes of clicks generated by a TDH-39 earphone measured in a 6 cm³ coupler, and as modified by the two hearing aids presented in Figure 1, measured in a 2 cm³ coupler.

CASE REPORTS

The following case studies illustrate the applications of this procedure.

Case 1. This 18-month-old female, referred to the Glenrose Hospital Audiology Clinic, was born at term by an uncomplicated delivery. Pregnancy was complicated by hemorrhage occurring four weeks prior to delivery. At birth preauricular tags were observed and a concern for hearing impairment was expressed, however there were no further investigations. Ultimately, the parents expressed concern when at 18 months the infant was still nonverbal. In behavioral testing she was very inconsistent. Acoustic reflexes were absent bilaterally with adequate middle ear function. Figure 3 illustrates unaided and aided auditory brainstem responses to clicks. The aided responses displayed were obtained with a Phonic Ear HC 880 postauricular hearing aid. Unaided responses to 85 dB and 90 dB clicks respectively were questionable bilaterally. The difference between aided responses is evident: well-defined typical brainstem response patterns were obtained from the right ear, down to 30 dB HL. The aided responses obtained from the left ear were poorly defined and threshold was determined to be 50 dB HL with the variable gain control of the hearing aid set to maximum. As suggested by these results, the right ear was aided and this female has been making steady progress with her aural rehabilitation program. She has also been followed regularly with behavioral audiometry. The consistency of her behavioral responses has been improving steadily and both a confirmation and a possible explanation of the electrophysiological results have been gradually emerging. Her aided behavioral pure-tone thresholds in sound field average 30-35 dB HL. Although tympanograms were within normal limits bilaterally, the results of recent behavioral audiometry under earphones and with bone conduction suggest the presence of a mixed hearing loss in at least one ear (bone-conducted pure-tone average = 45 dB HL). As masking could not yet be used reliably with this now 2½-year-old female the bone-conducted thresholds obtained are a reflection of hearing in the better ear. Since the right ear responded so much better to amplification than the left, it is most probably the source of those unmasked bone-conduction thresholds. An otological consultation has failed so far to provide an explanation of the air-bone gap.

Case 2. This nonverbal male was first referred to the audiology clinic at five years of age, when he and his family moved to Edmonton from overseas. Hearing impairment was suspected to be the cause for his failure to develop speech; however, one or two attempts to assess his hearing in his hometown had failed to yield any information. The pure-tone thresholds obtained at our clinic indicated a moderate bilateral hearing impairment and he was fitted with a Maico P-311* postauricular hearing aid (Fig. 4). Following several months of intensive speech training and little progress, it was decided to verify his behavioral thresholds (aided and unaided) by brainstem audiometry. Aided and unaided ABRs for this patient's left ear are shown at the bottom of Figure 4. It is evident that the behavioral and electrophysiological thresholds are in close agreement.

Case 3. A moderate bilateral sensorineural hearing impairment was diagnosed at three years of age in this 5-year-old female. She was fitted monaurally with a Danavox 775 PP† postauricular aid shortly thereafter. Brainstem audiometry was initiated at this stage to verify unaided and aided thresholds prior to the initiation of binaural amplification. Unaided and aided ABRs are shown in Figure 5. Aided click thresholds were determined to be 20 dB HL. The effect of turning up the variable gain control by one division is also shown: it consisted of an increase in the amplitude of wave V with no significant change in its latency.

Case 4. This male presented at birth with several anomalies (multiple anomalies of the spine, dislocated hip, a midline cleft of the hard palate and asymmetric irises) diagnosed as Klippel-Feil syndrome. Since this syndrome may also be associated with hearing impairment ranging from mild conductive to profound sensorineural,[6] he was referred to audiology and assessed at six days of age. Brainstem audiometry indicated a moderate hearing loss in the left ear (unfiltered clicks and 500 Hz tone pip thresholds 60 dB HL) and a severe-to-profound hearing loss in the right ear (click thresholds 90 dB). Tympanograms were within acceptable normal limits bilaterally.[7] A decision was made to initially aid the left (better) ear, therefore aided brainstem responses were also elicited. Figure 6 illustrates unaided and aided responses to unfiltered clicks. The aided responses were obtained with a Phonic Ear HC 810 postauricular hearing aid. The results shown in Figure 6 suggest that the hearing aid is providing adequate amplification: aided click thresholds are in the normal range.

DISCUSSION

The utilization of auditory brainstem responses to determine effectiveness of amplification is a logical extension of the audiometric applications of this technique. The case studies presented here clearly

*Maico Hearing Instr., Inc, Minneapolis.

†Danavox, Inc, Minneapolis.

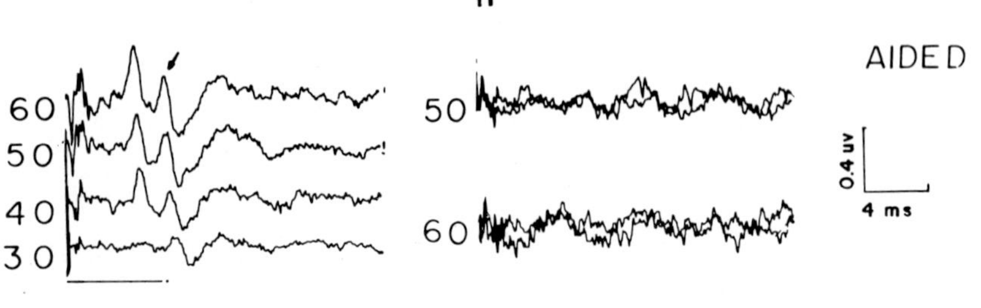

Fig. 3. (Case 1) Unaided and aided brainstem responses (clicks). In this and subsequent figures, click intensities in dB HL are listed on the left of the respective response trace. Right ear - Phonic ear HC 880, vol 6; left ear - Phonic ear HC 880, vol 9. The arrow indicates wave V.

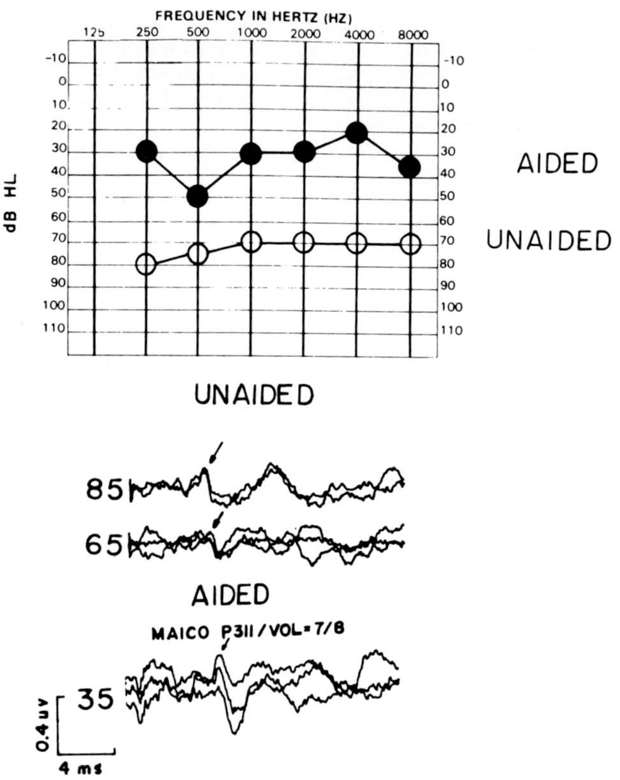

Fig. 4. (Case 2) Unaided and aided audiogram and brainstem responses. Arrows point to wave V.

demonstrate both the technical feasibility and the benefits of this procedure. The utilization of auditory brainstem responses to determine effectiveness of amplification has been recently considered to be problem-ridden.[8] A review of the earlier literature revealed one report which mentioned the use of the late cortical auditory evoked potentials to determine effectiveness of amplification in children.[9] While due to the limitations imposed by the nature of the late components of the auditory evoked re-

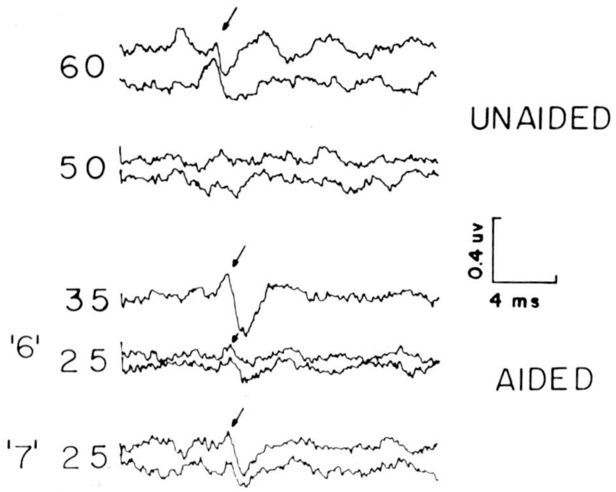

Fig. 5. (Case 3) Unaided and aided brainstem responses (clicks). The aided responses also illustrate the effect of turning up the variable gain control of the hearing aid by one arbitrary division ('6' to '7') with the stimulus intensity remaining constant (25 dB HL). Arrows point to wave V.

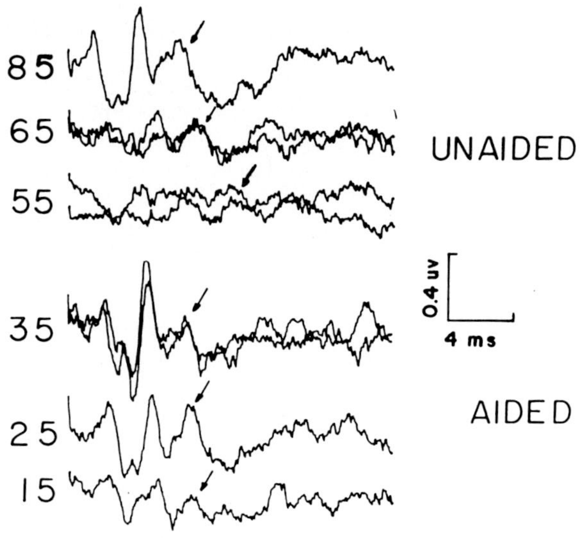

Fig. 6. (Case 4) Unaided and aided responses (clicks) from a 6-day-old male baby presenting with Klippel-Feil syndrome. Arrows point to wave V.

sponse (ie, dependency on stage of sleep and sensitivity to sedation) actual thresholds were not determined, improvements in aided vs unaided responses were clearly demonstrated by the authors, Rapin and Graziani.[9]

The advantages provided by measuring the early auditory brainstem responses (ie, low sensitivity to drugs[10] and close coincidence with behavioral thresholds) carry over to the measurement of aided responses. However there is one potential problem area associated with the aided ABRs: the contamination of recorded electrophysiological potentials by electromagnetic artifacts originating from prolonged "ringing" of the hearing aid by the transients utilized as stimuli. Clicks are brief enough and produce relatively little ringing (Fig. 1) to avoid this problem. When utilizing tone pips especially with powerful high gain aids, ringing lasting up to 20 ms was observed. Work is underway at present toward a solution of this problem.

Additional issues to be considered are changes in the frequency spectrum and temporal characteristics of the stimulus which may be introduced by specific hearing aids. Some examples are illustrated in Figures 1 and 2. Knowing the temporal modifications of the signal introduced by the hearing aid is relevant if one desires to measure the latencies of the aided responses, in order to specify an appropriate time reference. Knowing the modifications in the frequency spectrum of the stimulus will become more relevant with utilization of frequency-specific stimuli such as low frequency tone pips currently in use in brainstem audiometry.[5,8,11,12]

Since brainstem responses elicited by clicks reflect hearing sensitivity in the range of 2,000-4,000 Hz as a rule, this procedure provided information on the effects of amplification in that frequency range. Figure 5 illustrates among others the effect of turning up the variable gain control of the hearing aid (case 3) on the aided response. While wave V increased in amplitude, it failed to manifest the decrease in latency usually associated with an increase in click intensity. An increase in click intensity brings about an increase in the velocity of the traveling wave, the result being an activation of higher frequency basal regions. This fact and a decreased latency in synaptic transmission at higher stimulus intensities account for the inverse relationship between wave V latency and stimulus intensity.[13] The absence of this phenomenon in case 3 is probably due to hair cell damage in the basal high frequency region of the basilar membrane, which ruled out a response from this region.

The technique described in this communication has proved to be easy to use and successful with youngsters as long as the stimuli utilized were clicks, the patients remained motionless, preferably asleep, and provided that the earmolds were of good quality to avoid feedback. There are no more problems associated with this procedure than routinely encountered with brainstem audiometry. The four cases presented here are typical cases with some residual hearing where effectiveness of amplification could be demonstrated. They demonstrate that this procedure has the potential to assist in the early selection of suitable amplification and in predicting the feasibility of amplification.

ACKNOWLEDGMENTS — Many thanks to all staff audiologists at the Glenrose Hospital for their contributions and suggestions.

REFERENCES

1. Matkin ND. Hearing aids for children. In: Hodgson WR, Skinner PH, eds. Hearing aid assessment and use in audiologic habilitation. Baltimore: Williams and Wilkins, 1977:145-69.

2. Kileny P, Connelly C, Robertson C. Auditory brainstem responses in perinatal asphyxia. Int J Ped Otorhinolaryngol 1980; 2:147-59.

3. Mokotoff B, Schulman-Galambos D, Galambos R. Brainstem auditory evoked responses in children. Arch Otolaryngol 1977; 103:38-43.

4. Schulman-Galambos C, Galambos R. Brainstem auditory-evoked responses in premature infants. J Speech Hear Res 1975; 18:456-65.

5. Kileny P. The frequency specificity of tone pip evoked auditory brainstem responses. Ear and hearing (in press).

6. McLay K, Maran AGD. Deafness and the Klippel-Feil syndrome. J Laryngol Otol 1969; 83:175-84.

7. Keith RW. Middle ear function in neonates. Arch Otolaryngol 1975; 101:376-9.

8. Picton TW. The strategy of evoked potential audiometry. In: Gerber SE, Mencher GT, eds. Early diagnosis of hearing loss. New York: Grune and Stratton, 1978:279-307.

9. Rapin I, Graziani LJ. Auditory-evoked responses in normal, brain damaged and deaf infants. Neurology 1967; 17:881-94.

10. Goff WR, Allison T, Lyons W, Fisher TC, Conte R. Origin of short latency auditory evoked potentials in man. In: Desmedt JE, ed. Auditory evoked potentials in man. Psychopharmacology correlates of evoked potentials. Basel: S. Karger, 1977:30-44.

11. Davis H, Hirsch SK. The audiometric utility of brainstem responses to low-frequency sounds. Audiology 1976; 15:181-95.

12. Klein AJ, Teas DC. Acoustically dependent latency shifts of BSER (wave V) in man. J Acoust Soc Am 1978; 63:1887-95.

13. Picton TW, Woods DL, Baribeau-Braun J, Healey T. Evoked potential audiometry. J Otolaryngol 1977; 6:90-119.

Ann Otol 91:1982

MANAGEMENT OF PARANASAL SINUS SCHWANNOMAS

MARTIN A. SHUGAR, MD
HOLLYWOOD, FLORIDA
WILLIAM W. MONTGOMERY, MD EDWARD J. REARDON, MD
BOSTON, MASSACHUSETTS

Schwannomas arising in the nasal cavities and paranasal sinuses are rare entities, with only sporadic cases appearing in the world literature. The lesion most commonly arises in the ethmoid and maxillary sinuses, with two cases having been reported in the sphenoid sinus. There are no reported cases of frontal sinus schwannoma. Four illustrative cases are presented which demonstrate the clinical features. The radiological investigation should include plain films and anteroposterior and lateral polytomography. Computerized tomography appears to be useful in planning surgery. An operative approach is proposed which emphasizes a meticulous and complete removal of the lesion with preservation of adjacent structures and repair of any resultant dural defect.

INTRODUCTION

Schwannomas occurring in the head and neck are not uncommon with 25-35% of all reported schwannomas being found in this region.[1,2] By contrast, involvement of the nose and paranasal sinuses is quite rare, with only sporadic cases having been reported in the world literature.[2] Though the lesion is rare, schwannoma is still the most common of the peripheral nerve tumors occurring in the upper respiratory tract.[3]

Schwannomas are tumors of nerve sheath origin,[2] the lesion being derived from the Schwann cell surrounding neural tissue. In the nose and paranasal sinuses, these tumors arise from intranasal nerves, the ophthalmic and maxillary branches of the trigeminal nerve, and branches of the autonomic nervous system; the olfactory nerve is excluded from consideration as a site of origin as it contains no Schwann cells.[2] At the time of surgery, the nerve of origin is usually not identifiable.

Verocay described a nerve sheath tumor in 1908 which he believed was derived from the Schwann cell and possibly of ectodermal origin; in 1910, he termed the lesion a neurinoma.[4] In 1920, Antoni further elucidated the histopathology when he reported the two characteristic histologic forms: the palisading (compact stroma) type A pattern and the whorling (loose fiber) type B pattern[5] (Fig. 1A, B). Terplan and Rudofsky reported the first documented neurinoma involving the left nasal cavity and ethmoid sinuses in 1926.[6]

There are discrepancies in the reported prevalence of this lesion. This is undoubtedly due to confusion over terminology and the etiological classification of these tumors as evidenced by the variety of names used to refer to this lesion in the past. Though the terms neurinoma, neuroma, neurolemmoma, and neurilemmoma have all been used synonymously with schwannoma, the correct designation of this lesion based on histological and etymological criteria is schwannoma.[2,7] The terms neurinoma or neuroma, which are often used in connection with lesions of the internal auditory canal, are incorrect, as these lesions should by definition contain all elements of a nerve such as is found in a traumatic neuroma.[7] The precise and correct term is schwannoma.

Kragh et al reported 152 peripheral nerve tumors of the head and neck region at the Mayo Clinic; only 5 of these cases involved the nose and antrum.[8] A review of 176 cases of head and neck schwannomas occurring over a 10-year period at the Massachusetts Eye and Ear Infirmary and Massachusetts General Hospital revealed 148 internal auditory canal lesions. Twenty-eight other cases arose from other nerves in the jugular foramen, gasserian ganglion area, parasellar region, retrobulbar space, facial canal, parapharyngeal space, pterygomaxillary space, nasal fossa, oral cavity, forehead and mandible.[9] In 1972, Iwamura et al reviewed the world literature and found 45 cases of schwannomas of the nasal fossa and paranasal sinuses, with 7 occurring in the nasal cavity, 5 in the maxillary sinus, and 33 in the nose and ethmoid sinuses.[10] Robitaille et al critically reviewed the literature in 1975 and felt that only 13 of those cases could be substantiated as schwannoma based on available data.[11] Only one of their cases was associated with von Recklinghausen's disease. To date, there have been only two reported cases of sphenoid sinus schwannoma while none have been described in the frontal sinuses.[12]

Schwannomas are most often slow growing benign tumors; however, malignant variance does oc-

From the Department of Otolaryngology, Harvard Medical School and the Massachusetts Eye and Ear Infirmary, Boston.
Presented before the Massachusetts Eye and Ear Infirmary Alumni Association Meetings, June 12, 1980.
REPRINTS — William W. Montgomery, MD, Massachusetts Eye and Ear Infirmary, 243 Charles Street, Boston, MA 02114.

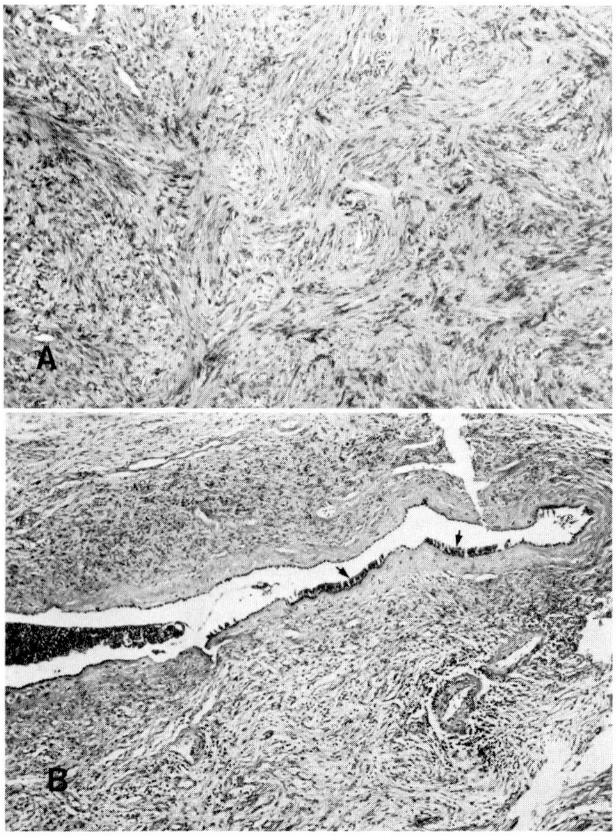

Fig. 1. A) Antoni type A pattern demonstrating palisading compact stroma. B) Antoni type B pattern. Note whorling loose fiber arrangement and respiratory epithelium (arrows). (H & E, x100)

cur. Ghosh et al reviewed 115 cases of malignant schwannoma.[13] Sixteen of these malignant tumors were found in the head and neck region with 30% being associated with von Recklinghausen's disease. The relationship with von Recklinghausen's disease carried a poor prognosis with a 5-year survival of 30% compared to an overall 5-year survival of 65.7%.

These tumors, whether benign or malignant, are radio-resistant with complete surgical resection being the prime mode of therapy.[11] The prognosis is excellent if the tumor is completely removed.[7,11]

Presented are four cases of schwannomas involving the paranasal sinuses which demonstrate the clinical features. The radiologic investigation and operative approach are discussed in detail.

CASE REPORTS

Case 1. A 16-year-old female complained of left nasal obstruction following an automobile accident eight years previously with progressive obstruction for three months prior to admission. Two years prior to admission the patient began to experience intermittent facial pain in the left molar and periorbital regions which had also increased in frequency and severity. There was no history of visual loss, diplopia, dental pain, facial paresthesias or epistaxis. Physical examination revealed a smooth mass in the left upper nasal vault and ethmoid areas.

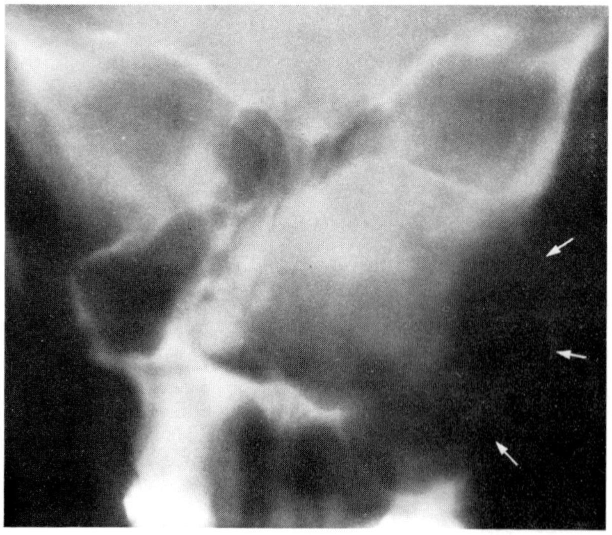

Fig. 2. (Case 1) Coronal polytomography showing large lesion involving the left maxillary sinus, extending into the left ethmoid sinus and nasal cavity. Note the eggshell thinning with no bony destruction (arrows).

Initial evaluation by a referring otolaryngologist included sinus plain films which showed a 6 cm diameter mass involving the left ethmoid and maxillary regions, displacing bone. This lesion was thought to be slowly expansile rather than a bony destructive process. Biopsy of the nasal mass by the referring physician revealed probable plexiform neurofibroma. Following polytomography of the sinuses (Fig. 2), the lesion was excised through a left Caldwell-Luc approach with a Denker extension and a left lateral rhinotomy/external ethmoidectomy. A soft yellow mass filled the entire left maxillary sinus and extended into the left nasal cavity, ethmoid sinus and pterygomaxillary fossa. The postoperative course was uncomplicated. There was no recurrence at three years. Final histological diagnosis was schwannoma of the left maxillary sinus.

Case 2. A 40-year-old female complained of progressive right

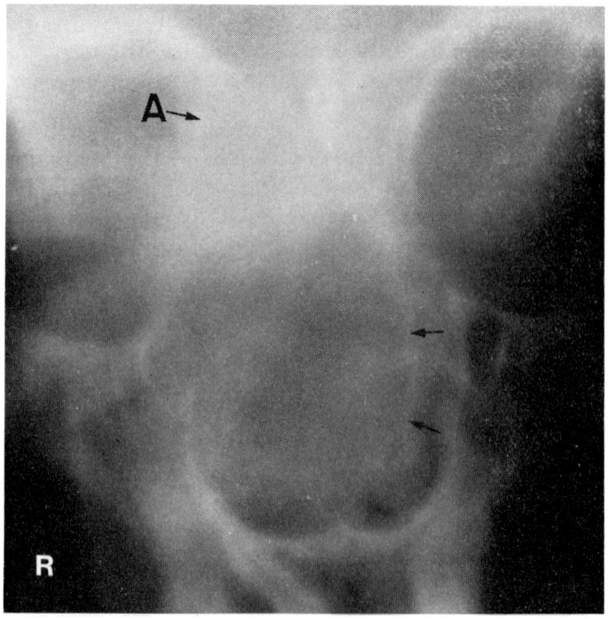

Fig. 3. (Case 2) Coronal polytomography demonstrating mass in right nasal cavity. Note the extreme displacement of nasal septum (arrows). A - Lamina papyracea.

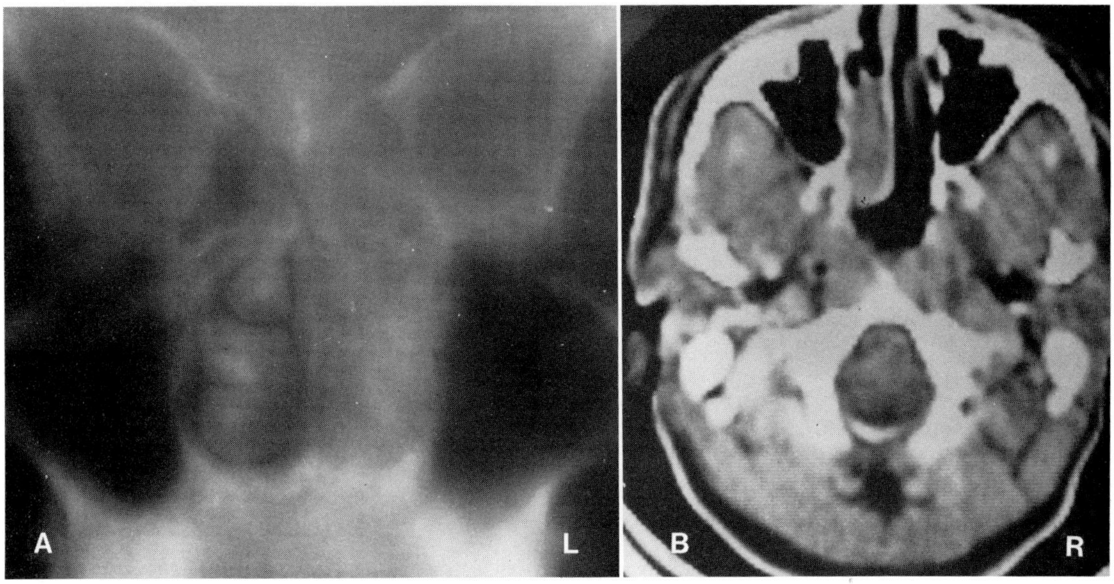

Fig. 4. (Case 3) A) Coronal polytomography showing lesion filling left nasal cavity with extension into ethmoid sinus. B) Axial CT scan demonstrating lesion in left posterior nasal cavity.

nasal obstruction with clear rhinorrhea, associated with right inner canthus and nasal labial fold swelling for nine months. She denied facial pain or paresthesia, visual loss, or epistaxis. Physical examination revealed expansion of the right inner canthus and nasal labial fold regions. Intranasal examination revealed a hard, rubbery, smooth, polypoid mass causing expansion of the right nasal cavity with protrusion into the right choana. There were no neurological deficits. Following plain films and polytomography of the sinuses (Fig. 3), the lesion was excised through a right lateral rhinotomy/external ethmoidectomy approach. A large (10 x 10 x 5 cm) tumor arose from the roof of the right ethmoid labyrinth and completely filled the right nasal cavity displacing the septum to the left. The maxillary and sphenoid sinuses were free of the tumor. The postoperative course was uneventful. The patient was symptom-free with good cosmesis and no recurrence at four years. Final histological diagnosis was schwannoma, right ethmoid sinus.

Case 3. A 41-year-old male complained of progressive left nasal obstruction of 2 years' duration. He denied facial pain or paresthesias, visual loss, diplopia or epistaxis. There was no history of trauma or sinusitis. Physical examination revealed a rubbery, grey-white mass filling almost the entire posterior left nasal cavity arising from the roof, and protruding into the left choana.

Following plain films, polytomography and computerized tomography of the sinuses (Fig. 4A, B), a biopsy of the left posterior nasal cavity was performed and revealed schwannoma. The tumor was excised through a left lateral rhinotomy approach with external ethmoidectomy. The lesion measured approximately 2.5 cm in diameter arising low in the ethmoid complex, and filled the posterior left nasal cavity and posterior ethmoid cells. The front wall of the sphenoid sinus was eroded with some extension of tumor into it.

The postoperative course was uneventful and there was no recurrence at 18 months. Final histological diagnosis was schwannoma, left ethmoid sinus (Fig. 1A, B).

Case 4. A 36-year-old female reported gradually increasing right nasal obstruction over a 3-year period. She denied facial pain, fever, visual symptoms or paresthesias.

Initial examination revealed a large polypoid mass filling the right nasal cavity, originating high in the vault and extending posteriorly. There was crusting of the lesion with slight purulent debris suggestive of a low grade secondary infection. She was treated with an appropriate antibiotic and was reexamined two weeks later at which time it was noted that the infection had subsided; however, the mass was unchanged in size. The antibiotics were discontinued but a few days later there was an abrupt onset of right eyelid swelling and discoloration. It appeared that the superinfection had recurred and that the lid swelling was secondary to ethmoid sinus obstruction by the lesion. Antibiotics were therefore reinstituted and thereafter there was rapid resolution of the lid-swelling and infection but the mass remained unchanged in size.

Routine sinus films, polytomography and computerized axial tomography revealed a lesion high in the nasal vault impinging onto the cribriform plate (Fig. 5A, B). There was no bony destruction or intracranial extension.

Biopsy of the right nasal mass was performed as an outpatient procedure by the referring physician. The lesion was noted to arise high in the nasal vault in the area of the cribriform plate and to extend laterally into the ethmoid cells. Excisional biopsy was performed by means of a snare technique to achieve a tissue diagnosis, promote drainage and to improve the airway.

The histological diagnosis was schwannoma. The patient did well thereafter and in follow-up there was no mass noted in the right nasal cavity, although a remnant of the lesion was noted to persist high in the nasal vault.

The definitive surgery was performed through a right lateral rhinotomy/external ethmoidectomy approach. The lesion measured 2.5 cm in diameter and arose high in the ethmoid labyrinth off the cribriform plate approximately 1 cm anterior to the sphenoid sinus (Fig. 6). The lesion had pushed the ethmoid cells laterally and was abutting the perpendicular plate of the ethmoid. The tumor was dissected off of the roof of the ethmoid labyrinth and was found to be attached by a stalk protruding through the dura at the junction of the middle turbinate and roof. Excision of this stalk left a small dural defect with a CSF leak. Frozen sections of a small portion of tissue which protruded through the dural defect revealed glial tissue. The dural defect was repaired with a lateral nasal wall mucosal flap, with no further leak noted.

The postoperative course was uneventful and there was no recurrence at 12 months. Final histological diagnosis was schwannoma, right ethmoid sinus.

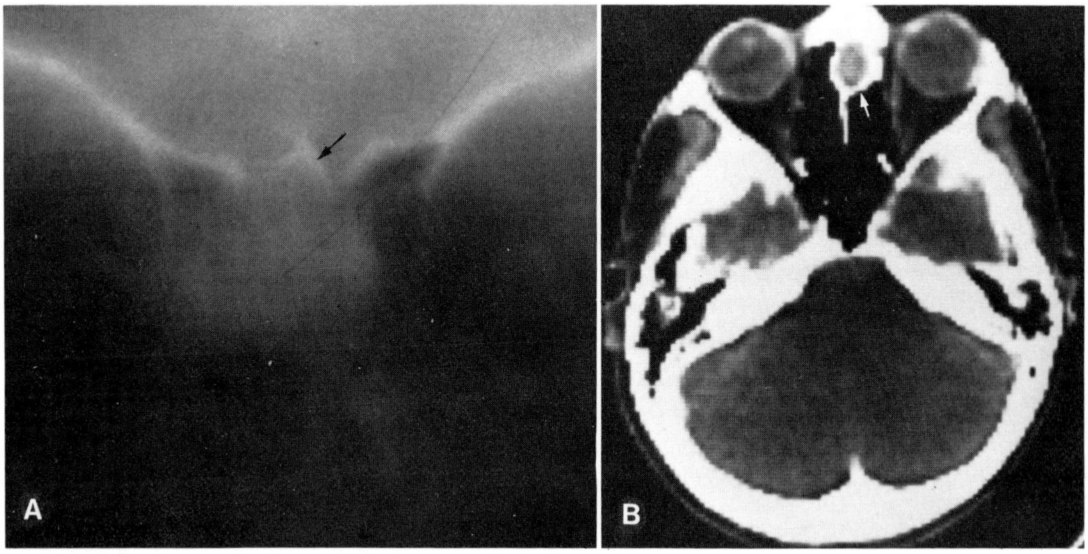

Fig. 5. (Case 4) A) Coronal polytomogram showing lesion high in nasal vault with impingement onto cribriform plate. Arrow - Crista galli. B) Axial CT scan showing lesion high in nasal vault (arrow).

DISCUSSION

Schwannomas of the paranasal sinuses are exceedingly rare and have no predilection for age, sex, or race.[12] These lesions are similar to other neurogenic tumors of the paranasal sinuses in producing varying signs and symptoms depending upon the involved anatomic site, nerve of origin and/or compression of adjacent nerves. Robitaille et al found that epistaxis was often associated with lesions of the ethmoid sinus and nasal fossae, while pain was more common with maxillary sinus tumors.[11] Epistaxis did not occur in the clinical presentation of any of our patients while nasal obstruction (9 months - 8 years) was the most common presenting complaint. Schwannomas of the sphenoid sinus may be associated with symptoms of diplopia (secondary to deficits of cranial nerves III, IV, VI) and deep retroorbital and/or occipital, frontal and bitemporal pain.[12] Symptoms of hypopituitarism may be evident if the lesion extends posteriorly to the hypophysis. Other common but less specific presenting signs and symptoms of paranasal sinus schwannomas are nasal airway obstruction, hyposmia, mucopurulent rhinorrhea, exophthalmos and facial swelling.

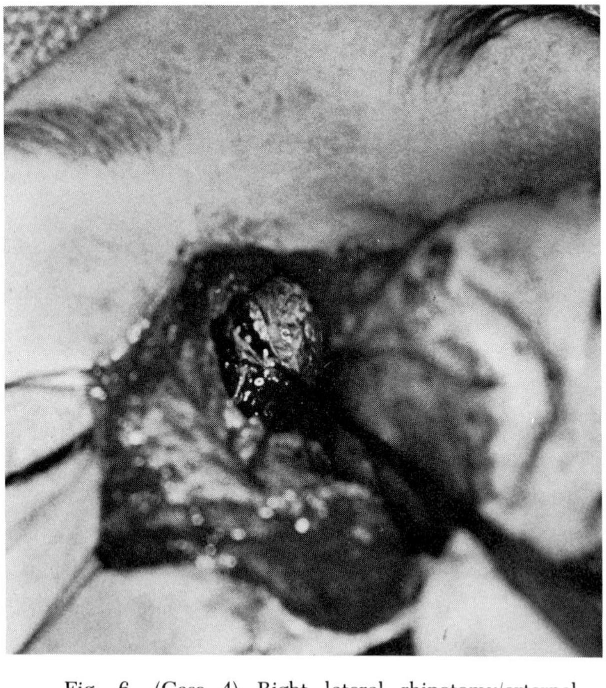

Fig. 6. (Case 4) Right lateral rhinotomy/external ethmoidectomy approach. Note lesion (tip of instrument) over cribriform plate region.

Nasal-ethmoid involvement by the lesion is most frequent, followed by maxillary sinus, intranasal and sphenoid sinus.[2] Our series showed a similar pattern with three nasal-ethmoid and one nasal-maxillary lesion. All of our patient's lesions were solitary tumors first presenting as a unilateral nasal mass. They were accordingly evaluated with the usual suspicion and caution. The tumor which presents as a nasal mass or polyp may clinically resemble an angiofibroma or fibrotic nasal polyp.[2,7] The lesion should also be differentiated from mucocele, ossifying fibroma, ameloblastoma, dentigerous cyst and other mesenchymal tumors.[9]

Schwannomas characteristically expand and thin the bony confines of cavities or foramina in the facial and paranasal sinus regions due to their slow growth.[9] These findings may be evident on plain films; however, laminography (A-P and lateral views) or computerized tomography are superior in delineating enlargement of these spaces.[9] Computerized tomography may reveal the soft tissue component of the lesion in regions where no air interface exists, such as the orbit, intracranial cavity, pterygomaxillary space and temporal fossa.[9] The demonstration of intracranial extension or proximity to the meninges by these techniques is most helpful in planning surgery, as removal of the tumor may result in a dural defect with CSF leak. Angiography is frequently performed to differentiate schwannoma from vascular lesions such as chemodectoma or meningioma which may clinically mimic them.[9] Enlargement of a vascular schwannoma may result in areas of cystic degeneration as the tumor outgrows its blood supply.

Schwannomas are occasionally richly vascularized and biopsy may therefore be complicated by severe bleeding in similarity to biopsy of an angiofibroma.[2,11] This complication did not occur in the three of our patients who were biopsied and the confirming histological diagnosis in two of them was helpful in planning surgery. Calcaterra et al contend that unless a vascular network consistent with angiofibroma is seen with angiography, a transnasal biopsy using biting forceps to obtain a small amount of tissue should be performed before definitive surgery.[12]

The definitive treatment of paranasal sinus schwannoma is complete surgical excision or, at least, decompression, due to the slow growth characteristic of this lesion. Radiotherapy should be reserved for palliation with malignant tumors or when surgery is impossible.[12] The operative approach should emphasize wide exposure with identification and preservation of adjacent structures. Lesions of the nasal fossa and ethmoid sinuses should be excised through a lateral rhinotomy/external ethmoidectomy approach with preservation of the infraorbital nerve and lacrimal apparatus. Maxillary sinus schwannomas may be approached through a Caldwell-Luc incision, with Denker extension if necessary. If the lesion is large or extends into the nose, ethmoid sinus or pterygomaxillary fossa, the addition of a lateral rhinotomy and/or external ethmoidectomy may prove helpful. Calcaterra et al believe that the nonmalignant sphenoid sinus schwannoma should be removed by an extracranial approach if possible, which offers less morbidity and wider exposure than the transcranial route.[12] They suggest a transantral approach with lateral eccentric extension for such lesions. They did not believe that base of skull erosion with mild-to-moderate extension into the middle cranial fossa was a contraindication to this approach. However, more extensive intracranial involvement necessitates an extradural craniotomy approach initially, followed by a transantral excision at the same sitting if the dura is not opened.[12] Here too, lateral rhinotomy and transethmoid modifications may be utilized depending upon tumor extent. When the tumor cannot be completely enucleated, decompression may be attempted and repeated if symptoms recur.

Excision of any ethmoid or sphenoid sinus schwannoma may result in a dural defect with a CSF leak. An increased index of suspicion of this complication occurring may be derived from the lesion's position as demonstrated by laminography and computerized tomography. If this complication is anticipated, fluorescein dye solution may be injected intrathecally preoperatively to facilitate detection of small dural defects created by tumor removal. A dural defect resulting from excision of a schwannoma should be repaired by the appropriate nasoseptal mucosal flap well described elsewhere.[14]

REFERENCES

1. Putney FJ, Moran JJ, Thomas GK. Neurogenic tumors of the head and neck. Laryngoscope 1964; 74:1037-59.

2. Batsakis JG. Tumors of the peripheral nervous system. 2nd ed. Baltimore: Williams and Wilkins 1979;313-33.

3. Ash JE, Beck MR, Wilkes JD. Atlas of tumor pathology, Section IV, fascicle 12. Tumors of the upper respiratory tract and ear. Washington, DC: Armed Forces Institute of Pathology, F-12-77-78, 1964.

4. Verocay J. Zur Kenntnis der "Neurofibrome." Beitr Pathol Anat Allg Pathol 1910; 48:1.

5. Antoni NRE. Über Ruckenmarkstumoren und Neurofibrome. München: JF Bergmann Verlag, 1920:413-23.

6. Terplan K, Rudofsky F. Über zwei neurogene Tumoren in der Nasen und Mundhohle. Z Hals-Nasen-Ohrenheilkd 1926; 14:260-8.

7. Kaufman SM, Conrad LP. Schwannoma presenting as a nasal polyp. Laryngoscope 1976; 86:595-7.

8. Kragh LV, Soule EH, Masson JK. Benign and malignant neurilemmomas of the head and neck. Surg Gynecol Obstet 1960; 3:211.

9. Weber AL, Montgomery WW. Neurolemmoma of maxillary antrum. Ann Otol Rhinol Laryngol 1978; 87:436-7.

10. Iwamura S, Sugiura S, Nomura Y. Schwannoma of the nasal cavity. Arch Otolaryngol 1972; 96:176-7.

11. Robitaille Y, Seemayer TA, Deiry AE. Peripheral nerve tumors involving paranasal sinuses: a case report and review of the literature. Cancer 1975; 35:1254-8.

12. Calcaterra TC, Rich R, Ward PW. Neurilemmoma of the sphenoid sinus. Arch Otolaryngol 1974; 100:383-5.

13. Ghosh BC, Ghosh L, Huvos AG, Fortner JG. Malignant schwannoma, a clinicopathologic study. Cancer 1973; 31:184-90.

14. Montgomery WW. Surgery of the upper respiratory system. 2nd ed. Philadelphia: Lea & Febiger, 1979; 1:175-208.

HUMORAL AND CELL-MEDIATED IMMUNITY IN PERIPHERAL BLOOD FOLLOWING INTRODUCTION OF ANTIGEN INTO THE MIDDLE EAR

ALLEN F. RYAN, PhD
M. TERRY HARTMAN, BA
PATRICK H. CLEVELAND, PhD
ANTONINO CATANZARO, MD

SAN DIEGO, CALIFORNIA

Serum levels of specific IgG and the sensitization of peripheral blood T-lymphocytes were measured in guinea pigs after single-dose antigenic sensitization by two routes: intratympanic and intradermal injection. Keyhole limpet hemocyanin (KLH) served as the antigen. Intratympanic injection of antigen resulted in much lower levels of circulating anti-KLH IgG than intradermal injection. When KLH was conjugated with alum to produce nonspecific inflammation and serve as an adjuvant, the intratympanic route was considerably enhanced, but remained much less effective than the intradermal route. Development of an IgG response was also somewhat less rapid following intratympanic than following intradermal administration. Marked sensitization of circulating T-lymphocytes was seen after intradermal injection of alum-precipitated KLH. A much weaker, though still positive, response was seen after intradermal injection of KLH alone and with the intratympanic injection of alum-precipitated KLH. No T-lymphocyte sensitization could be detected after intratympanic injection of KLH alone. It was concluded that the afferent limb of both humoral (IgG) and cell-mediated immunity was operative in the middle ear. Therefore, the middle ear does not represent an immunologically "privileged" site. On the other hand, the afferent limb from the middle ear appears to operate less effectively and rapidly than that from the dermis. This observation is consistent with observations in other mucosal systems.

INTRODUCTION

Immune responses in the middle ear (ME) are recognized to be an important factor in host defences against infection at this site.[1-3] Deficiencies in immune response have been postulated as contributing to the susceptibility of ME to infection early in life.[4,5] It has also been hypothesized that immune responses are a factor in the pathogenesis of such diseases of the ME as serous otitis media[6,7] and tympanosclerosis.[8]

Our understanding of the role of immunity in ME disease is hampered by the paucity of information available concerning immune responses at this site. Kastenbauer[9] found that previous sensitization of animal subjects with a skin graft enhanced the later rejection of incus homografts from the ME. Stewart and Helsop[10] detected specific, circulating antibodies after injection of allogeneic lymphocytes in the ME of animal subjects. Both of these studies demonstrate the existence of immune response to antigens placed in the ME. However, neither attempted to quantify immune responses or document their kinetics. The contributions of humoral versus cell-mediated immunity to ME immune responses are also unexplored.

As part of a series of experiments to characterize immunity at this site, we have assessed the systemic immune response to neoantigenic stimulation on the ME. Both humoral and cell-mediated responses were explored.

METHODS

Forty-five Hartley guinea pigs (200-400 g) served as subjects. The absence of ME pathology was assured by otoscopic observation and the presence of a normal Preyer reflex.

Keyhole Limpet Hemocyanin (KLH). KLH was purchased from Pacific Biomarine Supply Co., Venice, Calif, as an ammonium sulfate precipitate. The slurry was dialyzed extensively against phosphate-buffered saline (PBS) pH 7, then centrifuged at 4 C for 30 minutes at 1478 times gravity (XG). The supernatant was removed and recentrifuged at 37,000XG for 120 minutes. The precipitate was redissolved in PBS pH 6.4, filtered through 0.45 μ Millipore® filter, and stored at 4 C. KLH was found to be in the associated form on ultracentrifuge analysis. Associated KLH was used for immunization and in the lymphocyte transformation assay (1-10 μg/ml). The supernatant was unassociated KLH and was used as the antigen in the radioimmunoassay (RIA).

Alum precipitate was prepared using 10 mg KLH/ml. Ten percent $AlKSO_4$ was added dropwise to 1:2.5 by volume. Then 1N NaOH was added dropwise until pH 6.2 was reached. After incubation at room temperature for 30 minutes the suspension was centrifuged at 2300XG for 30 minutes, washed with cold saline twice, and resuspended in saline at 1 mg/0.1 ml.

Gamma Imaging. In order to document the fate of antigen introduced into the ME, associated KLH was labeled with ^{131}I. Lactoperoxidase was bound onto Sepharose® beads. Washed lactoperoxidase beads were added to 1 μCi ^{131}I, in the presence of 5 mg of associated KLH, $1x10^{-4}$M KI and $5x10^{-5}$M H_2O_2. The solution was rotated for 30 minutes at 21 C. Unreacted ^{131}I and beads were removed by passage through a P10 column (Pharmacia, Piscataway, NJ). Four guinea pigs were injected with labeled associated KLH and four subjects with labeled KLH as an alum precipitate. As controls, three guinea pigs were injected with a solution of $Na^{131}I$ in normal saline. Two animals were injected with $Na^{131}I$ solution postmortem. The distribution of the injected material was then monitored on a gamma camera for as long as activity exceeded background.

From the Division of Otolaryngology, Department of Surgery and the Pulmonary Division, Department of Medicine, University of California at San Diego Medical School. This study was supported by research grants from NIH-NINCDS 1, R01 NS-14389-01, and 5 K04 NS00176-01.

Presented in part before the Association for Research in Otolaryngology, St. Petersburg Beach, Florida, January 23, 1979.

REPRINTS — Allen F. Ryan, PhD, University of California Medical Center, San Diego, 225 West Dickinson Street, San Diego, CA 92103.

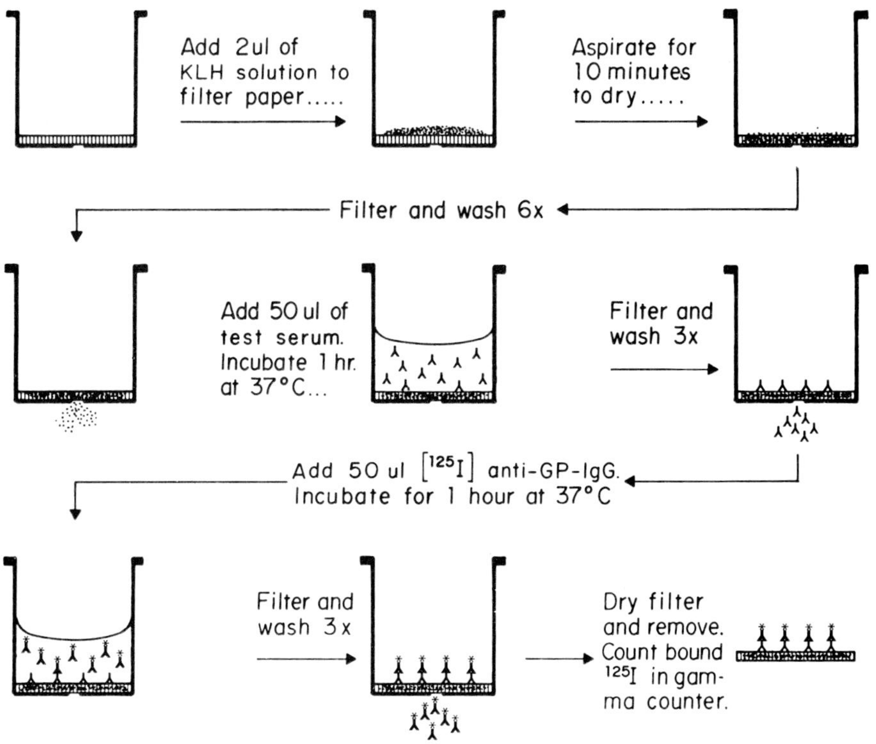

Fig. 1. Flow diagram of the immunofiltration technique employed in the RIA for anti-KLH IgG.

Experimental Plan. The remaining 32 subjects were divided into four equal groups. The first group was injected with 1000 μg of KLH intradermally (group ID). The second group received 1000 μg of KLH as an alum precipitate by intradermal injection (group IDA). The third group received 1000 μg of KLH by injection through the tympanic membrane (group IT), while the fourth group received 1000 μg of alum precipitated by KLH in intratympanic injection (group ITA).

At weekly intervals, beginning with the first week following administration of KLH, 3 ml of whole blood was centrifuged (1800 RPM, 7 minutes) to obtain plasma for immunoglobulin assay. Plasma was stored at −70 C. At the eighth week following KLH injection, 10-15 ml of whole blood was obtained and cells were harvested for a lymphocyte proliferation assay T-cell sensitization.

Anti-KLH Antibody Assay. Levels of anti-KLH IgG in plasma samples were measured using an immunofiltration technique described in detail by Cleveland et al[11]* using a 96-well filter manifold† in a solid-phase RIA. The assay is described schematically in Figure 1. Briefly, unassociated KLH (25 μg in 2 μl) was dried on each filter disc by 10 minutes of vacuum aspiration, which was found to bind 63% (±1%) of the KLH to the filter paper round. The filters were then rehydrated and washed six times with 300 μl of 0.3% gelatin, 0.01M PBS, pH 7.4 (gel buffer). Fifty microliters of control or immune serum diluted in gel buffer containing 1% bovine serum albumin (BSA) and 10% fetal calf serum (FCS) were added to triplicate filters containing KLH, and to triplicate filters without KLH, and incubated for two hours at 37 C. The serum was aspirated and the filters washed three times. Of the previously bound KLH, 74% (±1%) remained on the filter. Fifty microliters of rabbit antiguinea pig IgG (Cappel), ^{125}I-labeled as described for KLH, was added to each filter and incubated for two hours at 37 C. The unbound ^{125}I antiglobulin was then aspirated and the filters washed three times. Of the bound KLH, 72% (±3%) remained on the filter. The filters were then gamma-counted to measure the amount of bound ^{125}I antiglobulin. Nonspecific binding activity, determined by the amount bound to filters without KLH, was subtracted from the activity of the corresponding filters with KLH to obtain KLH-specific counts. At least four dilutions of each serum were analyzed in triplicate to determine serum titers.

Blocking tests were conducted to further define the specificity of the assay. After drying KLH on filters as above, the filters were incubated for 90 minutes with 50 μl of rabbit anti-KLH (Cappel), rinsed three times and incubated with serum of a guinea pig known to have a high anti-KLH titer. Bound guinea pig anti-KLH IgG was then measured by our standard assay. A second blocking test to determine specificity for guinea pig immunoglobulin was conducted by inserting in the standard assay an incubation with 50 μl of unlabeled rabbit antiguinea pig IgG after the test serum incubation and before incubation with ^{125}I-labeled rabbit antiguinea pig IgG.

To convert counts per minute to micrograms per milliliter, the sensitivity of each batch of ^{125}I-labeled rabbit antiguinea pig IgG was measured. Unlabeled rabbit antiguinea pig IgG was dried on filter paper, washed six times with gel buffer and incubated for one hour with various concentrations of guinea pig IgG (Cappel). Fifty microliters of ^{125}I-labeled rabbit antiguinea pig IgG was then added and incubated for two hours, rinsed three times in gel buffer, dried by vacuum aspiration and counted. The sensitivity of the labeled rabbit antiguinea pig IgG varied from 5 to 19 ng/500 cpm. These data were then applied to convert serum titers to serum levels of anti-KLH IgG, using 500 cpm as the standard.

Immunoelectrophoresis and RIA against guinea pig IgG, IgM and IgA showed the Cappel rabbit antiguinea pig IgG to be highly specific to IgG, with a slight (2-5%) reactivity to IgA and no detectable reactivity to IgM.

Lymphocyte Transformation Assay. T-lymphocyte sensitization was measured using a lymphocyte transformation response in a microtiter assay. Six to ten milliliters of heparinized blood was allowed to separate by sedimentation. The buffy coat was decanted, and white blood cells collected by centrifugation (1000

*Cleveland PH, Rickman DD, Oxman MN, et al. A rapid and simplified radioimmunoassay for soluble and small particulate antigens using a filter manifold. J Anat Biochem 1981. Submitted for publication.

†V&P Enterprises, San Diego, Calif.

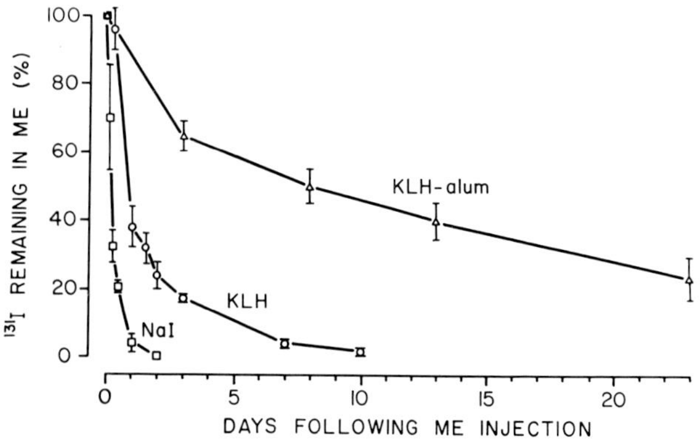

Fig. 2. Clearance of ^{131}I from the ME, after injection as NaI, conjugated to associated KLH, or conjugated to alum-precipitated KLH. Free iodide ions are removed quite rapidly, with most of the ^{131}I having been cleared by 24 hours after injection. When conjugated to associated KLH, ^{131}I cleared more slowly, with detectable activity still present in the ME 10 days after injection. ^{131}I conjugated to alum-precipitated KLH was still detectable in the ME 30 days after injection. All data points were obtained by gamma imaging the ME cavity. Each data point represents four subjects, except for the NaI points which represent three subjects. Vertical bars indicate one standard deviation about each mean.

RPM for 10 minutes) and washed in F10 culture medium.* Cell cultures in quadruplicate were normalized to 10^5 lymphocytes suspended in 50 μl of F10 medium enriched with 10% fetal calf serum; 0-50 μg/ml of KLH in 50 μl was added. Cultures were incubated in microtiter plates† at 37 C in a 10% CO_2 atmosphere for six days. Eighteen hours prior to termination, 4 μCi ^{3}H-labeled thymidine in 50 μl was added. Upon termination, cells were collected on filters in an M24 cell harvester§ and washed ten times with PBS. Beta scintillation counting of the harvested cells was quantitated on a Searle scintillation counter (Chicago, Ill). Counts per second were normalized by dividing counts from stimulated cultures by those from cultures which were incubated without KLH. The resultant ratio is discussed as the stimulation index.

RESULTS

Gamma Imaging of Antigen. As illustrated in Figure 2, when dissolved Na^{131}I was injected into the tympanic cavity, ^{131}I moved rapidly from the ME, with the great majority already having been cleared within 12 hours of injection. Cleared radioactivity appeared primarily in the gut. In subjects injected postmortem, little or no ^{131}I moved from the ME for up to 24 hours, demonstrating that this clearance is an active process.

^{131}I-labeled associated KLH left the ME at a much slower rate. However, within one week the majority of the activity had disappeared from the ME. As with Na^{131}I, cleared radioactivity appeared mostly in the gut.

Labeled alum-precipitated KLH showed far less movement over a four-week observation period. The activity which was lost could not be localized to any particular site and was presumed to have been excreted.

*Gibco, Grand Island, NY.

†Falcon, Oxnard, Calif.

§Biomedical Research Development Labs, Rockville, Md.

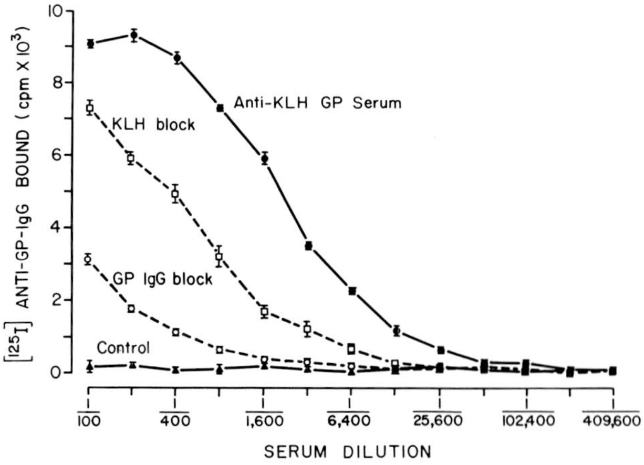

Fig. 3. Specificity of the RIA. ^{125}I-labeled rabbit antiguinea pig IgG bound to KLH after incubation with immune and control sera. All data are corrected for nonspecific activity. No KLH-specific activity is noted in control serum. Anti-KLH serum was obtained four weeks after immunization with KLH as an alum precipitate in the dermis and showed a high degree of anti-KLH activity. The KLH blocking curve was generated by incubating the KLH-filter paper with rabbit anti-KLH prior to incubation with the test serum. The guinea pig IgG blocking curve was generated by incubating the filter paper with unlabeled rabbit antiguinea pig IgG, after the test serum incubation but before incubation with ^{125}I-labeled rabbit antiguinea pig IgG. The blocking curves and control serum data indicate the specificity of the assay both for KLH and for guinea pig immunoglobulin.

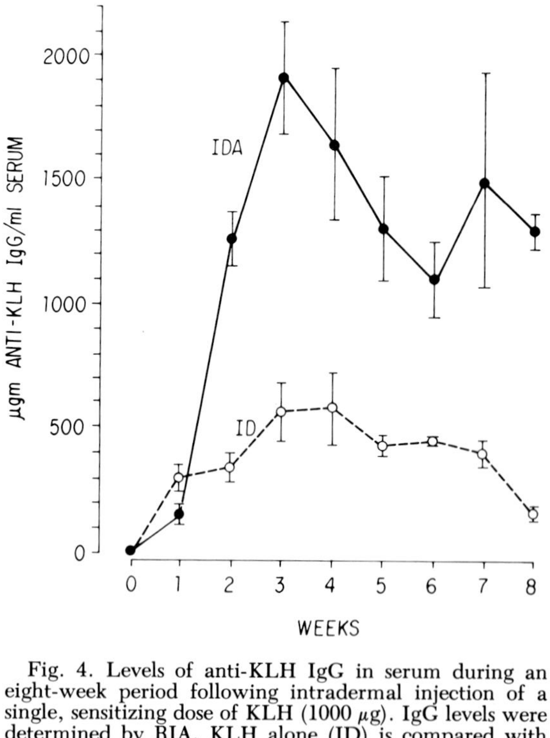

Fig. 4. Levels of anti-KLH IgG in serum during an eight-week period following intradermal injection of a single, sensitizing dose of KLH (1000 μg). IgG levels were determined by RIA. KLH alone (ID) is compared with alum-precipitated KLH (IDA). In this and in subsequent figures, each point represents the mean of observations from six subjects. Vertical bars represent one standard deviation of the corresponding mean. The serum samples from three subjects in group IDA were lost after week 6, which probably accounts for the sudden increase in mean value of serum KLH and in the standard deviation seen at week 7 in this group.

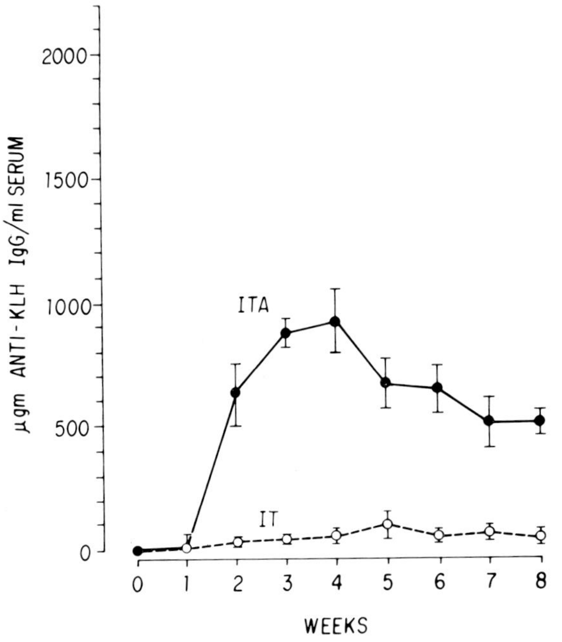

Fig. 5. Level of anti-KLH in serum during an eight-week period following intratympanic injection of the same dosage of KLH employed in the intradermal groups of Fig. 4. KLH alone (IT) is compared with alum-precipitated KLH (ITA). Note that the levels of anti-KLH IgG observed in serum after intratympanic injection of KLH are much lower than those observed after intradermal injection of the same antigen dose, especially in group IT. The response also develops more slowly, with no detectable antibody at one week in either intratympanic group.

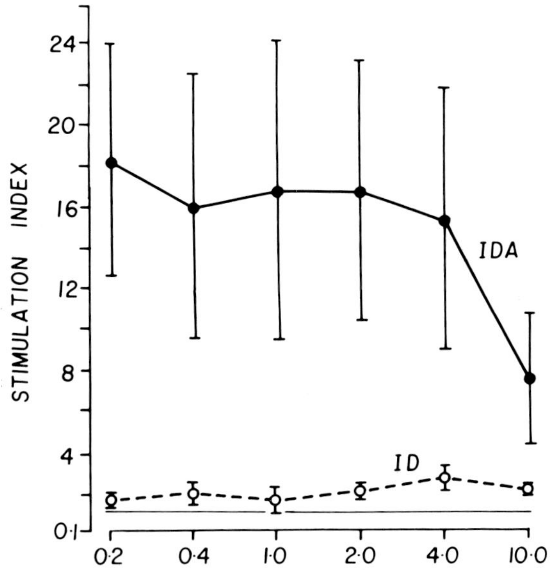

Fig. 6. Sensitization of peripheral blood T-lymphocytes measured eight weeks following intradermal sensitization with associated KLH alone (ID) and alum-precipitated KLH (IDA). T-cell sensitization was measured utilizing a microtiter lymphocyte transformation assay. Data are normalized as the ratio of ^{3}H-thymidine incorporation in stimulated and control cultures, so that a stimulation index of 1 signifies no response. The response is plotted against the stimulating dose of KLH used in each culture. Weak T-cell sensitization is observed in subjects which receive KLH alone. A powerful sensitization response was seen in subjects which received alum-precipitated KLH.

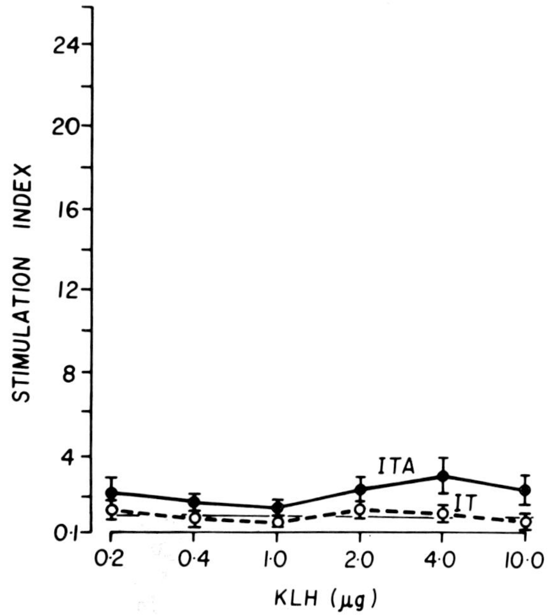

Fig. 7. Sensitization of peripheral blood T-lymphocytes measure eight weeks following intratympanic sensitization with aggregated KLH alone (ID) and alum-precipitated KLH (ITA). No T-cell sensitization was observed in the subjects which received KLH alone in the ME. Weak T-cell sensitization was observed after introduction of alum-precipitated KLH in the ME.

Specificity of the RIA. Nonspecific binding of IgG to the filter paper used in the immunofiltration assay was minimal and readily corrected by background subtraction. The specificity of the assay is illustrated in Figure 3. Normal guinea pig serum showed no specific activity against KLH. Serum from the immunized animal illustrated showed a high degree of anti-KLH activity, saturating the assay at a dilution of 1:400. The blocking curves demonstrate that it was possible to block the assay very effectively by covering either KLH sites or guinea pig IgG sites with specific antiserum.

Humoral Immune Response. The levels of anti-KLH measured in the sera of the intradermal groups of guinea pigs are illustrated in Figure 4. In prebleed samples obtained immediately before introduction of antigen, no detectable levels of anti-KLH antibody could be demonstrated. At one week postinjection, anti-KLH IgG at well above background levels was observed in group IDA. The concentrations rose rapidly between one and three weeks, reaching a peak of 1900 (± 450) g/ml of anti-KLH in group IDA, and 500 (± 270) μg/ml in group ID.

The humoral response observed in the subjects which received KLH by intratympanic injection is illustrated in Figure 5. No detectable anti-KLH IgG was measured in prebleed samples or at one week after antigen administration in either group. The concentration in serum rose rapidly between two and three weeks in group ITA, to a peak level of 900 (± 250) μg/ml, and gradually declining thereafter. Serum titers in group IT were detectable two weeks after injection but remained low throughout the eight-week period, never exceeding 50-100 μg/ml. There was no clear peak to the IgG response.

Cell-mediated Immune Response. Sensitization of T-cells to KLH was measured eight weeks postinjection. This interval is sufficient to allow development of cell-mediated immunity as demonstrated in other systems[12] and short enough to prevent missing a response by exceeding the half-life of the T-lymphocyte.[13] The results of the lymphocyte transformation assay in the intradermal groups is illustrated in Figure 6. A weak but positive ($p < 0.05$) transformation response was observed in group ID, indicating low-level sensitization of circulating T-lymphocytes. In contrast, a powerful response ($p << 0.01$) was seen in the subjects of group IDA. This indicates strong sensitization of circulating T-lymphocytes in this group to KLH.

The results of the transformation assay in the intratympanic groups is shown in Figure 7. No detectable response was observed in the subjects of group IT, which had received KLH alone in the ME, indicating a complete failure to sensitize circulating T-cells. In group ITA a weak but positive response ($p < 0.05$) was observed, similar to that seen in group ID.

To determine whether our failure to detect T-lymphocyte sensitization in group IT reflected an early or late development of sensitization, additional subjects were added to this group and sampled at intervals from 4 to 19 weeks postinjection. No lymphocyte transformation response was seen in any of these subjects.

DISCUSSION

Three major conclusions may be drawn from the results of this investigation. First, it is clear that both cell-mediated and humoral immune responses can be detected after introduction of antigen into the ME. That is, the ME is not an immunologically "privileged" site. Second, the immune responses detected in the circulation after ME sensitization are less vigorous than that seen after introduction of antigen into the dermis. Third, as with other sites, the use of an adjuvant markedly enhances immune response to antigen in the ME.

We have demonstrated both humoral and cell-mediated immune response after introduction of antigen into the ME. Therefore, the tympanic cavity cannot be regarded as an immunologically "privileged" site. This observation is in agreement with that of Stewart and Helsop.[10] They introduced allogeneic lymphocytes into the ME of animal subjects, and later observed specific, circulating antibodies utilizing a cytotoxicity assay. While demonstrating the existence of circulating antibodies after ME antigen introduction, Stewart and Helsop did not examine the kinetics of the response, nor did they identify the specific immunoglobulin which they detected.

Our data indicate that the nature of the immune response to antigen in the ME is different from that observed when exposure occurs via a parenteral route. This was not an entirely unexpected result, given the observations which have been reported from other mucosal systems. Repeated application of antigen to the oral mucosa of unsensitized animals has been shown to produce a relatively weak antibody response in serum.[14,15] Application of inactivated influenza virus to the nasal mucosa also resulted in very low serum titer.[16,17] On the other hand, application of formalin-activated *Pseudomonas aeruginosa* to the nasal mucosa produced serum antibody levels almost as high as in parenterally immunized animals.[18] This may reflect an enhancing effect of the potent bacterial inflammatory substances for which *Pseudomonas* is noted, and is consistent with our observations with alum-precipitated KLH.

Weak systemic immune response is not seen after application of antigen to all mucosae. Intratracheal application of killed influenza virus produced a brisk serum antibody response with maximum levels present within seven days.[17] Our data suggest that the ME mucosa responds in a manner more similar to oral and nasal mucosa than to tracheal mucosa.

The relatively weak IgG response and absence of T-cell response seen after ME administration of associated KLH may reflect the rapidity with which a single dosage of this antigen is cleared from the ME. However, antigen was present in the ME at detectable levels for at least one week following injection. Lim[19] has shown that horseradish peroxidase injected into the ME cavity is rapidly absorbed by the ME mucosa and can be found in draining lymph nodes within 30 minutes. During the week of antigen presence in the ME, apparently an insufficient quantity of associated KLH was absorbed by the mucosa and transported to draining lymph nodes to result in strong circulating immune responses. It can also be concluded that lymphocyte traffic into the ME and into contact with the antigen was insufficient in the absence of inflammation to allow detectable sensitization of calculating T-lymphocytes. Thus the accessibility of antigen introduced into the ME to the lymphocytes which determine circulating humoral and cell-mediated immune response is relatively poor when adjuvant is not present.

This situation is altered when KLH is conjugated to alum. The prolonged presence of KLH in the ME may contribute to enhanced immune responses. Alternatively, the inflammatory effects of alum, with increased vascularization and white blood cell traffic, could provide the enhancement. It seems likely that both factors play a role.

ACKNOWLEDGMENT — The authors wish to acknowledge the dedication and technical assistance of Sharon Batcher, James Marsh, Edda Roberts and Paul Goodwin, and Ruth Allen for preparation of the manuscript.

REFERENCES

1. Mogi G, Yoshida T, Honjo S, et al. Middle ear effusions — quantitative analysis of immunoglobulins. Ann Otol Rhinol Laryngol 1973; 82:196-202.

2. Bernstein JM, Tomasi TB, Ogra P. The immunochemistry of middle ear effusions. Arch Otolaryngol 1974; 99:320-6.

3. Mogi G, Maeda S, Yoshida T, et al. Immunochemistry of otitis media with effusion. J Infect Dis 1976; 133:125-36.

4. Sloyer JL, Howie VM, Ploussard JH, et al. Immune response to acute otitis media in children. I. Serotypes isolated and serum and middle ear fluid antibody in pneumococcal otitis media. Infect Immunol 1974; 9:1028-32.

5. Liu YS, Lim DJ, Lang RW, et al. Chronic middle ear effusions: immunochemical and bacteriological investigation. Arch Otolaryngol 1975; 101:278-86.

6. Hopp ES, Elevitch FR, Pumphrey RE, et al. Serous otitis media — an "immune" theory. Laryngoscope 1965; 74:1149-50.

7. Miglets A. The experimental production of allergic middle ear effusions. Laryngoscope 1973; 83:1355-85.

8. Schiff M, Poliquin JF, Catanzaro A, Ryan AF. Tympanosclerosis: a theory of pathogenesis. Ann Otol Rhinol Laryngol 1980; 89 Suppl 70.

9. Kastenbauer E. Tierexperimentelle Untersuchunger uber das immunologische Verhalten allogener Gehorknochelchen-Tranpantate. Arch Klin Exp Ohren Nasen Kehlkopfheilkunde 1972; 201:332-50.

10. Stewart IA, Heslop BF. The immunological status of allografts in the middle ear. Acta Otolaryngol (Stockh) 1979; 87:539-44.

11. Cleveland PH, Richman DD, Oxman MN, et al. Immobilization of viral antigens on filter paper for a ^{125}I staphylococcal protein A immunoassay: a rapid and sensitive technique for detection of herpes simplex virus antigens and antiviral antibodies. J Immunol Methods 1979; 29:369-86.

12. Curtis JE, Hersh EM, Harris JE, et al. The human primary immune response to keyhole limpet hemocyanin. Clin Exp Immunol 1970; 6:473-91.

13. Everett NB, Tyler RW. Lymphopoiesis in the thymus and other tissues. Int Rev Cytol 1967; 22:205-37.

14. Molinari JA, Ebersole JL, Platt D. Investigation of secretory immunoglobulins in saliva from germ free mice. Infect Immunol 1974; 10:1207-12.

15. Heremans JF. Peroral stimulation of IgA antibody formation in mice. In Dayton DH, ed. The secretory immunologic system. Bethesda: NICHD, 1969;309-24.

16. Waldman RH, Spencer CS, Johnson JE. Respiratory and systemic cellular and humoral immune responses to influenza virus vaccine administered parenterally or by nose drops. Cell Immunol 1972; 3:294-300.

17. Kasturi K, Hannoun C. Immune responses to influenza virus in rabbits after local immunizations. Ann Microbiol 1977; 128:97-117.

18. Reynolds HY. Pulmonary host defenses in rabbits after immunization with pseudomonas antigens. J Infect Dis 1974; 130:S134-S142.

19. Lim DJ. Functional morphology of the lining membrane of the middle ear and eustachian tube: an overview. Ann Otol Rhinol Laryngol 1974; Suppl 11:83:5-16.

GRANULOCYTE PROTEASES IN MIDDLE EAR EFFUSIONS

BRITT CARLSSON, MD
STOCKHOLM, SWEDEN

CHRISTER LUNDBERG, MD
STOCKHOLM, SWEDEN

KJELL OHLSSON, MD
MALMÖ, SWEDEN

Analyses of 20 middle ear effusions and plasma from 15 patients with serous otitis media demonstrated a marked local release of the granulocyte proteases, elastase, and collagenolytic neutral protease in the effusions. Furthermore, activation of C3 and complexes with antiplasmin were demonstrated. Complex formations between the granulocyte proteases and the protease inhibitors, α_1-antitrypsin, α_2-macroglobulin, and antileukoprotease were shown. A residual inhibitory capacity for α_1-antitrypsin and antileukoprotease was also demonstrated in the middle ear effusions.

INTRODUCTION

The presence of granulocytes in the middle ear effusions (MEE) of serous otitis media (SOM)[1,2] implies phagocytosis and hence an extracellular release of lysosomal enzymes.[3-5] If not inactivated, the proteolytic enzymes will cause tissue damage as well as activation of other enzyme systems, such as the complement[6,7] and fibrinolytic systems.[8] Sufficient amounts of protease inhibitors are therefore of importance for tissue protection and for regulating activation and inhibition of the enzyme systems involved in the inflammatory process. We have previously demonstrated[2] the main protease inhibitors of serum, α_1-antitrypsin, α_1-antichymotrypsin, and α_2-macroglobulin, as well as the low molecular weight protease inhibitor, antileukoprotease,[9] in MEE of SOM.

In the present work the middle ear specimens from our previous study[2] were further analyzed. The leukocyte proteases, elastase and collagenolytic neutral protease, were quantitated and the extent of complex formation between these proteases and their inhibitors studied. The primary inhibitor of plasmin, antiplasmin,[10] was assayed in order to determine whether the fibrinolytic system is engaged in SOM. Finally, the presence of C3 was determined and studied electrophoretically.

METHODS

Middle ear effusions were collected under general anesthesia by aspiration through a myringotomy in 20 ears of 15 patients with the diagnosis of SOM exceeding two months' duration and without signs of active ear infection.[2] High viscosity mucoid fluids that were nonpipettable were excluded from the study. The specimens were diluted 1:10 with 0.9% NaCl solution containing ethylenediaminetetraacetic acid (EDTA). Blood specimens from the same patients were collected simultaneously in 5 ml tubes containing EDTA. The diluted middle ear fluids and the blood specimens were centrifuged at 1000 g for five minutes and the supernatants recovered and stored at -18° C until studied.

Antisera. Specific antisera against granulocyte collagenolytic neutral protease and granulocyte elastase and antileukoprotease were prepared in our laboratory.[11-14] Rabbit antisera against α_1-antitrypsin, α_1-antichymotrypsin, α_2-macroglobulin and C3 are routinely produced in our laboratory. Rabbit antiserum against antiplasmin was provided by Collen.[10]

Protein Analyses. Quantitative assays of granulocyte collagenolytic protease and granulocyte elastase in MEE were performed with the single radial immunodiffusion technique of Mancini et al,[15] using 1 mm thick 1% (w/v) agarose gel containing 3% (w/v) polyethyleneglycol. Purified preparations of granulocyte collagenolytic protease[12] and granulocyte elastase[13] with known concentrations were used as standards. For reference purposes quantitative assays of granulocyte elastase in corresponding plasma specimens were studied with a radioimmunoassay technique developed in our laboratory.[16] This afforded a considerably higher sensitivity than the Mancini technique.

Quantitative analyses of C3 and antiplasmin in MEE and plasma were performed with electroimmunoassay as described by Laurell,[17] except the agarose gel was prepared with 0.8% (w/v) agarose. The agarose gel was prepared with 10% (w/v) Dextran for the analyses of antiplasmin. Analyses of MEE and paired plasma specimens were run in parallel. Pooled plasma from healthy blood donors was used as standard. For the analyses of C3, fresh plasma was used.

Changes in the electrophoretic homogeneity of C3 were studied with crossed immunoelectrophoresis according to Ganrot.[18]

Protease Inhibitor Complex Analyses. Protease inhibitor complexes containing α_1-antitrypsin, α_1-antichymotrypsin or antiplasmin were studied with crossed immunoelectrophoresis.[18] To help define the several α_1-antitrypsin components discovered, a modification of the crossed immunoelectrophoresis technique was used.[19] The residual inhibitory capacity of free α_1-antitrypsin in MEE was tested by incubating middle ear fluid with 3-10 μg of purified granulocyte elastase[13] for 15 minutes at room temperature prior to analyses by crossed immunoelectrophoresis.

Complexes of α_2-macroglobulin in MEE were studied by isoelectric focusing in a polyacrylamide gel followed by crossed immunoelectrophoresis with specific antiserum against α_2-macroglobulin, according to the method described by Ohlsson and Skude.[20]

From the Department of Otolaryngology, Södersjukhuset, Stockholm, and the Department of Surgery and Clinical Chemistry, Malmö General Hospital, Sweden. This investigation was supported by grants from the Swedish Medical Research Council (project no. B81-17X-03910-09C), the Swedish Association against Cancer (project no. 1300-B81-03XB), the University of Lund Medical Faculty, the Swedish National Association against Heart and Chest Diseases, the Swedish Association against Rheumatism, the Swedish Society of Medical Sciences, the Swedish Tobacco Company, the Foundation of Eir, the Foundation of King Gustav V, the Foundation of Greta and Johan Kock, the Foundation of Alfred Österlund, and the Foundation of Malmö General Hospital.

REPRINTS — Britt Carlsson, MD, Sturevägen 1, 182 74 Stocksund, Sweden.

TABLE 1. GRANULOCYTE PROTEASES IN MIDDLE EAR EFFUSION AND PLASMA

	MEE			Plasma			Ratio Mean Conc. MEE/mean Conc. Plasma
	No.	Range (g/ml)	Mean and SEM (g/ml)	No.	Range (g/ml)	Mean and SEM (g/ml)	
Granulocyte collagenolytic enzyme	20	37 - 307	120±16.5	NM	NM	NM	—
Granulocyte elastase	19	43 - 1420	315±80.3	15	51-257 x 10^{-3}	99±12.6 x 10^{-3}	3.2 x 10^{3}

SEM - Standard error of mean; Conc. — Concentration; NM - Not measured.

Complexes of antileukoprotease and granulocyte elastase were studied immunochemically after gel filtration of 450 μl middle ear fluid obtained by pooling all the middle ear specimens. Gel filtration of this pool was performed on a Sephadex G-50 column (0.9 x 70 cm) equilibrated with 0.05M TRIS-HCl buffer, pH 7.4, containing 0.5M NaCl. A constant flow of 8.5 ml per hour was maintained and 0.5 ml fractions were collected. The fractions eluted were analyzed using single radial immunodiffusion with specific antiserum against antileukoprotease. The fractions in which immunogenic free inhibitor was found were then pooled and concentrated in an Amicon cell with a Diaflo UM 2 membrane at 0° C to a volume of 300 μl. This pool was incubated with 300 μg granulocyte elastase for 30 minutes. After gel filtration of this material, the eluted fractions were again analyzed using single radial immunodiffusion with specific antiserum against antileukoprotease. The protein content in the eluted fractions of the gel filtrations was determined spectrophotometrically at 280 nm.

RESULTS

ENZYME CONTENT

Granulocyte collagenolytic protease was demonstrated in all studied MEE with a mean concentration of 120 μg/ml and a range of 37-307 μg/ml (Table 1).

Granulocyte elastase was detected in 19/20 middle ear specimens. The mean concentration in these 19 samples was 315 μg/ml with a range of 43-1420 μg/ml. The mean concentration of granulocyte elastase in the paired plasma was 99 x 10^{-3} μg/ml with a range of 51-257 x 10^{-3} μg/ml (Table 1).

C3 was detected in all MEE. The range of C3 in MEE compared to the corresponding plasma value of C3 was 45-153%, with a mean value of 75% (Table 2). In 18/20 specimens the concentration of C3 was below that of the corresponding plasma value. Crossed immunoelectrophoresis of MEE with specific antiserum against C3 showed cleavage products of C3 in all specimens (Fig. 1 b,c). Similar analyses of the corresponding plasma showed no changes in the electrophoretic homogeneity of C3 (Fig. 1a).

Inhibitor-Protease Complex Analyses. Crossed immunoelectrophoresis of all middle ear specimens with specific antiserum against α_1-antitrypsin revealed the following similar changes in the electrophoretic homogeneity of α_1-antitrypsin: 1) one component, approximately 80-85% of the total α_1-antitrypsin, in the α_1-area of native α_1-antitrypsin, 2) one in the α_2-region, and 3) one in the β_2-region. In 4/20 specimens a fourth component was demonstrated cathodal to the β_2-region (Fig. 2). Antiserum against the collagenolytic enzyme specifically precipitated the α_2-component (Fig. 3a). The component in the β_2-region was specifically precipitated by antiserum against granulocyte elastase (Fig. 3b). We were unable to identify the fourth component. When increasing amounts of granulocyte elastase were added to the middle ear specimens prior to crossed immunoelectrophoresis, an increase in the β_2-region and a decrease in the region of native α_1-antitrypsin were observed (Fig. 4).

Crossed immunoelectrophoresis with antiserum against α_2-macroglobulin following isoelectric focusing of 17/20 middle ear fluids showed the major portion of the α_2-macroglobulin to be in its free state, and less than 10% with an altered isoelectric point, indicating complex formation. In 3/20 specimens approximately 40% of the α_2-macroglobulin was in complex (Fig. 5).

TABLE 2. HUMORAL COMPONENTS IN MIDDLE EAR EFFUSION IN RELATION TO PATIENTS' OWN PLASMA CONCENTRATION (MEE/PLASMA x 100)

	C3	Antiplasmin
Range	45 - 153	32 - 127
Mean	75 ± 5.5*	70 ± 5.7*
Number	20	19

*Standard error of mean.

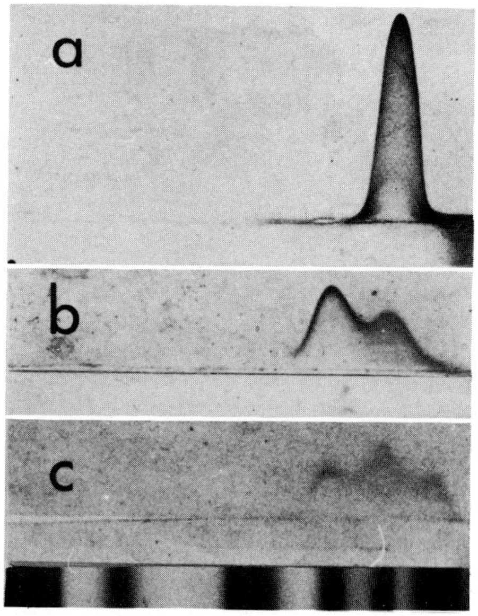

Fig. 1. Precipitate pattern on crossed immunoelectrophoresis with antiserum against C3 of a) patient plasma and b,c) specimens of MEE from two different patients. Agarose gel electrophoresis of plasma is given for reference.

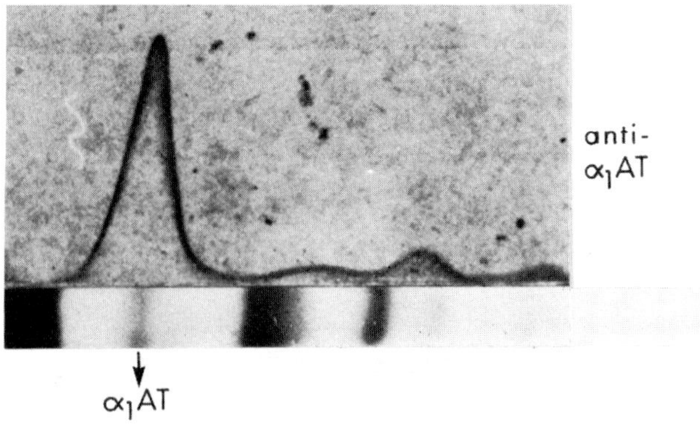

Fig. 2. Precipitate pattern on crossed immunoelectrophoresis of MEE with antiserum against α_1-antitrypsin (α_1-AT). Agarose gel electrophoresis of MEE is given for reference.

Crossed immunoelectrophoresis with antiserum against α_1-antichymotrypsin revealed no changes in electrophoretic mobility from that of free α_1-antichymotrypsin. However, in 5/20 specimens the precipitate showed three peaks within the area of "free" α_1-antichymotrypsin, indicating an electrophoretic inhomogeneity (Fig. 6 b,c).

Antileukoprotease from gel filtration of MEE was eluted in two separate volumes; one appeared within the void volume and one in a larger volume (fractions 54-67) corresponding to a lower molecular weight (Fig. 7A). Following a second gel filtration after the addition of elastase to the pooled fractions 54-67, the inhibitor was eluted exclusively within the void volume and no inhibitor was found in any larger volumes (Fig. 7B).

Antiplasmin in MEE was detected in 19/20 specimens. The range of antiplasmin in MEE compared to the paired plasma value was 32-127%, with a mean value of 71% (Table 2). Sufficient material was available for testing with crossed immunoelectrophoresis in only 10/20 specimens. These were tested using specific antiserum against antiplasmin.

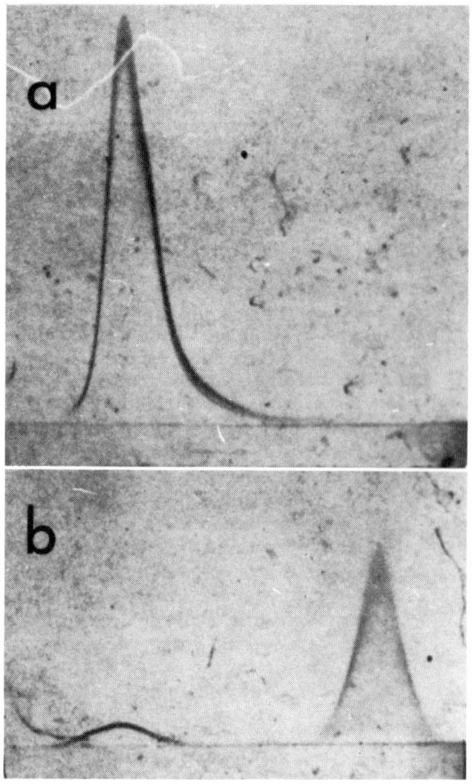

Fig. 4. Precipitate patterns on crossed immunoelectrophoresis of a specimen of MEE a) before and b) after the addition of 10 μg of granulocyte elastase with antiserum against α_1-antitrypsin.

Complex formation was suggested on the crossed immunoelectrophoresis pattern in 9/10 specimens (Fig. 8).

DISCUSSION

None of the patients had clinical signs of acute middle ear infection. Despite this, granulocyte collagenolytic neutral protease and granulocyte elastase were present in the effusions. Although desirable for reference purposes, determinations of

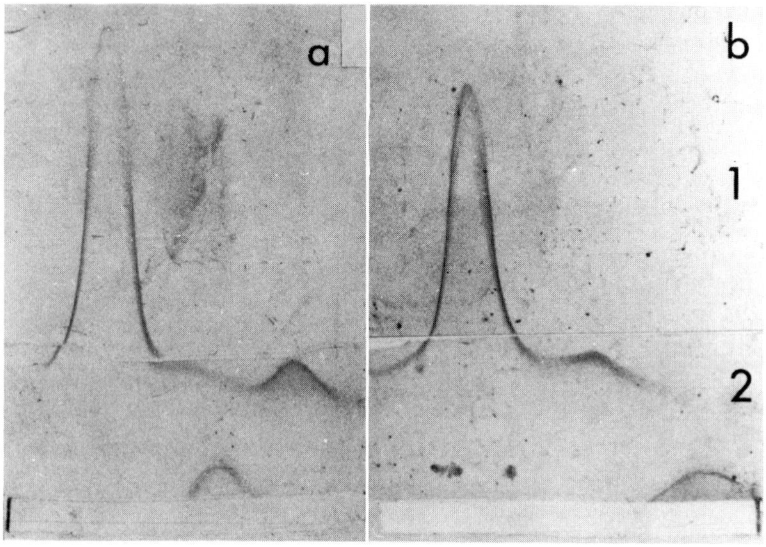

Fig. 3. Crossed immunoelectrophoresis of MEE. Part a_2 shows the pattern obtained with antiserum specific for collagenolytic neutral protease from human granulocytes. Part a_1 shows the precipitate pattern with antiserum against α_1-antitrypsin after precipitation with the anticollagenase antiserum (a_2). The α_2-peak of α_1-antitrypsin in complex was due to the collagenolytic enzyme, since it was specifically eliminated by the anticollagenase antiserum. b) Similar precipitation and arrangement to that of a), with the single exception that antiserum against elastase from human granulocytes replaced the antiserum against the collagenolytic enzyme (b_2). The peak with β_2 mobility was due to elastase-α_1-antitrypsin complex.

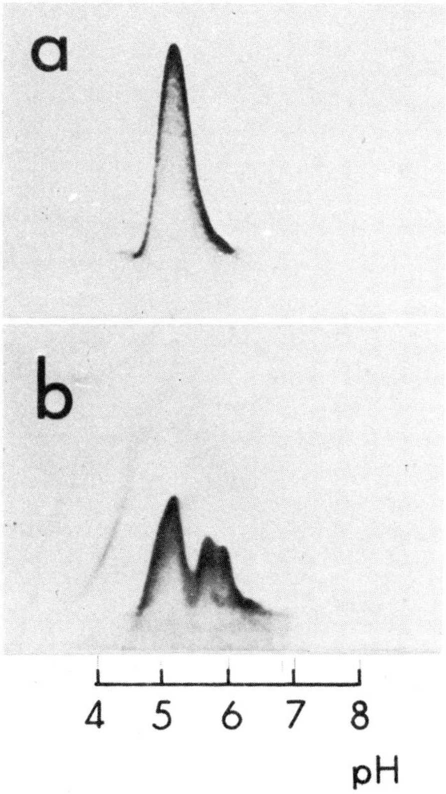

Fig. 5. Precipitate pattern on crossed immunoelectrophoresis following isoelectric focusing in polyacrylamide gel with antiserum against human α_2-macroglobulin of a) normal human plasma and b) a specimen of MEE. The altered isoelectric point in b) is attributed to the existence of α_2-macroglobulin in complex with enzyme.

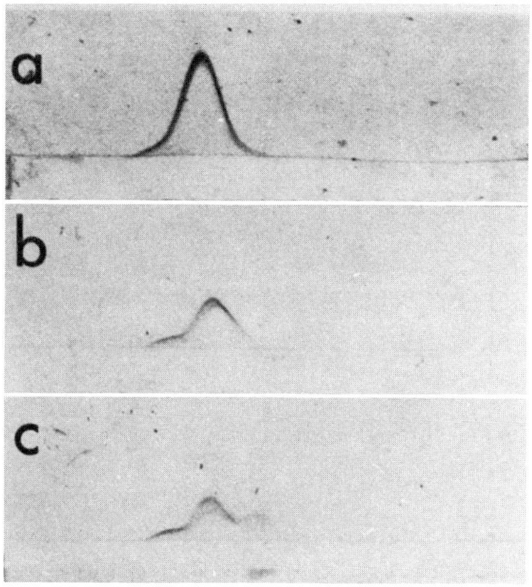

Fig. 6. Precipitate pattern on crossed immunoelectrophoresis with antiserum against α_1-antichymotrypsin of a) normal plasma and b,c) two specimens of MEE.

granulocyte collagenolytic neutral protease in corresponding plasma could not be performed due to a lack of a sufficiently sensitive assay method. However, the concentration of granulocyte elastase in the plasma of our patients was readily determined using an RIA technique developed in our laboratory. The concentrations were found to be within normal limits.[16] On comparison the mean granulocyte elastase concentration in MEE exceeded the mean plasma concentration by 3.2 x 10^3 times. This difference is most unlikely caused by the sampling procedure, since the plasma and MEE samples were treated identically. Our results rather imply a marked local release of granulocyte elastase in the MEE in SOM.

Granulocyte collagenolytic neutral protease and granulocyte elastase are known to activate the complement system via the alternate pathway.[7] This activation is independent of bacterial toxins and immuno complexes. In our study C3 was demonstrated in all MEE and activation of C3 was suggested by crossed immunoelectrophoresis, which is in accordance with previous reports.[21,22]

Plasmin, essential in the fibrinolysis, is also capable of activating C3.[23] This enzyme is specifically inhibited by antiplasmin present in plasma.[10] In our study this inhibitor was demonstrated in all but one of the studied middle ear specimens. Complex formation with plasmin was suggested by the presence of an antiplasmin component with retarded electrophoretic mobility similar to the plasmin-antiplasmin complex. Thus, our results indicate activation of the fibrinolytic system in SOM and that the activation of C3 in MEE may be effected both by granulocyte proteases and by plasmin.

In C3 activation fragments are formed which are chemotactic for granulocytes, thereby further granulocytes are attracted to the inflammatory site and a further release of granulocyte proteases may occur. If there is insufficient inhibition of granulocyte proteases and plasmin in the middle ear, a perpetuation of this inflammatory reaction could take place, even in the absence of antigen.[24]

Complexes between granulocyte proteases and α_1-antitrypsin were demonstrated in all MEE. The range of complexes, 15-20%, found for α_1-antitrypsin is rather rough as the immunoreactivity of the complexed α_1-antitrypsin differs considerably from the one of free α_1-antitrypsin. No indications of complexation with α_1-antichymotrypsin were found. The nonhomogenous peaks of α_1-antichymotrypsin found in five specimens were not consistent with complex formation with chymotrypsin-like granulocyte enzymes.[25]

Complexes between granulocyte proteases and α_2-macroglobulin were demonstrated in all MEE. No correlation between the concentration of proteases in MEE and the degree of complex formation with α_2-macroglobulin was found. The range of complexes found for α_2-macroglobulin, 10-40%, could be due to the relative insensitivity of the method used for detection of α_2-macroglobulin complexes.[20] Another possibility is that there were

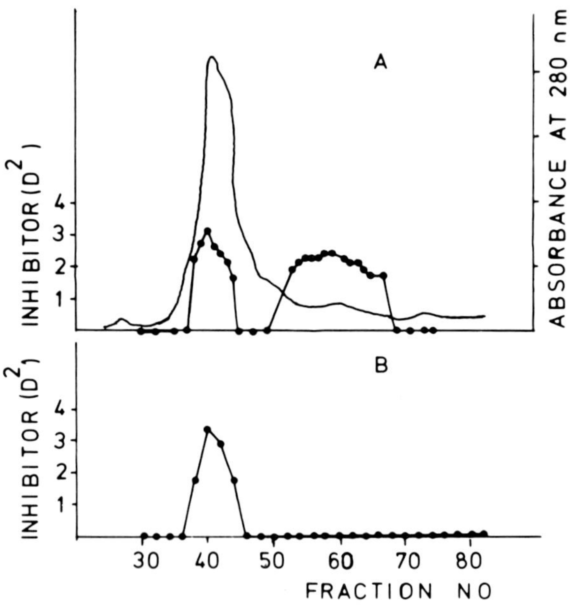

Fig. 7. Localization of antileukoprotease with single radial immunodiffusion, using antiserum against antileukoprotease. A) After gel filtration on Sephadex G-50 of pooled middle ear fluid. B) After addition of granulocyte elastase to fractions 54-67.

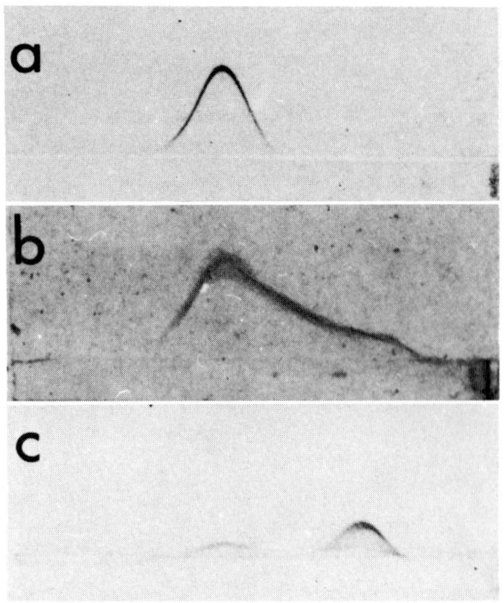

Fig. 8. Precipitate pattern on crossed immunoelectrophoresis with antiserum against antiplasmin of serum a) before and b,c) after activation of plasminogen with streptokinase (c) and of a specimen of MEE (b).

varying rates for the elimination of α_2-macroglobulin complexes in different ears secondary to the degree of inflammation. It has been observed in arthritic knee joints in the dog that the rate of elimination of α_2-macroglobulin complexes correlates directly with the degree of inflammatory reaction (Ekeroth L, personal communication).

Antileukoprotease forms stable complexes with elastase, but has no inhibiting effect on granulocyte collagenolytic protease.[14] Complex formation of this low molecular weight protease inhibitor in MEE was suggested on gel filtration, since the inhibitor was eluted in two separate volumes, indicating different molecular weights. From Figure 7 it appears that approximately one third of the inhibitor was complexed. However, this calculation does not take into account the probable reduction in the immunoreactivity of the inhibitor secondary to its complexed form, ie, the amount of antileukoprotease in complex with granulocyte elastase may be greater than what is illustrated in Figure 7.

The remaining inhibitory capacity in MEE was studied for α_1-antitrypsin and antileukoprotease. After addition of granulocyte elastase to the middle ear specimens, all of the noncomplexed antileukoprotease and the major part of α_1-antitrypsin were found complexed with elastase, as judged from the results of the gel filtration and crossed immunoelectrophoresis respectively. Thus, if granulocytes, as suggested[26] by their oxidative enzyme system, are able to inactivate α_1-antitrypsin this effect was limited in the MEE studied, despite the rather high content of granulocyte proteins. The results thus indicate an unsaturated capacity for enzyme inhibition in the middle ear fluid studied, but they do not exclude that tissue damage caused by granulocyte proteases may occur in the middle ear cavity, if the barrier of enzyme inhibition is locally exceeded.

REFERENCES

1. Palva T, Holopainen E, Karma P. Protein and cellular pattern of glue ear secretions. Ann Otol Rhinol Laryngol 1976; 85 Suppl 25: 103-9.

2. Carlsson B, Lundberg C, Ohlsson K. Protease inhibitors in middle ear effusions. Ann Otol Rhinol Laryngol 1981; 90:38-41.

3. Wright DG, Malawista SE. The mobilization of extracellular release of granular enzymes from human leukocytes during phagocytosis. J Cell Biol 1972; 53:788-97.

4. Ohlsson K. Collagenase and elastase released during peritonitis are complexed by plasma protease inhibitors. Surgery 1976; 79:652-7.

5. Ohlsson K, Olsson I. The extracellular release of granulocyte collagenase and elastase during phagocytosis and inflammatory processes. Scand J Haematol 1977; 19:145-52.

6. Johnson U, Ohlsson K, Olsson I. Effects of granulocyte neutral proteases on complement components. Scand J Immunol 1976; 5:421-6.

7. Taylor JC, Crawford IP, Hugli TE. Limited degradation of the third component (C3) of human complement by human leukocyte elastase (HLE): Partial characterization of C3 fragments. Biochemistry 1977; 16:3390-6.

8. Plow EF, Edgington TS. An alternative pathway for fibrinolysis. I. The cleavage of fibrinogen by leukocyte proteases at physiologic pH. J Clin Invest 1975; 56:30-8.

9. Schiessler H, Hochstrasser K, Ohlsson K. Acid-stable inhibitors of granulocyte neutral proteases in human mucous secretions: Biochemistry and possible biological function. In: Havemann K, Janoff A, eds. Neutral proteases of human poly-

morphonuclear leukocytes. Baltimore, Munich: Urban & Schwarzenberg, 1978: 195-207.

10. Collen D. Identification and some properties of a new fast-reacting plasmin inhibitor in human plasma. Eur J Biochem 1976; 69:209-16.

11. Ohlsson K, Olsson I. The neutral proteases of human granulocytes. Isolation and partial characterization of two granulocyte collagenases. Eur J Biochem 1973; 36:473-81.

12. Ohlsson K. Polymorphonuclear leukocyte collagenase. In: Wooley DE, Evanson JM, eds. Collagenase in normal and pathological connective tissues. Somerset: John Wiley & Sons Ltd, 1980: 209-22.

13. Ohlsson K, Olsson I. The neutral proteases of human granulocytes. Isolation and partial characterization of granulocyte elastase. Eur J Biochem 1974; 42:519-27.

14. Ohlsson K, Tegner H. Inhibition of elastase from granulocytes by the low molecular weight bronchial protease inhibitor. Scand J Clin Lab Invest 1976; 36:437-45.

15. Mancini G, Carbonara AO, Heremans JF. Immunochemical quantitation of antigens by single radial immunodiffusion. Immunochemistry 1965; 2:235-54.

16. Ohlsson K, Olsson A-S. Immunoreactive granulocyte elastase in human serum. Hoppe-Seyler's Z Physiol Chem 1978; 359:1531-9.

17. Laurell C-B. Electroimmuno assay. Scand J Clin Lab Invest 1972; 29 Suppl 124:21-37.

18. Ganrot PO. Crossed immunoelectrophoresis. Scand J Clin Lab Invest 1972; 29 Suppl 124:39-41.

19. Ohlsson K, Tegner H. Experimental pancreatitis in the dog. Demonstration of trypsin in ascitic fluid, lymph and plasma. Scand J Gastroenterol 1973; 8:129-33.

20. Ohlsson K, Skude G. Demonstration and semiquantitative determination of complexes between various proteases and human α_2-macroglobulin. Clin Chim Acta 1976; 66:1-7.

21. Veltri RW, Sprinkle PM. Secretory otitis media. An immune complex disease. Ann Otol Rhinol Laryngol 1976; 85 Suppl 25: 135-9.

22. Bernstein JM. Biological mediators of inflammation in middle ear effusions. Ann Otol Rhinol Laryngol 1976; 85 Suppl 25:90-6.

23. Ward PA. A plasmin-split fragment of C3 as a new chemotactic factor. J Exp Med 1967; 126:189-206.

24. Goldstein IM, Brai M, Osler AG, Weissmann G. Lysosomal enzyme release from human leukocytes: mediation by the alternate pathway of complement activation. J Immunol 1973; 111:33-7.

25. Ohlsson K, Åkesson U. α_1-Antichymotrypsin interaction with cationic proteins from granulocytes. Clin Chim Acta 1976; 73:285-91.

26. Matheson NR, Wong PS, Travis J. Enzymatic inactivation of human α_1-proteinase inhibitor by neutrophil myeloperoxidase. Biochem Biophys Res Commun 1979; 88:402-9.

≈

PAN AMERICAN ASSOCIATION OF OTORHINOLARYNGOLOGY AND BRONCHOESOPHAGOLOGY

The XVIII Congress of the Pan American Association of Otorhinolaryngology and Bronchoesophagology will be held November 2-6, 1982, in San Juan, Puerto Rico. Dr. Hans von Leden has been elected President of the Association.

Ann Otol 91:1982

COMPARATIVE ANATOMY OF EUSTACHIAN TUBE AND MIDDLE EAR CAVITY IN ANIMAL MODELS FOR OTITIS MEDIA

HAL J. DANIEL III, PhD
JACK E. BRINN, PhD
ROBERT S. FULGHUM, PhD
KATHRYN A. BARRETT, MS
GREENVILLE, NORTH CAROLINA

The comparative anatomy of the normal eustachian tube (ET) and normal middle ear cavity of three animal species (rat, gerbil, and chinchilla) is described relating to the usefulness of these animals as models for otitis media (OM). Routine histological and anatomical techniques and procedures were used. The gerbil and chinchilla, although of different sizes, are quite similar, having hypertrophied middle ear bullae, nearly vertical ET, and similar histology including seromucous glands draining directly into the ET. In contrast, the rat has a small bulla, a nearly horizontal ET, and a large concentration of goblet cells but few mucous glands in the ET. It appears that the chinchilla and the gerbil may serve as alternative models for OM research. Chinchillas and gerbils are relatively free of naturally occurring OM, while the rat has a high incidence of naturally occurring OM.

INTRODUCTION

Laboratory rats, gerbils, and chinchillas are frequently used as models for otitis media (OM) research.[1-8] The anatomy of the laboratory rat,[9] chinchilla,[10] and gerbil[11] auditory apparatus are well known but to date no comparative anatomical description of the middle ear (ME) cavity and eustachian tube (ET) of these laboratory animals has been published.

Comparisons of the epithelium of the ME cavity, ET, and nasopharynx as well as anatomical measurements of the angle and length of the ET were made for each species in this study. Measurements of the auditory bullae as they relate to skull size were also made.

Our studies show the gerbil, while physically smaller, has ME cavity and ET structural features quite similar to the chinchilla, while both of these animals differ considerably from the rat.

The collective results are discussed in light of recent research concerned with these structures and their respective functions as it was anticipated that appraisals could be made of the efficacy of the animals as models in future OM research. Based on these studies, we conclude that the chinchilla and the gerbil may possibly serve in many procedures as alternative animal models. As an alternative model the gerbil would be a useful starting model since it breeds rapidly and prolifically, and would allow more rapid development of inbred strains than could be achieved with chinchillas. Furthermore gerbils are more consistently available and less expensive to purchase, ship, and maintain than chinchillas.

METHODS

Bulla: Skull Comparisons. The mammalian auditory bulla encapsulates the entire ME. The size of the auditory bulla was defined for this study as the widest dimension in any one plane from any inferiorly based view. Total skull length was defined as the length from the anterior margin of the foramen magnum to the anterior margin of the upper incisor teeth. All measurements were obtained using microcalipers. Ten randomly selected macerated adult skulls of each species, Long-Evans hooded rat (*Rattus norvegicus*), Mongolian gerbil (*Meriones unguiculatus*), and chinchilla (*Chinchilla laniger*), were used for bulla:skull measurement data. Skulls were obtained from the skull collection of the Speech and Hearing Research Laboratory, East Carolina University. Fifty skulls from each species (50 rat, 50 gerbil, and 50 chinchilla skulls) were selected and assigned numbers 1 to 50. A Horton-Smith table of random numbers was then used to randomly select ten from each species.

Histological Methods. Histological preparations were the same for both rats and gerbils.[12,13] Five animals of each species were studied. Animals were anesthetized, and perfused with 0.9% NaCl followed by perfusion with 10% buffered (pH 7.4) formalin. The head was removed, decalcified in formic acid and sodium citrate solution, trimmed, and dehydrated in a graded series of ethanol. Specimens were cleared in xylene, embedded in paraffin, and cut 8 μm thick on a microtome. Coronal sections at 80 μm intervals were mounted and stained with hematoxylin and eosin (H & E, Harris).[12] Additional sections of the nasopharyngeal area (NP), ET, and middle ear cavity (MEC) were stained with Mayer's mucicarmine.[12]

The length of the ET was determined by adding the number of 8 μm sections from the osteum pharyngeum tubae auditivae to the osteum tympanicum tubae auditivae. The angle of the ET was estimated by using the length of the ET as the hypotenuse of a right-angle triangle. The angle formed by the hypotenuse and base of the triangle was determined to be the angle of the ET. In making this estimation it was assumed that each skull was sectioned in the same plane, as specimens were carefully positioned prior to sectioning. In addition to the external gross bulla:skull comparisons, internal measurements of the length, height, and width of the bulla of the three species were obtained from the histologic sections.

Microscopic observations were made to determine epithelial cell differences in various locations. Goblet cell and mucous duct

From the Department of Speech, Language, and Auditory Pathology, School of Allied Health, and the Departments of Microbiology and Anatomy, School of Medicine, East Carolina University, Greenville, North Carolina. Supported in part by Sigma Xi, East Carolina University Research Council, North Carolina United Way, and The Deafness Research Foundation.

REPRINTS — Hal J. Daniel III PhD, Dept. of Speech, Language, and Auditory Pathology, E.C.U. School of Allied Health, Greenville, NC 27834.

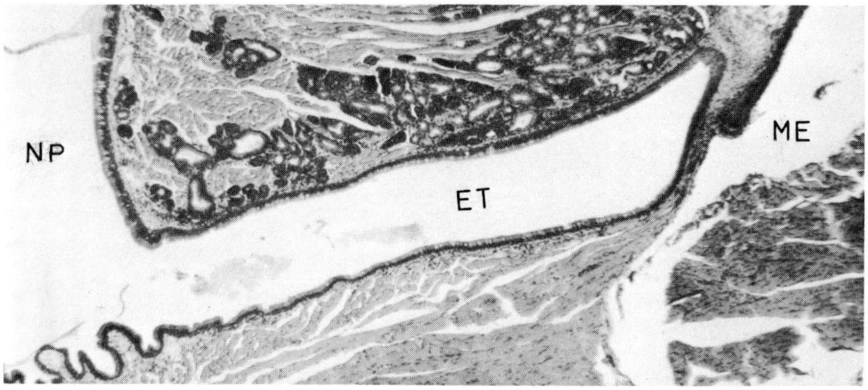

Fig. 1. Nasopharynx (NP), eustachian tube (ET), and middle ear (ME) cavity of the rat. Note cilia in the ET as compared to lack of cilia in the middle ear cavity. (H & E, x62.5)

counts were made on every other of the mounted and stained sections (every 160 μm).

Histological preparations for the chinchilla were completed in the Temporal Bone Histopathology Laboratory of the Department of Otolaryngology, University of Minnesota School of Medicine. Animals were perfused first with normal saline, then with Heidenhain Susa preservative.[13] Specimens were decalcified in 5% trichloroacetic acid (TCA), trimmed, dehydrated in a graded series of ethanol, and cleared in 50% ether-50% absolute ethanol. After embedding in celloidin (nitrocellulose), specimens were hardened in chloroform vapor, stored in 80% ethanol, and cut 20 μm thick. Coronal sections at 200 μm intervals were mounted and stained with H & E. Two exceptionally well-prepared chinchilla specimens were examined for this study.

RESULTS

Histology of the Rat ME and ET. The eustachian tube of the rat is lined by pseudostratified ciliated columnar respiratory epithelium throughout its length (Fig. 1). The cilia appear thicker and longer than those of the gerbil. Goblet cells are found on the dorsal aspect of the nasopharynx, continuing up the ET and in more abundance on the dorsal wall especially near the tympanic osteum. The epithelium of the ET upon approaching the MEC changes abruptly from tall pseudostratified ciliated columnar cells to nonciliated stratified squamoid cells (Fig. 2). The epithelium of the MEC consists of stratified squamous cells with no evidence of cilia or goblet cells, while an average of 54.5 goblet cells per 8 μm section was found in the ET.

Histology of the Mongolian Gerbil ME and ET. Figure 3 shows that the epithelium of the nasopharynx near the nasopharyngeal osteum of the ET in the Mongolian gerbil consists of respiratory epithelium being pseudostratified ciliated columnar cells with short, fine, evenly distributed cilia. The basement membrane is well demarcated from the underlying connective tissue. At approximately two thirds of the distance from the nasopharyngeal osteum to the tympanic osteum in the ET there is a cessation of ciliated epithelium (Fig. 4). At this point the cells become squamoid, varying in thickness from one to five layers.

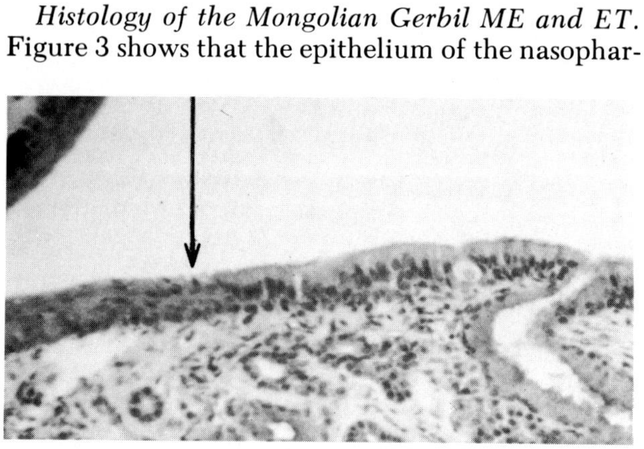

Fig. 2. View of the cessation (arrow) of cilia and goblet cells in the epithelium of the ET as it approaches the middle ear cavity in the rat. (Mayer's mucicarmine, x400)

Goblet cells are found along the epithelium of the nasopharynx but not beyond the pharyngeal osteum of the ET. There are, however, mucous glands in the medial side of the ET that open into the lumen of the ET (Fig. 3).

The stratified squamoid epithelium of the tympanic end of the ET continues into the MEC which is lined by these cells. The MEC is subdivided by trabeculae of bone, forming connecting chambers, and is lined by this squamous epithelium. There is no evidence of goblet cells or mucous glands in the normal ME of the Mongolian gerbil.

Histology of the Chinchilla ME and ET. The ET is lined for most of its length by respiratory epithelium (Fig. 5A) which is columnar at the nasopharyngeal end and decreases in height, becoming cuboidal (Fig. 5B) toward the tympanic end. The epithelium is ciliated for its entire length. The nasopharyngeal two thirds of the length of the tube receives short ducts from seromucous glands. Goblet cells are also found along the epithelium of the ET. The entire medial border of the tube is supported by hyaline cartilage, which forms an arch to support the lateral aspects of the tube as it turns laterally toward the MEC. The MEC is divided into connecting chambers by trabeculae of bone and is lined by a squamous epithelium which is for the most part simple.

Comparison of Skulls and Skull Measurements of the Rat, Gerbil, and Chinchilla. Inferior and lateral views of the rat (Fig. 6A, B), gerbil (Fig. 7A, B) and chinchilla (Fig. 8A, B) skulls are presented. Mean bulla and skull measurements of ten skulls of each species are contained in Table 1. Internal

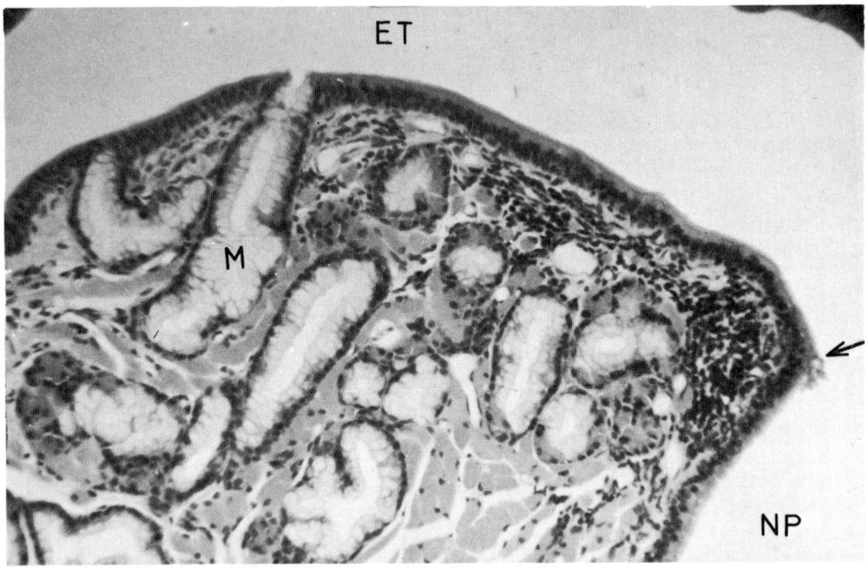

Fig. 3. Eustachian tube (ET) and nasopharynx (NP) of the gerbil showing pseudostratified ciliated columnar cells (arrow) at the orifice of the ET, and a mucous gland (M) opening into the ET. (H & E, x200)

measurements taken from the histological preparations of the auditory bulla for each species are presented in Table 2. Figure 9 is a highly schematic presentation of the relative bulla size, and the angle and length of the ET of each of the animals. The ET of the rat was found to be almost horizontal in comparison to the nearly vertical ET of the chinchilla and the gerbil. The ET of the rat is relatively long in an anterior-posterior direction paralleling an elongation of its skull in the anterior-posterior plane. The relatively long ET of the rat is in contrast to the extremely short and vertical tube of the gerbil, while that of the chinchilla is intermediate in length and the angle slightly more horizontal. The vertical elongation of the tube in the chinchilla is possibly related to the superior-inferior expansion and relatively narrower medial-lateral dimension of the chinchilla bulla.

The small rat bulla and the gerbil bulla are relatively ovoid in shape while that of the chinchilla is more elliptical. The dorsal attic area in the gerbil is more narrow laterally and the attic is divided into two separate chambers, the anterior and the posterosuperior chambers, that do not connect with each other. These each connect with the lower, wider, tympanic chamber of the bulla.

Figures 10 and 11 are comparative sketches (but not to equal scale) of the gerbil and chinchilla ME as coronal sections just posterior to the location of the inner ear. Figure 12 is a sagittal section of the gerbil showing the various chambers and landmarks in a manner similar to the drawings of the chinchilla by Browning and Granich.[10] Figure 13 is the sagittal section of the ME of the chinchilla by Browning and Granich.[10] More detailed descrip-

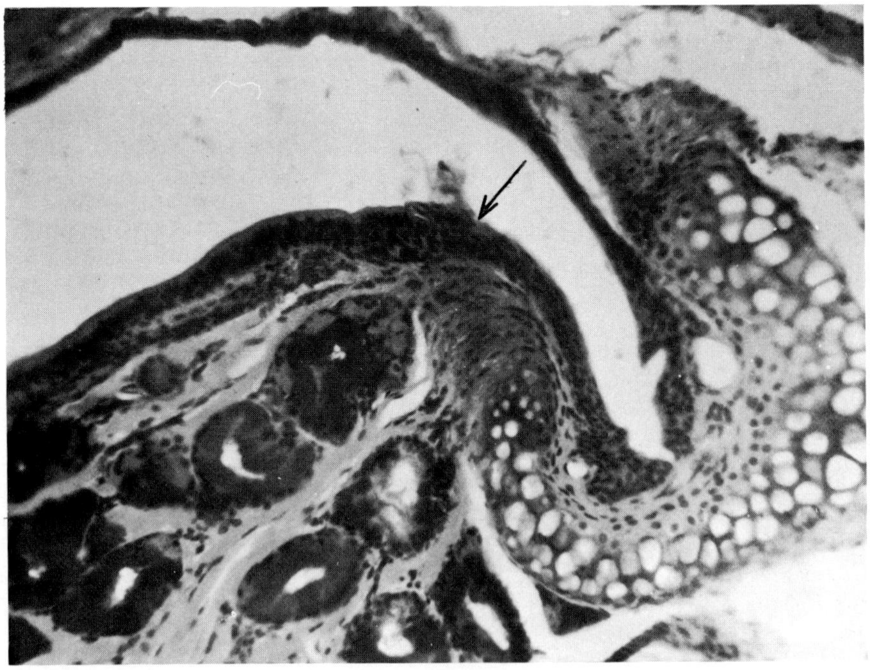

Fig. 4. Point (arrow) where the epithelium changes from ciliated columnar to nonciliated stratified squamoid cells in the ET of the gerbil. (Mayer's mucicarmine, x200)

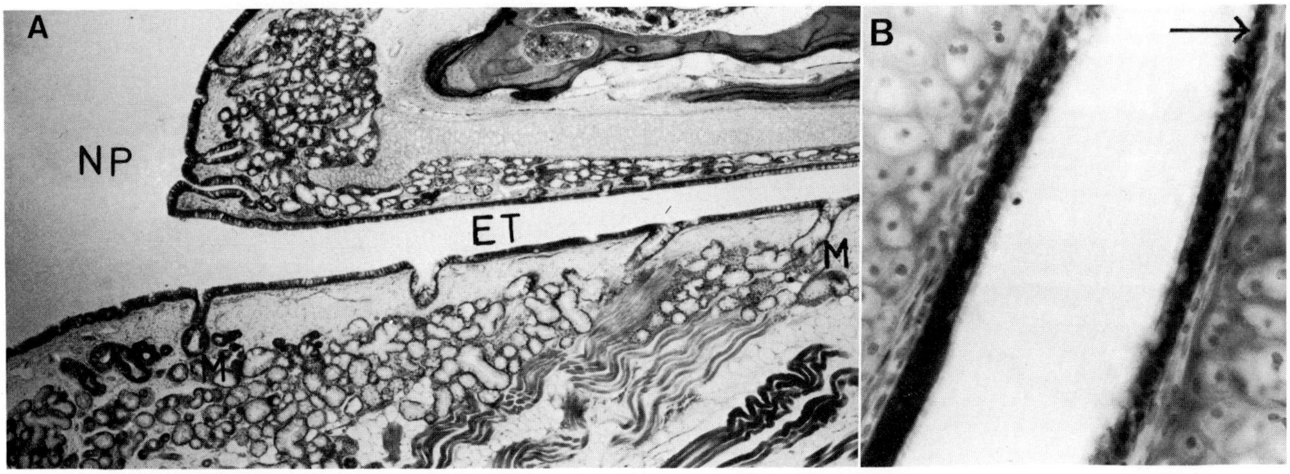

Fig. 5. A) Nasopharynx (NP) and eustachian tube (ET) in the chinchilla showing ciliated columnar epithelium and abundant seromucous (M) glands. (H & E, x40) B) ET of the chinchilla near the tympanic osteum. Note ciliated epithelium, its point of cessation (arrow), and goblet cells. (H & E, x400)

tions of the landmarks of the bullae of gerbilline rodents were recorded by Lay.[11] The anatomical information provided in Figures 10 through 13 is useful to investigators in developing laboratory techniques for inoculating and collecting specimens from the ME using the percutaneous routes used by Giebink et al.[14] The bone of the bulla of the chinchilla is very thin whereas that of the gerbil is somewhat heavier relative to the size of each bulla. In both of these animals the strength of the bullae is derived from the large but variable number of internal septa (Figs. 10-13).[10] In the chinchilla, the dorsal or cephalad portion of the bulla is subcutaneous[10] whereas in the gerbil the posterior superior chamber lies below muscle making palpation of the bone and injection of bacterial inoculum slightly more difficult. In the chinchilla, the external auditory canal is a tunnel located within the temporal bone. The lateral wall is continuous with and in the same plane as the mastoid and labyrinthine part of the bulla[10] resulting in an elongated S-shaped external auditory canal through which it is difficult to visualize the entire tympanic membrane. Similarly it is difficult to deliver inoculum to the ME or remove specimens by tympanocentesis without contamination of needles by the bacterial flora of the external auditory meatus. The gerbil (compare Figs. 7B and 8B; also Figs. 10 and 11) has a much smaller but less convoluted opening.

DISCUSSION

The high incidence of natural OM in the rat[1,2] may be related to its small auditory bulla and horizontal ET. It is well established that humans with small ME cavities,[15,16] more horizontal ET,[17] and greater goblet cell density[18,19] are otitis prone. Holmquist[20] has recently reported that the larger the mastoid, the greater the MEC ventilation. Furthermore, Andréasson[21,22] has shown a correlation between abnormally small mastoid air cell systems, impaired tubal function, and the incidence of chronic OM. In contrast, the hypertrophied auditory bulla, vertical ET, and tubal mucous gland structure of the chinchilla and gerbil may contribute to the observed lower incidence of natural OM in these animals.[3-5] In addition, Loesche[23] found in a postural behavioral study that laboratory gerbils spend significantly more nocturnal, diurnal,

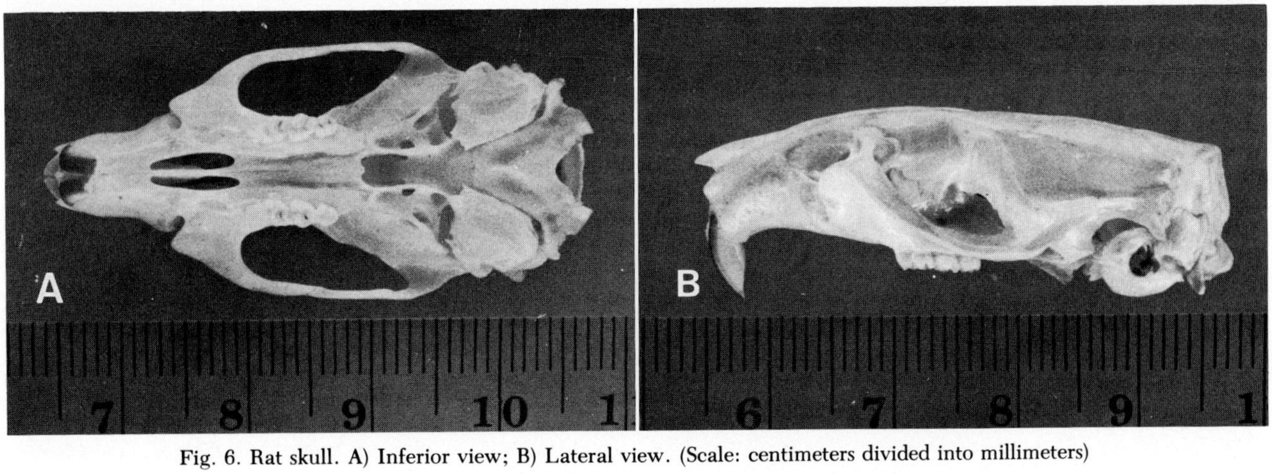

Fig. 6. Rat skull. A) Inferior view; B) Lateral view. (Scale: centimeters divided into millimeters)

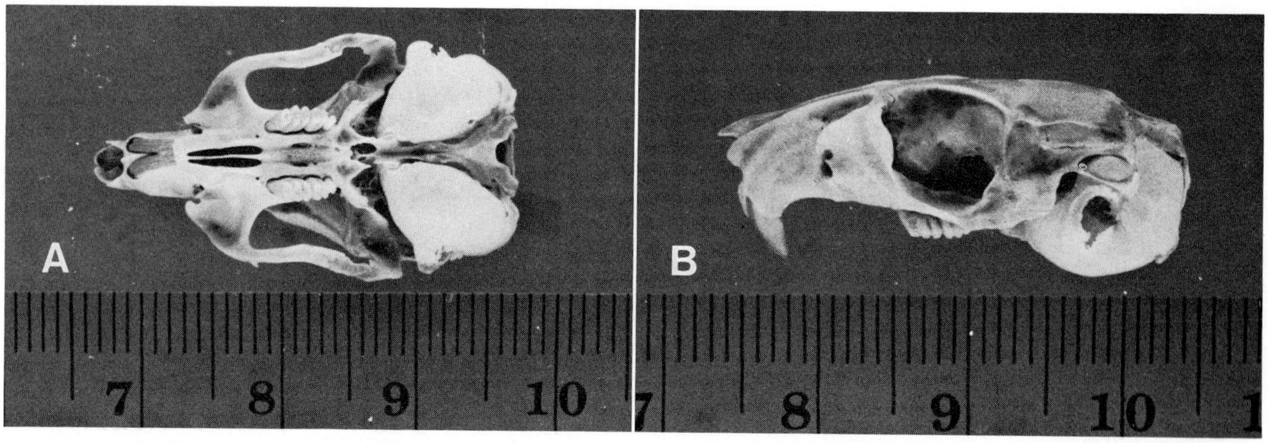

Fig. 7. Gerbil skull. A) Inferior view showing hypertrophied bulla as compared to rat (Fig. 6A). B) Lateral view showing hypertrophied bulla as compared to rat (Fig. 6B). Note that the dorsal bulla is much larger than that of rat but somewhat smaller than that of chinchilla (Fig. 8B).

and overall time in "optimal tubal ventilation positions" than do laboratory rats. These data are interesting in light of Sadé's[24] hypothesis that the lack of ventilation is the single most important factor in the chronicity of secretory OM, as well as Elner's[25,26] observations of the role of gas exchange in the normal human ME. These observations of MEC size and its potential for oxygenation in humans are not unlike our present data for laboratory animals. Although purely speculative at this point, it is possible that the seromucous glands of the gerbil and chinchilla may secrete immunoglobulins as has been reported for human salivary glands.[27] Such a mechanism would provide additional protection aganist bacterial invasion. Proof of the existence of these secretions would provide valuable insights into the understanding of OM.

It should also be pointed out that isolation of anaerobic bacteria in specimens obtained from laboratory rat effusions[4] could be partially related to that species' small, underventilated, and poorly drained MEC. It may follow, then, that the hypertrophied, better ventilated and drained MEC of the gerbil and chinchilla could be related to lower incidence of acute and chronic OM in these animals[3] and possibly to the low levels and transitory nature of the indigenous bacterial flora of the MEC of gerbils[28,29] and chinchillas (Fulghum et al, unpublished data).

TABLE 1. MEAN EXTERNAL MEASUREMENTS OF BULLA AND SKULL FOR EACH SPECIES*

	Skull (mm)	*SD*	*Bulla (mm)*	*SD*	*Skull: Bulla Ratio*
Rat	40	.48	6	.05	.15
Gerbil	28	.31	12	.08	.43
Chinchilla	55	.61	25	.20	.45

*Ten skulls for each species.

TABLE 2. INTERNAL MEASUREMENTS OF THE AUDITORY BULLA FOR EACH SPECIES

	Length (mm)	*Height (mm)*	*Width (mm)*
Rat	5	4	2.0
Gerbil	11	10	8.0
Chinchilla	23	25	6.5

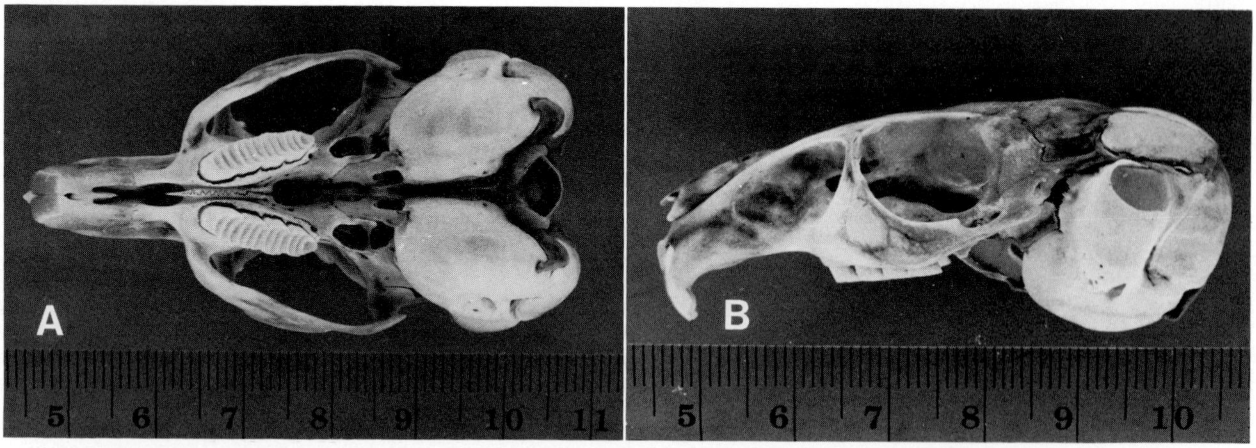

Fig. 8. Chinchilla skull. A) Inferior view showing the hypertrophied bulla as compared to rat (Fig. 6A) but similar in skull:bulla ratio to gerbil (Fig. 7A). B) Lateral view showing hypertrophied bulla with large cephalad bulla. Note the displaced auricular orifice of the external auditory meatus, resulting in an elongated S-shaped auditory canal, as compared to the rat and the gerbil.

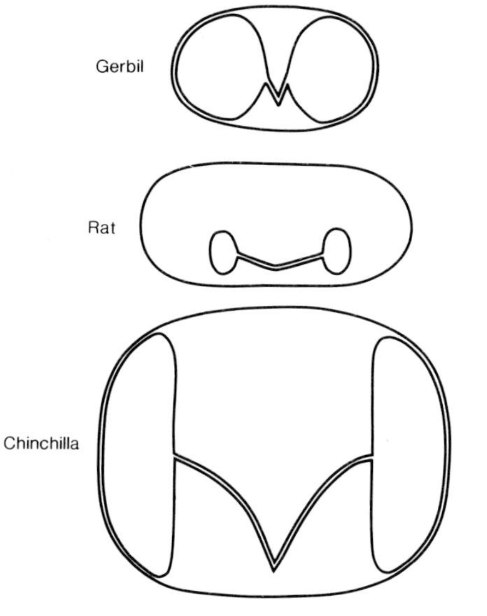

Fig. 9. Highly schematic drawing comparing rat, gerbil and chinchilla. Note hypertrophied bulla and more vertical ET of gerbil and chinchilla as compared to rat (see also Table 1). Measurements in millimeters are:

	Skull Width	*Skull Height*	*Tubal Length*	*Tubal Angle*
Rat	24	11	4.3	15°
Gerbil	18	11	1.8	81°
Chinchilla	31	26	5.6	75°

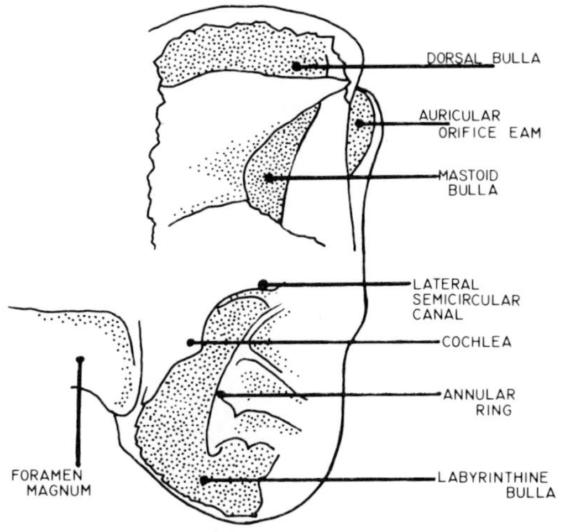

Fig. 11. Sketch of coronal section of chinchilla ME. Note the location of the auricular orifice of the external auditory meatus (EAM) and its relationship to the annular ring compared to the gerbil (Fig. 10).

Recent data from our laboratory show the indigenous microflora of the pharynx[29] and MEC[28] of the chinchilla and the gerbil do not normally include the common etiological agents of OM, although *Staphylococcus aureus* and *Staphylococcus epidermidis* are frequently found in the nasopharynx of gerbils.[29] Giebink et al[6] have previously shown chinchillas do not harbor *Streptococcus pneumoniae* but are susceptible to induced OM caused by this bacterium. Furthermore, we find the indigenous flora of the MEC of both chinchillas and gerbils to be sparse, variable, and transitory. We are currently involved in studies with monomicrobic and polymicrobic infections involving anaerobic bacteria[4] in both the chinchilla[5] and the gerbil in order to develop suitable animal models for anaerobic infections. The data to date indicate that both chinchillas and gerbils are susceptible to infections due to the anaerobic polymicrobic infections we reported in children[4] and to *S pneumoniae*.

The gerbil is a relatively new model for auditory research.[30,31] If its response to infection is as good as that of the chinchilla,[6-8] the Mongolian gerbil could be an alternative model for many aspects of OM research. Gerbils are much more consistently available and less expensive to purchase, ship, and maintain than chinchillas. Because of its rapid and prolific breeding, inbred strains have been developed, and additional inbred strains can be much more rapidly developed in gerbils than in chinchillas, making the gerbil an ideal "beginning model." Furthermore, gerbils meet the criteria of Lewis et al[8] for selection as an experimental model for OM research,

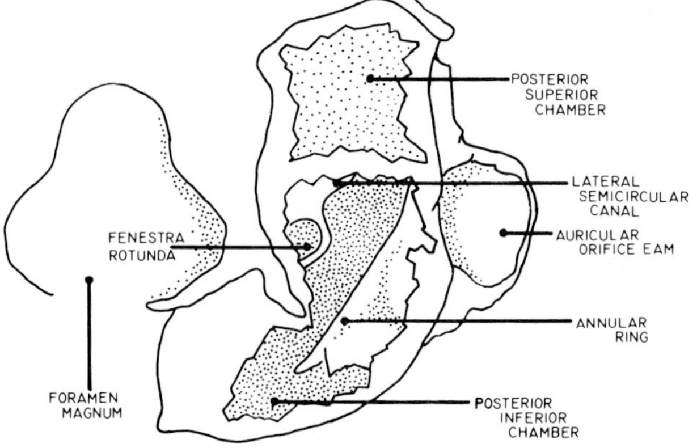

Fig. 10. Sketch of coronal section of gerbil ME.

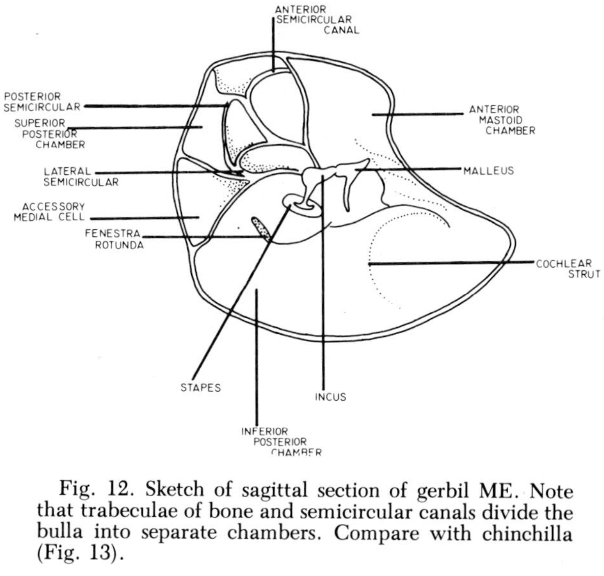

Fig. 12. Sketch of sagittal section of gerbil ME. Note that trabeculae of bone and semicircular canals divide the bulla into separate chambers. Compare with chinchilla (Fig. 13).

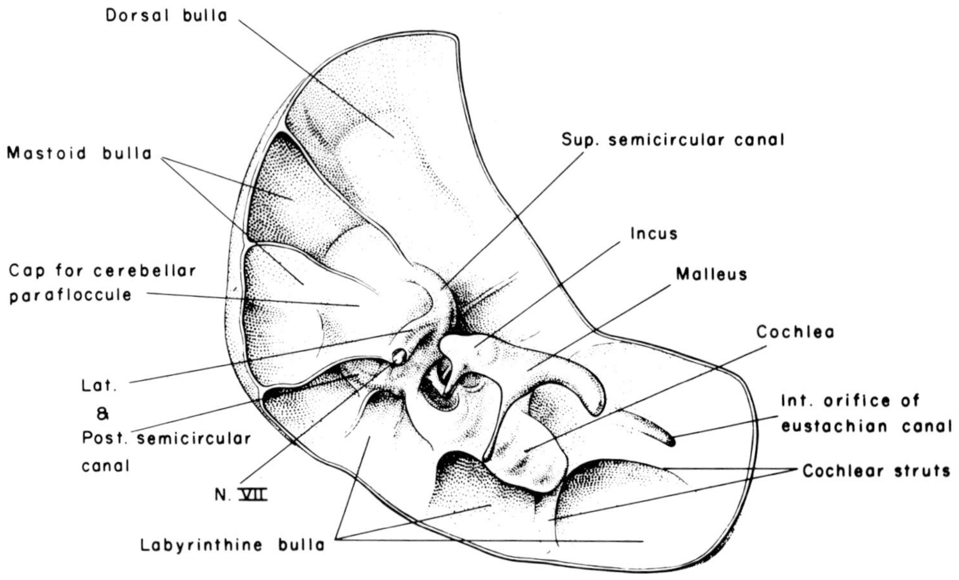

Fig. 13. Drawing of sagittal section of chinchilla ME. (Reproduced with permission.[10])

and much is known of the microbiology[28,29,32] and immunology[33] of the gerbil.

Because we conclude the rat is not a useful animal model for the study of induced ME disease of bacterial etiology, we have omitted detailed drawings of the ME gross anatomy. Details of the anatomy of this animal have been published elsewhere by Hebel and Stromberg.[34]

Finally, while inherent dangers exist in making anatomical and physiological comparisons across species, as we have done, the relationships we have encountered thus far have provided useful information not only about rats, gerbils, chinchillas, and humans, but also about the mammalian ME mechanism in general. An understanding of the similarities and differences of this system across species is a logical framework for studying its pathologies.

ACKNOWLEDGMENTS — The authors wish to thank Drs. William L. Meyerhoff and Donald A. Shea of the Department of Otolaryngology, School of Medicine, University of Minnesota, for the loan of three beautiful sets of slides of serially sectioned chinchilla temporal bones from which the histological descriptions of the chinchilla were made. We appreciate reviews of the manuscript by Drs. William Meyerhoff, Josef Miller, Brenda Lonsbury-Martin, and G. Lynis Dohm. The interest in our work and suggestions made by Dr. G. Scott Giebink were especially helpful and highly stimulatory to us in completing this work. The excellent technical assistance in our laboratories of Mary Margaret McDade and John Worthington is acknowledged with great appreciation. We thank Mr. Edward Friesch of the Carolinas Branch of the Empress Chinchilla Breeders Cooperative for arranging for gifts of chinchillas used in a portion of this work.

REFERENCES

1. Daniel HJ, Carmine FH, Cook RA. Otitis media in two strains of laboratory rats. J Aud Res 1971; 11:276-8.

2. Daniel HJ, Means LW, Dressel ME, Loesche PJ. Otitis media in laboratory rats. Physiol Psychol 1973; 1:7-8.

3. Means LW, Daniel HJ, Jordan LH, Loesche PJ. Nonsusceptibility to otitis media of the laboratory gerbil, *Meriones unguiculatus.* Physiol Psychol 1975; 3:229-30.

4. Fulghum RS, Daniel HJ, Yarborough JG. Anaerobic bacteria in otitis media. Ann Otol Rhinol Laryngol 1977; 84:198-202.

5. Loesche PJ, Daniel HJ, Smith NM, Worthington JM, Smith AM, Fulghum RS. Preliminary investigations into the inducement and detection of otitis media with anaerobic bacteria in chinchillas. ASM News 1980; 46:217.

6. Giebink GS, Payne EE, Mills EL, Juhn SK, Quie PG. Experimental otitis media due to *Streptococcus pneumoniae*: immunopathogenic response in the chinchilla. J Infect Dis 1976; 134:595-604.

7. Giebink GS, Berzins IK, Quie PG. Animal models for studying pneumococcal otitis media and pneumococcal vaccine efficacy. Ann Otol Rhinol Laryngol 1980; 89 Suppl 68:339-43.

8. Lewis DM, Schram JL, Meadema SJ, Lim DJ. Experimental otitis media in chinchillas. Ann Otol Rhinol Laryngol 1980; 89 Suppl 68:344-50.

9. Greene EC. Anatomy of the rat. Trans Am Philosophical Soc 1935; vol 27. New York: Hafner Publishing Company, 1955.

10. Browning GG, Granich MS. Surgical anatomy of the temporal bone in the chinchilla. Ann Otol Rhinol Laryngol 1978; 87:875-82.

11. Lay DM. The anatomy, physiology, functional significance and evolution of specialized hearing organs of gerbilline rodents. J Morphol 1972; 138:41-120.

12. Preece A. A manual for histologic technicians, 3rd ed. Boston: Little, Brown and Co, 1972.

13. Lillie RD. Histopathologic technic and practical histochemistry, 3rd ed. New York: McGraw-Hill, 1965.

14. Giebink GS, Schiffman G, Petty K, Quie PG. Modification of otitis media following vaccination with the capsular polysaccharide of *Streptococcus pneumoniae* in chinchillas. J Infect Dis 1978; 138:480-7.

15. Diamant M. Otitis and pneumatisation of the mastoid bone. Acta Otolaryngol (Stockh) 1940; 28 Suppl 41.

16. Diamant M. Otitis and the size of the air cell system. Acta Radiol 1940; 21:543.

17. Ingelstedt S. Chronic adhesive otitis. Acta Otolaryngol (Stockh) 1963; Suppl 188.

18. Tos M, Bak-Pederson K. Goblet cell population in the normal middle ear and eustachian tube of children and adults. Ann Otol Rhinol Laryngol 1976; 85 Suppl 25:44-50.

19. Tos M, Bak-Pederson K. Goblet cell population in the

pathological middle ear and eustachian tube of children and adults. Ann Otol Rhinol Laryngol 1977; 86:209-18.

20. Holmquist J. Aeration in chronic otitis media. Clin Otolaryngol 1978; 3:279-84.

21. Andréasson L. Correlation of tubal function and volume of mastoid and middle ear space as related to otitis media. Ann Otol Rhinol Laryngol 1976; 85:198-203.

22. Andréasson L. Correlation of tubal function and volume of mastoid and middle ear space as related to otitis media. Acta Otolaryngol (Stockh) 1977; 83:29-33.

23. Loesche PJ. Posture and otitis media in laboratory rats and gerbils, thesis. East Carolina University, Greenville, 1975.

24. Sadé J. The biopathology of secretory otitis media. Ann Otol Rhinol Laryngol 1974; 83 Suppl 11:59-70.

25. Elner A. Normal gas exchange in the human middle ear. Ann Otol Rhinol Laryngol 1976; 85 Suppl 25:161-4.

26. Elner A. Quantitative studies of gas absorption from the normal middle ear. Acta Otolaryngol (Stockh) 1977; 83:25-8.

27. Weiss L, Greep R. Histology, 3rd ed. New York: McGraw-Hill, 1977.

28. Gardner D. Identification of the normal flora in the tympanic bulla of the laboratory gerbil *(Meriones unguiculatus)*, thesis. East Carolina University, Greenville, 1977.

29. Thompson TA. Otitis media and the nasopharyngeal microflora of the Mongolian gerbil, *Meriones unguiculatus*, thesis. East Carolina University, Greenville, 1979.

30. Daniel HJ, Loesche PJ. The gerbil as a subject for auditory research. Presented at the meeting of the American Association for Laboratory Animal Research, Boston, 1975.

31. Daniel HJ, Loesche PJ. The gerbil as a subject for auditory research. Presented at the meeting of the American Speech and Hearing Association, Washington, DC, 1975.

32. Vincent AL, Rodrick GE, Sodeman WA Jr. The pathology of the Mongolian gerbil *(Meriones unguiculatus)*: a review. Lab Anim Sci 1979; 29:645-51.

33. Karavodin LM, Ash LR. Weak mixed lymphocyte culture response in the Mongolian gerbil *(Meriones unguiculatus)*. Lab Anim Sci 1977; 27:195-203.

34. Hebel R, Stromberg MW. Anatomy of the laboratory rat. Baltimore: Williams and Wilkins Co, 1976; 1-5, 8, 9, 148-52.

ADDENDUM

After this manuscript had been set in type an account of the microflora of the middle ear cleft and nasopharynx of the mongolian gerbil was published by us (Infect Immun 1981; 32:1113). A manuscript from our laboratory on experimental otitis media in gerbils and chinchillas with *Streptococcus pneumoniae*, *Hemophilus influenzae* and other aerobic and anaerobic bacteria is being revised for publication.

Ann Otol 91:1982

EXPERIMENTAL VIRAL INFECTIONS OF THE INNER EAR

III. VIREMIC SPREAD OF REOVIRUS TO HAMSTER EIGHTH NERVE GANGLION CELLS

LARRY E. DAVIS, MD

ALBUQUERQUE, NEW MEXICO

Rubella, cytomegalovirus, mumps, and rubeola viruses cause deafness in man and are believed to reach the inner ear through viremic spread. Although several experimental studies of viral infection of the inner ear have been described, all require the virus inoculum to reach the labyrinth directly rather than through hematogenous spread. In this model, reovirus, type 3, infected the cell bodies of cochlear and vestibular ganglia of infant hamsters following a viremia induced by intraperitoneal inoculation. This model provides the first experimental evidence for viremic spread to the inner ear.

INTRODUCTION

Viral infections have been associated with many abnormalities of auditory and vestibular functions. Rubella[1] and cytomegalovirus[2] infections of the fetus are important causes of congenital deafness. Other viruses including mumps[3,4] and rubeola[5] have been implicated as causes of postnatal acquired deafness. All of these viruses are believed to reach the inner ear through viremic spread.[6]

Experimentally, rubeola virus,[7,8] mumps virus,[7,8] herpes simplex virus,[8] vaccinia virus,[8] influenza virus,[7,8] Sendai virus,[9] and mouse cytomegalovirus[10] have been shown to infect the inner ear of the mouse or hamster. These animal studies have demonstrated that inner ear structures have differing selective vulnerability to infection by different viruses.[7,8] However, these models have all required that the virus be inoculated directly into the labyrinth or intracerebrally to reach the inner ear via the cochlear aqueduct. Intraperitoneal or intravenous inoculations of virus have not been successful in producing inner ear infections.

In the model presented, reovirus, type 3, was shown to infect cells of the inner ear by the viremic route following intraperitoneal inoculation.

METHODS

The Abney strain of reovirus, type 3,[11] grown in baby hamster kidney cells (BHK-21), had an infectivity titer of $10^{7.3}$ 50% tissue culture infectious doses ($TCID_{50}$) per milliliter in African green monkey kidney cells (CV-1). This virus pool was diluted 1:100 in balanced salt solution and each animal was given either 0.05 ml by intraperitoneal (ip) inoculation or 0.005 ml by intracerebral (ic) inoculation.

One hundred twenty-three Syrian golden hamsters (Engle Lab Animals, Farmersburg, Ind.) less than 48 hours of age received ip inoculations and 131 received ic inoculations. The suckling hamsters were then observed for signs of illness. Since hamsters are born immature and do not have functioning cochleas until the 20th postnatal day,[12] no obvious signs of auditory defect and disequilibrium could be observed. In initial studies, the animals were killed daily for the first nine days and examined for viral antigens. Subsequently, the majority of animals were killed on days 4-6, when immunofluorescence was the most intense for detailed studies of viral antigen distribution. A total of 88 animal heads were processed for immunofluorescent and histological evaluation. Fifty-eight animals had received ip viral inoculation.

In one experiment, 32 newborn hamsters were inoculated ip with 10^5 $TCID_{50}$ of virus. At 12-hour intervals, two to six animals were killed. From two animals at each time period, cardiac blood, brain and temporal cartilage (free of skin and jaw) were aseptically removed. Individual tissues were homogenized into 10% suspensions and assayed for virus by inoculating tenfold dilutions onto monolayers of CV-1 cells in tissue culture wells. The average of both tissue titers was then determined. Fourteen animal heads at varying 12-hour intervals were also processed for immunofluorescent evaluation of viral antigens in the brain and inner ears.

Optimal preservation of inner ear structures and viral antigens was achieved by fixation of the skinned head in 95% ethanol at 4 C and embedding in paraffin, as previously described.[8] Horizontal sections (4μm) of the head, including both inner ears and the brain, were cut on a rotatory microtome (American Optical, Buffalo, NY) at six to ten levels. At each level, three adjacent sections were made. One slide was stained with hemotoxylin and eosin, Lendrum inclusion body stain,[13] or acridine orange.[14] The second slide was stained with polyvalent reovirus antiserum made in goats (Scientific Resources Branch, Center for Disease Control, Atlanta, Ga.) and then fluorescein-conjugated rabbit antiserum to goat IgG (Cappel Laboratories, Cochranville, Pa.) in the indirect immunofluorescent staining procedure.[8] The third slide served as a control and received nonimmune goat serum and the same fluorescein-conjugated serum.

RESULTS

Animals that received ic viral inoculation began to feed poorly and became lethargic on day 3 and died on days 4 and 5. Animals that received ip viral inoculation became ill on day 4 and slowly died through day 9.

After ip inoculation of 10^5 $TCID_{50}$ of reovirus, virus was repeatedly isolated from blood except at 36 hours (Fig. 1). Recovery of virus from ear and

---

From the Veterans Administration Medical Center and the Department of Neurology, University of New Mexico School of Medicine, Albuquerque.
Supported by Research Service, Veterans Administration Medical Center, USPHS.
REPRINTS — Larry E. Davis, MD, Neurology Service, Veterans Administration Medical Center, 2100 Ridgecrest SE, Albuquerque, NM 87108.

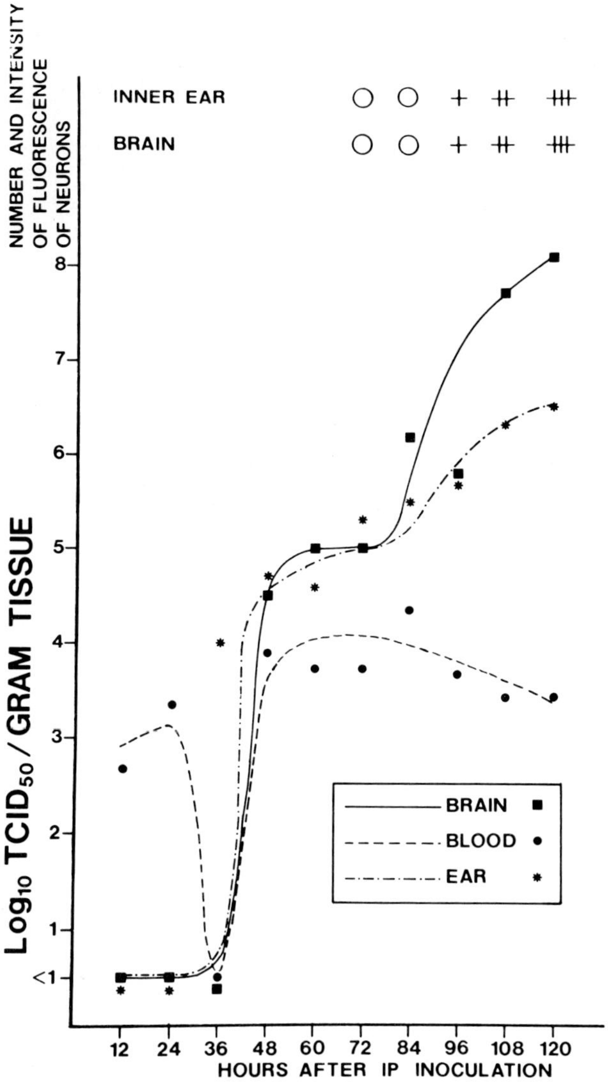

Fig. 1. Recovery of reovirus, type 3, from homogenates of brain, temporal cartilage, and whole blood of newborn hamsters after ip inoculation of 0.05 ml of stock virus. The intensity of fluorescence seen in neurons of the brain and inner ear and number of neurons with fluorescent staining recorded by time at top of graph (0 - No viral antigen, ⧻ - Maximal intensity and number of neurons that show fluorescence).

brain began at 36 and 48 hours respectively. Viral titers then paralleled the blood titer until 84 to 96 hours when they increased markedly over blood levels. The abrupt increase in brain and ear viral titers over the blood titer corresponded to the first appearance of fluorescent viral antigen within neurons of both tissues. No spread of viral antigen from neurons to nonneuronal cells occurred in either the inner ear or brain.

There was no difference in distribution of viral antigen in the inner ear between those animals who received ip versus ic inoculations. However, those animals who received the ic inoculation had a more intense encephalitis that accounted for their early deaths. Reovirus caused an infection of the cell bodies of the neurons in the cochlear and vestibular ganglia. After either route of inoculation, viral antigen was detected in the cytoplasm of the cell body of these neurons but not in their nerve processes (Figs. 2 and 3). Viral antigen was first detected four days after ip inoculation, reached maximal intensity and distribution 1-2 days later, and began to fade by seven days after inoculation. Detection of the viral antigen in the ganglion cells paralleled that seen within the brain (Fig. 1). After day 3, 84% of the animals who received the ip inoculation demonstrated viral infection of the inner ear and from 10 to 70% of the ganglia neurons contained viral antigens. Likewise, 87% of animals receiving ic inoculation developed inner ear infections. No viral antigen was detected within adjacent ganglion satellite cells or within the membranous labyrinth. In spite of intense fluorescent staining of adjacent cochlear and vestibular ganglia neurons, no staining of Corti's organ, macula, of the utricle and saccule, or the cristae of the semicircular canals was observed.

Histological examination of the inner ears demonstrated no inflammatory response to the infection. The organ of Corti, although immature, did not differ from age-matched control animals. The Lendrum stain demonstrated diffuse eosinophilic cytoplasmic staining of selected neuronal cell bodies in the cochlear and vestibular ganglia. Rare discrete eosinophilic inclusions also could be seen in these neurons. This staining pattern was similar to the neurons of the brain and differed from the large cytoplasmic inclusions that have been described.[14] Some ganglion neurons stained with acridine orange demonstrated diffuse green staining or occasional discrete green staining of the cytoplasm. No cytoplasmic inclusions, by Lendrum or acridine orange stains, were seen within the cochlea, saccule, utricle, or semicirclar canals.

DISCUSSION

In this study, ip inoculation of reovirus, type 3, resulted in a viremia that was detected as early as 12 hours after inoculation. Beginning at day 2, a sustained viremia occurred similar to an earlier report.[15] At day 4, fluorescent viral antigen was first detected within neurons of the brain and inner ear. The intensity of fluorescence and number of neurons with viral antigen in the brain and inner ear increased over time in parallel. The appearance of the viral antigen also correlated with the marked increase in viral titers in brain and ear above blood levels. This study did not determine the location of the primary viral infection and source of the early viremia but Papadimitriou has previously shown mesothelial cells of the peritoneal cavity to be the site of initial viral replication after ip injection.[16] Since viral antigen was not seen to spread from neurons to adjacent nonneuronal cells in either the brain or inner ear, this strain of reovirus appears to

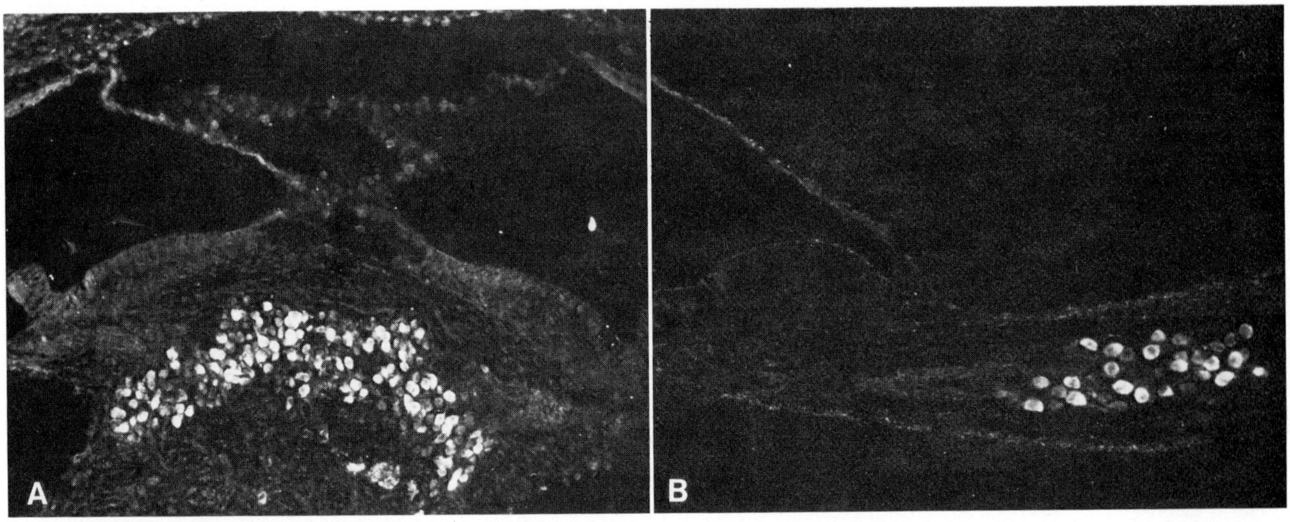

Fig. 2. Evidence of infection of cochlear ganglion neurons of an infant hamster six days after ip inoculation of the Abney strain of reovirus type 3. A) Cell bodies of cochlear ganglion neurons in the upper modiolus of the cochlea show specific fluorescent staining of the cytoplasm (x125). B) Cell bodies of neurons of the basal turn of the cochlea show specific fluorescent staining. In both figures the remaining areas of the cochlea, including the organ of Corti, show no specific fluorescent staining. (x200)

be very neurotropic. These observations demonstrate that the neurons of the brain and the ganglia of the inner ear were infected simultaneously by a viremia. There is no evidence to suggest that the eighth nerve ganglia became infected by viral spread from the brain.

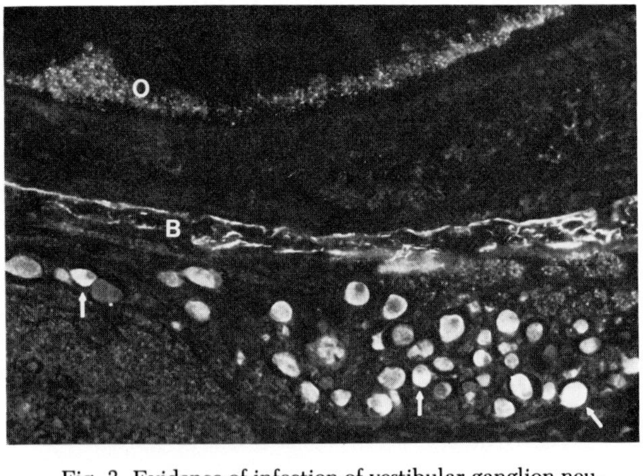

Fig. 3. Evidence of infection of vestibular ganglion neurons of an infant hamster six days after ip inoculation of the Abney strain of reovirus type 3. Specific fluorescent staining of the cytoplasm of neuronal cell bodies is present (arrows). Autofluorescence of otic capsule bone (B) and otoconia of the macula of the utricle (O) is also present. (x380)

Evidence of viral infection of the neurons in the eighth nerve ganglia was demonstrated by detection of viral antigen within neuronal cytoplasm by immunofluorescent and histological stains. Since reovirus RNA is double-stranded, it should stain greenish by acridine orange dye, and such green cytoplasmic inclusions have been reported in tissue culture cells infected with reovirus.[17] In this study, a similar but less discrete green cytoplasmic staining was seen in some neurons of the eighth nerve ganglia and brain.

Reoviruses are ubiquitous and found worldwide. They have been recovered from man and a wide variety of naturally infected mammals.[18] In small animals, most strains of type 3 reovirus have a striking tropism for neurons in the brain resulting in encephalitis.[13,19,20] In man, however, the majority of human infections are asymptomatic or associated with respiratory or diarrheal illness.[11,21] Yet, occasionally type 3 reovirus has caused encephalitis,[19,22,23] demonstrating that the virus is capable of infecting the human nervous system. At present, it is unknown whether reovirus plays a role in causing labyrinthitis and deafness in man.

ACKNOWLEDGMENT — I thank Mrs. Brenda Mitchell and Mr. Jerry Bartyzel for their help.

REFERENCES

1. Alford BR. Rubella-La Bete noire de la medicine. Laryngoscope 1968; 78:1623-59.

2. Myers EN, Stool S. Cytomegalic inclusion disease of the inner ear. Laryngoscope 1968; 78:1904-14.

3. Westmore GA, Pickard BH, Stern H. Isolation of mumps virus from the inner ear after sudden deafness. Br Med J 1979; 1:14-5.

4. Lindsay JR, Davey PR, Ward PH. Inner ear pathology in deafness due to mumps. Ann Otol Rhinol Laryngol 1960; 69:918-35.

5. Lindsay JR, Hemenway WG. Inner ear pathology due to measles. Ann Otol Rhinol Laryngol 1954; 63:754-61.

6. Lindsay JR. Profound childhood deafness: inner ear pathology. Ann Otol Rhinol Laryngol 1973; 82 Suppl 5:103-11.

7. Davis LE, Shurin S, Johnson RT. Experimental viral labyrinthitis. Nature 1975; 254:329-30.

8. Davis LE, Johnson RT. Experimental viral infections of the inner ear: I. Acute infections of the newborn hamster labyrinth. Lab Invest 1976; 34:349-56.

9. Shimokata K, Nishiyama Y, Ito Y, et al. Affinity of Sendai virus for the inner ear of mice. Infect Immunol 1977; 16:706-8.

10. Davis GL, Hawrisiak MW. Experimental cytomegalovirus infection and developing mouse inner ear. Lab Invest 1977; 37:20-9.

11. Rosen L, Houis JF, Masterota FM, Bell JA, Huebner RJ. Observations on a newly recognized virus (Abney) of reovirus family. Am J Hyg 1960; 71:258-65.

12. Stephens CB. Development of the middle ear and inner ear in the golden hamster. Acta Otolaryngol (Stockh) 1972; Suppl 296.

13. Margolis G, Kilham L, Gonatas NK. Reovirus type III encephalitis observations of virus-cell interactions in neural tissue. I. Light microscopy studies. Lab Invest 1971; 24:91-100.

14. Margolis G, Kilham L. Pathogenesis of intrauterine infections in rats due to reovirus type 3. II. Pathologic and fluorescent antibody studies. Lab Invest 1971; 24:101-9.

15. Stanley NF, Dorman DC, Ponsford J. Studies on the hepato-encephalomyelitis virus (HEV). Aust J Exp Biol Med Sci 1954; 32:543-62.

16. Papadimitriou JM. An analysis of the peritonitis in acute murine reovirus infection. Pathology 1979; 11:447-56.

17. Hsiung GD. Diagnostic virology: an illustrated handbook. New Haven: Yale University Press, 1973:46-7.

18. Rosen L. Reoviruses. In: Blair JE, Lennette EH, Truant JP, eds. Manual of clinical microbiology. Bethesda: American Society for Microbioloy, 1970:543-7.

19. Walters MN-I, Joske RA, Leak PJ, et al. Murine infection with reovirus. I. Pathology of the acute phase. Br J Exp Pathol 1963; 44:427-36.

20. Raine CS, Fields BN. Reovirus type III encephalitis — a virologic and ultrastructural study. J Neuropathol Exp Neurol 1973; 32:19-33.

21. Rodriguez WJ, Kim HW, Arrobio JO. Clinical features of acute gastroenteritis associated with human reovirus-like agent in infants and young children. J Pediatr 1977; 91:188-93.

22. Krainer L, Aronson BE. Disseminated encephalomyelitis in the human with recovery of hepatoencephalitis virus (HEV); pathologic and virologic report. J Neuropathol Exp Neurol 1959; 18:339-42.

23. VanTongern HAE. Familial infection with hepatoencephalomyelitis virus in the Netherlands: study on some properties of the infective agent. Arch Ges Virusforsch 1957; 7:429-48.

CARCINOMA OF THE ANTERIOR TONGUE

BRUCE LEIPZIG, MD
LITTLE ROCK, ARKANSAS

CHARLES W. CUMMINGS, MD
SEATTLE, WASHINGTON

CHUNG T. CHUNG, MD
SYRACUSE, NEW YORK

JONAS T. JOHNSON, MD
PITTSBURGH, PENNSYLVANIA

ROBERT H. SAGERMAN, MD
SYRACUSE, NEW YORK

We have reviewed 126 patients with squamous cell carcinoma of the anterior tongue. Our experience suggests that carcinoma of the anterior tongue is a highly aggressive disease. It is no less aggressive and dangerous than carcinoma of the posterior tongue. The clinically negative neck is a problem. Many clinical stage I and II cancers are, in fact, stage III when analyzed by the pathologist. This difficulty in clinical staging results in a significant management problem when stage III carcinomas are treated as stage I and stage II disease. Management, if it is to cure, must be aggressive. An adequate, wide surgical resection will control early carcinoma of the anterior tongue. Advanced cancers of the anterior tongue, clinical stages III and IV, should be widely excised; the cervical lymph nodes on the side of the primary lesion must be treated by surgery and radiation therapy. Treatment of the opposite side of the neck is indicated based on a high rate of metastases to contralateral lymph nodes in this series. Those patients treated with irradiation who had recurrence did so predominantly at the primary site of disease. Patients treated surgically tended to have recurrence in the regional cervical lymphatics.

The literature on the management of carcinoma of the tongue[1-7] reveals conflicting, confusing, and controversial results. Both surgeons and radiotherapists claim success with early lesions while neither group, either singly or in combination, is happy with the poor cure rate and quality of palliation for advanced cancer of the tongue.

Tumors of the anterior two thirds of the tongue are thought to have a more favorable prognosis, and their management is believed to be much less complicated than tumors of the tongue base. Our experience with a series of 126 patients having squamous cell carcinoma of the anterior tongue, each of whom has been followed for at least three years, challenges the view that carcinoma of the anterior tongue is a less aggressive disease. Anterior tongue cancers are extremely capricious lesions and need aggressive treatment. These cancers are no less dangerous than posterior tongue cancers. That base-of-tongue tumors are discovered at a later stage of disease probably is the source of the misconception that the base-of-tongue cancer is a more lethal disease.

An analysis of the cause of failure following treatment of tongue carcinomas emphasizes the fact that too many clinical stage I and II cancers, ie, with clinically negative neck examinations, are in fact stage III when the specimen is examined by the pathologist. The problem which results is that stage I and stage II treatment is given when the disease is, in fact, stage III.

METHODS

One hundred twenty-six patients were treated for squamous cell carcinoma of the anterior tongue during the 6½ years from June 1968 through 1974 at the State University of New York Upstate Medical Center (Table 1). The median age of patients at the time of diagnosis was 60 years. Women comprised 38% of those with tumors in the mobile tongue. All patients were followed for at least three years or until death, and none included in this series were lost to evaluation.

All patients studied were treated by one of three methods. Surgery, regardless of the procedure, was always performed with the intention of cure. Similarly, when radiotherapy was employed alone, a minimum tumor dose of 6,000 rads in six weeks was delivered to the primary tumor and both sides of the neck utilizing a megavoltage linear accelerator. Attempted salvage, either for persistence or recurrence of disease, usually used the treatment modality not yet employed in that patient, ie, surgical salvage for radiation failures and vice versa. A third treatment modality was undertaken as an interdepartmental cooperative program: preoperative radiation to a level of 5,000 rads in five weeks was followed, after a 4- to 6-week therapeutic interval, by a composite jaw-neck resection to include the primary cancer, a portion of the mandible and a radical neck dissection.

Reclassification of all patients was performed at the time of study utilizing data from the time of treatment planning. Staging was performed according to the guidelines of the American Joint Committee for Cancer Staging and End Results Reporting, 1976.

RESULTS

Stage I. Of the 30 stage I patients, 22 were treated initially with surgery and 8 with radiation therapy (Tables 2 and 3). Among those patients treated initially with surgery, 12 (55%) were cured. Three of eight patients (37%) treated with irradiation were cured. Analysis of the site of failure revealed several interesting facts. Eight of the ten patients in whom surgery failed had spread of their lesion to the regional lymphatic drainage of the neck which became clinically apparent after treatment of a primary tumor; three of those eight demon-

From the Departments of Otolaryngology of the University of Texas Medical Branch, Galveston, The University of Washington, Seattle, and the University of Pittsburgh; and the Department of Radiology, Division of Radiotherapy, Upstate Medical Center, Syracuse, New York.

REPRINTS — Bruce Leipzig, MD, Div. of Head and Neck Oncology, Dept. of Otolaryngology, Univ. of Arkansas for Medical Sciences, 4301 W. Markham, Slot 543, Little Rock, AR 72205.

TABLE 1. CARCINOMA OF ANTERIOR TWO-THIRDS TONGUE (N = 126)

Stage	*Patients* No.	*Patients* %
I	30	24
II	31	25
III & IV	65	52
Total	126	100

strated contralateral metastases. Disease in the remaining two surgical patients recurred locally. In other words, eight patients exhibited pathologic stage III disease despite clinical treatment as stage I. An attempt was made to salvage seven of the ten failures. Among these 7 patients, 4 were successfully salvaged, 3 by radical neck dissection and 1 with irradiation.

When radiotherapy was utilized initially, failure most often occurred at the site of the primary tumor. Only one patient among five radiation therapy failures was salvaged surgically, although an attempt was made in all five patients.

Stage II. Thirty-one patients were analyzed (Tables 2 and 3). Sixteen were treated primarily by surgery and 14 primarily with radiation therapy. About one third of each group was cured with initial treatment. One patient initially received combined treatment.

Ten of the surgically treated patients underwent hemiglossectomy. Four of these were cured with initial therapy; six had metastatic disease in the ipsilateral regional lymphatics and were treated with further surgery or radical radiotherapy to 6,000 rads. Nevertheless, all six of these patients expired of distant metastatic disease despite tumor control at the primary site and in the neck.

The remaining six patients underwent composite resection. One was cured initially; one developed extension to the contralateral neck which was controlled by irradiation. One had recurring disease at

TABLE 3. CARCINOMA OF ANTERIOR TWO-THIRDS TONGUE BY FIRST SITE OF FAILURE, STAGE, AND TREATMENT (N = 70)

Stage and Treatment	*First Site of Failure* Local	Regional	Distant	*Total*
Stage I				
Surgery	2	8*	0	10/22
Radiation	3	2	0	5/8
Stage II				
Surgery	1	7†	3	11/16
Radiation	8	1	1	10/14
Stage III				
Surgery	8	1	0	9/13
Radiation	22	5	0	27/31
Combined	2	3	3	8/13

*3/8 in contralateral neck.
†5/7 in contralateral neck (3 - alone, 2 - both).

the site of the primary tumor, but was medically unable to undergo further treatment. Three died of distant metastases without local recurrence.

Only 4 of the 14 patients treated by radiotherapy alone were controlled. Among the ten patients whose treatment failed, eight (80%) failed at the site of the original tumor. Surgery salvaged four of the nine patients in which it was attempted. Thus 8 of the 14 patients were controlled, yielding a total control rate of 59%.

One patient was treated with combined preoperative irradiation. He is without evidence of recurrent disease.

Stages III and IV. Sixty-five patients with advanced disease were studied. Overall survival was 30% with no one therapy showing an advantage (Tables 2 and 3).

A majority of these patients (31 of 57) were treated by radiotherapy because of the advanced state of their lesions and/or their poor medical condition. Control rates were poor with only 4 of the 31 patients so treated responding to the initial course of therapy; 17 of the 27 patients whose initial therapy failed were then operated on despite the initial judgment that an operation would not be tolerated.

TABLE 2. CARCINOMA OF ANTERIOR TWO-THIRDS TONGUE TREATMENT RESULT BY STAGE (N = 118)

Stage and Treatment	*No.*	*NED* No.	*NED* %	*Failed*	*Salvaged*	*Total NED* No.	*Total NED* %
Stage I							
Surgery	22	12	55	10	4*/7	16	70
Radiation	8	3	37	5	1†/5	4	50
Stage II							
Surgery	16	5	31	11	1⨎/6	6	40
Radiation	14	4	29	10	4∮/9	8	59
Combined	1	1		—		1	
Stage III & IV**							
Surgery	13	4	31	9	0/4	4	31
Radiation	31	4	13	27	6§/17	10	32
Combined	13	5	38	8	0/3	5	38

NED - No evidence of disease.
*3 - Radical neck dissection; 1 - Radiation therapy.
†1 - Radical neck dissection.
⨎ - Radiation therapy.
∮3 - Composite; 1 - hemiglossectomy.
§ - Composite.
**Results do not include 8 patients treated palliatively.

Six of these 17 patients were salvaged by radical surgery.

In contrast, initial surgery was more effective in controlling advanced disease in selected patients. Four of 13 patients (31%) were cured in this manner. Among nine failures, salvage was attempted with radical radiotherapy in four patients and was uniformly unsuccessful.

Planned composite resection after 5,000 rads radiotherapy added little to the control of advanced disease. Five of 13 patients were cured by combined therapy, but among the remaining 8 failures, none could be salvaged. Five of these eight patients had recurrent disease within the treatment field (site of primary tumor plus regional lymphatics), while three others succumbed to distant metastatic disease.

DISCUSSION

Control of carcinoma of the anterior two thirds of the tongue is closely related to both the extent of the primary tumor and the state of the regional lymph nodes.[6-8] Analysis of the site of failure of each treatment mode as well as the attempt of secondary treatment to eradicate this failure has confirmed the aggressive nature of this cancer. This challenges the concept of Martin[9] and others that these cancers are less aggressive than tongue base carcinomas.

Small localized lesions (stage I) should be highly curable with either radiation or surgery. In this series, only half (15/30) of our patients were cured by the initial treatment and an additional one third (5/15) were salvaged for a total cure rate of 67%. This reflects the inadequacy of clinical staging procedures; the depth of tumor invasion is important to determine the curability of the tumor.[7] Too many stage I and II cancers are, in fact, pathologic stage III. Aggressive management is mandatory for these patients since few were salvaged by secondary treatment. Radical neck dissection was most successful to cure metastatic disease in cervical lymphatics. Patients who were initially treated with radiotherapy failed predominantly at the site of primary disease, while in surgically treated patients, regional lymphatic extension was the main cause of failure. It is significant that one third of these recurrences were in the opposite side of the neck.

Local control following surgical excision of a small carcinoma (stage I) was very effective; of 22 patients treated in such a manner (wedge resection of the tongue), only 2 had recurring disease at the site of the primary lesion. Over 90% were locally controlled. Recurrence was common in the regional lymphatics.

Regardless of initial therapy, approximately one third of all patients with stage II carcinoma were cured. Patients treated primarily with surgery, as stage I patients, usually had recurring disease in the cervical lymphatics; the disease in five of seven patients recurred in the opposite side of the neck. This again emphasizes the fact that many clinical early-stage carcinomas of the anterior tongue are pathologically advanced carcinomas and should be treated accordingly.

Among stage II patients whose initial surgery was composite elective neck dissection with resection of the primary tumor and mandible, there were no recurrences at the surgical site. The message is that, despite inadequate staging, one should treat the N_0 neck with stage II carcinoma of the anterior tongue. One patient's disease metastasized to the opposite neck; three others succumbed to distant disease three to six years later. In contrast, six of the ten patients who were treated with hemiglossectomy alone had recurrent disease in the ipsilateral neck. The neck metastases were controlled in all six, employing radical radiotherapy and/or radical neck dissection. However, all six eventually died of distant metastases. This suggests that adequate treatment of the clinically negative neck is advisable in stage I and stage II disease because it often behaves as stage III disease. This could be accomplished by cervical lymphadenectomy or radiotherapy.

Advanced carcinoma was the only lesion for which planned combined therapy was attempted. This therapy was not more effective than either surgery or radiotherapy alone. Among 13 patients treated, 8 failed to respond to their treatment regimen. This poor control may be due to inadequate surgical extirpation, a pattern which was also present in patients treated with surgery alone. Margins at the site of the primary tumor were too close in several cases despite extensive procedures, and these patients had recurrence at the site of the primary tumor. An adequate procedure, guided by frozen section histologic examination of surgical margins in the operating room, should be more effective in controlling advanced carcinoma of the anterior two thirds of the tongue. This seems obvious, but is often neglected. This may require subtotal or total glossectomy and the patient should be so advised. Local recurrence was rare in patients whose margins were adequate histologically, and those who failed usually succumbed to distant metastases.

In those patients who received radical radiotherapy, 6 of 17 failures were controlled with adequate composite resection.

CONCLUSIONS

Despite early clinical diagnosis of carcinoma of the anterior two thirds of the tongue, the data support aggressive treatment of these tumors. Our experience suggests that carcinoma of the anterior tongue is as aggressive and dangerous as carcinoma of the posterior tongue. Management, if it is to cure, must be radical.

Stage I and II cancers are often actually stage III

cancers, with subclinical disease in the regional cervical lymphatics. Failure to recognize this fact may cause delayed treatment of neck disease and/or inadequate treatment of primary disease. Adequate surgery usually controlled primary local disease; neck metastasis was most often salvaged with a delayed radical neck dissection. Radiotherapy for cure of these early lesions was less successful to control local primary disease; observation with the expectation of surgical salvage was usually unsuccessful.

For clinically advanced lesions, there is no evidence that combined therapy is superior to surgery alone. Surgery should include a wide excision guided by histologic examination of the margins; the ipsilateral neck must be treated by surgery and radiation therapy. Radical radiotherapy for cure was seldom successful; radiation salvage did not work at all. Control of subclinical disease by radiotherapy in the contralateral neck is indicated based on its high rate of occurrence in these tongue carcinomas.

REFERENCES

1. Chu A, Fletcher GH. Incidence and causes of failure to control by irradiation the primary lesions in squamous cell carcinomas of the anterior two-thirds of the tongue and floor of mouth. Am J Roentgenol Radium Ther Nucl Med 1973; 117:502-8.

2. Lees AW. The treatment of carcinoma of the anterior two-thirds of the tongue by radiotherapy. Int J Radiat Oncol Biol Phys 1976; 1:849-58.

3. Maddox WA, Sherlock EC, Evans WB. Cancer of the tongue: review of thirteen years experience. Am Surg 1971; 37:642-5.

4. Spiro RH, Strong EW. Surgical treatment of cancer of the tongue. Surg Clin North Am 1974; 54:4-12.

5. Spiro RH, Strong EW. Discontinuous partial glossectomy and radical neck dissection in selected patients with epidermoid carcinoma of the mobile tongue. Am J Surg 1973; 126:554-6.

6. Mendelson BC, Woods JE, Beahrs OH. Neck dissection in the treatment of carcinoma of the anterior two-thirds of the tongue. Surg Gynecol Obstet 1976; 143:75-80.

7. Johnson JT, Leipzig B, Cummings CW. Management of T_1 carcinoma of the anterior tongue. Arch Otolaryngol 1980; 106:249-52.

8. Droulias C, Whitehurst JO. The lymphatics of the tongue in relation to cancer. Am Surg 1976; 42:670-4.

9. Martin HE. Surgery of head and neck tumors. New York: Hoeber-Harper, 1957.

COMBINED PECTORALIS MAJOR MYOCUTANEOUS FLAP WITH MEDIALLY BASED DELTOPECTORAL FLAP FOR CLOSURE OF LARGE PHARYNGOCUTANEOUS FISTULAS

ROBERT H. MAISEL, MD STEPHEN L. LISTON, MD

MINNEAPOLIS, MINNESOTA

The pectoralis major myocutaneous flap has become the new and heavily used tool for head and neck reconstruction. This flap is reliable, versatile and allows moving large blocks of skin and soft tissue quickly, with little morbidity to the donor site. This paper describes the concept of combining the pectoralis flap with an ipsilateral medially based deltopectoral flap, to reconstruct a large pharyngostome. The skin incisions must be correctly drawn and the flaps elevated in sequence to prevent interruption of blood supply to the deltopectoral flap. Using the techniques described in the paper, rapid rehabilitation with little morbidity can be achieved.

The pectoralis major myocutaneous flap represents a new concept in reconstructive head and neck surgery.[1] The idea of the myocutaneous flap was introduced as a latissimus dorsi flap for breast reconstruction at the turn of the century by Tansini.[2,3] The thought lay dormant until the 1950s when local myocutaneous flaps were used to reconstruct the palate,[4] the leg,[5] and the breast. McGregor,[6] working during the 1960s, described both an arterially based forehead skin flap and a groin flap, gaining his perception of these flaps from the medially based deltopectoral skin flap popularized by Bakamjian.[7] McGregor and Morgan pursued their ideas about flaps further and defined both axial and random pattern skin flaps.[8]

The surgical advantage of an axial flap, which has a recognizable arterial and venous circulation that the long axis of the flap can follow and which yields branches to the dermal-subdermal plexus, is clear. Such a flap has no length-to-width restriction, but is limited only by the length of the arterial pedicle. The pectoralis major muscle has a vascular path from the thoracoacromial (an axial segmental artery), which branches from the axillary artery.

Large flat-bellied muscles of the neck and torso (latissimus dorsi, trapezius and pectoralis major) represent available axial myocutaneous flaps and the skin over these flaps is fed by musculocutaneous perforating vessels from the deep segmental vessels. The gross and microscopic surgical anatomy of the pectoralis major muscle has been defined and the pectoralis branches of the thoracoacromial vessels traverse the deep surface of the pectoralis major on an axis from the acromion to the xiphoid, after they have pierced the clavipectoral fascia at the upper border of the pectoralis minor muscle.[9-11]

The pectoralis major myocutaneous flap can be elevated as an island flap and can be freed from its heads of origin at the medial half of the clavicle, the anterior sternum and adjacent upper six costal cartilages, and occasionally the aponeurosis of the abdominal external oblique muscle, to increase mobility. Similarly, its insertion into the humerus can also be interrupted.

The flap has become widely used and it performs admirably as a skin island flap used for skin coverage in the head and neck as well as for mucosal reconstruction in the pharynx and esophagus.

The workhorse flap of the past 15 years for head and neck reconstruction has been the medially based deltopectoral skin flap. This has been the standard technique for closure of large pharyngostomes or esophagostomes with anterior neck resurfacing. Many procedures have been conceived, from Wookey's[12] technique and other local flaps to the use of bilateral deltopectoral flaps.[13,14] The risk of failure and tissue necrosis from local flaps after neck dissection or heavy radiation mitigates against them. Bilateral medially based deltopectoral flaps require multiple procedures, and while successful, require extensive skin grafting and staging. We describe a combination of pectoralis major myocutaneous flap for the inner lining, and skin resurfacing with an ipsilateral medially based deltopectoral flap.

CASE REPORT

A 70-year-old male was seen for odynophagia with radiation of pain to the right ear. Indirect laryngoscopy showed an ulcerative, suprahyoid squamous carcinoma of the laryngeal surface of the epiglottis. Direct laryngoscopy and biopsy confirmed the size, location, and diagnosis. The patient had severe restrictive and obstructive pulmonary disease and full course x-ray therapy was elected for his treatment. At eight weeks postcompletion of x-ray therapy, residual tumor was obvious, and the pain had returned. No neck nodes were palpable. A wide-field laryngectomy was performed following confirmatory biopsy 12 weeks after x-ray therapy. The lesion at the time of surgery appeared to involve 50% of the epiglottis with invasion through to the lingual surface and with vallecular involvement.

From the Departments of Otolaryngology of the University of Minnesota and Hennepin County Medical Center, Minneapolis.

REPRINTS — Robert H. Maisel, MD, Hennepin County Medical Center, 701 Park Avenue South, Minneapolis, MN 55415.

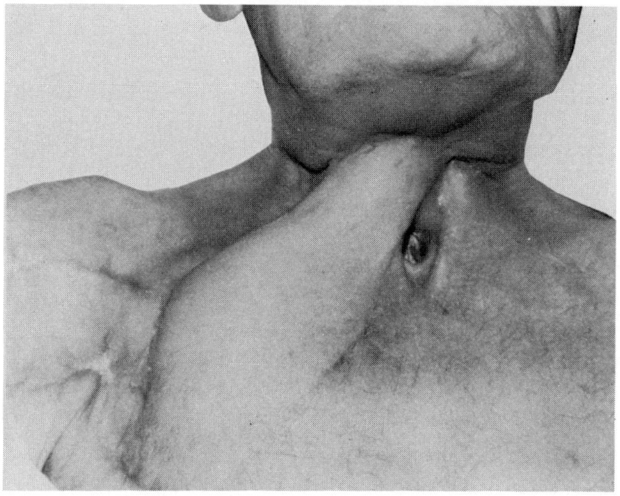

Fig. 1. Patient is shown 12 weeks after surgery with all wounds healed.

Healing was complicated by a pharyngocutaneous fistula evident on day 10 and treated by incision and drainage of the neck skin with midline diversion of the salivary stream. The wound was cleaned and debrided over the next 20 days in the hospital and the patient discharged with a 5-cm pharyngeal opening and an 8 x 10 cm skin dehiscence. Six weeks of home care demonstrated no shrinkage of the fistula and the patient was admitted for a combined right pectoralis major myocutaneous flap with a right medially based deltopectoral flap.

Early healing appeared excellent but at six days, a draining fistula was noted at the superior lateral junction of the flaps with the recipient bed. This area and a dehiscent 1-cm superior skin layer of the deltopectoral flap, where it met the recipient neck skin, were treated by debridement and continuous suction to the pharynx through the fistula for ten days. The patient was then discharged and the wounds closed by secondary intention over a period of three weeks. The neck is presently completely healed and the patient is swallowing and using a Blom-Singer tube for speech (Fig. 1).

DISCUSSION

This case addresses the versatility and survivability of the pectoralis major myocutaneous flap and indicates a new combination of available flaps. The pectoralis major flap appears to be the most suitable vascular regional flap,[1,11,15] and has survived in all cases when used by the present authors as well as in those described by the recent literature.[16] Failures have occurred secondary to the torsion of the pedicle and hematoma but the flap when carefully designed and correctly placed should survive in every case. The surgeon's attention to gentle handling of the tissues near the pedicle and meticulous attention to hemostasis with the use of suction drainage makes this flap successful. The skin edges frequently require secondary healing to grow satisfactorily to the heavily radiated recipient bed but with good local wound technique, excellent healing will occur and only a single procedure will be required.

The present case describes our use of the pectoralis major flap with deltopectoral flap to close a large pharyngocutaneous fistula with skin breakdown in a two-flap, single-staged operation which further confirms the value of this new flap to the head and neck surgeon.

The technique of the pectoralis major myocutaneous flap has been described elsewhere.[9-11,16] Our recommendation, which builds on the observation of Theogaraj et al,[11] is that when both a pectoralis major myocutaneous flap and a deltopectoral flap are considered either synchronously or metachronously, the skin incision should be outlined as shown in Figure 2. When used simultaneously the superiorly based skin island should begin from the inferior transverse line demarcating the deltopectoral flap. This is similar to Shumrick's concept of using the inferior limb of a Macfee neck dissection incision as the superior incision of a deltopectoral flap used for pharyngeal reconstruction.[17]

The pectoralis major flap can be used as a transfer for an island of skin with muscle as a secondary

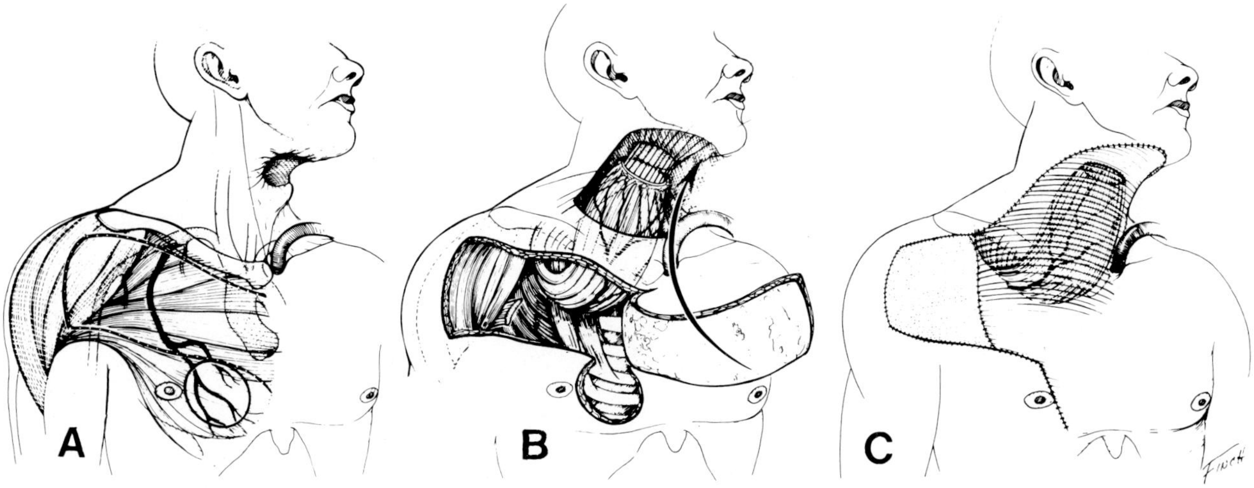

Fig. 2. A) The skin paddle of the myocutaneous pectoralis major flap is outlined immediately subjacent to the medially based deltopectoral flap. B) The skin and soft tissue around the pharyngocutaneous fistula is debrided to healthy tissue and prepared for receiving the sandwich graft. The latter is elevated and then the myocutaneous flap is developed and sutured, skin side inward, to the pharynx (arrow). C) It is then covered by the deltopectoral flap. The donor site is sutured closed with a split thickness skin graft to cover laterally where primary closure was difficult.

procedure after a deltopectoral flap since the incision for the former is merely a road to the muscle proximally, and the skin island of the pectoralis muscle flap is placed inferior to the deltopectoral incisions.

The reverse is probably not true since the axial (pectoral) part of the deltopectoral flap demands that no vertical incision of the chest skin and subcutaneous tissue cross the tissue to be included in the flap. Therefore, it is requisite in doing a combined flap or in performing a myocutaneous pectoralis major flap in a patient where a subsequent ipsilateral deltopectoral flap is to be considered[11] to outline the inferior transverse skin incision of the deltopectoral flap before initiating the shoulder-to-xiphoid incision recommended by Ariyan and Cuono.[1] This elevation permits full use of either flap without compromise and allows one side of the chest to be used for both layers of the closure of a large midline pharyngeal fistula or planned full-thickness pharyngeal and neck resection.

REFERENCES

1. Ariyan S, Cuono CB. Myocutaneous flaps for head and neck reconstruction. Head Neck Surg 1980; 3:321-45.

2. Tansini I. Nuovo processo per l'amputazione delta mammaella per cancro. La Riforma Medica 1896; 12:3-5.

3. Owens N. A compound neck pedicle designed for repair of massive facial defects: formation, development and application. Plast Reconstr Surg 1955; 15:369-89.

4. Bakamjian VY. A technique for primary reconstruction of the palate after radical maxillectomy for cancer. Plast Reconstr Surg 1963; 31:103-17.

5. Orticochea M. The musculo-cutaneous flap method: an immediate and heroic substitute for the method of delay. Br J Plast Surg 1972; 25:106-10.

6. McGregor IA. The temporal flap in intra-oral cancer: its role in repairing the post-excisional defect. Br J Plast Surg 1963; 16:318-35.

7. Bakamjian VY. A two-stage method for pharyngoesophageal reconstruction with a primary pectoral skin flap. Plast Reconstr Surg 1965; 36:173-84.

8. McGregor IA, Morgan G. Axial and random pattern flaps. Br J Plast Surg 1973; 26:202-13.

9. Ariyan S. The pectoralis major myocutaneous flap. A versatile flap for reconstruction in the head and neck. Plast Reconstr Surg 1979; 63:73-80.

10. Baek S, Biller HF, Krespi YP, Lawson W. The pectoralis major myocutaneous island flap for reconstruction of the head and neck. Head Neck Surg 1979; 2:293-300.

11. Theogaraj SD, Merritt WH, Acharya G, Cohen IK. The pectoralis major musculocutaneous island flap in single stage reconstruction of the pharyngoesophageal region. Plast Reconstr Surg 1980; 65:267-76.

12. Wookey H. Surgical treatment of carcinoma of the pharynx and upper esophagus. Surg Gynecol Obstet 1942; 75:499-506.

13. Ogura JH, Dedo HH. Repair of large pharyngostoma utilizing bilateral non-delayed regional pedicle flaps. Laryngoscope 1965; 75:588-600.

14. Petty CT, Theogaraj SD, Cohen IK. Secondary reconstruction of the cervical esophagus. Plast Reconstr Surg 1975; 56:70-6.

15. Ariyan S. Further experiences with the pectoralis major myocutaneous flap for the immediate repair of defects from excisions of head and neck cancer. Plast Reconstr Surg 1979; 64:605-12.

16. Maisel RH, Liston S. How I do it: the pectoralis major myocutaneous island flap. Laryngoscope 1980; 90:2051-6.

17. Shumrick DA. Reconstructive flaps in head and neck surgery. In: Paparella MM, Shumrick DA, eds. Otolaryngology, 2nd ed, vol. 3. Philadelphia: Saunders, 1980: 2878-92.

Ann Otol 91:1982

CHARACTERISTICS OF TISSUE PLASMINOGEN ACTIVATOR FROM PARANASAL MUCOUS MEMBRANE IN CHRONIC SINUSITIS

T. KOSUGI, MD

O. MATSUO, MD

H. MIHARA, MD

MIYAZAKI, JAPAN

K. HIRANO, MD

YOKOHAMA, JAPAN

M. HAMAYA, MD

SAITAMA, JAPAN

Tissue extract of paranasal mucous membrane from patients with chronic sinusitis was found to show a large lysis area on plasminogen-rich fibrin plates, but not on plasminogen-free fibrin plates. This indicates the existence of tissue plasminogen activator in the tissue extract. Further studies by the gel filtration technique showed that two plasminogen activators of different molecular weights were present in the tissue extract. The existence of tissue plasminogen activator with a low molecular weight has not previously been reported. This activator is labile at neutral pH at 37° C, but stable on fibrin under the above conditions. The molecular weight of this compound is lower than that of cytochrome c. It may be a compound which is proteolytically modified by proteases, ie, trypsin-like enzymes, existing in the paranasal mucous membrane tissue of patients with chronic sinusitis.

INTRODUCTION

Plasminogen activator has been reported to exist in various body fluids and organs. These include urine,[1,2] milk,[3] bile,[4] saliva,[5] tracheobronchial secretions,[6] tissue extracts of various organs,[7,8] and leukocytes[9] and macrophages[10,11] in the circulating blood. In the otorhinolaryngological field, large amounts of tissue plasminogen activator (TA) have been reported to exist in the nasal and paranasal mucous membranes.[12-14]

The present paper deals with TA from the paranasal mucous membrane of patients with chronic sinusitis, and attempts to clarify some of the biochemical properties of the TA which may play an important role in modifying the inflammatory responses.

METHODS

Acetone Powder Preparation from Paranasal Mucous Membrane. Paranasal mucous membrane surgically removed from 30 patients with chronic sinusitis was dissected into small pieces in a cold room (4° C), and washed many times with cold physiological saline to exclude contaminant blood and pus. The fragmented pieces of tissue were then centrifuged at 3,000 rpm at 4° C for 15 minutes. After discarding the supernatant, cold acetone was added to the precipitate in the proportion of 10 ml/1 g of tissue, and the mixture was homogenized for 15 minutes in the cold room with an Ultra homomixer (Nihon Seiki Kaisha Ltd.). The homogenate was then filtered through a filter paper and the retained fraction was dried in vacuo.

Extraction of TA from the Acetone Powder Preparation. Fifty milliliters of 2 M KCl was added to 3 g of the acetone powder, and the suspended solution was stirred for six hours at 4° C. After centrifugation at 3,000 rpm for 15 minutes, the supernatant obtained was diluted ten times with phosphate buffer (M/15, pH 6.8) for use as starting material in the subsequent investigations.

Reagents. Fibrinogen (Cohn's fraction I, bovine, Miles Laboratory) was dissolved in borate saline buffer (pH 7.8). Thrombin (bovine, Mochida Pharm. Co. Ltd.) was dissolved in physiological saline. Trypsin (lyophilized, 238 units/mg, Worthington Biochem. Co. Ltd.) was dissolved in phosphate buffer (M/15, pH 6.8). Papain (a sodium acetate suspension of the recrystallized powder, Sigma Biochem. Co. Ltd.) was dissolved in phosphate buffer (M/15, pH 6.8). Streptokinase (SK), (Kabikinase®, Kabi Laboratory) was dissolved in physiological saline. Lysine-sepharose (sepharose 4B substituted with L-lysine, Daiichi Pure Chem. Co. Ltd.) was prepared.

As synthetic inhibitors, N-α-p-tosyl-L-lysine chloromethyl ketone HCl (TLCK), p-chloromercuri-benzoic acid (PCMB) (Sigma Biochem. Co. Ltd.), and trans-4-aminomethylcyclohexane-1-carboxylic acid (t-AMCHA) (Daiichi Pharm. Co. Ltd.) were dissolved in phosphate buffer (M/15, pH 6.8). Sephadex® G-50 and G-200 (Pharmacia Fine Chem. Co. Ltd.) were swollen with phosphate buffer (M/15, pH 6.8).

Determination of Protease and Plasminogen Activator Activities in the Extract. To estimate the protease and plasminogen activator activities, standard fibrin plates (st. plates) and plasminogen-free fibrin plates (free plates) were used. The st. plates were prepared from plasminogen-rich fibrinogen and thrombin as described by Astrup and Müllertz.[15] Plasminogen-free fibrinogen was prepared by affinity chromatography using lysine-sepharose[16-18] and used to make the free plates as described by Astrup and Müllertz.[15]

Fractionation of the TA Preparation with Ammonium Sulphate. The TA preparation (starting material) was fractionated at 4° C by adding solid ammonium sulphate to 33% saturation. The solution was centrifuged at 3,000 rpm at 4° C for 15 minutes and the precipitate obtained was dissolved in phosphate buffer (M/15, pH 6.8). The supernatant was fractionated at 4° C by the addition of solid ammonium sulphate to 50% saturation according to Dixon's method.[19] Finally, the supernatant was fractionated at 4° C in ammonium sulphate at 75% saturation. The details of the fractionation procedures with ammonium sulphate are summarized in Figure 1.

Gel Filtration of the Above Fraction. Gel filtration for desalting the ammonium sulphate from the precipitate and for analyzing the molecular size of the TA was carried out according to

From the Department of Physiology, Miyazaki Medical College, Miyazaki, Japan; the Kouhoku Ear Nose and Throat Hospital, Yokohama, Japan; and the Department of Otorhinolaryngology, Saitama Medical College, Saitama, Japan.

REPRINTS — T. Kosugi, MD, Department of Physiology, Miyazaki Medical College, 5200 Kihara, Kiyotake-cho, Miyazaki-gun, Miyazaki-ken 889-16, Japan.

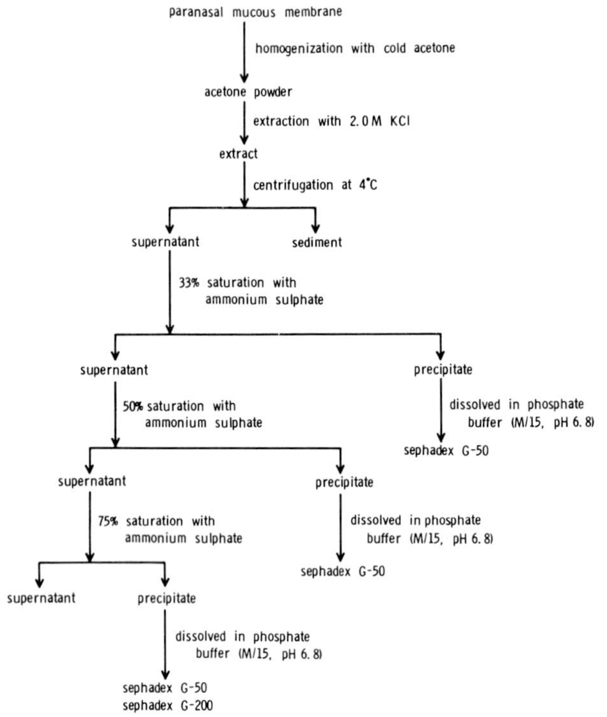

Fig. 1. Fractionation procedures of tissue extract with ammonium sulphate.

Flodin and Killander's procedure.[20] A 1.6 x 70 cm Sephadex G-200 column and a 2.6 x 40 cm Sephadex G-50 column were equilibrated with phosphate buffer (M/15, pH 6.8) at 4° C. The eluate was collected using an automatic fraction collector (LKB); 2.6 ml was collected in a test tube on Sephadex G-200 and 5.2 ml was collected in a test tube on Sephadex G-50. The protein concentration of the eluate was measured with a spectrophotometer (Hitachi) at 280 nm.

Determination of the Inhibitory Effect of Synthetic Inhibitors on the TA with Low Molecular Weight. The inhibitory activity of three synthetic inhibitors (t-AMCHA, TLCK and PCMB) on the TA with low molecular weight was estimated using st. plates containing the inhibitors at concentrations of from 10^{-7} to 10^{-2} M.

Estimation of the pH and Thermostability of the TA With Low Molecular Weight. The solution of low molecular weight TA was adjusted to pH 3-9 with 0.1 M HCl or solid TRIS (hydroxymethyl) aminomethane and the mixture was then heated for 30, 60 or 120 minutes at 37° C or 60° C. Solutions so treated were cooled to 0° C in ice water, neutralized to pH 7 and immediately applied to st. plates.

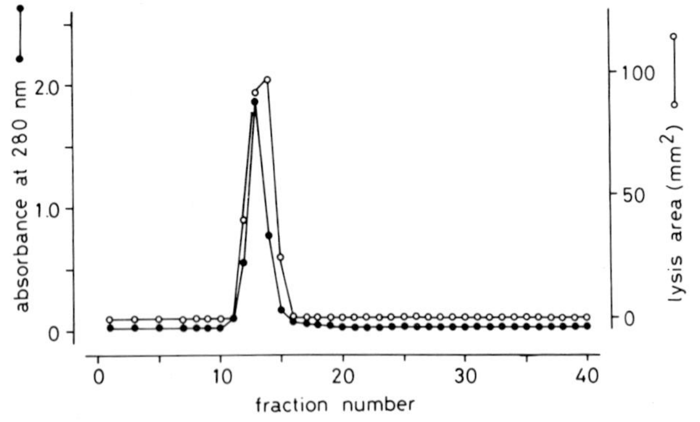

Fig. 2. Gel filtration of the 33% ammonium sulphate precipitate on Sephadex G-50. The activities of the fractions were determined by the standard fibrin (st.) plates.

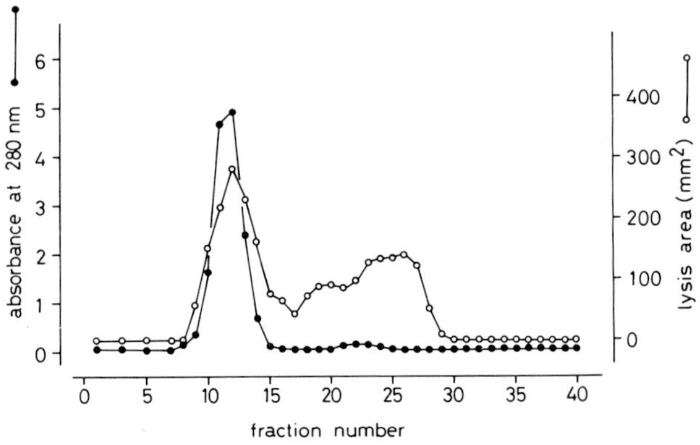

Fig. 3. Gel filtration of the 50% ammonium sulphate precipitate on Sephadex G-50. The activities of the fractions were determined by the st. plates.

RESULTS

Gel Filtration of Ammonium Sulphate Precipitates. When the fibrinolytic activities of the fractions were measured on st. plates, the 33% ammonium sulphate precipitate from the extract showed one peak of fibrinolytic activity on Sephadex G-50 gel (Fig. 2). However, the 50% and 75% ammonium sulphate precipitates revealed two peaks of activity on the same gels (Figs. 3 and 4). On the other hand, when the fibrinolytic activities of the fractions were measured on free plates, no fibrinolytic activities were observed in the 33%, 50%, and 75% ammonium sulphate precipitates.

Molecular Weight of the TA. The 75% ammonium sulphate precipitate presented two peaks of fibrinolytic activity on Sephadex G-200 gel (Fig. 5) as well as on Sephadex G-50 gel. The eluates containing compounds of high molecular weight showed the properties of plasminogen activator and SK-reactive activator (proactivator), but the eluates containing low molecular weight compounds showed the properties of plasminogen activator only (unpublished data). In the determination of

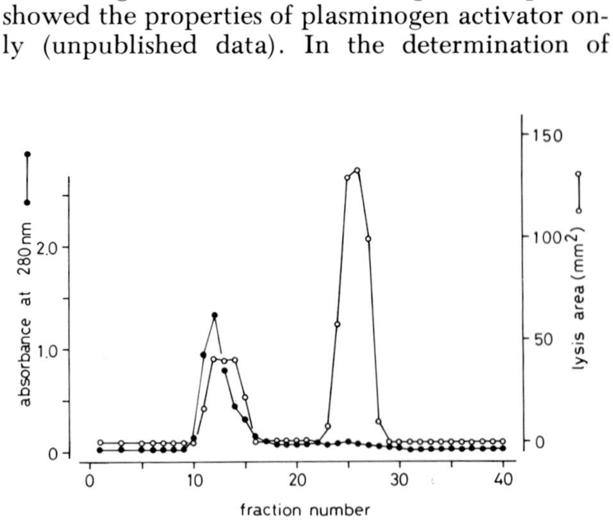

Fig. 4. Gel filtration of the 75% ammonium sulphate precipitate on Sephadex G-50. The activities of the fractions were determined by the st. plates.

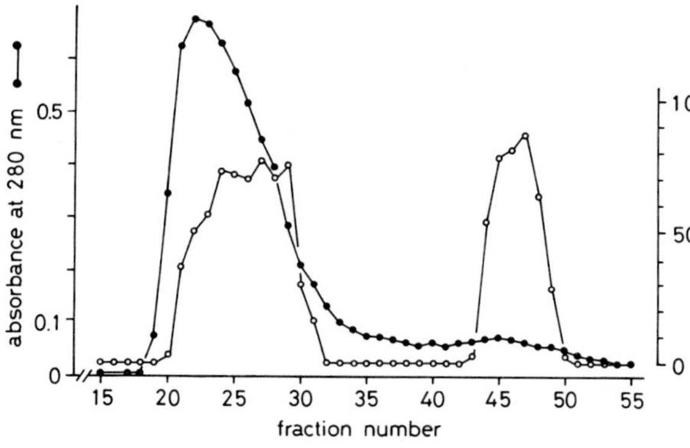

Fig. 5. Gel filtration of the 75% ammonium sulphate precipitate on Sephadex G-200. The activities of the fractions were determined by the st. plates.

molecular weight, the TA with low molecular weight eluated later than cytochrome c (Fig. 6).

Effect of Synthetic Inhibitors on the TA with Low Molecular Weight. At a 5 x 10^{-6} molar concentration, t-AMCHA inhibited the activity of the TA with low molecular weight most. At a 10^{-5} molar concentration, PCMB and TLCK did not inhibit the activity of the TA with low molecular weight (Fig. 7).

Stability of the TA with Low Molecular Weight. Maximum fibrinolytic activity was observed at pH 6.8 and a low level of fibrinolytic activity was observed at pH 3.0. As regards thermostability, the TA with low molecular weight was labile at 37° C, at pH 6.8 and 8.2. Almost all of the fibrinolytic activity was lost on heating at 60° C (Fig. 8).

DISCUSSION

Some of the characteristics of the TA in nondefatted paranasal mucous membrane from patients with chronic sinusitis have been described by Miura[21] and Okanishi.[22] Recently, however, extraction from defatted tissue has been reported to be ap-

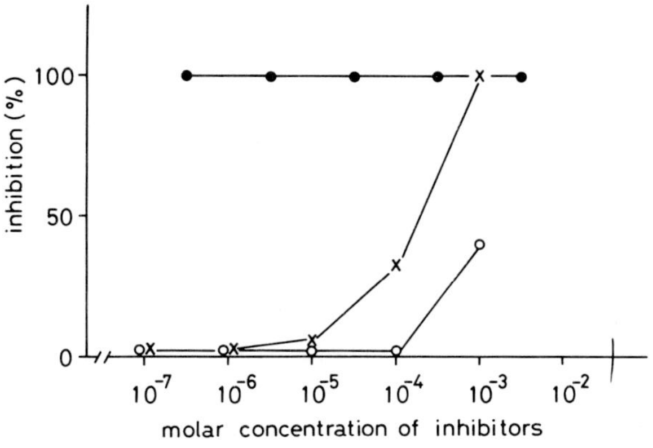

Fig. 7. Effect of synthetic inhibitors on the TA with low molecular weight. ● ———— ● - t-AMCHA; x————x - PCMB; ○————○ - TLCK.

propriate for the purification of TA, since if lipids contaminate the TA, the solubility of the TA should decrease leading to TA aggregation.[23] Accordingly, we made an acetone powder preparation from paranasal mucous membrane using the methods of Hijikata et al[24] and Bachmann et al.[25]

In the extract of the acetone powder preparation, fibrinolytic activity was detected on plasminogen-rich fibrin plates but not on plasminogen-free fibrin plates. Based on this result, it can be said that plasminogen activator is present in the extract but other proteolytic enzymes, including plasmin, are not. Furthermore, the TA preparation was purified partially on using the ammonium sulphate precipitation and gel filtration techniques to clarify some of the properties of the TA. On Sephadex G-50 gel, the precipitate prepared with 33% ammonium sulphate was found to contain only TA with a high molecular weight or SK-reactive activator (proactivator), whereas precipitates prepared with 50% or 75% ammonium sulphate contained two kinds of TA with different (high and low) molecular weights. Although the physicochemical properties of the TA with high molecular weight were not in-

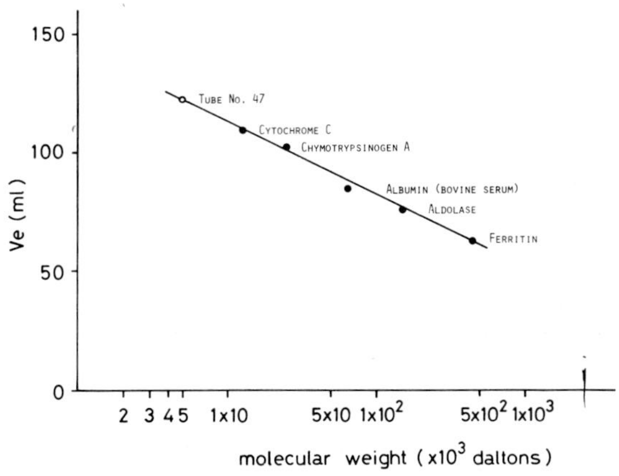

Fig. 6. Molecular weight determination of the tissue plasminogen activator (TA) with low molecular weight and some standard proteins using Sephadex G-200. Ve - Eluated volume.

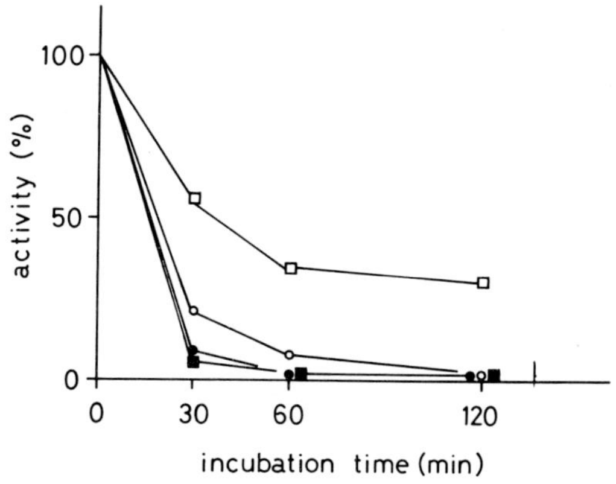

Fig. 8. Stability of the TA with low molecular weight. ○————○ - Heating at 37° C, pH 6.8; ●————● - Heating at 60° C, pH 6.8; □————□ - Heating at 37° C, pH 8.2; ■————■ - Heating at 60° C, pH 8.2.

vestigated in detail in the present study, it was thought that they might well be similar to those of the SK-reactive activator (proactivator) in antrochoanal polyps.[26] The physiocochemical properties of the TA with high molecular weight in the paranasal mucous membrane of patients with chronic sinusitis are now being studied further.

The TA with low molecular weight was found in the precipitates prepared with 50% or 75% ammonium sulphate on Sephadex G-50 and G-200. The molecular weight of this TA was less than that of cytochrome c (12,000 daltons), ie, some 5,000 to 10,000 daltons, based on determinations by gel filtration on Sephadex G-200.

The molecular weights of TA obtained from various organs have so far been determined by only a few investigators.[27-30] The general molecular weight range of the TA has been from 46,000 to 69,000 daltons. However, Cartwright reported that the molecular weight of TA from porcine parotid glands is 20,000 to 25,000 daltons.[31] Even so, the TA in the present paper clearly exhibits the lowest molecular weight so far determined.

The effect of synthetic proteinase inhibitors on the TA with low molecular weight was investigated using fibrin plates. At a concentration of 5×10^{-6} M, t-AMCHA inhibited the fibrinolytic activity of the TA strongly, but PCMB and TLCK showed no inhibition at a concentration of 10^{-5} M. These results indicate that the fibrinolytic enzyme with low molecular weight is not an SH-protease or a trypsin-like enzyme, but is a plasmin or plasminogen activator. In fact, because the fibrinolytic enzyme did not show a lytic zone on free plates, it can be concluded that this fibrinolytic enzyme is a plasminogen activator. Observations of the pH stability revealed that the TA with low molecular weight was similar in properties to the TA obtained from pig heart and ovary. However, observations of the thermostability showed that the TA with low molecular weight was extremely thermolabile, in contrast to other TAs so far reported.

It is suggested that TA with the above properties is produced by a mechanism involving proteases, ie, trypsin-like enzymes, at the locus of the chronic inflammation in the paranasal mucous membrane. Such proteases are thought to react with the TA of high molecular weight resulting in the production of TA with low molecular weight.

REFERENCES

1. Sgouris JT, Inman JK, McCall KB. The preparation of urokinase. Am J Cardiol 1960; 6:406-8.

2. Cellandar DR, Guest MM. The biochemistry and physiology of urokinase. Am J Cardiol 1960; 6:409-19.

3. Okamoto U, Nagamatsu Y, Matsumoto M. Studies on a plasminogen activating system in human milk: I. Isolation of plasminogen activator and proactivator from human milk, and estimation of their molecular weights. Acta Haematol Jpn 1974; 37:57-67.

4. Oshiba S, Ariga T. Purification and characterization of bilokinase, a biliary plasminogen activator, abstracted. Thromb Diath Haemorrh 1975; 34:319.

5. Albrechtsen OK, Thaysen JH. Fibrinolytic activity in human saliva. Acta Physiol Scand 1955; 34:138-45.

6. Kosugi T, Morimitsu T, Matsuo O, Mihara H. Fibrinolytic enzyme in tracheobronchial secretion of rats: existence of plasminogen activator. Laryngoscope 1980; 90:1045-51.

7. Astrup T, Sterndorff I. Fibrinolytic activity of tissue extracts and of trypsin. Nature 1952; 170:981.

8. Astrup T. Tissue activators of plasminogen. Fed Proc 1966; 25:42-51.

9. Henderson BW, Horwitz DL, Astrup T. Release of plasminogen activator from viable leukocytes of man, baboon, dog and rabbits. Exp Biol Med 1972; 141:634-8.

10. Vassalli JD, Reich E. Macrophage plasminogen activator induction by products of activated lymphoid cells. J Exp Med 1977; 145:429-37.

11. Werb Z. Biochemical action of glucocorticoids on macrophages in culture: specific inhibitor of elastase, collagenase and plasminogen activator secretion and effects on other metabolic functions. J Exp Med 1978; 147:1695-712.

12. Sasaki Y, Okamoto S, Ohwada K, Nishibata T. Some observations on a remarkable fibrinolytic activity in the extract of nasal tissues and related tissue. Keio J Med 1959; 8:235-46.

13. Sasaki Y. The electrophoretic analysis of the nasal fibrinolytic enzyme. Acta Otolaryngol (Stockh) 1968; 65:346-58.

14. Kosugi T, Matsuo O, Mihara H, Hamaya M. Study of plasminogen tissue activator in paranasal mucous membrane. J Jpn Rhinol Soc 1977; 16:92-3.

15. Astrup T, Müllertz S. The fibrin plate method for estimating fibrinolytic activity. Arch Biochem Biophys 1952; 40:346-51.

16. Matsuda M, Iwanaga S, Nakamura S. A simple, large scale method for preparation of plasminogen-free fibrinogen. Thromb Res 1972-1:619-32.

17. Matsumoto M, Igarashi M, Moroi M, Urita Y, Takuchi S, Asada T. Assay of plasma plasmin and plasminogen by affinity chromatography. J Med Soc Toho 1973; 20:83-7.

18. Deutsch D, Mertz E. Plasminogen, purification from human plasma by affinity chromatography. Science 1970; 170:1095-6.

19. Dixon M. A nomogram for ammonium sulfate solutions. Biochem J 1953; 54:457-8.

20. Flodin C, Killander J. Fractionation of human serum proteins by gel filtration. Biochim Biophys Acta 1963; 63:403-10.

21. Miura M. Activators and proactivator of fibrinolytic system in paranasal mucous membrane of man. Kobe J Med Sci 1965; 11:13-21.

22. Okanishi N. Fibrinolysis in nasal and paranasal mucous membrane. Pract Otol (Kyoto) 1975; 68:427-79.

23. Rijken D, Wijngaards G, Zaal-De Jong M, Welbergen J. Purification and partial characterization of plasminogen activator from human uterine tissue. Biochim Biophys Acta 1979; 580: 140-53.

24. Hijikata A, Fujimoto K, Kitaguchi H, Okamoto S. Some properties of the tissue plasminogen activator from the pig heart. Thromb Res 1974; 4:731-40.

25. Bachmann F, Fletcher A, Alkjaersig N, Sherry S. Partial purification and properties of the plasminogen activator from pig heart. Biochemistry 1964; 3:1578-85.

26. Kosugi T, Morimitsu T, Matsuo O, Mihara H. A protease-

antiprotease system in antrochoanal polyp. I. Evidence for the existence of proactivator. Arch Otorhinolaryngol (NY) 1979; 225:97-102.

27. Rickli E, Zaugg H. Isolation and purification of highly enriched tissue plasminogen activator from pig heart. Thromb Diath Haemorrh 1970; 23:64-76.

28. Cole E, Bachmann F. Purification and properties of a plasminogen activator from pig heart. J Biol Chem 1977; 252: 3729-37.

29. Ali S, Evans L. Purification of rabbit kidney cytokinase and a comparison of its properties with human urokinase. Biochem J 1968; 107:293-303.

30. Soszka T. Partial purification and some properties of the tissue plasminogen activator from the human myometrium. Thromb Res 1977; 10:823-32.

31. Cartwright T. Partial purification of a specific plasminogen activator from porcine parotid glands. Thromb Diath Haemorrh 1974; 31:403-14.

≈

NINTH CONGRESS OF THE EUROPEAN RHINOLOGIC SOCIETY — THIRD INTERNATIONAL SYMPOSIUM ON INFECTION AND ALLERGY OF THE NOSE AND PARANASAL SINUSES

The Ninth Congress of the European Rhinologic Society and the Third International Symposium on Infection and Allergy of the Nose and Paranasal Sinuses will be held in Stockholm, Sept. 5-8, 1982. For information write: Ninth ERS Congress 1982, c/o Reso Congress Service, S-105 24 Stockholm.

Ann Otol 91:1982

NASAL DECONGESTANT EFFECT OF PROPYLHEXEDRINE

LYLE H. HAMILTON, PhD

MILWAUKEE, WISCONSIN

Propylhexedrine was evaluated for its objective and subjective effectiveness and duration of action as an inhaled topical nasal decongestant. It was studied with and without aromatic oils in subjects with nasal congestion due to acute upper respiratory infection (URI) or to allergic rhinitis. A logarithmic transformation of nasal airway resistance (R_n) was performed to allow the application of standard statistical tests to R_n changes. Subjective rating scales for congestion and symptoms were analyzed by nonparametric statistical procedures. R_n was statistically decreased from control values for 120 minutes after propylhexedrine vapors. Responses were the same for subjects with URI and allergic rhinitis, and no effect of the aromatic oils could be demonstrated. A comparison of the relationship between objective and subjective assessments of congestion demonstrated that the subjective rating scale had reduced sensitivity and poor reliability when compared with the objective measurement of R_n.

Propylhexedrine, 1-cyclohexyl-2-aminopropane, is widely used as the active ingredient in topical nasal decongestant inhalers. Its effectiveness was demonstrated by Sulman[1] with 51 patients having sinusitis and nasopharyngitis. He reported more than a 75% shrinkage of the nasal mucosa in 49 patients and 50% shrinkage in the remaining two patients. The decongestant effect lasted 1 to 2 hours in most trials, with a persistence for 3 hours in one patient and for less than 45 minutes in five cases. To our knowledge, other data have not been published in the medical literature, and no previous studies have compared the response in objectively measured nasal airway resistance (R_n) with the subjective assessment of a change in nasal congestion following treatment with propylhexedrine.

This report describes the effectiveness and duration of action of propylhexedrine on nasal congestion due to a) ragweed pollen in sensitized individuals, and b) an acute upper respiratory infection (URI) in otherwise healthy normal individuals. Objective measurement of R_n and subjective ratings of the degree of congestion, other symptoms, and related side effects were measured prior to and up to four hours after administration of the medication.

METHODS

All subjects used in the study were otherwise healthy individuals between the ages of 12 and 57 years who were not under a physician's care and were not taking medication. Potential subjects were excluded if they were pregnant or nursing a child, had known hypersensitivity to or chronically used nasal inhalers, or had a control R_n less than 2 cm H_2O/L/s (considered to be the upper limit of the normal range). Subjects were classified as being congested due to allergy or URI on the basis of the history provided by the subject and the seasonal nature of allergy symptoms.

Three types of inhalers, two medicated and one placebo (blank), were used for the studies reported here. Fifteen subjects with URI and 15 subjects with allergic rhinitis used inhalers containing 250 mg of propylhexedrine + 250 mg of aromatic (menthol, camphor, methyl salicylate, bornyl acetate, lavender oil). An additional 25 subjects with URI used inhalers containing 250 mg propylhexedrine but no aromatics. Each group was compared with an equal number of volunteer subjects (40 with URI and 15 with allergic rhinitis) selected by random to use placebo inhalers containing only a blank wick, and tested in the same serial sequence as the subjects receiving propylhexedrine.

Nasal airway resistance was measured with a nasal airway resistance computer previously described by Hamilton and Christman.[2] The system is based on posterior rhinometry, in which nasal airflow is measured with a pneumotachometer mounted on a modified scuba mask, and the driving pressure is measured as the difference between pharyngeal and mask pressure. Voltage signals representing the ratio of pressure to flow, updated breath-by-breath, were recorded as R_n on a strip-chart recorder. The R_n for each subject was calculated as the mean of four values for inspiratory R_n at 0.5 L/s for each time period measured.

After the subjects met the criteria and were accepted into the study, they were instructed in the technique for the measurement of R_n and in the completion of a form (Table 1) which rated their subjective assessment of nasal congestion and reported any symptoms or side effects.

After at least 30 minutes in the laboratory, the first R_n measurement was recorded and the subjective rating form was completed. However, the criteria for remaining in the study depended on having R_n equal to or exceeding 2.0 cm H_2O/L/s at 0.5 L/s inspiratory flow at 0-time for the study, which was no sooner than one hour after coming to the laboratory.

Subjects who met the criteria at 0-time used their assigned inhalers under the supervision of laboratory personnel, and remained in the lounge and the laboratory where the measurements were made. Smoking of nonmentholated cigarettes was allowed in a designated area, but not within 15 minutes of a measurement, and with the subjects recording the number of cigarettes smoked.

Prior to each measurement of R_n, the subject completed the report form shown in Table 1. This procedure was followed at −30 minutes, 0-time, and 10, 30, 60, 90, 120, 180 and 240 minutes after using the placebo.

STATISTICAL ANALYSIS

To establish the existence of a normal distribution of the data to be analyzed, R_n values and some transformations of R_n were assessed for skewness at three time periods early in the study. The distribution of the logarithm of R_n was not skewed at any

From the Research Service, Wood Veterans Administration Medical Center, and the Department of Physiology, The Medical College of Wisconsin, Milwaukee. This investigation was supported by the Veterans Administration.

REPRINTS — Lyle H. Hamilton, PhD, Research Service/151A, Veterans Administration Medical Center, Wood, WI 53193.

TABLE 1. RATING SHEET USED BY THE SUBJECTS FOR SUBJECTIVE ASSESSMENT OF NASAL CONGESTION, RELATED SYMPTOMS, AND SIDE EFFECTS FROM THE MEDICATION

Registration No.	_ _ _	EXAMPLE: No. 1 0 0 1, No. 63 0 6 3, No. 117 1 1 7
Patient No.	_ _ _	
Study period	_ _ _	EXAMPLE: Fill in time that is announced: Minute 1 8 0 or hour 0 0 3
Nasal congestion	L _ R _	1 = Clear; 2 = Almost clear; 3 = Stuffy; 4 = Quite stuffy; 5 = Very stuffy; 6 = Completely blocked. Select the NUMBER which corresponds with the word which *best* describes how stuffy your nose is at this moment. Record for each nostril.
Headache	_	0 = None; 1 = Mild: Aware of discomfort, but not annoying; 2 = Uncomfortable and annoying
Nausea	_	0 = None
Nervousness	_	1 = Mild: Aware of discomfort, but not annoying
Drowsiness	_	2 = Moderate: Annoying, but not severe enough to alter daily routine
Dizziness	_	3 = Severe: Very uncomfortable
Other	_	("Other" may include smell, taste, burning, itching, or any other unspecified sensation which is distracting or *unpleasant*. Please specify the complaint if this box is used.
		Since the *last time* you were asked this question, indicate the number of times you have sneezed and blown your nose
Sneezes	_	
Nose blows	_	Sneezes 0 3 Nose blows 1 1
Cigarettes in last hour	_	

period examined, so all R_n values were transformed to their logarithms prior to the application of parametric statistical analyses. Data are presented as the geometric mean (antilogarithm of the mean of ln R_n) when R_n is reported (Fig. 1).

The change in R_n at each time period from the value at 0-time was calculated for such subjects. These paired-sample changes were tested for statistical significance by the Student *t* test. Unpaired analyses were necessary to compare the mean response of each group receiving propylhexedrine with the mean response of its corresponding placebo group at every time period. Such unpaired statistical analyses were also made between the responses of subjects with URI who were treated with propylhexedrine and those with allergic rhinitis who were similarly treated; between the URI subjects who received propylhexedrine plus aromatics and the URI subjects who received propylhexedrine without aromatics; and, finally, between the 55 subjects who received propylhexedrine and the 55 who received only the placebo treatment.

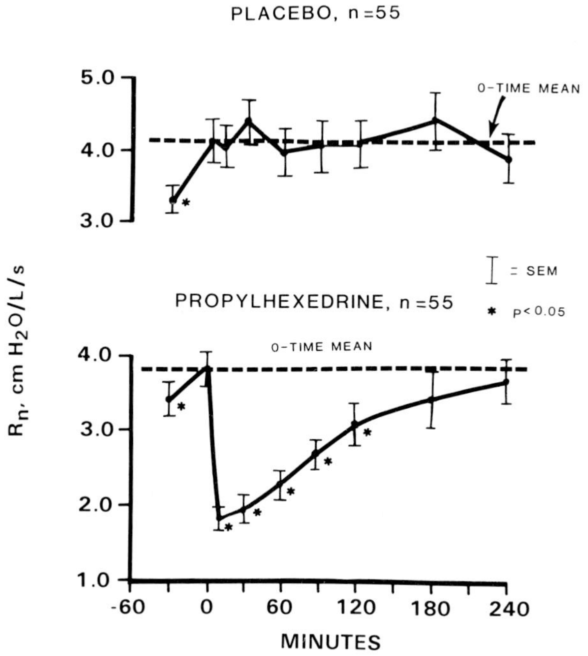

Fig. 1. Geometric mean values for R_n measured before and for four hours after administration of placebo or propylhexedrine in subjects with nasal congestion due to allergic rhinitis or upper respiratory infection. Vertical lines represent the antilogarithm of 1 SEM.

The subjective ratings for nasal congestion in each nostril were summed to provide a value called the "subjective congestion index" (SCI). The SCI and the reports of symptoms and side effects were evaluated by nonparametric statistical methods. The Wilcoxon Rank Sum test was used to compare the cumulative scores for each rating scale from all subjects receiving propylhexedrine with those from all subjects using the placebo inhaler. A comparison was also made of the cumulative scores for subjects reporting symptoms prior to, compared with only after, use of the propylhexedrine and placebo inhalers.

An assessment of the relationship between the objective and subjective evaluation of nasal congestion was made with a graphic display of individual values for SCI and R_n recorded during the study. These values and a comparison of the responses in SCI and R_n (expressed as a change from 0-time values for each measurement) are displayed as scattergrams in Figure 2.

RESULTS

Equilibration Period for R_n and Response to the Placebo. Figure 1 presents the geometric mean R_n values at each time period for all subjects who received the placebo (top) and all who received pro-

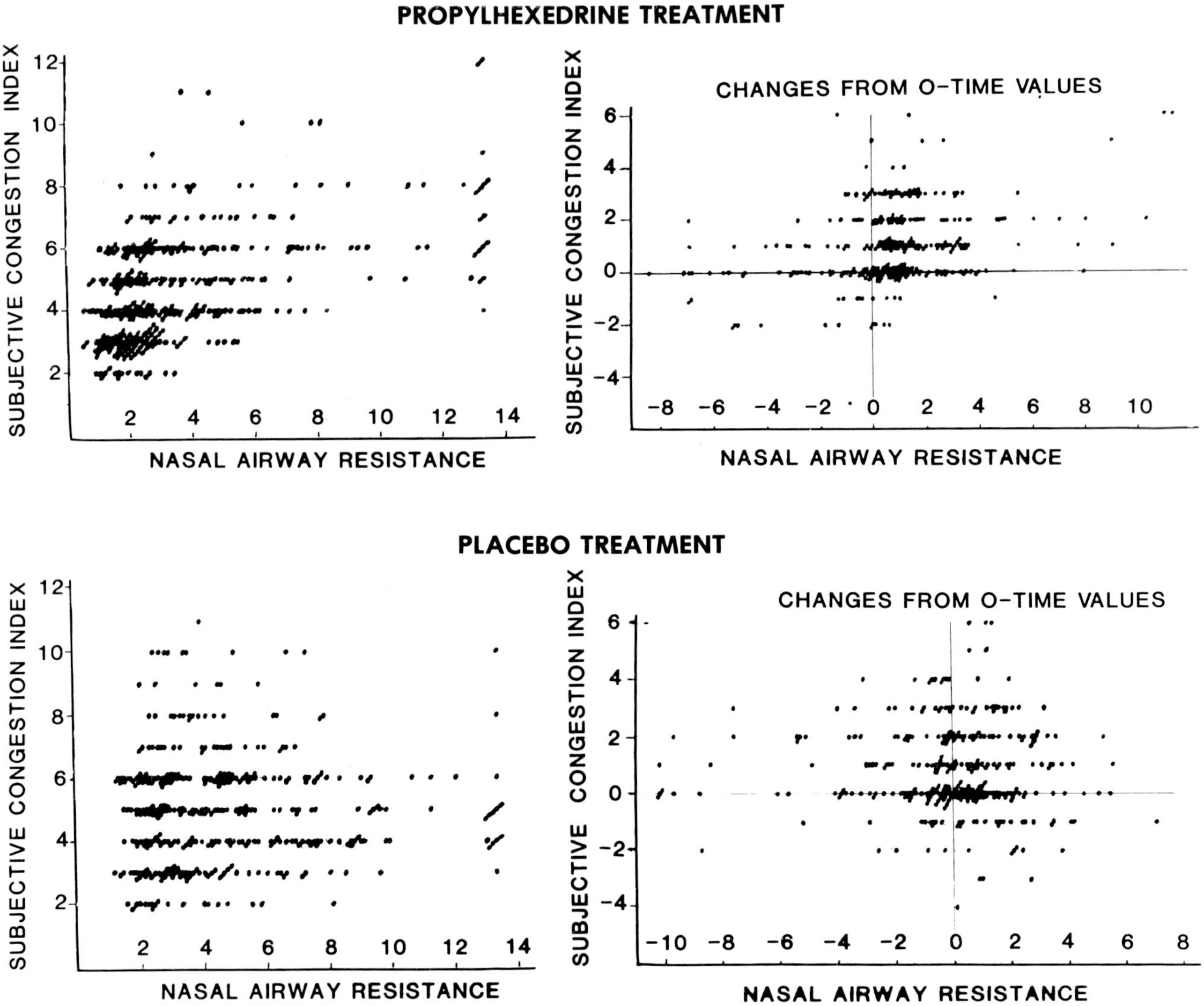

Fig. 2. Subjective (SCI) vs objective (R_n) measurement of nasal congestion. Scattergram plots of all SCI and R_n values from subjects receiving medication and those who used the placebo inhaler; and plots of the *responses* (changes from 0-time) for SCI and R_n in those same subjects who used the propylhexedrine and placebo inhalers.

pylhexedrine (bottom). The vertical lines represent the antilogarithm of 1 SEM. An asterisk identifies the points which are statistically different from the 0-time value, based on a change in R_n for each subject and the application of paired-sample statistics to the change in nasal patency.

Both groups of subjects had an increase in R_n between −30 minutes and 0-time. Paired-sample differences (ln of 0-time value minus ln of −30 minute value for each subject) were significant for the placebo group ($p<0.001$) and for the propylhexedrine group ($0.04<p<0.035$) during that time period. The R_n of the placebo group remained elevated after that, and did not fall significantly for the rest of the study period.

Effect of Propylhexedrine on R_n. The lower plot in Figure 1 represents the trend of geometric mean values for R_n for all subjects who received propylhexedrine. The decrease in R_n from the 0-time values remained statistically significant ($p>0.05$) for 120 minutes after use of the inhaler.

There was no difference between either the efficacy or the duration of effect between URI and allergic rhinitis subjects, or between URI subjects administered propylhexedrine plus aromatic and those treated with propylhexedrine alone.

Subjective Rating of Response to Propylhexedrine. A comparison of the objective response in nasal airway resistance (R_n) and the subjective assessment of SCI revealed that a relationship existed between them, but that R_n was not particularly deterministic of SCI.

Mean values for SCI scores at each time period for all subjects using propylhexedrine and placebo inhalers are presented in Table 2. When the effect of medication was compared to the effect of the placebo, there was no difference between the −30 minute and the 0-time rating. Although the scores

TABLE 2. SUBJECTIVE CONGESTION INDEX FOR SUBJECTS USING INHALERS

Time Period (min)	SCI Mean Value Propylhexedrine (n = 55)	Placebo (n = 55)	p
– 30	5.8	5.8	> 0.700
0-time	5.6	5.8	
10	4.2	5.3	< 0.005
30	4.1	5.0	< 0.005
60	4.5	4.9	0.067
90	4.4	4.8	> 0.400
120	4.4	4.7	> 0.300
180	4.8	4.7	> 0.600
240	4.8	4.5	> 0.100

p - Value is for no difference existing between the response (change from 0-time) to the placebo and the response to propylhexedrine at each time period.

were reduced from 0-time at all periods after treatment with either propylhexedrine or placebo, there was a sharper reduction in SCI for the subjects who received propylhexedrine than for those who used the placebo inhaler at 10 minutes and 30 minutes after treatment ($p < 0.005$), and the difference was still borderline ($0.1 > p > 0.05$) after 60 minutes. The lack of a difference later in the study reflected a gradually decreasing SCI score in the placebo group. This pattern of change in the subjective estimate of nasal congestion was not seen in the objective R_n measurements made at the same time (Fig. 1).

The scattergrams presented in Figure 2 show the poor relationship which was recorded between each R_n value and the corresponding SCI score. The relationships were plotted separately for subjects receiving propylhexedrine and those using the placebo inhaler in order to demonstrate graphically that large changes in R_n (in both groups) were not accurately reflected in any SCI scores, and that the pattern in the placebo group did not mask SCI changes following propylhexedrine. A tendency for a positive correlation could be observed by inspection of the scattergram.

Although there were statistically significant decreases in SCI scores at 10 and 30 minutes after treatment, and a nearly significant change after 60 minutes, its magnitude of response was small, and it showed a poor relationship to the objective R_n value measured at the same time.

Duration of Propylhexedrine Effectiveness. Propylhexedrine produced a statistically significant reduction in R_n for two hours in subjects congested by allergic rhinitis or upper respiratory infection. The duration of subjective relief, based on subjective ratings for nasal decongestion (SCI scores), was not as long as that for R_n. In fact, the subjective effect of propylhexedrine was limited to less than one hour, based on the statistical analysis of the SCI scores. Part of this was due to a temporal decrease in the perceived severity of congestion for those using the placebo, so the group differences did not remain significant.

Symptoms of Congestion and Side Effects of the Medication. Table 3 presents the scores accumulated at each time period in response to inquiries listed on the rating sheet (Table 1). The number of subjects responding positively to each category at some time during the study is recorded in the first column of numbers. The numbers listed in the other columns represent the sum of the ratings recorded by all subjects at that time period. A statistically significant difference ($p < 0.05$) in the accumulated scores between treatments was registered for drowsiness, nausea, headache, dizziness, and the number of cigarettes smoked during each period. A χ^2 analysis was performed on each entry on Table 1 to determine if there was an effect of treatment on the pattern with which symptoms were reported. No

TABLE 3. ACCUMULATED SCORES REPRESENTING SYMPTOMS AND SIDE EFFECTS

Condition Reported	No. of Subjects with Positive Responses	– 30	15	10	Time Period (min) 30	60	90	120	180	240
					Propylhexedrine (n = 55)					
Drowsiness*	22	21	15	9	5	7	9	8	8	12
Nervousness	15	16	9	10	10	9	8	6	6	5
Nausea*	11	8	8	9	10	8	8	7	7	8
Headache*	39	23	23	20	18	19	20	17	19	18
Dizziness*	5	1	2	3	3	2	2	3	3	2
Sneezes	33	40	11	9	13	11	9	15	29	69
Nose blows	48	82	49	39	35	33	38	57	67	69
Cigarettes*	26	36	22	19	24	34	30	31	41	42
					Placebo (n = 55)					
Drowsiness	30	33	26	22	23	21	21	20	20	18
Nervousness	16	13	10	7	7	6	3	4	4	3
Nausea	6	1	3	4	4	3	3	2	2	2
Headache	32	23	21	22	24	25	24	25	28	27
Dizziness	10	7	7	5	5	3	3	3	2	4
Sneezes	30	57	17	24	14	8	14	9	21	15
Nose blows	45	62	51	38	50	43	48	52	69	65
Cigarettes	16	18	13	9	8	16	15	19	24	25

*Significant ($p < 0.05$) difference in accumulated scores for individual subjects between propylhexedrine and placebo groups.

TABLE 4. INCIDENCE OF SYMPTOMS AND SIDE EFFECTS REPORTED BEFORE AND AFTER OR ONLY AFTER USE OF NASAL INHALER

	Number of Subjects with Positive Responses			
	Propylhexedrine		*Placebo*	
Observation	*Including Premedication Periods*	*Only Postmedication*	*Including Premedication Periods*	*Only Postmedication*
Drowsiness	17	5	25	5
Nervousness	14	1	16	0
Nausea	6	5	4	2
Headache	22	7	19	14
Dizziness	2	3	9	1
Sneezes	19	14	22	8
Nose blows	39	9	34	11
Cigarettes	23	3	13	3

differences in the distribution between the pretreatment and posttreatment incidence of positive responses was seen for drowsiness, nervousness, nausea, headache, sneezes, nose blows or the number of cigarettes smoked, but a significant χ^2 ($p<0.05$) was recorded for the pattern of dizziness reported. Ten of 55 subjects who used the placebo inhaler reported dizziness, with nine having positive responses prior to medication. Only five subjects receiving propylhexedrine reported dizziness, with two having positive responses prior to medication (Table 4).

A more careful analysis was made of the effect of propylhexedrine on the symptoms by comparing (nonparametric analysis) the accumulated scores recorded from 10 through 180 minutes for each subject having positive responses following placebo vs those with positive responses following propylhexedrine. No effect of the medication was seen on the accumulated scores for nervousness, nausea, headache, dizziness, sneezes, or nose blows. A significant difference ($0.05>p>0.025$) was seen for accumulated scores for drowsiness, in which the scores following placebo were higher than those following the administration of propylhexedrine during the period when the medication might have had an effect. Twenty-three subjects who received the placebo subsequently reported some drowsiness, as compared with 15 subjects receiving propylhexedrine. More significantly, subjects who received the placebo reported higher cumulative scores for drowsiness during the 10 to 180-minute period (mean = 5.3 points per subject) than those who received propylhexedrine (mean = 3.1 points per subject). These two differences (greater incidence of drowsiness and higher cumulative scores for subjects who received the placebo) accounted for the statistically significant effect of treatment on the subjective report of drowsiness during the period when propylhexedrine might have exerted an effect.

DISCUSSION

This study supported the report by Sulman[1] that propylhexedrine is an effective topical nasal decongestant, with an expected effectiveness of about two hours. Other information about the expected duration of action is not readily available because claims for its accepted efficacy and safety are largely based on unpublished data.[3] On the basis of subjective reports of relief, symptoms associated with URI or allergic rhinitis other than nasal congestion were not affected by the medication. The subjective assessment of nasal congestion and the change in nasal patency were poorly related to the objective measurements of R_n made using a nasal airway resistance computer.

No side effects of propylhexedrine were observed, with the possible exception of a slight, nonperceptible CNS stimulation or arousal. That possibility is based on the observations that, although propylhexedrine had no effect on the incidence or pattern of nervousness ("jitters") reported on the rating sheet, fewer subjects who received propylhexedrine were drowsy; and when drowsiness occurred, it was less severe than in subjects receiving placebo (Tables 3 and 4). This could be interpreted to mean that, if the difference was indeed related to the treatment, propylhexedrine prevented or reduced drowsiness in some patients, all of whom remained in the laboratory area with restricted activity for at least 5½ hours. The relatively long period of inactivity associated with this study, with the subject confined to the laboratory area, may have induced some of the drowsiness, but a more carefully designed study should be completed before drawing conclusions about a CNS-stimulating effect from the propylhexedrine inhaler.

A CNS-stimulating effect has been associated with accidental propylhexedrine poisoning of a child,[4] but acute poisoning in an adult was accompanied only by systemic (primarily pulmonary) complications.[5] To our knowledge, no previous indication of even a slight stimulating effect from the use of a propylhexedrine inhaler has been reported.

No effect of the aromatic additive on the response to propylhexedrine could be demonstrated by comparing the two groups of URI patients who used propylhexedrine (15 with and 25 without the aromatic). Because of the size of the study, no group received only the aromatic without propylhexedrine. Therefore, this study did not eliminate the possibility that the presence of an odor might have affected the response to the nasal decongestant, because propylhexedrine without the aromatics also had a distinct smell. However, the response to propylhexedrine without the aromatics was the same as the response when the aromatics were included.

Likewise, no difference was seen in the response to propylhexedrine (with or without aromatics) in URI patients when compared to the response in patients with allergic rhinitis. Similar magnitudes of response and similar durations of effectiveness were recorded for both groups.

These observations were the basis for combining all subjects into the active (propylhexedrine treatment) and placebo groups. The larger value for n (55) which resulted from doing so provided more confidence in the statistical statements about duration of effectiveness for propylhexedrine. Since the subjective assessment of the degree and duration of congestion were only generally correlated with R_n, the "clinical" effectiveness of the medication was less than its "statistical" effectiveness. The subjective assessment of the degree of congestion, or its change, is affected strongly by reference to the most recent previous assessment. This will favor the tendency to detect more reliably, and possibly to exaggerate, reports of change following sudden or large alterations, and to attenuate the perception of slow or gradual changes in nasal congestion. That may explain the pattern of decongestion reported following propylhexedrine administration.

In addition, SCI may reflect factors other than nasal congestion, eg, sinus congestion, headache, pharyngitis, etc, which will affect the subjective scoring. These factors may have changed during the study so there was a gradual decrease in SCI scores during the study, with no similar change in R_n for the placebo group. Thus, dependency on R_n accounts for only a small proportion of the SCI variability, and R_n must be judged to be not reliably deterministic of the subjective assessment of nasal congestion.

ACKNOWLEDGMENTS — Mr. N. T. Christman was responsible for the development and construction of the nasal airway resistance computer. Mrs. Judith A. Hoernke assisted in the collection of objective (R_n) and subjective (rating scales) data. Dr. John H. Kalbfleisch, Biostatistician, Research Service, Wood Veterans Administration Medical Center, and the Departments of Preventive Medicine and Physiology, The Medical College of Wisconsin, provided valuable advice and guidance concerning the statistical treatment of the data analyzed for this study. Support from Vick Divisions Research, New Rochelle, New York, and Smith Kline & French Laboratories, Philadelphia, is acknowledged and was appreciated. Support was also provided from the Medical Research Service, Wood Veterans Administration Medical Center.

REFERENCES

1. Sulman LD. A new volatile vasoconstrictor for relief of nasal congestion. Med Times 1945; 73:262-3.

2. Hamilton LH, Christman NT. Nasal airway resistance computer. Laryngoscope 1977; 87:1945-50.

3. Advisory Review Panel on Over-the-Counter Cold, Cough, Allergy, Bronchodilator and Antiasthmatic Products. Over-the-counter drugs: establishment of a monograph for OTC cold, cough, allergy, bronchodilator and antiasthmatic products. Federal Register 41:38402 (Sept 6) 1976.

4. Poster H. Uber eine Vergiftung mit dem Appetitzügler Propylhedrin, "Obesin," bei einem 3 jährigen Kinde. Arch Toxical 1965; 20:271-3.

5. Marsden P, Sheldon J. Acute poisoning by propylhexedrine, abstracted. Br Med J 1972; 1:730.

NASAL CYCLE AND POSTURAL VARIATIONS IN NASAL RESISTANCE

MAKOTO HASEGAWA, MD
TOKYO, JAPAN

The relationship between the nasal cycle and postural variations in unilateral nasal resistance (UNR) was observed in ten normal subjects. During the nasal cycle, postural variations in UNR were notable in congested nasal chambers; UNR at 0° from a horizontal plane was found to be higher than at greater angles. Postural variations in UNR in constricted sides of nasal chambers, however, were very slight. This phenomenon was observed in all ten cases. For total nasal resistance, postural variations were small. (Total nasal resistance was strongly influenced by UNR in constricted sides.) The nasal cycle may be induced by alternative changes in the sympathetic tone to the nasal mucosa, probably regulated by the hypothalamus.

INTRODUCTION

The phenomenon of the nasal cycle was first reported by Kayser[1] in 1895, and subsequently has been investigated by many authors.[2-8] The nasal cycle is the regular dilation and constriction of the cavernous veins in the mucosa of the chonchae and septum. During these cyclical changes of the nasal mucosa, one nasal chamber becomes more open and the other more engorged. Eccles[8] demonstrated that this phenomenon was possibly regulated by the hypothalamus, the autonomic center in the brain.

Postural variations in total nasal resistance (TNR: nasal airflow resistance through both nostrils) are greater in patients with allergic rhinitis than in normal subjects.[9-11] For both groups TNR is greater in a supine than a sitting position, but the difference is more marked in patients with allergic rhinitis.

The aim of this study was to learn why normal subjects have a slight increase in TNR in the supine position, how unilateral nasal resistance (UNR: nasal airflow resistance through one nostril) varies with positional changes of the head, and whether postural variations in UNR are influenced by the nasal cycle.

METHODS

Ten normal subjects (three males 39-54 years of age and seven females 20-51 years of age) were examined. None had a history of allergic rhinitis, asthma, chronic rhinitis, or septal deviations. UNR was measured through each nostril every 15 minutes, using anterior rhinomanometry. For this purpose, Mercury's nasal resistance meter NRI was modified to allow each nostril to be measured separately. UNR was recorded when nasal airflow was 0.25 l/s. TNR was calculated by the following formula:

$$\frac{1}{TNR} = \frac{1}{UNR(r)} + \frac{1}{UNR(l)}.$$

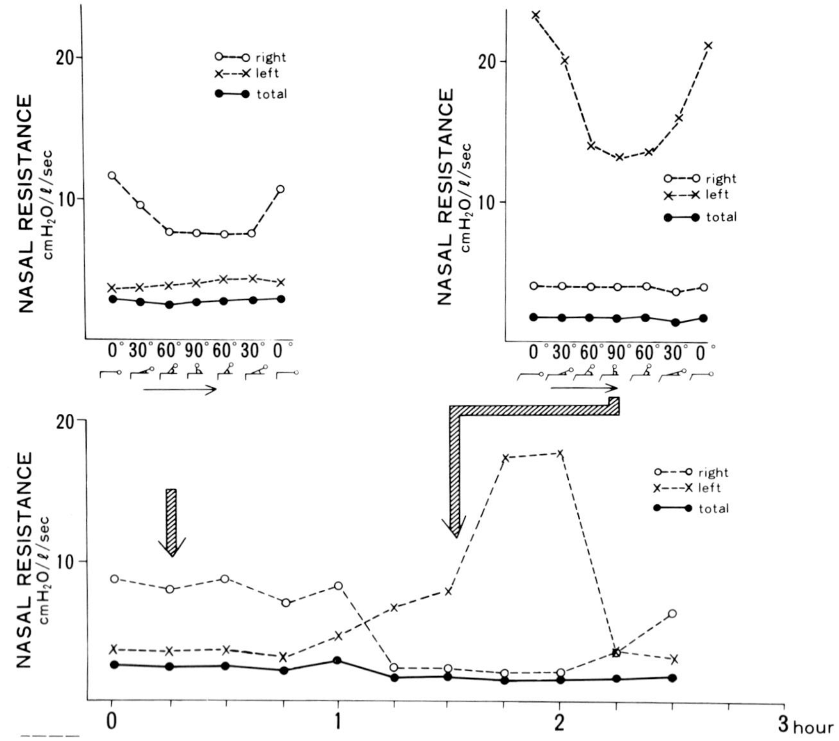

Fig. 1. (Case 1) Postural variations of UNR in a congested side of the nasal chambers in a 39-year-old male. The change in posture of the head was performed after the arrow.

From the Department of Otorhinolaryngology, Tokyo Medical and Dental University.
REPRINTS — Makoto Hasegawa, MD, Department of Otorhinolaryngology, Tokyo Medical and Dental University, 5-45 Yushima, 1-Chome, Bunkyo-ku, Tokyo, Japan.

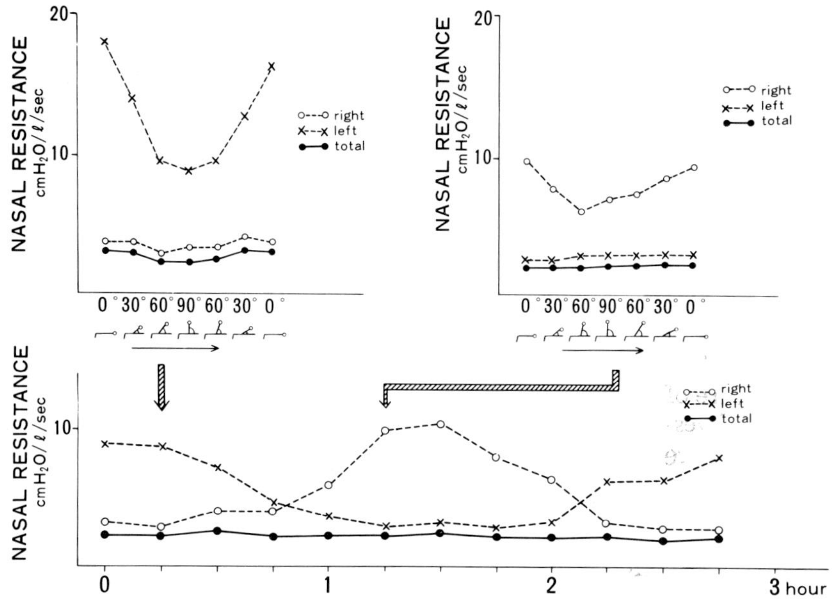

Fig. 2. (Case 2) Postural variations of UNR in a congested side of the nasal chambers in a 20-year-old female. The change in posture of the head was performed after the arrow.

Postural variations in UNR (cmH$_2$0/l/s) were observed at 0°, 30°, 60°, and 90° from a horizontal plane in each subject. Initial measurement was at 0°, followed by measurements at 30°, 60°, 90°, 60°, 30° and 0°. The subject was kept in each position for one minute before UNR was determined. Postural variations in UNR were examined twice during the observation of nasal cycle in each subject. One examination was carried out when the right nasal chamber revealed a higher UNR, and the other when the left nasal chamber revealed a higher UNR.

RESULTS

Postural variations in UNR were more marked in congested sides of the nasal chamber than in constricted sides (Figs. 1 and 2). This phenomenon was observed in all ten cases. UNR gradually decreased between 0° and 90°, and, conversely, increased between 90° and 0°. UNR at the angle of 0° was considerably higher than at greater angles (Fig. 3).

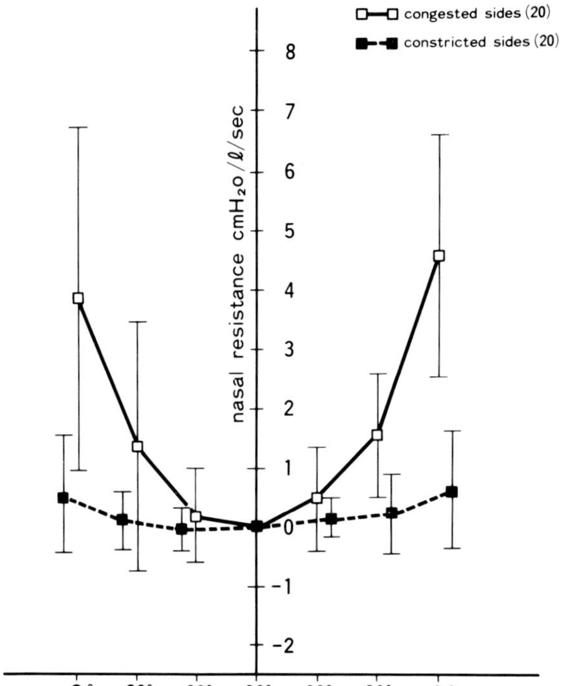

Fig. 3. Postural variations of UNR in congested sides (20) and constricted sides (20) of normal nasal chambers.

The postural variations in TNR were less than in UNR, since TNR was strongly affected by the UNR of a constricted side (Figs. 1 and 2).

DISCUSSION

Postural variations in TNR in patients with allergic rhinitis were first reported by Rundcrantz in 1964.[9] In 1969,[10] he reported that this phenomenon also occurred during a common cold. Hasegawa and Saito[11] found that postural variations in TNR were more remarkable in patients with allergic rhinitis than in normal subjects, and that these patients were improved by nasal insufflation of beclomethasone dipropionate. They reported that normal subjects also showed a slight increase in postural variations in TNR.

The present study shows that postural variations of UNR are strongly influenced by the nasal cycle. The procedure for measuring postural variations of UNR during the nasal cycle was carried out within 15 minutes. The determination of UNR to observe the nasal cycle was carried out regularly, every 15 minutes, without interruption. It was retrospectively demonstrated that this procedure was carried out during the same phase of the nasal cycle in all ten cases. If measurements were taken during the reverse stage of the nasal cycle when the dominant side changes from one to the other, the pattern of postural variations in UNR might have been modified.

TNR was not determined directly in this study, but was calculated to the formula noted above. To determine TNR directly, posterior rhinomanometry, which requires more time than anterior rhinomanometry, is necessary. For this reason, posterior rhinomanometry was not used. In this study TNR was strongly affected by UNR in constricted sides, as reported by Arbour and Kern.[12]

The mechanism of postural variations in nasal resistance has not yet been elucidated. Rundcrantz[9] suggested that vascular hypotonicity due to stimulation of parasympathetic nerve fibers was the cause in patients with allergic rhinitis. In this study, postural variations in UNR in constricted sides were absent or very slight, suggesting that the diameters of constricted vessels in the nasal mucosa were not significantly influenced by the change of posture of the head. Conversely, the diameters of dilated vessels in the nasal mucosa of the congested cavity were altered by the change of posture of the head.

Some of the factors which induce constriction in the nasal mucosa, eg, breath-holding, rebreathing, and exercise, are well known.[13,14] McCaffrey and Kern[15,16] demonstrated that a rise in Pco_2 stimulated chemical receptors in the body and induced an increase in sympathetic tone to the nose, and that constriction of the nasal mucosa consequently occurred.

Considering previous studies and the current study, it may be said that an increase in sympathetic tone to the nasal mucosa interrupts postural variations in UNR. Observed postural variations in UNR in a congested side may be caused by a decrease in sympathetic tone to the nasal mucosa. Thus the nasal cycle may be induced by alternative changes in sympathetic tone which are regulated by the hypothalamus.

REFERENCES

1. Kayser R. Die exacte Messung der Luftdurchgängigkeit der Nase. Arch Laryngol 1895; 3:101-20.

2. Heetderks DR. Observations on the reaction of normal nasal mucous membrane. Am J Med Sci 1927; 174:231-44.

3. Beickert P. Halbseitenrhythmus der Vegetativen Innervation. Arch Ohren Nasen Kehlkopfheilkd 1951; 157:185-9.

4. Stoksted P. The physiologic cycle of the nose under normal and pathologic conditions. Acta Otolaryngol (Stockh) 1952; 42:175-9.

5. Principato JJ, Ozenberger JM. Cyclic changes in nasal resistance. Arch Otolaryngol 1970; 91:71-7.

6. Dallimore NS, Eccles R. Changes in human nasal resistance associated with exercise, hyperventilation and rebreathing. Acta Otolaryngol (Stockh) 1977; 84:416-21.

7. Hasegawa M, Kern EB. The human nasal cycle. Mayo Clin Proc 1977; 52:28-34.

8. Eccles R. The central rhythm of the nasal cycle. Acta Otolaryngol (Stockh) 1978; 66:464-8.

9. Rundcrantz H. Posture and congestion of nasal mucosa in allergic rhinitis. Acta Otolaryngol (Stockh) 1964; 58:283-7.

10. Rundcrantz H. Postural variations of nasal patency. Acta Otolaryngol (Stockh) 1969; 68:435-43.

11. Hasegawa M, Saito Y. Postural variations in nasal resistance and symptomatology in allergic rhinitis. Acta Otolaryngol (Stockh) 1979; 88:268-72.

12. Arbour P, Kern EB. Paradoxical nasal obstruction. Can J Otolaryngol 1975; 4:333-7.

13. Tatum AL. The effect of deficient and excessive pulmonary ventilation on nasal volume. Am J Physiol 1923; 65:229-33.

14. Hasegawa M, Kern EB. The effect of breath holding, hyperventilation and exercise on nasal resistance. Rhinology 1978; 16:243-9.

15. McCaffrey TV, Kern EB. Response of nasal airway resistance to hypercapnia and hypoxia in the dog. Acta Otolaryngol (Stockh) 1979; 87:545-53.

16. McCaffrey TV, Kern EB. Response of nasal airway resistance to hypercapnia and hypoxia in man. Ann Otol Rhinol Laryngol 1979; 88:247-52.

Ann Otol 91:1982

INDICATIONS OF CONGENITAL PALATAL INCOMPETENCE BEFORE DIAGNOSIS

HUGHLETT L. MORRIS, PhD

LOIS J. KRUEGER, MA

ROBERT M. BUMSTED, MD

IOWA CITY, IOWA

Frequently the disorder of congenital palatal incompetence (CPI), in the absence of physiological evidence of clefting, is not discovered until after adenoidectomy. That is because the adenoidal pad served to mask the insufficiency of the velopharyngeal mechanism. Findings from this study indicate that early disorders in speech production, particularly nasalization of speech, is a useful predictor of CPI. Recommendations are made about methods for screening children before adenoidectomy or those suspected of having the CPI disorder.

Congenital palatopharyngeal incompetency (CPI) has been described in the literature from several points of view.[1-9] In general the term refers to the condition in which the patient demonstrates speech production patterns (nasal emission during consonants and hypernasal voice quality) that are typical of an unoperated cleft palate, but there is no cleft palate or history of one. The clinical findings clearly indicate that the physiologic disorder is velopharyngeal incompetence due to either a short palate, a palate with reduced mobility, or both. Although subject groups in some early studies and some clinical classifications of CPI included patients with bifid uvula or submucous cleft palate, contemporary use of the descriptive term CPI excludes those patients.

Not much information is available about the prevalence of CPI[9] but patients with the condition present clinically for diagnosis and treatment with sufficiently high frequency that the disorder deserves our attention. That is particularly the case in the matter of diagnosis.

There are exceptions, but in general the diagnosis of CPI is not made until the child is of school age, and sometimes only after disruption of the velopharyngeal mechanism following adenoidectomy. This disruption occurs because prior to the adenoidectomy the adenoidal pad compensates in the A-P dimension for the palatal deficit; after adenoidectomy the deficit becomes apparent in the form of persistent nasalized speech.[7,10] Clinicians have suggested that the same phenomenon can occur following normal adenoidal atrophy, but to date no reliable data have been reported in support of that contention. Perhaps the mechanism can compensate for very small increments in velopharyngeal port dimension, which would be the case with normal adenoidal atrophy, but it cannot compensate for a sudden and relatively large increment following adenoidectomy.

In many instances there are no obvious indications of the disorder until sustained nasalized speech follows adenoidectomy. At that point, the parents usually seek assistance from a center that specializes in orofacial disorders; the diagnosis is made and corrective surgery such as the pharyngeal flap,[11] nasopharyngeal pushback,[12] or Teflon® injection[13] is performed. The palatal lift dental prosthesis[14] has also on occasion been used satisfactorily for treatment of CPI. Generally, speech therapy is needed following either surgery or dental prosthesis. CPI frequently occurs in isolation but may also be part of a syndrome.[15,16]

Obviously there would be many advantages to the capability of diagnosis of the disorder before adenoidectomy or at an earlier age in childhood. Such early diagnosis would alert the surgeon, the speech pathologist, and the family to the likelihood of later difficulties in speech production. In some cases, perhaps, the adenoidectomy could be delayed, or a partial adenoidectomy performed. In those cases where full adenoidectomy is medically required, more adequate predictions about the eventual outcome could be made than are now possible.

Two investigators have addressed the issue of early diagnosis directly. Lubit[6] described several symptoms (mainly pertaining to speech production) that he considered useful in identifying CPI before adenoidectomy. Mason[7] reported findings of 110 children with CPI that might be useful in early diagnosis. His subjects included those with signs of clefting (bifid uvula and submucous cleft palate) and he identified those two findings as danger signals during the preoperative clinical examination. Other significant findings were the presence of

From the Department of Otolaryngology and Maxillofacial Surgery, University of Iowa, Iowa City.

REPRINTS — Hughlett L. Morris, PhD, Department of Otolaryngology, University Hospitals and Clinics, University of Iowa, Iowa City, IA 52242.

an anteriorly positioned soft palate dimple on elevation, indicating short effective length of the velum; midline translucency of the velum; short palatal length; and poor velar elevation. Thirty percent of the 110 subjects had radiographic evidence of anomalies of the upper cervical vertebra and cranial base. (He recommended x-ray examination only for those who showed oral symptoms of the disorder.)

The search continues, then, for symptoms of congenital palatopharyngeal incompetence that may be detected before the clinical diagnosis is made. The purpose of this study was to determine whether information collected by questionnaire from parents of CPI children would uncover any new clues about such early symptoms.

METHODS

Subjects were 49 patients who were identified from existing departmental records as having the diagnosis of CPI. Patients with oral signs of clefting, such as bifid uvula or submucous cleft palate, were excluded since these signs can be detected by physical examination alone and their value in predicting velopharyngeal incompetence is already known. In all 49 cases, the diagnosis of CPI had been made on the basis of speech pathology and physical examinations. No other criteria were used in subject selection.

Questionnaires were sent to the parents of each subject explaining the purpose of the study (in nontechnical language) and asking their assistance in providing information about certain aspects of the problem, the pregnancy, health history, speech history, and the time and circumstances of the diagnosis.

Twelve normal subjects and their families were used for comparison; they were selected at random from subjects known to the investigators for other nonmedical reasons. The same questionnaire, excluding items about the CPI disorders, was mailed to those parents.

Responses were obtained from 28 of the 49 CPI parents, and from all 12 parents of the normal controls. Ages of children under study ranged from 6 to 18 years for the CPI group, and from 6 to 16 years for the controls. Sex was almost evenly distributed in the two groups.

FINDINGS

For 18 of the 28 CPI children, the initial diagnosis was made between the ages of 4 and 10 years; for 3 children, the diagnosis was made before the age of 4, while 5 were detected after age 10 (no answer was given by two families). Problems with speech were reported as the major symptom by 26 of the 28 families; 15 of the 26 specifically cited nasal speech, and 3 reported speech that was difficult to understand. Ear infection was cited as the primary symptom for one CPI subject; parents of one CPI subject failed to answer that question. For ten CPI subjects, the diagnosis was reported to be made by the speech pathologist; seven families cited university hospitals and clinics as the major source of diagnosis with no specific profession named; other sources included local school personnel, the local physician, and members of the family. Fourteen of the 28 CPI children had adenoidectomy immediately before the diagnosis was made and all but one had some kind of physical management, primarily surgical, after the diagnosis was made. Nine of the 28 CPI children were reported to have had other physical problems, among them problems of hearing and motor development.

Differences in questionnaire responses between the CPI and normal groups were evaluated for statistical significance by either the two-sample t test (when distribution permitted) or by chi-square. No differences were found in birth order or twinning; mother's health before and during pregnancy (including incidence of illness such as rubella during early pregnancy); exposure to x-ray, falls, injuries, or emotional stress; drug or alcohol consumption during early stages of pregnancy; complications during delivery; problems in feeding (about which information we asked in considerable detail); early language development (as opposed to speech production); and the child's physical development and general health history (childhood diseases, frequency of colds, sore throats, etc).

Significant differences were obtained on 4 of the 25 questionnaire items. Birthweight for the CPI children was less (2.9 kg) than for the normal children (3.3 kg). Mothers of CPI children reported a higher incidence of cigarette-smoking during early pregnancy than did the normals. More CPI children had early speech that was difficult for the parents to understand (12 of 27, 1 "can't recall") than did the control parents (1 of 12). More CPI children were reported to have nasal speech as a young child (12 of 22, 6 "can't recall") than did the normals (1 of 11, 1 "can't recall").

DISCUSSION

We need to acknowledge the limitations to the sort of research design used in this investigation. It seems likely, for example, that more, and perhaps better, information could have been obtained in face-to-face interviews than by mailed questionnaires. Responses made by some informants were ambiguous and probably reflected lack of clarity in the questionnaire. The major design problem is the difference among families in remembering detail about circumstances of the pregnancy, birth, and early childhood of the child under study. One factor, of course, is time: the probability of forgetting detail is higher for parents of older children than for younger children. Another factor is the number of children in the family. Spriestersbach[17] previously considered these design difficulties with retrospective investigations and concluded that, in general, methodology like the one used here is satisfactory for most purposes. Consequently we are inclined to consider the obtained differences to be reliable findings. It is of course possible that a more precise data collection method would uncover more findings than our procedures.

The major finding that CPI children have speech production problems (many of them nasal in type) early in life is certainly not unexpected. Other studies have yielded similar findings, and clinical observation is also consistent with this notion as well. However, that was not the case for all subjects. Half of the CPIs did not have such a problem at that age level, or at least not to the extent that the parents noticed it. Rather, the problem was discovered during the preschool or early school years by the speech pathologist or some other specialist. The diagnosis for half the children was made after adenoidectomy; for the other 14 onset or recognition of the speech production problem was not associated with such surgery.

These findings leave several important unanswered questions. What was the nature of the early speech problems if they were not nasal, or were they nasal but not recognized or remembered as such by the parents? Was velopharyngeal status consistent during the period of time before diagnosis? If velopharyngeal status was not consistent, was the variation due to change in size of adenoidal pad? For those children reported to have nasalized speech, was the nasalization detectable from the early beginnings of speech production? Unfortunately design limitations of this investigation prevented acquisition of such information, but the questions direct attention to needs for future study.

The lack of significant findings in the area of early deglutition patterns is disappointing. Clinical impressions are that many CPI children demonstrate nasal leakage of milk during feeding at a very early age (birth to 2 or 3 weeks). Parents who report this observation indicate that the leakage is consistent and that the phenomenon is recognized as being clearly different from nasal regurgitation, which is more projectile in nature. Also the leakage is reported to cease during the first month of life. Apparently the infant learns to compensate somehow for the velopharyngeal incompetence, probably by raising the tongue against the palate during swallowing.

Several items on the questionnaire were designed to inquire about this feeding problem. The finding of no difference between CPI and control children indicates that the nasal leakage is no more characteristic of the CPI infant than the normal, or that the data collection procedure was not sufficiently precise or reliable to detect this possible difference.

The findings of lower birth weight and higher incidence of cigarette smoking in mothers are consistent with other data about these two factors.

RECOMMENDATIONS

It seems possible from these and other reported findings about CPI to summarize some clinical symptoms that indicate the possibility of congenital palatal incompetence. The clinical examination should include methodical search for the symptoms in cases where adenoidectomy is needed, or when the diagnosis of CPI is considered. If the symptoms are observed, the patient should be examined by a specialty team (cleft palate team, orofacial team) at a teaching hospital before the surgery or before the diagnosis is made. Following is an examination protocol for identifying symptoms.

1. Carefully observe the patient for any anatomic or physiologic signs of clefting, including bifid uvual, bony defect in the region of the posterior nasal spine of the hard palate, and/or a soft palate that appears unusually short or poorly mobile. We must note here that intraoral observations of palate length and mobility are not very reliable, so some false positives will be obtained from those aspects of the examination. However, it seems better to have false positives than the unexpected CPI! As we pointed out earlier, the findings of bifid uvula and bony defect of the hard palate are indications of a submucous cleft rather than CPI. However, they frequently are accompanied by velopharyngeal incompetence and are included here for the sake of completeness. Look also for anterior dimpling of the soft palate (described by Mason[7]) that seems to indicate abnormal physiology of the musculature of the soft palate. Radiographic evidence of vertebral abnormalities (also described by Mason[7]) can be a valuable indication of CPI. In addition lateral x-ray films of the nasopharynx allow evaluation of the depth of the nasopharynx and the size of the adenoid pad in patients who are difficult to examine clinically.

2. Look for signs of abnormal palatal innervation such as asymmetry of palatal elevation. Look also for signs of neurologic impairment, even so-called "soft" signs, in other parts of the body. Typically such signs are not part of the CPI disorder but may indicate a neurologic disorder which is responsible for the velopharyngeal dysfunction.

3. Ask questions about the incidence of cleft lip, cleft palate, or related orofacial abnormalities in the family.

4. If there are signs of neurologic dysfunction, determine the child's history and neurologic development which will give a more complete history. Referral to a neurologist may be needed.

5. Ask questions about early speech production (or make direct observations if the patient is young) that are directed toward nasalization of speech. Use lay terms in asking the questions, such as "talking through the nose." It is abnormal if the child is reported (or observed) to do so. Positive findings in the speech history should be followed by referral to a speech pathologist for further examination and diagnosis.

6. Ask questions about nasal leakage of milk or other liquids during feeding. In our opinion, the negative findings from this study do not preclude

the possibility that such information may be an important indicator of CPI.

7. If any or all of these symptoms are observed and adenoidectomy seems indicated in spite of them, the parents must be warned before the surgery about the possibility of CPI with hypernasal speech (velopharyngeal incompetence) postoperatively.

8. Be aware that patients with a normal velopharyngeal mechanism may develop temporary nasalized speech for only a day or two after adenoidectomy. This may occur while the patient adjusts to the new set of relationships in the nasopharynx. However, the normal patient typically adjusts rather quickly and shows normal oral speech within the first or second postoperative day. If the patient has nasalized speech several weeks after surgery, the chances are very high that it is a case of CPI. Additional surgery or dental prosthesis will be needed if normal oral speech production is the objective.

SUMMARY

By questionnaire, parents of 28 children with CPI were asked about pregnancy and delivery; speech, developmental, and health history; and the circumstances of the CPI diagnosis. A normal control group was used for comparison. CPI children had lower birth weights and, during early childhood, were more poorly understood by parents and more frequently had nasalized speech. In 50%, CPI diagnosis was made following adenoidectomy. Data and clinical findings indicate that possible predictors of CPI are unusually defective speech production, particularly characterized by nasalization, as a young child; a short or poorly mobile palate; anterior dimpling of the soft palate during elevation; radiographic abnormalities of the cervical vertebrae; neurologic abnormalities (developmental milestones or clinical examination); and nasal leakage of liquids as a very young infant. Temporary velopharyngeal incompetence and nasalized speech may occur in the normal patient following adenoidectomy but the disorder resolves in a day or two. Persistent nasalized speech following adenoidectomy indicates the likelihood of CPI; such a patient requires evaluation by a speech pathologist and possible surgical correction.

REFERENCES

1. Calnan JS. Diagnosis, prognosis, and treatment of palatopharyngeal incompetence with special reference to radiographic investigations. Br J Plast Surg 1956; 8:265-82.

2. Calnan JS. Permanent escape in speech after adenoidectomy. Br J Plast Surg 1971a; 24:197-204.

3. Calnan JS. Congenital large pharynx. Br J Plast Surg 1971b; 24:263-71.

4. Randall P, Bakes FP, Kennedy C. Cleft-palate type speech in the absence of cleft palate. Plast Reconstr Surg 1960; 25:484-95.

5. Blackfield HM, Miller ER, Owsley J, Lawson LI. Cinefluorographic evaluation of patients with velopharyngeal dysfunction in the absence of overt cleft palate. Plast Reconstr Surg 1962; 30:441-51.

6. Lubit EC. Before an adenoidectomy. Stop! Look! Listen! N Y State J Med 1967; 67:681-5.

7. Mason RM. Preventing speech disorders following adenoidectomy by preoperative examination. Clin Pediatr (Phila) 1973; 12:405-14.

8. Minami RT, Kaplan EN, Wu G, Jobe RP. Velopharyngeal incompetence without overt cleft palate. Plast Reconstr Surg 1975; 55:573-87.

9. Bradley DP. Congenital and acquired palatopharyngeal insufficiency. In: Bzoch KR, ed. Communication disorders related to cleft lip and palate. Boston: Little Brown and Company, 1979:77-89.

10. Morris HL. The speech pathologist looks at the tonsils and adenoids. Ann Otol Rhinol Laryngol 1975; 84 Suppl 19:63-6.

11. Smith JK, Huffman WC, Lierle DM, Moll KL. Results of pharyngeal flap surgery in patients with velopharyngeal incompetence. Plast Reconstr Surg 1963; 32:493-501.

12. Smith HW, Lee KJ. Nasopharyngeal pushback in treatment of velopharyngeal insufficiency. Arch Otolaryngol 1976; 102:83-6.

13. Smith JK, McCabe BF. Teflon injection in the nasopharynx to improve velopharyngeal closure. Ann Otol Rhinol Laryngol 1977; 86:559-63.

14. LaVelle WE, Hardy JC. Palatal lift prostheses for treatment of palatopharyngeal incompetence. J Prosthet Dent 1979; 42:308-15.

15. Cohen MM. Syndromes with cleft lip and cleft palate. Cleft Palate J 1978; 15:306-28.

16. Shprintzen RJ, Croft CB, Berkman MD, Rakoff SJ. Velopharyngeal insufficiency in the facio-auriculo-vertebral malformation. Cleft Palate J 1980; 17:132-7.

17. Spriestersbach DC. Psychosocial aspects of cleft palate. Iowa City: University of Iowa Press, 1973; 35-9.

Ann Otol 91:1982

VOCAL SYMPTOMS IN PARKINSON DISEASE TREATED WITH LEVODOPA

A CASE REPORT

W. SHAIN SCHLEY, MD
NEW YORK, NEW YORK

ELAINE FENTON, PhD
NEW YORK, NEW YORK

SEIJI NIIMI, MD
TOKYO, JAPAN

This is a report of a patient with unusually severe hoarseness in the absence of vocal fold pathology demonstrating Parkinson disease as one of the neurological diseases in which vocal symptoms occur. Although it is classifiably a severe, progressive, degenerative disorder, the popularity of pharmacotherapy for Parkinson disease during the past decade has resulted in improved functionality for an undetermined course of time in most patients. The classically described deterioration of speech and voice may develop in a variant manner difficult to distinguish as disease-related, as this case report illustrates. An explanation of the hoarseness based on dyssynchronous vocal fold motion related to the disease is suggested by the acoustic methods (spectrography, waveform analysis) used in this study, and supported by strobe light laryngoscopy. This conclusion is important because of the extremely high incidences of varying degrees of hoarseness reported in recent studies of Parkinson disease.

Parkinson disease, named after James Parkinson who first described it in 1817,[1] is a progressive degenerative neurological disease characterized by tremor and rigidity. The current method-of-choice in treatment is the administration of pharmacotherapy,[2] of which the best known medication is the popularized L-dopa, with or without peripheral metabolic inhibitors.

Consequences to communication of Parkinson disease have been reported, and both voice disorders[3-8] and upper articulatory tract dysarthria[9-14] have been noted. The attempt to relate speech disorders to adequate medication has been only partially successful,[15-17] but it is logical to assume some correlation. Although there is no direct evidence, anecdotal accounts of patients diagnosed as having Parkinson disease sometimes give indirect indication that the patient has had a long history of modest vocal dysfunction prior to any other symptom. It is tempting to speculate upon the occurrence of voicing anomalies as early-onset signs of Parkinson disease, and important to study vocal fold function in diagnosed patients, because the laryngologist may wish to include parkinsonism among other neurological diseases known to manifest hoarseness as part of the symptom complex.

CASE REPORT

The patient, born in 1898, began to manifest some symptoms during the last portion of his sixth decade, for which he consulted his family physician. At the age of 71 he was diagnosed as having idiopathic Parkinson disease on the basis of his appearance, gait and handwriting, and was successfully medicated with levodopa. The following year his physician recommended that he consult a laryngologist for a severe persistent hoarse voice. Indirect laryngoscopy was unsatisfactory; a possible right ventricular fold disorder was suspected. Direct laryngoscopy was performed due to the severity of his vocal symptoms. The vocal folds were clear and had normal mobility. A biopsy of both ventricular bands gave negative results. In the absence of other signs, a tentative diagnosis of dysphonia ventricularis was made. The patient remained severely hoarse during the next three years with no further indication of laryngeal pathology.

At the time he was seen by us, the patient was 76 years of age, an ambulatory medicated out-patient of the Parkinson's Disease Clinic. He manifested the severely rough hoarse voice that is generally associated with advanced vocal fold pathology. The vocal "fading" at the ends of phrases which is believed to be characteristic in parkinsonians was inconsistently present in mild degree. No upper articulatory tract dysarthria or dyskinesia was observed, although the patient's facial mask and postural symptoms were classic. He described himself as having a hoarse voice and reported that his voice was better during periods of effective medication and tended to worsen as medication wore off. Clinical observation over a one-year period did not validate this; although he may have experienced less effortful voicing during periods of effective medication, no external evidence of change in voicing was found. The patient's voice was audible but severely hoarse.

From the Departments of Otolaryngology and Neurology, New York Hospital-Cornell University Medical Center, and the Institute of Logopedics and Phoniatrics, Faculty of Medicine, University of Tokyo.

REPRINTS — W. Shain Schley, MD, F844-New York Hospital, 525 East 68th Street, New York, NY 10021.

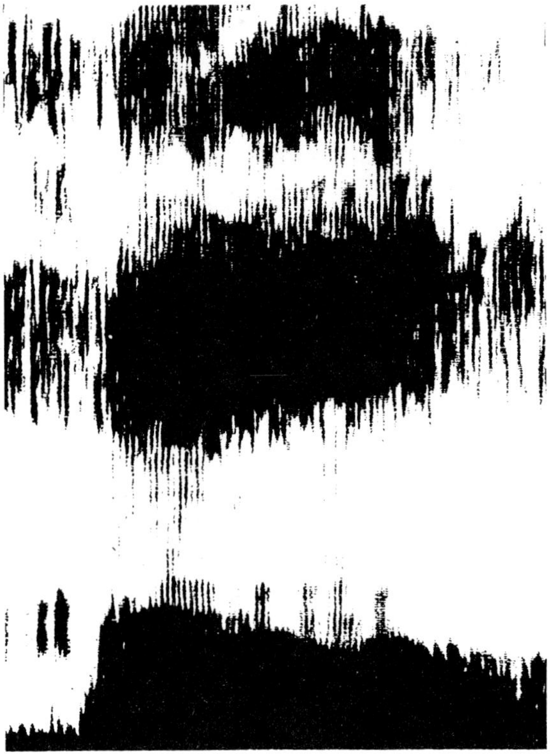

Fig. 1. Portion of a wide band spectrogram of patient saying the word "hayed," demonstrating striations and evidence of air leakage in upper portion. Calibration tone on left shows frequency scale in 1000 Hz. Intervals; approx. 600 ms sample. (Kay Sonograph 80-8000/540)

Five tape-recorded samples of oral reading and spontaneous conversation were made at intervals during the one-year period that the patient was followed in the Parkinson's Disease Clinic. Portions of these samples were subjected to acoustic analysis in an attempt to further investigate this patient's voicing disorder. Spectrographic analysis demonstrated obvious voicing anomalies, and some evidence of air leakage was found in the upper portions suggested by the indication of noise across the top of the spectrogram (Fig. 1). These signs in spectrograms are commensurate with vocal fold disorder of various etiology and were sufficiently severe to warrant further acoustic analysis as a method of investigation.

Waveform analysis demonstrated irregular pitch periods; as the scale is enlarged, the phenomenon becomes more obvious, and could be explained by an irregularity of the synchronous motion of the vocal folds. Such problems can be observed during the production of vowels. For example, five contiguous pitch periods gated out of the midpoint of /e/ in "rainbow" are all dissimilar in this patient (Fig. 2). The relationship between perceived hoarseness and irregular pitch periods is well known.[18] Figure 3 shows a waveform analysis of a normal speaker for comparison. All figures were prepared in accordance with standard techniques.[19,20]

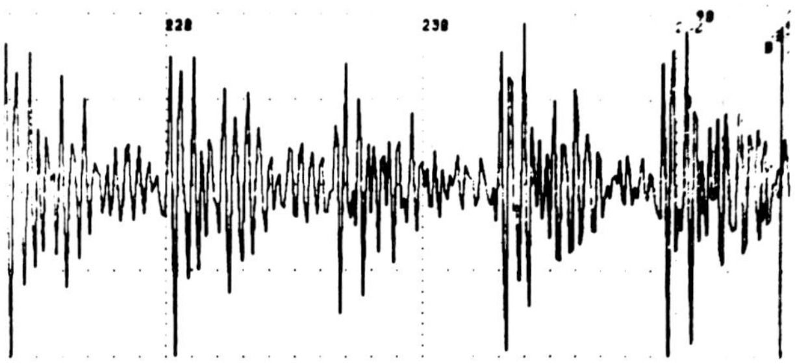

Fig. 2. Waveform analysis of five pitch periods gated out of patient's utterance of /e/ in "rainbow." Note that all five pitch periods are dissimilar.

DISCUSSION

This severely hoarse patient demonstrated voicing patterns on acoustic analysis which prompted further laryngeal study of idiopathic Parkinson disease. Seven cases were examined with the stroboscopic light on indirect laryngoscopy (for which this patient was not a candidate, as indicated above) in an effort to observe vocal fold function during phonation. A double-blind design was used, in which the laryngologists and neurologists examined sidedness of the disease entity. In six of the seven cases, sidedness was indicated as the same by both laryngological and neurological examinations; the seventh case was a bilaterally involved patient.

On the basis of these findings it was possible to hypothesize[21] that roughness of phonation in Parkinson disease patients is caused by assymetrical motion of the vocal folds as a manifestation of a pathological muscle condition characteristic of the disease entity, and is likely to occur in the absence of any specific laryngeal pathology.

It seems likely that this patient's hoarseness and the vocal symptoms displayed in acoustic analysis are due to dyssynchronous fold motion. It is possible that the air leakage demonstrated spectrographically (Fig. 1) may be due to a severe form of this disorder. Abnormality leading to irregular fold movement may not be obvious in visualization. For example, Hirano[22] has proposed that the movement

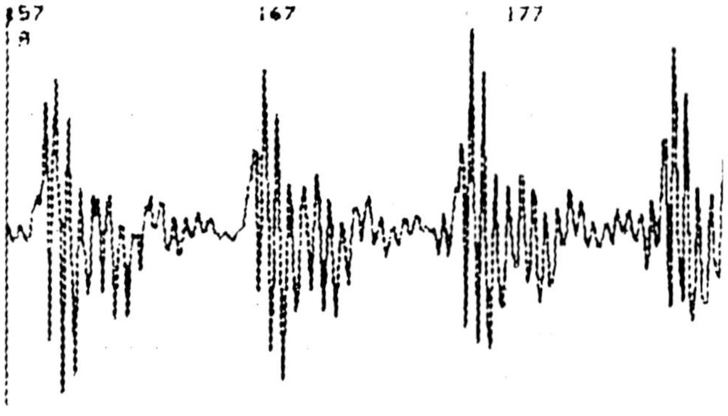

Fig. 3. Waveform analysis of a normal speaker demonstrating expected similarity between pitch periods of same sound, same utterance; compare to Fig. 2.

of the mucosal cover of the folds is important in producing the periodic wave perceived as normal voicing.

The presence of hoarseness in the patient and the absence of laryngeal pathology of the type which would produce a load on the vocal folds was especially striking but not wholly unexpected. A high incidence of voicing disorders among Parkinson disease patients has been reported in several recent studies;[8,23,24] this case study examines a severe instance in detail.

ACKNOWLEDGMENTS — The authors gratefully acknowledge F. Plum, MD, Neurologist-in-Chief, N.Y.H.; R. W. Sweet, MD; P. Papavasiliou, MD; and F. McDowell, MD. We are indebted to K. S. Harris, PhD, for helpful suggestions in the preparation of the manuscript. All acoustic displays were produced at the Haskins Laboratories with the kind assistance of T. Holwes, PhD, and F. Bell-Berti, PhD.

REFERENCES

1. Critchley McD, ed. James Parkinson, 1755-1824. London: Macmillan, 1955.

2. Cotzias G, McDowell R, eds. Developments in treatment for Parkinson's disease. New York: Medcom Medical Update Series, 1971.

3. Canter G. Speech characteristics of patients with Parkinson's disease. I. Intensity, pitch and duration. J Speech Hear Disord 1963; 30:221-9.

4. Logemann J, Boshes B, Fisher H. The steps in the degeneration of speech and voice control in Parkinson's disease. In: Parkinson's disease. Bern: Hans Huber, 1972; 2:101-12.

5. Darley F, Aronson A, Brown J. Differential diagnostic patterns of dysarthria. J Speech Hear Res 1969; 12:246-69.

6. Boshes B. Voice changes in Parkinsonism. J Neurosurg 1966; 1 Suppl 24:286-8.

7. Ludlow C. Acoustic study of speech in Parkinson's disease. J Acoust Soc Am 1976; 60 Suppl 1.

8. Fenton E, Harris K, Sweet R. Parkinson's disease: acoustic analysis of phonation. ASHA 1975; 17:607.

9. Blonsky E, Logemann J, Boshes B, Fisher H. Comparison of speech and swallowing function in patients with tremor disorders and in normal geriatric patients: a cinefluorographic study. J Gerontol 1975; 30:299-309.

10. Canter J. Speech characteristics of patients with Parkinson's disease. III. Articulation, diadochokinesis, and overall speech adequacy. J Speech Hear Disord 1965; 30:217-24.

11. Leanderson R, Meyerson B, Persson A. Lip muscle function in parkinsonian dysarthria. Acta Otolaryngol (Stockh) 1972; 74:350-7.

12. Morrison E, Rigrodsky S, Mysak E. Parkinson's disease: speech disorder and released infantile oroneuromotor activity. J Speech Hear Res 1970; 13:655-66.

13. Netsell R, Daniel B, Celesia G. Acceleration and weakness in parkinsonian dysarthria. J Speech Hear Disord 1975; 40:170-8.

14. Doshay L. Parkinson's disease: its meaning and management. Philadelphia: Lippincott, 1970.

15. Nakano K, Zubick H, Tyler H. Speech defects of parkinsonian patients. Neurology (Minneap) 1973; 23:865-70.

16. Rigrodsky S, Morrison E. Speech changes in parkinsonism during L-dopa therapy: preliminary findings. J Am Geriatr Soc 1970; 18:142-51.

17. Leanderson R, Meyerson B, Persson A. Effect of L-dopa on speech in parkinsonism: an EMG study of labial articulatory function. J Neurol Neurosurg Psychiatry 1971; 34:679-81.

18. Niimi S. Pulse train and tonality. Japan J Logopedics Phoniatrics Tokyo 1972; 13:2.

19. Lieberman P. Speech physiology and acoustic phonetics: an introduction. New York: Macmillan, 1977.

20. Borden G, Harris K. Research tools in speech science. Baltimore: Williams and Wilkins, 1980:215-43.

21. Fenton E, Niimi S, Harris K, Schley W. Stroboscopic investigation of larynges of Parkinson's disease patients. ASHA 1976; 18:670.

22. Hirano M. Phonosurgery: basic and clinical investigations. Otol (Fukuoka) (Jibito Rinsho) 1975; 21 Suppl 1.

23. Logemann J, Fisher H, Boshes B. Frequency and progression of speech and voice degeneration in Parkinson's disease. Parkinson's Dis Abstr 1972; 301-3.

24. Uziel A, Boke M, Cadilhac J, Passouant P. Les troubles de la voix et de la parole dans les syndromes parkinsoniens. Folia Phoniat 1975; 27:166-76.

A CASE OF CYSTICERCOSIS CEREBRI
NEUROTOLOGIC IMPLICATIONS

STEVEN J. MILLEN, MD
MILWAUKEE, WISCONSIN

JACK L. PULEC, MD
LOS ANGELES, CALIFORNIA

Cysticercosis is an unusual disease entity in the United States. A case is reviewed in which a young Mexican-American female presented to an otologist's office with a headache and vertigo. Her symptoms were a manifestation of a single larval cysticercus cyst which had become lodged in the fourth ventricle resulting in an obstructive hydrocephalus and a fatal course. The epidemiology of this disease traces the life cycle of the pork tapeworm from man, normally the definitive host, to the pig, the intermediate host. It is noteworthy that the disease cysticercosis in humans is a deviation from the parasite's normal life cycle in which man serves as the intermediate host. The literature is reviewed. The broad clinical spectrum of this disease's presentation can extend from a single headache to multiple nerve palsies and convulsions. The importance of radiographic evaluation complement fixation testing and CSF evaluation in making a diagnosis is stressed. There is no known medical treatment for this disease. Surgical procedures such as primary excision and shunts to relieve intracranial pressure have had mixed results. The prognosis depends on the location and the number of infesting larva. Special note is made of this disease's endemic status in Mexico and other Latin American countries and the role that this may play in medicine practiced in the southwest United States considering the ever-increasing immigration from this area.

INTRODUCTION

Two of the more perplexing diagnostic symptoms confronting the otolaryngologist today are the complaints of dizziness and headache. Both are common and initially often do not command the attention they merit. Their differential diagnoses are diverse and can lead a patient through an extensive array of diagnostic studies and treatments that frequently ends in frustration and dissatisfaction on the part of the patient and the physician, who is not prepared to deal with them in a systematic and thorough approach.

Although the majority of headaches evaluated may not represent a grave threat to the patient, it is important to evaluate this symptom with respect to the significant morbidity and mortality which may accompany it.

An unusual and tragic case of a patient who presented to an otologist's office with a headache and dizziness is presented to emphasize this problem and review the neurologic implications of the uncommon disease entity, cysticercosis cerebri.

CASE REPORT

The patient, a 23-year-old married Mexican-American female, was initially seen in June 1977 with a complaint of bilateral hearing loss of long duration. The otologic examination revealed dry, almost total pars tensa perforations bilaterally, and an audiogram showed a 40 dB conductive hearing loss bilaterally. A left tympanoplasty (using a homograft tympanic membrane) was performed under a local anesthetic on July 6, 1977.

Postoperatively the patient experienced a breakdown of her graft, and she began for the first time to complain of headaches. Evaluation including an ENG and petrous pyramid x-ray study was unremarkable. An internist was consulted for a general physical examination. No abnormalities were found.

The patient failed to return for follow-up until one year later in June 1978. At that time she complained of headaches and vertigo. The headaches were described as paroxsymal and occurred sporadically throughout the day. They were bilateral, began in the occipital area, and radiated to the frontal area. They had begun about one year previously but had been totally absent during a recent pregnancy, only to resume again three weeks following her delivery. There was no aura preceding the headaches. She was not on any medication, and her past medical history was unremarkable. Other symptoms included visual complaints of blurring and flashing of bright lights, perioral paresthesia, and paresthesias of the hands and feet; there was no motor weakness.

The vertigo was described as a rotatory sensation which began approximately 12 days prior to her return to the office. She felt it was positionally related with her right ear down, and was accompanied by nausea and vomiting.

The otologic examination revealed a dry left tympanic membrane perforation and a right tensor perforation with mucoid drainage. No mastoid tenderness was found. An immediate consultation for a general medical evaluation was obtained.

Work supported by Ear International, Los Angeles.
Presented at the meeting of the American Neurotology Society, Dallas, Texas, October 7, 1979.

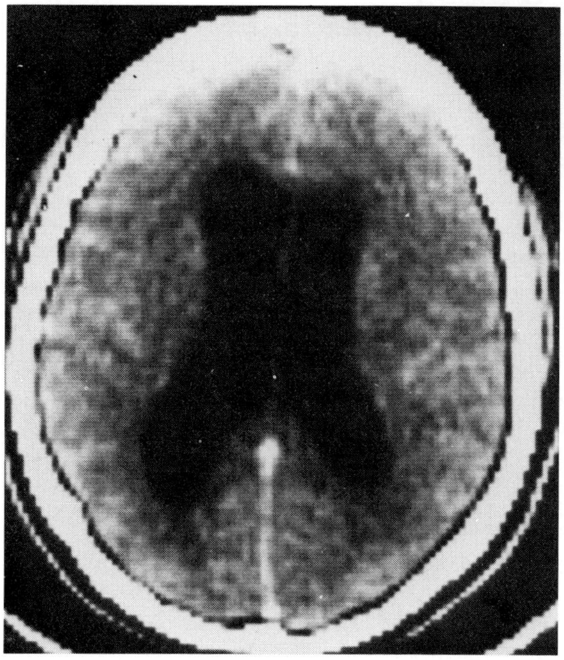

Fig. 1. CAT scan demonstrating marked hydrocephalus with dilatation of the lateral ventricles.

Upon follow-up examination the next morning the patient's symptoms of headache and vertigo appeared to have increased in severity. She was admitted to the hospital for further evaluation. At the time of admission she was alert, oriented, afebrile, with normal vital signs, but appeared in mild distress. The physical examination revealed patient discomfort on neck hyperextension, but none with flexion or rotation. The Kernig's and Brudzinski's signs were negative. All cranial nerves were intact, and the fundi appeared normal. Motor and sensory function were also unremarkable. As part of the patient's initial evaluation, a CAT scan was performed and showed marked hydrocephalus with dilatation of the third and lateral ventricles (Fig. 1). The remaining laboratory and radiologic studies including chest x-ray study, c-spine, skull films, CBC, and SMA-12 were unremarkable.

The initial management following neurologic and neurosurgical consultations was a medical regime to relieve the increased intracranial pressure. On the second day following admission, the patient's headaches increased in severity and she became lethargic, but she remained afebrile and the WBC remained normal. A lumbar puncture revealed clear CSF and an opening pressure of 160 mm H_2O. The CSF report showed 165 WBC, 91% polymorphonuclear leukocytes, and 9% lymphocytes, protein 48 mg% and sugar 56 mg%. The India ink prep was negative.

As the patient's condition continued to deteriorate she was transferred to the intensive care unit and preparations were made to perform a ventriculoperitoneal (VP) shunt. At this point she experienced a cardiac arrest but was resuscitated. The VP shunt was then performed as an emergency procedure. Postoperatively the patient required ventilatory assistance and vasopressors. Her pulmonary status was further complicated by a shock lung syndrome. Her condition deteriorated steadily, and following multiple cardiac arrests, the patient died one day postoperatively.

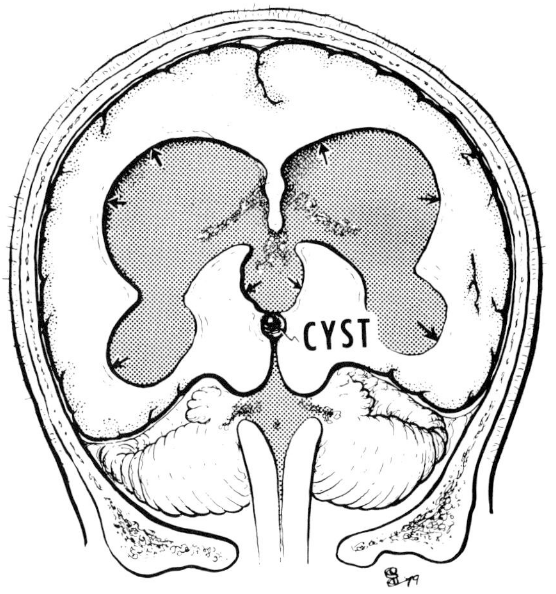

Fig. 2. Schematic diagram of the ventricular system demonstrating the cysticercosis cyst obstructing the fourth ventricle.

At the time of autopsy, intracranical findings included flattening of the cerebral convolutions and a pressure groove along the cerebral peduncles secondary to downward herniation of the brain. Gross sections of the brain showed the ventricles to be of normal size with the shunt tube in place. A small 2-3 mm soft mass was noted within the fourth ventricle (Fig. 2). On microscopic section this mass was found to be a cysticercosis cyst. There was no other evidence of disseminated parasitic disease.

DISCUSSION

Cysticercosis is a parasitic disease which results when the human serves as intermediate host in the life cycle of *Taenia solium*, the pork tapeworm. It is a common misconception that man acquires cysticercosis through the ingestion of poorly cooked pork. When one ingests pork infested with the larva of *T solium*, he becomes the definitive host within the life cycle, not the intermediate host. As the definitive host, he does not manifest the symptoms of cysticercosis, but rather develops an intestinal pork tapeworm. In the definitive stage of the life cycle, larvae are released from the ingested pork by digestion and attach to the gut wall of man, maturing into adult tapeworms within 5 to 12 weeks. The adult tapeworm periodically sheds proglottids, which are egg-bearing segments, and these pass in

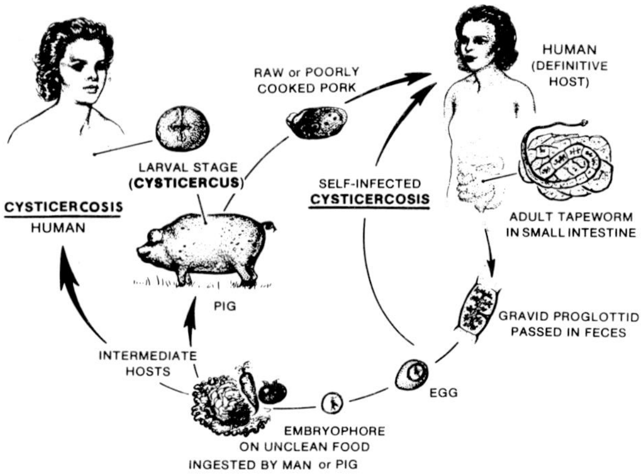

Fig. 3. The life cycle of the pork tapeworm *Taenia solium*.

the feces. When ingested by the pig, the ova have their shells dissolved and liberate mobile oncospheres which penetrate through the gut wall and enter into the mesenteric circulation. In 60 to 70 days these oncospheres continue to develop and each forms a hooked scolex surrounded by a fluid-filled bladder. This represents the larval stage and is known as cysticercosis.

In order for humans to serve as the intermediate host and therefore develop cysticercosis, it is necessary for them to ingest the ova of *T solium*, and not the larva found in infested pork. Contamination with ova may be accomplished either by direct consumption of fecally-contaminated food, anus-to-mouth contamination by hand, or regurgitation of the ova from the gastrointestinal tract (Fig. 3). Man can serve as both the definitive and intermediate host at one time, and 26% of patients with cysticercosis cerebri have been found to have an adult intestinal tapeworm.[1]

Cysticercosis cerebri is an uncommon disease entity in most of the United States.[2-7] However, this disease is endemic in areas of the world such as Central and South America, Eastern Europe, India, and the Far East. And important to the physician practicing in the southwestern United States is the reported incidence of cysticercosis in the Mexican population where it has been reported to account for 13-34% of all intracranial tumors[7-12] and has a reported incidence of 3.6% in general autopsies.[13]

The diagnosis of cysticercosis is difficult to make because of the infinite variety of symptoms with which it may present. Within the CNS its presentation has been separated into three clinical groups by Stepien and Chorobski.[14] The first group are those patients whose symptoms are similar to space-occupying lesions with manifestations of focal neurologic deficits, cranial nerve palsies, and obstructive hydrocephalus. The second group are those patients with diffuse cerebral signs and symptoms of increased intracranial pressure. And the third group are those patients whose cysts are located at the base of the brain causing a chronic basalar leptomeningitis, internal hydrocephalus and variable focal signs.

Probably the most common presentation includes the symptoms of increased intracranial pressure with severe headaches, nausea, and vomiting. Other less common presenting symptoms include cranial nerve abnormalities and visual field impairments. Seizures are frequent and usually of the Jacksonian type.[15] Psychic disturbances including amnesia, disorientation, confusion, and dementia may also be present. The association of headache, vertigo, nausea and vomiting, appearing periodically and usually after a rapid change in position, is suggestive of a cysticercosis cyst lying free in the fourth ventricle. This has been termed Burns' sign and was manifested in this case.[16,17]

Within the brain cysticercosis will show a predilection for the leptomeninges and ventricles and less commonly the brain parenchyma.[12] When present in the ventricles, it is most commonly found in the third or fourth ventricle,[8] as was the case with our patient. Clinically the symptoms of cysticercosis may present from a few months to 30 years after contact.[18] The average time from contact to symptom presentation in one large series was 4.8 years.[19] Cysticercosis cysts may remain viable within the CNS from three to six years.[20] This life span is somewhat longer than when they are present in the skeletal musculature, the most common area of localization. When the organism dies, a portion of its structure called a bladder may absorb fluid from the host and increase in size up to 5 cm in diameter.

In the case of ventricular cysts it is after the death of the organism with its resultant increase in size that symptoms frequently occur. Following the death of the organism the spinal fluid findings return to normal.[21] A review of the microscopic sections in our case revealed that the patient's symptom progression and terminal events were probably caused by an expanding cyst.

The diagnosis of cysticercosis is primarily based on radiologic findings and the CSF complement fixation test in conjunction with the appropriate historical presentation. The diagnosis may also be made by a biopsy of a subcutaneous nodule. Subcutaneous nodules have been reported to occur in 54% of cases.[18] Marlet has described an intradermal antigen which may be used for diagnosis.[22] The use of CT scanning is usually not helpful in demonstrating ventricular cysts because the cyst fluid and CSF have similar absorptive values.

One of the best aids to diagnosis is the spinal fluid evaluation. Commonly found are an elevated protein, a decreased sugar and a mild pleocytosis with eosinophilia. The complement fixation test is reported positive in 64-80% of cases.[21,23]

Radiologically a number of findings are present in cysticercosis. Calcification of the dead larva has been reported in from 11-19%.[1,8,15] Calcified larvae are found earlier and more commonly in muscle than in brain tissue, and almost every patient with a calcified cerebral cyst will have calcified muscular cysts. It is believed to take approximately ten years after infestation for calcification to occur.[18] Radiographic signs of intracranial hypertension have been reported in 72% of one series with 88 patients.[8] These changes include erosion of the dorsum sella, enlargement of the sella turcica, and widening of the cranial sutures.

There is no known medical treatment for cysticercosis. The use of steroids as an adjunct to surgery has been reported by Cabieses,[24] and several reports of radiotherapy have indicated good results.[14] However, the primary mode of therapy in patients with a single cyst acting as a cerebral tumor is surgery. Stepien and Chorobski reviewed 63 operative cases of this type and reported the following results: 28.9% recovered, 38.1% improved, 19% died, and 6.3% no change.[14,25]

Simms has discussed shunting of the CSF as an effective treatment for cysticercosis cerebri with aqueductal occlusion.[26] However, others feel that shunts usually fail when they become blocked with debris from the ventricles. A third ventriculostomy has been suggested by Tolosa as an alternative approach to the shunt in order to relieve intracranial pressure.[27]

The prognosis of cysticercosis as presented in a series of 284 patients reviewed by Dixon and Hargreaves showed a mortality of 8%.[1] It is apparent that the localization and numbers of larvae involved play a significant role in the mortality and morbidity. If the disease solely involves the brain parenchyma and the larvae are few in number, the disease may regress spontaneously.[23] The poorest prognosis has been found in those patients with hydrocephalus as was the case in our patient.

SUMMARY

A case of cysticercosis cerebri occurring in a young Mexican-American female has been presented and the epidemiology evaluation and treatment reviewed. The medical practitioner is reminded of the high incidence of this disease in the population of Mexico, Central and South America and the related significance of Mexican immigration into the southwestern United States.

REFERENCES

1. Dixon HBF, Hargreaves WH. Cysticercosis (*Taenia solium*): further 10 years' clinical study covering 284 cases. Q J Med 1944; 13:107-21.

2. Cohen B. Cysticercosis cerebri: a case report. South Med J 1962; 55:48-55.

3. Dent IH. Cysticercosis cerebri-cestode infestation of human brain: report of a case occurring in Louisiana. JAMA 1947; 164:401-5.

4. Greenspan G, Stevens L. Infection with cysticercus cellulosae: report of a case. N Engl J Med 1961; 264:741-54.

5. Haining RB, Haining RG. Cysticercosis cerebri. JAMA 1960; 172:2036-9.

6. Hoffman SF, Guthrie TH. Cerebral cysticercosis. South Med J 1975; 68:105-8.

7. White JC, Sweet WH, Richardson EP Jr. Cysticercosis cerebri: a diagnostic and therapeutic problem of increasing importance. N Engl J Med 1947; 256:479-86.

8. Dorfsman J. The radiological aspects of cerebral cysticercosis. Acta Radiol [Diagn] (Stockh) 1963; 1:836-42.

9. Lombardo L, Mateus JH. Cerebral cysticercosis in Mexico. Neurology 1961; 11:824-8.

10. Obrador S. Clinical aspects of cerebral cysticercosis. Arch Neurol Psychiatry 1948; 59:457-68.

11. Olive JI, Angulo-Rivero P. Panel discussion: cysticercosis of the nervous system. J Neurosurg 1962; 19:632-43.

12. Santin G, Varga JS. Roentgen study of cysticercosis of central nervous system. Radiology 1966; 86:520-8.

13. Costero L. Cisticercosis del sistema nervioso. Tratado de Anatomia Patologica Mexico, Atlanta, 1946:1485-95.

14. Stepien L, Chorobski J. Cysticercosis cerebri and its operative treatment. Arch Neurol Psychiatry 1949; 61:499-527.

15. Pupo PP. Cysticercosis of the nervous system: clinical manifestations. Rev Neuropsiquiatr 1964; 27:70-82.

16. Burns L. Neuropathie demonstration. Neurol Zentralbl 1906; 25:540.

17. Oppenheim H. Lehrbuch der Nervenkrankheiten für Arzie und Studierende. S. Karger, 1908:193.

18. Dixon HBF, Lipscomb FM. Cysticercosis: an analysis and follow-up of 450 cases. Privy Council, Medical Research Council Special Report, no. 299, London, Her Majesty's Stationery Office, 1961:1-57.

19. Carbajal JR, Palacios E, Azar-Kia B, Churchill R. Radiology of cysticercosis of the central nervous system including computed tomography. Radiology 1977; 125:127-31.

20. King JS, Hosobuchi Y. Cysticercus cyst of the lateral ventricle. Surg Neurol 1977; 7:125-9.

21. Goni PB. Panel discussion: cysticercosis of the nervous system: III. Clinical findings and treatment. J Neurosurg 1962; 19:641-3.

22. Marlet JM. Estudo de um antigeno intradermico para o diagnostico da cisticercose. Noa Preria. Rev Saude Publica 1974; 8:443-5.

23. Cardenas J. Panel discussion: cysticercosis of the nervous system: II. Pathological and radiologic findings. J Neurosurg 1962; 19:635-40.

24. Cabieses F. Panel discussion: cysticercosis of the nervous system. J Neurosurg 1962; 19:643.

25. Stepien L. Cerebral cysticercosis in Poland: clinical symptoms and operative results in 132 cases. J Neurosurg 1962; 19:505-13.

26. Simms NM, Maxwell RE, Christenson PC. Internal hydrocephalus secondary to cysticercosis cerebri: treatment with a ventriculoatrial shunt. J Neurosurg 1969; 30:305-9.

27. Olive J, Angulo-Rivero P. Cysticercosis of the central nervous system: I. Introduction and general aspects. J Neurosurg 1962; 19:632-43.

OBITUARY

SAMUEL ROSEN

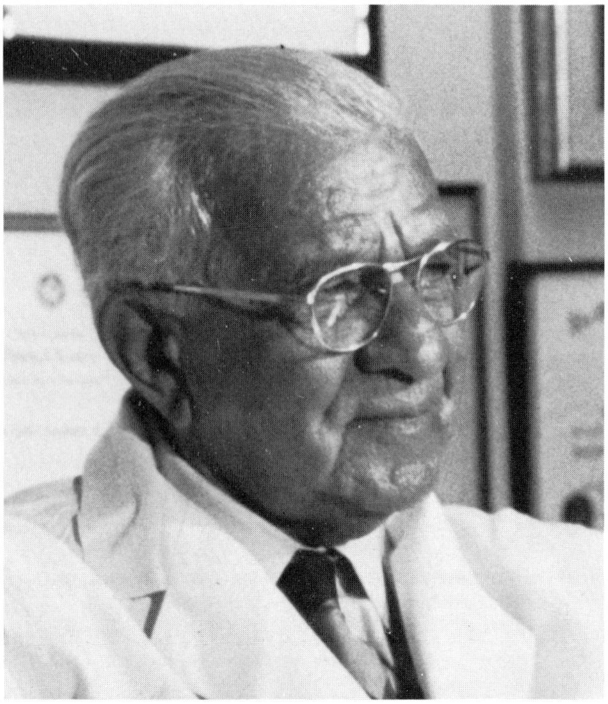

1898-1981

Sam Rosen was a remarkable man: an outstanding otologic surgeon, a serious student and clinical investigator, an enthusiastic and effective teacher, an indefatigable traveller, a liberal-minded world citizen, and a devoted husband.

Sam did not come by these unique characteristics easily. He was born into a poor immigrant family; his brother and sisters made major sacrifices in order to provide him with the financial assistance to attend college and medical school. He demonstrated superior intellectual and surgical aptitudes in his residency training, and was promptly selected by a prestigious otologist as his protege and his medical future seemed assured. He was on his way to a successful career as an otologic surgeon.

It would have been very simple for Sam to fit into the pattern of a successful Park Avenue consultant with the likely prospect of succeeding to the directorship of the otologic service of one of the major hospitals in New York. But Sam and his intelligent and lovely wife, Helen, were caring and concerned people who believed that a full and productive life meant total commitment, not only to medicine but to the humanitarian ideas and ideals in which they believed. They devoted their lives to the achievement of these goals.

Otology owes a great debt to Sam Rosen. He was devoted to his work and enjoyed his efforts to shed some light on the unexplained causes of deafness and vertigo. He lived to see worldwide appreciation of the role of the Rosen stapes mobilization procedure in the evolution of hearing rehabilitation; he derived great pleasure in watching his students and proteges all over the world build upon and improve his fundamental concepts.

For a large part of his adult life, Sam devoted himself to the dissemination of otologic information and to the gathering of research data in many areas of the world. Despite some resistance to these efforts and with considerable personal sacrifice, he made possible an interchange of knowledge and experience between members of the medical professions of the United States and some 40 other countries.

The Rosens became interested in China and the Chinese people in 1937. They were among the first Americans to be invited to visit that country. Most recently, they devoted themselves to establishing better communications between the United States and China. Sam and Helen led groups of otolaryngologic teachers to China, providing them with the opportunity to see and to understand the many contributions made by the Peoples Republic of China and their doctors, and to provide the Chinese medical profession with the most recent otolaryngological developments in the United States.

Sam was recognized and honored all over the world; a list of his honors, citations, gold medals and elections to honorary memberships is endless. In the United States, he was awarded the prestigious American Otological Society Award of Merit in 1971, and in 1980 he received the Presidential Citation of the American Academy of Ophthalmology and Otolaryngology.

Sam is survived by his wife, two children, Judith Ruben and Dr. John F. Rosen, and four grandchildren.

The world will miss Sam Rosen's enthusiastic medical leadership and his humanitarianism. Otolaryngology has lost a valued colleague. Many of us have lost a dear friend.

Ben H. Senturia, MD

COMBINED OTOLARYNGOLOGICAL SPRING MEETINGS

The Breakers, Palm Beach, Florida

1982 Preliminary Programs
(Subject to change and Council approval)

AMERICAN BRONCHO-ESOPHAGOLOGICAL ASSOCIATION

May 3-4, 1982

Observations on So-called Idiopathic Vocal Cord Paralysis. Paul H. Ward, MD, George Berci, MD.

Hereditary Abductor Vocal Cord Paralysis — A New Look at a Rare Disorder. Gregory Milmoe, MD, Kenneth M. Grundfast, MD.

Atlanto-Axial Instability Revisited — An Alert for Endoscopists, Martin L. Norton, MD.

Laryngeal Malignancies and Computerized Tomography: A Correlation of Tomographic and Histopathologic Sections, Joyce A. Schild, MD, Galdino E. Valvassori, MD, Mahmood F. Mafee, MD.

A New Tracheal Valve for Voice Production. Eric D. Blom, PhD, Mark I. Singer, MD, Ronald C. Hamaker, MD.

Factors in Successful Deglutition Following Subtotal Laryngeal Surgery. Toribio C. Flores, MD, Benjamin G. Wood, MD, Howard L. Levine, MD, Lawrence Koegel, Jr., MD, Harvey M. Tucker, MD.

The Complications of Tracheal Intubation. William M. Keane, MD, James Denneny, MD, Joseph P. Atkins, Jr., MD, Lee D. Rowe, MD.

Wegener's Granulomatosis of the Subglottic and Upper Trachea. Thomas J. McDonald, MD, H. Bryan Neel, III, MD, Richard A. DeRemee, MD.

Wegener's Granulomatosis Appearing Initially in the Trachea. Juan Carlos Arauz, MD, Rolando Fonseca, MD.

Anatomic Abnormalities in Obstructive Sleep Apnea. Dale Wilms, MD, William Conway, MD, Shiro Fujita, MD, Frank Zorick, MD, John Popovich, MD.

Brainstem Evoked Response Auditory in Adult Sleep Apnea. Nancy L. Snyderman, MD, Charles F. Reynolds, MD, Margareta Mǿller, MD, Jonas T. Johnson, MD.

Foley Catheter Removal of Esophageal Foreign Bodies: A Survey. W. Frederick McGuirt, MD.

A Simple Endoscopic Intubation Technique of a Malignant Esophageal Obstruction. Enje Th. Edens, MD, Jos. J. M. van Overbeek, MD.

Presentation of New Instruments.
1. Minimally Combustible Endotracheal Tube for Laser Surgery. Thomas Yarrington, MD.
2. Heat Sump Protection for Endotracheal Cuff. Francis LeJeune, MD.

Research Speaker: Dysphagia, Its Clinical and Basic Investigations. Tetsuzo Inouye, MD.

Research Essay Contest — First Prize: The Dynamics of Venturi Jet Ventilation Through the Operating Laryngoscope. Peak Woo, MD, Stephan Eurenius, BS. Second Prize (Paper Will Not Be Presented). Idiopathic Inflammatory Obstructive Tracheitis. J. T. Twiggs, MD, E. J. O'Connell, MD, R. L. Telander, MD, B. W. Pearson, MD, L. H. Weiland, MD, and J. C. McDougall, MD.

Seymour R. Cohen Award for Pediatric Laryngology and Bronchoesophagology, The Infant Larynx — Normal and Anomalous. John A. Tucker, MD.

Foregut Cysts in the Pediatric Age Group: Airway Problems — Diagnosis and Management. Seymour R. Cohen, MD, Kenneth A. Geller, MD, Jeffrey W. Birns, MD, Jerome W. Thompson, MD.

The Treatment of Recurrent Respiratory Papillomatosis (RRP) with Mumps Skin Test Antigen (MSTA). Allan B. Seid, MD, Thomas J. Fischer, MD, John E. Neely, MD, Robert I. Kaplan, MD, Ruth Bockhold, RN, Robin T. Cotton, MD.

Pediatric Tracheostomy: Experience During the Past Decade, Ralph T. Wetmore, MD, Steven D. Handler, MD, William P. Potsick, MD.

Home Care of Tracheostomies. R. J. Ruben, MD, L. Newton, MD, H. Chambers, MD, D. L. Jornsay, RN, PNP, C. A. Lawrence, MA, RN, J. Liquori, CSW.

Scanning Electron Microscopic Examination of Non-Beating Cilia. James P. Dudley, MD, Lance Eisner, James D. Cherry, MD.

Bronchoscopic Limited Lavage for Cystic Fibrosis Patients — An Adjunct to Therapy. Bruce F. Rothmann, MD, Lewis H. Walker, MD, Robert T. Stone, MD, Francois W. Seguin, MD.

Transtracheal Catheter Oxygen Delivery System. Henry J. Heimlich, MD.

Tracheobronchial Obstruction from Metastatic Malignancies from Distant Sites. Stanley M. Shapshay, MD.

Photoradiation Therapy in Local Control of Cancer of the Tracheobronchial Tree. Denis L. Cortese, MD, James H. Kinsey, PhD.

Caustic Indigestion in Children — A Review of 400 Cases. J. S. Adams, MD, H. G. Birck, Md.

Mediastinoscopy for Extra Thoracic Tumors Involving the Mediastinum. Louis W. Welsh, MD.

AMERICAN LARYNGOLOGICAL ASSOCIATION

May 4-6, 1982

Age-Related Changes in the Monkey Larynx. Charles W. Cummings, MD.

Office Telescopic Photography of the Larynx. Eiji Yanagisawa, MD.

A Classification and Approach to Patients With Functional Voice Disorders. James A. Koufman, MD.

Pathogenesis of Vocal Cord Polyps. Oskar Klein, MD.

Endoscopic Rehabilitation of the Airway in Laryngeal Paralysis. F. R. Kirchner, MD, FACS.

Predictive Factors of Success or Failure in Endoscopic Management of Laryngeal and Tracheal Stenosis. George T. Simpson, MD.

Present Diagnosis and Conservative Surgical Management of Condrosarcoma of the Larynx. Julius N. Hicks, MD.

Case Presentation of Chondrosarcoma of the Larynx. Francis LeJeune, Jr., MD.

Baker Lecture — "Subcertificiation in Otolaryngology: Now or Never." George F. Reed, MD.

An Extended Transantral Approach for Pterygomaxillary Tumors. Charles J. Krause, MD.

The Primary Management of Laryngeal Trauma. Steven D. Schaefer, MD, Robert G. Anderson, MD.

An Assessment of Intubation in Croup and Epiglottis. David E. Schuller, MD.

Laryngeal Paralysis in the Pediatric Patient. Seymour R. Cohen, MD.

Neonatal Tracheotomy. Gabriel F. Tucker, Jr., MD, Carol Roberts Gerson, MD.

Laryngeal Papilloma: Results of Treatment with the CO_2 Laser and Podophylum. Robert X. Jackler, MD, Herbert H. Dedo, MD.

Leukocyte Interferon in Patients with Juvenile Laryngeal Papillomatosis. Helmuth Goepfert, MD.

Single Stage Correction of the Twisted Nose. M. Eugene Tardy, MD.

Sarcoidosis of the Larynx. H. Bryan Neel, MD.

Incidence of Potential Complications Associated with the Crycothyrotomy. Ernest A. Weymuller, Jr., MD.

Nerve-Muscle Pedicle Reinnervation of the Larynx: Avoiding Pitfalls and Complications. Harvey M. Tucker, MD.

Surgery of the Inferior Nasal Turbinates. William H. Saunders, MD.

Correction of Posterior Glottic Incompetence Following Extended Partial Laryngectomy. Hugh F. Biller, MD.

Tracheosostomal Stenosis After Total Laryngectomy. Eugene N. Myers, MD.

Causes of Failure of Esophageal Speech. George A. Gates, MD.

Prognostic Factors Affecting Success of Duckbill Vocal Restoration. David E. Schuller, MD.

Primary Vocal Rehabilitation Using the Blom-Singer and Panje Voice Prosthesis. Michael D. Maves, MD, Raleigh E. Lingman, MD.

AMERICAN LARYNGOLOGICAL, RHINOLOGICAL AND OTOLOGICAL SOCIETY, INC.

May 4-6, 1982

Five Years Experience Using the Intact Canal Wall Tympanoplasty with Mastoidectomy for Cholesteatoma — Preliminary Report. Sam E. Kinney, MD.

Tinnitus Aurium: Fact . . . or Fancy. Clarence T. Sasaki, MD.

Human Histopathology of Cis-Platinum Ototoxicity. Steven D. Schaefer, MD.

Treatment of Tinnitus with Tocainide. Patrick J. Doyle, MD.

Adductor Spastic Dysphonia: Three Years After Recurrent Laryngeal Nerve Resection. Arnold E. Aronson, PhD.

Results of 300 Recurrent Nerve Sections for Spastic Dysphonia. Herbert H. Dedo, MD.

Thin-Needle Aspiration Biopsy Revisited. Mary Ann Smith Frable, MD.

Delayed Failure of Myocutaneous Flaps in Head and Neck Reconstruction. Hyun Cho, MD.

Modified Supraglottic Laryngectomy in the Resection of Extensive Malignant Neoplasms of the Base of Tongue and Pharyngeal Wall. Raleigh E. Lingeman, MD.

Lateral Laryngeal Suspension — A New Procedure to Minimize Swallowing Disorders Following Tongue Base Resection. Richard L. Goode, MD.

Laryngeal Transposition Flap for Reconstructing Large Oral Cavity Defects. Steven M. Sobol, MD.

Infratemporal Fossa Approach for Juvenile Angiofibromas and Other Parasellar Lesions. Prof. Ugo Fisch.

Tracheal Involvement in Laryngeal Papillomatosis. Haskins Kashima, MD.

The Composition and Function of the Nasal Valve. J. Haight, MD.

Symposium: The Nose: The Forgotten Organ. John J. Ballenger, MD, Moderator.

Survival Rates in 548 Patients with Multiple Neoplasms of the Upper Aerodigestive Tract. Jack L. Gluckman, MD.

CT Diagnosis of Head and Neck Cancers with Intact Mucosa. William Hanafee, MD.

Computed Tomography of Laryngeal Cancer with Histopathological Correlation. Carol R. Archer, MD.

Tracheo-Esophageal Party Wall. John A. Tucker, MD.

The Role of Conservative Surgery in the Management of Inverted Papilloma of the Nose. Hugh F. Biller, MD.

AMERICAN NEUROTOLOGY SOCIETY

April 30-May 1, 1982

Methodology for Assessment of Brainstem Auditory Evoked Potential Test Results. R. H. Nodar, MD.

Auditory Evoked Potentials, Impedance Measures and Diagnostic Speech Audiometry in Severe Head Injury: Serial Findings. J. W. Hall, MD, et al.

Velocity of Saccadic Eye Movements in Clinical Neurotology. J. Corvera-Bernadelli, MD.

Eye Velocity Pattern in Lesions in the Posterior Fossa. C. Wennmo, MD, et al.

Vestibular Plasticity. G. Melville-Jones, MD, Guest Speaker.

Downbeat Gaze Nystagmus — A Useful Clinical Diagnostic Sign. A. Katsarkus, MD, et al.

Isolated Vestibular Disturbances Following Head Trauma. M. Ziv, MD, et al.

Effects of Position Change on Optokinetic Nystagmus (OKN) and Optokinetic after Nystagmus (OKAN) in Man. W. LeLiever, MD, et al.

Cytoarchitecture of the Y Group. E. Mhoon, MD, et al.

Some Observations on the Localizing Significance of Ear-Dependent Positional Nystagmus. S. Althaus, MD, et al.

Autoimmune Reactivity in Cogan's Syndrome. G. Hughes, MD, et al.

Immunology of the Inner Ear. J. Harris, MD.

Vascular Mechanisms in Meniere's Disease. R. Gussen, MD.

Membrane Ruptures in Meniere's Disease. F. Linthicum, MD.

Acute Vestibular Neuritis Following Stapedectomy. K. Adour, MD.

Recent Advances in Medical and Surgical Management in Bell's Palsy. F. McGovern, MD.

Facial Paralysis in Children. M. E. Glasscock, III, MD, et al.

Histopathology of the Cochlea, Auditory Nerve, and Brainstem Auditory Nucleus Following Intracochlear Electrical Stimulation. T. Balkany, MD, et al.

Superior Ultra-Audiometric Hearing Associated with Genetic Hearing Loss. L. Bergstrom, MD, et al.

Head Shake Response as Prognostic Factor After Vestibular Lesions. M. Schiff, MD, et al.

Titration Streptomycin Therapy for Bilateral Meniere's Disease. M. Graham, MD, et al.

Tocainide and Tinnitus: Results of a Double-Blind Study. J. Nedzelski, MD, et al.

Sudden Deafness. U. Fisch, MD, Guest Speaker.

Panel: Vertigo. Moderator, H. Schuknecht. Panelists to be announced.

AMERICAN OTOLOGICAL SOCIETY, INC.

May 2-3, 1982

Cochlear and Otoconial Abnormalities in Capsular Otosclerosis with Hydrops. Lars-Goran Johnsson, MD, Joseph E. Hawkins, Jr., DSC, Roland C. Rouse, PhD, Fred H. Linthicum, Jr., MD.

Round Window Niche Surgery Singular Neurectomy: An Update. Richard R. Gacek, MD.

Experimental Study of the Fate of the Vestibular Nerve Following Labyrinthectomy: Surgical Implications. Harold F. Schknecht, MD.

Glomus Jugulare Tumors of the Temporal Bone, The Infratemporal Fossa Approach. Professor Doctor Ugo Fisch.

Cochlear Implantation in Children. William F. House, MD.

Speech and Language Development in a Parent Infant Total Communication Program. Robert J. Ruben, MD, Anita Dee, MD, Isabelle Rapin, MD.

Facial Nerve Anatomy — Normal and Variable. Bruce Proctor, MD, George T. Nager, MD.

Polytomography in Congenital Abnormalities of the Ear. J. William Wright, Jr., MD.

Panel: Congenital Anomalies of the Ear — Techniques, Complications and Controversies. Eugene L. Derlacki, MD, Moderator, Jack V. Hough, MD, James A. Crabtree, MD, George T. Nager, MD, Richard J. Bellucci, MD, Robert A. Jahrsdoerfer, MD.

The Normal Neonatal Brainstem Auditory Evoked Potentials. Marvin P. Fried, MD, Howard H. Zubick, PhD, Peter Feudo, Jr., Marshall Strome, MD.

Harmonic Acceleration Tests as a Measure of Vestibular Nystagmus Responses During Computerized Harmonic Accelera-Tests. Paul H. Ward, MD.

Comparison of Vestibular Subjective Sensation and Nystagmus Responses During Computerized Harmonic Acceleration Tests. Paul H. Ward, MD.

Computerized Tomographic Scanning with Air Contrast of the Internal Auditory Canal. Robert G. Anderson, MD, James Olson, MD, Marie Merkel, MD, Steven Schaefer, MD.

The Hindbrain Circulation and its Evaluation by Dynamic Computed Tomography. Galdino E. Valvassori, MD, Glen D. Dobben, MD.

The Anatomical Specificity of Central Vestibular Signs in Posterior Fossa Lesions. Arvind Kumar, MD, Mahmood Mafee, MD, Nicholas Torok, MD.

Stapedectomy — A Long-Term Report. John J. Shea, MD.

What Can Be Done for the Recruiting Ear? Maurice Schiff, MD, Robert E. Sandlin, PhD.

The Effect of Mastoid Cavity Modification on Middle Ear Sound Transmission. Richard L. Goode, MD.

The Homograft Tympanic Membrane After 12 Years. Roger E. Wehrs, MD.

Freeze-Dried Incus CrutchImplant. Mansfield F. W. Smith, MD.

Panel: Tympanoplasty: Indications and Pitfalls. James L. Sheehy, MD, Moderator, Gordon D. L. Smyth, MD, Harold F. Schuknecht, MD, Professor Doctor Ugo Fisch, James A. Crabtree, MD.

AMERICAN SOCIETY FOR HEAD & NECK SURGERY

May 5-6, 1982

45 Cases of Vertico-Fronto-Lateral Laryngectomy (Hemilaryngectomy): Indications, Techniques and Results. R. M. Mohr, MD, Quenelle, MD, D. A. Shumrick, MD.

Nasal Septal Cartilage Graft in Hemilaryngectomy. R. B. Butcher, MD.

Staging of Supraglottic Laryngeal Cancer — 1972 *vs* 1977. M. E. Johns, MD, E. Farrior, MD, J. C. Boyd, MD, R. W. Cantrell, MD.

Two Useful Adjuncts to Visceral Transplantation for Hypopharyngeal Malignancy. J. L. Freman, MD, K. Brondbo, MD, M. Osborne, MD, A. M. Noyek, MD, H. L. Shaw, MD, J. S. Chapnik, MD.

Modified Supraglottic Laryngectomy in the Resection of Extensive Malignant Neoplasms of the Base of Tongue and Pharyngeal Wall. E. C. Weisberger, MD.

Total Glossectomy — A Method of Reconstruction Eliminating Laryngectomy. H. F. Biller, MD, W. Larson, MD.

Reconstructing Using Fixation Plate — Proplast Prosthesis: A Preliminary Study. V. V. Strelzow, MD, J. Siddoway, MD, W. H. Friedman, MD.

The CO_2 Laser: Its Effects on the Facial Nerve. M. E. Goldman, MD, R. Ossoff, MD, C. Thomas, MD, M. Jabalon, MD.

Changing Patterns in Reconstruction Following Head and Neck Cancer Surgery. C. T. Yarington, Jr., MD, W. F. Larrabee, MD.

Reconstruction of the Hypopharynx and Cervial Esophagus. V. L. Schramm, MD, E. N. Myers, MD, J. T. Johnson, MD.

Muscle Flap Reconstruction of the Pharynx after Laryngectomy. M. I. Singer, MD, R. C. Hamaker, MD, W. W. Shockley, MD.

Thyroid Tumors, The Endocrinologist's Perspective. C. H. Hollenberg, MD.

Diagnostic Thyroid Imaging. A. M. Noyek, MD.

The Role of Needle Biopsy in the Management of Thyroid Tumors. R. C. Hamaker, MD.

Practical Anatomic Consideration in Thyroid Tumor Surgery. J. M. Lore, Jr., MD.

Surgical Decision-Making in Thyroid Tumors. H. F. Biller, MD.

The Management of Airway Involvement in Thyroid Tumors. V. G. Lawson, MD.

Vasopressin Secretion in Olfactory Neuroblastoma. V. S. Dayal, MD, R. Love, MD, R. T. Gregor, MD, J. R. Srigley, MD, A. W. P. Van Nostrand, MD.

Evaluation of Frozen Section in Major Salivary Gland Surgery. A. Hillel, MD, W. E. Fee, Jr.

The Use of Computed Tomography in Diagnosing Deep Neck Infections. G. E. Holt, MD, K. McManus, MD, R. Newman, MD, J. Potter, MD, P. P. Tinsley, MD.

Computerized Tomographic Assessment of Squamous Cell Carcinoma of the Head and Neck. S. Schaefer, MD, M. Merkel, MD, J. Diehl, MD, K. Maravilla, MD, R. Anderson, MD.

Digital Subtraction Video Angiography: Applications in Head and Neck Surgery. R. W. Miller, MD, S. W. Coulthard.

High Resolution and Dynamic Sequential Computerized Tomography in the Evaluation of Glomus Complex Tumors (Chemodectoma). M. F. Mafee, MD, G. E. Valvassori, MD, M. A. Shugar, MD, G. D. Dobben, MD.

Parathyroid Localization with CT Scanning. M. Friedman, MD, M. F. Mafee, MD, F. Berlinger, MD, H. Baim, MD, V. Shelton.

Multifactorial Analysis of the Staging Parameters for Cancer of the Laryngopharynx. J. R. Jacobs, MD, E. Spitznagel, MD, D. G. Sessions, MD, J. H. Ogura, MD.

Immunostimulation of Head and Neck Cancer Patients: in Vitro and Preliminary Clinical Experiences. J. T. Johnson, MD, B. Hirch, MD, B. S. Rabin.

Energy and Tissue Metabolism in Cancer Patients in Response to Nutritional Support. S. Edstrom, MD, E. Eden, MD, K. Bennegard, MD, K. Lundholm, MD.

Observations on Nerve-Muscle Preparation Reinnervation of the Paretic Larynx — An Evaluation of the Tucker Procedure. P. H. Ward, MD, G. Berci, MD.

Medullary Carcinoma of the Thyroid Gland. C. H. Hollenberg, MD, Guest Speaker.

Skull Base Surgery in Composite Resection. Y. P. Krespi, MD, G. A. Sisson, MD.

Local Excision and Radical Radiotherapy for Cancer of the Oral Tongue — A Preliminary Report. C. T. Chung, MD, R. R. Gacek, MD, R. H. Sagerman, MD, G. A. King, MD, D. D. Rabuzzi, MD, D. A. Leopold, MD.

High Fractional Dose Irradiation of Advanced Head and Neck Cancer. J. B. Weissberg, MD, H. Pillsbury, MD, C. T. Sasaki, MD, Y. H. Son, MD, J. J. Fischer, MD.

Effect of WR-2721 on Radiation-Induced Changes in Perfusion of Skin Flaps. R. A. Weisman, MD, A. L. Blumberg, MD, D. Brosseau, MD, D. G. Silverman.

Ultrasound-Induced Hyperthermia for Advanced Squamous Carcinoma of the Head and Neck: Progress Report. T. J. Ervin, MD, P. P. Lele, MD, D. Miller, MD, R. L. Fabian, MD, R. R. Weichselbaum, MD.

Innovative Regional Therapy for Head and Neck Cancer. S. R. Baker, MD, R. H. Wheeler, MD.

Predicting Postoperative Head and Neck Complications Utilizing Nutritional Assessment (The Prognostic Nutritional Index). T. C. Flores, MD, H. Levine, MD, R. Hooley, MD, T. Wheeler, MD, E. Steiger, MD.

The Management of Early Supraglottic Laryngeal Carcinoma by Irradiation with Surgery in Reserve. A. R. Harwood, MD.

Spectrum of Reconstruction for Mid-Facial Cutaneous and Soft Tissue Neoplasms. J. Jacobs, MD. S. Burres, MD, R. Stanley, MD, R. Mathog, MD.

A Comparative Analysis of Disability Resulting from Radical and Modified Neck Dissections. D. E. Schuller, MD, N. A. Reiches, MD, J. J. Conley, MD, R. C. Hamaker, MD, R. E. Lingeman, MD, E. C. Weisburger, MD, J. Y. Suen, MD, D. R. Kelly, MD, A. W. Miglets.

Rehabilitative Surgery for Aspiration — A Clinical Analysis. M. Strome, MD.

Surgical Management of Nasopharyngeal Angiofibroma. Wu Shan, MD.

Ann Otol 91:1982

BONE RESORPTION IN HUMAN CHOLESTEATOMAS

PAUL BRETLAU, MD
MARTIN B. JØRGENSEN, MD
CHRISTIAN H. SØRENSEN, MD
ERIK DABELSTEEN, DDS
COPENHAGEN, DENMARK

In vivo studies of different aspects of bone resorption in human cholesteatomas are described in the immunodeficient "nude" mice. Cholesteatoma membranes were transplanted into the middle ear cavities of the mice. After 21-28 days, growth of cholesteatoma tissue could be demonstrated in 8 of 13 animals. In 7 of these 8 animals bone resorption of the labyrinthine wall and ossicles could be demonstrated; resorption with acute inflammation was found in only two animals. The cellular mechanism in relation to bone resorption is discussed.

The mechanism of bone resorption in chronic otitis media, with or without cholesteatoma, has not yet been fully clarified. Clinical observations[1] show that bone resorption nearly always is found together with or is said to be a result of infection, or that the cholesteatoma itself is supposed to cause destruction by pressure. Our previous histopathological examinations[2,3] have shown that acute inflammation is not necessarily a part of the bone resorption picture in chronic otitis media, and that the cholesteatoma membranes with the subepithelial connective tissue play an important role.

In the otological liteature many investigators have produced cholesteatomas experimentally in different animals using different chemical and biological agents. The beautiful experimental work by Fernandez and Lindsay,[4] Friedmann,[5,6] and Rüedi[7] have all confirmed Habermann's immigration theory of the pathogenesis of epidermoid cholesteatoma. The question whether the mesenchyme plays an important role in formation of epidermoid cholesteatoma has been raised by Friedmann,[8] and lately Steinbach and Grüninger[9] showed that the connective tissue of the pars flaccida is a decisive factor in the genesis of cholesteatoma. In a recent paper[10] we have shown how immunodeficient "nude" mice could be used in studying human cholesteatomas in vivo. This paper presents the results of transplanting human cholesteatoma membranes into the middle ear cavities of nude mice.

MATERIAL AND METHODS

Human cholesteatoma membranes, including the subepithelial tissue, obtained during surgery from ten patients between 5 and 67 years of age were transplanted into the middle ear cavity of 13 Nu/Nu nude mice. The specimens were stored for transportation to the laboratory in tissue culture medium 1640 with penicillin, streptomycin and gentamicin and trimmed to 2 x 2 mm pieces before they were transplanted. Recipients were anesthetized intraperitoneally with Epontal, and an incision was made through the skin into the anterolateral region of the neck. The bulla on the right side was opened, the cholesteatoma tissue was placed into the middle ear cavity and the incision closed with a suture and Histoacryl.

The animals were followed clinically for 21-28 days, and after sacrificing, the head was fixed in 10% neutral formalin and processed for histological examination. After decalcification in formic acid and embedding in celloidin each animal head was cut horizontally in 15 μ sections and stained with hematoxylin and eosin. In this way both ear cavities were on the same slide and the unoperated ear served as a control (Fig. 1).

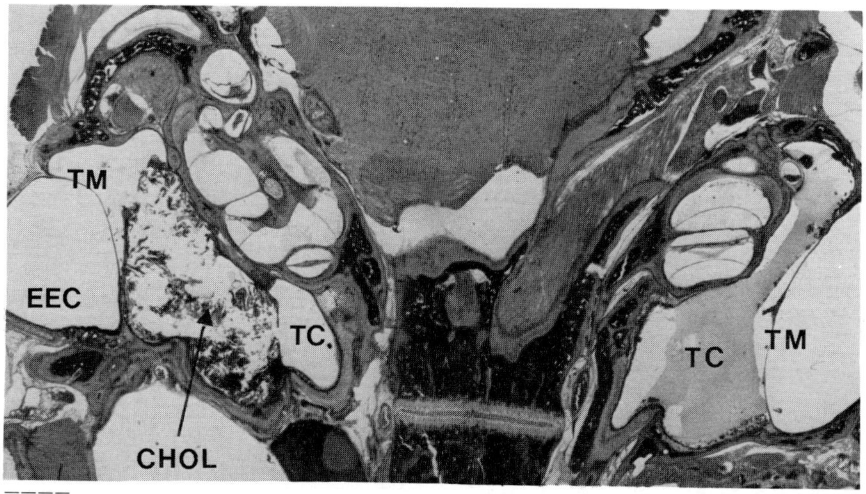

Fig. 1. Transplanted cholesteatoma membranes (arrow - CHOL) in the tympanic cavity (TC) on the right side of a nude mouse. EEC - External ear canal; TM - Tympanic membrane. (H & E, x 12)

From the University ENT Department, Gentofte Hospital; the Oto-pathological Department, Rigshospitalet; the Departments of Oral Diagnosis and Oral Pathology, The Royal Dental College; and the Department of Pathology, Community Hospital, Copenhagen.
REPRINTS - Paul Bretlau, MD, University ENT Department, Gentofte Hospital, DK 2900 Hellerup, Denmark.

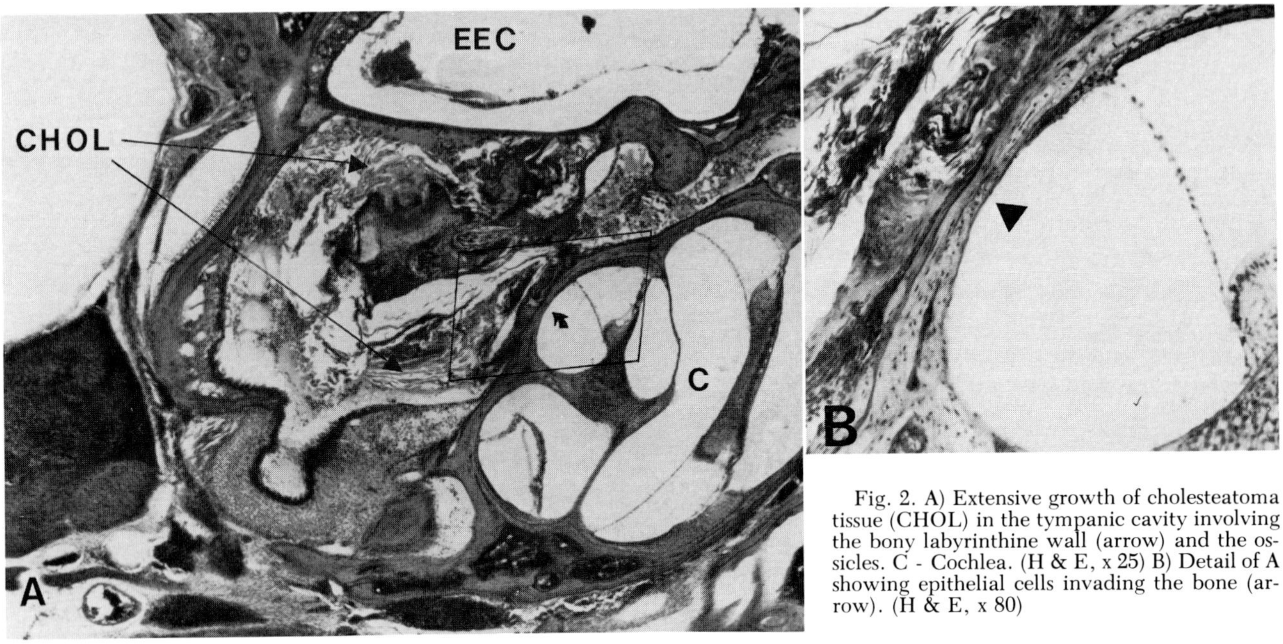

Fig. 2. A) Extensive growth of cholesteatoma tissue (CHOL) in the tympanic cavity involving the bony labyrinthine wall (arrow) and the ossicles. C - Cochlea. (H & E, x 25) B) Detail of A showing epithelial cells invading the bone (arrow). (H & E, x 80)

RESULTS

In 8 of 13 animals growth of cholesteatoma tissue in the middle ear cavity could be demonstrated; very often it filled most of the middle ear cavity (Fig. 2), indicating considerable growth from the original 2 x 2 mm transplanted pieces. In the remaining five animals one cholesteatoma was seen growing in the muscle tissue in close relation to the middle ear cavity and in four cases the cholesteatoma membranes failed to grow.

In analyzing the histological sections we have been mainly interested in inflammation and/or bone resorption (the table).

Inflammation. In the eight animals where the cholesteatoma grew as a tumor in the middle ear cavity, acute inflammation occurred in only three ears. In five animals without cholesteatoma growth, acute inflammation was found in three ears, probably as a result of the surgical procedure. In these cases most of the middle ear cavities were filled with granulocytes in pus.

Bone Resorption. In 7 of 8 mice showing cholesteatoma growth in the middle ear cavity it was possible to show a close relation between the cholesteatoma tissue and the bony labyrinthine wall or the ossicles (Fig. 2A). Epithelial cells producing keratin invaded the bone, resulting in destruction of the bony tissue, sometimes with epithelial cells placed deeply under the bony surface (Figs. 2B and 3). In the light microscope no multinuclear osteoclasts could be demonstrated, but instead mononuclear, noninflammatory cells were seen along the eroded bone in the middle ear cavity (Figs. 4 and 5). Bone destruction could be demonstrated in five animals with no sign of acute inflammation (the table). Bone destruction with inflammation could be seen in only two animals, and in these the bony destruction seemed to be more extensive than in the five animals without inflammation (Fig. 3). One animal, however, showed acute inflammation with no sign of bone destruction or resorption in spite of considerable growth.

In the observation period it was not possible to show any relationship between the activity and growth of the cholesteatoma and the patient's age.

DISCUSSION

In discussing bone resorption or bone destruction in chronic cholesteatomatous otitis media the most important factors are the subepithelial connective tissue reactions and the accompanying infection. Both the organic (collagen, water, mucopolysaccharides and protein) and the inorganic (calcium phosphate, carbonate, and citrate) parts of the bone have to be resorbed, and such resorption requires enzymatic activity derived from living cells. Prostaglandins,[11,12] collagenase,[13,14] and lysosomal enzymes[15] appear to be active. We have previously shown [15] that mononuclear cells in the subepithelial connective tissue can be identified at the bone resorption margin, and recently Gantz et al[16] have reported immunohistochemical and immunocytochemical evidence confirming the destructive proportions of granulation tissue.

In bone the mineral protects the collagen from denaturation and proteolytic attack; therefore a

HISTOLOGICAL FINDINGS IN NUDE MICE WITH TRANSPLANTED CHOLESTEATOMA (N = 13)

	Bone Resorption	*No Bone Resorption*	*Necrosis*	*Total*
Inflammation	2	1	3	6
No sign of inflammation	5	0	2	7
Total	7	1	5	13

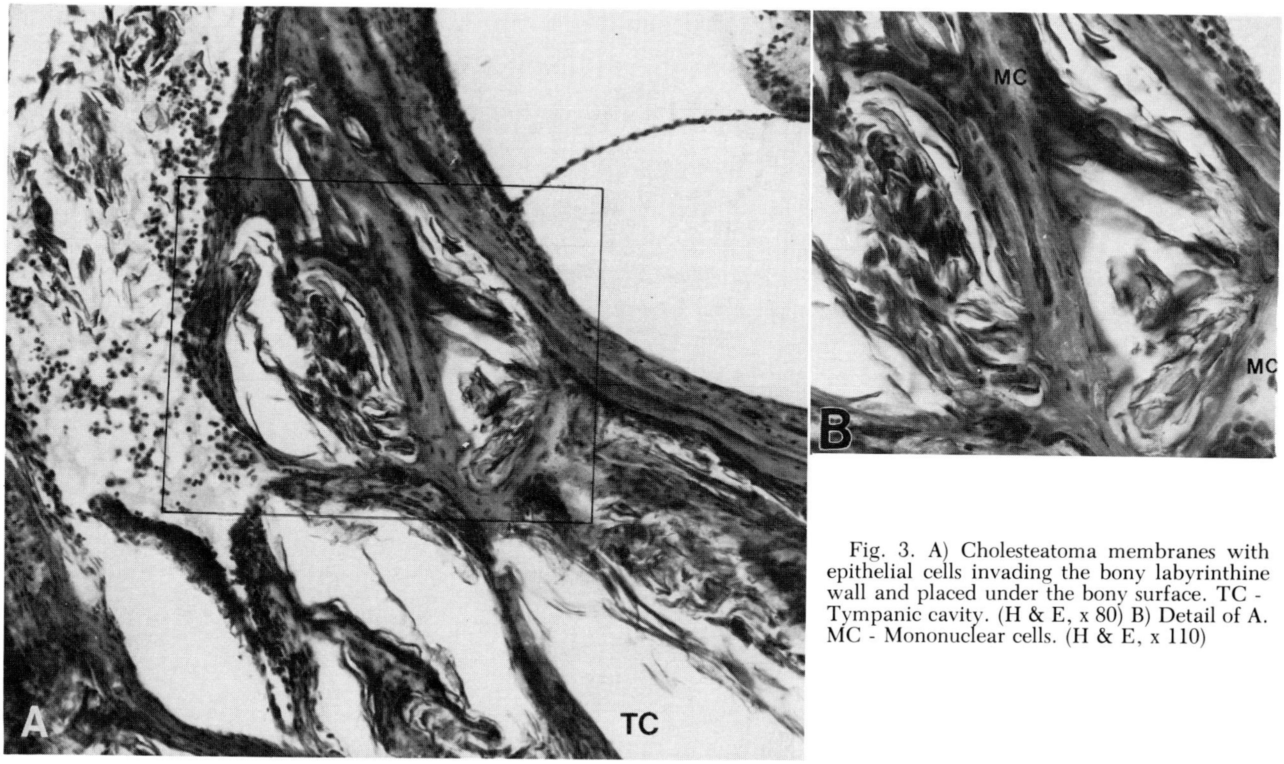

Fig. 3. A) Cholesteatoma membranes with epithelial cells invading the bony labyrinthine wall and placed under the bony surface. TC - Tympanic cavity. (H & E, x 80) B) Detail of A. MC - Mononuclear cells. (H & E, x 110)

mechanism for prior removal of mineral ions must be operative in both normal and pathological situations to permit degradation of the collagenous matrix. This process of demineralization must be closely followed by matrix resorption, since extensive denuding of the collagen has not been observed.[17] Under resorptive stimulus the bone cells produce considerable amounts of acid, mostly lactic, and to a lesser extent citric acid, due to glycolytic activity. The lowering of the pH makes the calcium phosphate salts of the mineral easily soluble. Removal of the decalcified collagen matrix may be accomplished by either a specific neutral protease (collagenase) or digestion by nonspecific lysosomal acid hydrolases after denaturation by local accumulation of metabolic acid. Cellular localization of collagenase identifies the organic component of bone resorption, whereas the cellular

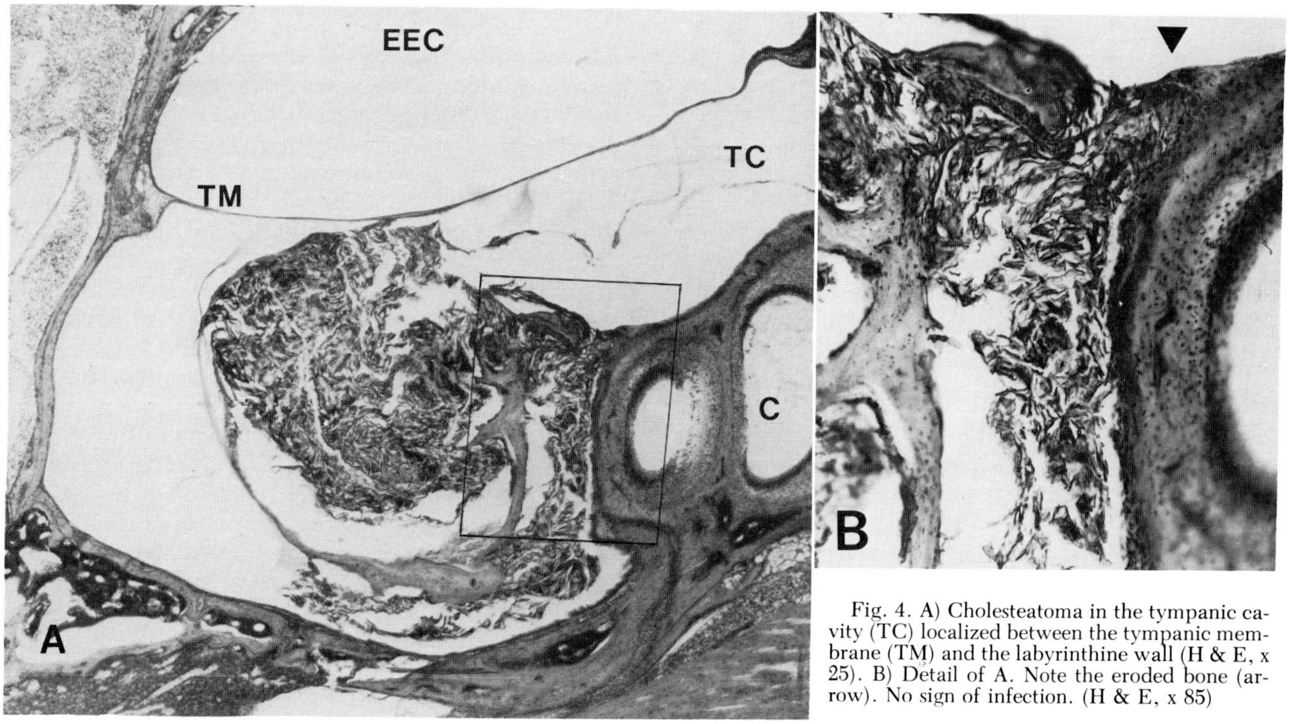

Fig. 4. A) Cholesteatoma in the tympanic cavity (TC) localized between the tympanic membrane (TM) and the labyrinthine wall (H & E, x 25). B) Detail of A. Note the eroded bone (arrow). No sign of infection. (H & E, x 85)

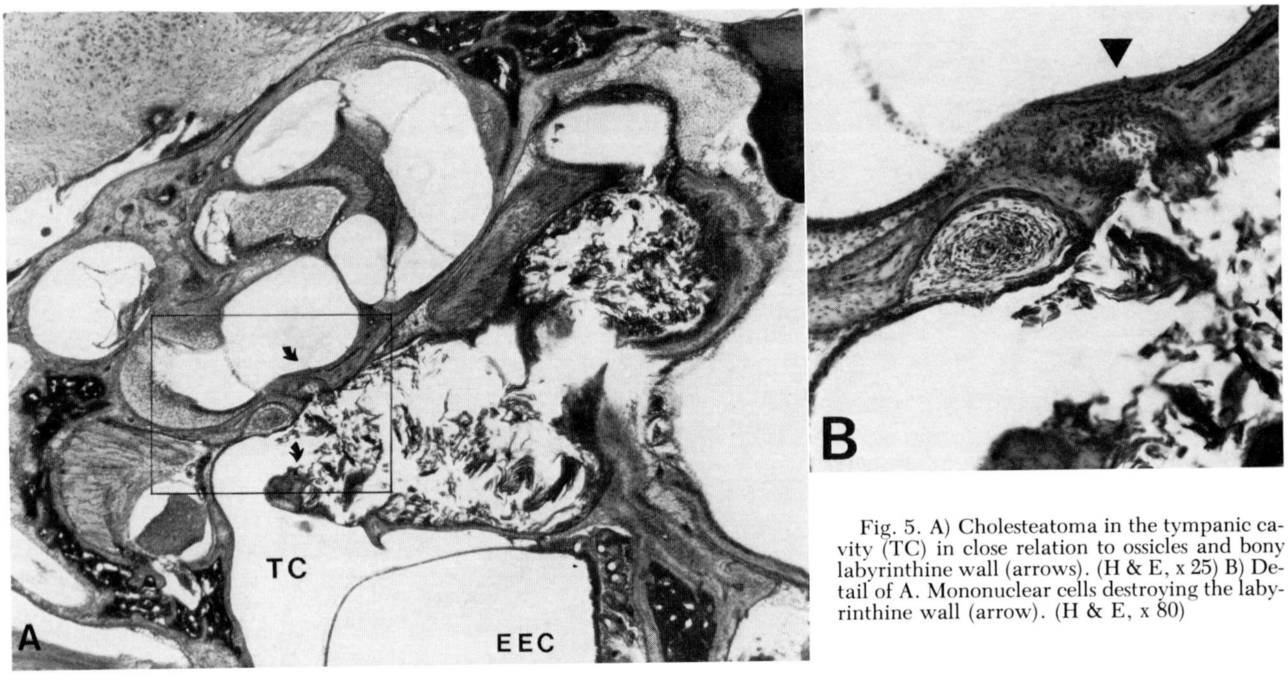

Fig. 5. A) Cholesteatoma in the tympanic cavity (TC) in close relation to ossicles and bony labyrinthine wall (arrows). (H & E, x 25) B) Detail of A. Mononuclear cells destroying the labyrinthine wall (arrow). (H & E, x 80)

localization of lysosomal enzymes delineates cells, most likely involved in both organic and inorganic phases of bone resorption. Both mechanisms have been shown to exist in chronic otitis media, where Abramson[13] and Abramson and Gross[14] have demonstrated collagenolytic activity at neutral pH in chronic otitis media, whereas we[15] have demonstrated that the marker enzyme for lysosomal activity, the acid phosphatase, is present in large quantities along the eroded bone in the middle ear, both intracellularly in mononuclear cells as well as extracellularly.

Regarding the question of which cell or cells are responsible for bone resorption, there are several possibilities. It is generally accepted that the multinuclear osteoclast with its lysosomal hydrolases, is capable of and responsible for normal bone resorption. The osteoclast with its well developed "ruffled border" has an extensive area of contact with the bone which enhances its resorption capacity. However, other cells have also been suggested as being capable of bone resorption. Several authors have presented evidence suggesting that the osteocytes are capable of bone resorption,[16,18] while Cameron[19] indicated that endothelial cells may be implicated. The role of the mononuclear histiocyte has previously been suggested by us.[15,20,21] Gantz et al[16] demonstrated collagenase activity in mononuclear inflammatory cells (macrophages, lymphocytes, and plasma cells); in this and in our previous works the multinucleated osteoclast in close relation to the resorbing zone in chronic otitis media was not demonstrated. This observation has also been made by Abramson et al[22] and Gantz et al,[16] who state that multinucleated osteoclasts were an infrequent finding in the area of bone resorption.

It has been demonstrated that inflammation, with or without infection, is a major factor in bone resorption.[1,16] In our work[15] we demonstrated that, on the microscopic level, there is no difference in the cellular picture whether cholesteatoma is present or not. But it must be emphasized that this does not exclude the possibility that the cholesteatoma may have an enhancing effect upon the resorptive process. We demonstrated a very high enzymatic activity in the squamous epithelium itself,[15] and it is likely that this may influence the amount of resorption present in cholesteatoma.

In a recent experimental investigation[10] we showed how transplanted cholesteatoma membranes subcutaneously continue to grow. In this study the epithelial cells not only continued to produce keratin, but in the majority of the animals the subepithelial tissue showed no sign of inflammation, and probably through mononuclear noninflammatory cells, acted upon the bony margin, resulting in resorption. This observation is contradictory to Sadé and Halevy,[1] who after a clinical study felt that squamous epithelium played no role in bone resorption. How do the epithelial cells influence bone resorption? This question has been investigated by Gantz et al[11] who found that granulation tissue from the subepithelial layer of the cholesteatoma is capable of chemically activating bone resorption in vitro, and that keratinized squamous epithelium of skin did not influence bone resorption. These authors demonstrated that it was prostaglandin that was the chemical mediator responsible for producing demineralization of the bone, thus playing an active role in localized bone resorption in chronic middle ear disease. Abramson and Huang[23] demonstrated that in animal experiments the presence of epithelium, though not crucial, greatly increases the incidence of cochlear fistulas, and they believe that the epithelium functions to maintain the connective tissue in a chronic inflammatory state. This is in agreement with our findings showing a more marked bone resorption in those animals who also showed acute inflammatory reaction, than in those without sign of acute inflammation. But our definite findings of bone resorption without inflammation seem to suggest that living epithelial cells with subepithelial tissue in themselves are capable of producing bone destruction, probably as a result of enzymatic activity. Can other cells be responsible for the bone resorption? It has recently been shown[24] that a factor released by lymphocytes can stimulate collagenase in vivo in rheumatoid synovial cells and thereby be involved in cartilage resorption. Lymphokines produced by T-lymphocytes may also be important for the initiation of inflammatory bone breakdown. But the nude mice have no thymus and are therefore lacking T-lymphocytes and a cell-mediated immune response. The absence of this system in the animal model seems to point to another cellular resorption mechanism, probably involving mononuclear cells.

In summary, both clinical and nonclinical research indicate that cholesteatoma and squamous epithelium directly and indirectly enhance bone resorption in chronic otitis media. Opinions about the effect, however, are conflicting, suggesting the need for further research. An animal model using nude mice with implanted living human cholesteatomatous tissue in the middle ear cavity can provide more information about the growth and activity of cholesteatomas. Identifying which cells and the kind of biochemical activity involved in bone resorption can probably tell us how to avoid complications in chronic otitis media, with or without cholesteatoma.

ACKNOWLEDGMENTS — The authors want to express their thanks to J. Rygaard, MD, Chief of the Department of Pathology, Community Hospital, Copenhagen, for his kind help and for laboratory facilities for the animals. The authors would also like to thank Jytte Kremer, Lise Solvbjerg, Lene Richter, and Bodil Collatz for their invaluable assistance in preparing the animals, histological sections, and photographs.

REFERENCES

1. Sadé J, Halevy A. The aetiology of bone destruction in chronic otitis media. J Laryngol Otol 1974; 88:139-43.

2. Thomsen J, Bretlau P, Kristensen HK. Bone resorption in chronic otitis media: a light microscopical and histochemical investigation of acid phosphatase activity. Acta Otolaryngol (Stockh) 1975; 79:400-4.

3. Thomsen J, Bretlau P, Jorgensen MB. Bone resorption in chronic otitis media: the role of cholesteatoma, a must or an adjunct? Clin Otolaryngol 1981; 6:179-86.

4. Fernandez C, Lindsay JR. Aural cholesteatoma: experimental observations. Ann Otol Rhinol Laryngol 1960; 70:1119-41.

5. Friedmann I. Epidermoid cholesteatoma and cholesterol granuloma: experimental and human. Ann Otol Rhinol Laryngol 1959; 68:57-79.

6. Friedmann I. The pathology of the ear. Oxford: Blackwell, 1974.

7. Rüedi L. Cholesteatoma formation in the middle ear in animal experiments. Acta Otolaryngol (Stockh) 1959; 50:233-42.

8. Friedmann I. The pathology of epidermoid cholesteatoma: human and experimental In: McCabe BF, Sadé J, Abramson M, eds. Cholesteatoma: first international conference. Birmingham: Aesculapius Publishing Co, 1977:10-22.

9. Steinbach E, Grüninger G. Experimental production of cholesteatoma in rabbits by using non-irritants (skin tolerants). J Laryngol Otol 1980; 94:269-79.

10. Bretlau P, Dabelsteen E, Holmstrup P. A method for studying cholesteatomas in vivo: with special attention to epithelial-mesenchymal interaction. Clin Otolaryngol 1981; 6:81-5.

11. Gantz B, Clancey C, Abramson M. Decalcification factors in granulation tissue and ear canal skin. In: McCabe BF, Sadé J, Abramson M, eds. Cholesteatoma: first international conference. Birmingham: Aesculapius Publishing Co, 1977:167-9.

12. Bernstein J, Hausmann E, Wright J. Middle ear disease release of soluble factor (S) stimulating bone resorption. In: McCabe BF, Sadé J, Abramson M, eds. Cholesteatoma: first international conference. Birmingham: Aesculapius Publishing Co, 1977: 152-61.

13. Abramson M. Collagenolytic activity in middle ear cholesteatoma. Ann Otol Rhinol Laryngol 1969; 78:112-24.

14. Abramson M, Gross J. Further studies on a collagenase in middle ear cholesteatoma. Ann Otol Rhinol Laryngol 1971; 80:177-85.

15. Thomsen J, Bretlau P, Jorgensen MB, Kristensen HK. Bone resorption in chronic otitis media. In: McCabe BF, Sadé J, Abramson M, eds. Cholesteatoma: first international conference. Birmingham: Aesculapius Publishing Co, 1977:136-48.

16. Gantz BF, Maynard J, Bumsted RM, Huang CC, Abramson M. Bone resorption in chronic otitis media. Ann Otol Rhinol Laryngol 1979; 88:693-700.

17. Krane SM, Dayer JM, Goldring SR. Aspects of bone resorption. In: McCabe BF, Sadé J, Abramson M, eds. Cholesteatoma: first international conference. Birmingham: Aesculapius Publishing Co, 1977:102-14.

18. Belanger LF. Osteocytic osteolysis. Calcif Tissue Res 1969; 4:1-12.

19. Camaron DA. Erosion of the epiphysis of the rat tibia by capillaries. J Bone Joint Surg (Br) 1961; 43:590.

20. Chevance LG, Bretlau P, Jorgensen MB, Causse J. Otosclerosis: an electronmicroscopic and cytochemical study. Acta Otolaryngol (Stockh) 1970; Suppl 272.

21. Bretlau P, Causse J, Jorgensen MB, Chevance LG. Histiocytic activity in otosclerotic bone. Arch Otorhinolaryngol (NY) 1971; 198:301-16.

22. Abramson M, Asarch RG, Litton WB. Experimental aural cholesteatoma causing bone resorption. Ann Otol Rhinol Laryngol 1975; 84:425-32.

23. Abramson M, Huang CC. Cholesteatoma and bone resorption. In: McCabe BF, Sadé J, Abramson M, eds. Cholesteatoma: first international conference. Birmingham: Aesculapius Publishing Co, 1977:162-6.

24. Dayer JM, Russel RG, Krane SM. Collagenase production by rheumatoid synovial cells: stimulation by a human lymphocyte factor. Science 1977; 195:181-3.

Ann Otol 91:1982

INNER EAR PATHOLOGY FOLLOWING INJURY TO THE EIGHTH CRANIAL NERVE AND THE LABYRINTHINE ARTERY

ISAMU SANDO, MD, DMS
PITTSBURGH, PENNSYLVANIA

AKIRA OGAWA, MD, DMS
TOKYO, JAPAN

BRUCE W. JAFEK, MD, FACS
DENVER, COLORADO

Inner ear pathology following surgical sectioning of the eighth cranial nerve and labyrinthine artery in humans is compared histologically to the pathology observed following severance of the eighth cranial nerve. The case in which both the eighth cranial nerve and the labyrinthine artery were surgically severed revealed severe pathologic changes in the cochlea, including complete loss of the organ of Corti and moderate pathologic changes in the fairly well-preserved vestibular end-organs. Interestingly, the endolymphatic sac appeared to be normal. However, the second case in which the eighth cranial nerve was sectioned but the labyrinthine artery was preserved revealed the organ of Corti and vestibular end-organs to be well preserved and normal. These findings suggest that the blood supply from the labyrinthine artery plays a major role in maintaining most of the structures in the inner ear except for the endolymphatic sac, and that the vestibular end-organs are more resistant than the organ of Corti to the effects of damage of the labyrinthine artery.

Experimental studies have been performed in animals to determine the effects of surgical lesions of the labyrinthine artery and eighth cranial nerve on the inner ear structures.[1-3] These studies concluded that, when the blood supply to the inner ear is obstructed, the organ of Corti and vestibular end-organs are the most vulnerable to degeneration and that such obstruction is followed by marked reparative changes in the inner ear.[1,2] In contrast, when only the eighth cranial nerve is sectioned, with the blood supply to the inner ear being preserved, the sensory organs of the cochlear and vestibular labyrinth are well preserved.[1,3]

To our knowledge, no reports have been published on the human inner ear comparing the histopathologic findings resulting from labyrinthine artery damage with those changes occurring in the inner ear as a result of eight cranial nerve damage. The purpose of this paper is to present and discuss the results of histopathological examinations of the inner ears of two patients in whom either the labyrinthine artery and eighth cranial nerve or only the eighth cranial nerve were injured. We will also compare the inner ear pathology present in these two patients to that seen in animals subjected to the experimental studies mentioned above.

CASE REPORTS

CASE 1

A 48-year-old female who had had a history of dizziness for a year was seen in January 1973. The patient stated that the dizziness was like a "woozy" feeling associated with a feeling of fullness in the back of her head and in her ears. She also noted tinnitus in the right ear along with gradual hearing loss in that ear for 20 years. The physical examination performed at that time revealed that the external ear and tympanic membrane were normal bilaterally. Detailed neurologic evaluation showed hypesthesia to pinprick in V_{1-3} on the right with a decreased right corneal reflex. A positive right Hitselberger sign was found. Tuning fork testing was consistent with a right sensorineural loss. Motor function was symmetrical with slightly hypoactive (1^+) reflexes throughout. Cerebellar testing showed a poor tandem gait with a tendency to fall to the right. There was a positive Romberg with a tendency to fall backward to the right. One observer noted left-beating nystagmus. There was no papilledema. The audiological examination of the affected (right) ear showed a severe degree of sensorineural hearing loss (Fig. 1) characterized by a flat threshold pattern. The average hearing loss in the speech frequency range was 58 dB without loudness recruitment. Her speech reception threshold was 55 dB and speech discrimination score was 52%. There was evidence of tone decay in the right ear. The results of all tests mentioned above were within normal limits for the left ear. Caloric testing (water irrigations at temperatures of 44° and 30°C) showed no response in the right ear and normal response in the left ear. There was no spontaneous or positional nystagmus. Stenver's views and plain films of the skull showed no enlargement of the internal auditory canals bilaterally. A pneumoencephalogram, however, demonstrated a "large" (4 cm) right CPA tumor growing mainly dorsally with severe displacement of the pons to the left and moderately severe indentation of the right side of the fourth ventricle. An angiogram showed deviation of the adjacent vessels, but no "tumor stain." The area of the tumor showed increased uptake with scanning following injection of technetium-99. Cerebral spinal fluid studies were not undertaken. A diagnosis of acoustic neurinoma in the right ear was made.

On February 21, 1973, a right suboccipital craniectomy was performed and the major part of the tumor was successfully freed from the right eighth cranial nerve in the posterior cranial fossa and the internal auditory canal. The tumor was moderately large in size, indenting the cerebellar peduncle and pons to the extent of 1-1.5 cm. During the operation, the tumor remaining inside the

From the Departments of Otolaryngology and Pathology, University of Pittsburgh School of Medicine, Eye and Ear Hospital of Pittsburgh; and the Department of Otolaryngology, University of Colorado Health Sciences Center, Denver. This study was supported by Research Grants NS 09293 and 13787 from the National Institute of Neurological and Communicative Disorders and Stroke. This paper was presented at the AAO/ARO Research Forum Meeting in Anaheim, California, September 27, 1980.

REPRINTS — Isamu Sando, MD, DMS, Director, Division of Otopathology, Department of Otolaryngology, Eye and Ear Hospital of Pittsburgh, 230 Lothrop Street, Pittsburgh, PA 15213.

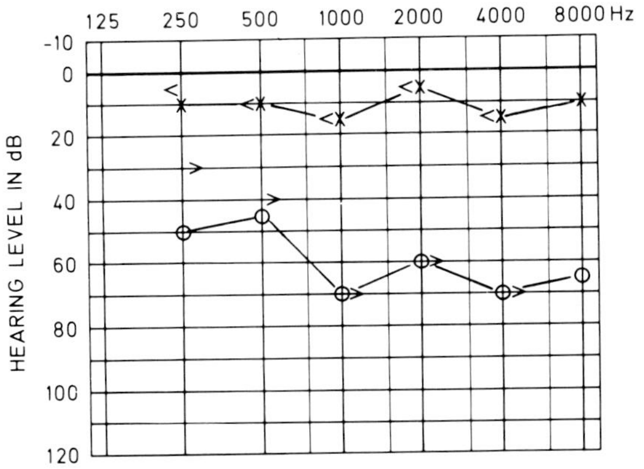

Fig. 1. (Case 1) Audiogram obtained 40 days before the operation for removal of an acoustic tumor and eight months prior to the patient's death. SRT: R 55 dB, L 10 dB. Discrim: R 52%, L 100%. Tone decay test: R(4000 Hz) - positive.

internal auditory canal was coagulated. Histological examination of the tumor confirmed it to be an acoustic neurinoma: the surgically removed specimen showed palisading of nuclei probably of Schwann cells. After the surgery, the patient's clinical course was characterized by recurrent episodes of seizure activity. These seizures were noted to be most frequent following events which precipitated hypoxia. On May 25 she had a seizure and respiratory arrest from which she was successfully resuscitated. Her course improved and she was discharged. However, she had severe reactive suicidal depression, and was hospitalized in a psychiatric hospital, where she had several episodes of respiratory distress. On September 8, 1973, she died in severe respiratory distress.

At the time of autopsy no recurrences of the acoustic neurinoma were evident. The temporal bones were removed from the refrigerated cadaver 13 hours after death, fixed in 10% formalin solution, decalcified, and embedded in celloidin. Serial horizontal sections were cut at 20μ thickness. Every tenth section was stained with hematoxylin and eosin and studied under a light microscope.

HISTOPATHOLOGICAL FINDINGS

Right Temporal Bone.

EXTERNAL AND MIDDLE EARS. The external auditory canal and the tympanic membrane were normal. In the facial canal the facial nerve, except for the geniculate ganglion cells and their nerve fibers, was severely degenerated. The other structures in the middle ear were essentially normal.

INNER EAR. No inflammatory round cell infiltration was observed. The most significant pathological finding in the cochlea was a total loss of the organ of Corti. In all turns of the cochlea the organ of Corti had been replaced by a single layer of squamous epithelium which overlay the basilar membrane (Fig. 2A-C). In the upper basal turn, dense connective tissue, which was separated from the scala media by a single layer of squamous epithelium, was observed to have replaced the organ of Corti; this tissue was confluent with the similar tissue which was seen to occupy the area of the spiral ligament (Fig. 2C). The tectorial membrane was absent (Fig. 2C), separated (Fig. 2B), or rolled and covered by squamous epithelium (Fig. 2D). The limbus demonstrated loss of the interdental cells in the upper basal turn. The stria vascularis was atrophic or absent in most of the turns (Fig. 2B, C). There was mild endolymphatic hydrops, particularly in the apical turn (Fig. 2A). A moderate amount of eosinophilic precipitate was present in both endolymphatic and perilymphatic spaces, particularly in the basal turn. In addition, fibrous connective tissue was present in the scala tympani in the upper basal turn, especially in the area where dense connective tissue had replaced the organ of Corti (Fig. 2C). The only cochlear nerve present consisted of a few nerve fibers to the upper cochlear turns. No intraganglionic spiral bundles were present. Fibro-osseous sclerosis was seen in Rosenthal's canal and in the vascular channels of the modiolus, particularly in the area close to the basal turn of the cochlea (Fig. 2A). The cochlear aqueduct and the inferior cochlear vein were normal.

In the vestibular system the maculae of the saccule (Fig. 2E) and the utricle and the cristae of the three semicircular canals were present but appeared to be atrophic. The epithelial lining of the endolymphatic sac appeared to be normal (Fig. 2F). Eosinophilic precipitate was present in the endolymphatic space in the saccule, common crus, superior semicircular canal, and endolymphatic sac. The vestibular aqueduct and the vein in the paravestibular canaliculus seemed to be normal.

INTERNAL AUDITORY CANAL. The orifice of the internal auditory canal was completely shielded by scar tissue which was confluent with the late stage of granulation tissue observed in the internal auditory canal. Inside the canal the seventh and eighth cranial nerve fibers were markedly decreased in number. Also present in the canal was a dense eosinophilic substance which appeared to be scar tissue replacing the cochlear nerve (Fig. 2G). No labyrinthine artery was evident, but a moderately large artery (89 μ in diameter) was seen to course from the geniculate ganglion area along the labyrinthine portion of the facial nerve to the internal auditory canal (Fig. 2H).

Left Temporal Bone.

EXTERNAL AND MIDDLE EARS. The external ear canal, the tympanic membrane, and the middle ear were normal.

INNER EAR. The organ of Corti was present and well preserved. The tectorial membrane, the limbus, the stria vascularis, the spiral ligament, and Reissner's membrane were normal. No endolymphatic hydrops was noted. In both endolymphatic and perilymphatic spaces neither fibrous connective tissue nor eosinophilic precipitate were observed. The spiral ganglion cells with their nerve fibers and intraganglionic spiral bundles were present. The cochlear aqueduct and the inferior cochlear vein were normal.

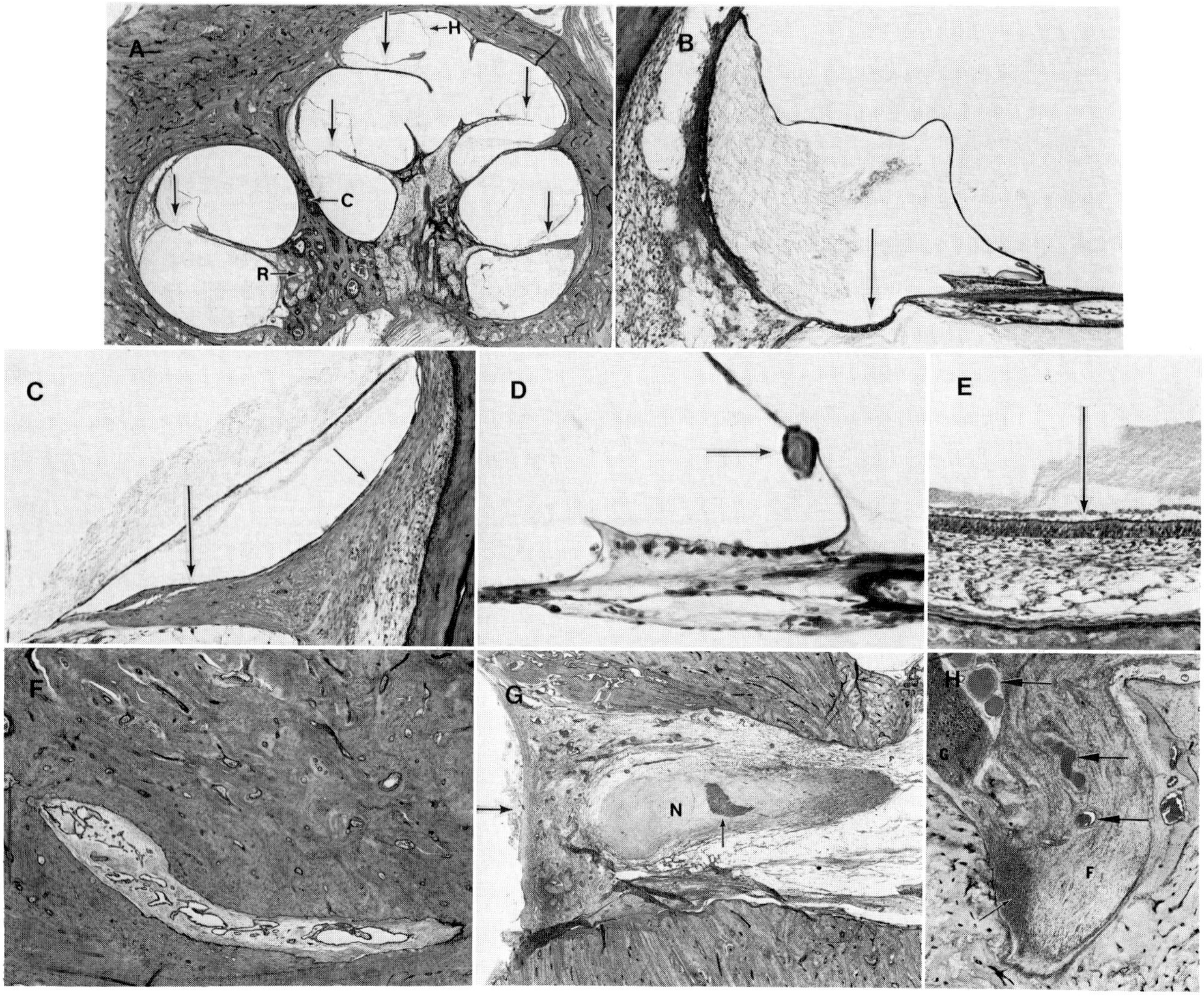

Fig. 2. (Case 1) Right ear. A) The organ of Corti is absent (arrows) in all cochlear turns. There is endolymphatic hydrops (H) in the apical turn. Spiral ganglion cells are absent. Fibro-osseous sclerosis is seen in Rosenthal's canal (R) and small vascular channels (C) of the modiolus. Some of the vessels seen in the modiolus may well have been preserved during surgery to eliminate totally the labyrinthine artery while some may have been newly formed in the course of the postoperative reparative process. Interestingly, a few nerve fibers to the apical turn remain in the internal auditory canal even though their ganglion cells and their nerve fibers in the osseous spiral lamina are absent. (H & E, x 11) B) Complete absence of the organ of Corti (arrow) and somewhat atrophic stria vascularis in the basal turn are evident. (H & E, x 50) C) Upper basal turn of the cochlea demonstrates absence of the organ of Corti (large arrow) and stria vascularis (small arrow). Dense connective tissue has replaced the organ of Corti and part of the spiral ligament. (H & E, x 60) D) The organ of Corti is absent and the tectorial membrane (arrow) is rolled and covered by a single layer of squamous epithelium. (H & E, x 130) E) Saccular macula (arrow) is well preserved. (H & E, x 82) F) Epithelial lining of the endolymphatic sac is well preserved. (H & E, x 17) G) The orifice of the internal auditory canal is sealed completely by a layer of scar tissue (large arrow). A dense eosinophilic substance (N), which appears to be scar tissue replacing the cochlear nerve, is seen in the internal auditory canal. There was a focal hemorrhage (small arrow) in the scar tissue. (H & E, x 10) H) An unusually large artery (large arrow), which takes its course from the geniculate ganglion area along the degenerated facial nerve (F) in the labyrinthine portion of the facial canal to the internal auditory canal, is observed. Note that the geniculate ganglion cells (G) and their nerve fibers (small arrow) appear to be normal. (H & E, x 15)

Vestibular end-organs were present and were well preserved. There were no eosinophilic precipitates in the endolymphatic and perilymphatic spaces. The endolymphatic sac, vestibular aqueduct, and vein in the paravestibular canaliculus were normal.

INTERNAL AUDITORY CANAL. The seventh and eighth cranial nerves, and the labyrinthine artery and its branches, were normal.

CASE 2

In May 1958 a 64-year-old male was seen for evaluation of intermittent attacks of pain in the left ophthalmic and maxillary divisions. These attacks were characterized by superimposed, paroxysmal, lightning-like stabs of pain, and had been occurring for a year. A diagnosis of tic douloureux was made. An audiogram made on May 15, 1958, showed a moderate, bilateral hearing loss characterized by a descending audiometric pattern. The average hearing loss in the speech frequency range was 40 dB in the left ear and 50 dB in the right ear (Fig. 3).

On May 22, 1958, the patient underwent surgery for partial sectioning of the left trigeminal sensory root through the posterior

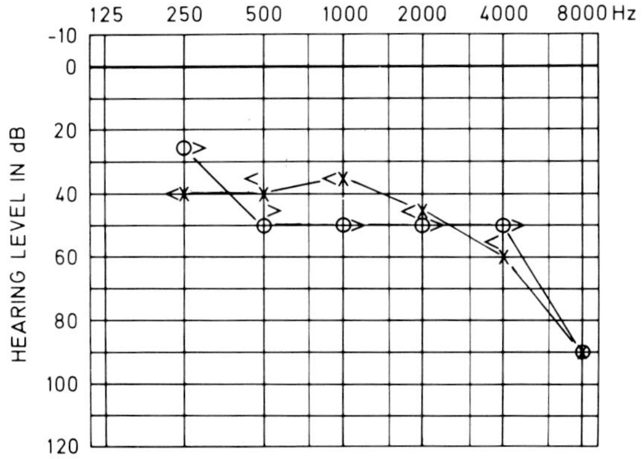

Fig. 3. (Case 2) Audiogram obtained 12 days before the operation for incomplete posterior fossa sectioning of the trigeminal sensory root.

cranial fossa; during this procedure it was necessary to section the left eighth cranial nerve. After the operation, the patient had a permanent total hearing loss in the left ear, disturbance of balance and gait, and a tendency to fall to the left.

On October 23, 1974, 16 years after the surgery just described, the patient died of an extensive acute myocardial infarct at the age of 80. The temporal bones were obtained and were processed and studied as detailed for case 1.

HISTOPATHOLOGICAL FINDINGS

Left Temporal Bone.

EXTERNAL AND MIDDLE EARS. No abnormalities were observed.

INNER EAR. All basic structures of the organ of Corti were easily identifiable (Fig. 4A, B), and a normal population of hair cells was present. The tectorial membrane was flattened but present throughout the cochlea. The stria vascularis and the spiral ligament in the lower turns appeared to be normal; however, these structures in the upper turns were somewhat atrophic. In the middle turn a dark blue-staining deposit was observed in the stria vascularis in a triangular space between the marginal cells and intermediate cells. The cochlear duct was collapsed, more predominantly in the lower turns than in the upper turns. In most turns the spiral ganglion cells and their nerve fibers were decreased in number, but this was less obvious in the apical turn. A few intraganglionic spiral bundle fibers were present in Rosenthal's canal of the basal turn; however, no spiral bundle fibers were noted in the remaining cochlear turns. The cochlear aqueduct was dupli-

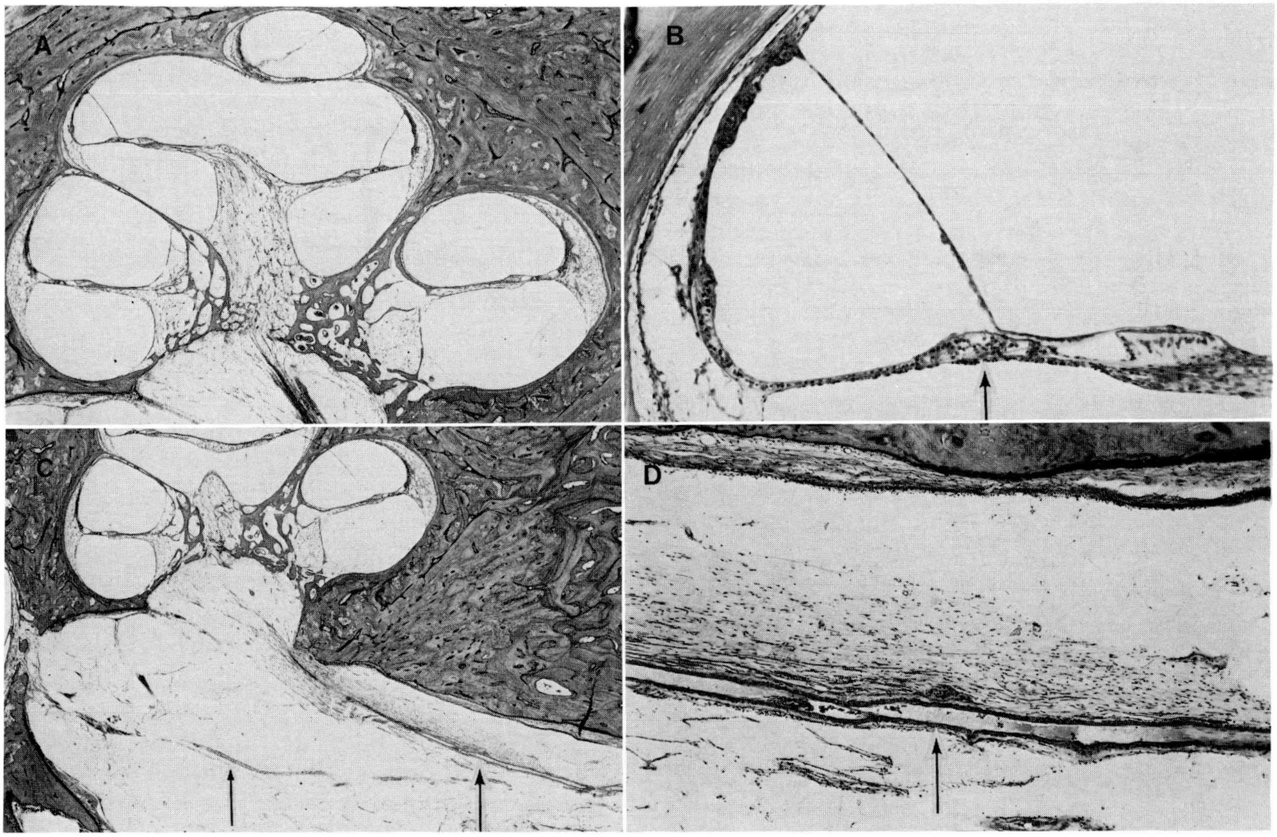

Fig. 4. (Case 2) Left ear. A) Most of the cochlear nerve in the modiolus is absent. Note that the organ of Corti is well preserved in all cochlear turns; however, Reissner's membrane is collapsed, especially in the lower turns. (H & E, x 12) B) Upper half of the second turn of the cochlea has a well preserved organ of Corti (arrow). In this particular area, a moderately atrophic stria vascularis, flattened tectorial membrane, and relatively collapsed Reissner's membrane are also seen. (H & E, x 64) C) Well-preserved labyrinthine arteries (small and large arrows) may be noted, coursing along with the degenerated cochlear and saccular nerves in the internal auditory canal. Large arrow - Main cochlear artery. Small arrow - Vestibulocochlear artery. (H & E, x 8) D) High-power view of the main cochlear artery (arrow) seen in C. (H & E, x 42)

cated for a portion of its course. The inferior cochlear vein was normal but for a short distance ran out of the otic capsule under the mucous membrane of the middle ear.

The maculae of the utricle and the saccule and the cristae of the three semicircular canals appeared to be normal. The epithelial lining of the endolymphatic sac was normal. However, an eosinophilic precipitate was observed in the endolymphatic space and some fibrous connective tissue was present in the subepithelial layer. The vestibular aqueduct and the vein in the paravestibular canaliculus were normal.

INTERNAL AUDITORY CANAL. Only a few fibers of the cochlear and vestibular nerves were present, but the facial nerve was normal. A striking finding was that the labyrinthine artery and its branches were well preserved and appeared to be intact (Fig. 4C, D).

Right Temporal Bone.

EXTERNAL AND MIDDLE EARS. It was impossible to evaluate the external ear and the middle ear because of the presence of preparation artifacts.

INNER EAR. The organ of Corti was well preserved, as were the hair cells. The cochlear duct was normal in contour. The stria vascularis was normal in the lower turns but somewhat atrophic in the upper turns. A dark blue-staining deposit was present between the marginal cells and the intermediate cells in the stria vascularis of the lower half of the middle turn. The spiral ligament was normal. In most of the cochlear turns there was a normal population of spiral ganglion cells and their nerve fibers; however, there was a loss of approximately 50 to 70% of those cells and nerve fibers in the lower half of the basal turn. The cochlear aqueduct and the inferior cochlear vein were normal. In the vestibular system the crista of the posterior semicircular canal was present and well preserved. Other vestibular end-organs could not be evaluated because of preparation artifacts. The endolymphatic sac, the vestibular aqueduct, and the vein in the paravestibular canaliculus were all normal.

INTERNAL AUDITORY CANAL. The seventh and eighth cranial nerves and the labyrinthine artery were normal.

DISCUSSION

Case 1 appears to be one of the few cases in which inner ear pathology following the surgical removal of an acoustic tumor has been studied.[4-6] In addition, it appears that the surgical lesion made in the internal auditory canal in this case was the most severe recorded.

The extensive pathology observed in the cochlea in this case is similar to that observed to occur in animals following obstruction of the labyrinthine artery;[2] for this reason we speculate that the pathology was the result of the surgical sectioning of the labyrinthine artery. However, the following factors could also have had an effect on the inner ear: 1) It is possible that prior to the surgery the tumor might have compressed arteries in the internal auditory canal resulting in impairment of the arterial blood supply to the cochlea.[7] 2) Severe degenerative changes in the cochlear nerve might have resulted from sectioning not only of the labyrinthine artery but also of the eighth cranial nerve.

In case 1, while severe cochlear pathology was present, the vestibular end-organs showed only moderate atrophic changes and were surprisingly well preserved. This same finding has been described in previous reports.[2,4,6] In this case it was impossible to detect any arterial blood supply from the intracranial side, although it was sought in the internal auditory canal, the vestibular aqueduct, and the paravestibular canaliculus.

However, a moderately large artery (89 μ in diameter) was seen to course along the degenerated facial nerve in the labyrinthine portion of the facial canal and to enter the internal auditory canal. This artery is much larger than the artery (25 μ average diameter) we observed in 18 normal cases.[8] In case 1, then, it appears that the vestibular end-organs were more resistant than the organ of Corti to the effects of damage to the labyrinthine artery. Indeed, it seems that these end-organs were preserved by the blood supply from an unusual intrameatal branch of the external carotid artery system, a branch which formed in the course of the postoperative reparative process.

Although the creation of a severe surgical lesion in case 1 was followed by a moderately prolonged ($6^1/_2$ months) postoperative survival period, there was no marked evidence of repair such as was seen in experimental animals: in the experiments, severe fibrosis and ossification were observed to fill the cochlear duct and the perilymphatic spaces five months after the labyrinthine artery had been surgically obstructed.[2] This lack of repair in human tissue may be explained by the fact that in this case blood came to be supplied to the inner ear from the external carotid artery system through the labyrinthine portion of the facial canal.

Kimura and Perlman[2] observed substances in the perilymphatic and endolymphatic spaces of animals they operated upon to create a labyrinthine artery obstruction. These substances seem to be similar to the eosinophilic precipitate seen in case 1. Perhaps the eosinophilic precipitate is the result of high levels of protein in these fluids, as reported by Silverstein and Makimoto.[3] However, it should not be assumed that the precipitate is the result of such obstruction or lesion, particularly when the precipitate is seen in the perilymphatic space. Such material may have formed secondary to processes associated with the development of the acoustic tumor.[9]

It is interesting that in case 1 the endolymphatic sac and the vestibular aqueduct were normal. This was also noted to be the case in animals in which the labyrinthine artery was obstructed.[2] It may be that in humans the arterial blood supply for the sac is from the posterior meningeal artery[10] and not from the labyrinthine artery, so that injury to the labyrinthine artery would not have any effect on the sac.

Case 2 appears to be the first instance in which the histopathological change in the inner ear brought by sectioning of the eighth cranial nerve only could be studied in man. In this case the cochlear nerve was found to be degenerated but the cochlear end-organs were well preserved; these findings are similar to those seen in animals after cochlear nerve sectioning.[1,2] We thus speculate that the changes observed in the human vestibular system which are similar to those seen in the cochlea are due to sectioning of the vestibular nerve.

The atrophy of the stria vascularis noted in the upper turns of the cochlea of case 2 and the absence of the cochlear nerve in the basal turn of the cochlea in case 2 could be associated with this patient's hearing loss which had been detected before the surgery. This pathology may also represent a combination of neural presbycusis and metabolic presbycusis as described by Schuknecht.[11] However, we are unable to explain the fact that the patient suffered a total hearing loss postoperatively and yet cochlear nerve fibers and the organ of Corti in the apical turn were present.

SUMMARY

We report a human temporal bone histopathological study comparing pathology of the inner ear following surgical sectioning of the eighth cranial nerve and the labyrinthine artery with the pathology resulting from damage only to the eighth cranial nerve.

The first case, in which both the eighth cranial nerve and the labyrinthine artery were surgically severed, revealed severe pathologic changes in the cochlear end-organ and moderate pathologic changes in the fairly well-preserved vestibular end-organs. Interestingly, the endolymphatic sac in the vestibular aqueduct was normal. On the other hand, the second case, in which the eighth cranial nerve was sectioned but the labyrinthine artery was preserved, revealed the organ of Corti and vestibular end-organs to be well preserved and normal. These findings suggest that the blood supply from the labyrinthine artery plays a major role in maintaining most of the membranous structures in the inner ear, except for the endolymphatic sac in the vestibular aqueduct, and that the vestibular end-organs are more resistant than the organ of Corti to the effects of damage to the labyrinthine artery.

An additional interesting finding was the observation in the first case of an unusually large artery running from the geniculate ganglion area, along the facial nerve in the labyrinthine portion of the facial canal, to the internal auditory canal. This artery was the only artery which could have supplied blood postoperatively to the inner ear, and this suggests that a compensatory arterial blood supply which draws blood from the external carotid artery system to supply the inner ear may be developed when the labyrinthine artery is severed.

Presently Dr. Ogawa is Assistant Professor in the Department of Otolaryngology, Tokyo Medical and Dental University, Japan.

ACKNOWLEDGMENTS — The authors wish to express their deep gratitude to Eugene N. Myers, MD, Professor and Chairman, Department of Otolaryngology, University of Pittsburgh School of Medicine, for giving helpful advice during the preparation of the paper. Appreciation is also expressed to Reisuke Saito, MD, for helping in the pathological interpretations, and to Shelly Frisch, Ellie Lee, and Ruth Anderson for their assistance in this study. Otolaryngology, Tokyo Medical and Dental University.

REFERENCES

1. Schuknecht HF, Woellner RC. An experimental and clinical study of deafness from lesions of the cochlear nerve. J Laryngol Otol 1955; 69:75-97.

2. Kimura R, Perlman HB. Arterial obstruction of the labyrinth. Part I. Cochlear changes. Part II. Vestibular changes. Ann Otol Rhinol Laryngol 1958; 67:1-36.

3. Silverstein H, Makimoto K. Superior vestibular and "singular nerve" section - animal and clinical studies. Laryngoscope 1973; 83:1414-32.

4. De Moura LRP. Inner ear pathology in acoustic neurinoma. Arch Otolaryngol 1967; 85:125-33.

5. Igarashi M, Jerger J, Alford BR, et al. Functional and histological findings in acoustic tumor. Arch Otolaryngol 1974; 99:379-84.

6. Suga F, Lindsay JR. Inner ear degeneration in acoustic neurinoma. Ann Otol Rhinol Laryngol 1976; 85:343-58.

7. Schuknecht HF. Pathology of the ear. Cambridge: Harvard University Press, 1974.

8. Ogawa A, Sando I. Spatial occupancy of vessels and facial nerve in the facial canal. Ann Otol Rhinol Laryngol (in press).

9. Schuknecht HF. The pathophysiology of angle tumors. In Wolfson RJ, ed. Vestibular system and its diseases. Philadelphia: University of Pennsylvania Press, 1966:428-38.

10. Bast TH, Anson BJ. The temporal bone and the ear. Springfield: Charles C. Thomas, 1949.

11. Schuknecht HF. Further observations on the pathology of presbycusis. Arch Otolaryngol 1964; 80:369-82.

BENIGN MUCOUS MEMBRANE PEMPHIGOID

RICHARD J. H. SMITH, MD

ROY B. SESSIONS, MD SAMUEL F. BEAN, MD

HOUSTON, TEXAS

Benign mucous membrane pemphigoid (BMMP) is a rare vesiculobullous disease capable of causing serious ocular and aerodigestive morbidity. The otolaryngologist must not be lulled to complacency by the adjective, benign. A case of complete laryngeal stenosis is presented and the clinical, histological and therapeutic aspects of BMMP are discussed.

Benign mucous membrane pemphigoid (BMMP) is one of a group of vesiculobullous diseases that present primarily in the oral cavity. The word "benign" should not lead to a sense of complacency on the part of the physician; through an autoimmune destructive process, serious ocular and aerodigestive sequellae can occur. It is our purpose to acquaint the otolaryngologist with BMMP, its morbidity, and the problems inherent in its management.

Since its description by Cooper[1] in 1857, BMMP has been called ocular pemphigus, pemphigus conjunctivae, pemphigus ocularis, and cicatricial pemphigoid. In 1911 Thost[2] separated it from its close counterpart, pemphigus, on clinical grounds, but it was not until 30 years later that Civatte[3] and Lever[4] described the histologic difference between the two diseases. Untreated pemphigus has a mortality of greater than 90%; deaths due to BMMP have not been reported.[5]

CASE PRESENTATION

In 1978 a 62-year-old female first noticed oral mucosal blisters which were at that time diagnosed as herpetic. The blistering continued for some months however; in addition, dyspnea associated with exertion began to develop. Over the ensuing 14 months she experienced increasing respiratory difficulty until emergency hospitalization and tracheostomy became necessary. Biopsies of the larynx and oropharynx showed the characteristic immunofluorescence of BMMP. Prednisone and azathioprine therapy resulted in subjective improvement, but a complete laryngeal stenosis developed. A recent laryngoscopy and bronchoscopy showed that while her oropharynx is free of disease, there is diffuse involvement of the tracheobronchial tree.

DISCUSSION

BMMP is a rare disease; it tends to afflict elderly females without showing any racial predilection.[6] The primary lesion is either a vesicle or bulla that appears in the oral cavity or conjunctiva.[7] Within 48 hours the blister ruptures and the raw denuded surface becomes covered by a fibrinous exudate. Usually reepithelialization and scarring follow. More than half of these patients have oral and conjunctival disease, although other mucous membranes can be involved. Lesions in the nasopharynx, esophagus, penis, vagina, and anal canal have been reported. Bean has also found a 30% incidence of cutaneous involvement in the areas of the face and neck.[8]

Even though oral lesions are generally located on the palate, they can and do occur on the buccal mucosa[9] (Fig. 1). Hypopharyngeal extension is unusual and laryngeal involvement a rarity. Fisher et al have reported two patients with laryngeal stenosis requiring tracheostomy.[10] Extensive disease of the trachea and bronchi has not previously been reported.

Ocular involvement causes irritation and burning in the eyes. Conjunctival inflammation (Fig. 2) follows the blister formation and, as synechiae form between the lid and bulbar conjunctivae, the blink reflex becomes impaired leaving the cornea unprotected. In 20% of cases, the cornea dries and becomes cloudy, resulting in secondary blindness.

In first describing the histopathology of the BMMP lesion, Lever was struck by the absence of acantholysis on light microscopy. Acantholysis, as exemplified by pemphigus, refers to the loss of intercellular desmosomal attachments of the epidermal cells that then assume a spheroid shape and float freely in the intraepidermal blister fluid. This does not occur in BMMP — the fact that prompted Lever to use the adjective, benign.[11] In BMMP, the blister is located below the epidermis and is associated with a nonspecific inflammatory infiltrate of lymphocytes, fibroblasts, and plasma cells. Immunologic studies[12-17] have shown that antibodies are present and attached to the basement membrane of the mucosa in the involved sites (Fig. 3). An invoked

From the Department of Otorhinolaryngology and Communicative Sciences, and the Department of Dermatology, Baylor College of Medicine, Houston.

REPRINTS — Roy B. Sessions, MD, 6501 Fannin, Houston, TX 77030.

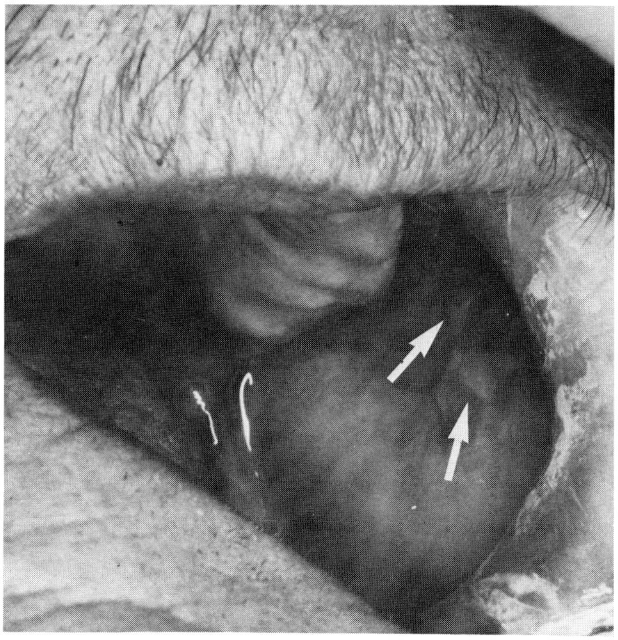

Fig. 1. Oral vesiculation in benign mucous membrane pemphigoid (arrows).

cytotoxic response results in edema and the clinically apparent bulla.

Blister formation to the degree found in BMMP that is limited to the mucous membrane is unusual; and this feature thereby limits the differential diagnosis. Bullous pemphigoid, similar histologically but more extensive clinically than BMMP, may present with oral lesions.[7] Widespread cutaneous involvement ultimately develops. Erythema multiforme is primarily a disease of the young and presents with hemorrhagic mucosal lesions and pathognomic target-like lesions. Dermatitis herpetiformis, or Buhring's disease, has grouped skin lesions reminiscent of herpes and rarely involves the mucous membranes. Lichen planus of the buccal mucosa is identifiable by an irregular lacelike whitening

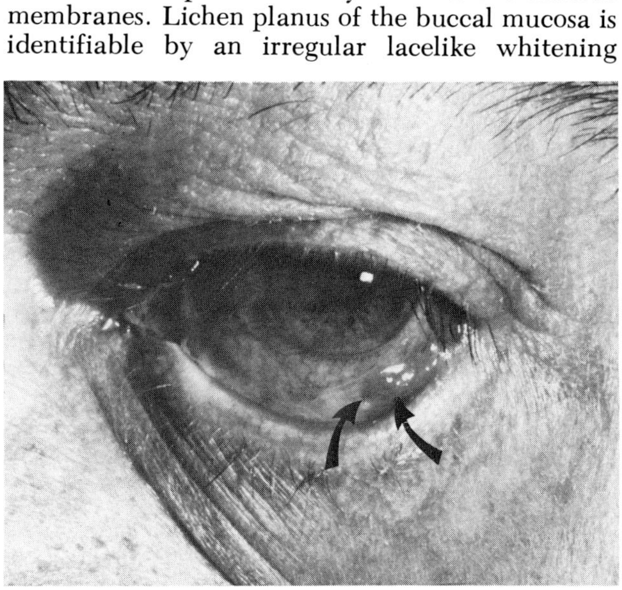

Fig. 2. Ocular involvement of the lid and bulbar conjunctivae (arrows).

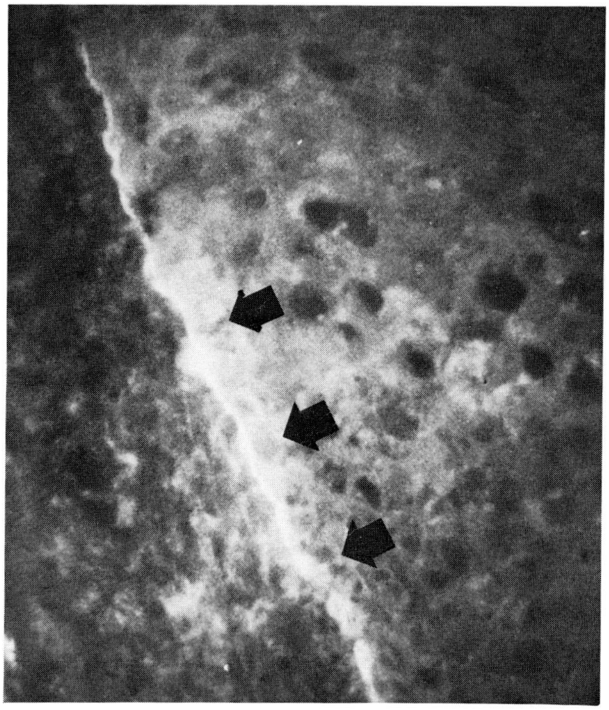

Fig. 3. IgG immunofluorescence in an oral mucosal lesion. IgG antibodies affixed to the basement membrane (arrows).

known as Wickham's striae. This is diagnostic in patients presenting with only oral involvement.[8] A small number of patients will have erosive or vesicular lesions on the oral mucosa that cause severe pain. However, the microscopic appearance of these varieties of lichen planus distinguishes this disease entity from BMMP.[11]

The treatment of BMMP is largely symptomatic. Corticosteroids play a major role.[9] Immunosuppressive agents such as methotrexate and azathioprine have also been used successfully. The greatest benefit seems to occur with a normal dosage of azathioprine, 100-200 mg/day, in conjunction with steroid administration. Repeated courses are often necessary. The reader is referred to the literature for a detailed description of the various treatment plans.[9,10]

Although a rare disease, because BMMP presents in the oral cavity, the burden is on the otolaryngologist to consider it in the differential diagnosis. One must not be lulled to complacency by the adjective, benign. This refers only to a histologic finding and has no significance in prognosticating the clinical course of the disease. Significant morbidity such as blindness and laryngeal stenosis can and do occur. It is of interest in the case that we have presented that cicatricial formation has obliterated the glottic aperture and although the disease is now quiescent above the glottic level, it is present in the trachea and bronchi. Whether or not the disease in the upper aerodigestive tract will again become active is unknown. To decannulate our patient would require treating the stenosis, but we have felt it prudent to refrain from surgery for a period of time. Perhaps her tracheal and bronchial lesions will heal and leave her free of active disease. Possibly she would then be a more suitable candidate for a surgical procedure.

REFERENCES

1. Cooper W. Pemphigus of the conjunctiva. Ophthalmol Hosp Rep 1857; 1:155.
2. Thost A. Der chronrische Schleimhauptem pemphigus der oberen Luftwege. Arch Laryngol Rhinol 1911; 25:459.
3. Civatte A. Le diagnostic des dermatoses bulleuses an laboratorie. Arch Belg Dermatol Syphiligr 1949; 5:273-5.
4. Lever WF. Pemphigus: a histopathologic study. Arch Dermatol 1951; 64:727-53.
5. Perry HO. Benign mucous membrane pemphigoid. In: Demis DJ, Dobson RL, McQuire J, eds. Clinical dermatology. Vol. 2. Hagerstown: Harper & Row, 1979; unit 6-13:1-4.
6. Gorlin R, Sedano H. Benign mucous membrane pemphigoid. J Dermatol Surg Oncol 1978; 4:504-5.
7. Bean SF. Cicatricial pemphigoid: a study of 15 cases. South Med J 1974; 67:1187-90.
8. Bean SF. Oral cicatricial pemphigoid. Trans Am Acad Ophthalmol Otolaryngol 1977; 84:530-3.
9. Foster M, Nally F. Benign mucous membrane pemphigoid (cicatricial mucosal pemphigoid): a reconsideration. Oral Surg 1977; 44:697-705.
10. Fisher I, Dahl MV, Christiansen TA. Cicatricial pemphigoid confined to the larynx. Cutis 1980; 25:371-3.
11. Ossoff R, Wolff AP. Vesiculobullous lesions of the upper aerodigestive tract. Otolaryngol Head Neck Surg 1979; 87:20-6.
12. Bean SF. Cicatricial pemphigoid. Arch Dermatol 1974; 110:552-5.
13. Rogers R, Jordon R. Immunopathology of oral mucosal inflammatory diseases. Clin Exp Dermatol 1977; 2:97-106.
14. Peck SM, Osserman KE, Weiner LB, Lefkovits A, Osserman BS. Studies in bullous diseases. N Eng J Med 1968; 951-8.
15. Chorzelski TP, Beutner EH. Factors contributing to occasional failures in the laboratory diagnosis of bullous pemphigoid by indirect immunofluorescence. Br J Dermatol 1972; 86:111-7.
16. Person JR, Rogers RS, Jordon RE. Cicatricial pemphigoid with circulating antibasement membrane antibodies. Dermatologica 1977; 154:90-7.
17. Rogers RS, Perry HO, Bean SF, Jordon RE. Immunopathology of cicatricial pemphigoid: studies of complement deposition. J Invest Dermatol 1977; 68:39-43.

≈

CONGRESS OF SKULL BASE STUDY GROUP

The First International Congress of Skull Base Study Group, an international interdisciplinary group interested in all problems of the skull base, will meet in Brussels, Belgium, June 10 through June 12, 1982. Those interested should contact Prof. P. Clement, MD. ENT Department, A.Z.-V.U.B., Laarbeeklaan-101, 1090 Brussels.

Ann Otol 91:1982

BASIC PRINCIPLES OF CHEMOTHERAPY IN THE TREATMENT OF METASTATIC HEAD AND NECK CANCER

SAMUEL W. NEEDLEMAN, MD

IOWA CITY, IOWA

For patients who fail to achieve control of head and neck cancer with local therapy, chemotherapy offers limited benefit at present. Better understanding of the phenomena which surround tumor cell killing by active agents should allow for the rational design of more effective programs. For example, as tumors grow larger, many cells cease to engage in DNA synthesis and are refractory to drugs like methotrexate. In such a case, alkylating agents might be more effective. Tritiated thymidine uptake and nuclear DNA fluorescence studies can be exploited to analyze the kinetic and metabolic behavior of tumor cells, and are described. For animal models these studies have allowed the design of "kinetic" regimens of enhanced efficacy. Methotrexate, hydroxyurea, cyclophosphamide, vinblastine, and cis-platinum have appreciable antitumor activity in head and neck carcinoma. Combining active agents in a rational sequence could be facilitated by kinetic analysis of a patient's tumor, giving rise to specific regimens with more cytoreduction, less toxicity and resistance, and ultimately, better survival.

INTRODUCTION

Currently, chemotherapy of head and neck carcinoma enjoys only modest success in causing tumors to remit and allowing patients to survive longer. However, continued investigations into the biology of the host-tumor interaction and mechanisms of tumor cell killing may lead to a better future for patients with these tumors. The focus of this discussion, then, will be a number of biologic considerations derived from observations in animal models and human tumors such as the lymphomas and acute leukemias. Since treatment of these tumors met with limited success initially, but has improved dramatically in recent years, it is conceivable that these concepts similarly will serve as a model for the development of more effective therapy of head and neck carcinoma.

Host-Tumor-Drug Relationship and the Response to Chemotherapy. A number of pharmacokinetic parameters such as activation, inactivation, binding to carrier proteins, excretion, and delivery of drug have obvious impact in the clinical response to even the most active agents. These considerations are beyond the scope of this discussion and are reviewed comprehensively elsewhere.[1] As well, the response to an agent given in an appropriate schedule seems to depend heavily on the proliferative status of tumor cell populations, which in turn seems to vary as a function of tumor burden. Thus, understanding the host-tumor relationship with the purpose of designing more effective schedules might be profitable.

The early pioneering work of Skipper et al in the L1210 leukemia model led to their statement of the log-kill hypothesis in 1964.[2] This holds that a constant fraction of the tumor cells will survive a given level of effective therapy irrespective to the size of the tumor. Thus, the greatest number of cells will be killed in large tumors, while small tumors should be curable if the same level of therapy is repeatedly applied until virtually every cell is killed. While the log-kill hypothesis holds well for the L1210 system, in clinical chemotherapy, a number of observations mitigate against it.

In 1977 Norton and Simon[3] suggested that tumor killing for a given level of effective therapy varies with the growth rate of the tumor. For L1210 or other tumors which follow logarithmic growth, growth fraction (GF) is large and stays constant. Thus, growth rate accelerates as the tumor grows, rendering large tumors sensitive. In contrast, for Gompertzian tumor growth (Fig. 1), which probably more accurately describes human tumors, GF is large initially, but progressively diminishes. Growth rate progressively increases reaching its maximum at about 37% of total volume and subsequently decreases, as decreased GF becomes significant. Consequently, large tumors, as well as very small tumors, have low growth rates and are relatively resistant to effective treatment.

Some have suggested that increasing cell death or slowed cell generation time are responsible for the deceleration of tumor growth and the plateau at the top of the Gompertzian curve.[4] However, as the tumors grow larger in mass, a greater proportion of cells become more distant from nutrient vessels, experiencing greater competition for oxygen and nutrients. Cells such as these reversibly lose their proliferative capacity[5] and remain dormant, decreasing GF. While cell death and slowing of generation

From the Department of Medicine, Division of Hematology-Oncology, University of Iowa Hospitals and Clinics, Iowa City. This work was supported by the American Cancer Society (CF 4768).

REPRINTS — Samuel W. Needleman, MD, Department of Medicine, University of Iowa, Iowa City, IA 52242.

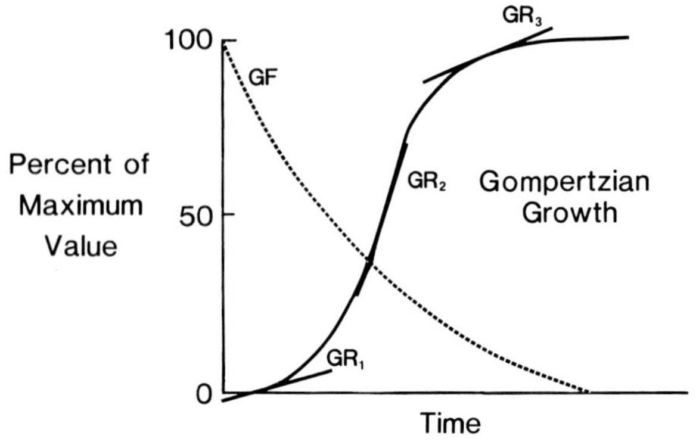

Fig. 1. Gompertzian tumor growth. Mass is shown as a function of time (——). Progressively declining growth fraction is shown as a function of time (_ _ _ _). Three growth rates are represented for small (GR_1), intermediate (GR_2) and large (GR_3) tumor burdens by tangent lines to the mass curve. GR_1 and GR_3 illustrate slow tumor growth rates for large and small tumor burdens. (Adapted from Norton and Simon.[3] From Needleman SW. Chemotherapeutic approaches to transitional cell carcinoma of the bladder. In: Bonney W, ed. Bladder cancer. Vol. 1. Baltimore: Williams and Wilkins, 1982. Reprinted with permission.)

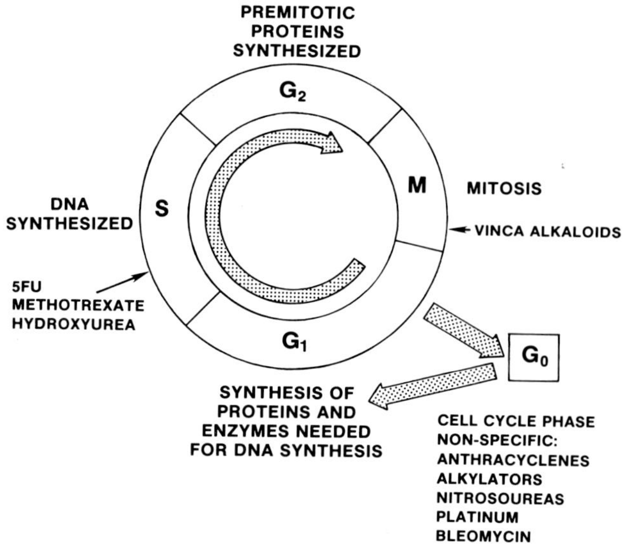

Fig. 2. Cell cycle and chemotherapy. The principal metabolic functions of the cell in various phases of the cell cycle and relationship of agents active in head and neck tumors to the cell cycle are indicated. (From Needleman SW. Chemotherapeutic approaches to transitional cell carcinoma of the bladder. In: Bonney W, ed. Bladder cancer. Vol. 1. Baltimore: Williams and Wilkins, 1982. Reprinted with permission.)

times doubtless contribute in part to the plateau in tumor growth, most investigators suggest that the majority of cells remain viable but dormant, and if they do go into the cell cycle, they do so with normal generation times.[6]

The therapeutic implication of the mechanism of slowed growth in the plateau phase is illustrated in Figure 2. A diagrammatic representation of the cell cycle, the principal metabolic functions of its various phases, and the agents with greatest activity against head and neck tumors are illustrated. Of note, is that after mitosis, the cell is quite inactive metabolically. Tumor cells seem to have a great capacity for staying in this state virtually indefinitely, and most authors designate this as G_o, functionally separate from the generation cycle.[6] Drugs like vinblastine and methotrexate are active only against cells in the generation cycle in a particular phase and are termed "cell-cycle-phase specific." Agents like BCNU and cyclophosphamide (Cytoxan) act throughout the generation cycle, and are termed "cell-cycle-phase nonspecific. Agents such as the nitrogen mustards and ionizing radiation exhibit cytolytic activity irrespective of the generation cycle and are termed cell-cycle nonspecific. While these latter agents may have some activity against cells in G_o, it is the relative resistance of the G_o population to chemotherapy that presents the clinician with a difficult problem.[7]

Techniques to Assess Kinetic Behavior of Tumors. The use of thymidine labeled with tritium (^{3}HTdR) has proved a powerful tool in assessing the proliferative activity of cells in tumors, as well as allowing calculation of cycle times and phase durations. Cells engaging in DNA synthesis incorporate ^{3}HTdR sufficient to give autoradiographic visualization without disturbing cell function. Labeling in vitro correlates well with labeling in vivo. By counting labeled cells per 100 total cells one hour after exposure to ^{3}HTdR and expressing the result as a percentage, one derives the Labeling Index (LI) which is a measure of the fraction of cells at the time of exposure to ^{3}HTdR which are in S phase (Fig. 2). LI is a crude indicator of the extent to which the cell population is invested in proliferative biochemistry. Since the fraction of cells in S phase is determined by the duration of S phase relative to the entire cycle, as well as the fraction of cells which are engaged in proliferation (GF), a high LI may reflect long S phase duration or a high GF. Alternatively, the two factors may obscure the LI, with opposing contributions. Thus, high LI has been reported to predict both favorable[8] and unfavorable[9] therapeutic outcomes. The Mitotic Index (MI) is the number of mitoses per 100 cells. It is similarly influenced by the GF as well as the duration of mitosis, and with similar limitations reflects the proliferative capacity of the population. Growth fraction (GF) is defined as the ratio of proliferating cells to total cells, and would provide a better handle on cell population kinetics in relation to the tumor burden. GF can be estimated by mathematical analysis of the percent labeled mitosis, or PLM curve.[10]

One can also exploit the PLM to calculate the duration of the cell cycle and its various phases. The PLM is determined by examining the tumor by light microscopy for a number of mitotic figures, usually 1,000. By autoradiography the corresponding mitoses are deemed labeled if isotope emission grains are noted over the nucleus. If the PLM is plotted

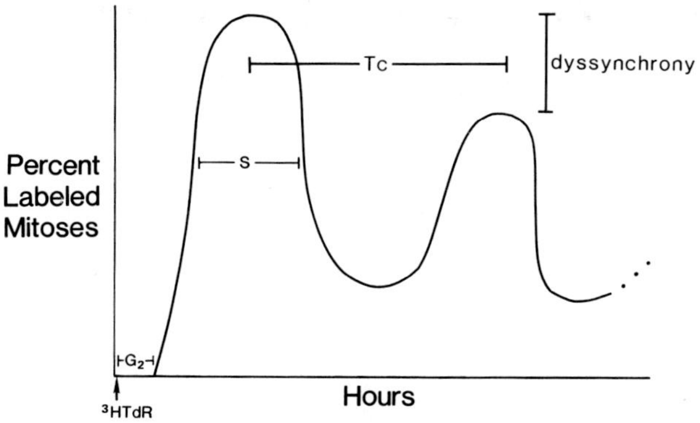

Fig. 3. PLM curve. Percent labeled mitoses determined by autoradiography is plotted as a function of time. (Adapted from Cronkite.[11] From Needleman SW. Chemotherapeutic approaches to transitional cell carcinoma of the bladder. In: Bonney W, ed. Bladder cancer. Vol. 1. Baltimore: Williams and Wilkins, 1982. Reprinted with permission.)

against time, a curve such as that depicted in Figure 3 is obtained. At the time of ^{3}HTdR pulse, all cells in S phase will pick up isotopes, but mitotic figures will not be labeled until cells that were just finishing S phase proceed through G_2 and enter mitosis. Thus, the time from pulsing to the first appearance of labeled mitoses approximates the duration of G_2. Similarly cells that were just beginning S phase will proceed through S and G_2 phases and will appear as the last labeled mitoses at time S + G_2 after the pulse, on the right shoulder of the first peak. The duration of the first peak then, approximates the duration of S phase (Ts). If the daughter cells of the first peak proceed synchronously through the cell cycle, an identical peak will appear one generation time (Tc) later. The degree to which the progeny cells lack synchrony will be manifest in dampening of subsequent peaks.[11]

A newer technique, nuclear DNA-content evaluation,[12] allows the estimation of the number of cells in a given phase of the generation cycle. Capitalizing on the development of technique ability to quantitate fluorescence in a single cell, tumors are labeled with a fluorescent reagent which binds to DNA. The amount of fluorescence then will correspond to the content of DNA. Cells in G_1 are diploid and have relatively little DNA, cells in G_2 are tetraploid and have the greatest content while cells in S phase have variable, intermediate content. This technique may provide more rapid and better resolution of kinetic data for heterogeneous, dysynchronous cell populations than the PLM curve.

Use of Kinetic Data in the Treatment of Head and Neck Tumors. It is theoretically possible to exploit these data in the design of treatment programs. Thus, where toxicity permits, the treatment would be repeated at intervals shorter than Tc, so that no cell could complete a cycle during the interim between therapies. Similar reasoning applies to the scheduling of S phase active agents at intervals shorter than Ts. A typical "kinetic" regimen then will initiate therapy with a cell-cycle-phase nonspecific agent like cyclophosphamide in order to reduce the tumor burden and "recruit" cells from the G_o pool into the generation cycle. A number of drugs like vincristine will reversibly arrest cells and then release them in synchrony; these synchronizing agents are generally employed after recruitment. At time M + G_1 ($= T_c$-[$T_s + TG_2$]) after synchronizing, cells would presumably enter S phase and be susceptible to S phase specific agents.[8]

TABLE 1. ACTIVE AGENTS IN HEAD AND NECK CARCINOMA

Drug	*Responders/Total*	*% Response*
Methotrexate	298/360	47
Hydroxyurea	7/18	39
Cytoxan	28/77	36
Vinblastine	10/35	29
Cis-platinum	10/38	26
Adriamycin	15/95	16
Bleomycin	24/158	15
5 Fluorouracil	18/118	15
Me CCNU	6/40	15
Vincristine	1/25	4

Adapted from Khandekar and Dewys.[18]

PLM curves suggest that recruitment and synchronization indeed take place when these manipulations are performed in animals, and treatment results are very good. In humans, however, the repeated biopsies needed to obtain PLM curves cannot be performed, except principally in patients with accessible, superficial tumors or bone marrow involvement. Thus, there are few actual calculations of cell cycle times for human head and neck and other carcinomas, but rather approximations from animal data are frequently used. This may at least in part explain the fact that in humans this approach has not yielded greater benefit.

A few studies have determined kinetic data on tumors from patients with head and neck cancer.[13-17] GF has ranged from 31-84%, Ts 11-34 hours, and Tc 25-88 hours. It is apparent from these data that tremendous variation from one tumor to another exists. Indeed, nuclear DNA-content analysis[15] suggests that within a single tumor there is significant kinetic heterogeneity. Using this technique as well as PLM curves, this study found a small proportion of G_o cells. Moreover, looking at patients who respond to or fail chemotherapy, these authors were not able to demonstrate any significant differences in kinetic parameters.[14] Results could perhaps be improved if the kinetic behavior of a tumor could be analyzed prior to treatment to allow design of a program relevant to that patient's tumor, rather than to a model or to another patient's tumor from which it may differ substantially.

Currently Available Chemotherapy for Head and Neck Tumors. Phase 2 single-agent response studies for head and neck cancer should be viewed with

TABLE 2. COMBINATION CHEMOTHERAPY REGIMENS IN METASTATIC HEAD AND NECK CARCINOMA WITH >40% RESPONSE RATES (15 OR MORE PATIENTS)

Investigator†	*Drugs*	*Response/Patients Evaluation (%)*	*Duration (mo)*
DeWell (1975)	CTX, VCR, MTX, PDN, 5 FU	14/32 (44)	MR = 2.2
Richman (1976)	BLE, ADR, CCNU, VCR, $HN_2 \pm$ BCG	15/32 (44)	MR = 4.2 MS = 5.2
Eisenberger (1980)	BLE, HOU	9/20 (45)	MR = 4.2
Huang (1980)[19]	BLE, MTX, VBL, CCNU	19/38 (50)	MS = 8.5
Yagoda (1975)	BLE, MTX	8/15 (53)	MR = 3.0
Cortes* (1980)	MTX, 5FU, BLE	22/40 (55)	R = 7-13
Costanzi* (1976)	BLE, MTX, HOU	10/17 (59)	MR = 2.0
Pitman (1979)	MTX, CDP	12/20 (60)	Not given
Livingston* (1976)	MTX, ADR, MCCNU, CTX, VCR, BLE	17/28 (61)	MR = 6.2 MS = 6.0
Kaplan (1979)	MTX, BLE, CDP	29/46 (63)	MR = 5.0
Price* (1975)	6 MP, BLE, VCR, ADR, MTX, HOU	19/24 (79)	Not given

Adapted from Khandekar and Dewys.[18]

*"Kinetic" design.

†Studies not referenced in the text are published in Proceedings of the American Association of Cancer Research and the American Society of Clinical Oncology for the year noted.

MR - Median duration of response; MS - Median survival; R - Remission duration; CTX - Cyclophosphamide; VCR - Vincristine; MTX - Methotrexate; PDN - Prednisone; 5 FU - 5 Fluorouracil; BLE - Bleomycin; ADR - Adriamycin; MCCNU, CCNU - Nitrosoureas; HN_2 - Nitrogen mustard; VBL - Vinblastine; 6 MP - 6 Mercaptopurine; HOU - Hydroxyurea; CDP - Cis-diammine dichloroplatinum; BCG - Bacillus Calmette-Guerin.

some caution in that they are compiled in many instances from a number of studies with different schedules, methods for gauging response, and programs of supportive care (Table 1). No attempt has been made to ascertain response of tumors for various sites. The measurement of lesions in this region can be especially difficult, making it hard to accurately assess responses. It is worth noting that the cell-cycle-phase specific agent, methotrexate, is the most active agent, which is in agreement with one kinetic study that found, contrary to what one might expect, no evidence for a large number of G_o cells.[15]

Combining active single agents has provided more effective, synergistic tumor control with only additive, nonoverlapping toxicity in other neoplasms. Table 2 is a partial list of the more promising combination programs for head and neck tumors.[18,19] Only studies from the English literature, with 15 or more evaluable patients, and a response rate of >40% have been included. Almost all patients had been previously treated with surgery and radiation. In most studies previous chemotherapy had not been given. While response rates appear high, most responses are partial, duration of response is short, and toxicity is considerable. Survival has probably not been significantly prolonged, and in some cases, one can seriously question whether the patient's symptoms have been palliated to the extent that toxicity is justified. It is of interest to note that 4 of the 6 best response rates were observed with kinetically designed programs.

While many patients' tumors show a gratifying, often dramatic response initially, the responses are regrettably short-lived. The response duration ranges from 8 to 24 weeks, and death soon follows the end of this period. This implies that head and neck cancers regularly develop cellular resistance. The mechanism for this is probably multifactorial. Tumors have been shown to decrease transport of drug, increase its catabolism, and/or decrease its activation in developing resistance. Biochemical adjustments such as increasing target or alternate pathway enzymes have been demonstrated. Enhancement of DNA repair enzymes has been shown in the development of resistance to drugs which act by causing damage to DNA.[20]

The Future. Obviously, the development of new drugs offers hope for the future. Top priority is given to agents which are nonmyelosuppressive. Clinical trials of preoperative and postoperative adjuvant chemotherapy, offering the hope of sterilizing clinically inapparent metastases and increasing surgical cure rates, are being initiated.

As new agents are developed and incorporated into combined modality regimens, our knowledge of the interaction of drugs with tumor cells continues to grow. Improved tools for studying kinetics from small tissues such as those obtained by biopsy may allow the design and scheduling of programs specific to each patient; this in turn would optimize response, aid in anticipating and circumventing the development of drug resistance, minimize toxicity, and play a significant role in improving the future for these patients.

REFERENCES

1. Mihich E. Pharmacologic principles and the basis for selectivity of drug action. In: Holland JF, Frei E, eds. Cancer medicine. Philadelphia: Lea & Febiger, 1974:650-74.

2. Skipper HE, Schabel FM, Wilcox WS. Experimental evaluation of potential anticancer agents XII on the criteria and kinetics associated with curability of experimental leukemia. Cancer Chemother Rep 1964; 35:1-111.

3. Norton L, Simon R. Tumor size, sensitivity to therapy and

design of treatment schedules. Cancer Treat Rep 1977; 61:1307-17.

4. Laird AK. Dynamics of growth in tumors and in normal organism. National Cancer Institute Monograph 1969; 30:15-28.

5. Tannock IF. The relation between cell proliferation and the vascular system in a transplanted mouse mammary tumor. Br J Cancer 1968; 22:258-72.

6. Steel GG, Lamerton LF. Cell population kinetics and chemotherapy. National Cancer Institute Monograph 1969; 30:29-50.

7. Gavosta F, Pileri A. Cell cycle of cancer cells in man. In: Baserga R, ed. The cell cycle and cancer. New York: Dekker Inc, 1971:124.

8. Burke PJ, Owens AH. Attempted recruitment of leukemia myeloblasts to proliferative activity by sequential drug treatment. Cancer 1971; 28:830-6.

9. Durie BG, Salmon SE, Moon TE. Pretreatment tumor mass, cell kinetics and prognosis in multiple myeloma. Blood 1980; 55:364-72.

10. Mendelsohn ML. The growth fraction: a new concept applied to tumors. Science 1960; 132:1496.

11. Cronkite EP. Kinetics of granulopoiesis. National Cancer Institute Monograph 1969; 30:51-62.

12. Bohm N, Spengher E. Fluorescence cytophotometry: a valuable method for the quantitation of nuclear feulgen-DNA. Histochemistry 1968; 16:100.

13. Bresciani F, Daoluzi R, Benassi M, et al. Cell kinetics and growth of squamous cell carcinoma in man. Cancer Res 1974; 34:2405-15.

14. Nervi C, Arcangeli G, Badaracco G, et al. The relevance of tumor size and cell kinetics as predictors of response in head and neck cancer. Cancer 1978; 41:900-6.

15. Nervi C, Badaracco G, Morelli M, et al. Cytokinetic evaluation in head and neck cancer by autoradiography and DNA cytofluorometry. Cancer 1980; 45:452-9.

16. Terz JJ, Curutchet HD, Lawrence W. Analysis of the cell kinetics of human solid tumors. Cancer 1971; 28:1100-10.

17. Tejada R, McKensie R, Leung I, et al. Cell kinetics of primary head and neck cancer. Proc Am Assoc Cancer Ress 1978; 19:212.

18. Khandekar J, Dewys WD. Chemoimmunotherapy of head and neck cancer. Am J Surg 1978; 135:688-95.

19. Huang AT, Lucas VS, Baughn SG, et al. A trial of chemotherapy for recurrent head and neck tumors. Cancer 1980; 45:2038-41.

20. Henderson JF, Brockman RW. Biochemical mechanisms of drug resistance in cancer chemotherapy. In: Pharmacological basis of cancer chemotherapy. Baltimore: Williams and Wilkins, 1975:629-42.

≈

THE 12th INTERNATIONAL COURSE OF OTOLARYNGOLOGY

The 12th International Course of Otolaryngology, dealing with the eustachian tube, will be held on November 22-24, 1982, in Barcelona. For further information contact J. Oliveras, MD, Secretary, Pl. Eusebio Guell 12-13, Barcelona 34, Spain.

BACTERIOLOGY OF THE MAXILLARY SINUS OF RHESUS MONKEYS

EUGENE D. SHAPIRO, MD
WILLIAM DOYLE, PhD
ELLEN R. WALD, MD
DALE ROHN, BA
PITTSBURGH, PENNSYLVANIA

Quantitative cultures of transantral aspirates of the maxillary sinuses of rhesus monkeys were performed to determine whether the sinuses have a normal bacterial flora. Of 13 sinus aspirate cultures 11 (85%) were sterile. The two positive sinus aspirate cultures had extremely low colony counts of the same bacteria present on the nasal mucosa prior to the sinus puncture. The maxillary sinuses of rhesus monkeys are sterile.

INTRODUCTION

The mucosa of the oropharynx and nasopharynx are heavily colonized with bacteria. The proximity and contiguity of the mucous membranes of the paranasal sinuses and the pharynx might lead one to expect that the sinuses, too, have a normal bacterial flora. However, the trachea and middle ear cavity, also contiguous with the pharynx, are generally considered to be sterile.[1,2]

Two early studies, in which the radiographically "normal" sinus contralateral to a diseased sinus was cultured, found the normal sinuses to be sterile.[3,4] More recently, three maxillary sinus aspirates from two asymptomatic human volunteers were reported to be sterile.[5] To further examine this question, an investigation was undertaken to determine whether the maxillary sinus of the rhesus monkey (*Macaca mulatta*) has a normal bacterial flora.

MATERIALS AND METHODS

Juvenile rhesus monkeys weighing 3-5 kg each were anesthetized with ketamine. Their nasal cavities were cleansed with a 10% povidone-iodine solution (Betadine) for five minutes. Cultures of the nasal mucosa before and after application of the Betadine were performed using a calcium alginate swab on a flexible aluminum shaft (Calgiswab) and were interpreted semiquantitatively (graded as 1+ to 4+). The maxillary sinus was then entered via the transantral route using a 16 gauge, 2.5-inch (6.25 cm) sterile needle attached to a 5 ml sterile syringe containing 2.5 ml of sterile nonbacteriostatic saline. The saline was gently instilled and fluid was then aspirated from the sinus and cultured quantitatively.

Nasal swabs and sinus aspirates were immediately cultured anaerobically by planting the specimens on anaerobic blood agar plates (Scott) and anaerobic KV agar plates (Scott) and incubated in a GasPak (BBL) anaerobic jar at 37°C for 48-72 hours. In addition, sinus aspirates were cultured aerobically by planting the specimens on trypticase soy agar with 5% sheep blood (BBL) and on chocolate agar (BBL) and inoculating tubes of trypticase soy broth (BBL) and Brewer thioglycolate media (Difco) with the specimens. Quantitative cultures were performed by planting a 0.001 ml aliquot of the sinus aspirate on chocolate and sheep blood agar using a calibrated loop. Nasal swabs were cultured aerobically by planting the specimens on trypticase soy agar with 5% sheep blood (BBL), MacConkey agar (BBL), Columbia CNA agar with sheep blood (BBL) and chocolate agar (BBL) and incubated with a 5% CO_2 atmosphere at 37°C. Plates were examined after 24 and 48 hours of incubation; broth tubes were held for ten days if no growth occurred on the solid media. Isolation and identification of all organisms were done using standard bacteriologic techniques.

RESULTS

Thirteen maxillary sinus punctures were performed on ten different animals; three animals had bilateral maxillary sinus punctures. Cultures obtained from nasal swabs following Betadine cleansing of the mucosa were either sterile or had a very light growth of the same organisms present on the initial nasal swab.

Of 13 sinus aspirates, 11 (85%) were sterile. One sinus aspirate grew two colonies of *Streptococcus pneumoniae;* the initial nasal swab of that animal also grew *S pneumoniae* although culture of the post-Betadine swab was sterile. The other culture-positive sinus aspirate grew three colonies of *Staphylococcus epidermidis* and one colony each of a *Micrococcus* species and an alpha streptococcus; each of these organisms was present on the nasal swab cultures of the animal both before and after Betadine cleansing.

DISCUSSION

S pneumoniae and nontypable *Hemophilus influenzae* are the bacterial species most often recovered in significant colony count from the maxillary sinuses of children and adults with acute sinusitis.[6,7] The predominant bacterial species in the nasopharyngeal and throat cultures did not correlate with the sinus aspirate cultures in these patients.[7]

Because invasion of the sinuses of healthy individuals can rarely be justified, careful studies of the

From the Departments of Pediatrics and Otolaryngology, University of Pittsburgh School of Medicine. This research was supported in part by the National Institutes of Health Grant #-PO1-DEO1697.

REPRINTS — Ellen R. Wald, MD, Children's Hospital of Pittsburgh, 125 DeSoto Street, Pittsburgh, PA 15213.

microbial flora of normal maxillary sinuses have not been performed. Consequently, it is unclear whether the bacteria recovered from presumably infected sinuses are normal resident flora or are organisms introduced into previously sterile sinus cavities. If there is a normal bacterial flora of the sinuses, it would be important to identify the common organisms and compare them with the bacteria recovered from the presumably infected sinuses.

Factors which impair normal sinus drainage, such as inflammation due either to viral infection or allergy, may potentiate infection by promoting multiplication of normal sinus flora. If the sinuses are normally sterile, then the infecting bacteria may be introduced by other factors, such as nose blowing or intermittent negative intrasinus pressure accompanied by impairment of mucociliary transport.

Few animal species other than humans have paranasal sinuses. The anatomy of the maxillary sinus of the monkey is reasonably similar to that of humans[8] and may provide an animal model for the study of sinus disease.

The results of this study indicate that most rhesus monkey sinuses are sterile. The two positive sinus cultures had extremely low colony counts suggesting nasal contamination rather than in situ colonization.

REFERENCES

1. Lees A, McNaught W. Bacteriology of lower respiratory tract secretions, sputum, and upper respiratory tract secretions in "normals" and chronic bronchitics. Lancet 1959; 2:1112-5.

2. Howie V. Natural history of otitis media. In: Wiet R, Coulthard S. Proceedings of the Second National Conference on Otitis Media. Columbus, Ohio: Ross Laboratories, 1979; 10.

3. Bjorkwall T. Bacteriologic examinations in maxillary sinusitis: I. Bacterial flora of the maxillary antrum; II. Bacterial findings in the normal (healthy) maxillary antrum. Acta Otolaryngol (Stockh) 1950; Suppl 83:33-58.

4. Bjuggren G, Kraepelien S, Lind J. Sinusitis in children at home and in day-nurseries. Ann Paediatr 1949; 173:205-21.

5. Evans E Jr, Sydnor J, Moore W, et al. Sinusitis of the maxillary antrum. New Engl J Med 1975; 293:735-9.

6. Harmony B, Sande M, Sydnor A Jr, Seale D, Gwaltney J Jr. Etiology and antimicrobial therapy of acute maxillary sinusitis. J Infect Dis 1979; 139:197-202.

7. Wald E, Milmoe G, Bowen A, et al. Acute maxillary sinusitis in children (abstract No. 198). In: Program and Abstracts 20th Interscience Conference on Antimicrobial Agents and Chemotherapy, New Orleans, September 1980. American Society for Microbiology, Washington, D.C., 1980.

8. Hartman C, Straus W Jr, eds. The anatomy of the rhesus monkey. New York: Hafner Publishing, 1971.

≈

AMERICAN AUDITORY SOCIETY

Interested professionals and researchers in the communicative disorders are invited to submit papers for the annual meeting of the American Auditory Society to be held in New Orleans, October 18, 1982. The theme for the program will be The Edge of Tomorrow: Today's Research, Tomorrow's Practice. Five copies of a 300-word abstract should be submitted by June 15, 1982, to LaVonne Bergstrom, MD, Division of Head and Neck Surgery, UCLA, 31-24, 1000 Veteran Ave., Los Angeles, CA 90024.

HEAD AND NECK CARCINOMA IN PATIENTS UNDER 40 YEARS OF AGE

PAUL J. CARNIOL, MD
BALA CYNWYD, PENNSYLVANIA

MARVIN P. FRIED, MD
BOSTON, MASSACHUSETTS

From 1965-1978 over 2,700 patients were admitted to the Massachusetts Eye and Ear Infirmary or the Massachusetts General Hospital with carcinoma of the oropharynx, larynx or nasopharynx; only 36 of these patients were less than 40 years of age. Twelve patients had oropharyngeal carcinoma, 13 patients had laryngeal or hypopharyngeal carcinoma, and 11 patients had nasopharyngeal carcinoma. Analysis of these patients indicates an increased incidence of head and neck cancer in younger females. In patients less than age 31 there was no significant social history which contributed to early onset of disease. The younger patients with nasopharyngeal carcinoma survived longer than patients of all ages with comparable neoplasms. The survival of patients with oropharyngeal, laryngeal and hypopharyngeal carcinoma is comparable to survival in patients of all ages with similar lesions.

The incidence of head and neck carcinoma in patients less than 40 years of age is relatively low. Many unanswered questions exist about this group of patients. Who are the affected patients? What types of disease do they have? How do they respond to therapy, especially compared to patients of all ages? Do they tend to develop second primaries? This study analyzes patients under 40 with oropharyngeal, laryngeal, hypopharyngeal and nasopharyngeal carcinoma treated at the Massachusetts Eye and Ear Infirmary and the Massachusetts General Hospital between 1965 and 1978.

METHODS

A review of all patients admitted to both institutions from 1965-1978 was performed. Over 2,700 patients were treated yet there were only 36 patients less than 40 years of age. Children are treated at both hospitals; however during this period there were no patients with carcinoma less than 14 years of age. Follow-up was obtained on all but two from the patients' records, the tumor registry, or the patients' current physicians. This follow-up ranged from 2 to 14 years with a mean of 6.4 years. All patients were staged retrospectively by the TNM system.[1]

Patient Population. The patients ranged in age from 14 to 39 years at the time of initial diagnosis. Six patients were less than 20, 3 were between 20 and 29, and 27 patients were between 30 and 39.

Overall there were 5 females and 21 males. In the second-decade group there were two females and four males. The third-decade group contained two females and one male. The fourth-decade group contained 11 females and 16 males.

Three of the patients with nasopharyngeal carcinoma were Chinese.

Among the nine patients less than 30 years of age there was no history of alcohol intake or cigarette smoking. Seventeen patients in the fourth decade group had a history of daily alcohol intake and smoking at least one pack of cigarettes daily. Three patients reported occasional alcohol consumption.

None of the patients had a second primary neoplasm at the time of presentation. Three later developed a second primary.

Duration of Symptoms. Patients presented with a history of symptoms from 1-18 months. Within this group there was no consistent relationship between the duration of symptoms, stage of disease, or cure rate.

RESULTS

Nasopharyngeal Carcinoma. Eleven patients had nasopharyngeal carcinoma. Nine of these had lymphoepitheliomas. There were three Chinese patients and they all presented with stage IV disease. Five of the patients were female.

All patients were treated with radiotherapy. The 19-year-old male patient received debulking cryosurgery prior to radiotherapy. One 31-year-old male developed a second nasopharyngeal neoplasm eight years after the first lesion.

As shown in Table 1, survival does not correlate with initial tumor stage. One patient had stage I disease and she died from metastatic disease. Five patients with stages II and III disease are alive without recurrence. Four of five patients with stage IV disease are alive without recurrence.

Laryngeal and Hypopharyngeal Carcinoma. Eleven patients had laryngeal carcinoma; two patients had pyriform sinus disease. The 14-year-old and two 17-year-old patients did not have a history of alcohol, smoking, or papillomatosis. The other ten patients had a history of daily alcohol intake and smoked an average of $1\frac{1}{2}$ packages of cigarettes daily. The 17-year-old male patient had a history of vocal abuse. The male to female ratio is 2.7:1. The stage of disease, therapy and average survival are shown in Table 2.

Of the three patients less than 20, one exsanguinated from carotid artery rupture after developing a postoperative fistula, and the other two are alive without recurrent disease.

Only three patients in the fourth decade group presented with advanced disease, stages III and IV.

From the Department of Otolaryngology, Harvard Medical School, Boston.
REPRINTS — Paul J. Carniol, MD, 705 Harvard Rd., Bala Cynwyd, PA 19004.

TABLE 1. CHARACTERISTICS OF PATIENTS WITH NASOPHARYNGEAL CARCINOMA (N = 11)

Age Group	*No. of Patients*	*Tumor Stage*	*Avg. Survival, NED (yr)*
10-19	2	III	9.0
	1	IV	5.0
20-29	1	I	Deceased from metastatic carcinoma
	2	II	3.0
30-39	1	III	5.0
	4	IV	3.2 (One deceased from metastatic carcinoma)

NED - No evidence of disease.

Two of these patients are deceased from metastatic disease. The rest of the patients survived without a recurrence. One patient developed a second neoplasm, ten years later, of the right maxilla.

Oropharyngeal Carcinoma. Twelve patients presented with oropharyngeal carcinoma. All of the patients were between 30 and 39. Seven are women and five are men. Eight patients had a history of both smoking and daily alcohol consumption; one patient had a history of alcohol intake only. Three patients had either extensive periodontitis and/or caries. Stage of disease, therapy and average survival are shown in Table 3.

Of the three patients with tongue carcinoma only one is alive over five years after initial presentation and over four years from her surgery without recurrence; she was treated with full-course radiation therapy following within a year of presentation by surgery for recurrent disease.

All of the patients with carcinoma of the floor of the mouth are without a local recurrence. One of these patients developed a squamous cell carcinoma of the lower esophagus treated with radiotherapy and was reported to be alive five years later but refused medical examination.

Four of five patients with oropharyngeal carcinomas at sites other than the tongue or floor of mouth are alive without recurrence. One patient refused surgery after developing a cervical nodal recurrence and was lost to follow-up.

DISCUSSION

Nasopharyngeal Carcinoma. Several characteristics of this group of patients are unusual. The male to female ratio is 1.2:1. In studies of patients of all ages, this ratio has consistently been over 2:1.[2-5] A study performed in Greece in patients under 30 also had a higher percentage of women than in older patients.[6]

Nine of 11 patients had a lymphoepithelioma. This is a higher incidence than has been reported for patients of all ages.[4,7-9] Of the 8 patients on whom at least a 3½ year survival is available, 6 are alive without recurrent disease. This is higher than has been reported for patients of all ages.[2-4,10]

The higher survival may be due to the predominant tumor type, lymphoepithelioma, which tends to be a more radiosensitive tumor. It may be due to improved radiotherapy techniques or better response to neoplasms and therapy in this younger group of patients.

Laryngeal and Hypopharyngeal Carcinoma. Laryngeal carcinoma is not common in patients less than 20 years old. Although a statistical survey has not been performed in the United States, Herold and Bockmuhl analyzed the patient population in East Germany,[11] and found a 0.5% incidence among all cases of laryngeal carcinoma.

Three of the patients in this study are less than 20 years of age. They differ from the other three patients in that they do not have a history of cigarette smoking or alcohol intake. They also did not have a history of papillomatosis and radiation therapy which have been associated with developing carcinoma of the larynx.[12] One of these patients does have a history of vocal abuse. In a study from Memorial Hospital 10% of the patients with laryngeal carcinoma had a history of vocal abuse.[13]

TABLE 2. CHARACTERISTICS OF PATIENTS WITH LARYNGEAL AND HYPOPHARYNGEAL CARCINOMA (N = 13)

Age Group	*Site*	*Stage*	*No. of Patients*	*Therapy*	*Avg. Survival, NED (yr)*
10-19	Glottic	I	1	Radiotherapy	9.0
	Glottic	II	1	Radiotherapy and surgery	Deceased, carotid rupture
	Glottic	III	1	Chemotherapy, radiotherapy and surgery	3.0
30-39	Glottic	I	2	Radiotherapy and cryosurgery	10.4
	Glottic	II	2	Surgery and radiotherapy	6.0
	Supraglottic	II	2	Surgery and radiotherapy	4.3
	Supraglottic	IV	1	Surgery	10.5
	Transglottic	III	1	Surgery and radiotherapy	Deceased, metastatic disease
	Pyriform sinus	II	1	Surgery and radiotherapy	10.8
	Pyriform sinus	IV	1	Surgery and radiotherapy	Deceased, metastatic disease

NED - No evidence of disease.

TABLE 3. CHARACTERISTICS OF PATIENTS WITH OROPHARYNGEAL CARCINOMA (N = 12)

Site	*Stage*	*No. of Patients*	*Therapy*	*Avg. Survival, NED (yr)*
Oral, tongue	II	1	Surgery and radiotherapy	4.0
Oral, tongue	III	1	Surgery and radiotherapy	Deceased, metastatic carcinoma
Oral, tongue	IV	1	Surgery and radiotherapy	Deceased, metastatic carcinoma
Anterior floor mouth	I	2	Radiotherapy	3.0
Anterior floor mouth	II	2	Radiotherapy	2.3
Buccal mucosa	I	1	Surgery	2.2
Retromolar trigone	II	1	Radiotherapy and surgery	14.0
Retromolar trigone	III	1	Radiotherapy and cryosurgery	Unknown, patient refused surgery for recurrent nodal disease
Tonsillar pillar	III	1	Radiotherapy	5.3
Palate	II	1	Radiotherapy	5.0

NED - No evidence of disease.

Most of the patients in this group presented with early stages of carcinoma. The disease-free survival is consistent with these early stages. All of the patients with stage I carcinoma are alive without recurrence. Four of 5 patients with stage II disease are alive without recurrence. Three patients presented with advanced stages of disease and two are alive. The three female patients presented with earlier stages of disease and they are all alive without recurrence.

Only two patients had hypopharyngeal disease; their survival is also as expected based on tumor stage at time of presentation.

Oropharyngeal Carcinoma. Seven of the 12 patients in this group are women. Other studies have indicated a rising incidence of carcinoma in women but not to this extent.[14-17] One study found that women tend to develop carcinoma of the floor of the mouth earlier than men. If this tendency to develop carcinoma earlier applies to all oropharyngeal sites, then together with the rising incidence in women, this could explain the prevalence of women in this group.

Disease-free survival correlates best with stage at presentation. All patients with earlier stages of disease had a good response to therapy. Only one may be deceased and that would be from a second neoplasm. Four patients presented with advanced lesions and only one has over a 5-year survival.

CONCLUSIONS

Of over 2,700 patients admitted between 1965 and 1978 with carcinoma of the nasopharynx, larynx, hypopharynx, and oropharynx, only 36 patients were under 40 years of age. Fifteen of these patients were female. The overall percentage of women is higher than reported for patients of all ages.

None of the patients less than age 31 had a history of smoking cigarettes or alcohol consumption.

Eleven patients had nasopharyngeal carcinoma. The predominant tumor type was lymphoepithelioma. Nine of the 11 patients are alive without recurrent disease. The percentage of disease-free survivors is greater than has been reported for patients of all ages.

Thirteen patients had laryngeal and hypopharyngeal carcinoma. Survival correlated best with initial stage of disease and is comparable to groups of patients of all ages.

Twelve patients had oropharyngeal carcinoma. Survival for this group of patients is comparable to that reported for patients of all ages with the same stage of disease.

Three of the 36 patients developed second primary carcinomas. Further long-term follow-up would help delineate whether patients who develop carcinoma at an earlier age have a greater tendency to develop a second primary.

REFERENCES

1. American Joint Committee for Cancer Staging and End-Results Reporting. Manual for staging of cancer 1978. Chicago: American Joint Committee, 1978.

2. Chao G. Nasopharyngeal carcinoma. J Laryngol Otol 1974; 88:145-58.

3. Hoppe RT, Goffinet DR, Bagshaw MA. Carcinoma of the nasopharynx: eighteen years experience with megavoltage radiation therapy. Cancer 1976; 32:2605-12.

4. Strong EW. Carcinoma of the tongue. Otolaryngol Clin North Am 1979; 12:107-14.

5. Urdaneta N, Fischer JJ, Vera R, Gutierrez E. Cancer of the nasopharynx. Cancer 1976; 37:1707-12.

6. Papavasilov C, Pavlativ M, Pappas S. Nasopharyngeal cancer in patients under the age of thirty years. Cancer 1977; 40:2312-6.

7. Kirchner JA, Owen JR. Five hundred cancers of the larynx, and pyriform sinus: results of treatment of radiation and surgery. Laryngoscope 1977; 87:1288-303.

8. Lowry LD. 269 Laryngeal carcinomas. Arch Otolaryngol 1973; 98:147-51.

9. Southwick HW. Cancer of the tongue. Surg Clin North Am 1973; 53:145-7.

10. Little JB, Schulz MD, Wang CC. Radiation therapy for cancer of the nasopharynx. Arch Otolaryngol 1963; 77:67-70.

11. Herold HJ, Bockmuhl F. Uber die Haupigkeit, Geschlechts-un Alterverteilung de Kehlkopfkarzinoms. Z Laryngol Rhinol 1966; 45:785-9.

12. Robbett WF. Juvenile laryngeal papillomatosis: the relation of irradiation to malignant degeneration in this disease. Ann Otol Rhinol Laryngol 1965; 74:1149-61.

13. Daly CJ, Strong EW. Carcinoma of the glottic larynx. Am J Surg 1975; 130:489-92.

14. Ballard BR, Suess GR, Picken JW, Green GW, Shedd DP. Squamous cell carcinoma of the floor of the mouth. Oral Surg 1978; 45:568-79.

15. Byers RM. Squamous cell carcinoma of the oral tongue in patients less than thirty years of age. Am J Surg 1975; 130:475-8.

16. Farr HW, Arthur K. Epidermoid carcinoma of the mouth and pharynx 1960-1964. J Laryngol Otol 1972; 86:243-53.

17. Harrold CC. Management of cancer of the floor of the mouth. Am J Surg 1971; 122:487-93.

≈

COLLAGENASE ACTIVITY IN SQUAMOUS CELL CARCINOMA OF THE HUMAN PAROTID GLAND

CHENG-CHUN HUANG, PhD

ANDREW BLITZER, DDS, MD MAXWELL ABRAMSON, MD

NEW YORK, NEW YORK

A collagenase obtained from a single squamous cell carcinoma of human parotid gland was purified to homogeneity by procedures including precipitation with ammonium sulfate, gel filtration, ion-exchange chromatography with DEAE-cellulose, and extraction from polyacrylamide gel after electrophoresis. The parotid tumor collagenase had a molecular weight of approximately 68,000 and appeared similar to other mammalian collagenases in many respects such as action on collagen and response to common collagenase inhibitors. Analysis of specimens of various human parotid gland tumors revealed that the levels of collagenase activity were higher in squamous cell carcinoma than in nonsquamous tumors. A high level of collagenase activity from squamous cell carcinoma suggests that collagenase may promote local connective tissue destruction associated with tumor invasion and lymph node metastasis.

INTRODUCTION

Several investigators have demonstrated collagenase activity in various human and animal tumors.[1-4] In our previous study, we compared the histology of squamous cell carcinomas of the oral cavity and of the larynx with their collagenase activities. The more active tumors appeared to contain more loosely arranged connective tissue structure with a higher concentration of capillary buds.[5] The level of collagenase activity was found to be higher at the edge of the tumor than in the center.[6] These observations suggest that collagenase activity causing local destruction of adjacent connective tissue may promote the invasive properties of the malignant tumors.

Squamous cell carcinomas of the parotid gland probably arise from squamous metaplasia of the epithelial lining of the ducts. These squamous cell carcinomas infiltrate surrounding structures and grow rather rapidly with a high incidence (approximately 50%) of regional lymph node metastasis.

In our present study, we analyzed levels of collagenase activity in various types of human parotid gland tumors and purified a collagenase obtained from a single squamous cell carcinoma of the human parotid gland in order to characterize its biochemical properties.

METHODS

Preparation of Tumor Collagenase. The specimens of human parotid tumors were obtained from the University of Iowa Hospital (Iowa City), the Veterans Administration Hospital (Bronx) and Columbia Presbyterian Medical Center (New York). The parotid tumor specimens were cut into 1 cu mm pieces; rinsed in Hank's balanced salt solution containing 100 units of penicillin, 100 μg of streptomycin, 0.25 mg of Fungizone/ml; and cultured in Dulbecco's modified Eagle medium in Falcon plastic flasks at 37°C under O_2/CO_2 (95:5, v/v). The media were changed daily for four days. All media were collected and stored at −20°C before assay. The culture medium from a large squamous cell carcinoma specimen was dialyzed against water with several changes, lyophilized and stored at −20°C before purification. The following purification steps were performed at 4°C.

Ammonium Sulfate Precipitation. The dry crude human parotid tumor collagenase was dissolved in 0.05 *M* TRIS-HCl (pH 7.6), 0.005 *M* $CaCl_2$ to a concentration of 15 mg protein/ml. Any insoluble material was removed by centrifugation. Solid ammonium sulfate was added slowly to achieve 60% saturation. The resulting precipitate was collected by centrifugation at 10,000 x gravity for 20 minutes and redissolved in the TRIS buffer containing 0.2 *M* NaCl.

Chromatography. Gel filtration of the ammonium sulfate enzyme preparation was carried out in a Sephadex G-150 column (1.6 x 100 cm), equilibrated with the TRIS buffer containing 0.2 *M* NaCl (5 ml fractions; flow rate, 30 ml/hr). The eluates were assayed for collagenase activity. Active fractions were pooled and concentrated to a small volume with Amicon UM-10 membrane. Ion-exchange chromatography was carried out in a DEAE-cellulose column (2.6 x 25 cm) equilibrated with the TRIS buffer. The column was eluted stepwise with increasing ionic strength of sodium chloride (3 ml fractions: flow rate 25 ml/hr). The eluates were monitored for protein and collagenase activity.

Molecular weight determination was conducted by gel filtration through a Sephadex G-150 column (1.6 x 100 cm). The protein standards were γ-globulin (160,000), albumin (68,000), ovalbumin (45,000), chymotrypsinogen (25,000) and cytochrome C (12, 400).

Assay Procedures. Collagenase activity was determined by enzymatic release of soluble radioactivity from reconstituted ^{14}C collagen fibrils (20,000 cpm/mg). The radioactive collagen was extracted from guinea pig skin with sodium chloride and purified by the method of Gross.[7] The reconstituted collagen fibrils were prepared from the solution of ^{14}C collagen by mixing 0.05 ml of 0.4% radioactive collagen (4,000 cpm) with 0.05 ml TRIS buffer and allowed to gel at 37° overnight. Aliquots (0.01-0.10 ml) of the enzyme were added to the collagen gels for assay with incubation at 37°C for four hours. Protein was determined by the method of Lowry et al.[8]

From the Department of Otolaryngology and the Cancer Center, Institute of Cancer Research, Columbia University, College of Physicians and Surgeons, New York. This investigation was supported by NCI research grant CA 22907 and NINCDS Teacher-Investigator Development Award NS-00932.

REPRINTS — C-C. Huang, PhD, Department of Otolaryngology, Columbia University, New York, NY 10032.

TABLE 1. COLLAGENASE ACTIVITIES OF PAROTID TUMORS

Tissue Specimen	*Cpm/mg* of Tissue*
Squamous cell carcinoma	256
Squamous cell carcinoma	285
Squamous cell carcinoma	352
Malignant mixed tumor	0
Malignant mixed tumor	30
Malignant mixed tumor	80
Benign mixed tumor	10
Adenocarcinoma	54

*Collagenase activity expressed as cpm ^{14}C collagen degraded/mg tissue in a 4-hr assay at 37°C.

Inhibition Studies. The inhibitors used and their final concentrations were as follows: fetal calf serum, 1:10 and 1:40 dilution; 5 x 10^{-3} *M* and 5 x 10^{-2} *M* cysteine; and 1 x 10^{-2} *M* and 4 x 10^{-2} *M* EDTA. All assays were conducted at pH 7.6.

Electrophoresis Methods. The homogeneity of human parotid tumor collagenase was examined by polyacrylamide gel electrophoresis according to the method of Davis[9] using a 7.5% gel. The gel was stained with Coomassie Brilliant Blue R 250. The collagen-degraded products were subjected to electrophoresis in 7.5% polyacrylamide gels according to the method of Nagai et al.[10] The reaction mixtures containing 100 μg collagen and 20μg purified tumor collagenase in 0.1 ml TRIS buffer were incubated at 26°C for eight hours and, after adding one drop of acetic acid, were denatured by heating at 45°C for five minutes.

For determination of molecular weight, polyacrylamide gel electrophoresis in the presence of sodium dodecylsulfate (SDS) was performed by the method of Weber and Osborn[11] using 10% polyacrylamide gels. The protein standards were albumin (68,000), glutamate dehydrogenase (57,000), glyceraldehyde phosphate dehydrogenase (37,000), myokinase (27,000), β-lactoglobulin (17,500) and cytochrome C (12,500). The molecular weights were plotted against the electrophoretic mobilities relative to bromophenol blue in a semilogarithmic diagram.

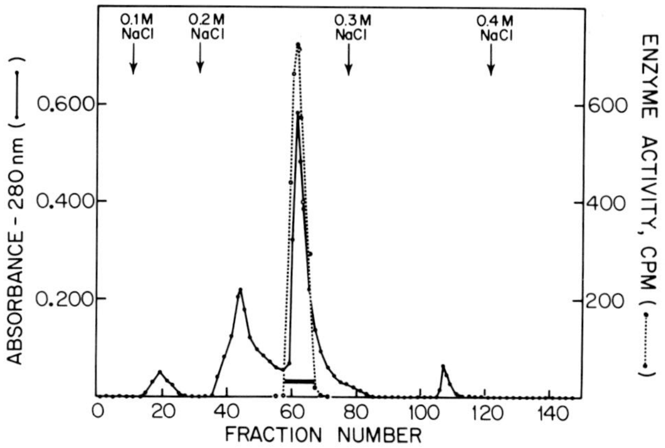

Fig. 2. Ion-exchange chromatography in DEAE-cellulose of the concentrated human parotid tumor collagenase from gel filtration. The sample (61 mg protein) was applied to a DEAE-cellulose column (2.6 x 25 cm). The column was then eluted stepwise with increasing ionic strength of sodium chloride as shown (3 ml fractions; flow rate, 25 ml/hr). An aliquot (0.05 ml) from each fraction was used for collagenase activity assay.

RESULTS

Collagenase Activity of Parotid Tumors. Specimens of eight parotid tumors were analyzed for the levels of collagenase activity. Squamous cell carcinomas of the parotid gland produced much higher levels of collagenase activity than nonsquamous tumors (Table 1).

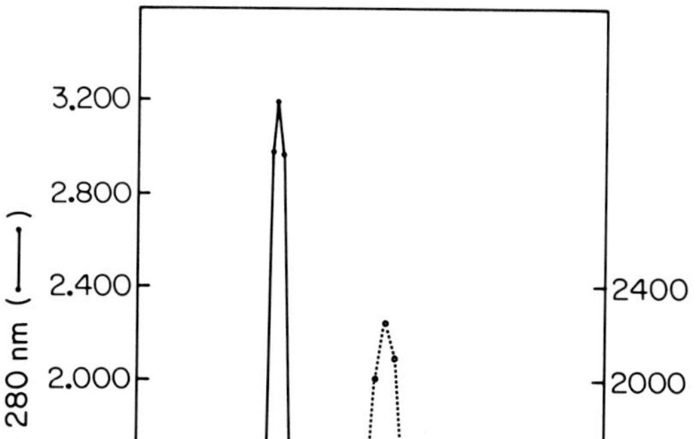

Fig. 1. Gel filtration in Sephadex G-150 of human parotid tumor collagenase. The sample (216 mg protein) was applied to a Sephadex G-150 column (1.6 x 100 cm) and the column was eluted with 0.05 *M* TRIS-HCl, (pH 7.6) 0.2 *M* NaCl, 0.005 *M* $CaCl_2$ (5 ml fractions; flow rate, 30 ml/hr). An aliquot (0.1 ml) from each fraction was used for collagenase activity assay.

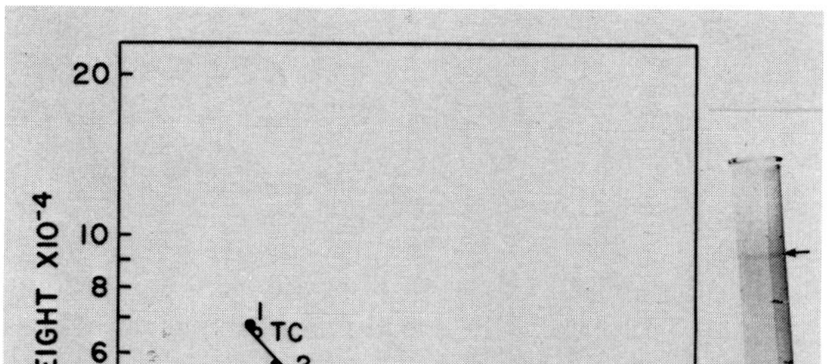

Fig. 3. Determination of the molecular weight of human parotid tumor (TC) by SDS-polyacrylamide gel electrophoresis. The protein standards were as follows: albumin (1), glutamate dehydrogenase (2), glyceraldehyde phosphate dehydrogenase (3), myokinase (4), β-lactoglobulin (5), and cytochrome C (6). The arrow indicates the collagenase band (20 μg protein) on the gel.

TABLE 2. PURIFICATION OF PAROTID TUMOR COLLAGENASE

Purification Step	Total Protein (mg)	Specific Activity* (units/mg protein)	Total Activity (units)	Recovery (%)
Crude enzyme	526.0	0.90	473	100
$(NH_4)_2SO_4$	216.0	1.84	396	83
Sephadex G-150	61.0	5.66	345	73
DEAE-cellulose	13.6	7.87	107	22
Polyacrylamide gel	0.9	25.80	23	5
Sephadex G-150	0.3	66.70	20	4

*Specific activity refers to μg collagen degraded/min/mg protein.

Purification of Human Parotid Tumor Collagenase. The ammonium sulfate enzyme preparation was eluted by gel filtration through a Sephadex G-150 column (Fig. 1). The enzyme activity was separated into one major peak and one small peak. Only the major peak was further purified. Ion-exchange chromatography of the parotid tumor collagenase was performed in a DEAE-cellulose column (Fig. 2). Collagenase activity was eluted with 0.2 *M* NaCl. The active fraction was further purified by extraction from polyacrylamide gel after electrophoresis and gel filtration through a Sephadex G-150 column. The purified tumor collagenase showed a single protein band on polyacrylamide gel with (Fig. 3) or without sodium dodecylsulfate. The yield and purification of human parotid tumor collagenase are summarized in Table 2.

Molecular Weight of Human Parotid Tumor Collagenase. The molecular weight of the parotid tumor collagenase was estimated between 32,000-35,000 using gel filtration through a Sephadex G-150 column. However, the molecular weight of 68,000 was obtained from SDS-polyacrylamide gel electrophoresis (Fig. 3).

Action of Collagenase on Soluble Collagen. At 26°C, the parotid tumor collagenase degraded the collagen molecule and produced fragments corresponding to the size of three fourths the original molecule. The denatured products of the enzyme-collagen reaction mixture on polyacrylamide gel demonstrated one new band below the original β band and another two new bands below the original α bands.

Effect of Inhibitors. Enzymatic activity of human parotid tumor collagenase was inhibited by fetal calf serum, cysteine and EDTA (Table 3).

DISCUSSION

The present study demonstrated the release of high levels of collagenase activity in the culture of squamous cell carcinomas of human parotid gland incubated in serum-free medium. A collagenase obtained from a single squamous cell carcinoma has been purified to homogeneity by procedures including precipitation with ammonium sulfate, gel filtration through Sephadex G-150, ion-exchange chromatography with DEAE-cellulose, and extraction from polyacrylamide gel after electrophoresis. Ion-exchange chromatography and gel electrophoresis caused a marked loss of collagenase activity (Table 2).

TABLE 3. EFFECT OF INHIBITORS ON HUMAN PAROTID TUMOR COLLAGENASE

Inhibitor	Concentration	Activity (cpm)	Inhibition (%)
None		2240	
Serum	1:10	218	91
	1:40	516	77
Cysteine	50 m*M*	870	61
	5 m*M*	1080	52
EDTA	40 m*M*	404	82
	10 m*M*	692	69

The purified human parotid tumor collagenase appears to be similar to other mammalian collagenases in many respects, such as action on collagen and response to common collagenase inhibitors (Table 3). However, the parotid tumor collagenase similar to rabbit VX-2 carcinoma collagenase[4] is less sensitive to cysteine than other mammalian collagenases.

The human parotid tumor collagenase has a molecular weight of 32,000 based on gel filtration or 68,000 determined by SDS-polyacrylamide gel electrophoresis. The molecular weight for collagenase derived from SDS-polyacrylamide gel electrophoresis seems to be more reliable than that derived from gel filtration. This low value for a molecular weight of collagenase derived from gel filtration is possibly due to the anomalous interaction between collagenase and Sephadex beads.

Analysis of human parotid tumor specimens showed that the squamous cell carcinoma produced much higher levels of collagenase activity than other parotid tumors such as benign and malignant mixed tumors and adenocarcinoma (Table 1). This is consistent with our previous report[12] and that of other investigators[1], indicating that the level of collagenase activity in squamous cell carcinoma is much higher than that of nonsquamous tumors. The squamous cell carcinomas used in the present study showed invasion of the dermis and had lymph node metastases. These data suggest that collagenase of squamous cell carcinoma of the parotid gland might play a significant role in local host connective tissue destruction associated with tumor invasion. Malignant mixed tumors and adenocarcinoma are both locally aggressive and have a rather high incidence of regional metastases, approximately 20%. These nonsquamous tumors, having very low levels of collagenase activity, might invade host tissue through action of other enzymatic systems. Specification of the types of enzymatic systems requires further exploration.

Our previous work[13] and that of others[14] have shown that collagenase is produced by tumor connective tissue stroma and not by the epithelial tumor cells. Parotid tumor cells may release a chemical mediator such as prostaglandin E_2 which is capable of stimulating the tumor connective tissue stroma to produce collagenase for breakdown of host connective tissue. Our recent work of rat prostate squamous cell carcinoma has demonstrated that prostaglandin E_2 is capable of stimulating the synthesis of collagenase (Huang CC, unpublished data). Collagenase produced by the tumor connective tissue stroma suggests that collagenase production may be a wound response of the host to the presence of tumor cells. Tumors can be considered as nonhealing wounds in that the high production of collagenase may occur, resulting in the destruction of connective tissue at the margin of tumors. Active wounds have shown higher collagenase activity than the normal tissues but less than that seen in tumors.[6]

The squamous cell carcinoma specimens of parotid gland used in the present study showed ulceration with necrosis and chronic inflammation. This suggests the possibility that collagenase could be also derived from macrophages and leukocytes in response to inflammatory effects of tumor, since these inflammatory cells have been shown to produce collagenase.[15] More work is required to understand the mechanism and regulation of collagenase production and the interaction between tumor cells and host.

ACKNOWLEDGMENTS — The authors thank the pathologists of the University of Iowa Hospital (Iowa City), the Veterans Administration Hospital (Bronx), and Columbia Presbyterian Medical Center (New York) for supplying the clinical and histologic data. The authors also thank Doris Look for her help in the preparation of this manuscript.

REFERENCES

1. Dresden MH, Heilman AS, Schmidt J. Collagenolytic enzymes in human neoplasms. Cancer Res 1972; 32:993-6.

2. Hashimoto K, Yamanishi Y, Dabbous MK. Collagenase of human skin basal cell epithelioma. Cancer Res 1972; 32:2561-7.

3. Huang CC, Wu CH, Abramson M. Collagenase activity in cultures of rat prostate carcinoma. Biochim Biophys Acta 1979; 570:149-56.

4. Dabbous MK, Roberts AN, Brinkley B. Collagenase and neutral protease activities in cultures of rabbit VX-2 carcinoma. Cancer Res 1977; 37:3537-44.

5. Abramson M, Schilling RW, Huang CC, Salome RG. Collagenase activity in epidermoid carcinoma of the oral cavity and larynx. Ann Otol Rhinol Laryngol 1975; 84:158-63.

6. Schilling RW. Collagenase activity in epidermoid carcinoma of the oral cavity and larynx, thesis, University of Iowa, Iowa City, 1974.

7. Gross J. Studies in the formation of collagens: I. Properties and fractionation of neutral salt extracts of normal guinea pig connective tissue. J Exp Med 1958; 107:247-66.

8. Lowry OH, Rosebrough NJ, Farr AL, Randall RJ. Protein measurement with the folin phenol reagent. J Biol Chem 1951; 193:265-75.

9. Davis BJ. Disc gel electrophoresis of enzymes. Ann N Y Acad Sci 1964; 121:404-27.

10. Nagai Y, Gross J, Piez KA. Disc electrophoresis of collagen components. Ann N Y Acad Sci 1964; 121:494-500.

11. Weber K, Osborn M. The reliability of molecular weight determinations by dodecyl sulfate polyacrylamide gel electrophoresis. J Biol Chem 1969; 244:4406-12.

12. Huang CC, Blitzer A, Abramson M, Wu CH. Collagenase and protease activities in head and neck tumors. Otolaryngol Head Neck Surg (in press).

13. Huang CC, Abramson M, Schilling RW, Salome RG. Collagenase activity in tumors of the head and neck. Otolaryngology 1976; 82:138-41.

14. Reddick ME, Bauer EA, Eisen AZ. Immunocytochemical localization of collagenase in human skin and fibroblasts in monolayer culture. Clin Res 1973; 24:481.

15. Wahl LM, Wahl SM, Mergenhagen SE, Martin GR. Collagenase production by lymphokine-activated macrophages. Science 1975; 187:261-3.

TETRACYCLINE BONE LABELING

An Improved Technique Using Incident Fluorescence

Rinaldo F. Canalis, MD Juan Lechago, MD, PhD

Los Angeles, California

A simple modification of the tetracycline bone labeling techique, based on the use of incident fluorescence, is introduced. The method has proven effective in the study of osteoneogenesis in bone grafts assisted by a soft tissue pedicle. The results obtained are highly specific, with new bone showing as a yellow band against blue background. The degree of fluorescence appears to be related to that of osteoneogenesis and correlates well with histological findings of the same specimens when examined by conventional light microscopy. The main advantages of this new technique over currently used methods are 1) avoidance of the time-consuming thinning procedure; 2) ability to study bone and surrounding soft tissues simultaneously; and 3) one-to-one comparison and documentation of the results of fluorescence and histological examination of the same specimen.

Milch et al[1] reported in 1957 on the process of uptake and fixation of tetracyclines by bone in vivo. Since then the use of these antibiotics has become standard practice for the study of bone formation and, to this date, the original labeling technique has remained essentially unaltered.

Microscopic observation of tetracycline-labeled bone is currently based on the use of transmitted fluorescence. This technique is time-consuming and does not allow for the simultaneous study of bone and related soft tissues. In this communication we introduce a modification based on the use of incident fluorescence which permits the expeditious study of new bone formation in association with surrounding muscle and skin.

METHODS

Experimental Design. During the past three years, the tetracycline labeling technique described below was used in several experiments directed to a better understanding of the fate of pedicle-assisted bone grafts and involved a total of 20 canines.[2-4] A typical experimental model consisted of a cutaneous or muscular pedicle in continuity with a bone graft supported by its periosteal attachments and the recipient area (bone or muscle). The pedicles had an average length of 3.5 cm and an average diameter of 2 cm. The bone grafts were rounded or rectangular with an average area of 8.3 $cm.^2$ The thickness of these grafts varied between 1.1 cm and 2.2 cm. The grafts were removed from the experimental animals 10 to 220 days after transfer.

Administration of Tetracycline. Demethylchlortetracycline hydrochloride (Declomycin) was used because of its higher fluorescence relative to other antibiotics of the tetracycline group. Two doses of 75 mg/kg were administered intramuscularly, the first two weeks and the second two days preceding removal of the specimens.

Preparation of the Specimen. Specimens were removed by excising them in conjunction with a generous amount of surrounding tissue. They were fixed for ten days or more in 10% buffered formalin and then examined under the operating microscope. A typical specimen, measuring approximately 4 x 2 x 2 cm, was then reduced by careful dissection to a composite block, approximately 2 x 2 x 1 cm, containing the bone implant sandwiched between the pedicle and the recipient tissue. Using a thin laryngeal saw, 2.5 cm in diameter (Storz 77840), the specimen was first divided into two halves perpendicular to the bone graft, and then a 1 mm thick slice was sawed off the center of each half.

Incident Fluorescence Technique. Specimens were examined by incident fluorescence using a Zeiss Photomicroscope III equipped with an epifluorescence condenser III RS and an HBO 50 mercury lamp. Two settings were used: A) a blue interference exciter filter set at 455-490 nm, and FT 510 chromatic beam splitter, and a LP 520 orange barrier filter; and B) a BP 405/5 and a BP 405/14 violet exciter filter, and FT 420 chromatic beam splitter and an LP 418 colorless UV barrier filter. Color microphotographs were taken at magnifications ranging between x16 and x40, using Kodak Ektachrome 200 or 400 ASA daylight film.

Histologic Examination. After fluorescence examination and photographic documentation, all specimens were decalcified, embedded in paraffin, sectioned, and stained with hematoxylin and eosin. The sections were examined and photographed with the same Zeiss photomicroscope utilized for fluorescence work, but this time using transmitted bright field microscopy with a halogen lamp as source of illumination.

RESULTS

Under incident fluorescence tetracycline-labeled bone showed as a bright yellow band where the marker had been incorporated during osteogenesis (Figs. 1-3). The two fluorescence systems utilized yielded different results. System A, with an excitation wavelength of 455-490 nm, showed bright yellow fluorescence with a blue background.

Whereas the tetracycline-induced fluorescence was brighter and more abundant with system A, the presence of a blue background conferred much higher specificity to the results obtained with system B. The latter system was clearly superior and was adopted as the standard procedure on which are based the observations and illustrations presented here.

From the Division of Head and Neck Surgery and the Department of Pathology, Harbor/UCLA Medical Center, Torrance, and UCLA School of Medicine, Los Angeles. This research was supported in part by Grant GR-2201 by the Professional Staff Association, Harbor/UCLA Medical Center, Torrance.

REPRINTS — Rinaldo F. Canalis, MD, Division of Head and Neck Surgery (Otolaryngology), Harbor/UCLA Medical Center, 1000 West Carson Street, Torrance, CA 90509.

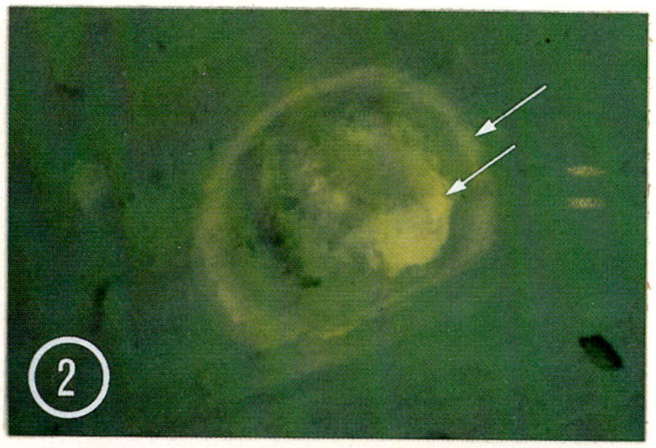

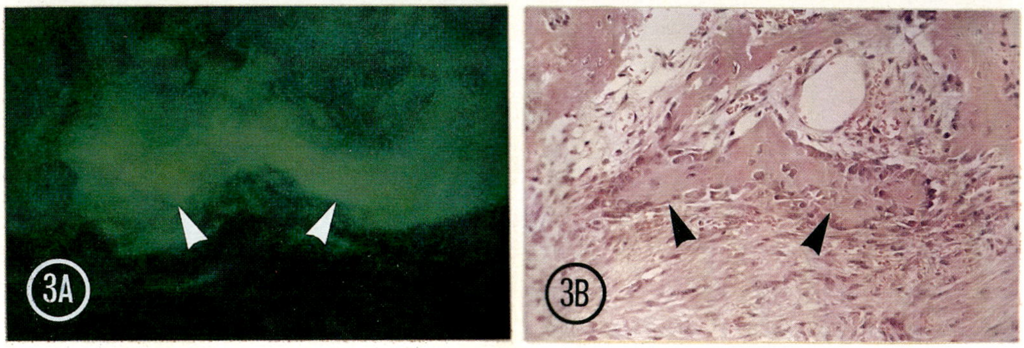

Fig. 1. Osteocutaneous graft in the forehead of an adult dog removed six weeks after implantation and 14 days after intramuscular tetracycline injection. An area of new bone formation is seen as a bright yellow band at the interface between the bone below and the vascularized pedicle above. (x48)

Fig. 2. Osteocutaneous graft in the forehead of an adult dog removed 16 weeks after implantation and 14 weeks and 2 days after tetracycline injection. Under incident fluorescence two distinct bright yellow rings (arrows) point the site of ongoing new bone formation. (x120)

Fig. 3. Osteomuscular flap implanted in the soft tissues of the neck in an adult dog, removed 4 weeks after implantation and 2 weeks after tetracycline injection. A) Under incident fluorescence, a roof-shaped area of new bone formation can be identified as an area of green-yellow fluorescence (arrowheads). B) A deeper section from the same area shows a similarly shaped portion of newly formed bone (arrowheads) rimmed by numerous osteoblasts. (H & E, x200)

The intensity of fluorescence appeared to be directly related to the degree of osteoneogenesis, allowing the distinction of areas of new bone formation from stable and inert areas. The technique was sensitive enough to show unequivocal areas of fluorescence, even in very early new bone formation (ten days). The double injection method, used to obtain an approximate measure of the rate of new bone formation, consistently produced a double ring which was easily identifiable and measurable (Fig. 2).

When comparing the tetracycline-induced fluorescence localization with conventional light microscopy of the same specimens, it was possible to identify with accuracy the areas of tetracycline uptake and their relationship to surrounding structures, including soft tissues (Fig. 3).

DISCUSSION

The tetracycline molecule has the capacity to chelate with several biologically active ions such as calcium, magnesium, iron and copper.[5] The antibiotic, when present in the bloodstream, tends to deposit in areas where new bone is mineralizing following the same pattern as calcium. Once deposited in newly mineralized matrix, tetracycline remains fixed in situ for a prolonged but as yet unspecified period of time.

According to Frost et al[5] tetracycline incorporated to bone matrix during osteoneogenesis, when excited with an ideal wavelength range of 420 to 460 nm, emits fluorescent light with a peak emission wavelength between 480 and 660 nm. Of the two systems we utilized, system A, with an excitation wavelength ranging between 455 and 490 nm and a barrier filter set for a maximum wavelength of 510 nm, clearly gives the better yield. Yet the presence of abundant bright background is troublesome and makes it difficult to assess clearly the presence of small tetracycline deposits. System B, on the other hand, with an excitation range up to 405 nm and a barrier filter set for a maximum wavelength of 418 nm, provides a much lower yield of fluorescence. This system, however, results in a much subdued blue background which enhances greatly the fluorescence present and provides a reasonably sensitive setting for the detection of relatively small deposits of tetracycline in bone. In spite of being theoretically less suitable, system B proved to be more sensitive than system A. A hypothetical explanation for the discrepancy between our findings and those of Frost et al[5] is that the use of incident, as opposed to transmitted, fluorescence results in excitation of superficially located and probably hydrated tetracycline deposits. Tetracycline in aqueous solution has a peak excitation range between 390 and 450 nm, well within the capacity of our system B.

So far, all the procedures for tetracycline bone labeling have involved the use of transmitted fluorescence, which in turn necessitates the preparation of bone specimens of no more than 50 μm in thickness. This approach has several disadvantages: 1) filing and polishing bone specimens to a thickness of 50 μm is a delicate, tedious, and time-consuming procedure; 2) as it is done by hand, this step often results in a specimen of uneven thickness, thus precluding reliable quantitative assessment of tetracycline deposition; 3) a relatively small mechanical imprecision may result in the loss of a valuable, perhaps irreplaceable specimen; 4) soft tissues cannot be effectively incorporated into such thin specimens to be viewed under fluorescence microscopy; 5) it is virtually impossible to study 50 μm thick bone specimens with the resolving power provided by conventional light microscopy.

The method we have been using involves the utilization of incident fluorescence provided by a system analogous to that originally developed by Ploem.[6] This approach has several definite advantages over those using transmitted fluorescence: 1) As the incident fluorescent illumination is provided by the microscope objective lens, there is no need to use a bone specimen thin enough to allow the passage of light. Therefore, the problems derived from tedious polishing of the specimen, uneven thickness of bone, and possible loss through accidental breakage are eliminated. 2) Soft tissues surrounding bone can be easily incorporated into the specimen. This is a very desirable feature when emphasis is placed on the study of vascularized bone grafts, as it allows for a better understanding of the role of each portion of the graft in its eventual survival. 3) Since the total thickness of the specimens utilized by incident fluorescence can be between 0.3 and 1 mm or more, it is quite feasible, after appropriate observation and photographic documentation, to process the very same specimen and the surrounding soft tissues for routine light microscopy. Since the specimens are prepared for histological study immediately after fluorescence evaluation, microphotographs of fluorescence and routine histological slides of the same tissue sections may later be compared at identical magnification. This has proven to be especially valuable in the assessment of early new bone formation.

ACKNOWLEDGMENT — Thanks are given to Tatiana Astroza for the typing of the manuscript.

REFERENCES

1. Milch RA, Rall DP, Tobie JE. Bone localization of the tetracyclines. J Nat Cancer Inst 1957; 19:87-93.

2. Canalis RF, Saffouri M, Mirra J, Ward PH. The fate of pedicle osteocutaneous grafts in mandibulo-facial restoration. Laryngoscope 1977; 87:895-908.

3. Canalis RF, Hemenway WG, Ward PH. The role of periosteum on the fate of pedicle osteocutaneous grafts. Ann Otol Rhinol Laryngol 1979; 88:642-6.

4. Canalis RF. Further observations on the fate of pedicle osteocutaneous grafts. Otolaryngol Head Neck Surg 1979; 87:763-7.

5. Frost HM, Villanueva BA, Roth H, Stanisavljevie S. Tetracycline bone labeling. J New Drugs 1961; 1:206-16.

6. Ploem JS. The use of a vertical illuminator with interchangeable dichroic mirrors for fluorescence microscopy with incident light. Z Wissensch Mikrosk 1967; 68:129-42.

Ann Otol 91:1982

SUDDEN DEAFNESS DUE TO INFECTION BY *MYCOPLASMA PNEUMONIAE*

ELIAHU SHANON, MD
CHAIM REDIANU, MD
DANIEL ZIKK, MD
EMANUEL EYLAN, MD

TEL AVIV, ISRAEL

A case is described of sudden unilateral deafness associated with *Mycoplasma pneumoniae.* The hearing function of the patient returned to normal on the third day of treatment with tetracycline. *M pneumoniae* is a common causative agent of protean respiratory disease and the true incidence of hearing loss in these cases may be higher than reflected by the occasional reports. Therefore, appropriate laboratory studies should be included in the evaluation of sensorineural loss associated with diverse infections of the respiratory tract. Prompt diagnosis facilitates the administration of specific treatment. However, the actual contribution of tetracyclines to restoration of hearing cannot be assessed.

INTRODUCTION

Mycoplasma pneumoniae is a common etiological factor in a variety of respiratory diseases. Eaton atypical pneumonia represents 10-20% of all cases of pneumonia in the United States (400,000 per year). The peak incidence of infection with *M pneumoniae* is at the age of 10 years and the disease is less common below 5 years and above 40 years of age.[1] Involvement of the nervous system was observed in 5% of mycoplasmal pneumonia cases; meningoencephalitis, cerebellitis, myelitis, and cranial nerve palsies are described.[2-5] Other extrarespiratory symptoms include myositis, arthritis, myocarditis, and pancreatitis.[1] In the auditory system, otitis externa, myringitis bullosa, and serous otitis media may occur.[6,7] Reports on sensorineural hearing impairment are scarce. The clinical picture is that of sudden deafness and tinnitus, unilateral or bilateral, with signs of recruitment but no decay. The hearing loss may be temporary or permanent.[8-10] The diagnosis of an infection by *M pneumoniae* is based on serological tests, and/or isolation of the microorganism. Active infection is indicated by a fourfold or greater complement fixation titer rise between the acute and convalescent phase sera. Cold agglutinins are associated temporarily with clinical illness, prevail during the second week of the disease, and disappear within six weeks. Cold agglutinins are present in half of the *M pneumoniae* cases and may be positive in other conditions as well.[1,3]

CASE REPORT

An $11\frac{1}{2}$-year-old female was admitted because of sudden deafness in her left ear associated with tinnitus, fever, vertigo, and malaise of 2 days' duration. Physical examination was unremarkable, her eardrums were intact. Audiological tests (Fig. 1A) indicated a profound hearing loss in the left ear and normal hearing in the right ear. Caloric stimulation showed hypoactivity of the left labyrinth. Radiography of the chest and routine laboratory tests of blood and urine were noncontributory. Recording of brainstem potentials at a stimulation rate of ten clicks per second showed intact N_1 through N_5 responses in the right ear. Brainstem transmission time (BSTT or the N_1-P_5 interval) was 4.9 ms (normal adult value: 4.7 ± 0.1 ms). Cochlear microphonics were intact. In the left ear only N_1 and N_{4-5} complexes could be clearly recorded. BSTT was prolonged (5.08 ms) and cochlear microphonics appeared to be abnormal. Stress test[11] at a stimulation rate of 50 clicks per second showed intact responses in the right ear. In the left ear only residual N_1 and N_5 responses were observed and BSTT was found to be markedly prolonged (Fig. 2). Several days following admission a productive, hacking cough supervened and on radiography a homogenous infiltration was observed in the left hilar region. The tentative diagnosis of an atypical pneumonia was made and doxycycline was administered by mouth. On the third day of therapy the patient's body temperature returned to normal, she stopped coughing, and her hearing function improved markedly. The affected left ear showed recruitment (Fig. 1B).

Serological studies showed rising titers of complement fixation antibodies against *M pneumoniae* from 1:8 to 1:64 a week later. Follow-up two weeks later indicated decreasing antibody titers to 1:16.

PATHOLOGY AND PATHOGENESIS

Mycoplasma pneumoniae attaches to the cell membrane of the respiratory tract epithelium. The agent is rarely isolated from the central nervous system or blood and it is possible that clinical symptoms are mediated by an indirect mechanism, toxic or immunologic.[12,13] Some mycoplasmas, eg, *Mycoplasma neuroliticum*, produce an exotoxin. Other species release cytotoxic factors from lymphocytes. However, there is no evidence that *M pneumoniae* is capable of doing so.[1,12,13] Immunologic mediation of some symptoms is suggested by the fact that antibodies against *M pneumoniae* are cross-reactive with myocardium and brain tissue.[2,3] The pathogenesis of the hearing loss is poorly understood. The cochlea appears to be involved primarily and it is

From the Department of Otolaryngology and the Institute of Microbiology, Ichilov Medical Center, Sackler School of Medicine, University of Tel Aviv.

REPRINTS — Eliahu Shanon, MD, Department of Otolaryngology, Ichilov Medical Center, Tel Aviv, Israel.

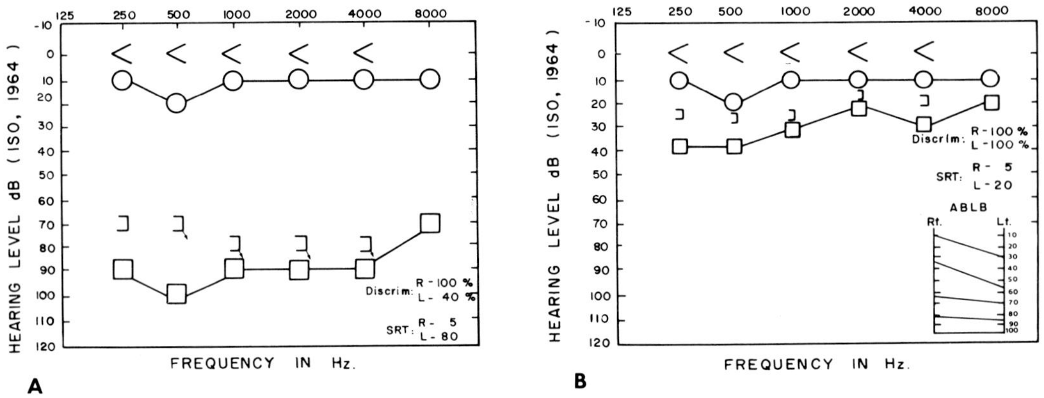

Fig. 1. Pure tone audiograms. A) Profound hearing loss in the left ear on admission: < - Right bone, unmasked; O - Right air, unmasked;] - Left bone, masked; □ - Left air, masked. B) Improved hearing in the left ear on the third day of therapy.

usually affected during the first week of the disease. The main pathological findings in *M pneumoniae* infections are changes in the cerebral capillary endothelium, edema, occlusion of the lumen, and thromboembolic phenomena.[1] However, perusal of the literature did not disclose descriptions of changes in the temporal bone.

M pneumoniae lacks a rigid cell wall and the clinical syndromes due to this microorganism are viral-like in nature. It is thus plausible that analogous findings may be sought for similar clinical states in some viral affections.

Schuknecht et al[14] studied temporal bones from six patients with sudden deafness associated with pneumonia, acute pharyngitis, or common cold. The salient findings were atrophy of the stria vascularis, organ of Corti, and tectorial membrane. In a case of herpes zoster oticus, Friedman[15] has described what may possibly represent an earlier reversible phase of similar pathological process — round cell aggregation of the perivascular, perineural, and intraneural areas of the cochlea and in the auditory nerve. Late in the disease process, about 15 weeks after onset, fibrosis and osteogenesis set in.[16] An irreversible state has been reached.

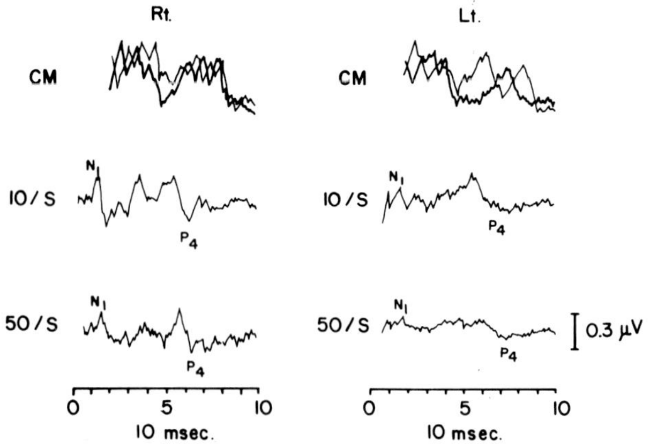

Fig. 2. Cochlear microphonics (CM) and brainstem responses recorded at 10 and 50 clicks per second.

DISCUSSION

There have been few reports on the temporal association of sudden deafness with an infection by *M pneumoniae*. Van Dishoeck[8] was the first to describe this clinical picture in a mother and son. The mother manifested tinnitus and sudden unilateral sensorineural hearing loss with recruitment and without decay. The hearing loss persisted. In her son a temporary impairment of the hearing function was observed. Additional sporadic cases were described.[9,10] However, it is possible that the true incidence of hearing loss due to *M pneumoniae* may be higher than the scarce reports suggest. This possibility is supported by the study of Jaffe.[10] He reviewed 47 cases of sudden deafness of viral origin. In seven patients *M pneumoniae* was isolated from nasopharyngeal swabs and in an additional ten patients serologic diagnosis was established (complement fixation and cold agglutinins).

The patient described in this report manifested hearing loss and vertigo. The hearing loss was probably of cochlear origin and deficient cochlear microphonics were elicited. The recorded aberrations in auditory brainstem potentials (ABP) may be predominantly related to the hearing loss rather than a neurological dysfunction in the brainstem proper. A follow-up study of cochlear microphonics and ABP was not feasible.

The clinical implication of this study is that appropriate serological and microbiological studies should become a part of the diagnostic test battery employed in the evaluation of the sensorineural hearing losses associated with a viral-like infection. An effective agent against *M pneumoniae* is available and hearing loss may be a reversible phenomenon is these patients. The actual value of such treatment in restoring hearing function cannot be assessed.

REFERENCES

1. Clyde WA. Neurological syndromes and mycoplasmal infection. Arch Neurol 1980; 37:65-6.

2. Lind K, Zoffmann H, Larsen SO, Jessen O. *Mycoplasma pneumoniae* infection associated with affection of the central nervous system. Acta Med Scand 1979; 205:325-32.

3. Lerer RJ, Kalavsky SM. Central nervous system disease associated with *Mycoplasma pneumoniae* infection: report of five cases and review of the literature. Pediatrics 1973; 52:658-68.

4. Jachuck SJ, Thorpe CG, Clark F, Foster JB. A brainstem syndrome associated with *Mycoplasma pneumoniae* infection — a report of two cases. Postgrad Med J 1975; 51:475-7.

5. Hodges GR, Fass RJ, Saslaw S. Central nervous system disease associated with *Mycoplasma pneumoniae* infection. Arch Intern Med 1972; 130:277-82.

6. Foy HM, Kenny GE, McMahan R, et al. *Mycoplasma pneumoniae* pneumonia in an urban area: five years of surveillance. JAMA 1970; 214:1666-72.

7. Rifkind D, Chanock R, Kravetz H, Johnson K, Knight V. Ear involvement (myringitis) and primary atypical pneumonia following inoculation of volunteers with Eaton agent. Am Rev Respir Dis 1962; 85:479.

8. Van Dishoeck HAE. Viral infection in two cases of sudden perceptive deafness. Acta Otolaryngol (Stockh) 1963; Suppl 183:30-3.

9. Rowson KEK, Hinchcliffe R, Gamble DR. A virological and epidemiological study of patients with acute hearing loss. Lancet 1975; 1:471-3.

10. Jaffe BF. Viral causes of sudden inner ear deafness. Otolaryngol Clin North Am 1978; 11:63-9.

11. Shanon E, Gold S, Himelfarb MZ. Assessment of functional integrity of brain stem auditory pathways by stimulus stress. Audiology 1981; 20:65-71.

12. Archer DB. Pathogenic mechanisms of mycoplasmas. Nature 1974; 277:268.

13. Rothstein TL, Kenny GE. Cranial neuropathy, myeloradiculopathy and myositis: complication of *Mycoplasma pneumoniae* infection. Arch Neurol 1979; 36:476-7.

14. Schuknecht HF, Kimura RS, Naufal PM. The pathology of sudden deafness. Acta Otolaryngol (Stockh) 1973; 76:75-97.

15. Friedmann I. Cochlear pathology in viral disease. Adv Otorhinolaryngol 1973; 20:155-77.

16. Lindsay JR. Profound childhood deafness: inner ear pathology. Ann Otol Rhinol Laryngol 1973; 82 Suppl 5:88-111.

≈

PAN AMERICAN ASSOCIATION OF OTORHINOLARYNGOLOGY AND BRONCHOESOPHAGOLOGY

The XVIII Congress of the Pan American Association of Otorhinolaryngology and Bronchoesophagology will be held November 2-6, 1982, in San Juan, Puerto Rico. Dr. Hans von Leden has been elected President of the Association.

Ann Otol 91:1982

BIOFEEDBACK REHABILITATION IN SEVENTH NERVE PARALYSIS

MIGUEL ANGEL CORRAL-ROMERO, MD ANDRÉS BUSTAMANTE-BALCÁRCEL, MD

MEXICO CITY, MEXICO

Patients with facial paralysis do not always attain satisfactory recovery through surgery or medical treatment. It was decided that patients could be reeducated by biofeedback training. The method was applied in ten patients; important improvements were achieved. It was concluded that this technique could be useful when the problem is of sufficient importance.

Patients with facial paralysis do not always attain satisfactory recovery through surgery or medical treatment. Many patients with partial recovery of the motor function (paresis), mass movements or contractures attend facial paralysis clinics. Among the efforts for solving these problems has been the use of a mime professor to teach the patients to control face movement.[1] Good results were obtained with this method. Taking this into consideration it was decided that patients could be reeducated by means of biofeedback training. Biofeedback[2] has been described as "a method of teaching one to learn to exert conscious control over areas of the body which previously were thought to be outside of the conscious mind. Instruments are used which will sense and amplify impulses coming from parts of the body which one wishes to alter."

METHODS

Of the 957 patients of the Facial Paralysis Clinic of the National Institute of Neurology, we selected 10. These patients were chosen from those with at least a one-year evolution and no total recovery. All of them showed significant emotional distress and were willing to participate in an experimental program through to its conclusion.

The diagnoses of the ten patients are presented in Table 1. The duration of facial paralysis was more than 1 year in 3 patients, more than 2 years in 3 patients, and more than 5 years in 4 patients.

A general method is used to reeducate the patient and in some cases other techniques to solve a specific problem are also applied (Table 2).

TABLE 1. DIAGNOSIS AND DURATION OF ILLNESS

	Time of Evolution
Bell's paralysis	
Case 1	1 yr 7 mo
Case 2	17 yr
Case 3	2 yr
Case 4	6 yr
Case 5	1 yr
Case 6	1 yr 1 mo
Cholesteatoma	2 yr
Congenital	11 yr
Postneurinoma with hypoglossofacial anastomosis	2 yr (postanastomosis)
Cause undetermined	22 yr

TABLE 2. SPECIFIC PROBLEMS

	No. of cases
Facial asymmetry during relaxation	3
Profound nasolabial fissure on abnormal side	3
Incomplete palpebral occlusion	3
Asymmetric smile	9
Mass movement	4

The first step is to explain to the patient the facial muscle anatomy; with this information, he or she can better cooperate by moving the muscles as requested by the instructor. The patient is asked to try to move the damaged side in front of a mirror. To succeed in this task, it is necessary to cover the normal side in such a way that the patient only sees the damaged side in the mirror; pieces of paper are placed on the face so the patient can see precisely if he has achieved the movement as desired (Fig. 1).

The patient is taught to appraise the movement so he can rate it daily. Once a week the instructor evaluates the performance of

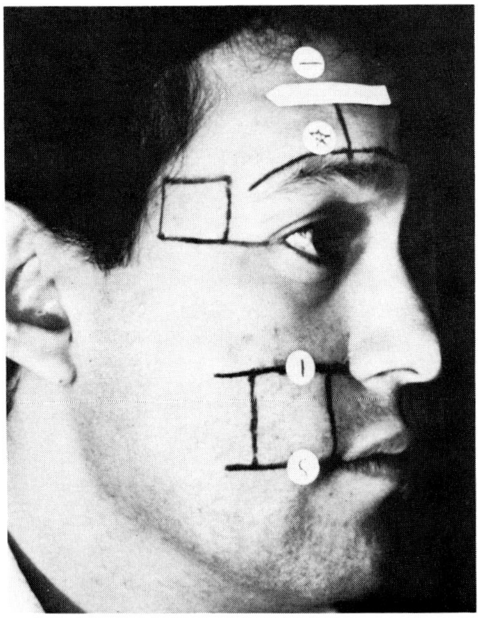

Fig. 1. Lines on the face of the patient are drawn so as to be seen correctly in a mirror. He tries to move the lines on the face as instructed to see if he has achieved the desired movement.

From the Neurology and Neurosurgery National Institute (Facial Paralysis Clinic), México City.

Presented at the meeting of the American Neurotology Society, Los Angeles, California, March 30, 1979.

REPRINTS — Miguel Angel Corral-Romero, MD, Servicios Otorrinolaringologicos, S.C., Av. Ejercito Nacional No. 615 904, Mexico 5, D.F., Mexico.

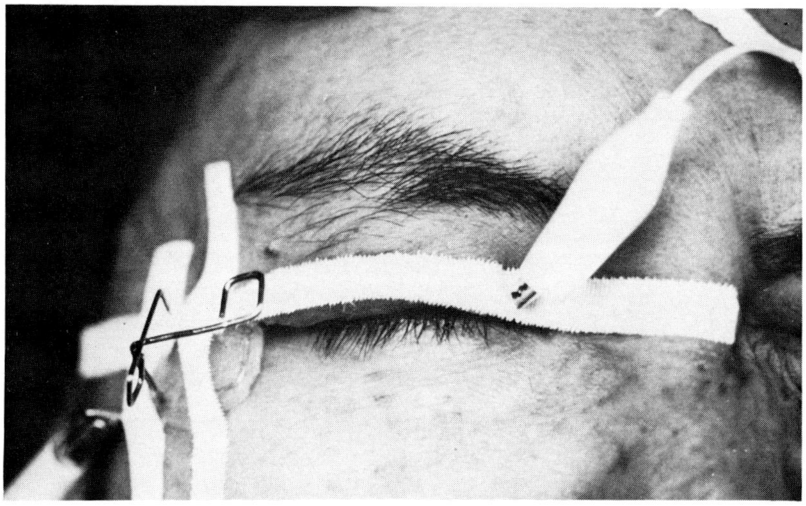

Fig. 2. Electrodes placed on the eyelids. When they come in contact they produce a sound which allows the patient to know he has closed the eye.

the exercise and explains the patient's errors. As an incentive for children, it is advisable to reward them whenever intermediate goals are reached. The patient is asked to perform the exercise as many times a day as he can; to ask for a maximum effort, it is necessary to know each patient's working capacity.

OBJECTIVES

Asymmetry in Nasolabial Fissure. The objective in asymmetry in nasolabial fissure is to strengthen the movements opposing the nasolabial fissure. This problem is corrected by inflating the cheeks; one way of achieving it is by playing a trumpet.

Elimination of Mass Movements. For the elimination of mass movement, the patient is instructed to place the palm of his hand on his cheek in such a way that when he closes his eye or blinks, he can monitor the existence of movement on his cheek.

Asymmetry in Smile. To achieve a symmetric smile it is necessary for the patient to learn to inflate and deflate the muscles of the damaged side in front of a mirror.

Incomplete Palpebral Closure. An electrode is placed upon each eyelid in such a manner that, when the lids are moved, the wires touch, producing an acoustic signal which informs him he has succeeded in performing the exercise (Fig. 2). Small amounts of air or water are also applied so that the uncomfortable sensation provokes the palpebral closure. When the patient has performed the exercises adequately, he is asked to carry them out in his normal environment.

RESULTS

Patients achieved very important improvements in all cases of facial asymmetry during relaxation, reducing the nasolabial fissure and mass movements (Fig. 3 A, B).

Of the 9 patients with smile asymmetry, 6 achieved important improvements, while 3 reached only partial improvement in relation to base line conditions. When the exercise was suspended in three patients with incomplete palpebral occlusion, a reversal of the previous result and even a regression to the initial level took place. At the reinitiation of the treatment the patients succeeded in closing their eyes in a permanent manner (Fig. 4 A, B). The improvement was measured by means of the displacement of painted lines on the face before and after the process of reeducation. Furthermore, the patients felt that improvement in their faces has been considerable.

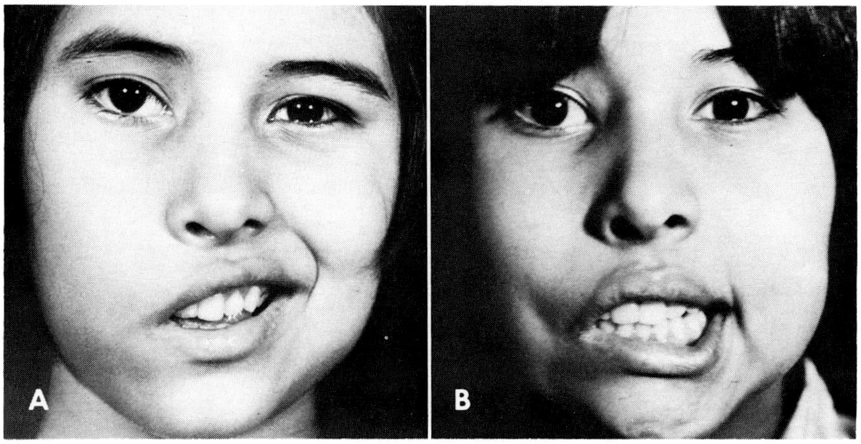

Fig. 3. Patient, 12 years old, diagnosed as having congenital paresis. A) Specific problem is asymmetry of the smile. B) Asymmetry of the smile is less after six months of biofeedback training.

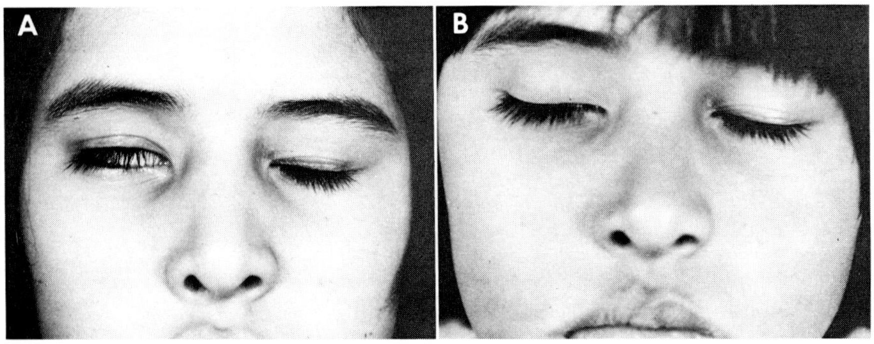

Fig. 4. Same patient as in Fig. 3. A) Incomplete palpebral closure. B) After two months of biofeedback training for palpebral closure.

DISCUSSION

The results obtained through biofeedback training prove that in many cases of incomplete facial recovery there exists sufficient innervation in the muscles to enable improvement of the motion. Besides ipsilateral innervation, it is possible that the facial musculature may be reinnervated other than by regeneration of the affected facial nerve. Reviewing this subject, the possibilities of alternate routes such as the contralateral facial nerve, trigeminal and sphenopalatine nerves had been pointed out.[3] Biofeedback training is possible which will allow the brain to use the ipsilateral facial nerve and also alternate routes to control the facial muscles.

It has been considered that mass movement is the result of the regeneration of the axons which lose their normal disposition and experience intercrossings. If the above is true, there is not sufficient reason to believe that the patient cannot learn to control this defect to the point that the facial movement can come close to being normal.

In other words, it is possible to replace a spontaneous facial expression by a controlled inhibited expression.

CONCLUSION

The biofeedback training could be a useful method for the improvement of those patients with sequelae of facial paralysis and it should be tried when the problem is of sufficient importance so that the effort which this procedure requires can be worthwhile.

REFERENCES

1. DeVriese PP, Bron KJ. Non-surgical rehabilitation of expression. In: Fisch U, ed. Facial nerve surgery. Amstelveen: Kugler Medica Publications BV, 1977:290-4.

2. House WJ. Treatment of severe tinnitus with biofeedback training. Laryngoscope 1978; 88:406-12.

3. Baumel JJ. Trigeminal-facial nerve communications: their function in facial muscle innervation and reinnervation. Arch Otolaryngol 1974; 99:34-44.

STANDARDIZATION OF ACOUSTIC REFLEX LATENCY

A STUDY IN HUMANS AND NONHUMAN PRIMATES

CHARLES A. MANGHAM, JR, MD, MS

PATRICIA A. BURNETT, MS   ROGER C. LINDEMAN, MD

SEATTLE, WASHINGTON

Acoustic reflex latency can be prolonged in subjects with an acoustic tumor. Before reflex latency becomes employed clinically, methods for latency measurement should be standardized to reduce variability. In this investigation, the temporal characteristics of reflex latency were examined in humans and in monkeys. A method of latency determination that minimizes variability is described.

INTRODUCTION

Acoustic reflex latency, the dead time between stimulus onset and the onset of the acoustic reflex, is increased in auditory nerve and in brainstem disorders.[1-4] Several investigators have used a clinical electroacoustic impedance bridge to measure reflex latency as part of an audiometric battery for site of lesion testing.[3,5-7] Before latency becomes routinely employed, methods for latency measurement should be standardized to improve interexaminer confidence levels.

There are several sources of variability for impedance bridge measurement of reflex latency. These include the following factors:

Impedance Bridge. The bridge contributes its intrinsic dead time to reflex latency and also limits the rate of rise of the output signal. These contributions and limitations vary among bridge models.[8-10]

Stimulus Parameters. Reflex latency varies with stimulus intensity,[11,12] stimulus frequency,[13-14] and stimulus rise time.[15] These variables should be easily standardized since their respective influence on latency has been previously described.

Polarity. On commercially available impedance bridges an acoustic reflex typically causes a downward deflection indicating a decrease in admittance (the reciprocal of impedance)[16] as shown in the reports of Clemis and Sarno[7] and Gersdorff.[17] However, most investigators report their data with the deflection upward indicating an increase in impedance.[1-3,8,14,15,18-20] This difference in display is confusing. In keeping with the format of most investigators we show acoustic reflexes as changes in impedance rather than admittance.

Reflex Pattern at Onset. Intersubject variability exists in the form of the reflex tracing at onset (Fig. 1).[20,21] Some normal subjects have a monotonic reflex while others exhibit a biphasic reflex.

The present study examines the latter source of variability in reflex latency measurement. Investigators vary in their methods for measurement of latency in this apparent dichotomy of responses. Some measure latency from stimulus onset to "L_X," the first impedance change, without regard to whether the impedance change is positive or negative (Fig. 1).[3,14,15,20] Others measure latency to "L_Y," the first positive impedance change.[7] A third group measures latency to "L_Z," the point where amplitude reaches 10% of maximum positive amplitude from base line.[22,23]

Absence of a standard for latency measurement results in interexaminer variability. In addition, intraexaminer variability occurs if the method for latency determination does not give comparable values in both monotonic and biphasic reflexes.

Given this problem, we addressed the question: What are the temporal relationships of the various latency measurements in monotonic and biphasic acoustic reflexes? With this information, we hoped to derive a method of latency measurement that would yield comparable values in both monotonic and biphasic reflexes. The study was done in both humans and in monkeys to further evaluate any limitations in comparing impedance data among human and nonhuman primates in future investigations.

METHODS

Subjects. Eight male monkeys ranging from 3 to 7 kg were studied. These included two crab-eating macaque *(Macaca fascicularis)* and six rhesus *(Macaca mulatta)* monkeys. All subjects had normal eardrums to microtoscopy and normal type A tympanograms.

From the Section of Otolaryngology and Facial Plastic Surgery, The Mason Clinic, and the Department of Otolaryngology, University of Washington, Seattle. This investigation was supported in part by NIH grants NS 08181, RR 00558, and the William G. Reed Laboratory for Research in Otolaryngology, the Virginia Mason Research Center, Seattle.

Presented in part at the Research Forum at the meeting of the American Academy of Otolaryngology, Dallas, October 7-11, 1979.

REPRINTS — Charles A. Mangham, Jr., MD, The Mason Clinic, 1100 Ninth Ave., PO Box 900, Seattle, WA 98111.

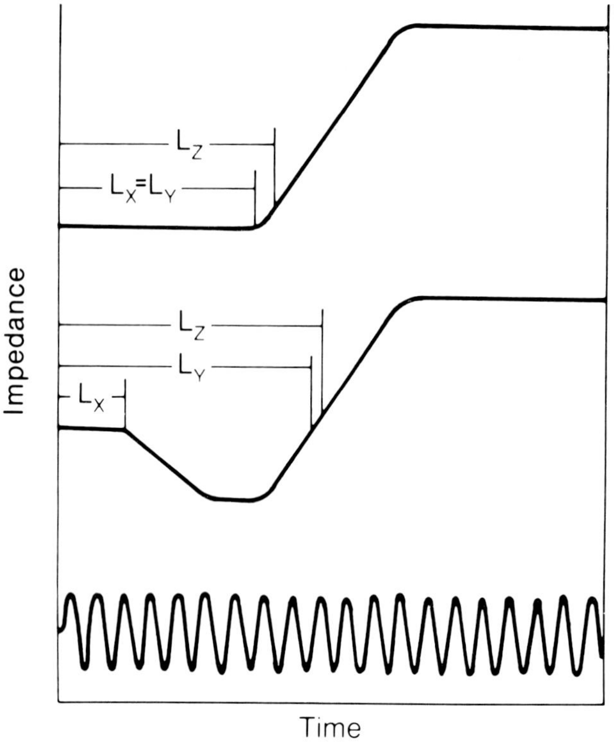

Fig. 1. A monotonic reflex (upper tracing) and a biplasic reflex (middle tracing) are schematized in response to a sinusoidal stimulus (lower tracing). The measurements of latency are: L_X, to the first change in impedance; L_Y, to the first positive deflection; and L_Z, to 10% of maximum amplitude.

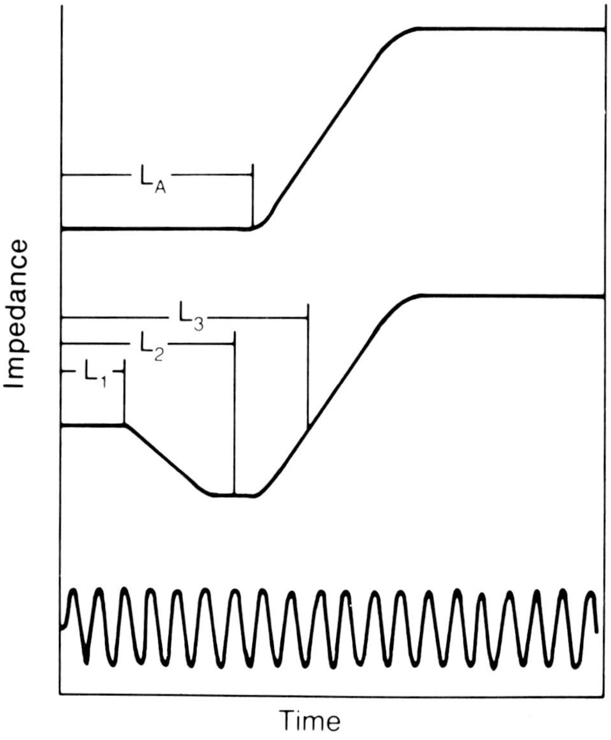

Fig. 2. A monotonic reflex (upper tracing) and biphasic reflex (middle tracing) are schematized in response to a tone stimulus (lower tracing). The measurements of latency are: L_A, to the first positive deflection; L_1, to the first negative deflection; L_2, to the center of the negative dip; and L_3, to the beginning of the positive deflection.

Eight humans, two males and six females, volunteered for the study. Each subject gave his (her) informed consent. All subjects denied a history of an otological disorder and had normal eardrums to microtoscopy. The subjects had auditory thresholds less than or equal to 15 dB re: ANSI-1969[24] at octave intervals from 0.25 to 8 kHz, and normal type A tympanograms. Ages ranged from 26 to 34 with a mean of 29 years.

Procedure. During testing, the unanesthetized monkeys sat in a standard primate restraint chair. All eight monkeys had a stainless steel head brace surgically fixed to the cranium at four points. A stabilization bar on the chair was coupled to the head brace to restrict movement sufficiently to permit testing the acoustic reflex. Both monkeys and humans were tested in a sound-attenuated room.

A programmable frequency synthesizer (Rockland 5100) and an externally triggered switch (Murray Sachs') generated the stimulus. The stimulus had a rise-fall time of 5 ms. The output intensity was regulated by an attenuator (Hewlett-Packard 350-D), an amplifier (Dynakit Mark IV) and a transformer (United Transformer Corp). The signal was delivered to the monkey's ear by a speaker (Beyer-Dynamic) held by a circumaural rubber cushion 32 mm deep (adapted from Pfingst et al[25]). The humans held the speaker and cushion assembly against their auricle.

The output of the speaker was monitored by a 1.27 cm condenser microphone (Brüel and Kjaer 5134) with a 0.2 cm probe tube located 0.2 cm from the speaker housing. The output of the microphone system was measured by a wave analyzer (General Radio 1900). The output voltage of the wave analyzer was converted to sound pressure level (SPL) in decibels re: 20μPa (method of Pfingst et al[25]).

Scalar acoustic impedance was measured in the ear contralateral to the stimulus by monitoring a 0.22 kHz probe tone with an electroacoustic impedance bridge (Madsen ZO-72). The direct current offset in the bridge output was canceled by use of a differential amplifier (Tektronix 3A9). Both the bridge and tone switch outputs were continuously monitored during test sessions on a storage oscilloscope (Tektronix 564) and recorded on magnetic tape with an FM instrumentation recorder (Hewlett-Packard 3960).

Pure-tone stimuli were presented for five seconds at a rate of 4s/minute. Intensity was randomly varied in 5 dB steps and across frequency at octave intervals from 0.5 to 8 kHz.

Reflex amplitude, latency, and rise time were measured offline from taped data with a storage oscilloscope and a clinical averaging computer (Nicolet CA-1000). The trigger for the oscilloscope, averaging computer, and time marker for analysis was derived from the recorded tone switch signal.

The electronic delay of the impedance bridge circuitry for a square wave stimulus ranged from 11-40 ms with a median of 12 ms (modification of the method of Niswander and Ruth[10]). Delays greater than 13 ms occurred when movement of the bridge balance meter in response to internal noise was in the direction opposite that of the stimulus. This variability was reduced by signal averaging. The bridge latency was sufficiently short so that valid reflex latency measurements were made in all cases.

The time constant for the rate of rise of the bridge output[10] for a pure-tone stimulus was 36 ms. This time constant was sufficiently short to follow acoustic reflex transients in most subjects. However, some had response transients equal to or less than the bridge time constant making rise-time measurements of limited meaning in these subjects.

Reflex latency was measured by either of two methods (Fig. 2). The median dead time for the bridge, 12 ms, was subtracted from each measurement. For a monotonic reflex, latency was measured from stimulus onset until "L_A," the first detectable rise in impedance. For a biphasic reflex, latency "L_1," was measured from stimulus onset until the first detectable fall in impedance.

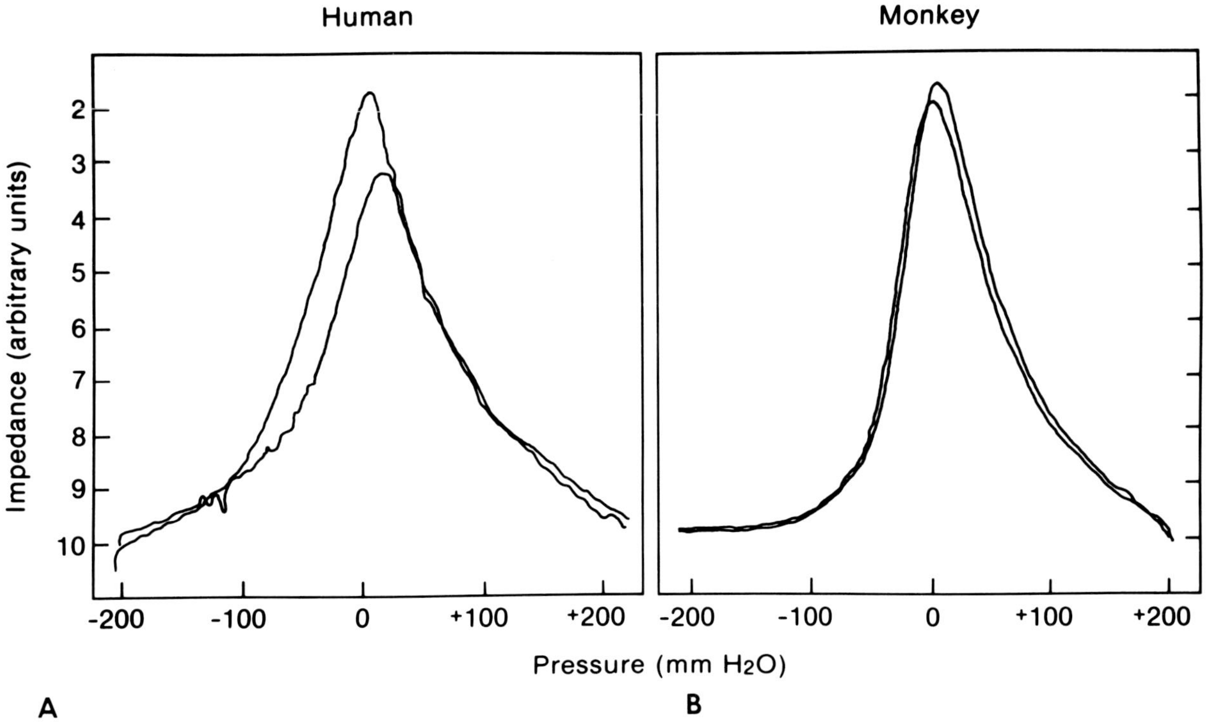

Fig. 3. A) Representative human tympanogram. B) Representative monkey tympanogram. The probe tone for each was 0.22 kHz.

Latency "L_2" was measured from stimulus onset until the middle of the nadir of the negative deflection. Latency "L_3" was measured from stimulus onset until the return to base line.

Acoustic reactance and resistance, components of the middle ear impedance vector, can be derived if external canal volume[8] and phase angle of the reflected probe tone are known.[26] However, the Madsen ZO-72 bridge provides no phase information, making vector impedance determination impossible. Given this limitation, we elected to express the amplitude of the acoustic reflex in arbitrary units inversely proportional to the bridge output voltage. The units are related to total scalar acoustic impedance of the external and middle ear. Changes in total impedance cannot be attributed to a unique shift in reactance or resistance.

Statistical Analysis. The Wilcoxon Rank Sum Test was applied to the data summarized in the table to examine the null hypothesis that the individual latency measurements were drawn from populations having identical distributions.[27] Any $p < 0.05$ was considered significant and the null hypothesis was rejected.

RESULTS

Representative human and monkey tympanograms displayed amplitude maxima of comparable magnitude (Fig. 3). The two monkey species under investigation, rhesus and macaque, had tympanograms similar to those in Figure 3. This contrasts with diminished amplitude peaks for a 0.22 kHz probe tone reported in squirrel monkeys.[28]

The human and monkey subjects had comparable reflex thresholds from 0.5 to 4 kHz (Fig. 4). These observations have been previously reported.[28,29]

Latency in monkeys varied more than in humans. This variability was reduced by averaging. Mean latency data from one monkey with relatively stable responses were compared with averaged data from four humans (Fig. 5A). Latency decreased asymptotically with increasing stimulus intensity.[11-13] The monkeys differed from the humans in that long latent periods, frequently in excess of one second, occurred near reflex threshold.

Mean latency for biphasic reflexes was measured at three loci (Figs. 2 and 5B). The width of the neg-

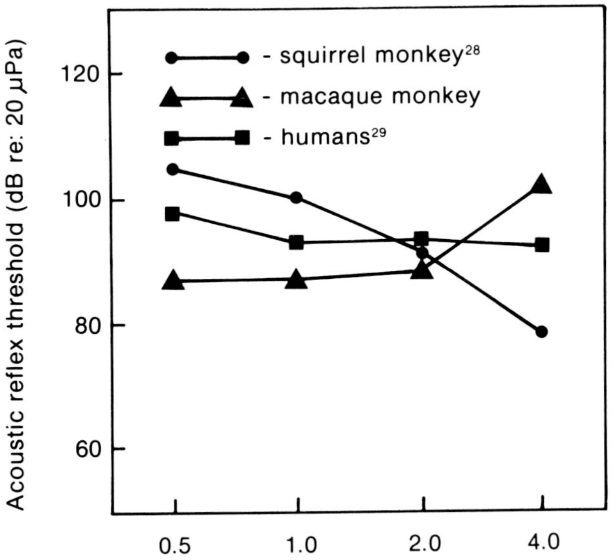

Fig. 4. Mean acoustic reflex thresholds for squirrel monkeys (n = 7), macaque monkeys (n = 5), and young adult humans.

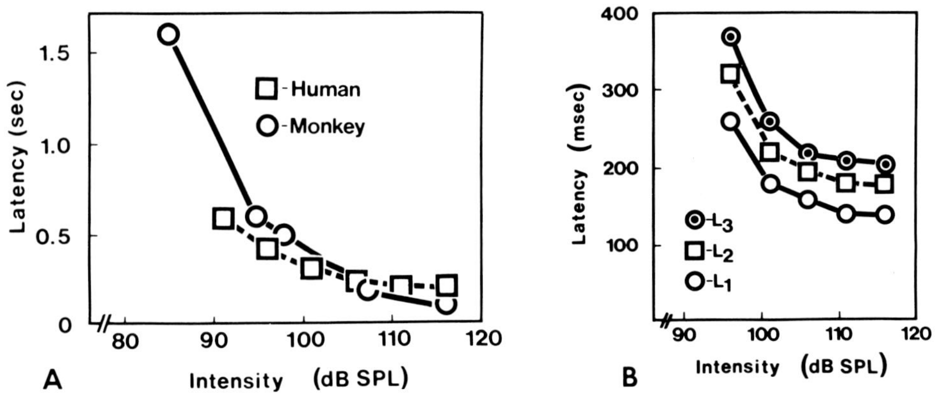

Fig. 5. Latency versus intensity function. A) Monotonic reflexes; data points are averages of at least ten responses for one monkey and four humans. The stimulus is a 1 kHz tone. Reflex threshold was 86 dB SPL for the monkey and a mean of 91 dB SPL for the humans. B) Biphasic reflexes; data points are averages of at least ten responses for two human subjects. The stimulus is a 1 kHz tone. Mean reflex threshold was 92 dB SPL.

ative dip, as determined by the intervals L_1-L_2, L_1-L_3, and L_2-L_3, showed no systematic change with intensity.[21] This characteristic also occurred in our monkey subjects.

A human who displayed a monotonic reflex at one intensity and at one frequency would typically display a monotonic relex at other intensities and other frequencies. In contrast, the monkey showed considerable variability. For example, consecutive stimuli at the same frequency and the same intensity may elicit a monotonic reflex on one occasion and a biphasic reflex on the next.

Intrasubject comparisons between monotonic and biphasic reflexes were made in four monkeys. Reflexes of comparable steady state amplitude collected from three test sessions greater than 48 hours apart were grouped for analysis. Sampling was done in this manner in an effort to avoid the effects of threshold adaptation. The findings in one representative monkey are displayed in the table. The data show that the mean latency L_A for monotonic reflexes lies between the mean latency L_2 and mean L_3 for biphasic reflexes. Because of intrasubject variability, the relationship $L_2 < L_A < L_3$ was not significant at the $p < 0.05$ level. However, the relationship $L_1 < L_A$ was significant ($p < 0.01$). Similar findings were observed in the three other monkeys.

The relationship between monotonic and biphasic reflexes was examined in another light (Fig. 6). What appears to be a monotonic reflex on the upper tracing with amplification is actually a biphasic reflex with a small initial negative dip. Latency L_A for the monotonic reflex in the upper tracing falls between L_2 and L_3 in the lower tracing. If L_A is projected from the upper tracing down to the lower tracing, L_A occurs at the first detectable increase in impedance in both traces. This finding was observed in all subjects. These data confirm the temporal relationship $L_2 < L_A < L_3$ indicated in the table.

By averaging many acoustic reflexes, subtle negative dips were observed in subjects initially judged to have monotonic reflexes (Fig. 7). All human and monkey subjects exhibited sufficient variability such that with the use of averaging and/or magnification a negative dip could be demonstrated in all 16 cases. For human subjects, the depth of the negative dip ranged from 2 to 30% of the steady state amplitude.

LATENCY MEASUREMENTS FOR MONOTONIC AND BIPHASIC REFLEXES FROM ONE MONKEY*

Form of Reflex at Onset	*Sample Size*	*Locus of Latency Measurement*†	*Mean Latency (ms)*	*Standard Deviation (ms)*
Monotonic	8	L_A	245	58
Biphasic	11	L_1	154	42
		L_2	226	33
		L_3	272	44

*Stimuli were 1-kHz tones at 117 dB SPL re: 20 μPa. Reflex threshold was 81 dB SPL.

†Loci ilustrated in Fig. 2.

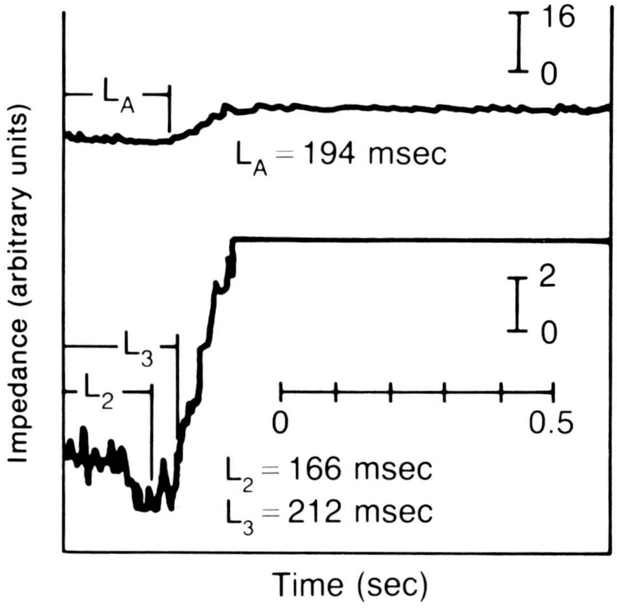

Fig. 6. Top, a single monkey acoustic reflex for 0.5 kHz tone at 107 dB SPL. Bottom, same as above with amplitude magnified x8. At this magnification, the system was driven to saturation 405 ms after stimulus onset.

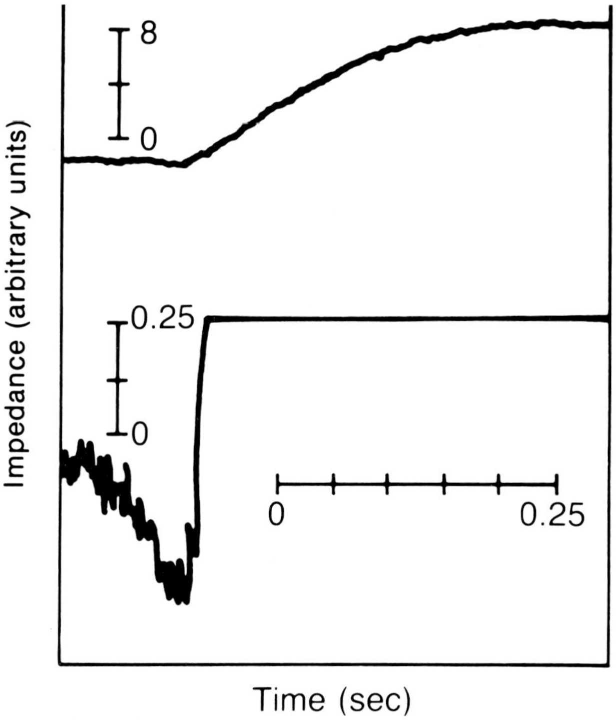

Fig. 7. Computer average of ten human acoustic reflexes from one subject (top). The stimulus was a 1 kHz tone at 107 dB SPL. Bottom, same as above except amplitude magnified x32. At this magnification, the system was driven to saturation 130 ms after stimulus onset.

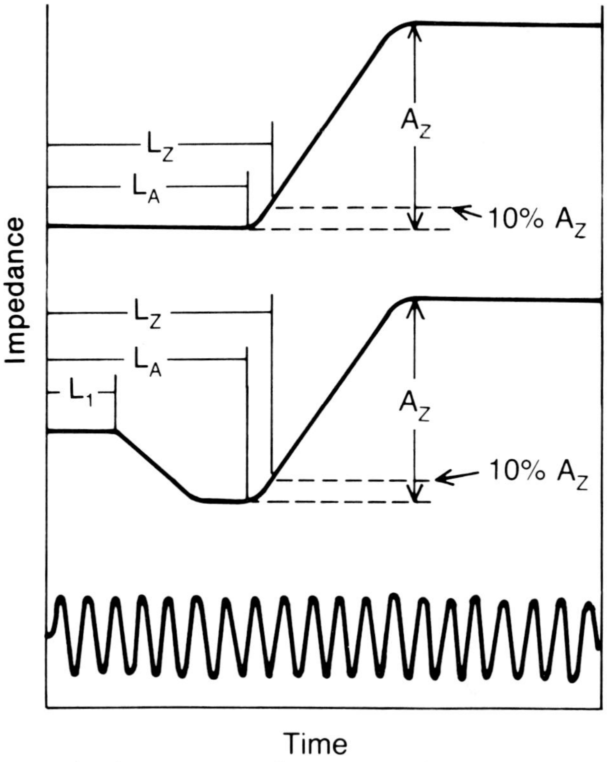

Fig. 8. Monotonic reflex (upper) and biphasic reflex (middle) are schematized in response to a tone stimulus (lower). The latency measurements are: L_1, to the first negative change in impedance; L_A, to the first positive change in impedance; and L_Z, to 10% of maximum amplitude.

DISCUSSION

Although the monkey acoustic reflexes were more variable, the physiological acoustic similarities between man and monkey have demonstrated that the monkey is a suitable animal model for studying the acoustic reflex. In this investigation, both subjects had comparable tympanograms, acoustic reflex thresholds, reflex latency versus intensity functions, and frequently exhibited biphasic acoustic reflexes. The biphasic reflex, under further investigation in our laboratories, is independent of tensor tympani function. This conflicts with a hypothesis based on human cadaver studies.[20] The origin of the biphasic reflex will be the subject of a future publication.

This investigation examined the temporal relationships of four latency measurements (L_1, L_2, L_3, and L_A). Ideally, latency should reflect the minimum dead time between stimulus onset and the onset of the response. When measuring the latency of the acoustic reflex, the first detectable intra-aural muscle effect on impedance occurs at L_1 (Fig. 8). However, L_1 cannot be measured in monotonic reflexes. Therefore, L_1 is unsuitable as a standard measurement of reflex latency.

We recommend that latency be measured at L_A, the shortest latency common to monotonic and biphasic reflexes. Determining latency at L_A is facilitated by use of an averaging computer. The computer tends to flatten the nadir of the negative dip which accentuates the transition from the trough to the positive wave (Fig. 6). Furthermore, the memory capability of the computer permits amplitude magnification so that the transition at L_A is easy to define in both monotonic and biphasic responses.

Although more time-consuming, an alternative method is to measure latency at L_Z, 10% of maximum amplitude (Fig. 8). Note that maximum amplitude (A_Z) should be referred to the amplitude at L_A rather than base line. This will assure equivalent latency determinations in monotonic and biphasic reflexes.

As a word of caution, a bridge used for latency determination measurement should have its latency and time constant sufficiently short to follow acoustic reflex transients. In subjects with rapid onset responses, latency measurements may only be possible at L_1 or L_A. Latency at L_Z would be invalid if the reflex onset transient is less than the bridge time constant.

SUMMARY

Before acoustic reflex latency determination becomes a clinical routine, measurements should be comparable among subjects. We recommend utilizing an averaging computer to measure latency at the first detectable rise in impedance in both monotonic and biphasic reflexes.

ACKNOWLEDGMENTS — We, the authors, thank Don Anderson and Josef M. Miller, PhD, for their efforts on our behalf.

REFERENCES

1. Colletti V. Some stapedius reflex parameters in normal and pathological conditions. J Laryngol Otol 1974; 88:127-37.

2. Bosatra A, Russolo M, Poli P. Modifications of the stapedius reflex under spontaneous and experimental brain stem impairment. Acta Otolaryngol (Stockh) 1975; 80:61-6.

3. Strasser DH. Contralateral and ipsilateral acoustic reflex latency measures in various otologic pathologies, thesis. University of Utah, Salt Lake City, 1975.

4. Mangham CA, Miller JM. Experimental acoustic neuroma effects on the stapedius reflex in monkeys. Trans Am Acad Ophthalmol Otolaryngol 1977; 84:ORL432-40.

5. Mangham CA, Miller JM. A case for further quantification of the stapedius reflex. Arch Otolaryngol 1979; 105:593-6.

6. Mangham CA, Lindeman RC, Dawson WR. Stapedius reflex quantification in acoustic tumor patients. Laryngoscope 1980; 90:242-50.

7. Clemis JD, Sarno CN. The acoustic reflex latency test: clinical application. Laryngoscope 1980; 90:601-11.

8. Kaplan HJ, Gilman S, Dirks DD. Dynamic properties of acoustic reflex adaptation. Trans Am Acad Ophthalmol Otolaryngol 1976: 82; ORL368-74.

9. Morgan DE, Gilman S, Dirks DD. Temporal integration at the "threshold" of the acoustic reflex. J Acoust Soc Am 1977; 62:168-76.

10. Niswander PS, Ruth RA. A discussion of some temporal characteristics of electroacoustic impedance bridges. J Am Aud Soc 1979; 5:151-5.

11. Metz O. Studies on the contraction of the tympanic muscles as indicated by changes in the impedance of the ear. Acta Otolaryngol (Stockh) 1951; 39:397-405.

12. Dallos PJ. Dynamics of the acoustic reflex: phenomenological aspects. J Acoust Soc Am 1964; 36:2175-83.

13. Moller AR. Intra-aural muscle contraction in man, examined by measuring acoustic impedance of the ear. Laryngoscope 1958; 68:48-62.

14. Ruth RA, Niswander PS. Acoustic reflex latency as a function of frequency and intensity of eliciting stimulus. J Am Aud Soc 1976; 2:54-60.

15. McPherson DL, Thompson D. Quantification of the threshold and latency parameters of the acoustic reflex in humans. Acta Otolaryngol (Stockh) 1977; Suppl 353.

16. Feldman AS, Wilber LA. Introduction. In: Feldman AS, Wilber LA, eds. Acoustic impedance and admittance. Baltimore: Williams and Wilkins, 1976:1-7.

17. Gersdorff MCH. Modifications du reflexe acoustico-facial chez l'homme en fonction de l'age, par etude impedancemetrique. Audiology 1978; 17:260-70.

18. Habener SA, Snyder J. Stapedius reflex amplitude and decay in normal hearing ears. Arch Otolaryngol 1974; 100:294-7.

19. Norris TW, Stelmachowicz P, Bowling C, Taylor DJ. Latency measures of the acoustic reflex. Audiology 1974; 13:464-9.

20. Love JT, Stream RW. The biphasic acoustic reflex: a new perspective. Laryngoscope 1978; 88:298-313.

21. Hung IJ, Dallos P. Study of the acoustic reflex in human beings: I. Dynamic characteristics. J Acoust Soc Am 1972; 52:1168-80.

22. Borg E. Dynamic characteristics of the intra-aural muscle reflex. In: Feldman AS, Wilber LA, eds. Acoustic impedance and admittance. Baltimore: Williams and Wilkins, 1976:236-99.

23. Liden G, Nilsson E, Laaskinen O, Roos BE, Miller J. The stapedius reflex and motor reaction time: a parallel investigation of the effect of drugs. Scand Audiol 1974; 3:73-80.

24. American National Standard Specifications for Audiometers. ANSI S3.6-1969. New York: American National Standards Institute Inc., 1970.

25. Pfingst BE, Hienz R, Kimm J, Miller J. Reaction time procedure for measurement of hearing: I. Suprathreshold functions. II. Threshold functions. J Acoust Soc Am 1975; 57:421-36.

26. Berlin CI, Cullen JK. The physical basis of impedance measurement. In: Jerger J, ed. Handbook of clinical impedance audiometry. Acton: American Electromedics Corp, 1975; 1:1-20.

27. Wilcoxon F. Individual comparisons by ranking methods. Biometrics 1945; 1:50-83.

28. Jerger J, Mauldin L, Igarashi M. Impedance audiometry in the squirrel monkey. Arch Otolaryngol 1978; 104:214-24.

29. Jerger J, Jerger S, Mauldin L. Studies in impedance audiometry. Arch Otolaryngol 1972; 96:513-23.

Ann Otol 91:1982

OXATOMIDE IN THE TREATMENT OF CHRONIC ALLERGIC RHINITIS

E. VANNIEUWENHUYSE, MD
BOOM, BELGIUM

W. DE PROOST, MD
HERENTALS, BELGIUM

F. DEGREEF, MD
SINT-TRUIDEN, BELGIUM

J. CALLIER, MD
SINT-NIKLAAS, BELGIUM

Fifty-six patients with chronic allergic rhinitis were selected for a randomized double-blind study comparing oxatomide with a placebo. At the end of the 1-month treatment period symptoms had disappeared or were markedly improved in 81% of the oxatomide-treated patients compared with only 17% of the placebo group. Therapeutic control was achieved in most patients with a dose of 30 mg bid. Improvements were characterized by a reduction in the number, duration and severity of episodes of rhinitis. Oxatomide also significantly reduced the requirements of patients for additional antiallergic medication. No significant side effects were reported.

INTRODUCTION

Oxatomide is a new antiallergic drug with novel properties.[1,2] Oxatomide inhibits mast cell mediator release in response to IgG- and IgE-mediated hypersensitivity states by preventing mast cell degranulation.[3,4] Oxatomide also inhibits the attachment of different mediators of allergic reactions to smooth muscle cell receptor sites.[3,5]

Three independent controlled studies have shown oxatomide to be superior to both placebo and the widely used antihistamine drug diphenhydramine in the treatment of seasonal allergic rhinitis (hay fever).[6-8]

The present trial was designed to evaluate oxatomide in the treatment of patients with chronic allergic rhinitis, defined as a condition occurring throughout the year in frequent attacks with short remissions and without obvious seasonal relationship. Particular attention was paid to the influence of oxatomide on the frequency as well as the severity of rhinitis "attacks," ie, recurrence of symptoms.

METHODS

Fifty-six patients who had suffered from chronic allergic rhinitis for a median time of three years took part in the study (Table 1). Four patients were asthmatic and three were hay fever sufferers but rhinitis was not associated with polyposis. The majority of patients presented with a history of allergic rhinitis supported either by the presence of eosinophilia (8 patients) or by positive skin tests (38 patients) using inhalant allergens (house dust, house dust mites, pollen, mold spores, wool, and cat epithelium). No evidence was found of food allergy. Seven subjects were admitted into the trial solely on the basis of a history of clinical symptoms while three others responded positively to more than one of the diagnostic tests (skin test, eosinophilia, radioallergosorbent test).

At the first visit patients withdrawn from previously used antiallergic drugs were randomly assigned to oxatomide (30 mg) or identical-looking inert tablets. The initial dose was two tablets taken daily, one in the morning and one in the evening. This dose was doubled after the first week of treatment if improvement was insufficient. Patients were allowed a maximum of three tablets 2.5 mg isopropamide iodide + 10 mg cinnarizine + 50 mg norephedrine hydrochloride (Rinomar) a day for the supplementary symptomatic control of rhinitis only if the double-blind medication was ineffective. At the end of the trial, the patient's responses were rated as being "excellent" (rapid disappearance of symptoms), "good" (marked reduction of complaints), "moderate" (slight but definite improvement) or "insufficient" (virtually no improvement).

TABLE 1. PATIENT CHARACTERISTICS

Characteristics	*Oxatomide Group (n = 27)*	*Placebo Group (n = 29)*	*Total Population (n = 56)*	*Statistical Intergroup Comparison*†
Sex				
Males	14	14	28	F
Females	13	15	28	F
Age (yr) Median (range)	32 (13-52)	40 (11-72)	33 (11-72)	MW
Weight (kg) Median (range)	64 (35-76)	62 (34-78)	62.5 (34-78)	MW
Duration of chronic allergic rhinitis (yr)* Median (range)	3 (1->20)	4 (3 mo->20)	3 (3 mo->20)	MW
Concomitant allergic diseases				
Patients with hay fever	2	1	3	F
Patients with asthma	1	3	4	F

*Only one patient had suffered allergic rhinitis for less than a year.

†F - Fisher test; MW - Mann-Whitney *U* test; no significant differences were found.

REPRINTS — E. Vannieuwenhuyse, MD, Tuyaertstraat 51, B-2650 Boom, Belgium.

TABLE 2. RESULTS OVER ENTIRE OBSERVATION PERIOD

	Oxatomide Group (n = 27)		*Placebo Group (n = 29)*		
	Median	*Range*	*Median*	*Range*	*P**
% of days with complaints	55.20	(2.7-100)	92.90	(44.8-100)	<0.01
% of days with Rinomar	27.60	(0-79.3)	69.00	(6.9-100)	<0.001
Mean individual Rinomar consumption†	0.31	(0-1.1)	0.90	(0.28-2.6)	<0.001
Mean individual severity score∫					
All complaints	1.80	(0.7-4.1)	3.40	(1.5-8.9)	<0.001
Sneezing	0.55	(0.28-1.38)	0.98	(0.34-2.58)	<0.001
Watery nasal discharge	0.45	(0.07-1.38)	1.00	(0.35-2.05)	<0.001
Nasal congestion	0.48	(0-1.79)	0.93	(0.14-2.08)	<0.001
Eye itching§	0	(0-0.76)	0	(0-1.18)	NS
Lacrimation§	0	(0-0.55)	0	(0-2.0)	NS

*Mann-Whitney *U* test.
†Sum of all tablets taken by each patient/no. days patient was in study.
∫Sum of scores for each patient/no. days patient was in study. 0 - Absent; 1 - Mild; 2 - Marked; 3 - Severe.
§Complaints present in less than ten patients of either group at the start.

To allow a detailed evaluation of the treatment patients were requested to keep a daily record of the severity of their condition. Five symptoms of rhinitis (sneezing, watery nasal discharge, nasal congestion, eye itching, and lacrimation) were graded as being absent (0), mild (1), marked (2), or severe (3). To correct for some differences in the duration of follow-up, the total number of complaint-free days for each patient was expressed as a percentage of the duration of the total observation period. The study took place out of the pollen season to ensure that symptoms were not mistaken for those caused by hay fever.

RESULTS

Twenty-seven patients were treated with oxatomide. Twenty-nine received the placebo; three who experienced insufficient symptomatic relief discontinued treatment after 11, 12, and 21 days respectively. All patients were followed up for 27 to 31 days except one in the placebo group who was treated for 40 days. Patient characteristics (Table 1) at the start of the trial were comparable between the two groups ($p>0.05$, Mann-Whitney *U* test and Fisher exact probability test).

At the end of the first week of treatment the starting dose was doubled by 72% of the placebo-treated patients compared with only 26% of the oxatomide group. This difference was statistically significant and favored active treatment ($p<0.001$, Fisher exact probability test). Moreover, two of the seven oxatomide-treated subjects who doubled their dosage showed an "excellent" or "good" result at the end of the study.

When assessed over the 1-month treatment period oxatomide was superior to the placebo in increasing the number of complaint-free days, in reducing the number of days of administration and the mean daily dosage of Rinomar, and in alleviating the symptoms of rhinitis (Table 2). The onset of action of oxatomide was fairly rapid with significant intergroup differences in symptom severity being observed in the placebo-treated patients which were slower in onset and less marked and may be partly explained by their high daily intake of Rinomar tablets (the figure and Table 3).

Statistically significant intergroup differences in favor of oxatomide were also demonstrated when the drug was evaluated on the basis of its ability to shorten the duration of attacks of rhinitis, and to reduce both the severity of symptoms and the requirement for concurrent medication during these episodes (Table 4).

The results of the global assessments made at the end of the study are shown in Table 5. Good or excellent responses were obtained for 81% of the oxatomide group against only 17% of the controls.

Therapeutic improvements were observed in the absence of significant side effects: one oxatomide-treated patient reported slight drowsiness and another, who also took about one Rinomar tablet daily, reported fatigue.

TABLE 3. RINOMAR CONSUMPTION*

	Time (days)																											
	1	2	3	4	5	6	7	8	9	10	11	12	13	14	15	16	17	18	19	20	21	22	23	24	25	26	27	28
Placebo group																												
PAT	21	25	27	24	22	21	22	24	21	19	17	15	15	17	21	15	17	16	13	18	16	18	11	18	17	14	14	16
TAB	1.3	1.5	1.3	1.3	1.2	1.3	1.3	1.2	1.2	1.1	0.9	0.8	0.7	0.8	1.0	0.8	0.9	1.0	0.7	0.9	1.0	0.9	0.7	0.9	1.0	0.8	0.7	0.7
Oxatomide group																												
PAT	15	20	22	18	11	7	8	12	11	7	6	8	8	11	8	6	5	6	6	4	4	7	6	9	4	2	4	3
TAB	0.8	0.9	1.0	0.8	0.5	0.3	0.3	0.5	0.6	0.3	0.3	0.4	0.5	0.5	0.3	0.3	0.2	0.2	0.2	0.1	0.1	0.3	0.2	0.4	0.2	0.1	0.2	0.1

PAT - No. of patients taking Rinomar tablets; TAB - Mean no. of Rinomar tablets taken in the group.
*The patient distribution of total Rinomar consumption in each group was comparable ($p>0.05$, Mann-Whitney *U* test).

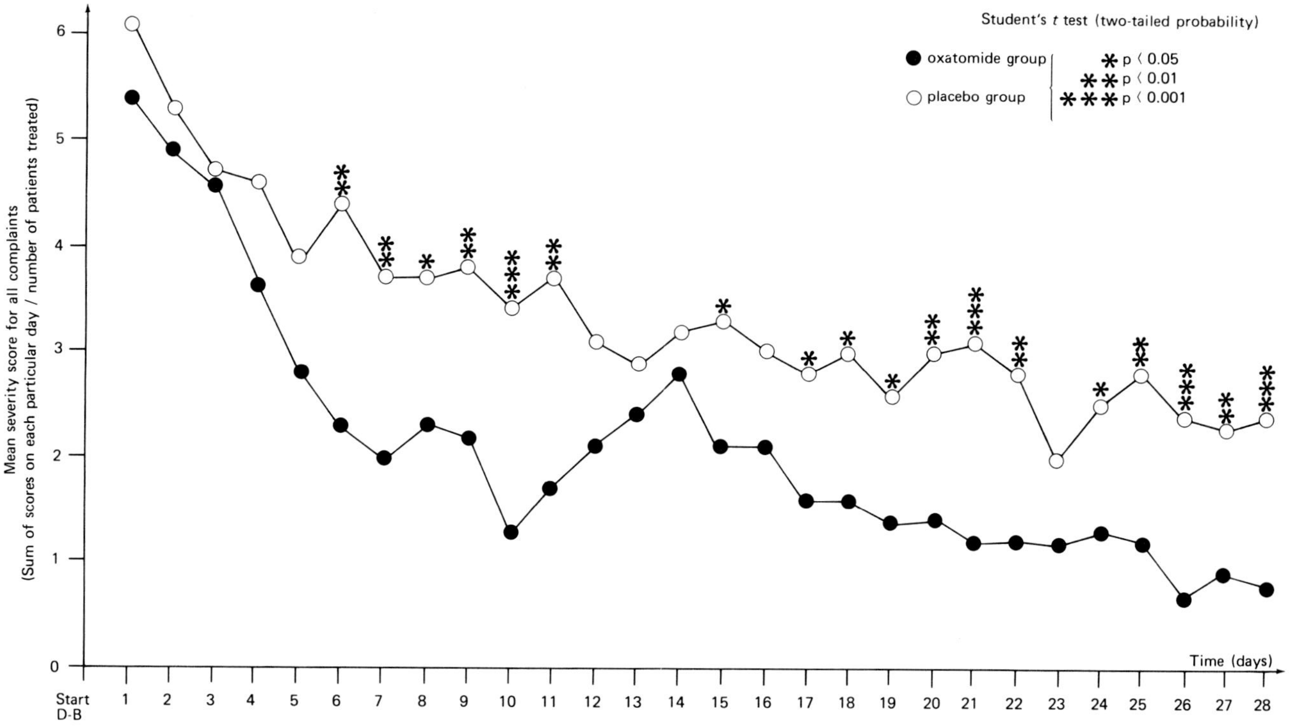

Changes in symptom severity and Rinomar administration in patients with chronic allergic rhinitis.

DISCUSSION

For the symptomatic control of chronic allergic rhinitis the administration of antihistamines or sodium cromoglycate fails to provide adequate relief in a significant number of patients. In the present study investigating the use of oxatomide, a new antiallergic drug combining the mast cell stabilizing properties of sodium cromoglycate with the receptor-blocking properties of the antihistamines,[3] adequate clinical control was obtained in all 27 patients assigned to active treatment. Moreover, in 81% clinical responses were graded as marked or excellent.

For the majority of patients symptoms were controlled by a dose of 30 mg bid and therapeutic improvements, manifest as a reduction in the number, duration, and severity of rhinitis attacks, became fully established after only six days of treatment.

Oxatomide thus appears to offer an advantage over other drugs used to treat allergic rhinitis.

TABLE 4. RESULTS CONCERNING THE ATTACKS

	Oxatomide Group (n = 27)		*Placebo Group (n = 29)*		
	Median	*Range*	*Median*	*Range*	*P**
Individual mean daily no. of Rinomar tablets during attacks	1.00	(0-2.2)	1.40	(1-3)	< 0.001
Individual mean severity score of all complaints during attacks	3.30	(2.2-6.1)	3.60	(2.7-8.9)	<0.05
Duration of the first attack (days)	8.00	(1-29)	16.00	(3-31)	<0.05
Duration of first attack-free period (days)	2.00	(0-15)	1.00	(0-7)	<0.01
Individual mean duration of all attacks (days)	3.70	(2.2-29)	11.30	(1.9-3.1)	<0.05
Individual mean duration of all attack-free periods (days)	3.25	(0-15)	1.25	(0-4.0)	0.001

*Mann-Whitney *U* test

TABLE 5. GLOBAL EVALUATION

Rating	*Oxatomide Group (n = 27)*	*Placebo Group (n = 29)*	*p**
Excellent	6	0	
Good	16	5	
Moderate	5	14	<0.001
Insufficient	0	10	

*Mann-Whitney *U* test

REFERENCES

1. Emanuel MB, Towse GDW. Oxatomide a new drug combining anti-allergic and anti-spasmogenic properties. Drugs of Today 1980, in press.

2. De Cree J, Hörig Ch, Verhaegen H. Oxatomide, a new antiallergic drug, in the treatment of various allergic diseases. Cur Med Res Opin 1980; 6:380-5.

3. Awouters F, Niemegeers CJE, Van den Berk J, et al. Oxatomide, a new orally active drug which inhibits both the release and the effects of allergic mediators. Experienta 1977; 33:1657-9.

4. Borgers M, De Brabander M, Van Reempts J, Awouters F, Janssen PAJ. Morphological evaluation of oxatomide, a new antiallergic drug, in guinea pig anaphylaxis. Int Arch Allergy Appl Immunol 1978; 56; 507-16.

5. Van Nueten JM, Xhonneux R, Janssen PAJ. Preliminary data on antiserotonin effects of oxatomide, a novel anti-allergic compound. Arch Int Pharmacodyn Ther 1978; 232:217-20.

6. De Beule R, Vannieuwenhuyse E, Callier J, et al. Double-blind placebo-controlled clinical evaluation of oxatomide (R 35 443), a novel potent anti-allergic drug in the treatment of hay fever. Acta Allergol 1977; 32:278-89.

7. Ferrière A. Oxatomide in the treatment of hay fever: a double-blind comparison with diphenhydramine and a placebo. Janssen Research Products Information Service, Clinical Research Report N° R 35 443/15 (August 1978).

8. Van der Bijl WJF, Cordier R, van Dishoeck EA, DeProost W, Vannieuwenhuyse E. A double-blind comparison of oxatomide (R 35 443) and diphenhydramine in the treatment of hay fever. Laryngoscope 1980; 90:145-51.

≈

Ann Otol 91:1982

COMPARISON OF NORMAL EUSTACHIAN TUBE FUNCTION IN THE RHESUS MONKEY AND MAN

ERDEM I. CANTEKIN, PhD
WILLIAM J. DOYLE, PhD
CHARLES D. BLUESTONE, MD
PITTSBURGH, PENNSYLVANIA

Employing inflation-deflation and forced-response tests, the eustachian tube (ET) function was evaluated in six adult human subjects with traumatic perforations of the tympanic membrane and otherwise negative otologic histories; and 15 juvenile or adult rhesus monkeys with freshly created myringotomy perforations of the tympanic membrane and otherwise documented normal middle ears. The study findings demonstrated that the rhesus monkey ET functions as a scaled down model of the ET of man, exhibiting a shorter tubal dilation duration and a lesser capacity to pass air. When ET function in the two species was compared using a dimensionless measure expressing the tubal dilation efficiency, the operational biomechanics of both systems were found to be almost identical. These observed functional homologies between man and the rhesus monkey ET systems suggest that the rhesus monkey is a suitable animal model in which to study the pathogenesis of otitis media with effusion, stemming from ET dysfunction.

INTRODUCTION

In the quest for a better understanding of the pathogenesis of otitis media with effusion, several species of animals were studied in order to create a suitable animal model. The choice of the rhesus monkey (*Macaca mulatta*) as an animal model is substantiated by the observed morphological and anatomical homologies in the middle ear-eustachian tube (ET) system between man and the rhesus monkey.[1-4] Using this animal model, the causal relationship between ET dysfunction and otitis media with effusion was demonstrated.[5-7] Concurrent studies of anatomy[2] and physiology[8] of the paratubal muscles have shown that the tensor veli palatini muscle is the only dilator of the ET. Results of gas absorption studies in the rhesus monkey middle ear have implied that the mechanisms for the development of high negative middle ear pressure commonly observed in humans with ET dysfunction may be entirely different from the currently supported hypothesis.[9]

The present investigation was conducted in order to expand our understanding of normal ET function in man. The aim of the present study was to compare the normal ET function of a group of rhesus monkeys to a group of human subjects without otitis media and show a functional-anatomical congruency. Such a demonstration will better define the interrelationships between structure and function, thus rationalizing the use of the rhesus monkey

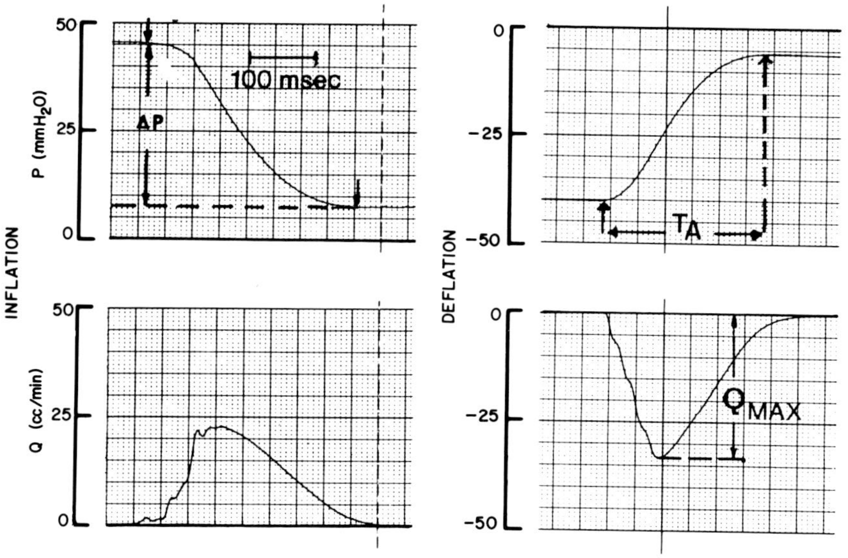

Fig. 1. An example recording of the inflation-deflation test in the human subject. The upper traces show middle ear pressure (P) and the lower traces show the simultaneous flow measurement (Q) through the ET. Flow direction is taken as positive when air is evacuated from the middle ear cavity. The equilibration attempt by swallowing for applied positive middle ear pressure (inflation) and for negative middle pressure (deflation) are depicted. The duration of active tubal dilation (T_A) is defined as the elapsed time between two consecutive steady pressure levels. Also, middle ear pressure drop per swallow ($\triangle P$) and maximum flow rate (Q_{MAX}) through the ET are shown.

From the Department of Otolaryngology, University of Pittsburgh School of Medicine, and Children's Hospital of Pittsburgh. Supported in part by Grant Number NS 13735 of the National Institutes of Health.

Presented at the Research Forum, Eighty-fourth Annual Meeting of the American Academy of Otolaryngology, Dallas, October 6, 1979.

REPRINTS — Erdem I. Cantekin, PhD, Department of Otolaryngology, Children's Hospital, 125 DeSoto Street, Pittsburgh, PA 15213.

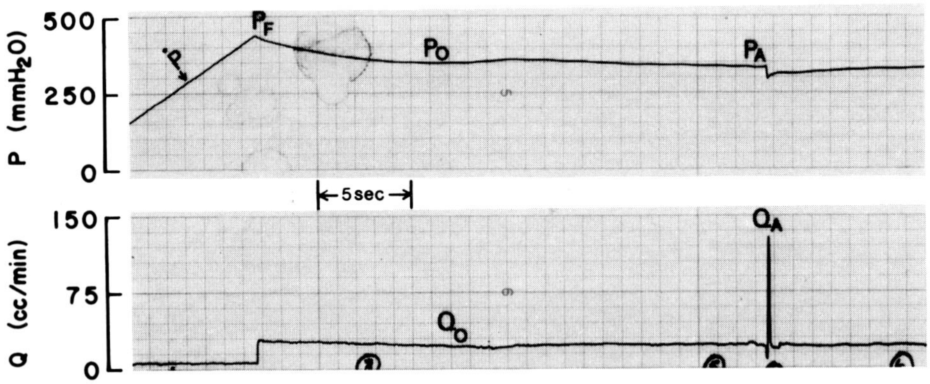

Fig. 2. An example recording of forced-response test in the rhesus monkey. Using a constant flow pump, the middle ear is inflated with fixed pressure rate ($\dot{P}$) and the ET is forced open (P_F). The lower trace shows the abrupt change in flow rate (Q) during forced opening. The pump maintains a constant flow rate. The pressure reaches a steady level (P_O), and flow rate through the ET stabilizes (Q_O). The pressure to flow ratio at this steady-state is taken as the passive resistance. The spike in the flow trace with a corresponding drop in pressure shows active tubal dilation during swallowing. The ratio of pressure before the drop (P_A) to the maximum flow rate during swallowing (Q_A) is defined as the active resistance.

animal model to study the pathogenesis of otitis media with effusion.

METHODS AND MATERIALS

ET function was assessed in six adult human subjects (mean age 29 years) with traumatic perforations of the tympanic membrane and otherwise negative otologic histories, and in 15 juvenile or adult rhesus monkeys (2-6 kg) with freshly created myringotomy perforations of the tympanic membrane and otherwise documented normal middle ears. Each human subject was tested on three different occasions within a 2-week period whereas each rhesus monkey was tested 3 to 8 times during a 6-month study period. The animals were alert and awake, sitting in a primate restraining chair during the testing procedure.

ET function testings were conducted employing a manometric system designed to monitor the pressure and airflow rate.[10] A positive displacement constant flow pump was used to induce variable rate positive and negative pressures in the middle ear. The airflow rate was monitored by a laminar flow element. A differential pressure across the laminar flow element and the upstream and downstream pressures were measured by pressure sensors, fed into signal conditions and displayed on an oscillograph.

Tubal function was assessed using two tests: the inflation-deflation test and the forced-response test. Figure 1 shows an example of recordings from the inflation-deflation test where the subject's ability to equilibrate applied positive and negative middle ear pressure by swallowing was determined. At the beginning of the test, the middle ear pressure was altered to a preset value of positive or negative pressure. Pressure and flow rates were recorded during each swallow from which three characteristic parameters were subsequently computed: T_A (duration of active tubal dilation), Q_{MAX} (maximum airflow rate through the ET), and $\triangle P$ (change in middle ear pressure after tubal opening).

An example of the recording obtained during the forced-response test is shown in Figure 2. The middle ear was inflated with a constant flow rate, thereby forcing the tube to open passively. Following this, the pump continued to deliver a constant airflow rate, thus maintaining a steady stream of air passing through the tube. The passive tubal resistance was then determined. The subject was then instructed to swallow in order to assess the active dilation of the tube. This process was repeated using a different constant flow rate. Usually, the flow rate was doubled for each

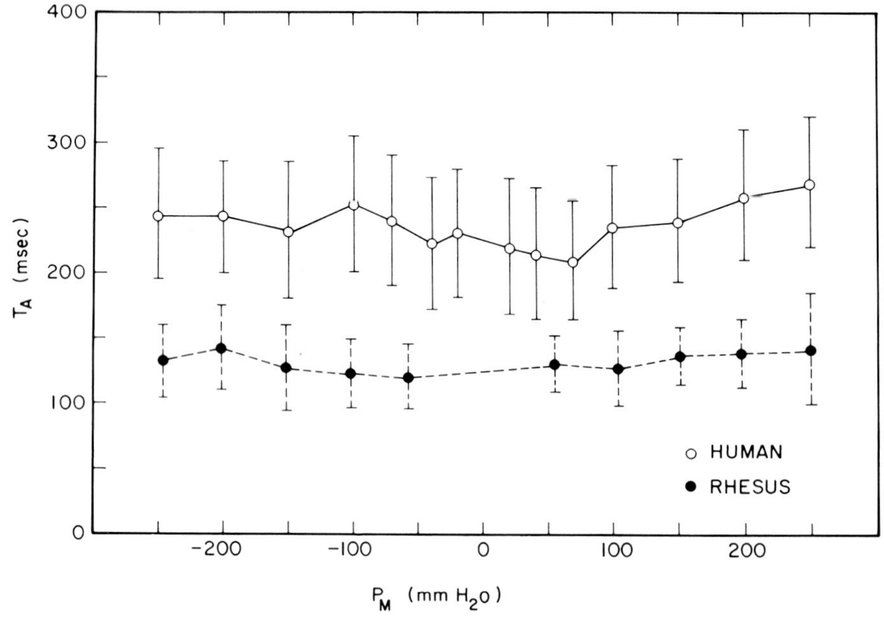

Fig. 3. Duration of active tubal dilation (T_A) as a function of applied middle ear pressure (P_M) during the inflation-deflation test. Data points are the group means and error bars indicate one standard deviation of the mean in this and all subsequent figures.

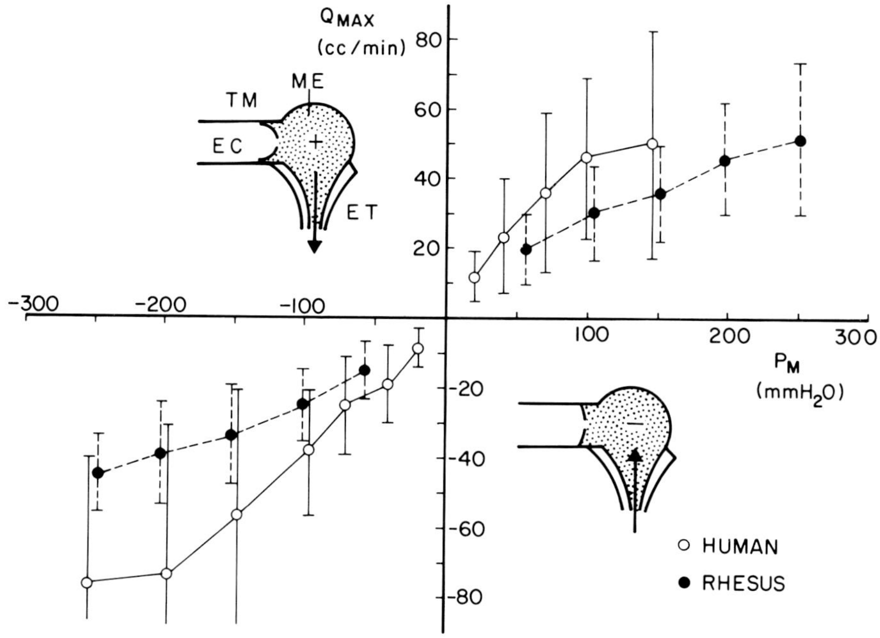

Fig. 4. Maximum airflow rate through the ET (Q_{MAX}) as a function of applied middle ear pressure (P_M) during the inflation-deflation test. The diagrams show airflow out of and into the middle ear. EC - Ear canal; TM - Tympanic membrane; ME - Middle ear; ET - Eustachian tube.

subsequent test. The maintenance of a steady stream of air through the tube allows for the determination of passive resistance which reflects tubal distensibility and for the assessment of the effect of tensor veli palatini muscle action on tubal dilation independent of intraluminal mucus forces.

During this test and for each contant flow rate, three parameters of tubal function were determined: P_F (forced opening pressure), R_O (passive tubal resistance which is the ratio of middle ear pressure to airflow rate during the steady-state flow conditions [P_O/Q_O]), and R_A (active tubal resistance, which is the ratio of middle ear pressure to maximum airflow rate during the active dilation by swallowing [P_A/Q_A]).

RESULTS

The inflation-deflation test findings are summarized in Figures 3-5. In both study populations, each subject could completely equilibrate both applied positive and negative middle ear pressures. Figure 3 shows the relationship between applied middle ear pressure and the duration of tubal dilation, which was independent of the applied middle ear pressure level within the range of pressures employed. The group average values depicted in this figure demonstrate that tubal opening duration was about 100 ms shorter in the rhesus monkey than in man. The maximum airflow rate through the ET as a function of middle ear pressure is shown in Figure 4. The group average values of airflow rate in the rhesus monkey were always smaller than the values recorded in man, indicating that active tubal opening in the monkey induces a relatively smaller dilation. In both species, the flow rate showed a linear dependence on the middle ear pressure. Figure 5

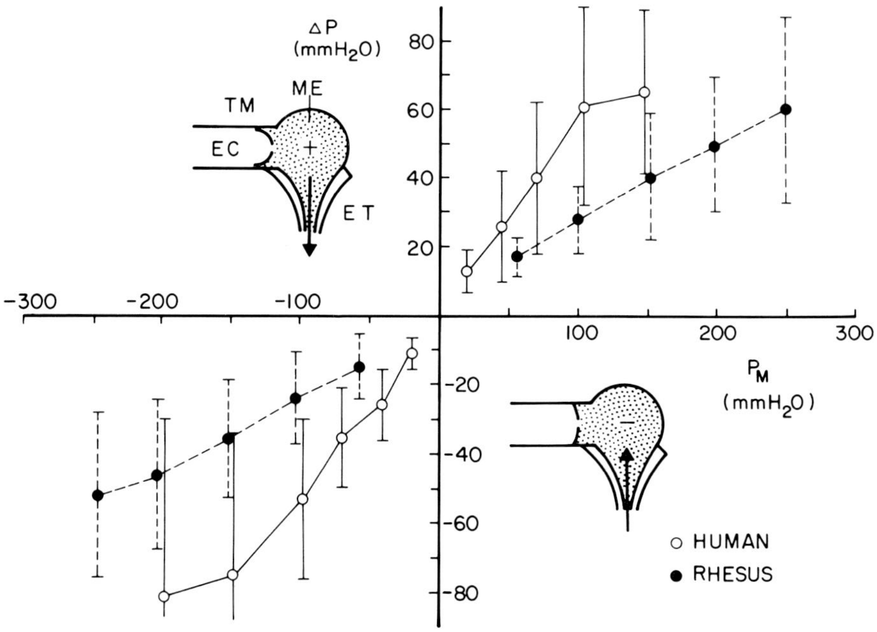

Fig. 5. Change in middle ear pressure (△P) after active tubal opening as a function of applied middle ear pressure (P_M) during the inflation-deflation test.

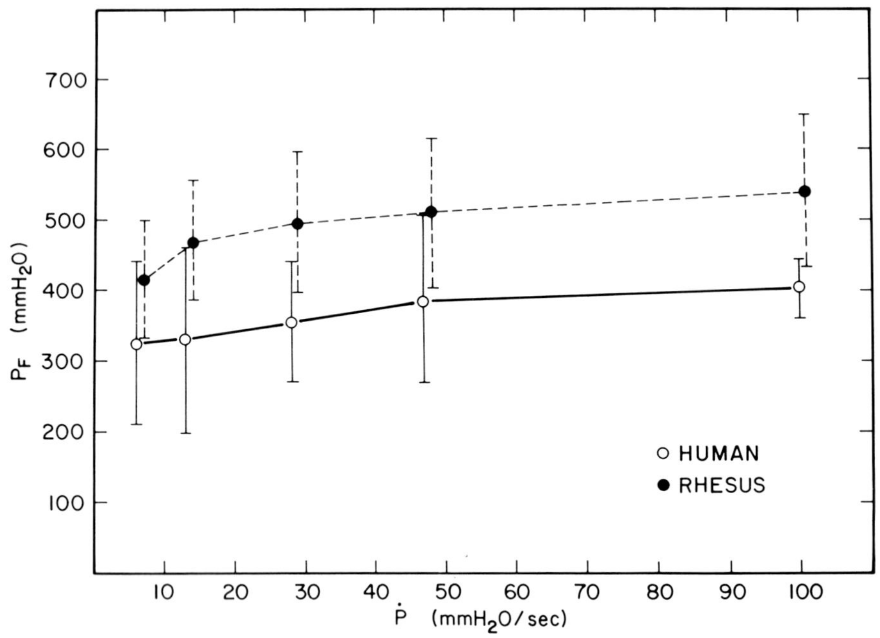

Fig. 6. Relationship between forced-opening pressure (P_F) and application rate of middle ear pressure ($\dot{P}$).

shows a similar linear dependence of the change in the middle ear pressure after each tubal opening on the applied middle ear pressure level. Again, the recorded values in the rhesus monkey were smaller than those recorded for man over all values of middle ear pressure.

During the forced-response test, and prior to the maintenance of a constant flow of air through the tube, the ET was forced open due to an overpressure in the middle ear. Figure 6 shows the relationship between the rate of middle ear inflation and the forced-opening pressure. Both species showed a dependence of the forced-opening pressure on the inflation rate. This dependence was more pronounced in the rhesus monkey for the lower inflation rates. In general, regardless of the inflation rate, the rhesus monkey forced opening pressures were greater than the values obtained for man. The active and passive tubal resistance findings for both species are shown in Figure 7. The top frame shows the flow rate dependencies of passive tubal resistance for both species. The average values for the rhesus monkey were always larger than those recorded for man. However, the similarities in shape of these two curves suggest that the resistance differences in the two tubal systems can be attributed to differences in lumen size or cross-sectional area. The bottom frame shows the independence of active tubal resistance on flow rate in both species. Again, for all values of applied constant flow rate, the rhesus monkey exhibited a higher active resistance, indicating that during swallowing, the active dilation of the rhesus monkey tube is not as great as the dilation observed in man.

A measure of tubal dilation efficiency (R_O/R_A) was computed by obtaining the ratio of passive resistance to active resistance, which normalizes the geometric differences. Figure 8 shows the tubal dilation efficiency as a function of applied constant flow rate. The values obtained for the group averages of both species overlap. This figure demonstrates that when the tubal system of the rhesus

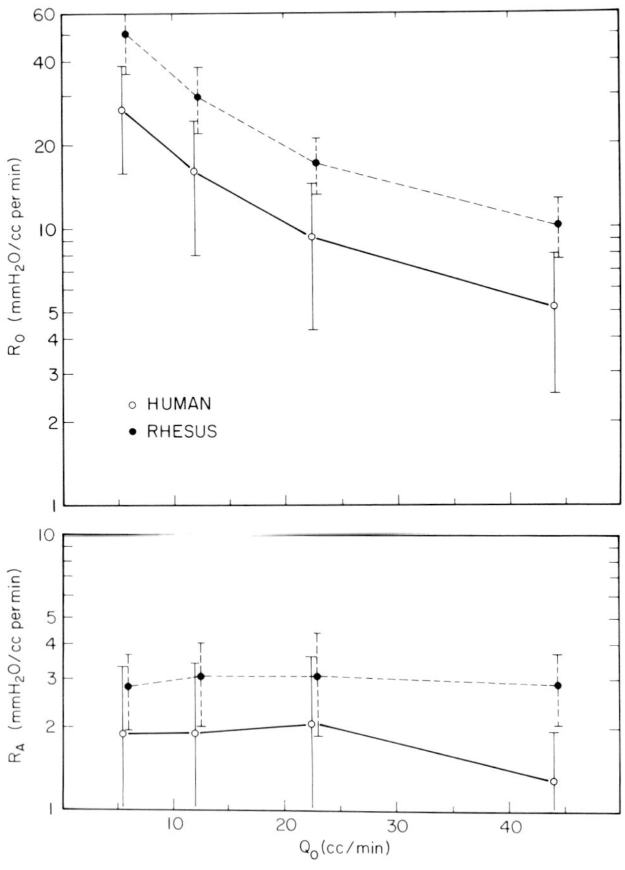

Fig. 7. Passive tubal resistance (R_O) (top) and active tubal resistance (R_A) (bottom) as a function of steady-state airflow rate (Q_O).

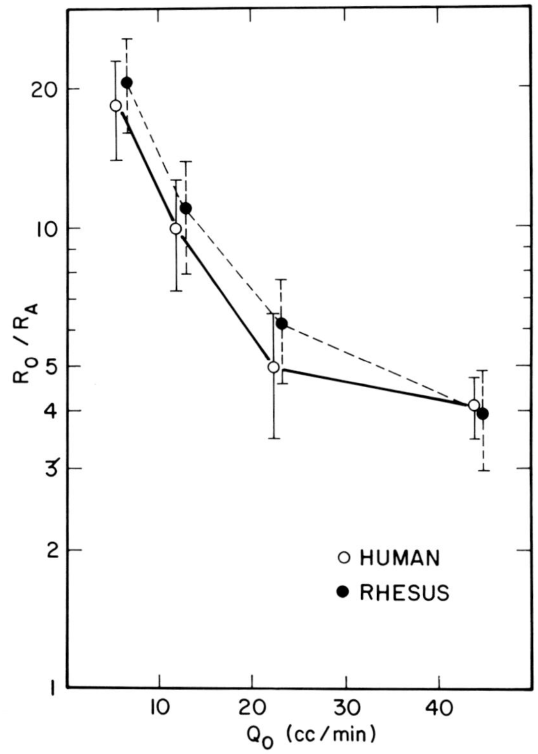

Fig. 8. The ratio of passive tubal resistance to active tubal resistance (R_O/R_A) or tubal dilation efficiency as a function of steady-state airflow rate (Q_O).

monkey is compared with the tubal system of man in a normalized fashion, the physiological functioning of the ET is almost identical within the confines of the evaluation methods employed in this investigation.

DISCUSSION

The inflation-deflation test findings indicate that the rhesus monkey ET functions as a scaled-down model of the ET of man exhibiting a shorter tubal dilation duration and a lesser capacity to pass air. The middle ear pressure independence of tubal dilation duration and the linear dependencies of both the flow rate and the change in the middle pressure level after each tubal opening on the applied pressure level suggest that the ET works as a flow-limiting device.

Airflow through the ET during active dilation may depend on two temporal events related to tubal mechanics: the lateral displacement of the ET wall due to tensile forces exerted by the contracting tensor veli palatini muscle, and the return of the lateral wall to the resting closed position due to elastic recoil as determined by the compliance of the ET. Tubal compliance is a loosely defined entity which can be viewed as a composite parameter encompassing the mass, pressure, and elasticity of the extramural tissue as well as the stiffness of the tubal walls. During lateral displacement of the ET wall (the first event), the airflow rate increases since after the initial opening, the medial and lateral walls of the ET are further separated. The lumen reaches its most distended position when the maximum airflow is observed. Usually, the lumen remains maximally dilated for some milliseconds, indicating a continuing active lateral pull of the tensor veli palatini muscle. Following this, the airflow rate monotonously decreases during the passive closing phase. This phase is probably dependent on tubal compliance. Observed differences in the duration of tubal dilation between the two species studied may stem from the differences in duration of closing and can be explained by the morphological differences reported recently.[2] The rhesus ET has a lumen cross-sectional area smaller than that of man and thus requires a shorter travel time for the lateral wall to return to the resting closed position. Further, as the majority of the rhesus monkey ET is supported wholly or in part by the bullar structure, it is probably less compliant than that of man which is supported by bone only in the protympanic portion. This may be manifested as a stronger elastic recoil, which will result in a faster tubal closing time. The shorter duration of tubal dilation observed in the rhesus monkey may be explicable by the additive effects of these two morphological observations.

These functional-anatomical correlates are further supported by the findings of the forced-response test. The rhesus monkey ET exhibits forced-opening pressures and passive tubal resistance values larger than the values obtained for man, which are congruent with the expectations of a stiff ET with a small lumen.

Although there are metric differences in tubal function between the two species, the operational mode of ET mechanics is the same as illustrated by Figures 3 through 7. This functional similarity is best illustrated when ET function in these two species is compared in a normalized fashion (Fig. 8). The normalization process is based on the assumption that the flow conditions during the forced-response test can be modeled as a Hagen-Poiseuille flow between two parallel plates; in this case the "plates" are the lateral and medial walls of the ET lumen. For this flow condition, the expression relating the pressure drop to the flow rate is given by the following equation:

$$Q = \frac{2}{3} \frac{\triangle P B^3 W}{\mu L}$$

which can be adapted to express the passive and active ET resistances by rearranging the terms:

$$R_O = \frac{\triangle P}{Q_o} = \frac{3}{2} \frac{\mu L}{B_o{}^3 W}, \text{ and}$$

$$R_A = \frac{\triangle P}{Q_A} = \frac{3}{2} \frac{\mu L}{B_A{}^3 W}$$

where $\triangle P$ is the pressure difference between the middle ear and the nasopharynx, μ is the viscosity of air, L is the functional length of the ET, W is the superoinferior height of the tubal lumen, B_O is the mediolateral lumen width during constant flow rate Q_O, and B_A is the mediolateral lumen width during active dilation. From the slit-like lumen at rest, it can be assumed that tubal dilation occurs in the mediolateral axis and therefore changes in variables L and W are negligible during active and passive resistance evaluations. Therefore, the ratio of passive to active resistance can be expressed as:

$$\frac{R_o}{R_A} = \frac{B_A^3}{B_o^3}$$

This simply expresses the ratio of the dilation levels of the lumen during these two conditions in a dimensionless form.

This ratio can be used as a measure of tubal dilation efficiency since it expresses the level of the lateral wall movement due to muscle pull (B_A) at different passive dilation conditions (B_O). As depicted in Figure 8, the dilation efficiency decreases with increasing constant flow rate. With larger flow rates, the lumen is already distended considerably; therefore the active muscle pull induces relatively smaller lateral displacements. When ET function in the two species is compared using this measure, the data points are almost identical, suggesting that both systems operate in the same manner.

Therefore, in conclusion, the rhesus monkey is ideally suitable for physiological modeling in studies of the middle ear-eustachian tube system. Investigations of tubal mechanics using this model will enable us to increase our understanding of the physiology and pathophysiology of tubal dysfunction in man in relation to the pathogenesis of otitis media.

REFERENCES

1. Doyle WJ, Rood SR. Anatomy of the auditory tube and related structures in the rhesus monkey (*Macaca mulatta*). Acta Anat 1979; 105:209-25.

2. Doyle WJ, Rood SR. Comparison of the anatomy of the eustachian tube in the rhesus monkey (*Macaca mulatta*) and man: implications for physiologic modeling. Ann Otol Rhinol Laryngol 1980; 89:49-57.

3. Rood SR, Doyle WJ. Interspecific study of the eustachian tube/middle ear system. Trans Am Acad Ophthalmol Otolaryngol 1979; 32:55-61.

4. Saad MM, Doyle WJ, Gest TR. The morphology of the middle ear in the rhesus monkey (*Macaca mulatta*). Acta Anat 1982 (in press).

5. Cantekin EI, Bluestone CD, Saez CA, Doyle WJ, Phillips DC. Normal and abnormal middle ear ventilation. Ann Otol Rhinol Laryngol 1977; 86 Suppl 41:1-15.

6. Cantekin EI, Phillips DC, Doyle WJ, Bluestone CD, Kimes KK. Effect of surgical alterations of the tensor veli palatini muscle on eustachian tube function. Ann Otol Rhinol Laryngol 1980; 89 Suppl 68:47-53.

7. Doyle WJ, Cantekin EI, Bluestone CD, Phillips DC, Kimes KK, Siegel MI. A nonhuman primate model of cleft palate and its implications for middle ear pathology. Ann Otol Rhinol Laryngol 1980; 89 Suppl 68:41-6.

8. Cantekin EI, Doyle WJ, Reichert TJ, Phillips DC, Bluestone CD. Dilation of the eustachian tube by electrical stimulation of the mandibular nerve. Ann Otol Rhinol Laryngol 1979; 88:40-51.

9. Cantekin EI, Doyle WJ, Phillips DC, Bluestone CD. Gas absorption in the middle ear. Ann Otol Rhinol Laryngol 1980; 89 Suppl 68:71-5.

10. Cantekin EI, Saez CA, Bluestone CD, Bern SA. Airflow through the eustachian tube. Ann Otol Rhinol Laryngol 1979; 88:603-12.

Ann Otol 91:1982

SEMICIRCULAR CANAL STRUCTURE DURING POSTNATAL DEVELOPMENT IN CAT AND GUINEA PIG

I. S. CURTHOYS, PhD

SYDNEY, AUSTRALIA

R. H. I. BLANKS, PhD

IRVINE, CALIFORNIA

C. H. MARKHAM, MD

LOS ANGELES, CALIFORNIA

The gain of the vestibulo-ocular reflex in the cat continues to increase for some time after birth. The reason for this increase is not presently known and one possibility is that it occurs because the cat semicircular canals increase in size. The present study examined this possibility by measuring the radii of curvature *(R)* of individual semicircular canals and the angular relationships of the semicircular canal planes within a labyrinth in cats and guinea pigs during postnatal growth. It was found that the labyrinths do move apart substantially during postnatal development in both species, but neither the planar relations nor the radii of curvature change significantly during postnatal development. The stability of semicircular canal structure during postnatal skull growth indicates that postnatal developmental changes in canal-related function, such as increased gain in the vestibulo-ocular reflex, in these species are probably due to receptor cell or neural maturational factors.

INTRODUCTION

Recently it has been shown that the gain or sensitivity of the cat vestibulo-ocular reflex (VOR) to sinusoidal rotatory stimulation increases gradually during development and does not attain adult values until about 60 days after birth.[1] There are a number of possible causes for such a change ranging from maturation of central neural connections to postnatal growth of semicircular canal dimensions.

Considering the latter possibility, Fernández and Valentinuzzi[2] reported a postnatal developmental increase in the radius of curvature *(R)* of the cat semicircular canals. Since in the torsion pendulum model of canal operation *R* partially determines VOR gain,[3] one might explain the development-dependent VOR increase on this basis. One aim of this study was to establish for the cat and the guinea pig whether structural changes during postnatal development indeed occur. This aim was achieved by measurements of *R* of the semicircular canals in cats and guinea pigs at various stages of growth.

In addition, the angular relationships between the planes of the semicircular canals within the labyrinth were also measured in both species during development. This relationship determines the pattern of neural activity from the three canals reaching the brainstem in response to any given head movement.[4] If there were changes in these angular interrelationships during postnatal growth, then the same head movement would cause different patterns of neural input at different ages. Such a result might require some development-dependent restructuring of VOR pathways to achieve the appropriate compensatory eye movements.

Two methods of measurement, ROTA and reticle, were used to determine *R* in neonatal and adult cats and guinea pigs, and the former method was also used to examine the angular relations of the semicircular canals to each other.

METHODS

ROTA Computer Measurement Technique. Data for computer processing were obtained from seven cats and five guinea pigs. The animals were selected to have as broad a range of age and size as possible. Body weights ranged from 115 to 3200 g for the cats and from 66 to 818 g for the guinea pigs. The neonatal weights for both species were about average.[5-7] In all skulls the distances from the rostral edge of the foramen magnum to the incisors (skull length) and between zygomatic arches (skull breadth) were recorded.

The animals were killed by an overdose of pentobarbital, and all soft tissue was removed from the skulls which were then dried. When required, dental cement was applied to the cranial sutures to prevent dislocation during the cleansing process. The osseous semicircular canals were exposed using a lateral approach and the lateral-most portions of bone were removed from each canal with a dental drill.[8] Each skull was placed in a Kopf stereotaxic apparatus. Because of the very small size of neonatal skulls, the head-holding device of the stereotaxic apparatus was modified so that both neonatal and adult skulls were held in stereotaxic horizontal.[9,10]

Using techniques which have been described elsewhere[8,9,11] the stereotaxic x, y, and z coordinates of series of points along the medial wall of each osseous canal were measured with a fine stylus attached to a micromanipulator. These data were processed by computer, yielding the coefficients of the plane best fitting each canal. The data points from each canal were rotated by computer (ROTA technique) and were printed on computer pa-

From the Department of Psychology, University of Sydney, Sydney, Australia, the Department of Anatomy, Division of Otolaryngology, University of California, Irvine, and the Department of Neurology, School of Medicine, University of California, Los Angeles. This research was supported by grants from the National Health and Medical Research Council of Australia, by the U.S. Public Health Service grant NS-06658 and NASA; and by career development award EY00160 and research grant EY03018 from the National Eye Institute.

REPRINTS — I. S. Curthoys, PhD, Department of Psychology, University of Sydney, Sydney N.S.W. 2006, Australia 692-3570.

per in such a way that the sheet of computer printout corresponded exactly to the plane best fitting the canal. Calculations using the planar coefficients yielded the angles between the canal planes in each labyrinth. The stereotaxic coordinates of the centers of the semicircular canals were also determined. Calculations gave the distance between contralateral canals enabling the documentation of the manner in which the canals move apart during growth.

The radii of curvature of the horizontal *(Rh)*, anterior *(Ra)*, and posterior *(Rp)* semicircular canals were determined from the magnified ROTA technique printouts of the data.[12] Three widely spaced data points were selected and the intersection of the perpendicular bisectors of these points defined the center of the circle of which the semicircular canal was an arc. The radius of this arc was recorded as the ROTA measure of radius of curvature for *Ra* and *Rp*.[13] In these canals the original data points closely followed the line of attachment of the membranous ducts to the osseous canals, and so the values of *Ra* and *Rp* from the osseous canals are a close approximation to the radii of curvature of the membranous ducts. However, in the horizontal canal the membranous duct is attached to the lateral wall of the osseous canal, and this wall was removed during the dissection. In order to compensate for the fact that the data points along the osseous horizontal canal were not taken along the line of attachment of the membranous duct, a correction factor was added to the ROTA *Rh* measurements. The corrected data should be a close approximation of the radii of the horizontal membranous ducts. This correction factor is equal to the cross-sectional radius of the horizontal bony canal and is 0.2 mm for the cat and 0.26 mm for the guinea pig.[13] Although it is possible that this correction factor may itself change during postnatal development, only the one value appropriate for each species was added to all horizontal canal radii measured by ROTA. Since this constant value was added to all *Rh* data from a given species, it should have no effect on the slope of any growth-dependent size changes in *Rh*.

Reticle Measurement of R. In order to confirm the radii of curvature measures from ROTA, another independent method of measuring *R* was used on another sample of cat and guinea pig labyrinths. These data were obtained from 12 cats, ranging in weight from 115 to 3800 g and seven guinea pigs ranging from 42 to 815 g. Each animal was killed by an overdose of pentobarbital and the head fixed for two weeks with 10% formalin. The temporal bones of these animals were dissected and all measurements were made with the skull wet with fixative or Ringer's solution. This dissection technique allowed about 180° of each canal arc to be measured rather than an average of 140° in the ROTA approach.[10]

Measurement of the diameter of each canal was done by viewing the canal through an Olympus operating microscope fitted with an eyepiece reticle consisting of a series of concentric circles. These were optically superimposed on the arc of the canal and the measure of 2*R* was the diameter of the reticle circle best fitting the arc of the canal. Measures were made at 31 magnification and the skull was manipulated until the canal plane was perpendicular to the line of sight.

In order to confirm that the reticle technique is sensitive enough to detect any growth-dependent changes in *R*, 48 rat labyrinths were dissected and the *Rh* of each measured using the reticle technique. The 26 animals, ranging in weight from 5.4 to 380 g, were killed by an overdose of pentobarbital and the horizontal semicircular canal was exposed using only Ringer's solution for irrigation. The rat was used in this test since Clark[14] has shown the rat *Rh* continues to increase during the early stages of postnatal development.

RESULTS

Statistical Analysis. Because of the variability of the measurements between labyrinths, statistical methods were used to decide whether there were systematic changes in orientation or size of the semicircular canals as a function of age. We have used correlation coefficients (r) and regression coefficients (B) as indicators of the relation between two variables. Correlation coefficients can range between +1 and −1; a positive value of r indicates the two variables are directly related, a negative r indicates they are inversely related, and a zero r indicates no relationship. With small numbers of observations, as in the present study, nonzero values of r can be obtained by chance even when the two variables are in fact unrelated. To avoid erroneous conclusions based on these spurious correlations, only r values statistically significantly different from zero were studied. The criterion of statistical significance was 0.05 (the probability had to be less than 0.05 that the r value occurred by chance) and in the present study this criterion was usually met if the r value was greater than +0.7 or less than −0.7.

The regression coefficient (B) gives the slope of the regression line best fitting the plot of the two variables, ie, the changes in skull breadth for a unit change in skull length. The standard error of the regression coefficient (SE) is the variation of data points around the regression line. In every case both variables were transformed by a logarithmic transformation as is usually done in studies of the growth of bodily characteristics.[7]

Two indices of growth were available: body weight and skull length. Although these two indices are directly and strongly correlated (correlation coefficients of 0.99 for both cat and guinea pig) it is possible that a growth-dependent relationship may be shown with one variable and not the other. Therefore two sets of statistical analyses were performed separately relating each variable first to skull length and second to body weight. The results of the two sets of analyses were very similar; both showed exactly the same pattern of significant correlations. Since the correlations were usually slightly higher with skull length than with body weight, only the results of the skull length analyses are presented in the table.

The values in the table can be interpreted as follows. The two variables, skull length and skull breadth, are directly and strongly correlated as indicated by correlation coefficients of 0.99 for both cat and guinea pig (row a). The regression coefficients (B) of 1.06 and 1.13 in cat and guinea pig respectively indicate increase in skull length is significantly associated with a proportional change in skull breadth.

Despite the results of these statistical analyses it is possible that structural changes may occur only early in postnatal development and might escape detection in an overall statistical analysis. To insure that no such changes had occurred, the data were examined graphically. Separate graphs were drawn relating each variable to skull length and to body weight. Again the results of the two graphic analy-

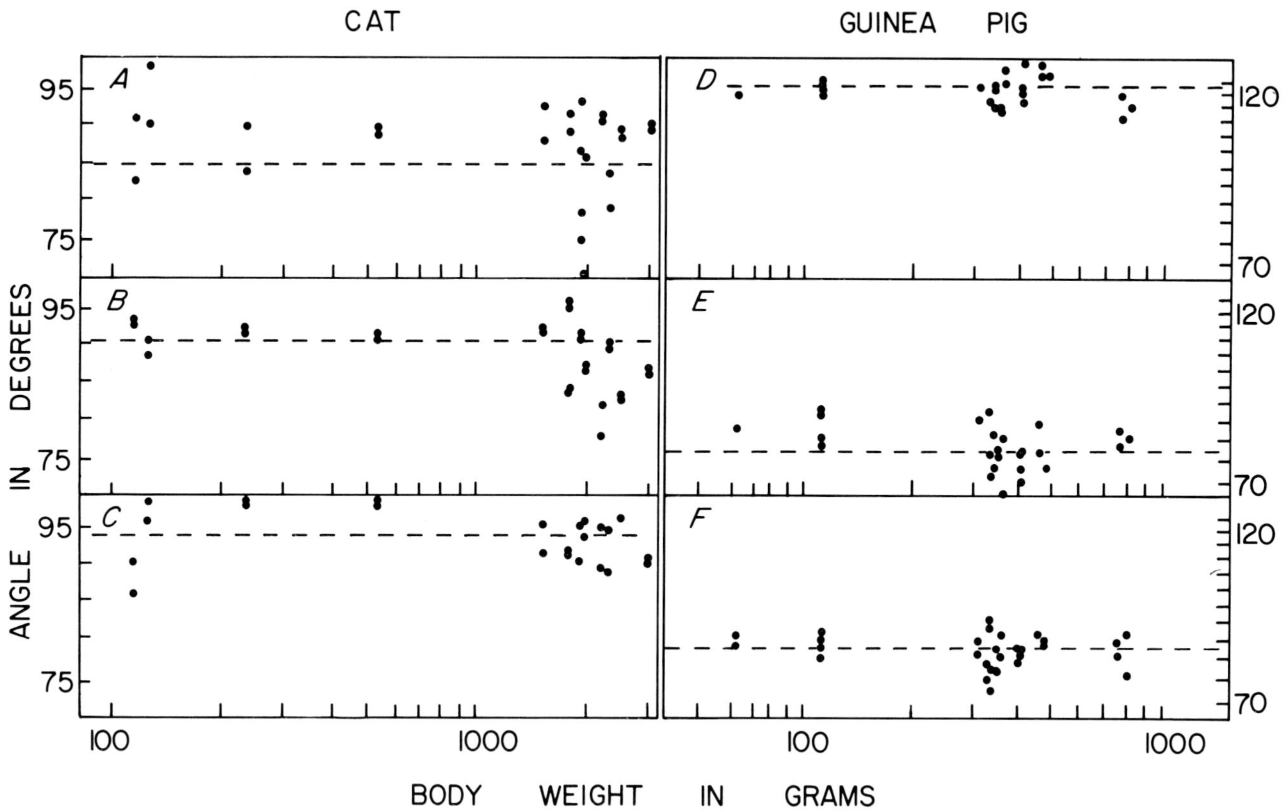

Fig. 1. Angles between canal planes at different stages of postnatal development for cat and guinea pig. Shown are the angles between the planes of A) and D), the horizontal and anterior canals; B) and E) the anterior and posterior canals; C) and F) the horizontal and posterior canals. The broken line in each graph is the mean of the adult population of the particular parameter.

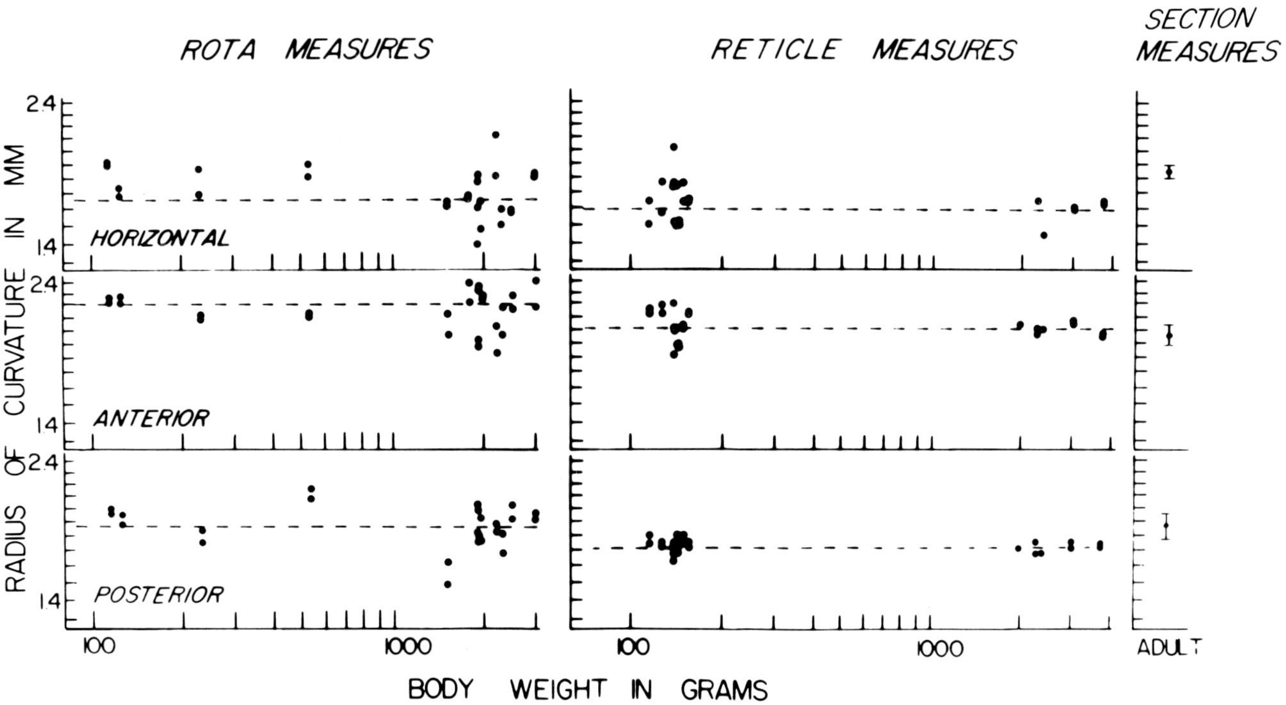

Fig. 2. Measures of the radii of curvature of the cat horizontal, anterior, and posterior semicircular canals during development. Left figures show measures using ROTA technique; center figures show measures using reticle technique on a different sample of cats. The section measures (right figures) are from an earlier study[12] and are measures made from serial sections from fixed, decalcified temporal bone from adult animals. The broken lines are the adult means of each set of measurements; the vertical bars in the section graphs show two-tailed 95% confidence intervals.

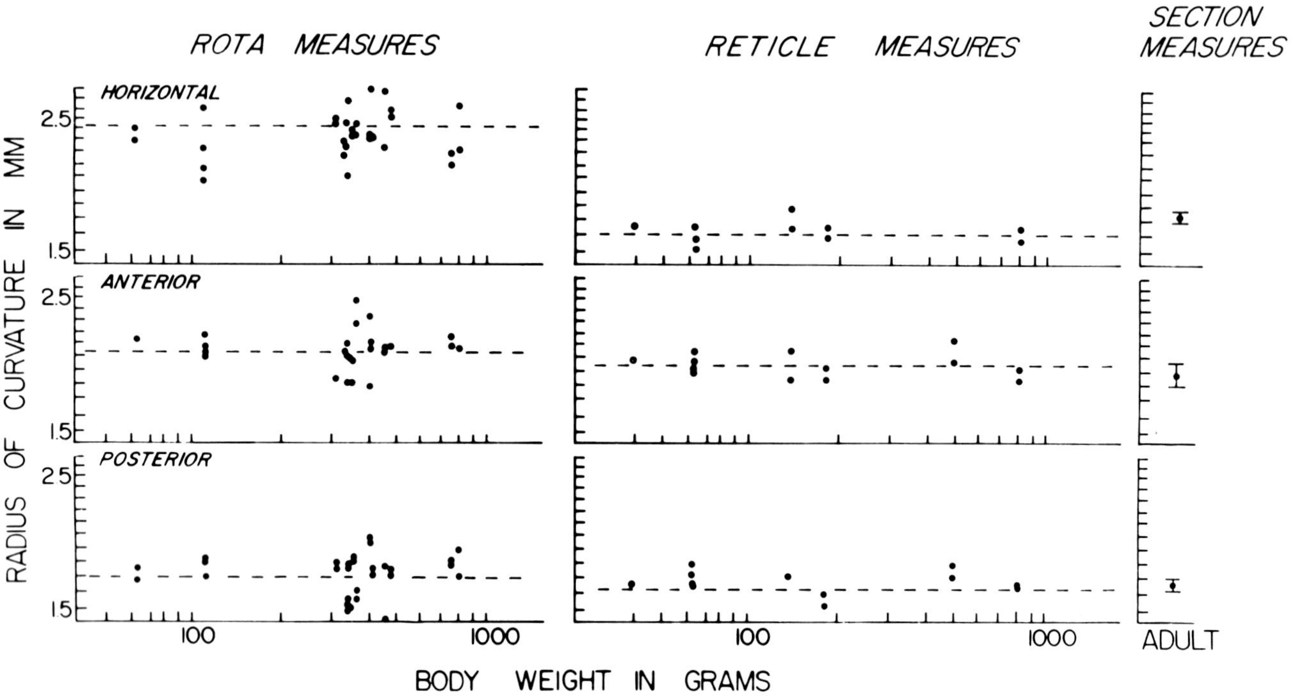

Fig. 3. Measures of the radii of curvature of guinea pig horizontal, anterior, and posterior canals during development. All conventions are the same as for Fig. 2.

ses were very similar and for convenience only the graphs showing the data relative to body weight are shown in Figures 1, 2, and 3. The broken lines in these figures indicate the adult means of the various parameters where "adult" refers to the means of the values from animals greater than 1000 g for the cat data and 150 g for the guinea pig data.

Postnatal Migration of Labyrinths. As the skull grows with age, the petrous temporal bones undergo a lateral displacement. In the adult cat, the shift between the centers of the horizontal, anterior, and posterior canal pairs (labyrinthine centers) averaged 11.2 mm (a 70% increase from birth) and in guinea pigs 3.55 mm (a 35% increase from birth). Correlation and regression coefficients for these parameters are given in the table. The correlation coefficients are very high, indicating a very close relationship between these distances and skull length. Each regression coefficient is statistically significant, and its value is the slope of the line relating the interaural distance to skull length.

Angular Interrelationships. Tests of the relationship between canal planes within the labyrinth and skull length yielded small correlation coefficients which were not statistically significant (the table, rows b-d). These results indicate that there are no detectable changes between canal planes during postnatal growth. That result is confirmed by inspection of Figure 1 which shows that the angles between canals in newborn animals are virtually identical to the angles between canals in adults. The sole exception is the angle between the anterior and posterior canal planes where the statistical analysis indicated a systematic change during growth.

Radii of Curvature. Tests of the relationship between radii of curvature *(R)* and skull length also yielded small correlation coefficients which were not statistically significant. These results were obtained with the two independent measuring techniques of *R*, ROTA (table, rows h-i) and reticle (table, rows k-m). These tests indicate that there are no detectable changes in *R* of any canal during postnatal growth. That result is confirmed by inspection of Figures 2 and 3 which shows for each canal that the radii of curvature of newborn animals are virtually identical to the radii of adult animals. The broken lines in Figures 2 and 3 indicate the

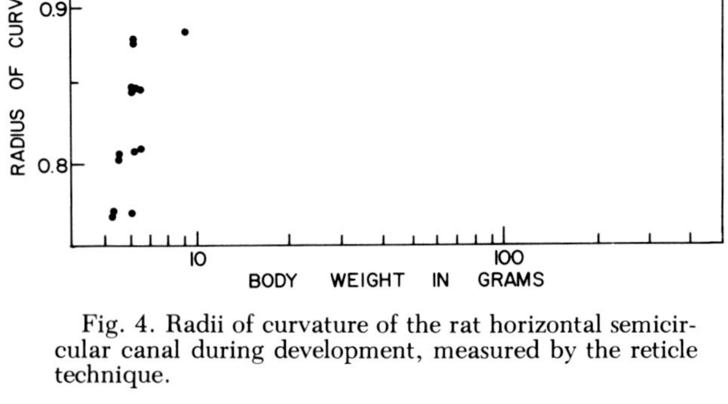

Fig. 4. Radii of curvature of the rat horizontal semicircular canal during development, measured by the reticle technique.

CORRELATION AND REGRESSION COEFFICIENTS FOR REGRESSIONS OF LABYRINTHINE MEASURES RELATED TO SKULL LENGTH

Regression of Each of the Following Related to Skull Length	Cat r	Cat B	Cat SE	Cat n	Guinea Pig r	Guinea Pig B	Guinea Pig SE	Guinea Pig n
a. Skull breadth	0.99*	1.06*	0.04	13	0.99*	1.13*	0.04	15
b. Angle between horizontal canal plane and anterior canal plane	-0.27	-0.06	0.04	26	-0.08	-0.02	0.06	25
c. Angle between anterior canal plane and posterior canal plane	-0.45	-0.07*	0.02	26	-0.33	-0.15	0.09	25
d. Angle between horizontal canal plane and posterior canal plane	-0.10	-0.02	0.03	26	-0.15	-0.05	0.06	29
e. Distance between centers of horizontal canals	0.98*	0.61*	0.03	13	0.93*	0.46*	0.05	15
f. Distance between centers of anterior canals	0.98*	0.64*	0.04	13	0.88*	0.42*	0.08	15
g. Distance between centers of posterior canals	0.98*	0.68*	0.05	13	0.90*	0.53*	0.07	15
h. ROTA *R* of horizontal canal	-0.34	-0.10	0.06	26	0.17	0.10	0.10	30
i. ROTA *R* of anterior canal	-0.17	-0.04	0.04	26	0.01	0.01	0.10	25
j. ROTA *R* of posterior canal	-0.21	-0.06	0.05	26	0.04	0.02	0.08	29
k. Reticle *R* of horizontal canal	-0.17	-0.04	0.05	22	-0.08	-0.01	0.06	10
l. Reticle *R* of anterior canal	-0.13	-0.02	0.03	24	-0.01	-0.01	0.06	13
m. Reticle *R* of posterior canal	-0.29	-0.02	0.01	24	-0.01	-0.01	0.06	12

r - Correlation coefficient; B - Regression coefficient; SE - Standard error of the regression coefficient; n - Number of the data pairs.
*Statistically significant ($p<0.05$).

adult means. Figures 2 and 3 also show in the far right panel means and 95% confidence intervals for measures of *Rh, Ra* and *Rp* obtained from histological studies from fixed and decalcified temporal bones of adult cats and guinea pigs from an earlier study.[10]

Growth of R in the Rat. In contrast to the cat and guinea pig, the value of *Rh* in the rat, measured with the reticle method, increased from birth (when the animal weighed about 5 g) to about ten days of age (when the animal weighed about 17 g).[15] At about this time, *Rh* has attained full adult size. The relationship between rat *Rh* and skull length was statistically significant showing that rat *Rh* does increase during growth (regression coefficient = 0.24, standard error = 0.04, $p<.001$). That result is confirmed by inspection of Figure 4 and demonstrates that the reticle method is sensitive enough to detect subtle developmental changes in *R*.

DISCUSSION

Radii of Curvature. The radii of curvature were measured in neonatal and adult guinea pigs and cats by two quite different techniques, ROTA and reticle, and no maturational changes were found for these species. The accuracy of ROTA and reticle leading to this conclusion is supported by a third method of measuring canal radii in which measurements were made from low-power magnifications of serial sections of fixed and decalcified temporal bones.[10] These values, made in adult cats and guinea pigs, are very similar to the values in adult animals using ROTA and reticle (Figs. 2 and 3, far right column).

There is reasonably good agreement between ROTA and reticle in neonatal and adult cats and guinea pigs and in the histological sectioning technique in adults (Figs. 2 and 3). The major exception is that *Rh* in guinea pigs as measured by ROTA is distinctly larger ($\overline{x}$ 2.4 mm) than for reticle ($\overline{x}$ 1.6 mm) or for the sectioning technique ($\overline{x}$ 1.75 mm). The reason for this erroneously large ROTA value is that the horizontal canal in the guinea pig has a markedly elliptical shape, rather than being circular. The ROTA data points for the guinea pig were taken from the shallow part of the ellipse, so the circle fitted to these points will be an overestimate of the true radius of curvature.

Close inspections of Figures 2 and 3 will reveal that the ROTA means are 0.1-0.2 mm larger than the reticle means for all *R*s, except *Rh* discussed above. If this represents a trend or systematic difference, it may be because the ROTA measures were made on arcs of the canals of about 140°, while the reticle values were obtained from arcs of about 180°.

The number of guinea pigs studied by the reticle technique was small, but encompassed a wide range of animal weights. The smallest guinea pig was premature and consequently smaller than average guinea pig birth weight. Yet, even in this animal the size of the canals was close to the mean adult size.

A major question in cases of such a null result is whether the techniques used have adequate power to detect any postnatal changes which may occur. This question was resolved by using the reticle technique to measure postnatal changes in the rat whose canals are reported to increase in diameter after birth.[14] Reticle measures in rats showed an increase in *Rh* with age (Fig. 4) which are statistically significant. We conclude that the reticle technique does have adequate power to detect postnatal changes in R; and since they were not detected in the cat and guinea pig, we conclude that the size of the semicircular canals does not change during postnatal development in cat and guinea pig.

In contrast to this conclusion, Fernández and Valentinuzzi[2] indicated that cat R continues to increase during life. They substituted weights of the smallest (1.7 kg) and largest (3.9 kg) adult cats they studied in an empirical formula which Jones and Spells[16] had established as relating R to body mass for mammals of *different* species:

$$\log_{10} = 0.1157 \log_{10} \underline{m} + 2.2466$$

where $\underline{m}$ is body mass in kilograms. This calculation yielded predicted radii of curvature of 1.8 mm for a 1.7 kg cat and 2.1 mm for a 3.9 kg cat.[2] These values were close to the radii of curvature they had measured in their animals, and they concluded that the Jones and Spells[16] formula applies *within* the species of cats during postnatal growth; in other words, canal R continues to increase during postnatal development. The discrepancy between their conclusion and ours probably lies in the very restricted range of adult cat weights they studied; their extreme values were 1.7 and 3.9 kg compared to our sample which ranged from 0.115-3.8 kg.

The consequences of using a restricted weight range can also be seen in our cat ROTA data where for the three canals the ROTA R of the largest adult is larger than the ROTA R of the smallest adult (Fig. 2). Had we studied only these particular largest and smallest adult skulls we would have agreed with Fernández and Valentinuzzi. However the measurement of other adult animals in the present study and more importantly the measurement of very young animals clearly shows that the data from these particular animals are chance variations and that there is no systematic postnatal developmental change in R. Furthermore the variability of our data is small enough so that even small systematic increases in the magnitude of R would have been detected, and indeed an increase of only 0.3 mm was clearly detected by the reticle method in the rat data.

Is there a "best" method to measure R? Measures of R from temporal bone serial histologic sections require extensive reconstruction and it is therefore an indirect method. The ROTA method is also indirect and tends to be based upon a somewhat smaller arc of the semicircular canal than reticle and to provide values which were consistently larger than those provided by the reticle method. The reticle technique is simple, direct, and powerful. Departures from circularity are observed and their effect can be minimized. It would seem that as long as the semicircular canals are approximated as a circle in mathematical treatments of canal operations, rather than exact specifications of canal shape, the measure provided by reticle is simplest and least subject to error.

Angular Relations Between Canal Planes. The present regression analysis between ipsilateral pairs of canals are remarkably constant throughout the postnatal period, despite the increasing mass of the temporal bone and the lateral migration of the labyrinths within the skull (see below). In the two species studied, only one angular relationship in the cat was found to change during postnatal growth. This was the angle between the planes of the anterior and posterior canals in the cat, which decreased from $90.2° \pm 2.51°$ in two neonates ($n = 4$ angles) measured to a mean of $87.0° \pm 4.23°$ (standard deviation) in the adult ($n = 16$). Keeping in mind that as a canal is tipped out of the plane of angular acceleration the force acting in the plane of the canal decreases in a cosine fashion, the angular difference of 3.2° correponds only to a 0.2% reduction ($\cos 3.2° = 0.998$) in the plane component of the applied stimulus. Physiological investigations of cat primary afferents[17] indicate that an angular difference of this size is too small to be functionally significant.

The constancy in angular interrelationships suggests it is not necessary to postulate any development-dependent mechanism to decode instantaneous head position in order to produce appropriate compensatory responses in these species.

Labyrinth Migration in the Skull. Although the angular interrelationships and canal radii remain fixed in both species during postnatal growth, the two labyrinths do move apart by an average of 70% in cats and 35% in guinea pigs. The functional significance, if any, of such labyrinth migration remains to be established.

In the literature we found reports suggesting there are probably only small changes in canal size and planar relationships within the labyrinth in the human during postnatal growth.[18,19] Hadziselimovic[20] concluded that some rotation of the whole temporal bone occurs during early human life. Sato[21] referred to similar small changes in the "inclining angles" of the human posterior canal. Bellocq[22] has noted that human canal R changes minimally during postnatal growth. Regarding growth of the labyrinth in the human fetus, Anson[18] has commented, "In the short period of approximately five months (4½ to 25 weeks) the otocyst gives rise to a membranous labyrinth of full size and adult form."

Functional Significance of Canal R. With maturation in the cat, there is a gradual increase in gain of the VOR as measured during sinusoidal oscillation. Adult values are achieved at about 60 days after birth.[1] Since R does not change in the cat, this increase in gain of the VOR would appear to be due to changes in receptor cells or first-order vestibular afferents,[23-25] or vestibular nucleus neurons,[26] or the commissural system between the vestibular nuclei,[27] or a combination of these.

In the rat, the situation is different. The present investigation, confirming that of Clark,[14] shows that the horizontal semicircular canal of the rat continues to grow after birth, reaching adult size about ten days after birth. In the rat, postnatal developmental changes in VOR gain have not yet been measured. However, postnatal developmental changes in the gain of rat primary and secondary vestibular neurons have been measured.[28-30] Even in these peripheral elements in the VOR system there is an early increase in gain when the canal radius is increasing, in line with the expectation from the torsion pendulum model. However, the gain of rat secondary vestibular neurons continues to increase for at least 35 days after birth,[30] long after the canals have reached their full adult size (ten days after birth, Fig. 4). Again, as in the cat, factors other than canal radius size must be operating to cause this later increase in gain although canal size is probably a factor in determining the early increase in gain.

Finally, further evidence that canal radius is not of major importance in determining the development of VOR gain comes from studies of species where *R* increases but VOR gain remains constant. In fish the semicircular canals continue to increase in size throughout life[31-36] in contrast to the early development and typical postnatal stability of the mammalian semicircular canal structure.[37-40] Yet despite the continuous increase in *R* of the pike canals ten Kate was unable to detect any concomitant changes in the gain of the pike VOR during development.[31]

CONCLUSION

In the cat and guinea pig structural changes in canal radius of curvature and angular interrelationships during postnatal development are less than structural differences between individuals. We conclude that in these species such factors do not determine postnatal changes in the gain of the vestibulo-ocular reflex. Factors such as receptor and afferent neuron maturation[23-25] and maturation of central connections[26] would appear to be the major cause of any postnatal changes in VOR gain.

ACKNOWLEDGMENTS — Computing assistance was obtained from the Health Sciences Computing Facility, UCLA, sponsored by NIH Special Research Resources Grant RR-3. We are grateful to Dr. Peter Wenderoth for discussions and statistical advice and to Jan Curthoys for her continuing assistance.

REFERENCES

1. Flandrin JM, Courjon JH, Jeannerod M. Development of the vestibulo-ocular response in the kitten. Neurosci Lett 1979; 12:295-9.

2. Fernández C, Valentinuzzi M. A study on the biophysical characteristics of the cat labyrinth. Acta Otolaryngol (Stockh) 1968; 65:293-310.

3. Wilson VJ, Melvill Jones G. Mammalian vestibular physiology. New York: Plenum Press, 1979.

4. Curthoys IS, Blanks RHI, Markham CH. Semicircular canal functional anatomy in cat, guinea pig and man. Acta Otolaryngol (Stockh) 1977; 83:258-65.

5. Bessesen AN, Carlson HA. Postnatal growth in weight of the body and of the various organs in the guinea pig. Am J Anat 1923; 31:483-521.

6. Draper RL. The prenatal growth of the guinea pig. Anat Rec 1920; 18:369-92.

7. Nelson NS, Cooper J. The growing conceptus of the domestic cat. Growth 1975; 39:435-51.

8. Blanks RHI, Curthoys IS, Markham CH. Planar relationships of semicircular canals in the cat. Am J Physiol 1972; 223:55-62.

9. Curthoys IS, Curthoys EJ, Blanks RHI, Markham CH. The orientation of the semicircular canals in the guinea pig. Acta Otolaryngol (Stockh) 1975; 80:197-205.

10. Curthoys IS, Blanks RHI, Markham CH. Semicircular canal functional anatomy in cat, guinea pig and man. Acta Otolaryngol (Stockh) 1977; 83:258-65.

11. Blanks RHI, Curthoys IS, Markham CH. Planar relationships of the semicircular canals in man. Acta Otolaryngol (Stockh) 1975; 80:185-96.

12. Curthoys IS, Markham CH, Curthoys EJ. Semicircular duct and ampulla dimensions in cat, guinea pig and man. J Morphol 1977; 151:17-34.

13. Curthoys IS, Blanks RHI, Markham CH. Semicircular canal radii of curvature (R) in cat, guinea pig, and man. J Morphol 1977; 151:1-16.

14. Clark DL. Correlative postnatal vestibular development. Report RF 2988. Columbus: Ohio State University Research Foundation, 1973.

15. Curthoys IS, Webber SCA. Techniques for acute single neuron recording in newborn rats. Physiol Behav 1977; 19:689-92.

16. Jones GM, Spells KE. A theoretical and comparative study of the functional dependence of the semicircular canal upon its physical dimensions. Proc Roy Soc Lond [Biol] 1963; 157:403-19.

17. Blanks RHI, Estes MS, Markham CH. Physiologic characteristics of vestibular first order canal neurons in the cat: II. Response to constant angular acceleration. J Neurophysiol 1975; 38:1250-68.

18. Anson BJ. The labyrinths and their capsule in health and disease. Trans Am Acad Ophthalmol Otolaryngol 1969; 73:17-38.

19. Elliott GB, Elliott KA. Some pathological, radiological and clinical implications of the precocious development of the human ear. Laryngoscope 1964; 74:1160-71.

20. Hadziselimovic H. Contribution to knowledge of the bony labyrinth and interfenestral axis in certain mammals and man. Acta Anat (Basel) 1968; 70:54-65.

21. Sato T. Vergleichende Untersuchungen über die Bogengänge des Labyrinthes beim Neugeborenen und beim erwachsenen Menschen. Z Ohrenheilkd 1903; 42:137-56.

22. Bellocq P. Sur les changements qui se produisent au niveau du labyrinthe osseux au cours de la croissance chez l'homme et sur les causes qui les determinent. C R Assoc Ant 1923; 18:71-8.

23. Brument N, Pujol R, Sans A, Marty R. Maturation epitheliale des recepteurs dans l'oreille interne de chat. C R Soc Biol (Paris) 1969; 163:688-92.

24. Romand R, Sans A, Romand MR, Marty R. The structural maturation of the stato-acoustic nerve in the cat. J Comp Neurol 1976; 170:1-16.

25. Favre D, Sans A. Embryonic and postnatal development of different innervation of cat vestibular receptors. Acta Otolaryngol (Stockh) 1979; 87:97-107.

26. Sans A, Chat M. Maturation post-natale des noyaux vestibulaires chez le chat: etude histologique par la methode de Golgi Cox. Brain Res 1976; 111:13-30.

27. Markham CH, Yagi T, Curthoys IS. The contribution of the contralateral labyrinth to second order vestibular neuronal activity in the cat. Brain Res 1977; 138:99-109.

28. Curthoys IS. The development of function of horizontal semicircular canal primary neurons in the rat. Brain Res 1979; 167:41-52.

29. Curthoys IS. The vestibulo-ocular reflex in newborn rats. Acta Otolaryngol (Stockh) 1979; 87:484-9.

30. Lannou J, Precht W, Cazin L. The postnatal development of functional properties of central vestibular neurons in the rat. Brain Res 1979; 175:219-32.

31. Ten Kate JH. The oculo-vestibular reflex of the growing pike: a biophysical study, thesis. Rijksuniversiteit te Groningen, Netherlands, 1969.

32. Ten Kate JH. The mechanics of the growing semicircular canal. J Exp Biol 1973; 58:351-62.

33. Howland HC, Masci J. The phylogenetic allometry of the semicircular canals of small fishes. Z Morphol Tiere 1973; 75:283-96.

34. Howland HC, Masci J. The functional allometry of semicircular canals, fins and body dimensions in the juvenile centrarchid fish, *Lepomis gibbosus* (L.). J Embryol Exp Morphol 1973; 29:721-43.

35. Gray O. An introduction of the study of the comparative anatomy of the labyrinth. J Laryngol Otol 1951; 65:681-703.

36. Werner CF. Wachstum und Formvariation des Labyrinths in ihrem Verhaltnis zu gehirn und Schadel. I bei Rochen (Raja batis und Raja Clavata). Anat Anz 1927; 63:225-37.

37. Girard L. Le plan des canaux horizontaux considere comme plan horizontal de la tete. Bull Mem Soc Anthropol Paris 1923; 14:14-33.

38. Perez F. Craniologie vestibienne, ethnique et zoologique. Bull Mem Soc Anthropol Paris 1922; 13:16-32.

39. Altmann F. Normal development of the ear and its mechanics. Arch Otolaryngol 1950; 52:725-66.

40. Turkewitsch BG. Zur Anatomie des Gehororgans der Vogel. Z Anat Entwicklungsgesch 1934; 103:551-608.

≈

CASSELBERRY AWARD

The American Laryngological Association announces that it will receive essays or theses relating to the art and science of laryngology and rhinology for consideration of the Casselberry Award for 1981-82. The Award is open to physicians, interns, residents and graduate students in laryngology and rhinology in the Americas and scientists in the field in laryngology and rhinology. For information write to: William M. Trible, MD, Secretary, American Laryngological Association, 1234 19th Street, NW, Washington, DC 20036.

VATERITE OTOCONIA IN TWO CASES OF OTOCONIAL MEMBRANE DYSPLASIA

CHARLES G. WRIGHT, PhD
DALLAS, TEXAS

ROLAND C. ROUSE, PhD
LARS-G. JOHNSSON, MD
ANN ARBOR, MICHIGAN

ARTHUR G. WEINBERG, MD
DAVID G. HUBBARD, MD
DALLAS, TEXAS

Scanning electron microscopy, electron microprobe analysis, and x-ray powder diffraction were used to study temporal bone specimens obtained at autopsy from an infant with Potter syndrome and from a second trimester fetus, which was the product of an elective abortion. The mothers of both the infant and fetus were juvenile-onset rheumatoid arthritis patients who took prostaglandin inhibitors during pregnancy. The infant's external ears were low set and the left ear canal was stenotic. The vestibular maculae on the left were covered by aberrant otoconia composed of vaterite. In the right inner ear, otoconia were entirely absent, although the gelatinous otoconial membranes were intact. Only the left saccule and right utricle from the fetus were studied; both contained vaterite crystals similar to those in the infant. In addition, apatite was present in the fetal utricle, apparently lying on the macula beneath the vaterite otoconia.

INTRODUCTION

The otoconial membranes, which overlie the vestibular maculae, are made up of sheets of gelatinous material covered by calcareous crystals called otoconia. It is now well established that the otoconia (and otoliths) of almost all vertebrates are composed of calcium carbonate ($CaCO_3$) together with an admixed organic fraction usually termed the otoconial matrix.[1,2] In mammals, the inorganic mineral material is normally present in the form of calcite, which is the trigonal polymorph of calcium carbonate.[1]

Recent studies of the vestibular apparatus have combined electron microscopy with microanalytic techniques to provide new data on development and structure of the otoconial membranes of man as well as a variety of experimental animals.[3-6] In addition, information is now becoming available regarding alterations of the otoconia in association with human ear pathology. Degeneration of saccular otoconia has, for example, been described in connection with aging by Johnsson and Hawkins[7] and by Ross et al.[4] There also exists evidence that otoconia may be morphologically altered in some cases of otitis media.[8] Moreover, congenital absence of otoconial crystals in a human infant was recently described by Wright et al.[9]

In this report, we present two cases in which anomalous otoconia, composed of vaterite (the hexagonal polymorph of $CaCO_3$), were found in inner ear specimens. One of these was an infant with Potter syndrome; the other was a second trimester fetus, which was the product of a prostaglandin-induced abortion. In both instances the mothers were juvenile-onset rheumatoid arthritis patients, who took prostaglandin synthetase-inhibiting drugs during pregnancy.

METHODS

Preparation of Specimens. Temporal bone specimens were taken from the newborn infant at autopsy. The middle ears were opened, the stapes gently removed from each of the oval windows, and the inner ear structures fixed by perilymphatic perfusion with 1% veronal acetate-buffered osmium tetroxide (pH 7.4) approximately 12 hours postmorten. After partial dehydration in 50% ethyl alcohol, whole-mount preparations of the inner ear sensory organs were obtained by microdissection.[10] These specimens were subsequently processed for light or scanning electron microscopy (SEM). The vestibular maculae were taken stepwise to 100% alcohol, critical point dried, and sputter coated with gold-palladium. All material was removed from alcohol and dried within 36 hours after it was obtained at autopsy.

The fetus was one of several specimens from which fresh, unfixed otoconia were taken for SEM in connection with another study. The microdissection was carried out in saline. Saccular otoconia were obtained from the left ear and utricular otoconia from the right ear. The samples were air dried and coated with gold.

Electron Microscopy and Analytical Procedures. Preparations from the infant were studied with a JEOL JSM 35 scanning electron microscope operated at an accelerating voltage of 15 kV. The fetal specimens were examined using a JEOL JSM U3 instrument at 15 and 25 kV. Qualitative chemical analyses of the fetal otoconia were made with a Kevex solid state x-ray detector coupled to a Tracor Northern Scientific Model 710 multichannel analyzer.

In both cases, identification of the crystal samples was made by

From The Callier Center for Communication Disorders, University of Texas at Dallas; Kresge Hearing Research Institute, University of Michigan, Ann Arbor; Department of Pathology and Pediatrics, Children's Medical Center and The Behavioral Research Center, Dallas. This investigation was supported by USPHS research grants NS 16236, NS 11672, NS 12706, NS 05065, DE 034443, and Program Project Grant NS 05785. Support was also provided by the Research Fund of the American Otological Society, Inc., and by the Leland Fikes Foundation, Dallas.

REPRINTS — Charles G. Wright, PhD, The Callier Center for Communication Disorders, 1966 Inwood Road, Dallas, TX 75235.

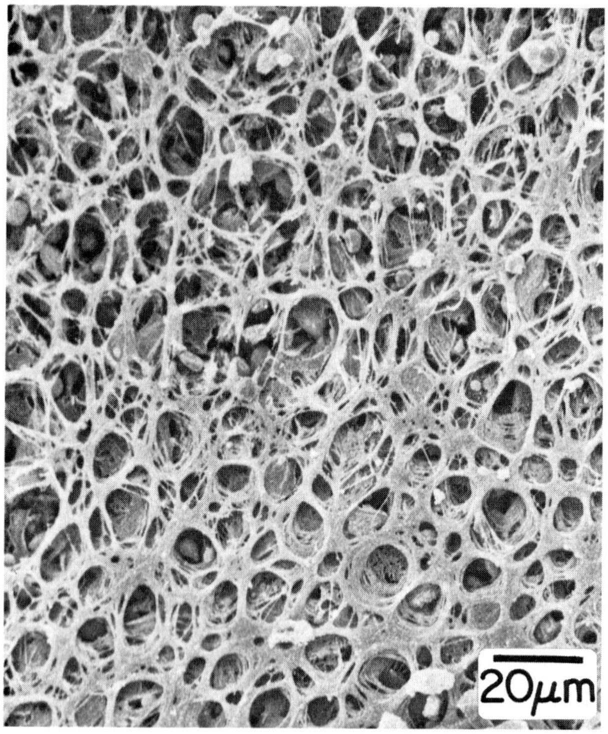

Fig. 1. (Case 1) Central portion of the otoconial membrane from right utricle of infant with Potter syndrome. Globules of organic material are visible within the gelatinous meshwork of the membrane; however, no otoconial crystals were present.

x-ray diffraction. Small pieces of each otoconial mass were glued to the tips of glass fibers and mounted in a 114.6 mm diameter Debye-Scherrer camera. Since the crystallites were already small enough to give good powder photographs, the usual reduction of the samples to powders by grinding was unnecessary. This was fortunate because grinding may induce artifactual phase transformations in vaterite, yielding a mixture of vaterite, calcite, and aragonite.[11]

CASE REPORTS AND RESULTS

Case 1. The 2,750 g female infant was born to a 34-year-old mother after a gestation of approximately 36 weeks. The fetal membranes were said to be ruptured at the time of delivery; thus the presence of oligohydramnios could not be confirmed in the obstetric record. During pregnancy the mother had taken three prostaglandin synthetase inhibitors for treatment of juvenile-onset rheumatoid arthritis. These drugs included aspirin (6 tablets/day), sulindac (300 mg/day), and indomethacin (dosage unspecified in clinical history). There was no family history of congenital defects of the kidneys, heart, or other organs. From the time of birth, the infant showed profound respiratory insufficiency and respiratory failure resulted in death at 12 hours postpartum.

At autopsy, phenotypic features typical of Potter syndrome were noted. The mandible was small, the ears were low set and posteriorly rotated, and the feet had a rocker-bottom configuration. Bilateral cataracts were also present. No preauricular or cervical fistulae were noted. The infant had bilateral

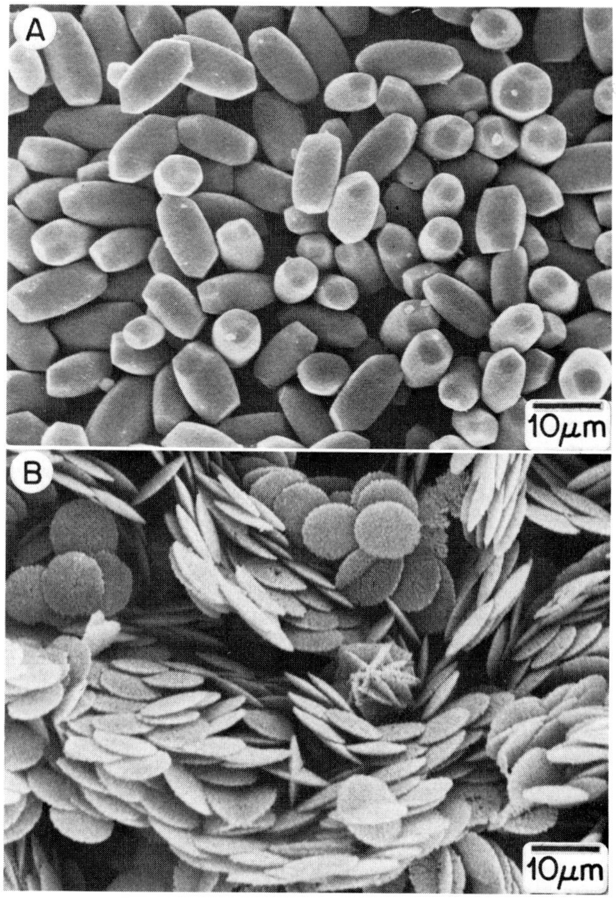

Fig. 2. A) Normal saccular otoconia from a young adult. B) (Case 1) Aberrant saccular otoconia, composed of vaterite, from left labyrinth.

pulmonary hypoplasia and microscopic examination revealed hyaline membrane disease. Both kidneys were completely dysplastic, the left ureter was atretic, and the bladder was hypoplastic. The labia majora were prominent; however, no abnormalities were found in the vagina, uterus, fallopian tubes, or ovaries.

The left external ear canal was stenotic and the tympanic annulus was narrowed so that the tympanic membrane was slightly reduced in surface area. Otherwise, both middle ears were normal. Careful study revealed no abnormalities of the cochlear structures (including the stria vascularis) or the semicircular canals.

Immediately after the temporal bones were opened and before fixative was introduced into the labyrinth, the contents of both vestibules were examined through the open oval windows with the aid of an operating microscope. No otoconia were seen on either the saccular or utricular macula of the right side. On the left, a thin layer of crystals covered the saccular neuroepithelium; it was possible to see that otoconia were also present on the macula of the utricle.

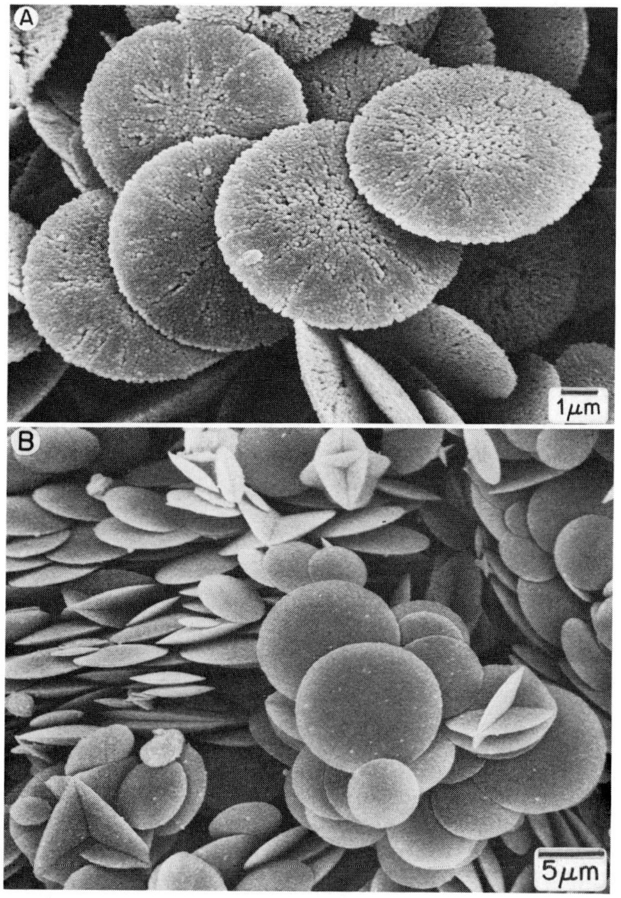

Fig. 3. (Case 1) A) Higher power view of crystals from left saccule. These lenticular vaterite otoconia appear to be composed of numerous tiny spherules. B) Vaterite crystals from left utricle.

Microdissection confirmed the total absence of otoconia on the right side. However, the gelatinous layers of the otoconial membranes were intact on both maculae. Figure 1 shows a portion of the bare gelatinous otoconial membrane of the right utricle. In small areas where the gelatinous layer was incomplete, normal-appearing stereocilia bundles were noted on the maculae.

Scanning electron microscopy revealed that the left saccular and utricular maculae were each covered by a thin layer of discoid, biconvex crystals (Figs. 2 and 3). The wafer-like, lenticular crystals in the saccule varied from approximately 4 to 10 μ in diameter and had an eroded or pitted appearance suggestive of partial dissolution. These crystals were strikingly different from normal otoconia in morphology (Fig. 2) and many of them appeared to be structurally nonhomogeneous, being lenticular aggregates of numerous tiny spherulites (Fig. 3A). The utricular crystals, on the other hand, had smooth surfaces and ranged from approximately 2 to 10 μ in width. Intergrowth of two or more adjacent crystals, resulting in intricate and sometimes bizarre patterns (Fig. 3B), was more frequently seen in the utricle than in the saccule.

X-ray diffraction analyses were done on crystal samples from both maculae. In each case, powder diffraction patterns characteristic of calcium carbonate in the form of vaterite were obtained. Unit cell parameters of the utricular crystals were refined by least-squares using the Debye-Scherrer data and an NBS silicon (a = 5.43088 Å) internal standard. The values obtained were a = 7.138 (1) and c = 16.989 (4) Å (numbers in parentheses are standard deviations times 1,000). These figures differ slightly from those determined by Meyer[12] for synthetic vaterite (a = 7.151 and c = 16.941 Å, average of three) with a silicon standard; however, the differences are probably not significant.

Regarding the overall condition of the saccule and utricle, it should be mentioned that the myelinated innervation supplying the maculae of both sides had a normal light-microscopic appearance and no obvious defects of the neuroepithelia were evident. However, except for observation of stereocilia bundles in a few areas, it did not prove possible to make any detailed evaluation of the macular neuroepithelia.

Case 2. The 284 g female fetus included in this study was the product of an elective prostaglandin-induced abortion at approximately 20 weeks of gestation. The mother was a 23-year-old primipara who had juvenile-onset rheumatoid arthritis which apparently converted to systemic lupus erythematosus at age 21. During the pregnancy she took 15 aspirin tablets and 15 mg of prednisone daily.

The fetus showed well-balanced growth with no external malformations and normal visceral anatomy, including normal kidneys. The membranous labyrinths had normal shape; however, the condition of the cochlear hair cells and vestibular neuroepithelia could not be determined.

As in the Potter syndrome infant, it was found that both the saccular and utricular otoconia of the fetus were thin biconvex lenses (Fig. 4). These crystals ranged from 1 to 15 μ in diameter with little size difference between saccular and utricular samples. Some of the saccular otoconia appeared to be in various stages of degeneration, with the dissolution process beginning in the central portion of the lens and proceeding outward (Fig. 4B).

Upon x-ray diffraction analysis the saccular otoconia gave a pure vaterite pattern, while the utricular sample contained a mixture of vaterite and apatite $[Ca_5(PO_4,CO_3)_3\ (OH,F,Cl)]$. Since only lenticular crystals were observed by SEM, we infer that the apatite was buried under the lenses. In fact, when a fragment of the otoconial mass was scanned and chemically analyzed by microprobe in cross section, some amorphous-looking material in the central portion produced a strong phosphorus signal not given by the lenses.

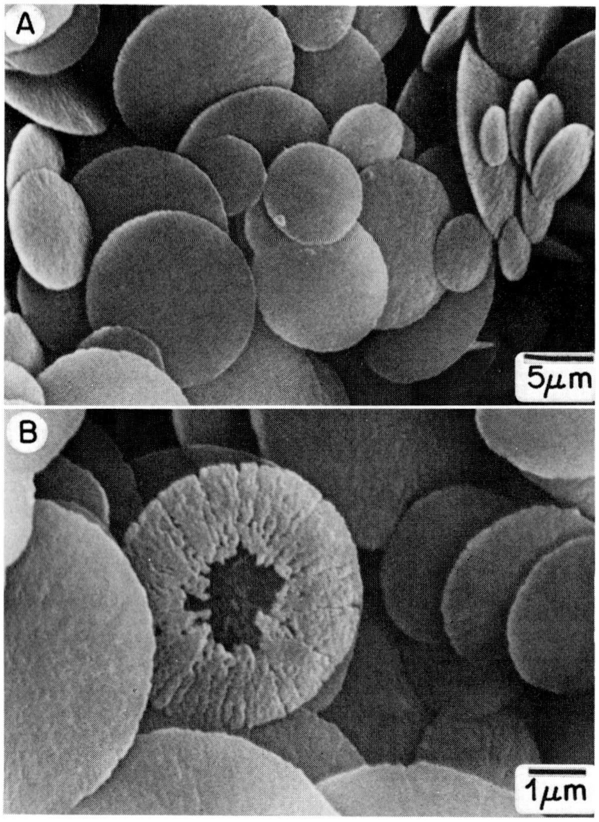

Fig. 4. (Case 2) A) Vaterite crystals from utricle. B) Otoconia from fetal saccule illustrating dissolution of the central part of a vaterite crystal.

The qualitative chemical composition of the vaterite crystals, obtained by energy-dispersive x-ray analysis, resembles that of normal human otoconia.[4] The x-ray emission spectrum of the lenses from the fetus indicated major calcium, minor phosphorus, and a trace of magnesium. The phosphorus was probably a constituent of the organic matrix material of the crystals. The magnesium, on the other hand, was almost certainly a minor substituent for calcium in the vaterite structure.

DISCUSSION

At present, relatively little information is available concerning alterations of the otoconial membranes in association with inner ear pathology; this is particularly true in regard to developmental defects of the vestibular apparatus. In fact, the cases described here are among the first reported instances of congenital otoconial dysplasia in human material.

The absence of crystals in the right inner ear of the infant was noted at the time the temporal bones were opened for fixation; it cannot, therefore, be attributed to fixation or storage artifact. Moreover, it is very unlikely that either the absence of otoconia or the presence of vaterite represents a postmortem artifact, since long postmortem delays before fixation of human and experimental animal specimens have never produced such effects.[4,9]

Although there were no otoconia in the infant's right labyrinth, the gelatinous otoconial membranes were intact on the saccular and utricular maculae. This condition is like that found in a case recently reported by Wright et al[9] in which there was bilateral, congenital absence of otoconia. It is also a morphological parallel to the agenesis of otoconial crystals which occurs in several species of genetically defective experimental animals such as the pallid mouse.[13,14]

In the left inner ear of the infant, and in the fetus, the vestibular maculae were covered by crystals composed of vaterite. Of the three naturally occurring polymorphs of $CaCO_3$ (calcite, aragonite, and vaterite), vaterite is the rarest and least stable.[15] Though seldom found in geological systems, vaterite is synthesized by a variety of animals. It is, for example, present in the spicules of certain tunicates,[16] on the surfaces of the egg capsules of ampullarid snails,[17] and in the egg shells of the nonparasitic cuckoos.[18] It is also formed during repair and regeneration of the shell in some species of mollusks.[19] Prior to this report, the only known occurrences of vaterite in man were in urinary,[20] biliary,[21] and pancreatic[22] calculi, where it has been noted as a fine-grained constituent of unknown morphology.

During his extensive phylogenetic studies on the composition of vertebrate otoliths, Carlström[1] found that vaterite is normally formed in the vestibular organs of certain primitive fish, including the gar, bowfin, and bichir. In these species, lenticular vaterite crystals are associated with the large aragonite (orthorhombic $CaCO_3$) otoliths which overlie the macular neuroepithelia. Aberrant otoliths consisting of vaterite have been reported to occur occasionally in a teleost fish, the cod,[23] which like other teleosts normally synthesizes aragonite. Among birds and mammals the otoconia are normally composed exclusively of calcite[1] and developmental studies have shown that vaterite is not an intermediate in the formation of calcite during the fetal period.[24]

Both vaterite and apatite were present in the fetal utricle, with the apatite apparently lying beneath the mass of vaterite crystals. The spatial relationship of the two minerals implies that precipitation was episodic, the sequence being apatite followed by vaterite. The existence of two such chemically dissimilar phases on the otoconial membrane indicates that significant changes in composition of the endolymph occurred before and during the course of precipitation. In particular, the presence of apatite implies a much higher phosphate concentration than the approximately 0.8 m*M* of normal endolymph.[25] However, a high phosphate concentration would prevent precipitation of any form of calcium carbonate until after removal of most of the phosphate from solution by calcium phosphate formation.[26] The predicted precipitation sequence is therefore apatite, vaterite in agreement with observation.

Although we can only speculate on the composition of the endolymph during the time of apatite formation, the presence of a phosphate rather than a carbonate phase does suggest a major homeostatic disturbance of the inner ear fluids. Johnsson and Hawkins[27] have found, for example, that apatite may be formed in the human vestibular labyrinth when the integrity of the membranous wall or the neuroepithelia is severely compromised.

The overall issue of pathogenesis in the present cases is complicated by a variety of potentially significant factors including renal pathology, maternal disease, and drug treatment during pregnancy.

The fascinating immunological, anatomical, and physiological relationships between the inner ear and the kidney have been the focus of considerable attention during recent years[28,29] and several cases in which renal and ear anomalies were combined with other congenital defects have been reported.[30] Our Potter syndrome case represents another instance in which ear defects have been associated with renal abnormalities as part of a constellation of multiple anomalies. In this case, the family history did not suggest a hereditary basis for the observed anomalies.

Both mothers in our study had juvenile-onset rheumatoid arthritis; in the mother of the fetus the arthritis converted to systemic lupus approximately two years before her pregnancy. We are aware of no evidence that connective-tissue disease in the mother might play any direct role in producing developmental defects like those described here. It is, however, well known that the incidence of fetal wastage in mothers with systemic lupus is quite high.[31] In addition, abnormal IgG antibodies from the mother do cross the placenta and have been implicated in congenital heart block in infants born to mothers with lupus and/or rheumatoid arthritis.[31,32] Histological study of specimens from cases of fatal congenital heart block has revealed extensive connective tissue disease of the cardiac conduction system.[33]

Another factor which must be considered is the possibility that the drug treatment these patients received played a pathogenic role. This is particularly true with regard to aspirin administration. In addition to being ototoxic in adult animals,[34] salicylates have been shown to produce skeletal defects[35] in mammalian fetuses and have been implicated in developmental anomalies in man.[36,37]

In view of the otoconial defects described above, it is of special interest that salicylates are inhibitors of acid mucopolysaccharide synthesis during fetal development.[38] Sulfated acid mucopolysaccharides are thought to be essential compounds in the synthesis of the organic otoconial matrix.[39] There is, in fact, evidence that a genetic abnormality in mucopolysaccharide metabolism is a critical factor in the agenesis of otoconia which occurs in animals such as the pallid mutant mouse.[40]

In connection with possible pharmacological influences, it should also be noted that the nonsteroid prostaglandin inhibitors indomethacin and sulindac may cause tinnitus and dizziness as side effects in patients receiving these drugs for arthritis treatment.[41,42]

Crystallization of calcium carbonate in biological systems usually occurs in association with an organic matrix. Although the composition of the organic material in mammalian otoconia is not yet known, the structure of the organic otolith matrix of a wide phylogenetic range of fish species has been determined by Degens et al.[43] They found the material to be a protein with a high acidic amino acid content and a molecular weight of approximately 150,000. Using mollusks as experimental models, Wilbur and Watabe[19] have shown that the structure of the proteinaceous matrix material can determine which of the three calcium carbonate polymorphs will be laid down by a given species. We might therefore hypothesize that the otoconial anomalies in our cases were the result of defects in the synthesis of matrix material essential for formation of calcite otoconia. Such defects might prevent deposition of $CaCO_3$ completely or result in production of a matrix suitable only for crystallization of vaterite.

As an alternate hypothesis, it is possible that the formation of vaterite in these cases was due entirely to alterations in physicochemical properties of the endolymph rather than to matrix defects. Which of the polymorphs of $CaCO_3$ precipitates from aqueous solution in vitro is influenced by conditions which include temperature, pH, and the degree of supersaturation prevailing during crystal nucleation and growth.[44] It is known, for example, that a high degree of supersaturation with respect to calcium carbonate is especially favorable to the formation of vaterite[45] and, in fact, lenticular vaterite crystals resembling the anomalous otoconia described here have been produced synthetically.[46] The possibility of altered endolymph composition has been mentioned above in connection with the presence of apatite in the fetus. Analogous (and perhaps related) abnormalities in the physicochemical properties of the labyrinthine fluid environment may have promoted the crystallization of vaterite in both cases we studied.

At present, we clearly lack sufficient information to determine whether drug treatment or other factors, such as the presence of maternal collagen disease, played a part in producing the anomalies described in this report; nor can we make firm conclusions regarding the basic mechanism responsible for the deposition of vaterite. It is our hope, however, that the etiology of such developmental defects will be further clarified in the course of future case studies and/or experimental animal work.

ACKNOWLEDGMENT — The authors wish to thank Mason Barr, Jr., MD, Director, Teratology Unit, University of Michigan Medical School, for consultation during this study.

REFERENCES

1. Carlström D. A crystallographic study of vertebrate otoliths. Biol Bull 1963; 125:441-63.

2. Lim DJ. Formation and fate of the otoconia. Ann Otol Rhinol Laryngol 1973; 82:23-35.

3. Ross MD, Peacor D. The nature and crystal growth of otoconia in the rat. Ann Otol Rhinol Laryngol 1975; 84:22-36.

4. Ross MD, Johnsson L-G, Peacor D, Allard LF. Observations on normal and degenerating human otoconia. Ann Otol Rhinol Laryngol 1976; 85:310-26.

5. Lim DJ. Fine morphology of the otoconial membrane and its relationship to the sensory epithelium. Scan Electron Microsc 1973; 3:929-35.

6. Salamat MS, Ross MD, Peacor DR. Otoconial formation in the fetal rat. Ann Otol Rhinol Laryngol 1980; 89:229-38.

7. Johnsson L-G, Hawkins JE Jr. Sensory and neural degeneration with aging, as seen in microdissections of the human inner ear. Ann Otol Rhinol Laryngol 1972; 81:179-93.

8. Wright CG, Hubbard DG. Observations of otoconial membranes from human infants. Acta Otolaryngol (Stockh) 1978; 86:185-94.

9. Wright CG, Hubbard DG, Graham JW. Absence of otoconia in a human infant. Ann Otol Rhinol Laryngol 1979; 88:779-83.

10. Hawkins JE Jr, Johnsson L-G. Microdissection and surface preparations of the inner ear. In: Smith CA, Vernon JA, eds. Handbook of auditory and vestibular research methods. Springfield: CC Thomas, 1976:5-52.

11. Gammage RB, Glasson DR. The effect of grinding on the polymorphs of calcium carbonate. J Colloid Interface Sci 1976; 55:396-401.

12. Meyer HJ. Struktur und Fehlordnung des Vaterits. Z Kristallogr 1969; 128:183-212.

13. Lyon MF. Absence of otoliths in the mouse: an effect of the pallid mutant. J Genet 1953; 51:638-50.

14. Lim DJ, Erway LC. Influence of manganese on genetically defective otolith. A behavioral and morphological study. Ann Otol Rhinol Laryngol 1974; 83:565-81.

15. Turnbull AG. A thermochemical study of vaterite. Geochim Cosmochim Acta 1973; 37:1593-601.

16. Lowenstam HA, Abbott DP. Vaterite: a mineralization product of the hard tissues of a marine organism (Ascidiacea). Science 1975; 188:363-5.

17. Meenakshi VR, Blackwelder PL, Watabe N. Studies on the formation of calcified egg-capsules of ampullarid snails: I. Vaterite crystals in the reproductive system and the egg capsules of Pomacea paludosa. Calcif Tiss Res 1974; 16:283-91.

18. Board RG, Perrott HR. Vaterite, a constituent of the eggshells of the nonparasitic cuckoos, *Guira guira* and *Crotophagi ani.* Calcif Tiss Int 1979; 29:63-9.

19. Wilbur KM, Watabe N. Experimental studies on calcification in molluscs and the alga *Coccolithus huxleyi.* Ann NY Acad Sci 1963; 109:82-112.

20. Gibson RI. Descriptive human pathological mineralogy. Am Mineral 1974; 59:1177-82.

21. Sutor DJ, Wooley SE. A statistical survey of gallstones in eight countries. Gut 1971; 12:55-64.

22. Lagergren C. Calcium carbonate precipitation in the pancreas, gallstones and urinary calculi. Acta Chir Scand 1962; 124:320-5.

23. Palmork KH, Taylor MEU, Coates R. The crystal structure of aberrant otoliths. Acta Chem Scand 1963; 17:1457-8.

24. Veenhof VB. The development of statoconia in mice. Amsterdam: Akademie van Wetenschappen, 1969.

25. Rauch S. Biochemie des Hororgans. Stuttgart: Georg Thieme Verlag, 1964.

26. Bachra BN, Trautz OR, Simon SL. Precipitation of calcium carbonates and phosphates. I. Spontaneous precipitation of calcium carbonates and phosphates under physiological conditions. Arch Biochem Biophys 1963; 103:124-38.

27. Johnsson L-G, Hawkins JE Jr. Hydrops and cupulolithiasis as seen in microdissections of human temporal bones. In: Pulec JL, ed. Meniere's disease. Palisades Publishing Co (in press).

28. Quick CA, Fish A, Brown C. The relationship between cochlea and kidney. Laryngoscope 1973; 83:1469-82.

29. Arnold W, Weidauer H, Seelig HP. Experimenteller Beweis einer gemeinsamen Antigenizität zwischen Innenohr und Niere. Arch Otorhinolaryngol 1976; 212:99-117.

30. Bergstrom L, Thompson P, Wood RP. New patterns in genetic and congenital otonephropathies. Laryngoscope 1979; 89:177-94.

31. Esscher E, Scott JS. Congenital heart block and maternal systemic lupus erythematosus. Br Med J 1979; 1:1235-8.

32. McCue CM, Mantakas ME, Tingelstad JB, Ruddy S. Congenital heart block in newborns of mothers with connective tissue disease. Circulation 1977; 56:82-90.

33. Lev M, Silverman J, Fitzmaurice FM, Paul MH, Cassels DE, Miller RA. Lack of connection between the atria and the more peripheral conduction system in congenital atrioventricular block. Am J Cardiol 1971; 27:481-90.

34. Hawkins JE Jr. Drug ototoxicity. In: Keidel WD, Neff WD, eds. Handbook of sensory physiology. Vol 5. Berlin: Springer Verlag, 1976:707-48.

35. Kimmel CA, Wilson JG, Schumacher HJ. Studies on metabolism and identification of the causative agent in aspirin teratogenesis in rats. Teratology 1971; 4:15-24.

36. McNiel JR. The possible teratogenic effect of salicylates on the developing fetus. Clin Pediatr (Phila) 1973; 12:347-50.

37. Benawra R, Mangurten HH, Duffell DR. Cyclopia and other anomalies following maternal ingestion of salicylates. J Pediatr 1980; 96:1069-71.

38. Larsson KS, Boström H. Teratogenic action of salicylates related to the inhibition of mucopolysaccharide synthesis. Acta Pediatr Scand 1965; 54:43-8.

39. Erway LC, Hurley LS, Fraser AS. Congenital ataxia and otolith defects due to manganese deficiency in mice. J Nutr 1970; 100:643-54.

40. Shrader RE, Erway LC, Hurley LS. Mucopolysaccharide synthesis in the developing inner ear of manganese-deficient and pallid mutant mice. Teratology 1973; 8:257-66.

41. Woodbury DM, Fingl E. Analgesic-antipyretics, antiinflammatory agents, and drugs employed in the therapy of gout. In: Goodman LS, Gilman A, eds. The pharmacological basis of therapeutics. 5th ed. New York: McMillan, 1975:325-58.

42. Huff BB, ed. Physicians' desk reference. 33rd ed. Oradell: Medical Economics Co, 1979.

43. Degens ET, Deuser WG, Haedrich RL. Molecular structure and composition of fish otoliths. Mar Biol 1969; 2:105-13.

44. Lippman F. Sedimentary carbonate minerals. New York: Springer-Verlag, 1973.

45. Girou A, Roques H. Etude des conditions de précipitation à 30°C des différentes variétés allotropiques des $CaCO_3$ en fonction du degré de sursaturation. C R Acad Paris Sci 1969; 268: 1244-7.

46. Meyer HJ. Bildung und Morphologie des Vaterits. Z Kristallogr 1965; 121:220-42.

≈

AMERICAN BOARD OF OTOLARYNGOLOGY
SPECIAL ANNOUNCEMENT

The American Board of Otolaryngology will give the written examination Sunday, September 12, 1982, at the Palmer House, Chicago. Registration will be on Saturday, September 11, 1982, at 5:00 PM at the Palmer House. It is estimated that the examination will conclude at 6:00 PM Sunday. Deadline for application is May 1. For the new application forms, contact George F. Reed, MD, Secretary-Treasurer, American Board of Otolaryngology, 220 Collingwood, Suite 130, Ann Arbor, MI 48103.

BONY AUDITORY TUBE AND OTITIS MEDIA WITH EFFUSION

R. BRUCE DUNCAN, FRACS

PALMERSTON NORTH, NEW ZEALAND

The author has for 25 years manually probed the malleus handle for indications of middle ear pathology. Dissection of the bony auditory tube (BAT) and isthmus comprised 120 fresh autopsy and 26 anatomically prepared temporal bones. The semicanal lamina was not completely ossified in all infants and children and 52% of adults. The tensor tympani muscle was edematous and prolapsed into the superior portion of the BAT in eight ears with otitis media with effusion. Infants and children have the tendon of the tensor tympani muscle inserting into the neck of the malleus at an angle of 60° or greater, possibly explaining the relatively large muscle bulk. It is suggested from these autopsy findings that the BAT and isthmus lumen is a functional 2-way channel for air superiorly and mucus streaming inferiorly. Manual palpation of the cartilaginous auditory tube in infants did not suggest malacia.

INTRODUCTION

Rosen's epochal probing of the stapes in 1955 suggested malleus handle probing.[1] I had already been sectioning the tensor tympani muscle (TTM) to prevent contractions disturbing middle ear grafts the prior year. The independent movements of the malleus handle and the membranous drum during pneumatic otoscopy did not conform to the then accepted "ex vacuo" theory. A retracted drum was seen with a normal handle position or vice versa. In 1962, five marine engineers from an ocean-going ferry were examined one hour after finishing the engine room shift. All had marked malleus handle retraction[2] and when asked to do the Valsalva maneuver, commented on how easy this was to perform while working in noise. I anesthetized their malleus handles with Bonain's solution (equal parts of cocaine, phenol and menthol) and on probing they were fixed, yet the pars tensa moved with the Valsalva maneuver. I assumed that the TTM had retracted the handle and opened the auditory tube in some way that was independent of the then accepted view. In 1966, I began probing the malleus handle before myringotomy to predict the presence of otitis media with effusion (OME) and the state of pathological change in the middle ear cleft. The reliability of this test (Duncan RB, unpublished data) initiated a program of TTM and semicanal lamina (SCL) dissection in fresh cadavers and preserved temporal bones. The results supported my hypothesis that the belly of the TTM could cause partial obstruction of the bony auditory tube (BAT).

METHODS

The material comprised 120 fresh cadaver and 26 anatomically prepared temporal bones. A 4x loupe was used for bones in cadavers and a 9x microscope for removed fresh and prepared bones. The exposure of the TTM and SCL begins with removal of the tegmen tympani and exposure continues anteromedially to the sphenoid. The TTM is separated from the tensor veli palatini muscle (TPM), along with the attachments to the sphenoid, and then dissected posteriorly so that the tendon remains attached to the malleus neck (Fig. 1). This method avoids damage to the posterior margin of the SCL. Particular care is needed when the bony SCL is absent. After thorough examination of the SCL, the bony auditory canal, ossicles, and extent of mastoid pneumatization, a portion of the sphenoid wing and base are removed to palpate the cartilaginous auditory tube (CAT).

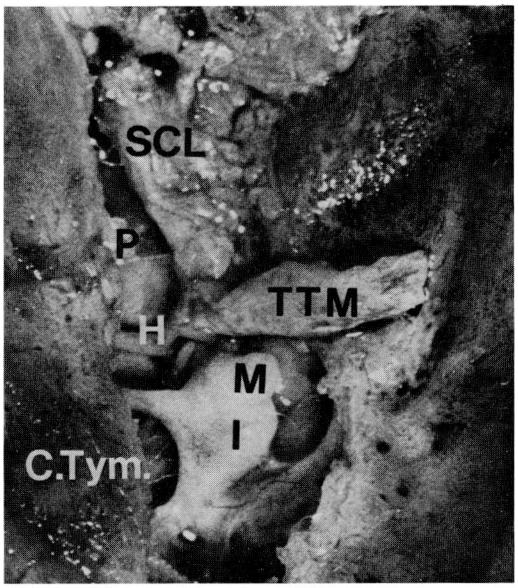

Fig. 1. Right cadaver ear, age 5½ months. SCL - Semicanal lamina, unossified; P - Floor of protympanum; TTM - Body of tensor tympani muscle dissected and laid laterally to expose malleus handle (H). M - Malleus; I -Incus; C. Tym. - Chorda tympani nerve.

RESULTS

The tegmen tympani was thin or not completely ossified in infants but thin to very thick in adults with occasional air cells. The roof of the TTM canal varied from a thin membrane in infants to thin or thick compact bone with red marrow in adults. Peritubular cells were seen in this area. The TTM appears relatively larger in the infant and occupies the width of the SCL, which appears relatively nar-

From the Department of Otolaryngology, Palmerston North Hospital, New Zealand.

REPRINTS — R. Bruce Duncan, FRACS, 233 Broadway Avenue, Palmerston North, New Zealand.

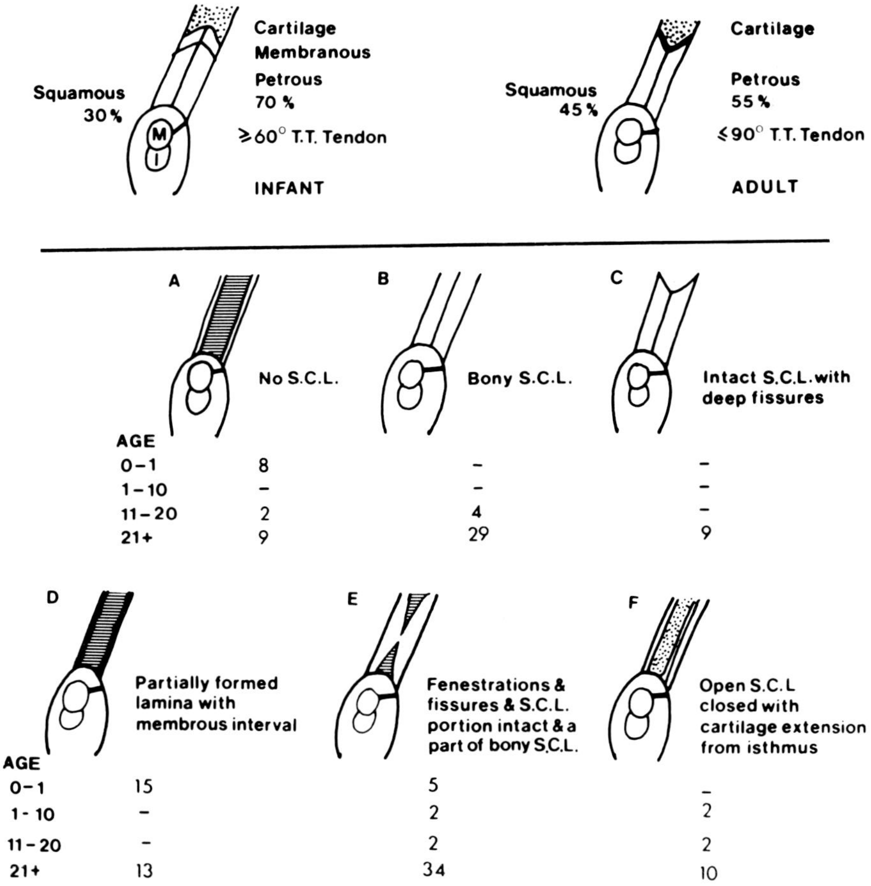

Fig. 2. A-F) The semicanal laminae (S.C.L.) grouped by age and variation. A series of 146 temporal bones are represented in the Figure as the left ear. Isolated ossifications occurred at the isthmus and protympanum. Sq. S.C.L - Squamous SCL; T. Tymp. M. - Tensor tympani muscle; Pet. S.C.L. - Petrous SCL.

rower. The cochleariform process or trochlea was often sited anteriorly to the malleus neck. This altered the direction of the tendon of the TTM which inserted into the malleus neck at an angle of 60° or greater. The narrower angle of insertion could result in poor leverage compared to the 90° angle of insertion in the adult. This may explain the relatively large TTM body bulk. I suggest that with growth the SCL lengthens and widens and the trochlea moves posteriorly so that the angle of insertion widens to 90° in the adult. I observed at autopsy that when the angle of insertion was 60° to 80°, retraction with forceps of the detached TTM body in the same anteromedial direction as its canal increased the rigidity of the posterosuperior quadrant of the drum by 5 to 8 g using a mechanical pressure gauge. When the TTM tendon is detached from the malleus and the muscle body is freed from the SCL up to the isthmus, posterolateral retraction with forceps in the plane of the TTM canal caused slight to moderate elevation of the thin fibrous lamina of the baby's isthmus roof. I realize these two manipulations are artificial because the body of the TTM has short muscle fibers attached to the walls of the semicanal and also inserted into the central tendon.[3] If elevation of the isthmus roof of infants does occur in life, I surmise that tubal function would be improved in the primitive head-up position of nursing and carrying.

Four children at autopsy had OME and an edematous TTM prolapsing through a thin fibrous SCL and obstructing the wider superior portion of the BAT lumen.[4] The inferior portion was not obstructed by the TTM. Chronic tubal inflammation and infection may involve the relatively large TTM of infants and children when the SCL and isthmus are closed by a fibrous membrane. These four children died of leukemia, hydrocephalus and meningitis, a fall to his death by a retarded child, and drowning in a bath by an epileptic female. Eight children between the ages of 1½ and 10 months died from sudden infant death syndrome (SIDS). All had OME mucoid but no TTM prolapse. The possibility of postmortem swelling of the TTM body producing the prolapse was excluded by finding the condition in certain BATs with OME. The eight children who died of SIDS and had associated OME did not have TTM prolapse. Normal BATs with SCL dehiscences did not show any tendency to TTM prolapse.

Figure 2 shows the variations of the components of the SCL. The medial or petrous lamina supports most of the TTM belly and contributes half to two thirds of the SCL. The lateral or squamous lamina fuses with the medial lamina often producing ridges or grooves, but deficiencies occur which are more frequent at the protympanum area. Wide deficiencies of the whole length of the SCL were closed by a variable thickness fibrous lamina which was often

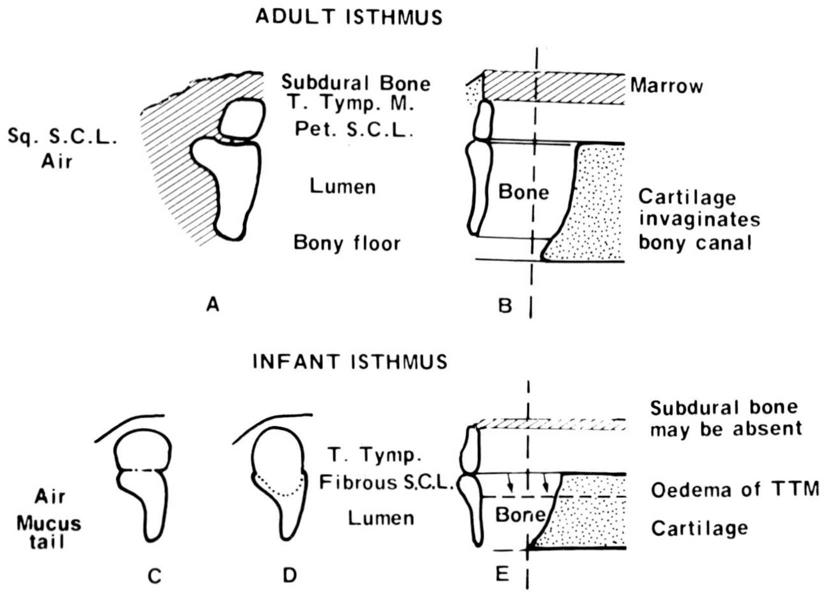

Fig. 3. A-E) Schematic concept of the adult and infant isthmus and the suggested effect of tensor tympani muscle.

fenestrated and incomplete, or an extension of cartilage from the lateral cartilaginous lamina of the CAT. Incomplete bony SCL formation was frequent, affecting the lateral more than the medial lamina. All babies and children had a fibrous SCL and roof of the isthmus. The age group 1-10 years is poorly represented with two autopsies, so no conclusions can be made on the growth of the SCL during this very important period. More evidence is urgently required. The isthmus roof of infants and adults varied considerably (Fig. 3). Separate cartilage and bony rests occur in the fibrous SCL. An adult specimen had a separate bony rest 2.5 mm x 1.5 mm lying in the fibrous protympanum SCL. I speculate that this may represent a first arch remnant.[5]

The cartilaginous lateral lamina medial to the fibrous isthmus roof in infants is thin in contrast to the marked thickness of this lamina in adults. The attachment of cartilage to bone is very strong in adults and usually incomplete inferiorly, but three complete annular attachments were seen. Although some specimens had been involved in high-speed motorcycle accidents, there was no rupture of this junction. There are no reports of traumatic rupture in the literature. The roof of the infant's BAT is the SCL with a relatively large TTM occupying the whole width. In the adult the BAT widens and the SCL and TTM occupy the medial two thirds of the roof and the lateral third is related superiorly to the middle fossa. Possible explanations of the gap in the isthmus roof between the SCL and the lateral lamina of the CAT is the rate of basicranial growth in width, the need for a flexible isthmus roof in childhood, and the more recent phylogeny of the lateral lamina. I have insufficient material to determine when the lateral lamina fuses with the medial lamina of the SCL. The SCL can be closed by a cartilaginous lamina. I could find no adequate description of the SCL in the fetus.

Dissection of fresh normal cadaver BATs by removing the SCL revealed mucus lying in the narrow inferior portion of the tube and air, not bubbles, in the wider superior lumen, despite the variation in head position prior to autopsy. The floor of the bony canal at the protympanum has deep peritubal cells which always contained pooled mucus. The lumen of the medial bony auditory canal and isthmus junction is roughly comma-shaped on cross section (Fig. 3), suggesting a superior air transmitting channel and an inferior cleft-shaped mucus channel, or a two-way functional lumen. Radiological demonstration of the thin SCL was attempted on three adults with drum perforations and two prepared adult temporal bones which were later dissected and shown to have well-ossified SCL. The SCL cannot be demonstrated by conventional views or tomography or the use of fluid contrast media.[6] The CAT in infants and children was exposed and manually palpated to detect loss of spring (malacia). Comparison by age, period since death and presence or absence of OME did not suggest malacia. Mastoid pneumatization was assessed visually and was considered to be within normal limits in all infants and children. One sclerotic adult mastoid had large well-developed peritubal cells.

CASE REPORTS

Case 1. An autopsy on July 25, 1977, revealed a white stillborn infant who had the TTM lying under the dura with no bony cover. The SCL and isthmus roof were thin fibrous membranes. The TTM tendon inserted into the malleus neck at 65°.

Case 2. An autopsy was performed on December 30, 1977, on a white female, aged 16, who had died in a bath during an epileptic fit. The SCL was membranous and the edematous TTM prolapsed into the bony canal lumen. There was OME (glue) throughout all air cells and spaces and drum retraction pockets of both ears.

Case 3. On September 20, 1980, an autopsy was performed on a white male, aged six months, who had died of SIDS. The dura was stripped to reveal a cartilaginous surface with areas of thin bone, which was removed to expose a poorly developed TTM with normal thickness tendon inserting at a 65° angle. The SCL and isthmus were thin fibrous membranes; OME (glue) was found throughout all air cells and spaces of both ears.

DISCUSSION

"Little is known about how air is propelled through the tube or how much passes either in health or in disease."[7] The BAT has attracted little comment in the literature of OME because it has been assumed that functional obstruction occurred in the CAT. The SCL is considered a bony structure throughout life. The isthmus is a functional obstruction because of the narrow lumen in infants (2 - 4mm by 0.5 - 2 mm) and the angulation between the BAT and CAT. Bluestone et al[8] commented on the radius and length of the isthmus in children and demonstrated that radio-opaque fluid will enter and leave the cartilaginous tube on swallowing.[9] Autopsies of patients with OME show no evidence of auditory tube obstruction, swollen mucosa or pathology.[10,11] Schuknecht and Kerr[12] reported autopsy findings on 400 adult ears with chronic otitis media; 51 ears had complete obstruction of the bony auditory canal. These reports do not comment on the structures considered in this study, as the methods were different.

The membranous isthmus roof and TTM attachment suggests that infants have an additional valve-like effect from elevation of the isthmus roof. TTM may have a pumping action during swallowing.[8] This study suggests the TTM fixes the malleus handle to stop drum flap, elevates the isthmus before or as the TPM opens the cartilaginous tube. Inflammation of the TTM and its prolapse through a membranous SCL would negate this activity and the chronic tonic contraction would maintain handle retraction. A degree of functional obstruction in the BAT could give a false impression of obstruction or floppiness in the CAT.[9] Studies[13] on air passage through the normal and inflamed auditory tube assume there is no functional obstruction in the BAT. The present techniques of auditory tube function[7] cannot assess BAT and CAT functions separately.

The consistent finding at autopsy of stratified air and mucus in the BAT suggests the lumen has 2-way channels, the wider superior transmitting bubbles of air and the narrower inferior transmitting mucus. This cross-sectional shape is not continued into the CAT, but the inferiorly placed compound mucous glands and convoluted mucosa may encourage mucus streaming in this area. The present concept is mixed air and mucus occupying the whole lumen, but this was not seen even in postmortems performed a few hours after death and despite the variation in head position of cadavers prior to dissection. The movement of air superiorly and mucus inferiorly in opposite directions would facilitate air entry and mucus transport. Passage of radio-opaque fluid may not be a measure of the air channel.[6] Air entry would not occur with swallowing but could be forced via either channel if the other had a temporary obstruction. Tensor tympani muscle edema and prolapse could occur with acute otitis media and resolve with the infection but persistent swelling would perpetuate chronic OME. Increased autopsy reporting will determine the possibility and frequency of TTM prolapse. If TTM edema and prolapse are present in some chronic OME, they could hinder the clearance of thick mucus and increase the resistance to air entry. I demonstrated that positional otitis media[14] from bottle feeding could be reduced by head and body elevation. Rundcrantz[15] showed that the head should be elevated at 20° for optimum auditory tube function. This head position could facilitate the suggested 2-way flow in the BAT. Some findings of this study may be additional pieces of the jigsaw of OME.

REFERENCES

1. Rosen S, Bergman M. Mobilization of the stapes for otosclerotic deafness. Arch Otolaryngol 1955; 61:197-206.

2. Roydhouse N. A survey of engine room noise in the RNZN. NZ Med J 1968; 67:133-40.

3. Candiollo L. The control mechanism of the middle ear transmission system: the middle ear muscles. Beltone Institute for Hearing Research, Chicago, 1967; 20:13-41.

4. Bluestone CD, Wittel R A, Paradise J L, Felder H. Eustachian tube function as related to adenoidectomy for otitis media. Trans Am Acad Ophthalmol Otolaryngol 1972; 76:1325-39.

5. Strickland E, Hanson J, Anson B. Branchial sources of the auditory ossicles in man. Arch Otolaryngol 1962; 76:20-35.

6. Compare W. Radiologic evaluation of the eustachian tube. Otolaryngol Clin North Am 1970; 31:45-9.

7. Sadé J. Eustachian tube function. In: Sadé J, ed. Secretory otitis media and its sequelae. New York: Churchill Livingstone, 1979: 212-52.

8. Bluestone CD, Berry QC, Andrus WS. Mechanics of the eustachian tube as it influences susceptibility to and persistence of middle ear effusions in children. Ann Otol Rhinol Laryngol 1974; 83 Suppl 11:27-34.

9. Bluestone CD, Paradise JL, Berry QC. Physiology of the eustachian tube in the pathogenesis and management of middle ear effusions. Laryngoscope 1972; 82:1654-70.

10. Sadé J. Pathology and pathogenesis of serous otitis media. Arch Otolaryngol 1966; 84:297-305.

11. Harja J, Jokinen K, Seppala A. Temporal bone findings in the late stage of secretory otitis media. J Laryngol Otol 1977; 91:127-31.

12. Schuknecht H, Kerr A. Pathology of the eustachian tube. Arch Otolaryngol 1967; 86:497-502.

13. Ingelstedt S. Physiology of the eustachian tube. Ann Otol Rhinol Laryngol 1976; 85 Supp 25:156-60.

14. Duncan RB. Positional otitis media. Arch Otolaryngol 1960; 72:454-63.

15. Rundecrantz H. The effects of position change on eustachian tube function. Otolaryngol Clin North Am 1970; 3:103-10.

AN INEXPENSIVE EFFECTIVE CRYOPROBE FOR PALLIATIVE CARE

NIGEL R. T. PASHLEY, MB, FRCS(C)
ANN ARBOR, MICHIGAN

Cryotherapy has been shown to be an effective method of palliation for recurrent head and neck tumors. Commercially produced cryotherapy units, however, are extremely expensive; a factor that is significant for otolaryngologists in other than large academic centers where utilization justifies such an expenditure. A simply constructed, effective, and inexpensive cryoprobe is described which can be used by any practitioner in the care of recurrent head and neck tumors.

Cryotherapy is an effective method of palliation for recurrent head and neck tumors,[1] particularly for cavitary lesions, eg, in the maxilla or oral cavity. The application of multiple freezes with near-normal thaw cycles has been shown[1] to provide a good tumor kill provided there is a fast freeze to at least −30 C. This can be achieved only with a liquid nitrogen probe which, if commercially produced, is very expensive. A simply constructed, clinically effective cryoprobe which could be available to any practitioner is described.

METHOD

A commercially available Teflon® rod 3/4 in (1.9 cm) in diameter was first cut to a length of 30 cm (12 in), and on a lathe the diameter was reduced to 1.3 cm (1/2 in) on one end for a distance of 1.3 cm (1/2 in). The rod was bent to a gentle curve using heat. A solid copper rod of the same diameter was rounded on one end using the lathe. The metal rod was then cut to 5 cm (2 in) in length and a 1.3 cm (1/2 in) diameter hole drilled in the flat end to a depth of 1.3 cm (1/2 in).

A steel pin was inserted through a previously drilled hole in the copper and Teflon rods so that a tight joint was obtained. The protruding pin was flattened flush to the copper rod (Fig. 1).

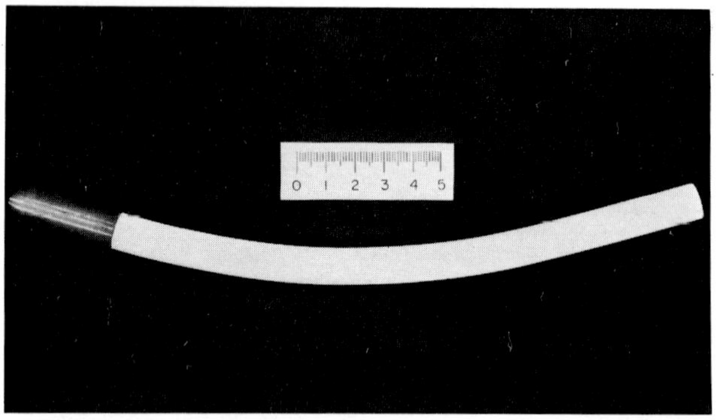

Fig. 1. A simply constructed cryoprobe approximately 20 cm (7.9 in) in length.

Liquid nitrogen, which is available in most clinical laboratories or which can be preordered and delivered to the operating room, is placed in a Dewar flask, and the metallic tip of the probe is immersed until boiling stops (the isothermal point). With the patient under general anesthesia, the probe is directly applied to the treatment area and a small quantity of saline is applied to the tissue/probe interface. This provides a good seal and insures maximal contact. Ice, being a good conductor of cold, insures the formation of a good ice ball. Freezing is continued for 3-5 minutes and the probe is not moved during this time.

To remove the probe it is twisted slightly or irrigated with warm saline to free it. The cycle is then repeated allowing a natural thaw to occur between freezings.

DISCUSSION

A simply constructed, inexpensive, effective cryoprobe is described, bringing this technology within the grasp of every otolaryngologist. For palliative care, cryosurgery provides effective debulking, cleansing of the surface of necrotic tumors, and pain relief by thermally induced sensory neuropraxia.

The probes can be constructed with varying diameters and curves to adapt to individual circumstances and allow for immersion in a container of liquid nitrogen. Further studies at this institution are under way with thermocouples in tissue to determine the distance from the probe tip of effective freeze, which on clinical grounds extends in a ball the diameter of the probe distance in all directions within the tissue.

REFERENCES

1. Neel NB. Cryosurgery for the treatment of cancer. Laryngoscope 1980; 90 Suppl 23.

From the Department of Otolaryngology, University of Michigan Medical Center, Ann Arbor.
REPRINTS — Nigel R. T. Pashley, MB, FRCS(C), Department of Otolaryngology, University of Michigan Medical Center, Ann Arbor, MI 48109.

LATENCY OF AUDITORY NERVE RESPONSE IN NEONATES ONE TO EIGHT HOURS OLD

A. RUBINSTEIN, BA H. SOHMER, PhD

JERUSALEM, ISRAEL

Recording the response of the auditory nerve (W_1) in neonates can contribute to the diagnostic distinction between audiological-otological versus neurological pathology. If W_1 latency were subject to relatively rapid shortening in the hours directly after birth, inconsistencies in the literature might be clarified. The purpose of this research was to study W_1 in neonates one to eight hours old in order to determine if significant latency changes occur during this period. Auditory nerve-brainstem responses were recorded in 40 full-term neonates and in 12 normal adults. W_1 latency in 1- to 3-hour-old neonates was 1.81 ± 0.28 ms and 1.77 ± 0.18 ms in 7- to 8-hour-old neonates. This difference was not significant. In adults, W_1 latency was significantly shorter (1.36 ± 0.06 ms). These findings indicate that auditory nerve latency is about 0.43 ms longer at birth than in the adult and that the latency does not shorten significantly during the first hours after birth.

INTRODUCTION

It has been demonstrated in recent years that auditory nerve-brainstem responses (ABR) can serve as an important diagnostic tool even in the newborn population.[1,2] A major parameter in the differential diagnosis between audiological-otological versus neurological pathology is the absolute latency of wave 1 (W_1) and the comparison of the latency of this wave with the latency of one or more of the waves following it. Since wave 1 reflects the compound action potential of the eighth nerve, its latency represents the transmission time of the stimulus through the outer, middle, and inner ear and of the response through the peripheral segment of the eighth nerve. If the latency of later waves is longer than usual while the latency of wave 1 is within normal limits, then the central or brainstem transmission time (BTT) will be prolonged and a neurological disorder may be suspected.[3] If the later waves are delayed while wave 1 is delayed by the same degree, the BTT will be normal suggesting a peripheral (conductive) problem.[4] If both W_1 and the BTT are long, both an audiological and neurological problem may be suspected.

To make a proper diagnosis it is critical to know the expected latency of W_1 in the normal neonatal population. Presently, the literature is mixed regarding this issue.[5-8] However, if W_1 latency were subject to relatively rapid shortening in the hours directly after birth, inconsistencies in the literature might be clarified. Mean latencies reported by different groups would then differ depending on the specific postnatal age makeup of the experimental group (eg, number of babies a few hours old versus a few days old).

It is the purpose of this paper to determine the latency of W_1 in neonates within the first eight hours after birth and to determine if significant changes occur during this period.

METHODS

This study was conducted on 40 neonates who were normal with respect to gestational age (38-41 weeks), birth weight (2,830-4,300 g) and Apgar scores (9-10 after five minutes). Otoscopic examination was performed on all subjects but no evidence of significant conductive pathology was noted. ABR recordings were obtained between one and eight hours after birth while the infants lay in their bassinets in a room adjacent to the neonatal nursery. Sixteen of the neonates (32 ears) were tested at least twice, 1-3 hours and 7-8 hours after birth, while the remaining infants were tested once during the 8-hour period. Recording electrodes were applied to the earlobe and to the scalp at a point about 2 cm anterior to the vertex. A ground electrode was applied to either the contralateral ear or a finger. A small portable electric response audiometer system (Micro-Shev C-ERA-100; Microshev, Inc., Philadelphia) operated by a relatively untrained individual was used to obtain ABR responses. The preamplifier was optically isolated in order to insure maximum subject safety. Electrode condition, contact and degree of subject relaxation were monitored prior to the test and excessively noisy responses during the test were automatically rejected.

Alternating polarity clicks, 75 dB HL in intensity (based on the subjective thresholds of 12 adults with normal hearing) were applied separately to each ear at a repetition rate of 10/s. In eight newborns, rates of 20 and 40/s were used as well. Between one and three replications of each trace were performed, depending upon the clarity of W_1. The electrical activity was band pass filtered with 3 dB points at 200 Hz and 2.2 kHz, amplified, and the responses to 1,024 clicks were averaged. The latency and amplitude of W_1 were measured by means of a cursor from the multiple display of repeated runs on the screen. Finally, a built-in chart recorder printed out the response traces.

For comparison with neonatal recordings, ABR recordings were made in 12 adults (24 ears) in response to the same stimulus and using the same instrument as with the neonates. Means and standard deviations of W_1 latencies were calculated separately from measurements taken during the time periods 1-3 hours and 7-8 hours. A paired t test was performed on the data obtained from neonates tested both at 1-3 and 7-8 hours. Clear repeatable response peaks could not be identified in the recordings made on five of the neonates.

From the Department of Physiology, Hebrew University-Hadassah Medical School, Jerusalem, Israel. This study was supported in part by A. Leitman, New York.

REPRINTS — H. Sohmer, PhD, Department of Physiology, Medical School, P.O.B. 1172, Jerusalem, Israel.

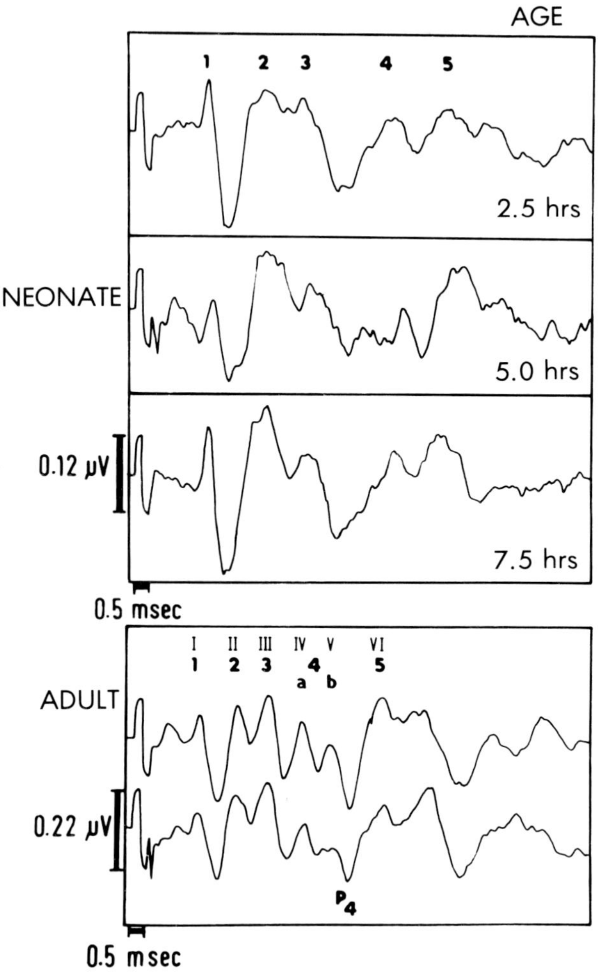

Fig. 1. ABR recordings in one neonate and one adult. The neonate recordings cover a span of 7½ hours after birth. The adult recordings are two successive replications. Response waves are labeled using the two systems in use today.

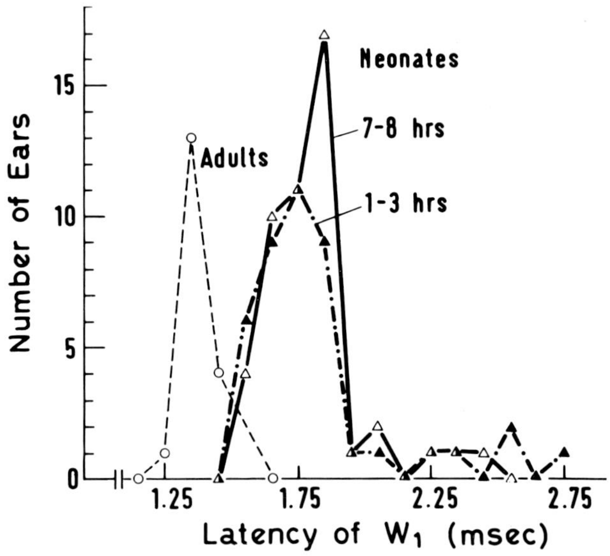

Fig. 2. Histograms of latency of the auditory nerve response in 1- to 3-hour-old neonates, 7- to 8-hour neonates, and adults. Note the almost complete overlap of the latencies in the two neonatal groups and the fact that the modal value (17 ears with a latency between 1.8 and 1.89 ms) in the 7- to 8-hour group is even longer than that in the 1- to 3-hour group (11 ears with a latency between 1.7 to 1.79 ms). Adult latency values are distinctly shorter.

In order to determine the prevalence and latency of the other component waves, the results from one testing session of one ear were chosen for comparison. The choice was based on the session and ear which demonstrated waves with the sharpest peaks and largest amplitude. These latency measurements were performed by hand from the chart recorder traces on completion of data collection.

RESULTS

In a typical example of the responses obtained from one newborn tested 2½, 5, and 7½ hours after birth, waves 1, 2, 3 and 4 (complex IV-V) are evident (Fig. 1). Representative recordings from an adult (two traces from the same adult) are shown as well.

Latency of the auditory nerve response in the age groups studied is given in Table 1. Even though a small decrease in average latency is seen between the 1- to 3-hour neonates and the 7- to 8-hour neonates, this difference was barely significant ($p < .05$) in the neonates studied during both periods (paired t test), and was not significant in the grand total groups (1.81 ± 0.28 ms in 1- to 3-hour neonates and 1.77 ± 0.18 ms in 7- to 8-hour neonates). The absence of significance is further demonstrated in the histograms of Figure 2 which show that the modal value of W_1 latency in the 7- to 8-hour neonatal group is longer than the modal value in the 1- to 3-hour group. In comparison, the latency of W_1 in the adult group was significantly shorter (1.36 ± 0.06 ms). Thus, the neonatal W_1 latencies are between 0.41 to 0.45 ms longer than in adults.

Mean latencies and standard deviations of the other component waves over the neonatal age period studied (1-8 hours) appear in Table 2. Waves 4a (IV) and 4b (V) were computed separately where possible. Brainstem transmission time (BTT) was determined by subtracting W_1 latency from P_4 as described elsewhere.[3] Wave 3 was found to be the most common (97.5%), followed by wave 1 (95%) and wave 4 (IV-V complex, 90%). Wave 2 was

TABLE 1. LATENCY OF AUDITORY NERVE RESPONSE IN NEONATES AND ADULTS

	Neonates 1-3 h (ms)	*No. of Ears*	*Neonates 7-8 h (ms)*	*No. of Ears*	*p*	*Adults (ms)*	*No. of Ears*
Paired	1.84±0.31	32	1.76±0.21	32	0.05		
Total	1.81±0.28	42	1.77±0.18	48	NS	1.36±0.06	24

NS - Not significant.

TABLE 2. LATENCY OF AUDITORY NERVE-BRAINSTEM RESPONSE IN NEONATES 1-8 HOURS OLD (N = 50 EARS)

	Wave Latency (ms)							
	1	*2*	*3*	*4 (IV-V)*	*4a (IV)*	*4b (V)*	P_4	*BTT*
Average	1.79	3.17	4.36	6.87	6.12	6.94	7.54	5.85
SD	0.23	0.23	0.23	0.31	0.47	0.31	0.35	0.34

SD - Standard deviation; BTT - Brainstem transmission time; P_4 - Trough following wave 4b.

present in 82.5% of those tested, which is higher than the 60% reported by Goldstein et al,[7] and may be due in part to the relatively large number of traces obtained on most of the neonates. Only small increases in latency as a function of click repetition rate were found.

DISCUSSION

The results of this study indicate that reliable ABR can be obtained consistently from full-term neonates even as early as 1-3 hours after birth.

One of the response parameters studied was BTT which is a measure of the time interval between the auditory nerve response and a response from a more rostral region of the brainstem.[3] Some investigators use wave V (4b) as an end-point of this measurement.[5-7] We prefer to use the trough following this wave (which we call wave P_4) since the exact form taken by the IV-V complex is highly variable in normal subjects,[9] while wave P_4 is highly consistent (provided a relatively high low-pass recording filter is used). (It is for this reason also that we prefer to use the 4a-4b nomenclature rather than IV, V.) Therefore, in order to compare the BTT values obtained with these two different end-points, the time interval between end-points must be used (about 0.65 ms) and when this is done, close agreement is found between the value of BTT in this study and results of other research.

Several investigations have studied wave latencies in full-term neonates. Values for W_1 range from 1.64 ms[7] and 1.7 ms[6] to 2.12 ms[5,10] and 2.25.[8] Because variations in experimental design (eg, age makeup, click repetition rate, and click intensity) may be responsible for differences in absolute latency values, a comparison can be improved by using as a reference the adult value for W_1 latency reported by each investigator (assuming that identical stimulus and recording conditions were used). The adult values reported are quite similar: 1.4 ms,[11,12] 1.51, 1.53, and 1.57 ms.[5,7,10] Unfortunately, the largest absolute neonate W_1 value, as obtained by Despland and Galambos[8] (2.25 ms), cannot be compared in this manner because no adult value is provided. Goldstein et al[7] show the smallest difference for W_1 latency between neonate and adult subjects (0.1 ms), while Salamy and McKean[5] and Salamy et al[10] show the largest (0.55-0.6 ms). The results of this study reveal a mean difference of no more than 0.45 ms (1- to 3-hours-old).

The main purpose of this study was to determine whether the contradictions in the literature concerning the latency of W_1 in neonates might not be a result of differences in the age makeup of the neonatal samples studied by each group together with a rapid latency shortening soon after birth. Thus, Despland and Galambos,[8] Salamy and McKean,[5] and Salamy et al,[10] who found the longest latencies (2.25 and 2.12 ms respectively) may have studied a younger population while Goldstein et al[7] and Starr[6] (1.64 and 1.7 ms respectively) perhaps studied an older neonatal group.

The results of this study do not support this hypothesis. First of all, even though the sample studied here was obviously younger than that used in the other studies, the latency values found (1.81 ms for 1- to 3-hours-old and 1.77 ms for 7- to 8-hours-old) were closer to the shorter values reported by Goldstein et al[7] and Starr et al.[6] In addition, the overall difference between the latencies in the 1- to 3-hour group and the 7- to 8-hour group (an average difference of only 0.078 ms) was not significant. This finding does not support the notion of a tendency toward a rapid decrease in latency within the period studied. In addition, the results of this study have shown that the literature discrepancies on this point of W_1 latency do not seem to be due to differences in click intensity or repetition rate used by the different groups. Small decreases in click intensity and small increases in click repetition rate lead to very small prolongations of W_1 latency so that it is unlikely that the particularly longer W_1 latencies reported by Salamy and McKean[5] and Salamy et al[10] (2.12 ms) and by Despland and Galambos[8] (2.25 ms) are due to the stimulus intensities and repetition rates which they used.

The age range of the subjects in the above studies included neonates up to the age of approximately four days, and it is likely that the W_1 latency shortens slightly during this period since in another study we have found that W_1 latency in 3-month-old infants is about 0.10 ms shorter than in neonates. It would have been ideal to follow the same children beyond eight hours through their first few days of life but this was not feasible. In any case this would not lead to values closer to the relatively long latencies (2.12 and 2.25 ms) reported[5,8,10] since, if anything, the latencies would be even shorter in older neonates. Also, inclusion of older neonates in the study would lead to a smaller difference in W_1 latency between such older neonates and adults. Even then, it does not seem likely that the very short neonate-adult latency difference (0.1 ms) reported by Goldstein et al[7] can be explained in this way.

The issue of W_1 latency inevitably raises the question concerning the relative maturity of the peripheral auditory system at birth. The results of this study (a very gradual decrease in W_1 latency) support the contention that maturity is almost but not quite complete at birth but does not shed light on the site of this incomplete development. Neonates have been shown to have normal tympanograms,[13,14] making the possibility of a significant conductive loss unlikely, while postmortem study of neonatal cochleae reveal hair cells which appear to be completely developed.[15] This question requires further study.

REFERENCES

1. Leiberman A, Sohmer H, Szabo G. Cochlear audiometry (electrocochleography) during the neonatal period. Dev Med Child Neurol 1973; 15:8-13.

2. Schulman-Galambos C, Galambos R. Brainstem evoked response audiometry in newborn hearing screening. Arch Otolaryngol 1979; 105:86-90.

3. Fabiani M, Sohmer H, Tait C, Gafni M, Kinarti R. A functional measure of brain activity: brainstem transmission time. Electroencephalogr Clin Neurophysiol 1979; 47:483-91.

4. Sohmer H, Cohen D. Responses of the auditory pathway in several types of hearing loss.In: Ruben RJ, Elberling C, Salomon G, eds. Electrocochleography. New York: C. C. Thomas, 1976:431-7.

5. Salamy A, McKean CM. Postnatal development of human brainstem potentials during the first year of life. Electroencephalogr Clin Neurophysiol 1976; 40:418-26.

6. Starr A, Amlie RN, Martin WH, Sanders S. Development of auditory function in newborn infants revealed by auditory brainstem potentials. Pediatrics 1977; 60:831-9.

7. Goldstein PJ, Krumholz A, Felix JK, Shannon D, Carr RF. Brainstem evoked response in neonates. Am J Obstet Gynecol 1979; 135:622-8.

8. Despland PA, Galambos R. The auditory brainstem response (ABR) is a useful diagnostic tool in the intensive care nursery. Pediatr Res 1980; 14:154-8.

9. Chiappa KH, Gladstone KJ, Young RR. Brainstem auditory evoked responses: studies of wave form variations in 50 normal human subjects. Arch Neurol 1979; 36:81-7.

10. Salamy A, McKean CM, Pettett G, Mendelson T. Auditory brainstem recovery processes from birth to adulthood. Psychophysiology 1978; 15:214-20.

11. Leiberman A, Sohmer H, Szabo G. Standard values of amplitude and latency of cochlear audiometry (electro-cochleography) response in different age groups. Arch Klin Exp Ohren Nasen Kehlkopfheilkd 1973; 203:267-73.

12. Starr A, Achor LV. Auditory brainstem responses in neurological disease. Arch Neurol 1975; 32:761-8.

13. Keith RW. Impedance audiometry with neonates. Arch Otolaryngol 1973; 97:465-7.

14. Keith RW. Middle ear function in neonates. Arch Otolaryngol 1975; 101:376-9.

15. Johnsson LF, Hawkins JE Jr. Sensory and neural degeneration with aging as seen in microdissections of the human inner ear. Ann Otol Rhinol Laryngol 1972; 81:179-93.

Ann Otol 91:1982

FUNCTIONAL PATENCY OF THE COCHLEAR AQUEDUCT

BJÖRN CARLBORG, MD
DURHAM, NORTH CAROLINA

BARBARA DENSERT, MD
MALMÖ, SWEDEN

OVE DENSERT, MD
MALMÖ, SWEDEN

The perilymphatic (P_P) and cerebrospinal fluid (P_{CSF}) pressures were investigated in relation to pressure variations in the ear canal, middle ear and intracranial compartment before and after occlusion of the cochlear aqueduct (CA). Experiments using intracranial infusion showed that the CA was responsible for a perfect hydrodynamic balance between the CSF and the perilymph. There are indications of additional pressure release factors but their capacities were not sufficient to prevent the appearance of a longstanding and substantial pressure gradient following occlusion of the CA. A gradual P_P build-up, from zero to its original level after the CA was opened and occluded, indicated perilymph production within the labyrinth. Investigation of pressure transfer from the ear canal and middle ear to the perilymph showed that the CA was the major pressure release route from the cochlea. Occlusion of the CA reduced the compliance of the inner ear and severely reduced the pressure release capacity. In such a situation the inner ear is almost incapable of equilibrating ambient pressure changes.

INTRODUCTION

The pressure-regulating mechanisms of the inner ear have been receiving increasing attention since numerous reports indicate that inner ear symptoms can be induced by changes in ambient pressure,[1-4] or by high intensity, low frequency pressure waves.[5-7] Densert et al[8] demonstrated experimentally that the inner ear function of patients with Menière's disease can be influenced by ambient pressure changes. However, the pathogenesis of inner ear disorders caused by variations in ambient pressure is not fully understood.

Experimental investigations on the transmission of low frequency pressure changes from the middle ear to the perilymphatic fluid performed by Densert et al[9] demonstrated an almost direct transmission of pressure to the inner ear. However, the pressure stabilization in the perilymph was not a homogenous process. One pressure release factor, probably the cochlear aqueduct (CA), seemed to be responsible for the major part of the inner ear pressure regulating capacity.

The patency of the CA in lower mammals is generally accepted.[10,11] In man, however, the aqueduct is considered to be closed in some individuals, whereas an open communication through the aqueduct has been demonstrated in others.[12-14] Efforts have been made to determine the fluid flow through the CA by measuring the perilymph outflow from a perforation in the cochlea.[15,16] Kellerhals[16] reported that about one-fifth of the perilymphatic fluid was derived from a CSF influx via the CA, whereas the remaining part was derived from the ultrafiltration process within the labyrinth. Studies on the CSF and perilymphatic pressures have demonstrated that the CA was responsible for the functional relationship existing between these two fluid systems.[17-19] However, it is not fully understood how the patency of the CA affects the pressure regulation of the inner ear. The purpose of this study was therefore to analyze the effect of experimental occlusion of the CA on 1) the functional communication between the CSF and the perilymphatic fluid; 2) the transmission of pressure changes from the external ear canal and the middle ear to the perilymphatic fluid; and 3) the pressure-regulating capacity of the inner ear.

METHODS

Fifteen cats weighing 2 to 3.5 kg were used. The animals underwent tracheostomy and were ventilated with a respirator. Ears with signs of chronic infection or middle ear effusion were excluded.

Perilymphatic pressure (P_p) was measured in the vestibule via a canal drilled through the temporal bone using an extra-aural approach. A metallic cannula, inside diameter (ID) 0.8 mm, with a short adapter, was screwed into the canal and sealed. The ear canal and the middle ear cavity were left intact.[20]

Cerebrospinal fluid pressure (P_{CSF}) was measured in one of the lateral ventricles via a metallic cannula (ID 1 mm) with a short adapter. A similar metallic cannula was inserted into the opposite lateral ventricle and connected to an automatic syringe pump for intracranial infusion (Sage Instruments, Cambridge, Mass.).

The pressure sensor of a Millar microtip transducer PC 360 5F (Millar Instruments, Inc., Houston, Tex.) was inserted into each adapter for measuring the P_P and P_{CSF}. The total fluid volume in the measuring systems was about 12 and 25mm,[3] respectively.

External ear canal pressure changes (P_{EC}) were applied and measured via two polyethylene tubes (PE 190) fitted into a rubber stopper that was inserted and sealed in the ear canal.

Middle ear pressure changes (P_M) were applied and measured in the tympanic bulla via two polyethylene tubes (PE 190) in a rubber stopper that was fitted into a predrilled perforation in the

From the Departments of Otolaryngology and Experimental Research, Malmö General Hospital, University of Lund, Malmö, Sweden. This investigation was supported by grants from Segerfalkska Stiftelsen and Tysta Skolan, Sweden.

REPRINTS — Björn Carlborg, MD, Division of Otolaryngology, Duke University Medical Center, Box 3805, Durham, NC 27710.

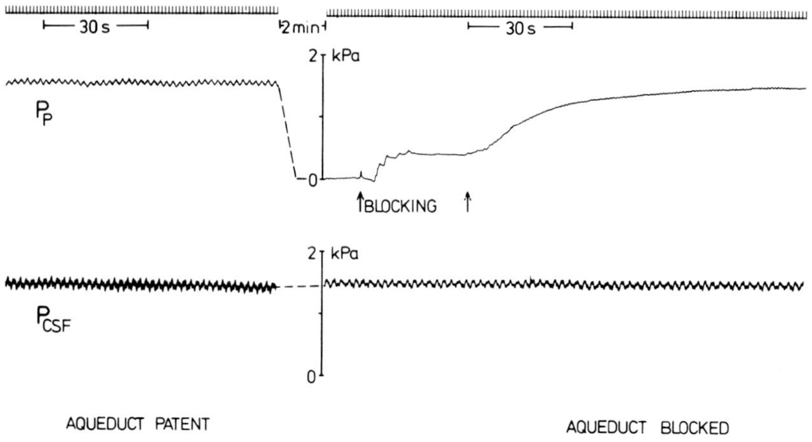

Fig. 1. Recordings of the perilymphatic (P_P) and cerebrospinal fluid (P_{CSF}) pressures before, during (arrows) and after blocking of the cochlear aqueduct. When the cochlear aqueduct is divided the P_P drops to zero. When the aqueduct is blocked there is a spontaneous pressure build-up in the perilymph and a reduction of respiratory fluctuations.

bulla. The P_{EC} and P_M were measured with Millar microtip pressure transducers.

Pressure changes applied to the external ear canal and middle ear were generated with a source of variable air pressure. Low-pass filtered pressure steps were produced with a rise time of 20 and 80 ms, respectively (equivalent to a corner frequency of about 18 Hz and 4 Hz[9]). The amplitude of the pressure steps was changed stepwise within the range of 0 to ± 5kPa (37.6 mm Hg) and was kept constant for about 30 s. In a few experiments very slow pressure changes were applied with rise times of about 0.25-0.5 kPa/s (1.9-3.8 mm Hg/s).

Pressure stimulation was first applied to the ear canal and then to the middle ear. The first series of experiments was performed to study the initial peak change in P_P as well as the subsequent pressure release process. The time constants of this process were determined by extrapolation of the rate of pressure release.[9]

The CA was then blocked via an approach through the opening previously made in the tympanic bulla. The CA was exposed posteriorly and medially to the round window by means of a diamond drill, and was completely transected and blocked with amalgam. The inferior cochlear vein was encountered in some animals. A rubber stopper (4 x 3 mm) with two polyethylene tubes was fitted to make an airtight seal with the opening made in the bulla. In this way middle ear pressure changes could be applied when the CA was blocked. Thus, with the CA blocked, the same series of pressure changes as mentioned above could be applied to the middle ear and ear canal. The tympanic cavity was sealed during ear canal pressure stimulation and ventilated in between. Continuous measurements of the P_P and P_{CSF} were performed before, during, and after the opening and occlusion of the CA.

Intracranial infusion of artificial CSF[21] was performed at a rate of 0.15-0.3 ml/minute before and after occlusion of the CA. In this way the communication between the CSF and the perilymphatic fluid was investigated.

After the series of experiments was completed the tympanic membrane and tympanic cavity were inspected with an operating microscope for signs of hemorrhage or other damage.

The T test for paired observations indicated that differences were significant at the $p<0.05$ level. Pressure measurements are given in kilopascals (kPa) according to the International System of Units, 1 kPA = 7.5 mm Hg.

RESULTS

Functional Communication Between the CSF and the Perilymphatic Fluid Systems. Before blockage of the CA no significant difference was seen between the mean perilymphatic and CSF pressure ($p>0.05$). The pressure level ranged from 0.2-1.8 kPa between the individual animals.

The opening of the CA caused leakage of some fluid, and a sudden fall in the P_p to the zero level as well as a complete disappearance of the pulse and respiratory induced pressure variations previously seen. The CSF pressure remained unchanged (Fig. 1). Even though the CA was completely transected, the P_P spontaneously started to rise. This might be interpreted as a partial obstruction of the periotic duct caused by debris or swelling of traumatized endothelial cells, since the P_P again fell rapidly to zero when the duct was manipulated with a needle.

In three animals the inferior cochlear vein was exposed. Compression of the vein caused an immediate and transient rise in the P_P.

After blockage of the CA the P_P gradually rose to its original level, usually within one minute (Fig. 1). Provided the experimental conditions were kept stable no significant different was found in the P_P level before and after blockage of the CA in six animals ($p>0.05$). The respiratory induced pressure variations were substantially reduced but could still be detected using high amplification of the pressure recordings. No major change was observed in the amplitude of the pulse pressure variations.

When the CA was patent, infusion of artificial CSF into the lateral ventricle caused a simultaneous and equal rise in the P_P and P_{CSF}. When the infusion was stopped the P_P and P_{CSF} reached their peak values and leveled off simultaneously indicating the existence of a direct communication.

Following blockage of the CA, intracranial infusion produced quite a different pressure response in the perilymph indicating that the communication between the two fluid compartments was severely reduced. The cerebral spinal fluid pressure reacted as before (Fig. 2). The P_P appeared to respond simultaneously with the CSF pressure; however, the rise of the P_P was much slower and reached only a fraction of the rise seen in the P_{CSF}. When the infusion was stopped the P_{CSF} reached its peak and leveled off, while the P_P continued to rise, sometimes several minutes, before it reached its maximum lev-

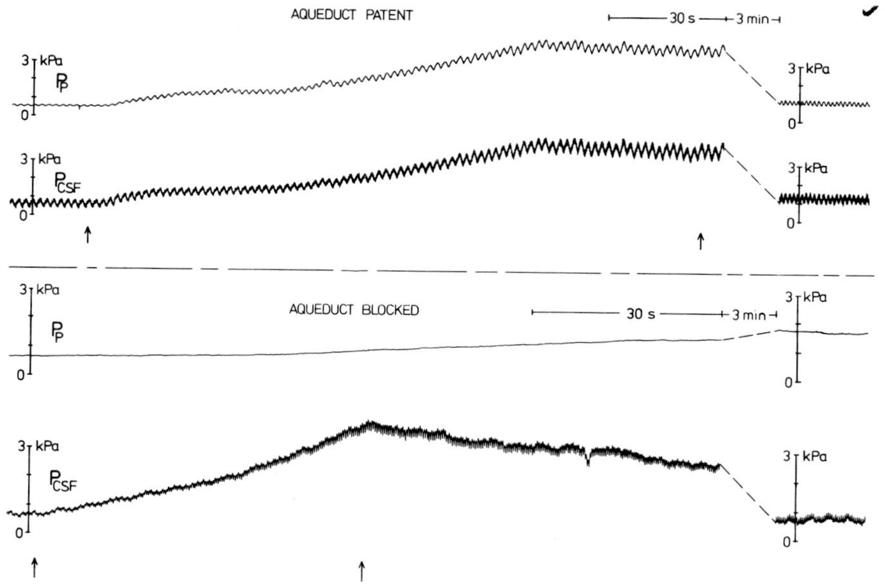

Fig. 2. Pressure recordings during intracranial infusion when the cochlear aqueduct is patent (top) and blocked (bottom). When the aqueduct is patent the change in perilymphatic (P_P) and CSF pressure (P_{CSF}) is approximately equal. When the aqueduct is blocked the rise in P_P is much slower than in the P_{CSF}, and a considerable and long-lasting pressure gradient is seen between the perilymph and CSF. (Arrows indicate beginning and end of intracranial infusion).

el. The subsequent fall in P_P was equally slow as the previous rise. Thus, each change in CSF pressure induced a significant and long-standing pressure gradient between the CSF and the perilymphatic fluid when the CA was blocked.

Transmission of Pressure Steps From the Ear Canal and Middle Ear to the Perilymphatic Fluid. The perilymphatic pressure reacted without any observable time lag to changes in pressure in the middle ear and the ear canal (Fig. 3). The initial perilymphatic peak values ($\triangle P_P$) were plotted as a function of the applied pressures in the middle ear ($\triangle P_M$), before and after blockage of the CA (Fig. 4). Before blockage of the CA an asymmetry was seen in the amplitude of the perilymphatic response to high positive and negative pressure steps, ie, significantly higher perilymphatic pressure peaks ($\triangle P_P$) were seen in response to a positive stimulus than to a negative one ($p<0.05$). After occlusion of the aqueduct no significant asymmetry ($p>0.05$) was found (Fig. 4).

The initial perilymphatic peaks ($\triangle P_P$) were plotted as a function of the applied pressures in the ear canal ($\triangle P_{EC}$) in six animals before and after occlusion of the CA (Fig. 5). With the middle ear cavity intact the transfer function did not show any essential differences when the CA was patent or blocked. The limitation in pressure transmission, seen at stimulus levels exceeding about 3 kPa, remained unchanged and so did the asymmetry of the amplitude of the perilymphatic peaks in response to positive and negative pressure stimuli.

The eustachian tube was not forced open by the applied pressure levels. This was checked by continuous pressure recordings.

Pressure-Regulating Capacity of the Inner Ear. Pressure changes similar to those given above were applied to the external ear canal and to the middle ear. When the CA was patent the initial perilymphatic peak ($\triangle P_P$) was followed by a stabilization of the P_P to the original level despite a constant pressure stimulus level. The form of this pressure stabilization process differed somewhat between cats (Figs. 3 and 6). A quantitative measure of this difference was obtained by comparing the values of the time constants of the stabilization process. The initial time constant, T_1, was generally dominant and represented the major and rapid part of the

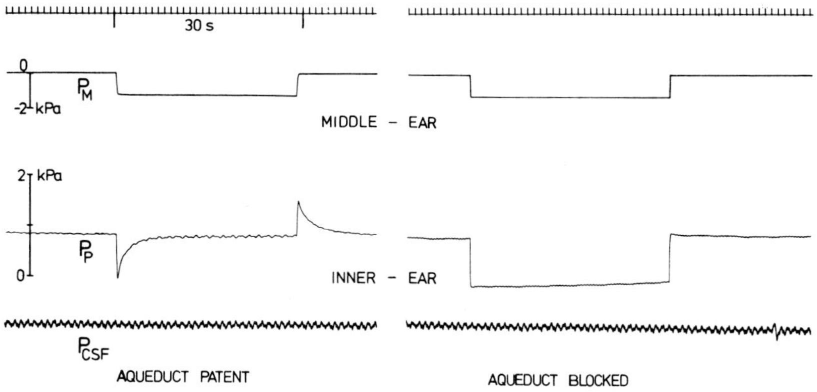

Fig. 3. Application of a negative pressure step to the middle ear (P_M) produces an immediate change in perilymphatic pressure (P_P). Pressure recordings before and after blockage of the cochlear aqueduct. Note the rapid pressure release process when the aqueduct is patent and the extremely slow pressure release when the aqueduct is blocked. No change is seen in the CSF pressure.

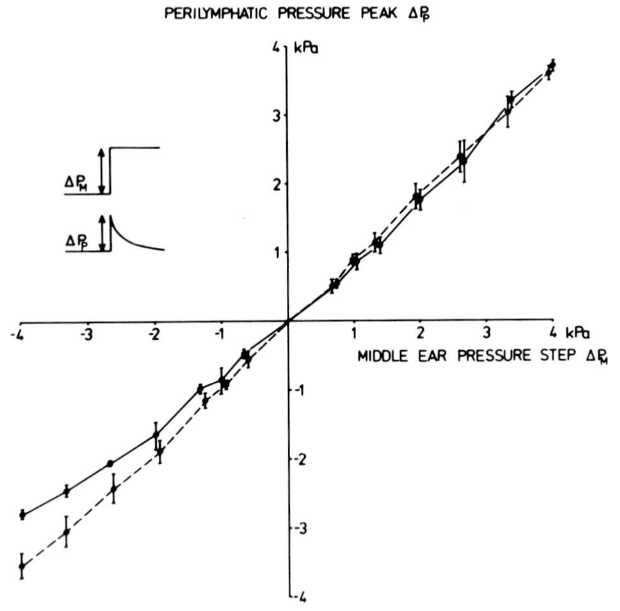

Fig. 4. Transfer functions obtained from pressure applications in the middle ear, before and after occlusion of the cochlear aqueduct. The graph shows the mean values ± 1 SD of the initial perilymphatic peaks ($\triangle P_P$) as a function of middle ear pressure steps ($\triangle P_M$) in six cat ears. ——— - Cochlear aqueduct patent; ----- - Cochlear aqueduct blocked.

pressure stabilization. A second time constant, T_2, which was longer and sometimes difficult to calculate, indicated a much slower pressure release process. The value of T_1 was, to some extent, decreased with increasing stimulus pressure, thus indicating the amount of compliance of the inner ear.

When the CA was blocked the form of the perilymphatic pressure stabilization became completely different. Most often one very long, sometimes infinite time constant (T′) was observed, indicating the very small remaining pressure release capacity in addition to that of the CA (Figs. 3 and 6). T′ showed no dependency on the applied stimulus pressure level in the ear canal and middle ear, indicating a reduced compliance in the system (see table). By comparing the T^1 and T′ a measure was obtained of the difference in pressure release capacity before and after occlusion of the CA. A 20-fold to infinite increase of the major time constant was seen when the aqueduct was blocked. Thus, after the initial perilymphatic peak ($\triangle P_P$) seen in response to a pressure stimulus in the ear canal or middle ear, the P_P remained practically constant despite a continuation of the stimulus pressure for several minutes. The form of the P_P response was thus similar to that of the stimulus pressure (Figs. 3 and 6).

Animals showing a short initial time constant (T_1) could almost completely compensate pressure changes with a rise time of about 0.25-0.5 kPa/s due to the pressure release via the CA (Fig. 7). When the aqueduct was blocked there was a severe impairment to the pressure-regulating capacity and consequently the inner ear was affected by any change in the stimulus pressure throughout the duration of the stimulus.

DISCUSSION

Investigation of the perilymphatic pressure (P_P) as a function of a pressure variations outside the cochlea, eg, variations in the vascular and CSF pressures as well as pressure changes in the ear canal and middle ear, have previously been reported by our group.[9,20,22]

Blockage of the CA in the present study provided an opportunity to directly follow and evaluate the significance of the patency of the CA for inner ear pressure-regulating abilities as well as for the functional communication between the perilymphatic and CSF systems.

The most widely accepted view on the origin of the perilymphatic fluid seems to be that of a combination of CSF influx via the CA and ultrafiltration within the cochlea.[13-16,23] The theory of a CSF

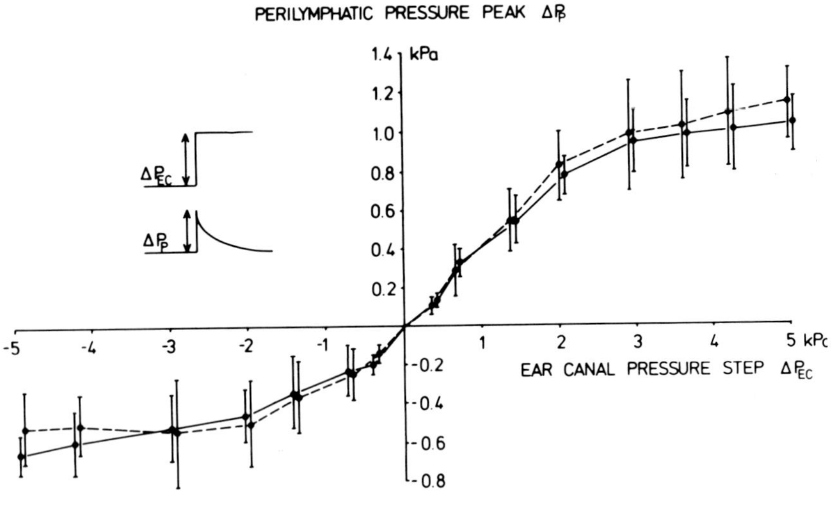

Fig. 5. Transfer functions obtained from pressure applications in the ear canal, before and after occlusion of the cochlear aqueduct. The graph shows the mean values ± 1 SD of the initial perilymphatic peaks ($\triangle P_p$) as a function of ear canal pressure steps ($\triangle P_{EC}$) in six cat ears. ——— - Cochlear aqueduct patent; ----- - Cochlear aqueduct blocked.

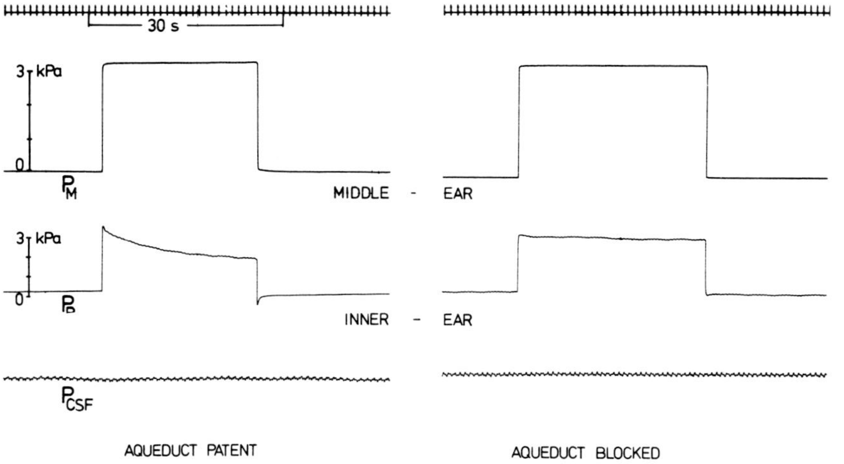

Fig. 6. Recordings of the change in perilymphatic pressure (P_P) produced by pressure steps applied to the middle ear. The slow perilymphatic pressure release process (left) indicates poor patency of the cochlear aqueduct (even before it is blocked). With the aqueduct blocked there is hardly any pressure release at all. No change is seen in the CSF pressure.

influx is supported by investigations with tracer substances in animals,[11,15,24,25] and by histological examinations of human temporal bones after fatal subarachnoid hemorrhage.[14] However, Lindsay et al[10] and Schuknecht and Seifi,[11] who occluded the CA in cats and found normal inner ear structures, concluded that the perilymph volume can be preseved in spite of blockage of the aqueduct. A local perilymph production theory is also supported by Silverstein et al,[26] who demonstrated an increase in protein concentration in the perilymph following blockage of the CA. In the present investigation transection and subsequent occlusion of the CA was performed during continuous measurement of the perilymphatic and CSF pressures. A fall in the P_P to zero when the CA was opened was followed by spontaneous rapid rise in P_P to its original level when the aqueduct was blocked. This indicates a local production of perilymph within the labyrinth and that the production of perilymph is sufficient to maintain a pressure equilibrium without supply of CSF via the CA. It also suggests that the CA may function as a two-way communication for exchange of fluid with elimination of waste products from the perilymph. When the rate of the pressure build-up from the suggested perilymph production (Fig. 1) was compared to the rate of the P_P rise, seen on intracranial infusion after obstruction of the aqueduct (Fig. 2), the latter process was by far the slower. The perilymphatic pressure rise after intracranial infusion might be explained by an increase in perilymph production initiated by the

VALUES OF THE MAJOR TIME CONSTANT OF THE PERILYMPHATIC PRESSURE RELEASE PROCESS BEFORE (T_1) AND AFTER (T') BLOCKAGE OF THE COCHLEAR AQUEDUCT IN THREE CATS

	Cochlear Aqueduct Patent						*Cochlear Aqueduct Blocked*					
	T_{1EC}			T_{1M}			T'_{EC}			T'_M		
	19/79	*23/79*	*1/80*	*19/79*	*23/79*	*1/80*	*19/79*	*23/79*	*1/80*	*19/79*	*23/79*	*1/80*
$+\triangle P$												
0.33	2.0	5.0	2.5				>600	110	>600			
0.67	2.0	4.0	2.5	4	8	5	>600	110	>600	>600	>600	350
1.00				4	8	5				>600	>600	310
1.34	1.5	3.0	2.0	3	9	5	600	110		>600	>600	350
2.00	1.0	2.5	1.7	2	8	4	600	110	>600	600	>600	350
2.66				2	7	3				600	>600	330
3.00	1.0	2.5	1.7				600	110	>600			
3.50	1.0	2.5	1.7	2	7	3	600	110	>600	600	>600	330
4.00	1.0	2.5	1.7	2	7	4	600	110	>600	600	>600	350
5.00	1.0	2.5	1.7				600	110	>600			
$-\triangle P$												
0.33	0.7	2.0	1.7				500	270	>600			
0.67	0.7	2.0	1.7	0.8	2.0	0.7	500	300	>600	500	>600	210
1.00				0.8	2.0	0.7				500	>600	210
1.34	0.5	1.7	1.0	0.8	1.5	0.4	500	340	>600	500	>600	210
2.00	0.5	1.5	1.0	0.5	1.5	0.4	500	340	>600	500	>600	210
2.66				0.5	1.5	0.4				500	>600	210
3.00	0.5	1.5	0.5				500	340	>600			
3.50				0.5	1.5	0.4				500	>600	210
4.00	0.5	1.5	0.5	0.5	1.5	0.4	500	340	>600	500	>600	210
5.00	0.5	1.5	0.5				500	340	>600			

T_{EC} - Time constant in response to ear canal pressure stimuli; T_M Time constant in response to middle ear pressure stimuli; $\triangle P$ - Stimulus pressure level (kPa).

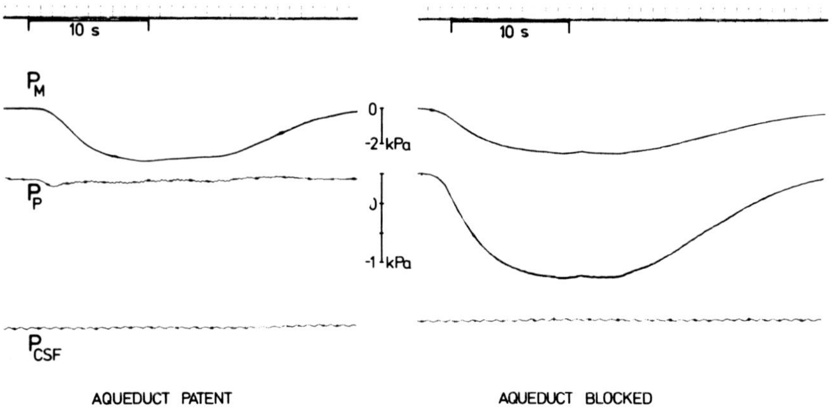

Fig. 7. Recording of the perilymphatic pressure (P_P) in response to a slow change in middle ear pressure (P_M). The small and temporary change in P_P, when the aqueduct is patent, indicates an immediate pressure release via the aqueduct. When the aqueduct is blocked, no pressure release is seen, and the P_P directly follows the change in middle ear pressure. The CSF pressure is shown at the bottom.

pressure gradient induced between the perilymph and CSF compartments. Another plausible theory is that additional routes for CSF influx exist when the CA is blocked, but that they only make a very slow contribution to the pressure equilibrium between the two fluid systems. Histological investigations have demonstrated that the perivascular and perineural spaces may serve as such additional routes.[10,25,27,28] Beentjes[19] reported a sustained decrease of the labyrinthine pressures, often to zero, when the CA was blocked. Kerth and Allen,[17] Martinez,[18] and Beentjes[19] reported that a blocked CA prevented any rise in intracochlear pressure during intracranial infusion. Furthermore, contrary to our findings, they also reported a complete absence of breathing fluctuations in the perilymphatic fluid.[18,19] No definite explanation can be offered for the discrepancy between these findings in previous reports and those made in the present investigation. It is, however, possible that the differences can be attributed to the different experimental methods used. The substantially reduced P_P reactions, seen when the CA was blocked, can easily be overlooked when using an open manometer system,[17] or when any fluid leakage is present in the system. Beentjes[19] measured the labyrinthine pressures some time after the CA was blocked, using a measuring system with about a 1000-fold larger volume displacement (according to his report) than we used in the present investigation.

The pressure-regulating capacity of the inner ear was evaluated by determining the rate of the pressure release process in the perilymph. This was done using low frequency pressure stimulation to the ear before and after occlusion of the CA. The rate of the pressure release process varied among animals before blockage of the aqueduct. Occlusion of the aqueduct always resulted in a severe impairment of the pressure-regulating capacity of the inner ear, demonstrated by a 20-fold to infinite increase of the time constants for the pressure release process. This indicates that a variability of the patency of the CA exists among animals and also that the CA is the major pressure-regulating factor of the inner ear. Additional pressure-regulating factors (eg, perivascular, perineural spaces, changes in perilymph production and resorption) seem to exist but their contribution seems to be very limited. It was further demonstrated that increasing stimulus levels to the ear could increase the rate of the pressure release when the CA was patent but not when it was occluded. This indicates that the CA plays the major role in the compliance of the inner ear.

Investigation of the pressure transfer from the ear canal and middle ear to the perilymphatic space was performed using pressure stimuli with a rise time of 20 and 80 ms (corner frequency 4-18 Hz[9]). It was shown that the patency of the CA generally did not influence the amplitude of the initial perilymphatic response. The reason seems to be that the rise time of the stimuli exceeded that at which an immediate pressure release occurred via the patent CA. However, negative pressure stimuli in the middle ear were an exception because a significantly higher initial perilymphatic peak ($\triangle P_P$) was observed when the CA had been occluded. This indicates that negative pressure stimuli could be compensated for to a small extent when the CA was patent as illustrated by the differences in the transfer functions before and after occlusion of the CA (Fig. 4). The reason for this may be that pressure stimulation in the middle ear produced a much greater perilymphatic peak than did a corresponding pressure stimuli in the ear canal. Furthermore, fluid is more easily forced through the CA from the subarachnoid space to the cochlea (during negative pressure stimulation) than in the opposite direction (during positive pressure stimulation). An anatomical basis for this finding may be the difference in shape of the subarachnoid and cochlear openings of the aqueduct.[10,29] Previously we have demonstrated that the perilymphatic pressure response to infrasound stimulation was reduced when the frequency of the infrasound was reduced below about 1 Hz.[30] In the present study it was shown that a patent CA could almost completely protect the inner ear from pressure changes when the ear canal or middle ear was exposured to pressure changes with a very long rise time

(0.25-0.5 kPa/s). However, a blocked CA will drastically reduce the pressure-regulating capacity, thus leaving the inner ear with little protection against pressure changes regardless of the rise time and also incapable of equilibrating pressure changes induced from the ear canal and middle ear. The inner ear is therefore likely to be more vulnerable to ambient pressure changes when the CA is obstructed.

The present study concerned acute experimental conditions and it is conceivable that long-time obstruction of the CA may increase the efficiency of the existing minor pressure release routes. This point needs to be addressed by future experiments.

REFERENCES

1. Goodhill V, Harris I, Brockman SJ, Hantz O. Sudden deafness and labyrinthine window ruptures. Ann Otol Rhinol Laryngol 1973; 82:2-12.

2. Tjernström Ö. Alternobaric vertigo: an experimental study in man of vertigo due to atmospheric pressure changes, thesis, Malmö, Sweden, 1974.

3. Freeman P. Rupture of the round window membrane. Otolaryngol Clin North Am 1978; 11:81-93.

4. Simmons FB. Fluid dynamics in sudden sensorineural hearing loss. Otolaryngol Clin North Am 1978; 11:55-61.

5. Gavreau V. Infrasound. Sci J 1968; 4:33-7.

6. Von Gierke HE, Nixon CW. Effects of intense infrasound on man. In: Tempest W, ed. Infrasound and low frequency vibration. London: Academic Press, 1976:115-50.

7. Evans MJ. Physiological and psychological effects of infrasound at moderate intensities. In: Tempest W, ed. Infrasound and low frequency vibration. London: Academic Press, 1976:97-113.

8. Densert O, Ingelstedt S, Ivarsson A, Pedersen K. Immediate restoration of basal sensorineural hearing (Mb Menière) using a pressure chamber. Acta Otolaryngol (Stockh) 1975; 80:93-100.

9. Densert O, Carlborg B, Stagg J. Transmission of low frequency pressure steps to the perilymphatic fluid. Acta Otolaryngol (Stockh) 1981; 91:55-64.

10. Lindsay JR, Neff WMD, Schuknecht HF, Perlman HB. Obliteration of the ductus endolymphaticus and their accompanying venous channels. Acta Otolaryngol (Stockh) 1953; 43:176-89.

11. Schuknecht HF, Seifi AE. Experimental observations of the fluid physiology of the inner ear. Ann Otol Rhinol Laryngol 1963; 72:687-712.

12. Palva T, Dammert K. Human cochlear aqueduct. Acta Otolaryngol (Stockh) 1969; Suppl 246.

13. Rask-Andersen H, Stahle J, Wilbrand H. Human cochlear aqueduct and its accessory canals. Ann Otol Rhinol Laryngol 1977; Suppl 42:1-16.

14. Holden HB, Schuknecht HF. Distribution pattern of blood in the inner ear following spontaneous subarachnoid haemorrhage. J Laryngol Otol 1968; 87:321-9.

15. Kellerhals B. Quantitative assessment of perilymph sources. ORL 1976; 38:193-7.

16. Kellerhals B. Perilymph production and cochlear blood flow. Acta Otolaryngol (Stockh) 1979; 87:370-4.

17. Kerth JD, Allen W. Comparison of the perilymphatic and cerebrospinal fluid pressures. Arch Otolaryngol 1963; 77:581-4.

18. Martinez DM. Simultaneous measurements of endolymphatic and perilymphatic fluid pressures before and during anaphylaxis and associated changes in cerebrospinal fluid, venous and arterial pressures. Acta Otolaryngol (Stockh) 1968; Suppl 238:1-53.

19. Beentjes BIJ. On the pressure of the endolymphatic, the perilymphatic and the cerebrospinal fluid with data on the endolymphatic membranes, thesis. Amsterdam: North-Holland Publishing Co, 1970.

20. Carlborg B, Densert O, Stagg J. Perilymphatic pressure in the cat: description of a new method for study of the inner ear hydrodynamics. Acta Otolaryngol (Stockh) 1980; 90:209-17.

21. Pappenheimer JR, Heisey SR, Jordan EF, Downer J de C. Perfusion of the cerebral ventricular system in unanesthetized goats. Am J Physiol 1962; 203:763-74.

22. Carlborg B. On experimental and physiological variation of the perilymphatic pressure in the cat. Acta Otolaryngol (Stockh) 1981; 91:19-28.

23. Arnold W. Zur Frage der Produktion und Resorption der Perilymphe (Lymphabfluss des Innenohres). Laryngol Rhinol Otol (Stuttg) 1974; 53:774-90.

24. Kimura RS, Schuknecht HF, Ota CY. Blockage of the cochlear aqueduct. Acta Otolaryngol (Stockh) 1974; 77:1-12.

25. Arnold W, v Ilberg C. Verbindungswege zwischen Liquor und Perilymphraum. Arch Klin Exp Ohren Nasen Kehlkopfheilkd 1971; 198:247-61.

26. Silverstein H, Davies GD, Griffin WL. Cochlear aqueduct obstruction changes in perilymph biochemistry. Ann Otol Rhinol Laryngol 1969; 78:532-41.

27. Angelborg C. Distribution of macromolecular tracer particles (Thorotrast) in the cochlea: an electron microscopic study in guinea pig. Acta Otolaryngol (Stockh) 1974; Suppl 31:19-41.

28. Sando I, Wood RP, Masuda Y, Hemenway WG. Perilymphatic communication routes in guinea pig cochlea. Ann Otol Rhinol Laryngol 1971; 80:826-34.

29. Lempert J, Meltzer PE, Wever EG, Lawrence M, Rambo JHT. Structure and function of the cochlear aqueduct. Arch Otolaryngol 1952; 55:134-45.

30. Krukowski B, Carlborg B, Densert O. Nonlinear aspects of infrasonic pressure transfer into the perilymph. Hear Res 1980; 2:207-12.

Ann Otol 91:1982

EVIDENCE FOR PRESYNAPTIC PARASYMPATHETIC RECEPTORS ON NASAL BLOOD VESSELS

RICHARD T. JACKSON, PhD
ATLANTA, GEORGIA

Noradrenergic synapses in the heart and several blood vessels have been shown to possess prejunctional receptors that modulate the release of norepinephrine from the synapse. The present experiment attempted to find evidence for presynaptic receptors for acetylcholine that modulated norepinephrine release. From the evidence obtained, it appears that the acetylcholine released from nasal parasympathetic fibers does not directly affect the smooth muscle of nasal blood vessels. Acetylcholine does, however, appear to inhibit the release of norepinephrine from nasal sympathetic nerve terminals. It appears that any nasal vasodilation produced by nasal parasympathetic fibers is caused by acetylcholine acting on an inhibitory, presynaptic, muscarinic receptor on the sympathetic nerve terminals. Acetylcholine would exert its control over nasal vessels by regulating the degree of sympathetic neurotransmitter release.

INTRODUCTION

It is commonly assumed that autonomic control of nasal blood vessels is by reciprocal innervation of the smooth muscle of nasal blood vessels by both sympathetic and parasympathetic nerve fibers. Postganglionic sympathetic fibers join the muscle at a synapse. The presynaptic complex releases norepinephrine (NE) which crosses the synaptic cleft, combines with a receptor on the muscle, induces contraction of the muscle, and results in vasoconstriction. Parasympathetic fibers form a similar synapse. Here the presynaptic complex releases acetylcholine (ACh) which crosses the cleft, combines with a muscarinic receptor on the muscle, induces muscle relaxation and vasodilation. Thus the blood flow at any time is the result of the combined effects of both systems.

However, animal nasal experiments with one of the prime neurotransmitters, ACh, produced equivocal results.[1-4] Administration of NE produced a quick, large, dose-related constriction of nasal vessels, often at doses that have little effect on blood pressure. Administration of ACh however, usually produced small dilation responses or none, and these are overshadowed by blood pressure changes. Whereas it was quite simple to demonstrate a pharmacological block of the effects of NE with antagonists like phenoxybenzamine, it was difficult or impossible to demonstrate a block of ACh effects with atropine. The equivocal behavior of nasal blood vessels to ACh prompted the author to look for other mechanisms.

In the last few years, pharmacologists have demonstrated that the presynaptic complex of sympathetic neurons contains several different kinds of receptors that modify the output of NE from the neurons.[5-9] It has been shown that the presynapse contains alpha receptors, responsive to the NE released from the synapse, that act to inhibit the release of NE. This negative feedback loop appears to regulate sympathetic effects, especially after higher neuronal activity. Besides alpha receptors, there is evidence in some adrenergic tissues for the existence of cholinergic receptors on the presynaptic complex, eg, the heart and several blood vessels.[6,7,9] Data show that in the heart presynaptic adrenergic tissue is inhibited by activation of a muscarinic receptor in addition to the effects caused by parasympathetic innervation of nodal tissue.[6-8] Thus, slowing of the heart rate could result not only from cholinergic effects on nodal tissue but also from cholinergic effects on the adrenergic synapse. Besides the heart, several isolated vascular tissue preparations have been shown to possess presynaptic, muscarinic receptors that inhibit NE release from sympathetic nerve endings.[9] With this in mind, I attempted to determine if nasal vascular tissue gave evidence that its sympathetic nerve endings possessed presynaptic, muscarinic receptors that affected NE release.

METHODS

An in vitro preparation of dog nasal blood vessels was used in this study. The responses of this preparation to drugs and electrical stimulation have been described previously.[10,11] The reader should be aware that this is an en masse blood vessel preparation. Nasal mucosa contains no contractile tissue except the smooth muscle of the blood vessels. Since mucosa contains various types of vessels (small arteries, capillaries, small veins), the recorded responses are the result of the activity of all vessel muscle.

The isolated nasal mucosa exhibits an increase in tension (contracts) when treated with common alpha adrenergic drugs such as NE, methoxamine, xylometazoline, ephedrine, phenylephrine and pseudoephedrine. These drugs are well-known vasoconstricting agents. It thus seems appropriate to relate and equate the contraction of the mucosa to vasoconstriction. Common vasodilating drugs such as acetylcholine, isoproterenol, nitroglycerine and histamine relax this tissue. It seems appropriate to relate this response to vasodilation or to interference with vasoconstriction. These relationships appear more secure because when these drugs

From the Division of Otolaryngology, Emory University School of Medicine, Atlanta.
REPRINTS — Richard T. Jackson, PhD, 441 Woodruff Memorial Bldg., Emory University, Atlanta, GA 30322.

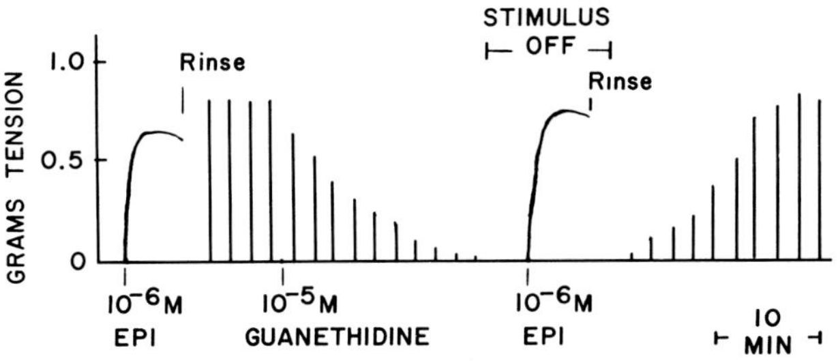

Fig. 1. Reduction of the electrically-induced response of the nasal mucosa by guanethidine. The response (increased tension) to epinephrine (EPI) is followed by four control responses to electrical stimulation. After the introduction of guanethidine, the responses to electrical stimulation are virtually abolished. The nasal smooth muscle still responds to EPI. Rinsing restores the electrically-induced responses.

are tested on nasal tissue in vivo, they induce the appropriate response.[12,13]

Electrical stimulation of this isolated nasal mucosa preparation causes a contraction of the tissue.[11] The mechanism of "field stimulation" is via stimulation of sympathetic nerve remnants still remaining on nasal blood vessels in the isolated mucosa. This mechanism has been shown by responses to guanethidine[11] and is demonstrated in this study (Fig. 1).

Two pieces of dog nasal septal mucosa were placed in muscle baths containing 10 ml of bicarbonate-buffered Ringer's solution. The bath solution was gassed with a 95% oxygen - 5% carbon dioxide mixture. A tension of 0.5 g was applied to the tissue and it was allowed to equilibrate for about 15-30 minutes. The mucosa was attached by a string to a force transducer and the tension changes were recorded. Electrical stimulation of this tissue or the introduction of vasoconstricting agents causes the mucosa to contract. Electrical stimuli were generated by a Grass S4 stimulator. The timing of the stimuli was regulated by two interval timers. Two 16-gauge wires (insulated except at the tip) were introduced into the muscle bath; one above and one below the tissue. The stimulus was usually five seconds in duration at a level of 20 to 40 V and frequency of 5 Hz. A 2-minute interval was allowed between stimulations.

Vasoactive drugs were introduced via a side port in the muscle bath. Vasoconstricting agents induced a contraction of the mucosa. Vasodilating agents reduce the electrically stimulated contraction or induce relaxation in a tissue previously contracted by a constricting agent.[11]

RESULTS

It has previously been shown that electrical stimulation of the isolated nasal mucosa causes a contraction of the nasal blood vessels.[11] The size of the contraction is related to the strength and duration of electrical stimulation (Fig. 2): Figure 2A shows the effect of varying the frequency of stimulation; Figure 2B shows the effect of varying the voltage of the stimulation while keeping the other parameters constant. The experiments that follow were performed with constant stimulus parameters. Thus, after the initial equilibration period, the responses to stimulation would be expected to be constant for the time interval of the experiment.

Guanethidine interferes with this electrically-induced contraction (Fig. 1). It reduces or abolishes the response to electrical stimulation but does not reduce the response of the nasal smooth muscle to exogenous epinephrine (or NE). Thus the postsynaptic receptors are not blocked. The inhibition is

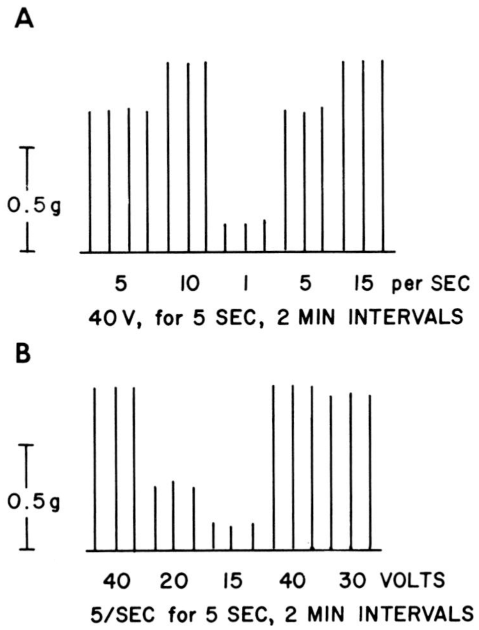

Fig. 2. Tracings of contractions of the nasal mucosa induced by varying the stimulus parameters of electrical stimulation. A) Frequency of stimulation was varied while the voltage (40V), duration (5 sec) and interval (2 min) were held constant. B) Voltage was varied while the frequency, duration and interval were held constant. The size of the contraction is related to the strength and duration of electrical stimulation.

reversible. Guanethidine is known to interfere with the terminal neuronal stores of sympathetic transmitter. Transmitter (NE) uptake, storage, and release mechanisms are affected and this results in a reduction in transmitter release from the nerve terminal following nervous activity.[14] Electrical stimulation of isolated nasal mucosa induces a release of NE from sympathetic nerve terminals which in turn acts on the smooth muscle of nasal vessels and causes contraction (Fig. 1).

When acetylcholine (ACh) is added to the muscle bath during electrical stimulation, the contraction

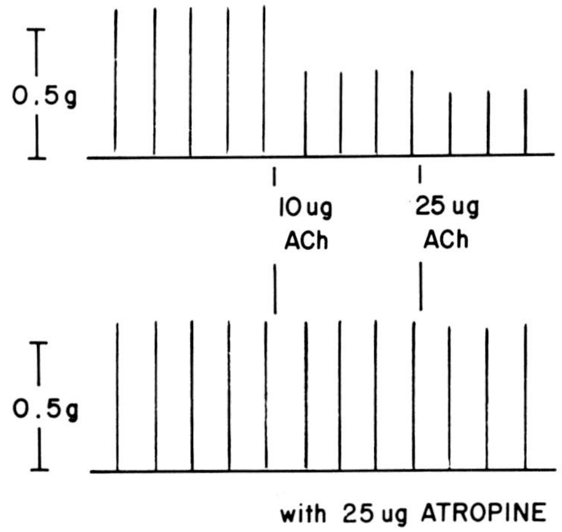

Fig. 3. Effect of acetylcholine (ACh) and atropine on electrically-induced responses. The introduction of ACh quickly reduces the responses. Atropine blocks this effect. Stimulus interval is two minutes.

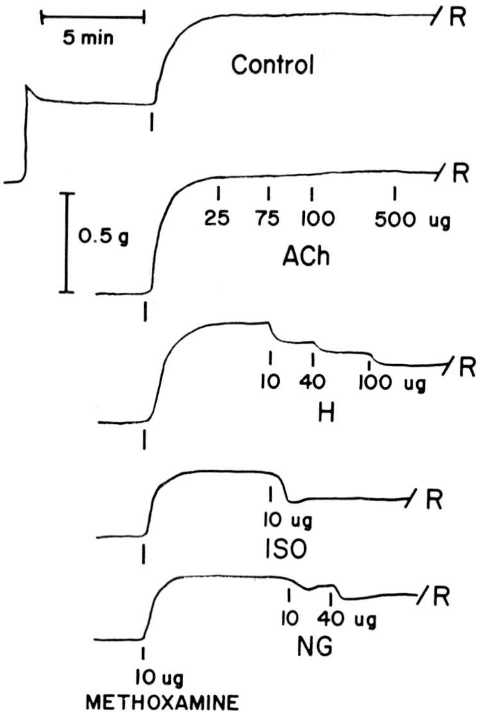

Fig. 4. The effect of vasodilating agents on the contraction induced by methoxamine. ACh does not relax the contracted muscle. Histamine (H), isoproterenol (ISO) and nitroglycerine (NG) relax the contracted muscle. Rinsing with 30 ml of Ringer's solution (R) is indicated.

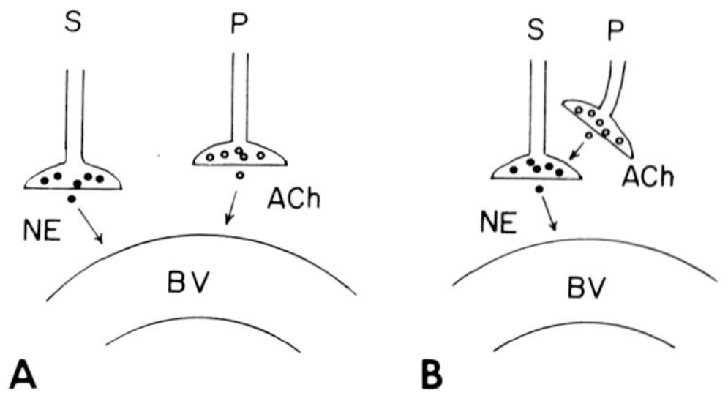

Fig. 5. Two schemes of autonomic innervation of nasal blood vessel (BV) smooth muscle. A) Postganglionic sympathetic (S) and parasympathetic (P) fibers terminate separately on the muscle. The tone of the muscle is the result of the combined effects of the two neurotransmitters norepinephrine (NE) and acetylcholine (ACh). B) Tone of the muscle is mainly determined by the continuous release of NE. The action of ACh is to inhibit this release by varying degrees.

is inhibited in a dose-related manner. Atropine blocks this effect of ACh (Fig. 3). The effect of ACh is rapid in onset and reversed by rinsing. The response to electrical stimulation is not affected by hexamethonium. The latter drug is a ganglionic blocking agent which competes with ACh for receptor sites on postsynaptic membranes. These results, coupled with the response to guanethidine, imply that ACh is either inhibiting the release of NE from the sympathetic terminal on nasal vessels or serving as a physiological antagonist of NE by acting directly on the smooth muscle and causing it to relax, ie, a postsynaptic effect.

An attempt was made to show an effect of ACh on the postsynaptic smooth muscle receptor. When ACh was introduced into the muscle bath in the absence of electrical stimulation, no relaxation occurred even though the muscle was under a tension of 0.5 g. The nasal smooth muscle was then contracted with 10 μg of methoxamine. This produces a sustained contraction (Fig. 4, top). The companion piece of nasal septal mucosa was treated with methoxamine and then treated with four doses of ACh. There was no sign of relaxation of the contraction, even at high doses of ACh. Similarly, the methoxamine-contracted mucosa was treated with lower doses of three other common vasodilating agents: nitroglycerine, histamine, and isoproterenol. The smooth muscle relaxed in a dose-dependent manner. If postsynaptic receptors for ACh were present on the muscle, a similar dose-dependent relaxation due to ACh would be expected.

DISCUSSION

Two points emerge from these results. ACh, the neurotransmitter of the parasympathetic nervous system, inhibits the muscle contraction resulting from the sympathetic sequence of neuronal activity, release of NE and attachment of NE to the muscle receptor. Second, ACh appears not to relax the muscle itself even though other vasodilating agents do have this effect under the same test conditions.

In recent years, pharmacologists have demonstrated the existence of receptor-coupled mechanisms at nerve terminals through which transmitter release may be modified.[5] Thus NE released from noradrenergic nerve terminals acts on prejunctional alpha receptors, causing an inhibition on further transmission. Besides prejunctional alpha receptors, some tissues exhibit prejunctional receptors for dopamine, ACh, prostaglandins and others.[8]

Pharmacologists have amended their views on the mechanisms of reciprocal innervation. Data for the heart, eg, show the presence of presynaptic muscarinic inhibition of adrenergic activity in addition to parasympathetic innervation of nodal tissue.[6,8] Instead of direct sympathetic and parasympathetic innervation of the heart (Fig. 5A), ACh may affect the release of NE (Fig. 5B). The mechanism of ACh regulation, according to Muscholl et al,[15] is that excitation of presynaptic muscarine receptors decreases the availability of calcium necessary for NE release.

The evidence reported in this paper suggests that the autonomic innervation of nasal blood vessels is indirect (Fig. 5B). Parasympathetic nerve activity probably has no direct effect on the smooth muscle of nasal blood vessels. The parasympathetic system can only modulate (inhibit) sympathetic activity going to the muscle cell. This implies that if there is no sympathetic activity, there will be no evidence of change with parasympathetic stimulation.

The author is aware that another interpretation of these data is possible. It may be that nasal blood vessels have postjunctional muscarinic receptors in addition to those postulated to be prejunctional. If so, the experimental design or the sensitivity of the system precluded their discovery.

Several workers have shown that the sympathetic neurons always seem to be active on nasal blood vessels.[16,17] As a consequence, cutting the sympathetic supply to the nose results in nasal congestion,[12] as does inhibition of sympathetic activity by reserpine-like drugs. A patent nasal airway due to continuous sympathetic activity is the preferred basal condition. It seems more efficient to modulate or interrupt this activity when necessary rather than keep both autonomic systems active and depend upon the combined effect for the basal condition.

REFERENCES

1. Malm L. Vasodilation in the nasal mucosa of the cat and the effects of parasympatholytic and beta adrenergic blocking agents. Acta Otolaryngol (Stockh) 1973; 76:277-82.

2. Eccles R, Wilson H. The autonomic innervation of the nasal blood vessels of the cat. J Physiol 1974; 238:549-60.

3. Anggard A. The effects of parasympathetic nerve stimulation on the microcirculation and secretion in the nasal mucosa of the cat. Acta Otolaryngol (Stockh) 1974; 78:98-105.

4. Gadlage R, Behnke EE, Jackson RT. Is the vidian nerve cholinergic? Arch Otolaryngol 1975; 101:422-5.

5. Westfall TC. Local regulation of adrenergic neurotransmission. Physiol Rev 1977; 57:659-728.

6. Stark K. Regulation of norepinephrine release by presynaptic receptor systems. Rev Physiol Biochem Pharmacol 1977; 77:1-124.

7. Muscholl E. Presynaptic muscarine receptors and inhibition of release. In: Paton DM, ed. The release of catecholamines from adrenergic neurons. Oxford: Pergamon Press, 1979:87-110.

8. Rand MJ, Majewski H, Medgett IC, McCulloch MW, Story DF. Prejunctional receptors modulating autonomic neuroeffector transmission. Circ Res 1980; 46 Suppl 1:70-6.

9. Endo T, Starke K. Bangerter A, Taube HD. Presynaptic receptor systems on the noradrenergic neurones of the rabbit pulmonary artery. Naunyn Schmiedebergs Arch Pharmacol 1977; 296:229-47.

10. Jackson RT. A new in vitro method of drug assay of nasal blood vessels. Arch Otorhinolaryngol 1979; 225:33-8.

11. Jackson RT. An in vitro technique for testing nasal vasodilating agents. Otolaryngol Head Neck Surg 1980; 88:434-8.

12. Rooker DW, Jackson RT. The effects of certain drugs, cervical sympathetic stimulation and section on nasal patency. Ann Otol Rhinol Laryngol 1969; 78:403-14.

13. Jackson RT. Pharmacologic responsiveness of the nasal mucosa. Ann Otol Rhinol Laryngol 1970; 79:461-7.

14. Weiner N. Drugs that inhibit adrenergic nerves and block adrenergic receptors. In: Gilman AG, Goodman LS, Gilman A, eds. The pharmacological basis of therapeutics. 6th ed. New York: Macmillan and Co, 1980:198-201.

15. Muscholl E, Ritzell H, Rossler K. Presynaptic muscarinic control of neuronal noradrenaline release. In: Langer SZ, Starke K. Dubocovich ML, eds. Presynaptic receptors. New York: Pergamon Press, 1979:287-91.

16. Franke FE. Sympathetic control of the dog's nasal blood vessels. Proc Soc Exp Biol Med 1966; 123:544-7.

17. Malcomson KG. The vasomotor activities of the nasal mucous membrane. J Laryngol Otol 1959; 73:73-98.

≈

NINTH CONGRESS OF THE EUROPEAN RHINOLOGIC SOCIETY — THIRD INTERNATIONAL SYMPOSIUM ON INFECTION AND ALLERGY OF THE NOSE AND PARANASAL SINUSES

The Ninth Congress of the European Rhinologic Society and the Third International Symposium on Infection and Allergy of the Nose and Paranasal Sinuses will be held in Stockholm, Sept. 5-8, 1982. For information write: Ninth ERS Congress 1982, c/o Reso Congress Service, S-105 24 Stockholm.

Ann Otol 91:1982

TYPHOID FEVER AND COCHLEOVESTIBULAR LESIONS

J. RAMÓN ESCAJADILLO, MD

GUILLERMO ALATORRE, MD　　ARTURO ZÁRATE, MD

MEXICO CITY, MEXICO

Six cases of pathologically confirmed cochleovestibular lesions due to typhoid fever are presented. The lesions occurred between the second and third weeks of the disease (5 of 6 cases), in the left ear more commonly than in the right (4 of 6 cases), and in females more often than in males (5 of 6 cases). Some of the lesions were reversible. Factors believed to be significant for development of these lesions include host susceptibility, endotoxins, arteritis, and ischemia.

INTRODUCTION

Since Bretonneau described intestinal lesions caused by typhoid fever in 1820,[1] a considerable literature has developed concerning the physiopathology, diagnosis, and treatment of these kinds of lesions. Studies of typhoid-related lesions in the inner ear, however, are much less common. Only a few isolated reports suggest that cochlear lesions can be produced by endotoxins of the typhoid bacillus.[2,3] Hirasugi[3] further suggests that such lesions can be reversible. This article presents six additional cases of cochleovestibular lesions due to typhoid fever.

METHODS

The Hospital for Infectious Diseases of the La Raza Medical Center, Mexican Institute of Social Security, sent us 40 patients with the diagnosis of typhoid fever confirmed by isolation of *Salmonella typhi* in the bone marrow, blood, and feces. Extensive histories were obtained for each patient with emphasis on otologic problems, noise exposure, and ingestion of ototoxic drugs. Hearing levels, tinnitus, and dizziness were evaluated at the onset of typhoid fever, and monitored during treatment (Tables 1 and 2). Otoscopy, tonal studies (Amplaid 300 audiometer), speech discrimination tests (Ampex recorder), and noninstrumental vestibular tests were completed for all patients. For patients with cochleovestibular symptoms, Bekesy audiometry (Amplaid Bekesy) and electronystagmograms (Tracoustics Electronystagmograph) also were obtained.

Twenty-three (57.5%) of the 40 patients studied were female and 17 (42.5%) were male. The age range was 17-45 years (average 26.7 years). Fifteen (37.5%) of these patients had cochlear and/or vestibular lesions; of these, nine had histories of otologic problems prior to the onset of typhoid fever and thus were not included. Of the remaining six presented below, the average age was 34.1 years; five were female.

CASE REPORTS

Case 1. A 45-year-old female presented with headache, diarrhea, and gastric pain of one-week's duration, but without fever. *S typhi* was isolated; Widal reactions were positive (1:640) and the leukocyte count was 2,900. Ampicillin was given, 500 mg every four hours for 15 days.

During the second week of the disease, dizziness, hearing loss, and bilateral tinnitus developed. Otoscopic examination was normal.

TABLE 1. OTOLOGIC HISTORY OF PATIENTS WITH COCHLEOVESTIBULAR LESIONS (n = 15)

History	*No. of Patients*
Family deafness	1
Chronic otitis media	1
Chronic noise exposure	4
Hearing loss prior to onset of typhoid fever	3
No otologic history	6

Audiologic studies revealed bilateral superficial-to-moderate sensorineural hearing loss, with a descent of acute tones (greater on the left side), pain with the speech discrimination test at 100 dB (Fig. 1A), and a bilateral type 2 Bekesy audiogram. Electronystagmography (ENG) showed nystagmic movements to the right and intermittently to the left; the pendular tracing showed nystagmoid movements; optokinetic nystagmus (OKN) was normal. Caloric stimulation revealed bilateral vestibular depression, predominantly on the left side.

When the patient was seen three months later (Fig. 1B), the hearing loss had advanced to a bilateral moderate sensorineural loss with left-side predominance. The speech discrimination test showed that the pain level persisted at 100 dB. Although the dizziness had resolved, ENG revealed that the bilateral vestibular depression continued.

Case 2. A 45-year-old female patient presented with diarrhea and gastric pain, headache, and fever of one month's duration. *S typhi* was isolated; Widal reactions were positive (1:320) and the leukocyte count was 4,500. Ampicillin was given, 500 mg every four hours for 15 days.

During the third week of the disease the patient experienced a feeling of fullness in both ears, tinnitus, and instability. Otoscopic examination was normal. The audiologic study showed sensorineural hearing loss, superficial-to-moderate on the left side, and superficial for acute frequencies on the right side. Speech discrimination regressed in the left ear (Fig. 2A). The Bekesy audiogram could not be evaluated due to a misunderstanding of the test. ENG showed no spontaneous nystagmus, and the pen-

TABLE 2. OTOLOGIC SYMPTOMS OF TYPHOID PATIENTS (n = 6)

Symptoms	*No. of Patients*
Tinnitus	3
Dizziness	5
Hearing loss	3
Fullness in ear	1

From the Department of Otolaryngology, La Raza Medical Center, Mexican Institute of Social Security, Mexico City.

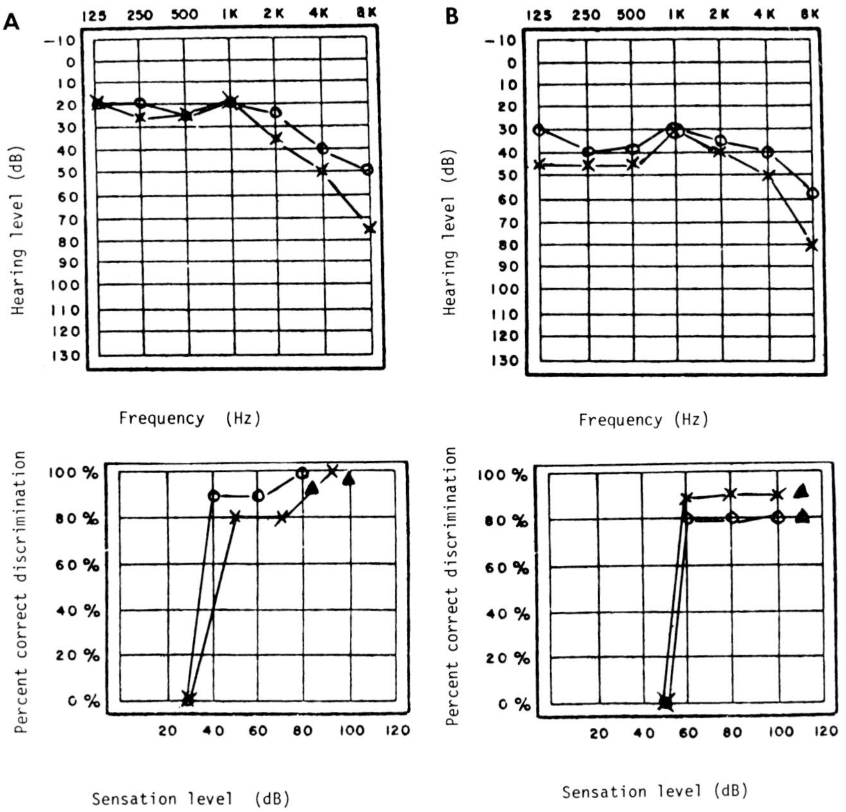

Fig. 1. (Case 1) Audiograms of a 45-year-old female. A) March 5, 1979; B) June 9, 1979. o - Right ear; x - Left ear; ▲ - Pain level.

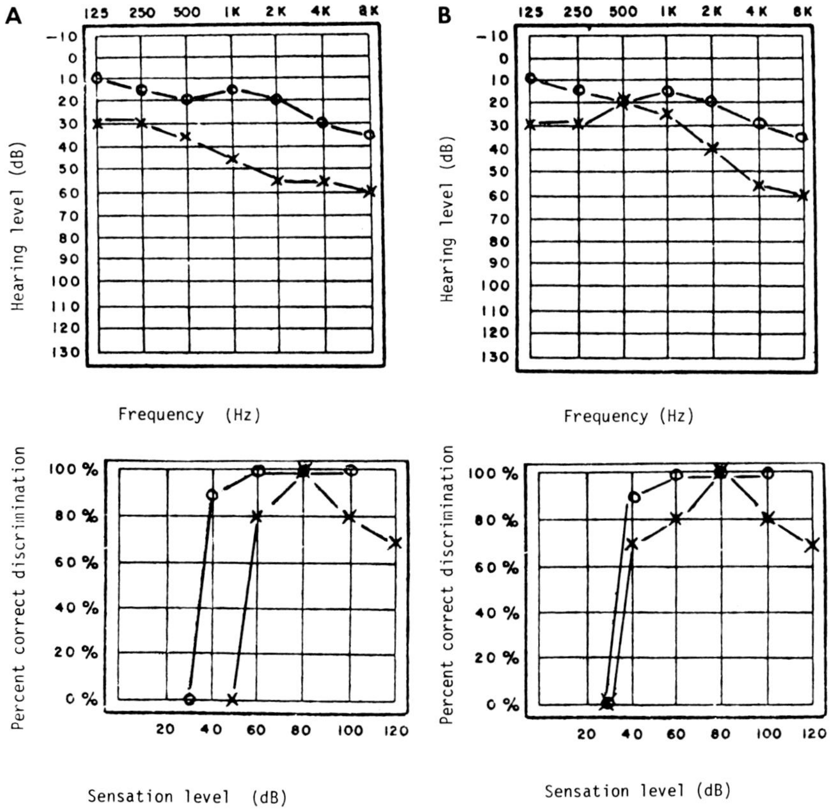

Fig. 2. (Case 2) Audiograms of a 45-year-old female. A) June 2, 1979; B) September 9, 1979.

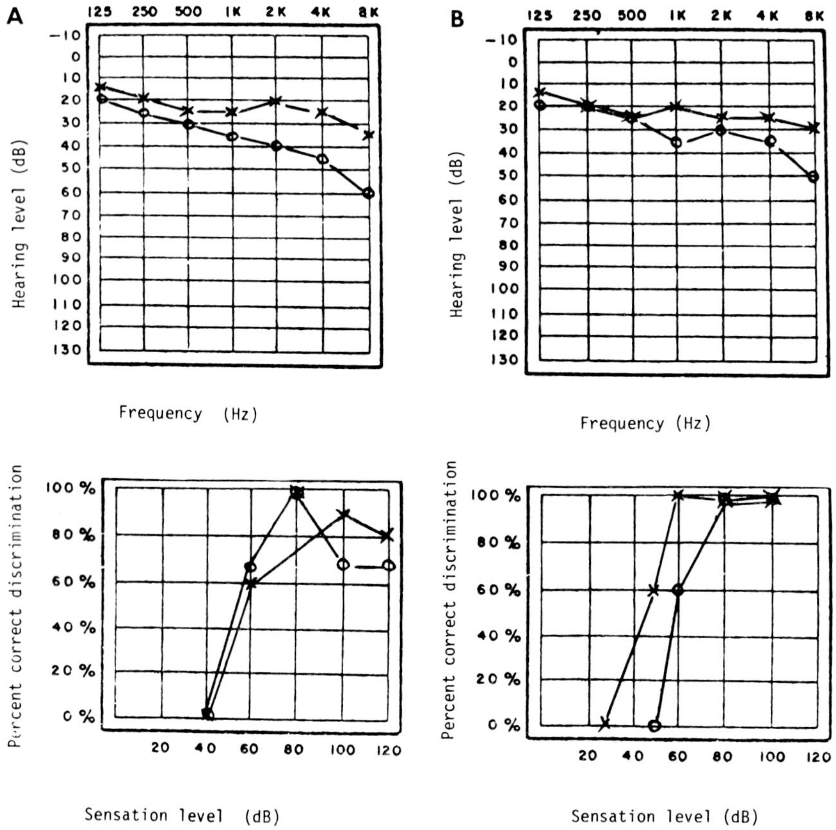

Fig. 3. (Case 3) Audiograms of a 19-year-old male. A) August 1, 1979; B) October 17, 1979.

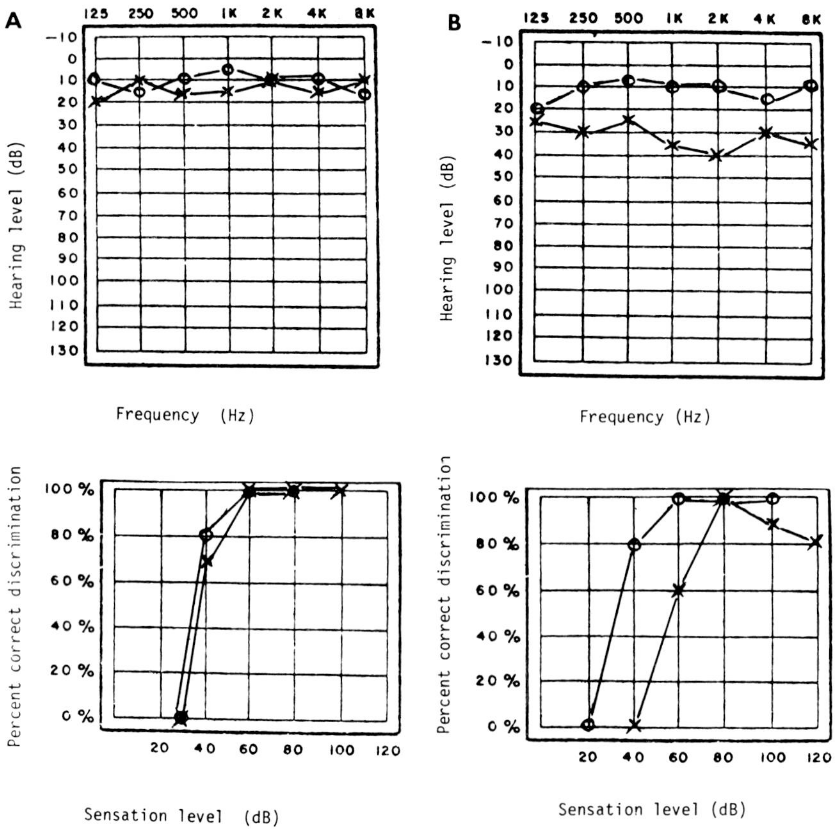

Fig. 4. A) (Case 4) Audiograms of a 24-year-old female, August 17, 1979. B) (Case 5) Audiograms of a 20-year-old female, January 4, 1980.

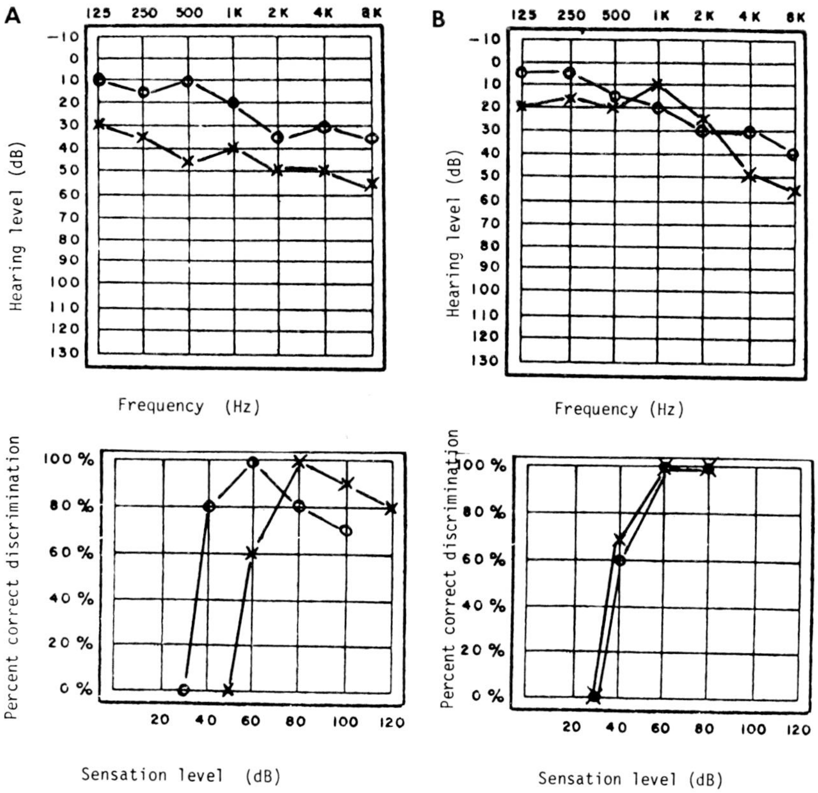

Fig. 5. (Case 6) Audiograms of a 48-year-old female. A) January 5, 1980; B) July 3, 1980.

dular tracing was normal. OKN was depressed with a rotating drum to the left. Caloric stimulation revealed left vestibular paresis.

When the patient was seen three months later (Fig. 2B), she showed a 15 dB improvement in hearing at medium frequencies in the left ear; hearing in the right ear remained unchanged. The patient's instability had resolved; the speech discrimination results and ENG were essentially unchanged.

Case 3. A 19-year-old male presented with epistaxis, headache, diarrhea, gastric pain, and fever of two weeks' duration. *S typhi* was isolated; the leukocyte count was 4,900. Chloramphenicol and ampicillin were given, 500 mg every six hours for 15 days.

During the third week of the disease, hearing loss, bilateral tinnitus, and instability which increased with abrupt head movements developed. Otoscopic examination was normal. Audiologic studies revealed sensorineural hearing loss, superficial in the left ear, moderate in the right ear, bilateral regression in speech discrimination (Fig. 3A), and type 2 Bekesy audiograms in both ears. ENG showed first degree nystagmus to the left; spontaneous nystagmus remained unchanged with positional testing; pendular tracing showed additional nystagmoid movements; OKN eased to the left.

Caloric stimulation revealed bilateral paresis with right predominance.

When the patient was seen three months later (Fig. 3B), he had gained 10 dB at 2, 4 and 8 Hz, and 5 dB at 250 and 500 Hz in the right ear. The left ear was unchanged. Speech discrimination tests involved no recruitment. The vestibular test revealed an improvement in the caloric response in the left ear.

Case 4. A 24-year-old female patient presented with frontal headache, diarrhea, gastric pain, and fever of seven days' duration. *S typhi* was isolated; leukocyte count was 5,000. Ampicillin was given, 500 mg every four hours for 15 days.

During the second week of the disease, dizziness and other symptoms relative to the autonomic nervous system occurred.

Otoscopic examination was normal. Audiologic tests revealed normal hearing and a bilateral type 1 Bekesy audiogram (Fig. 4A).

ENG showed second degree spontaneous nystagmus to the right; the pendular tracing showed additional nystagmus. OKN was well organized, and eased to the right. Caloric stimulation revealed left vestibular paresis.

Case 5. A 20-year-old female presented with continuous gastric pain and fever of five days' duration. *S typhi* was isolated; Widal reaction was positive (1:320); leukocyte count was 4,900. Chloramphenicol was given, 500 mg every four hours for 15 days.

During the eighth day of the disease dizziness and instability developed, without hearing alterations. Otoscopic examination was normal.

Audiologic studies revealed left superficial sensorineural hearing loss, and a left type 2 Bekesy audiogram; speech discrimination tests (PI-PB) showed regression on the left side (Fig. 4B).

Case 6. A 48-year-old female presented with fever, diaphoresis, headache, and arthralgia of seven days' duration. *S typhi* was isolated; leukocyte count was 3,000. The patient was treated with trimetroprim and sulfametoxasol for 15 days.

During the second week, bilateral hearing loss and dizziness related to fever developed. Otoscopic examination was normal. Audiologic tests revealed superficial bilateral sensorineural hearing loss from 1,000 dB in the right ear, and superficial-to-moderate in the left ear, and type 2 Bekesy audiogram. Speech discrimination tests showed bilateral phonemic regression (Fig. 5A). ENG was normal. Further tests six months later (Fig. 5B) revealed improved hearing in the left ear (30 dB) as well as the disappearance of phonemic regression and recruiting in the Bekesy tests.

RESULTS

The six patients studied had normal otoscopic profiles and the following clinical symptoms (Table

2): hearing loss (3), feeling of fullness in the ear (1), tinnitus (3), and dizziness (5). In 3 cases symptoms occurred during the second week of the disease; in 2 cases, during the third week; and in 1 case, during the first week. This means that cochleovestibular symptoms developed between the second and third weeks of the disease in 5 of the 6 patients. This corresponds with the onset of other complications of typhoid fever, which are well documented in the literature.[4-7]

DISCUSSION

Typhoid fever, caused by the Gram-negative bacterium *Salmonella typhi*, is widely distributed over the world.[8] Susceptibility, however, is related to environment as well as to individual resistance.[1,4,9] *S typhi* is not related to race or sex.[8,10]

The bacillus is transported through the intestinal epithelium by means of local macrophages, probably to lymphatic sites;[8] it travels through the thoracic duct into the bloodstream, and is carried primarily to the liver, spleen, Peyer's patches, and bone marrow. Some *S typhi* bacteria are phagocytosed by reticulum-endothelial cells,[11] and some are able to reproduce and return to the bloodstream. The most important clinical symptoms of the disease appear during the second septicemic phase.[10,12]

The following factors contribute to the symptomatology: endotoxins, pyrogen, a significant vessel response to catecholamines with pressor and vasomotor changes in the microcirculation, and increased serotonins. These factors explain the arteritis which accompanies typhoid fever.[10-14]

Endotoxins cause degeneration of the organ of Corti.[2,14] Majlesi et al[15] cultured *S typhi* in a mastoid abscess which appeared after a case of typhoid fever, and their findings indicate that this bacillus, by itself, is capable of producing cochleovestibular lesions.

Since 5 of the 6 patients in this study were female, it is possible that women may be predisposed to cochleovestibular lesions. Vestibular symptoms prevailed over cochlear lesions, and the left ear was more affected (71.1%) than the right. The risk of cochleovestibular lesions increases when leukocyte counts are below 5,000, a characteristic of four of our cases.

Follow-up tests were made on 4 of the 6 patients: in 1 the hearing loss became slightly worse, 2 improved, and 1 revealed no cochlear alterations. Dizziness disappeared in 3 of the 4 patients, but vestibular paresis remained.

CONCLUSIONS

1. Studies which describe focal lesions with necrosis and an increased response to pressor substances which cause arteritis[8,10,13] suggest that ischemia plays an important role in the development of cochleovestibular lesions produced by typhoid fever. The cochlear branch of the internal auditory artery, as well as the rear vestibular artery, can suffer damage.

2. Cultures of *S typhi* have been reported to produce cochleovestibular lesions.

3. There appears to be an inverse relationship between the extent of the lesion and leukocyte count.

Since our data lack statistical significance, their value at this time is chiefly descriptive. Further investigations are needed to explain deafness due to typhoid fever.

ACKNOWLEDGMENTS — We want to thank Dr. Leticia Tijerina de Sánchez, audiologist on our service, for revising this manuscript.

REFERENCES

1. Anderson WAD. Pathology. 5th ed. St. Louis: CV Mosby Co, 1966: 219-22.

2. Davis H, Silverman RS. Hearing and deafness. 4th ed. New York: Holt, Rinehart & Winston, 1978: 123.

3. Hirasugi Y. A case report of sensory-neural hipoacusia with typhoid fever. Otolaryngology (Tokyo) 1978; 50:533-7.

4. Hornick RB, Greisman SE, Woodward TE, DuPont HL, Dawkins AT, Snyder MJ. Typhoid fever: pathogenesis and immunologic control. N Engl J Med 1970; 283:686-737.

5. Vázquez V, Calderón JE, Rodríguez RS. Chloramfenicol resistant strains of *Salmonella typhosa*. N Engl J Med 1972; 286:1120-4.

6. Yugoslav Typhoid Commission. A controlled field trial of the effectiveness of acetone dried and inactivated heat fenol inactivated typhoid vaccines in Yugoslavia. Bull WHO 1964; 30:623-8.

7. Besudo D, Olarte J, Mendoza M, et al. Aislamiento de Salmonella typhi resistente a altas concentraciones de cloramfenicol. Pr XXXV Reunión Reg AIP, Vista Hermosa, Mor, Mexico, August, 1972.

8. Calderón JE. Conceptos clíncos de Infectología pediátrica. 1st ed. Mexico City: IMAN, 1973: 295-315.

9. Aimon HG, Miller RC. Ampicillin in the treatment of chronic typhoid carriers. N Engl J Med 1966; 274:807-15.

10. Beltrán F, Franco A, Contreras CM. Algunos aspectos de la perforación intestinal en la fiebre tifoidea. Revisión de 206 casos. Bol Med Hosp Inf Mex 1960; 17:745-63.

11. Kumate J, Benavides UL, Pérez NJ. Pathological physiology of salmonellosis. J Infect Dis 1956; 98:1-9.

12. Heredia D, Besudo D, Calderón JE, et al. Estudio de un brote epidémico de fiebre tifoidea en Ciudad Netzahualcóyotl, Estado de México. Salud Pública Mex 1967; 9:375-90.

13. López F. Trombosis tifoídica de la arteria silvana. Bol Med Hosp Infect Mex 1944; 1:20-3.

14. Corvera Bernardelli J. Neurotología clínica. 1st ed. Mexico City: Salvat Editores, 1978: 223-4.

15. Majlesi H, Naderi A, Farough H. Mastoid abscess in a patient with typhoid fever. Asian Med J 1977; 20-8, 59-60.

BINOCULAR COUNTERROLLING DURING SUSTAINED BODY TILT IN NORMAL HUMANS AND IN A PATIENT WITH UNILATERAL VESTIBULAR NERVE SECTION

SHIRLEY G. DIAMOND, BA

CHARLES H. MARKHAM, MD NOBUHIKO FURUYA, MD

LOS ANGELES, CALIFORNIA

Two normal persons and a patient with unilateral vestibular nerve section were held motionless for ten minutes in the upright position, at 60° tilt right ear down, and at 60° tilt left ear down. In addition, one normal subject was held for ten minutes at each of 30, 60, and 90° tilt left ear down. Photographs were taken of both eyes every ten seconds. Measurements of ocular counterrolling during these trials revealed torsional eye movements in all positions, including the upright, even though the head and body were stationary. Variations in torsion in the upright position ranged up to 2.75°. At the tilt positions, variations ranged up to 4°. Disconjugate movements were seen in all subjects in all positions. There were no significant differences in measurements of ocular counterrolling during static tilt between the normal subjects and the patient with the vestibular nerve section, in contrast to measures obtained during slow velocity dynamic testing.

During the century or so in which ocular counterrolling (OCR) has been studied, several investigators have noted considerable variation in measurements taken at a given angle of tilt in the same subject on different occasions. A review of studies noting this phenomenon[1] pointed out the difficulty of knowing whether this variability, seen under conditions of tilt sustained for varying periods of time, was due to the uncertainty of the methods of measurement or whether the counterrolling reflex is itself subject to spontaneous fluctuations. In contrast, other workers have referred to the "persistent, static nature of counterrolling with sustained head tilt,"[2] and it is this latter assumption which prevails in present-day studies.

Investigations in our laboratory of OCR during dynamic tilt[3-6] included observations made during several 30-second stationary intervals interspersed in the dynamic portions of the trials. These observations were provocative in failing to confirm either the static notion or the decay reported in some early studies.[7,8] The results of these static observations were reminiscent of the variability reported in a study in which subjects were tilted for eight hours, but whose heads were permitted to move between the short intervals of photography.[9] A systematic sequence of observations during stationary tilt over a longer period of time, with the head restrained for the entire duration of study, seemed likely to clarify the question of how stable the OCR reflex is when the subject is held in a tilted position. Our studies of dynamic tilt had shown significant differences in OCR between normal humans and patients who had unilateral eighth nerve sections, and the question of whether static tilt would similarly reveal differences was also of interest.

METHODS

Subjects. Three persons who had earlier undergone dynamic OCR testing served as subjects. LM, a 31-year-old male, and DS, a 23-year-old female, were normal individuals with characteristically normal dynamic profiles. JR was a 55-year-old male who had had a left-sided acoustic neuroma removed under direct vision with a binocular operating microscope 12 years earlier, a procedure in which his left superior vestibular nerve was sectioned and the inferior portion preserved. Caloric testing at 30, 44, and 0°C demonstrated all the features of a nonfunctioning left horizontal semicircular canal. His dynamic profile was characteristic of other patients with unilateral vestibular nerve sections. The dynamic profiles of LM and JR may be seen elsewhere.[3]

Subjects were securely strapped into a large motor-driven tilting apparatus. The centers of the pupils were aligned horizontally, the head positioned and stabilized by a bite bar. The upper part of the face, encompassing both eyes, was photographed with a single lens reflex camera rigidly attached to the rotating device. The tilting apparatus, as well as photographic and measurement methods, are described in detail elsewhere.[4]

Experiment 1 (0° for 10 minutes). Subjects were carefully aligned in the upright position, with lap and shoulder belts and bite bar maintaining the head motionless. Photographs were taken every 10 seconds for 10 minutes.

Experiment 2 (60° left ear down for 10 minutes, 60° right ear down for 10 minutes). DS and JR were tilted at a constant velocity of 3°/s to 60° left ear down with photographs taken at each 10° of tilt. Subjects were held at 60° for 10 minutes, with photographs at each 10 seconds. At the end of 10 minutes they were brought back to the upright position at the same velocity. After some minutes rest, the procedure was repeated at 60° right ear down.

Experiment 3 (30°, 60°, and 90° left ear down for 10 minutes each). LM was tilted to 30°, 60°, and 90° left ear down on separate trials and photographed at each 10° of tilt. He was brought to each tilt position at a velocity of 3°/s, and was held there for 10 minutes while photographs were taken every 10 seconds, and then returned to the upright position.

In all experiments, subjects' eyes were continuously monitored by the investigator through the camera viewfinder.

From the Reed Neurological Research Center, UCLA School of Medicine, Los Angeles.

REPRINTS — Charles H. Markham, MD, UCLA School of Medicine, Department of Neurology, Reed Neurological Research Center, Los Angeles, CA 90024.

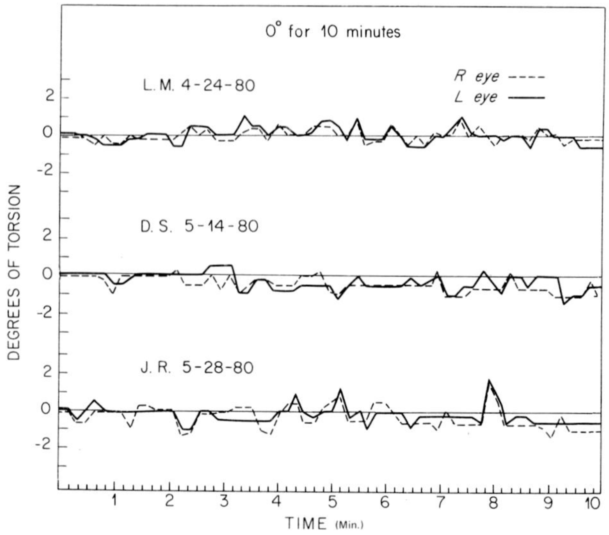

Fig. 1. Two normal subjects, LM and DS, and a patient with left vestibular nerve section, JR, were held motionless for 10 minutes in the upright position. Photographs of both eyes were taken each 10 seconds. Torsional variations in the normal subjects ranged up to 1.5°; in the patient they ranged up to 2.75°. Note some disconjugate eye movement in all subjects.

RESULTS

Experiment 1. Torsional eye movements were seen in all three subjects while they were held motionless in the upright position (Fig. 1). Variations during the 10 minutes in which 61 OCR measurements were taken ranged up to 1.5° in LM and DS, and to 2.75° in JR.

Disconjugate movement was defined as the two eyes moving in different *directions* (regardless of amount of difference), eg, right eye moving clockwise 0.5° while the left eye was unchanged would be classified disconjugate; right eye moving clockwise 0.5° while left eye moved clockwise 1° would not. Disconjugate movements were seen in all three subjects. LM had 23% of observations disconjugate, DS, 43%, and JR, 45%. Differences between subjects were not significant (*t* tests).

Experiment 2. When held for 10 minutes at 60° left ear down and 60° right ear down, both DS and JR showed considerable variability in amplitude of OCR (Fig. 2). In the left ear down mode, OCR measured in DS ranged from 1.5 to 5.5° in the right eye and 1 to 5° in the left eye, with differences of 4°. Amplitude appeared to decay over time; 40% of the observations were disconjugate. In the right ear down mode, amplitude ranged from 3 to 5.75° in the right eye, a difference of 2.75°. In the left eye it ranged from 2.5 to 5.5°, a difference of 3°. Amplitude appeared to increase over time; 43% of eye movements were disconjugate.

JR in the left ear down mode showed amplitude of 1 to 3.5° in the right eye, a difference of 2.5°. The left eye ranged from 0.5 to 3.5°, a difference of 3°. No trend to increasing or decreasing amplitude over time was evident. Disconjugate movements were seen in 45% of observations. In the right ear down mode, JR showed amplitude ranging from 1 to 4.5° in the right eye, a difference of 3.5°. In the left eye, amplitude ranged from 1 to 4.75°, a dif-

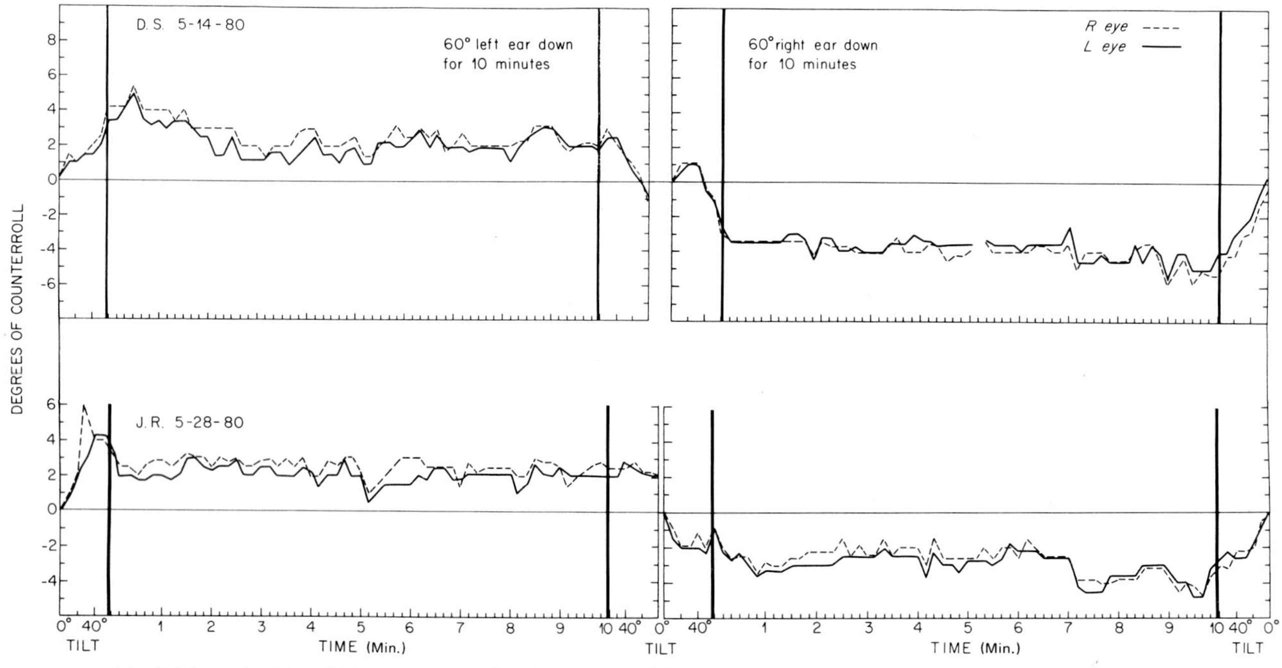

Fig. 2. Normal subject (DS, upper tracing) and patient with left vestibular nerve section (JR, lower tracing) were tipped to 60° left ear down, held for 10 minutes, and brought back to upright. Later the procedure was repeated for 60° right ear down. During the static portions, torsional variations in DS ranged up to 4° left ear down and 3° right ear down. In JR variations ranged up to 3° left ear down and 3.75° right ear down. Amount of disconjugate eye movement did not appear to differ in the two subjects. Note the smoother tracings of DS compared to JR in the tilt portions.

ference of 3.75°. Amplitude tended to increase over time; 30% of eye movements were disconjugate.

In brief, the static studies showed no significant difference by *t* tests between DS, the normal subject, and JR, the patient with the unilateral vestibular nerve section.

Examining the dynamic portion of each trial, DS's eyes were seen to move smoothly from 0 to 60° tilt, and back again to the upright. On the other hand, JR's eyes moved irregularly, and in returning to the upright position from left ear down tilt, failed to respond to the movement of the chair, maintaining their torted position during and after the return to the upright position. These brief observations were consistent with our earlier findings that OCR under dynamic conditions differed in normals and in persons with vestibular lesions.[3]

Experiment 3. Results of this experiment were similar to those reported above. All three tilts, 30, 60, and 90°, showed instability of OCR in normal subject LM when he was held at each of these positions for 10 minutes. At 30° left ear down, amplitude ranged from 3.5 to 6.5° in the right eye, a difference of 3°. The left eye ranged from 4 to 7.5°, a difference of 3.5°; 23% of eye movements were disconjugate.

At 60° left ear down, amplitude in the right eye ranged from 6 to 8.5°, a difference of 2.5°. In the left eye, it ranged from 6.5 to 9.25°, a difference of 2.75°; 35% of eye movements were disconjugate.

At 90° left ear down, amplitude in the right eye ranged from 6 to 8.75°, a difference of 2.75°. In the left eye, it ranged from 7 to 9.25°, a difference of 2.25°; 47% of eye movements were disconjugate. No trend to increasing or decreasing amplitude over time was observed in any of the three static positions. Eye movements during dynamic portions were smooth and conjugate.

No nystagmus, torsional or otherwise, was observed in any of the studies by the investigator continuously monitoring the subjects' eyes through the camera viewfinder.

DISCUSSION

It is significant but not surprising that no differences were evident in this study between OCR in normal subjects and in the patient with the unilateral vestibular nerve section. This lack of difference is consistent with the findings reported in an earlier study of normal persons and labyrinthine-defective subjects[9] in which OCR during static tilt was examined. The conflicting results of the numerous studies which attempted to find differences in OCR between normal persons and patients with vestibular lesions, reviewed elsewhere,[3] are more easily understood when it is seen that they too were almost invariably static in design, and examined amplitude of OCR as the main or sole parameter. The OCR

VARIABILITY SCORES

	Dynamic 60°		*Static 60°*	
	Mean	*(SD)*	*Mean*	*(SD)*
JR, patient with VNS	3.00°	(1.376)	3.19°	(0.554)
DS, normal subject	0.78°	(0.432)	3.44°	(0.657)

VNS - vestibular nerve section.

observed under conditions of dynamic tilt, ie, during constant velocity, appears to differentiate between normal persons and those with vestibular problems, and the whole pattern of response rather than only amplitude is a richer vein to explore.[3,4]

To illustrate the difference between the two paradigms, we examined the data obtained from DS, the normal subjects, and JR, the patient with previous unilateral vestibular nerve section, when they had earlier undergone dynamic testing. For this comparison we confined our examination to the instances in which the subjects had passed through 60° tilt during a protocol in which they were tipped at a constant velocity of 3°/s to 90° right ear down, back past upright to 90° left ear down, back to upright (trial 1) and the procedure repeated without stopping (trial 2). This protocol enabled us to extract eight data points at 60° for each eye in each subject. A variability score was calculated in the following manner: the mean and standard deviations of the differences in degrees of amplitude between trial 1 and trial 2 at each 60° position was determined for each eye for each subject. Another variability score was derived for the 60° static tilt studies of these two persons by determining the mean and standard deviations of the maximum differences in degrees of amplitude observed in each eye in both directions of tilt. The results of this examination are seen in the table. The differences in dynamic scores is significant ($p < 0.05$, *t* test), while the static scores failed to differentiate the normal person from the patient with the unilateral vestibular nerve section.

What is the difference between dynamic OCR, which appears to allow differentiation between normal subjects and those with vestibular nerve sections, and static testing which does not? One possibility is that otolith receptors or their central connections in normal persons are more influenced by prior position or direction of travel than is the case in the unilaterally labyrinthectomized patient. Tilt in a downward direction, for example, may stimulate a different population of directionally-sensitive hair cells than does tilt back to upright. The normal subject, having bilaterally symmetric input to regulate OCR, might reasonably be expected to have a less variable response to directional influences than would the patient in whom the stabilizing reciprocal input from a reverse utricle is lacking.

Other factors to be considered in defining the difference between the static and dynamic OCR studies include the influence of the semicircular canals.

The acceleration and deceleration in the dynamic studies were calculated at $0.21°/s^2$. This value should be compared to the mean $0.65°/s^2$ threshold of tonically firing vestibular neurons to horizontal acceleration (lowest threshold $0.23°/s^2$);[10] and to the mean $0.10°/s^2$ threshold of the oculogyral illusion (lowest threshold $0.05°/s^2$) and mean $0.29°/s^2$ threshold of perception of rotation (lowest threshold $0.09°/s^2$).[11] Regardless of the thresholds of angular acceleration, the OCR during portions of the dynamic studies which were conducted totally under constant velocity did not differ from comparable observations during the times in which acceleration and deceleration occurred. In the static studies, in which subjects were brought to the tilt position at 3°/s with a terminal deceleration of $0.21°/s^2$, we observed no systematic decay of OCR that might be expected if canal transients had been evoked. We concluded that the canals made no contribution to either study.

Was visual input providing some optokinetic influence under dynamic conditions? In the standard dynamic protocol, the central portion of the visual field was occupied by the camera which rotated with the subject; peripheral vision was unobscured. Two normal subjects who had undergone several tests in the standard dynamic protocol were also tested under a hood of black velvet which eliminated all peripheral visual stimuli. The OCR profiles of both subjects under this condition did not differ from their profiles in the standard condition. On the basis of this, we ruled out any optokinetic influence to explain the difference between the dynamic and static studies.

Drowsiness is known to diminish eye movements, and while the subjects in the dynamic study easily remained alert during the less than five minutes that study required, the sustained tilt of ten minutes was clearly boring to them. Yet we found no systematic decrease in amplitude or increase in instability over time in the static study. Hence a difference in alertness in the two studies is not sufficient to explain the difference in results.

A more promising conjecture involves the role of phasic and tonic neurons in utricular responses.[12,13] Both are known to be active during dynamic tilt, while in the static position only the tonic units fire. If the role of the phasic units is to record the extent and direction of changes in position, the bilateral input may be more vital than is the case in the tonic units, whose role may be the reporting of no change, a task requiring less information and handled adequately by one utricle. Possibly other commissural influences are at work as well.

The other major finding of this study is that ocular counterrolling is *not* a stable, unvarying response to head tilt, maintained at a steady conjugate level as long as tilt is maintained. On the contrary, it appears to be a continuously varying to-and-fro torsional movement occurring not only in a tilted position but also when the individual is upright. The torsional movements recorded when the subjects were held steady were not visible to the observer through the camera viewfinder. From this we infer that the spontaneous torsion is either slower or a lesser magnitude than saccades or nystagmus, both of which are clearly visible when they occur.

The question arises, what mechanisms are responsible for OCR when the shear force exerted on the utricle is constant? Possibly spontaneous changes in extraocular muscle tone may account for some of the variability, although this is unlikely to be the entire explanation since the variability appears immediately after tilt is assumed and does not increase over time, as might be expected if fatigue were a factor. A failure of combined primary nerve afferents from the otoliths to supply a stable tonic discharge is another possibility. In addition, other CNS influences acting presynaptically or on secondary vestibular neurons may be partially responsible. Still other possibilities include respiration or blood vessel pulsations causing vibration sufficient to dislodge otoconia even though the head was held motionless.

Present efforts in our laboratory center on automating the measurement of OCR, using a continuous record of videotape in addition to the discrete 35 mm photographs. The videotape method potentially allows many more observations per unit of time, making those several issues more easily studied.

REFERENCES

1. Howard IP, Templeton WB. Human spatial orientation. London: John Wiley & Sons, 1966.

2. Nelson JR, Cope D. The otoliths and the ocular countertorsion reflex. Arch Otolaryngol 1971; 94:40-50.

3. Diamond SG, Markham CH. Binocular counterrolling in humans with unilateral labyrinthectomy and in normal controls. In: Cohen B, ed. Vestibular and oculomotor physiology: International meeting of the Bárány Society. Ann NY Acad Sci 1981; 374:69-79.

4. Diamond SG, Markham CH, Simpson NE, Curthoys IS. Binocular counterrolling in humans during dynamic rotation. Acta Otolaryngol (Stockh) 1979; 87:490-8.

5. Diamond SG, Markham CH. Ocular counterrolling during constant velocity roll in normal humans and in patients with unilateral VIII nerve sections. Neurosci Abstr 1979; 5:63.10.

6. Markham CH, Diamond SG. Asymmetries in binocular counterrolling in humans during dynamic rotation. In: Proceedings of Space Motion Sickness Symposium, November 1978, Lyndon B. Johnson Space Center, Final Report. Houston: General Electric Co, 1978.

7. Fischer MH. Messende Untersuchungen über die Gegenrollung der Augen und die Lokalisation der scheinbaren vertikalen bei seitlicher Neigung des Gesamtkörpers bis zu 360°: II. Mitteilung. v.Graefs Arch Ophthal 1930; 123:476-508.

8. Mulder ME. Over parallele Rolbewegingen der Oogen. Acad Proefschrift physiol Laborat te Utrecht 1874; 3:168 ff.

9. Miller EF, Graybiel A. Ocular counterrolling measured during eight hours of sustained body tilt. Houston: NASA (CR-127034, N72-26058), 1972.

10. Shimazu H, Precht W. Tonic and kinetic responses of cat's vestibular neurons to horizontal angular acceleration. J Neurophysiol 1965; 28:991-1013.

11. Clark B, Stewart JD. Comparison of sensitivity for the perception of bodily rotation and the oculogyral illusion. Percept Psychophysics 1968; 3:253-6.

12. Fujita Y, Rosenberg J, Segundo JP. Activity of cells in the lateral vestibular nucleus as a function of head position. J Physiol 1968; 196:1-18.

13. Lowenstein O, Roberts TDM. The equilibrium function of the otolith organs of the thornback ray (Raja clavata). J Physiol 1950; 110:392-415.

≈

ANNOUNCEMENT

Hallowell Davis, MD, of Central Institute for the Deaf, St. Louis, Missouri, was honored with the Award of Merit of the Association for Research in Otolaryngology at the Association's Midwinter Meeting in St. Petersburg, Florida, in January 1982.

X-Ray Study Of The Month

RHABDOMYOSARCOMA OF THE NASOPHARYNX

ROLAND EAVEY, MD

ALFRED L. WEBER, MD

GERALD HEALY, MD

BOSTON, MASSACHUSETTS

PATIENT

This 7-year-old female developed left facial pain three weeks prior to admission. Treatment with antibiotics for "sinusitis" was unsuccessful. Her voice became increasingly hyponasal and she complained that "her throat felt small." She was referred to the Children's Hospital Medical Center in no acute distress. A hyponasal voice was evident. The left ear demonstrated a hemotympanum; tuning fork tests were consistent with a left-sided conductive hearing loss. A mass was present posteriorly in the left nasal cavity. The soft palate was displaced inferiorly and toward the right. No neck masses were present. Hyperesthesia was noted in the distribution of the mandibular branch of the trigeminal nerve (V2).

Diagnosis. The nasopharynx was evaluated under general anesthesia; a necrotic mass filled the entire left side from the posterior choana to the posterior wall. The left eustachian tube orifice was also involved. A nasopharyngeal biopsy from another hospital prior to admission to the Children's Medical Center was interpreted as a rhabdomyosarcoma.

RADIOGRAPHIC FINDINGS

Figure A reveals a large mass in the nasopharynx (asterisk) extending to the oropharynx with displacement of the soft palate inferiorly and anteriorly (arrows).

A lateral tomographic section (Fig. B) through the midsagittal plane of the nasopharynx reveals bone destruction involving the floor of the sphenoid sinus (arrow) and adjacent basisphenoid (arrowhead). The cortical outline of the sella is partially eroded (open arrow).

An anteroposterior tomographic section (Fig. C) reveals complete destruction of the left pterygoid bone and plates (asterisk), the left wall of the sphenoid sinus together with erosion of the adjacent left middle fossa (asterisk). A large soft tissue mass is noted in the nasopharynx extending laterally into the parapharyngeal soft tissues.

An axial CT section (Fig. D) demonstrates extension of the left nasopharyngeal mass into the adjacent parapharyngeal space with obliteration of the fat plane between the medial and lateral pterygoid muscles (short arrows) (note destruction of the pterygoid bone and posterior-medial wall of the antrum, asterisk); see normal medial and lateral pterygoid muscles on the right (long arrows).

DISCUSSION

Rhabdomyosarcoma ranks as the most common soft tissue neoplasm in the head and neck region in children. It can occur at any age throughout life, but the incidence drops strikingly after the first decade. This tumor demonstrates a notable predisposition for whites and shows a slightly higher frequency in males. The tumor arises from pluripotental mesenchymal cells with a capacity for aberrant differentiation. Histologically, three types of rhabdomyosarcoma exist: 1) embryonal, 2) pleomorphic, and 3) alveolar. The childhood form of tumor almost exclusively exists as the embryonal type which resembles developing muscle tissue in a 7-10-week fetus.

The head and neck region is the most commonly involved body site even considering the extremities and the pelvis. Within the head and neck region, the most frequent site is the orbit. The nasopharynx, however, was first in frequency in one rhabdomyosarcoma series,[2] and this site often surfaces in children as a common location for tumors of other various types. Rhabdomyosarcoma metastasizes by direct invasion, hematogenous spread, and through lymphatic involvement. The direct invasion route poses a special hazard to the meninges if the tumor resides in the nasopharynx. Evidence for meningeal contamination can be assessed by evaluating cranial nerve involvement and signs of increased intracranial pressure. A lumbar puncture can determine increased pressure as well as provide cytologic specimens.

The hematogenous and lymphatic modes of

From the Department of Otolaryngology and the Department of Radiology, Massachusetts Eye and Ear Infirmary; the Department of Pediatrics, Massachusetts General Hospital; and the Department of Otolaryngology, Children's Hospital Medical Center, Boston.

REPRINTS — Alfred L. Weber, MD, Department of Radiology, Massachusetts Eye and Ear Infirmary, 243 Charles Street, Boston, MA 02114.

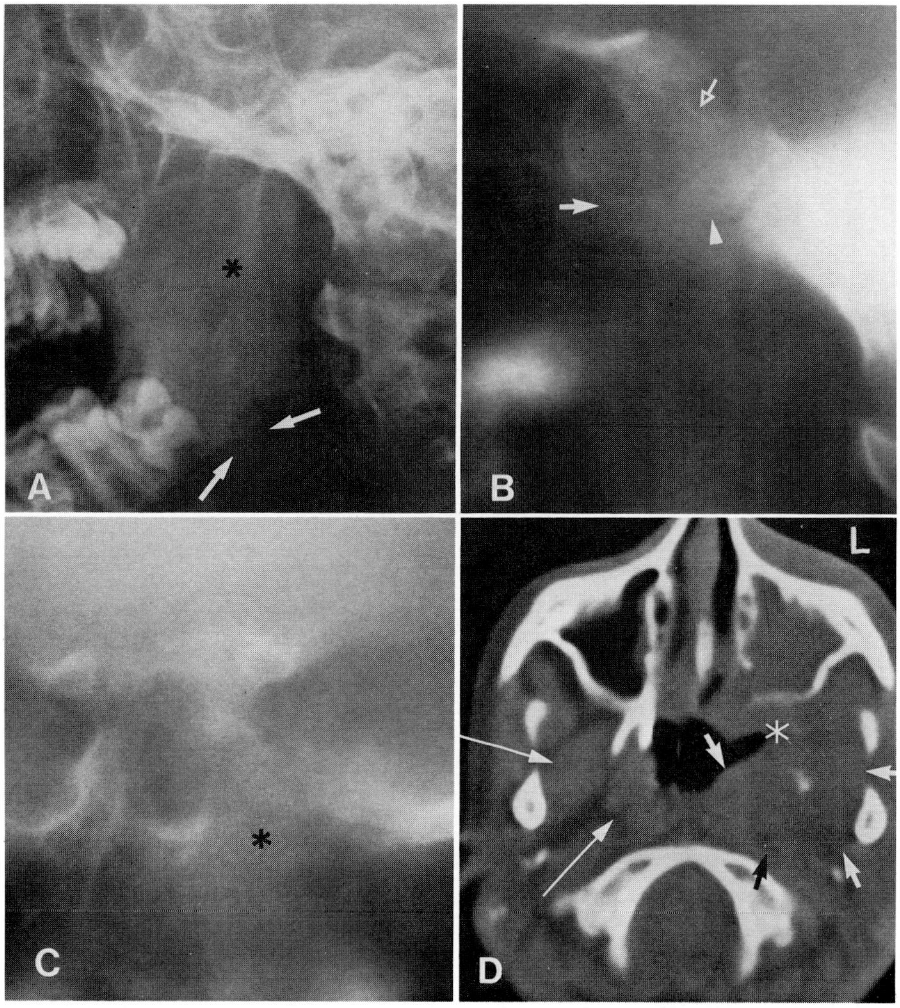

spread, once devastating, are now relatively contained by newer treatment methods. Hematogenous metastases have a predilection for the lung and bone marrow, however. Lymphatic spread with therapy has recently been reduced to a low incidence of 3%.

Treatment of this tumor consists of radiation therapy (5,000 to 6,000 rads) and chemotherapy with vincristine, actinomycin D and cyclophosphamide (VAC). Survival rates for rhabdomyosarcoma have increased dramatically. In 1962, Dito and Batsakis[2] reported an 8% survival after five years for head and neck rhabdomyosarcomas in the same time period. Recently, Healy et al reported a 75% NED (no evidence of disease) with a mean follow-up of 27 months.[4]

Radiographic evaluation for diagnosis and demonstration of the extent of the tumor plays an important role. Conventional sinus films will often show a mass in the nasopharynx. For detailed evaluation of the size, extent and bone destruction, anteroposterior, lateral, and basal tomographic sections are useful. Tomography, however, does not satisfactorily demonstrate extension of the tumor into the parapharyngeal space, orbits, pterygopalatine fossa, and intracranial cavity. The invasion of tumor into these structures is best evaluated by axial and coronal computerized tomographic sections.[5] Some rhabdomyosarcomas show hypervascularity by angiography and contrast enhancement on the CT scan following infusion with contrast material.

Computed tomographic findings of rhabdomyosarcoma, however, are not pathognomonic. Craniofacial malignancies such as lymphoma, carcinoma, as well as benign lesions may present as mass lesions with bone destruction. Tumor extent is evaluated by combining clinical, conventional, radiographic and CT examinations.

ACKNOWLEDGMENT - Special thanks is extended to Karen M. Easter for her research assistance in preparing this paper.

REFERENCES

1. Batsakis J. Tumors of the head and neck. 2nd ed. Baltimore: Williams and Wilkins, 1979: chap 14.

2. Donaldson S, Castro J, Wilbur J, Jesse R. Rhabdomyosarcoma of the head and neck in children. Cancer 1973; 31:26-35.

3. Dito W, Batsakis J. Rhabdomyosarcoma of the head and neck: an appraisal of the biological behavior in 170 cases. Arch Surg 1962; 84:582-8.

4. Healy G, Jaffe N, Cassady J. Rhabdomyosarcoma of the head and neck: diagnosis and management. Head and Neck Surg 1979; 1:334-9.

5. Reney R, Zimmerman R, Bilaniuk L, et al. Management of craniofacial sarcoma in childhood assisted by computed tomography. Int J Radiat Oncol Biol Phys 1979; 5:529-34.

OBITUARY

FRENCH K. HANSEL

1893-1981

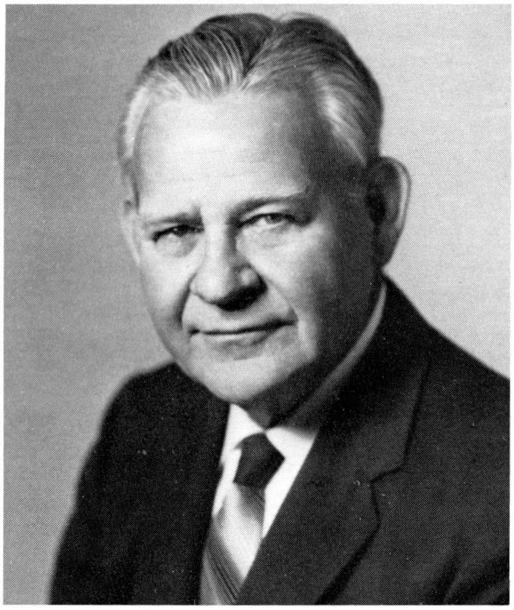

Dr. French K. Hansel was born on January 25, 1893, in Fidelity, Illinois. He received his MD degree from St. Louis University and did his residency in ear, nose and throat at the Mayo Clinic. He financed his education through high school, college and medical school by waiting tables, working in foundries and doing clerical work. He was a star on St. Louis University's first basketball team in 1915. He was affiliated with the Department of Otolaryngology at Washington University School of Medicine, St. Louis, where he studied cytology of nasal secretions and developed the specialized stain (Hansel's stain) which permitted rapid cytologic differential diagnosis of nasal secretions. His concern and disappointment with the extensive and frequently repetitive nasal surgery practiced at that time led him to explore alternative medical solutions for some of the acute rhinologic problems which were encountered. He believed that the routine use of antibiotics was far in excess of their need in the treatment of infections.

Early in his career, Dr. Hansel became disenchanted with the then current treatment of allergy, the "maximal dose" therapy, which often produced severe constitutional reactions. He developed and utilized the low or "optimal dose" therapy based on the principle of the introduction of that amount of allergen or antigen which will produce tolerance. This principle is used in clinical allergy by members of the American Society of Ophthalmologic and Otolaryngologic Allergy. Dr. Hansel also advanced the use of sublingual therapy, incorporating small amounts of offending substances in rapidly dissolving tablets in an effort to potentiate the effects of injections.

For many years he made accurate pollen counts from plates exposed outside his office, which were reported daily to the news media.

Dr. Hansel became a teacher at Washington and St. Louis Universities, author, editor, organizer of specialty allergy units, clinical investigator, botanist and pathologist. He published *Allergy of the Nose and Paranasal Sinuses* in 1936. His second text, *Clinical Allergy*, published in 1953, was a revision of the earlier book.

He conducted private courses in his office for those interested in allergy. In 1935, with approximately 40 students, he participated in the formation of the American Society of Ophthalmologic and Otolaryngologic Allergy. The Hansel Foundation, organized in 1948, received an estimated 2000 otolaryngologists for allergy training. It has been estimated that Dr. Hansel taught at least 3000 more otolaryngologists in instructional courses presented over 36 years as a member of the American Academy of Ophthalmology and Otolaryngology. He was one of the organizers of the American College of Allergists and was its second president. He was honored as a Fellow Distinguished in 1975 and received the Award of Merit in 1977. He was the editor of the *Annals of Allergy* from 1943 to 1954. In 1940, Dr. Hansel received the prestigious Casselberry Award from the American Laryngological Association, and in 1980 he was awarded a Presidential Citation as the "Father of Otolaryngologic Allergy" by the American Academy of Otolaryngology.

In collaboration with Jack Anderson, MD, he coauthored *Allergy and Immunity in Otolaryngology* in 1959. After his retirement, he continued his studies. He will be remembered by his colleagues and by his grateful patients for his willingness to assist them at all times.

Edward A. Westaver, DO

Clinical Otolaryngology

By *Vijay S. Dayal*. Hard cover, illustrations, indexed, 325 pp, 1981. J. B. Lippincott Co, Philadelphia-Toronto. Price $24.50

This is a brief and concise survey of the field intended for medical students and junior residents in otolaryngology which with some modification I believe will take its place as a standard textbook in otolaryngology. The writing is clear and the print attractive. Sprinkled through the volume are numerous line drawings which are so well done and so clear that teachers of otolaryngology would do well to emulate them at the blackboard. In each of the seven parts of the book covering the specialty regionally is a particularly useful section for students detailing the important features of history-taking, physical examination, and investigations. The best handled parts of the book are those covering the nose and sinuses, larynx, pharynx, and bronchoesophagology. I sorely missed a section on plastic and reconstructive surgery which would point out to students this is an integral part of our specialty. In the section on the neck there is no mention of deep fascial space infections. There are a few errors such as misnaming the areal ratio of the ear, the hydraulic ratio, and virtually dismissing brainstem evoked response audiometry as "of limited clinical use." A test that is at least 95% accurate in the detection of acoustic neuromas cannot be taken lightly. On balance however the pluses far outweigh the minuses. The index is especially well done.

BRIAN F. MCCABE, MD
Iowa City, Iowa

Psychophysical, Physiological and Behavioural Studies in Hearing

Edited by *G. van den Brink* and *F. A. Bilsen*. Hard cover, black and white illustrations, indexed, 480 pages, 1980. Delft University Press, Delft, The Netherlands. Price $42.50.

This book contains the proceedings of the 5th International Symposium on Hearing, which took place in April, 1980 in the Netherlands. These symposia have been held at varying intervals since 1969 and are intended to provide a forum for an international exchange of new research in the anatomy, physiology and psychology of hearing.

There are 67 papers, many of which include the discussion which followed from other participants. Some of the comments, because of their length, detail, and spirit, could also be considered articles. They are not edited transcripts of discussions, but rather written and often illustrated expansions or corrections of points made by the presenter.

The book is divided into seven sections. The first is entitled "Cochlear Functioning"; here the importance of Kemp's finding of stimulus-evoked acoustic emissions arising from the cochlea is reflected in the amount of research and discussion that it has generated. Theorists must now deal with the evidence indicating that active as well as nonlinear biomechanical processes may be involved in cochlear frequency analysis.

Section II comprises papers on "Frequency and Time Resolution." The dominant topic here is the assessment, both psychophysically and physiologically, of the frequency selectivity of both healthy and damaged auditory systems. Still unresolved, but discussed often in this symposium, is the question of proper psychoacoustic techniques for measuring auditory frequency analysis.

Section III is devoted to papers concerned with "Lateral Suppression and Distortion Products," two phenomena resulting from the nonlinearity inherent in normal cochlear functioning that have received much research attention recently.

The papers in Section IV address the dynamic-range problem, which, simply put, is how to account for a 100 dB range in loudness with neural responses that saturate within a 40 dB range. While several insightful approaches are offered, the puzzle has yet to be solved.

Papers in Sections V and VI deal with "Pitch Perception" and "Binaural Hearing." In neither section is there a dominant theme to the research questions that were addressed. Rather, the papers represent the range of experimental techniques and theoretical insights that have been applied in these two areas of auditory research.

Finally, Section VII contains four interesting papers on interrelations among measures of quiet threshold, masking, and speech perception. These studies, and others recently, have sought to describe the poor speech-reception performance of some hearing-impaired persons by loss in frequency resolution, or other factors, in addition to the audibility problem imposed by the elevated thresholds. These four papers point up well the difficulty, due to overwhelming interindividual differences, in finding simple relations among psychoacoustic measures of hearing impairment.

In all, this is a lively and interesting collection of papers. The problems with the book are those that can be expected of a record of proceedings of this kind. The papers are necessarily brief and sometimes, particularly in comments, results and provocative conclusions are put forth with so few details of procedure that the statements tend to tease rather than inform. Also, although most papers are of very high quality, a few others either carry very little news or present unreasonable conclusions from the data.

Whereas preceding symposia in this series included a few papers that gave an overview of an area of research, there is little here for the nonspecialist. Those who are active in research on hearing certainly should examine this volume for new work in their field. Others, who ordinarily care only to keep sight of the forest, will want to wait for a good summary article to come along to learn about the goings-on in the trees.

PATRICK M. ZUREK, PhD
St. Louis, Mo

Controversy in Otolaryngology

Edited by *James B. Snow, Jr.* Hard cover, black and white illustrations, indexed, referenced, 561 pages, 1980. WB Saunders, Philadelphia. Price $40.00.

This is a unique book. The preface states that this is ". . . a forum for the analysis and discussion of several of the most important areas of controversy in clinical otolaryngology." The book is divided into 23 chapters or "problems" each introduced by an editor's statement of the problem as he sees it followed by his instructions and questions for the discussants. Each problem has two or more essayists and each submitted his paper without knowing who was taking the alternative point of view, and without reading the contrary expression. Twelve of the chapters are then concluded by an editorial comment on the views expressed. Although the editor states that no attempt has been made to describe the field of otolaryngology, the controversies discussed include otology, allergy, rhinology, laryngology, head and neck surgery, facial plastic and reconstructive surgery, maxillofacial surgery, bronchoesophagology, and pediatric otolaryngology.

My criticisms of the material presented are few and reflect personal biases. For example, in the chapter, "Canal Up versus Modified Radical or Radical Mastoidectomy for Cholesteatoma," I would have preferred stronger emphasis of the fact that the majority of adults with chronic otitis media have sclerotic mastoids and in these people a well performed modified radical procedure results only in a large ear canal rather than a troublesome cavity.

The problem of Menière's disease is discussed quite narrowly (sacculotomy versus vestibular nerve section). Its incidence is such that a wider discussion would seem appropriate in this forum.

I thoroughly enjoyed this book. Dr. Snow's questions to each essayist are comprehensive and reflective of the concerns (or what should be the concerns) of every practitioner facing these problems. The list of contributors represents a comprehensive cross section of our field. This is a valuable addition to our library.

JEROME C. GOLDSTEIN, MD
Albany, NY

LETTER TO THE EDITOR

Dear Editor,

In his admirable account of the congenital ear deformity first described by a gentleman of Bologna in 1791,[1] Professor Schuknecht correctly points out that this author translated his name as well as his work into medieval Latin and that the name in the title is in the genitive form.[2] The only record we have of this man is the name at the head of the article, however, and it is only an assumption that he was known to his contemporaries as Carlo Mondini; a very reasonable assumption as there are about 50 Mondinis in the current Bolognese telephone directory (The Italian Embassy, London, personal communication, 1980). It is a pity that we do not know more of the life and work of this clever and learned anatomist, who must also have been a practicing otologist, as he states in his paper that he had occasion to test the deafness of his patient quite often while the boy was still healthy. Mondini made other temporal bone dissections and his paper makes fascinating reading. He tried to demonstrate the lesion causing deafness in albino cats and dogs but as this is an end-organ (Scheibe) type with a normal labyrinth he was of course unable to do so.

Mondini's description of the bony labyrinth of the deaf boy is detailed and precise, and corresponds well with his accurate macroscopic diagrams. As almost any deformity of the bony labyrinth is nowadays labeled as some type of "Mondini dysplasia," an account of the findings would seem pertinent. The oval and round windows and all semicircular canals and their openings into the vestibule are described as normal in size and position. The vestibule was larger than normal, and the cochlea is described as having $1\frac{1}{2}$ instead of $2\frac{1}{2}$ turns of the spiral and ending in an apical cavity. Neither the cochlear aqueduct nor the internal auditory meatus are mentioned in the text, but the latter is well shown in the diagrams and appears normal in size and shape. The acoustic nerve is described as having a normal appearance as far as the cochlea and vestibule. One of the most interesting features, however, seems to have escaped attention. The vestibular aqueduct was very large, lacked a medial bony covering, and was seven lines wide at the medial end and one line wide and larger than the opening for the crus commune at the vestibular end. As a line is one-twelfth inch these figures represent approximately 2 mm and 15 mm respectively. There was little difference between the two sides and these large vestibular aqueducts would therefore seem very similar to those described by Valvassori and Clemis,[3] and in fact the lateral tomograms published by these authors show a remarkable similar bony structure to Mondini's Figures 1 and 2. It is surprising that Mondini only gets a mention at the very end of the paper.

Mondini's precise description of the abnormality of the bony cochlea is closely paralleled by that of Alexander[4] whose histological study shows an apparently normal basal turn with a distal sac. In this type of dysplasia some hearing is therefore possible, and we have in several cases noted the presence of some cochlear function with deficiency of the apical part of the modiolus shown by tomography. This phenomenon has been observed by others.[5,6] Moreover we are not convinced that this type of lesion is prone to develop a cerebrospinal fluid fistula via a dilated cochlear aqueduct, as is so often stated. It would seem logical that where a scala communis replaces the helicotrema there would be a direct route from cochlear aqueduct to oval window, but we have consistently failed to demonstrate a dilated cochlear aqueduct tomographically. In our opinion a true Mondini dysplasia is not prone to develop a CSF fistula spontaneously but may do so as a result of surgical interference with the stapes.

There is a more severe dysplasia which, although almost always labeled as a Mondini dysplasia, should be differentiated from it on management grounds if nothing else, as this lesion is incompatible with any cochlear function but carries a very real risk of developing a *spontaneous* CSF fistula.[7] There is a generalized dilatation and dysplasia of the labyrinth which is abnormally wide at the junction of the vestibule and cochlea. The cochlea is an amorphous sac lacking a modiolus, and the internal auditory meatus narrows at its lateral end. The route of the fistula is from internal auditory meatus to the abnormal labyrinth, oval window and middle ear, via dehiscences in the lamina cribrosa. This defect has been observed directly through the oval window[8] and posterior fossa contrast studies have demonstrated the route.[9] We have now studied the tomograms of 17 such cases, 6 of whom developed a spontaneous fistula.

Studies of anencephalic ears reveals a great range of developmental abnormalities of the cochlea[10] and it seems very likely that a similar range can occur in isolation, making the traditional classifications rather pointless. Undoubtedly the commonest congenital anomaly of the bony labyrinth is the short, dilated, lateral semicircular canal which can occur in isolation with normal cochlear function. It is for instance not uncommonly found in the Treacher Collins syndrome, a condition in which the bony cochlear structure and cochlear function are almost always normal.[11] To call this anomaly "Mondini dysplasia of the vestibular system"is illogical, confusing and far removed from the original account.

REFERENCES

1. Mundinus C. Anatomica surdi nati sectio. Bononiensi scientarium et artium instituto atque academia commentarii. Bononiae, 1791, VII, 419-28.

2. Schuknecht HF. Mondini dysplasia: a clinical and pathological study. Ann Otol Rhinol Laryngol 1980; 89 Suppl 65.

3. Valvassori EG, Clemis JD. The large vestibular aqueduct syndrome. Laryngoscope 1980; 88:723-8.

4. Alexander G. Zur pathologie und Pathologischen Anatomie der Kongenitalen Taubheit. Arch Klin Exp Ohren Nasen Kehlkopfheilkd 1904; 61:183-219.

5. Mundnich K. The dysplasias of the middle and the inner ear in different types of malformation. Proc R Soc Med 1974; 65:1197-9.

6. Paparella MM, Elfiky FM. Mondini's deafness. Arch Otolaryngol 1972; 95:134-40.

7. Phelps PD, Lloyd GAS. Congenital deformity of the internal auditory meatus and labyrinth associated with cerebrospinal fluid fistula. Adv Oto-Rhino-Laryngol 1978; 24:51-7.

8. McNab Jones RF, Fairburn B. Spontaneous cerebro-spinal fluid otorrhoea. J Laryngol Otol 1977; 91:897-902.

9. Carter BL, Wolpert SM, Karmody CS. Recurrent meningitis associated with an anomaly of the inner ear. Neuroradiology 1975; 9:55-61.

10. Friedmann I, Wright JLW, Phelps PD. Temporal bone studies in anencephaly. J Laryngol Otol 1980; 94:929-44.

11. Phelps PD, Poswillo D, Lloyd GAS. The ear deformities in mandibulofacial dysostosis. Clin Otolaryngol 1981; 6:15-28.

Yours sincerely,

P.D. Phelps, FRCS, FRCR
G.A.S. Lloyd, DM, FRCR
P.C. Windle-Taylor, MA, FRCS
P.J. Emery, FRCS

The Royal National Throat Nose and Ear Hospital
Gray's Inn Road, London W.C.1. 8EE

INFORMATION FOR AUTHORS

Send manuscripts by first-class mail to Editor Brian F. McCabe, MD, University of Iowa Hospitals, Iowa City, IA 52242, or to Co-editor Ben H. Senturia, MD, 4949 Forest Park Blvd., St. Louis, MO 63108. Original manuscripts which deal with clinical and scientific aspects of otolaryngology, bronchoesophagology, head and neck, maxillofacial and plastic surgery, audiology, speech pathology and related specialties will be considered for publication. It is understood that manuscripts will not have been published elsewhere.

MANUSCRIPTS. Papers should be limited to a maximum of 15 double-spaced typewritten pages including tables and references, so as not to exceed the permitted maximum of 6 typeset pages. This allows for one page of illustrations. If a manuscript of slightly greater length is approved by the Editorial Board all typeset pages in excess of 6 will be charged to the authors at the publisher's cost of $125 per page. An **original of the manuscript** and one set of **original illustrations** should be provided for reproduction. **Two clear copies** of the manuscript and illustrations should be submitted for review. Manuscripts should be typewritten on white bond paper (8½ x 11 in). Use double spacing throughout with margins of at least one inch. Each manuscript component should begin on a new page in the following sequence: title page, abstract and key words, text, acknowledgments, references, tables and legends for illustrations. Number pages consecutively in the upper right hand corner beginning with the title page.

COPYRIGHT. In compliance with the Copyright Revision Act of 1976, all manuscripts must be accompanied by a letter containing the following statement before they will be reviewed for publication: "In consideration of the *Annals of Otology, Rhinology & Laryngology* taking action in reviewing and editing my (our) submission the author(s) undersigned hereby transfers(s), assign(s) or otherwise convey(s) all copyright ownership to the Annals Publishing Company in the event such work is published in the *Annals of Otology, Rhinology & Laryngology.*" We regret that manuscripts not accompanied by such a letter will be returned.

TITLES of manuscripts should be concise and informative and worded to facilitate indexing.

RUNNING HEAD. An abbreviated form of the title, to be used at the top of each page, should be provided by the author.

GENERIC NAMES should be used in the text whenever possible.

REFERENCES should be numbered consecutively in the order in which they are first mentioned, and cited in the text in arabic numerals in superscript. The number of references should not exceed 30. Use the style of references given in *Uniform Requirements for Manuscripts Submitted to Biomedical Journals.* Include in the reference list manuscripts accepted but not yet published; designate the journal followed by "in press" in parentheses. Manuscripts submitted but not yet accepted should be referred to as "unpublished data" in parentheses in the text. Primary references only should be used and must be verified by the author(s) against the original documents. Examples of correct forms of references are given below.

Journal Article

(List all authors when six or fewer; when seven or more, list only first three and add "et al.")

Ketchum LD, Smith I, Robinson DW, et al. The treatment of hypertrophic scar, keloid and scar contracture by triamcinolone acetonide. Plast Reconstr Surg 1966; 38:209-18.

Books and Other Monographs

Personal Author(s)

Payne SW, Olson MA. The esophagus. Philadelphia: Lea and Febiger, 1974: 1-3.

Corporate Author

American Medical Association Department of Drugs. AMA drug evaluations. 3rd ed. Littleton: Publishing Sciences Group, 1977.

Chapter in Book

Belsey R. Diaphragmatic hernia. In: Jones FA, ed. Modern trends in gastroenterology. London: Butterworths: 1952:128-78.

ILLUSTRATIONS should be original drawings, glossy photographs or halftones. Line drawings should be in black on white paper. Letters, numbers and symbols should be clear and even throughout, and of sufficient size that when reduced for publication, each item is still legible. Titles and detailed explanations of illustrations must be listed on a separate sheet, not on the illustrations themselves. Each figure should have a label pasted on the reverse indicating the number of the figure, the names of the authors, title of the paper; the top of the figure should be indicated. Cite each figure in the text in consecutive order. If a figure has been published, acknowledge the original source and submit written permission from the copyright holder to reproduce the material. Actual publication cost of illustrations will be charged to the author. Color illustrations are acceptable for publication; cost estimates for color separations and printing will be provided upon request.

TABLES should be on separate sheets, numbered consecutively, each headed by a concise title. Place explanatory matter in footnotes. Cost of setting tables will be charged to the author.

MEASUREMENTS should be expressed in the metric system. Audiograms must be plotted according to ISO standards.

ABSTRACTS should contain not more than 150 words and should state the purposes of the study, primary procedures, main findings and the principal conclusions, emphasizing new and important aspects of the investigation.

PERMISSIONS. Materials taken from other sources must be accompanied by a written statement from both senior author and publisher giving permission to the *Annals* for republication. If permission for publication is required by the author's institution, such clearance should be provided. Written permission of subjects is required for identifiable photographs of individuals.

SUPPLEMENTS. A manuscript too long for inclusion in the *Annals* may be published as a supplement if approved by the Board of Editors. All costs must be borne by the author; estimates of cost will be provided upon request. Early publication of supplements is often possible since supplements are produced independently of the regular *Annals* issues.

PROOFS accompanied by prints of the illustrations will be sent to the first author and should be returned within 48 hours. Changes in galley proofs initiated by the author will be charged to the author.

AUTHOR RESPONSIBILITY. All accepted manuscripts are subject to copy editing. The author is responsible for all statements in his work, including changes made by the copy editor which were approved by the author on the proofs.

REPRINTS. Rates are quoted when the proofs are sent. Orders must be signed by the author and returned with the proofs.

These requirements are in accord with *Uniform Requirements for Manuscripts Submitted to Biomedical Journals* (Lancet 1979; 1: 428-30).

THE GIANT APICAL AIR CELL SYNDROME
A NEW ENTITY

ERIC M. KRAUS, MD

BRIAN F. MCCABE, MD

IOWA CITY, IOWA

A new entity, the giant apical air cell syndrome, is presented and its surgical management is described. The syndrome triad consists of a giant apical air cell, spontaneous CSF rhinorrhea, and recurrent meningitis. Constant pounding of the brain against the dura overlying the giant air cell eventually causes dural rupture and CSF leak. The giant apical air cell communicates with the eustachian tube creating a direct route for CSF to leak from the subarachnoid space into the nasopharynx. The syndrome is best diagnosed by polytomography of the petrous apex, surgical exploration, and careful dissection using the operating microscope. Dye or contrast studies are no longer necessary. Extracranial surgical management is preferable to the intracranial approach. Tympanomastoidectomy is performed with obliteration of the eustachian tube, middle ear, and mastoid. In this manner, the subarachnoid space is separated from the nasopharynx, preventing further episodes of meningitis. A detailed knowledge of the regional anatomy and the application of basic surgical principles should enable the temporal bone surgeon to accurately diagnose and manage most CSF fistulae.

The giant apical air cell syndrome consists of the triad of 1) a giant air cell of the petrous apex, 2) nontraumatic CSF rhinorrhea, and 3) recurrent meningitis. To our knowledge, the syndrome has not been previously described although it has been morphologically noted in the radiological literature. We feel that it has occurred prior to our report but has gone unrecognized as a cause of either spontaneous CSF rhinorrhea or of recurrent meningitis. However, it is important to recognize as an entity because, as evidenced by our case report, it is difficult to seal from a middle cranial fossa approach. The most effective method of eliminating the repeated meningitis is to separate the subarachnoid space from the nasopharynx by completely sealing the eustachian tube. To accomplish this, the best surgical approach is tympanomastoidectomy and cavity obliteration.

CASE REPORT

The patient was the product of a full term, uncomplicated pregnancy. During the first years of life, she experienced numerous sore throats and upper respiratory infections which remitted in 1961 after uncomplicated tonsillectomy and adenoidectomy at age five years. During 1962, she had two episodes of pneumonia requiring hospitalization. In May and September 1963, she was treated with penicillin and gammaglobulin for cough, intermittent rhinorrhea, and fever. In October 1963, she developed culture-negative meningitis treated with penicillin and chloramphenicol. She then experienced repeated episodes of pneumococcal and *Hemophilus influenzae* meningitis in November 1963 and January 1964. Chest, thoracic, lumbosacral, skull and mastoid films were "normal," including views of the sella turcica and optic foramina. An electroencephalogram was normal, and she was begun on prophylactic penicillin. In early 1964, the patient's mother noted clear fluid draining from her daughter's left nostril. A Pantopaque myelogram was thought to show a defect in the left basisphenoid suture. An intrathecal indigo carmine test was negative. Five months later, September 1964, a left temporal craniotomy was performed. The trigeminal nerve was reported to be entering Meckel cave "through an aperture in bone rather than under a sleeve of dura." The opening was packed with fibrin clot, Gelfoam, and temporalis muscle. Postoperatively, she developed a moderate amnestic and sensory aphasia which resolved. For eight months, she remained asymptomatic.[1] In May 1966, she was again hospitalized for recurrent pneumococcal meningitis. A pneumoencephalogram, repeat Pantopaque myelogram, and an intrathecal radioactive iodinated serum albumin (RISA) test failed to elucidate any abnormalities. While on prophylactic antibiotics, she developed her sixth episode of meningitis one year later. In January 1967, she underwent a second left temporal craniotomy. A 10 by 6 mm opening was found near the left petrous apex and was thought to represent an enlarged Meckel cave aperture. Rolled oxycel gauze was packed into the aperture, and the dura was closed. Postoperatively, she had a left facial paresis, a dead left ear, and neuropraxia of cranial nerves V, IX, X, and XII. All the nerves improved except V, VII, and VIII. Penicillin prophylaxis was continued because of persistent left rhinorrhea which was most marked during eating. A food allergy was implicated, and she was placed on pyrrobutamine (Co-Pyronil) and dust/feather precautions without success. For the next two years, she had repeated episodes of mild meningitis culminating in clinical meningitis during December 1968 and March 1969. Repeat skull, cervical spine, and mastoid films were negative. Skull laminograms were reported to show no bony defects. Two pneumoencephalograms showed a dilated left temporal horn. A repeat EEG contained no focal abnormalities. For the next ten years, she continued to have intermittent left sided rhinorrhea but no meningitis while maintained on 200,000 units of penicillin daily.

However, her ninth episode of meningitis occurred in April 1979. Sinus films showed a discrepancy in the height of the left orbit (56 mm) as compared to the right orbit (51 mm). The superior and lateral left orbital walls showed thinning suggestive of an expansile tumor. Polytomograms of the temporal bones and ethmoid sinuses were reported to be normal. Computerized axial tomography with and without contrast of the head and orbits revealed a normal left orbit and a lucent left temporal area along the posterior portion of the temporal lobe. The abnormality was consistent with either a surgical defect or an abscess of the left temporal lobe. Cisternography using 0.5 mC of ytterbium169 diethylene triamine pentacetic acid showed more uptake on sphenoid pledgets (left = 1,565 counts/2 min; right = 1,409 counts/2 min) than cribriform pledgets (left = 608 counts/2 min; right = 483 counts/2 min). A posterior fossa myelogram showed no filling of the left middle cranial fossa or spilling of Pantopaque above the rostral clivus. In April 1979, a third left temporal craniotomy was performed. A skull defect containing two small

From the Department of Otolaryngology and Maxillofacial Surgery, University of Iowa Hospitals, Iowa City.

REPRINTS — Eric M. Kraus, MD, Department of Otolaryngology and Maxillofacial Surgery, University of Iowa Hospitals, Iowa City, IA 52242.

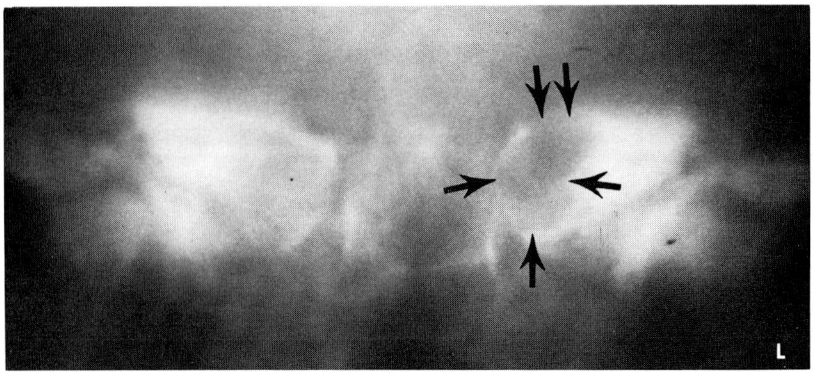

AP tomogram of patient's temporal bone demonstrating the giant air cell (arrows) of the left petrous apex. Note that the bony roof of the giant air cell is absent (double arrow).

holes and an invaginated tuft of arachnoid was found on the anteromedial aspect of the left petrous bone. The arachnoid was removed, and a second large hole was found medial to the gasserian ganglion. A small piece of brain was removed, and the hole was "reidentified on the lateral posterior aspect." After opening overlying dura, fibrous tissue was found filling part of the defect. The bony hole was covered by a pericranial graft held in place by overlying brain. She had an uncomplicated postoperative course and remained free of symptoms for 19 months.

In November 1980, she was admitted for her tenth episode of meningitis. During otolaryngologic consultation, no CSF could be found on either otologic or nasal examination but review of temporal bone polytomograms showed a giant air cell of the left petrous apex which had not been previously appreciated (figure). The defect was confirmed on CAT head scan. The bony roof of the giant air cell was absent. It was postulated that her recurrent meningitis was being caused by a communication between the subarachnoid space and the nasopharynx via the giant apical air cell and the left eustachian tube. A left tympanomastoidectomy was performed with the goal of sealing the left eustachian tube and obliteration of the resulting radical mastoidectomy cavity.

At the time of tympanomastoidectomy, a dehiscence of the medial wall of the middle ear was found 5 mm anterior to the cochleariform process and cochlea. The defect contained ruptured, pulsating durarachnoid membrane. The medial wall of the tympanum anterior to the cochlea was absent, as well as the lateral one half of the bony eustachian tube. Copious CSF was found in the mesotympanum coming through the durarachnoid defect. The eustachian tube mucosa was then elevated and inverted, and the eustachian tube was plugged with fascia. The tympanic membrane and malleus were removed, and the middle ear and mastoid were obliterated with fat. A drain was not placed.

Since operation, the patient has experienced two upper respiratory infections but no further episode of meningitis.

PATHOPHYSIOLOGY

The pneumatization process of the temporal bone and the petrous apex has been well described by Anson and Donaldson.[2] Apical cells develop from peritubal, perilabyrinthine, posterosuperior, posteromedial, and subarcuate cell tracts. They attain their maximum size by age 5-6 years. Therefore, after age 6 years, one may be at risk to develop a CSF leak caused by a giant apical air cell. Our patient was 7 years old at the time of her initial episode of meningitis. Parisier and Birken have reported the average age of meningitis associated with spontaneous CSF otorrhea to be 6.4 years.[3]

As the giant apical air cell enlarges, its roof is subjected to constant dural pounding caused by physiologic brain pulsation. The bony air cell roof resorbs, and the overlying dura ruptures into the giant air cell as it is steadily stretched over an area larger than it can cover and a depth greater than it can reach. CSF then leaks from the air cell into the nasopharynx via the eustachian tube. The abnormal communication between the subarachnoid space and nasopharynx permits retrograde contamination and recurrent meningitis until the pathway is surgically interrupted.

DISCUSSION

Giant apical air cells are uncommon, and the syndrome described is rare. To date, a similar case has not been reported. Dubois and Roub have described the tomographic features of giant apical air cells of the petrous apex.[4] In a retrospective analysis of 1600 temporal bone polytomes, they identified 15 patients (0.94%) whose petrous apices contained a single, nonseptated apical air cell with a diameter of at least 1.5 cm. Our patient's air cell measured 1.5 by 2 cm. All giant air cells examined were located posteromedially to the carotid canal and could be distinguished from destructive lesions of the petrous apex, with the exceptions of primary cholesteatomas and acoustic neuromas, by their location, low radiodensity, uninterrupted margins, and regular shape. None of their patients were reported to have CSF leaks or recurrent meningitis, but it is true that these were morphologic rather than clinical reports. Thus the incidence of meningitis in these patients is not known.

Multiple reports of spontaneous, normal pressure CSF fistulae may be found in the literature.[5-13] Kaufman et al have described four cases of CSF rhinorrhea each involving defects in the anteromedial middle cranial fossa floor.[5] They attributed the development of fistulae to the "pulsatile forces of the CSF and brain" causing dural thinning, bone erosion, and the rupture of meningoceles or meningoencephaloceles. Although no cases of meningitis were reported, these patients may well have had a variety of the giant apical air cell syndrome. Multiple fistulae could occur if the petrous apex was well pneumatized. Even though bony fenestrations might develop, they may be filled with tufts of herniated arachnoid and/or brain. In such instances, there would be no CSF leak or meningitis. Similarly, Brisman et al described two patients with CSF rhinorrhea and middle cranial fossa defects.[10] One patient presented with spontaneous meningitis and was found to have a dural defect at the fenestration site. The other patient had a middle fossa encephalocele plugging the defect; he had psychomotor seizures but no meningitis. No comments concerning the presence of giant apical air cells were made.

Once the possibility of a spontaneous CSF leak is entertained, the fistula must be precisely localized. CSF may leak from all three cranial fossae — anterior fossa via the frontal sinus, cribriform plate, or fovea ethmoidalis; the middle fossa through the sphenoid sinus, or a giant apical air cell; and the posterior fossa via the eustachian tube. After careful history and physical examination, the safest and most reliable modality to accurately locate the fossa containing the fistula is polytomography. The fossa is then best explored from below rather than from above utilizing the operating room microscope to enhance the subtle differences between tissues.

Because we have been able to locate each of 15 small anterior and middle cranial fossa fistulae using polytomography, the microscope, and careful dissection, we have given up the use of RISA or other intrathecal/intraventricular agents such as fluorescein, methylene blue, indigo carmine, or Pantopaque. These substances may be neurotoxic and are nonspecific localizers. Test results are subject to misinterpretation which may lead to unfounded conclusions. New generation CAT scanners combined with various contrast materials may aid in diagnosing intracranial fistulae.[14]

If a dural defect is found with an underlying bony dehiscence, the dura should be repaired or grafted, and *the cavity should be filled with tissue in order to support the dura.* Covering a durarachnoid dehiscence with fascia alone is unsatisfactory, as refistulization may occur, as abundantly demonstrated by this case report. As with most air-containing cavities, complete obliteration should be performed by filling the space with autogenous tissue-flaps, or free muscle or fat. When available, flaps are always superior to grafts, and deficient tissue should be replaced by like tissue.[15] Packing is then used to hold the tissue in place until complete healing has occurred. After three temporal craniotomies, a temporalis flap was not available in our case. Obliteration was accomplished by an abdominal fat graft. Calcaterra has reported similar techniques.[16,17]

Finally, congenital as well as neoplastic and traumatic conditions should be considered in the differential diagnosis of “spontaneous” CSF rhinorrhea and recurrent meningitis. Congenital causes include cribriform plate aplasias, idiopathic oval window fistulae, sella turcica fistulae, nasal encephaloceles, meningoceles, meningomyeloceles, persistent craniopharyngeal canal, and Mondini dysplasia. Mondini deformity may occur alone or may be associated with Pendred syndrome, Klippel-Feil syndrome, trisomy, DeGeorge syndrome, teratogenic drugs, and maternal infection.[18,19] Neoplasms to be considered are pituitary adenomas and craniopharyngiomas, acoustic neuromas, cerebellar gliomas, III ventricle tumors, meningiomas, pinealomas, osteomas, and nasopharyngeal carcinoma. Osteomyelitis must be ruled out especially in diabetics or immunocompromised individuals.

REFERENCES

1. Pribram HFW, Hass AC, Nishioka H. Radiographic localization of a spontaneous cerebrospinal fluid fistula. J Neurosurg 1966; 24:1031-3.

2. Anson BJ, Donaldson JA. Surgical anatomy of the temporal bone. 3rd ed. Philadelphia: WB Saunders 1981;405-11.

3. Parisier SC, Birken EA. Recurrent meningitis secondary to idiopathic oval window CSF leak. Laryngoscope 1976; 86: 1503-15.

4. Dubois PJ, Roub LW. Giant air cells of the petrous apex: tomographic features. Radiology 1978; 129:103-9.

5. Kaufman B, Nulsen FE, Weiss MH, Brodkey JS, White RJ, Sykora GF. Acquired spontaneous, nontraumatic normal-pressure cerebrospinal fluid fistulas originating from the middle fossa. Radiology 1977; 122:379-87.

6. Ommaya AK, DiChiro G, Baldwin M. Pennybacker JB. Non-traumatic cerebrospinal fluid rhinorrhoea. J Neurol Neurosurg Psychiatr 1968; 31:214-25.

7. O'Connell JEA. Primary spontaneous cerebrospinal fluid rhinorrhoea. J Neurol Neurosurg Psychiatr 1964; 27:241-6.

8. Kaufman HH. Nontraumatic cerebrospinal fluid rhinorrhea. Arch Neurol 1969; 21:59-65.

9. Grahne B. Spontaneous cerebrospinal fluid rhinorrhoea. Acta Otolaryngol (Stockh) 1970; 70:383-91.

10. Brisman R, Hughes JEO, Mount LA. Cerebrospinal fluid rhinorrhea. Arch Neurol 1970; 22:245-52.

11. Anderson WM, Schwarz GA, Gammon GD. Chronic spontaneous cerebrospinal rhinorrhea. Arch Intern Med 1961; 107:723-31.

12. Morley TP, Wortzman G, in discussion. Raaf J. The importance of the lateral extensions of the sphenoidal sinus in post-traumatic cerebrospinal rhinorrhoea and meningitis. J Neurosurg 1965; 22:331-2.

13. Stool S, Leeds NE, Shulman K. The syndrome of congenital deafness and otic meningitis: diagnosis and management. J Pediatr 1967; 71:547-52.

14. Schaefer SD, Diehl JT, Briggs WH. The diagnosis of CSF rhinorrhea by metrizamide CT scanning. Laryngoscope 1980; 90:871-5.

15. McCabe BF. The osteo-mucoperiosteal flap in repair of cerebrospinal fluid rhinorrhea. Laryngoscope 1976; 86:537-9.

16. Calcaterra TC, Rand RW. Tympanic cavity obliteration for cerebrospinal otorhinorrhea. Arch Otolaryngol 1973; 97: 388-90.

17. Calcaterra TC. Extracranial surgical repair of cerebrospinal rhinorrhea. Ann Otol Rhinol Laryngol 1980; 89: 108-16.

18. Schuknecht HF. Mondini dysplasia: a clinical and pathological study. Ann Otol Rhinol Laryngol 1980; 89 Suppl 65: 3-23.

19. Paparella MM. Mondini's deafness: a review of histopathology. Ann Otol Rhinol Laryngol 1980; 89 Suppl 67:1-10.

Ann Otol Rhinol Laryngol 91:1982

THE PRICE OF PRESERVATION OF HEARING IN ACOUSTIC NEUROMA SURGERY

MIRKO TOS, MD JENS THOMSEN, MD, PhD

COPENHAGEN, DENMARK

Translabyrinthine surgery for acoustic neuroma was introduced in Denmark in 1976, and the results of the first 100 operations are presented. Two deaths occurred, unrelated to the translabyrinthine surgery. Postoperatively, 75% of the patients had normal facial function, while function was reduced in 15% and abolished in 10%. The series represents 85% of all acoustic neuromas operated in Denmark, with 30 new neuromas being diagnosed each year, derived from a population of 5.1 million. The overall postoperative results are compared with the available results from suboccipital removals of acoustic neuromas, and are clearly in favor of the translabyrinthine approach. It is concluded that centralization of acoustic neuroma surgery is necessary, that all acoustic neuromas regardless of size can be removed by the translabyrinthine approach and that the discussion about the hypothetical preservation of hearing by applying the suboccipital approach is being made without solid grounds. To adduce the theoretical chance of preserving hearing in a very small percentage of patients as an argument in favor of the suboccipital approach appears quite irrelevant, and the price of attempting this with the suboccipital approach is too high.

Removal of acoustic neuromas via the translabyrinthine approach[1] is undoubtedly one of the greatest advances within the field of otosurgery. During recent years, many clinics have reported on large groups of patients[1-10] with far better postoperative results than were formerly obtained by the suboccipital approach. It has therefore been assumed that the translabyrinthine approach would gradually become the preferred method of operation everywhere, although there is keen competition in many places between the two approaches, and thereby between neurosurgery and otosurgery, not least because the neurosurgeons have improved their results of the suboccipital approach since the introduction of the operating microscope.[11-19] This is the reason why the translabyrinthine approach has not been introduced in several countries and why, in most countries, more tumors are still being removed via the suboccipital approach than via the translabyrinthine approach.

During recent years, one important argument for preferring the suboccipital approach has been the possibility of preserving hearing, although reports of this are scarce. Smith et al[20] found residual hearing in 3 out of 10 patients with tumors smaller than 2 cm. The postoperative discrimination scores were 60%, 48% and 80%, respectively. Cohen[21] reports preservation of hearing in 3 out of 6 patients with tumors smaller than 2 cm. Others[11,22,23] have reported a few cases with slight residual hearing, which, however, was not audiometrically verified.

Based on the results from the first 100 patients with acoustic neuromas operated via the translabyrinthine approach, we find it reasonable to discuss whether the price paid by some patients is not too high in order that others may have the predominantly theoretical possibility of preserving a slight residual hearing, which very often is useless for the patient. In Denmark, 80-90% of all acoustic neuroma surgery has gradually become centralized to one surgical team, and in view of this, we wish to discuss the importance of such a centralization.

METHODS AND MATERIAL

Since the introduction of the translabyrinthine approach in Denmark in January 1976, and the subsequent establishment of an otoneurosurgical cooperation, 100 patients with acoustic neuromas have been operated on up until April 1980, according to the following principles:

1. All tumors regardless of size were operated on by otologists using the translabyrinthine approach.
2. If complete removal was impossible, the size of the tumor was reduced, the facial nerve was dissected free and marked, and 1-2 weeks later the neurosurgeons removed the tumor remnant via the suboccipital approach.

At the time of operation, 47% of the patients were between 40 and 60 years of age, 17% were over 60 years and 36% were under 40 years old. The oldest patient was 73 years old. There was no significant relationship (x^2 test $p>0.05$) between the age of the patient and the size of the tumor, and the very large tumors were found with the same frequency among young and old patients. The size of the tumor was determined according to the classification by House.[1] Only one tumor was intrameatal and did not protrude into the cerebellopontine angle; 41 of the tumors were medium-sized with an extrameatal diameter of up to 25 mm; 22 tumors were large with an extrameatal diameter of 26-40 mm, and 36 tumors were very large with a diameter between 40 mm and 80 mm.

RESULTS

In the first year, we were unable to remove completely the very large tumors, not even those of 3 cm (Table 1). During the second year, already half of the tumors could be removed and during the third

From the ENT University Clinic, The Gentofte Hospital, Copenhagen.

REPRINTS — Mirko Tos, MD, Københavns Amts Sygehus I Gentofte, ENT-Dept., Niels Andersens Vej 65, 2900 Hellerup, Copenhagen, Denmark.

TABLE 1. NUMBER AND EXTRAMEATAL SIZE OF ACOUSTIC TUMORS NOT AMENABLE FOR TOTAL TRANSLABYRINTHINE REMOVAL (JANUARY 1976-APRIL 1980)

Year	*Total No.*	*No. >4 cm*	*Suboccipital Operation*	*Size (cm)*
1976	10	3	4	3-6
1977	19	6	3	5-6
1978	30	10	2	6
1979	24	10	0	4-7
1980	17	7	0	4-8
Total	100	36	9	

year we removed 80% of the tumors. Since May 1978, all tumors have been removed completely via the translabyrinthine approach, the largest of these measuring 7 and 8 cm in diameter. An example is depicted in the figure, showing a CT scan of a patient with a very large tumor, before and after translabyrinthine removal.

Mortality. Two patients died. A 50-year-old male died two months after the suboccipital operation,[24] and a 73-year-old male died one day after the translabyrinthine operation. The latter had a 6-cm tumor and pronounced pressure symptoms that could not be relieved by a ventricle shunt, and the operation had to be performed on vital indication. Because of his age, total removal was not attempted. The operation went smoothly and the patient was awake after the operation and had normal function of the facial nerve. One hour later, however, he became unconscious with dilated pupils. The wound was immediately reopened and the tumor remnant removed. The autopsy showed an extensive cerebral hemorrhage in the temporal lobe from the medial cerebral artery and no subarachnoidal hemorrhage. The short interval between the two events makes a causal relation probable, although a coincidental cerebral apoplexy cannot be excluded.

TABLE 2. RELATION BETWEEN TUMOR SIZE AND TIME INTERVAL BEFORE RETURNING TO PREVIOUS NORMAL LIFE AND WORK

Tumor Size (mm)	*No.*	*1 mo*	*3 mo*	*6 mo*	*1 yr*	*Death*
Intrameatal	1	1				
1-25	41	32	6	2	1*	
26-40	22	15	7			
40-80	36	17	14	1	2	2
Total	100	65	27	3	3	2

*Retired at age 64.

Postoperative CSF Leak. In 11% of the patients postoperative CSF leak occurred via the eustachian tube. In 6% it stopped spontaneously within one week, and in 4% within two weeks. In one patient, who had CSF leak after physical stress six days after discharge from the hospital, the dura defect was closed with fascia lata four weeks after operation. There was no significant relationship between the size of the tumor and postoperative CSF leak ($p > 0.05$). Meningitis occurred in 4%, all of whom had postoperative CSF leak. No sequelae were found following treatment with antibiotics. Prophylactic antibiotic treatment was used in only the first 13 patients.

Length of Hospital Stay and Postoperative Life. The postoperative stay in the hospital was less than 10 days for 55% of the patients, 10-15 days for 19%, and more than 16 days for 26%; 94% were discharged to their homes.

Apart from one patient who retired at age 64 all patients returned to their normal life and work; most of them started working within the first month (Table 2). Nearly half of the patients with very large tumors resumed their preoperative life within one month.

Cerebellar Symptoms. Prior to the operation, 29% of the patients had one or more cerebellar

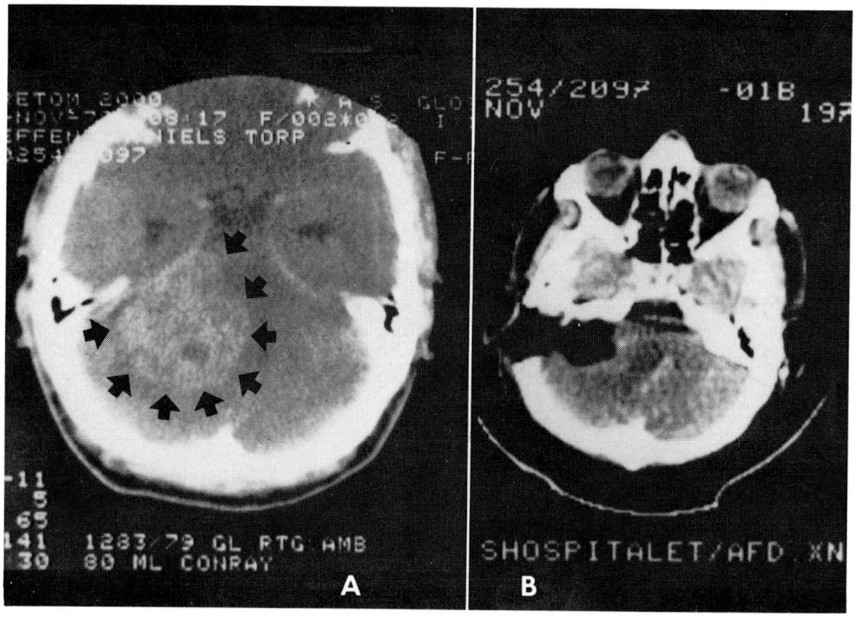

CT scan of very large acoustic neuroma A) before and B) after total removal by translabyrinthine approach. The direct access to the tumor after removal of the bone is clearly illustrated.

TABLE 3. CEREBELLAR SYMPTOMS IN 100 ACOUSTIC NEUROMAS

Symptom	Tumor size (mm) Intra-meatal (N = 1)	1-25 (N = 41)	26-40 (N = 22)	>40 (N = 36)	Total preop (N = 100)	Total postop (N = 100)
1. Romberg	—	2	2	11	15	1
2. Gait disturbance	—	7	5	25	37	1
3. Dysdiadochokinesis	—	3	3	10	16	4
1 + /or 2 + /or 3–	—	8	6	25	39	5
		←	p<0.01	→		p<0.01

symptoms (Table 3) that were significantly related to the size of the tumor ($p<0.01$). Postoperatively, only 5% of the patients had cerebellar symptoms, which is a significant improvement ($p<0.01$).

Trigeminal Nerve Symptoms. Involvement of the trigeminal nerve (Table 4) either in the form of reduced sensibility of cornea and/or of the face, occurred preoperatively in 29% — the relation to tumor size was significant ($p<0.01$) — and postoperatively in 4%. The postoperative reduction in the symptoms from the trigeminal nerve was significant ($p<0.01$).

Pathological Optokinetic Nystagmus. An indication of considerable pressure on the pons, pathological optokinetic nystagmus was found in 3% of the patients, which is a significant reduction ($p<0.01$).

In 28 patients with very large tumors removed via the translabyrinthine approach, the postoperative symptoms from cerebellum, the trigeminal nerve or optokinetic nystagmus were significantly less frequent ($p<0.05$) than in 9 patients in whom the tumor was removed secondarily via the suboccipital approach (Table 5). One of the mentioned symptoms was present in 6 patients (21%) with very large tumors who had translabyrinthine surgery and in 7 patients (78%) who had suboccipital surgery. Among 63 patients with tumors smaller than 40 mm, only one patient (2%) had one of the mentioned symptoms postoperatively.

TABLE 4. INVOLVEMENT OF THE TRIGEMINAL NERVE RELATED TO TUMOR SIZE

Decreased Sensation	Tumor size (mm) Intra-meatal (N = 1)	1-25 (N = 41)	26-40 (N = 22)	>40 (N = 36)	Total preop (N = 100)	Total postop (N = 100)
Corneal	—	3	2	18	23	1
Facial	—	2	1	12	15	1
Corneal + facial	—	—	—	9	9	2
Corneal and/or facial	—	5	3	21	29	4
		←	p<0.01	→		p<0.01

TABLE 5. PREOPERATIVE AND POSTOPERATIVE SYMPTOMS FROM EITHER THE CEREBELLUM, TRIGEMINAL NERVE OR OPTOKINETIC NYSTAGMUS

Operation Group	No.	Size in mm Median (range)*	Symptoms Preop +	Preop –	Postop +	Postop –
Translabyrinthine						
≤40 mm	63	23	20			20
		(0-40)		43	1	42
>40 mm	28	55	24		6	18
		(41-80)		4		4
Suboccipital	9	51	7		6	1
		(30-70)		2	1	1
Total	100		51	49	14	86

*Median of all sizes - 35 mm.

Function of the Facial Nerve. The facial nerve was anatomically preserved in 93% of the patients (Table 6). The day after the operation, the function of the facial nerve was normal in half of the patients, reduced in one fourth and abolished in the remaining one fourth. This percentage distribution remained unchanged at the follow-up investigations at six weeks, one month and three months after the operation. However, it did not concern the same patients, as the function improved in some patients and deteriorated in others.

In the 59 patients first operated on, the function of the facial nerve was registered at the follow-up investigation one year after the operation; in the other 41 patients it was registered at the last control visit 1 to 7 months after the operation (Table 6). The function of the facial nerve was normal in 67%, reduced in 17%, and abolished in 16% of the patients. When related to the size of the tumor, normal function was found in the patient with an intrameatal tumor, in88% of patients with medium-sized tumors, in 77% with large tumors, and in only 36% with very large tumors, which is significantly lowest ($p<0.01$). Since the function of the facial nerve was still improving in the latest operated patients, we have reason to believe that 75% of patients will have normal, 15% reduced and 10% abolished function of the facial nerve one year after the operation (Table 6).

In patients secondarily subjected to the suboccipital operation, the facial nerve function was poorer than in patients with large tumors removed via the translabyrinthine approach, since no one had normal function in the first group against 43% in the other group.

The four patients subjected to a 12th-7th nerve anastomosis had a reasonable tonus, while only 1 patient out of 4 subjected to cross-face transplantation of nervus surralis had beginning clinical function one year later.

Ten patients had abolished or reduced function of the facial nerve preoperatively. These had a poorer postoperative function than patients with a normal preoperative function. Excluding those pa-

TABLE 6. POSTOPERATIVE FUNCTION OF THE FACIAL NERVE

Tumor Size (mm)	*Total No.*	*Anatomically Preserved*	*Postoperative Function* Normal	*Postoperative Function* Partial Paresis	*Postoperative Function* Total Paralysis	*Anastomosis*
Intrameatal	1	1	1			
1-25	41	40	36	3 + 1*	1	
26-40	22	22	17	1 + 1*	1 + 2*	1 XII-VII
>40	36	30	13	6 + 5*	10 + 2*	3 XII-VII 4 cross-face
Total	100	93	67	10 + 7*	12 + 4*	8

*Will probably improve.

tients who had preoperative involvement of the facial nerve and those who were operated suboccipitally, a total of 79% had a completely normal function of the facial nerve after the translabyrinthine approach (Table 7). Since the function of the facial nerve was improving in 11% at the last follow-up, we expect to find normal function in 85%, abolished function in 5%, and reduced function in 10%. It is interesting to note that by the translabyrinthine approach in patients with large tumors (26-40 mm in diameter), normal function of the facial nerve occurred almost as frequently as in patients with medium-sized tumors (Table 6).

In patients with very large tumors, we are unable to obtain high percentages of normal postoperative function of the facial nerve with the translabyrinthine approach, although they are considerably higher than those obtained with the suboccipital approach.

Hematoma in the cerebellopontine angle occurred in two patients. In one patient it was diagnosed by computer tomography performed because of a somewhat slow postoperative recovery; it was evacuated one week later by the translabyrinthine approach. The other patient had profuse bleeding and edema of cerebellum after removal of three fourths of the tumor which precluded removal of the remnant. Four months later, the tumor remnant was removed via the translabyrinthine approach, which resulted in development of a hematoma that was evacuated one week later.

DISCUSSION

When evaluating acoustic neuroma surgery, the most relevant question is, what are the *total* results in a country or in a large geographical area? The second question is, which type of operation yields the best results: the translabyrinthine or the suboccipital approach? This must be indicative of whether or not attempts to preserve hearing can at all be considered an argument for the suboccipital approach. The following summary is based on five years of experience with acoustic neuroma surgery.

TABLE 7. POSTOPERATIVE FACIAL NERVE FUNCTION AFTER TRANSLABYRINTHINE OPERATION IN 82 PATIENTS WITH NORMAL PREOPERATIVE FUNCTION OF THE FACIAL NERVE

Tumor size (mm)	*Total No.*	*Normal* No.	*Normal* %	*Diminished* No.	*Diminished* %	*Abolished* No.	*Abolished* %
Intrameatal	1	1	100	—	—	—	—
1-25	39	37	95	2	5	—	—
26-40	21	18	86	1	5	2*	10
>40	21	9	43	5*	24	3 + 4*	33
Total	82	65	79	3 + 5*	10	3 + 6*	11

*Will probably improve.

1. In the treatment of patients with large acoustic neuromas, cooperation with neurosurgeons is essential. This applies to the preoperative treatment, eg, insertion of a ventricle shunt to relieve the increased intracranial pressure (which was performed in 11 patients in this study), as well as to the postoperative follow-up of the patients.

2. Centralization of the acoustic neuroma surgery is definitely necessary in order to improve the total results. This has been possible to a high degree in Denmark, and during the last three years 80-90% of all patients with acoustic neuromas have been operated on by us using the translabyrinthine approach. Especially in a country like Denmark, with a total population of 5.1 million inhabitants, such a centralization is important since just a little more than 30 patients are diagnosed and operated on yearly. If these operations were to be performed in different places, it would impair the results, regardless of the approach used. Likewise, the total results would be impaired by a strict differentiation between the use of the two methods, eg, the translabyrinthine approach for small and the suboccipital for the large tumors, or, vice versa, the suboccipital for the small tumors, in an attempt to preserve hearing, and the translabyrinthine approach for the large tumors.

3. All acoustic neuromas, regardless of size, can be removed by the translabyrinthine approach,[1-3,8] although there are many technical problems with the large tumors (Table 1). Since such operations very often are prolonged, it is essential that two otosurgeons take turns, which, furthermore, is a great advance for didactic reasons.

4. The results obtained with the translabyrinthine approach[1-10] have so far been considerably better than those obtained with the suboccipital approach.[11-19] This applies both to the mortality rate and to the function of the facial nerve, as also dem-

onstrated in the present study. It can thus be concluded that the price of preserving hearing via the suboccipital approach would be too high.

5. In addition to the mortality rate and the function of the facial nerve, the total evaluation of the patient should include other sequelae as well as the ability to resume a preoperative way of life. These parameters have only to a minor degree been evaluated in the literature on suboccipital acoustic neuroma surgery,[19] but they are considerably more important for the patient than preservation of a slight residual hearing. As shown in Table 1, 65% of the patients resumed normal work within the first month and the preoperative cerebellar symptoms (Table 3), as well as symptoms from the trigeminal nerve (Table 4), were significantly reduced. The great advantage of the translabyrinthine approach over the suboccipital approach is avoidance of pressure on the cerebellum.[1-3] Also, postoperative ataxia probably occurs more frequently following the suboccipital approach than following the translabyrinthine approach, as was the case in this study (Table 5).

In an older study from Denmark, comprising 125 acoustic neuromas operated via the suboccipital approach from 1957 to 1972, the postoperative condition was good in 27%; acceptable in 33%, who were able to take care of themselves; poor in 18%, who needed help in their daily lives; and 25% died.[25] Since then the results have improved immensely, but exact documentation for the total postoperative course following the suboccipital approach is often lacking in the literature, and it ought to be included in the total evaluation of the two surgical approaches. So far, the best neurosurgical study[17] reports poorer results than those obtained in most of the published studies using the translabyrinthine approach, including the present one. Postoperative hydrocephalus, which has not been reported after the translabyrinthine approach,[1-3] occurs frequently after the suboccipital approach.

6. Reports of improved or preserved hearing in patients with tumors larger than 2 cm so far have not been published. In our study, only three patients with tumors smaller than 25 mm had preoperative hearing that was worth saving, ie, a speech audiometric index (SRT) better than 50 dB and a discrimination score of more than 80%. Even if it were possible to preserve this hearing, it would do more harm than good in patients with normal contralateral hearing (which was demonstrated in all of our patients). In von Recklinghausen disease, with bilateral neuromas, no one as yet has been able to preserve hearing, not even by the middle cranial fossa approach.[26] In cases of small or medium-sized tumors, it is most often no problem to preserve the acoustic nerve, but this does not imply preservation of hearing, one of the reasons being that the vascular supply is the same as for the tumor and must be severed. Another considerable risk in attempting to preserve hearing by the suboccipital approach is that the tumor in the fundus of the internal acoustic meatus must be left behind, as drilling out the remaining 2-3 mm posteriorly in the meatus makes preservation of hearing impossible.[26] So, to adduce the theoretical chance of preserving hearing in a very small percentage of patients as an argument in favor of the suboccipital approach appears quite irrelevant to us.

In patients with intrameatal tumors that do not protrude out of the meatus, Brachmann[26] was able to preserve hearing in 10 out of 17 patients using the middle cranial fossa approach, but even in these cases, he prefers the translabyrinthine approach if hearing does not exceed 50 dB. In the present study, there was only one patient with an intrameatal tumor (Table 2) and he had a preoperative hearing of 80 dB.

7. Today, translabyrinthine surgery is to a higher extent centralized to certain centers than is the suboccipital operation. Reports published in recent years on suboccipital surgery have seldom comprised more than 100 patients.[13,14,18] Considerably more reports have been published on the translabyrinthine approach.[2,3,5,7,10,27,28] If we take the yearly incidence in Denmark of 30 acoustic neuromas in a population of 5.1 million inhabitants and apply this to bigger countries, it gives a yearly incidence of 1,308 neuromas in North America, 368 in Germany, 336 in England, and 318 in France. House's study, from one of the places where acoustic neuroma surgery is most concentrated, comprises 500 patients who were operated during a period of seven years (from 1968 to 1975) which corresponds to 71 tumors a year. From 1975 to 1977, a further 300 patients have been operated, corresponding to 100 operations a year.[3] The total number of translabyrinthine operations per year performed in other centers in North America that have published results[4-6,8,27] and from clinics that have not published their results but are known to perform this operation probably does not exceed 200 a year. This means that only one fourth of all acoustic neuromas in North America are removed via the translabyrinthine approach.

Based on neurosurgical publications, which comprise relatively small numbers of patients, it must be assumed that by far the majority of suboccipital operations in North America are strongly decentralized, which in itself must give rather poor total results.

In England, King and Morrison[10] have published the largest study of 150 patients, corresponding to 15 patients a year. In France, Sterkers[28] reported on 126 patients, 15 a year. In Germany, results from more than 100 patients have not been published. Also in Europe, three fourths of acoustic neuromas are operated by neurosurgeons at numerous neurosurgical departments, of which there are about 1 department/1 million inhabitants. Still using our incidence of 30 tumors/5.1 million inhabitants, each neurosurgical department should on an average operate about 6 tumors a year. Evidently, the results from such small groups of patients must be poorer than those obtained in centers specializing in this type of surgery. A survey on a national basis will in all probability show poorer results with the suboccipital approach than are evident from the scarce neurosurgical publications during recent years.[11-19] On the basis of these calculations, it must be concluded that the price of attempting to preserve hearing with the suboccipital approach is very high, perhaps even too high.

REFERENCES

1. House WF. Transtemporal bone microsurgical removal of acoustic neuromas. Arch Otolaryngol 1964; 80:599-76.

2. House WF. Acoustic neuroma. Arch Otolaryngol 1968; 88; 586-91.

3. House WF, Luetje CM. Acoustic tumors. Vol. 2. Baltimore: University Park Press, 1979.

4. Montgomery WW. Surgery for acoustic neuroma. Ann Otol Rhinol Laryngol 1973; 82:428-41.

5. Glasscock ME, Hays JW. The translabyrinthine removal of acoustic and other cerebellopontine angle tumors. Ann Otol Rhinol Laryngol 1973; 82:415-27.

6. Maddox HE. The lateral approach to acoustic tumors. Laryngoscope 1977; 87:1572-8.

7. Morrison AW. Translabyrinthine surgical approach to the internal acoustic meatus. J Roy Soc Med 1978; 71:269-73.

8. Glasscock ME, Hays JW, Jackson CC, Stennerson RL. A one-stage combined approach for the management of large cerebellopontine angle tumors. Laryngoscope 1978; 88:1563-76.

9. Palva T, Troupp H. Recent experience in the surgery of acoustic neurinomas. Acta Otolaryngol (Stockh) 1979 Suppl 360: 48-50.

10. King TT, Morrison AW. Translabyrinthine and transtentorial removal of acoustic nerve tumors. J Neurosurg 1980; 52: 210-6.

11. Rand RW, Kurze TL. Micro-neurosurgery in acoustic tumors (suboccipital transmeatal approach). Trans Am Acad Ophthalmol Otolaryngol 1967; 71:682-94.

12. Smith MFW, Miller RN, Cox DJ. Suboccipital microsurgical removal of acoustic neuromas of all sizes. Ann Otol Rhinol Laryngol 1973; 82:407-14.

13. Hullay J, Tomits GH, Gombi R, Velok G. Experiences with radically operated acoustic tumors. Acta Neurochir (Wien) 1975; 32:69-72.

14. MacCarty CS. Acoustic neuroma and the suboccipital approach. Mayo Clin Proc 1975; 50:15-6.

15. Rhoton AL. Suboccipital microsurgical approach to acoustic neuromas. In: Silverstein H, Norrell H, eds. Neurologic surgery of the ear. Birmingham: Aesculapius; 1977:220-34.

16. Erickson DL, Ausman JI, Chou SN. Prognosis of seventh nerve palsy following removal of large acoustic tumors. J Neurosurg 1977; 47:31-4.

17. DiTullio MV, Malkasian D, Rand R. A critical comparison of neurosurgical and otolaryngological approaches to acoustic neuromas. J Neurosurg 1978; 48:1-12.

18. Yasargil MG. Mikrochirurgie der Kleinhirnbrückenwinkel-Tumoren. In: Plester D, Wende S, Nakayama N, eds. Kleinhirnbrückenwinkel-Tumoren. Berlin: Springer-Verlag, 1978: 215-57.

19. Ochiai C, Masuzawa H, Manaka S, Sano K, Kitamura K, Komatsuzaki A. Supine-lateral approach versus sitting operation — statistical analysis of brainstem, cranial nerve and cerebellar function in 165 acoustic neurinomas. Neurol Med Chir (Tokyo) 1979; 19:629-35.

20. Smith MFW, Clancy TP, Lang JS. Conservation of hearing in acoustic neurilemmoma excision. Trans Am Acad Ophthalmol Otolaryngol 1977; 84:704-9.

21. Cohen NL. Acoustic neuroma surgery with emphasis on preservation of hearing. Laryngoscope 1979; 89:886-96.

22. Rand RW, Kurze TL. Preservation of vestibular, cochlear, and facial nerves during microsurgical removal of acoustic tumors. J Neurosurg 1968; 28:158-61.

23. Buchheit WA, Gastaldo JA. The posterior approach to acoustic tumors. Preservation of hearing. In: Silverstein H, Norrell H, eds. Neurologic surgery of the ear. Birmingham: Aesculapius; 1977: 263-6.

24. Thomsen J, Tos M, Harmsen Å, Riishede J, Thornval G. Surgery of acoustic neuromas. Preliminary experience with a translabyrinthine approach. Acta Neurol Scand 1977; 56:277-90.

25. Thomsen J. Suboccipital removal of acoustic neuromas. Result of 125 operations. Acta Otolaryngol (Stockh) 1976; 81: 406-14.

26. Brachmann DE. Middle cranial fossa approach. In: House WF, Luetje CM, eds. In: Acoustic tumors, Vol. 2. Baltimore: University Park Press; 1979: 15-41.

27. Clemis JL, Mastricola PG. Special audiometric test battery in 121 proved acoustic tumors. Arch Otolaryngol 1976; 120: 654-6.

28. Sterkers JM. Neurinome de l'acoustique et autres tumeurs de l'angle et du conduit auditif interne. Ann Otolaryngol (Paris) 1979; 96: 373-86.

Ann Otol Rhinol Laryngol 91:1982

WARTHIN'S TUMOR, A MULTIFOCAL DISEASE

JOEL M. A. SHUGAR, MD
PETER M. SOM, MD
HUGH F. BILLER, MD
NEW YORK, NEW YORK

Of all salivary gland neoplasms Warthin's tumor is the only lesion which is truly multicentric. The most common presentation of these multiple lesions is bilateral solitary masses. We present the first reported case of bilateral multiple tumors occurring simultaneously. The embryology of the salivary glands as it relates to the pathogenesis of this tumor is discussed. The differential diagnosis of the multinodular parotid gland is reviewed.

An unusual tumor consisting of both lymphoid and parotid ductal elements was first described by Albrecht and Artz in 1910.[1] Warthin reported two cases of this lesion in 1929[2] and coined the term "papillary cystadenoma lymphomatosum." This entity, now commonly referred to as Warthin's tumor, is the second most common benign lesion of the parotid gland and represents about 6% of all parotid neoplasms.[3] Whereas most major salivary gland tumors occur as solitary lesions, Warthin's tumors have been reported to occur as bilateral lesions and/or multiple unilateral tumors.[4-13] We present a case of multiple Warthin's tumors occurring in each parotid gland at the same time. This simultaneous bilateral multicentric presentation is the only such case found in a review of the literature. It is the purpose of this paper to present this case and discuss the resulting clinical implications of Warthin's tumor in the differential diagnosis of the multinodular gland.

CASE REPORT

A 56-year-old white male was found on routine head and neck examination to have multinodular lesions of both parotid glands. Each gland had three distinct masses to palpation, all of which were firm, nontender and measured 2-3 cm in diameter. The patient had no associated symptoms and claimed to have had these lesions for many years. The other salivary glands and the lacrimal glands were normal. He was otherwise in good health and specifically had no symptoms of xerostomia or arthritis. A chest film was normal. Because of the multinodular bilateral involvement the patient was clinically felt to have Mikulicz's disease or a systemic granulomatous disease such as sarcoidosis. A CT sialogram was performed which revealed multiple benign-appearing lesions which were confined to the parotid gland (Fig. 1). There was no infiltration of the surrounding tissues. The punctate and globular sialographic changes of the autoimmune diseases were not seen (Fig. 2). An excisional biopsy of one of the lesions in the tail of the left gland was diagnostic of Warthin's tumor. In order to confirm that the contralateral gland was involved with Warthin's tumors and that the remaining masses in the left parotid gland were of similar histology, a Tc^{99} parotid scan was performed. It revealed bilateral intense parotid uptake consistent with this diagnosis (Fig. 3). The benign nature of the lesion was explained to the patient and he declined further surgery unless the lesions increased in size.

DISCUSSION

Warthin's tumor usually presents as an asymptomatic solitary slow-growing mass in the tail of the parotid gland.[11] Only 10% of the patients complain of pain, pressure or a more rapidly enlarging mass.[3] The tumor is essentially benign with malignant transformation being extremely rare.[14] Facial nerve involvement is extremely rare. Eighty percent of the patients are in the fourth to seventh decades and there is a 5:1 male predominance.[3] It is very rare to find this tumor in a noncaucasian.[11] Gross examination reveals an encapsulated roundish tumor that is either cystic or semisolid. Usually a brownish mucoid fluid exudes from the freshly cut surface. Solid areas are gray and may have small white nodules which represent lymphoid follicles.

Microscopically, a tubulopapillary-cystic epithelial pattern is seen within lymphoid tissue or a lymph mode. The epithelium is a double layer of oxyphilic finely granular cells. This appearance is due to an abundance of mitochondria as determined by special stains and electron microscopy.[3]

The currently accepted theory of the pathogenesis of Warthin's tumor is that it has its origin from heterotopic salivary gland ductal tissue within lymph nodes which are either included in or lie adjacent to the parotid gland.[3] Embryologically the parotid gland arises from a loose arrangement of cells and encapsulation occurs late in its development. This unique situation allows an admixture of developing lymphoid and parotid tissue which results in inclusion of salivary ducts in the developing lymph nodes. The subsequent formation of the glandular capsule then separates the intraparotid and extraparotid nodes, some of which contain ductal elements that may give rise to Warthin's tumor either within the parotid gland or its adjacent lymph nodes.

Unequivocal evidence for this pathogenesis was provided by Azzopardi[15] who reported a case of

From the Departments of Otorhinolaryngology and Radiology, Mount Sinai Medical School, City University of New York.
REPRINTS — Peter M. Som, MD, Department of Radiology, The Mount Sinai Hospital, One Gustave L. Levy Place, New York, NY 10029.

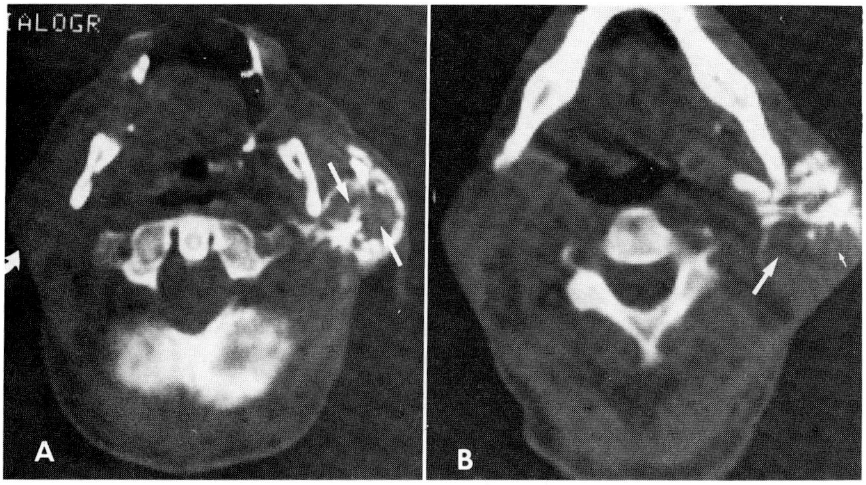

Fig. 1. Axial CT scan performed immediately after sialogram. A) Contrast material in the left parotid gland with two discrete masses seen within gland (straight arrows). Margins with adjacent parotid tissue are smooth. Note fullness in right parotid region (curved arrow). B) Scan at different level reveals third large mass in posterior portion of deep lobe (large arrow) and lower margin of lateral mass seen in A (small arrow).

multiple unilateral Warthin's tumors with one lesion, within a lymph node, showing clear transition from ductal elements to Warthin's tumor. The embryogenesis of this lesion further explains why approximately 20% of Warthin's tumors present as an extraparotid neck mass.[7]

The submaxillary and sublingual glands develop as compact entities and encapsulation occurs early, preventing the mixing of salivary and lymphoid tissue. Thus Warthin's tumor originates exclusively from the parotid gland or its immediate environs.[11]

The intermingling of salivary and lymphoid tissue occurs diffusely, throughout both parotid glands. Since one such site can lead to the development of a Warthin's tumor, the potential is present to have multiple tumors develop either unilaterally and/or bilaterally. That this is, in fact, the case is exemplified by reported cases demonstrating multicentricity.[4-13] Although the most common clinical presentation of a Warthin's tumor is that of a solitary mass in the tail of the superficial lobe, the most common presentation of a multifocal occurrence is bilateral solitary tumors. Other less common presentations are 1) a solitary lesion on one side and multiple tumors on the other side, 2) unilateral multiple lesions and 3) bilateral multiple tumors. In the vast majority of cases of bilateral involvement,

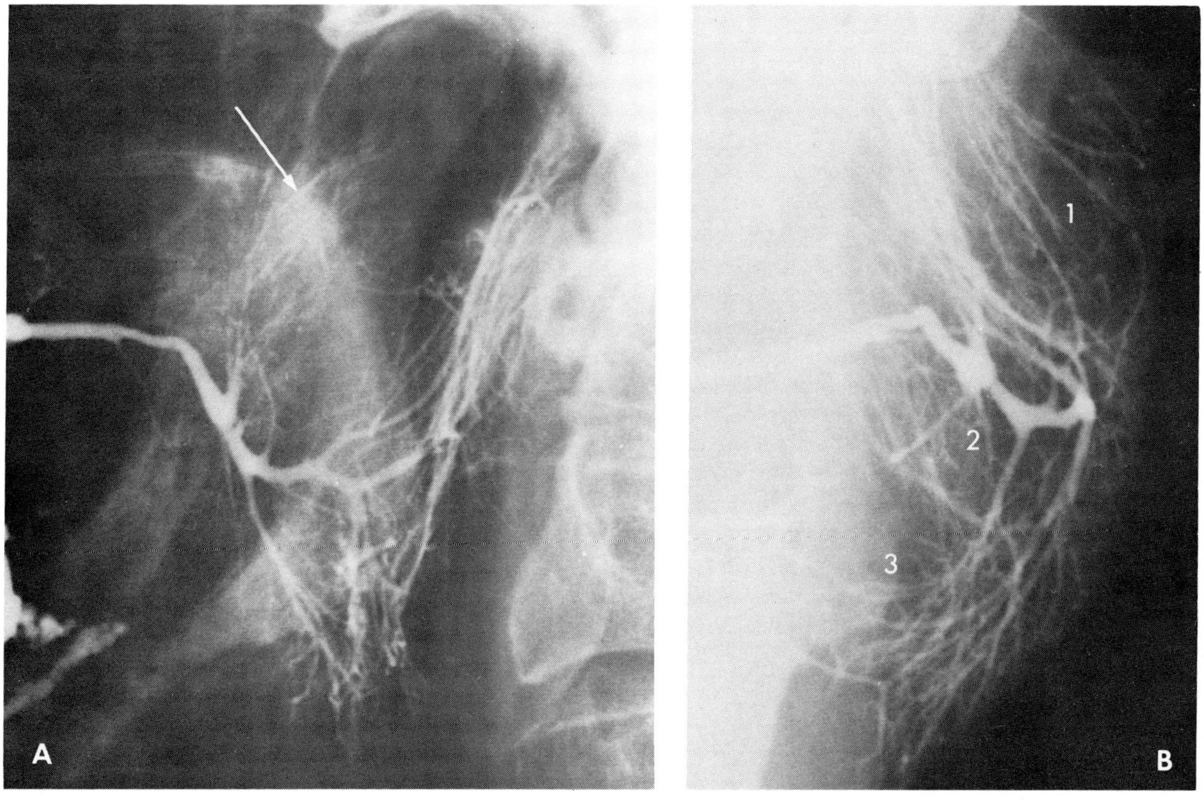

Fig. 2 A) Lateral sialogram film reveals displacement of upper pole parotid ducts around mass lesion (arrow) with crowding of posterior ducts. B) Oblique frontal sialogram film reveals three masses (1, 2, 3), each displacing parotid ducts around them.

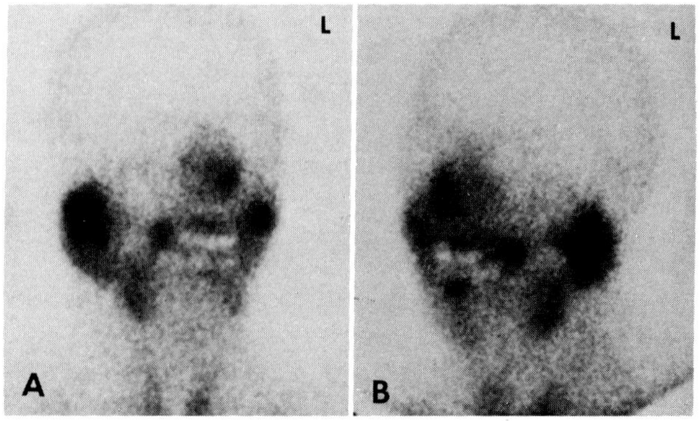

Fig. 3. A) Right and B) left oblique views of a Tc^{99} parotid scan reveal bilateral intense uptake of isotope.

the second lesion usually occurs as a separate entity manifesting itself months to years after the initial lesion.[8,12] The commonly quoted statistic of a 6% bilateral occurrence[4,16] of Warthin's tumor gives an erroneously low impression of the multicentric nature of this tumor. There are several reasons justifying the above statement.

1. This statistic does not include cases of multiple lesions occurring in the same gland.
2. A second lesion in the opposite gland may be falsely reported as a single entity because the time interval between it and the first lesion was so long that the patient had changed doctors or the charts were lost.
3. A second lesion in the same gland may be reported as a "recurrence" while in fact it represents a second primary.[5]
4. Only one lesion may be grossly visible and if the salivary gland is not examined histologically, microscopic foci of tumor may be missed. This was demonstrated by a *retrospective* study in which the pathology slides of the salivary glands containing Warthin's tumor were reviewed.[10] Thirty percent of the specimens were found to have gross and microscopic evidence of multiple lesions. Patey[17] designed a *prospective* study scrutinizingly examining involved parotid glands. The salivary glands were serially sectioned and the slides studied for microscopic foci of tumor. In this study multiple lesions were the rule rather than the exception with 4 out of 5 glands demonstrating more than one lesion. The finding of occult Warthin's tumors in radical neck dissection specimens emphasizes the slow evolution of this lesion resulting eventually in grossly detectable disease.[7] This further supports the concept that the incidence of this lesion is higher than indicated by clinical or gross examination of the specimen alone. Even microscopic examination of a few slides through the area of the lesion is not adequate in this regard and it seems necessary to perform serial sections of the entire portion of the removed parotid gland in order to give reliable statistics of multicentricity.
5. It is conceivable that the involved gland may have only one Warthin's tumor and that the contralateral gland has only microscopic foci of tumor which clinically may not manifest themselves because of their slow growth potential.

Despite the benign nature of Warthin's tumor there is a significant postoperative recurrence rate of 12%.[13] This is higher than for the benign mixed tumor and can be explained by the frequency of multiple lesions. Thus, unless the tumor is violated at the time of surgery, the term "recurrence" is actually a misnomer because the subsequent lesion actually represents a second primary and not residual tumor or spilled tumor cells.

A superficial parotidectomy should be the procedure of choice for removal of Warthin's tumor in order to remove multicentric foci of disease.[10] A total parotidectomy is theoretically a more complete operation, but because of its greater morbidity it should be reserved for cases in which there is palpable evidence of tumor in the deep lobe at the time of surgery. The only indication for a local resection of a palpable tumor would be a Warthin's tumor occurring in the neck away from the main gland itself.

Most salivary gland lesions are single lesions unless recurrent and Warthin's tumor is the only neoplasia which is primarily multifocal.[5,18] This places Warthin's tumor in a unique position and it must be included in the differential diagnosis of the multinodular parotid gland. The other entities to consider are the autoimmune diseases, the granulomatous diseases and rarely neurofibromatosis, lymphoneoplasms and metastases. Isolated case reports describe the rare coexistence of two different types of salivary gland tumors.[9] Differentiation between these diseases may be further accomplished by a combined clinicoradiographic approach. The clinical presentations have all been well described. Radiographically the conventional sialogram will identify the autoimmune diseases by a pathognomonic uniformly diffuse punctate or globular appearance. All the remaining lesions usually appear as multiple, discrete space-occupying masses which displace the adjacent parotid ducts around them. The CT-sialogram increases the sensitivity of the roentgen procedure by allowing easier detection of occult disease. Rarely the lymphoneoplasms and metastases may show frank sialographic changes of malignancy. These include abrupt ductal cutoff, lack of parenchymal filling, irregular pooling of the sialographic contrast material within the tumor and rarely parotolymphatic backflow can be seen.

A Tc^{99} scan will show progressive glandular uptake in those tumors which contain oncocytes. These include Warthin's tumor and the rare oncocytoma. Because this latter tumor is not a multicentric lesion, it is not included in the differential diagnosis of the multinodular gland. Thus, if the clinicoradiographic findings are those of a multinodular parotid gland a positive Tc^{99} scan will establish the diagnosis of multifocal Warthin's tumors.

REFERENCES

1. Albrecht H, Artz L. Beitrage zur Frage der gewebsverirrang papillare Cystadenoma in Lymphdrusen. Z Pathol 1910; 4: 47-69.

2. Warthin AD. Papillary cystadenoma lymphomatosum. J Cancer Res 1929; 13:116-25.

3. Batsakis JG. Tumors of the head and neck. 2nd ed. Baltimore: Williams and Wilkins Co, 1979:54-6.

4. Hales B, Hansen JE. Bilateral simultaneous Warthin's tumor in a woman. South Med J 1977; 70:157-8.

5. Breck LD, Maguda TA. Papillary cystadenoma lymphomatosum (Warthin's tumor): a multicentric benign tumor. Laryngoscope 1967; 77:1840-8.

6. Shaw HJ, Friedmann I. Bilateral adenolymphoma of the parotid salivary gland associated with tuberculosis. Br J Surg 1959; 46:500-5.

7. Dietert SE. Papillary cystadenoma lymphomatosum (Warthin's tumor) in patients in a general hospital over a 24-year period. Am J Clin Pathol 1975; 63:866-75.

8. Greeley PW, Gleason MC, Curtin JW. Papillary cystadenoma lymphomatosum (Warthin's tumor). Plast Reconstr Surg 1958; 21:223-32.

9. Turnbull AD, Frazell EL. Multiple tumors of the major salivary glands. Am J Surg 1969; 118:787-9.

10. Blatnik DS, Kurtin JB, Lehman RH. Multicentricity of Warthin's tumors. Wis Med J 1976; 75:61-3.

11. Chaudrey AP, Gorlin RJ. Papillary cystadenoma lymphomatosum (adenolymphoma). A review of the literature. Am J Surg 1958; 95:923-31.

12. Kavka SJ. Bilateral simultaneous Warthin's tumors. Arch Otolaryngol 1970; 91:302.

13. Foote FW, Frazell EL. Tumors of the major salivary glands. Sec IV, fasc 11. Washington DC: Armed Forces Institute of Pathology Atlas of Tumor Pathology, 1954; 129-33.

14. Kessler E, Koznizky MD, Schindel J. Malignant Warthin's tumor. Oral Surg 1977; 43:111-5.

15. Azzopardi JG, Tsun HL. The genesis of adenolymphoma. J Pathol Bacteriol 1964; 88:213-8.

16. Thackery AC, Lucas RB. Atlas of tumor pathology. Tumors of the major salivary glands. 2nd Series, Fasc 10. Washington DC: Armed Forces Institute of Pathology, 1974; 40-55.

17. Patey DH, Thackery AC. The treatment of parotid tumor in the light of a pathological study of parotid material. Brit J Surg 1958; 45:477-87.

18. Gaynor EB, Hershberg R. Unilateral multiple tumors of the parotid gland. J Laryngol Otol 1976; 90:295-8.

≈

AMERICAN ACADEMY OF PEDIATRICS SECTION ON OTOLARYNGOLOGY AND BRONCHOESOPHAGOLOGY

The American Academy of Pediatrics Section on Otolaryngology and Bronchoesophagology Meeting will take place on Monday, October 25, 1982 (closed session), and Tuesday, October 26, 1982 (open session). The meeting will be held at the Sheraton-Center Hotel in New York City. For further information please contact Dr. Lyon Greenberg, Program Chairman, 980 Western Avenue, Albany, NY 12203.

F4

Ann Otol Rhinol Laryngol 91:1982

DEAFNESS IN CRYOGLOBULINEMIA

YASUYA NOMURA, MD
SHIGEO MORI, MD
MINEKO TSUCHIDA, MD
TERUHISA SAKURAI, MD

TOKYO, JAPAN

We present a histopathological study of a 44-year-old female with essential cryoglobulinemia. She had suffered from purpura and ulcer in winter, bilateral tinnitus and progressive hearing loss. An audiogram taken a week before her death showed bilateral total deafness. In the cochlea of the left temporal bone, the organ of Corti was either missing or present as a mound. The stria vascularis was atrophic throughout the cochlea. The tectorial membrane showed drooping and encapsulation. Reissner membrane was in the normal position. Eosinophilic precipitate was noted in the scala media at the site where Reissner membrane bulged. The spiral ganglion cells were well preserved. In the lower basal turn, there was fibrosis and ossification intermingled in the scala tympani. Ossification was most marked near the basal end. The semicircular canals and vestibule were almost totally ossified and fused with surrounding bone. There was a small, cyst-like structure in the vestibule containing eosinophilic fluid. Our findings indicate that the deafness was the result of circulatory disturbance due to cryoglobulinemia. To our knowledge, this is the first cryoglobulinemia case in which temporal bone findings are reported.

Circulatory disturbances in the inner ear can produce gradual or sudden sensorineural hearing loss, depending on the changes of the circulatory systems involved. The morphological and physiological aspects of inner ear changes attributable to experimental arterial or venous flow disturbances have been well documented.[1-4] However, there is little histopathological evidence proving that alterations in cochlear circulation result in sensorineural hearing loss. In leukemia, hemorrhage in the cochlea is a relatively common finding[5] and human temporal bone studies revealed sudden deafness to be attributable to vascular origin.[6,7]

Cryoglobulinemia can produce circulatory disturbances in the extremities with occasional sensory neuropathy and deafness.[8-10] We now present histopathological findings on an essential cryoglobulinemia patient with bilateral slowly progressive hearing loss and eventual total deafness.

CASE REPORT

A 44-year-old woman visited a local hospital in March 1960 with the chief complaint of purpura and petechiae in the lower extremities. Subsequently, these symptoms worsened every winter. In 1965, arthralgia appeared in all joints after the birth of an apparently normal child. In 1968, a diagnosis of cryoglobulinemia was made, because refrigeration of her serum (4°C) resulted in a whitish precipitate which could be resolved by exposure to warm temperature. After further examinations, the diagnosis was essential cryoglobulinemia of mixed type (IgG-IgA) and the patient received predonine, inositol hexanicotinate and vitamin C. In 1972, she was admitted for two months to University of Tokyo Hospital because of exacerbation of ulcers on the lower extremities. Admission examination revealed the serum cryoglobulin level to be 150 mg/dl; the cryoglobulin was of mixed type (IgG and IgA); cryocrit was less than 2%. C-reactive protein was strongly positive, ASO x 1250; the patient was RA-negative and the direct Coombs test returned negative results. ESR was 105 (1°); serologic tests for syphilis were negative.

In March 1972, she first noted tinnitus and hearing loss of the left ear. During each subsequent winter and spring, the symptoms worsened. Funduscopic findings were bleeding and grade III (Keith-Wagener) hypertension. Dizziness appeared in January 1978 and as her hearing loss was progressive, she was fitted with a hearing aid in August 1978. However, her hearing deteriorated to the point where the hearing aid was useless.

In September 1978, the patient was brought to our department on a stretcher. The chief complaint was deafness. Upon inspection, the eardrums were normal; audiograms were indicative of total bilateral deafness. There was no spontaneous nystagmus; the nasal septum had a perforation about 1 cm in diameter. One week later, she expired of bronchopneumonia.

Postmortem findings revealed systemic vasculitis in several organs, and there were rather massive changes in the kidneys, liver and colon. The morphological features of the arteritis were somehow different from those of typical periarteritis nodosa. The involved arteries were medium to small. The inflammatory cell reaction was rather mild, and infiltrating cells were exclusively lymphocytes, lacking in neutrophil leukocytes. Intimal hyperplasia and adventitial fibrosis were the most common

From the Department of Otolaryngology and the Department of Pathology, Faculty of Medicine, University of Tokyo. This study was supported by a Research Grant for Specific Diseases from the Ministry of Health and Welfare, Idiopathic Sensorineural Hearing Loss Research Committee of Japan.
REPRINTS — Yasuya Nomura, MD, Department of Otolaryngology, University of Tokyo, 7-3-1 Hongo, Bunkyo-ku, Toyko 113, Japan.

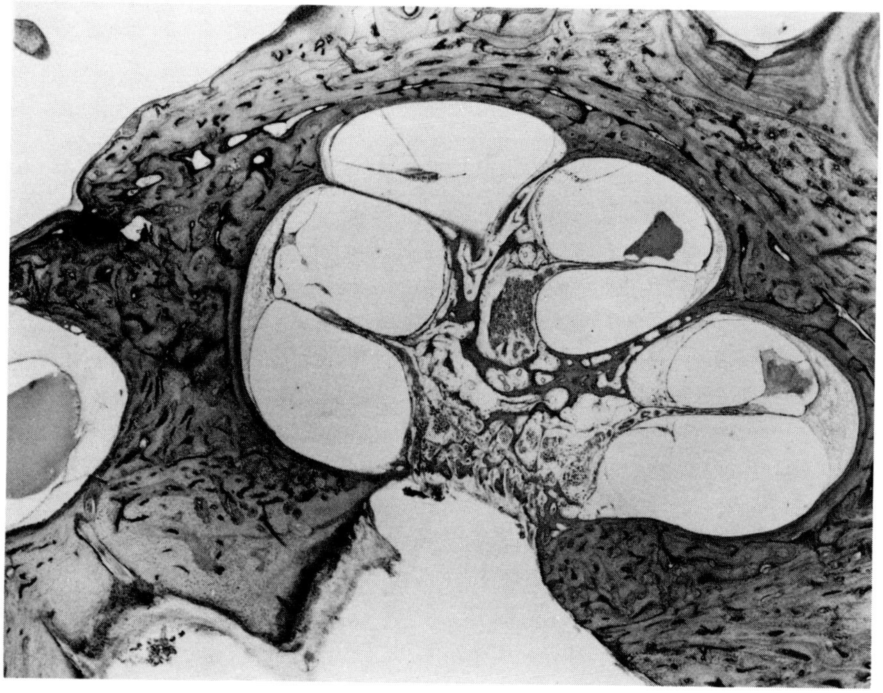

Fig. 1. Midmodiolar section of the left cochlea showing an eosinophilic precipitate in the scala media of the upper middle turn. Organ of Corti is either missing or present as a mound. Stria vascularis is atrophic throughout the cochlea. Spiral ganglion cells are fairly well preserved.

findings. Few arteries took the form of necrotizing arteritis, while acidophil amorphous mass deposition in the intima and microthrombi in affected arteries were common. Due to vasculitis of the arcuate and interlobar arteries, the kidneys manifested nephrosclerosis with a peculiar, coarse granular surface. In the colon, several small ulcers were found; these were attributable to vasculitis of the mucosa.

The left temporal bone was removed five hours postmortem and immediately fixed in a 10% formalin solution. Horizontal, 20 μm-thick sections were prepared according to the conventional celloidin embedding method. Every tenth section was stained with hematoxylin and eosin and used for study.

TEMPORAL BONE FINDINGS

Cochlea. In all cochlear turns, the organ of Corti was either missing or noted as a mound on the basilar membrane (Fig. 1).

The spiral ganglion cells were relatively well preserved. The nerve fibers within the osseous spiral lamina were densely populated. There were degenerative changes of the tectorial membrane with drooping into the inner sulcus. In some areas, this membrane was spherical and encapsulated (Fig. 2). The limbus revealed a loss of interdental cells.

The stria vascularis was atrophic throughout the cochlea and eosinophilic precipitate containing floating macrophages was found in the scala media of the upper middle turn (Fig. 3A). Reissner membrane revealed bulging at the site of the precipitate in the scala media. In the scala media of the upper basal turn, heavy concentrations of proteinaceous exudate with fibrin-like crystals and occasional mononuclear cell infiltration were present (Fig. 3B). In some sections, strial cells with stalks protruded into the precipitate at the junction of Reissner membrane and the atrophic stria.

There was marked ossification of the scala tympani of the lower basal turn (Fig. 4). The round window was completely closed by bony tissue. Toward the apex, the bony tissue decreased gradually; approximately 7 mm from the basal end, the scala tympani was mainly occupied by connective tissue with melanocytes.

There were few blood vessels in the spaces of the modiolus and no vasculitis was noted. However, some lymphocytic infiltration around the small modiolar artery was present (Fig. 5). The number

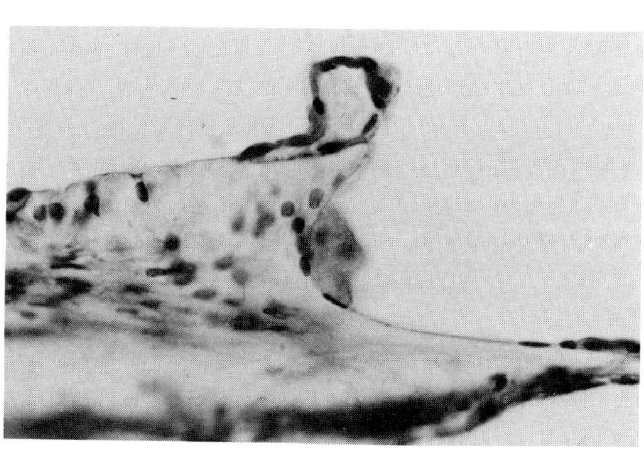

Fig. 2. Partial drooping of the tectorial membrane into the inner sulcus. Remainder of the membrane is encapsulated on the limbus which shows atrophy of the interdental cells. No inner sulcus cells are seen.

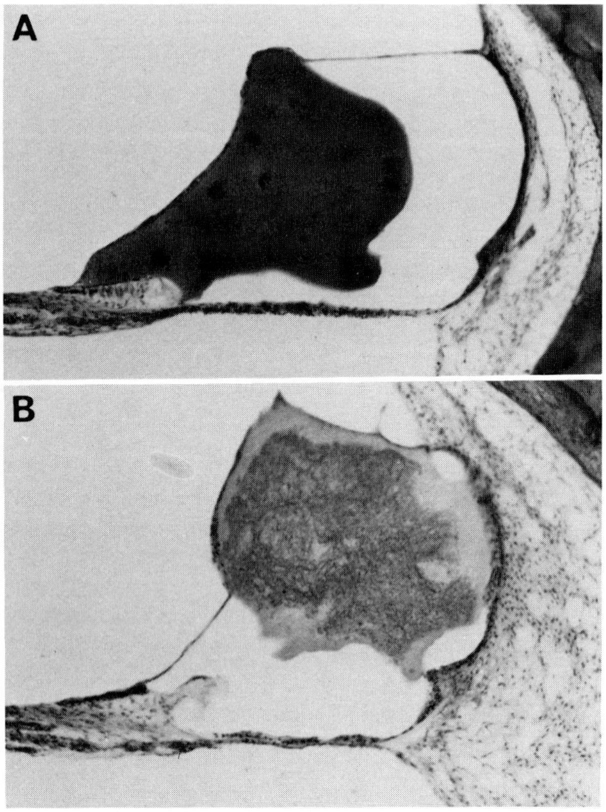

Fig. 3. A) Eosinophilic precipitate in the scala media of the upper middle turn. Note the scattering of macrophages containing brownish pigment. Strial cells are also observed. Reissner membrane shows bulging. B) Heavy concentrations of proteinaceous exudate with fibrin-like crystals and occasional mononuclear cell infiltration in the scala media of the upper basal turn.

of small vessels in the interscalar septum and spiral ligament was markedly decreased. No capillaries were observed in the atrophic stria. The diameter of the inferior cochlear vein seemed to be decreased. The cochlear aqueduct was normal. The temporal bone was devoid of nerves and blood vessels in the internal auditory meatus.

Vestibule and Semicircular Canals. There was remarkable ossification in the vestibule and semicircular canals (Fig. 6). The sensory epithelium of the maculae and cristae was completely missing. Spaces of the vestibule and canals were almost completely occupied by bony tissue adjacent to which there was connective tissue with melanocytes. In the vestibule, a space containing eosinophilic fluid with scattered histiocytes was seen. This space, lined by a single cell layer and surrounded by connective tissue, may represent the original endolymphatic space although it was not in the normal position. The vestibular nerves of the superior and inferior division showed a marked loss of fibers. The vestibular aqueduct, the paravestibular canaliculus and the endolymphatic sac appeared almost normal.

DISCUSSION

According to the immunoglobulin constituents, cryoglobulin is classified as pure or mixed monoclonal or polyclonal cryoglobulin.[11] Pure monoclonal cryoglobulin is of four types: IgG, IgM, IgA, and Bence-Jones type. It has been found in some patients with multiple myeloma, macroglobulinemia, malignant lymphoma, collagen- and liver disease.

Of the three mixed monoclonal cryoglobulin types (IgM-IgG, IgA-IgG, and IgG-IgG), IgM-IgG is most common. In the IgM-IgG type, IgM has the character of anti-IgG antibody. While IgM and IgG alone do not show precipitation at low temperature, admixed they do. Mixed type cryoglobulin has been found in some patients with macroglobulinemia, multiple myeloma, and malignant lymphoma. Barnett et al[12] reported that essential cryoglobulinemia can be diagnosed by excluding 19 diseases.

The characteristic clinical signs and symptoms of cryoglobulinemia are purpura, arthralgia and Raynaud-like symptom in the lower extremities. Proteinuria, hematuria, oliguria and edema may ap-

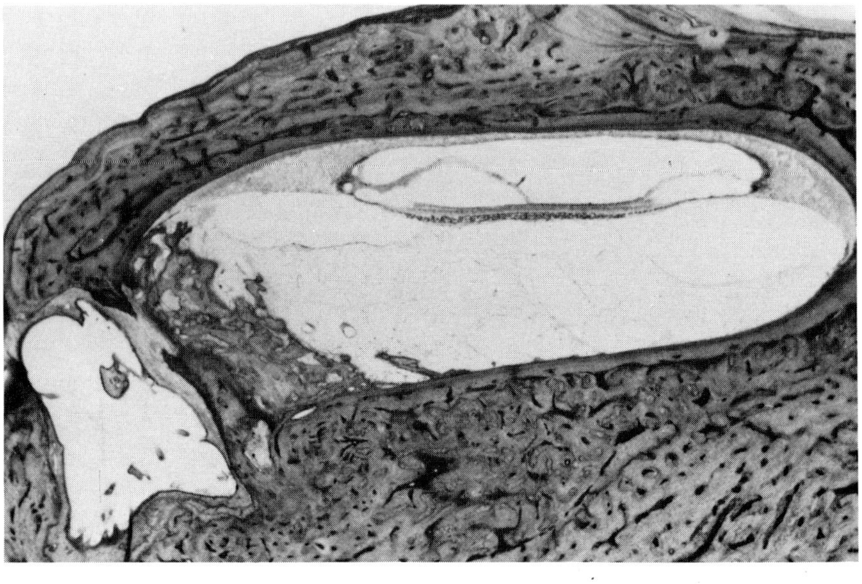

Fig. 4. Ossification and fibrosis in the scala tympani of the lower basal turn. Note the marked ossification at the basal end.

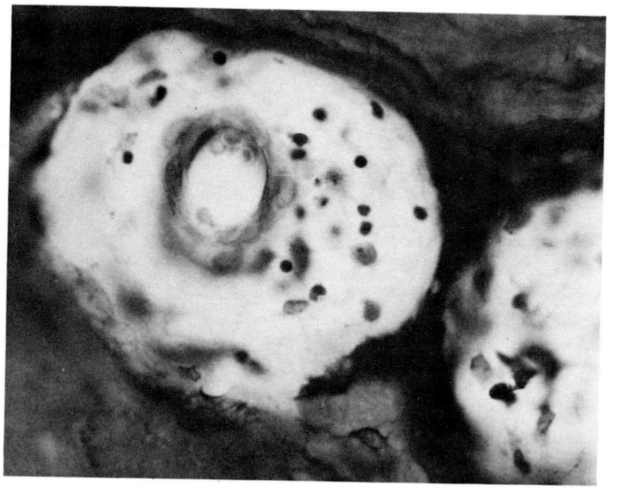

Fig. 5. Modiolar blood vessel. Some lymphocytic infiltration in the perivascular tissue is present.

pear suddenly and the acute renal insufficiency may be fatal. In cryoglobulinemia, the histopathologic changes essentially consist of diffuse glomerulonephritis. Swelling of the endothelium, leukocytic infiltration, mesangial proliferation, and thickening of the glomerular basement membrane are common findings. Precipitation of immune complex in the glomeruli has been suggested as the cause of glomerulonephritis.[13]

Barr et al[8] were probably the first to report tinnitus and progressive deafness as symptoms of cryoglobulinemia and similar findings have subsequently been documented.[9,10]

Patients with macroglobulinemia, some of whom are known to have cryoglobulin, occasionally manifest cochlear and vestibular disorders. Ronis et al[14] reported two patients whose symptoms were related mainly to the eighth nerve function; however, overall the incidence of involvement of the eighth nerve function is low. According to Logothetis et al,[15] of 182 macroglobulinemia patients with neurologic manifestation, 9 (5%) showed vestibular involvement and 7 (4%) suffered hearing loss.

Our patient had a 6-year history of gradually progressing bilateral hearing loss and dizziness. Based on her signs and symptoms, the hearing loss was thought to be due to cryoglobulinemia-induced circulatory disturbance of the inner ear.

The symptoms of cryoglobulinemia are explicable by the physicochemical properties of cryoglobulin. Although the mechanism by which cryoglobulin is formed has not yet been elucidated, the immunoglobulin responsible for cryoglobulin formation seems to be characterized by its conjugation under low temperature conditions. Blood viscosity is markedly increased by the presence of cryoglobulins. Meltzer and Franklin[16] reported a case in which the viscosity of the serum was 20 times that of normal serum.

When the extremities are exposed to cold, intravascular cryoglobulin precipitation occurs, leading to circulatory disturbance and eventually, to thrombus formation. Histamine and other vasoactive chemical mediators are released locally and they increase the permeability of the blood vessels. As a consequence, perivascular infiltration may result.

Alternatively, cryoglobulin formation may be the result of antigen-antibody reaction. In mixed type cryoglobulin, individual immunoglobulins do not produce a precipitate even under low-temperature conditions. However, upon admixing, precipitation occurs at low temperatures. This phenomenon is thought to be ascribable to antigen-antibody reaction rather than agglutination.

Mixed type cryoglobulin may combine with complement to produce an immune complex, as sug-

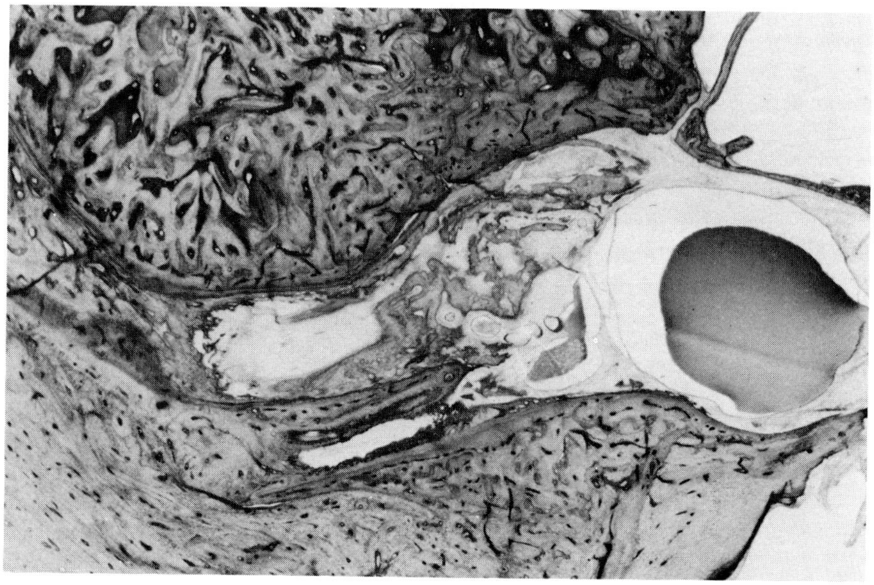

Fig. 6. Pathologic changes in the vestibule and lateral canal. Lateral canal is almost completely ossified. A mixture of fibrosis and new bone and eosinophilic precipitate are noted in the vestibule. The endolymphatic duct and paravestibular canaliculus seem normal.

gested by the finding that the level of complement in circulating blood decreases as tissue injury proceeds in patients with mixed type cryoglobulinemia.[16,17] There is some evidence supporting the hypothesis that the immune complex plays a role in producing the symptoms. For example, upon immunofluorescence study, immunoglobulin precipitates are noted on the vascular wall. The dermal and renal pathology in mixed type cryoglobulinemia is similar to that in serum sickness. These observations support the contention that antigen-antibody reaction is responsible for the development of the symptoms.

The inner ear may be involved in systemic vascular diseases. Periarteritis nodosa is a systemic disease which involves the small elastic arteries of particular organs. Involvement may also be widespread. Gussen[18] and Jenkins et al[19] reported involvement of the inner ear in periarteritis nodosa, although such involvement is rare.

Nomura and Kitamura[20] reported a case of pulseless disease with perforation of the nasal septum in which bilateral abrupt sensorineural hearing loss was observed. Their temporal bone study revealed a clear-cut separation of the normal organ of Corti toward the apex and the complete lack of hair cells in the basal turn. However, these workers were unable to histopathologically establish a causative relationship between the pulseless disease and the sensorineural hearing loss.

Not only diseases of the vascular walls, but also those of the blood and its constituents may produce changes in the inner ear. Hearing loss in the course of leukemia may be due to hemorrhage in the inner ear or to labyrinthitis.[5]

Different vascular experiments on the inner ear produced different types of pathology.[1-3] The major histopathological change brought about by the sudden blockage of the arterial supply was the disintegration of the organ of Corti within a few hours. Finally, fibrosis and ossification of the cochlear duct and the perilymphatic space resulted and the lesion spread toward the apex from the basal turn.

Gussen[6] reported a patient experiencing sudden deafness. Temporal bone study indicated that the deafness was of vascular origin. Pathologically, the cochlea, saccule and posterior ampulla were involved. These changes were consistent with vascular embarrassment of the temporal bone; in addition, the posterior vestibular artery was thought to be involved.

Belal[7] reported two cases of sudden deafness. The temporal bones, removed 1 and 12 years after the episode, showed fibrosis and new bone formation within the cochlea. Sacrifice of the internal auditory artery, either by middle fossa or translabyrinthine removal of the acoustic tumors, resulted in ossification of the cochlea. One of his patients manifested ossification of the entire cochlea one year after tumor removal.

Based on the distribution of the arterial supply to the inner ear in our patient, the ossified areas were supplied by the anterior and posterior vestibular artery and by the vestibulocochlear artery. The main cochlear artery may not have been occluded, because except for the lower basal turn, the cochlea showed neither fibrosis nor new bone formation in the perilymphatic space.

Under pathological conditions, the tectorial membrane of human temporal bones shows varying changes such as detachment, atrophy, fragmentation, and encapsulation. In endolymphatic viral labyrinthitis, the tectorial membrane is encapsulated on the limbus.[21-26] In Gussen's patient, the tectorial membrane was either depressed into the inner sulcus, fragmented or encapsulated on the limbus.[6]

Similarly, in our patient, one portion of the tectorial membrane drooped, and another was encapsulated. This suggests that the existing circulatory disturbance in the cochlea was also responsible for these changes of the tectorial membrane. Swelling of this membrane and its detachment from the spiral limbus was a unique finding in arterial obstruction experiments.

The absence of the stria vascularis is associated with a marked decrease in the endolymph volume of the pars inferior.[27] Despite atrophic stria vascularis, in our case, there was no evident decrease of endolymph in Reissner membrane. Rather, in some areas where the endolymph in the scala media showed eosinophilic staining, the membrane was bulged. The altered endolymph may have maintained a high osmotic pressure and, therefore, a high endolymph volume in the scala media.

Endolymph staining is occasionally found in patients with sensorineural hearing loss of unknown etiology, and increased protein concentrations result in eosinophilic staining.[27] The results of our study indicate that the eosinophilic endolymph in the scala media was brought about by a circulatory disturbance of the inner ear.

The endolymphatic duct and sac and the paravestibular canaliculus showed no lesions in our patient. Kimura and Perlman[1] also noted that the endolymphatic sac is not directly affected by arterial lesions.

Despite the complete loss of hair cells, the ganglion cell population in our patient was at an almost normal level. This observation contrasts with that made in acute arterial obstruction of the labyrinth in the latter case; the ganglion cells showed degeneration in an early stage of obstruction.[2] In profoundly deaf patients, Kerr and Schuknecht[28] found that the spiral ganglion cells were either fairly well preserved, even in the presence of severe atrophy of the organ of Corti, or markedly decreased. In one of their patients who suffered sudden, complete and permanent hearing loss, vascular occlusion was presumed as the etiological factor. There were a few ganglion cells at the basal end where the organ of Corti was completely missing.

REFERENCES

1. Kimura R, Perlman HB. Arterial obstruction of the labyrinth. Part I. Cochlear changes. Ann Otol Rhinol Laryngol 1958; 67:5-24.

2. Kimura R, Perlman HB. Arterial obstruction of the labyrinth. Part II. Vestibular changes. Ann Otol Rhinol Laryngol 1958; 67:25-40.

3. Perlman HB, Kimura R, Fernandez C. Experiments on temporary obstruction of the internal auditory artery. Laryngoscope 1959; 69:591-613.

4. Kimura R, Perlman HB. Extensive venous obstruction of the labyrinth. Ann Otol Rhinol Laryngol 1956; 65:332-50.

5. Schuknecht HF. Pathology of the ear. Cambridge: Harvard University Press, 1974.

6. Gussen R. Sudden deafness of vascular origin: a human temporal bone study. Ann Otol Rhinol Laryngol 1976; 85:94-100.

7. Belal A Jr. Pathology of vascular sensorineural hearing impairment. Laryngoscope 1980; 90:1831-9.

8. Barr DP, Reader GG, Wheeler CH. Cryoglobulinemia. I. Report of two cases with discussion of clinical manifestations, incidence and significance. Ann Intern Med 1950; 32:6-29.

9. Lucey HC, Leigh E, Hoch H, Marrack JR, Johns RGS. Study of a case of purpura associated with bone changes and formation of a gel in the serum on cooling. Br J Exp Pathol 1950; 31:380-9.

10. Huchinson JH, Howell RA. Cryoglobulinemia: report of a case associated with gangrene of the digits. Ann Intern Med 1953; 39:350-7.

11. Grey HM, Kohler PF. Cryoimmunoglobulins. Semin Hematol 1973; 10:87-112.

12. Barnett EV, Bluestone R, Cracciolo A, Goldberg LS, Kantor GL, McIntosh RM. Cryoglubulinemia and disease. Ann Intern Med 1970; 73:95-107.

13. Verroust P, Mery J-P, Morel-Maroger L, Clauvel J-P, Richet G. Glomerular lesions in monoclonal gammopathies and mixed essential cryoglobulinemias IgG-IgM. Advances in Nephrology. Year Book 1971; 161-94.

14. Ronis ML, Rojer CL, Ronis BJ. Otologic manifestations of Waldenström's macroglobulinemia. Laryngoscope 1966; 76: 513-23.

15. Logothetis J, Silverstein P, Coe J. Neurologic aspects of Waldenström's macroglobulinemia. Arch Neurol 1960; 3:564-73.

16. Meltzer M, Franklin EC. Cryoglobulinemia — a clinical and laboratory study. II. Cryoglobulins with rheumatoid factor activity. Am J Med 1966; 40:837-56.

17. Brouet J-C, Clauvel J-P, Danon F, Klein M, Seligmann M. Biological and clinical significance of cryoglobulins. A report of 86 cases. Am J Med 1974; 57:775-88.

18. Gussen R. Polyarteritis nodosa and deafness. A human temporal bone study. Arch Otorhinolaryngol (NY) 1977; 217: 263-71.

19. Jenkins HA, Pollak AM, Fisch U. Polyarteritis nodosa as a cause of sudden deafness. A human temporal bone study. Am J Otolaryngol 1981; 2:99-107.

20. Nomura Y, Kitamura K. Abrupt (sharp cut) type sensorineural hearing loss — a human temporal bone study. Auris Nasus Larynx (Tokyo) 1979; 6:13-21.

21. Lindsay J. Sudden deafness due to virus infection. Arch Otolaryngol 1959; 69:13-8.

22. Lindsay J, Hemenway W. Inner ear pathology due to measles. Ann Otol Rhinol Laryngol 1954; 63:754-71.

23. Lindsay J, Davey P, Ward P. Inner ear pathology in deafness due to mumps. Ann Otol Rhinol Laryngol 1960; 69:918-35.

24. Beal DB, Hemenway WG, Lindsay JR. Inner ear pathology of sudden deafness. Arch Otolaryngol 1967; 85:591-8.

25. Schuknecht HF, Kimura R, Naufal PM. The pathology of sudden deafness. Acta Otolaryngol (Stockh) 1973; 76:75-97.

26. Sando I, Harada T, Loehr A, Sobel JH. Sudden deafness: histopathologic correlation in temporal bone. Ann Otol Rhinol Laryngol 1977; 86:269-79.

27. Schuknecht HF, McNeill RA. Light microscopic observations on the pathology of endolymph. J Laryngol Otol 1966; 80: 1-10.

28. Kerr A, Schuknecht HF. The spiral ganglion in profound deafness. Acta Otolaryngol (Stockh) 1968; 65;586-98.

LONGITUDINAL STUDY OF THE EFFICACY OF AMPICILLIN IN THE TREATMENT OF PNEUMOCOCCAL OTITIS MEDIA IN A CHINCHILLA ANIMAL MODEL

JOHN S. SUPANCE, MD
PITTSBURGH, PENNSYLVANIA
WILLIAM J. DOYLE, PhD
PITTSBURGH, PENNSYLVANIA
GABRIEL MARSHAK, MD
REHOVOT, ISRAEL
ERDEM I. CANTEKIN, PhD
PITTSBURGH, PENNSYLVANIA

A chinchilla animal model was used to determine the effects of early antibiotic treatment with ampicillin on the local and systemic protective mechanisms during pneumococcal acute otitis media with effusion (AOME). The right bullae of 74 chinchillas were inoculated with 170 colony-forming units (CFU) of *Streptococcus pneumoniae* type 7F, and animals were randomly assigned to 1 of 2 groups: early (24 hours postinoculation) and late (12 days postinoculation) initiation of ampicillin treatment. During the first challenge, 52 chinchillas died within a 1-month period, apparently from suppurative complications of AOME. Following the resolution of AOME in their right ears, all surviving animals were challenged for the second time by bilateral bullar inoculations using 130 CFU of the same organism. All 10 animals in the early ampicillin treatment group developed severe bilateral AOME, whereas only 3 of the 12 animals in the late ampicillin treatment group developed a recurrence of AOME in the right ear. Significantly, 8 of the 12 animals in this group developed severe left AOME. These findings suggest the presence of a local middle ear defense system and support the results of previous similar studies in which *S pneumoniae* types 3 and 6A were used. The results of the present study also suggest that in the chinchilla the early administration of a systemic antibiotic (ampicillin) interferes with this defense mechanism.

INTRODUCTION

The advent of antimicrobial therapy has altered the natural course of acute otitis media with effusion (AOME) as manifested by an overall decline in the incidence of suppurative complications and an apparent increase in the persistence and recurrence of otitis media with effusion. The pathogenesis of recurrent AOME has been investigated recently from the immunologic point of view, using an animal model. Evidence for a local middle ear protection mechanism has been reported in two recent longitudinal studies of AOME which used the chinchilla animal model.[1,2] The design of each of these studies involved repeated inoculation of the middle ear with a specific pneumococcal serotype, type 3 or type 6A, followed by documentation of the middle ear status by various techniques. The results showed that, following the initial challenge, the ipsilateral middle ear was resistant to subsequent challenges with homologous organisms, but the contralateral, previously unchallenged, ear was not afforded protection. These findings suggested the presence of a local middle ear protection mechanism that is dependent on previous exposure to the same bacterium. Lewis et al[1] reported that the early administration of ampicillin rendered this local protection mechanism ineffective.

In order to complement and to verify the results reported by Lewis et al[1] we used a different pneumococcal serotype (type 7F), which is purported to be highly antigenic in the chinchilla,[3] to study the efficacy of ampicillin in the treatment of pneumococcal otitis media. The hypothesis of the present investigation was that early treatment with ampicillin of pneumococcal AOME may interfere with the necessary antigenic stimulation required to activate the local protection mechanism to prevent recurrent homologous infection.

MATERIALS AND METHODS

Seventy-four healthy 1- to 2-year-old chinchillas (*Chinchilla laniger*) culled from breeding stock because of defective fur and weighing 400 to 500 mg each were utilized in this study. The strain of *S pneumoniae* supplied was type 7F. Pneumococcal growth and preparation methods as described by Giebink et al[3-5] were followed. Virulence of the organisms was maintained by passage through the chinchilla. Aliquots of prepared stationary-phase bacteria were frozen in a glycerin buffered albumin suspension at −70° C. An aliquot of frozen pneumococcal suspension was thawed and diluted in sterile saline to the desired concentration of approximately 150 CFU immediately prior to each inoculation. The inoculation procedure, the assessment of middle ear status, the determination of pneumococcal antibody levels, and the methods used to culture middle ear specimens were reported previously.[2]

An overview of the present study design is depicted in Figure 1. The challenge 1 phase of the study, lasting 40 days, represents the period from the initial to the second inoculation. Prior to challenge 1, the condition of the middle ears of each animal was documented by tympanometry and otomicroscopy for two weeks. Seventy-four animals with documented normal middle ears bilaterally were challenged via transbullar inoculation of 170 CFU *S pneumoniae* type 7F into their right ears. Subsequent to inoculation, the animals were divided into two groups: group A (those treated early with antibiotics) and group B (those treated late

From the Department of Otolaryngology, University of Pittsburgh School of Medicine, and Children's Hospital of Pittsburgh. Supported in part by a grant from the National Institute of Neurological and Communicative Disorders and Stroke 1-PO1-NS-16337. Presented at the Meeting of the Association for Research in Otolaryngology, St. Petersburg Beach, Florida, January 19, 1981.

REPRINTS — John S. Supance, MD, Children's Hospital of Pittsburgh, 125 DeSoto Street, Pittsburgh, PA 15213.

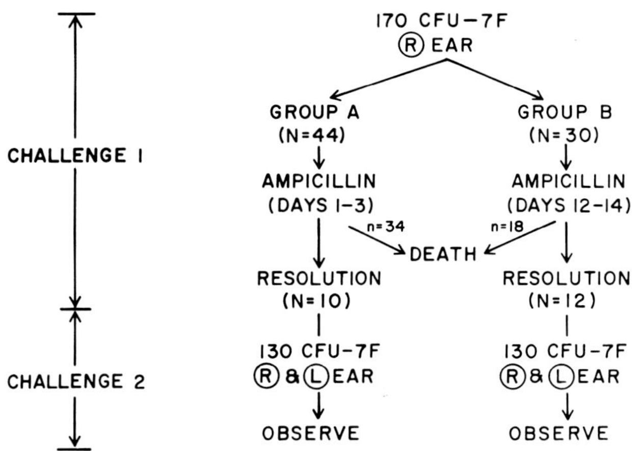

Fig. 1. Overall experimental design of the study in which chinchilla middle ears were challenged with *S pneumoniae* type 7F. The goal of the study was to determine how early and late administration of antibiotics would affect a hypothesized middle ear protection mechanism.

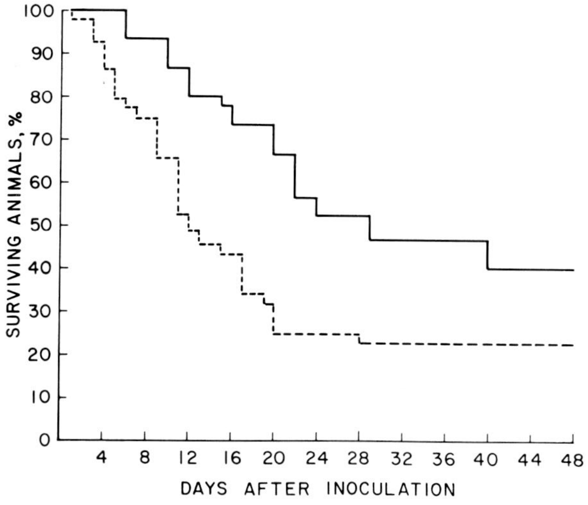

Fig. 2. Life-table analysis of chinchilla mortality in the course of AOME: a study of the effects of antibiotic treatment administered early (group A, N = 44, depicted by interrupted line) or late (group B, N = 30, depicted by solid line).

with antibiotics). Group A consisted of 44 animals; each animal received ampicillin, 50 mg/kg IM three times daily for three days, initiated 24 hours following inoculation. Group B consisted of 30 animals that received the same dose and duration of ampicillin therapy starting 12 days after inoculation. This dosage of ampicillin has been shown to maintain therapeutic serum levels in the chinchilla.[2] Two weeks following otomicroscopic and tympanometric confirmation of the resolution of the AOME of the right ears, the right and the left bullae of all surviving animals were inoculated with 130 CFU *S pneumoniae* type 7F (challenge 2).

Throughout the study, the condition of the middle ears was evaluated by tympanometry and otomicroscopy every other day. Tympanometry was done using the compliance mode of the electroacoustic impedance bridge because of the extreme hypercompliance of the tympanic membrane in the chinchilla. Flat tympanograms were used to document the presence of a middle ear effusion. This method was validated in a previous study.[2] Otomicroscopic diagnosis was considered to be positive when the observer reported hyperemia of the tympanic membrane, suggestive of impending infection, or when the tympanic membrane was noted to be opaque, bulging, or characterized by a fluid level, indicating obvious effusion. Each right middle ear was cultured directly through the bullar opening on days 1, 4, and 10 in challenge 1; both middle ears were similarly cultured on day 8 of challenge 2. Before each culture, direct inspection of the middle ear, using the microscope to determine the presence or absence of effusion, was performed through the bullar opening. Serum and middle ear effusion antibodies to the capsular polysaccharide type 7F *S pneumoniae* were measured by Schiffman using a radioimmunoassay technique[6]; the antibody concentrations were expressed in nanograms of pneumococcal antibody nitrogen per milliliter (ng Ab N/ml). Serum specimens were collected by percutaneous cardiac aspirations on the day of inoculation and 14 days postinoculation during challenges 1 and 2, as well as on the eighth day postinoculation during challenge 1. Middle ear effusion specimens were obtained from group B animals eight days after inoculation during challenges 1 and 2.

RESULTS

The mortality encountered during the challenge 1 phase of this study was unexpectedly high, as illustrated in the life-table analysis depicted in Figure 2. Overall, 52 of 74 animals (70%) died prior to challenge 2 due to sepsis or meningitis or both. During challenge 1, the overall mortality was different for the two groups; 34 of the 44 animals (77%) that received early antibiotic treatment (group A), and 18 of the 30 animals (60%) that received late antibiotic treatment (group B) died. Twenty-two animals (50%) in group A died within 12 days of the initial right bullar inoculation, whereas 50% mortality was observed 29 days after inoculation in group B animals.

The discrepancy in the incidence of disease and rate of mortality between the two groups was unexpected and remains unexplained. However, similar findings were encountered in the chinchilla model of AOME secondary to *S pneumoniae* type 6A.[2] In order to rule out the possibility that morbidity could be due to the antibiotic treatment alone, the toxicity of ampicillin was studied in a group of ten chinchillas which were not involved in the pneumococcal experiments. Each animal received ampicillin, 50 mg/kg IM three times daily for three days. Animals were weighed on a daily basis and the group was observed for ten days. There was no mortality and no weight loss during this observation period, suggesting that the mortality observed in the pneumococcal experiments was not due to the ampicillin therapy.

The findings of the study are summarized in Table 1 with respect to four independent methods of middle ear assessment (tympanometry, otomicroscopy, bullar inspection, and middle ear culture). In group A surviving animals during challenge 1, the incidence of right AOME approached 30% and was noted within 3 to 9 days after inoculation, with resolution of the effusion within 9 to 15 days. The overall incidence of AOME in group B animals was higher than the incidence observed in group A animals. In group B, 9 of the 12 surviving animals had

TABLE 1. INCIDENCE OF ACUTE OTITIS MEDIA WITH EFFUSION IN CHINCHILLAS AS DIAGNOSED BY FOUR INDEPENDENT METHODS DURING TWO CHALLENGES OF MIDDLE EAR WITH *S PNEUMONIAE* TYPE 7F

			Challenge 1				*Challenge 2*							
			Right Ear				*Right Ear*				*Left Ear*			
		N	*T*	*O*	*I*	*C**	*T*	*O*	*I*	*C*	*T*	*O*	*I*	*C*
Group A (Early antibiotics)	S	10	3	3	3	4	10	10	10	10	10	10	10	10
	NS	34	7	12	6	7	—	—	—	—	—	—	—	—
Group B (Late antibiotics)	S	12	9	10	10	8	3	2	2	5	8	7	5	8
	NS	18	16	17	16	14	—	—	—	—	—	—	—	—

*Culture findings with *S pneumoniae* growth are reported as positive diagnosis.

T - Tympanometry; O - Otomicroscopy; I - Bullar inspection; C - Middle ear culture; S - Animals surviving challenge 1; NS - Animals not surviving challenge 1.

developed right AOME as documented by tympanometry within two to six days after inoculation. In this group the resolution of the disease was observed within 16 to 29 days after inoculation. Overall, the early antibiotic treatment animals (group A) had a lower incidence of AOME and shorter duration than did the animals that received late antibiotic treatment (group B). Five animals in group B had bilateral AOME. The onset of AOME was delayed in the left ear in comparison to the onset of the disease in the right ear. Of these animals, only one survived and was subsequently entered into the second phase of the study (challenge 2). In group A, only one animal developed bilateral AOME and this animal died 19 days after inoculation.

Due to the high mortality rate encountered over the course of challenge 1, only 22 animals were available for challenge 2. Following bilateral transbullar inoculations with 130 CFU *S pneumoniae* type 7F, all animals (N = 10) in group A developed bilateral AOME within two to six days. However, of the 12 surviving animals in group B, only 3 developed bilateral AOME and an additional 5 animals developed AOME only in the left ears according to tympanometric and middle ear culture findings. The onset of AOME occurred within four to ten days after the inoculation. In group B animals, only 3 of the 12 previously challenged right middle ears (25%) had AOME, whereas 8 of the 12 previously unchallenged left ears (66.7%) had AOME during challenge 2.

Table 2 shows the serum antibody concentrations of *S pneumoniae* type 7F. At the beginning of the study, the serum antibody levels for all animals (N = 74) were determined; however, only the levels for the surviving animals are presented and will be discussed. At the beginning of challenge 1, all ten animals in group A had detectable serum antibody levels (5-58 ng AB N/ml). Fourteen days following inoculation, only two animals evidenced an appreciable rise in these levels. Similarly, all 12 animals in group B had detectable serum antibodies to 7F (3-202 ng Ab N/ml). However, by day 14, five of these animals had considerable increases in serum antibody levels.

At the start of challenge 2, two animals in group A had detectable serum antibody levels (8 and 104 ng Ab N/ml); the remaining eight animals evidenced zero concentration values (below the sensitivity of the radioimmunoassay technique) on the day of the second inoculation. By day 14 of this challenge, five animals in group A had elevated serum antibody levels. Three animals in group B had elevated serum antibody concentrations on the day of the second inoculation and five animals had zero concentration values. By day 14, the same three animals still had elevated serum antibody concentrations.

Eight days after inoculation during challenges 1 and 2, attempts were made to determine middle ear effusion antibody concentrations of *S pneumoniae* type 7F in group B animals. Of the 12 survivors, 4 had detectable 7F antibody levels of 6, 6, 9, and 24 ng Ab N/ml for the specimens obtained during challenge 1, and insignificant antibody levels (0-5 ng Ab N/ml) were measured in the five middle ear effusion specimens obtained during challenge 2.

TABLE 2. SERUM ANTIBODY CONCENTRATIONS* OF *S PNEUMONIAE* TYPE 7F DURING TWO CHALLENGES OF THE MIDDLE EARS OF SURVIVORS

	Challenge 1			*Challenge 2*	
	Day 0	*Day 8*	*Day 14*	*Day 0*	*Day 14*
	32	22	26	0	—
	58	21	17	0	—
	4	6	6	0	63
Group A	17	18	20	0	42
(n = 10)	7	141	692	104	55
(early	12	—	0	0	—
antibiotics)	8	—	8	8	151
	8	—	0	0	0
	6	—	0	0	—
	5	—	58	0	58
	38	277	496	56	3
	202	344	363	63	60
	14	20	573	670	293
	9	123	491	99	248
Group B	39	87	—	379	550
(n = 12)	10	9	22	16	2
(late	23	13	20	9	21
antibiotics)	5	10	8	0	—
	6	9	8	0	—
	6	7	8	0	—
	3	7	8	0	—
	22	11	16	0	—

*Concentrations are in nanograms of pneumococcal antibody nitrogen per milliliter (ng Ab N/ml).

DISCUSSION

The present study was designed as a longitudinal study of the influence of systemic ampicillin on middle ear protection in pneumococcal-induced AOME in the chinchilla. Lewis et al[1] and Marshak et al[2] have demonstrated the importance of a local protection mechanism in the chinchilla middle ear and have postulated that the lack of sufficient antigenic stimulation, resulting from the early administration of antibiotics, may deprive the middle ear of the necesary local antigenic stimulation required for the acquisition of this protective response.

In the present study, *S pneumoniae* type 7F was chosen as the pathogen because past studies have shown it to be highly immunogenic in the chinchilla.[3,5]

As designed, the present study is bounded by two experimental parameters: the duration of exposure to the live pathogen, and the type of protection afforded the middle ear: local (middle ear-induced) or systemic, or both. Ampicillin administered 24 hours following transbullar inoculation (group A) shortened the duration of exposure to the pathogenic bacteria when compared to group B animals. Rapid sterilization of the middle ear cleft of group A animals resulted in either no AOME or a milder and more abbreviated course of the disease. However, on subsequent homologous challenges, these ears developed AOME congruent with that reported for previously unchallenged ears. In contrast, group B animals which received delayed antibiotic therapy developed a protracted AOME on the initial challenge, but with a subsequent homologous challenge, the incidence of AOME was significantly reduced in the previously challenged ears.

The results for group B animals are similar to those previously reported by Marshak et al[2] and suggest that prolonged exposure to a pathogenic organism produces local protection to a second challenge. Little to no protection is afforded to the contralateral middle ear. The results for group A animals show that protection does not develop if the middle ear cleft is rapidly sterilized by early antibiotic therapy.

The mechanism of this protection is not known but data provided on the concentration of serum and middle ear antibodies do not support an antibody-mediated protection. Giebink[3,5] found mean concentrations of antibody to the capsular polysaccharide of *S pneumoniae* type 7F in serum of chinchillas before vaccination with homologous organisms to vary between 2.5 and 25.3 ng Ab N/ml, which approximates the baseline levels measured at the onset of the present study. Chinchillas systemically vaccinated with *S pneumoniae* 7F and with elevated levels of serum 7F antibody (ie, that seroconverted) had a significantly lower incidence of middle ear infection following nasal colonization than those that failed to seroconvert.[3] Analysis of the data from the animals in group B in challenge 2 shows that of the 5 animals that demonstrated an appreciable increase in serum antibody levels by day 14 in challenge 1, none developed right AOME while 2 had left AOME in challenge 2. However, of the remaining 7 animals that failed to show an increase in serum antibody levels, only 3 developed right AOME and 6 evidenced left ear disease. Of the 10 survivors in group A, 2 had evidence of a large increase in serum antibody levels in challenge 1, yet all animals in challenge 2 had overwhelming bilateral ear disease. Thus, this study does not substantiate the hypothesis that serum antibodies to *S pneumoniae* type 7F play a dominant role in the protection of the middle ear from infection. Furthermore, the levels of antibody detected in the middle ear effusions of group B animals during challenges 1 and 2 were quite low, and differ from previously reported findings.[3]

In summary, this study of AOME *in the chinchilla* showed that:

1. 170 CFU *S pneumoniae* type 7F induced AOME is associated with high mortality (approximately 70%).
2. A local middle ear defense system has been demonstrated supporting previous findings with *S pneumoniae* type 3 and type 6A.
3. Early administration of ampicillin may alter this local middle ear defense system.
4. A weaker systemic defense response is suggested.
5. This study supports the hypothesis that in the chinchilla the early administration of ampicillin (which is one of the current drugs of choice for AOME in humans) may interfere with the local defense system of the middle ear, rendering the host more susceptible to subsequent infections.

ACKNOWLEDGMENTS — The authors are indebted to Gerald Schiffman, PhD, Department of Microbiology and Immunology, SUNY Medical Center, Brooklyn, New York, for performing radioimmunoassays and for supplying the *S pneumoniae* type 7F; to Dale Rohn and Randy Boyles for technical assistance; to William G. Doyle for his supply of chinchillas; and to Suzanne Stewart and Sandra Arjona, who assisted in the preparation of this manuscript.

REFERENCES

1. Lewis DM, Schram BS, Meadema SJ, Lim DJ. Experimental otitis media in the chinchilla. Ann Otol Rhinol Laryngol 1980; 89 Suppl 68:344-50.

2. Marshak G, Cantekin EI, Doyle WJ, Schiffman G, Rohn DD, Boyles R. Recurrent pneumococcal otitis media in the chinchilla: a longitudinal study. Arch Otolaryngol 1981; 107:532-9.

3. Giebink GS, Berzins IK, Schiffman G, Quie PG. Experimental otitis media in chinchillas following nasal colonization with type 7F *Streptococcus pneumoniae:* prevention after vaccination with pneumococcal capsular polysaccharide. J Infect Dis 1979; 140:716-23.

4. Giebink GS, Payne EE, Mills EL, Juhn SK, Quie PG. Ex-

perimental otitis media due to *Streptococcus pneumoniae:* immunopathogenic response in the chinchilla. J Infect Dis 1976; 134:595-604.

5. Giebink GS, Schiffman G, Petty K, Quie PG. Modification of otitis media following vaccination with the capsular polysaccharide of *Streptococcus pneumoniae* in chinchillas. J Infect Dis 1978; 138:480-7.

6. Schiffman G, Douglas RM, Bouner MJ, Robbins M, Austrian RA. A radioimmunoassay for the study of immunologic antibody response to pneumococcal vaccines. I. Method for the radioimmunoassay of anticapsular antibodies and a comparison with other techniques. J Immunol Methods 1980; 33:133-44.

≈

NINCDS NOTES*

CONFERENCE PROCEEDINGS IDENTIFIES VOCAL PATHOLOGY ASSESSMENT TECHNIQUES

A report, *Proceedings of the Conference on the Assessment of Vocal Pathology*, edited by NINCDS staff members Christy L. Ludlow, PhD, and Molly O. Hart, MS, stresses the need for objective, reliable and valid procedures for assessing voice disorders. Procedures that improve the transfer of patient data between clinics, between investigators, and during treatment evaluation are emphasized. The conference, which attempted to bridge the gap between laboratory and clinical needs in vocal pathology, was organized by the NINCDS Communicative Disorders Program and held at the National Institutes of Health in April 1979. The proceedings (ASHA Report No. 11) are available from the American Speech-Language-Hearing Association, 10801 Rockville Pike, Rockville, MD 20852.

SHINGLES PAMPHLET

Shingles, a virus infection that begins in the sensory neurons and affects the nervous system, is the subject of a new pamphlet published by NINCDS. *Shingles: Hope through Research* explores the origins and consequences of a disorder in which individuals with weakened immune systems are attacked by varicella zoster. The pamphlet describes the symptoms of shingles — including a painful rash and possible eye damage — and the medications being tested against the condition. The effects of shingles during pregnancy are also discussed, along with prospects for prevention of the illness. Copies of this pamphlet can be obtained from the Office of Scientific and Health Reports, NINCDS, Building 31, Room 8A06, 9000 Rockville Pike, Bethesda, MD 20205; (301) 496-5751.

TEACHER INVESTIGATOR, RESEARCH CAREER DEVELOPMENT AWARDS

Following the January 1982 meeting of the National Advisory Neurological and Communicative Disorders and Stroke Council, NINCDS made seven new Teacher Investigator Development Awards and four Research Career Development Awards. The deadlines for receiving applications for RCDAs and TIDAs are October 1, February 1, and June 1 of each year. Additional information on these training awards can be obtained from Dr. John W. Diggs, Deputy Director, Extramural Activities Program, NINCDS, NIH, Bethesda, MD 20205; (301) 496-4188.

RESEARCH TRAINING FOR MINORITIES

The National Institute of Neurological and Communicative Disorders and Stroke continues to offer research and research-training opportunities to minority scientists and institutions through several cooperative National Institutes of Health programs. To increase minority participation in the basic and clinical neurosciencies, the NINCDS will make awards to qualifying individuals and institutions through NIH's Minority Biomedical Support (MBS) and Minority Access to Research Career (MARC) programs. Further information on the requirements of the MBS and MARC programs can be obtained from Mr. Levon O. Parker, Equal Opportunity Officer, NINCDS/NIH, Building 31, Room 8A22, 9000 Rockville Pike, Bethesda, MD 20205; (301) 496-5332.

NEUROLOGICAL DISORDERS PROGRAM PUBLICATION

NINCDS Neurological Disorders Program activities during fiscal year 1981 have been summarized for the neuroscience community in a new publication. The 100-page *Fiscal Year 1981 Neurological Disorders Program* report provides a detailed overview of the program's recent biomedical research efforts, involving the awarding of over $78 million for research grants, research training and contracts. The publication outlines NDP's organization, budget, operation and accomplishments from October 1, 1980, to September 30, 1981. The report covers the current state of NINCDS-supported extramural research in such areas as convulsive, demyelinating and sclerosing infectious and neuromuscular disorders, as well as diseases of early life and aging. Significant advances in research are also reported. Single copies of the publication are available on request from the Neurological Disorders Program, Federal Building, Room 714, Bethesda, MD 20205; (301) 496-5679.

CT CONSENSUS STATEMENT

Single, free copies of the National Institutes of Health *Consensus Development Statement on Computed Tomographic Scanning of the Brain* are now available. The report is a product of a consensus development conference sponsored by the NINCDS in November 1981. To obtain the report, contact Michael J. Bernstein, Director of Communications, Office for Medical Applications of Research, Building 1, Room 214, NIH, Bethesda, MD 20205.

*This information is prepared monthly by the Office of Scientific and Health Reports, National Institute of Neurological and Communicative Disorders and Stroke, National Institutes of Health, Building 31, Room 8A06, Bethesda, MD 20205; (301) 496-5751.

Ann Otol Rhinol Laryngol 91:1982

OCCURRENCE OF ADDITIONAL PRIMARY NEOPLASMS IN PATIENTS WITH LARYNGEAL CARCINOMA IN ISRAEL (1960-1976)

EHUD DEVIRI, MD
ISAAC ELIACHAR, MD
ARIE BARTAL, MD
RUTH STEINITZ, MD
MOSHE GOLDSHER, MD, MSc
ELIEZER ROBINSON, MD
HAIFA, ISRAEL

One thousand-six-hundred and sixty cases of laryngeal cancer were diagnosed in Israel during the years 1960-1976. In 98 of these cases another primary cancer accompanied the laryngeal carcinoma. Patients whose second primary cancer was basal or squamous cell carcinoma of the skin were not included in this study. Therefore, the results reported here deal with 84 patients. The prevalence of multiple primary cancer in patients with laryngeal carcinoma was found to be 5%. Lung cancer is the other primary tumor accompanying laryngeal carcinoma most frequently (29% of the additional tumors) followed by colorectal and bladder cancers. Most of the additional tumors (83%) appeared in a metachronic form with an average time interval of six years. In most metachronic tumors laryngeal carcinoma appeared as the first tumor (86%). Eighty percent of the patients were dead by August 1978. The majority (74%) succumbed due to the additional tumor and only 4% died of laryngeal carcinoma.

INTRODUCTION

The interest in multiple primary cancer (MPC) has been increasing since the first patients were described by Billroth.[1] It is a well-established fact that patients who were cured of their initial malignant disease or who have a controlled tumor have a higher likelihood of developing a second neoplasm than the normal population. This possibility ranges between 1-34%.[2-9]

Laryngeal carcinoma is a relatively curable disease by surgery, radiation, or both. Patients develop additional primary tumors simultaneously or metachronously at a rate of 4-5%.[10,11] Few nationwide studies concerning the incidence of MPC associated with laryngeal cancer have been reported. The understanding of tumor associations and time, type, and patient relationship may cast further light on the etiology and pathogenesis of solitary and multiple neoplastic processes.

The Israeli population is composed of various ethnic groups from many countries. Most solid tumors and chronic lymphatic leukemias have been reported to occur more frequently in European-born Jews than Asian- and African-born Jews.[12-15] Laryngeal cancer, however, is known to occur more often in Asian- and African-born Jews than European-born patients.[12]

The purpose of this study was to investigate the incidence of additional primary tumors associated with laryngeal cancer, the tumor-to-tumor association, and the tumors' time relationship during a period of 16 years in Israel. This work is carried out in collaboration with the cancer registry of the Ministry of Health, as all cancers diagnosed in Israel are supposed to be reported to this Center.

METHODS

One thousand-six-hundred and sixty patients with laryngeal carcinoma were reported to the Israel Cancer Registry during the years 1960-1976. Of 98 patients who were registered to have additional primary cancer, 14 patients with basal cell and squamous cell carcinoma of the skin were excluded because this tumor type is not fully reported to the Cancer Registry. The remaining 84 patients entered the study.

The data accumulated at the Israel Cancer Registry in Jerusalem and clinical charts of the hospital medical archives and/or oncology clinics were reviewed. Complete information on the patients including the year of birth (from which age at time of diagnosis is calculated), sex, country of origin, time interval between the tumors, histology, stage, treatment, and day of death were checked. The latter was confirmed in the Israel population registry as corrected up to August 1978. Ethnic groups were divided into: 1) Jews born in Europe, 2) Jews born in Asia or Africa, 3) Israel-born Jews, 4) non-Jews born in Israel.

The criteria used for the diagnosis of further primary tumors were those of Warren and Gates.[16] Tumors appearing during a time interval of less than six months were considered as metachronous tumors.

Comparison of age and survival distribution in the various groups was done by the Student's t test. The sequence of appearance of the additional tumors in relation to the laryngeal carcinoma was computed by the Chi-square $(X)^2$ statistic.

RESULTS

This study has shown that prevalence of MPC among laryngeal carcinoma patients in Israel between 1960-1976 was 5% (84 of 1,660 patients). Sixty-three of the patients (75%) were Jews of European origin, mainly from Poland and Rumania. Sixteen were of Asian and African origin, and the others were Israel-born Jews (2 patients) or non-Jews (3 patients) (Fig. 1).

From the Department of Otolaryngology and the Northern Israel Oncology Center, Rambam Medical Centers and the Faculty of Medicine, Technion-Israel Institute of Technology, Haifa; and the Israel Center for Registration of Cancer and Allied Diseases, Jerusalem.

REPRINTS — Moshe Goldsher, MD, Department of Otolaryngology, Rambam Medical Center, Israel Institute of Technology, Haifa, Bat-Galim, Israel.

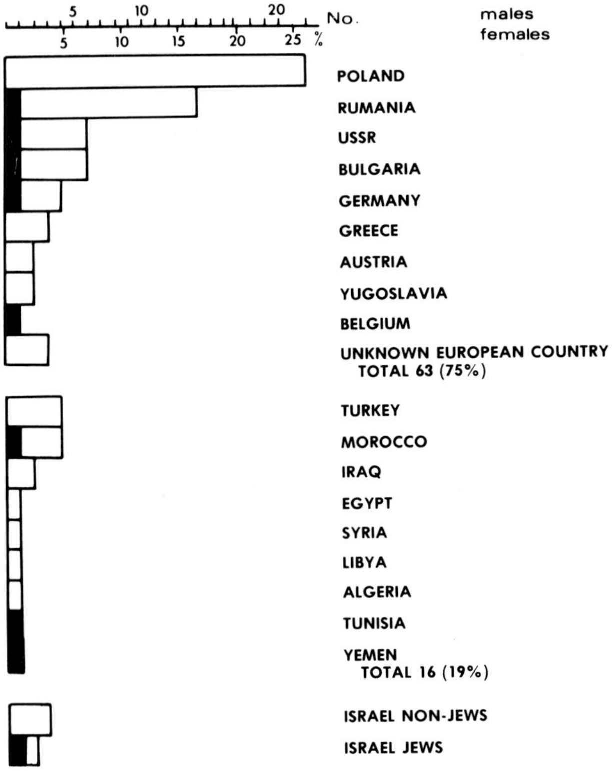

Fig. 1. Distribution of patients according to ethnic groups.

The male-to-female ratio among the patients was 8:1. The mean age of diagnosis of the first tumor (which in most of the cases was laryngeal carcinoma) was 61 years (median 62, range 33-92 years) (Fig. 2). There are no significant differences in distribution of age between males and females, or among the various ethnic groups ($p>0.05$). The mean age of diagnosis of the second primary cancer was 66.5 years (median 65.5, range 36-96 years) with no significant differences among sexes or ethnic groups.

The 84 patients had 86 additional primary tumors (Table 1). Two patients (2.4%) had three primary neoplasms each (clinical data are summarized in Table 2). The most frequent additional tumors were: lung 29%, colorectal 16% and bladder 9% (Table 1). In 14 patients (17%) the tumors appeared synchronously (Fig. 3). The types of tumors appearing synchronously are shown in Table 1. In 3 of 7 patients, laryngeal and stomach tumors appeared synchronously, but due to the small number of patients no statistical evaluation could be performed.

Among the metachronous tumors laryngeal carcinoma appeared as the first tumor in 60 patients (86%). The mean time interval between diagnosis of the tumors was 5.5 years (median 5 years, range 6 months-12 years (Fig. 3). Metachronous colorectal tumors appeared at a significantly higher rate before laryngeal cancer than other additional tumors ($p<0.05$) (Table 1).

The mean survival time following diagnosis of the additional tumor was 2 years (range 21 years, median 1 year). The 5-year survival of patients who subsequently developed lung carcinoma was 8% (mean lifetime 6 months, range up to 10 years). The 5-year survival of patients with an additional colorectal cancer was found to be 43% (age range to 81 years).

Eleven patients (13%) were alive in August 1978. Sex, age at diagnosis of the tumors, and ethnic distribution were not significantly different in the surviving patients than in those who died. Of the 54 patients whose cause of death is known, 40 (74%) died because of the additional tumor and only 2 patients (4%) died because of laryngeal carcinoma.

DISCUSSION

The occurrence of MPC in patients with laryn-

TABLE 1. DISTRIBUTION OF ADDITIONAL TUMORS ACCORDING TO SEX, ANATOMIC SITE AND SEQUENCE OF APPEARANCE

Site	Male No.	Male %	Female No.	Female %	Total No.	Total %	Metachronous Laryngeal Tumors First (No.)	Second (No.)	Total No.	Synchronous Tumors No.
Lung	23	29.8	2	22.2	25	29.0	21	2	23	2
Colon-rectum	13	16.9	1	11.1	14	16.2	9	5	14	
Urinary bladder	8	10.4			8	9.3	7		7	1
Stomach	5	6.5	2	22.2	7	8.1	4		4	3
Head and neck	5	6.5			5	8.8	2	2	4	1
Esophagus	4	5.2			4	4.7	4		4	
Prostate	4	5.2			4	4.7	3		3	1
Breast and ovary	1	1.3	3	33.3	4	4.7	4		4	
Leukemia	3	3.9			3	3.5	2		2	1
Lymphoma	2	2.6			2	2.3	—	2	2	
Thyroid	1	1.3	1	11.1	2	2.3			—	2
Melanoma	1	1.3			1	1.2	—		—	1
Kidney	1	1.3			1	1.2	1		1	
Chest wall	1	1.3			1	1.2	1		1	
Origin unknown	5	6.5			5	3.8	3		3	2
Total	77	100.0	9	99.9	86	100.0	61	11	72	14

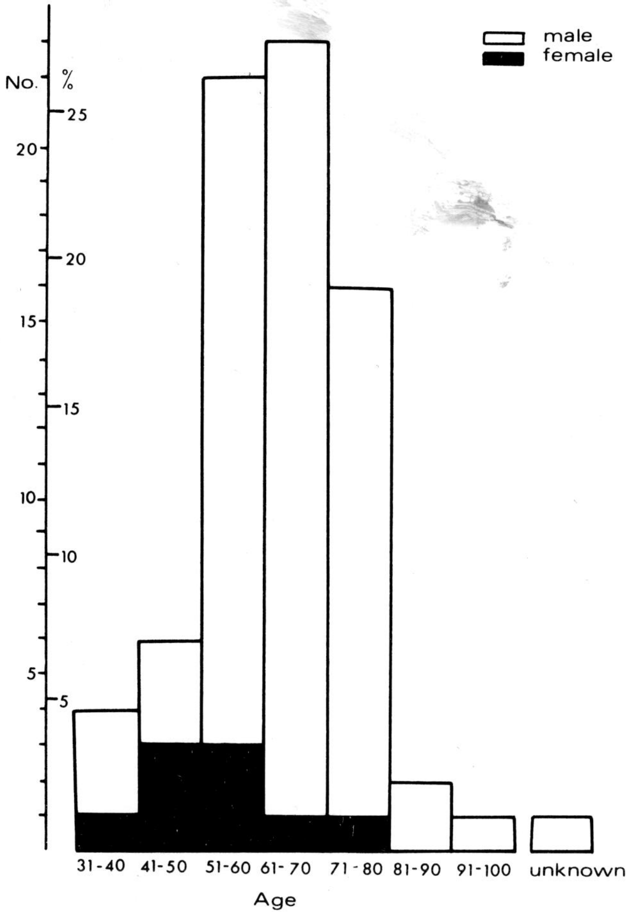

Fig. 2. Distribution of patients according to sex and age at diagnosis of first tumor.

geal carcinoma was found to be 5%. The occurrence of an additional malignant tumor in cancer patients has been reported to be 1-34%.[2,9] According to Ballantine[11] additional primary cancers appear in 5% of laryngeal carcinoma patients. Brown[10] found that 3.8% of laryngeal carcinoma patients subsequently developed another primary neoplasm; when excluding skin cancers, this rate dropped to 2.8% (lower than the rate found by us of 4.4%). The male to female ratio in our study was 8:1 (75 males vs 7 females) as compared to that reported by Brown of 59:2.[10]

In Israel cancer is more frequent among Jews of European origin than in those of Asian and African origin.[12-15] One of the exceptions is laryngeal cancer which is more frequent among Jewish males of Asian and African origin than among those of European origin (annual incidence of 6.1:100,000 vs 4.2:100,000 respectively.[12] The incidence of MPC, including laryngeal cancer, is higher among males of European origin than among those of Asian or African origin (0.4:100,000 vs 0.2:100,000) ($p < 0.05$). This is an important observation. Maybe the reason is that as the incidence of most malignant neoplasia is higher in patients born in Europe, the tendency to develop a second primary tumor is also higher in this group.

In Israel, among chronic lymphatic leukemia patients, a 12.5% rate of MPC was found. Most of the patients are of European origin.[13] A different incidence of MPC among various ethnic groups living in New Mexico was reported by Bordin et al[17] who found 4% of MPC among Anglo-Saxons compared to 2.4% in the Spanish and 1% in the Indian populations.

Despite the fact that head and neck tumors tend to be multicentric[2,7,11] we found that 60% of the additional tumors (excluding skin carcinomas) appeared in organs other than the head and neck, respiratory or upper digestive systems.

Schottenfeld et al[6] reported 518 additional primaries developed in 9,415 patients with cancer of the respiratory system and upper digestive tract. Seventy-five percent had additional tumors in the respiratory and upper digestive system, 20% had skin cancers, and 7% only had neoplasms somewhere else. Brown[10] reported 65 additional tumors appeared in 1,600 laryngeal carcinoma patients (4%). Excluding tumors of the skin there remained 48 additional tumors of which 75% were in the head and neck, respiratory, and upper digestive system and only 25% were elsewhere.

Fig. 3. Time interval between diagnosis of laryngeal carcinoma and additional primary tumor.

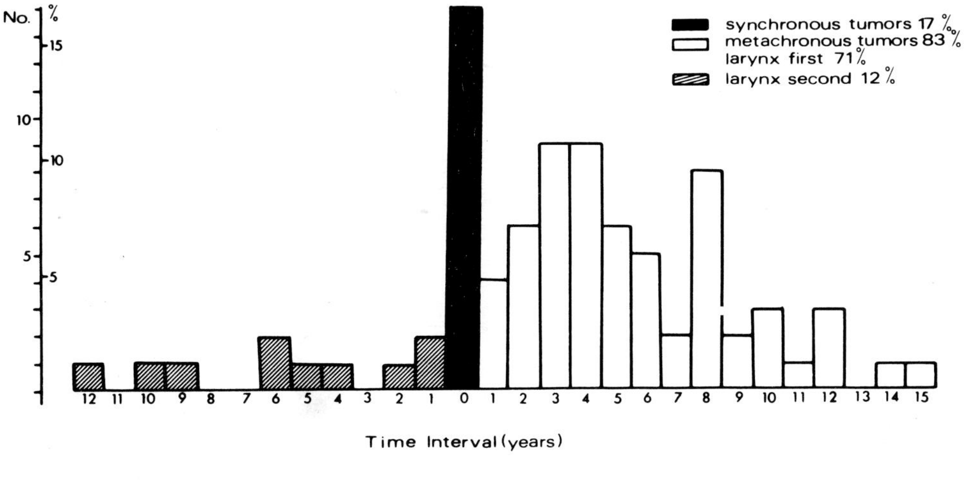

TABLE 2. PATIENTS WITH THREE PRIMARY MALIGNANT TUMORS EACH

Sex	Patient 1 — Male	Patient 2 — Male
Age laryngeal carcinoma diagnosed	56	47
Age additional tumor 1 diagnosed	58	38
Age additional tumor 2 diagnosed	81	59
Country of origin	Yugoslavia	Unknown European country
History of smoking	Present	Unknown
Other diseases	Emphysema and chronic bronchitis	Basal cell carcinoma of the skin
Sequence of laryngeal carcinoma	First	Second
Stage of laryngeal carcinoma	Unknown	II
Region of laryngeal carcinoma	Unknown	Vocal cords
Treatment of laryngeal carcinoma	Radiation	Radiation
Site of additional tumor 1	Prostate	Colon
Histology of additional tumor 1	Adenocarcinoma	Unknown
Treatment of additional tumor 1	Resection	Resection and radiation
Metastases from additional tumor 1	None	None
Site of additional tumor 2	Lung	Rectum
Histology of additional tumor 2	Squamous cell carcinoma	Adenocarcinoma
Treatment of additional tumor 2	Unknown	Not treated
Metastases from additional tumor 2	Liver lymph nodes adrenal	Unknown
Age at death	81	59
Cause of death	Lung cancer	Unknown

Look[18] showed that the only tumor appearing at a significantly higher rate after larynx carcinoma is lung cancer. Berg et al[5] found that the frequency of lung, pancreas, and colorectal cancers was significantly higher after diagnosis of larynx carcinoma.

The appearance of lung and laryngeal cancer in the same patient was first reported by Schall and Jesberg,[19] followed by many others.[5,20-28] According to Ferlitto[20] 10-15% of laryngeal carcinoma patients are predisposed to develop lung cancer. Two of 25 patients with lung carcinoma associated with laryngeal carcinoma appeared synchronously in other reports; 16-83% of laryngeal and lung carcinoma in the same patient appeared synchronously.

Gluckman reports an incidence of 9.2% synchronous second primaries in the upper digestive and respiratory systems.[29] Brown[10] found that 13% of the additional primary tumors associated with laryngeal cancer appeared synchronously. In the present study we found a rate of 17%.

In 86% of the metachronous tumors, laryngeal carcinoma was diagnosed first, possibly due to the fact that life expectancy after the treatment of laryngeal carcinoma is longer than that of most other tumors.

Campbell and Wante[4] and Moertel[30,31] found a higher frequency of a third primary neoplasm in patients with two primary tumors than in patients with one additional primary tumor. This is prominent in head and neck cancers. Cahan et al[32] reported that 30% of patients with MPC in the head and neck region had over three primary tumors. Odette et al[33] found the rate of 17%. In contrast, Brown[10] found the rate 3% of laryngeal carcinoma patients with MPC to be not higher than the frequency of an additional primary tumor in laryngeal carcinoma patients. In this study the frequency of a third tumor in patients with laryngeal carcinoma and associated with another primary tumor patient was found to be 2.4%.

Multiple primary malignancies in the upper aerodigestive tracts are explained by the diffuse effect of carcinogens on wide areas of the mucosa. Smoking and alcohol singularly[34] or in combination,[35] when applied extensively though not equally onto the epithelial tissues, are bound to bring about focal malignant changes surrounded by multiple additional cancerous foci or areas with premalignancy. This pathogenic process is best termed "field of cancerization" or "condemned mucosa syndrome."[36] Multiple multicentric neoplasms must therefore be anticipated throughout the epithelium likewise exposed to carcinogenic agents, following the diagnosis of one primary tumor. Due to lack of appropriate data we could not define the connection of carcinogens with the multiple tumors in our patients.

The recognition of the potential development of multifocal or multiple primary malignant lesions in the aerodigestive tract has led to improved close follow-up of patients with primary tumors in these organs.[37,38] It is accepted today that the complete evaluation of every such patient should include panendoscopy, including laryngoscopy, pharyngoscopy, nasopharyngoscopy, bronchoscopy and esophagoscopy with thorough examination of the oral and nasal mucosa.[30]

REFERENCES

1. Billroth T. Chirurgische Klinik: Wein 1871-1876: BEBST Ein gesammt Bericht veber die chirurgischen Kliniken in Zuerich und Wein waehrend der Jahre 1870-1876. Erfahrungen auf dem Gebiete der praktischen Chirurgie. Berlin: A. Hirschwald, 1879: 258.

2. Harrison LH, Nordon JM, Resnick MI, Myers RT. Metachronous quadruple malignant neoplasms: a case report and review of the literature. NC Med J 1976; 35:241-5.

3. Cleary JB, Kazarian KK, Mershimer WL. Multiple primary cancer. Am J Surg 1975; 686-90.

4. Campbell LU, Wante AL. Multiple primary malignant neoplasms. Arch Surg 1969; 99:401-5.

5. Berg JW, Schottenfeld D, Ritter F. Incidence of multiple primary cancer II. Cancer of the respiratory and upper digestive system as multiple primary causes. J Natl Cancer Inst 1970; 263-74.

6. Schottenfeld D, Gantt RC, Wynder EL. The role of alcohol and tobacco in multiple primary cancers of the upper digestive system, larynx and lung. Prev Med 1974; 3:277-93.

7. Wynder EL, Dodo U, Bloch BM, Gnatt RC, Moore OS. Epidemiologic investigation of multiple primary cancer of the upper alimentary and respiratory tracts. Cancer 1969; 24:730-9.

8. Baker HW. The natural history of head and neck cancer and its conventional therapy. Laryngoscope 1978; 88 Suppl 8:64-5.

9. Hyman GA. Increased incidence of neoplasm in association with chronic lymphatic leukemia. Scand J Haematol 1969; 6:99-104.

10. Brown M. Second primaries in cases of cancer of the larynx. J Laryngol Otol 1978; 92:991-6.

11. Ballantine JC. Diseases of the ear, nose and throat. 3rd ed. London: Butterworth, 1971.

12. State of Israel, Ministry of Health, Israel Cancer Registry. Cancer in Israel. Facts and figures, 1967-1971. Sept 1977.

13. Mass M, Modan B. Epidemiological reports on neoplastic disorders in Israeli migrant population IV. Cancer of the colon and the rectum. J Natl Cancer Inst 1969; 42:529-36.

14. Tulchinski D, Modan B. Epidemiological survey of gastric cancer in Israel. Harefuah 1966; 71:340-5.

15. Bartal A, Bentwich Z, Manny M, Izak G. Ethnical and clinical aspects of chronic lymphocytic leukemia in Israel. Acta Hematol 1978; 60:161-71.

16. Warren S, Cates O. Multiple primary malignant tumors. Am J Cancer 1932; 16:1358-414.

17. Bordin GM, Key CR, McQuade CE, Kutviri DH, Hugness WB, Brilinski DD. Multiple primary cancers. Relative risk in New Mexico's triethnic population. Cancer 1977; 40:1793-800.

18. Look GB. Comparison of single and multiple primary cancers. Cancer 1966; 19:959-66.

19. Schall LA, Jesberg N. Unusual laryngeal lesions. Ann Otol Rhinol Laryngol 1947; 56:904-10.

20. Ferlitto A, DiBonnito L. Primary cancer of the larynx associated with primary lung cancer. ORL 1976; 38:230-45.

21. Goorwitch J. Consecutive primary cancer of bronchus and larynx. JAMA 1973; 113:375-7.

22. Knudsen RJ, Hatch HB, Ochsner A, LeJeune FE. Multiple carcinomas of the lung and upper respiratory tract. Dis Chest 1965; 48:140-4.

23. Sakula A. Multiple primary carcinomas of the respiratory tract: primary carcinomas of larynx followed by primary carcinomas involving two lungs consecutively. Br J Dis Chest 1974; 68:128-36.

24. Sherman JA, Staley CJ, Shields TW. Double primary carcinoma tumors of larynx and lungs. Arch Surg 1967; 94:550-8.

25. Titche L. Carcinoma of the larynx following carcinoma of the lungs. Arch Otolaryngol 1966; 83:598-601.

26. Perez PE, Bernatz E, Devine MD, Wooner LB. Associated primary endolaryngeal carcinoma and bronchogenic carcinoma. JAMA 1961; 177:596-9.

27. Holinger PH, Johnston KL, Jesnsik RJ, Hurzeler D. Laryngeal and bronchial cancer: a study of double primary malignancy. Ann Otol Rhinol Laryngol 1961; 70:475-89.

28. Goldsher M, Bartal A. Laryngeal carcinoma association with multiple additional tumors. Harefuah 1978; 95:215-6.

29. Gluckman JL. Synchronous multiple primary lesions of the upper digestive system. Arch Otolaryngol 1979; 103:597-8.

30. Moertel CG. Multiple primary malignant neoplasms, historical aspects. Cancer 1977; 40:1786-91.

31. Moertel CG. Incidence and significance of multiple malignant neoplasms. Ann NY Acad Sci 1964; 114:896-921.

32. Cahan WC, Castro FB, Rosen PP, Strong EW. Separate primary carcinomas of the esophagus and head and neck region in the same patient. Cancer 1976; 39:85-9.

33. Odette J, Szymanowski RT, Nichols RD. Multiple head and neck malignancy. Trans Am Acad Opthalmol Otolaryngol 1977; 84:805-13.

34. Moor C. Ciagarette smoking and cancer of the mouth, pharynx & larynx. JAMA 1971; 218:553-8.

35. Rothman K, Keller A. The effect of joint exposure to alcohol & tobacco on risk of cancer in mouth & pharynx. J Chronic Dis 1972; 25:711-6.

36. Slaughter DP, Southwick HW, Smejkal W, et al. Field cancerization in oral stratified squamous epithelium. Cancer 1953; 6:963-8.

37. Goldsher M, Bartal A, Eliachar I, Robinson E. Laryngeal carcinoma associated with multiple additional primary tumors. Arch Otolaryngol 1977; 103:550-2.

38. Bartal A, Goldsher M, Eliachar I, Mekori T, Robinson E. Cellular immunity in patients with laryngeal cancer developing additional primary malignant tumors. Ann Otol Rhinol Laryngol 1979; 88:311-5.

Ann Otol Rhinol Laryngol 91:1982

ACCURACY OF AUDITORY BRAINSTEM EVOKED RESPONSE WITH HEARING LEVEL UNKNOWN

LEE E. SMITH, MD

F. BLAIR SIMMONS, MD

STANFORD, CALIFORNIA

We reported a comparison of auditory brainstem response (ABR)-estimated hearing levels with hearing levels by pure-tone audiogram for 84 ears of 42 children. Their average age was 34 months at the time of ABR and 73 months for the audiogram. Thus, all of these children were managed clinically on the basis of their ABR results. The ABR accurately predicted the pure-tone average (PTA) in 76% and was in error by no more than about ±10-12 dB in another 18%.

INTRODUCTION

There is a certain amount of guesswork in estimating hearing thresholds of young and multihandicapped children. Auditory brainstem response (ABR) has eliminated some of this, but how much? This report reviews the precision of ABR in predicting pure-tone average thresholds (PTA), 500, 1,000, and 2,000 Hz, in a group of 42 children whose hearing levels were unknown at the time of ABR testing. In other words, in these children ABR was the definitive test. Months or years later, each child had a pure-tone audiogram — which was compared with the earlier test. We felt the addition of this type of study to the ABR literature was needed to validate the use of ABR in typical pediatric clinical situations, ie, when behavioral tests are ambiguous or unavailable.

Jerger and Mauldin[1] evaluated the accuracy of ABR for predicting the PTA (1-4 Hz) in patients 7 to 83 years old when the PTA was already known. They found the PTA (1-4 Hz) was most accurately predicted by multiplying the ABR threshold by 0.6, regardless of audiometric configuration. In addition, they stated that the standard error of such predictions was large (15-16 dB), limiting the success of using ABR alone. Mokotoff et al[2] suggested ABR was an accurate tool for evaluation of "difficult to test" pediatric patients. Their study used impedance audiometry to obtain corroborative data, but only in anecdotal cases were follow-up pure-tone (PT) thresholds obtained. Schulman-Galambos and Galambos[3] have also suggested that ABR is a reliable method of determining threshold hearing levels in newborns, but again without PT audiometric confirmation. Jerger et al[4] compared ABR, impedance, and behavioral audiometry in normal and handicapped pediatric populations. They found greater than 84% correlation among these tests using three broad hearing level ranges: 0-40 dB, 50-90 dB, and greater than 90 dB. Our study provides long-term PT audiometric follow-up data in all cases, comparing ABR thresholds with PTAs using the currently accepted hearing level categories of Goodman.[5]

METHODS

Subjects: Subjects in this study were referred for ABR testing for one of the following reasons: they had failed screening tests such as Crib-O-Gram and Behavioral Audiometry; they were difficult to test because of age or multiple handicaps; and they had speech and language retardation and "unknown hearing thresholds" in which the differential diagnosis was typically between hearing loss, mental retardation, and autism. The study group consisted of 84 ears in 42 subjects, 19 female and 23 male. They ranged in age from 3 to 144 months (at the time of ABR testing); the mean age was 34.4 months. Fortunately, there was a variety of PT thresholds against which to evaluate the ABR estimates. These included 10 normal, 2 mild, 5 moderate, 4 moderately severe, 10 severe, and 53 profound losses by follow-up audiogram.

Procedure: The ABRs were obtained using conventional band pass filter settings of 300 - 3,000 Hz, TDH-39 earphones, and conventional recording techniques, usually with sedation of children older than six months.

These subjects were followed until such time as a reliable PT audiogram was obtained, typically 2 to 3 years later at 4- to 7-years old. The shortest time between ABR and PT audiogram was one month, the longest was five years, and the average time 39.5 months.

The originally reported wave V threshold was used as the ABR predictor of the PTA in the following manner: if there was no response to the 100 dB HL click (the most intense stimulus typically used), the child's hearing loss was called profound; a wave V threshold between 75-100 dB was severe; 65-75 dB, moderately severe; 55-65 dB moderate; 40-55 dB, mild; and a less than 40 dB threshold was called normal. These categories are 10-15 dB higher than when the same descriptors are applied to threshold ranges for PT audiograms. We presumed that the true PT threshold would probably be 10-15 dB better than the ABR threshold. In order to delineate the most accurate correction factor, we also calculated the PTA using Jerger's factor of 0.6 x ABR.

RESULTS

The results of the PTA predictions from the ABR are illustrated in the figure. The PTA was accurate-

From the Division of Otolaryngology-Head and Neck Surgery, Stanford University Medical Center, Stanford, California.

Presented at the meeting of the American Neurotology Society, May 8, 1981, Vancouver, British Columbia.

REPRINTS — Lee E. Smith, MD, Division of Otolaryngology-Head and Neck Surgery, Stanford University Medical Center, 300 Pasteur Drive, Stanford, CA 94305.

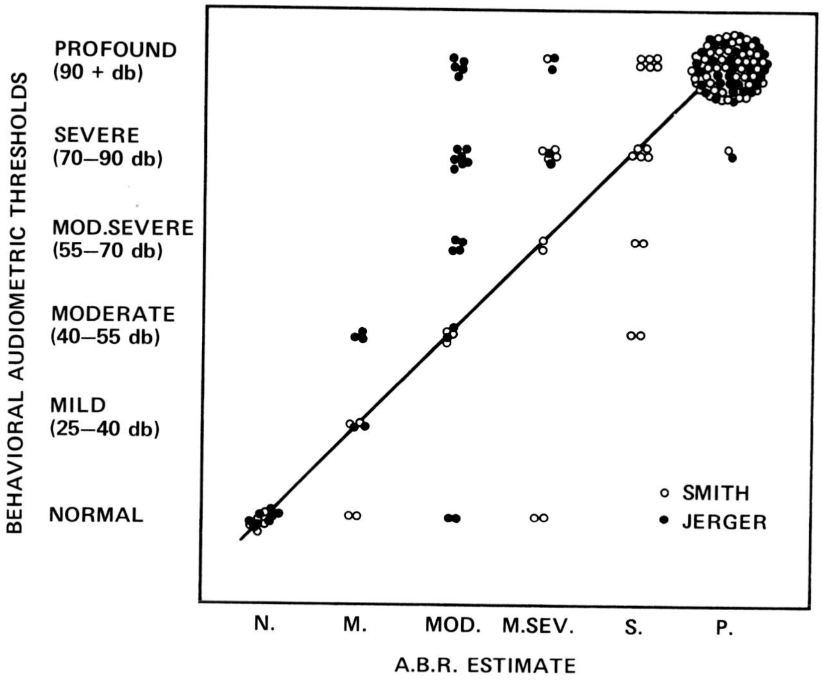

Comparison of wave V ABR estimates of the PTA 500-2,000 Hz with those obtained by follow-up (typically 2-3 years later) pure-tone audiogram. ABR - Brainstem response audiometry; N - Normal; M - Mild; Mod -Moderate; MSEV - Moderately severe; S -Severe; P - Profound. (Jerger data adapted from Jerger and Mauldin.[1])

ly predicted, using our scale categories, in 76% of subjects, and was accurate ± one category in another 18%. Jerger's correction factor applied to these data resulted in 70% correct predictions and 12% ± one category correct predictions. Neither of these differences is particularly striking, but what is impressive is the difference in those children whose threshold estimates were off by more than one category. Our predictions were off in more than one category in five patients (6%), while Jerger's predictions were off in 16 patients (19%). This difference is accounted for by the tendency of Jerger's factor to overcorrect the wave V threshold when predicting the PTA in those patients with severe and profound hearing loss, and some response on ABR. In other words, in patients with wave V thresholds of 80-100 dB Jerger's factor would predict a moderately severe hearing loss although most of these patients had severe to profound losses on follow-up PT audiogram.

SUMMARY

Our data suggest that ABR is an accurate method for estimating the PTA 500 - 2,000 Hz in young and multihandicapped children, when conventional audiometric testing is unavilable or the results ambiguous. The correction factors for converting wave V thresholds to an estimated behavioral threshold used herein appear to be more accurate than previously published methods.

REFERENCES

1. Jerger J, Mauldin L. Prediction of sensorineural hearing level from the brain stem evoked response. Arch Otolaryngol 1978; 104:456-61.

2. Mokotoff B, Schulman-Galambos C, Galambos R. Brain stem auditory evoked responses in children. Arch Otolaryngol 1977; 103:38-43.

3. Schulman-Galambos C, Galambos R. Brain stem evoked response audiometry in new born hearing screening. Arch Otolaryngol 1979; 105:86-90.

4. Jerger J, Hayes O, Jordan C. Clinical experience with auditory brain stem response audiometry in pediatric assessment. Ear Hear 1980; 2:19-25.

5. Goodman A. Reference zero levels for pure tone audiometer. ASHA 1965; 7:262-3.

Ann Otol Rhinol Laryngol 91:1982

DISTRIBUTION OF ANTILEUKOPROTEASE IN UPPER RESPIRATORY MUCOSA

ULLA FRYKSMARK, MD
ÅSA POLLING, BSc

KJELL OHLSSON, MD
HANS TEGNER, MD

MALMÖ, SWEDEN

Human respiratory tract secretions contain enzyme inhibitors derived from plasma and a low molecular weight, acid-stable protease inhibitor, antileukoprotease. The distribution of antileukoprotease in normal upper respiratory tract mucosa has been studied using an immunohistologic technique. The inhibitor was localized to the serous parts of the submucosal glands of the maxillary sinus and the trachea but was not demonstrable in mucous glands and goblet cells. It is concluded that the antileukoprotease found in respiratory tract secretions is produced locally in the submucosal serous glands.

INTRODUCTION

Antileukoprotease is a potent inhibitor of human leukocyte elastase[1,2] and chymotrypsin-like cationic proteins.[2,3] It accounts for about 90% of the protease-inhibiting capacity of human bronchial secretions.[4] The remainder of the inhibiting capacity is mainly accounted for by α_1-antitrypsin and α_1-antichymotrypsin.[4] Antileukoprotease has not been found in plasma using an immunodiffusion technique.[1] However, using a new radioimmunoassay for the inhibitor, we have recently found antileukoprotease in human serum in a concentration of about 125 μg/l.[5]

Antileukoprotease was originally localized to mucosal and submucosal structures of the upper airways in our laboratory with an indirect immunoperoxidase technique.[6] The results obtained did not allow detailed analyses as to cell localization of the inhibitor. The purpose of the present investigation tion was therefore to establish more exact localization for the inhibitor by applying recent improvements of an immunohistologic technique. The method basically utilizes immune complexes of peroxidase with rabbit antibody against peroxidase (PAP) according to Sternberger.[7]

METHODS AND MATERIALS

MATERIALS

Materials used in this study are as follows: 3.3-diaminobenzidine-tetrahydrochloride from BDH Chemicals Ltd, Poole, England; Pertex, from Histolab, Bethlehem Trading Ltd, Gothenburg, Sweden; swine-antirabbit IgG, PAP and normal swine serum from Dako Immunoglobulins, Copenhagen; Shiffs reagents from Merck, Darmstadt, Germany; and pepsin from Sigma Chemical Co, Stockholm. Monospecific rabbit antiserum against the low molecular weight inhibitor from bronchial secretions was prepared as described earlier.[1] A sample of the antiserum was absorbed with antileukoprotease isolated as described earlier[8] for use with the controls.

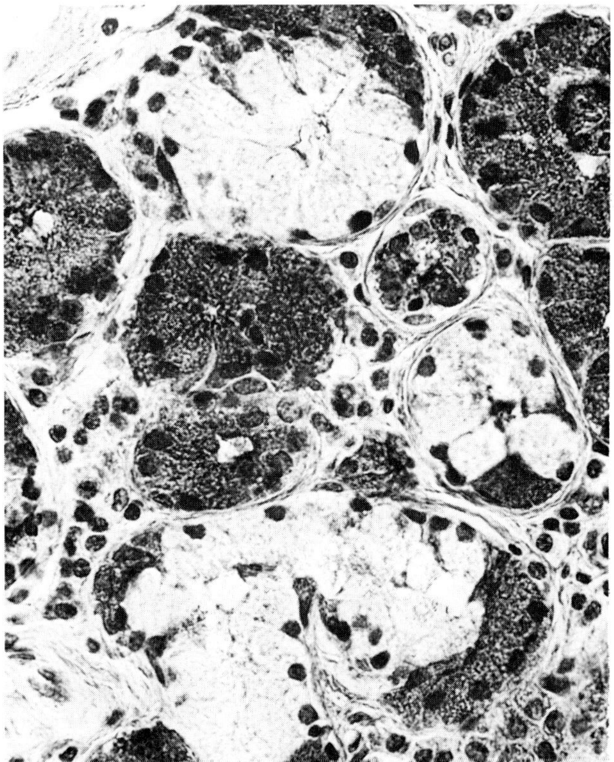

Fig. 1. Seromucous gland of tracheal mucosa. Positive (black) staining of the serous glands, semilunary surrounding the negative mucous glands. (Panchrome green filter, x 450)

From the Departments of Otorhinolaryngology, Experimental Research, Clinical Chemistry, and Surgery; University of Lund, Malmö General Hospital, Malmö, Sweden. This investigation was supported by grants from the Swedish Medical Research Council (project no. B81-17X-03910-09C), the Medical Faculty, University of Lund, the Swedish Society against Cancer (project no. 1300-B81-03XB), the Foundation of Malmö General Hospital against Cancer, the Swedish Association against Heart and Chest Diseases, the Swedish Association against Rheumatism, the Foundation of Thorsten and Elsa Segerfalk, the Foundation of Torsten and Ragnar Söderberg, and the Swedish Tobacco Company.

REPRINTS — Kjell Ohlsson, MD, Department of Experimental Research, Malmö General Hospital, S-214 01 Malmö, Sweden.

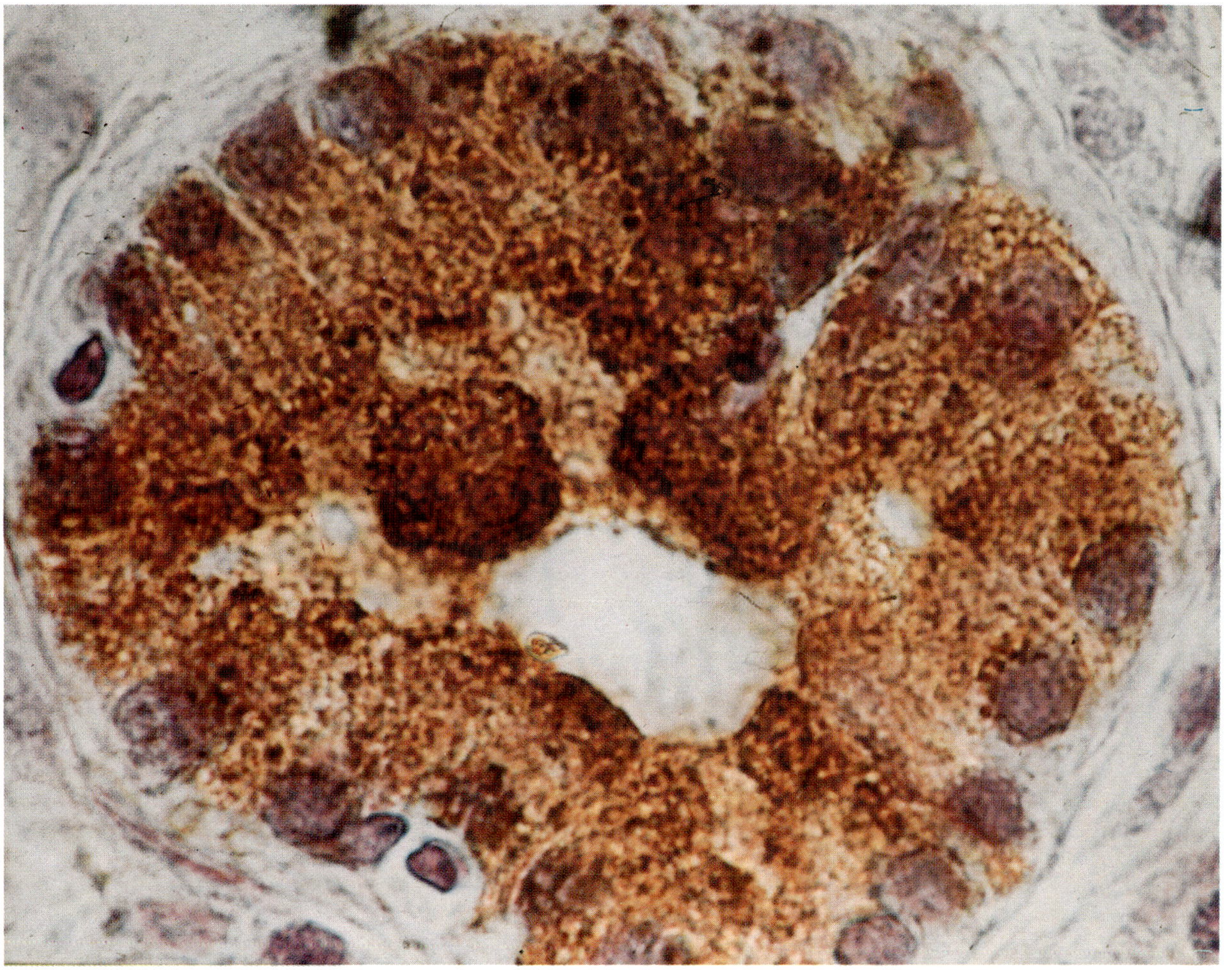

Fig. 2. Positive (brown) staining for antileukoprotease in serous gland cells of tracheal mucosa. (x 1250)

Tissue Sections. Human tracheal mucous membranes were taken at operation from three patients undergoing tracheostomy. Maxillary sinus mucosa was obtained from three patients undergoing surgical correction of facial deformities.

METHODS

The fixation and immunological staining procedures were adopted and slightly modified from earlier publications[7,9,10] as follows:

1. Tracheal and maxillary sinus mucosa were fixed immediately in buffered formalin solution for more than 24 hours and then imbedded in histowax.

2. Sections were cut at 5 μ, mounted on glass slides, dewaxed and hydrated by washing for 2-3 minutes in xylene, ethanol 99.5%, and ethanol 96% and Tris-buffer successively. The Tris-buffer (0.05*M* Tris-HC1, pH 7.6 containing 0.15*M* NaC1) was used for all serum dilutions and washings. Washing was performed in three changes of the Tris-HC1 buffer, each for 30 minutes.

3. Sections were incubated for 30 minutes at 37°C in a solution of pepsin (4 mg/ml in 0.01*M* HC1) to reduce background staining.[10]

4. Endogenous peroxidase activity was blocked by incubation with a 0.3% solution of hydrogen peroxide in methanol for 30 minutes.

5. To further reduce nonspecific background staining, sections were treated for 10 minutes with normal, nonimmune swine serum, diluted 1:20.[9]

6. Specific antiserum to antileukoprotease in seven different dilutions (1:20, 1:50, 1:100, 1:200, 1:500, 1:1000, 1:2000) was applied for 30 minutes. Controls were incubated with the same dilutions of the specific antiserum, which had been previously absorbed to purified antileukoprotease.

7. Sections were treated with swine-antirabbit IgG, diluted 1:20, for 30 minutes.

8. Peroxidase-antiperoxidase (PAP) complex was then added for 30 minutes in a dilution of 1:20.

9. The sections were developed with diaminobenzidine (0.6 g/l) and hydrogen peroxide (0.01%) for 5-10 minutes.

10. After counterstaining with the PAS-method or hematoxylin, sections were dehydrated and mounted in Pertex. All steps were carried out at room temperature and in a humidified chamber.

RESULTS AND DISCUSSION

The high concentrations of antileukoprotease found in bronchial secretions[4] suggested local production of the inhibitor. In a previous study using an immunoperoxidase method, we found positive staining of the seromucous glands of the tracheal mucosa and also of the ciliated epithelium indicating a mucosal production site of antileukoprotease.[6] To localize the productive site more specifically, we combined a more sophisticated immunoperoxidase method with PAS staining. To reduce background staining, we incubated sections first in pepsin and then in swine serum, also higher dilutions of antiserum were used and the sections were washed more thoroughly. The most suitable dilutions of our

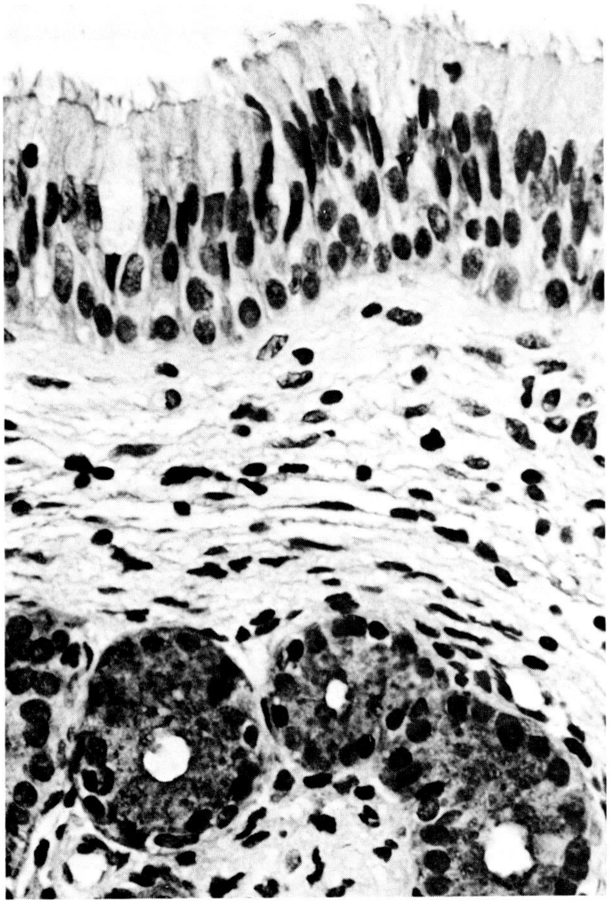

Fig. 3. Maxillary sinus mucosa. Positive (black) staining for antileukoprotease in serous gland cells. Ciliated epithelium with goblet cell negative. (Panchrome green filter, x 450)

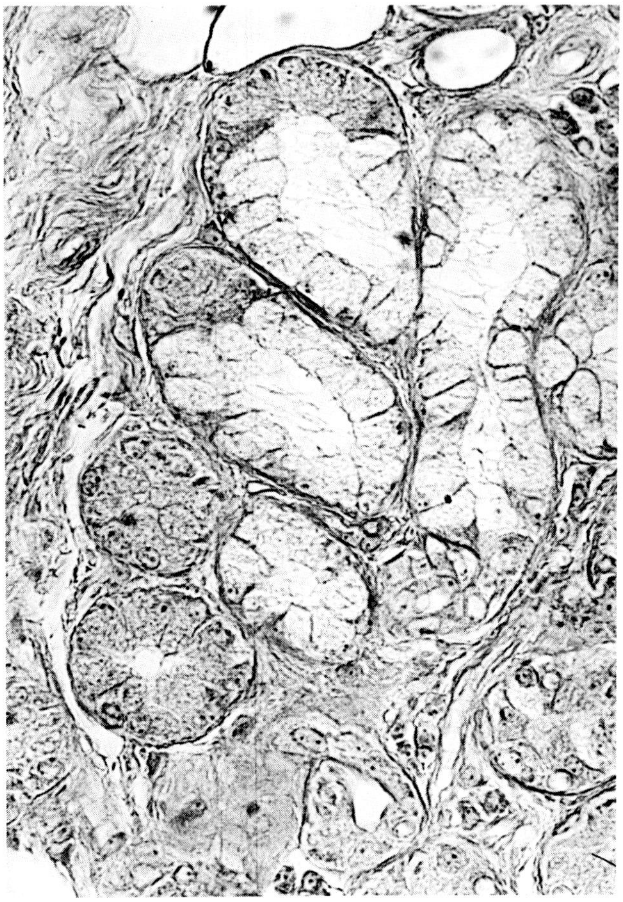

Fig. 4. Control. Serous and mucous gland cells of tracheal mucosa incubated with specific antiserum previously absorbed with antileukoprotease showing no positive staining. (Panchrome green filter, x 450)

antiserum were 1:1000-1:2000. Sections prepared with this method showed no background staining.

Morphological detail in all sections examined was excellent. Positive brown staining for antileukoprotease contrasted well with the blue hematoxylin or the pink PAS counterstains. Positive staining for antileukoprotease was confined to the serous parts of the seromucous glands of both tracheal (Figs. 1 and 2) and maxillary sinus mucosa (Fig. 3). The PAS-positive cells contained no demonstrable antileukoprotease nor did any cell of the ciliated epithelium (Fig. 3). In control sections handled in the same way but incubated with the specific antiserum previously adsorbed with antileukoprotease, the positive staining was completely abolished confirming the specificity of the reaction for antileukoprotease (Fig. 4). The present results strongly indicate that antileukoprotease found in bronchial secretions is produced in the respiratory tract mucosa by the submucosal serous glands. This conclusion is supported by the absence of any demonstrable immunologic cross-reactivity with plasma proteins.[5] Preliminary studies of the immunoreactive antileukoprotease found in serum show that this protein has a molecular weight of about 10,000, indicating a noncomplexed inhibitor.

It remains to be proven, although it seems most likely, that antileukoprotease found in serum is derived mainly from the respiratory tract. The same inhibitor appears to be produced in vesicula seminalis and in the uterine cervical mucosa. However, given the size differences between the respiratory and other sources, it seems likely that the respiratory tract is the main source of serum antileukoprotease.[2]

REFERENCES

1. Ohlsson K, Tegner H. Inhibition of elastase from granulocytes by the low molecular weight bronchial protease inhibitor. Scand J Clin Lab Invest 1976; 36:437-45.

2. Schiessler H, Hochstrasser K, Ohlsson K. Acid-stable inhibitors of granulocyte neutral proteases in human mucous secretions: biochemistry and possible biological function. In: Havemann K, Janoff A, eds. Neutral proteases of human polymorphonuclear leukocytes. Baltimore-Munich: Urban & Schwarzenberg Inc, 1978: 195-207.

3. Tegner H, Ohlsson K, Olsson I. The interactions between a

low molecular weight protease inhibitor of bronchial mucus and chymotrypsin-like cationic proteins of granulocytes. Hoppe-Seyler's Z Physiol Chem 1977; 358;431-3.

4. Tegner H. Quantitation of human granulocyte protease inhibitors in non-purulent bronchial lavage fluids. Acta Otolaryngol (Stockh) 1978; 85:282-9.

5. Ohlsson K. Interactions between granulocyte proteases and protease inhibitors in the lung. Bull Europ Physiopath Resp 1980; 16:209-22.

6. Tegner H, Ohlsson K. Localization of a low molecular weight protease inhibitor to tracheal and maxillary sinus mucosa. Hoppe-Seyler's Z Physiol Chem 1977; 358:425-9.

7. Sternberger LA, Hardy PH Jr, Cuculis JJ, Meyer HG. The unlabelled antibody enzyme method of immunochemistry, preparations and properties of soluble antigen-antibody complex (horseradish peroxidase-antihorseradish peroxidase) and its use in identification of Spirochetes. J Histochem Cytochem 1970 a; 18:315-33.

8. Ohlsson K, Tegner H, Åkesson U. Isolation and partial characterization of a low molecular weight acid stable protease inhibitor from human bronchial secretion. Hoppe-Seyler's Z Physiol Chem 1977; 358:583-9.

9. Mason DY, Taylor CR. The distribution of mucoamidase (lysozyme) in human tissues. J Clin Pathol 1975; 28:124-32.

10. Reading M. Reduction of background staining. J Clin Pathol 1977; 30:88-90.

≈

THIRD INTERNATIONAL SYMPOSIUM ON RECENT ADVANCES IN OTITIS MEDIA WITH EFFUSION

The Third International Symposium on Recent Advances in Otitis Media with Effusion will be held May 17-20, 1983, at Hotel Bahia Mar in Fort Lauderdale, Florida. Those interested in participating or attending the meeting should contact Dr. David J. Lim, Dept. of Otolaryngology, The Ohio State University College of Medicine, 456 Clinic Drive, Columbus, OH 43210. F5

EARLY- AND MIDDLE-AER COMPONENTS TO CLICKS AS RESPONSE INDICES FOR NEONATAL HEARING SCREENING

HELENE A. FRYE-OSIER, MS
JUDITH E. HIRSCH, PhD
ROBERT GOLDSTEIN, PhD
KATHLEEN WEBER, LPN

MADISON, WISCONSIN

Early- and middle-component-averaged electroencephalic responses (AER) to monotic clicks at 60, 40 and 20 dB normal hearing level were elicited from 18 carefully selected normal neonates. Grand-composite AERs of the responses from all 18 babies showed stimulus-related configurations at all three stimulus levels. AERs for individual babies were more frequently identified as stimulus-related when poststimulus activity beyond 10 ms was included in response-identification procedures than when only the first 10 ms was observed.

The importance of screening the hearing of newborn babies who are at risk for congenital hearing loss has had extensive endorsement.[1-3] Similar endorsement is being given to the importance of screening the hearing of neonates who are at risk for survival because of the high incidence of hearing loss in this population.[4,5] Increasing interest also is being expressed in those babies born with mild to moderate hearing losses.[6-10]

Because hearing impairments of varying magnitude are common in young children,[11] it is desirable to reconsider earlier calls for routine hearing screening of all neonates. Any routine procedure should screen out mild to moderate and unilateral hearing impairments as well as the severe losses.

The most popularly used behavioral observation procedure of the past[12] or a frequently recommended objective, automated procedure,[13] both of which are simple and economical, are not sufficiently sensitive for screening a broad range of hearing impairments. In addition, these procedures are not applicable for follow-up hearing evaluation. Thus, if a difference in hearing is found during follow-up, one cannot be certain that the difference represents a true change in hearing or is just an artifact of differences in test procedures.

Electroencephalic procedures, on the other hand, are proving sensitive to mild and moderate hearing impairments and are usually applied in a way to detect unilateral hearing losses. Further, they can be applied, with negligable variations, on older infants and children during follow-up examination in the same way they were applied to neonates.

Others[4,5,14,15] have reported promising results with electroencephalic audiometry with wave V of the early or brainstem components (first 10 ms) of the averaged electroencephalic response (AER) as the response index. Our observations with the early components are consonant with those reported by others. However, our experience[16-19] with the middle components (10-80 ms) of the AER suggests that they may be an equally sensitive index for neonatal hearing screening. The purpose of the present study was to compare early and middle component AERs to the same clicks in the same normal neonates before considering a single response index, or combination of indices, for routine screening of the hearing of all normal and high-risk neonates.

METHODS AND MATERIALS

SUBJECTS

We selected babies who were not high-risk for congenital hearing loss according to the five criteria established by the Joint Committee on Infant Hearing Screening and who had not experienced hypoxia or neonatal sepsis.[20,21] Eighteen babies meeting our criteria served as subjects. They ranged in age from 43-168 hours (mean of 77 hours). We allowed at least 24 hours to elapse for the pediatric and nursing staff to detect subtle abnormalities that may not have been apparent at birth. All 18 babies were described by their pediatricians as normal term infants. Estimated gestational age ranged between 38-41 weeks (mean of 39.7 weeks). Fifteen of the births were normal, spontaneous vertex presentations; three were caesarian sections. One- and 5-minute apgar scores were 8-10. Other babies who met all of the hearing and physical criteria were not tested if the nursery staff expressed any concern about a baby's normality even if the nurses or aides could not define the basis for their misgivings. No baby selected by these same rigid criteria for previous studies has yet been reported to us as having a hearing loss or other communicative disorder.

PROCEDURES

Stimulus Conditions. Clicks were generated by a 0.1 ms electric pulse delivered to an electrically-shielded earphone (Telex, TDH-49). The polarity of the pulse was constant throughout the study. The clicks were presented monotically at 10/s at 60, 40 and 20 dB re normal adult thresholds (nHL) for the same clicks. Only one ear was tested. An equal number of right and left ears was used. Each resulting AER consisted of responses to 1500 clicks at each level. A silent control of 1500 samples was also obtained. The four conditions were repeated.

From the Department of Communicative Disorders, University of Wisconsin, Madison. This investigation was supported by Public Health Service Research Grant NS09278 from the National Institute of Neurological and Communicative Disorders and Stroke, Grant Number 6-191 from the March of Dimes Birth Defects Foundation, a grant from the Nicolet Instrument Corporation, and Grant Number 181230 from the Graduate School Research Committee of the University of Wisconsin.

REPRINTS — Robert Goldstein, PhD, University of Wisconsin, Department of Communicative Disorders, 1975 Willow Drive, Madison, WI 53706.

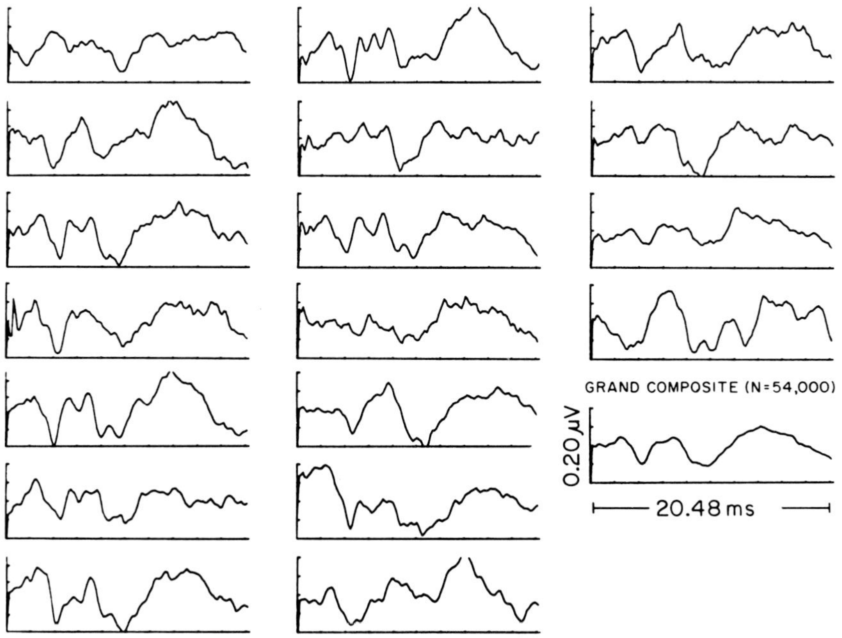

Fig. 1. Composite early component AERs (2 x 1500 = 3000 sweeps per trace) for the 60 dB nHL click from each of the 18 normal neonates who were subjects in this study. The grand-composite AER (18 x 3000 = 54,000 sweeps per trace) is in the lower right.

The earphone and its cushion (MX-41/AR) were set in an acoustic enclosure (Audiocup) to reduce some of the ambient noise during the test. A piece of cotton gauze was placed over the earphone with a hole cut at the position of the earphone diaphragm. The gauze prevented contact of the shielding against the baby's ear or face. Hearing levels were established in the same acoustic environment on normal-hearing young adults with the same shielded earphone and enclosure and with a gauze separator.

Recording Conditions. Electroencephalic activity was recorded between silver disc electrodes (Grass E5SH) attached to the vertex and to the mastoid ipsilateral to the stimulated ear. A third electrode on the forehead served as the ground. Interelectrode impedances were 5000 Ω or less.

Electroencephalic activity was amplified (Hewlett-Packard 8811A) 20,000 times. The passband of the amplifier was 1.5-3000 Hz with 6 dB/octave skirts. The amplified activity was routed in parallel to an FM tape recorder (Hewlett-Packard 3960A) and to a filter (Krohn-Hite 3342R). At the tape speed of 15 ips the recording passband was DC-5000 Hz with a low-pass roll-off of 18 dB/octave. All data reported were derived from off-line analysis of the FM tapes.

The electroencephalic activity routed through the filter was filtered through a passband of 20-3000 Hz and further amplified ten times. The filtered and amplified activity was fed into a signal averager (Nicolet 1070) for visual monitoring of ongoing activity and of accumulating AER. The signal averager was set to reject any sample containing any point greater than 9.4 μV at the head.

Electroencephalic activity was recorded with the baby positioned comfortably on the lap of the attending nurse. The earphone with its acoustic enclosure and gauze protector was placed over the baby's ear. Care was taken to avoid collapse of the ear canal. Most babies slept throughout the test session although a few cried or moved actively during portions of the session.

Data Analysis. The analog FM tape recordings of the amplified electroencephalic activity were analyzed through a computer-based system (Nicolet MED 80). Preliminary investigations of tape-recorded activity from neonates and adults played through various filter passbands led to the selection of different passbands for looking at the early or brainstem activity (first 10 ms poststimulus): 40-3000 Hz for neonates and infants and 100-3000 Hz for older children and adults. The lower high-pass cutoff for neonates reflects the greater proportion of low-frequency energy in their early-component AERs than in the equivalent AERs from adults. The high-pass slope of the filter (Krohn-Hite 3342R) had a linear roll-off of 48 dB/octave with a 40 Hz cutoff. Above that, the passband was flat until about 850 Hz. The roll-off then gradually increased so that at 3000 Hz the attenuation was 18 dB. The tape-recorded activity also was amplified ten times through the filter. For middle-component AERs, the recorded activity was filtered without additional amplification with a passband of 25-85 Hz with a linear 48 dB/octave roll-off on both sides of the band. The poststimulus-onset analysis window was 80 ms.

Visual comparison of the early- and middle-component AERs indicated more clearly identifiable middle-component AERs, especially at 20 dB nHL. Wave V, the most identifiable aspect of the early-component AERs, appeared to be too close to the end of the 10 ms analysis window to be a useful landmark. Therefore, we replayed the recorded electroencephalic activity through an extended analysis window of 20 ms even though, by definition,[22] the 10-20 ms portion of the window is part of the middle components. Wave V is a more prominent landmark in the 20 ms traces and the following negative and positive waves of the middle components also contribute to waveform identification.

We examined both the individual AERs (N = 1500) and the composites of the two replications of each condition (N = 3000). For both early- and middle-component AERs, the composites were slightly freer of background noise and their characteristic configurations were more easily identified, particularly for the 20 dB nHL condition. In the next section, therefore, we display only the composite AERs.

RESULTS

The early-component AERs from all 18 babies for the 60 dB nHL clicks are shown in Figure 1. Although there are obvious differences between babies, attributed mainly to differences in the uncancelled noise background, there are more commonalities than differences. The trace in the lower right of the figure is the grand-composite AER across all 18 babies. If individual differences were great, the grand-composite would be much smaller and, perhaps, even a straight line.

Figure 2 shows the middle-component AERs to the identical clicks. Again, similarities between the 18 babies are greater than are the differences as attested by the grand-composite AER in the lower right.

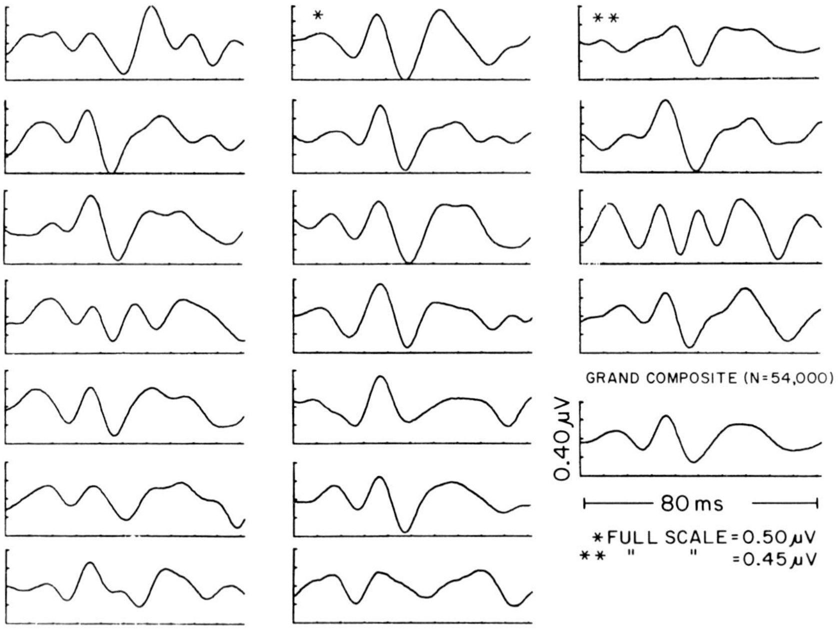

Fig. 2. Composite middle-component AERs (2 x 1500 = 3000 sweeps per trace) for the 60 dB nHL click for each of the normal neonates who were subjects in this study. The grand-composite AER (18 x 3000 = 54,000 sweeps per trace) is in the lower right.

The grand-composite early- and middle-component AERs at each intensity level and for the silent control are shown in Figure 3. The systematic reduction of peak amplitudes with reduction in signal level is apparent in both sets of AERs. Some of the peaks in the silent control traces are as large as those of the 20 dB nHL trace. However, the configurations of the silent control traces do not resemble those of the 60 dB and 40 dB nHL traces whereas the 20 dB nHL trace closely resembles those derived with stronger signals. Figure 3 also indicates that, at least as a group, the neonates show both early- and middle-component responses down to 20 dB nHL.

Naturally, individual neonates do not show as clean or as definable traces as are seen in the grand composite AERs. For most of them, however, the responses are identifiable by inspection. In Figure 4A, the middle components are as identifiable at the three levels as are the middle components in the

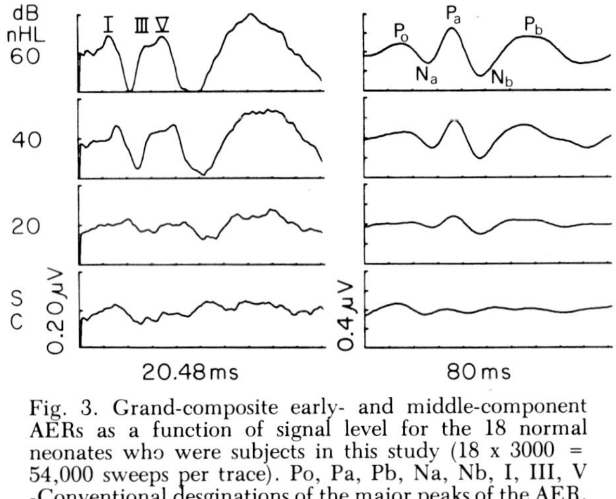

Fig. 3. Grand-composite early- and middle-component AERs as a function of signal level for the 18 normal neonates who were subjects in this study (18 x 3000 = 54,000 sweeps per trace). Po, Pa, Pb, Na, Nb, I, III, V -Conventional desginations of the major peaks of the AER. SC - Silent control.

grand composite AERs (Fig. 3). The early components in Figure 4A for this particular baby are not quite so definable. The early- and middle-component AERs in Figure 4B also are easily identified. However, the silent control AERs could be misinterpreted as responses to a low sensation-level signal. Figure 4C displays the poorest of the 18 babies in terms of either early- or middle-component identification. This baby was physically active and cried during much of the test session.

Several objective computer-analysis techniques were used to score the early and middle AERs to determine at what levels the AERs had exceeded the minimal criteria for response. The criteria were based on amplitude measures at fixed latency values determined from the grand-composite AERs.[23] Peak latencies used to score the silent control AERs were derived by extrapolating the latency-intensity functions for the respective peaks to -10 dB nHL.[23] An AER was considered to be a response if its value exceeded the positive value of two standard deviations of the scores for the silent control AERs. Various combinations of peaks were used for each time zone to help ascertain which of the peaks appeared to be contributing most to response identification.

Neither the early-component waves nor the middle-component waves, in any combination, was distinctly superior to the other in identifying responses to the low-level signals or in rejecting silent-control AERs as responses. We did note, however, that the early-component scoring indices that incorporated peaks beyond wave V identified more signal-related AERs as responses than did the scoring indices, including wave V alone, that did not use peaks between 10-20 ms. These latter waves are part of the middle-component time zone as defined by Picton et al.[22]

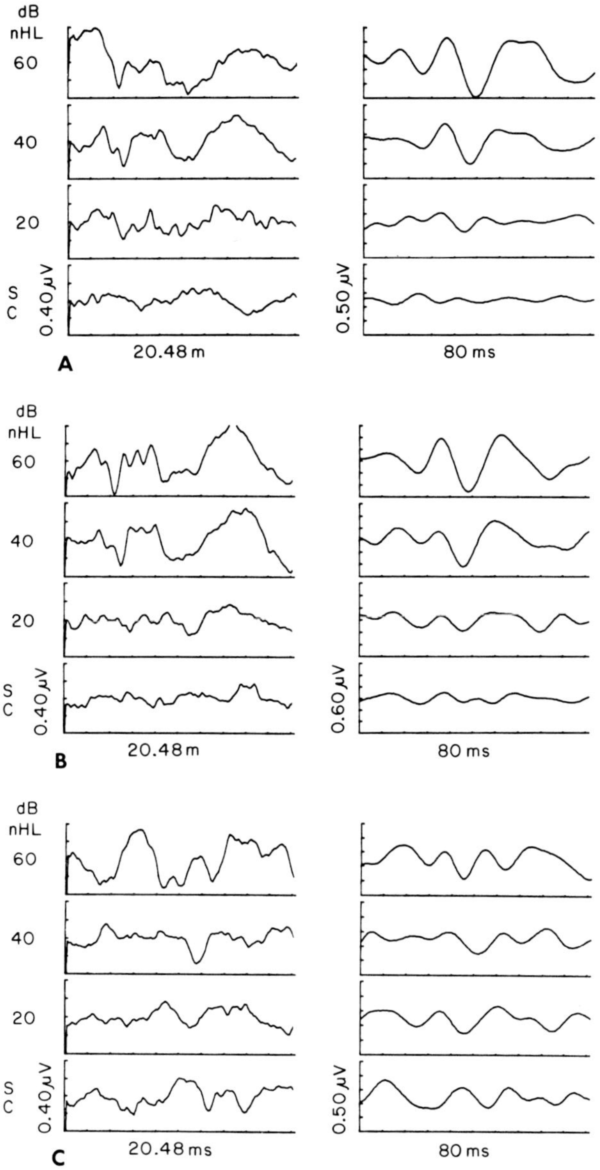

Fig. 4. Composite early- and middle-component AERs (2 x 1500 = 3000 sweeps per trace). A) Normal neonate A. Silent control traces do not appear response-related. B) Normal neonate B. Silent control traces could possibly be mistaken as a response-related configuration resulting from a weak (ie, less than 20 dB SL) but audible click. C) Normal neonate C. This baby was physically active and cried during much of the test session.

DISCUSSION

As a group (cf grand-composite AERs in Fig. 3), the 18 carefully selected normal neonates showed both early- and middle-component AERs indicative of response for the 60, 40 and 20 dB nHL clicks. Does the waveform for the 20 dB nHL click reflect positive contributions from all 18 babies or do only some of the babies contribute all of the response-related componentry overriding the physiologic noise from all 18 babies? Figures 1 and 2 display the AERs for the 18 individual babies for the 60 dB nHL clicks. The morphology of individual AERs does reflect that of the grand-composite AERs. Moreover, no subgroup of individual AERs shows drastic differences in waveform or amplitude which would skew the grand-composite AER to represent that subgroup. The signal-to-noise ratio for 20 dB nHL did not allow as easy a visual comparison between configurations of the individual AERs and the corresponding grand-composite AER. Nevertheless, inspection of the traces revealed nothing to suggest that AERs from only a subgroup of neonates influenced the configurations of the grand-composite AERs for 20 dB nHL shown in Figure 3.

Constraints of a research study on normal babies precluded adequate structuring of experimental conditions. For example, we could not test all of the babies at times when they would sleep quietly enough for us to be more nearly certain that lack of a response-related AER configuration for the 20 dB signal meant that the signal was not at or above threshold. Our inability to regulate the acoustic environment meant that we did not always have ambient noise levels low enough for us to be certain that the 20 dB nHL clicks were not being partially or totally masked, or that all babies were being tested in the identical noisy background.

It can be questioned why one would want to screen with a 20 dB nHL signal when inferences about normality of threshold might be derived from early-component peak latencies in an AER to a 60 dB nHL click. Such inferences may be safe and acceptable if threshold sensitivity is normal or if there is a conductive hearing loss. However, some evidence has been reported[24] that 60 dB nHL latencies may be normal in the presence of a sensory-neural hearing loss less than 60 dB if there is loudness recruitment. More importantly, extrapolation to threshold from suprathreshold early-component latencies depends on a narrow range of latencies. In neonates, the reported latency ranges and standard deviations[5,15] for wave V are large for extrapolation purposes. Also, change of latency as a function of age is most rapid shortly after birth.[5,14,15] Therefore, one would have to be certain of the gestational age, a measure which has its own considerable range of uncertainty, before the reference latency for 60 dB nHL could be determined.

It can also be questioned why at 20 dB nHL only 1500 samples were taken for each AER or 3000 for the composite of the two replications. During the time it took to accumulate 1500 samples at 10 per second to be certain that middle components were being encompassed, could not many more samples of early-component activity have been accumulated at a considerably faster rate (eg, 50 per second) thus assuring a more clearly-identifiable wave V? No easy answer can be given to this question but one can be offered on the basis of the grand-composite AERs. The grand-composite AERs were based on 54,000 samples. For 60 dB nHL and 40 dB nHL such a number is certainly sufficient to produce clean, robust AERs not much smaller than the individual AERs from which they were derived. It is not likely, therefore, that increasing the individual sample size to 7500 (or 15,000), for example, would have significantly improved the identifiability of wave V at 20 dB nHL. In the meantime extremely fast rates with correspondingly smaller analysis windows limit or even preclude the use of the following middle-component waves for response identification.

The most important middle-component activity for response-identification purposes appears to occur within the first 60 ms following click onset. If one limited the analysis window to 60 ms, then stimulus rates could be increased to about 15 per second allowing for an abbreviated test time without sacrificing the opportunity of seeing both early- and middle-component peaks to the identical stimuli.

We are not recommending any one scoring procedure at this time because the power of a scoring system cannot be validated on the population from which the scoring criteria were derived. The various objective scoring systems should be applied to equivalent but different populations of neonates before that decision is reached. Further, we are reluctant to recommend a specific objective scoring procedure based on the data reviewed because we are not convinced that we have identified the best way of recording and displaying the response-related electroencephalic activity. More recent experience in our laboratory suggests that it may be advantageous to filter all of the electroencephalic activity through only one passband and to display both early- and middle-component peaks in the same time window. The choice of filter passband, slope, and the nature of the filter itself will affect the relative prominence of each of the peaks; and, unless a phase-shiftless filter is used, even the apparent latency of some of the peaks will be affected.

New objective, automated scoring criteria will have to be derived for any new recording procedure. Ideally, the scoring criteria should be derived on a new population of normal neonates tested under acoustic conditions more favorable than were possible for this study.

ACKNOWLEDGMENTS — The study would not have been possible without the gracious cooperation of the Medical and Surgical Foundation and the nursery staff of Madison General Hospital and of the parents who permitted their babies to participate as subjects.

REFERENCES

1. Gerber SE. High risk registry for congenital deafness. In: Jaffe BF, ed. Hearing loss in children. Baltimore: University Park Press, 1977a:74-7.

2. Hodgson WR. Tests of hearing — birth through one year. In: Martin FN, ed. Pediatric audiology. Englewood Cliffs, New Jersey: Prentice-Hall, 1978:174-200.

3. Northern JL, Downs MP. Hearing in children. 2nd ed. Baltimore: Williams and Wilkins, 1978.

4. Galambos R, Despland PA. The auditory brainstem response (ABR) evaluates risk factors for hearing loss in the newborn. Pediatr Res 1980; 14:156-63.

5. Schulman-Galambos C, Galambos R. Brain stem evoked response audiometry in newborn hearing screening. Arch Otolaryngol 1979; 105:86-90.

6. Brooks DN. Otitis media and child development: design factors in the identification and assessment of hearing loss. Ann Otol Rhinol Laryngol 1978; 87:29-46.

7. Holm VA, Kunze LH. Effect of chronic otitis media on language and speech development. Pediatrics 1969; 43:833-9.

8. Katz J. The effects of conductive hearing loss on auditory function. ASHA 1978; 20:879-86.

9. Needleman H. Effects of hearing loss from early recurrent otitis media on speech and language development. In: Jaffe BJ, ed. Hearing loss in children. Baltimore: University Park Press, 1977:640-9.

10. Ventry IM. Effects of conductive hearing loss: fact or fiction. J Speech Hear Dis 1980; 45:143-56.

11. Downs MP. The expanding imperatives of early identification. In: Bess FH, ed. Childhood deafness. New York: Grune and Stratton, 1977:95-106.

12. Downs MP, Sterritt GM. A guide to newborn and infant hearing screening programs. Arch Otolaryngol 1967; 85:15-22.

13. McFarland WH, Simmons FB, Jones FR. An automated hearing screening technique for newborns. J Speech Hear Dis 1980; 45:495-503.

14. Morgon A, Salle B. A study of brain stem evoked responses in prematures. Acta Otolaryngol (Stockh) 1980; 89:370-5.

15. Starr S, Amlie RN, Martin WH, Sanders S. Development of auditory function in newborn infants revealed by auditory brainstem potentials. Pediatrics 1977; 60:831-9.

16. McRandle CC, Smith MA, Goldstein R. Early averaged electroencephalic responses to clicks in neonates. Ann Otol Rhinol Laryngol 1974; 83:695-703.

17. Goldstein R, McRandle CC. Middle components of the averaged electroencephalic response to clicks in neonates. In: Hirsh SK, Eldredge DH, Hirsh IJ, Silverman SR, eds. Hearing and Davis: essays honoring Hallowell Davis. St. Louis: Washington University Press, 1976:445-56.

18. Wolf KE, Goldstein R. Middle-component AERs to tonal stimuli from normal neonates. Arch Otolaryngol 1978; 104:508-13.

19. Wolf KE, Goldstein R. Middle component AERs from neonates to low-level tonal stimuli. J Speech Hear Res 1980; 23:185-201.

20. Gerber SE. Newborn and diagnostic screening tests. In: Jaffe BJ, ed. Hearing loss in children. Baltimore: University Park Press, 1977b:78-8.

21. Mencher GT, ed. Early identification of hearing loss. Basel: S. Karger, 1976.

22. Picton TW, Hillyard SA, Krausz HI, Galambos R. Human auditory evoked potentials. I. Evaluation of components. Electroenceph Clin Neurophysiol 1974; 36:179-90.

23. Vivion MC, Wolf KE, Goldstein R, Hirsch JE, McFarland WH. Toward objective analysis for electroencephalic audiometry. J Speech Hear Res 1979; 22:88-102.

24. Galambos R, Hecox KE. Clinical applications of the auditory brain stem response. Otolaryngol Clin North Am 1978; 11:709-22.

VOCAL QUALITY, ARTICULATION AND AUDIOLOGICAL CHARACTERISTICS OF CHILDREN AND YOUNG ADULTS WITH DIAGNOSED ALLERGIES

BARBARA M. BAKER, PhD

LOUISVILLE, KENTUCKY

CLAUDE D. BAKER, PhD

NEW ALBANY, INDIANA

HA THANH LE, MD

ELIZABETHTOWN, KENTUCKY

This study details vocal quality, articulation errors, and hearing disorders in 80 children and young adults with diagnosed allergies. Results indicated that almost 50% had abnormalities in vocal quality and/or articulation and 13% had reduced auditory acuity. Vocal quality disorders showed a significant relationship to bronchial asthma in association with other allergic reactions. All subjects with diminished hearing had allergic rhinitis either singly or in combination with another disorder. Findings suggest that bronchial asthma and allergic rhinitis are related to the development of vocal quality disorders and that allergic rhinitis is associated with misarticulations and diminished hearing. The presence of speech sound omissions in allergic rhinitis patients above age 8 may predict the presence or previous history of fluctuating hearing loss.

INTRODUCTION

Allergic individuals are often characterized by factors which may affect vocal, articulatory and auditory mechanisms. These factors may include 1) chronic cough, 2) throat clearing, 3) edema of the mucous membranes of the nose, pharynx and vocal cords, 4) enlarged adenoids, 5) otitis media, and 6) a high incidence of vocal cord lesions.[1-5] These allergic individuals may be more susceptible to developing disorders of vocal quality, articulation and hearing.[3] Nasal allergies originating early in development may contribute to poor nasal ventilation and eventually produce underdevelopment of the nasal sinuses. This condition in turn may produce improper development of the maxilla and palatine bones resulting in formation of a long narrow dental arch and a high domed palate. Consequently, many of the structural features related to proper speech production may be affected, eg, malocclusion of the dental arches.

The problems caused by allergies in children and young adults are often compounded by the multiplicity of complaints involved. For example, the chief presenting complaint of a young patient may be bronchial asthma. However, the patient may have previously experienced gastroenteritis, followed by the development of rashes and urticaria.[3] The allergic attack may move into the upper respiratory tract and produce allergic rhinitis and serous fluid in the middle ear, with concomitant diminished hearing. At any point in this process, the allergic patient may be referred to a speech-language pathologist or audiologist for evaluation and therapy. These specialists should recognize the multiplicity of factors involved in dealing with allergic patients.

Allergies have also been indicated in the development of vocal quality and articulation disorders. For example, Senturia and Wilson[2] found that there was frequently a history of allergic rhinitis in children with vocal quality disorders and Szanton[6] suggests that allergic hearing loss may affect the quality of speech development and production.

Although the relationship of allergies to vocal quality disorders, voice deviation and hearing loss has been reported repeatedly, few, if any, studies have detailed these hypothesized relationships. We found instead many studies suggesting additional work in these areas. For example, Szanton and Szanton[7,8] state that studies of allergic disease may establish etiologic conditions for many presently inexplicable problems of speech and language deviations. Yairi et al[9] note the need for more information on the influence of allergies and other factors on phonatory disorders, and Baynes[10] suggests that the high incidence of chronic hoarseness in children is an area for continued work. Therefore, the lack of definitive information in this area warrants research into the vocal quality and articulation characteristics of allergy patients.

The purposes of this study are to describe the vocal quality, articulation and hearing characteristics of a group of children and young adults with diagnosed allergies, and to determine whether specific allergies resulted in specific vocal quality and/or

From the Program in Communicative Disorders, Department of Surgery, University of Louisville School of Medicine, and the Department of Biology, Indiana University Southeast, New Albany.

REPRINTS — Barbara M. Baker, PhD, Department of Surgery, University of Louisville School of Medicine, 530 South Jackson St., Louisville, KY 40202.

TABLE 1. VOCAL QUALITY, AUDITORY AND FLUENCY DISORDERS AND ARTICULATORY ERRORS IN PATIENTS WITH ALLERGIES IN LOUISVILLE (N = 80)

Experimental Parameter	*No. with Disorder*	%
Vocal quality disorders	36	44.75
Articulatory errors	39	48.75
Vocal quality and articulatory errors	17	21.25
Auditory acuity disorders	11	13.75
Fluency disorders	0	0.00

misarticulation errors. The ultimate goal of research of this type is to ascertain if specific articulation and/or vocal quality errors may be used as diagnostic or predictive tools in the diagnosis and treatment of allergy patients.

METHODS

Subjects. Eighty patients were selected randomly from those being treated for allergic disorders at Norton-Children's Hospital, Louisville. All medical intervention was withheld for approximately 48 hours before assessment.

All patients were at least 8 years old ($\bar{x} = 12.1$, range 8 to 23) and possessed adequate oral structures and mobility as determined by a standard oral mechanism evaluation. Since adequate articulation is normally achieved by age 8, the articulation errors presented by this sample were assumed to be related to deviancy rather than lack of articulation maturation.[11]

Each patient had a complete history and physical examination, routine and specific laboratory tests and allergy skin tests. The history and physical examination were complete but emphasized problems related to upper and lower respiratory systems, eyes, ears, skin and gastrointestinal tract. Laboratory tests consisted of a complete blood count, nasal smear, quantitative immunoglobulins, chest x-ray films and, if necessary, x-ray films of sinuses and finding sweat chloride value. If the patient was shown to be allergic, skin tests for allergies to inhalants and food were done initially with scratch tests using 1:20 weight/volume concentration extracts. Patients' allergies were diagnosed as being seasonal and/or perennial allergic rhinitis, asthma, exercise-induced asthma, serous otitis media, eczema, food allergy or other allergic disorders. The use of symptomatic treatment and/or immunotherapy depended on clinical manifestations, laboratory tests, allergy skin tests, environmental control and avoidance.

Speech, Language and Hearing Assessment. Each patient was administered the Fisher-Logemann Test of Articulation Competence, which was originally determined on subjects representing a wide range of dialectic, socioeconomic and foreign language backgrounds. In this test, the patients were instructed to name stimulus pictures as the examiner pointed to them. Based on the patients' responses, articulation errors were phonetically transcribed on a standard form. The phonetic transcription was then analyzed according to error type and phoneme classes.

Patients' speech samples, for vocal quality analysis, were tape-recorded in a quiet room as they read aloud a selected passage. Microphone-to-mouth distance was standardized at 30.5 cm. The examiner then made a perceptual judgment of vocal quality according to the parameters of frequency, intensity and resonance.

To determine speech fluency, each patient read a selected passage, then produced spontaneous speech elicited from picture stimuli. A perceptual judgment was made by the examiner according to methodology outlined by Johnson et al.[12]

In addition to speech-language analysis, each patient was given pure tone air and bone conduction assessment on a Beltone portable audiometer, calibrated to the four standard frequencies of 1,000, 2,000, 4,000 and 6,000 Hz.[13]

After data collection, a nonparametric chi square analysis was employed to analyze the relation between vocal quality or misarticulations and specific allergic disorders.

TABLE 2. CHI SQUARE VALUES FOR ALLERGIES AND VOCAL QUALITY DISORDERS

Allergic Disorder	*Vocal Quality Disorder*	*Chi Square Value*
Bronchial asthma	Mouth breathing	10.56*
Bronchial asthma & allergic dermatitis	Hyponasality, voiced inhalations, difficult breathing	10.56*
Bronchial asthma, allergic dermatitis & food allergy	Breathiness, breathiness & hyponasality	39.49†
Bronchial asthma, atopic dermatitis & allergic rhinitis	Hoarseness, low vocal intensity	80.00†
Allergic rhinitis & urticaria	Low vocal intensity & breathiness	12.48†

*Significant at $p \leq 0.01$.
†Significant at $p \leq 0.001$.

The observed frequencies of specific allergic disorders and misarticulations were cast into a 2 x 2 contingency table to test the null hypothesis of no difference between the two groups. The alternative hypothesis was that a specific allergic disorder or disorders were significantly related to certain types of misarticulations or vocal quality disorders. The region of rejection consisted of all x^2 values so large that the probability associated with their occurrence was equal to or less than $\alpha = 0.05$. If a significant difference was obtained, it was concluded that the specific allergic disorder was found more frequently in conjunction with a specific misarticulation or vocal quality disorder.

RESULTS

In this population of 80 individuals, almost 50% of the subjects had vocal quality and/or articulatory errors (Table 1); 21% had both vocal quality and articulatory errors, 11 patients had reduced auditory acuity; no evidence was found of a fluency disorder (Table 1).

When the vocal quality disorders were broken down to type of disorder, most patients exhibited hoarseness (10%), breathiness (7.5%), hyponasality (6.25%) or low vocal intensity (3.75%), with most of the remaining patients having a combination of these disorders.

The significant chi square values listed in Table 2 indicate that bronchial asthma, either singly or in conjunction with other disorders, was related to vocal quality disorders in 6 of 7 patients. Allergic rhinitis, the only significant value not involving bronchial asthma, was significantly related to low vocal intensity accompanied by breathiness.

The articulation error analysis revealed a total of 136 errors distributed among 80 errors in blacks and 56 in whites. The errors ranged from 1-17 with a mean number of 1.7 errors for all patients.

All 11 patients with hearing loss at the time of the evaluation had allergic rhinitis either singly or in association with another disorder (Table 3). The range of the conductive type of hearing loss was 15 to 40 dB. This was found consistently across all subjects in the low frequency range of 250 to 500 cps.

TABLE 3. RELATIONSHIP OF HEARING LOSS TO ALLERGY DISORDER AND VOCAL QUALITY AND MISARTICULATIONS

Subject No.	*Diagnosed Allergy*	*Misarticulations No.*	*Misarticulations Type*	*Type of Vocal Quality Disorders*
1	AR, BA	0	—	—
2	AR	8	S	—
3	AR	4	1 S, 3 Om	Low frequency
4	AR, U, AD	0	—	—
5	AR	8	S	Hoarse
6	AR, ATD	1	Om	—
7	AR	4	3 S, 1 Om	—
8	AR	1	Om	Hoarse
9	AR, BA	2	S	—
10	AR, BA	1	S	—
11	AR, BA	2	1 S, 1 Om	Low intensity
N = 11	AR, BA, U, AD, ATD	31	24 S, 7 Om	Low intensity, low frequency, hoarseness

AR - Allergic rhinitis; BA - Bronchial asthma; U - Urticaria; AD - Allergic dermatitis; ATD - Atopic dermatitis; S - Substitutions; Om - Omissions.

Four of the subjects had a 15 dB hearing loss in all frequencies tested. Two subjects exhibited a 20 dB loss at 4,000 and 8,000 Hz. Nine of the 11 patients had articulation errors; 4 of the 11 had accompanying vocal quality disorders (Table 3). Case history analysis revealed that the two patients with neither disorder had essentially normal hearing with a slight hearing loss at higher frequencies.

In addition, the types of allergies were compared to misarticulations by the use of a chi square test. These test results indicated that allergic rhinitis occurring either singly or in conjunction with other disorders was related to 16 of 18 significant misarticulations. Omission errors were all in the final position and included the sounds s, z, j. The substitution errors were associated with a fronting phenomenon, ie, the tongue was placed in an anterior position within the oral cavity. Perhaps swollen tissue within the respiratory tract thrust the tongue in a forward position for breathing purposes; therefore, resulting in a compensatory speech pattern. An example of the substitution errors is t substituted for ch (t/ch); s/sh; z/sh; and f/th. Bronchial asthma and bronchial asthma associated with other disorders had only two significant misarticulations. Three of the five patients with allergic rhinitis and misarticulations also had a hearing loss. Specifically, the three significant speech sound omission relationships involved a hearing loss.

DISCUSSION

The percentage (44.75%) of vocal quality disorders is between five and ten times greater than the percentage (6%) found in mass screenings in the St. Louis metropolitan area.[2] Although the type of vocal disorders was not discussed, the authors note that a family history of allergy occurred in over 25% of the children with diagnosed vocal quality disorders. Significantly, however, a history of respiratory infection or allergic rhinitis occurred frequently in children with vocal quality disorders. These authors suggest that chronic allergic rhinosinusitis may predispose a child to recurrent hoarseness and/or eventual development of benign lesions of the true vocal cords because of the inflammatory changes that produce hoarseness, breathiness, whisper and stridency. In a related study, Yairi et al[9] found a high incidence of nasal allergies in children with chronic hoarseness.

In this study, bronchial asthma was associated with the most frequently found vocal quality disorders suggesting that both bronchial asthma and allergic rhinitis result in vocal quality disorders. Allergic rhinitis in conjunction with the other disorders was associated with hoarseness, breathiness and low vocal intensity.

The specific cause of the disorders was not the subject of this investigation; however, it is generally recognized that allergic reactions often result in either localized or edematous swellings.[3] If the respiratory tract is involved, the vocal cords also may develop edema and inflammation.[4]

These factors are potentially important for the speech-language pathologist and otolaryngologist in the evaluation and management of vocal quality disorders. If chronic or persistent hoarseness is the reason for therapy, the possibility of allergy as the cause should be evaluated carefully, along with other causes of edema such as disease, trauma, medication and hormonal imbalance. The importance of analyzing these factors is aptly summarized by Moore,[14] who states that the remediation of voice disorders encompasses more than voice assessment and vocal exercises.

The data obtained in this study on error categories of substitutions and distortions are similar to that of Templin[15] for normative data. Omission errors (15% of total), however, were about three times higher than the 5% recorded for children 8 years of age. As noted in the results section, these increased values are also related to the incidence of hearing loss in subjects with allergic rhinitis. The presence of speech sound omissions in allergy patients 8 years of age or older may be indicative of a fluctuating hearing loss and/or other causative factors.

The finding of allergic rhinitis in association with diminished hearing and misarticulations is not surprising since the literature is replete with reports of allergic rhinitis affecting the eustachian tube and middle ear.[1,5,7] Allergic rhinitis can result in diminished hearing and, when chronic, lead to the development of serous otitis media. It has been estimated that serous otitis may occur in 66% of children who have allergic rhinitis.[7] The presence of fluid in the middle ear causes a conductive hearing loss which may range as high as 20-30 dB.[16] It is difficult to detect this type of hearing loss because it is often transient and fluctuating.[6] If this fluctuating hearing loss is present in the early years when articulation is developing, delayed or faulty speech may result.[7] Thus, it is not uncommon for a young child with allergic rhinitis to have a history of delayed speech development.[6]

These results may imply that children with allergic rhinitis should receive audiological analysis as well as articulation analysis. In addition, it might be appropriate for children producing misarticulations to receive impedance screening. The audiogram obtained by use of impedance audiometry is useful in determining whether there is current hearing loss. If impedance audiometry had been used in this study to test hearing levels, the incidence of auditory pathology might have been higher because some children can pass a pure tone screening at 25 dB HL and still possess symptomatology of otitis media.

An articulation analysis may be suggestive of a previous hearing loss or a fluctuating hearing loss. The key factor in the analysis would be the presence of numerous substitutions and omissions in children 8 years of age or older. Substitutions and omissions are characteristic of immature articulation. This could suggest the possibility of a fluctuating hearing loss even with a normal audiogram.

REFERENCES

1. Halpern SR. Nasal allergy in children. Eye Ear Nose Throat Mon 1961; 40:259-62.

2. Senturia BH, Wilson FB. Otorhinolaryngic findings in children with voice deviations. Ann Otol Rhinol Laryngol 1948; 77:1027-41.

3. Clemis JD, Derlacki EL. Allergy of the upper respiratory tract. Otolaryngol Clin North Am 1970; 3:265-76.

4. Pang LQ. Allergy of the larynx, trachea, and bronchial tree. Otolaryngol Clin North Am 1974; 7:719-34.

5. Draper WL. Allergy in relationship to the eustachian tube and middle ear. Otolaryngol Clin North Am 1974; 7:749-55.

6. Szanton VL. Allergy and serous otitis media. W Va Med J 1967; 63:108-10.

7. Szanton VL, Szanton WC. Hearing disturbances in allergic children. J Asthma Res 1966; 4:25-9.

8. Szanton VL, Szanton WC. Allergic paracusis: new allergic syndrome. NY State J Med 1962; 62:3112-5.

9. Yairi E, Currin LH, Bulian N, Yairi J. Incidence of hoarseness in school children over a 1 year period. J Commun Disord 1974; 7:321-8.

10. Baynes RA. An incidence study of chronic hoarseness among children. J Speech Hear Disord 1976; 31:172-6.

11. Templin MC. Developmental aspects of articulation. In: Wolfe WD, Goulding DJ, eds. Articulation and learning. Springfield: Charles C Thomas, 1973:51-82.

12. Johnson W, Darley FL, Spriesterbach DC. Diagnostic methods in speech pathology. New York: Harper & Row, 1963.

13. Northern JL, Downs MP. Hearing in children. Baltimore: Williams & Wilkins, 1978.

14. Moore GP. Organic voice disorders. Englewood Cliffs: Prentice-Hall, 1971.

15. Templin MC. Certain language skills in children, their development and interrelationships. Institute of child welfare monograph, No. 26. Minneapolis: University of Minnesota Press, 1957.

16. Rapp, DJ, Fahey DJ. Chronic otitis and allergy. J Asthma Res 1973; 10:193-218.

MALLEUS HANDLE PROBE

A MIDDLE EAR DIAGNOSTIC PROCEDURE

R. BRUCE DUNCAN, FRCS, FRACS

PALMERSTON NORTH, NEW ZEALAND

Manual probing of the malleus handle (MH) of 477 patients suggests a protective middle ear reflex with a variable tonic contraction of the tensor tympani muscle (TTM). The degree and type of MH retraction suggests three stages of progressive middle ear inflammation. Prediction accuracy of 250 myringotomy findings was 60% with impedance audiometry and 92% with MH probing. Mechanical pressure gauge readings (grams) of 202 ears correlated with finger pressure estimations. The TTM tendons were sectioned in ten children with persisting otitis media with effusion (OME) and seven obtained benefit. The three diagnostic methods, pneumatic otoscopy, impedance audiometry and MH probing, assess similar and separate perimeters and are complementary. Malleus handle probing alone detects attic loculation of OME, 54 of 954 ears (5.6%). It extends the diagnostic range to the TTM activities.

INTRODUCTION

I began sectioning the tensor tympani muscle (TTM) tendon to free the malleus handle (MH) for middle ear reconstruction surgery in 1955. Rosen's paper on stapes mobilization described probing of the stapes.[1] This suggested routine MH probing at the commencement of ear surgery. The range of movement and resistance to MH probing often correlated with drum scarring, retraction pockets, middle ear adhesions and tympanosclerosis. Its use was limited in otosclerosis. During 1962, five marine diesel engineers were examined one hour after finishing their shift. All drums were retracted and on probing the MH was fixed. Topical anesthesia was used. The Valsalva maneuver was easily performed with movements of the pars tensa. The TTM had retracted the MH and also facilitated air entry during the Valsalva maneuver. I began routine MH probing prior to myringotomy for otitis media with effusion (OME) in 1968. MH probing predicted OME changes with a practical degree of accuracy. I suspected TTM tonic contraction from the inflammation of OME. I began a dissection program of the bony auditory tube (BAT), TTM and semicanal lamina (SCL) in fresh and preserved temporal bones. The results of dissection of 146 temporal bones are reported elsewhere.

METHODS

Adult MHs are probed with a disposable or metal instrument (Fig. 1) in the office using a topical anesthetic. Bonain solution (equal parts of cocaine phenol and menthol) or iontophoresis of 2% lidocaine are the preferred anesthetics. General anesthesia is required for young or nervous children. MH probing is followed by myringotomy if required. The disposable probe (Jefferson Products Ltd, PO Box 10-010, Wellington, NZ) is placed on the MH, 1 or 2 mm above the umbo and slowly increasing finger pressure is exerted. Movement of the MH is accompanied by a change of light reflection from the drum surface, movement of the MH and lateral process of the malleus. During 1980 a mechanical pressure gauge with a detachable sterile metal probe recorded the force applied. The angle and shape of the detachable probe was identical to the manual probe. The drum epithelium would not tolerate pressures over 70 g. The results were converted to force on the MH using the formula: Force grams on MH = gauge "give-way" force x cosine 35°. It is estimated that the error is less than 10%.

The normal MH yields slowly to a probing force of 10 to 18 g and the displacement medially can be seen and felt (Fig. 2A). The MH returns promptly to the preprobing position. Occasionally the normal MHs of children and adults require considerable force before yielding, up to 45 g. Restricted MH movements (Fig. 2B) are felt as a gradual yielding resistance to a force of 40 to 58 g, with a reduction of medial displacement because there is already some retraction from the TTM and protective reflex. The MH will return slowly to the preprobe position of retraction or remain retracted after probing for 6 to 48 hours. The fixed handle (Fig. 2C) is rigid on probing and will not yield to a force of 65-70 g. Probing has rarely produced an ecchymosis on the MH. I have not detected any MH delayed erosion or granulation ulcer in approximately 2200 probings. Audiograms before and after MH probing have not shown any acoustic trauma.

The survey comprised 477 patients seen during a 3-year period (Table 1). The first subgroup is a control of 82 children with normal ears who had general anesthesia for other procedures. The second subgroup of 96 patients had the MH give-way force measured by a pressure gauge. The third subgroup of 125 patients had impedance audiometry (Madson ZS76/1 and 220 Hz) recorded before operation. Prediction of the middle ear pathology using impedance audiometry and MH probing were compared with findings at myringotomy (Table 2). Most children were in the 4 to 8 age group, but ages did range from 2 to 14. Anterior myringotomy and occasionally incision of the anterior or posterior membrana flaccida was performed. Loculated mucus may be present in an aerated middle ear after anterior myringotomy. Some degree of MH retraction is always present with OME. A 20 gauge suction needle with a 2 mm foot is introduced and cautiously placed behind the posterior quadrants of the drum. It is then moved to behind the anterosuperior quadrant. If loculation is suspected in Prussak space or the attic, incision of the membrana flaccida anteriorly or posteriorly is performed. The quantity of mucus aspirated is greater than the capacity of Prussak space and must be supplemented from other attic loculations. An air-filled mesotympanum may discharge mucus when dependent, so re-examine after completing myringotomy on the other ear. Mucus in the auditory tube of an air-filled mesotympanum may be detected escaping from the torus in the mirror view of postnasal space. The position of the MH is the balance of force between the TTM tonic contraction and the resistance of the drum

From the Department of Otolaryngology, Palmerston North Hospital, Palmerston North, New Zealand.

REPRINTS — R. Bruce Duncan, FRCS, FRACS, 233 Broadway Avenue, Palmerston North, New Zealand.

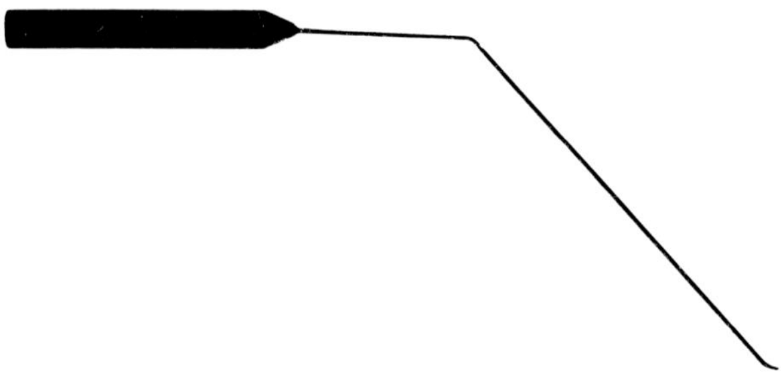

Fig. 1. Malleus handle probe.

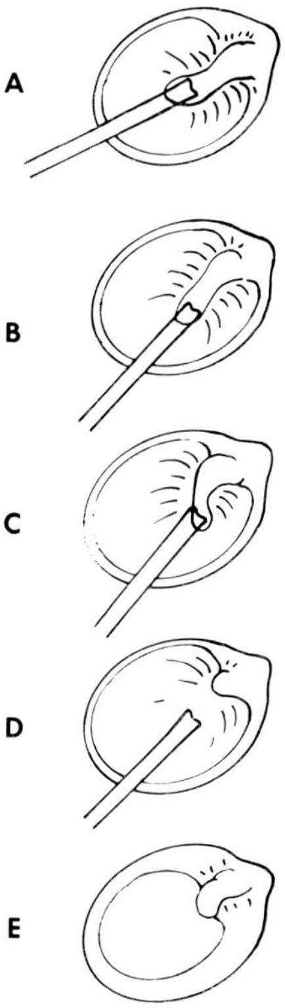

	Handle	Middle Ear	Procedure
A	Normal mobile and returns; rarely fixed	Air Air	Nil Nil
B	Restricted movement; slow return	Air or trace of fluid	Nil unless long-standing
C	Fixed; no return	Fluid; if not suspect compartment fluid	Venting tube Venting tube
D	Fixed or freely mobile when located in edematous drum; probe cautiously	Fluid; mucopus	Venting tube
E	Fixed or very mobile	Dry or attic infected fluid	Suction probe attic fluid

Fig. 2. Malleus handle probing technique and interpretations. A) Normal handle. B) Restricted movement. C) Fixed handle. D) Edematous drum. E) Central perforation and handle stump.

and ossicular ligaments. Serous effusion appears to provoke less TTM contraction force than a mucoid effusion. The MH-measured give-way force has some correlation with finger pressure groupings and the state of the middle ear. This is a practical guide because the use of pressure gauges during normal operating conditions is cumbersome.

RESULTS

The two groups of 325 normal mobile ears, 34.2% of the total survey, had 3 middle ears with a trace of effusion (Table 1). Subgroup of 198 ears had the MH probed with a mechanical pressure gauge and included 6 ears with ossicular fixation and normal middle ears. There were 43 (22.4%) normal ears, 12 (6.2%) had normal ears and slight retraction, 52 (27.1%) had air with a trace of effusion and 76 (39.6%) had middle ear effusion. The third subgroup, 125 patients (Table 2), had impedance audiometry on admission or within 1-4 days of operation (92%). The remainder were country patients with a time lag of 5-21 days before operation. The prediction error was 40% for tympanometry and 6% for MH probing. When both methods were combined the error improved to 3%. The C type tympanogram (Jerger) was the main cause of impedance prediction failure. Probe failures were 72 ears or 7.6%. The causes of MH probing prediction failures were:

1. Loculation of OME, in particular Prussak space and possibly attic loculation. Occasionally there was air in the mesotympanum with a thick layer of tenacious mucoid effusion on the promontory and on the undersurface of the myringotomy incision.

2. An edematous drum with no handle landmarks may be assessed as mobile because the fixed handle is not located by the probe (Fig. 2D).

3. The patient had not been adequately sedated before anesthesia, ie, a struggling, crying child may empty much of the middle ear effusion but still have a retracted handle.

4. Chronic OME with localized drum edema and a "floppy" MH suggests TTM atony, with a poor prognosis.

TENSOR TYMPANI MUSCLE

The TTM and tensor veli palatini muscle (TPM) are digastric.[2] The TTM evolved as a tubal and temporal muscle.[3] In man the temporal portion has disappeared, leaving the tubal portion as a spindle-shaped muscle occupying the semicanal. The tubal muscle is vestigial in the dog and cat which have the temporal muscle arising from a fossa on the medial wall of the middle ear.[4] The results of studies on the TTM activity of these animals may not apply to man. The TTM contains two types of striated muscle and is supplied by the autonomic system and trigeminal nerve.[5] Tetanic contraction of the TTM occurs as a startle, fatigable reflex from stimulation of the orbital skin or lingual nerve.[6] The tonic contraction is complex and regulates middle ear capacity by retracting or relaxing the MH and drum. The tympanic glomus bodies may form part of this pressure regulating system.[7] The TTM assists the TPM in opening the auditory tube.[8] Autopsy findings suggest it has an effect on the flexible isthmus roof of infants.[9] I surmise from clinical and autopsy evidence that there is an additional protective reflex initiated by inflammation of the auditory tube and middle ear. This reflex causes TTM tonic contraction with retraction of the MH and opening of the isthmus until resolution of the process occurs. The protective reflex may be abolished by chronic inflammation presumably of the TTM belly causing a floppy MH in an edematous drum. The TTM is relatively larger in the infant and I suggest this is because of the action on the isthmus roof, a narrow SCL and poor leverage of the TTM tendon inserting

TABLE 1. PATIENTS GROUPED BY FINGER SENSATION AND MECHANICAL PRESSURE GAUGE WITH MIDDLE EAR DISEASE* (N = 477)

Handle Mobility	*Middle Ear Condition*	*Finger Pressure*	*Pressure Gauge No.*	*Pressure Range(g)*	*Pressure Average(g)*
Mobile control	Normal	164			
Mobile	Air	158	43	12-25	16.5
	Trace of effusion	3*	1		24.4
Very slight restriction	Air	52	12	25-36	28.9
	Trace of	15	6	25-54	36.0
	effusion	6*	—		
Restricted movement	Air	42*	7	36-49	46.0
	Trace of fluid	45	14	30-54	45.0
	Effusion	2	1		42.5
Very slight movement	Air	12	—		
	Trace of effusion	59	12	42-61	52.5
		28	10	48-67	50.0
Fixed	Air	9*	2	48-61	54.0
	Trace of effusion	57	19	42-67	61.0
		289	65	49-73	64.0
Excluded		13	6		
Total		954	198		

*Probe diagnostic failures - 7.6%.

at 60° or greater angle into the neck of the malleus.[9] The autopsy evidence of TTM prolapse into the BAT lumen suggests that chronic tubal inflammation may involve the large TTM of children when the SCL and isthmus are closed by a thin membrane. The edematous TTM obstructs the superior portion of the BAT lumen but not the inferior. Chronic inflammatory obstruction may lead to adhesions and submucosal fibrosis of the BAT. Eight fresh cadaver ears had edematous obstructing TTM, a fibrous SCL and OME.[9] It is suggested that adults with SCL dehiscences could suffer a degree of edema and prolapse of the TTM after descent from altitude or ascent from scuba diving.

LOCULATION OF MIDDLE EAR EFFUSION

OME may be loculated in Prussak's space, the attic and between tympanic folds. This localized effusion and inflammation causes TTM retraction of the MH. The MH is fixed on probing and myringotomy reveals air in the middle ear and inflamed, often polypoid, mucosa on the promontory. Impedance audiometry is unable to detect loculated OME. The membrana flaccida is cautiously incised anteriorly or posteriorly and if mucus is released, a fine venting tube (VT) is placed anteriorly. The VTs extrude in three to nine months but Sadé[10] reports a longer duration. Loculation of OME was detected in 54 attics (5.6%). Loculated OME did not resolve with

TABLE 2. PREDICTION IN 250 MYRINGOTOMIES IN 125 PATIENTS IN WHICH IMPEDANCE AND MALLEUS PROBING USED

Impedance and probe correct	142	56.8%
Impedance incorrect, probe correct	91	36.4%
Impedance correct, probe incorrect	8	6.0%
Impedance incorrect, probe incorrect	7	
Drum perforated no impedance, probe correct	2	0.8%
	250	100.0%

simple myringotomy, and if it is present or there is a clinical suspicion of it, a VT is placed. At follow-up visits the degree of handle retraction usually indicates the stage of recovery.

CASE REPORT

An 8-year-old female had been bottle fed in a propped position and had developed positional otitis media. Adenotonsillectomy at age $3^1/_2$ gave no relief and VTs were inserted a year later. Profuse discharge persisted and after three months the VTs were extruded. The patient was first seen at age 5 and an allergic workup produced improvement in nasal function and reinsertion of the VTs was performed three months later. The ears continued to discharge intermittently and the VTs were extruded at age 6. Three months later the TTM tendons were sectioned and VTs replaced. Ear discharge became less frequent and the VTs were removed at age 7. The hearing has averaged 20 dB loss for the last two years and during the last year the Valsalva maneuver does not cause MH movement.

Comment. Profuse drainage from the ears followed insertion of VTs at age $4^1/_2$ and this continued until the TTM tendons were sectioned. Improvement in drainage and hearing was rapid, although the child was reaching the age when spontaneous improvement could be expected.

Obstruction of the air channel of the BAT is a diagnosis by exclusion. If OME persists despite repeated insertions of VTs, then a section of the TTM tendon should be contemplated before cortical mastoidectomy and inspection of the aditus. It is technically impossible to denervate the TTM and piecemeal removal would be hazardous. Ten children with OME had TTM tendon section, with clinical restoration of tubal function in 7, partial in 1, and 2 failures. Cortical mastoidectomy was later performed on the failures.

INTERPRETATION OF MALLEUS PROBING RESULTS

MH probing responses reflect three continuing stages of progressive middle ear disease. Intermittent OME has a degree of fixed handle on palpation, but after myringotomy with or without VT insertion, there is a return to normal handle position within 6 to 48 hours. The second stage is chronic OME with sustained TTM contraction. It is several days following myringotomy and VT insertion before the handle returns to the normal position. A persistence of retraction suggests OME loculation in the middle ear or obstruction and inflammation is continuing in the auditory tube. The third stage is a fixed retracted handle that does not return to the normal position after myringotomy and VT insertion. This is observed at follow-up visits and indicates that there is developing contracture and atrophy of the TTM. The infrequent occurring floppy handle and edematous drum with OME is the substage between 2 and 3. Recovery to a normal position following myringotomy and VT insertion (Fig. 2B) is always uncertain. The MH may not return to a normal position following resolution of OME because of 1) loss of the collagenous middle third of the membrana tensa, 2) middle ear adhesions and, I surmise, 3) changes to the ossicular ligaments and 4) changes in the TTM and tendon.

DISCUSSION

The TTM adjusts the drum to varying air capacity of the middle ear cleft. Contraction of the TTM expelling excess air occurs in the normal ear.[11] Bluestone et al[12] suggest a TTM pumping action to adjust middle ear pressure. Loud noise trauma and inflammation of the middle ear cleft cause tonic TTM contraction which disrupts pressure adjustments. Persisting MH retraction suggests a protective middle ear reflex. The reflex involves TTM tonic contraction, probably aided by elastic fibers in its attachment to the semicanal and the intramuscular tendons. This tonic contraction may spread to similar muscle fibers in the TPM restricting its tubal activity.

The politzerization and Valsalva maneuvers do not cause a retracted MH to move when air entry occurs. The membrana tensa movement may give an illusion of handle movement. These maneuvers cause a slight movement of the MH in a normal drum. "Ex vacuo" theory assumes MH retraction is passive. Retraction or bulging of the membrana tensa occurs in OM and OME but MH is retracted. Pneumatic otoscopy and impedance audiometry assesses the damaged or intact membrana tensa. Probing assesses the MH and tensor tympani protective reflex. Jerger[13] observed that impedance audiometry is not accurate in predicting fluid in the mesotympanum. Studies[14,15] assessing impedance and myringotomy confirm this finding. Orchik et al[16] suggest another screening technique is necessary. MH probing is suggested because it is complementary to impedance audiometry and when the two are combined gave a prediction accuracy of 97%. Wullstein[17] describes OME loculation but not the clinical signs. This important condition is easily missed if malleus probing is omitted. Restricted access to the attic via Prussak space and early rejection of VTs are problems, but the procedure is worth performing. Section of the TTM tendon to treat BAT obstruction remains to be evaluated. Loculated effusion in the attic is identified by MH probing. The procedure may reduce the incidence of this sinister condition and also the number of "dry hole" myringotomies.

REFERENCES

1. Rosen S, Bergman M. Mobilization of the stapes for otosclerotic deafness. Arch Otolaryngol 1955; 61:197-206.

2. Lupin AJ. The relationship of the tensor tympani and tensor palati muscles. Ann Otol Rhinol Laryngol 1969; 78:792-6.

3. Pye A, Hinchcliffe R. Comparative anatomy of the ear. Scientific foundations of otolaryngology. Chicago: Year Book Medical, 1976; 194-5.

4. Miller ME, Christensen GC, Evans HE. Anatomy of the dog. Philadelphia: WB Saunders, 1968.

5. Candiollo L. The control mechanism of the middle ear transmission system: the middle ear muscles. Beltone Institute for Hearing Research, Chicago, 1967; 20:14-41.

6. Russolo M, Semerara A. Value of the isolated tensor tympani muscle reflex elicited by electrical lingual stimulation. Audiology 1977; 16:373-9.

7. Sadé J. Secretory otitis media and its sequelae. New York: Churchill Livingstone, 1979: 246.

8. Holborow C. Eustachian tubal function: changes throughout childhood and neuromuscular control. J Laryngol Otol 1975; 89:47-55.

9. Duncan RB. The bony auditory tube and otitis media with effusion. Ann Otol Rhinol Laryngol, 1982 (in press).

10. Sadé J. Secretory otitis media and its sequelae. New York: Churchill Livingstone, 1979:262.

11. Ingelstedt S. Physiology of the eustachian tube. Ann Otol Rhinol Laryngol 1976; 85 Suppl 25:156-60.

12. Bluestone C, Berry Q, Scott Andrus W. Mechanics of the eustachian tube as it influences susceptibility to and persistence of middle ear effusions in children. Ann Otol Rhinol Laryngol 1974; 83 Suppl 11:33.

13. Jerger J. Clinical experiences with impedance audiometry. Arch Otolaryngol 1970; 92:311-24.

14. Haughton P. Validity of tympanometry for middle ear effusions. Arch Otolaryngol 1977; 103:505-13.

15. Grimoldi S. Value of impedance. J Laryngol Otol 1976; 90:141-52.

16. Orchik D, Dunn J, McNutt L. Tympanometry as a predictor of middle ear effusion. Arch Otolaryngol 1978; 104:4-6.

17. Wullstein SR. Histopathological alterations of the mucosal folds in chronic otitis media. Acta Otolaryngol (Stockh) 1976; 81:197-9.

EFFECTIVENESS OF MIDDLE EAR ELECTRICAL STIMULATION FOR ACTIVATING CENTRAL AUDITORY PATHWAYS

BEN M. CLOPTON, PhD MARTHA M. BOSMA, BSc

SEATTLE, WASHINGTON

Electrical stimulation of afferent auditory elements through electrodes placed in the middle ear was investigated in acute guinea pig preparations. Thresholds for auditory activation were current-dependent for low frequencies (< 1 kHz) and charge-dependent at higher frequencies. Threshold currents were 3-5 times those for intracochlear stimulation. Mechanisms of activation were examined with removal of cochlear fluids and injection of neomycin, Xylocaine, saline, and artificial perilymph with different calcium concentrations. Neurons of the spiral ganglion are indicated as mediators of this stimulation.

Intense interest in the amelioration of profound hearing loss has led to both clinical and experimental investigation of alternatives for electrically activating surviving peripheral elements. Most implanted electrode arrays in human patients have consisted of one or more electrodes introduced into the scala tympani through the round window.[1,2] Variations include placements through the lateral wall of the cochlea and in the eighth nerve at the modiolus.[3-6] All of these approaches compromise the integrity of the cochlea, thereby threatening the survival of remaining hair cells and spiral ganglion neurons as well as increasing the possibility of postoperative complications. Invasion of the cochlea may also be detrimental to the later use of improved implantation techniques and devices for a patient.

There is no consensus, at present, about the greater utility of multichannel as opposed to single-channel implant devices. While it can be assumed to be advantageous to stimulate selectively separate fiber groups near the round window of the afferent neural array, there is a clear indication that few excitable elements will survive in the basal turn of many candidates for cochlear prostheses.[7-10] Unpredictable survival of these elements would prevent the reliable activation of independent channels with a prosthesis inserted into the scala tympani. In addition, the dynamic range for restricted stimulation is small due to current spread,[11] so it is likely that relatively massive stimulation of remaining afferent fibers occurs in many cases. Single-channel, middle ear implants are thus attractive in light of current limits on the efficacy and possible long-term side effects of intracochlear, multichannel stimulation.

It has in fact been argued, primarily by investigators in England,[11,12] that activation of cochlear elements by electrodes placed in the middle ear has significant advantages at the present time over implants that invade the cochlea. Some patients have been implanted with electrodes near the round window with promising results.[12] The current paper reports investigations with guinea pigs where systematic variation in the placement of electrodes in the middle ear and other experimental manipulations were used to better define this avenue of auditory stimulation. The manipulations included monopolar versus bipolar square-wave stimulation, change in the frequency of sinusoidal stimulating waveforms, removal and replacement of cochlear fluids, and the introduction of an ototoxic agent and a local anesthetic. The aim was to provide an initial survey of the middle ear stimulation technique in order to increase understanding of this form of stimulation.

METHODS

Experimental Animals and Surgical Procedures. One dozen pigmented guinea pigs ranging in weight from 250-350 g were used for these experiments. A presurgical dose of atropine sulfate (0.8 mg/kg) was given IP, and surgical anesthesia was accomplished with IM injections of ketamine hydrochloride (Vetelar, 100 mg/kg) and xylazine hydrochloride (Rompun, 20 mg/kg). Anesthesia was maintained with a 4:1 mixture of Vetelar (100 mg/ml) and Rompun (20 mg/ml) administered IM. The head was stabilized by attaching a small bolt to the rostral skull with dental acrylic and stainless steel screws threaded into the bone. A small silver-wire electrode was placed on the brachium of the inferior colliculus contralateral to the experimental ear for recording electrically evoked responses at the collicular level. A reference silver electrode was placed in brain tissue rostral to the collicular site. The bulla surrounding the middle ear was opened and the middle ear cavity widely exposed.

Electrode Placements. Both bipolar and monopolar stimulation techniques were used. Monopolar stimulation was between an electrode on the cochlea and a hemostat on a neck muscle. Stimulating electrodes were made of platinum-iridium wire coated with Teflon. The wire was 0.127 mm in diameter with one end flamed to produce a small ball about 0.5 mm in diameter, the Teflon insulation extending to the ball. The electrodes were held by micromanipulators for positioning with the aid of a Wild operating microscope. The electrodes were positioned at various points on the medial surface of the middle ear, each placement

From the Department of Otolaryngology, School of Medicine, University of Washington, Seattle. This work was supported by a grant from NIH.

REPRINTS — Ben M. Clopton, PhD, Department of Otolaryngology, School of Medicine, University of Washington, Seattle, WA 98195.

being photographed with a Wild camera attached to the operating microscope. Projection of the photographic transparencies later provided documentation of the exact placement of the electrodes to supplement descriptions recorded during the experiment.

Stimulation Parameters. All stimulation waveforms were of constant current generated by a stimulator producing 1 μA of output current for 1 mV of input voltage.[13] Both single-cycle sinusoidal and monophasic square pulses of variable duration and polarity were employed as stimulating waveforms. The presentation rate was 10/s. These transient stimuli allowed the recording of evoked potentials on the brachium after the end of the associated artifact. The use of single cycles of a sinusoid permitted neural thresholds to be related to the frequency of stimulation. Polarity reversals were used to investigate differential sensitivities to direction of current flow. The sinusoidal stimuli covered up to six octaves from 250 Hz to 16 kHz in octave steps, and the duration of square waves ranged from 25 to 1600 μs through doubling, a 200 μs duration being used in most cases. Care was taken to keep DC baseline stimulation levels to a minimum, usually less than 1 μA. Current through the electrodes was monitored as voltage across a 1 kΩ resistor in series with the output of the stimulator with a high-impedance oscilloscope.

Cochlear Manipulations. Cochlear manipulations included the removal of fluids in the scala tympani and scala vestibuli by gentle suction at the round window after opening the oval window, the introduction of neomycin sulfate to destroy hair cells, the addition of a 2% Xylocaine solution to inactivate neural elements, and the manipulation of the concentration of calcium in artificial perilymph used to replace the perilymph that was removed. A saturated solution of neomycin sulfate was introduced into the cochlea by injection of 0.1 cc through the round window or by perfusion of 0.5 cc through aspiration at the round window of fluid introduced at the oval window. The neomycin was left in the cochlea at least 30 minutes before stimulation. Lidocaine (Xylocaine hydrochloride, 2% solution) was perfused through the cochlea and left for 15 to 20 minutes before testing. Physiological saline or artificial perilymph[14] was sometimes introduced into a cochlea after perilymph had been aspirated from the scalae as a control procedure for fluid replacement. The concentration of calcium in the artificial perilymph varied from none present to twice normal, normal being 1.3 m*M*. In addition to estimating thresholds to the stimulation of the middle ear surfaces after these various manipulations, some cochleas were opened with a Kerr drill so as to expose the turns of the cochlea and allow stimulation of the spiral lamina or, with further exposure, the eighth nerve in the modiolus.

Evoked-Potential Thresholds. The evoked tract potential at the brachium of the inferior colliculus is a sensitive indicator of activation at the contralateral ear. It has the advantage of having 2 to 4 times the amplitude of brainstem potential recorded from the vertex with a less complex, usually triphasic waveform. This potential was averaged with a dwell time of 40 μs for 10.24 ms after a stimulus onset with a Nicolet Med-80 computer. Thresholds were estimated manually by adjusting the amplitude of the electrical stimulation using a Hewlett-Packard 350D attenuator and determining the intensity at which the evoked potential was just detectable against the background noise on the cathode-ray computer display. Because of the high signal-to-noise ratio and very rapid rise in response magnitude with stimulus intensity, this determination could usually be independently replicated to within ± 2 dB. It was found that threshold estimates were stable for averages of 50 or more stimulus presentations, so an automated, repeating sequence of 50 response averages provided a basis for manually adjusting stimulus intensity to threshold.

RESULTS

Waveforms. The thresholds of evoked potentials had a predictable relationship to the frequency of single-cycle sinusoids. Bipolar stimulation between the apex and base of a normal cochlea was characterized by an increase in threshold intensity with frequency (Fig. 1). This growth was 3-4 dB/octave for frequencies between 250 and 2,000 Hz and 4.5-7 dB/octave for frequencies from 2,000 to 16,000 Hz. A slope of 6 dB/octave would conform to threshold mechanisms responding proportionately to the amount of charge delivered. The departure from this slope at frequencies below 2,000 Hz was apparent in all normal cochleas. The artifact produced by electrical stimulation sometimes precluded the collection of data at frequencies below 500 Hz, 250 Hz being the lowest frequency practical for data collection.

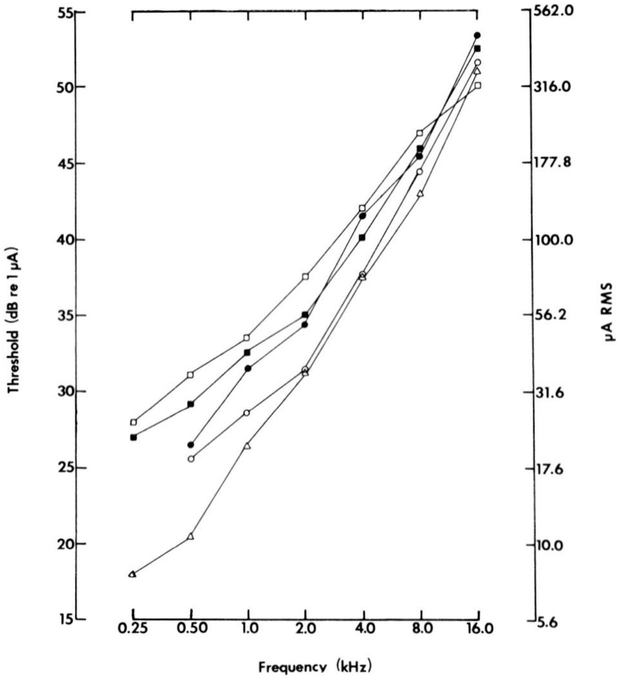

Fig. 1. Relationship of electrical threshold for neural activation to the frequency of a single-cycle sinusoid. Neural activation was measured as a tract response at the brachium of the inferior colliculus contralateral to the ear stimulated. Stimulation was between 2 electrodes, 1 at the apex and 1 just caudal to the round window. The results from five normal cochleas are shown to illustrate the variability in thresholds encountered between animals. Electrical artifact prevented collection of data at 250 Hz for two preparations. RMS - Root-mean-square.

The relationship of threshold to the duration of monopolar square pulses agreed with the sinusoidal results. For pulses with durations from 25 to 200 μs, the threshold decreased by approximately 4.8 dB for each doubling (Fig. 2). For durations in excess of 200 μs up to 1,600 μs, the threshold dropped by approximately 2.3 dB for each doubling. Because of the especially rich frequency content of monopolar square pulses, it is impractical to speak of a major frequency component but a doubling of duration shifts all components upward by one octave for every halving of the duration.

Figure 3 illustrates the relationships between the charge per pulse required for threshold and the frequency of a sinusoid or duration of a pulse. Long-

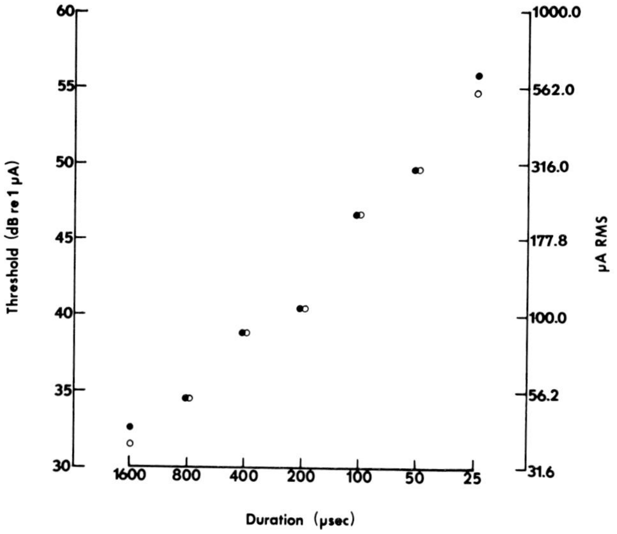

Fig. 2. Threshold for electrical activation versus duration of a monophasic pulse delivered through bipolar, base-apex electrodes. Little difference was seen in this preparation for the thresholds of neural activation between the two directions of current passage. These results are in agreement with those for single-cycle sinusoids. RW - Round window. Current direction: ○ - Apex to RW, ● - RW to apex.

duration pulses and low-frequency sinusoids have lower thresholds relative to the rate at which charge is passed through an electrode (current). High-frequency sinusoids and short-duration pulses clearly tend to be more efficient in evoking a response relative to the amount of charge delivered in a single pulse. In short, the stimulation process shifts from charge dependence toward current dependence as the frequency of sinusoids decreases below 1 kHz or the duration of monopolar square pulses exceeds 200 μs.

Extracochlear Electrode Position. Electrode placement on the outer surface of the cochlea and surrounding middle ear loci accounted for variations in threshold of up to 20 dB and more. The polarity of monophasic pulses delivered to monopolar electrodes also had significant effects for some preparations. Although many electrode placements were not characterized by polarity effects on threshold, 3 dB changes in threshold were common with polarity reversals and some sites showed polarity effects of 8 to 10 dB. Anodal monophasic pulses were usually more effective than cathodal pulses over most of the surface of the cochlea (Fig. 4). While some individual variability was seen, minimum thresholds were associated with the second and third turns of the cochlea. A focus of lowest thresholds was invariably seen near the center of these turns or near the apex. Foci of low thresholds were also common on the surface of the first turn or near the round window. Monopolar maps (Fig. 4) were used as initial guides for the placement of bipolar electrodes. Differences in threshold between the monopolar stimulation to a distant reference and bipolar stimulation for two electrodes on

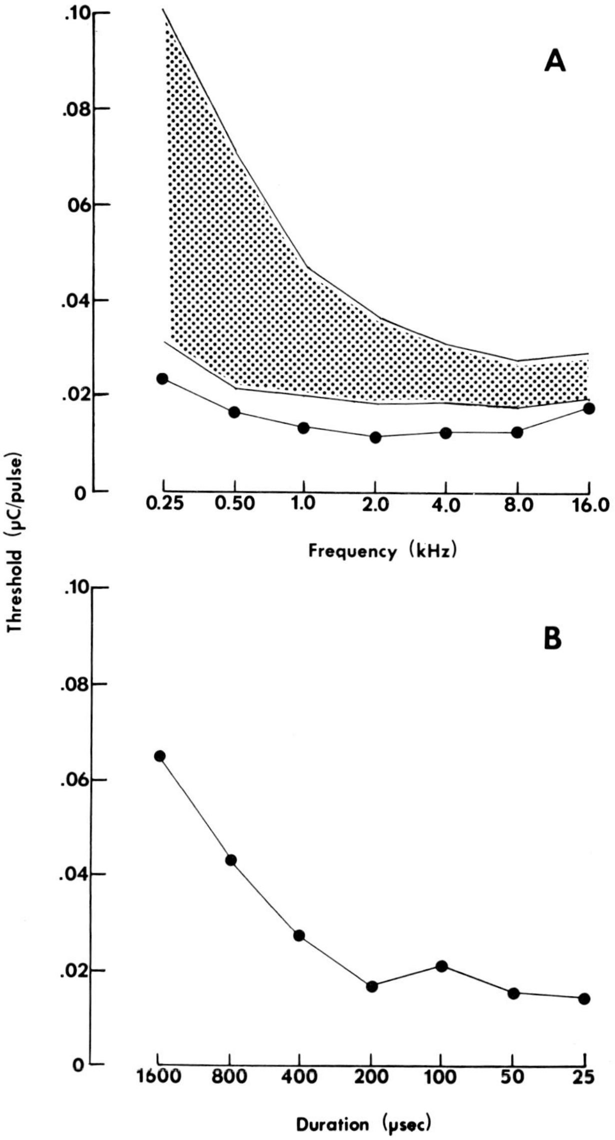

Fig. 3. Relationship between the charge transferred per pulse required for neural activation and the frequency or duration of a stimulus. A) The range of thresholds for normal cochleas to single-cycle sinusoids shown as shaded. The lower line indicates the averaged reduced thresholds for three cochleas after the removal of perilymph. B) The relationship of threshold, expressed as charge per pulse, to the duration of a square-wave stimulus is similar to that seen for single-cycle sinusoids. While duration cannot be strictly related to frequency because of the rich frequency content of the monophasic pulses, the similarity in the relationships suggests a common mechanism that is primarily dependent on the amount of charge delivered at higher frequencies with a decrease in effectiveness for this charge delivery or utilization at lower frequencies resulting in a current-dependent relationship.

the surface of the cochlea were often in excess of 5 dB. Figure 5 illustrates thresholds for various bipolar placements. Exploration with bipolar pairs on a number of animals revealed that a highly effective placement of bipolar electrodes was between the apex of the cochlea and a point just caudal to the round window at the vestibule. This base-apex bipolar placement was used in many preparations for

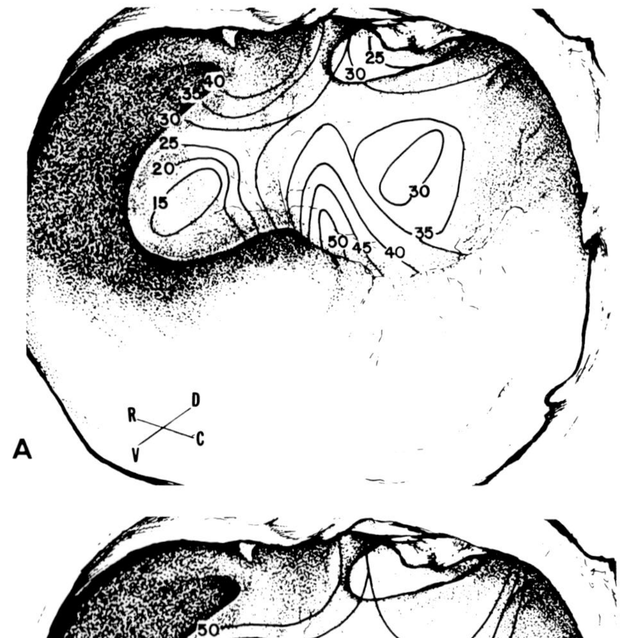

Fig. 4. Threshold contour maps for A) anodal and B) cathodal monophasic, monopolar square pulses of 200 μs duration. Thresholds are in peak μA. At most loci, anodal stimuli were more effective, but caudal to the round window and at sites off the outer surface of the cochlea points were often most effectively stimulated by cathodal pulses. R - Rostral; D - Dorsal; V - Ventral; C - Caudal.

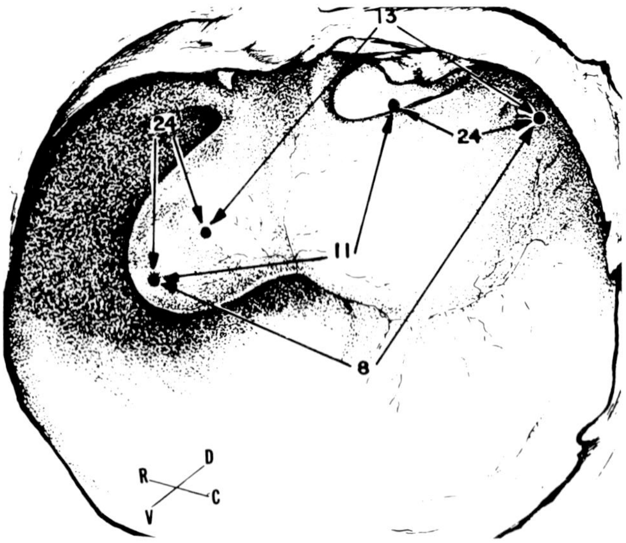

Fig. 5. Thresholds in μA for some placements of bipolar electrodes in one animal. The stimulus was a 200 μs square pulse of the optimal polarity. The threshold for the most distant pair for single-cycle sinusoids was 10 μA at 4 kHz, and 2 μA at 500 Hz. R, D, V, C - as in Fig. 4.

the investigation of the effects of cochlear manipulations. Thresholds to low-frequency, sinusoidal stimuli at 250 or 500 Hz were commonly in the range of 10 to 30 μA root-mean-square (RMS) for the normal cochlea with this electrode arrangement (Fig. 1).

Cochlear Manipulations. The removal of perilymph by aspiration through the round window after removal of the oval window had a profound effect on the threshold for electrical stimulation. At low frequencies of stimulation, thresholds dropped 10 to 15 dB relative to those for the normal cochlea. At 250 Hz, thresholds of less than 5 μA RMS were commonly seen under this condition corresponding to a charge per pulse of 0.02 μC or less (Fig. 3A). The effect was of lesser magnitude at higher frequencies, when expressed as current, resulting in an increase in the slope of the frequency response function after the perilymph was removed (Figs. 6 and 7). Replacement of the perilymph with physiologic saline did not restore thresholds to the normal range. After removal of perilymph, replacement by physiologic saline resulted in only a few decibels of threshold rise at low frequencies with an increasingly greater effect at higher frequencies.

The replacement of perilymph with an artificial perilymph having no calcium elevated thresholds to within 4 dB of normal, and the addition of calcium to approximately normal concentration reproduced essentially normal thresholds. If the calcium concentration was twice normal, thresholds up to 5 dB above normal were obtained at some frequencies. These results implicate the ionic environment provided by the perilymph as influencing activation of afferent auditory pathways by electrical stimulation.

The introduction of neomycin sulfate into the perilymph or the perfusion of the perilymphatic spaces with a neomycin sulfate solution led to a disappearance of cochlear microphonics evoked by sound stimuli within a few minutes, but slightly lower thresholds to electrical stimuli were obtained. Various sequences of introducing neomycin into the perilymph, perfusing neomycin through the perilymph spaces, and removal of perilymphatic fluids before and after these procedures did not change the relative effects. An ear filled with perilymph and treated with neomycin had thresholds near but slightly below normal, and an ear with the perilymphatic fluid removed had lower thresholds than an ear without the perilymphatic fluid removed regardless of whether it had been treated with neomycin.

The local anesthetic Xylocaine produced a rise in

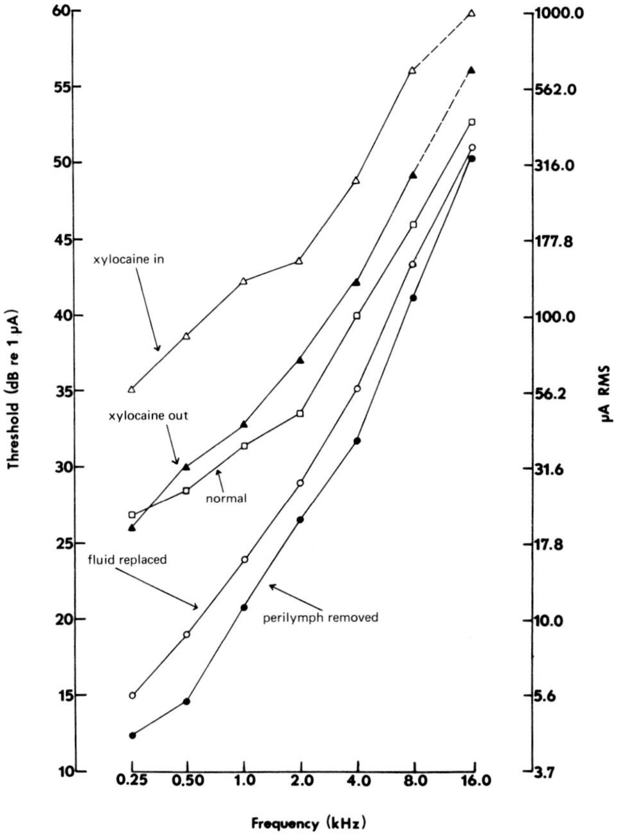

Fig. 6. Thresholds versus frequency of single-cycle sinusoids under various conditions of cochlear manipulation in one animal. Removal of perilymph decreased thresholds at lower frequencies by up to 14 dB. Replacement of the perilymph with physiological saline did not restore thresholds to their original higher levels. The introduction of Xylocaine into the perilymphatic space elevated thresholds to approximately 8 dB above normal after 30 minutes, and the removal of the Xylocaine solution in the perilymphatic space reduced thresholds to near normal within 15 minutes.

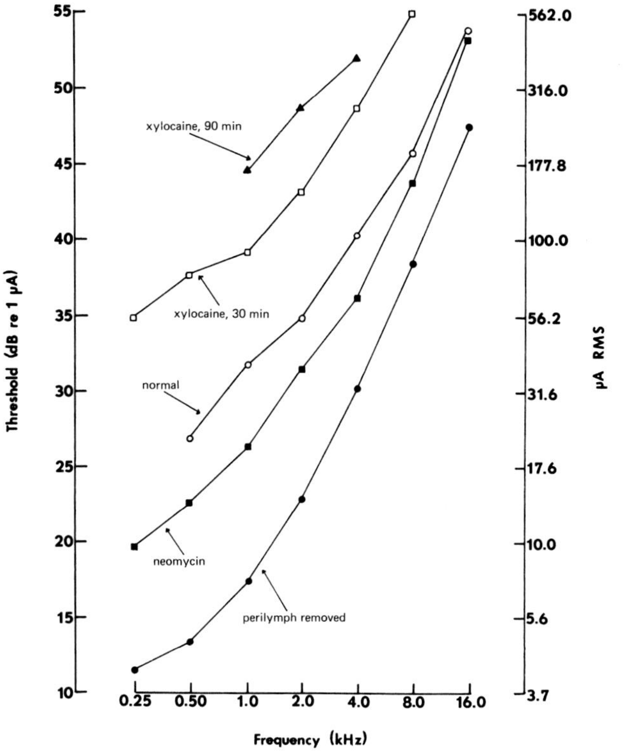

Fig. 7. Electrical thresholds versus frequency of single-cycle sinusoids under conditions of cochlear manipulation in one animal. The introduction of neomycin sulfate into the perilymph reduced thresholds to a few dB below normal, and the removal of perilymph further lowered thresholds in agreement with the results seen in Fig. 6. Thirty minutes after the introduction of Xylocaine, thresholds were elevated up to 10 dB above the thresholds for the originally normal cochlea. One and a half hours after the introduction of Xylocaine, thresholds were 13 dB above normal and difficult to obtain at many frequencies.

thresholds relative to control thresholds that increased with time. An immediate rise of 5 to 10 dB was seen which did not increase further for approximately 30 minutes. After that, a rise to very high thresholds was seen over the next two hours if the Xylocaine solution was left in the perilymphatic spaces. Removal of the Xylocaine solution resulted in a drop in threshold (Fig. 6). This effect was immediate and probably corresponded to the drop associated with removal of perilymph without introduction of Xylocaine.

Extracochlear Versus Intracochlear Stimulation. For three animals, the external wall of the cochlea was removed with a fine Kerr burr and the spiral lamina exposed. Thresholds for direct stimulation of the spiral lamina at a number of sites were 10 to 14 dB lower relative to stimulation of the outside of the normal cochlea near that point on the spiral lamina. The effect of entering the cochlea and directly stimulating the spiral lamina corresponded closely to that resulting from removal of the perilymph. Exposure and direct stimulation of the eighth nerve did not produce lower thresholds than were seen for direct stimulation of the spiral lamina or for stimulation of the entire cochlea with perilymph removed. The relationship of threshold to frequency of the stimulating waveform with internal stimulation was directly comparable to that for external stimulation with the perilymph removed.

DISCUSSION

Electrical stimulation of the middle ear in the guinea pig activates afferent auditory pathways somewhat less efficiently than direct stimulation of the spiral lamina or the eighth nerve. The loss of efficiency is not great, however, the required increase in current being 3 to 5 times that for stimulation inside the cochlea. The absolute threshold values remain well within theoretical limits for nongassing of the platinum electrodes in this experiment,[15] so tissue damage is unlikely at near-threshold currents for the frequencies used.

Electrical activation of the cochlea by means of middle ear stimulation is probably mediated by the depolarization of ganglion cells within the spiral lamina. This interpretation is suggested by four observations in this experiment. First, removal of perilymph from the cochlea significantly reduced the threshold for electrical activation. The perilymph appears to provide alternate current pathways that usually reduce the effectiveness of extracochlear stimulation. This observation suggests that the neural elements activated are within the cochlea, ie, the hair cells or the spiral ganglion cells. The second observation was that neomycin does not elevate the threshold for such stimulation, indeed it slightly reduces it, indicating that structures on the basilar membrane are not necessary for the mediation of the response to electrical stimulation. The relatively rapid effects of introducing a local anesthetic into the cochlea after neomycin destruction of basilar membrane structures is the third piece of evidence that implicates the spiral ganglion cells or their processes which lie near enough to be affected rather immediately by this local anesthetic. Fourth, and finally, similar reasoning applies in explaining these effects of manipulation of the calcium content of artificial perilymph on thresholds. None of these observations point to the mediation of this response by distant neural elements such as those in the cochlear nucleus. Previous studies are in agreement with this conclusion.[16] In spite of the implication that spiral ganglion cells mediate electrical activation in this case, it cannot be concluded that hair cells and dendrites of spiral ganglion cells on the basilar membrane do not contribute to the response when they are intact. It is only possible to say that they are not essential for the mediation of electrical activation.

Depolarization of neural membranes appears to be the basis for electrical activation of the deafened cochlea. Based on previous theoretical considerations and empirical evidence, some of the major results of this experiment can be explained in terms of membrane properties. Hill et al[17] and, more recently, Guttman and Hachmeister[18] have described the frequency-dependent characteristics of axons. The responses of squid and frog axons are very similar to those observed in the present experiment. The threshold for electrical stimulation varies as a function of frequency, and the ionic environment of the nerve membrane, especially the concentration of external calcium, affects the electrical threshold. Electrical activation of the cochlea, as with the nonmammalian axons, is apparently mediated through mechanisms that are charge-dependent at higher frequencies and current-dependent at lower frequencies. Sinusoidal stimuli below 1 kHz and square pulses with durations of more than 200-400 μs become increasingly less charge-efficient in activating afferent impulses. Based on the work with squid and frog axons it can be expected that lower frequencies of cochlear stimulation would produce a threshold minimum at 50-200 Hz with a rise as DC stimulation was approached.[17,18]

The presence of perilymph in the scala vestibuli and scala tympani appears to influence electrical activation of the cochlea in two ways. As mentioned previously, the perilymph provides alternate current pathways that reduce the effectiveness of extracochlear stimulation. This conclusion is indicated by the significant drop in threshold when the perilymph is removed, and the partial restoration of normal thresholds when saline is reintroduced. Secondly, the perilymph provides a biochemical environment that influences the process of electrical stimulation. Replacement of the perilymph with saline is not associated with normal thresholds to electrical stimulation. Artificial perilymph with a normal concentration of calcium must be present.[19] Neomycin introduced into the cochlea causes a slight decrease in thresholds that is probably associated with its well known destructive effects on structures of the basilar membrane.[20] Neomycin introduced directly into the cochlea of monkeys destroys structures on the organ of Corti (Sutton D, et al, unpublished observations). Spontaneous activity normally associated with an intact hair cell system may partially mask electrically introduced activation. Destruction of elements on the basilar membrane would eliminate this activity and result in a reduction of the threshold to electrical stimulation. This experimental observation agrees with the clinical finding that patients with probable loss of hair cell function are much more likely to respond to electrical stimulation of the middle ear in comparison to patients with normal hair cell function.[21]

A number of implications arise from these observations for the application of middle ear stimulation in the deaf. The first is that stimulation outside the cochlea, if appropriately done, can be a relatively effective way to stimulate fibers of the eighth nerve. While polarity effects are possible, the use of biphasic, symmetrical waveforms will largely obviate their consideration. A more important factor is the effect of charge balance and maximum charge density at the electrodes, which are likely to be major parameters in the determination of tissue damage and the electrode destruction. The charge density for the limit of gassing for platinum electrodes is least at low frequencies, an argument against the use of longer duration pulses. Other factors not investigated here include the effective dynamic range over which suprathreshold stimuli can be introduced before discomfort is encountered. Middle ear stimulation has been reported[11,12] to be associated with low pain thresholds and consequent small dynamic ranges in some human patients.

Electrical stimulation of the surface of the cochlea in the middle ear does provide activation of a cochlea where structures on the basilar membrane can be assumed to be inoperative. The threshold for activation is not elevated after basilar membrane elements are destroyed. It is thus likely that neurons of the spiral ganglion or their associated processes are easily stimulated by electrical currents introduced from outside the cochlea. The experimental evidence of this investigation supports the exploration of middle ear stimulation as an avenue for activation of eighth nerve fibers.

ACKNOWLEDGMENT — The authors wish to thank Mark Malone and Marion Odubiyi for their help in preparing illustrations.

REFERENCES

1. House WF, Urban J. Long term results of electrode implantation and electronic stimulation of the cochlea in man. Ann Otol Rhinol Laryngol 1973; 82:504-17.

2. Michelson RP. Electrical stimulation of the human cochlea: a preliminary report. Arch Otolaryngol 1971; 93:317-23.

3. Chouard CH, MacLeod P. Implantation of multiple intracochlear electrodes for rehabilitation of total deafness: preliminary report. Laryngoscope 1976; 86:1743-51.

4. Hansen CC, Lauridsen O. Electrical stimulation of the inner ear. Nord Med Tidskr 1975; 9:20-5.

5. Simmons FB, Epley JM, Lummis RC, et al. Auditory nerve: electrical stimulation in man. Science 1965; 148:104-6.

6. Simmons FB. Electrical stimulation of the auditory nerve in man. Arch Otolaryngol 1966; 84:2-54.

7. Johnsson L-G, House WF, Linthicum FH. Bilateral cochlea implants: histological findings in a pair of temporal bones. Laryngoscope 1979; 89:759-62.

8. Johnsson L-G. Sequence of degeneration of Corti's organ and its first order neurons. Ann Otol Rhinol Laryngol 1974; 83: 294-303.

9. Bredberg G. Cellular pattern and nerve supply of the human organ of Corti. Acta Otolaryngol (Stockh) 1968; Suppl 236:1-135.

10. Otte J, Schuknecht HF, Kerr AG. Ganglion cell populations in normal and pathological human cochleae. Implications for cochlear implantation. Laryngoscope 1978; 88:1231-46.

11. Thornton ARD, ed. A review of artificial auditory stimulation. Medical Research Council Working Group Report; Institute of Sound and Vibration Research, University of Southampton, 1977.

12. Fourcin AJ, Rosen SM, Moore BCJ, et al. External electrical stimulation of the cochlea: clinical, psychophysical, speech-perceptual and histological findings. Br J Audio 1979; 13:85-107.

13. Spelman FA, Pfingst BE, Miller JM. A constant current stimulator for use with chronic cochlear implants. Proceedings of the San Diego Biomedical Symposium, 1978:1-3.

14. Fex J, Adams JC. X-bungarotoxin blocks reversibly cholinergic inhibition in the cochlea. Brain Res 1978; 159:440-4.

15. Brummer SB, Turner MJ. Electrical stimulation with Pt electrodes: II. Estimation of maximum surface redox (theoretical non-gassing) limits. IEEE Trans Biomed Eng 1977; BME 24:440-3.

16. Clopton BM, Spelman FA, Miller JM. Estimates of essential neural elements for stimulation through a cochlear prosthesis. Ann Otol Rhinol Laryngol 1980; 89 Suppl 66:5-7.

17. Hill AV, Katz B, Solandt DY. Nerve excitation by alternating current. Proc R Soc Lond [Biol] 1936; 121:74-133.

18. Guttman R, Hachmeister L. Effect of calcium, temperature, and polarizing currents upon alternating current excitation of space-clamped squid axons. J Gen Physiol 1971; 58:304-21.

19. Konishi T, Kelsey E. Effects of calcium deficiency on cochlear potentials. J Acoust Soc Am 1970; 47:1055-62.

20. Leake-Jones PA, O'Reilly BF, Vivion MC. Neomycin ototoxicity: ultrastructural surface pathology of the organ of Corti. Scan Electron Microsc 1980; 3:427-34.

21. Brackmann D. Multichannel electrical stimulation in man. In: Merzenich MM, Schindler RA, Sooy FA, eds. Electrical stimulation of the acoustic nerve in man. San Francisco: Velo-Bind, 1974:129-31.

Ann Otol Rhinol Laryngol 91:1982

MONOPHASIC EXTRASKELETAL MANDIBULAR FIXATION IN HEAD AND NECK SURGERY

STEVEN D. SCHAEFER, MD

GEORGE A. WESSBERG, DDS

STEUART L. HEATON, MD

DALLAS, TEXAS

Stabilization, reconstruction, and rehabilitation of certain mandibular fractures or continuity defects may be facilitated by external skeletal fixation. The utilization of a convenient and inexpensive monophasic extraskeletal fixation appliance in select instances of mandibular trauma or head and neck surgery is described herein and illustrated with case reports.

INTRODUCTION

Mandibular continuity is generally essential to optimal masticatory function.[1] Loss of an intact lower arch, especially in the body or symphysis due to severe trauma or elective resection, compromises mastication and/or facial esthetics.[2] Therefore, the primary goal in the management of individuals with a comminuted mandibular fracture or a surgically-induced continuity defect is to secure the proximal and distal segments of the mandible in their proper positions. Anatomical stabilization of this arch preserves normal facial esthetics and occlusion while osseous repair occurs following fractures, or until secondary reconstruction with bone grafting is completed, or until mature fibrosis of the defect ensues and physical rehabilitation is achieved.[3,4]

Stabilization of the mandible is most often accomplished by the application of arch bars and wiring the teeth into proper occlusion. However, when prolonged intermaxillary fixation is necessary, subsequent shortening of the muscles of mastication further compromises the postoperative rehabilitation. The requirement of prolonged mandibular immobilization is an indication for some method of extraskeletal pin fixation. The combination of arch bars and intermittent elastic therapy with a rigid extraskeletal fixation appliance permits functional rehabilitation of the masticatory muscles, preserves the normal occlusal relationship, and provides continuity to the mandible where a portion is comminuted or included in an ablative procedure. Although preservation of occlusal relations is not a significant consideration in edentulous patients, insuring masticatory function and providing continuity to the mandible is important. Functional rehabilitation is particularly difficult when the mandible and muscles of mastication are included in the radiotherapy field.

Several methods of rigid internal or external skeletal fixation have been reported. Placement of stainless steel Steinman pins or Kirschner wires between the proximal and distal segments of the edentulous mandible have often proven effective if the area is *not* irradiated.[5,6] In 1942, Converse and Waknitz employed a Roger Anderson appliance for external skeletal fixation of the mandible.[7,8] Shortly thereafter, Morris developed a similar biphasic appliance specifically for mandibular and maxillofacial injuries.[9] Recently, a more convenient and less expensive monophasic appliance has been developed for stabilization of the mandible and is the topic of this report.[10]

METHODS

Application of a monophasic extraskeletal fixation appliance to the mandible follows closure of the surgical wound in the head and neck oncology patient. When dentition is to be preserved and a bone graft or osseomyocutaneous flap used, maxillary and mandibular arch bars should be applied before or at the time of surgery. The edentulous patient, or one in whom no reconstruction of the mandibular continguity is planned, requires only the monphasic appliance. In the fracture patient, initial application of arch bars insures proper occlusal and anatomical relationships.

Placement of the appliance begins with a small percutaneous puncture over the mandibular segments in the selected areas of pin placement. The pins should be spaced 2.5 cm apart and 2.5 cm from the mandibular defect between the inferior border and the inferior alveolar canal. Threaded Steinman pins (Houmet Corp.) 2.8 to 4.0 mm in diameter are inserted through the soft tissues and the outer and inner cortices of the mandible with a manual pin driver (Fig. 1). Palpation of the lingual surface of the mandible during pin placement will alert the surgeon when the proper depth is attained. Following insertion the stability of each pin is assessed manually before it is cut 5 cm from the skin surface. This pin length allows for soft tissue edema without necrosis and permits easy removal with a pin cutter in the future. Two pins are placed in each segment. A large plastic endotracheal tube (Portex No. 10 or 11) is trimmed to remove the pilot tube and cuff, and cut to extend 2 cm beyond the most distant stainless steel pins. The dentulous patients are placed into intermaxillary fixation at this time and the mandibular segments are properly oriented by palpation or direct inspection (open reduction in fracture cases) in

From the Departments of Otolaryngology and Surgery (Oral Surgery), University of Texas Health Science Center at Dallas.

REPRINTS — Steven D. Schaefer, MD, Department of Otolaryngology, University of Texas Health Science Center at Dallas, 5323 Harry Hines Boulevard, Dallas, TX 75235.

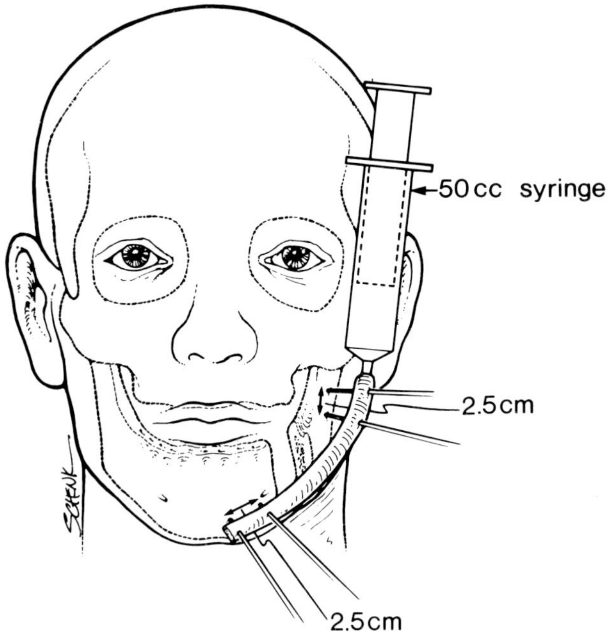

Fig. 1. Placement of monophasic extraskeletal fixation appliance in continuity defects.

both dentate and edentulous patients. The endotracheal tube is molded to accommodate all pins and the inner surface is marked where they intersect. Holes slightly larger than the pins are cut with a No. 15 blade and the tube is placed securely over all of the pins. A petroleum-based ointment (Vaseline) is spread over the plastic tube, exposed pins, and skin surface. The mandibular segments are properly positioned and 25 cc of autopolymerizing acrylic (Cranioplast) is mixed and placed into a 50 cc catheter-tip syringe. When the acrylic attains a "creamy" state it is injected into one end of the endotracheal tube until the material reaches the opposite end. The plastic tube is held securely as well as the segments of the mandible (via clamps to the pins or manually) until the "solid" state is reached. However, while the acrylic is in the "rubber" state an assistant can peel the excess material from the lubricated surfaces. When the acrylic has cured (approximately 10 minutes) the tube can be released and antibacterial ointment placed around the pins at the skin surface.

CASE REPORTS

Over the past three years 17 patients have undergone monophasic extraskeletal mandibular fixation following resection or fracture of the lower dental arch at the University of Texas Health Science Center at Dallas affiliated hospitals. Representative cases are presented.

Case 1. Segmental Resection of Mandibular Body. A 53-year-old female presented to Parkland Memorial Hospital with a complaint of sore throat of several months' duration. The clinical examination revealed a large left tonsillar lesion. Panendoscopy and biopsy demonstrated a $T_3N_2M_0$ poorly differentiated squamous cell carcinoma of the left pharyngeal tonsil, soft palate, and pharyngeal wall. Metastatic workup was negative. Surgical management of the tumor included left radical neck dissection, partial glossectomy, partial pharyngectomy, and a 4 cm resection of the mandibular body (Fig. 2 A). The surgical wound was closed primarily and the monophasic appliance was placed to provide stability to the mandible (Fig. 2 B). A complete odontectomy was accomplished postoperatively in preparation for tumoricidal radiation therapy (5,500 rads to the primary and supraclavicular neck areas). There were no complications associated with the monophasic appliance or the radiation. With further postoperative follow-up limited to four months, a satisfactory cosmetic and functional result was achieved (Fig. 2 C).

Case 2. Segmental Resection of Mandibular Symphysis. A 64-year-old male was referred to the Dallas Veterans Administration Hospital for a $T_3N_2M_0$ squamous cell carcinoma of the floor of mouth. Preoperative evaluation, including panendoscopy, was otherwise unremarkable. The patient underwent an en bloc resection of the primary, including the mandible from midbody to midbody, bilateral neck dissection, and a medial-based deltopectoral flap reconstruction. Following closure of the surgical wound, a monophasic appliance was applied. At six weeks after the initial surgery, 5,500 rads was begun to the primary and to the supraclavicular nodes. The appliance was removed at this time. Although no attempt was made to reconstruct the mandibular defect, cosmesis was good due to fixation of the mandibular segments which prevented contracture during the initial healing phase (Fig. 3). The only adverse effect of the procedure was loss of good oral sphincter competence with the mouth open. This patient was followed over 30 months until his death from pulmonary metastasis. Prior to death, there was no evidence of local or regional recurrent disease, and no change esthetically or functionally of the lower arch.

Case 3. Mandibular Fracture with Chronic Osteomyelitis. A 34-year-old female presented to Parkland Memorial Hospital emergency room with an open, complete right mandibular angle fracture. She underwent open reduction and internal fixation with intermaxillary wiring (Fig. 4). She failed to return until six weeks following routine discharge from the hospital. She then had an open and draining intraoral wound, a mobile fracture, and apparent bony sequestra. The infection did not respond to removal of the transosseous wire, three weeks of frequent irrigations, inter-

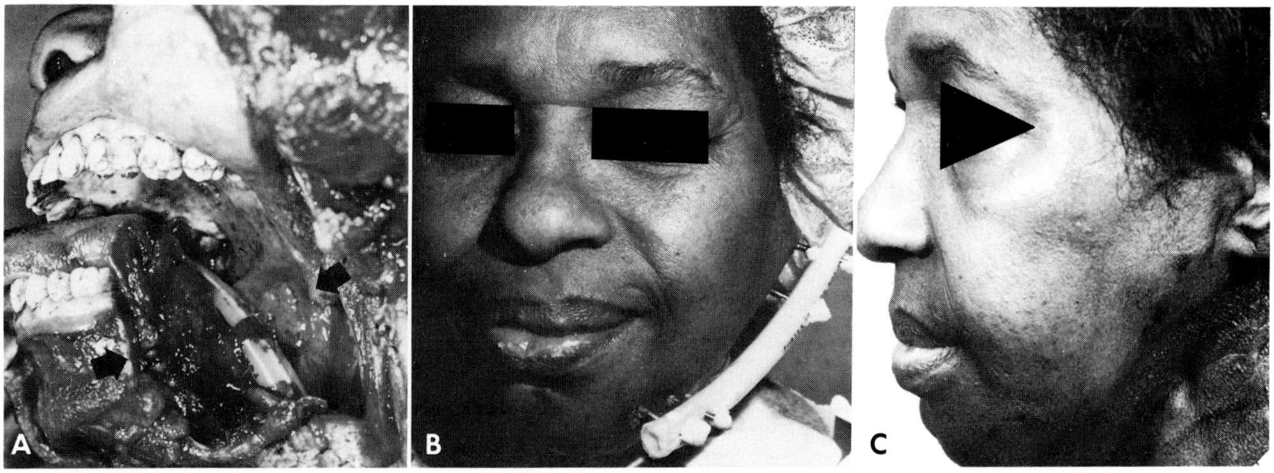

Fig. 2. (Case 1) A) Surgical defect (arrows). B) Early postoperative with fixation device applied. C) Four months after surgery.

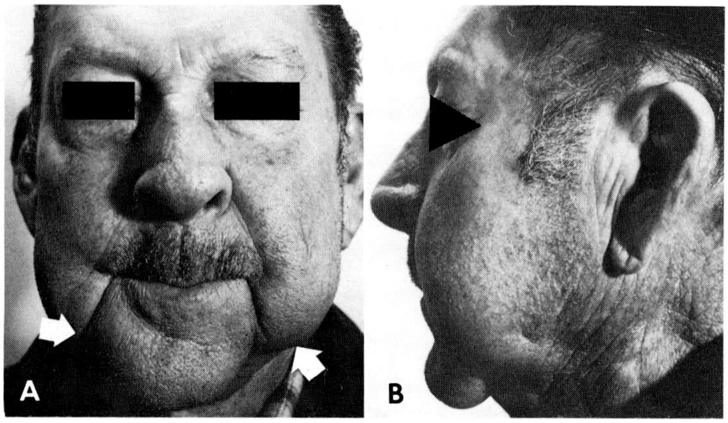

Fig. 3. (Case 2) Two years postoperative. A) Arrows - site of anterior mandibular resection. B) Despite shortening of mandibular projection, patient has reasonable profile.

maxillary fixation, and systemic antibiotic therapy. A sequestrectomy was then performed with buccal saucerization via a submandibular approach. The segments of the mandible were stabilized with a monophase appliance while the teeth were in fixation. Intermaxillary wires were removed to permit active physiotherapy of the masticatory muscles during the prolonged recovery period, but elastic bands were employed intermittently to preserve occlusal relations. The skeletal fixation was removed eight weeks following placement, leaving the patient with adequate osseous stability and good mandibular movement.

Case 4. Comminuted Mandibular Body Fracture. A 22-year-old male presented to John Peter Smith Hospital emergency room with multiple gunshot wounds to the abdomen, thorax and face. Facial injuries consisted of minor soft tissue lacerations and severely comminuted fractures of the left mandibular body and angle (Fig. 5). However, hypothermia during the initial laparotomy prevented primary treatment of the open mandibular fractures. Subsequently, *Pseudomonas aeruginosa* infection developed in the fracture site despite frequent wound irrigation and systemic antibiotic therapy. Six days later his physical status improved and the young man was returned to the operating room for treatment of his facial injuries. Excessively mobile teeth were removed, the wounds thoroughly irrigated, arch bars applied and the right teeth placed into temporary intermaxillary fixation. A monophasic appliance was placed because there was excessive comminution of the left mandibular body, missing teeth in the proximal segment, and a persistent *Pseudomonas* wound infection. Extraskeletal fixation stabilized the left ascending ramus, provided continuity to the mandible and permitted release of intermaxillary fixation for frequent oral and wound irrigation. A notch was cut in the endotracheal tube to create a right angle bend to include all of the pins in the acrylic bar. Thereafter, the patient's clinical course was unremarkable.

In the entire series of 17 patients, complications have included facial hematoma (1), wound infection around a pin (1), and intraoral perforation of the lingual mandibular mucosa (2). None of these was a serious problem or altered the patient's recovery. In one patient, a sternocleidomastoid-clavicle-myocutanous flap failed, unrelated to the external appliance. The flap, including the clavicle, was removed and the oral defect closed with a tongue flap. Recovery was uneventful and despite resection of the mandibular body, cosmesis and function were near normal because

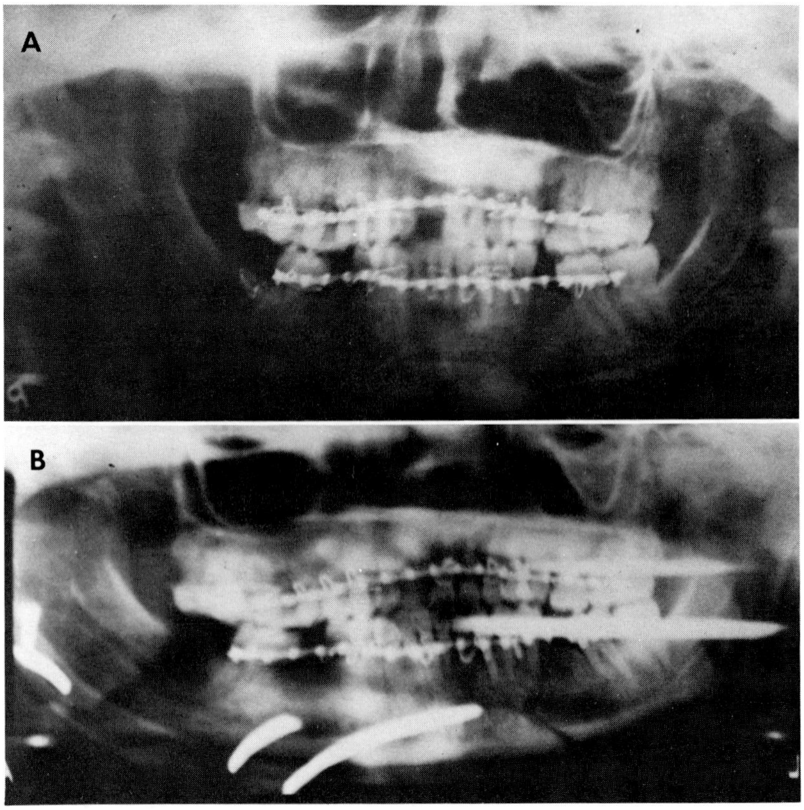

Fig. 4. (Case 3) Radiographs demonstrating A) malunion in right mandibular angle fracture, and B) pin fixation following sequestrectomy.

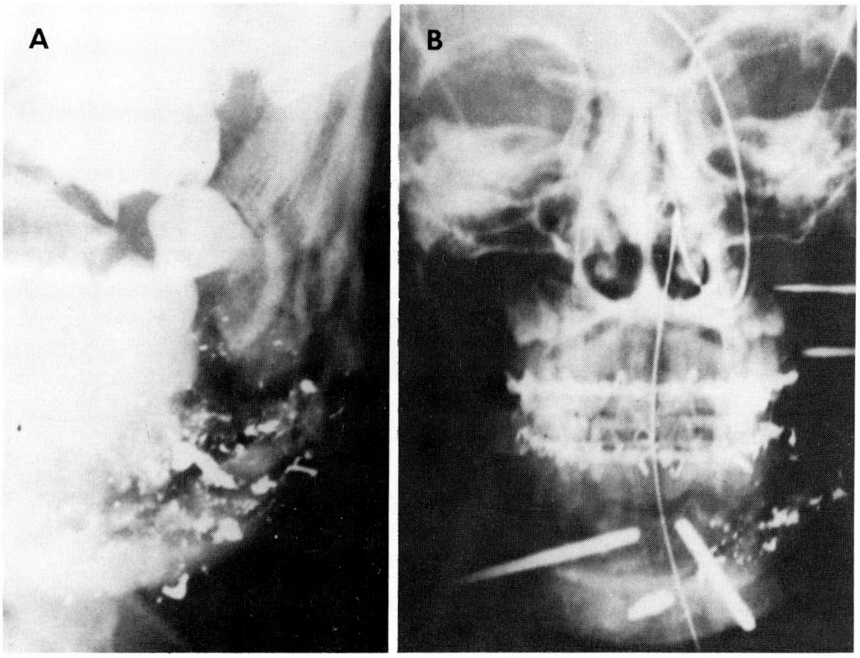

Fig. 5. (Case 4) A) Radiographs revealing grossly comminuted left mandibular body and angle fracture. B) Radiograph showing fractured mandible stabilized with pin fixation.

the appliance was left in place for six weeks postoperatively. There have been no facial nerve or salivary gland injuries.

DISCUSSION

The monophasic extraskeletal fixation appliance is so named because its application involves only one phase. There are no connecting rods which must be applied, and subsequently removed in the second phase or step, as in the biphasic technique.[9] The fabrication of a monophasic device arose from the use of flexible plastic conduits filled with a polymer joining Steinman pins for extraskeletal fixation of extremity fractures by orthopedic surgeons. This simple and effective method was termed "hot links." The "hot links" principle was adapted for the mandible because the component parts are disposable and commonly available in the operating room. The indications for this appliance are numerous.

In oncology patients with surgical mandibular contiguity defects, extraskeletal fixation permits immediate postoperative stability of the lower dental arch. Early stability is essential to prevent mobility of the resected segments and success of a primary bone graft.[3] In the patient who is not felt to be a candidate for immediate reconstruction, the monophasic appliance fixates the mandibular segments in proper anatomic position during the initial healing phase (six weeks on the average) with surprisingly good long-term functional and esthetic results. Surgical trauma to the periosteum adjacent to the mandibular defect during placement of the appliance is minimal. In fact, our institution has over five years' experience using extraskeletal fixation after mandibular resection in radiotherapy patients, without any complications attributed to the appliance.

The obvious success and simplicity of arch bars limit the indications for extraskeletal fixation. However, as seen in cases 3 and 4, such management is clearly useful in posttraumatic osteomyelitis and comminuted mandibular fractures involving the angle. The edentulous mandible with an unstable fracture that normally requires open reduction, internal fixation and intermaxillary splints, may be managed by this technique when intermaxillary fixation is not indicated. Unlike open reduction with wiring or compression plates, extraskeletal fixation does not strip the periosteum away from the fracture site. Preservation of periosteum is essential to bony union in the atrophic edentulous lower arch since this is the site of bone formation in the older patient.

Potential complications associated with the use of extraskeletal fixation involve injury to nerves, blood vessels, teeth and salivary glands. Damage to the facial nerve can be avoided by making the percutaneous stab incisions just through the skin and allowing the Steinman pin to displace the nerve as it rotates through the subcutaneous tissues toward the

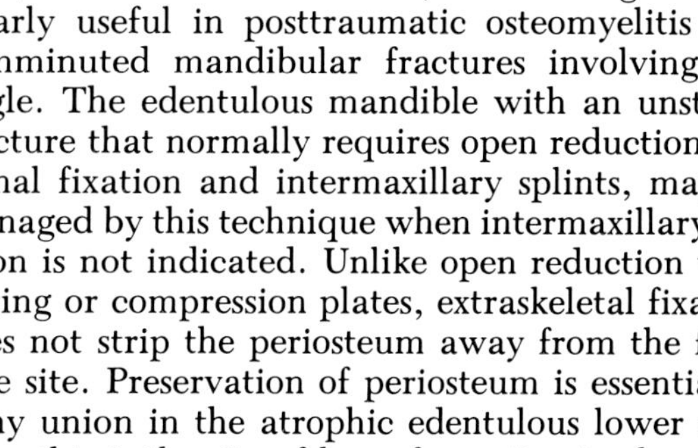

Fig. 6. Facial photograph illustrating right-angle bend of fixation device which may be necessary when pins are placed in ascending ramus of mandible.

mandible. Damage to the inferior alveolar nerve is usually transient. Dental trauma resulting from errant pin placement is usually observed closely during the period of fixation, but not treated until symptoms arise. Salivary fistulas secondary to pin placement into a gland are uncommon, but when they occur, resolve spontaneously or respond to pressure following removal of the pin.

Secondary infection may arise from intraoral communication with a pin, an abscessed tooth, or retrograde from the skin surface and cause a pin to become loose. Inadequate placement through the lingual cortex, insufficient pin size, or necrosis of bone surrounding a pin can result in mobility of the appliance. When a pin becomes loose during fixation, it may be cut free from the acrylic bar and replaced or a supplementary pin can be placed, under local anesthesia, and secured to the bar with autopolymerizing acrylic.

Extraskeletal fixation was employed without complications in these four cases to provide prolonged continuity or stability to fractured or partially resected mandibles. As noted previously, morbidity for this series of 17 patients has been limited to facial hematoma and minor wound infection. The monophasic appliance permitted mandibular function during the period of myofibrositis induced by infection or irradiation and minimized scar contracture across continuity defects to maintain optimal facial esthetics and occlusal relationships during healing. The monophasic appliance was selected for use in these cases because the component parts are conveniently available, the device is quickly applied by experienced surgeons, and the cost of the disposable materials is minimal.

REFERENCES

1. Jackson MJ. Maxillofacial prosthetic rehabilitation of the patient with head and neck cancer. Otolaryngol Clin North Am 1980; 13:541-50.

2. Adesman K. Principles, concepts and practices in maxillofacial prosthodontics. In: Lefkowitz W, ed. Proceedings of second international prosthodontic congress. St. Louis: CV Mosby, 1979: 237-40.

3. Alonso MR, Bailey B. Reconstruction of the mandible. Otolaryngol Clin North Am 1972; 5:501-11.

4. Spiessel B, Prein J, Schomoker R. Anatomic reconstruction and functional rehabilitation of mandibular defects after ablative surgery. In: Spiessel B, ed. New concepts in maxillofacial bone surgery. New York: Springer-Verlag, 1976: 160-3.

5. Saskins JA, Ertugral G, Rush BF. Tolerance to stainless steel prostheses in patients after postradiation hemimandibulectomy. Am J Surg 1969; 117:375-6.

6. Kodsi MS, Culf NK, Hulnick SJ, Cramer LM. Reconstructive management of the mandible in the treatment of head and neck cancer. In: Anderson R, Hoopes JE, eds. Symposium on malignancies of the head and neck. St. Louis: CV Mosby, 1975: 198-203.

7. Anderson R. An ambulatory method of treating fractures of the shaft of the femur. Surg Gynecol Obstet 1936; 62:865-8.

8. Converse JM, Waknitz FW. External skeletal fixation in fractures of the mandibular angle. J Bone Joint Surg 1942; 24: 154-60.

9. Morris JH. Biphase connector, external skeletal splint for reduction and fixation of mandibular fractures. Oral Surg 1949; 2:1382-98.

10. Wessberg GA, Schendel SA, Epker BN. Monophase extraskeletal fixation. J Oral Surg 1979; 37:892-6.

HAIR-CLIP TYPE PISTON ARTIFICIAL STAPES AND THE SAFETY AUGER

TUNG MIN-SHENG, MD

ZHENGZHOU, HENAN PROVINCE, PEOPLE'S REPUBLIC OF CHINA

A hair-clip artificial stapes prosthesis was used in the surgical treatment of otosclerosis in 22 ears. In nine patients followed an average of 15 months the air-bone gap stabilized at 6-7 dB. Further advantages of the prosthesis design and technique are that they minimize the risk of ischemic necrosis and perilymphatic fistula formation.

Successful surgical treatment of otosclerosis was first achieved by Lempert[1] in the early 1940s. A decade later Rosen[2] mobilized an ankylosed stapes, but Shea[3] and Shea et al[4] made probably the first attack on stapes surgery which gave consistently successful results. Since then, in an effort to evolve simpler techniques and improved results, many new methods have been introduced. Although results are improving, particular hazards and difficulties remain. In this paper observations on the following problems are presented, along with instruments and techniques developed by the author:

1. Trauma to the inner ear.
2. Necrosis and securing the prosthesis.
3. Perilymphatic fistula.
4. Long-term results.

INNER EAR TRAUMA

Otosclerotic thickening of the footplate usually occurs at the margin, especially the anterior portion. The central portion frequently is so thin that it looks like a dark blue dimple. In such cases it is quite easy to perforate the footplate with a needle. Control of the depth of the perforation, however, is not so easy, and injury to the membranous labyrinth can result, or a small fragment of bone may drop into the labyrinth. In response to these technical problems, a prism-shaped pointed auger was designed (Fig. 1A). The safety feature is a ring attached 1.2 mm from the auger tip. The ring is approximately 0.3 mm wide; the diameter of the auger head ranges from 0.6-0.75 mm.

The technique is to place the auger point perpendicular to the center of the footplate, along the posterior border of the long process of the incus. With two fingers holding the auger, the shaft is rotated with clockwise and counterclockwise motions. In this way a hole can be precisely drilled to receive the piston. If the footplate is thick, the arrowhead auger (Fig. 1B) is used to thin out the bone to a disc shape before drilling with the pointed auger. With these instruments a diamond-head electrical burr is not necessary.

SECURING THE PROSTHESIS AND NECROSIS

Today various kinds of artificial piston prostheses are available, including those with a circular hook, Teflon ring, and half-circle wire. Hooks require special forceps for fixing the wire tightly to the long process of the incus. The problem with this procedure is the entailed risk of shutting off the blood supply in the mucous membrane covering the incus, and thus increasing the possibility of ischemic necrosis of the lenticular process. The hair-clip piston artificial stapes (Fig. 2) is different from many prostheses in that instead of encircling the long process it clips onto it on two sides, thus avoiding the main vessels and lessening the danger of necrosis.

PERILYMPHATIC FISTULA

Douek[5] reported that perilymphatic fistula following a stapes operation commonly resulted from

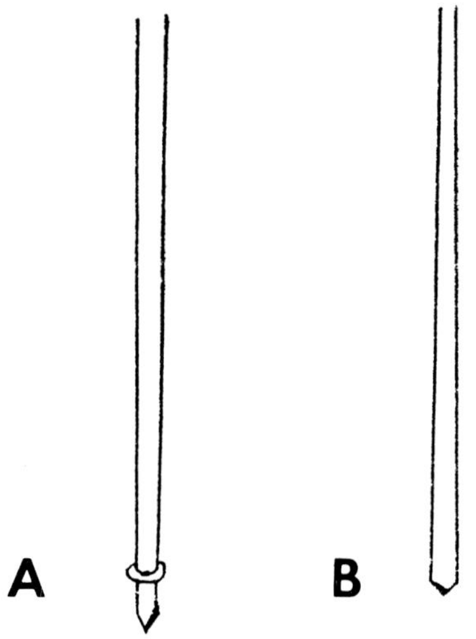

Fig. 1. Two types of hand augers used in operations for the treatment of otosclerosis. A) Prism-shaped pointed auger with safety ring. B) Arrowhead auger.

From the ENT Department, The Teaching Hospital of Henan Medical College, Zhengzhou, Henan Province, People's Republic of China.

REPRINTS — Tung Min-Sheng, MD, ENT Department, The Teaching Hospital of Henan Medical College, Zhengzhou, Henan Province, People's Republic of China.

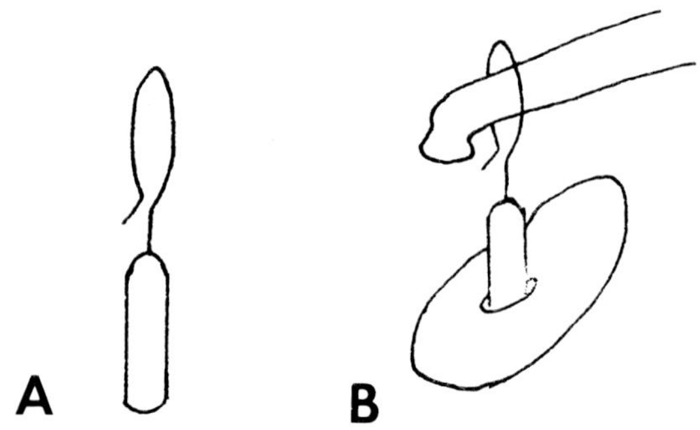

Fig. 2. Artificial prosthesis. A) Hair-clip piston artificial stapes. B) Hair-clip prosthesis in position.

an irregular and/or overly large hole drilled in the footplate. If the piston is loose, perilymph may leak out around it. Or, adhesions may pull the piston to one side so that a perilymph fistula forms directly from the gap, or a sleeve-like fistula might occur. With the safety hand auger a smooth hole can be drilled which is just slightly larger than the piston. With the hole diameter 0.6-0.75 mm, a piston 0.55 mm in diameter fits tightly and the risk of a fistula forming is minimal.

SURGICAL PROCEDURE

Local anesthesia (1 ml of 2% Xylocaine) is administered and the middle ear exposed in the usual manner. The superstructure is fractured. The safety auger is inserted perpendicular to and in the center of the footplate with the shaft of the auger just along the posterior side of the long process of the incus. The hole is drilled by hand, as described above. Alligator forceps is used to insert the piston into the vestibule through the plate hole and then smoothly slip the clip onto the long process of the incus.

LONG-TERM RESULTS

From 1976 to 1979 operations were performed on 22 ears (13 males, 5 females) using the technique described. In these patients the air-bone gap averaged 9.4 dB two weeks after the operation. In nine cases followed for 6-38 months (average follow-up 15 months) improvement in the air-bone gap was greater (6.8 dB). Subjectively, patients reported that their hearing was best one month postoperatively, and remained stable thereafter.

REFERENCES

1. Lempert J. Fenestra non-ovalis: a new oval window for the improvement of hearing in cases of otosclerosis. Arch Otolaryngol 1941; 34:880-912.

2. Rosen S. Mobilization of the stapes to restore hearing in otosclerosis. NY J Med 1953; 53:2650-3.

3. Shea JJ Jr. Fenestration of the oval window. Ann Otol Rhinol Laryngol 1958; 67:932-50.

4. Shea JJ, Sanabria F, Smyth GDL. Teflon piston operation for otosclerosis. Arch Otolaryngol 1962; 76:516-21.

5. Douek E. Perilymph fistula. J Laryngol Otol 1975; 89: 123-30.

≈

BILATERAL MIDDLE EAR CARCINOMAS ASSOCIATED WITH WALDENSTRÖM'S MACROGLOBULINEMIA

GERALD B. BROOKES, FRCS

LONDON, ENGLAND

A case of bilateral middle ear squamous cell carcinomas with concurrent Waldenström's macroglobulinemia is described. An increased incidence of malignant tumors occurring in patients with this potentially fatal, chronic lymphoproliferative disorder is well recognized, but the association with an otological tumor has not previously been reported. The relationship between the two conditions is discussed.

INTRODUCTION

Primary neoplasia of the middle ear cleft and mastoid bone is a rare condition. The incidence compared to the frequency of other aural pathology presenting to otologists is about 1 in 4,000 to 1 in 20,000.[1-6] Squamous cell carcinoma is by far the most common malignant tumor in this site, accounting for 75-90% of all malignancies.[5-11] Only two previous cases of bilateral middle ear carcinomas have been reported.[8,12] Lederman's case has been included in two subsequent series.[9,13] Middle ear carcinomas associated with a contralateral external auditory meatus malignancy have also been recorded.[12,14] A case is described in which following presentation of a second middle ear carcinoma, further investigation led to the diagnosis of concurrent Waldenström's macroglobulinemia (MG). An increased incidence of malignant tumors occurring in patients with this condition is well recognized,[15,16] but the association with an otologic tumor has not previously been reported.

CASE REPORT

A 62-year-old female presented to the London Hospital in 1961 with a history of bilateral intermittent otorrhea and deafness since early childhood. Medical advice was sought following the recent onset of right otalgia and positional vertigo. There was no family history of neoplasia nor of previous exposure to known carcinogens. On examination active chronic suppurative otitis media (CSOM) with granular aural polyps was present in the right ear, with quiescent left CSOM. Clinically, facial nerve function was intact, and there was no cervical lymphadenopathy. On surgical exploration, a polypoid tumor replacing the tympanic membrane and filling the mesotympanum with extension into the eustachian tube and erosion of the posterior bony meatal wall was found. Histologically the tumor was moderately well-differentiated squamous cell carcinoma with associated inflammatory changes (Fig. 1A), and evidence of carcinoma in situ (Fig. 1B). Following an extended radical mastoidectomy, the patient was treated with 5,500 rads of telecobalt radiotherapy, and complete tumor eradication was achieved. She remained well and free of disease at 16 years posttreatment.

In 1980 the patient was referred again with a 6-week history of left otalgia, throbbing tinnitus and vertigo. She reported recent weight loss and lethargy. Examination now revealed active left CSOM with an aural polyp protruding through an anterior marginal perforation. First degree spontaneous right nystagmus was noted, while facial nerve function was normal. There was no cervical or generalized lymphadenopathy, nor hepatosplenomegaly. At surgery, a vascular tumor was found filling the posterior mesotympanum, extending into the aditus and eroding bone of the deep posterior meatal wall. A formal radical mastoidectomy was carried out. Histologically this tumor was also a moderately well-differentiated squamous cell carcinoma, with associated carcinoma in situ features (Fig. 2). The pathological appearance was very similar to that of the earlier contralateral tumor. Ten days postoperatively the patient developed a transient facial palsy, and was once again referred for a course of radical telecobalt radiotherapy. In view of the rarity of bilateral middle ear carcinomas and the associated systemic symptoms, full medical and immunological assessment was undertaken.

RESULTS

General Assessment. Hemoglobin 12 g/dl; white blood count 7.2/nl; lymphocyte count 1,280/cu ml; platelet count normal; ESR (Westergren) 121 mm/hr; serum calcium (corrected) 2.52 mmol/l (upper limit of normal); alkaline phosphatase 104 units/1 (upper limit of normal); serum inorganic phosphate 0.74 mmol/l; serum albumin and protein assays normal. Radiological skeletal survey showed mild osteoporosis but no osteolytic lesions.

Immunological Assessment. Immunoglobin assay (normal range in parentheses): IgG 6.37 g/l (7-19); IgM 30 g/l (0.45-1.8); IgA 0.45 g/l (0.9-4.5). Immunoelectrophoresis: monoclonal protein of IgM kappa specificity. Bence Jones proteinuria: negative. Bone marrow examination: no abnormal or excess plasma cells; lymphocytes comprise 40% of the nucleated cell count. Lymphocyte subpopulation counts: normal T-cell count but significantly reduced B-cell count. Lymphocyte transformation studies to phytohemagglutinin (PHA), tuberculoprotein (PPD) and pokeweed mitogen (PWM) revealed normal T and B cell responses, and no clear evidence of deficient immunity.

Diagnosis. Waldenström's MG without secondary immunoincompetence.

From the Department of Otolaryngology, The London Hospital, Whitechapel, London.

REPRINTS — Gerald B. Brookes, FRCS, Department of Otolaryngology, The London Hospital, Whitechapel, London E1 1BB, England.

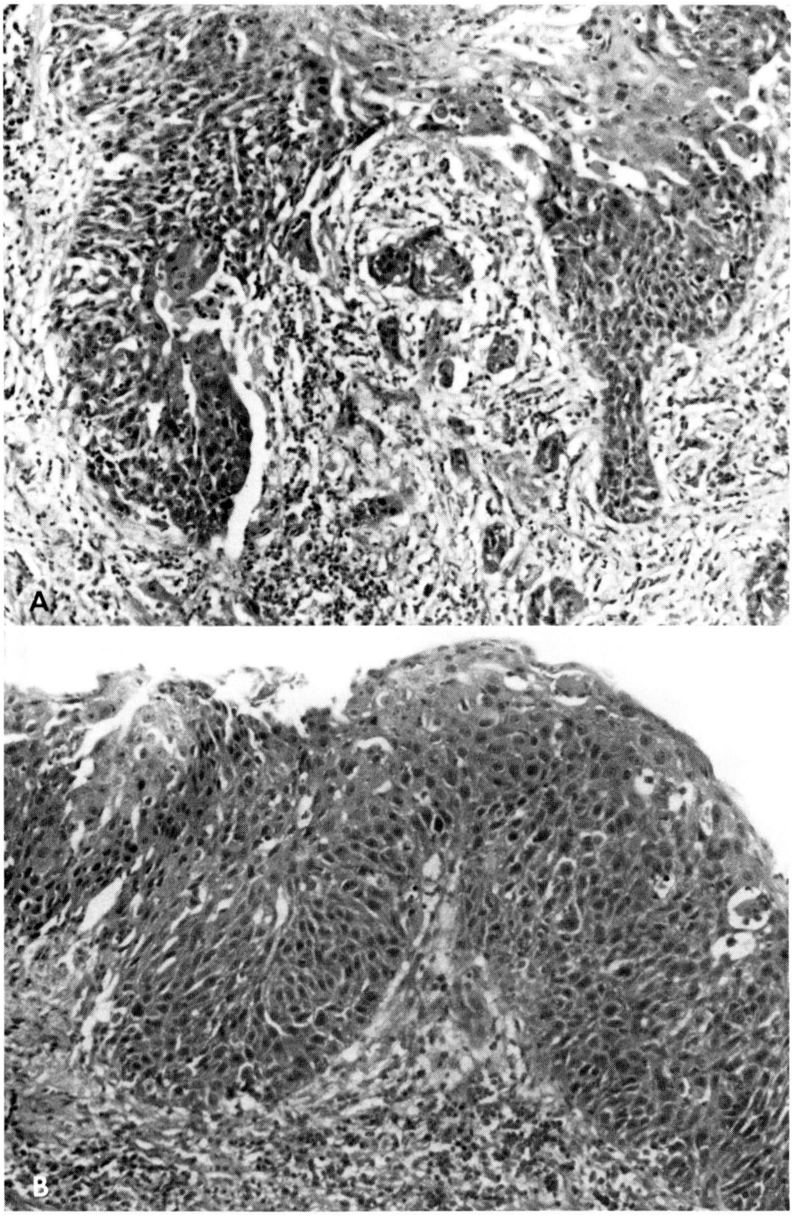

Fig. 1. A) Histological section of right middle ear tumor showing moderately well-differentiated squamous cell carcinoma (H & E, x120). B) Different histological section of right middle ear epithelium showing carcinoma in situ features (H & E, x200).

Course. As the patient's only symptoms were mild anemia, lassitude and slight weight loss, the progress of her MG was closely monitored but no active treatment was given. Seven months postradiotherapy the left mastoid cavity was stable and tumor-free. The IgM level remained raised at 22.5 g/l, and the ESR significantly elevated. Blood viscosity values were slightly raised at 2.9 cps (normal range 1.3-2 cps), but were too low to cause symptoms. It was concluded that the MG was only of a slowly progressive nature.

DISCUSSION

Macroglobulinemia was first described by Waldenström in 1944.[17] It is an uncommon chronic lymphoproliferative disorder involving the B-lymphocyte system,[16,18-20] which has a wide spectrum of possible presentations. Clinical features may include weight loss, anemia, lymphadenopathy, bone marrow infiltration by pleomorphic lymphoid cells, hepatosplenomegaly, peripheral neuropathy and central nervous system abnormalities.[16,20] All patients show an increased production of monoclonal gammaglobulin of IgM type. The main differences in symptomatology from multiple myeloma are an absence of localized bone resorption, pathological fractures and renal disease. Classical Bence Jones proteinuria is rare. The clinical course may be dominated by immunological effects from the abnormal gammaglobulin in the form of autoimmune hemolytic anemia, or increased sensitivity to cold. More common manifestations are caused by the raised high molecular weight plasma protein levels which produce a hyperviscosity syndrome in about one third of patients, with an increased tendency to both thrombosis and hemorrhage.[16,20] Secondary suppression of the other immunoglobulins may pro-

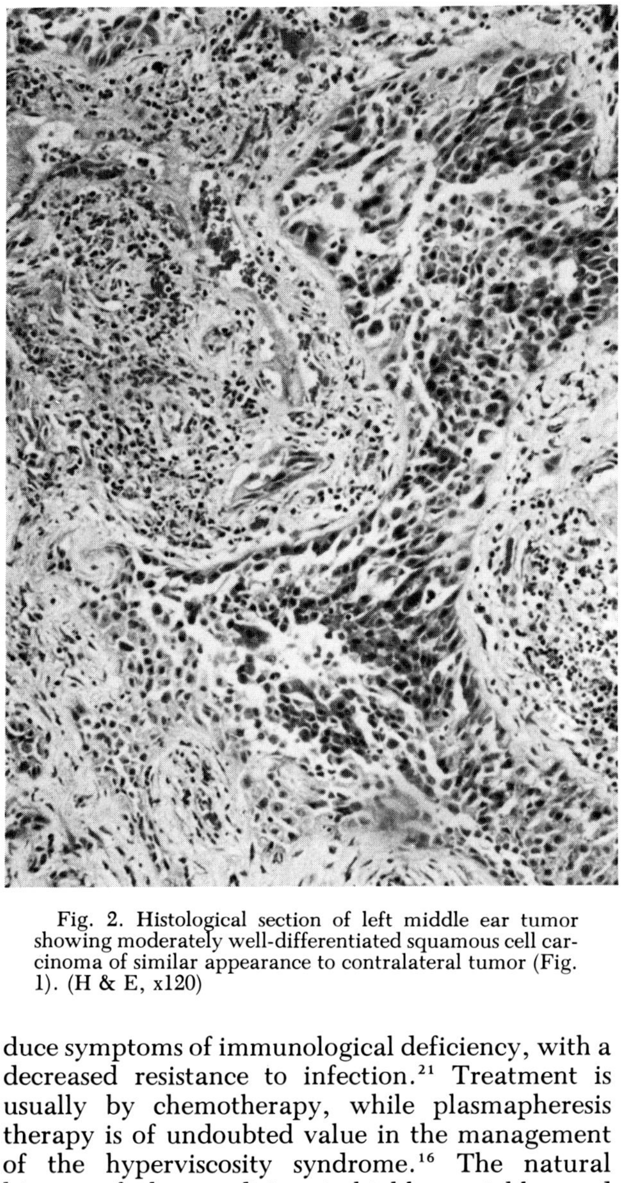

Fig. 2. Histological section of left middle ear tumor showing moderately well-differentiated squamous cell carcinoma of similar appearance to contralateral tumor (Fig. 1). (H & E, x120)

duce symptoms of immunological deficiency, with a decreased resistance to infection.[21] Treatment is usually by chemotherapy, while plasmapheresis therapy is of undoubted value in the management of the hyperviscosity syndrome.[16] The natural history of the condition is highly variable, and about 20% of patients require no specific treatment for long periods.[20]

The possibility of a relation between Waldenström's MG and cancer was discussed as early as 1953 by Schaub.[22] In 1954 Kappeler and his coworkers had traced 18 cases with malignant disease of 146 with Waldenström's MG in the literature.[23] Hällén found an incidence of 33% in his own series of 27 patients who had concurrent or previously diagnosed cancer,[15] while Mackenzie and Fudenberg reported a 60% tumor incidence in 40 patients.[16] Many of these tumors were of epithelial origin. However, it has proved difficult to delineate the precise relationship between the two conditions. Figure 3 illustrates possible theoretical mechanisms which may account for the association between Waldenström's MG and middle ear neoplasia.

Although a primary malignant disorder of the B-cell lymphatic system has long been assumed, the cause of MG remains unknown. The evidence for the presence of antibody activity in these abnormal proteins, which has been reviewed by Ritzman et al,[24] suggests that some forms of MG occur as a result of antigenic stimulation. This theory was first suggested by Osserman and Takatsuki[25] and has been documented in patients in response to a wide variety of chronic infections.[24] In a similar manner tumor-specific antigens may also stimulate excessive immunoglobulin production. Thus Mackenzie and Fudenberg have proposed the hypothesis that the monoclonal IgM proteins in MG are antibodies to either a tumor-specific antigen, or to microorganisms related to tumor induction, or may be produced inappropriately by the tumor itself.[16] They explored these possible relationships by immunofluorescent techniques in four patients, but were unable to demonstrate either tumor antigens which reacted with the specific macroglobulins, or significant tumor IgM production, so that these theories remain unsubstantiated.

It is well recognized that foreign antigens usually cause a general increase in immunoglobulin concentrations so that other factors must exist for specific IgM to be produced. Several reports describe the familial occurrence of MG or asymptomatic IgM paraproteinemia in the relatives of patients with the disease.[26-28] The frequency of abnormal immunoglobulin assays in these familial studies were substantially greater than those found in normal subjects,[15,29] so that there may well be a hereditary basis for the uncontrolled synthesis of the abnormal paraproteins in this condition. In the present case, it is possible that the longstanding chronic middle ear suppuration, extending over 40 years, provided the antigenic stimulus for macroglobulin formation in such a susceptible individual (Fig. 3C).

The increased tumor incidence in Waldenström's MG may result from a secondary immunodeficiency, caused by suppression of the other immunoglobulins following bone marrow infiltration (Fig. 3A). The increased incidence of tumors in subjects whose immune responses are suppressed is well documented. Such evidence supports the concept of immunological surveillance against tumor cells, which was proposed by Thomas in 1959,[30] and later developed by Burnet.[31] Thus immunosuppression predisposing to malignant transformation may be artificially induced by neonatal thymectomy or administration of antilymphocytic serum in experimental animals.[32-34] In addition there is a significantly increased incidence of malignant neoplasms in humans with hereditary immunodeficiency syndromes,[35] and in immunosuppressed recipients of organ allografts.[36-39] It has been suggested that human cancers occur characteristically at the extremes of life because the immune system is either maturing or is weakened by thymic atrophy.[31] Immunosurveillance breakdown could theoretically

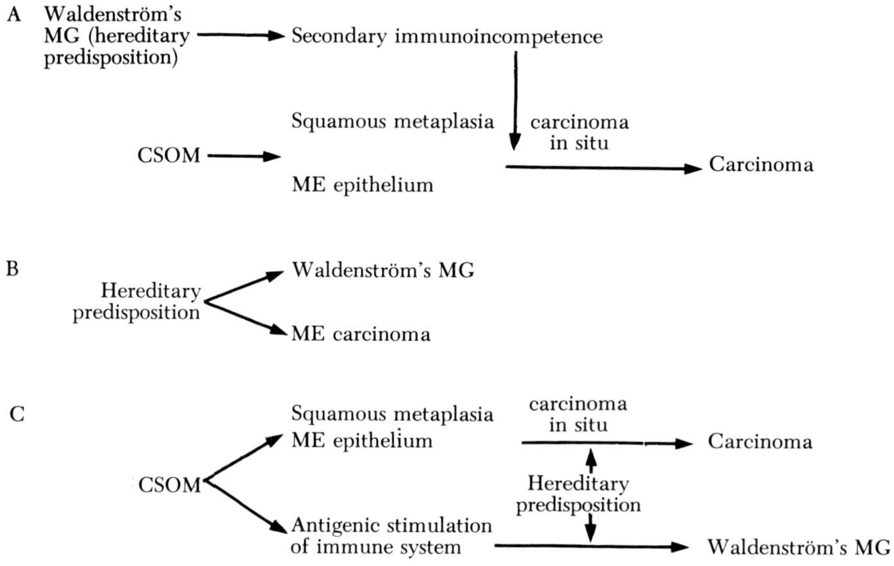

Fig. 3. A-C) Possible mechanisms to explain the association between Waldenström's macroglobulinemia (MG) and middle ear neoplasia. ME - Middle ear; CSOM - Chronic suppurative otitis media; ↓ - Facilitates.

explain the malignant transformation of metaplastic middle ear epithelium, which has arisen in response to chronic infection. However, the bone marrow was not extensively infiltrated in the present case, so that there was no significant associated immunological dysfunction.

A history of active CSOM of many years' duration is frequently present in patients with middle ear tumors, and has been incriminated as an important etiological agent.[5-11,40] Bradley and Maxwell first suggested that squamous metaplasia of the columnar or cuboidal epithelium of the tympanic cavity may result from chronic infection, and proceed to malignant transformation.[5] Lederman compared the development of carcinoma of the middle ear to the development of epitheliomas in relation to chronic sinuses in bone,[8] while Lodge et al drew an analogy with Marjolin's ulcer.[40] Carcinoma in situ changes have been described in association with middle ear carcinomas.[10,13] This histological feature, which was present bilaterally in the present case, offers support for the theory of tumor induction by chronic irritation. However,the paradoxically few middle ear neoplasms that are diagnosed, compared to the very large number of patients with chronically discharging ears, indicates that other factors must be involved in tumor pathogenesis. An underlying hereditary predisposition may be important in this respect.

Thus, the primary pathological process of active CSOM in a susceptible individual may account both for the development of bilateral aural carcinomas and concurrent Waldenström's MG due to chronic antigenic stimulation of the immune system (Fig. 3C).

In conclusion, it is recommended that patients with neoplastic or longstanding chronic suppurative otorhinolaryngological diseases who report systemic symptoms warrant full medical and immunological investigation. An underlying disorder may be diagnosed which could adversely influence the effects of primary therapy. In addition, serious medical conditions may be identified and evaluated at an early and possibly curative stage. In the case presented, Waldenström's MG, a potentially fatal lymphoproliferative disorder has been diagnosed in association with very rare bilateral middle ear carcinomas. Although not in an aggressive phase, recognition of the coexistent paraproteinemia will enable close long-term surveillance for possible future complications.

ACKNOWLEDGMENTS — The author would like to thank Mr. Peter McKelvie, Consultant Surgeon at the London Hospital, for permission to report details of a patient under his care, and the Histopathology Department for preparing the illustrations.

REFERENCES

1. Robinson GA. Malignant tumours of the ear. Laryngoscope 1931; 41:467-73.

2. Schall LA. Neoplasms involving the middle ear. Arch Otolaryngol 1935; 22:548-53.

3. Peele JC, Hauser GH. Primary carcinoma of the external auditory canal and middle ear. Arch Otolaryngol 1941; 34: 254-66.

4. Towson CE, Shoftstall WH. Carcinoma of the ear. Arch Otolaryngol 1950; 51:724-38.

5. Bradley WH, Maxwell JH. Neoplasms of the middle ear and mastoid. Report of 54 cases. Laryngoscope 1954; 64:533-56.

6. Lewis JS. Cancer of the ear. Laryngoscope 1960; 70: 551-79.

7. Boland J, Paterson R. Cancer of the middle ear and external auditory meatus. J Laryngol Otol 1955; 69:468-78.

8. Lederman M. Malignant tumours of the ear. J Laryngol Otol 1965; 79:85-119.

9. Tucker WN. Cancer of the middle ear; a review of 89 cases. Cancer 1965; 18:642-50.

10. Friedmann I. Pathology of the ear. Oxford: Blackwell Scientific Publications, 1974; 145-225.

11. Conley J, Schuller DE. Malignancies of the ear. Laryngoscope 1976; 86:1147-63.

12. Juby HB. Bilateral malignant disease of the middle ear. J Laryngol Otol 1957; 71:700-2.

13. Michaels L, Wells M. Squamous cell carcinoma of the middle ear. Clin Otolaryngol 1980; 5:235-48.

14. Schmidt PH, Verdonk GJ. Bilateral carcinoma of the ear. J Laryngol Otol 1967; 81:567-9.

15. Hällén J. Discrete gammaglobulin (M-) components in serum. Acta Med Scand 1966; 179 Suppl 462:1.

16. Mackenzie MR, Fudenberg HH. Macroglobulinaemia: an analysis of 40 patients. Blood 1972; 39:874-89.

17. Waldenström J. Incipient myelomatosis or essential hyperglobinaemia with fibroinogenopenia: new syndrome? Acta Med Scand 1944; 117:216-47.

18. Bachmann R. The diagnostic significance of the serum concentration of pathological proteins (M-components). Acta Med Scand 1965; 178:801-8.

19. Hobbs JR. Paraproteins, benign or malignant? Br Med J 1967; 3:699-704.

20. Alexian R. Plasma cell neoplasms. Medicine 1975; 2: 1700-12.

21. Fahey JL, Scoggins R, Utz JP, Szwed CF. Infection antibody response in gammaglobulin components in multiple myeloma and macroglobulinaemia. Am J Med 1963; 35:698-705.

22. Schaub F. Gleichzeitiges Vorkommen von Makroglobulinämie Waldenström und von malignen Tumoren. Schweiz Med Wchnschur 1953; 83:1256-7.

23. Kappeler R, Krebs A, Riva G. Kliniker Makroglobulinämie Waldenström: Beschreibung von 21 fällen und ubersicht der literatur. Helv Med Acta (Basel) 1958; 25:54-101.

24. Ritzmann SE, Loukas D, Sakai H, Daniels JC, Levin WC. Idiopathic (asymptomatic) monoclonal gammopathies. Ann Intern Med 1975; 135:95-106.

25. Osserman EF, Takatsuki K. Considerations regarding pathogenesis of the plasmacytic dyscrasias. Semin Hematol 1964; 4:28-52.

26. Seligmann M, Danon F, Mihaesco C, Fudenberg HH. Immunoglobulin abnormalities in families of patients with Waldenström's macroglobulinaemia. Am J Med 1967; 43:66-83.

27. Williams RC, Erickson JL, Polseky HF, Swain WR. Studies of monoclonal immunoglobulins (M-components) in various kindreds. Ann Intern Med 1967; 67:309-27.

28. Kalff MW, Hijmans W. Immunoglobulin analysis in families of macroglobulinaemia patients. Clin Exp Immunol 1969; 5:479-98.

29. Axelsson U, Bachmann R, Hällén J. Frequency of pathological proteins (M-components) in 6,995 sera from an adult population. Acta Med Scand 1966; 179:235-47.

30. Thomas L. Reactions to homologous tissue antigens. In: Lawrence HS, ed. Cellular and humoral aspects of the hypersensitive state. London: Cassell, 1959: 539.

31. Burnet FM. Immunological surveillance in neoplasia. Transplant Rev 1971; 7:3-25.

32. Allison AC, Taylor RB. Observations on thymectomy and carcinogenesis. Cancer Res 1967; 27:703-7.

33. Balner H. Immunosuppression and neoplasia. Rev Eur Etud Clin Biol 1970; 15:599-604.

34. Wagner JL, Haughton G. Immune suppression by antilymphocytic serum and its effect on tumours induced by 3-methylcholanthane in mice. J Nat Cancer Inst 1971; 46:1-10.

35. Gatti RA, Good RA. Occurrence of malignancy in immunodeficiency diseases. Cancer 1971; 28:89-98.

36. McKhann CF. Primary malignancy in patients undergoing immunosuppression for renal transplants. Transplantation 1969; 8:209-12.

37. Starzl TE, Penn I, Putnam CW. Iatrogenic alterations of immunologic surveillance in man and their influence on malignancy. Transplant Rev 1971; 7:112-45.

38. Walder BK, Robertson MR, Jeremy D. Skin cancer and immunosuppression. Lancet 1971; 2:1282-3.

39. Penn I. Malignancies in recipients of organ transplants. John Hopkins Med J 1974; Suppl 3:211-21.

40. Lodge WO, Jones HM, Smith MEN. Malignant tumours of the temporal bone. Arch Otolaryngol 1955; 61:535-41.

Ann Otol Rhinol Laryngol 91:1982

EFFECTS OF CONDUCTIVE HEARING LOSS ON AUDITORY BRAINSTEM RESPONSE

THERESE J. MCGEE, PhD

JACK D. CLEMIS, MD

CHICAGO, ILLINOIS

The purpose of this paper is not to propose that auditory brainstem response (ABR) be utilized for the assessment of conductive losses, but to define the effects of conductive hearing loss on the ABR when such a complication occurs. Conductive losses attenuate cochlear stimulation. Since wave V latency is inversely related to stimulus intensity, the magnitude of the conductive loss should be a predictor of the wave V latency delay. In this study, ABR wave V latencies from patients with known conductive losses due to canal occlusion, middle ear effusion, ossicular fixation and chain interruption were compared with latency values calculated from the magnitude of the loss. In those patients with occlusion of the external auditory canal and middle ear effusion, the shift of the wave V latency-intensity function correlated well with the air-bone gap. This correlation was poor for patients with ossicular chain disorders. In mixed hearing losses, the increased wave V latency due to the conductive component may totally mask an increase in latency caused by a retrocochlear component.

INTRODUCTION

The purpose of hearing assessment is to determine the existence of hearing loss, its characteristics, and the magnitude of any loss across frequency. Such determinations are relatively straightforward in the adult and older child. With special pediatric audiometric techniques, there is little problem testing the cooperative child. But in the newborn, infant, mentally-retarded, or uncooperative patient, these determinations are considerably more difficult to obtain.

The use of auditory brainstem response (ABR) testing in the diagnosis of hearing loss in the latter group has gained widespread acceptance in the past few years. Auditory brainstem responses, as described by Jewett[1] and Sohmer and Feinmesser[2], have been shown to be reliable indicators of peripheral auditory function. The 7-peaked response can be obtained with surface electrodes. The wave V marker can be recorded to within 10 dB of behavioral threshold. The test does require that the patient be resting quietly to reduce undesired background physiological "noise" that can contaminate these measures. However, the responses are not adversely affected by sleep state, sedation, or general anesthesia, if such measures are necessary.[3]

In view of the increased utilization of ABR testing and the frequent occurrence of conductive losses in children, it is important to understand the effect of conductive hearing loss on ABR results. The present study therefore was designed to determine 1) whether conductive losses can be differentiated from cochlear and retrocochlear losses with ABR measurements; 2) whether the various components

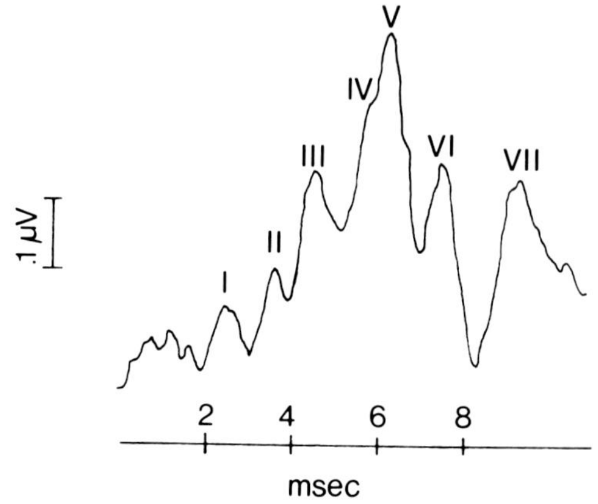

Fig. 1. Normal ABR elicited by 1024 sweeps of a 2000 Hz tone pip. (Signal level = 80 dB HL, repetition rate = 20 pips/s.)

of mixed losses can be delineated, and 3) whether conductive losses of different etiologic types give similar ABR results.

It is important to point out that the purpose of this paper is not to propose that ABR be utilized in the assessment of conductive hearing loss when other, simpler assessment methods are available, but rather to define the effects conductive hearing losses have on the ABR.

PROPERTIES OF THE ABR FROM NORMAL LISTENERS

In a normal listener, a click stimulus at an intensity of 70 dB HL will elicit a 7-peaked response within the first ten milliseconds after stimulus onset (Fig. 1). The response is quite small in amplitude, less than a microvolt, and digital signal averaging techniques are needed to make the response discer-

From the Department of Speech and Audiology, Hines VA Hospital, the Department of Otolaryngology and Maxillofacial Surgery, Northwestern University School of Medicine, and the Department of Otolaryngology, Mercy Hospital and Medical Center, Chicago.

This research was supported by the American Hearing Research Foundation, Kiwanis International Foundation and Mercy Hospital and Medical Center.

REPRINTS — Jack D. Clemis, MD, Mercy Hospital and Medical Center, Stevenson Expressway at King Drive, Chicago, IL 60616.

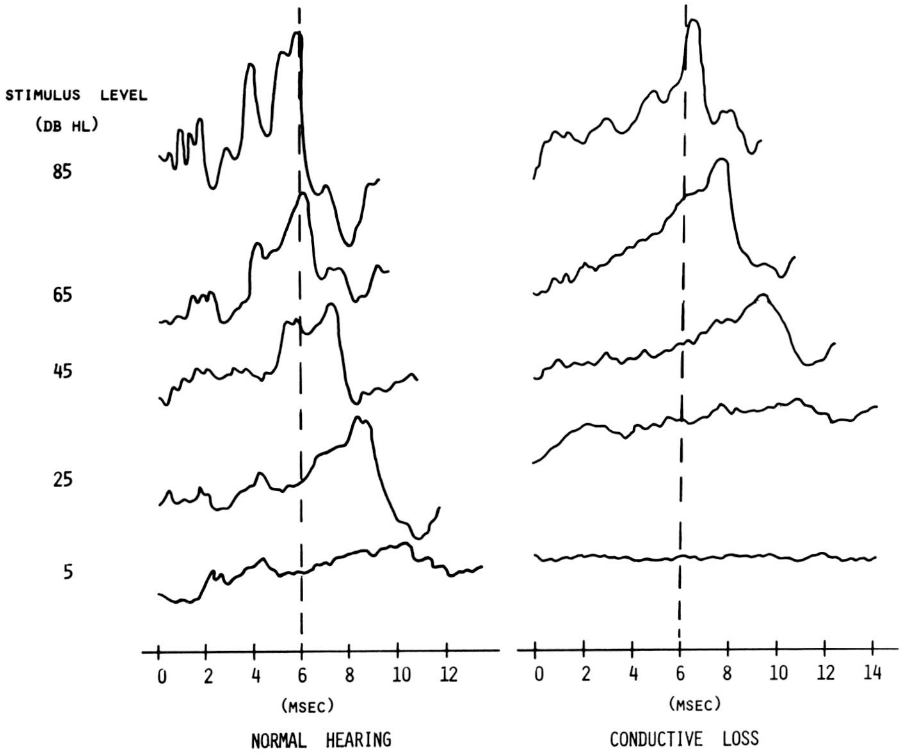

Fig. 2. Comparison of ABR responses from a normal-hearing subject and a person with a 20 dB conductive loss.

nible. The fifth peak (wave V) is the largest and most reliable of the seven. It is therefore used as a marker for both threshold and site of lesion testing.

Tone pips with a rise time of one millisecond or less may also be used to elicit the ABR. They have narrower frequency spectra than do clicks and, therefore, provide better information on frequency specificity. However, due to the fast rise time, tone pips have significantly more spectral spread than do standard audiometric tone bursts.

EFFECT OF SITE OF LESION ON THE ABR

In general, for a given signal level, latency values for wave V are longer than normal in conductive and retrocochlear lesions, but essentially normal for cochlear losses.[4-6] There are some exceptions to this rule in cochlear losses. Some delay in latency may be observed when the stimulus is very close to the patient's threshold. However, when the stimulus intensity is increased, the latencies rapidly approach normal values in a recruitment-like pattern. Patients with severe cochlear losses may not show this "recruitment" effect, and their ABR latencies will then be delayed when compared to normal values. In addition, when the ABR is elicited by a click or by a high frequency tone pip, patients with high frequency cochlear losses may show increased latency values.

The longer latency seen with retrocochlear damage is probably due to desynchronized neural firing or a selective effect on the high frequency fibers.[6,7] These delays are observed with both tone pip and click stimuli[8,9] and can vary from rather small delays of 0.3 ms to very large prolongations of 3.0 ms or more. This property of ABR is very reliable, making ABR one of the most efficient special auditory tests in the differential diagnosis of vestibular schwannomas and other lesions affecting the auditory nerve.

Latency values are inversely related to stimulus intensity (Fig. 2). Thus, if a conductive loss attenuates cochlear stimulation, then it is to be expected that is will increase wave V latency values. This observation has been previously reported, but only on very few subjects in each report.[10-12] Additionally, it has been suggested that these increased latency values can be predicted by the magnitude of the conductive component. This is a point that has not been supported by the studies of Mendelson et al,[13] Clemis and Mitchell,[8] and Yamada et al.[5] In the Mendelson et al series, comparative audiometric data for most subjects was unavailable. Technical factors probably biased the results of Clemis and Mitchell, and Yamada et al may have shown poor correlation because of the dissimilar stimuli used in the study (ie, click for ABR and tone bursts for assessing audiometric thresholds).

METHODS

Audiometric and ABR results were obtained from 22 subjects with normal hearing (threshold better than 10 dB HL) and from 23 patients (32 ears) with various conductive disorders: occlusions of the external auditory canal, middle ear effusion, otosclerosis, and various ossicular chain disorders (Table 1). Ages ranged from 3 to 76 years. All patients were cooperative and able to respond reliably on conventional audiometric tests. Air and bone conduction thresholds obtained by conventional audiometry were carefully documented and the differences between the air and the

TABLE 1. PATIENTS AND THEIR DISORDERS

Disorder	No. of Subjects	No. of Ears
External canal occluded	3	5
Middle ear effusion	11	15
Otosclerosis	6	7
Ossicular discontinuity	4	5
Total	23*	32

*One patient, with an ossicular discontinuity in the right ear and a fluid-filled left middle ear, is included in two categories.

bone conduction thresholds (air-bone gap) were calculated. The audiometric data were obtained by qualified audiologists not associated with this laboratory. Thus, those performing the ABR testing had no prior knowledge of the audiometric results.

Of the five ears with occlusions of the external auditory canal, all had bone conduction thresholds better than 10 dB HL. Of the 15 ears of patients with middle ear effusion, 13 had bone conduction thresholds better than 15 dB HL, and two had thresholds of 30-40 dB Hl. Of the 12 ears of patients with ossicular chain disorders, 5 had bone conduction thresholds better than 20 dB HL, while 7 had bone conduction of 25-35 dB HL.

In all ABR tests, electrode sites were prepared by an alcohol cleansing, electrode paste was rubbed into the skin, and silver, silver-chloride electrodes were applied. The active electrode was placed at the vertex, the reference at the ipsilateral mastoid, and the ground at the forehead. Resistance was measured and ascertained to be less than 5 kohms for each electrode pair.

Patients reclined in a hospital cart during the test. Children under age ten were sedated with chloralhydrate. Adults were sometimes given diazepam to aid in relaxation. Testing was carried out only while the patient's ongoing physiological activity was less than 10 uV.

Responses were elicited by tone pips with a one millisecond rise-decay time and no plateau, for a total duration of two milliseconds. Frequencies of 1000, 2000, and 4000 Hz were used. Responses were amplified at a gain of 10^5 and filtered with a band-pass of 100 to 3000 Hz and a roll-off of 6 dB/octave. The ongoing activity was monitored on an oscilloscope. The responses were averaged on a Tracor-Northern NS-570 digital signal averager.

Figure 3 demonstrates the procedure for determining an estimate of the conductive loss from the patient's latency-intensity function. For each patient the ABR wave V latencies were plotted with the mean wave V latencies of the normal subjects. The degree of attenuation in the signal level which would produce the observed shift in the patient's latency-intensity function was then

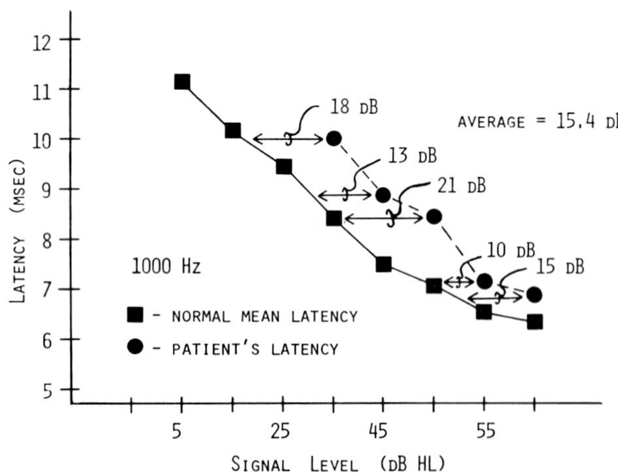

Fig. 3. Demonstration of the determination of the latency-intensity function (LIF) shift in order to estimate the degree of conductive loss.

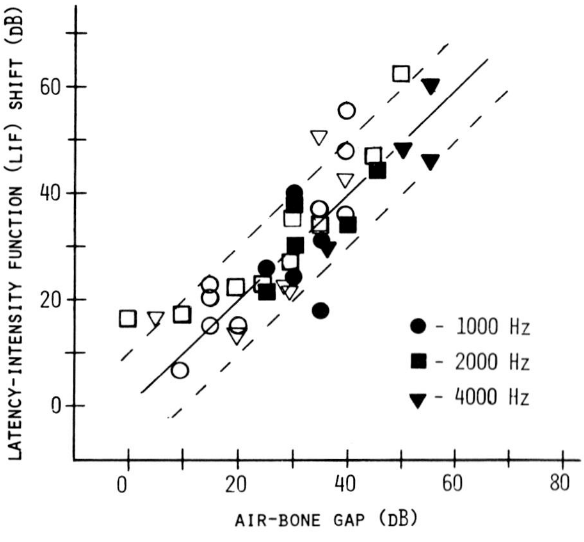

Fig. 4. LIF shift vs air-bone gap: losses induced with earplugs (closed symbols), and middle ear effusion (open symbols).

measured. These values were averaged over all points on the latency-intensity function to produce a mean latency-intensity function (LIF) shift value (in dB units).

RESULTS

In Figures 4 and 5, the wave V LIF shift versus the air-bone gap has been compared. Solid lines mark the calculated values and the dashed lines denote a region plus or minus 10 dB. Patients with hearing losses produced with earplugs and patients with middle ear effusion show a very good agreement between LIF shift and air-bone gap (Fig. 4). Virtually all of the points fall within 10 dB of the calculated line. However, for patients with ossicular chain disorders, the LIF estimate tends to be larger than the air-bone gap (Fig. 5).

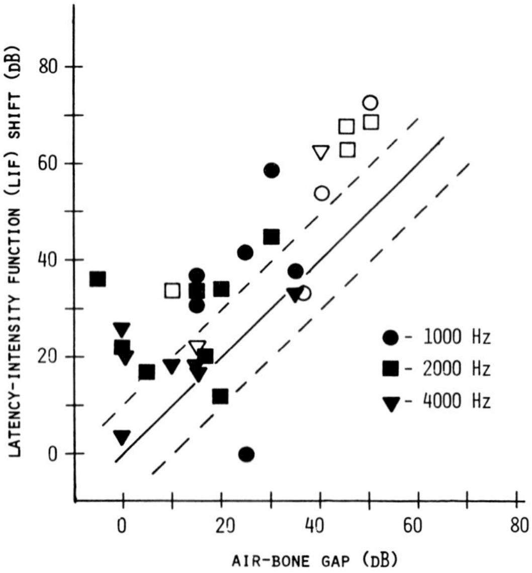

Fig. 5. LIF shift vs air-bone gap: ossicular chain disorders. Closed symbols - otosclerosis; open symbols - ossicular discontinuity.

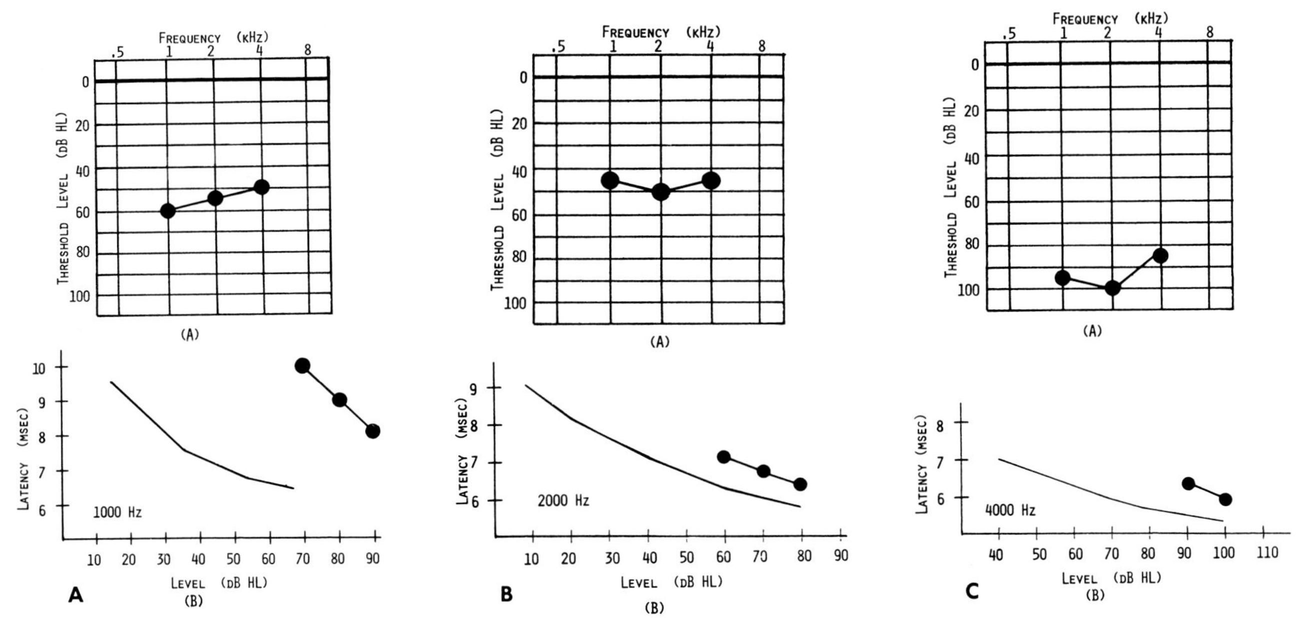

Fig. 6. ABR results. A) Case 1 (right ear only; B) Case 2; C) Case 3. (A) - Wave V thresholds; (B) - Patient's wave V latencies denoted by closed circles (●——●); lower line indicates normal mean wave V latencies.

DISCUSSION

The results from the first two groups support the hypothesis that increased ABR latency in conductive loss is due to a simple reduction in signal level. That reduction is equal to the amount of conductive component which is accurately measured by the air-bone gap.

The lack of agreement between LIF shift and air-bone gap for the third group could be due to either of two factors: 1) the latencies are affected by cochlear or retrocochlear components in the hearing loss, or 2) the air-bone gap is not an accurate measure of the amount of sound reduction caused by the conductive component.

With respect to the first possibility, 7 of 12 ears of these subjects displayed some elevation of the bone conduction threshold, but there was no evidence that the elevation was due to retrocochlear damage in any patient. In all seven cases, the bone conduction thresholds were better than 35 dB, and thus would not indicate the type of cochlear loss that would result in a latency delay.

Alternatively, the bone conduction thresholds may be affected by a mechanical artifact. In the case of otosclerosis, Carhart[14] has shown that a significant improvement occurs in the bone conduction threshold after corrective surgery. He concluded that presurgical bone conduction thresholds are elevated by purely mechanical factors which are alleviated with surgery (Carhart notch phenomenon).

If this is also the case for the patients in this study with ossicular chain disorders, then the air-bone gap will underestimate the sound reduction caused by the conductive component, while the wave V LIF shift will reflect the actual sound reduction.

The accuracy of the LIF shift in estimating the conductive component of a hearing loss is evident from these results, at least for conductive losses that do not involve abnormalities of the ossicular chain. The extent of the clinical usefulness of these data can be illustrated by the following cases:

Case 1. A 3-month-old infant with Treacher-Collins syndrome was referred for audiologic assessment. The otoscopic examination indicated an atretic right external auditory canal and a normal left tympanic membrane. The ABR results indicated bilateral symmetrical wave V thresholds of 50 to 60 dB HL, an LIF shift of 55 to 60 dB when compared to a normal wave V latency-intensity function (Fig. 6A). Comment: It was concluded that this child has a right congenital atresia and a left congenital ossicular chain fixation. Considering the age of this child, surgical intervention will probably not be done for several years. The ABR results not only served to reassure the parents and physician that the auditory sensorineural apparatus is intact, but also picked up a large conductive loss on the left side that may have been missed by inspection alone, and therefore provided the indication for early habilitation through amplification.

Case 2. A hyperactive, uncooperative 3-year-old child with a severe language delay was referred for an evaluation using ABR. The wave V thresholds were 45 to 50 dB HL, and the LIF shift was 20 dB (Fig. 6B). Impedance testing revealed flat tympanograms bilaterally. Comment: This child has a mixed hearing loss of 45 to 50 dB HL, flat in the mid-frequency range, with a conductive component of approximately 20 dB.

Case 3. A mentally retarded child was referred for an ABR evaluation. Wave V thresholds showed a profound loss and the LIF shift was 30 dB (Fig. 6C). Impedance measurements indicated flat tympanograms bilaterally. Comment: Severe-to-profound sensorineural hearing loss with a conductive component of not more than 30 dB. This conclusion is based on speculative interpretation of all the data. The magnitude of the loss is too great to be purely conductive and the magnitude of the LIF shift is small, supporting this conclusion. However, the sensorineural loss may be severe enough in itself to cause an increase in latency. Impedance audiometry and otoscopy supported the diagnosis of a conductive component to the loss in this case.

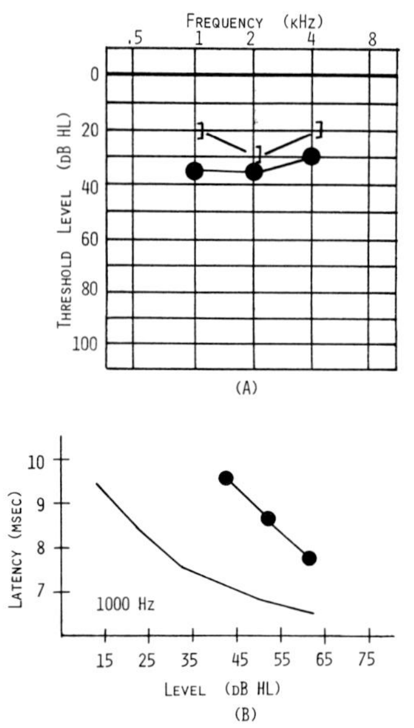

Fig. 7. (Case 4) (A) - Audiometric thresholds and (B) -ABR wave V latencies.

Case 4. A man with otosclerosis is suspected of having a vestibular schwannoma. His air-bone gap at 1000 Hz was 15 dB. The ABR wave V LIF shift was 35 dB at this frequency (Fig. 7). Similar results were obtained at 2000 and 4000 Hz. Comment: The ABR results have added nothing to the diagnostic picture in this case since an LIF shift larger than the air-bone gap is characteristic of otosclerosis.

Eggermont et al[7] discuss at length the use of the difference between the latencies of waves I and V as a diagnostic tool for the detection of retrocochlear damage. A delay in both peaks with a normal wave I-V interval is an indication of peripheral damage, while a prolonged wave I-V interval would indicate retrocochlear damage. The difficulty that we have had with this measure is that in many cases wave I is difficult to discern. In the present study, for 15 of the 32 ears tested, the wave I-V interval was normal. For 17 ears, no wave I could be recorded. This percentage might be improved by using more intense stimuli at a lower repetition rate, or by using electrocochleographic methods to obtain the wave I latency value.

Unless the wave I latency is determined, even a minor conductive component can severely complicate the detection of retrocochlear damage with ABR. Selters and Brackmann[6] report that this situation rarely occurs, but the coexistence of schwannoma and otosclerosis has been documented[15] and must be considered. If the air-bone gap and the LIF shift correlate well in cases of pure conductive loss, then it would be tempting to merely use the air-bone gap to extrapolate the amount of latency delay due to the conductive component. Unfortunately, some patients with vestibular schwannoma show very small latency delays of only 0.3 to 0.4 ms. The precision of an air-bone gap to LIF extrapolation would need to be very fine for a clinician to sort out such a small retrocochlear component from the total delay.

Of course, if the patient had a retrocochlear disorder which produced a large latency delay and his conductive loss was due to a disorder not involving the ossicular chain (for which the air-bone gap and LIF shift correlate well), then the components could be sorted out. However, it should be remembered that if the conductive loss involves the ossicular chain, then the air-bone gap will not be a reliable indicator of the amount of LIF shift due to the conductive component. For such a case, it is essential to obtain a measure of the wave I latency.

CONCLUSIONS

1. For patients with occlusion of the external auditory canal or middle ear effusion, the shift of the wave V latency-intensity function correlates well with the audiometric air-bone gap.

2. For patients with ossicular chain disorders, the increase in wave V latency from the conductive loss is larger than would be expected from the audiometric air-bone gap. It is speculated that this is due to a mechanical artifact affecting bone conduction thresholds.

3. When conductive and retrocochlear hearing loss coexist, and no wave I can be recorded, the increased wave V latency due to the conductive component may totally mask a delay caused by the retrocochlear component, unless the retrocochlear delay is fairly large. Wave V latency measurement alone is particularly useless in this regard when the conductive loss is due to an ossicular chain disorder.

ACKNOWLEDGMENTS — We wish to thank Cynthia Sarno, MA, and the physicians and audiologists of Otologic Professional Associates and Mercy Hospital and Medical Center, Chicago, for their help with this study.

REFERENCES

1. Jewett D. Volume-conducted potentials in response to auditory stimuli as detected by averaging in the cat. Electroenceph Clin Neurophys 1970; 28:609-18.

2. Sohmer H, Feinmesser M. Cochlear and cortical audiometry. Israel J Med Sci, 1970; 6:219-23.

3. Gibson WPR. Essentials of Clinical Electric Response Audiometry. London: Churchill-Livingstone, 1978.

4. Galambos R, Hecox KE. Clinical applications of the auditory brainstem response. Otolaryngol Clin North AM 1978; 11: 709-22.

5. Yamada O, Yagi R, Yamane H, Suzucki J. Clinical evaluation of the auditory evoked brainstem response. Aurix-Nasus-Larynx 1975; 2:97-105.

6. Selters WA, Brackmann DE. Acoustic tumor detection with brainstem electric response audiometry. Arch Otolaryngol 1977; 103:181-7.

7. Eggermont JJ, Don M, Brackmann DE. Electrocochleography and auditory brainstem electric responses in patients with

pontine angle tumors. Ann Otol Rhinol Laryngol 1980; 89 Suppl 75.

8. Clemis JD, Mitchell C. Electrocochleography and brainstem responses used in the diagnosis of acoustic tumors. J Otolaryngol 1977; 6:447-59.

9. Clemis JD, McGee TJ. Brainstem electric response audiometry in the differential diagnosis of acoustic tumors. Laryngoscope 1979; 89:31-42.

10. Yoshie N. Auditory nerve action potential responses to clicks in man. Laryngoscope 1968; 78:198-215.

11. Yoshie N, Ohashi T. Clinical use of cochlear nerve action potential responses in man for differential diagnosis of hearing losses. Acta Otolaryngol (Stockh) 1969; Suppl 252:71-87.

12. Hieber T, Hecox KE, Cone B. Brainstem auditory evoked potentials in patients with congenital atresia. Laryngoscope 1979; 89:1151-8.

13. Mendelson T, Salamy A, Lenoir M, McKean C. Brainstem evoked potential findings in children with otitis media. Arch Otolaryngol 1979; 105:17-20.

14. Carhart R. Clinical application of bone conduction audiometry. Arch Otolaryngol 1950; 51:798-808.

15. Clemis JD. The co-existence of acoustic neuroma and otosclerosis. Laryngoscope 1973; 83:1959-85.

≈

THE 12th INTERNATIONAL COURSE OF OTOLARYNGOLOGY

The 12th International Course of Otolaryngology, dealing with the eustachian tube, will be held on November 22-24, 1982, in Barcelona. For further information contact J. Oliveras, MD, Secretary, Pl. Eusebio Guell 12-13, Barcelona 34, Spain.

≈

NATIONAL HEARING ASSOCIATION

The Scientific Advisory Committee of the National Hearing Association solicits your research project for funding. Submit to: Wallace Rubin, MD, Chairman, Scientific Advisory Committee, 3333 Kingman St., Metairie, LA 70002.

Ann Otol Rhinol Laryngol 91:1982

CORTICAL, SUBCORTICAL, AND BRAINSTEM DYSFUNCTION: A CORRELATION IN DYSLEXIC CHILDREN

LOUIS W. WELSH, MD
MICHAEL HEALY, MA
JOHN J. WELSH, MD
BERNARD COOPER, PhD

JENKINTOWN, PENNSYLVANIA

A group of dyslexic students was examined by a central auditory test (CAT) battery including competing sentences, binaural fusion, filtered speech, and compressed speech. Auditory evoked brainstem responses (BSER) were measured in conjunction with the CAT data. The auditory tests indicate a high degree of failure in those areas requiring sophisticated integration, coordination, and identification of the modified speech stimuli. The BSER did not identify a significant abnormality. The cortical and subcortical areas of integration are proposed as the multicentric sites of impairment in the hearing function found in dyslexic students.

The goal of this paper is an evaluation of the cortical, subcortical, and brainstem disturbances in audition which are found in dyslexic students.

Students with perceptual defects may have, in addition, a hearing disorder which further compromises their function. The hearing impairment might not be suspected when the perceptual disorder, such as a reading problem, is so marked as to depress the awareness of other problems. The recognition of a concomitant hearing loss is necessary so that an appropriate educational environment and an individualized curriculum for achievement may be programmed. The initial purpose of this paper is to present a concept of hearing imperception through sophisticated challenges currently called Central Auditory Tests (CAT) in students classified as dyslexics.

A group of 20 children has been evaluated by the auditory evoked brainstem response (BSER) method and psychological parameters in conjunction with the CAT battery. The results and comparison of the data derived from two of these approaches are presented. The psychological evaluation has assumed such dimension that the authors will present this material in a separate publication. Localization of the site of the defect is postulated based upon the analysis of the data.

Dyslexia may be classified as a type of minimal brain dysfunction (MBD). The defects of this MBD are described in behavioral and perceptual-cognitive concepts. While the behavioral factors indeed contribute greatly to the utilization of the cognitive capabilities, this relationship and its contribution to scholarly achievement are beyond the scope of the current investigation.

The perceptual-cognitive aspects are multiple. Some defects include problems in memory, auditory perception, spatial relation, right-left disorientation, reversals and transposition of letters, and difficulty with auditory synthesis and discrimination.[1]

The magnitude of dyslexia is enormous; the number of students so classified may include 2 to 5% of the school population.[2] Extrapolated across the millions of children of school age, the total number may be staggering. As a sequel to the numerical problem is the fact that academic facilities are limited according to the financial structure of the community. Supportive services such as reading, counseling, writing techniques, and psychiatric therapy, when available, add great burdens to the parents and educational system. Identification of these students can be delayed until late in an academic career at which point the success of the special support programs may be markedly impaired.

In brief, several statements can be proposed about dyslexia. Early identification implies greater academic gain due to special assistance. The potential number of students so involved may be overwhelming. Specially oriented remedial education is expensive and with limited availability. With this background of general information, we proceed to the topic of hearing disability.

METHODS

The subjects are gathered from a school for dyslexics, clearly identified as such by educational, neurological, and psychological parameters. The ages are limited, with one exception (age 7), from 10 to 13 inclusive, in order that as homogeneous a group as possible be evaluated for purposes of internal and external comparison. By contrast with a previous report[2] in which selection for entrance into the project was based upon categorization of "dyslexia" alone, this group of 20 individuals can be classified as cooperative and motivated to participate in the study. There is no evidence of a hyperkinetic behavior pattern. None of the students at the time of the study were on tranquilizers or other forms of mood elevators or depressors, factors not necessarily present in the earlier study. The audiologic studies and the auditory evoked

Presented at the meeting of the American Neurotology Society, Vancouver, British Columbia, May 8, 1981.
REPRINTS — Louis W. Welsh, MD, 179 Washington Lane, Jenkintown, PA 19046.

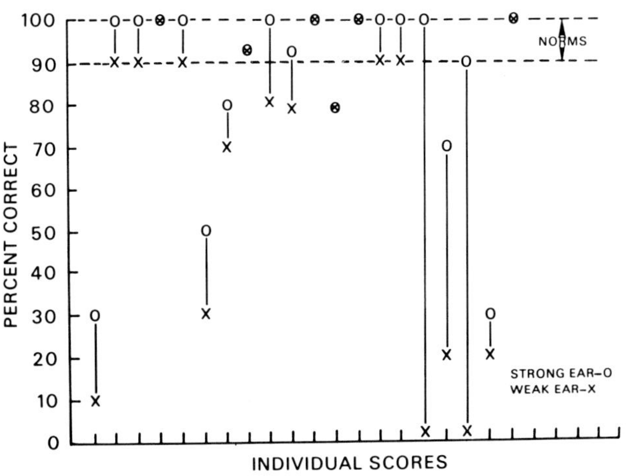

Fig. 1. Competing sentence test scored by strong and weak ears. A failure is defined as a score under 80%. Seven of the 20 subjects fell below normal range in one or both ears.

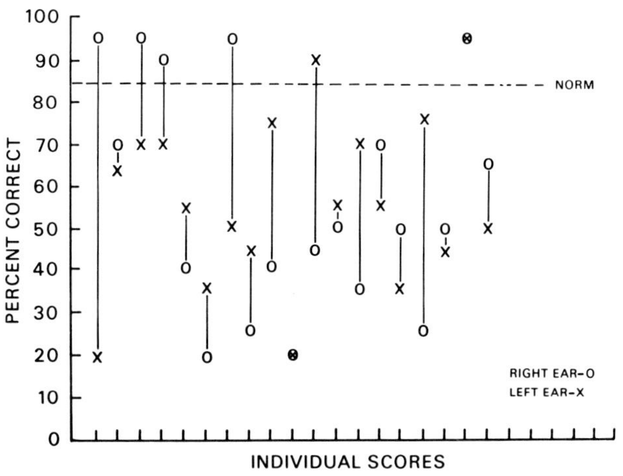

Fig. 2. Binaural fusion test. Normal value is approximately 85% correct. Seventeen of the 20 subjects fell below the 70% score considered to be within the failure range.

potentials are completed in a single exposure with periods of relaxation provided as needed. The psychological investigations are initial requirements for entrance into the academic program and later, on entry into the investigation, special batteries are employed for additional information.

The technical material of the test was presented in a previous publication. Specific requirements include a 2-channel audiometer (Maico MA 24B) with tape deck attachments for the special studies, a quiet environment which complies with ANSI standards, and accurately calibrated earphones.[2]

The CAT battery includes competing sentences, binaural fusion, filtered speech, and compressed speech. We have deleted the rapidly alternating speech perception test, supposedly a measure of brainstem capability for integration of fragmented speech, due to the high level of success in the previous report.[2] The assumption based upon these data is that the brainstem is not functionally deficient in dyslexia.

The auditory evoked responses are collected and recorded by a Teledyne TA-1000 unit which consists of a preamplifier signal conditioner, signal processor (analog computer), stimulus generator, oscilloscope, and x-y recorder. We have elected the 2 kHz stimulus at a rate of 20/s. The cumulative responses of 2,000 impulses were averaged and played on the oscilloscope and later recorded on permanent tape. The test is repeated several times to produce a consistently identifiable and reproducible pattern of latency and intensity.

RESULTS

Results of the CAT battery (four tests) are reported followed by the auditory evoked response data. Comprehensive data for three students are presented to identify a pattern of hearing and reading disability in addition to a performance profile characterized as an attentional deficit.

Competing Sentences. The site of lesion is presumbed to be in the posterior portion of the temporal lobe. The technique of the test is quite simple; different sentences are presented in each ear simultaneously at 35 and 50 dB (SL). The listener repeats the primary message at the lower intensity and intelligibility is scored as the percent correct. The test is reversed and scored accordingly. The higher value is recorded as the strong ear and the lower as the weak ear (rather than right-left). The normal values for ages 10 to 13 approach closely 100% in each ear. For our critique, a value less than 80% (scored in 10% increments) is considered to be a failure, whether the strong or weak ear.

A failure was evident in 7/20, or 35% (Fig. 1). One of this group is slightly depressed below normal (80/70), and the remaining 6 fail with surprisingly low values in each instance where the weak ear responds from 0 to 30% with an anticipated value of 90%. In addition, the strong ears in 3 of the 6 are under 50%.

Binaural Fusion. The area for integration of frequency-fragmented speech is considered to be the brainstem. The test is structured upon separation of the speech stimuli in two frequency bands, 500 to 700 Hz and 1,900 to 2,100 Hz. The simultaneous reception of these otherwise unintelligible sounds is merged through the brainstem and integrated into a composite form and presented to the central auditory centers for identification. The normal value of fusion is approximately 85% in the right and left ears for children age 10.

The authors define failure of this auditory challenge at a level below 70%, allowing 15% from the normal for range of variation. Employing this criterion, we observe a high rate of failure in 17/20 (Fig. 2). The range of failure is particularly outstanding since 16 of the 40 ears scored below 50% and 8 under 40%. There was no mean evidence of dominance; in 9 individuals the right ear scored higher than the left, and in 9 other students the left was superior; finally there were two examples of balanced hearing. The mean values for 20 individuals are 51% accuracy for the right ears and 56% for the left ears.

Filtered Speech. The test is based on evidence which correlates lesions in the temporal lobe with failure to accurately identify distorted words. The test stimuli are modified by filtration above 500 Hz

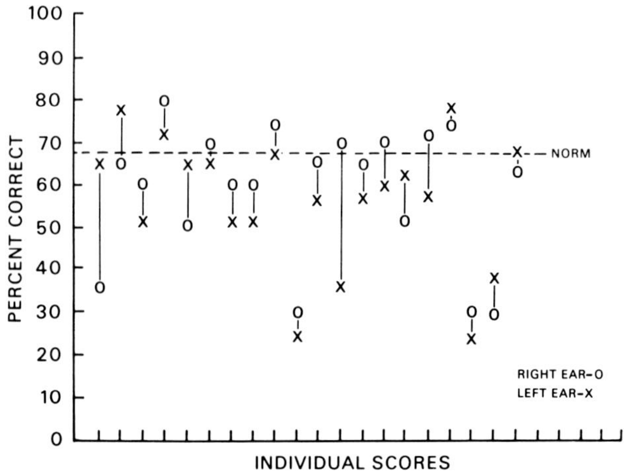

Fig. 3. Low pass filtered speech, monaural challenge with distorted speech. Ten of the 20 subjects were below the mean value of 58%.

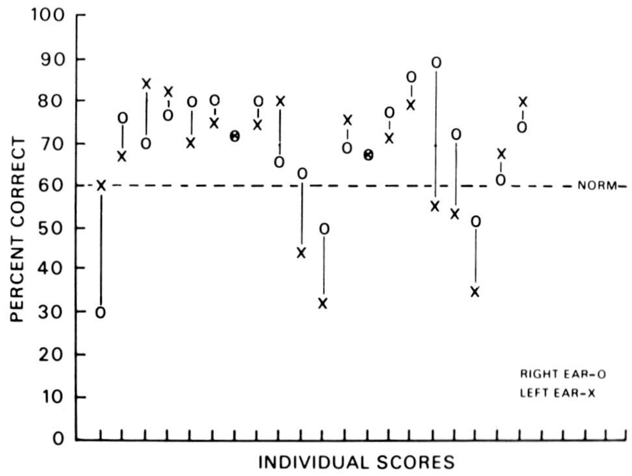

Fig. 4. Compressed speech test shortens the available time for word identification. Six of the group (30%) scored less than 60% correct, suggestive of a disturbance in the higher auditory pathways.

with an attenuation of 19 dB per octave band. The normative data indicate approximately 70% accuracy for age 10 (Fig. 3).

Failure of the test is defined as a value under 58%. Employing this criterion, we identified 10 of 20 whose ability to recognize speech in a distorted fashion was markedly impaired. A separate subgroup of three individuals is below 40% in both ears, a striking clinical failure. The remaining individuals are, on an average, moderately impaired with a mean in the middle 50% correct bracket; only 10 to 15% are below the normal mean.

Compressed Speech Test. This test relies upon the temporal distortion of the speech signal. The intelligibility scores indicate an inverse relationship to increasing compression. A direct ratio exists between intelligibility and intensity of stimulus as well as age (within a limited range). Consequently for the cerebral processing of an auditory stimulus, the individual requires a quantity of time for the reception of information and stimulus identification. Normal data presented by Beasley et al[3,4] indicate equal values for right and left ear with increasing time compression from 0 to 70%. The correct speech scores modified by compression were not affected until 40%; thereafter there was a gradual decrease in values until 70% when a rapid loss in discrimination became evident. Gradual increases in sensation levels from 8 to 32 dB again indicate equal right and left ear scores; consequently there is no apparent ear dominance.

Evidence presented by Bocca and Calearo[5] suggests the application of distorted speech tests for evaluation of the higher auditory pathways in the presence of normal peripheral organ studies. Further data by Calearo and Lazzaroni[6] using temporally compressed material indicated the temporal lobe as the site of the auditory defect with the score clearly lower in the ear contralateral to the site of the lesion.

For this study, the compression value is 60%, and 32 dB SL the common intensity of presentation. Each ear is tested separately with 25 words from the PB-K work list.

The normal data presented by Beasley[3] for 8-year-old students, which is nearest our test group age, indicate 92% accuracy at 32 dB sensation level, 0% compression, and approximately 80% correct at 30% compression, and 60% at 60% compression.

We have arbitrarily identified a failure of the test as a level below the norm, ie, 60% (Fig. 4). A clear indication of central auditory disturbance is apparent with a failure rate of 30%. Dominance is suggested by right ear scores in 7/12, 4 marginally or clearly left dominant and 1 subject indeterminate.

The relative importance of each test in the battery is depicted by the percentage of individual failure in each of the four components (Fig. 5). An intertest variation is evident, though, by the difference in score of each test.

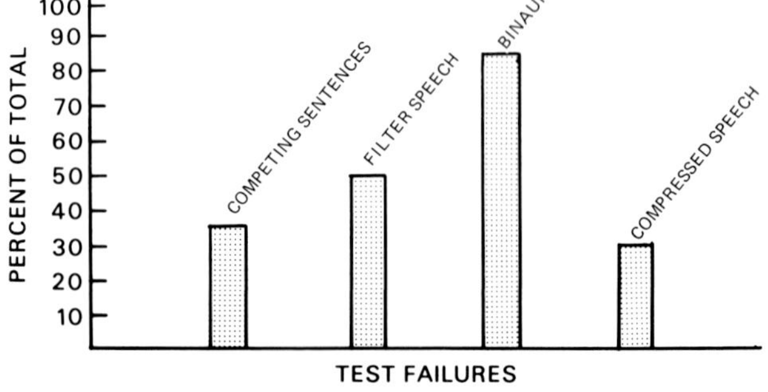

Fig. 5. Failure rate for each of the four central tests, extending from a low of 30% in the compressed speech test to the high of 85% in binaural fusion data.

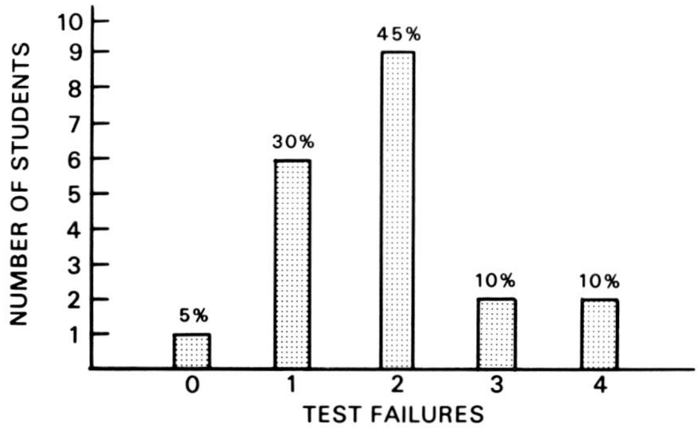

Fig. 6. Composite values of central auditory test failures. Approximately half of the group failed 2 tests, 20% either 3 or 4, and 30% a single test.

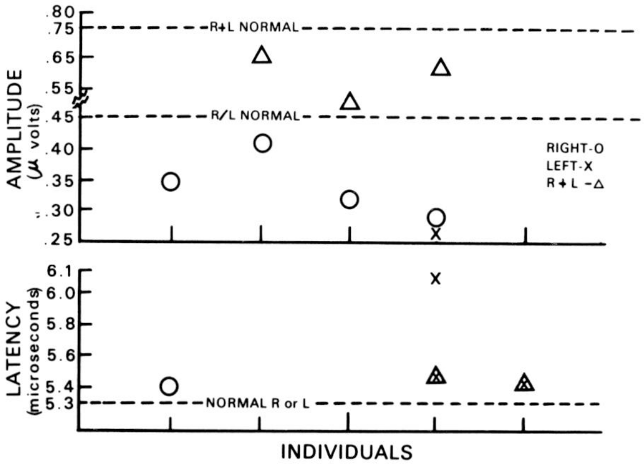

Fig. 7. Brainstem evoked auditory response. Data from five individuals are graphed to illustrate the minor variation from normal. Only two subjects exceeded the latency norm by 0.1 ms, probably within normal range. A third value of 6.1 ms is grossly abnormal. Minor variations in amplitude are also encountered.

The binaural fusion test is the most sensitive indicator of auditory disturbance in this dyslexic group; 80% score less than the normal value. Filtered speech with a 50% passing rate reveals a major disturbance in distorted monaural speech identification. The competing sentence and the compressed speech tests score in the proximity of one-third failures, a mild indicator of a central disturbance.

The success of the individual student in solving the auditory challenge is presented in Figure 6. Forty-five percent of the group failed two tests and 10% failed each of 3 and 4 segment challenges.

Auditory Evoked Responses. The data are analyzed according to the amplitude of the microvoltage responses in waves I and IV-V, from the right and left ears measured individually and the combined right-left response of simultaneous bilateral stimulation. Latency periods are presented by a similar method of unilateral and bilateral recording. Amplitude ratios IV-V/I are considered in the final data but are of little statistical value. Analysis of the information indicates that only 1 of the 20 individuals exceeded the normal latency values (by 0.2 ms) in one or more phases of the test and 4 were below the normal values for amplitude.

We shall not present the individual values of the 15 students who evidently fell within the normal range. Accordingly, the abnormal data of this segment are presented for comparison with the normal, abstracted from a group of individuals free from auditory impairment and aural disease as well as reading impairment (Fig. 7).

The values for amplitude of wave I have been deleted from the final report since the wave is often low and variable in configuration. The significant areas of abnormality appear in prolonged latencies, occasionally unilateral or due to simultaneous binaural stimulation. The amplitude of waves IV-V is diminished in several individuals. The failure of the auditory evoked response test appears most certain when both the latency and amplitude values are abnormal; this event occurs in 1/20 or 5% of the total group. At this point, we can clearly indicate that the data for the BSER do not identify a disorder in transmission in the brainstem.

There are three students who deserve an in-depth inspection, since in many ways they can be portrayed as fairly characteristic of the group as a whole yet with individual personality facets and idiosyncracies.

CASE REPORTS

Case 1. This 12-year-old male was admitted to a special education program following a psychological evaluation at age 6 years. This analysis was initiated after his teachers observed poor achievement in the reading readiness tests, an abnormal resistance to educational goals, and poor coordination and ungainly motor activity.

The psychological and performance tests indicated a bright but learning-disabled child, based upon language and visual-motor difficulty.

The central auditory tests are:

	R/L	Normal Values R/L
Competing sentence	100/0	90/90
Low pass filtered speech	72/58	66 mean
Binaural fusion	25/75	85 mean
Compressed speech	88/56	60 mean

At age 12 this student failed 3 of the 4 tests which would indicate difficulty in understanding speech when competing conversation is present, problems in central fusion when less than intelligible speech sounds are presented, and a minor loss in speech identity when the stimulus is accelerated in time. These auditory factors in conjunction with the identified visual-motor and language difficulties contribute further to academic interference.

Case 2. The second individual is the junior of two brothers referred for special testing due to a discrepancy between the intellectual scores and school achievement. The teacher described "poor visual memory, poor work habits, and difficulty paying attention" among other less evident problems. The school counselor further commented upon the child's attitude as disorganized and distractable, and noted difficulty keeping pace with grade-level work.

The central auditory test scores are:

	R/L	Normal Values R/L
Competing sentence	90/0	98/68 mean
Low pass filtered speech	30/24	64 mean
Binaural fusion	50/60	75/75 average
Compressed speech	56/36	60 mean

The amplitude of the wave V falls within normal range, unilateral greater than 0.46 μV and 0.75 μV respectively.

The psychological tests included WISC-R which indicated that this young man is functioning within the very superior range of intellectual development. Weakness was evident in long-term auditory memory, oral arithmetic skills, and hand-eye motor rapid coding skills. The Bender test suggested significant visual-motor integration problems and depressed scores on aural-written, plus reversals of written words.

The central test group indicates failure of each segment, though the range of the weak ear in competing sentences may test to 0% by established norms. The mean value is 68%, and the authors suggest either a very low normal score or, more likely, in combination with the other data, a failure. Filtered speech results are less than half the normal, fusion scores are depressed, and finally the compressed speech values are moderately abnormal.

Case 3. The third student is a 10-year-old male, the brother of student No. 2.

This young man was characterized through the psychological interview and by his teacher as having poor coordination, being easily distracted, and having difficulty sitting still.

The central auditory scores are:

	R/L	Normal Values R/L
Competing sentence	20/30	90/90
Low pass filtered speech	28/36	66 mean
Binaural fusion	95/95	85 mean
Compressed speech	60/64	60 mean

The amplitude and latency values of the auditory evoked brainstem responses are normal.

The WISC-R presented a very superior intellect and some weakness in orally presented arithmetic and coding skills. His achievement was rated overall as satisfactory in school in spite of the defects noted in distractability and coordination.

There are two major areas of deficit in the CAT battery, competing sentences and low passed filtered speech, giving evidence of a major impairment in auditory stimulus suppression and recognition of a distorted speech stimulus.

DISCUSSION

From the CAT battery we observe that 95% of the students failed at least one segment of the test. More than half of the group was unsuccessful in 2, 3 or 4 tests, while only 30% scored below normal in one phase of testing.

We reviewed the test data and propose certain clinical interpretations based upon these results. The competing sentence test is composed of simultaneous binaural stimuli with the test object lower in sensory intelligibility due to the relatively diminished intensity of presentation. Depressed scores would suggest an internal competitive state with less efficiency in the "weak ear" through the subcortical association fibers to the cortical auditory regions. Support for this contention is based upon normal monaural speech discrimination, the normal data in the rapidly alternating speech perception test effecting bitemporal stimulation, and previous research by the authors with discrimination scores in the presence of ipsilateral and contralateral white noise. We do not consider this test an indication of a potential split-brain individual particularly since the mean value of the weak ear is 66% versus the strong at 86%. Furthermore, the failure cases are characterized by extremely low scores in each ear more suggestive of defective transmission or integration and/or comprehension of stimuli in the presence of a competitive input.

The binaural fusion test integrates the frequency bands of speech which are presented dichotically. While the brainstem has been considered to be the site of the stimulus merger prior to cortical presentation, we question this hypothesis particularly in view of the apparently normal transmission of the electrical response through the brainstem. The high rate of failure (85% in this group) indicates an apparent lack of integration. We also observe that the fragmented stimuli, when presented as a monaural integrated stimulus, are readily identified in either ear with a high degree of success. Therefore, the monaural system from end-organ to auditory cortex functions in a competent manner. As a consequence the dissociation of stimuli must occur prior to the terminus and either represent a delay in subcortical transmission or be so modified as to yield a distorted response.

Filtered speech illustrates a modification of stimulus due to attentuation of the essential identifying components with a normal temporal duration. The verbal image is so distorted as to challenge the auditory identification-recognition mechanism. We can postulate that the complex sound package is sufficiently incomplete that a partially deranged transmission mechanism or reception center fails to provide the incoming data for proper interpretation. About half the students fail this test. There are three samples, however, where the scores of each ear are below 35%. In the absence of auditory dominance (ie, significant increase over weak side) and in the instance of bilaterally depressed values, it would suggest that the transmitted information as a whole, whether in the cortical or subcortical regions, is inadequate for normal function. Through a cross reference with associated failures in other segments of the CAT battery, we note a high correlation with the binaural fusion test data of the ten individuals who failed both segments. A correlation with other segments is not evident in the CAT battery.

The compressed speech test is a monaural challenge with accurate frequency representation though diminished in the time of presentation. This burden on cortical identification of the speech stimulus is not too stressful for the dyslexic group since 70% fall within or near the normal mean data. As suggested in elderly individuals with phonemic regression,[6] delay in transmission across the neuronal synapses or in the cortical region is a possible cause of failure in this test. Referring again to the BSER data which fail to identify delay in the brainstem neuronal transmission, we suggest that the site of the lesion when present be above the midbrain in the subcortical or in the association system. There is no correlation between the few who failed the compressed speech test and specific values in other components of the battery.

An interesting theoretical synthesis can be formulated by incorporating the data from the binaural fusion and filtered speech tests where a high failure rate occurs in each study. In each instance poor discrimination probably represents an inadequate stimulus for identification whether in coding as in filtered speech or in total composition as in fusion. Temporal sequencing of the monaural monosyllabic word is not a factor in distorted speech but may play an essential role in the dichotic frequency fragmented study. Further, the values do not suggest dominance. It is difficult to propose a discrete cortical lesion from a test battery in which the right ear exceeds the left in two tests and vice versa, the left dominates in the remaining two over the right, particularly in view of the localization for hearing of speech in the left brain.

At this time the BSER measures the electrical components secondary to auditory stimulation. As such it parallels the behavioral responses of the normal hearing. We cannot correlate with absolute certainty a normal BSER pattern and normal hearing, yet with the current state of the art the authors and others have measured pure tone thresholds within 15 dB by monitoring the brainstem with attenuated pure tone stimulation. Only future expansion of this technique will support the validity of the contention that the normal panorama of latency and amplitude equates to normal speech transmission. In the interim, further investigation is suggested in the time frame beyond 10 ms.

We might ask rhetorically whether the organic foundation for dyslexia is a common anatomical location occurring in a consistent area of the brain and thereby producing a more or less stereotyped individual pattern. Educators, psychologists, and psychiatrists are well aware of the heterogeneity of this group with varying degrees of academic disability, personality and behavioral instability, and need for supportive care. The organic disability of reading disturbances and the evident hearing failure of synthesis, reconstruction, and environmental auditory competition suggest multiple areas of functional disturbances.

Based upon the central battery which indicates a wide spectrum of auditory disturbance in anatomically disparate regions of the brain, the authors suggest the probability of a diffuse neural disturbance for this disorder of dyslexia.

SUMMARY

A battery of four central auditory tests was presented to a group of dyslexic students with normal hearing by pure tone and speech discrimination scores. The ages of the students extended from 10 to 13 inclusive but for one individual age 7 years. Ninety-five percent failed at least one segment of the battery. The binaural fusion test indicated the greatest degree of difficulty with 85% of the group significantly below the normal values. Filtered speech testing identified 50% of the group who were unable to pass this segment. The competing sentence as well as the compressed speech tests were below the normal values in about one third of the investigated students.

A composite of the individual test scores indicates that about half failed two sections of the CAT battery and 10% each were below normal in three or four components.

The auditory evoked brainstem response did not provide evidence of significant impairment in the auditory induced neuronal response evaluated by latency and amplitude.

A correlation of the CAT battery and the BSER does not implicate the brainstem nor the inner ear as the source of the hearing disability in dyslexia.

Specific examples of educational and psychological assessments in conjunction with the central evaluation of audition are presented to illustrate the comprehensive perceptual and behavioral disorders of the dyslexic students.

REFERENCES

1. Wenden PH. The minimal brain dysfunction syndrome. Annu Rev Med 1975; 26:45-62.

2. Welsh LW, Welsh JJ, Healy MP. Central auditory testing and dyslexia. Laryngoscope 1980; 90:972-84.

3. Beasley DS, Maki JE, Orchik DJ. Children's perception of time compressed speech on two measures of speech discrimination. Speech Hear Disord 1976; 41:216-25.

4. Beasley DS, Schwimmer S, Rintelmann WF. Intelligibility of time: compressed CNC monosyllables. J Speech Hear Res 1972; 15:340-50.

5. Bocca E, Calearo C. Central hearing processes. In: Jerger, J, ed. Modern developments in audiology. New York: Academic Press, 1963.

6. Calearo C, Lazzaroni A. Speech intelligibliity in relation to the speed of message. Laryngoscope 1962; 67:410-9.

ALEXANDER'S LAW: A MODEL AND RESULTING STUDY

M. J. DOSLAK, PhD
LINCOLN, NEBRASKA

L. F. DELL'OSSO, PhD
CLEVELAND, OHIO

R. B. DAROFF, MD
CLEVELAND, OHIO

Recently we developed an analog model to simulate Alexander's law in nystagmus secondary to dysfunction of a semicircular canal. Alexander's law is based on the observation that the amplitude of the nystagmus grows with increasing gaze in the direction of the fast phase and diminishes with gaze in the opposite direction. To investigate the assumptions made in the model, we conducted quantitative experimental studies on the effect of gaze on caloric-induced nystagmus in human subjects. A weak stimulus (water at 26.5°C and 240 ml/min) was administered for several minutes which caused the development of jerk nystagmus. Both the average slow phase velocity and frequency reached a steady state at about three minutes after the start of irrigation and remained stable until the flow of water was stopped. To investigate the effect of gaze, each subject was asked to hold gaze at various positions from center, to the right, to the left, and to repeat the cycle. Results indicated that the slow phase velocity of the nystagmus was greatest in the direction of the fast phase and decreased approximately linearly with gaze in the other direction in accordance with Alexander's law. Frequency was not a function of gaze. We speculate as to the biological advantages of the brainstem neural circuitry responsible for Alexander's law.

B - Central bias, EOM - Extraocular muscles, FφS - Fast phase stimulator, G - Summed gaze and tone signals, G_r, G_l - Right gaze, left gaze, LC - Left canal, LLR - Left lateral rectus, LVN - Left vestibular nuclei, NI - Neural integraters, Θ_D - Desired angle gaze, Θ_E - Eye (gaze) angle, OMN - Ocular motor nuclei, PG - Pulse generator, RC - Right canal, RMR - Right medial rectus, RPG - Right pulse generator, RVN - Right vestibular nuclei, SSC - Semicircular canals, SφM - Slow phase modulator, SV - Slow phase velocity, T - Central tone signals, TD - Total duration of the nystagmus beat.

INTRODUCTION

In 1912 Alexander[1] made the observation that the intensity of nystagmus grows as gaze is increased in the direction of the fast phase and diminishes with gaze in the opposite direction (Fig. 1); it later became known as Alexander's law. He categorized nystagmus into three degrees: First — present only during gaze in the direction of the fast phase; second — present during gaze straight ahead but increased in the direction of the fast phase; third — present in all fields of gaze but greatest in the direction of the fast phase.

Despite the long and almost universal recognition of Alexander's law by clinicians, there has been no serious attempt to explain the phenomenon. This prompted us to develop an analog computer model utilizing relevant brainstem anatomy and physiology in an effort to simulate Alexander's law in nystagmus secondary to dysfunction of a semicircular canal.[2] The model behaved in accordance with Alexander's law with total and partial unilateral canal dysfunction. To investigate the assumptions of the model and to quantitate the details of Alexander's law, we performed studies of variation with gaze of caloric-induced nystagmus in normal human subjects.

MODEL

The model represents the brainstem mechanisms that determine the gaze-dependent slope variation of the slow phase of vestibular nystagmus. We did not explicitly model the generation of the fast phases; they were assumed to occur with a constant frequency. A model has been proposed by other investigators for fast phase generation.[3]

A neural configuration, consistent with the known anatomy and physiology on which our model was based, is shown in Figure 2. The vestibular nuclei (right, RVN; left, LVN) transfer excitatory signals contralaterally and inhibitory signals ipsilaterally to the neural integrators (NI). Prior to synapsing with the integrators, these signals are

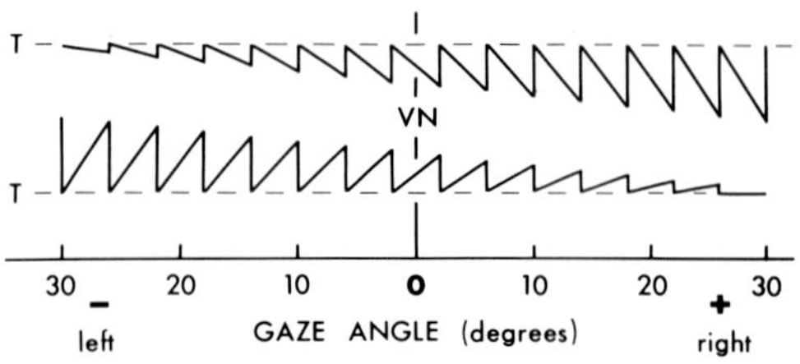

Fig. 1. Diagram of right- (upper) and left-beating (lower) vestibular nystagmus variations with gaze. T indicates target position.[2]

From the Ocular Motor Neurophysiology Laboratory, VA Medical Center, and Department of Neurology, Case Western Reserve University, School of Medicine, Cleveland. This study was supported in part by USPHS grant IT 32 EY-07021-05.

Presented at the meeting of the American Neurotology Society, Palm Beach, Florida, April 12, 1980.

REPRINTS — L. F. Dell'Osso, PhD, Ocular Motility (127A), VA Medical Center, Cleveland, OH 44106.

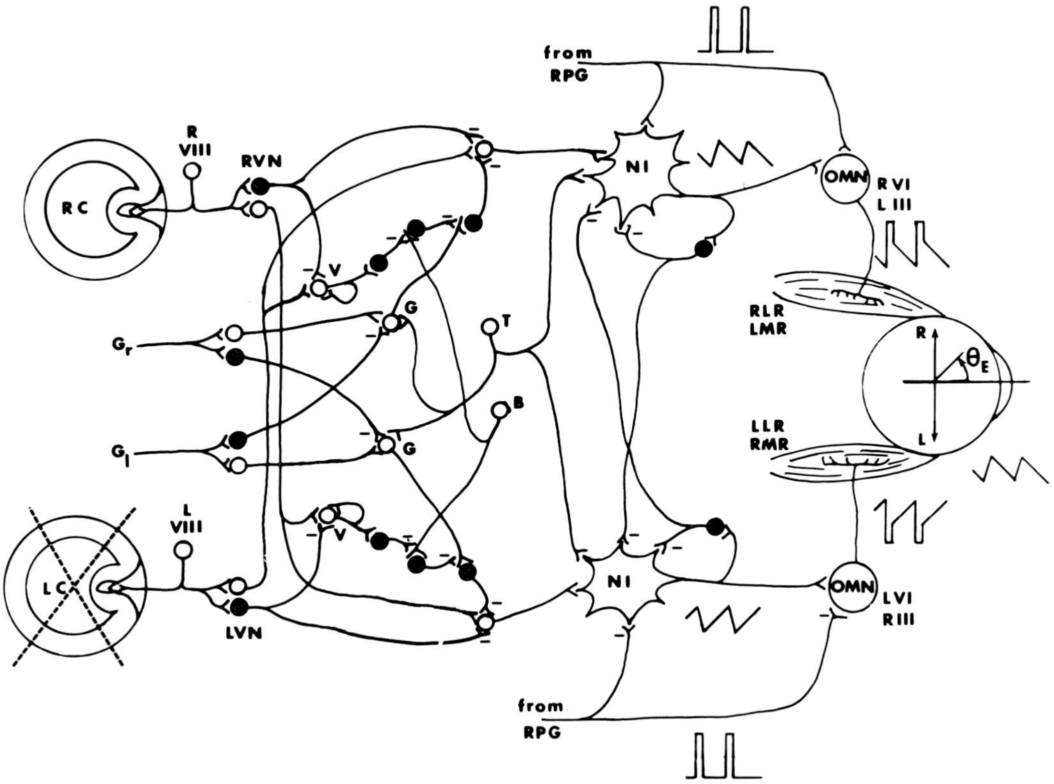

Fig. 2. A possible "wiring diagram" suggested by the model. The upper half of the diagram corresponds to the right side of the brainstem and the lower half to the left side. Open circles represent excitatory neurons; filled circles represent inhibitory neurons. Dysfunction of the left semicircular canal is signified by a large X through LC. C - Canal; R - Right; L - Left; VN - Vestibular nuclei; VIII - Eighth nerve nuclei; NI - Neural integrator; PG - Pulse generator; OMN - Ocular motor nuclei; LR - Lateral rectus; MR - Medial rectus; G - Gaze signals; T - Central tone; B - Central bias; V - Vestibular signals.[2]

modulated by desired right and left gaze (G_r, G_l) and central tone (T) signals. The evidence for a central T signal has been presented previously[2] and is related to the interconnections of the brainstem neural integrators. When no imbalance between vestibular nerve activity from each side is present, the summed gaze and tone signals (G) are prevented from influencing vestibular activity by means of the presynaptic inhibition supplied by a postulated central bias (B). When an imbalance of vestibular activity occurs, this inhibitory bias is turned off by additional presynaptic inhibition. Such inhibition of inhibitory signals is not unusual and has been documented in other areas of neurophysiology.[4] Also shown are the ocular motor nuclei (OMN) and the eye muscles. With dysfunction of the left canal (LC), the right canal (RC) provides increased stimulation of the left lateral rectus (LLR) and right medial rectus (RMR) causing the eyes (represented here as one eye) to drift to the left. Intervening saccadic pulses from the right pulse generator (RPG) move the eyes back to their predrift position. The waveforms shown represent changes in the neural firing frequencies and eye position (Θ_E).

Our model, which was implented on a Systron-Donner SD-80 analog computer, is described by the functional block diagram shown in Figure 3. Neural signals from the semicircular canals (SCC) pass to the vestibular nuclei (VN) before being integrated by the NI. The NI outputs then lead to stimulation of the extraocular eye muscles (EOM) via the OMN. The position of the eyes is represented by Θ_E.

In order to include a gaze-dependent variation, however, we added a slow phase modulator (SΦM) which modulated vestibular nuclei activity with desired gaze (Θ_D) and constant T. In this manner we

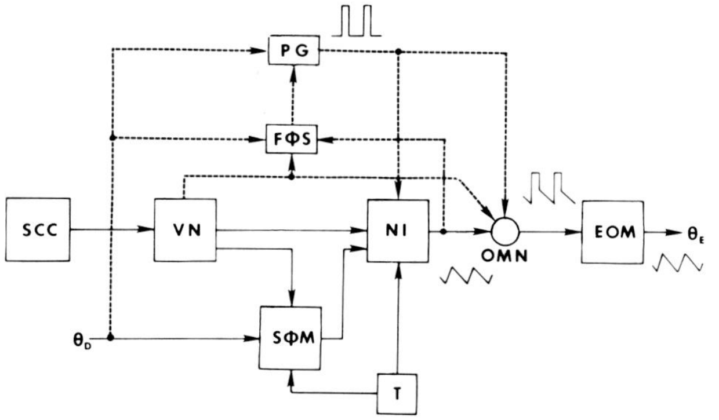

Fig. 3. Functional block diagram of the model. Solid lines represent slow phase generation; dashed lines represent fast phase aspects. SCC - Semicircular canal; VN - Vestibular nuclei; NI - Neural integrators; OMN - Ocular motor nuclei; EOM - Extraocular muscles; Θ_D - Desired gaze angle; Θ_E - Eye (gaze) angle; PG - Pulse generator; FΦS - Fast phase stimulator; SΦM - Slow phase modulator; T - Central tonic input.[2]

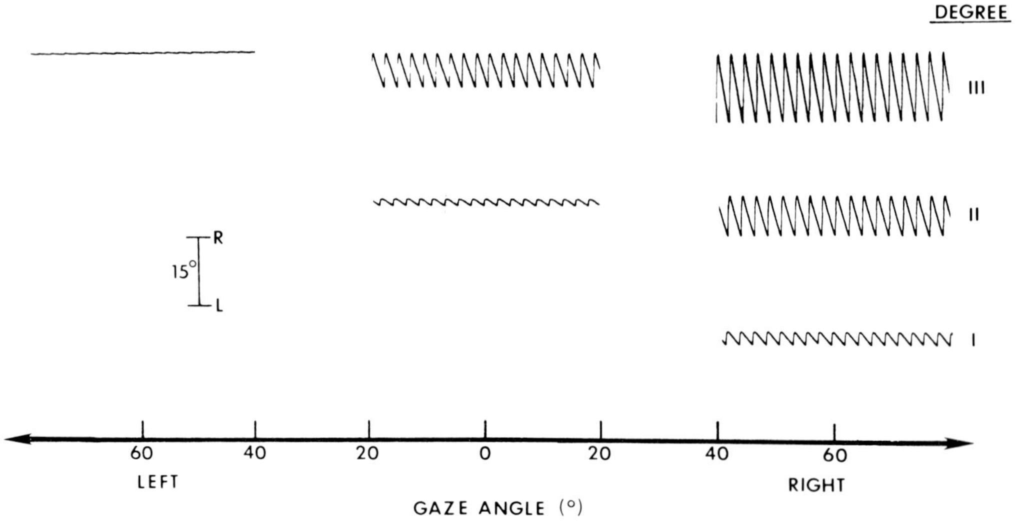

Fig. 4. Recordings of the outputs from the model with various parameter settings to stimulate three degrees of nystagmus (I-III) variation with gaze.[2]

were able to simulate the variation of slow phase velocity with canal imbalance and desired gaze. The fast phase stimulator (FΦS) and pulse generator (PG) are connected by dashed lines to illustrate that they were not *explicitly* modeled, although their role in the fast phase of the vestibular nystagmus was represented. The waveforms shown indicate both neural firing frequencies and the resulting nystagmus of the eyes.

When simulating normally functioning semicircular canals with equal spontaneous activity from the two sides, the model produced no nystagmus. When simulating total impairment of the canal on one side with gaze directed maximally in the opposite direction, the model produced large amplitude (arbitrarily chosen to be 15°) nystagmus with linear slow phases directed toward the "lesioned" side and fast phases in the opposite direction (corresponding with observed clinical phenomenology). As gaze was adjusted from far contralateral to ipsilateral, the nystagmus gradually diminished to zero. This is shown in Figure 4 as third degree nystagmus (by Alexander's classification). When one canal output was only partially reduced and the other normal, the nystagmus was smaller in amplitude and was absent in ipsilateral or in both ipsilateral and center gaze, as indicated by the second and first degree labels in Figure 4. As an initial simplifying assumption, the frequency of the nystagmus was held constant at 3.33 Hz.

Figure 5 illustrates the quantitative relationship between the amplitude of the nystagmus, the angle of desired gaze, and the amount of canal dysfunction measured as the percentage of its normal spontaneous activity. The linear property of these curves is a result of our simple interpretation of Alexander's law, ie, the amplitude of third degree nystagmus increases linearly with increasing gaze in the direction of the fast phase. The parallel property of the curves is again the result of our approximation of the linear variation of nystagmus with canal deficit (as measured above). This is not meant to imply that the vestibular function (VOR) of a canal is directly related to its spontaneous activity.

The model provoked some interesting questions: 1) Is the relationship between the amplitude of the

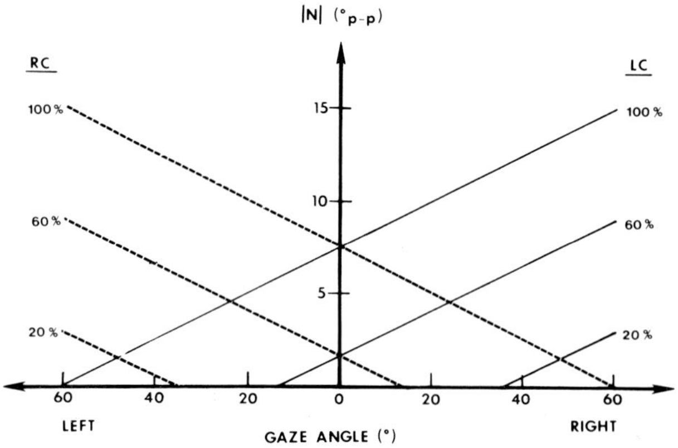

Fig. 5. Plots of variations of nystagmus amplitude as a function of gaze angle and the amount of simulated semicircular canal dysfunction. LC - Left canal; RC - Right canal.[2]

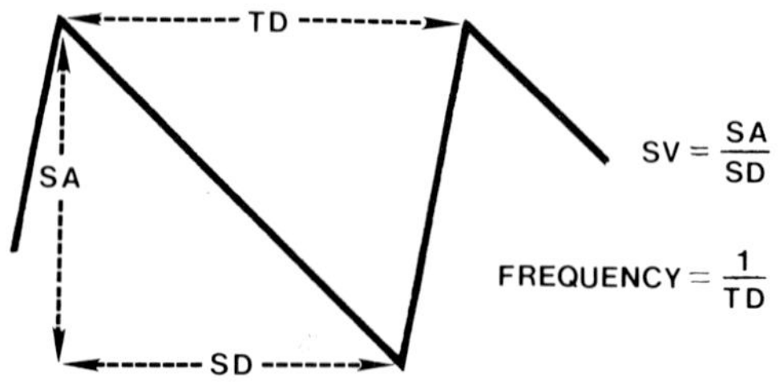

Fig. 6. Sketch of nystagmus waveform showing parameters measured. SA - Slow phase amplitude; SD - Slow phase duration; TD - Total duration of the nystagmus beat.

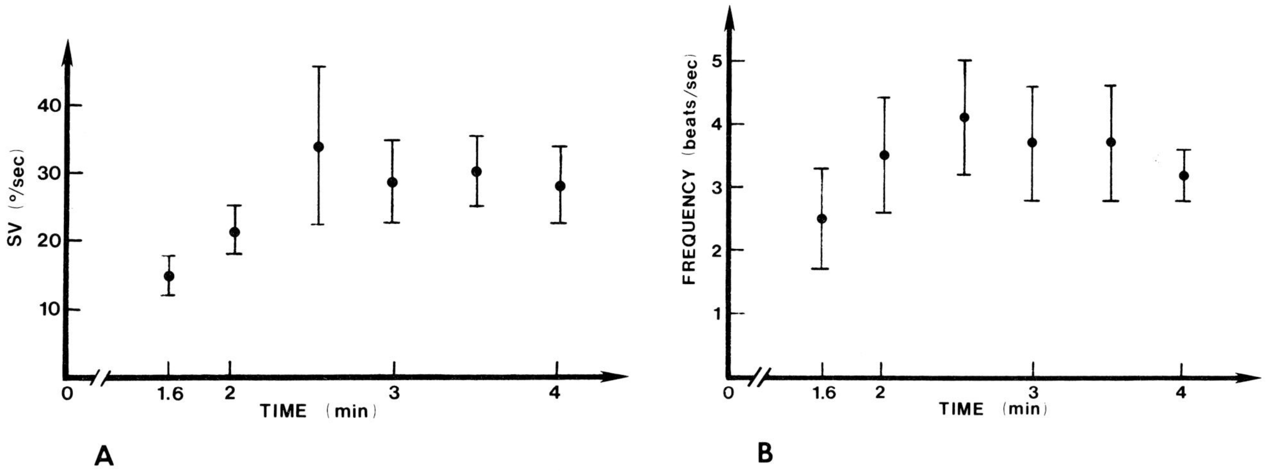

Fig. 7. (Subject 1) A) Time course of the nystagmus slow phase velocity (SV), while holding center gaze during constant irrigation. Each filled circle and error bar represents the SV mean and standard deviation, respectively, of 10 sampled beats. The position on the time axis is the mean time of occurrence of the 1C samples. B) Time course of the nystagmus frequency, while holding center gaze during constant irrigation. Each filled circle and error bar as in A.

nystagmus and the desired gaze angle actually linear? 2) For a given angle of gaze, is the nystagmus amplitude a linear function of canal deficit? 3) How does the nystagmus frequency vary with gaze? Consequently, studies of calorics on normal subjects were initiated in our laboratory to answer these questions and to provide additional direction for our modeling.

METHODS

Caloric-induced horizontal nystagmus was monitored, using an infrared technique, as a function of gaze in seven normal male subjects between the ages of 18 and 34; the infrared system was linear within ± 20°. The subjects were not patients, had no clinical ocular motor complaints, and made normal eye movements during calibration. The subjects were in complete darkness (except during calibration) and were in a reclined sitting position with the coronal plane of the head at 60° from the vertical. Blinks were detected with a vertical electro-oculographic recording of one eye. During calibration, each subject was asked to look at small spots located on the ceiling (at a distance of approximately 20 m) at gaze angles of 0°, ±20°, and ±25°.

The time courses of the slow phase velocity (SV) and frequency of one subject holding center gaze during continuous irrigation were calculated to establish when and if adaptation had occurred. The intent in this study was to first get our subjects into the adapted plateau region and then study the effect of gaze on the SV.

Cold water (26.5°C and 240 ml/min) was delivered continuously for several minutes to the external auditory meatus of the subject's left ear; right-beating linear nystagmus was thus induced. After the nystagmus reached a constant amplitude, the subject was asked to look at his best estimate (since it was dark) of various angles of right and left gaze while receiving constant corrective feedback as needed from the experimentor. Usually gaze variations originated at 20° right, proceeded to 20° left in a stepwise manner, returned to 20° right, and then the cycle was repeated at least once. In this way many beats at various gaze angles were recorded. Calibration was then rechecked after the experiment. The slow phase velocity and frequency of every third, fourth, or fifth beat, depending on the total number of beats recorded from a particular subject, were calculated (Fig. 6). The individual amplitudes and durations were determined graphically.

RESULTS

The time courses of both the SV and frequency for subject holding center gaze are shown in Figure 7A,B respectively. Notice the peak at 2½ minutes and the subsequent plateau region in each figure.

Results from all the subjects are shown in Figure 8. The heavy solid line is the mean of the SV regression lines for subjects,[3,5-7] eliminating three special

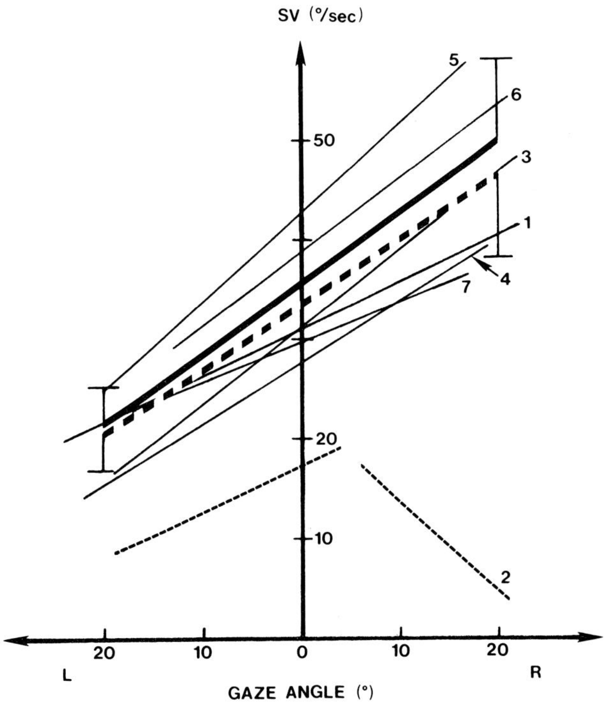

Fig. 8. Plots of nystagmus slow phase velocity (SV) versus gaze angle for each of the subjects tested. Each subject's data are represented as a linear regression. The heavy solid line is the mean of the individual curves of four subjects (3, 5-7). The heavy dashed line is the mean of the individual curves of six subjects (1, 3-7). The error bars are standard deviations.

STATISTICAL INFORMATION FOR FIGURES 9-13

Subject	Age	Sample Size	Data Starts (s)*	Data Ends (s)*	Frequency (Mean)	(SD)
1	34	53	137	290	3.80	1.41
2	18	66	120	290	1.95	0.83
3	34	52	65	138	2.91	0.62
4	30	56	180	345	3.08	1.40
5	30	69	180	350	3.34	1.10
6	27	43	180	360	3.01	0.87
7	22	51	180	450	3.05	1.41

*After the start of irrigation.

cases discussed below. The heavy dashed line is the mean of the SV regression lines for six subjects, excluding the markedly different data for subject 2. In all cases, frequency was not a function of gaze; the means were 3.08 and 3.2 beats/second corresponding to the above groupings of four and six subjects respectively. The table presents individual data for each of the subjects.

The data for subject 3 was best fit by a regression line (Fig. 9). The subject made multiple sweeps of rightward and leftward gaze during the time the nystagmus was recorded. The frequency was not a function of gaze. These results were characteristic of most of the subjects tested. The data of subjects 1, 4 and 2 are unique and will be presented separately.

Figure 10 describes data for subject 1 which were consistent with Alexander's law with one sweep of gaze from right to left (dots), but not on the return to right gaze (x's). The frequency derived from the

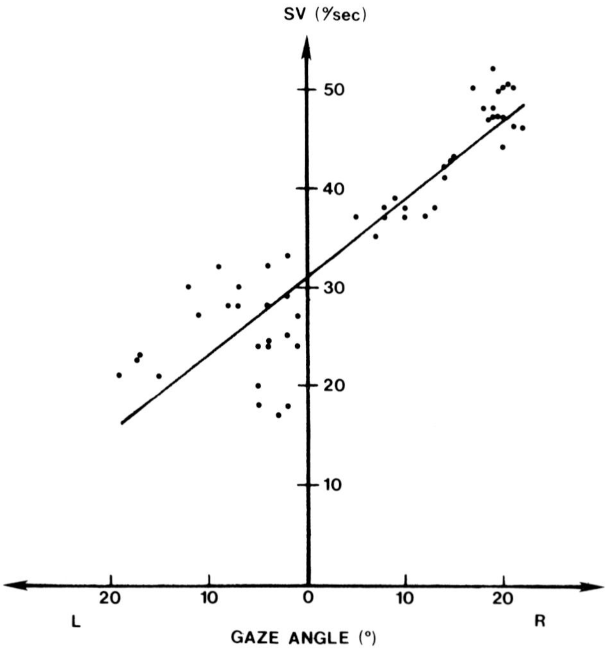

Fig. 9. Plot of slow phase velocity (SV) as a function of gaze angle (shown by dots) for the sampled nystagmus beats from subject 3 with multiple sweeps of gaze from one side to the other. The solid line is a linear regression with a = 31.25, b = 0.77, r = 0.91. In this and all subsequent figures, a and b are parameters in the equation SV = a (gaze angle) + b; r is the correlation coefficient.

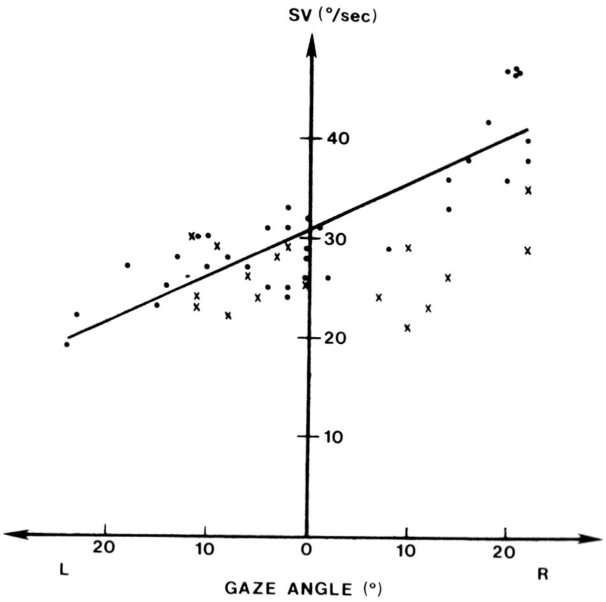

Fig. 10. Plot of slow phase velocity (SV) as a function of gaze angle for the sampled nystagmus beats from subject 1. The dots represent 36 beats occurring between 137 seconds and 242 seconds for one sweep of gaze starting at the right and ending at left gaze. The x's represent 17 beats occurring between 244 seconds and 290 seconds for the return to right gaze. The solid line is a linear regression (a = 30.95, b = 0.47, r = 0.87) of the data shown by dots. A linear regression on the other data had a value of r equal to only 0.3.

beats, referred to by the dots, was not a function of gaze.

Data for subject 4 are consistent with Alexander's law with one sweep of gaze from right to left (dots), but not for other sweeps of gaze (Fig. 11). The data shown by the dots were recorded during a time in the middle of all the data recorded. Frequency was not a function of gaze.

Subject 2 demonstrated "hemifield reciprocity"[11] (Fig. 12). With multiple rightward and leftward sweeps of gaze, results were consistent with Alexander's law at center and left gaze but *not* during right gaze where the opposite occurred. Frequency was not a function of gaze; the mean value (1.95) was the smallest of all subjects' mean frequencies (table).

DISCUSSION

For all subjects the data were obtained when we felt reasonably sure that the SV was not a function of time, ie, the system was in steady-state; this time was usually greater than 2½ minutes after the start of irrigation, based on the SV adaptation characteristic of subject 1. The frequency change also followed a similar time course. The SV time course is consistent with data in the literature.[5-8] The time course of the frequency does not appear to be documented elsewhere.

The data for subject 3 (Fig. 9) began 65 seconds after commencement of irrigation. These data,

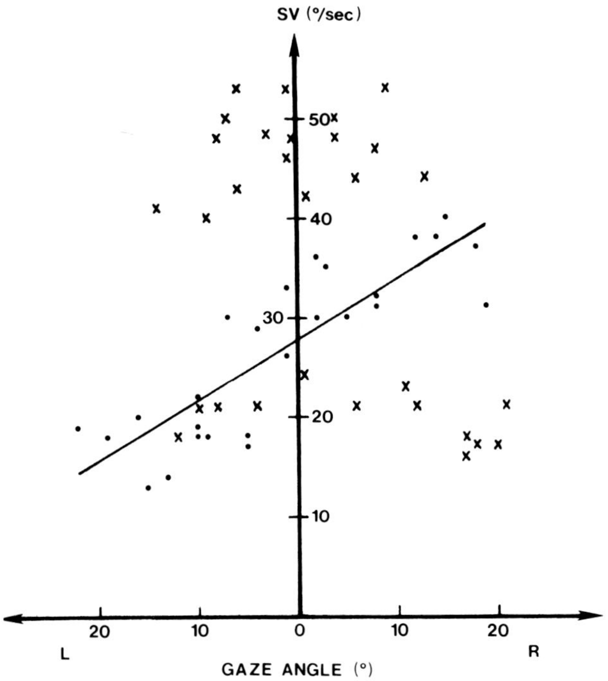

Fig. 11. Plot of slow phase velocity (SV) as a function of gaze angle for the sampled nystagmus beats from subject 4. The dots represent 26 beats occurring between 210 seconds and 300 seconds for one sweep of gaze from right to left. The x's represent 30 beats occurring from 180 seconds to 210 seconds and 300 seconds to 345 seconds. The solid line is a linear regression (a = 27.61, b = 0.61, r = 0.84) of the data shown by dots.

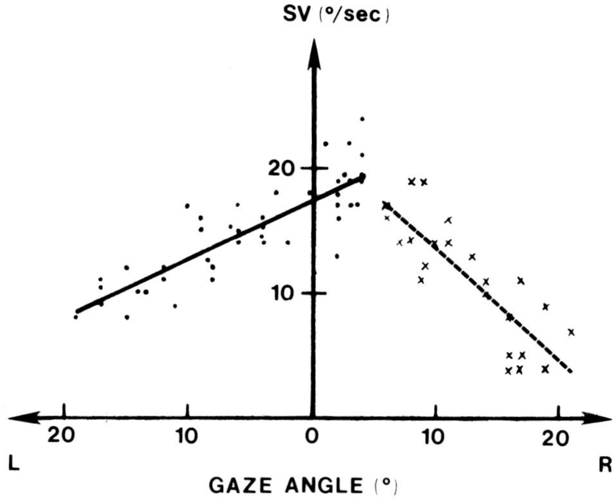

Fig. 12. Plot of slow phase velocity (SV) as a function of gaze angle for the 66 sampled nystagmus beats from subject 2 with multiple sweeps of gaze from one side to the other. The solid line is a linear regression (a = 17.46, b = 0.47, r = 0.85) of data, shown by the dots, from 43 samples. The dashed line is a linear regression (a = 22.51, b = 0.89, r = 0.84) of data, shown by x's from 23 samples.

nonetheless, had the best fit to a linear regression line and followed Alexander's law. It is probable that the SV for this subject reached a steady state prior to the beginning of the data. Otherwise the SV would have increased as gaze was changed from the far right, to center, and to the left. Also, since the SV path was retraced with multiple right and left sweeps of gaze, and since the nystagmus first appeared much sooner than average, the subject's SV and frequency were most probably adapted.

The SV data for subject 1 (Fig. 10), on returning from left to right gaze, did not conform to the SV line established when gaze initially changed from right to left. The reduced SV on returning to right gaze was possibly due to a minor fluctuation of the SV, even when it has adapted.[5] Other possibilities are diminished attention of the subject or variation of the caloric stimulus.

The SV data for subject 4 (Fig. 11) had high values initially for variations of gaze and did not follow Alexander's law. However, for a subsequent gaze variation from right to left, Alexander's law was obeyed. With the return of gaze to the right, Alexander's law was again violated. These inconsistencies may have been due to fluctuations in the adapted state, late-occurring adaptation, fluctuations in the subject's mental state, or variation of the applied stimulus.

The SV data for subject 2 (Fig. 12) were unique. In addition to being considerably smaller than for the other subjects, they were in agreement with Alexander's law for center and left gaze but *not* for right gaze. This "hemifield reciprocity" has not, to our knowledge, been reported in patients with pathological vestibular end-organ nystagmus. Interestingly, the slope of the SV versus gaze line in left gaze was similar to the slopes of the corresponding lines for all the other subjects. Since this entire SV line was followed quite well with multiple right and left sweeps of gaze, we feel that the decrease of SV with rightward gaze is a biological anomaly.

The SV data for the remaining three subjects (5-7) were quite similar to the data from subject 3. Their mean is shown by the heavy solid line in Figure 8. The SV data for two of the special cases mentioned above (subjects 1 and 4) are very similar to that of the four mentioned above (3, 5-7). In fact, the mean SV line for subjects 2, 3-7 compares very closely with the mean SV line for subjects 3, 5-7.

Figure 13 is a superposition of the mean SV line for subjects 3, 5-7 and the initial results from the model (with amplitude converted to SV). The induced vestibular nystagmus SV was linear within ± 20° of gaze, as we assumed in the model; the magnitudes of the actual and model SVs were also in close agreement. The linear extrapolations beyond ± 20° are merely to simplify comparison with the model; this region needs further investigation. It is not known what extent of canal deficit is needed to mimic the caloric-induced third degree nystagmus. In each subject, the effective degree of deficit produced was probably different as a result of biological variation and different thermal conduc-

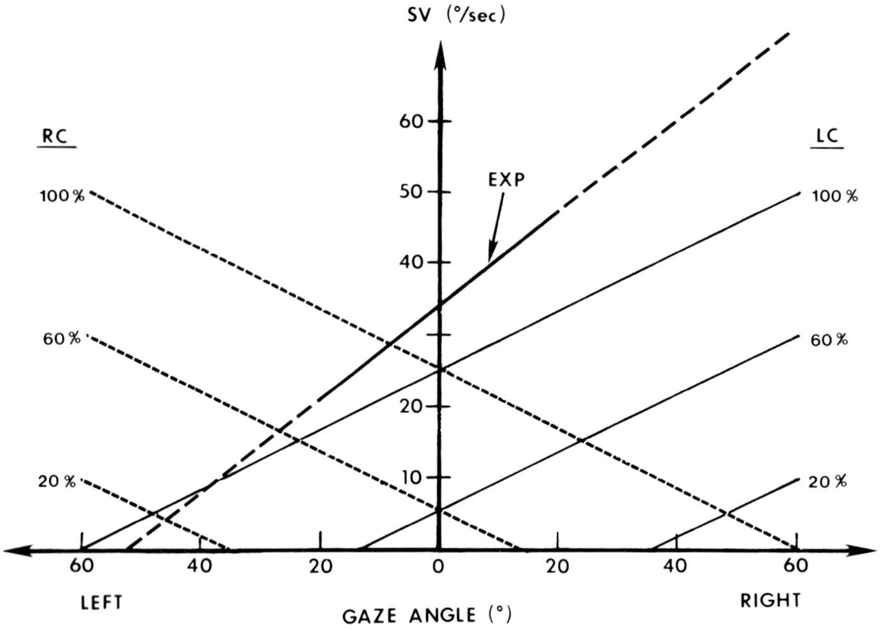

Fig. 13. Superposition of the experimental data (utilizing the heavy solid line in Fig. 8) upon the model data. The amounts of simulated semicircular canal dysfunction are indicated. LC - Left canal; RC - Right canal.

tivity properties of the meatus and petrous bone. This probably accounts for the intersubject differences in SV (Fig. 8). The fact that the slopes were quite similar and the lines were nearly parallel but separate, supports another assumption of the model. The mean frequency (3.2 Hz) of the nystagmus for all the subjects (except no. 2) tested was both constant (not a function of gaze) and also of similar magnitude to the frequency (3.33 Hz) assumed in the model. The parameters in the model can now be adjusted slightly so that the SV slopes and the frequencies are equivalent to those obtained experimentally.

The phenomenon which constitutes Alexander's law is the natural consequence of our brainstem neural circuitry. What might be the biological benefits of having a neural network so constituted? We speculate that it might be to enhance the vestibulo-ocular reflex (VOR) and, in pathological vestibular states, to minimize nystagmus. With head rotation, the eyes deviate in the direction of the fast phase.[9] The SV would therefore be greatest with the eyes deviated in that direction. Consequently, the gain of the VOR (SV/rotation velocity) would be greatest, thereby maximizing the performance of this reflex. In clinical cases of labyrinthine dysfunction, the eyes usually deviate in the direction of the affected side,[10] *away* from the fast phase of the resulting nystagmus. Thus, the SV of the nystagmus and the visual impairment would be minimized.

ACKNOWLEDGMENTS — The authors thank Iris Rothchild and James Birkett for their technical assistance, and Paul Shipkin, MD, for his consultation.

REFERENCES

1. Alexander G. Die Ohrenkrankheiten im Kindesalter. In: Pfaundler M, Schlossmann A, eds. Handbuch der Kinderheilkunde. Leipzig: Vlg. FCW Vogel, 1912: 84-96.

2. Doslak MJ, Dell'Osso LF, Daroff RB. A model of Alexander's law of vestibular nystagmus. Biol Cybern 1979; 34:181-6.

3. Chun KS, Robinson DA. A model of quick phase generation in the vestibulo-ocular reflex. Biol Cybern 1978; 28:209-21.

4. Davidoff RA. Synaptic transmission in the mammalian central nervous system. Weekly update. Neurol Neurosurg 1978; 1:24.

5. Bock O, Koschitzky HV, Zangemeister WH. Vestibular adaptation to long-term stimuli. Biol Cybern 1979; 33:77-9.

6. Barnes GR, Benson AJ. Adaptation in the caloric response. In: Hood JD, ed. Vestibular mechanisms in health and disease. London: Academic Press, 1978; 254-62.

7. Baertschi AJ, Johnson RN, Hanna GR. Theoretical and experimental determination of vestibular dynamics in caloric stimulation. Biol Cybern 1975; 20:175-86.

8. Cawthorne T, Cobb WA. Temperature changes in the perilymph space in response to caloric stimulation in man. Acta Otolaryngol (Stockh) 1954; 44:580-8.

9. Honrubia V, Baloh RW, Lau CG, Sills AW. The patterns of eye movements during physiologic vestibular nystagmus in man. Trans Am Acad Ophthalmol Otolaryngol 1977; 84:339-47.

10. Jung R, Mittermaier R. Zur objectiven Registrierung und Analyse verschiedener Nystagmusformen: Vestibularer, optokinetischer und spontaner Nystagmus in ihren Wechselbeziehungen. Arch Klin Exp Ohren Nasen Kehlkopfheilkd 1939; 146:410-39.

Ann Otol Rhinol Laryngol 91:1982

FAMILIAL LARYNGEAL ABDUCTOR PARALYSIS WITH PRESUMED AUTOSOMAL DOMINANT INHERITANCE

G. MORELLI, MD
B. TESTA, MD
C. MESOLELLA, MD
V. VENTRUTO, MD
F. COSTA, MD
B. SANTULLI, MD
NAPLES, ITALY

The etiology of Gerhardt's syndrome is uncertain. With the present work the authors present a hereditary form of this syndrome, which was found in three subsequent generations with autosomal dominant transmission.

INTRODUCTION

Paralysis of the dilatators of the glottis, known as Gerhardt's syndrome,[1] has been the object of attention by many authors and clinically its nosology has been determined. However, there is still uncertainty about its etiology.

In the past a luetic etiology of the lesion was suggested. Possible causes have been attributed to diseases of the central nervous system, both irritative and dystrophic (amyotrophic lateral sclerosis, multiple sclerosis, epidemic encephalitis, poliomyelitis); to acute viral infections and vascular encephalopathies; and to toxic agents (lead, nicotine, alcohol).[2] The cases now showing an evident etiology are assumed to be cryptogenetic forms. In fact, statistics show a high percentage of cases, especially among young people, in which the syndrome cannot be related to any recognized etiological agent. The present study documents a familial form of the affection, and suggests the possible genetic nature of the syndrome, at least in some cases.

CLINICAL OBSERVATION

The family was partially studied in the past,[3,4] and its pedigree is shown in Figure 1. There are five recognized affected subjects in three subsequent generations. Apart from respiratory troubles they all show a normal phenotypic aspect and normal psychic development. Two of them have congenital clubfoot.

Three adult subjects were treated surgically for asphyxia, one by cordectomy and two by arytenoidopexy. For the other two, the respiratory conditions have not required surgical treatment at present. The age at the onset of the respiratory problems varied from case to case. The oldest (58 years) was treated by cordectomy about 20 years ago and two of his children (Fig. 1, III 4 and III 5) were treated by arytenoidopexy at 18 and 16 years of age respectively. Two other children (Fig. 1, III 2 and III 3) died from asphyxia, one at birth and the other a little later, before a diagnosis was made. The laryngeal picture in all subjects examined showed bilateral paralysis with the vocal cords in adduction (paralysis of the posterior cricoarytenoid muscles). The laboratory data, the EEG and the neurologic findings were inconclusive. Furthermore all the patients had normal results on audiometric tests. The karyotype test was normal.

DISCUSSION

In the family examined the hereditary feature of the syndrome seems evident. The presence of affected individuals of different sex in three subsequent generations suggests autosomal dominant inheritance. In the third generation, all the siblings were affected. However, in relation to the variable expression of the gene in terms of age at onset and severity of disease, it should be noted that nongenetic factors also may have had an important role.

As to the pathogenesis we agree with Plott,[5] according to whom the dysgenesis should be searched out at the nuclear level and, more precisely, in the median portion of the nucleus ambiguus where are found the cells from which depart the fibers for the posterior cricoarytenoid muscles. The dysgenesis would affect this portion of the nucleus ambiguus bilaterally. The possibility that the lesions can compromise other regions of the supranuclear nervous system must be excluded. In fact it seems unlikely that the dysgenesis may have affected the corticobulbar tracts involving only the fibers of the posterior cricoarytenoid nucleus.

Publications on the inheritance of Gerhardt's syndrome are very rare.[6] The family described by Plott[5] as well as the patients reported by Walters and Fitch[7] were all males with suggested x-linked recessive or male limited autosomal dominant in-

From the Istituto di Clinica Otorinolaringoiatrica i Facoltá di Medicina, Universitá di Napoli, and Servizio di Genetica Medica, Ospedale Cardarelli, Napoli.

REPRINTS — G. Morelli, MD, Via D. Cotugno 3, Istituto di Clinica Otorinolaringoiatrica, Naples, Italy.

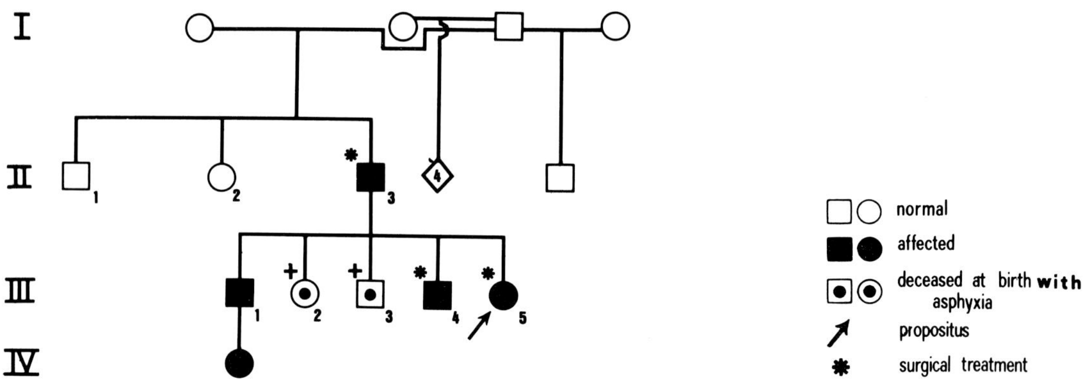

Fig. 1. Pedigree of family.

heritance. The syndrome was associated with mental deficiency and mild deafness. In the family reported here, all the affected subjects show normal psychic and intellectual development with no compromise of auditory function. This strongly suggests the presence of heterogeneity in this disorder. It is therefore desirable that more contributions be published, leading, in the future, to a better knowledge of the hereditary aspects of the disease.

SUMMARY

The authors report a familial congenital paralysis of the laryngeal abductors in seven members of three subsequent generations. The affected subjects showed the disease at different ages, and the seriousness of the respiratory troubles also varied among individuals. Two of them died from asphyxia (one at birth); three were treated surgically as adults (one by cordectomy, two by arytenoidopexy). In the other two the disease is not very serious at present and does not require surgical treatment. In all the subjects the clinical tests and all the laboratory data are inconclusive. The pedigree is compatible with autosomal dominant transmission. The present work suggests that 1) Gerhardt's syndrome is possibly a heterogeneous disorder, and 2) the inheritance pattern, in the rare familial cases, seems to be autosomal dominant, although multifactorial inheritance cannot be excluded.

REFERENCES

1. Gerhardt C. Encephalitis: Stimmbandlahmung ohne Stimmveranderung. Arch R Path Anat (Berl) 1863; 27:309.

2. Cervellera G, Salonna F, Bartoli E. Problemi clinici e patogenetici delle paralisi laringee. Atti LI Congr Naz, Soc Ital Laring Otol Rin Padova, 1963.

3. Massei V, Tortora R. Considerazioni su tre casi di Sindrome di Gerhardt. Ann Laringol 1965; 64:537.

4. Mesolella C, Costa F, Morelli G. Sindrome di Gerhardt a carattere familiare. Presented at the LXIV Congr Naz Soc, Ital ORL e Chir Cervico-facciale, Santa Margherita Ligure, 1977.

5. Plott D. Congenital laryngeal-abductors paralysis due to nucleus ambiguus dysgenesis in three brothers. N Engl J Med 1964; 271:593-7.

6. McKusick VA. Mendelian inheritance in man. 5th ed. Baltimore: Johns Hopkins, 1978:776.

7. Walters GV, Fitch N. Familial laryngeal abductor paralysis and psychomotor retardation. Clin Genet 1973; 4:429-33.

TRACHEOESOPHAGEAL FISTULA
A COMPLICATION OF FOREIGN BODY

M. N. OBIAKO, MD
ENUGU, NIGERIA

The case presented is one in which a coin in the esophagus resulted in a tracheoesophageal fistula. It is of interest not only because the occurrence is unusual, but also because the coin remained in the esophagus for an extraordinarily long period before the condition became symptomatic. The various factors responsible for the delay in getting medical help, including the nonavailability of medical services in many parts of Nigeria, are discussed.

CASE REPORT

A 9½-year-old male was referred from a mission hospital in one of Nigeria's 19 states with a diagnosis of foreign body in the esophagus complicated by tracheoesophageal fistula. Comprehensive radiological studies accompanied the patient. A lateral chest x-ray film revealed a coin in the midthoracic esophagus (Fig. 1). Barium x-ray film showed barium in the lower lobe of the right lung, implying an esophagotracheobronchial fistula (Fig. 2). The history was inadequate and the exact time the foreign body was swallowed cannot be determined.

The first symptom noticed was coughing at about age two years (1972). The patient was treated for this until 1974 when chest x-ray films revealed a coin in the chest. The attendant doctor referred the patient to a specialist center for further management. The parents did not do as the doctor directed; instead they took their son home where it was agreed at the village level that the coin would find its way out with the feces. For this reason the patient received no medical attention for four relatively symptom-free years. The coughing started again some time in 1978 and culminated in May 1980 in hemoptysis and hematemesis. On June 25, 1980, he turned up at a hospital with a letter from his school headmaster threatening to dismiss him from school as a case of suspected pulmonary tuberculosis.

On examination the patient appeared small for his age, obviously undernourished, dehydrated, and clinically anemic. He was febrile (38.8° C) with normal pulse rate (100/minute). The chest wall was not deformed, although reduced air entry throughout the anterior chest wall was noted. Dullness to percussion marked the right (R) lower zone posteriorly. Reduced air entry was noted in the left (L) lower zone posteriorly and the R lower zone anteriorly and posteriorly. Bronchial breath sounds were heard in the L middle zone and R midparasternal border, and expiratory rhonchi in the R middle zone posteriorly. Laboratory studies produced the following values: hematocrit, 66.5%; WBC 10,200/cu mm, with 67% polymorphs, 30% lymphocytes, and 3% eosinophils; sedimentation rate (Westergren) 20 mm/hour. Sputum was purulent, tuberculosis test negative (albuminose-free tuberculin), and Paragonimus ova absent. Clinical findings were obviously related to the barium swallow finding.

The patient was placed on systemic Amplicox as well as hematinics. He also received dextrose and normal saline intravenously. Feeding by mouth was restricted to occasional semifluids which now and again resulted in paroxysms of coughing and choking. After two weeks there was marked improvement in his general condition although he still had frequent episodes of

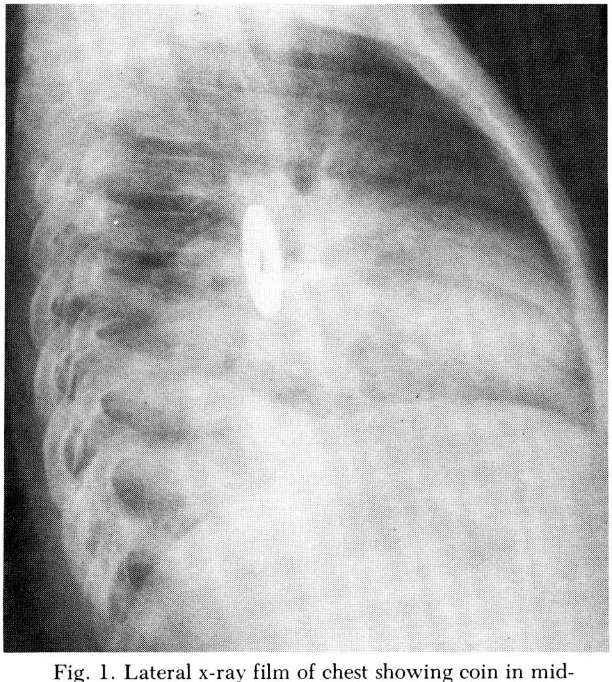

Fig. 1. Lateral x-ray film of chest showing coin in midthoracic esophagus.

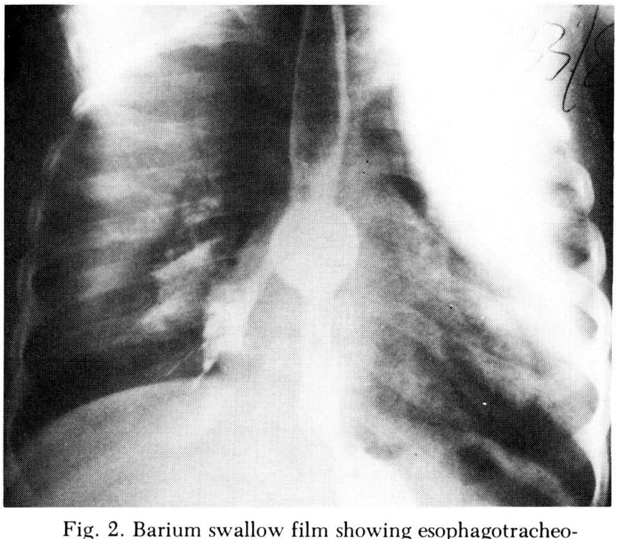

Fig. 2. Barium swallow film showing esophagotracheobronchial fistula (right).

From the Department of Otolaryngology, University of Nigeria Teaching Hospital, Enugu.
REPRINTS — M. N. Obiako, MD, Department of Otolaryngology, University of Nigeria Teaching Hospital, P.M.B. 1129, Enugu, Nigeria.

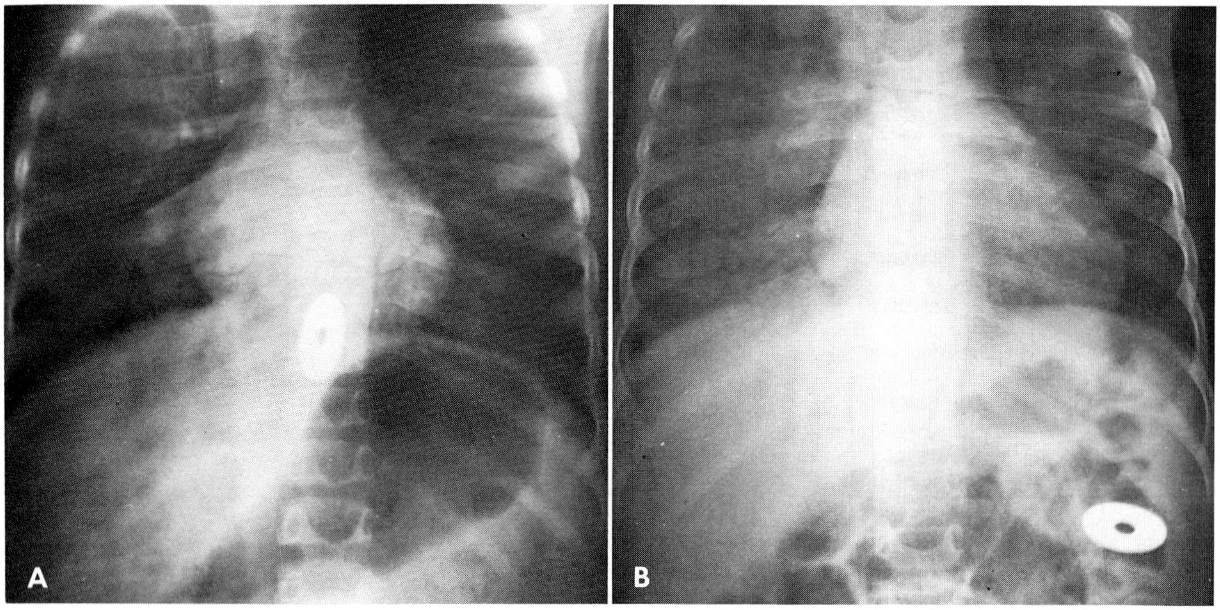

Fig. 3. AP x-ray films of chest and abdomen showing A) coin at cardioesophageal junction, and B) foreign body in the colon 2 days after film in A.

hemoptysis and hematemesis. It was, however, considered safe to subject him to esophagoscopy under general anesthesia, and endoscopic extraction of the foreign body was attempted. The esophageal lumen was filled with blood mixed with pus oozing from areas of ulceration and periesophageal abscess. Passing the esophagoscope provoked even more bleeding from the ulcerated areas of the esophagus. In spite of constant suction the coin could not be seen; apparently it had been dislodged and pushed further down during the procedure. An x-ray film taken during the operation showed the coin at the cardioesophageal junction (Fig. 3A). It continued to move (Fig. 3B) and was passed four days after the operation. The patient lost a large quantity of blood. He was kept on antibiotics and one week after the procedure he was cautiously introduced to a meal of semifluids. At first soft foods produced violent coughing, but this gradually eased off, the bleeding stopped, and the patient was up and about.

DISCUSSION

This case of tracheoesophageal fistula due to a foreign body is presented because of its other unusual but rather interesting aspects. It is noteworthy that the foreign body was a coin, which reportedly is the most common foreign body found in children.[1-7] The assertion that poor children who are left to feed themselves at an early age are more liable to swallow foreign bodies[8] than others is here supported. The patient is 1 of 9 children from a very poor family. The coin remained in the esophagus for well over seven years, an unusually long period which surpasses by over two years a case reported previously.[9] Foreign bodies in the air and food passages usually give dramatic and alarming symptoms which prompt patients to seek immediate medical help. When the impacted foreign body is a coin, however, the patient may remain asymptomatic for a long time. Some foreign bodies in the throat have been found by accident.[10-12] This patient started coughing at the age of about two years (1972) and continued until 1974 when, in the course of symptomatic treatment, the diagnosis of coin in the chest was made. Although the coin was not extracted, he seemed to be symptom-free until 1978 when he started coughing again. The period is so unusually long that there can be some doubts as to whether the patient was actually asymptomatic at that time. The fact that he is very small for his age (115 cm, 17 kg) suggests that he may be undernourished due to dysphagia.

The various forms of congenital tracheoesophageal fistula and esophageal atresia and their management are well documented.[13-14] Acquired tracheoesophageal fistulas, on the other hand, are far less frequent and most often associated with malignant diseases. Other causes of acquired fistulas include infectious diseases of the esophagus, trachea, or pleura, such as tuberculosis, syphilis, actinomycosis, suppurative esophagitis, nontuberculous empyema, esophageal diverticula and esophagomalacia.[15] Traumatic perforation of the esophagus as well as intrapleural surgical procedures for nonmalignant diseases have caused tracheoesophageal and esophagopleural fistulas.[16-17] Acquired tracheoesophageal fistula as a result of a foreign body seems to be relatively infrequent; this literature search revealed only one similar case, a fistula due to a piece of bone which lodged in the anterior esophageal wall[18] and perforated it. The coin, on the other hand, caused a breakdown of the esophageal wall by the localized inflammatory reaction.[19]

Many factors would appear to be responsible for the delay in getting medical help and thereby preventing this serious complication. In 1974 when a diagnosis of coin in the chest was made, the attending doctor directed the patient to a specialist center for further management. The parents did not do as directed, most certainly because of financial constraints. The patient is 1 of 9 children and the father a poor farmer. Specialist centers in otolaryngology are few and far between in Nigeria. Often one has to travel hundreds of kilometers and spend a lot of money to get to such a center. It must have been a big relief to the parents when, at the village level, they were assured that the coin would probably be passed. The fact that the patient was asymptomatic at the time further management was recommended must have made it difficult for them to understand or believe the doctor. On the other hand, the decision at the village level must have looked quite reasonable. The patient started coughing again in 1978, four years after the diagnosis of coin in the chest was made, and long after the details of that episode must have been forgotten. They did not relate the cough to the foreign body. Upper respiratory tract infection with a cough is a common phenomenon which villagers usually treat with a cough mixture from the local market.

Another factor responsible for the delay is the absence of cheap medical services in many areas of Nigeria. Private hospitals are beyond the reach of the poor. Medical centers are ill-equipped, poorly staffed, and mostly without drugs. General hospitals are not accessible because of transportation problems and even at the hospitals one may spend a week without seeing a doctor. Patients, therefore, go to a hospital as the last resort after quacks and self-medication have failed. This is why many patients seen in hospitals are in late or terminal stages of their illnesses. In the case reported, hemoptysis and hematemesis were not considered serious enough for the parents to seek medical help. It was, instead, the threat by the headmaster to expel their son from school because of suspected pulmonary tuberculosis that at last compelled them to go to the hospital.

REFERENCES

1. Miles-Foxen EH, Groves J. Foreign bodies in Oesophagus. In: Ballantine J, Grove J, eds. Scott-Brown's textbook of diseases of ear-nose-throat. 3rd ed. London: Butterworths, 1971:223-8.

2. Baraka A, Bikhazi G. Oesophageal foreign bodies. Br Med J 1975; 1:561-3.

3. Sawney KL, Roa PB, Ayyaswamy R. Foreign bodies in pharynx and oesophagus. Indian J Otolaryngol 1973; 25:47-50.

4. Rickham PP. Ingested foreign bodies in childhood. Ann R Coll Surg Engl 1971; 48:25.

5. Davidoff E, Towne JB. Ingested foreign bodies. NY State J Med 1975; 75:1003-7.

6. Brooks JW. Foreign bodies in the air and food passages. Ann Surg 1972; 175:720-32.

7. Okafor BC. Foreign body in the larynx — clinical features and a plea for early referral. Niger Med J 1976; 6:470-2.

8. Jackson C, Jackson GL. Diseases of the air and food passages of foreign body origin. Philadelphia: Saunders, 1936.

9. Okafor BC. Lung abscess secondary to esophageal foreign body. Ann Otol Rhinol Laryngol 1978; 87:568-70.

10. Wright FW, Ramsden PD. Chronic foreign body in the oesophagus. Br J Clin Pract 1974; 28:413-7.

11. Funnel G, D'arcy F. Failure to thrive. J Laryngol Otol 1976; 90:883-6.

12. Morioka WT, Maisel RH, Smith TW, Cantrell RW. Unexpected radiographic findings related to foreign bodies. Ann Otol Rhinol Laryngol 1975; 84:627-30.

13. Haller JA Jr. Tracheoesophageal fistula and esophageal atresia. In: Schwartz SE, Lillehei RC, Spencer FC, Storer EH, Shires GT. Textbook of principles of surgery. 2nd ed. New York: McGraw-Hill, 1974:1516-21.

14. Stephens HB. H-type tracheoesophageal fistula complicated by esophageal stenosis. J Thorac Cardiovasc Surg 1970; 59:325-9.

15. Clagett OT, Payne JH, Moersch HG. Acquired esophagotracheobronchial fistula. Surg Gynecol Obstet 1946; 82:87-90.

16. Hughes FA Jr, Fox JR Jr. Acquired nonmalignant esophagotracheobronchial fistula: report of 2 cases. J Thorac Surg 1954; 27:384-9.

17. Takaro T, Walkup HE, Okano T. Esophagopleural fistula as a complication of thoracic surgery. J Thorac Cardiovasc Surg 1960: 40:179-93.

18. Murtagh JA, Tyson MD. Esophagobronchial fistula: a result of foreign body. N Engl J Med 1940; 222:494-5.

19. Ellis FH Jr, Payne S. Esophageal perforation. In: Schwartz SI, Lllehei RC, Shires GT, Spencer FC, Storer EH. Textbook of principles of surgery. 2nd ed. New York: McGraw-Hill, 1974:1029-32.

OTITIS MEDIA SECONDARY TO AMPICILLIN-RESISTANT *HEMOPHILUS INFLUENZAE*

AN UPDATE

RICHARD H. SCHWARTZ, MD
WILLIAM J. RODRIGUEZ, MD, PhD
WAHEED N. KHAN, MD
WASHINGTON, DC

During a 2-year period ending December 1978, we encountered 27 cases of otitis media secondary to ampicillin-resistant *Hemophilus influenzae*. This represents 19% of the 139 *Hemophilus* isolates obtained by tympanocentesis. In agreement with data from Huntsville, Alabama, Boston, and Pittsburgh, we estimate that as of 1978, approximately 4% of all cases of acute otitis media are caused by this pathogen.

Disease caused by ampicillin-resistant strains of *Hemophilus influenzae* was first reported in 1974.[1-3] Currently, 10 to 20% of systemic and upper respiratory tract disease in many parts of the United States and of the world is associated with this ampicillin-resistant pathogen.[4,5] In an earlier communication, we summarized our experience with *H influenzae* as a cause of acute otitis media.[6] The purpose of this report is to update our experience.

METHODS AND MATERIALS

During a 2-year period ending December 1978, middle ear cultures were obtained from 444 children with acute otitis media. (Otitis media is defined as fullness or bulging of the tympanic membrane with loss of ossicular landmarks.) Ages ranged from 1 month to 17 years; 50% of these children were less than 24 months of age. The study population was composed of predominantly middle class, suburban children seen in a private pediatric office. These 444 children represented about 18% of all cases of otitis media seen by one pediatrician who collected the middle ear specimens. Myringotomy was performed as described in a recent article by one of the authors.[7] Standard microbiological methods were used in this study with modifications as previously described.[8] Using a simplified chromogenic cephalosporin technique, representative *Hemophilus* colonies growing in proximity to the ampicillin disc were tested for β-lactamase production.[9] Minimum inhibitory concentration (MIC) for all strains was determined at a reference laboratory using an agar dilution method.

RESULTS

Middle ear cultures were obtained from 444 children during the 2-year study. The table depicts the results of the cultures for each year of the study. There were approximately equal numbers of *Streptococcus pneumoniae* (29%) and *H influenzae* (31%) isolated from the middle ear. We were unable to recover a pathogenic isolate from 34% of the middle ear specimens. This is in accordance with the findings of other investigators. Group A streptococci were isolated from 3% of the series.

Whereas in 1977, 11 of 70 (16%) *H influenzae* recovered from the middle ear were ampicillin-resistant, in 1978, 16 of 69 (23%) were ampicillin-resistant. All the isolates were resistant to ampicillin by the disc sensitivity method. All strains produced β-lactamase (a penicillinase enzyme), and of the isolates available for MIC 90% were confirmed resistant by this method and had MIC of ≥ 3.12 μg/ml. The proportion of all *Hemophilus* recovered from middle ear aspirates did not differ significantly from that of *S pneumoniae*.

DISCUSSION

Since 1970 at least six reports presented data on the microbiology of acute otitis media.[10-15] In these studies, *H influenzae* was isolated from the middle ear in 25-30% of children who presented with signs of acute otitis media. While there have been several individual case reports of ampicillin-resistant strains of *H influenzae* as a cause of otitis media,[1,3] only two previous reports contain substantial numbers.[6,16] Syriopoulou et al have reported that 16% of middle ear isolates obtained in Boston and Huntsville, Alabama, were *H influenzae* ampicillin-resistant.[17] C. Bluestone (personal communication), on the other hand, estimates that 3% of children with acute otitis media seen at Pittsburgh Children's Hospital have ampicillin-resistant strains of *H influenzae* recovered from their middle ear. In our previous report, we had estimated that 8% of all cases of otitis media in our area are caused by these ampicillin-resistant organisms.[8] Our initial estimate, based on the first eight months of 1977, may have been too high. A certain element of bias may have existed due to our selection method, since children seen at the initial acute visit who had a noticeable bulging of the tympanic membrane with concomitant intensified fever or pain, and those children who had

From the Department of Child Health and Development, The George Washington School of Medicine and the Health Sciences, and the Microbiology and Infectious Disease Sections, Research Foundation of Children's Hospital, National Medical Center, Washington, DC.

REPRINTS — William J. Rodriguez, MD, PhD, Children's Hospital Nat. Med. Ctr., 111 Michigan Avenue NW, Washington, DC 20010.

MICROBIOLOGY OF ACUTE OTITIS MEDIA

Number of Myringotomies		*H Influenzae* Sensitive to Ampicillin	*H Influenzae* Resistant to Ampicillin	Pneumococcus	Group A β Hemolytic Streptococcus	No Growth	Other*
1977	270	59	11	83	6	100	11
1978	174	53	16	46	6	49	4
Totals	444	112 (25%)	27 (6%)	129 (29%)	12 (3%)	149 (34%)	15 (3%)
		31% (sensitive + resistant)					

*Includes 5 polymicrobic infections, *H influenzae*, in addition to *S pneumoniae*, and a number of *Neisseria* species and *Pseudomonas*.

failed to improve objectively after a course of ampicillin or amoxicillin, were more likely to undergo diagnostic paracentesis. If one were to aspirate consistently only those patients who failed to improve, a greater yield of *H influenzae* could have resulted. Of the 720 cases of acute otitis media seen by only one member of the group in 1978, 174 (24%) underwent myringotomy. Sixteen of 174 (9%) yielded ampicillin-resistant *Hemophilus* from the middle ear aspirate. However, in 1977, when we used less restrictive criteria for performing myringotomies, cultures from only 4% of such myringotomies yielded ampicillin-resistant *H influenzae.*

Recent treatment with ampicillin or amoxicillin in a child presenting with signs of a bulging, yellow-colored drumhead is likely to be associated with ampicillin-resistant *H influenzae*. Given such a clinical situation, we have been able to obtain *H influenzae* from at least 35% of the children.

REFERENCES

1. Tomeh MO, Starr SE, McGowen JE Jr, et al. Ampicillin-resistant Haemophilus Type B infection. JAMA 1974; 229:295-7.

2. Controni G, Rodriguez W, Pumphrey R, et al. Otitis media due to ampicillin-resistant Haemophilus influenzae. Lancet 1974; 2:1398.

3. Schiffer M, Schneerson R, MacLowry J, et al. Otitis media due to ampicillin-resistant Haemophilus influenzae. Lancet 1974; 2:257.

4. Scheifele DW. Ampicillin-resistant Haemophilus influenzae in Canada: nationwide survey of hospital laboratories. CMA Journal 1979; 121:198-202.

5. Morbidity and Mortality Weekly Report. June 22, 1979; 28:277-9.

6. Schwartz R, Rodriguez W, Khan W, Ross S. The increasing incidence of ampicillin-resistant Haemophilus influenzae: a cause of otitis media. JAMA 1978; 239:320-3.

7. Schwartz RH. New concepts in otitis media. American Family Physician 1979; 19:91-8.

8. Schwartz R, Rodriguez WJ, Mann R, et al. The nasopharyngeal culture in acute otitis media: a reappraisal of its usefulness. JAMA 1979; 241:2170-3.

9. O'Callaghan CH, Morris A, Kirby SM, et al. Novel method for detection of beta-lactamase by using a chromogenic cephalosporin substrate. Antimicrob Agents Chemother 1972; 1:283-8.

10. Howard JE, Nelson JD, Clahsen J, Jackson LH. Otitis media of infancy and early childhood: a double blind study of 4 treatment regimens. Am J Dis Child 1976; 130:965-70.

11. Kamme C, Lundgren K, Mardh PA. The aetiology of acute otitis media in children. Scand J Infect Dis 1971; 3:217-23.

12. Herberts G, Jeppsson PH, Nylèn O, et al. Acute otitis media: aetiological and therapeutic aspects. Pract Oto-Rhino-Laryngol 1971; 33:191-202.

13. Brook I, Anthony BF, Feingold SM. Aerobic and anaerobic bacteriology of acute otitis media in children. J Pediatr 1978; 92:13-5.

14. Branefors-Helender P, Nylèn O, Jeppsson PH. Acute otitis media: a bacteriological study. ORL 1972; 34:281-95.

15. Howie VM, Ploussard JH. Bacterial etiology and antimicrobial treatment for otitis media. South Med J 1971; 64:233-8.

16. McLina SE, Daly JF, Jones JE. Cephalexin monohydrate suspension: treatment for otitis media. JAMA 1975; 234:171-3.

17. Syriopoulou V, Scheifele D, Smith AL, et al. Increasing incidence of ampicillin resistance in Haemophilus influenzae. J Pediatr 1978; 92:889-92.

CONDITIONED MIDDLE EAR MUSCLE TINNITUS

A CASE REPORT

MARY E. COLLARD, MA

CYNTHIA A. WAGNER, MS — FRED R. TINGWALD, MD

CLEVELAND, OHIO

A case of bilateral middle ear muscle contraction tinnitus associated with eye blinks is presented. It is hypothesized that the association represents a conditioned middle ear muscle response.

Williams[1] reported an unusual case of unilateral fluctuating tinnitus due to stapedial muscle contraction synchronous with eye blinks, following traumatic seventh nerve injury. Exploratory tympanotomy confirmed the stapedial contraction, and lysis of the stapedial tendon relieved the annoying change in tinnitus which was associated with eye blinks. We would like to relate our experience with another case of tinnitus due to middle ear muscle contraction occurring with eye blinks.

A 32-year-old female presented with complaints of itching ears, ear pressure, nasal congestion, and a rushing noise in the ears every time she blinked. The periodic rushing tinnitus became extremely annoying whenever she tried to relax quietly. The otolaryngological examination was entirely normal except for a septal deviation, the apparent cause of frequent congestion. Her medical history was entirely negative for any episode of facial palsy or neurological disorder. Audiological evaluation indicated normal pure-tone thresholds, word discrimination, tympanometry, and reflex thresholds bilaterally. Large changes in impedance occurred with eye blinks, without any detectable facial or neck tension or movement. The impedance change was equal in both ears, and did not occur when eyes remained closed and relaxed, with a conscious effort made not to blink (Fig. 1). No etiological explanation could be made for this reaction.

The patient was seen a year later, with no change in the tinnitus. The audiological results were again normal, except for the large impedance changes associated with blinking. In counseling the patient, the tinnitus was explained as probably a result of contraction of one of the middle ear muscles, though it was unknown why the contraction occurred with blinking. It was also mentioned that some people can contract their middle ear muscles voluntarily.[2-4]

Four months later the patient returned with the report that since learning of the possibility of voluntary middle ear muscle contraction, she had discovered that, if she concentrated, she was able to prevent the rushing tinnitus that had been associated with eye blinks. It sometimes still occurred if she

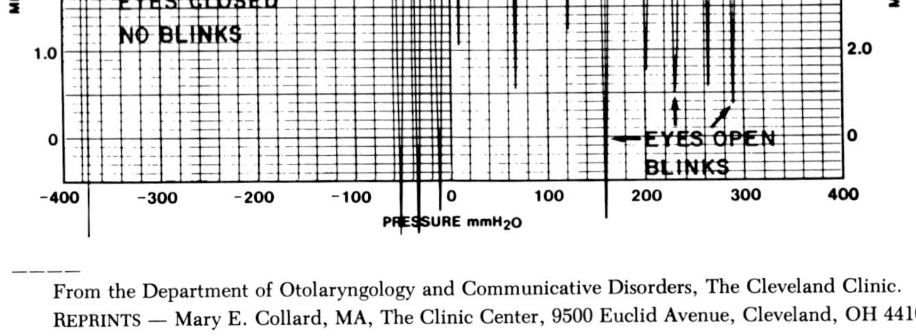

Fig. 1. Tympanogram. Recording of impedance with and without blinking.

From the Department of Otolaryngology and Communicative Disorders, The Cleveland Clinic.

REPRINTS — Mary E. Collard, MA, The Clinic Center, 9500 Euclid Avenue, Cleveland, OH 44106.

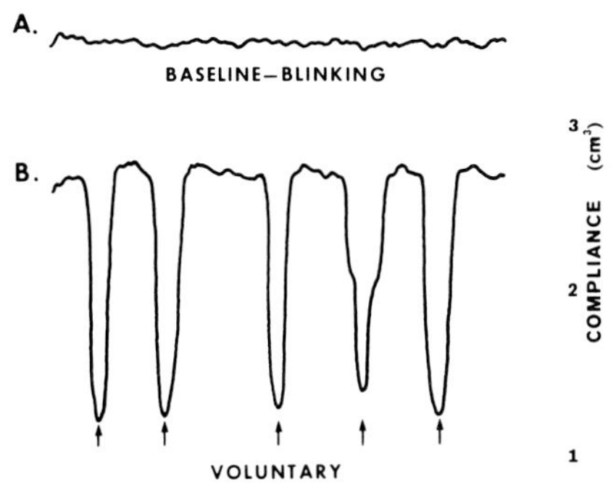

Fig. 2. A) Recording of baseline impedance while patient blinks. B) Recording of impedance changes with voluntary middle ear muscle contraction, without blinking.

was not making an effort to stop it. Impedence recording demonstrated complete voluntary control; she could blink without impedance change (Fig. 2A) or could produce a large impedance change at will (Fig. 2B). Three months later, another visit with the patient elicited a subjective impression that her control of the tinnitus was still good. Repeat tests again resulted in normal tympanometry and impedance changes very similar to those seen in Figure 2.

Otological examination during voluntary middle ear muscle contractions indicated that the tympanic membrane was being drawn inward by the contraction. Tensor tympani muscle contraction is suggested in this patient because of the inward tympanic membrane movement and the fact that the impedance change seen with voluntary contraction was larger than that demonstrated by maximum acoustic stimulation.[4]

A normally voluntary response can be conditioned to occur involuntarily by pairing of an unconditioned stimulus and a conditioned stimulus in behavioral conditioning paradigms. The normal acoustic middle ear muscle reflex in cats has been conditioned to occur in response to a visual stimulus alone, which was first paired with an acoustic stimulus.[5]

Our patient related to us her belief that she learned to contract her middle ear muscles in an attempt to relieve the pressure sensation in her ears. The following sequences are hypothesized:

1. Behavioral attempt to relieve pressure→leads to→middle ear muscle contraction.
2. Behavioral attempt to relieve pressure and simultaneous blink→leads to→middle ear muscle contraction.
3. Eye blink→leads to→middle ear muscle contraction.

It is thought that the attempt to clear pressure became associated with blinks by frequent simultaneous occurrence as in the second step above, and that her problem represents a conditioned middle ear muscle response. Counseling the patient and self-modification of her behavior allowed alleviation of her tinnitus complaint without necessity for any other treatment.

REFERENCES

1. Williams JD. Unusual but treatable cause of fluctuating tinnitus. Ann Otol Rhinol Laryngol 1980; 89:239-40.

2. Reger SN. Effect of middle ear muscle action on certain psycho-physical measurements. Ann Otol Rhinol Laryngol 1960; 69:1179-98.

3. Smith HD. Audiometric effects of voluntary contraction of the tensor tympani muscles. Arch Otolaryngol 1943; 38:369-72.

4. Metz O. The acoustic impedance measured on normal and pathological ears. Acta Otolaryngol (Stockh) 1946; Suppl 63.

5. Simmons FB, Galambos R, Rupert A. Conditioned response of middle ear muscles. Am J Physiol 1959; 197:537-8.

SIMULTANEOUS ROUND AND OVAL WINDOW FISTULAE IN A CHILD

NIGEL R. T. PASHLEY, MB, FRCS(C)

DENVER, COLORADO

Sudden hearing loss from simultaneous rupture of both oval and round windows, occurring in the only hearing ear of a child, is described. The condition was surgically managed with recovery of hearing. Of particular note was the presence of air aspirated into the labyrinth at the time of membrane rupture, which has not previously been described. The possible mechanisms and some clinical correlates associated with anatomic predisposition to such rupture are discussed.

Simultaneous rupture of both oval and round windows of the inner ear associated with aspiration of air into the labyrinth has not previously been reported. This paper describes such a case managed by prompt surgical intervention resulting in recovery of hearing. An attempt is made to explain the findings and occurrence of this phenomenon.

CASE HISTORY

A $4^1/_2$-year-old male presented to the Pediatric Otolaryngology Division of the Department of Otorhinolaryngology at the University of Michigan with a history of stable, profound, sensorineural hearing loss in his left ear since birth. The parents had been told that this was a congenital loss and he had developed speech and language normally. Auditory thresholds and discrimination scores in his right ear had been normal throughout his life.

Ten days prior to admission, he had slipped while playing, bumping his head lightly on a padded sofa. There was no loss of consciousness or dizziness, but an immediate complaint to his mother of a buzzing noise in *both* ears. An audiogram was performed at another center and showed slight depression of hearing levels in all frequencies in the right (and only hearing) ear and no change in the depressed thresholds of the left ear. During the ensuing week some difficulties in understanding speech were noted by the parents and a further audiogram showed an additional 10-dB drop in pure-tone thresholds with a fall in speech discrimination abilities from 96% to 92%.

The child was again seen at the University of Michigan where a complete physical examination revealed no abnormal findings other than the hearing loss (Fig. 1). He had a negative fistula test and no Hennebert sign despite testing with the impedance bridge, Frenzel glasses, and electronystagmography. No caloric testing was performed.

Following admission, thorough serologic and biochemical evaluations were performed revealing no abnormal findings. Thin-section laminography of both ears, obtained in anteroposterior and lateral projections, revealed the startling finding of a completely air-filled posterior semicircular canal (Fig. 2). Due to technical problems, posterior sections in the anteroposterior mode could not be completed and further x-ray studies were obtained two days later in this mode revealing resorption of the gas. No ossicular, cochlear, or vestibular labyrinthine abnormality was seen.

Clinically, there appeared to be a fluctuation in the sensorineural level of hearing in the right ear. In particular, it was noted that it was more difficult to communicate with the patient in the morning, but that in the afternoon he could understand speech well. This was documented by serial audiograms which showed a depression of all pure-tone levels and speech testing in the morning (SRT 45 dB, discrimination 86%) and an elevation in the afternoon (SRT 35 dB, discrimination 96%). This was consistent throughout two days. Further vestibular testing revealed no spontaneous nystagmus throughout the period of observation.

The hospitalization was complicated at this point by the onset of chicken pox from which the child made an uneventful recovery during the course of a week. Following recovery from this unrelated infectious disease, he was taken to the operating room with a working diagnosis of a perilymphatic fistula and a tympanotomy was performed. A general anesthetic, supplemented by local anesthesia, was required. The findings revealed a malformation of the round window niche such that the round window appeared to be a funnel-shaped hole approximately three times normal size and extending deeply into the temporal bone. In its depths, perilymph could be seen welling out of this region and it appeared

From the Department of Otolaryngology, University of Colorado, Denver.

REPRINTS — Nigel R. T. Pashley, MB, FRCS(C), University of Colorado Health Sciences Center, Department of Otolaryngology, 4200 East Ninth Avenue, Box B210, Denver, CO 80262.

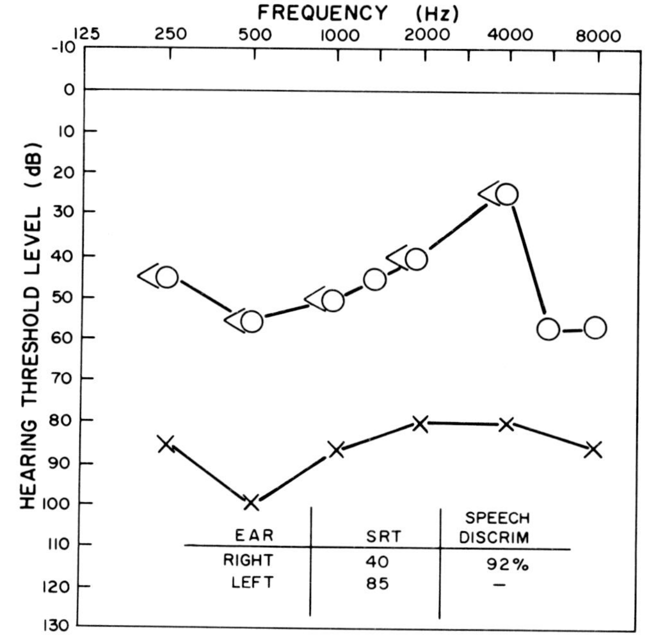

Fig. 1. Audiogram on day of admission to the hospital showing a profound hearing loss in the left ear, unchanged from previous tests, and an irregular sensorineural loss in the right ear not apparent on previous tests.

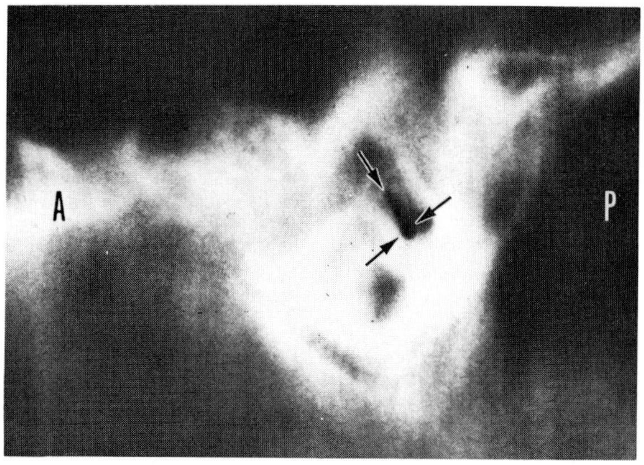

Fig. 2. Lateral laminographic x-ray film of the right ear. The posterior semicircular canal (arrows) appears in stark contrast due to air within the canal. A - Anterior; P -Posterior.

that the round window membrane did not lie in its normal axis but had been ruptured and was completely visible to the operating surgeon (Fig. 3).

Following routine exposure of the oval window, a malformation of the stapes crura was seen. The anterior crus lay in normal position, but the posterior crus joined the footplate almost at its center point. The posterior half of the footplate, therefore, could easily be seen under a normal stapedius tendon and centrally within this half was a dehiscence with a thin layer of mucous membrane overlying it. Fluid was not observed leaking from this dehiscence (Fig. 3). Following gentle scarification of the mucosa in the region of both round and oval windows, fat from the posterior earlobe was placed under the stapedius tendon anteriorly and under the crura and was reinforced with Gelfoam. The round window niche was similarly plugged and fortuitously a large central bony trabeculum bridging the window secured this fat in place. The tympanotomy flap was then replaced.

Postoperatively, a 512-Hz tuning fork lateralized to the operated ear and the patient could converse easily with his parents. He said that his hearing felt improved. The buzzing tinnitus, which he had noticed in the operated ear, had disappeared.

On the first postoperative day an audiogram was obtained showing almost normal sensory thresholds and a conductive hearing loss compatible with a tympanotomy having been performed. In further serial audiograms the air-bone gap had closed with resolution of blood and serum from the middle ear space (Fig. 4). Hearing was at this time stable.

The patient suffered an identical dramatic hearing loss in the right ear 3½ months following exploration and repair of the simultaneous round and oval window fistulae. Audiometry revealed a "carbon-copy" sensorineural hearing loss when compared to his previous loss. No radiologic study was undertaken.

Right tympanotomy and repair of a smaller recurrent round window perilymph leak were performed. The previous repair with lobular fat was intact except inferiorly in the round window niche where the atrophied fat membrane was adherent to the tympanic membrane. The impression was that this dense adherent membrane had retracted outward and allowed a further perilymphatic leak. The fistula was repaired with layered temporalis fascia.

Five days postoperatively an audiometric study revealed sensory levels within normal limits in the operated ear and a 20 dB air-bone gap with normal discrimination score. Spontaneous very rapid fluctuation in pure-tone levels with changes in discrimination were observed for ten days after the repair. These occurred within minutes and sometimes during audiometric testing.

Oral diuretics (hydrochlorothiazide) were tried without effect and although a glycerol or urea test was considered it was felt that fluctuation within minutes from normal (postoperative result) to preoperative levels precluded any significance being drawn from a rise in hearing level.

Two months postoperatively the patient could use the telephone and converse normally without a hearing aid. He is presently being closely followed by another surgeon and documented fluctuation in hearing has continued to occur infrequently. Exploration of the other ear and an endolymphatic sac

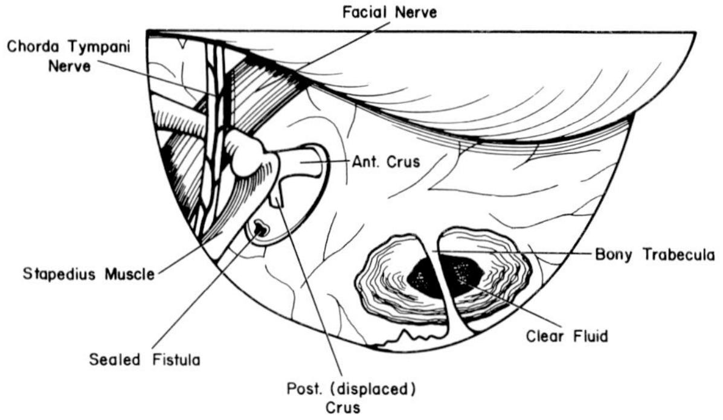

Fig. 3. Artist's drawing demonstrating malformations of both windows seen during exploration of the right ear.

procedure to attempt to stabilize the only hearing ear are being considered.

DISCUSSION

Spontaneous perilymphatic fistulae in children have been reported as presenting with meningitis or sudden hearing loss with or without vestibular symptoms. Spontaneous fistulae have also been recognized associated with mild physical exertion, although no specific reports in children of sudden hard physical exertion or barotrauma have been documented. Reported fistulae due to trauma have occurred in adults. In an excellent review of reported cases in children, Grundfast and Bluestone[1] indicate that 2 of 5 cases had congenital malformations of either the oval or round window. Their description of these anomalies occurring individually corresponds very closely to the malformations observed in our patient.

Although the pathogenesis of spontaneous perilymphatic fistula is unknown, three physiologic processes are accepted as important in the genesis of such fistulae. These are the so-called implosive, the explosive, and the mechanical-predisposition types of injury. Pashley and Shapiro in 1978[2] reported the last type of rupture, describing an anatomic defect in the stapes which they felt predisposed the oval window to rupture in an overloaded region of the footplate. Clinically, their case was noteworthy for its paucity of clear vestibular symptoms or signs. Although bilateral hypofunction was seen with caloric testing, the fistula test was negative and no consistent spontaneous nystagmus was found. Furthermore, there was no complaint or sign of vertigo from the patient. Similarly, negative fistula test results and an absence of vertigo were found in the two cases of congenital malformation of a window reported by Grundfast and Bluestone.[1]

In this case vestibular symptoms and signs were absent also, which contrasts with reports of many authors of implosive or explosive types of fistulae in which vestibular signs and symptoms were definitely present and occasionally resolved following repair of the fistula. This case provides a clinical correlate not previously documented and may lend support to the assertion by Goodhill[3] and Simmons[4] that rupture of a window may cause excessive stress on the intracochlear membranes. If the stress causing the initial window rupture is slight (mechanical predisposition), then the force transmitted through the intracochlear fluids will be less and the fluid wave exerted on the intracochlear membranes will be decreased. (A sudden implosive or explosive injury would normally cause a massive wave with dire consequences for the intracochlear and labyrinthine membranes and great potential for vestibular symptoms and hearing loss.) Theoretically, an improved prognosis for hearing might be anticipated in the mechanical predisposition group; this is demonstrated by Pashley and Shapiro[2] and in this case report.

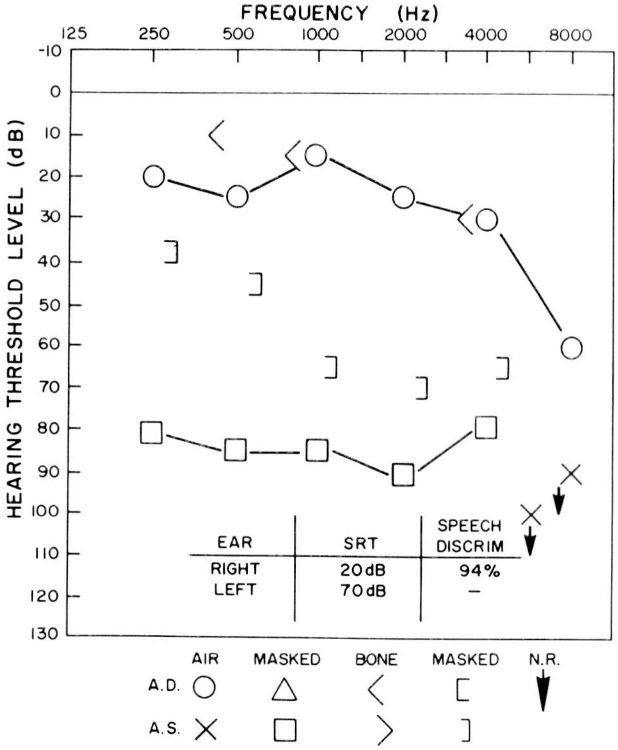

Fig. 4. Audiogram three months following exploration and repair of the simultaneous round and oval window fistulae in the right ear. A small air-bone gap remains but the sensory responses are restored and maintained at levels present on the audiogram performed at another center two years prior to the sudden rupture. A conductive hearing loss is present in the opposite (left) ear in the lower frequencies suggesting the presence of an identical anatomic anomaly. An exploration of this ear is under consideration.

It is radiologically apparent that a massive fluid shift associated with a surge of air into the labyrinth occurred in our patient, which is surprising without vestibular symptoms or signs. It is the author's postulate that air aspirated into the labyrinth entered the vestibule via one window in an implosive fashion, possibly associated with a Valsalva maneuver during a minor fall. The air then passed from the vestibule into the posterior semicircular canal when the head was positioned face down for the x-ray film. For air to enter in this manner, and not displace the intracochlear membranes in a catastrophic manner, a "pop-off" system for the pressure generated must be in effect. Such a release valve may be created when the second window is simultaneously ruptured. Massive fluid shift within the closed system would then be possible without significant intracochlear membrane injury. Goodhill[5] has suggested the term "aerodynamic implosive fistula" for this type of injury. The relatively minor initiating event in our case would further emphasize a subcategory of patients predisposed to such injuries.

When anatomic defects render the oval or round window susceptible to rupture, perilymphatic fistulae in children may occur without antecedent physical exertion or significant barotrauma. These children have little in the way of vestibular symptoms, and may recover hearing if the fistula is surgically repaired.

In the more recently reported congenital window ruptures, and in this report, the children had partial or complete unilateral sensorineural hearing loss prior to sudden loss of hearing in the only hearing ear. There is reason to suspect, therefore, that some unilateral, otherwise asymptomatic, sensorineural hearing losses in children may be due to previous, undiagnosed spontaneous fistulae, perhaps associated with the stress of birth, with relatively minor head trauma or with abnormal pressure fluctuations within the cochlea. As yet, no satisfactory diagnostic test or combination of tests exists for perilymphatic fistulae other than the clinical acuity of the otolaryngologist and an exploratory tympanotomy. There is a need to develop a noninvasive diagnostic test.

REFERENCES

1. Grundfast KM, Bluestone CD. Sudden or fluctuating hearing loss and vertigo in children due to perilymph fistula. Ann Otol Rhinol Laryngol 1978; 87:761-71.

2. Pashley NRT, Shapiro R. Spontaneous perilymphatic fistula. J Otolaryngol 1978; 7:110-8.

3. Goodhill V. Labyrinthine membrane ruptures in sudden sensorineural hearing loss. Proc R Soc Med 1976; 69:565-72.

4. Simmons FB. Fluid dynamics in sudden sensorineural hearing loss. Otolaryngol Clin North Am 1978; 11:55-61.

5. Goodhill V. Leaking labyrinth lesions, deafness, tinnitus and dizziness. Ann Otol Rhinol Laryngol 1981; 90:99-105.

≈

DEAFNESS RESEARCH FOUNDATION

The Deafness Research Foundation invites applications for 1983 grant support of research projects directed to any aspect of the ear, eg, investigation of function, physiology, biochemistry, genetics, anatomy or pathology. Grant support is given for one year, in an amount that cannot exceed $10,000, but can be renewed for one or two additional years. The deadlines for applications for 1983 grant support are as follows: first-year applications postmarked by July 15, 1982; renewal applications postmarked by August 15, 1982. For applications and for any additional information contact: Director of Medical Affairs, The Deafness Research Foundation, 55 East 34th St., New York, NY 10016.

≈

PAN AMERICAN ASSOCIATION OF OTORHINOLARYNGOLOGY AND BRONCHOESOPHAGOLOGY

The XVIII Congress of the Pan American Association of Otorhinolaryngology and Bronchoesophagology will be held November 2-6, 1982, in San Juan, Puerto Rico. Dr. Hans von Leden has been elected President of the Association.

INTRINSIC MALIGNANT SCHWANNOMA OF THE LARYNX

A CASE REPORT

HOWARD L. DELOZIER, MD

BURLINGTON, VERMONT

The first case of an intrinsic laryngeal malignant schwannoma is reported. The diagnosis of a malignant schwannoma is difficult to establish without gross evidence of its origination in a nerve. Although surgery remains the mainstay of treatment, a combination of surgery and radiotherapy appears promising. The prognosis in most cases is poor, with death usually resulting from persistent or locally recurrent disease.

INTRODUCTION

The incidence of nonepithelial laryngeal malignancies is extremely low. Krajina[1] reviewed over 6,000 malignant laryngeal tumors and reported the incidence of sarcoma to be 0.32%. Ferlito[2] in 1976 reported an incidence of 0.5% of nonepithelial malignancies over a 5-year period at the University of Padua. Thomas[3] reviewed over 850 primary laryngeal tumors from 1968-1977 at the Royal National Throat, Nose, Ear Hospital and found of 708 malignant neoplasms only 7 were of nonepithelial origin, an incidence of approximately 1%.

Although Michaels[4] alludes to one case of malignant transformation of a primary schwannoma of the larynx, a review of the literature reveals this patient to be the first reported case of a primary malignant schwannoma of the larynx.

CASE REPORT

A 46-year-old male had a left supraglottic mass excised at an outlying Vermont hospital in 1970. The pathology report was equivocal with the final diagnosis being fibrosarcoma.

The patient was lost to follow-up until April 1978, when he presented with a left neck mass. The mass was locally excised, and a histologic diagnosis of embryonal rhabdomyosarcoma was reported. It was intended for the patient to have postoperative radiation therapy, but he was lost to follow-up. The following year the patient reappeared with a recurrence of his neck mass and upper airway obstruction. An urgent tracheostomy was performed, and direct laryngoscopy revealed severe distortion of the left supraglottic larynx. The patient was subsequently transferred to the Medical Center Hospital of Vermont for further evaluation.

On examination, the patient had an 11 x 5 cm firm, slightly mobile, nonpulsatile mass involving the entire anterior cervical triangle, with fixation to the larynx. There was bulging of the left floor of the mouth and base of tongue, secondary to tumor compression.

Laryngeal tomograms revealed distortion of the supraglottic larynx bilaterally with obliteration of the left ventricle and no subglottic extension. A barium swallow showed complete obliteration of the left pyriform sinus and no distal esophageal disease. The CAT scan (Fig. 1) demonstrated the contiguous involvement of the neck mass and laryngeal disease. It also showed the mass to extend superiorly in the lateral pharyngeal space without apparent involvement of the base of the skull. A carotid arteriogram revealed the carotid system to be displaced posteriorly and laterally (Fig. 2). Pulmonary tomograms and bone scan demonstrated no evidence of metastatic disease. Direct laryngoscopy revealed bulging of the left aryepiglottic fold, false cord, and obliteration of the left ventricle. The left true cord was paralyzed. There was impingement of the neck mass into the lateral hypopharyngeal wall with obliteration of the left pyriform sinus. A biopsy of the left false vocal cord yielded embryonal cell rhabdomyosarcoma.

In April 1979, the patient underwent a total laryngectomy and left radical neck dissection. At the time of surgery, the tumor was found to involve the entire left glottic and supraglottic larynx. It extended to the base of the skull and completely infiltrated the internal jugular vein at the level of the mandible. The 10th, 11th and 12th cranial nerves were engrossed by tumor and were sacrificed in the en bloc removal of the mass.

Light microscopy of the resected specimen revealed increased cellularity and invasion of the surrounding fibrous tissue (Fig. 3A). The tumor displayed two distinct histologic patterns. The

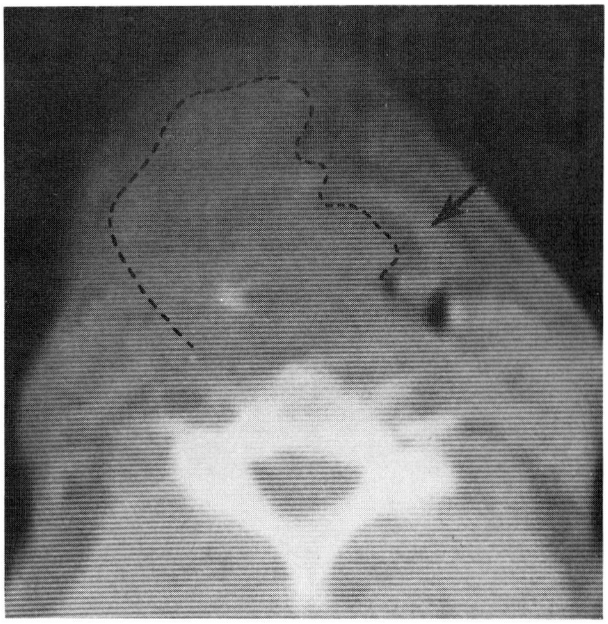

Fig. 1. CAT scan demonstrating contiguity of the neck mass with endolarynx (dotted line). Arrow - Contralateral lamina of thyroid cartilage.

From the Division of Otolaryngology, University of Vermont, Burlington.

REPRINTS — Howard L. DeLozier, MD, Division of Otolaryngology, University of Vermont, 1 S. Prospect Street, Burlington, VT 05401.

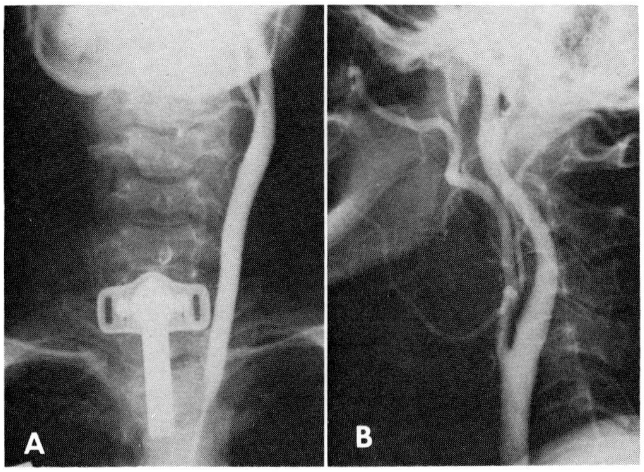

Fig. 2. Left carotid ateriogram. A) Lateral and B) posterior displacement of carotid system.

first was a loosely cellular myxoid pattern, and the other a more palisading configuration (Fig. 3B). The cells were small and spindle-shaped with large nuclear to cytoplasmic ratio. There was little nuclear pleomorphism and approximately 4 mitoses/10 high-power microscopic field.

Due to the clinically aggressive nature of the mass and its histologic appearance, a diagnosis of low-grade malignant schwannoma was made. Electron microscopy was of no help in establishing the diagnosis.

The patient underwent 5800 rads of postoperative radiotherapy and remained free of disease for seven months. Recurrent disease was then noticed submucosally along the left lateral pharyngeal wall and retromolar trigone area.

The patient subsequently received both intravenous and intra-arterial adriamycin therapy, which failed to inhibit progressive enlargement of the tumor. Following an unsuccessful trial of localized radiotherapy, the patient expired ten years after his initial presentation.

DISCUSSION

Malignant schwannomas (neurogenic sarcomas) are more frequently found outside the head and neck, ie, in the extremities, the chest wall, or the abdominal wall. In the head and neck, they originate most often from the brachial plexus, the sympathetic chain, or from the main trunk or branches of the cranial nerves. In this case, the tumor most likely originated from the peripheral branch of the superior laryngeal nerve, with subsequent growth in the supraglottic area (a common location for benign intrinsic laryngeal schwannomas).

There appears to be no age predilection for these tumors, although a slight female predominance has been noted.[5] An association between neurofibromatosis and neurogenic sarcoma has been reported with the incidence varying from 5 to 50%.[6-8] Sarcomatous change occurs more frequently in males and in the more deeply located tumors.[5]

Although symptoms may be caused by direct neuronal involvement, ie, pain, paresthesia, and secondary muscular atrophy, they are usually attributable to local expansion of the mass, such as air-

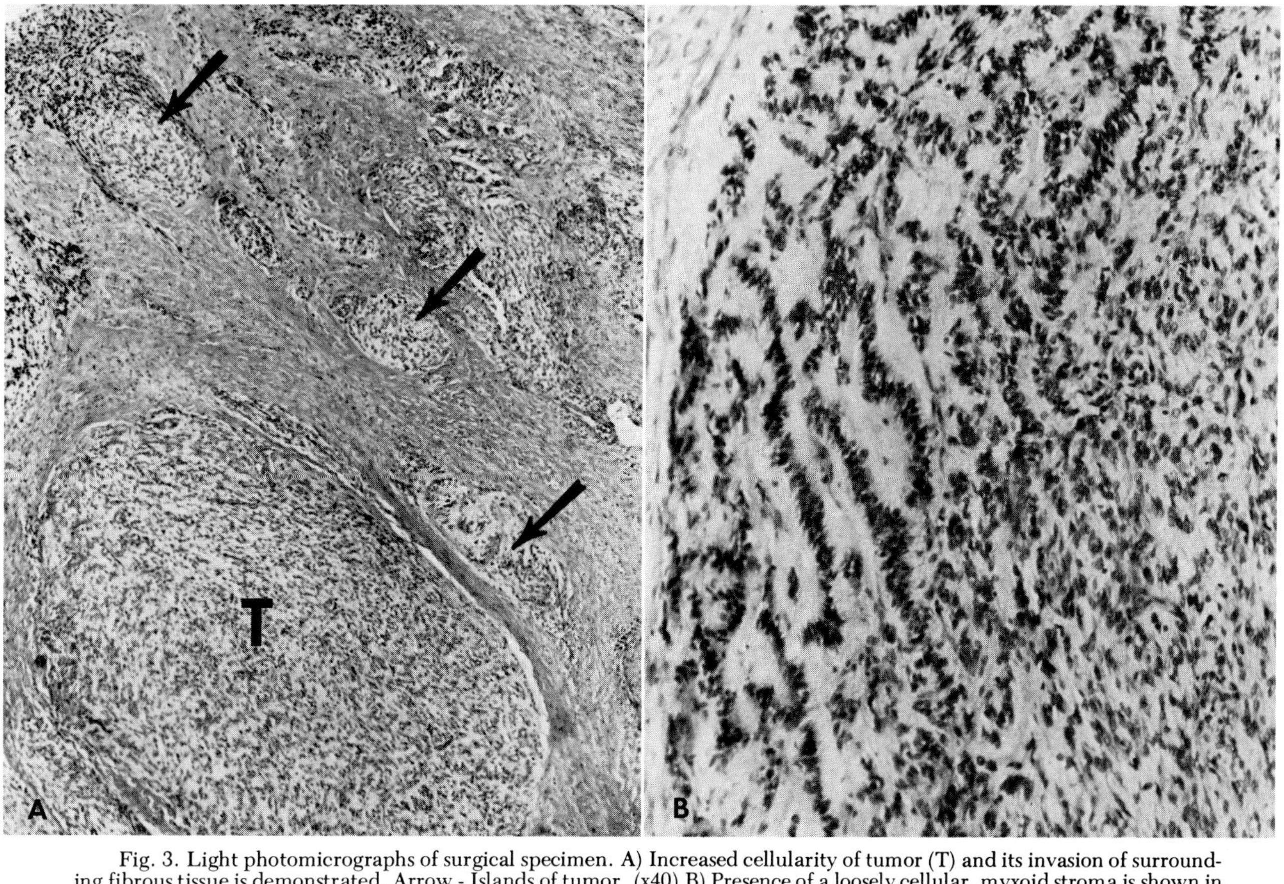

Fig. 3. Light photomicrographs of surgical specimen. A) Increased cellularity of tumor (T) and its invasion of surrounding fibrous tissue is demonstrated. Arrow - Islands of tumor. (x40) B) Presence of a loosely cellular, myxoid stroma is shown in association with an area of palisading. (x100)

way obstruction in this patient. Clinically, these tumors are firm, although necrosis and cystic degeneration can cause varying degrees of softness. They are usually circumscribed and frequently extensively invade the surrounding tissues. Lymphatic spread is uncommon, while blood-borne metastases to the chest, bone, brain, and liver are more routinely found.

Histologically, malignant schwannomas are comprised of spindle cells with various degrees of pleomorphism. They tend to be very cellular and palisading is sometimes evident. The mitotic rate is usually low, with greater than 5 mitoses/10 high-power field representing a high grade of malignancy.[9]

Because of the extensive pleomorphism, these tumors may be easily confused with other soft tissue sarcomas that may encroach on or infiltrate a nerve for various distances. The use of special stains to demonstrate a characteristic "straight wire" pattern of reticular fibers is of questionable value in documenting a neurogenic origin in a soft tissue sarcoma.[5] In fact, there have been no criteria established by which a primary neurogenic sarcoma can be differentiated from a fibrosarcoma without gross evidence of its origination in a nerve trunk; therefore, many investigators[5,6,10] would adhere to a strict dependence on the nature and degree of involvement of the nerve. In the present case, the mass had been resected twice prior to the patient being referred to our institution. With the size of the mass, the scarring from the previous surgical procedures, the degree of soft tissue invasion, and with the supraglottic locus of origin (the nerve of origin being extremely small this far peripherally), it is not surprising that the classical pattern of tumor growth inside an identifiable nerve trunk was not observed. Furthermore, it is not surprising that on the basis of the initial surgical specimen, the diagnosis was fibrosarcoma. A review of the ensuing slides revealed poor specimen sampling, containing mainly degenerated tissue, making any diagnosis difficult. It was not until the last surgical specimen was reviewed that the characteristic pattern of a malignant schwannoma could be found among the myoid stroma.

Traditionally, wide surgical excision has been the modality of choice in the treatment of these tumors, while radiation therapy has been felt to be ineffective.[8,10] However, the recent experience of Goepfert et al[11] and Hutcherson et al[12] argue in favor of the combination of surgery with postoperative full course radiotherapy.

The prognosis for malignant schwannomas of the head and neck is poor, with death usually resulting from persistent or locally recurrent disease. In Kragh et al's[13] series 50% of the patients and 67% in D'Agostino et al's[10] series died within three years. Of the six patients in Hutcherson et al's[12] series that had a significant period of follow-up, 50% died within one year, and only one of these six patients is currently alive and free of disease. With multiple surgical procedures, radiation therapy and chemotherapy, our patient survived for ten years; nevertheless, he still expired of his locally recurrent tumor.

In conclusion, malignant schwannomas of the head and neck are difficult tumors to diagnose and to cure. Although wide surgical excision remains the mainstay of treatment, evidence is accumulating in favor of the combination of surgery plus postoperative radiotherapy.

ACKNOWLEDGMENTS — The author would like to thank Dr. John Batsakis, Chairman of the Department of Pathology at the Maine Medical Center, and Dr. Thomas Trainer, Chairman of the Department of Pathology at the Medical Center Hospital of Vermont, for their counselling and repeated consultations regarding the histopathology of the specimen.

REFERENCES

1. Krajina Z. Laryngeal sarcoma. Can J Otolaryngol 1975; 4:303-6.

2. Ferlito A. Histological classification of larynx and hypopharyngeal cancers and their clinical implications. Pathological aspects of 2,052 malignant neoplasms diagnosed at the ORL Department of Padua University from 1966 to 1976. Acta Otolaryngol (Stockh) 1976; 342:1-88.

3. Thomas RL. Non-epithelial tumours of the larynx. J Laryngol Otol 1979; 93:1131-41.

4. Michaels L. Neurogenic tumors, granular cell tumor, and paraganglioma. Can J Otolaryngol 1975; 4:319-27.

5. Batsakis J. Tumors of the peripheral nervous system. In: Batsakis J. Tumors of the head and neck. Baltimore: Williams and Wilkins, 194:231-49.

6. Stout A. The peripheral manifestation of the specific nerve sheath tumor (neurilemoma). Am J Cancer 1935; 24:751-96.

7. Preston F, Walsh W, Clark T. Cutaneous neurofibromatosis (von Recklinghausen's disease): clinical manifestations and incidence of sarcoma in 61 male patients. Arch Surg 1952; 64:813-27.

8. Conley J. Neurogenic tumors in the neck. Arch Otolaryngol 1955; 61:167-80.

9. Hajdu S. Tumors of the peripheral nerves. In: Hajdu S. Pathology of soft tissue tumors. Philadelphia: Lea and Febiger, 1979:427-82.

10. D'Agostino A, Soule E, Miller R. Primary malignant neoplasms of nerve (malignant neurilemomas) in patients without manifestations of multiple neurofibromatosis (von Recklinghausen's disease). Cancer 1963; 16:1003-14.

11. Goepfert H, Lindberg R, Sinkovics J, et al. Soft tissue sarcoma of the head and neck after puberty: treatment by surgery and postoperative radiation therapy. Arch Otolaryngol 1977; 103:365-8.

12. Hutcherson R, Jenkins H, Canalis R, et al. Neurogenic sarcoma of the head and neck. Arch Otolaryngol 1979; 105:267-70.

13. Kragh L, Soule E, Masson J. Benign and malignant neurilemmomas of the head and neck. Surg Gynecol Obstet 1960; 111:211-8.

ANEURYSMAL BONE CYST OF THE SPHENOID IN A CHILD

CHARLES P. KIMMELMAN, MD

WILLIAM P. POTSIC, MD LUIS SCHUT, MD

PHILADELPHIA, PENNSYLVANIA

The aneurysmal bone cyst is a vascular lesion which destroys and expands bone. We report a case of an aneurysmal bone cyst of the sphenoid sinus which resulted in loss of vision due to compression of the optic chiasm. Staged intracranial and extracranial procedures were used to remove the lesion. Aneurysmal bone cysts are very rare in the sphenoid sinus, and this is the first reported case occurring at that site in a child.

INTRODUCTION

Because of its central location in the skull, the sphenoid bone and its contained sinus serve as a conduit for vital neural and circulatory elements. Consequently, the manifestations of sphenoid lesions may be protean. Since sphenoid disease per se is relatively rare, the physician should, from time to time, review and study these cases to maintain cliniical acumen. Our case represents a most unusual sphenoid lesion hitherto unreported in a child.

CASE REPORT

A 10-year-old male was seen at the Children's Hospital of Philadelphia in January 1976 for decreasing vision in the left eye. Physical examination at that time revealed normal extraocular motility without proptosis. Sensation in the ophthalmic and maxillary divisions of the fifth nerve was intact. No bruits were present over the globe or skull. There was pallor of the optic discs, more pronounced on the left. Central scotomas were present in both

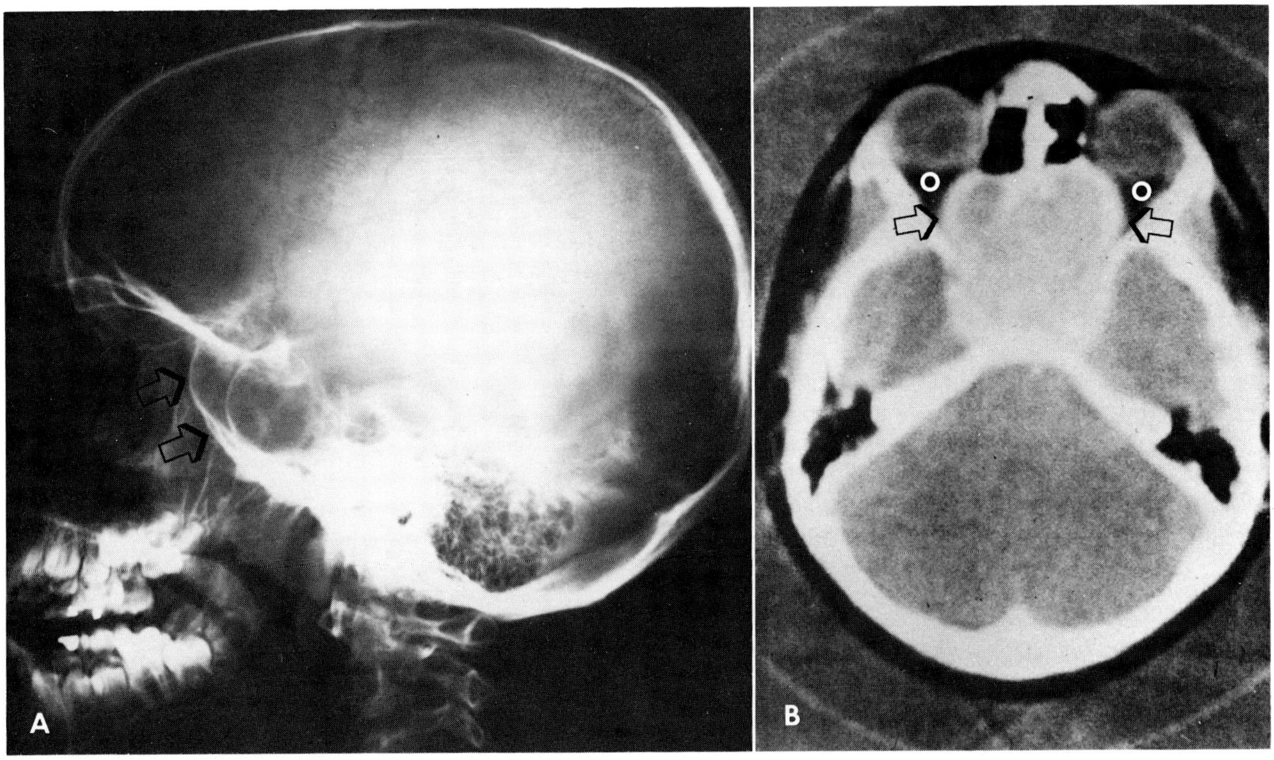

Fig. 1. A) Lateral skull x-ray film revealing expansion of the sphenoid sinus (arrows). B) Computed tomogram of the skull demonstrating expansile sphenoid mass (arrows) encroaching on orbits (O).

From the Departments of Otorhinolaryngology and Human Communication and Neurosurgery, Children's Hospital of Philadelphia and the University of Pennsylvania School of Medicine, Philadelphia.

REPRINTS — William P. Potsic, MD, Children's Hospital of Philadelphia, 34th and Civic Center Boulevard, Philadelphia, PA 19104.

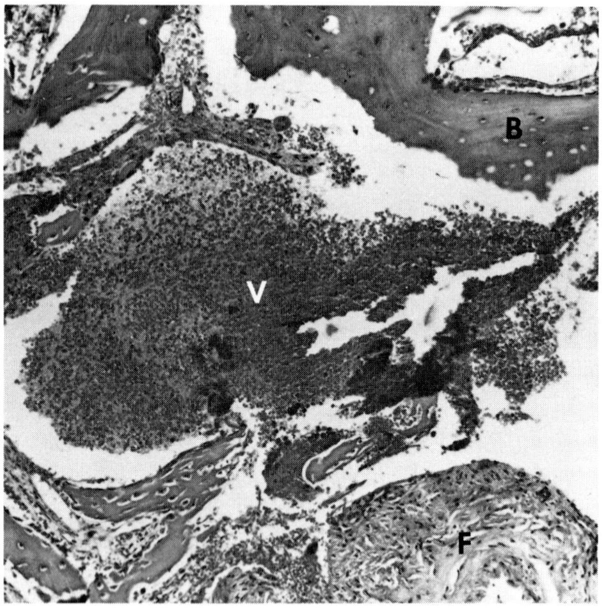

Fig. 2. Excised tissue from the nasopharynx reveals large vascular spaces (V) surrounded by fibrous tissue (F) within bone (B) consistent with aneurysmal bone cyst.

eyes. There was a soft tissue mass filling the nasopharynx and causing obstruction to air flow. The rest of the physical examination was normal.

Roentgenography of the skull showed a soft tissue mass expanding the sphenoid sinus and extending intracranially. The right maxillary sinus, nasopharynx, and posterior nasal cavity were similarly involved (Fig. 1A). A computed tomogram revealed an enlarged sphenoid sinus containing a soft tissue density which enhanced with the injection of Conray (Fig. 1B). The lesion extended into the right maxillary sinus and into the medial portion of the orbits. It also extended superiorly to produce destruction and deformity of the sella.

On January 12, 1976 a bifrontal craniotomy was performed; as much of the mass as possible was removed from the sella, carotid arteries and optic chiasm. The tissue was thought to be a giant cell tumor or giant cell granuloma. On February 6, 1976 a transpalatal and transantral approach was used to remove tumor from the nasopharynx, sphenoid sinus, and posterior walls of both maxillary sinuses. The blood loss was approximately 1000 ml. The patient tolerated the procedure well and was discharged on February 13, 1976. Histopathologic examination of the tissue removed at the second operation revealed aneurysmal bone cyst (Fig. 2).

There was some decrease in vision over the course of a week following discharge, and oral dexamethasone was given. This resulted in improvement of vision by March 16, 1976. The steroids were then tapered and stopped several weeks later.

In April 1976 the patient was evaluated at the National Eye Institute. The vision was 20/50 bilaterally. The consensus of the pathologists was that the lesion was an aneurysmal bone cyst.

Since that time there has been no progression of the lesion. At the last examination there was no evidence of further visual loss; the central scotomas remain.

DISCUSSION

Although it is more common in the extremities and spine, the aneurysmal bone cyst may nonetheless occur in the sphenoid bone. This lesion is a cystic, vascular osseous tumor which destroys and expands bone. It is not a true neoplasm.[1] Jaffe and Lichtenstein first described the lesion in 1942 in the extremities.[2] Histologically there are irregular enlarged vascular channels separated by septae of fibrous tissue containing prominent giant cells. An associated giant cell tumor may be present, and this makes the diagnosis difficult in lesions of the skull and jaws.[3] The histologic differential diagnosis also includes fibrous dysplasia, ossifying hematoma, and cavernous hemangioma of bone.

There are several phases of development of this lesion. The initial phase consists of osteolysis and periosteal elevation. In the second phase there is progressive bony destruction. Next is the phase of stabilization, giving the classic radiologic picture of an expanded tumor with a distinct bony shell. Finally there is the healing phase, as the tumor progressively ossifies.[1]

The etiology is unknown, but it may include such factors as trauma or alteration in osseous hemodynamics. Some pathologists question the existence of aneurysmal bone cyst as a pathologic entity.[4] In the head and neck aneurysmal bone cysts have been described in the maxilla, mandible, cranium, orbital roof, temporal bone, and sphenoid bone.[3,5-10]

Radiographic evaluation is critical in the evaluation of an aneurysmal bone cyst. Conventional roentgenograms of the sinuses may reveal bony destruction, opacification, expansion of sinus or sella, or abnormal calcification. A more detailed view of bony changes is obtained with multidirectional polytomography. Computed tomography with enhancement further defines the anatomic process.

Surgical excision is the treatment of choice for aneurysmal bone cysts. There are several routes in addition to the transpalatal, which was employed in this patient. The availability of the operating microscope and the use of intraoperative fluoroscopy have improved the ability to safely perform rhinologic approaches, such as the transseptal sphenoidotomy. Other routes include the transantral and transethmoid, which suffer from the obliquity of the approach as well as an external scar in the latter.[11,12] In the past radiation therapy in doses of 2000 rad has been recommended in cases where surgery is difficult.[1] However, it is generally best to refrain from the use of radiation for benign disease.

REFERENCES

1. Dabska M, Buraczewski J. Aneurysmal bone cyst. Pathology, clinical course, radiologic appearance. Cancer 1969; 23:371-89.

2. Jaffe HL, Lichtenstein L. Solitary unicameral bone cyst. Arch Surg 1942; 44:1004-25.

3. Yarington CT, Abbott J, Raines D. Aneurysmal bone cyst of the maxilla. Arch Otolaryngol 1964; 80:313-17.

4. Edling NP. Is the aneurysmal bone cyst a true pathologic entity? Cancer 1965; 1127-30.

5. Cacdac MA, Malis LI, Anderson PJ. Aneurysmal parietal bone cyst. J Neurosurg 1972; 37:237-41.

6. Costantini FE, Iraci G, Benedetti A, Melanotta PL. Aneurysmal bone cyst as an intracranial space-occupying lesion. J Neurosurg 1966; 25:205-7.

7. Fite JD, Schwartz JF, Calhoun FP. Aneurysmal bone cyst of the orbit. Trans Am Acad Ophthalmol Otolaryngol 1968; 72: 614-18.

8. Odeku EL, Mainwaring AR. Unusual aneurysmal bone cyst. J Neurosurg 1965; 22:172-76.

9. Jeremiah BS. Aneurysmal bone cyst of the temporal bone. J Int Coll Surg 1965; 43:179-83.

10. Delorit GJ, Summers GW. Aneurysmal bone cyst of the sphenoid sinus. Trans Am Acad Ophthalmol Otolaryngol 1975; 80:438-443.

11. Calcaterra TC, Rand RW. Current adjuncts for surgery of the sphenoid sinus and pituitary gland. Laryngoscope 1976; 86: 1692-98.

12. Konrad HR, Canalis RF. Transpalatal approach to deeper cranial structures. Laryngoscope 1977; 87:165-70.

≈

INTERSPECIALTY FACIAL SURGERY CONGRESS FOR AESTHETIC, CANCER AND RECONSTRUCTIVE SURGERY

The IFSCACRS will be held at the Waldorf-Astoria in New York, April 27-30, 1983. This Congress is sponsored by the International Oculoplastic Society. For more information contact Pierre Guibor, MD, IFSC Secretary, 630 Park Avenue, New York, NY 10021; (212) 734-1010. F1

≈

FOURTH WORLD CONGRESS ON BRONCHOESOPHAGOLOGY

The Fourth World Congress on Bronchoesophagology will take place at the Foresta Conference Center in Stockholm, Sweden, June 20-23, 1983. This Congress is arranged by the International Bronchoesophagological Society, Swedish Otolaryngological Society and Swedish Society for Pulmonary Diseases. During the meeting, the Congress will update the knowledge within bronchology and esophagology. Further information may be obtained by writing IBES Congress 1983, c/o RESO Congress Service S-105, 24 Stockholm, Sweden, or Dr. Stig Haglund, Secretary of the Congress, Dept. of Otolaryngology, Karolinska Sjukuset, S-104 01 Stockholm 60, Sweden. F2

PATHOLOGY CONSULTATION

MALIGNANT MIXED TUMOR

JOHN G. BATSAKIS, MD
PORTLAND, MAINE

Definitions of salivary gland tumors embraced by the term "malignant mixed tumors" have undergone considerable refinement in the past 30 years. Features such as incomplete encapsulation, epithelial cellularity, and recurrences no longer serve as justifications for a connotation of malignancy or "semi-malignancy."[1] It is now generally agreed that a high recurrence rate for mixed tumors is primarily the result of inadequate primary surgery removal.[2] A myxoid stromal dominance in the tumor is also more often associated with recurrence than is an epithelial dominance.

Definable, life-consuming malignancy is, however, associated with mixed tumors and generically malignant mixed tumor exists in *three* clinical and histological forms (Fig. 1).[3]

The overall frequency of these malignant mixed tumors is not high: less than 2% of all mixed tumors. The great majority of these malignant mixed tumors are carcinomas arising in or from a mixed tumor, the so-called *carcinomas ex pleomorphic adenoma.*

The other two histological variants are only rarely encountered and contain both components of a mixed tumor: epithelial and mesenchymal. In one variant there is a synchronous and biphasic malignant neoplasm: in effect a carcinosarcoma whose metastases contain both carcinoma and sarcoma.[3] A most unusual variant is the metastasizing mixed tumor. This lesion can be defined as a histologically benign mixed tumor that inexplicably manifests distant metastases. The metastatic deposits (most often in lungs and bones) deviate only minimally from the benign appearance of the primary mixed tumor. An infiltrative growth pattern and mitotic activity have been found in some of the eight examples of this form of malignant mixed tumor recorded in the literature through 1978.[4] Recurrences and surgical manipulations of the tumors may play a role in their hematogenous spread.

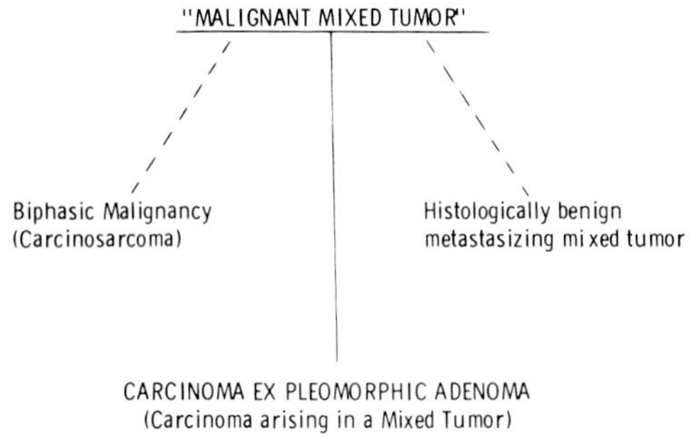

Fig. 1. The three forms of tumors encompassed by the term "malignant mixed tumor." Nearly 99% of such lesions are carcinomas ex pleomorphic adenoma.

Given the rarity of the two preceding forms, when one speaks of a malignant mixed tumor he is referring to the *carcinomatous* development of malignancy in a mixed tumor; carcinoma ex pleomorphic adenoma (carcinoma arising in a mixed tumor).[1,6] The latter, in turn, presents in two clinical settings. Most often the carcinoma arises in a mixed tumor of long duration: either as a consequence of no treatment or because of recurrences. The risk of carcinomatous transformation can be said to increase with the age of the tumor. Support for this hypothesis has been given by microspectrophotometric DNA analysis wherein there is a difference in the DNA content between morphologically benign pleomorphic adenomas with short and with long preoperative duration of the tumor.[5] A less common clinical presentation is malignancy appearing at the first surgical excision following a short preoperative time period.

Carcinoma ex pleomorphic adenoma may arise in any salivary tissue with the parotid gland most often, and the mucous glands of the upper respiratory tract the least often involved. Table 1 presents the salivary gland distribution of these lesions as presented in four series.[1,7-9]

The gross appearance of a malignant change presents valuable clues to its existence. The tumor usually appears encapsulated but with areas of cap-

TABLE 1. SALIVARY GLAND DISTRIBUTION OF CARCINOMA EX PLEOMORPHIC ADENOMA

Authors	*Parotid*	*Submandibular*	*Minor Glands*
Eneroth et al[1]	31	3	—
LiVolsi and Perzin[7]	23	6	18
Spiro et al[8]	107	23	16
Gerughty et al[9]	16	5	1

From the Department of Pathology and Laboratory Medicine, Maine Medical Center, Portland, Maine.
REPRINTS — John G. Batsakis, MD, Department of Pathology and Laboratory Medicine, Maine Medical Center, Portland, ME 04102.

sular invasion or outright disruption. The cut surface bears a resemblance to the benign counterpart with the exception of areas of softening, necrosis and hemorrhage. Any of these gross features should alert the pathologist to the fact that he is not dealing with an ordinary mixed tumor and should be the stimulus for additional sectioning.

For conclusive diagnosis, remnants of the benign mixed tumor should be histologically evident. The type of carcinoma most often observed is a ductal carcinoma, often with epidermoid areas. Carcinomas such as adenoid cystic, mucoepidermoid, and acinous cell only rarely evolve from a benign mixed tumor. LiVolsi and Perzin[7] have added an additional histological entity: carcinoma in situ or preinvasive carcinoma ex pleomorphic adenoma. This lesion demonstrates no capsular invasion or extension into adjacent salivary stroma.

The prognosis of a patient with carcinoma ex pleomorphic adenoma is poor, with nearly no survivors in 20-year determinate survival studies.[1,6] Spiro et al,[8] dealing with carcinoma at major and minor salivary gland sites, record net or determinate "cure" rates at 5-, 10-, and 15-year intervals of 40, 24, and 19% respectively. Local recurrence is almost invariably the reason for treatment failure and distant metastasis, which occur with a higher incidence than lymph node involvement, occur in nearly one third of patients with uncontrolled primary disease.[8]

REFERENCES

1. Eneroth C-M, Blanck C, Jakobsson PA. Carcinoma in pleomorphic adenoma of the parotid gland. Acta Otolaryngol (Stockh) 1968; 66:477-92.
2. Conley J, Clairmont AA. Facial nerve in recurrent benign pleomorphic adenoma. Arch Otolaryngol 1979; 105:247-51.
3. Batsakis JG. Tumors of the head and neck. 2nd ed. Baltimore: Williams and Wilkins, 1979.
4. Chen KTK. Metastasizing pleomorphic adenoma of the salivary gland. Cancer 1978; 42:2407-11.
5. Eneroth C-M, Zetterberg A. Malignancy in pleomorphic adenoma. A clinical and microspectrophotometric study. Acta Otolaryngol (Stockh) 1974; 77:426-32.
6. Moberger JH, Eneroth C-M. Malignant mixed tumor of the salivary glands: special reference to the histologic structures in metastases. Cancer 1968; 21:1198-1211.
7. LiVolsi VA, Perzin KH. Malignant mixed tumors arising in salivary glands. I. Carcinomas arising in benign mixed tumors: a clinicopathologic study. Cancer 1977; 39:2209-30.
8. Spiro RH, Huvos AG, Strong EW. Malignant mixed tumor of salivary origin. A clinicopathologic study of 146 cases. Cancer 1977; 39:388-96.
9. Gerughty RM, Scofield HH, Brom FM, Hennigar GR. Malignant mixed tumors of salivary gland origin. Cancer 1969; 24:471-86.

Ann Otol Rhinol Laryngol 91:1982

X-RAY STUDY OF THE MONTH

HYPERTELORISM IN NASAL AND PARANASAL SINUS POLYPOSIS

ALFRED L. WEBER, MD
WILLIAM R. WILSON, MD WILLIAM W. MONTGOMERY, MD
BOSTON, MASSACHUSETTS

PATIENT

This 13-year-old female has had a lifelong history of complete nasal obstruction. In early childhood she developed asthmatic bronchitis and required frequent hospitalizations for status asthmaticus. Allergy skin testing demonstrated sensitivity to dust, mold, feathers, and tree pollen. Despite antigenic therapy for four years, she required steroids for control of her asthma. She has no known aspirin sensitivity and evaluation for cystic fibrosis was negative.

At age 12 years she was first seen at the Massachusetts Eye and Ear Infirmary and noted to have total nasal occlusion with polyps and marked hypertelorism. Laboratory studies revealed an eosinophil count of 248 cells/mm^3 and a serum IgE level of 35 IU/ml.

The patient's mother has asthma, but no nasal polyps. No other family member has hypertelorism.

RADIOGRAPHIC FINDINGS

The Water's projection (Fig. 1 A) of the paranasal sinuses reveals complete opacification and slight dilatation of the maxillary antra with some thinning of the bony walls laterally and medially. There is distension and opacification of both nasal cavities and thinning of the bony outline.

A Caldwell projection (Fig. 1 B) demonstrates a marked diffuse increase in density of the ethmoid sinuses and frontal sinus, with hypertelorism.

On the lateral projection (Fig. 1 C) polypoid tissue is seen in the anterior half of the nasopharynx and there is complete opacification of the sphenoid sinus.

An AP polytome study (Fig. 1 D) of nasal cavities and paranasal sinuses was done when nasal obstruction recurred after surgery. This reveals complete reopacification of the sinuses and nasal cavities. Note the dilatation of both ethmoid sinuses with thinning and lateral displacement of the medial wall of both orbits.

DIAGNOSIS

The patient underwent bilateral intranasal ethmoidectomy and sphenoidectomy in March 1976. Within six months the polyps had recurred and were again causing nasal obstruction. In the next two years, three intranasal ethmoidectomies were necessary. Currently, she is stable and is receiving topical intranasal steroids (beclomethasone diproprionate).

DISCUSSION

Nasal polyps are uncommon in children,[1] their frequency increasing with age. The etiology of nasal polyps is not clear. Cystic fibrosis and aspirin intolerance are predisposing conditions for the formation of nasal polyps,[2] but patients with these diseases represent only a small proportion of the total population with nasal polyps. Allergy and infection are most frequently suggested as the primary factors contributing to the formation of nasal polyps. Settipane and Chafee noted asthma in more than 70% of their polyp patients.[2]

Polyps may be sessile or pedunculated. The extent of polyposis may range from a single polyp in the nasal cavity or ethmoid sinus to diffuse polyposis involving all paranasal sinuses and causing complete obstruction of both nasal cavities, frequently accompanied by chronic sinus infections, anosmia, and at times chronic otitis media. Nasal polyps that extrude through the choanae most often arise from the maxillary antrum and may extend into the nasopharynx as a single choanal polyp or as multiple bilateral masses. Mucoceles may develop in patients with multiple polyposis, especially in the ethmoid sinuses and supraorbital ethmoid sinus extensions.[3]

Radiologically, single polyps are characterized by a homogeneous sharply-defined round tissue density arising from the antral wall or in the nasal fossa. In marked nasal and paranasal polyposis there is opacification and expansion of the nasal and sinus cavities and thinning of the bony walls. Fluid levels are rarely seen. The ethmoid cell partitions are commonly lost and there is considerable thinning of the medial wall of both orbits. Marked expansion of

From the Department of Radiology, Massachusetts Eye and Ear Infirmary, Boston.
REPRINTS — Alfred L. Weber, MD, Department of Radiology, Massachusetts Eye and Ear Infirmary, 243 Charles St., Boston, MA 02114.

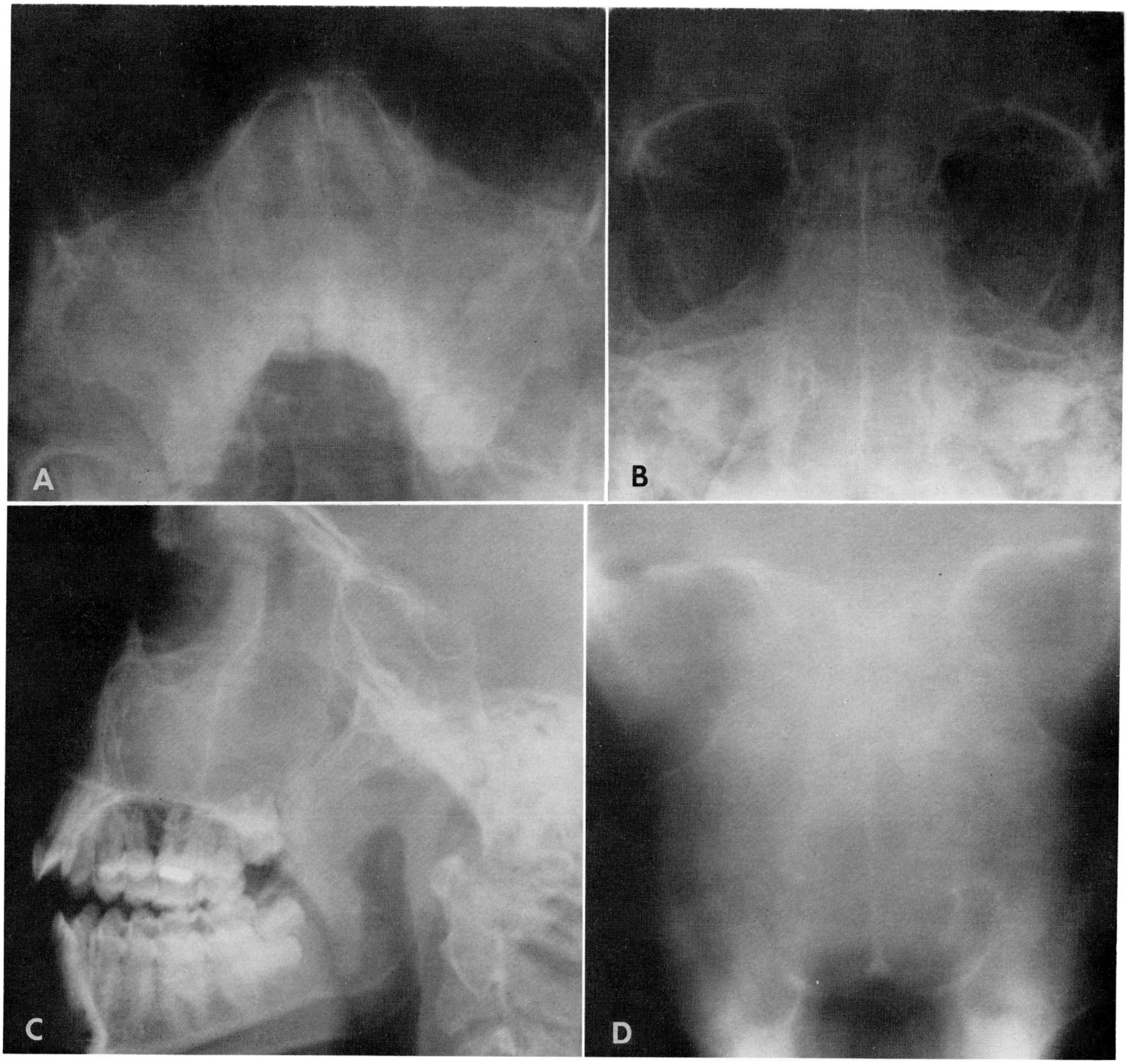

Fig. 1.

the ethmoid sinuses in a small child may produce hypertelorism, as observed in this patient. Nasal polyps are seen on conventional sinus films only when polyposis is extensive. For detailed evaluation of the extent of polypoid disease, polytomography of the nasal cavities and sinuses is very useful.

Surgery is indicated when there is severe nasal obstruction or chronic sinus infection and pain. Simple polypectomy should be tried first, but intranasal or external ethmoidectomy may be required if polyps recur. Malignant degeneration has not been reported in patients with polyposis.

ACKNOWLEDGMENT — Special thanks to Paula R. Griswold for her assistance in preparing this case.

REFERENCES

1. Lanoff G, Daddono A, Johnson E. Nasal polyps in children: a ten year study. Ann Allergy 1973; 31:551-4.

2. Settipane GA, Chafee FH. Nasal polyps in asthma and rhinitis. J Allergy Clin Immunol 1977; 59:17-21.

3. Weber AL, Klein TR. Ethmoid mucopyocele. Ann Otol Rhinol Laryngol 1979; 88:438-9.

BOOK REVIEWS

Prostaglandin Synthetase Inhibitors: New Clinical Applications

Edited by *Peter Ramwell.* Hard cover, black and white illustrations, 410 pp, 1980. Alan R. Liss, Inc, New York. Price $34.00

The prostaglandins (PGs) have been extensively studied in many centers during the past several decades. In his opening remarks, the editor emphasized the importance of prostaglandins by saying that the prostaglandins are now recognized as one of the four major classes of endogenous substances with high biologic activities, along with steroids, biologic amines and polypeptides. One reason that the PGs are so important is that they are easily synthesized by all body tissues. Furthermore, about a third of the drugs in the pharmacopoeia interact with the PG system.

The clinical importance of PGs became obvious by the discovery in 1971 that aspirin and other nonsteroidal anti-inflammatory agents inhibit the PG synthetase pathway.

This multiauthored volume, which is the first in the new proposed series on prostaglandins and related lipids, is devoted to the clinical application of PG synthetase inhibitor (PGSI). The book includes reviews on research in the biochemistry of the PG system, the pharmacokinetics of PGSI and potential clinical uses of PGSI. The potential clinical uses of PGSI discussed in the book encompass diverse areas such as inflammation, pain, bone resorption, cancer, thrombosis, hypertension, shock, renal functions, dysmenorrhea, premature labor, closure of the ductus arteriosus.

Special interests for an otolaryngologist may be found in the sections dealing with inflammation, disorders of the bone and cancer. This book will also serve as an introduction to prostaglandin research for those who want to learn about this fascinating subject.

As do most collections of articles, the book suffers from the variability in style and quality of presentations by various authors. It may be too broad in scope for many readers.

This book represents the state of the art in PGSI research and constitutes a welcome addition in the library of serious clinicians and researchers interested in PGs.

TIMOTHY T. K. JUNG, MD
Minneapolis, Minnesota

The Voice and its Disorders, Fourth Edition.

By *Margaret C. L. Greene.* Hard cover, black and white illustrations, indexed, bibliography, 446 pp, 1980. J. B. Lippincott Co, Philadelphia. Price $47.50.

This revised edition of *The Voice and its Disorders* remains one of the most complete clinically instructive scholarly texts on vocal pathology and management in the literature to date. Twenty-two years after its first edition, Greene updates the areas of surgical advances (pseudoglottis reconstruction in postlaryngectomy, surgical approaches to spastic dysphonia, posterior palatal repair in cleft palates and new approaches to papillomata), hormone related voice disorders, singing as a vocal technique, and pro and con approaches to breathing as an effective clinical technique. She adds to the sections on treatment strategies, which include excellent case studies, and outlines rehabilitative programs for specific vocal disorders. She utilizes primarily European scientific studies with only a respectable representation of the best in American contributions. Throughout the new edition, Greene's clinical philosophy is reiterated as 1) "... therapy is more art than science," 2)"... it transcends scientific explanation and embraces the personality of the therapist," and 3) "... developments in surgery and electronic microprocessors linked to the relatively new concept of biofeedback ... pose a real threat to traditional speech therapy." Although most American voice clinicians and scientists would agree that therapy is substantially a personal technique or "art," few view with "depressing outlook" the advent of scientific and technological advances in clinical instrumentation.

The text is divided into two major parts: Normal Voice and Voice Disorders. Part One, Normal Voice, is a sufficient review of the anatomy and physiology of the vocal instrument although several omissions in American research, notably Thomas Hixon's work in respiratory parameters of speech and the work of Thomas Shipp, John Michel and David Brewer, are unfortunate. Chapter 4, dealing with articulation and resonance, seriously omits any sufficient discussion of the function of the lateral pharyngeal walls in velopharyngeal closure as enhanced by the work of Skolnick, McCall and Minfie. There is no presentation of the work of Warren in the area of air flow and air pressure dynamics of velopharyngeal closure as it is able to predict adequate cross-sectional area of nasal-oral port for speech production.

This portion of the text makes valuable contributions in a section entitled "Vocal Synthesis" which is a glossary-type prose that outlines an excellent conceptual framework of viewing phonation. Chapter 6 is worth mentioning because it deals with a timely subject of "infancy and senescence" in normal voice evolution. While the chapter is comprehensive and timely it lacks depth of scientific reports from the other side of the Atlantic.

Part Two, entitled Voice Disorders, is outstanding because it is both a comprehensive and indepth presentation of assessment and rehabilitative techniques in the total area of vocal pathologies. Greene subdivides the disorders of voice into six categories of symptomatology rather than by organic versus functional or etiologic taxonomy. She presents six basic disorder areas: hyperkinetic dysphonias, psychogenic disorders, disorders of pitch, disorders of resonance, dysarthrophonia (upper motor neuron lesions) and laryngeal palsy (lower motor neuron lesions). She also deals specifically with some less common disease states such as chronic hyperplastic laryngitis, papillomata, tuberculosis of the larynx, and others. In two separate chapters she presents laryngeal carcinoma and its management as distinct forms of vocal disorder in appraisal and treatment. These last three chapters are excellent contributions and well updated.

The highlight of the text is clearly the presentation of hyperkinetic dysphonia (the most common form of vocal abuse) which occupies four separate chapters and 60 pages of the entire text. The author convincingly defends the necessity for breathing techniques in most voice disorders, with a valuable discussion of both American and European investigators (pro and con). She then outlines her own time-honored approach to breath control and abdominal support in phonation.

This superbly written scholarly book is a valuable teaching and reference text for the laryngologist interested in phonation and vocal rehabilitation. The substantial European emphasis in its references and approach is a positive feature commending it to every American library in vocal pathology.

RICHARD M. MERSON, PhD
St. Louis, Missouri

Audiology, Education and the Hearing-Impaired Child

By *Fred H. Bess* and *Freeman E. McConnell.* Hard cover, black and white illustrations, indexed, 321 pp, 1981. C. V. Mosby Co, St. Louis. Price $16.95.

Authors cite the separateness of audiology and education of hearing-impaired children as prompting this book. The primary readers are audiologists involved in managing hearing-impaired children and teachers who consider audiology important in teaching such children. Otolaryngologists will have only peripheral interest. Authors are primarily clinicians and do a better job of bringing audiology to the educator than the reverse. Despite a number of texts on this same theme recently, Bess and

McConnell, who represent different generations concerned with hearing-handicapped children, have made an important contribution. This book's best use is probably in the training of audiologists and teachers. It is refreshing for its unity in having the text written by only two authors, rather than following the popular trend for edited texts of chapters by numerous authors. Although there is some reference to the experience of the authors, the book borrows heavily from other publications cited throughout the text.

The text is quite readable with fine diagrams, illustrations and photographs. A special feature is inclusion of "vignettes" that are sometimes case histories, sometimes suggested forms or outlines. About half of the chapters are "standards" for comprehensiveness, but Chapters 2, 5, 7, 8, 9 and 11 are the real contributions, wrestling with the issues at the core of the problems of utilizing hearing for the education of hearing-impaired children.

DONALD R. CALVERT, PhD
St. Louis, Missouri

Breathing, Speech, and Song

By *Donald F. Proctor.* Hard cover, black and white illustrations, indexed, 159 pages, 1980. Springer-Verlag Inc., New York. Price $19.80.

This text is written primarily for the student of voice. It provides a collection of essays describing the anatomy and physiology of voice production in man. The author surveys the issue of voice mechanics from a very unique position as a clinical laryngologist and a student of voice himself. While the attempt to combine science with art is an especially noble one, the author, in my opinion, necessarily falls short of his intended goals because of the diversity of fields addressed. Certainly for the student of laryngology, the discussions of anatomy and physiology are superficial at best. In addition, guidelines for the laryngologist in the treatment of voice disorders appear fragmented and anecdotal. The textbook is, unfortunately, flawed by numerous spelling and typescript errors. Photographs are difficult to interpret without appropriate labeling to guide the reader.

For the student of voice, the description of anatomy and physiology may in fact be too complex and technical to provide meaningful interpretation and significance to the art of singing. For him also, the guidelines of treatment in voice disorders might appear unstructured and for the most part anecdotal.

In general, the strength of this text lies in its attempt to fuse the scientific interests of a singer with the art of singing itself. Whether it successfully accomplishes this is unfortunately open to question.

CLARENCE T. SASAKI, MD
New Haven, Connecticut

Progress in Clinical Neurophysiology, Volume 8, Spinal and Supraspinal Mechanisms of Voluntary Motor Control and Locomotion

Edited by *J.E. Desmedt.* Hard cover, black and white illustrations, indexed, 374 pp, 1980. S. Karger, Basel, New York. Price $82.75

This is a state of the art collection of monographs by multiple authors. Both animal and human investigations are described. The general subject areas include sensory input and spinal connectivities in motor control, segmental circuits involving interneurons and motoneurons, muscle vibration and motor control in man, and motor control mechanisms in postural and locomotor activities. The editorial quality is excellent. The reviews provide useful conceptual insights in relation to current research efforts. Overall the book comprises a useful reference for investigators and graduate students. For the clinician there may be some useful insights in regard to the status of studies of proprioceptive and vestibular mechanisms in relation to posture and movement.

WILLIAM M. LANDAU, MD
St. Louis, Missouri

Reconstruction of the Head and Neck

Edited by *Malcolm A. Lesavoy.* Hard cover, black and white illustrations, indexed, 319 pp, 1981. Williams and Wilkins, Baltimore. Price $43.00.

As the author states in his preface, this book is not intended to be a comprehensive review of constructive surgery of the head and neck. Rather, it addresses reconstructive problems in a regional and segmental fashion, illustrating only selected and favored techniques.

The book is divided into 16 chapters, each dealing with the reconstruction of a different region within the head and neck. The majority of the authors are plastic surgeons of whom over half are from southern California.

For the most part, the discussion of reconstructive techniques is kept quite simple; greater detail can be found in many other surgical texts. While not true for all, in most chapters there is little written about the indications and contraindications, advantages and disadvantages, and alternatives concerning particular reconstructive procedures. In general, each author discusses his preferred methods for attacking specific reconstructive problems.

Despite these shortcomings, the book provides a delightful and fairly informative overview of reconstructive concepts in the head and neck. As always, certain chapters are better than others; in general the book is well written and easy to read and follow. The illustrations and case photographs are clear. Because of the rather simple regional style and organization, it serves as a nice first book for general physicians, residents and students interested in the subject. It is a worthy contribution which can be recommended to the seasoned reconstructive surgeon only as an adjunct to a complete library on head and neck and reconstructive surgery.

STEVEN M. SOBOL, MD
New York, New York

Verbal Dyspraxia in Clinical Practice

By *Betty Hill.* Hard cover, black and white illustrations, appendix, 80 pp, 1978. University Park Press, Baltimore. Price $9.95.

This monograph attempts to outline treatment programs for the restoration of articulation skills in patients with cerebral lesions and clinically described as exhibiting some form of apraxia of speech. Ms. Hill, a senior speech pathologist at the Royal Talbot Rehabilitation Hospital in Melbourne, Australia, reports the results of a 10-year investigation with as many as 100 to 150 patients with some form of apraxia.

The report is not well organized, and gives no detailed description of her population or any quantification system to identify therapy progress. Ms. Hill specifies her own unique four major varieties of dyspraxia: dyspraxia with global aphasia, afferent dyspraxia, efferent dyspraxia, and efferent dyspraxia with adynamia. Only afferent and efferent dyspraxia are well defined and differentiated in the text while the other two forms are clouded, evidently by forms of severe aphasic syndromes that are not specified by any standard aphasia examinations.

The book does present some valuable outlines of articulation sequence drills moving from isolated consonants to syllables of increasing strength for the afferent types of dyspraxia, and utilization of rhyming techniques with carrier phrase verbal fill-in drills for the efferent dyspraxic. The appendix offers some helpful facilitating phrases following phonemic similarities. The area of interest, dyspraxia, although in need of further treatment in the literature is not improved much by this text. I cannot recommend it as a valuable book in a professional library.

RICHARD M. MERSON, PhD
St. Louis, Missouri

BOOKS RECEIVED

Basic Industrial Hearing Conservation

David F. Barr and Richard K. Miller. Black and white illustrations, hard cover, glossary, appendix, 125 pages, 1979. The Fairmont Press, Inc., Atlanta, $26.95.

Guide to Noise Control Literature

Richard K. Miller. Hard cover, 148 pages, 1980. The Fairmont Press, Inc., Atlanta, $24.95.

Concepts in Cancer Care. A Practical Explanation of Radiotherapy & Chemotherapy for Primary Care Physicians

Jay Scott Cooper and Donald J. Pizzarello. Black and white illustrations, indexed, hard cover, 257 pages, 1980. Lea & Febiger, Philadelphia, $16.50.

Neurological Surgery of the Ear, Volume II

Herbert Silverstein and Horace Norrell. Black and white illustrations, indexed, hard cover, 396 pages, 1979. Aesculapius Publishing Co., Birmingham, $60.

Otolaryngology, 3 volumes, 2nd edition

Michael M. Paparella and Donald A. Shumrick. Volume I: Basic Sciences and Related Disciplines ($70); Volume II: The Ear ($55); Volume III: Head and Neck ($70), hard cover, indexed, black and white illustrations, 3020 pages, 1980. W.B. Saunders Co., Philadelphia, $185 the set.

The Voice and Its Disorders, 4th edition

Margaret C.L. Green. Black and white illustrations, indexed, hard cover, bibliography, 446 pages, 1980. J.B. Lippincott Co., Philadelphia, $47.50.

Evoked Potentials

Edited by Colin Barber. Black and white illustrations, indexed, hard cover, 603 pages, 1980. University Park Press, Baltimore, $34.50.

External Ear Malformations: Epidemiology, Genetics, and Natural History

Michael Melnick and Nitnos C. Myrianthopoulos. Index, black and white illustrations, hard cover, 128 pages, Alan R. Liss, Inc., New York, $18.

Physiology and Pathophysiology of Eustachian Tube and Middle Ear

Edited by G. Münker and W. Arnold. Index, black and white illustrations, soft cover, 244 pages, Georg Thieme Verlag, Stuttgart.

Scott-Brown's Diseases of the Ear, Nose and Throat, 4 volumes, 4th edition.

Edited by John Ballantyne and John Groves. Volume I: Basic Sciences, 760 pages, $115. Volume II: The Ear, 978 pages, $145. Volume III: The Nose and Sinuses, 480 pages, $69.95. Volume IV: The Pharynx and Larynx, 626 pages, $99.95. Black and white illustrations, index, hard cover. Butterworths, Woburn, Mass., $400 the set.

Hearing Aid Assessment and Use in Audiologic Habilitation, 2nd edition

Edited by William R. Hodgson and Paul H. Skinner. Black and white illustrations, indexed, hard cover, 303 pages, 1981. Williams & Wilkins, Baltimore, $32.

Neuronal Mechanisms of Hearing

Josef Syka and Lindsay Aitkin. Black and white illustrations, indexed, hard cover, 1981. Plenum Press, New York, $45.

IN MEMORIAM

BEN H. SENTURIA, MD

November 3, 1910 — July 7, 1982

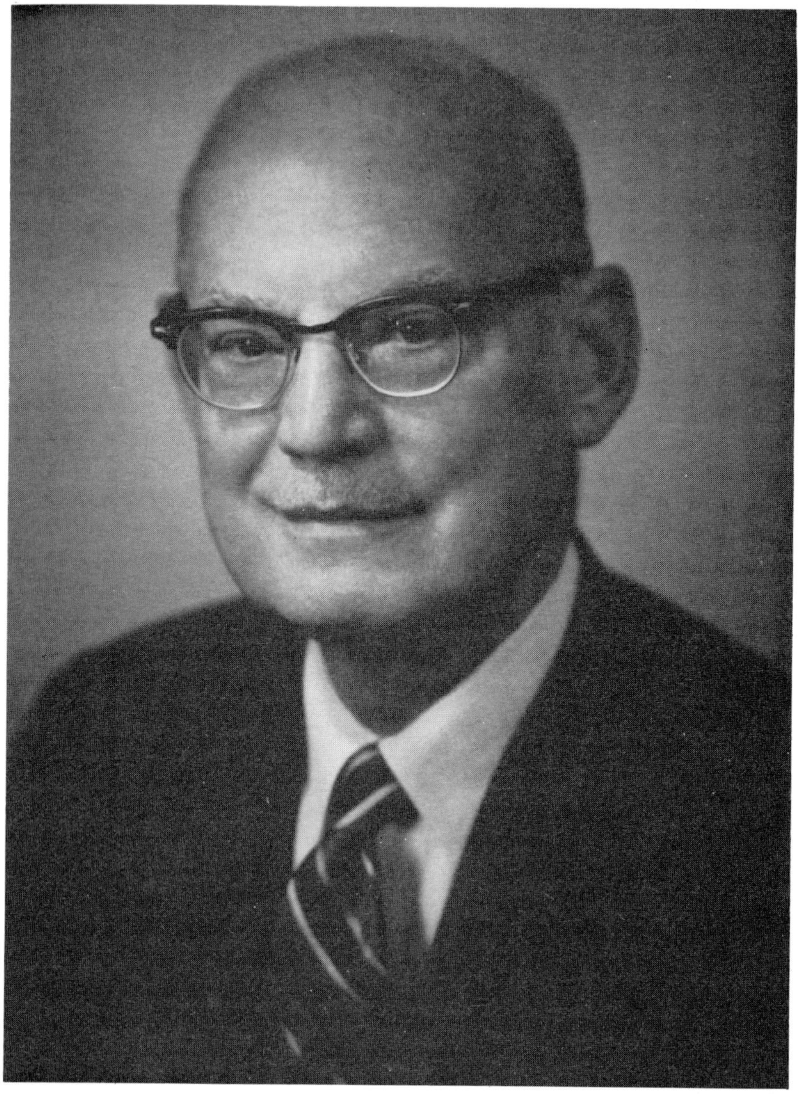

BEN H. SENTURIA, MD
Editor 1966-1982

TRIBUTE

It was with great personal sadness that, two days after the fact, I learned of Ben Senturia's passing. From the northern waters of Lake Huron, communication with the progressing situation had been poor. This was frustrating; the final news was crushing. We feel acutely the great void of having lost a friend — and a model, a mentor, an astute advisor as well — a truly selfless person who always gave more than he expected in return. As his close associate for almost 15 years, I learned he was all of these, and at the same time he was warm, humorous and always forgiving. His family, friends and associates must now do what he surely would wish us to do: take up our tasks in his stead and carry them out with him as our example. This we will do, for we can never forget him.

Brian F. McCabe, MD
Editor

OBITUARY

BEN H. SENTURIA, MD

Ben Harlan Senturia was born in St. Louis, was graduated from Washington University in 1931 with an AB degree, and received an MD from Washington University School of Medicine in 1935 with membership in the Alpha Omega Alpha honorary medical society. Upon completion of his residency in otolaryngology at McMillan Hospital (1935-1938), he was appointed to the Faculty of Washington University School of Medicine and to the staffs of Jewish, Barnes and Children's Hospitals in St. Louis.

During his service in the U.S. Air Force (1942-1945) Dr. Senturia was assigned to the Research Section of the School of Aviation Medicine where he conducted major investigations in infections of the external ear and in noise-induced hearing loss. Following his military service he returned to Washington University. At the McMillan Hospital Department of Otolaryngology, Dr. Senturia taught medical students and graduate students and conducted major research programs. His research in external otitis resulted in two textbooks and over 80 scientific papers, many of which were presented at national and international scientific meetings. In addition to his extensive basic and clinical investigations on external otitis, he conducted a number of significant studies on secretory otitis media and in a number of other otologic areas. In 1979 he was named Professor Emeritus of Clinical Otolaryngology at Washington University.

In addition to his teaching and research activities at Washington University and its affiliated hospitals, Dr. Senturia carried on an extensive practice. He also worked at the Central Institute for the Deaf with its founder, the late Dr. Max Goldstein, and later with Dr. Richard Silverman, now Emeritus Director of the Institute. Assuming the Directorship of the Department of Otolaryngology at The Jewish Hospital of St. Louis in 1952, Dr. Senturia retained this post until 1972 when he was named Director Emeritus. During those years Dr. Senturia served on the Medical Executive Committee, the Joint Conference Committee, the House Staff and Education Committee, and the Research Committees.

In 1958 Dr. Senturia was selected by Dr. Arthur Proetz to be the Associate Editor of the *Annals of Otology, Rhinology & Laryngology*, a position he held until Dr. Proetz's death in 1966, when Dr. Senturia became Editor of the *Annals*.

From 1963 to 1973 Dr. Senturia served as Chairman of the Committee on Otolaryngic Pathology of the American Academy of Otolaryngology. He was the Academy's First Vice President from 1971 to 1972, a former member of its Council, and inspired a teaching collaboration between the American Academy of Otolaryngology and the Armed Forces Institute of Pathology.

Dr. Senturia was President of the American Otological Society, Inc, from 1972-1973, and also served as Secretary and Chairman of the Board of Trustees of the Research Fund of the Society, the special committee responsible for distributing funds for otological research. In 1976 Dr. Senturia was the Society's Guest of Honor and in 1980 he received its prestigious Award of Merit.

The St. Louis Otological Foundation was organized in 1949 by a number of Dr. Senturia's patients who desired to contribute to his research and teaching activities. Dr. Senturia served as its President from 1949-1967, when he became its Director of Research. The Foundation established a Lectureship in Dr. Senturia's honor in 1976 and sponsors an annual Foundation Lecture by an outstanding otologic scientist before a combined meeting of the St. Louis Ear, Nose and Throat Club, the Central Institute for the Deaf, and the Departments of Otolaryngology at Washington University, St. Louis University School of Medicine and The Jewish Hospital of St. Louis.

Dr. Senturia had been ill for some time but insisted on continuing his clinical activities. Not surprisingly, the cardiac arrest leading to his final illness occurred in the clinic while he was examining the ears of a 16-month-old child. Dr. Senturia, the beloved, kind, caring physician, the brilliant research scientist, and the dedicated, meticulous editor of this journal from 1966 to 1982, died on July 7, 1982. Surviving him are his wife, Nancy, whom he married in December 1942; his son, Ben H. Jr; and his daughter, Alice.

The late Abraham Joshua Heschel once wrote, and I believe it applies to Ben Senturia, "The deepest wisdom man can attain is to know that his destiny is to aid, to serve . . . this act of giving . . . is reciprocity on man's part . . . for the gift of life."

Victor Goodhill, MD

EIGHTH DANIEL C. BAKER, JR, MEMORIAL LECTURE

SUBCERTIFICATION: A DILEMMA FOR OTOLARYNGOLOGY—HEAD AND NECK SURGERY

GEORGE F. REED, MD

SYRACUSE, NEW YORK

The issue of subspecialization and subcertification has been one of great concern for many years and has recently received increased attention, especially in our specialty of Otolaryngology—Head and Neck Surgery. The problem being faced by the various specialties and their boards is not so much that of subspecialization, since this has definitely occurred in most of the specialties and today is an accepted fact. More specifically, the problem is that of subcertification, or some form of recognition of the subspecialist's advanced training, knowledge and expertise. This matter is indeed creating a serious dilemma, not only for Otolaryngology—Head and Neck Surgery but for most of the specialties. On the one hand, the specialists are concerned about fragmentation of the parent specialty while, on the other hand, there is a growing demand for recognition by those individuals who feel that they have acquired special competence in their areas of subspecialization.

My main purpose in this presentation is to express some personal thoughts on the subject of subcertification. Before doing so, however, I would like to review some of the common arguments for and against subcertification.

On the positive side, a number of points can be considered. As in all aspects of medical education, research, and patient care, the ultimate consideration must be that of improved patient care. In this regard, if one accepts the fact that specialization has improved patient care, then certainly subspecialization can be expected to do likewise. If this be the case, such subspecialization should be recognized by some form of subcertification to protect the public interest. It can be well argued that passage of time inevitably produces new knowledge and new technologies in various areas of our presently accepted specialties. It can also be argued therefore that those who concentrate their activities in these fields should have some form of recognition or subcertification by the nationally accepted certifying bodies — namely, the Boards. Another point on the positive side is that, since many fields of subspecialization cross specialty lines, subcertification provides the opportunity for diplomates of one specialty board to compete with the diplomates of competing boards in the delineation of hospital privileges and in the third party reimbursement process. There is also concern that, if subcertification is not provided by the Boards in the American Board system, certification might be provided by other organizations with lesser standards than those presently utilized. This would certainly be to the detriment of the public interest.

Now, what of the arguments against subcertification? It can be argued that increasing subspecialization will increase the cost of medical care. This has generally been the case in the past, wherein specialists usually expect higher fees than generalists. It can be assumed that subspecialization will produce the same phenomenon of increased fees. However, the mere fact of recognition of subspecialities by subcertification should not by itself have any significant impact upon increasing the cost of care by virtue of increased fees.

The cost of care probably would be increased by virtue of the fact that subspecialization, spurred by subcertification, usually results in increased training requirements, increased cost to the institution providing the training and to the physician involved by decreased income during training. Ultimately these costs are passed on to the patient. Another argument frequently given by the presently recognized parent specialties is that of fragmentation with resultant erosion of the status of the parent specialties and their specialty boards. It is felt by many that this could result in a diminution of the status of the individual who possesses certification from the general discipline but does not possess subcertification in the subspecialty area. Indeed, it is this subtraction from the globality of the general or parent discipline which gives rise to the greatest fears of subcertification — that lack of a certificate in a discipline's subspecialty might deny one the privilege of practicing that subdiscipline by restriction of hospital privileges to only those possessing

Dr. Reed is currently Secretary-Treasurer of the American Board of Otolaryngology.

Presented at the meeting of the American Laryngological Association, Palm Beach, Florida, May 1-2, 1982.

REPRINTS — George F. Reed, MD, 750 E. Adams Street, Syracuse, NY 13210.

such subcertification. There are also fears that the possession, or lack thereof, of a certificate of special competence might influence the amount of reimbursement by third party payers and also increase the risk of malpractice judgments to those who do not possess the special certificate.

Thus, in reviewing the pros and cons of subcertification, we find many valid reasons favoring some form of certification of special expertise. In contrast, the main fears appear to be those of fragmentation on the part of organized medicine, and those of potential restriction of hospital privileges and the increased threat of malpractice susceptibility on the part of individuals.

Now I would like to exercise the privilege, which is inherent in a lecture of this type, of expressing some of my personal thoughts regarding subcertification. I have given a great deal of thought to this subject over the past few years — frequently with mixed emotions. I now definitely believe that the arguments in favor of subcertification outweigh those against it.

As far as fragmentation is concerned, I really consider this to be a nonproblem. Fragmentation in the specialties has already occurred in the form of subspecialization and certainly this will not be compounded by the recognition of subspecialists by some form of certifying process. I think we must recognize that what we are experiencing at present is merely an extension of that which occurred when the present specialties and Specialty Boards were initiated a number of years ago. We are merely undergoing a further evolution of that specialization process in the form of subspecialization, with the need for accompanying subcertification. We should accept this evolutionary process rather than fight it. We must accept the fact that the need to recognize special knowledge, special training, special expertise, and extra achievements by some form of certification process is pervasive, inexorable, and unavoidable.

At the present time, the 23 Specialty Boards which operate under the umbrella of the American Board of Medical Specialties do issue some 25 special certificates in various subspecialties, either through the mechanism of conjoint boards, subboards, or certificates of special competence. In my opinion, the best mechanism is that of the primary board issuing certificates of special qualifications to individuals who can demonstrate possession of such special qualifications in subspecialty areas within the domain of their primary board. It is time for this process to be expanded. Indeed, the American Boards have a responsibility to recognize special knowledge and expertise if they are to continue to fulfill their role of serving and protecting the public.

OFFICE TELESCOPIC PHOTOGRAPHY OF THE LARYNX

EIJI YANAGISAWA, MD, FACS
NEW HAVEN, CONNECTICUT

After testing many different procedures for photographing the larynx in the office, the author found that telescopic photography is a most effective and reliable method. Four currently available right-angle laryngeal telescopes were reviewed and are discussed with regard to their results, along with the author's method of office telescopic photography.

Accurate photographic documentation of the larynx is of considerable value for teaching, permanent records, proper diagnosis and management of various laryngeal disorders. Yet there is no single reliable method of still photography of the larynx which laryngologists can easily employ at the office.

Ever since the first documentation of the successful office laryngeal photography by Thomas French of Brooklyn, New York, in 1882, many different methods of laryngeal photography have been described. They include 1) indirect laryngoscopic photography,[1-3] 2) direct laryngoscopic photography,[4-7] 3) microscopic photography,[8-15] 4) telescopic photography[16-21] and 5) fiberscopic photography.[22,23]

The purpose of this paper is twofold: first, to review four currently available right-angle laryngeal telescopes of different makes with regard to their results and, second, to present the author's method of office telescopic photography of the larynx which has proven to be satisfactory.

EQUIPMENT

RIGHT-ANGLE (LATERAL) TELESCOPES

Berci-Ward Indirect Laryngopharyngoscope with Hopkins Telescope (8702D, Karl Storz Endoscopy-America, Inc). This endoscope (Fig. 1-a) consists of two parts, a telescope and a light-conducting tube, which can be locked together with a bayonet socket. The telescope contains a series of fixed glass cylinders replacing the interspace between the lenses in the more conventional endoscopes and producing a set of small air-lenses between them. This construction is reported to bring about a wider view angle in relation to the diameter of the optics.[18,19]

The telescope measures 28.3 cm in length and 4.5 mm in diameter. Its front lens diameter is 2.2 mm (Fig. 2A-a). The rectangular outlets, one on each side of the lens, measure 1 mm x 3 mm (Fig. 2B-a)

There are two different sizes of light-conducting tubes, one of a smaller diameter for visual examination and flash photography only, and one of a larger diameter intended for cinephotography but also useful when the available light source is insufficient. The larger light-conducting tube has two connections for the fiber light cables so that either two separate cables or the two distal ends of a Y-shaped cable can be attached. In both tubes the light outlet is shaped into two rectangular areas on each side of the front lens.[19] In this study only the smaller tube (outer diameter 8.5 mm) was used.

The instrument has an antifog airflow system by means of a small air channel made by a groove along the inner aspect of the light-conducting tube and the telescope.

Laryngoscope with Hopkins Telescope (8704D, Karl Storz). This instrument (Fig. 1-b) is quite similar to KS 8702D but has a built-in focusing capability and the entire larynx can be seen within one single viewing field in 4x magnification. One can focus the larynx at different distances like a telephoto lens and can photograph the magnified view of the larynx to fill the entire slide.

The instrument measures 24.4 cm in length and 7.6 mm in outer diameter. Its front lens diameter is 3 mm (Fig. 2A-b). The rectangular light outlet on each side of the lens measures 1 mm x 7 mm (Fig. 2B-b). It also has an antifog device.

Stuckrad Magnifying Laryngoepipharyngoscope (Richard Wolf Medical Instruments Corp). This instrument (Fig. 1-c) consists of a telescope, a light-transmission system and an antifog device, but they cannot be taken apart.[19]

A fiberoptic cable, which also includes an air tube for the antifog device, is fixed to the instrument. Connections for changing the fiberoptic cables (and air tubes) are available. The instrument includes a plastic handle. The telescope has a relatively low weight as it contains groups of lenses in-

From the Section of Otolaryngology, Department of Surgery, Yale University School of Medicine, and the Section of Otolaryngology, Department of Surgery, Hospital of St. Raphael, New Haven, Connecticut.

Presented at the meeting of the American Laryngological Association, Palm Beach, Florida, May 1-2, 1982.

REPRINTS — Eiji Yanagisawa, MD, 98 York Street, New Haven, CT 06511.

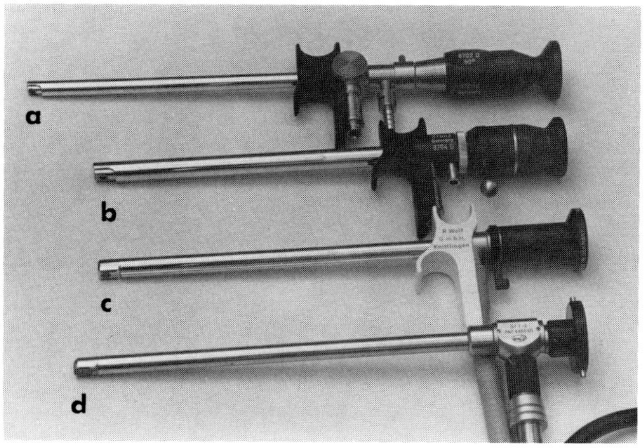

Fig. 1. Four right-angle laryngeal telescopes. a) Berci-Ward Hopkins telescope (Karl Storz 8702D), b) Hopkins magnifying telescope (Karl Storz 8704D), c) Stuckrad magnifying laryngoepipharyngoscope (Wolf), and d) Nagashima SFT-1 laryngoscope, Note that Berci-Ward telescope is longest while other three are about same length. Also note that Stuckard and Nagashima telescopes have integrated light cable which would prevent loss of light transmission at connection.

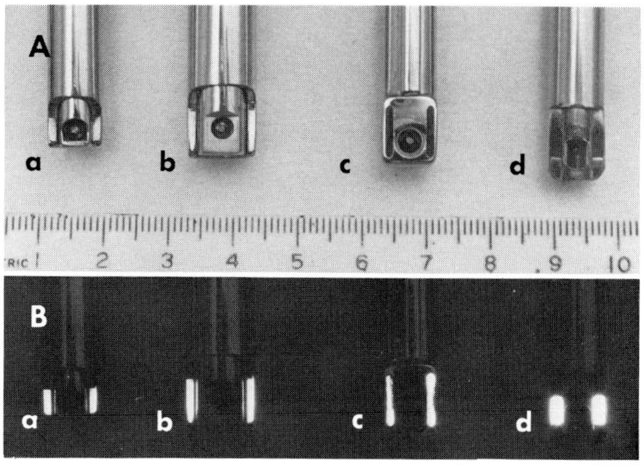

Fig. 2. A) Close-up view of tip of each telescope. B) Tips showing light-transmission outlets. a - Hopkins telescope 8702D, b - Hopkins telescope 8704D, c - Stuckrad telescope, and d - Nagashima SFT-1 laryngoscope. Note difference in sizes of lens openings and light-transmission outlets.

stead of glass rods. With the aid of a knob, it is possible to change the relationship of these lenses to each other, which results in a change of magnification and focus of the object under observation. This construction should not be confused with a zoom lens, which can change the angle of view continuously and without influencing the focus,[19] but it does have a zoom lens effect.

The light transmission opens at two rectangular outlets on each side of the front lens of the telescope (Fig. 2A-c, B-c). It measures approximately 1 mm x 8 mm. The length of the telescope is 24.3 cm and its outer diameter is 9-10 mm. The antifog device consists of an air-conducting narrow metal tube, permanently fixed to the instrument and opening immediately behind the front lens.[19]

Laryngoscope (SFT-1, Nagashima Medical Instrument Co, Tokyo). This laryngoscope is a single integrated unit composed of a telescope and a light-transmission system (Fig. 1-d). It measures 24.5 cm in length and 9 mm in outer diameter. The angle of the prism at the tip of the laryngoscope is 70°, providing a right-angled view of the larynx. The rectangular outlets on each side of the lens offer well-balanced illumination of the viewing field (Fig. 2B-d). Each measures approximately 2 mm x 4 mm. The front lens diameter measures 4 mm x 3 mm[22] (Fig. 2A-d).

The telescope is connected to the 100-mm attachment lens on the SLR camera (Fig. 3B) and its fiber-optic light cable to a xenon light source.

Light transmission of the Nagashima laryngoscope was excellent and provided brighter definition of the image than other endoscopes we tried. The reasons for this appeared to be the wide diameter of the telescope, the newer optical lens system it employed, integration of the light cable into the telescope without a connecting joint and a higher number of fibers in the light-transmission system. The laryngoscope requires no additional light cable nor a special photographic sheath.[20] The Nagashima telescope has been found to be very effective for video-recording of laryngeal disorders.[20]

CAMERA

Olympus OM2 SLR camera with a 1-9 focusing screen and autowinder was used (Fig. 3B). For the Nagashima telescope, a Nagashima 100-mm attachment lens was used (Fig. 3B-b). This produced a photographic image 13 mm in diameter on the finished slide. Since the image was rather small for viewing, a 2X teleconverter (Fig. 3B-c) was placed between the 100-mm attachment lens and the camera body to produce a finished image size of 28 mm in diameter. For the Hopkins and Stuckrad telescopes, a 100-mm Zuiko lens and the quick-connect camera adapter (Fig. 3B-a) were used. Ektachrome ASA 400 color film was chosen after trying many different films.

LIGHT SOURCES

Xenon Cold Light Fountain (487C, Karl Storz). This xenon illuminator (Fig. 4), which produces approximately 6000 K ("instant sunlight"), 300 W, was used for all four telescopes with special adapters.

Dual Mode Flash and Examining Light System (maximum output 100 W-seconds with three-power steps 110/240 V AC; Karl Storz, KSFG). This light source was used for Hopkins telescopes only because the Y-shaped light cable for the dual flash and examining light system was not available for Nagashima and Stuckrad telescopes with integrated light cables.

Fiber Light Flash Generator (proximal type, 5005, R. Wolf, WFG). This fiber light projector

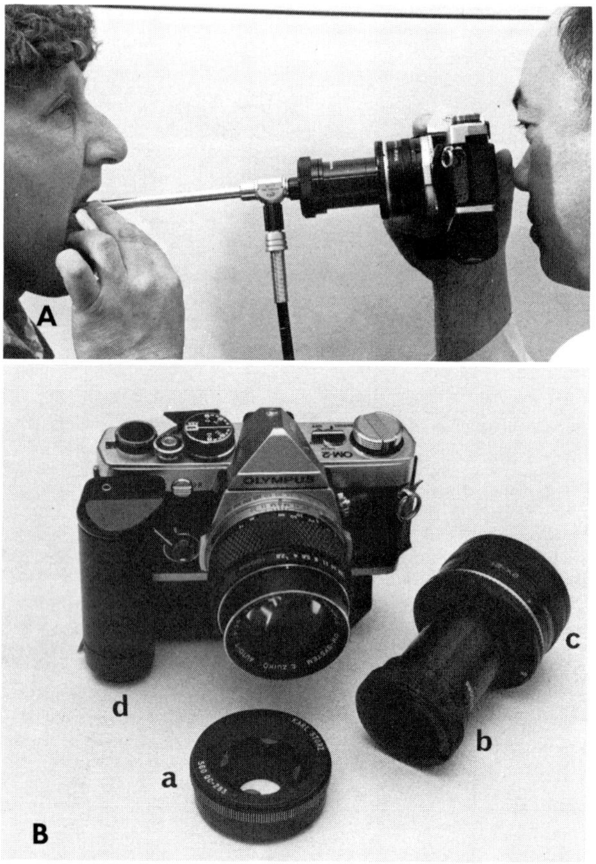

Fig. 3. Still telescopic photography. A) Nagashima telescope is connected to attachment lens for SLR camera. Examiner holds camera in one hand and inserts scope into mouth while holding patient's tongue with other hand. Larynx is centered on camera screen and picture is taken. B) Olympus OM2 SLR camera with autowinder, 1-9 focusing screen (not shown) and 100-mm Zuiko lens. a - Karl Storz quick-connect camera adapter, b - Nagashima 100-mm attachment lens, c - Vivitar 2X teleconverter, d - Autowinder.

and photographic light source combined in one unit was used for all four telescopes. The system of transmitting the light for observation as well as the electronic flash through the one cable makes it possible to take photographs with the small telescopes as well. The second light outlet permits simultaneous lighting of another instrument. Both diagnostic lights have a variable intensity control. The proximal flash has a 3-stage intensity control for photographic applications.

METHOD

The Olympus OM2 camera equipped with a 1-9 focusing screen, 100-mm Zuiko lens, automatic winder and Ektachrome ASA 400 color film is set at automatic mode with the aperture wide open (f 2.8) and the lens distance at infinity.

The patient and examiner sit facing each other. The soft palate and the posterior half of the tongue are topically anesthetized with 2% tetracaine hydrochloride (Pontocaine) solution. The telescope is connected to the camera via the adapter (the quick-connect adapter for KS 8702D, KS 8704D and Stuckrad telescopes and the Nagashima 100-mm attachment lens for the Nagashima telescope).

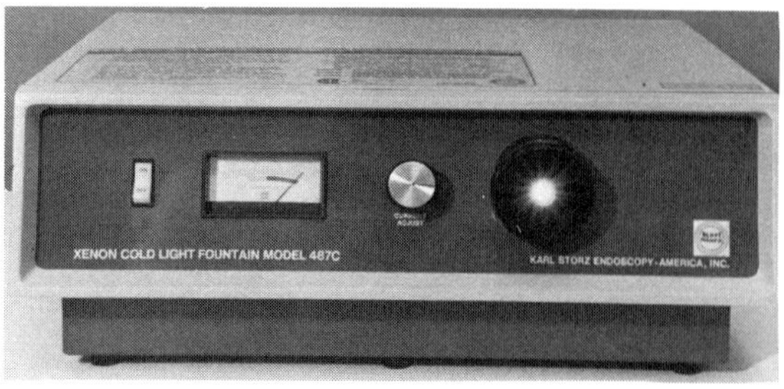

Fig. 4. Xenon cold light fountain (Karl Storz 487C).

The fiberoptic light cable of the telescope is connected to the xenon illuminator. The tip of the telescope is dipped in warm water and dried to prevent fogging of the lens during the photography. The xenon illuminator is turned on and set in the high filming mode (22A).

The examiner holds the camera in one hand and inserts the telescope into the mouth while holding the patient's tongue with the other hand. When the laryngeal image is viewed and centered on the focusing screen, a series of photographs of the larynx both on phonation and at rest are taken in rapid succession using the autowinder of the camera.

To find out if there are any differences between those pictures taken with the xenon light source and those taken with the electronic flash, laryngeal pictures were also taken using 1) the Karl Storz dual mode flash generator 558, and 2) the Wolf fiber light flash generator.

RESULTS

More than 1000 laryngeal photographs were taken using four different telescopes and three different light sources. Representative pictures of various laryngeal conditions taken with different methods are shown in Figure 5. Ektachrome ASA 400 color film was used for all the pictures shown.

The Berci-Ward Hopkins 8702D laryngoscope (Karl Storz) was very easy to use. The image was in focus from 4.5 cm to infinity. With the xenon illuminator at 22A, pictures were in focus in most cases. The final picture was 2.6 mm in diameter and ready for projection. Approximately 80% of the pictures taken were of satisfactory quality.

The Karl Storz Hopkins 8704D laryngoscope was difficult to focus during photography and required a great deal of cooperation on the part of the patients and skill on the part of the examiner. Since the operator had to hold the camera with one hand and manipulate the focusing knob of the telescope with the other hand, it was necessary for the patient to hold the tongue him- or herself. However, when adequately taken, picture quality was excellent and the enlarged view of the larynx filled the entire frame of the slide. Satisfactory results were obtained in approximately 40% of pictures taken.

The Stuckrad laryngoscope (Wolf) was also difficult to focus and required skill and practice on the part of the examiner and cooperation on the part of the patient. It was possible to change the magnification during examination and a detailed excellent view of the larynx could be obtained. The picture filled the entire frame of the slide. Satisfactory

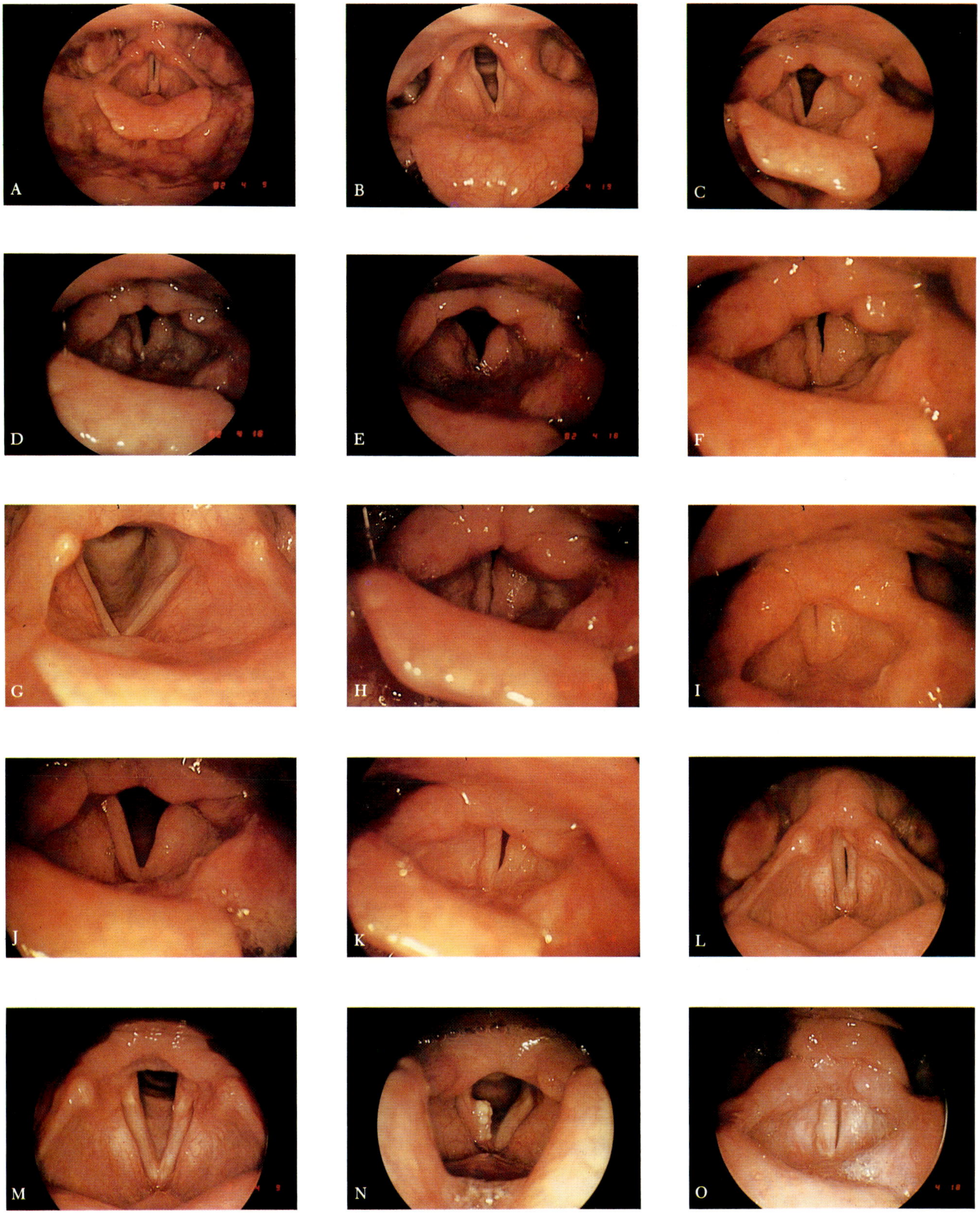

Fig. 5. Photographs of various laryngeal conditions taken with four different telescopes and three different light sources. A) Normal larynx on phonation (KS 8702D, Xenon f 2.8). B) Normal larynx on respiration (KS 8702D, Xenon f 2.8). C) Cancer of larynx after radiotherapy (KS 8702D, Xenon f 2.8). D) Cancer of larynx after radiotherapy (KS 8702D, KSFG f 2.8). E) Cancer of larynx after radiotherapy (KS 8702D, WFG f 2.8). F) Cancer of larynx after radiotherapy (KS 8704D, Xenon f 2.8). G) Normal larynx at rest (KS 8704D, KSFG f 2.8). H) Cancer of larynx after radiotherapy (KS 8704D, WFG f 2.8). I) Cancer of larynx after radiotherapy on phonation (Stuckrad, Xenon f 2.8). J) Cancer of larynx after radiotherapy on respiration (Stuckrad, Xenon f 2.8). K) Cancer of larynx after radiotherapy (Stuckrad, WFG f 2.8). L) Normal larynx on phonation (Nagashima, Xenon). M) Normal larynx on respiration (Nagashima, Xenon). N) Cancer of larynx (Nagashima, Xenon). O) Cancer of larynx after radiotherapy (Nagashima, WFG).

results were obtained in approximately 40% of the pictures taken.

The Nagashima SFT-1 laryngoscope was the easiest laryngoscope to manipulate because of its fixed focus. The size of the picture on a final slide when the 2X teleconverter was used was 28 mm in diameter. To visualize the anterior commissure, the tip of the laryngoscope had to be inserted deeply and tilted toward the examiner. Satisfactory results were obtained in approximately 80% of pictures taken.

When the flash generator — either Karl Storz or Wolf — was used, sharpness and color quality somewhat improved. However, recycling time was slow (4-5 seconds) and it took a much longer time to photograph the larynx. Repeated reinsertion of the telescope was necessary to take an adequate number of pictures. Use of the flash generator did not significantly change the success rate of each method.

CONCLUSIONS

1. The Berci-Ward 8702D telescope (Karl Storz) was the most satisfactory of those telescopes tested by the author when used with the xenon illuminator and Ektachrome ASA 400 film. It is recommended for general still photography of the larynx in the office.
2. The Nagashima SFT-1 telescope was the easiest to use and gave very satisfactory results. It is recommended for still and video photography of the larynx because of its excellent light transmission.
3. The Karl Storz 8704D telescope and the Stuckrad were difficult to use for photography, but were very useful for obtaining detailed enlarged views of the larynx. They are recommended for those otolaryngologists who are photographically oriented.
4. Use of the Olympus OM2 camera with a 1-9 focusing screen and automatic winder and xenon illuminator will make office telescopic photography of the larynx less complicated and more effective and pleasant.

REFERENCES

1. French TR. On photographing the larynx. Trans Am Laryngol Assn 1882; 4:32-5.
2. French TR. On a perfected method of photographing the larynx. NY Med J 1884; 4:655-6.
3. Padovan IF, Christman NT, Hamilton LH, Darling RJ. Indirect microlaryngoscopy. Laryngoscope 1973; 83:2035-41.
4. Holinger PA. Photography of the larynx, trachea, bronchi and esophagus. Trans Am Acad Ophthalmol Otolaryngol 1942; 46: 153-6.
5. Ferguson GB, Crowder WJ. A simple method of laryngeal and other cavity photography. Arch Otolaryngol 1970; 92:201-3.
6. Rosnagle R, Smith HW. Hand-held fundus camera for endoscopic photography. Trans Am Acad Ophthalmol Otolaryngol 1972; 76:1024-5.
7. Holinger PA, Brubaker JD, Brubaker JE. Open tube, proximal illumination mirror and direct laryngeal photography. Can J Otolaryngol 1975; 4:781-5.
8. Kleinsasser O. Microlaryngoscopy and endolaryngeal microsurgery. Philadelphia: WB Saunders Co, 1968.
9. Tardy ME, Tenta LT. Laryngeal photography and television. Otolaryngol Clin North Am 1970; 3:483-92.
10. Jako GJ, Strong S. Laryngeal photography. Arch Otolaryngol 1972; 96:268-71.
11. Alberti PW. Still photography of the larynx — an overview. Can J Otolaryngol 1975; 4:759-65.
12. Olofsson J, Ohlsson T. Techniques in microlaryngoscopic photography. Can J Otolaryngol 1975; 4:770-80.
13. Strong MS. Laryngeal photography. Can J Otolaryngol 1975; 4:766-9.
14. Hirano M. Phonosurgery, basic and clinical investigations. Otologia (Fukuoka) 1975; 21 Suppl 1:239-440.
15. Yanagisawa E, Eibling DE, Suzuki M. A simple method of laryngeal photography through the operating microscope. "Macrolens technique". Ann Otol Rhinol Laryngol 1980; 89: 547-50.
16. Gould WJ. The Gould laryngoscope. Trans Am Acad Ophthalmol Otolaryngol 1973; 77:139-41.
17. Ward PH, Berci G, Calcaterra TC. Advances in endoscopic examination of the respiratory system. Ann Otol Rhinol Laryngol 1974; 83:754-60.
18. Berci G, Calcaterra T, Ward PH. Advances in endoscopic techniques for examination of the larynx and nasopharynx. Can J Otolaryngol 1975; 4:786-92.
19. Hahn C, Kitzing P. Indirect endoscopic photography of the larynx — a comparison between two newly constructed laryngoscopes. J Audio V Media Med 1978; 1:121-30.
20. Yanagisawa E, Casuccio JR, Suzuki M. Video laryngoscopy using a rigid telescope and video home system (VHS) color camera. Ann Otol Rhinol Laryngol 1981; 90:346-50.
21. Saito S, Isogai Y, Fukuda H, et al. A newly developed curved laryngoscope. J Jpn Bronchoesophagol Soc 1981; 32:328-31.
22. Sawashima M, Hirose H. New laryngoscopic technique by use of fiber optics. J Acoust Soc Am 1968; 43:168-9.
23. Brewer DW, McCall G. Visible laryngeal changes during voice study. Ann Otol Rhinol Laryngol 1974; 83:423-7.

Ann Otol Rhinol Laryngol 91:1982

LARYNGEAL SARCOIDOSIS
REPORT OF 13 PATIENTS

H. BRYAN NEEL III, MD, PHD THOMAS J. MCDONALD, MD
ROCHESTER, MINNESOTA

Of 220 patients with sarcoidosis of the head and neck region, representing 9% of 2,319 patients with sarcoidosis seen at the Mayo Clinic from 1950 through 1981, we identified 13 who had laryngeal sarcoidosis. Edematous, pale, diffuse enlargement of the supraglottic structures was the most common laryngeal manifestation. The diagnosis is made by a group of clinical, radiologic, and laboratory findings, confirmed by the finding of noncaseating granuloma on biopsy. Sarcoidosis is a disease with frequent remissions and exacerbations and generally burns itself out; glucocorticoids may be indicated in particularly severe disease. When laryngeal sarcoidosis is suspected, the laryngologist should collaborate with other clinicians in a thorough evaluation of the patient.

Sarcoidosis is a chronic idiopathic granulomatous disease which may involve one or more of any number of organs, including those in the head and neck region.[1-6] Symptoms are generally mild in spite of extensive tissue involvement. The disease tends to progress slowly and is characterized by many relapses and remissions; ultimately, after years, the disease "burns out."

Epidemiologic studies have given no clues about the cause or pathogenesis of the disease, but it appears to be a host response to an unknown stimulus, possibly an infectious agent; an autoimmune disease or one of abnormal immunoregulation; or a response to chemical factors, such as zirconium and beryllium.[5,7] Many patients are not able to develop and maintain delayed-type hypersensitivity, have reduced lymphocyte blastogenesis, possess circulating immune complexes, and have a variety of other immunologic perturbations. The immunologic perturbations may be prerequisites to the development of the disease, but they are more likely a secondary rather than a primary phenomenon. In short, cell-mediated immunity is diminished and humoral immunity is heightened.

Microscopically, the granulomas are composed principally of epithelioid cells; occasionally there are a few giant cells and varying numbers of lymphocytes and plasma cells. There is no necrosis, that is, no caseation. The microscopic morphology becomes more fibrous and more hyalinization is seen in the late stages of the disease. The diagnosis is established by the exclusion of a variety of other disorders. Special staining techniques are required to exclude the presence of tubercle bacilli and fungi, and tissue should be cultured to substantiate this. The diagnosis is finally established by the consolidation of information derived from a thorough history, a physical examination, various laboratory tests, and interpretation of microscopic and culture examinations of tissue.

MATERIALS AND METHODS

From 1950 through 1981, 2,319 patients with sarcoidosis were seen at the Mayo Clinic. In this group 220 patients (9%) had clinically apparent manifestations in a variety of sites in the head and neck region. The anatomic locations of disease in the head and neck (and the approximate incidence in percent) were as follows: eye/lacrimal glands (40%), skin (26%), nose (13%), central or peripheral nervous system (6%), larynx (6%), salivary glands (4%), neck nodes (4%), and middle ear (1%). Thirteen patients with laryngeal involvement were identified, and one of these patients was seen before 1950. Most of the patients were from the north central part of the United States. There were ten females and three males. Their ages ranged from 12 to 67 years, with a mean of 40 years and a median of 47 years. Detailed case reports of 6 of these 13 patients were published previously.[8]

FINDINGS

Symptoms and Signs. Some combination of hoarseness, dysphagia, and dyspnea was quite common (table). The symptoms were as follows: hoarseness (9 patients), dysphagia (7), dyspnea (7), stridor (1), weak voice (1), sensation of a lump in the throat (1), and mild pain in the throat (1). In one patient, no symptoms related to the head and neck were noted, and sarcoidosis in the larynx was an incidental finding at bronchoscopy.

Appearance and Location in the Larynx. Sarcoidosis was found only in the supraglottic larynx in 11 patients and only in the subglottic larynx in 2. The true vocal cords were normally mobile in all except one patient, who had unilateral vocal cord paralysis following thyroid surgery several years before the diagnosis of sarcoidosis of the larynx was made.

The appearance of the larynx was strikingly characteristic in all of the patients with supraglottic involvement. The supraglottic larynx was chronically edematous and pale pink, and there was diffuse en-

From the Department of Otorhinolaryngology, Mayo Clinic and Mayo Foundation, Rochester, Minnesota.
Presented at the meeting of the American Laryngological Association, Palm Beach, Florida, May 1-2, 1982.
REPRINTS — H. B. Neel III, MD, Mayo Clinic, Rochester, MN 55905.

SUMMARY OF FINDINGS IN PATIENTS WITH LARYNGEAL SARCOIDOSIS (N = 13)

Age	Sex	*Laryngeal Disease** *Symptoms*	*Site*	*Clinical or Microscopic Evidence of Disease in Other Sites*	*Sequential Treatment and Response*	*Years Observ.*
20	F	Hoarseness Dyspnea	Supraglottic	Migratory polyarthritis, relapsing fever, erythema nodosum	Tracheotomy for 3 yr; spontaneous remission and decannulation	1941-62
33	F	Hoarseness Dyspnea Dysphagia	Supraglottic	Recurring erythema nodosum; angioedema of hands, feet, and lips; edematous, granular posterior pharyngeal wall, biopsy positive; central nervous system; peripheral neuritis of upper extremity	Tracheotomy for 2 yr; spontaneous remission and decannulation. Tracheotomy, removal of polypoid tissue, irradiation; decannulation 5 yr later and normal larynx. Tracheotomy for 3 mo for polypoid swelling; spontaneous remission and decannulation	1921-45
43	F	Dyspnea Hoarseness Dysphagia	Supraglottic	None (transient Horner's syndrome of questionable significance)	Injection of hydrocortisone acetate into larynx, tracheotomy; normal 1 mo later and decannulation	1955-63
47	F	Dysphagia Dyspnea	Supraglottic	None	None	1958-60
50*	F	Dysphagia	Supraglottic	Skin rash of arms, biopsy positive; nasal crusting and obstruction; hilar nodes; extensive pulmonary fibrosis	Systemic ACTH; some improvement. Subsequently died from complications of pulmonary sarcoidosis (no autopsy)	1944-56
56	M	Dyspnea Stridor	Subglottic	None	Tracheotomy. Laryngofissure — excision of thickened subglottic tissue, skin grafting; excellent airway and decannulation. Died from cancer of kidney	1955-58
12	M	Hoarseness Nocturnal dyspnea	Supraglottic	Relapsing fever; malaise; nasal obstruction; arthritis; splenomegaly; right sudden (cochlear) hearing loss; facial skin rash, biopsy positive; pale edema of uvula, pharyngeal pillars, and posterior pharyngeal wall	No change in larynx. Prednisone given in 1975 and larynx cleared	1966-75
39	F	Hoarseness	Supraglottic	None	Oral prednisone intermittently; improvement. Injection of Kenalog into larynx 1981; further improvement	1980-81
19	M	Hoarseness Dysphagia	Supraglottic	None	Tracheotomy for more edema after biopsies. Hydrocortisone acetate (x1) and Depo-Medrol (x6) injected into larynx; no change	1974-77
67	F	Hoarseness Sensation of lump and mild pain in throat	Supraglottic	None	Depo-Medrol injected into larynx; no change	1961-66
54	F	Hoarseness	Subglottic	Cough, relapsing fever, hilar nodes, and lung parenchyma; mediastinoscopy positive	Prednisone; no effect on larynx	1974-82
47*	F	None	Supraglottic	Relapsing fever; bloody rhinorrhea and septal perforation, nasal biopsy positive; marked pale thickening of mucosa of trachea and throughout bronchi, biopsy positive	Prednisone; no change. Irradiation of toe and trachea; marked improvement	1963-73
38	F	Hoarseness Weak voice Dyspnea Dysphagia	Supraglottic	None (scalene node biopsy positive, but chest roentgenograms negative)	Tracheotomy. Hydrocortisone acetate injected into larynx; shrinkage and decannulation	1963-76

*All patients had laryngeal biopsies except the two indicated by asterisks.

largement of the supraglottic structures (figure). This appearance is pathognomonic of supraglottic laryngeal sarcoidosis. The rim of the epiglottis was full and rounded, and it had a turban-like thickening. There occasionally were either reddened or granular areas, and this was the characteristic appearance of the subglottic region in the patients with subglottic laryngeal sarcoidosis. It should be emphasized that the true cords appeared normal in all cases except one; and indeed, even in that patient, the upper edges of the true cords were normal, but there was reddened thickening of the anterior-inferior portions of the true vocal cords, reflecting more extensive subglottic disease. This did not impair vocal cord mobility but caused severe hoarseness.

We want to emphasize too that the edematous, pale, diffuse enlargement of the supraglottic structures was the most common laryngeal manifestation of sarcoidosis, and, in fact, is considered pathogno-

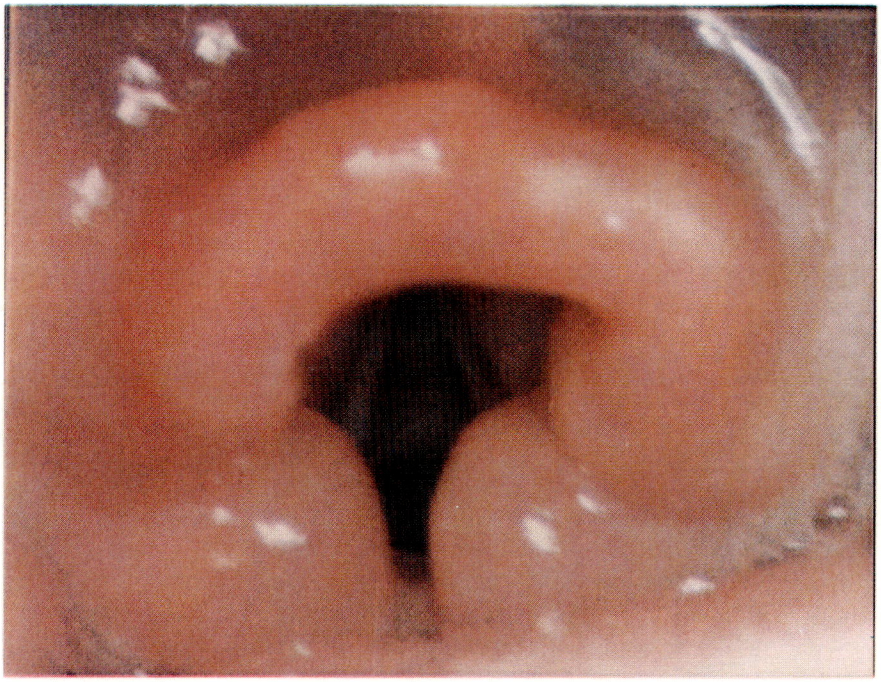

Typical appearance of laryngeal sarcoidosis. Supraglottic structures are edematous, pale pink, and diffusely enlarged, epiglottis is turban-like, and true cords are normal.

monic of sarcoidosis of the larynx (figure).

Biopsy. Biopsy of the larynx was carried out in 11 of the patients, and noncaseating granulomas were identified in all. Two patients who did not have laryngeal biopsies had the typical supraglottic appearance found in all of the patients with supraglottic sarcoidosis. One of these patients had a skin rash on the arms, and biopsy showed noncaseating granulomas. This patient also had nasal crusting and obstruction, the typical hilar nodes seen in sarcoidosis, and pulmonary fibrosis. The other patient had relapsing fever, bloody rhinorrhea, a septal perforation, a nasal biopsy that contained noncaseating granulomas, and marked, pale thickening of the mucosa of the trachea and bronchi, which also contained noncaseating granulomas. The diagnosis of systemic sarcoidosis was secure in both of these patients.

Several of the patients had biopsies of other organs, the results of which are described in the table.

Isolated Laryngeal Sarcoidosis. Of 6 patients with no obvious evidence of systemic sarcoidosis, 5 had the typical supraglottic appearance of sarcoidosis and biopsies that showed noncaseating granulomas; 1 patient had subglottic involvement and biopsies that revealed noncaseating granulomas. One other patient had no clinical evidence of systemic sarcoidosis, but a random scalene node biopsy showed noncaseating granulomas, although the chest roentgenograms were negative.

We feel comfortable with the diagnosis of isolated laryngeal sarcoidosis if the patient has had a careful history, thorough physical examination, laboratory tests, roentgenograms, biopsies of the larynx which show noncaseating granulomas in combination with the typical laryngeal appearance, and a long period of observation.

Laryngeal Sarcoidosis and Systemic Disease. In seven patients there were definite systemic manifestations as well as evidence of laryngeal sarcoidosis. These manifestations were skin involvement (5 patients), relapsing fever (4), migratory polyarthritis (2), pale edema and thickening of pharyngeal mucosa (2), granular nasal membranes and crusting (2), and central nervous system involvement (1). Three of these patients also had evidence of lung changes on roentgenograms, and two had obvious hilar nodes.

Duration of Observation. Six patients were observed for 9 to 24 years, three for 5 to 8 years, two for 3 to 4 years, and one for 1 to 2 years.

Sequential Treatment and Response. An outline of the sequence of treatment and response is shown in the table. Four patients had systemic cortisone; 4 patients had laryngeal injections of cortisone; 1 patient had both systemic and laryngeal cortisone; 1 patient had a laryngofissure, excision of the sarcoid tissue, and subglottic skin grafting; 1 patient had external radiation; and 2 patients had no treatment at all.

Tracheotomies for airway obstruction were necessary in six patients. Five patients had one tracheotomy, and one patient had three tracheotomies because of intermittent exacerbations of the laryngeal disease.

DISCUSSION

The diagnosis of sarcoidosis is made by assembling a constellation of clinical, radiologic, and laboratory findings (DeRemee RA, Zinsmeister AR, unpublished material).[5,7-10] The diagnosis is confirmed by the finding of noncaseating granulomas in biopsy material. Antigen of reliable consistency for Kveim testing is difficult to procure, and so this test is of more theoretic than practical importance.[5]

About 9% of our patients with sarcoidosis had fairly striking clinical manifestations in the head and neck region. Because the manifestations of the disease are so protean, patients initially seek consultation from a variety of specialists; however, a large proportion of the presenting manifestations can involve structures in the head and neck region. The generalist may see the patient because of dyspnea, lymphadenopathy, or rash; the neurologist, because of nerve palsy (eg, VII), encephalopathy, seizures, or meningitis; the ophthalmologist, because of red eye (uveitis), dry eye (lacrimal), or blurred vision; the dermatologist, because of erythema nodosum, rash, or lesions in scars; and the otorhinolaryngologist, because of hoarseness, dysphagia, or dyspnea. When the diagnosis of sarcoidosis is suspected, the laryngologist should collaborate with other clinicians to do a thorough physical examination as well as pulmonary, ocular, and dermatologic evaluations. Basic laboratory studies usually consist of serum calcium levels, protein electrophoresis, electrocardiogram, chest roentgenogram, pulmonary function tests, serum angiotensin-converting enzyme determination, and perhaps in some instances gallium scans. Levels of angiotensin-converting enzyme often parallel the clinical course, and increases often antedate exacerbations of the disease.[9] The diagnosis is confirmed by biopsies of one or more diseased organs, namely, skin, eyes, lymph nodes, lung, salivary glands, larynx, liver, or bone marrow, and by culture of the biopsy material to exclude the presence of tuberculosis or fungal infections.

When the laryngologist is confronted with a patient who has typical laryngeal appearance of sarcoidosis, he or she must rule out lymphoma and other malignant neoplasms, cartilaginous tumors, benign myomatous polypoid thickening of the larynx due to smoking, and specific infections such as tuberculosis, syphilis, histoplasmosis, coccidioidomycosis, blastomycosis, and actinomycosis, along with such entities as amyloidosis and lipoid proteinosis. Myxedema, previous irradiation to the neck, and a variety of systemic connective tissue diseases should also be excluded. In the very rare patient with subglottic sarcoidosis, the causes of nontraumatic nonneoplastic subglottic stenosis should be excluded, namely, relapsing polychondritis, amyloidosis, and Wegener's granulomatosis.[11]

Laryngeal sarcoidosis can occur as an isolated phenomenon. As stated by Devine,[8] "a careful history may reveal evidence that the disease is or has been systemic, has involved other organs in the past, may do so in the future, and often requires long-term follow-up to reveal its true, chronic relapsing systemic nature." Gallium-67 citrate scans may help define clinically inapparent granulomatous inflammation in other organs, such as the lacrimal and salivary glands.[12]

It is difficult to recommend any specific treatment. The indications for the use of systemic glucocorticoids are controversial, and their effects are difficult to assess because, by nature, sarcoidosis is a disease with frequent spontaneous remissions and exacerbations. In general, systemic glucocorticoids are recommended for the treatment of active ocular disease, persistent hypercalcemia and nephrocalcinosis, central nervous system disease, myocardial involvement, chronic skin lesions, progressive pulmonary disease, and certainly impending laryngeal obstruction (DeRemee RA, Zinsmeister AR, unpublished material).[5,7,10] In this series of patients, cortisone was injected into the larynx on one or more occasions in 4 patients and led to improvement of the appearance of the larynx in 2 and no change in 2 others. In one patient, subglottic skin grafting led to a favorable outcome and an excellent airway. A recent report described a successful outcome after supraglottic laryngectomy for supraglottic sarcoidosis in one patient, who has remained free of symptoms for 20 months after surgery.[13]

REFERENCES

1. Weisman RA, Canalis RF, Powell WJ. Laryngeal sarcoidosis with airway obstruction. Ann Otol Rhinol Laryngol 1980; 89:58-61.

2. Weiss JA. Sarcoidosis in otolaryngology: report of eleven cases. Evaluation of blind biopsy as a diagnostic aid. Laryngoscope 1960; 70:1351-98.

3. Carasso B. Sarcoidosis of the larynx causing airway obstruction. Chest 1974; 65:693-5.

4. Miglets AW, Viall JH, Kataria YP. Sarcoidosis of the head and neck. Laryngoscope 1977; 87:2038-48.

5. Hanno R, Callen JP. Sarcoidosis: a disorder with prominent cutaneous features and their interrelationship with systemic disease. Med Clin North Am Sept 1980; 64:847-66.

6. Trible WM. Sarcoidosis of the larynx. Arch Otolaryngol 1958; 68:382-3.

7. Mitchell DN, Scadding JG. Sarcoidosis. Am Rev Respir Dis 1974; 110:774-802.

8. Devine KD. Sarcoidosis and sarcoidosis of the larynx. Laryngoscope 1965; 75:533-69.

9. DeRemee RA, Rohrbach MS. Techniques in the evaluation of sarcoidosis. Semin Respir Med 1981; 3:54-6.

10. Bower JS, Belen JE, Weg JG, Dantzker DR. Manifestations and treatment of laryngeal sarcoidosis. Am Rev Respir Dis 1980; 122:325-32.

11. Djalilian M, McDonald TJ, Devine KD, Weiland LH. Nontraumatic, nonneoplastic subglottic stenosis. Ann Otol Rhinol Laryngol 1975; 84:757-63.

12. Lauver JW, Gooneratne NS. Lacrimal, parotid and mediastinal uptake of gallium 67 in sarcoidosis. Br J Radiol 1979; 52:582-4.

13. Haar JG, Chaudhry AP, Kaplan HM, Milley PS. Granulomatous laryngitis of unknown etiology. Laryngoscope 1980; 90: 1225-9.

Ann Otol Rhinol Laryngol 91:1982

LARYNGOTRACHEAL INVASION BY THYROID CARCINOMA

MICHAEL FRIEDMAN, MD
VICKI K. SHELTON, MD
EMANUEL M. SKOLNIK, MD
FREDERICK G. BERLINGER, MD
MOHAMMAD ARAB, MD
CHICAGO, ILLINOIS

Laryngotracheal invasion by well-differentiated thyroid carcinoma is an uncommon occurrence. Recommendations for therapy have primarily included total laryngectomy or shaving of the tumor from laryngeal or tracheal cartilages. Clear guidelines have not been established for the applicability of partial laryngeal resections. In a retrospective analysis of patients with thyroid carcinoma, 13 patients had airway invasion. Of the five patients with laryngeal involvement, three were treated by a partial laryngeal resection. An experimental study was undertaken to determine more precisely the amount of cricoid cartilage which could be resected without reconstruction. Varying amounts of cricoid cartilage were resected. The results indicate that 25% of the cricoid cartilage may be resected without appreciable airway narrowing. On the basis of the retrospective analysis and experimental study, we feel a partial laryngeal resection is possible in most cases of airway invasion by thyroid carcinoma.

INTRODUCTION

Laryngotracheal invasion by well-differentiated thyroid carcinoma is an uncommon occurrence. Reports in the literature vary from 1% to approximately 13%.[1-5] However, of those patients who eventually succumb to thyroid carcinoma, local recurrence is the most common postmortem finding.[6] Residual tumor involving either the laryngeal or tracheal cartilages results in a high incidence of local recurrence and potential for airway invasion.[7]

Surgical management of patients with thyroid cancer invading the airway has primarily been total laryngectomy. Clark et al,[8] in an analysis of 218 patients, noted that laryngectomy had been required in 5. He felt that if the larynx or trachea were invaded, these structures should be removed. Schindel[4] performed a total laryngectomy in 8 of 225 patients with thyroid carcinoma. Djalilian et al,[2] in a review of 2000 cases, found seven patients had undergone a total laryngectomy while two other patients underwent a partial laryngeal resection. Lawson et al,[9] on the other hand, reported on 6 patients with airway invasion, 5 of whom had local control of their disease with conservation surgery. It was his feeling that if the lesion was surgically amenable to a conservation procedure, this should be performed.

Although partial laryngeal resections for patients with thyroid carcinoma invading the larynx have been used successfully, clear guidelines have not been established. The indications for partial laryngectomy, both with intraluminal invasion as well as minimal cartilage destruction, have not been elucidated. Through a retrospective study of thyroid carcinoma treated at the University of Illinois and affiliated hospitals and an experimental animal study, an attempt is made to clarify the criteria for partial laryngeal resection.

RETROSPECTIVE STUDY

A total of 190 patients with thyroid carcinoma were treated at the University of Illinois and affiliated hospitals between 1950 and 1980. Thirteen patients with well-differentiated tumors had airway invasion, an incidence of 6.8%. Five of these patients had extension of the thyroid neoplasm into the larynx or subglottic space, while the remainder had varying degrees of tracheal invasion.

Surgical therapy used in treating these five patients included one total laryngectomy and three partial laryngectomies. One patient, whose lesion was thought to be amenable to a partial laryngeal resection, refused surgery. Patients with tracheal invasion were treated with various procedures (Table 1). One patient's tumor was deemed unresectable due to massive tracheal, mediastinal, and esophageal invasion and was treated with radiation therapy. Two patients required anterior resection of five and six tracheal rings. These tracheal defects were reconstructed with bilateral sternocleidomastoid flaps. A tracheostomy, performed at the lower margin of the reconstruction, was removed in less than two weeks in both patients. Neither patient developed notable tracheal stenosis over extended follow-up periods (16 and 18 years).

Of these 13 patients, 8 are alive with no evidence of disease; 5 have either died or are alive with disease present (Table 2). Although a 15-year follow-up period is not available for all 13 patients with

From the Departments of Otolaryngology-Head and Neck Surgery (Friedman, Shelton, Skolnik and Arab) and Medicine (Berlinger), University of Illinois College of Medicine and University of Illinois Hospital, and the Departments of Otolaryngology (Friedman) and Medicine (Berlinger), Illinois Masonic Medical Center, Chicago.

Presented at the meeting of the American Laryngological Association, Palm Beach, Florida, May 1-2, 1982.

REPRINTS — Michael Friedman, MD, Department of Otolaryngology-Head and Neck Surgery, 1855 W. Taylor St., Chicago, IL 60612.

TABLE 1. TREATMENT OF TRACHEAL INVASION

Treatment	*No. Patients*
Window resection	3
Resection with reconstruction	3
Tracheal resection, partial esophagectomy	1
Radiation*	1

*Massive tracheal, mediastinal, esophageal invasion.

airway invasion, it is apparent that the type of surgical procedure performed had a marked effect on the survival rate. In those patients where a wide excision of tumor was accomplished, survival was increased. Inadequate surgical resection in our series resulted in uncontrolled disease in 100% of patients.

CASE REPORTS

Case 1. A 63-year-old male had a 1.5 x 2-cm mass in the left lobe of the thyroid fixed to the larynx. Direct laryngoscopy and bronchoscopy showed no mucosal abnormality. He underwent left thyroid lobectomy and isthmusectomy, at which time the mass was found to be adherent to the cricoid. Tumor was shaved off the cricoid, leaving residual disease on the cartilage. The pathologic diagnosis was mixed papillary follicular carcinoma.

Two years postoperatively, the patient returned with a recurrent neck mass fixed to the larynx, again with no intraluminal signs or symptoms.

On radioactive iodine (^{131}I) scanning the tumor displayed no uptake. The surgical service treated the mass with external radiation, which resulted in moderate shrinkage of the tumor mass.

Six years postoperatively, the patient was again admitted with an increase in size of the neck mass. The patient also complained of hemoptysis but had no hoarseness. Several enlarged neck nodes were present, in addition to the mass adherent to the larynx. The surgical service performed a radical neck dissection and partial removal of the mass adherent to the cricoid.

Eight years after initial presentation, the patient returned with massive hemoptysis. His voice remained normal. Bronchoscopy revealed an intraluminal subglottic tumor, following which a total laryngectomy was performed.

He was subsequently evaluated by one of us (MF) for voice rehabilitation. Twelve years after initial presentation (four years after laryngectomy), he is free of disease.

COMMENT. The pathologic specimen (Fig. 1A) revealed, both grossly and microscopically, that approximately 25% of the anterolateral aspect of the cricoid cartilage was involved with tumor.

Case 2. A 60-year-old female had a thyroid nodule. She underwent a thyroid lobectomy and isthmusectomy at which time tumor was noted to be adherent to the cricoid and was not completely removed. On referral to another institution, she underwent a second neck exploration. Additional tumor was removed, but residual tumor remained adherent to the cricoid. Pathologic diagnosis was mixed papillary follicular carcinoma.

She was rehospitalized seven years after initial presentation with a large anterior neck mass and hoarseness. Partial removal of the tumor was again performed, and she subsequently was treated with ^{131}I.

One year later she returned with an extensive neck mass. The CT scan showed invasion of the cricoid and thyroid (Fig. 2A-C). The patient was then referred to one of us (MF). The patient underwent a partial subglottic resection, removing approximately 25% of the lateral aspect of the cricoid and thyroid cartilages. The recurrent laryngeal nerve was resected since it was involved with tumor.

TABLE 2. SURVIVAL STATUS FOR 13 PATIENTS

Interval Since Diagnosis	*NED*	*AWD*	*DOD*
<5 years			2
< 10 years	2	1	1
< 15 years	3		
> 15 years	3	1	

NED - No evidence of disease; AWD - Alive with disease; DOD - Dead of disease.

COMMENT. Reconstruction involved soft tissue closure of the defect. In view of the numerous previous surgical explorations and the postradiation treatment, reconstruction with cartilage, bone graft, or flap was not considered advisable.

Postoperatively, the patient was decannulated in ten days. She healed with minimal subglottic narrowing. She has a cord paralysis but an adequate airway. She is active without any shortness of breath, and she is currently free of disease two years after surgery.

Case 3. A 50-year-old female had a thyroid nodule, treated with a thyroid lobectomy and isthmusectomy. The diagnosis was a mixed papillary follicular carcinoma. Six years postoperatively, she presented with right cervical adenopathy, at which time she underwent a right radical neck dissection. Ten years postoperatively the patient presented with left cervical adenopathy, and underwent a left radical neck dissection. Twelve years after the first surgery, she had extensive recurrent neck disease and pulmonary metastasis. The recurrent neck disease was excised and she was treated with ^{131}I.

Subsequently, she had progressive enlargement of a neck mass adherent to the thyrohyoid membrane. Twenty years after initial presentation, she was admitted with airway obstruction and severe dysphagia. Examination revealed an extensive supraglottic mass obstructing the airway and requiring emergency tracheotomy. She underwent a supraglottic laryngectomy and partial pharyngectomy. Decannulation was accomplished seven days postoperatively. At present she eats normally and has a normal airway.

COMMENT. Although any treatment in a patient with pulmonary metastasis is palliative, this can be long-term. Removal of the local disease causing severe airway obstruction with a partial laryngectomy as opposed to a total laryngectomy is certainly optimum palliation.

EXPERIMENTAL STUDY

Review of the literature and analysis of our cases illustrate the need for several questions to be answered. In cases of minimal laryngeal involvement, how much can be removed without sacrificing function? In cases of more massive involvement, at what point of resection is some method of reconstruction essential?

An experimental model was designed to mimic possible areas of subglottic laryngeal involvement with thyroid carcinoma. Since other sites of laryngeal involvement fit into standard categories of partial laryngectomy, these were not studied.

Six mongrel dogs underwent preoperative soft tissue neck x-ray studies to establish the presence of a normal subglottic airway. The six dogs then had partial subglottic laryngectomies with varying amounts of resection. The amounts of resection ranged from a minimum of 25% cricoid resection (Fig. 3A,B) with preservation of the recurrent laryngeal nerve to a maximum resection of 50% of

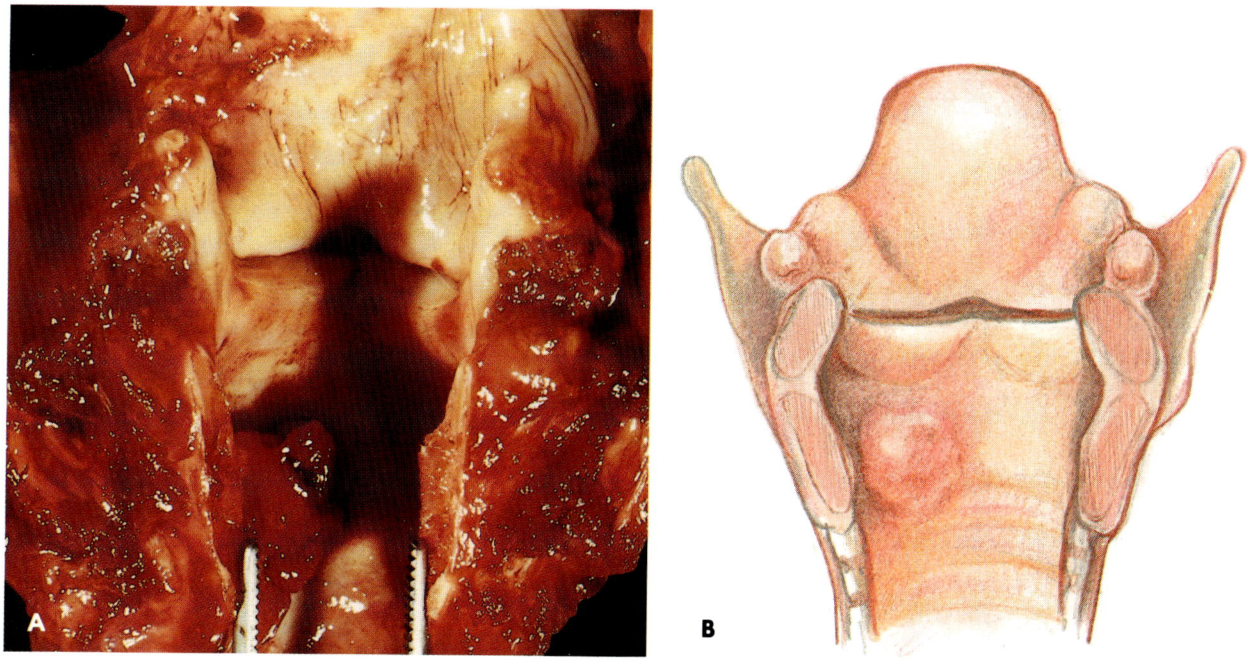

Fig. 1. (Case 1) A) Pathologic specimen showing intraluminal subglottic involvement by tumor. B) Sketch illustrating area of involvement found in pathologic specimen.

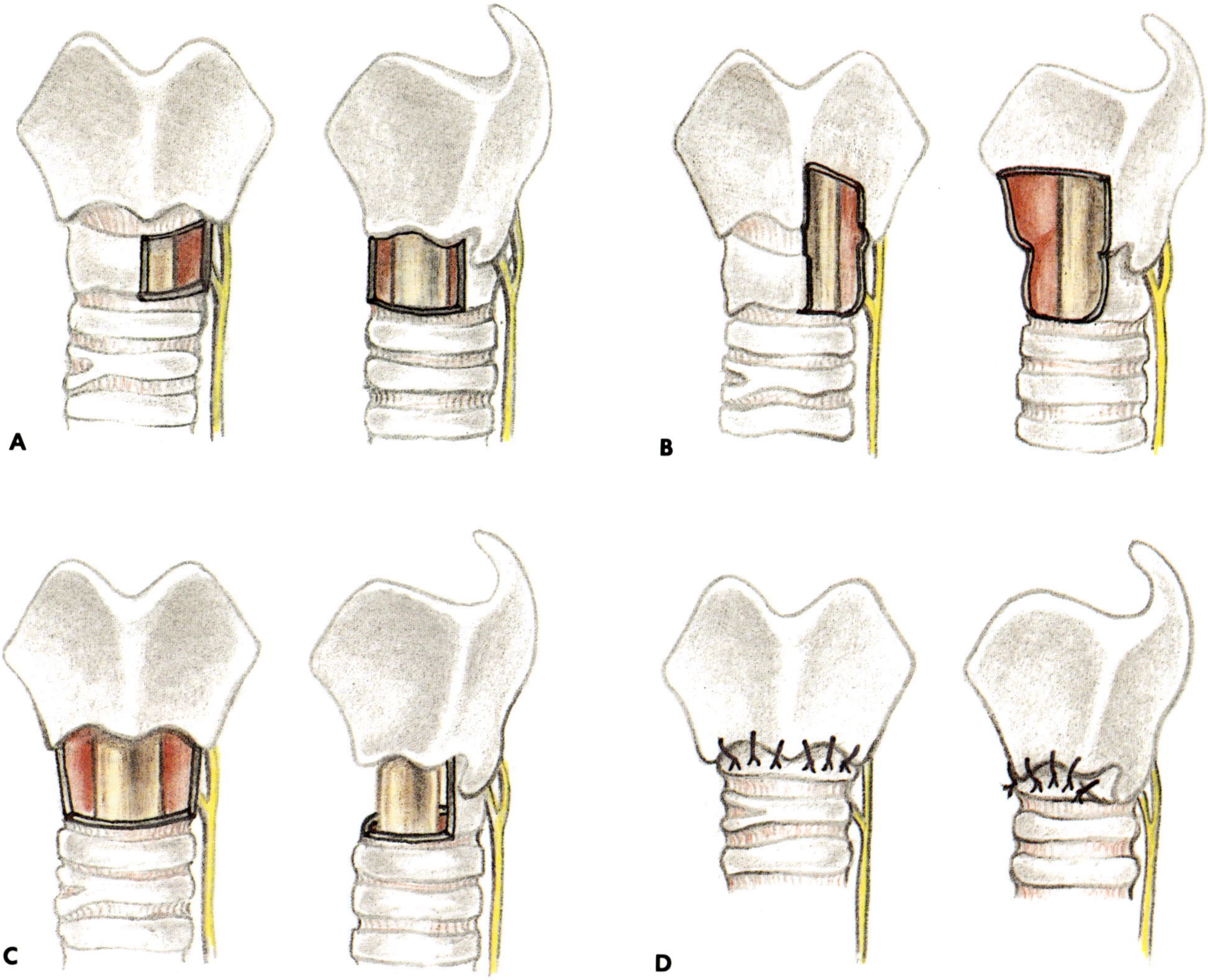

Fig. 3. Anterior and lateral views of reconstructions following partial subglottic laryngectomies. A) (Dog 1) Cricoid resection, 25%. B) (Dog 2) Cricoid and thyroid resection, 25%. C) (Dog 4) Cricoid resection, 50%. D) (Dog 6) Thyrotracheal anastomosis.

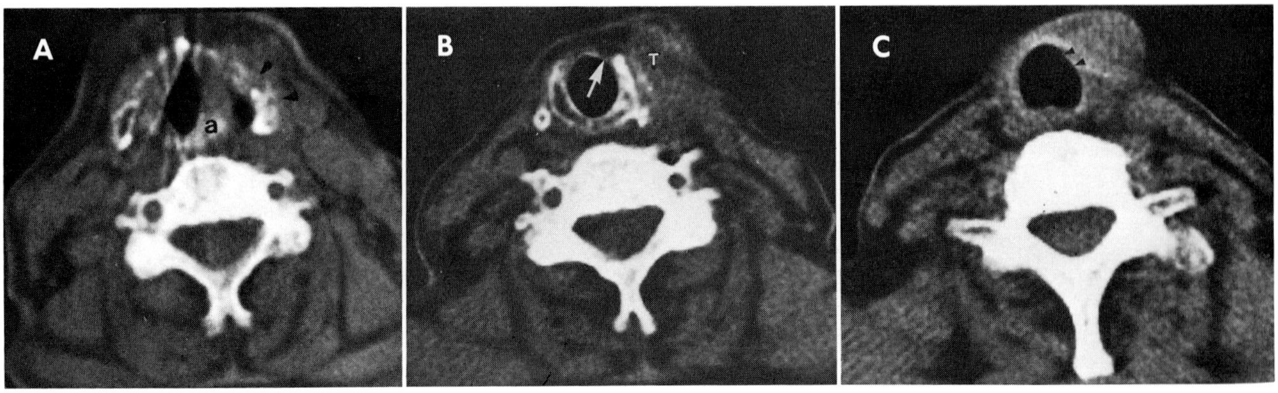

Fig. 2. (Case 2) A) Tumor eroding right thyroid cartilage (arrows) and extending onto aryepiglottic fold (a). B) Deformity of the cricoid cartilage (arrow) adjacent to the tumor (T). C) Subglottic airway invasion by the tumor (arrows).

the cricoid (Fig. 3C). Table 3 indicates the exact sites of resection.

Five of the six dogs had resections without reconstruction. Each of these dogs had closure of the subglottic defect with available soft tissue (strap muscles). None of the dogs had tracheotomies performed at the time of surgery. One of the dogs with 50% resection of cricoid and thyroid developed massive subcutaneous emphysema and bilateral pneumothoraces postoperatively. This dog died and was therefore not available for follow-up study. Because the dog had no stridor or evidence of upper airway collapse, the early death was thought to be due to a technical error in closure.

Dog 6 had a 50% resection of the anterior cricoid ring extending from the right cricothyroid joint to the left cricothyroid joint with identification and preservation of both recurrent laryngeal nerves. Primary thyrotracheal anastomosis was performed (Fig. 3D).

Dogs were evaluated at 2 weeks, 4 weeks and 8 weeks by soft tissue neck x-ray films and direct laryngoscopy and bronchoscopy. At the time of this writing, 8-week results were available. The dogs are being kept alive for long-term follow-up.

RESULTS

Five dogs were available for 2-month follow-up. None of the dogs had stridor at any time. Dog 1, which had a 25% resection of the cricoid, had a normal bark and normal endoscopic findings at two months. No narrowing, granulation tissue or scarring was detected. Soft tissue x-ray views (Fig. 4A,B) of the subglottic airway were unchanged compared to the preoperative x-ray views.

TABLE 3. PERCENTAGE AND SITE OF RESECTION OF CANINE LARYNGES

Dog	*Percentage Resection*	*Site*
1	25	Cricoid
2	25	Cricoid and thyroid
3	25	Cricoid and thyroid plus recurrent nerve transection
4	50	Cricoid
5*	50	Cricoid and thyroid
6	50	Cricoid†

*Dog 5 died in early postoperative course due to technical errors.
†With primary thyrotracheal anastomosis.

Dog 2, which had resection of 25% of the cricoid and 25% of adjacent thyroid cartilage, also had normal endoscopic and radiographic findings.

Dog 3 had an identical procedure to dog 2, except that the recurrent laryngeal nerve was resected as well. Postoperatively he had a breathy bark and vocal cord paralysis, with an adequate airway. Endoscopically, there was no subglottic narrowing.

Dog 4, with a 50% resection of cricoid, had a normal bark and no stridor. Endoscopy at two

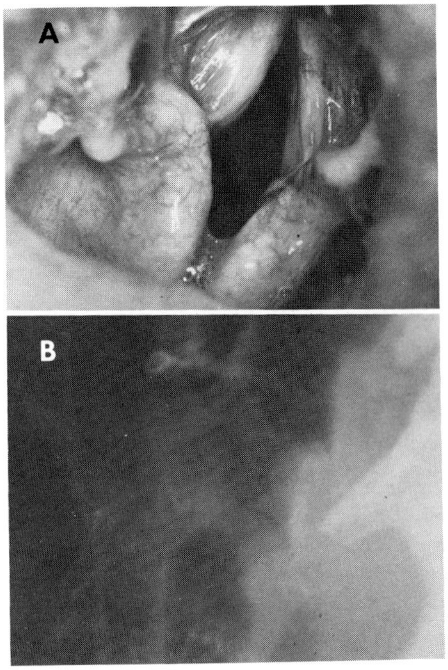

Fig. 4. (Dog 1) A) Postoperative endoscopic view showing normal subglottic larynx. B) Postoperative lateral neck x-ray film showing normal subglottic larynx.

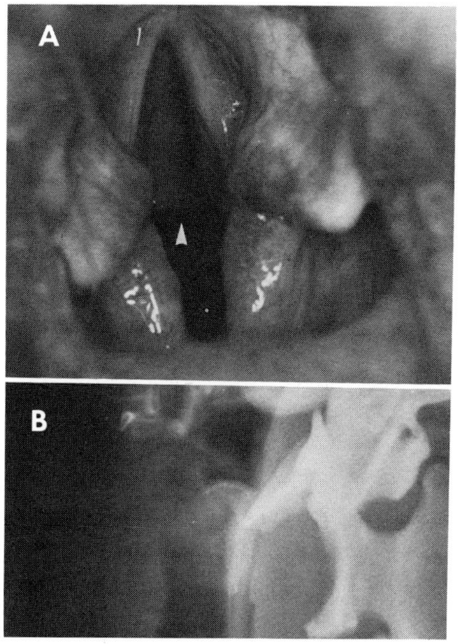

Fig. 5. (Dog 4) A) Postoperative endoscopic view showing enhanced subglottic narrowing (arrow). B) Postoperative lateral x-ray film confirming subglottic narrowing.

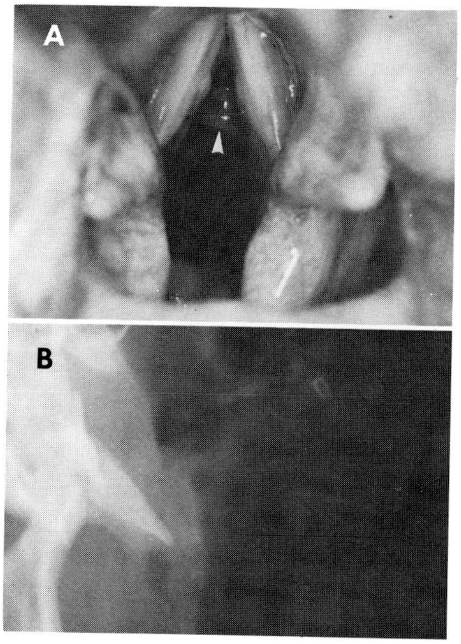

Fig. 6. (Dog 6) A) Postoperative endoscopic view showing mild moderate granulation tissue (arrow) without scar tissue formation. B) Postoperative lateral x-ray film showing no subglottic narrowing.

months, however, revealed subglottic narrowing and a marked amount of granulation tissue. X-ray examination confirmed the narrowed subglottis (Fig. 5A,B).

Dog 6, with the primary thyrotracheal anastomosis, had a mild amount of granulation tissue at two months. However, there was neither endoscopic nor radiographic evidence of narrowing (Fig. 6A,B).

Although none of the dogs developed stridor, we believe this is partially due to the large size of the canine larynx. Any evidence of narrowing present at two months in the experimental dog would be likely to suggest development of significant stenosis in the human. Procedures in which no narrowing could be detected at two months should result in an adequate postoperative airway. Long-term findings will be studied.

DISCUSSION

Patients with thyroid carcinoma invading the airway present difficult problems to the thyroid surgeon. The nature of the disease itself contributes considerably to the quandary of how to manage these patients. Unlike patients with squamous cell carcinoma of the head and neck, patients with invasive thyroid carcinoma can survive a long time with clinically evident disease, whether the disease is local or metastatic.

Treatment of thyroid carcinoma at the initial presentation remains controversial. Total thyroidectomy or total lobectomy and isthmusectomy for well-differentiated thyroid carcinoma have proponents. Universally accepted, however, are two basic principles of surgery for thyroid carcinoma. First, all gross tumor should be removed. Second, wide margins are not necessary and normal structures should not be sacrificed.

Adhering to these principles in cases of airway invasion by the thyroid carcinoma presents a surgical dilemma. Since the site of airway invasion in most cases is the subglottic space, no standard form of partial laryngectomy is applicable. Therefore, either tumor has been shaved off the laryngeal and tracheal cartilages in cases of marginal invasion, or total laryngectomy has been performed in cases of more extensive invasion.

The results of retrospective analysis as well as the experimental animal study indicate that less radical surgery may be performed in some cases of intraluminal invasion of thyroid carcinoma. Conversely, more extensive surgery may be necessary in patients with cartilage invasion, but no intraluminal involvement.

Although 3 of 5 patients with laryngeal invasion were treated with partial laryngectomy, retrospective analysis suggests that all 5 lesions were amenable to a partial laryngeal resection. Invasion into the subglottic airway did not necessarily dictate that a total laryngectomy need be performed. These patients may be managed with a subtotal subglottic resection. Animal studies and clinical findings indicate that up to 25% of the cricoid cartilage anterolaterally may be resected without appreciable airway compromise. More extensive resections of the cricoid cartilage would require reconstruction. Criteria for subglottic partial laryngectomy include adequate removal of disease, minimal functional change, and an acceptable risk of complications.

In those patients with cartilage involvement not extending intraluminally, a more extensive resection than shaving the cartilage is required. Removal of the involved cartilage should be performed. Resection of the cricoid cartilage can be treated as outlined. In cases of tracheal invasion, it is possible in many cases to resect portions of the tracheal rings without reconstruction. In those patients with minimal resections, closure of the defect with soft tissue is adequate.

Patients with extensive subglottic involvement may require resection of the entire anterior arch of the cricoid. In those patients, a primary thyrotracheal anastomosis is the preferable method of treatment. Gerwat and Bryce[10] and Pearson et al[11] have described the operative technique. Preservation of the cricothyroid joint stabilizes the larynx and protects the recurrent laryngeal nerves (if they are not involved with tumor).

Many techniques for reconstruction of tracheal and laryngeal cartilages have been used. These include the hyoid flap or graft,[12,13] rib graft,[14,15] and septal cartilage graft.[16,17] Circumferential tracheal resection has also been well described.[18-20] Primarily, these techniques have evolved from treatment of subglottic stenosis and traumatic airway injuries but are applicable in the treatment of airway invasion secondary to thyroid carcinoma.

Patients with thyroid carcinoma have unique limitations in reconstruction. Previous surgery, devascularized strap muscles and supporting structures and irradiation all tend to decrease the chance for successful graft or flap reconstruction. For these reasons, we strongly consider two alternatives. In minimal resections, reconstruction with soft tissue has been shown to be adequate. In extensive resections, primary anastomosis is the preferable method of treatment.

Our series reconfirms the importance of removal of gross disease. In those patients in whom an inadequate surgical resection was performed, 100% had uncontrollable disease and eventually died from their thyroid carcinoma. Residual disease predisposes the patient to local recurrence with airway invasion, possibly requiring extensive surgery.

CONCLUSIONS

On the basis of these observations we have reached the following conclusions.

1. Thyroid carcinoma invading the airway can usually be treated by partial laryngeal or tracheal resection.
2. Total laryngectomy may be required in cases of massive involvement.
3. Up to 25% of the cricoid cartilage may be resected without reconstruction.
4. Resection of a portion of the thyroid cartilage does not seem to alter the subglottic airway.
5. Primary thyrotracheal anastomosis is useful for reconstruction of patients requiring resection of the entire anterior cricoid arch.
6. Partial laryngeal or tracheal resection should be considered even in cases with no intraluminal involvement when the cartilage is involved. Gross tumor should not be left behind.

ACKNOWLEDGMENT — Mary McEnery, RN, assisted in this study.

REFERENCES

1. Cody H, Shah J. Locally invasive, well-differentiated thyroid carcinoma: 22 years' experience at Memorial Sloan-Kettering Cancer Center. Am J Surg 1981; 142:480-3.

2. Djalilian M, Beahrs O, Devine K, Weiland L, DeSanto L. Intraluminal involvement of the larynx and trachea by thyroid cancer. Am J Surg 1974; 128:500-4.

3. Frazell E, Foote FW. Papillary cancer of the thyroid: a review of 25 years of experience. Cancer 1958; 11:895-921.

4. Schindel J. Surgery of malignant tumors of the thyroid gland: a review of 15 years' experience with 225 cases. Ann Otol Rhinol Laryngol 1971; 80:61-6.

5. Breaux E, Guillamondegui O. Treatment of locally invasive carcinoma of the thyroid: how radical? Am J Surg 1980; 140: 514-7.

6. Silverberg S, Hutter R, Foote F. Fatal carcinoma of the thyroid: histology, metastases, and causes of death. Cancer 1970; 25:792-802.

7. Friedman M, Skolnik E, Baim H, Becker S, Katz A, Mantravadi R. Thyroid carcinoma. Laryngoscope 1980; 90: 1991-2003.

8. Clark RL, Ibanez M, White E. What constitutes an adequate operation for carcinoma of the thyroid? Arch Surg 1966; 92:23-6.

9. Lawson W, Som ML, Biller HF. Papillary adenocarcinoma of the thyroid invading the upper air passages. Ann Otol Rhinol Laryngol 1977; 86:751-5.

10. Gerwat J, Bryce DP. The management of subglottic laryngeal stenosis by resection and direct anastomosis. Laryngoscope 1974; 84:940-57.

11. Pearson FG, Cooper JD, Nelems JM, VanNostrand AWP. Primary tracheal anastomosis after resection of the cricoid cartilage with preservation of recurrent laryngeal nerves. J Thorac Cardiovasc Surg 1975; 70:806-16.

12. Alonso W, Druck N, Griffith C, Sumner H, Ogura J. Cricoid arch replacement in dogs: further studies. Arch Otolaryngol 1975; 101:42-5.

13. Alonso W, Druck N, Ogura J. Clinical experiences in hyoid arch transposition. Laryngoscope 1976; 86:617-24.

14. Cotton R. Management of subglottic stenosis in infancy and childhood. Ann Otol Rhinol Laryngol 1978; 87:649-57.

15. Cotton R, Evans J. Laryngotracheal reconstruction in children. Ann Otol Rhinol Laryngol 1981; 90:516-20.

16. Toohill R. Autogenous graft reconstruction of the larynx and upper trachea. Otolaryngol Clin North Am 1979; 12:909-17.

17. Toohill R. Panel discussion: the management of advanced laryngotracheal stenosis: composite nasal septal graft in the management of advanced laryngotracheal stenosis. Laryngoscope 1981; 91:233-7.

18. Grillo H. Tracheal reconstruction: indications and techniques. Arch Otolaryngol 1972; 96:31-9.

19. Dedo H, Fishman N. Laryngeal release and sleeve resection for tracheal stenosis. Ann Otol Rhinol Laryngol 1969; 78: 285-96.

20. Montgomery W. Suprahyoid release for tracheal anastomosis. Arch Otolaryngol 1974; 99:255-60.

NINCDS NOTES*

NATIONAL ADVISORY COUNCIL ADDS NEW MEMBERS

Three new members were recently appointed to the National Advisory Neurological and Communicative Disorders and Stroke Council. The appointees are Dr. Kenneth N. Stevens, C. J. LeBel professor of electrical engineering and computer science at the Massachusetts Institute of Technology; Jerome H. Stone, a manufacturing executive and president of the Alzheimer's Disease and Related Disorders Association (ADRDA) and Dr. John M. Tew, Jr., chairman of the Section on Neurosurgery and director of the graduate education program in neurological surgery at Good Samaritan and Christ Hospitals in Cincinnati. The new appointees will serve on the council until October 1985.

TEACHER INVESTIGATOR, RESEARCH CAREER DEVELOPMENT AWARDS ANNOUNCED

The deadlines for receiving applications for RCDAs (Research Career Development Awards) and TIDAs (Teacher Investigation Development Awards) are October 1, February 1 and June 1 of each year. Additional information on these training awards can be obtained from Dr. John W. Diggs, Deputy Director, Extramural Activities Program, NINCDS, NIH, Bethesda, MD 20205. Following the May 1982 meeting of the National Advisory Neurological and Communicative Disorders and Stroke Council, NINCDS made eleven new TIDA awards and three RCDA awards.

NEW PAMPHLET EXAMINES HEARING LOSS

Hearing loss, a disorder affecting an estimated 16 million Americans, is examined in a new NINCDS pamphlet, *Hearing Loss: Hope Through Research*. The publication addresses the causes, treatments, and prevention of hearing loss, and reviews the role of the NINCDS research programs in each of these areas. An illustrated explanation of the anatomical basis for different hearing disorders is provided, and current methods for detecting hearing impairment are discussed. The pamphlet also deals with the special communication problems of people who have hearing problems from birth. The pamphlet describes new hearing device technology and different language systems for aiding communication. In addition, it lists a number of voluntary health organizations concerned about the problems of the hearing-impaired. Single copies (Government Printing Office stock no. 017-049-00126-3) may be obtained from the Office of Scientific and Health Reports, NINCDS, Building 31, Room 8A16, 9000 Rockville Pike, Bethesda, MD 20205.

*This information is prepared monthly by the Office of Scientific and Health Reports, National Institute of Neurological and Communicative Disorders and Stroke, National Institutes of Health, Building 31, Room A816, Bethesda, MD 20205; (301) 496-5751.

AGE-RELATED CHANGES IN THE EPITHELIUM OF THE MONKEY LARYNX

M. P. STEARNS, FRCS
LONDON, ENGLAND

C. W. CUMMINGS, MD, FACS
SEATTLE, WASHINGTON

An experiment was designed to measure the area of subglottic squamous epithelium in a group of 14 adult monkeys. The animals were much older than any so far available for medical research. The larynges were strained using pyronin Y, which stains respiratory epithelium magenta and squamous epithelium pale pink. The areas of squamous epithelium inferior to the free margin of the vocal cord were measured. The results showed that the subglottic epithelium increased with age ($r = +0.61$, $p = <0.05$). This finding may have importance in the staging of laryngeal carcinoma.

INTRODUCTION

The first mention of the epithelium of the larynx in the scientific literature was by Galen[1] in the second century AD. In the late 19th century there was much controversy over the origins of the various types of epithelium in the larynx. This followed Tourneux's[2] writing that the free margin of the vocal cords was covered with stratified squamous epithelium and the adjacent areas with ciliated epithelium. The argument was whether the squamous epithelium was derived from physiological or pathological metaplasia. Kanthack[3] supported the physiological mechanism and Heymann[4] argued the case for pathological metaplasia.

A search of the literature fails to reveal the transition point from squamous to respiratory epithelium in the subglottic region. This area may have some importance in the staging and pathogenesis of laryngeal cancer as respiratory epithelium in the larynx has a rich lymphatic, whereas squamous epithelium does not. It is noteworthy that the UICC TNM[5] classification divides laryngeal carcinomas into supraglottic, glottic and subglottic, but does not specify where lies the division between the lower two regions. Stell et al[6] suggested that the division between glottis and subglottis should be the dividing line between squamous and respiratory epithelium. Kirchner and Som[7] suggested the upper border of the cricoid, and Ogura and Mallen,[8] a line 1 cm below the free edge of the cord.

A measure of the size of the squamous-lined subglottis and the area of transition therefore may be of importance. The purpose of this study was to try to establish whether the area of the squamous epithelium inferior to the free margin of the vocal cord was constant or whether it varied with age. The study was carried out on a group of rhesus monkeys.

MATERIALS AND METHOD

A group of 14 rhesus monkeys was used for the study. This was from one of the oldest primate colonies of experimental animals. Their age range was from 4 to 31 years (mean 15 years). The group included two 24-year-olds and three 31-year-olds. These latter animals might be expected to show some of the age changes seen in centenarian humans.

The larynges were removed, washed and subsequently fixed in 10% formol saline.

The epithelium of the larynges was stained using pyronin Y (Kodak). This dye stains ribonucleic acid.[9] After washing each larynx, it was suspended in a 4% aqueous solution of pyronin Y for one minute. The specimen was then washed to remove excess dye. Pyronin Y stains respiratory epithelium magenta and the squamous epithelium is left a pale pink color. This was confirmed histologically.

The specimens were split sagitally into two equal parts. They were then placed between two sheets of clear plastic (Perspex). The outline of the hemilarynx was then traced onto cellophane paper using a felt tip indelible marking pen. The areas of squamous and respiratory epithelium were recorded. These techniques have been fully described by Stell et al.[10]

The tracings of the larynges thus obtained were transferred to graph paper. This enabled the areas under study to be measured. These results were recorded and correlated with the animal's age.

RESULTS

It was found that the area of squamous epithelium inferior to the free margin of the vocal cord edge increased with age (table). Using the method of least squares, an r value for squamous epithelium in relation to age was obtained ($r = +0.61$, $p = <0.05$). No islands of squamous epithelium were seen in the respiratory epithelium-lined subglottic area.

CONCLUSIONS

The results show that in the group of animals studied, the area of squamous epithelium increases in size with advancing age. This appears to con-

From the ENT Department, Guy's Hospital, London, and the Department of Otolaryngology-Head and Neck Surgery, University of Washington, Seattle.
Presented at the meeting of the American Laryngological Association, Palm Beach, Florida, May 1-2, 1982.

AGE, SEX, AND SUBGLOTTIC SQUAMOUS EPITHELIALIZED AREA FOR EACH ANIMAL

Age (yr)	*Sex*	*Area of Subglottic Squamous Epithelium (sq mm)*
4	M	10
4	M	17
4	M	10
8	F	23
8	F	30
8	F	21
13	F	8
13	F	26
13	F	13
24	M	22
24	M	32
31	F	22
31	F	27
31	F	50

$n = 14$, $r = +0.61$, $p = <0.05$.

tinue even after skeletal growth has ceased. It is interesting to note that Pautow[11] in 1934 in a descriptive histological study stated that the laryngeal squamous epithelium increased with age, but did not support his statement with any data.

These animals were free of many of the factors that might be expected to contribute to pathological metaplasia such as tobacco smoke or air pollution, although local factors such as local and pulmonary infection could not be excluded. The results tend to support, therefore, Kanthack's[3] suggestion that a physiological metaplasia is involved. Hopp[12] in 1955 stated that occasional islands of squamous epithelium are seen in the subglottic region in the adult human larynx, but that these were rare and due to pathological change. We did not note any islands of squamous epithelium in our specimens. This may have been due to a lack of a pathological stimulus.

If one is able to draw any parallel with the human larynx, then the finding that the area of squamous epithelium beneath the free edge of the vocal cord increases in proportion to age may have importance in the staging of laryngeal tumors. These findings support Stell et al's[6] contention that for staging purposes the glottis should include the area of squamous epithelium below the vocal cords.

ACKNOWLEDGMENTS — I wish to thank Professor Josef Miller for his help with obtaining specimens and with the histology. I would also like to thank Dr. Roger Davies of Washington State University, Pullman, who made the specimens available.

REFERENCES

1. Galen. Opera omnia. Vol. 3. Kühn KG, ed. Leipzig: Cnobloch 1821-33. 1823:525, 551, 555, 586.

2. Tourneux MF. Sur le developpement de l'epithelium et des glands du larynx et de la trachee chez l'homme. Seances Soc Biol Paris 1885; 2:250-2.

3. Kanthack AA. Studien uber die Histologie der Larynxschleimhaut. Arch Pathol Anat Berlin 1889; 118:137-47, 273-94, 326-42.

4. Heymann R. Beitrag zur Kenntniss des Epithels und der Drüsen des menschliches Kehlkopfes im gesunden und kranken Zusande. Virchows Arch 1889; 118:320-48.

5. Union international contre le cancer. TNM classification of malignant tumours. Geneva, 1978.

6. Stell PM, Gregory I, Watt J. Morphometry of the epithelial lining of the human larynx. I. The glottis. Clin Otolaryngol 1980; 5:389-95.

7. Kirchner JA, Som ML. Clinical significance of a fixed vocal cord. Laryngoscope 1971; 81:1029-44.

8. Ogura JH, Mallen RW. Carcinoma of the larynx: diagnosis and treatment. Postgrad Med 1963; 34:493-8.

9. Brachet J. La localisation des acides pentasenucléiques dans les tissus animaux et les oeufs d'amphibiens en voie de développement. Arch Biol 1942; 53:207-57.

10. Stell PM, Gregory I, Watt J. Techniques for demonstrating the epithelial lining of the larynx. J Laryngol Otol 1972; 86: 589-94.

11. Pautow NA. Histologische Altersveranderungen an der Schleimhaut der Kehlkopfes. Z Hals Nasen Ohrenheilk. 1934; 37: 77-86.

12. Hoppe ES. The development of the epithelium of the larynx. Laryngoscope 1955; 65:475-99.

Ann Otol Rhinol Laryngol 91:1982

CLASSIFICATION AND APPROACH TO PATIENTS WITH FUNCTIONAL VOICE DISORDERS

JAMES A. KOUFMAN, MD P. DAVID BLALOCK, MA

WINSTON-SALEM, NORTH CAROLINA

Functional voice disorders result from vocal misuse or abuse; they are more easily recognized than other psychosomatic disorders because the clinician is able to visualize the laryngeal structure and function. If those structures appear normal, then an aberration of voice quality can be assumed to be functional. Functional dysphonia with prolonged aberrant vocal usage may lead to development of secondary pathological lesions of the larynx, which, although true pathological entities, must be recognized as resulting from the underlying and preceding functional disorder. In this report, we present a classification of and an approach to the diagnosis and treatment of functional voice disorders. On the basis of our clinical experience with 52 patients, we distinguished five types of functional voice disorders: type 1, hysterical aphonia/dysphonia; type 2, habituated hoarseness; type 3, falsetto voice; type 4, vocal abuse; and type 5, postoperative dysphonia. Forty-eight of the 52 patients (92%) were followed for a median period of 16 months (range 2-51 months). Therapy yielded excellent results in patients with types 1, 2 and 3; good results with types 4 and 5.

INTRODUCTION

A voice disorder is termed "functional" when it is primarily due to abuse or misuse of the anatomically and physiologically intact vocal apparatus. The underlying cause may be obscure or obvious, but prolonged abuse may result in the development of nodules, polyps, ulcers, or granulomas of the vocal cords.

The purpose of this paper is to present a classification and approach to treatment of functional voice disorders. The proposed system abandons the use of terms such as hypokinetic and hyperkinetic and focuses on the underlying mechanism and the clinical presentation. Although we present five clinically discrete groups (types), we have only limited data on some of the types and may not have identified other types or subtypes of voice disorders that can be termed truly functional.

MATERIAL AND METHODS

The medical records of 52 patients with a diagnosis of functional voice disorder were reviewed and yielded the data for this report. All patients were private patients seen by the senior author (JAK) from July 1978 through December 1981.

There were 39 female and 13 male patients (female to male ratio, 3:1). Their median age was 42 years (range: 6-76 years); seven patients were younger than 16 years. The median duration of symptoms before the patients were seen was 7 months (range 1-216 months); twelve patients (23%) had had a preceding bout of viral laryngitis.

To have been diagnosed as having a functional voice disorder, a patient had to have had a poor voice and a normal mirror laryngoscopy or had to have demonstrated patterns of vocal abuse with associated *secondary* pathological lesions. Patients with unilateral lesions or a lesion attributed to smoking, or with altered laryngeal physiology due to trauma or systemic illness (specifically, reflux esophagitis, thyroid disease, postinflammatory polyps, and spastic dysphonia) were specifically excluded from the study group. The voice problems were classified into one of five types by the senior author (Table 1). The criteria for each classification were as follows:

Type 1. Hysterical Aphonia/Dysphonia

1. Onset: sudden.
2. Indirect laryngoscopy: normal.
3. Often associated with a discrete precipitating event.
4. No history of prior laryngitis.
5. Associated symptoms: none.
6. Voice quality:
   a. Aphonia or whisper.
   b. Pitch-locked (if any voice present).
   c. Stable dysfunction (not intermittent or fluctuant).

Type 2. Habituated Hoarseness

1. Onset: persistence of hoarseness (for months or years) usually following an acute episode of laryngitis.
2. Indirect laryngoscopy; normal (except for occasional plica ventricularis).
3. Associated symptoms: none.
4. Not associated with a discrete precipitating event but frequently associated with "secondary gain."
5. Voice quality:
   a. Breathy, raspy, diplophonia, plica ventricularis (or a combination).
   b. Pitch-locked.
   c. Stable dysfunction (not intermittent or fluctuant).

Type 3. Falsetto

1. Onset: developmental or sudden.
2. Indirect laryngoscopy: normal.
3. Associated symptoms: none.
4. Voice quality:
   a. Abnormally high-pitched.
   b. Pitch-locked.
   c. Stable dysfunction (not intermittent or fluctuant).

Type 4. Voice Abuse

1. Onset: usually long-standing, intermittent or fluctuant dysphonia.

From the Section on Otolaryngology, Department of Surgery, Bowman Gray School of Medicine of Wake Forest University, Winston-Salem, North Carolina.

Presented at the meeting of the American Laryngological Association, Palm Beach, Florida, May 1-2, 1982.

REPRINTS — James A. Koufman, MD, Section on Otolaryngology, Bowman Gray School of Medicine, 300 S. Hawthorne Rd, Winston-Salem, NC 27103.

2. Vocal abuse resulting from:
   a. Overuse.
   b. Pitching the voice abnormally low.
   c. Abnormal muscular tension in the larynx and neck muscles.
   d. Any combination thereof.
3. Indirect laryngoscopy: normal or associated with "secondary" vocal nodules, polyps, ulcers, or granulomas.
4. Associated symptoms: throat pain coincident with the dysphonia (worse after voice strain).
5. Voice quality:
   a. Variable dysphonia.
   b. Hard glottal attack.
   c. Not pitch-locked.
   d. Intermittent and/or fluctuant dysfunction.

Type 5. Postoperative Dysphonia

1. Onset: severe dysphonia secondary to vocal abuse after operation.
2. Indirect laryngoscopy: normal or plica ventricularis, ulcers, or granulomas.
3. Associated symptoms: throat pain coincident with dysphonia (worse after voice strain).
4. Voice quality:
   a. Variable dysphonia.
   b. Hard glottal attack.
   c. Not pitch-locked.
   d. Frequent plica ventricularis.

All patients had undergone a complete otolaryngological examination and 40 patients had been evaluated by a speech pathologist. Eight of the patients underwent a neuropsychological evaluation which included an interview with a trained psychologist and a Minnesota Multiphasic Personality Inventory (MMPI). A neuropsychological evaluation was carried out in selected cases, both for research as well as for clinical purposes. (Such an evaluation may not be necessary for most patients with functional voice disorders; rather, referral to a psychologist or psychiatrist may suffice when referral is indicated.)

Treatment consisted of voice therapy alone in 67% of patients, voice therapy and operation in 17%, and voice therapy and psychiatric therapy in 6%. Five patients (10%) had been counseled but had received no formal therapy; it had not been recommended for 2 patients, and had been refused by 3 patients. The therapeutic procedures employed are discussed later.

Follow-up examinations of all 52 patients were carried out by the authors. "Late" follow-up (in March 1982) was also obtained by telephone interviews with 48 of the patients (92%). The results were judged by the authors as follows: *excellent* — voice normal without recurrent episodes of aphonia or dysphonia during the follow-up period; *good* — voice usually normal, but relapse occurred at least once during the follow-up period; *poor* — voice unimproved or improved but still poor.

Statistics. Due to the small sample size, medians and ranges rather than means were used. Statistical significance of the observed differences in the results of treatment in patients with type 1, 2, 4 and 5 disorders and type 4 subgroups was computed using the chi-square and ANOVA methods.

TABLE 1. CLASSIFICATION OF FUNCTIONAL VOICE DISORDERS

Type	*Disorder*	*% of Patients (n = 52)*
1	Hysterical aphonia/dysphonia	10
2	Habituated hoarseness	28
3	Falsetto voice	2
4	Vocal abuse*	52
5	Postoperative dysphonia*	8

*Only type 4 and 5 disorders are associated with pathological abnormalities of the larynx. Lesions were present in 60% of the type 4 patients (nodules — 13, polyps — 3, granulomas — 1) and lesions (nodules) were present in one type 5 patient (20%). These 18 cases represented 35% of the 52 patients.

RESULTS

Hysterical aphonia/dysphonia (Type 1). Four female patients and one male patient (10%) had exhibited hysterical conversion reactions. Each presented with a sudden loss of voice: two were aphonic and three whispered softly. In all, the vocal loss was stable and not fluctuant, and the dysphonia (if a voice was present) was "pitch-locked." The median duration of symptoms before presentation was two months (range: 0.5-17 months).

Complete voice restoration was accomplished with voice therapy during the initial visit in four patients, and after two therapy sessions in the fifth patient. Neuropsychiatric evaluation including MMPI was recommended to each of these patients, but only one patient agreed to be tested (a 45-year-old male with multiple somatic complaints and severe dysphonia; MMPI results showed elevated scales 1, 3, and 8 consistent with the diagnosis of hysteria).

The four female patients have remained asymptomatic with normal voices (median follow-up period: 16 months; range: 3-34 months). The male patient continues to have occasional relapses, and psychiatric therapy is in progress.

Habituated Hoarseness (Type 2). Thirteen female and two male patients (28%) were classified as having habituated hoarseness. The female to male ratio in this group was twice that of the overall group (6.5:1). The median age was 38.7 years (range: 14-76 years); the median duration of symptoms at presentation was 11 months (range: 2-24 months). In 12 of the 15 patients (80%), the dysphonia had begun with a bout of viral laryngitis. Three patients who denied having had laryngitis were included in this group because of the chronicity of their hoarseness and because, in all other respects, they resembled type 2 patients.

Indirect laryngoscopy had yielded normal findings in 10 patients; 3 patients had had false vocal cord voice and 2 had had mild Renke's edema.

Voice therapy and counseling were the only forms of therapy employed in this group. All 15 patients regained a completely normal voice, 12 (80%) doing so on the initial visit. Neuropsychological evaluation with counseling was suggested for three patients; however, only one patient was actually evaluated. Only 1 of the 15 patients has had recurrence of her hoarseness (median follow-up period: 16 months; range: 1-50 months).

Falsetto Voice (Type 3). Only one patient fell into this category, a 53-year-old female who had suddenly developed an abnormally high voice one year before we saw her. Her voice was restored with voice therapy, and she was referred for psychological evaluation and counseling because the neuro-

TABLE 2. TYPE 4 RESULTS OF TREATMENT ACCORDING TO SUBTYPE AND SEX

	Results		
	Excellent	*Good*	*Poor*
TFS			
M	3/7 (44%)	2/7 (28%)	2/7 (28%)
F	4/5 (80%)	1/5 (20%)	—
Nodules			
M	1/2 (50%)	—	1/2 (50%)
F	5/10 (50%)	3/10(30%)	2/10 (20%)
Polyps			
F	1/3 (33%)	2/3 (67%)	—
Granuloma			
M	1/1 (100%)	—	—

TFS - Tension-fatigue syndrome.

psychological evaluation had revealed a high psychosomatic score and possible impending psychological decompensation. Her voice is normal at 5-months follow-up.

Voice Abuse (Type 4). Of the 52 patients, 27 (52%) were classified as vocal abusers. The female to male ratio was 1.7:1. Sixteen (60%) had developed vocal nodules, polyps, or granulomas, and the remaining 11 (40%), who had had normal mirror laryngoscopic examinations, were classified as having musculoskeletal tension disorders, hereafter referred to as "tension fatigue syndrome." All nine of the patients in the entire study group who used their voices professionally were in this type 4 group. The median duration of symptoms for these 27 patients was 18 months (range: 2-216 months).

The results of treatment according to subclass and sex are shown in Table 2. Follow-up ranged from 1 to 38 months (median: 17 months). The best results were obtained in women with tension fatigue syndrome; the worst results in men with tension fatigue syndrome. However, the 5 patients with poor results had received no treatment (2 males with tension fatigue syndrome and 1 female with nodules had refused therapy, and no therapy was recommended for 2 children with nodules).

A chi-square test of the differences observed in results between male and female patients as well as between the subclasses revealed that none was statistically significant.

The nine patients in the entire series who were treated surgically all had type 4 disorders. All were women, three of whom had polyps and six of whom had nodules. The final results of operation were excellent in six patients (67%) and good in three patients (33%). (Of the 9 patients treated surgically by one of the authors, 3 developed transient postoperative plica ventricularis, which was responsive to voice therapy in every case).

The overall results for type 4 subjects were: excellent — 56%; good — 26%; and poor — 18%.

Postoperative Dysphonia (Type 5). Four patients had presented with severe dysphonia following operations at other institutions: bilateral vocal cord stripping in three patients, unilateral vocal cord stripping in one patient. One of the 4 had had severe dysphonia of the tension fatigue syndrome type; 1, a child, had developed recurrent nodules within six months of operation; and the other 2 patients employed a false vocal cord voice. The median duration of symptoms before presentation was three months (range: 1-6 months). Combining these four patients who had presented with type 5 disorders with the four type 4 patients who had developed type 5 disorders after operative treatment provided a group comprising 15% of the study population.

In this group, 5 of the 8 patients (63%) employed false vocal cord voices postoperatively. Late follow-up of those eight patients showed 50% with excellent results, 25% with good results, and 25% with poor results. The median follow-up period was 12 months (range: 6-28 months). These results are similar to the results observed in type 4 dysphonias.

Neuropsychological Evaluation. Four patients from group 4 and one patient each from the other groups had neuropsychological evaluations. The MMPI was interpreted as "psychosomatic" (classic conversion "V"; elevated 1, 3 scales) for 6 of the 8 patients, while two of the scores were normal. Evaluations suggested psychiatric disturbances in three patients (for which psychiatric referral was made); none of the patients were psychotic.

The neuropsychological evaluations were recommended for the few patients (15%) who were felt to be unresponsive to voice therapy due to psychological factors and for patients who seemed to display obvious psychopathological behavior. Further study is needed to clarify the contributing psychological factors in order to achieve a better understanding of the most effective therapeutic approach.

Comparative Results of Treatment: Types 1-5. The results of treatment for each type suggest that the overall prognosis in the functional voice disorders is dependent upon the presence or absence of pathological lesions of the larynx (Table 3). A statistical analysis of the differences in results of the individual types was not possible due to the small numbers in some of the groups. However, when the "non-lesion types" (types 1, 2, and 3) were grouped and compared with the grouped "lesion types" (types 4 and 5), the difference in the results of therapy was significant at a $p < .01$ level.

DISCUSSION

Arnold and Pinto,[1] Arnold[2,3] and Aronson[4] have contributed toward the classification of functional voice disorders; however, no unifying classification has been presented in the medical literature, despite the available data on many such disorders. Hysterical mutism, aphonia and dysphonia, for example,

TABLE 3. FUNCTIONAL VOICE DISORDERS: RESULTS BY TYPES (1-5)

Type	Results: Excellent (%)	Good (%)	Poor (%)
1	4/5 (80%)	1/5 (20%)	—
2	12/13 (92%)	1/13 (8%)	—
3	1/1 (100%)	—	—
4	15/27 (56%)	7/27 (26%)	5/27 (18%)
5	1/4 (25%)	1/4 (25%)	2/4 (50%)
	*4/8 (50%)	*2/8 (25%)	*2/8 (25%)

*Type 5 results including four type 4 patients who also had developed postoperative dysphonia.

are well-described[3-7] and are easily recognized, but are considered to be clinically discrete disorders. Polyps, nodules, contact ulcers, and granulomas, all well-known sequelae of vocal abuse, tend to be reported as separate entities rather than together as a single group.[8-10] Indeed, all the components of the classification presented here are well-known, but are seldom considered in the context of a common etiology.

Hysterical Aphonia/Dysphonia (Type 1). Carter[5] studied 100 cases of hysterical conversion reaction, excluding cases with diffuse or complicated symptoms, and noted that aphonia was, indeed, the most common conversion symptom (29%). In his series, 70% of patients were females, and while initial therapy successfully restored the voice in 100% of patients, follow-up of 27 patients 4 to 6 years later showed that only 68% had maintained a restored voice; 28% were improved; and 4% were unimproved. However, Carter concluded that "hysterical aphonia by itself is a symptom of only mild mental disassociation and has a very good prognosis."[5]

Habituated Hoarseness (Type 2). In Carter's series of patients with hysterical conversion reactions, many had aphonia following viral laryngitis.[5] Aronson has also suggested that "conversion aphonias and dysphonias are often triggered by cold or flu and associated laryngitis."[4] However, it is useful to separate the true hysterical conversion reaction from postviral chronic hoarseness: first, because more significant psychopathology may be associated with the true conversion reactions; second, because the long-term prognosis is probably better for the patient with postviral chronic hoarseness; and third, because the underlying cause is different for each group. In conversion reactions, the hysterical symptom (aphonia) is unconsciously selected and is usually of symbolic significance.[4-7] In postviral habituated hoarseness, on the other hand, the patient has simply made a chronic adaptation to an acute dysfunction, usually with some secondary gain.

Falsetto Voice (Type 3). Falsetto voice is uncommon, but is easily recognized. The larynx appears normal but the voice is disproportionately and inappropriately high-pitched. Correction is almost uniformly achieved by suggestion and reassurance.

It is likely that patients with falsetto voice can be divided into two subcategories. The first includes adolescents with preadolescent voices (mutational falsetto), and the second includes adults with acute onset falsetto (probably representing hysterical conversion reactions).

Vocal Abuse (Type 4). Unlike the first three types discussed which are associated with vocal misuse, this type is associated with functional abuse. Type 4 patients are prone to developing vocal nodules, polyps, ulcers, granulomas and lesions unassociated with the other functional types.

Other vocal abusers experience intermittent tension, fatigue, hoarseness and throat pain (the tension fatigue syndrome) without producing histopathological changes in the larynx. Patients in this group seem to be exclusively adult and are predominantly male. They are frequently ambitious, aggressive, hard-driving persons, and some are overly masculine, employing a fundamental voice pitch that is excessively low.[4] Our data and that in the literature suggest that tension-fatigue syndrome is the only functional voice disorder other than screamer's nodules that is more common in male patients. While type 4 females may develop tension-fatigue syndrome, they seem more prone to developing nodules or polyps. Children who abuse their voices are most prone to develop nodules.

Postoperative Dysphonia (Type 5). Some patients who undergo an endolaryngeal operation return to the surgeon's office for follow-up with severe dysphonia. These patients demonstrate a violent glottal attack, which represents a vain attempt to produce a normal voice. Some may speak with a false vocal cord voice or may even have developed postoperative ulcers or granulomas of the vocal cords. (We do not consider false vocal cord voice a distinct disorder type, even though 8 of the 52 patients (15%) in this series presented with or developed false vocal cord voice. Five of the 8 patients had developed postoperative plica ventricularis and 3 had had postviral laryngitis. Arnold[1] suggested that false vocal cord voice was a secondary form of "laryngitis" resulting from a primary vocal disorder. The data from this study also suggest that false vocal cord voice may simply be a compensatory mechanism associated with painful speaking, and that habituation is common. False vocal cord voice may, therefore, represent a symptom only and not a disorder entity.)

Postoperative dysphonia seems to occur in patients who either are not adequately prepared preoperatively or are noncompliant with postoperative voice conservation measures. Thus we believe that the incidence of postoperative dysphonias may be reduced by preoperative vocal reeducation of certain surgical patients.

Approach to Patients with Functional Voice Disorders. In laryngology, when the voice is disproportionately poor compared to the laryngeal findings, a functional voice disorder should be suspected. Since prompt voice restoration is the best confirmation of the diagnosis, the clinician should proceed with therapy as soon as the diagnosis is made, and avoid labeling the patient as psychosomatic, even though that may be the case. Since most patients seem to accept the concept that dysfunction may be the result of stress, the clinician should suggest it. Such an explanation serves three purposes: First, the patient is reassured that many normal persons have functional problems; second, the clinician suggests that he or she is willing to help; and third, the clinician implies that the patient will have a role in the therapeutic process.

Prompt vocal restoration may be achieved through techniques that encourage the patient to use any other voice, eg, falsetto; the clinician then works with the patient to extend incrementally the phonatory signal until a normal voice is achieved (asking the patient to cough, to clear his or her throat, or to meow like a kitten are effective maneuvers). If the clinician is successful in reestablishing the patient's voice, he or she should still refer the patient to a speech pathologist, who can reinforce the initial success. When the clinician is unsuccessful, he or she must be careful not to risk alienating the patient by expressing displeasure in the patient's response.

The speech pathologist employs relaxation techniques such as deep abdominal breathing, and repeats those methods already tried by the otolaryngologist. Biofeedback is another useful tool in the treatment of functional voice disorders, and a Vocal-2 Visible Training System or Fundamental Frequency Indicator may be employed. In resistant cases, a portable audiometer can be used to produce white noise masking.

Type 4 patients vary widely in terms of age, occupation, duration of symptoms, and motivation. Voice therapy remains the cornerstone of treatment, but the proportion of noncompliant patients resistant to such therapy is notably higher in this group than in the others.

Voice therapy techniques for type 4 patients are similar to those used in type 1, type 2, and type 3 patients, with the exception that the primary focus is on reducing or eliminating vocal abuse. Techniques toward this end include charting vocal behavior on a daily basis and voice taping for playback purposes, which are important because they reinforce the patient's awareness of normal versus abusive vocal patterns. Relaxation exercises and efficient use of the breath stream are also emphasized.

Postoperative dysphonia (type 5) patients may represent a special variety of type 4 patients. Postoperative dysphonia patients tend to be hostile and are poorly motivated. They are inclined to blame the surgeon for the poor result if not preoperatively counseled, and they may be resistant to therapy.

Routine preoperative voice therapy may be indicated for every vocal abuse patient with a surgical lesion. The patient should be forewarned that a hard glottal attack or any vocal abuse in the postoperative period may result in severe dysphonia and possibly even lead to the development of new lesions.

Patient motivation is the key to a successful therapeutic outcome in the functional voice disorders, and some patients with functional voice disorders may actually prefer dysphonia to a normal voice. This preference is especially common in those who use their voices professionally. Some use a "character" voice; in others (the late Louis Armstrong, for example), vocal abuse had led to the development of a uniquely individual voice quality. Patient motivation should therefore be evaluated in each case before formulation of a treatment plan.

Neither our experience nor that reported in the medical literature suggests the need for routine psychiatric therapy in patients with functional voice disorders. Such referral should be made whenever failure of treatment is thought to be due to psychological factors, or whenever a significant psychopathological condition is suspected.

CONCLUSIONS

1. A functional voice disorder should be suspected whenever a patient's dysphonia seems out of proportion to the laryngeal findings.
2. Chronic (habituated) hoarseness resulting from an acute viral laryngitis may be a discrete functional syndrome with an excellent prognosis.
3. Hysterical aphonia, habituated hoarseness and falsetto voice are more easily treated than the vocal abuse and postoperative dysphonia syndromes.
4. Voice therapy is essential for patients with functional voice disorders and particularly preoperatively for vocal abusers with surgical lesions.

REFERENCES

1. Arnold GE, Pinto S. Ventricular dysphonia: new interpretation of an old observation. Laryngoscope 1960; 70:1608-27.

2. Arnold GE. Vocal nodules and polyps: laryngeal tissue reaction to habitual hyperkinetic dysphonia. J Speech Hear Dis 1962; 27:205-17.

3. Arnold GE. Disorders of laryngeal function. In: Paparella MM and Shumrick DA, eds. Otolaryngology. Vol 3. Philadelphia: W. B. Saunders Co, 1980:2470-88.

4. Aronson AE. Psychogenic voice disorders. In: Aronson, AE. Clinical voice disorders: an interdisciplinary approach. New York: Decker, 1980:127-54.

5. Carter AB. The prognosis of certain hysterical symptoms.

Br Med J 1949; 1:1076-9.

6. Heaver L. Psychiatric observations on the personality structure of patients with habitual dysphonia. Logos 1958; 1:21-6.

7. Ljungberg L. Hysteria: a clinical, prognostic and genetic study. Acta Psychiatr Neurol Scand 1957; Suppl 112.

8. Harma R, Sonninen A, Vartiainen E, Haveri P, Vaisanen A. Vocal polyps and nodules. Folia Phoniatr 1975; 27:19-25.

9. Fitz-Hugh GS, Smith DE, Chiong AT. Pathology of three hundred clinically benign lesions of the vocal cords. Laryngoscope 1958; 68:855-75.

10. Preacher GM. Vocal therapy for contact ulcers of the larynx. A follow-up of 70 patients. Laryngoscope 1961; 71:37-47.

≈

INTERSPECIALTY FACIAL SURGERY CONGRESS FOR AESTHETIC, CANCER AND RECONSTRUCTIVE SURGERY

The IFSCACRS will be held at the Waldorf-Astoria in New York, April 27-30, 1983. This Congress is sponsored by the International Oculoplastic Society. For more information contact Pierre Guibor, MD, IFSC Secretary, 630 Park Avenue, New York, NY 10021; (212) 734-1010.

≈

FOURTH WORLD CONGRESS ON BRONCHOESOPHAGOLOGY

The Fourth World Congress on Bronchoesophagology will take place at the Foresta Conference Center in Stockholm, Sweden, June 20-23, 1983. This Congress is arranged by the International Bronchoesophagological Society, Swedish Otolaryngological Society and Swedish Society for Pulmonary Diseases. During the meeting, the Congress will update the knowledge within bronchology and esophagology. Further information may be obtained by writing IBES Congress 1983, c/o RESO Congress Service S-105, 24 Stockholm, Sweden, or Dr. Stig Haglund, Secretary of the Congress, Dept. of Otolaryngology, Karolinska Sjukuset, S-104 01 Stockholm 60, Sweden.

Ann Otol Rhinol Laryngol 91:1982

PATHOGENESIS OF VOCAL CORD POLYPS

OSKAR KLEINSASSER, MD

MARBURG, WEST GERMANY

Polyps of the vocal cords are a separate entity occurring nowhere else in the larynx or in the human body. Gelatinous and telangiectatic, but mainly transitional types of polyps can be discriminated. Histological, histochemical and electron microscopic investigations on a series of polyps show that an alteration of the permeability of blood vessels may be of importance, allowing the extravasation of edema fluid, fibrin or erythrocytes. Following this, reactive processes develop with the formation of labyrinthine vascular spaces. This process is very similar to the organization of a thrombus. Since polyps occur mainly in people who use their voices very intensively, and develop at the site of maximum muscular and aerodynamic forces exerted during phonation, vocal cord polyps are considered a sequela of a phonotrauma.

Polyps of the vocal cords are by far the most common benign lesions of the larynx. Polyps are a separate entity which can be discriminated easily from other forms of so-called laryngeal nodules; for instance, the true singer's nodules occurring in women only, the screamer's nodules in children of both sexes, and the polypoid corditis or Reinke edema. True polyps arise only on the vocal cords and in no other part of the larynx. Neither can polyps or analogous or even similar lesions be found anywhere else in the human body.

In a series of 900 vocal cord polyps which were removed by endolaryngeal microsurgery at the Clinic of Otolaryngology and Head and Neck Surgery of the University of Marburg 76% of the patients were males and 24% females. Most of the patients were between 30 and 50 years of age — the men averaged 40, the women 38 years; none of the patients were younger than 20 years of age. Of all these patients, 80-90% were smokers. Many of them reported that they had used or abused their voices professionally or habitually. Ten percent of the polyps were multiple and bilateral; 5% were multiple and unilateral.

Microlaryngoscopically two extreme types can be recognized: one of these is the glassy translucent gelatinous form; the second is the telangiectatic polyp. In some early lesions of the telangiectatic type a blister or convolute of capillaries can be seen. In more advanced forms there appear grape- or even raspberry-like convolutes of blood vessels which become more and more pedunculated. But most common are transitional forms with a nucleus of tortuous vessels embedded in a gelatinous substance covered by squamous epithelium.

Polyps have been called products of inflammation, allergic or immunologic processes or the results of trauma. Since none of these theories appeared plausible, we performed histological and histochemical investigations on a series of 100 consecutive vocal cord polyps. In addition, with the assistance of Professors H. Frenzel and W. Hort (Institute of Pathology, University of Düsseldorf), ten additional polyps were examined by electron microscopy.[1]

In the polyps which appear gelatinous macroscopically and histologically the stroma is very loose and edematous (Fig. 1A). Between the sparse collagen fibers lie blood vessels which have mostly a narrow lumen and relatively thick walls. Often cell-free sinus-like spaces lined with endothelial cells develop; in other areas within the stroma lake-like areas filled with a slightly basophilic fluid appear (Fig. 2 A), condensating sometimes to plaques of an eosinophilic material (Fig. 2B).

Some of the telangiectatic polyps are tightly filled with a dense nearly homogenous eosinophilic material around irregularly arranged vascular spaces. Most common are mixed forms consisting of a vascular nucleus surrounded by loose fluid-rich tissue (Fig. 1C).

Going further into the details of this vascular nucleus we find the deposits of the eosinophilic materials primarily around the walls of the vascular spaces, arranged either in larger or multiple small plaques. These eosinophilic deposits sometimes appear to be penetrated or organized by newly developing vascular sinuses. In this way some pictures remind one of a vascular labyrinth or even a renal glomerulus (Fig. 3A, B). These vascular labyrinths are lined with endothelial cells. In some cases bud-like endothelial proliferations and newly formed vessels show that the organization of these deposits is a very active process (Fig. 4A, B).

By histochemistry and electronmicroscopy we could identify these deposits as fibrin.[1] We were

From the Clinic of Otolaryngology, Head and Neck Surgery, Philipps-University, Marburg (Lahn), West Germany.

Presented at the meeting of the American Laryngological Association, Palm Beach, Florida, May 1-2, 1982.

REPRINTS — Prof. Dr. O. Kleinsasser, Univ-ENT-Clinic, Deutschhausstr 3, D-3550 Marburg (Lahn), West Germany.

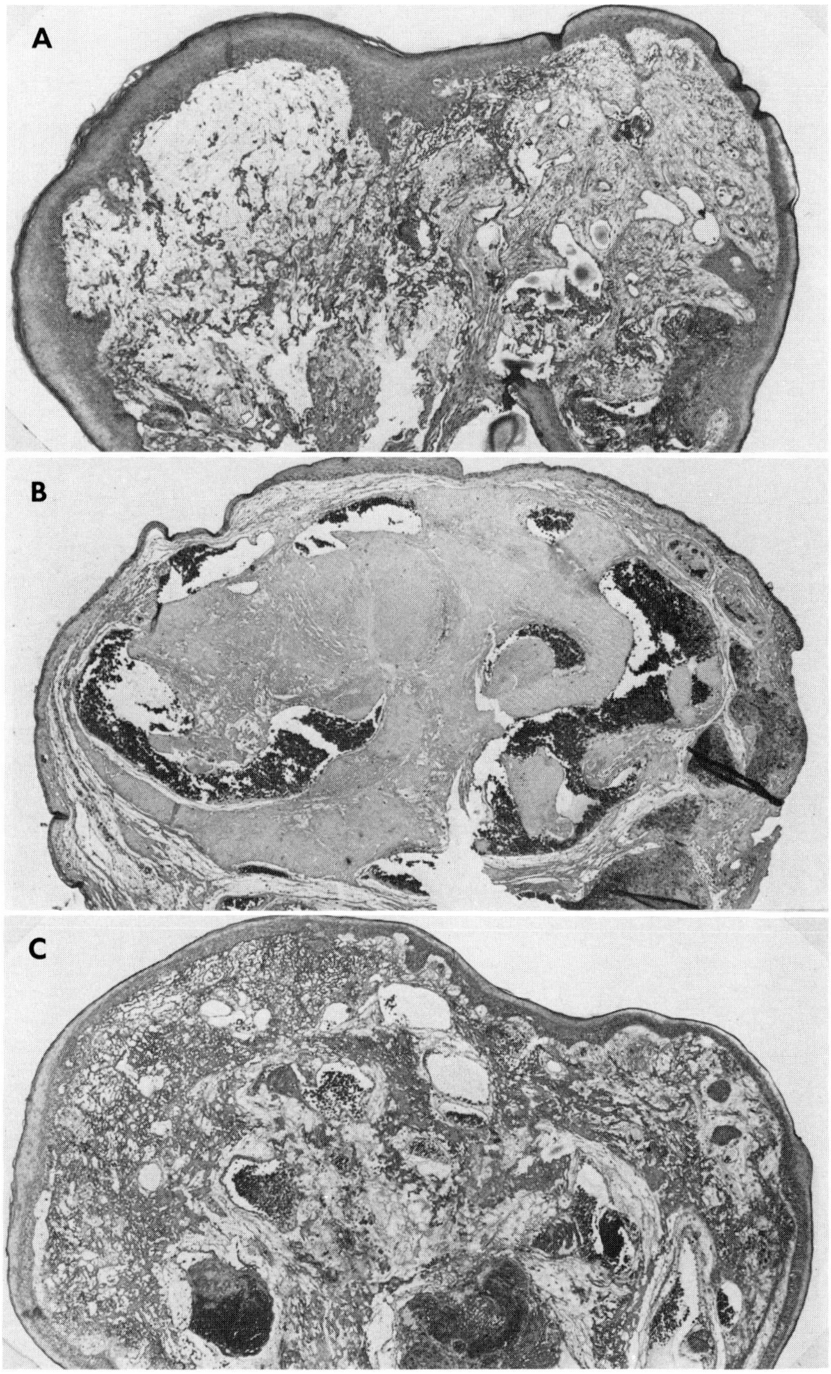

Fig. 1. A) Gelatinous type of vocal cord polyp. Polyp is filled with edema fluid in loose stroma, with several dilated vessels in right part. B) "Nucleus" of these telangiectatic polyps consisting of dense eosinophilic material and dilated vascular spaces. C) Most common "mixed type" vocal cord polyp containing vascular spaces of different configuration, deposits of dense eosinophilic material with edema. (x25)

especially interested in the vascular walls. In the gelatinous polyps the blood vessels were largely identical to the blood vessels of the normal vocal cords. Only seldom could a small gap be found between neighboring endothelial cells. The outer layers of the basal membrane were irregular and often incomplete, and mixed with the delicate collagen fibers of the loose stroma. Thereby the impression is given of a relatively thick vessel wall. In the telangiectatic parts of a polyp we often found gaps in the vascular walls permitting the extravasation of erythrocytes.

Summarizing the results of the morphological investigations our interpretation of the pathogenesis of vocal cord polyps is as follows. In the beginning of the process damage to the walls of the submucous capillaries of the vocal cords takes place. Coiled vessels and sinusoid vessels can appear. Depending on the extent of the damage an increased permeability of the vascular walls develops. Either a thin fluid permeates or a compact fibrin insudation emerges.

The reaction of this fibrin precipitation on the neighboring blood vessels and the connective tissue leads finally to a vascularization of the fissures between the fibers of the fibrin deposits. These pic-

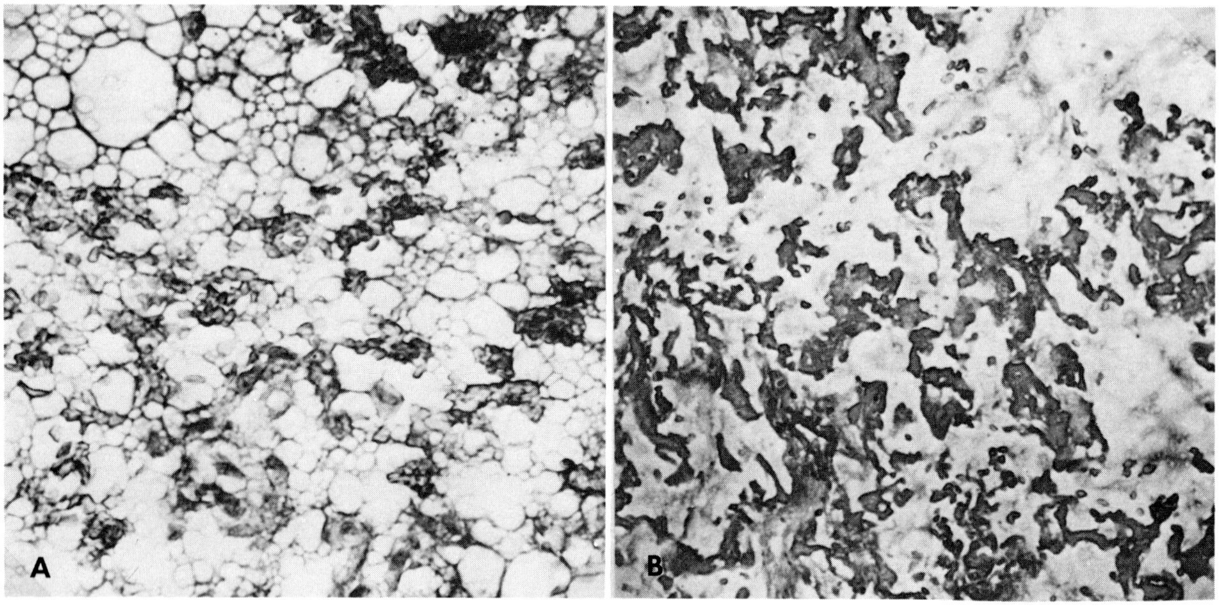

Fig. 2. A) Exudation of a thin fluid in a gelatinous polyp. B) In another case within the mucoid material more dense eosinophilic deposits appear which could be identified as fibrin. (x100)

tures are very similar to the organization of a thrombus. Gaps in the endothelial-lined sinus-like blood vessels cause the further efflux and the deposition of more blood constituents, and allow the increase in size of a polyp. Gelatinous and telangiectatic polyps have presumably the same formal genesis, since the slimy edema and the fibrinous secretions obviously are only expressions of a different permeability of the vascular walls.

Coming back from histopathogenesis to clinical observations: polyps develop with few exceptions on the middle of the surface of the vocal muscle. This is the place where the maximal aerodynamic and muscular forces hit one another during phonation, and most of our patients report an intensive use of their voices. Etiologically the human vocal cord polyps therefore could be considered as the results of a phonotrauma.

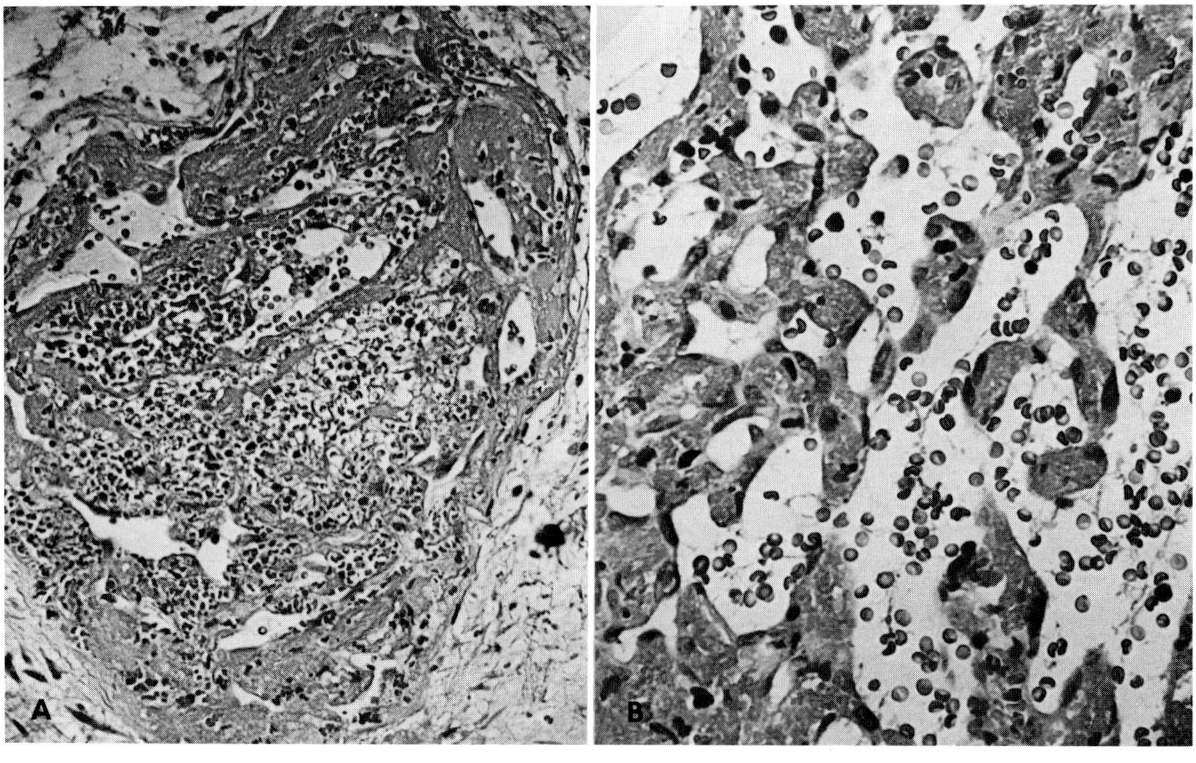

Fig. 3. A) Glomerulus-like labyrinth which develops during organization of a fibrin deposit (x80). B) Sponge-like labyrinth of vascular spaces lined with endothelial cells in the process of organization of a fibrin deposit (x400).

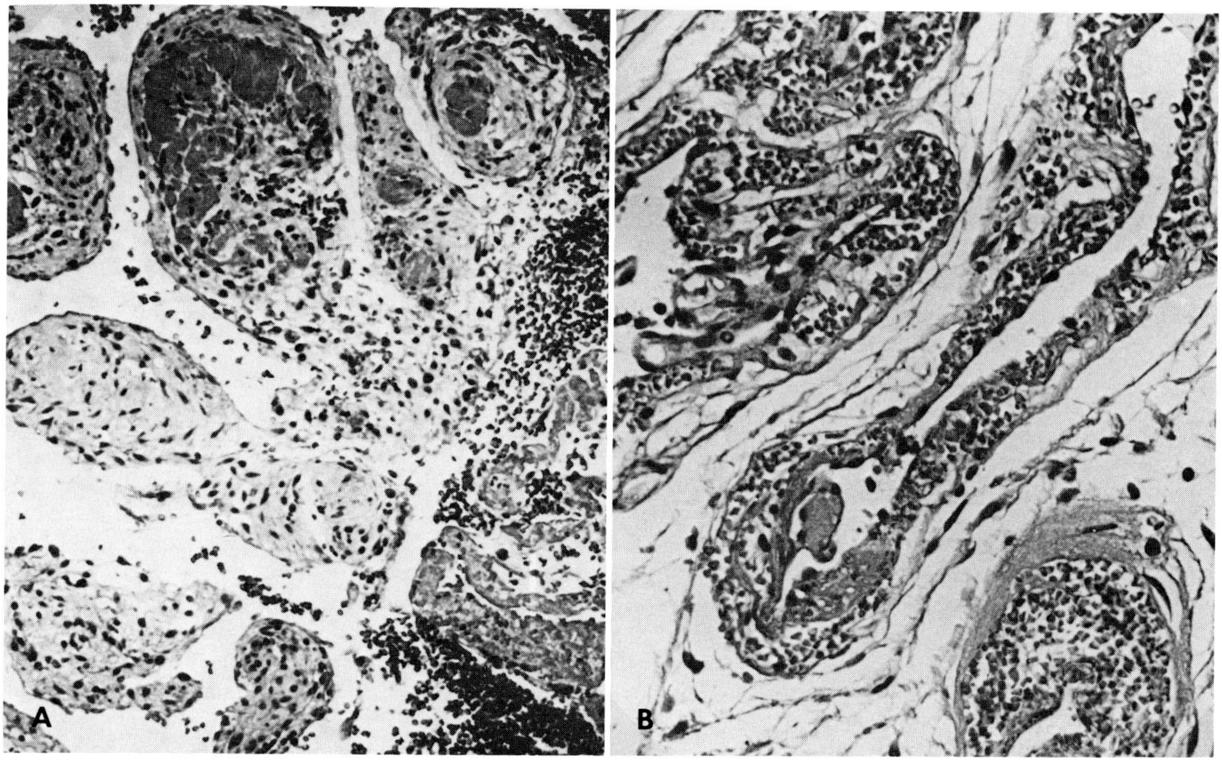

Fig. 4. A) Bud-like endothelial proliferations as a part of the organization process (x100). B) Newly formed vascular spaces in a mainly gelatinous polyp (x200).

REFERENCES

1. Frenzel H, Kleinsasser O, Hort W. Licht- und elektronenmikroskopische Untersuchungen am Stimmlippenpolypen des Menschen. Virchows Arch Pathol Anat Histol 1980; 389:189-204.

ENDOSCOPIC REHABILITATION OF THE AIRWAY IN LARYNGEAL PARALYSIS

FERNANDO R. KIRCHNER, MD, FACS

KANSAS CITY, KANSAS

This paper deals with the three most commonly encountered laryngeal problems that are related directly or indirectly to laryngeal paralysis. These problems are compromised airway secondary to excessive injection of Teflon paste, abductor paralysis of the vocal cords and posterior commissure laryngeal webs.

The dissecting microscope plus the use of focal heat, whether applied by the microcautery[1-5] or the laser beam, for surgical purposes has greatly expanded the field of endoscopic surgery. This report is based on two observations previously reported by the author. 1) The anatomical compartment occupied by the thyroarytenoid muscles may be surgically used to enlarge the airway by removing the fibers of this muscle and lateralizing the vocal ligament. 2) The posterior commissure is an important part of the airway since the arytenoids constitute about one fourth to one third of the anterior posterior diameter of the glottic aperture.

The purpose of this presentation is to describe three simple endoscopic techniques that have been used and the results that have been obtained in the rehabilitation of the airway in patients with 1) unilateral adductor paralysis with compromised airways secondary to excessive injections of Teflon; 2) bilateral abductor paralysis of the vocal cords; 3) revision surgery after arytenoidectomies that fail to produce adequate airway because of the formation of posterior commissure web.

EXCESSIVE INJECTION OF TEFLON

Teflon particles suspended in glycerin when injected in adequate amount into the thyroarytenoid muscle produce an indolent and stable granuloma.[6] This technique has been widely used as an augmentation procedure to accomplish the medial displacement of a laterally paralyzed vocal cord to improve voice and cough. Variable degrees of airway obstruction ensue, however, when the amount of Teflon is grossly increased and the site of injection improperly selected.

In the past several years 11 patients with airway obstruction after Teflon injection, including 2 with indwelling tracheostomies, have been successfully rehabilitated using the microcautery and simple endoscopic approaches. The anatomical distortion encountered in most of them has been either exophytic bulges or large intramural distortion producing imbrication of one cord upon the other or a combination of these two forms.

While the simple excision of the exophytic bulge with the microcautery was sufficient to rehabilitate the first group of patients, it required the excision of a block of infiltrated tissue and drainage to produce the improvement in the second group of patients.

LATERALIZATION OF VOCAL CORDS

The technique of lateralization of vocal cords has been used in 22 patients with bilateral abductor cord paralysis. All of these procedures were carried out with the aid of the microcautery, using routine endoscopic approaches.

The treatment consisted in the segmental removal of the thyroarytenoid muscle fibers adjacent to vocal ligament down to the conus elasticus medially and the thyroid cartilage laterally (Fig. 1A, B). This surgical excision is easily carried out with microcautery. The resultant surgical defect is then closed after lateralizing the vocal cord by means of two sutures of No. 2 Prolene that are introduced into the endolarynx above and below the vocal ligament through the lumen of two hypodermic needles (Fig. 1C). The splicing of these two sutures is always performed on the outside after extracting them from the endolarynx through the laryngoscope with the aid of a laryngeal alligator forceps. Adequate tension adjustments of these sutures on the surface of the neck are very important to prevent the sutures from injuring the laterally displaced vocal ligament. This adjustment and permanent fixation is easily accomplished by crimping lead sinkers around these sutures upon a padded button. Occasionally it is necessary to resect with a cup forceps an outstanding vocal process when this portion of the arytenoids protrudes into the airway after the vocal ligament has been lateralized. Three weeks later the stitch is removed via direct laryngoscopy.

Presented at the meeting of the American Laryngological Association, Palm Beach, Florida, May 1-2, 1982.

REPRINTS — Fernando R. Kirchner, MD, 155 South Street, Suite 270, Kansas City, KS 66102.

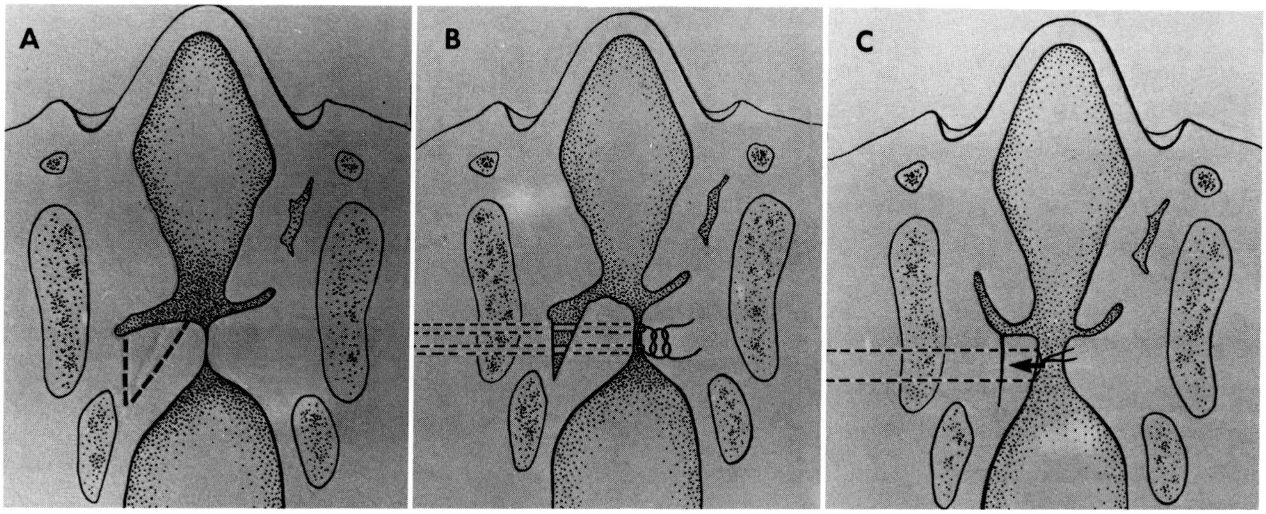

Fig. 1. A) Longitudinal section of larynx demonstrating the compartment occupied by the thyroarytenoid muscle. B) In the lateralization of the vocal ligament a wedge of thyroarytenoid muscle is removed with the microcautery. C) Closure of the defect produced is accomplished with two sutures introduced into the larynx through lumen of hypodermic needles.

Experience gained with these 22 patients has demonstrated that in order to produce a functional airway two requisites are necessary: first, lateralization of the vocal ligament of at least 5 mm, and in addition an anterior posterior diameter of the glottic opening, in the adult, of no less than 22-27 mm in length.

It is important to mention that the voice quality of these 22 patients changed to a more whispery coarse type after the lateralization of the vocal ligament was achieved. All of them, however, preferred this change rather than the alternative of chronic glottic obstruction or the inconveniences of wearing a tracheostomy tube.

REVISION SURGERY AFTER ARYTENOIDECTOMY

The following revision procedures have been successfully used in six patients whose airways remained impaired in spite of arytenoidectomies. The cause of failure of these initial procedures was found to be produced by a posterior cicatricial web that reduced by about one third the anterior posterior diameter of the airway in spite of an apparent adequate lateralization of the vocal cord. In three of these patients the reconstitution of the posterior commissure was accomplished in a rather simple fashion since the web obliteration yielded to a linear incision with minimal epithelial denudation. To avoid reformation of the web, however, a piece of reinforced Silastic sheeting was inserted into the surgical crevice and held in place by two parallel sutures, introduced into the larynx by two transfixion sutures using Keith needles from the right surface of the neck to the left surface with endoscopic guidance and visualization.

In the remaining three patients the scarred tissue was found to be broader and thicker in nature and, therefore, a wider incision became mandatory. A split-thickness skin graft was coadapted to the Silastic sheeting in order to provide the necessary epithelial coverage because of the extension of the epithelial denudation, which, when measuring the two surfaces, amounted to more than one square centimeter. The sutures and Silastic sheeting were removed six weeks later.

REFERENCES

1. Kirchner FR, Toledo PS. Microcauterization in otolaryngology. Arch Otolaryngol 1974; 99:198-202.

2. Kirchner FR, Duff WE. Treatment of laryngeal and ear strictures by microcauterization. Laryngoscope 1974; 84:1326-31.

3. Kirchner FR. Microcauterization in pediatric patients. Trans Am Acad Ophthalmol Otolaryngol 1975; 80:325-55.

4. Kirchner FR. Endoscopic lateralization of the vocal cords in abductor paralysis of the larynx. Laryngoscope 1979; 89;1779-83.

5. Kirchner FR. Suturing techniques in endolaryngeal surgery. Laryngoscope 1981; 91:1860-4.

6. Kirchner FR, Toledo PS, Svoboda DJ. Studies of the larynx after Teflon injection. Arch Otolaryngol 1966; 83:350-4.

Ann Otol Rhinol Laryngol 91:1982

PREDICTIVE FACTORS OF SUCCESS OR FAILURE IN THE ENDOSCOPIC MANAGEMENT OF LARYNGEAL AND TRACHEAL STENOSIS

GEORGE T. SIMPSON, MD, MPH

M. STUART STRONG, MD　　GERALD B. HEALY, MD

STANLEY M. SHAPSHAY, MD　　CHARLES W. VAUGHAN, MD

BOSTON, MASSACHUSETTS

Stenosis of the larynx and/or trachea presents perplexing problems. No one technique has proved totally satisfactory in the management of all varieties of stenosis. Recent reports have described the successful use of the CO_2 laser in the endoscopic management of stenosis of the larynx and trachea. Failures of this technique need emphasis to assure appropriate selection of therapeutic method. Retrospectively, 49 cases of laryngeal stenosis, 6 cases of tracheal stenosis and 5 cases of combined laryngeal and tracheal stenosis were studied (total 60 patients) following treatment at the Boston University Affiliated Hospitals. Follow-up ranged from 1 to 8 years. Multiple procedures were required in 35 laryngeal patients. Of the laryngeal patients 39 were successfully managed (average number of procedures in successful cases 2.18). Of 11 tracheal patients with combined laryngeal and tracheal procedures, 3 were successfully managed (average number of procedures in successful cases 6). Failures in laryngeal stenosis included four patients in whom an adequate airway was not established though voice was present while maintaining tracheostomies. Thirteen patients failing endoscopic management required open surgery with good result. Factors associated with poor result or failure include circumferential scarring with cicatricial contracture, scarring wider than 1 cm in vertical dimension, tracheomalacia and loss of cartilage, previous history of severe bacterial infection associated with tracheostomy, and posterior laryngeal inlet scarring with arytenoid fixation. In these circumstances, multiple procedures, more extensive alternative open surgical techniques, or maintenance of tracheostomy were necessary. In successful cases only three or fewer procedures on average were required. The factors associated with failure or success of endoscopic methods in the management of laryngotracheal stenosis, including use of the CO_2 laser and soft Silastic stents, are analyzed.

INTRODUCTION

Stenosis of the larynx and trachea can present perplexing problems. While not new, these clinical entities now most often result from different causes than previously. Caustic ingestions are far less frequent, and the infectious diseases associated with stenosis are now infrequent. New knowledge of physiology and advances in applied technology have allowed prolonged life-support efforts with artificial ventilatory support mechanisms. These methods, unfortunately, are sometimes associated with subsequent laryngeal and tracheal stenosis following airway trauma. High speed motor vehicle accidents produce crushing injuries to airway structures. New surgical techniques, such as cryosurgery and the laser, if used inappropriately, without adequate skill or precautions, may severely injure airway structures.

Whatever the cause, the clinical problems are the same. The surgeon facing them must select the most effective method, but on what factors should he base his decision?

The methods available for the surgeon's selection are of two general categories. Endoscopic methods include traditional dilatation and newer techniques utilizing stents and laser excision of stenotic areas, all having the advantage of lessened morbidity and hospitalization. Open surgical methods involve excision of stenotic lesions followed by reconstruction, but require perhaps greater costs in time and resources, with greater potential morbidity. Both methods can be effective if used properly.

In an effort to understand what factors may be associated with the successful use of endoscopic methods in the management of laryngeal and tracheal stenosis, we undertook a study of a series of cases managed endoscopically. Specifically, the factors which appeared associated with failure were sought.

MATERIALS AND METHODS

Sixty patients undergoing endoscopic treatment for laryngeal, tracheal or combined laryngotracheal stenosis between 1974 and 1981 at Boston University Affiliated Hospitals and whose records were available for review were subjected to retrospective analysis. Follow-up was from 1 to 8 years. The patients' ages ranged from two months to 72 years. The series included 49 cases of laryngeal stenosis, 6 cases of tracheal stenosis and 5 cases of combined laryngeal and tracheal stenosis. Laryngeal stenosis cases were further classified into supraglottic (6 cases), glottic (12 cases), and subglottic stenosis (31 cases) for analysis.

Of the 6 supraglottic stenosis patients, 4 followed supraglottic laryngectomy, 1 developed with Crohn's disease, and 1 followed blunt trauma.

Glottic stenosis was present in 12 patients and resulted from endolaryngeal intubation in 5. Congenital webs were present in two

From the Department of Otolaryngology, Boston University School of Medicine.

Presented at the meeting of the American Laryngological Association, Palm Beach, Florida, May 1-2, 1982.

REPRINTS — George T. Simpson, MD, Department of Otolaryngology, Boston University School of Medicine, 720 Harrison Avenue, Boston, MA 02118.

SUCCESSES AND FAILURES IN ENDOSCOPIC MANAGEMENT

	No. of Cases	*Successes No. %*	*Average No. of Endoscopic Procedures to Success*	*Failures No. %*	*Failures Successfully Treated with Open Surgery*	*Failures with Good Voice but Tracheostomy*
Laryngeal						
Supraglottic	6	4 (66.7)	1.25	2 (33.3)	1*	1
Glottic	12	9 (75.0)	1.66	3 (25.0)	2	1
Subglottic	31	25 (80.6)	2.44	6 (19.4)	4	2
Subtotal	49	38 (77.5)	2.11	11 (22.4)	6	4
Tracheal	6	2 (33.3)	6.0	4 (66.7)	3	1
Laryngeal & tracheal	5	1 (20.0)	1.0	4 (80.0)	4	2
Total	60	41 (68.3)		19 (31.7)	13 (21.7)	7 (11.7)

*Deceased.

patients. Postsurgical webbing, partial laryngectomy (vertical hemilaryngectomy), rheumatoid arthritic cricoarytenoid joint fixation, ideopathic cricoarytenoid joint ankylosis, and post-traumatic arytenoid fixation each produced one case of glottic stenosis.

Thirty-one patients had subglottic stenosis; 25 of these were secondary to endotracheal intubation. High tracheotomy produced two cases and two followed blunt trauma. Median thyrotomy for endolaryngeal surgery resulted in one case of subglottic stenosis. One patient had ideopathic subglottic stenosis for which no etiology could be identified.

All six cases of tracheal stenosis followed prolonged intubation and tracheotomy for respiratory assistance, as did all five cases of combined laryngeal and tracheal stenosis.

Florid bacterial infection associated with tracheotomy was identified as a precipitating factor in four patients with combined stenosis and one patient with subglottic stenosis.

One patient with combined stenosis and one with subglottic stenosis were each found to have retained nonabsorbable suture fragments from previous open surgeries present in the stenotic area.

Forty-five patients had tracheotomies present at the time of initial presentation: 4 with supraglottic stenosis, 3 with glottic stenosis, 29 with subglottic stenosis, 5 with tracheal stenosis, and 4 patients with combined laryngeal and tracheal stenosis.

All patients underwent endoscopic examination and treatment under inhalation general anesthesia provided via tracheostomy tube, when present, venturi ventilation, or ventilating bronchoscope, as necessary. Laryngeal exposure was provided by using Jako-Pilling laryngoscopes suspended by the Boston University-Pilling gallows or the Lewy suspension apparatus. Carbon dioxide surgical lasers (25-50W) coupled to Zeiss operating microscopes were employed to vaporize scar or granulation tissue, divide fibrotic bands, or excise redundant supraglottic tissue, this being sent for histologic examination.

Silastic stents were employed in 39 patients. One supraglottic stenosis patient had a solid Silastic stent suspended by a single transfixation wire for six weeks. A single sheet of reinforced Silastic was secured between the vocal folds of two glottic stenosis patients with webs (one anterior, the other posterior), suspended by wire in the Kleinsasser method.[1]

Of the 31 cases of subglottic stenosis 27 (87.1%) had soft Silastic roll stents secured in the subglottic area by the Evans method,[2] remaining from 2 to 6 weeks. Similar type roll stents were used in four cases of tracheal stenosis and four cases of combined laryngeal and tracheal stenosis.

Dilatation was employed in four cases each of tracheal and combined laryngeal and tracheal stenosis. No laryngeal stenosis patients underwent dilatation.

For purposes of analysis, successful patients were defined as those with good airway and voice and without tracheostomy, and not requiring further endoscopic manipulation of their airway either by laser excision or ablation, or by dilatation. Cases were classified as failures of endoscopic management if open surgical procedures were necessary, if continued tracheostomy was required for airway maintenance even with a good voice, or if recurrent endoscopic procedures were necessary to maintain voice or airway.

In successful cases, the numbers of endoscopic procedures required to produce the desired result were studied. All failures were then analyzed to determine pre-existing or concurrent factors which seemed contributory to the failure.

RESULTS

Forty-one cases (68.3%) of laryngeal, tracheal, or combined laryngeal and tracheal stenosis were successfully managed by endoscopic techniques (table). Nineteen cases (31.7% of the total) were classified as failures. Eleven laryngeal stenosis cases (22.4%), 4 tracheal stenosis cases (66.7%) and 4 with combined stenoses (80%) resulted in failure. A total of 13 cases (21.7%) required open surgery: 6 laryngeal (12.2%), 3 tracheal (50%) and 4 combined stenosis (80%). The remainder of the failures maintained tracheostomies with good voices.

Supraglottic Stenosis. Of 6 patients with supraglottic stenosis, 4 (66.7%) were managed endoscopically with success. The average number of endoscopic procedures required for a successful result was 1.25.

The two failures both had recurrent stenosis. One died of metastatic cancer, probably from the original supraglottic primary, but autopsy could not be obtained to confirm this. The other patient retained a tracheotomy with good voice. Both failures had reformation of cicatricial scarring in the supraglottic area. Both had tracheostomies present and one had five endoscopic procedures without success. Both were adults. No infection was associated with their endoscopic or previous (supraglottic laryngectomy) surgery. No stents had been employed in either failure.

Glottic Stenosis. Among 12 patients with glottic stenosis 9 (75%) achieved a successful result. This required an average of 1.66 endoscopic procedures. Three of the 9 had glottic webs, 3 had fibrotic bands between the vocal processes (postintubation),

2 had cricoarytenoid ankylosis and 1 had had a previous vertical hemilaryngectomy.

Three cases (25%) were failures, 2 requiring open surgery and 1 with good voice but maintaining a plugged tracheostomy and not desiring decannulation (but listed as a failure). Two of the failures had posterior fibrotic webbing resulting from prolonged endotracheal intubation in one patient and a traumatic intubation in the other. This webbing reformed after removal reproducing arytenoid fixation. The third failure occurred in the patient with arytenoid fixation following blunt trauma who underwent unsuccessful arytenoidectomy, but required a subsequent open procedure. In contrast, both patients with arytenoid fixation from rheumatoid arthritis and from idiopathic cause underwent successful arytenoidectomies using the laser. All three failures had tracheostomies as opposed to none of the successful cases. None of the glottic stenosis patients had a bacterial infection, scars that were circumferential or wider than 1 cm in depth, or history of cryosurgery. All failures were adults. None of the failures had had a stent.

Subglottic Stenosis. Thirty-one patients presented with subglottic stenosis; of these, 25 (80.6%) were managed endoscopically with a successful result, requiring an average of 2.44 endoscopic procedures. In 21 of these 25 cases (84%), soft Silastic stents were employed. Twenty of the successfully managed cases of subglottic stenosis followed endotracheal intubation (80.6%), while 2 had resulted from blunt trauma and 2 from high tracheotomy. One followed tracheotomy and median thyrotomy for a benign laryngeal lesion.

Six cases of subglottic stenosis (19.4%) were failures to endoscopic management methods. Four required open surgical procedures with successful result. One continues with plugged tracheostomy awaiting growth and one continues with functioning tracheostomy with a good voice.

Five of the 6 cases of failure (83.3%) had a tracheostomy on initial presentation but 29 of the total 31 cases of subglottic stenosis (93.5%) had tracheostomies similarly present. Five of the six cases of failure (83.3%) had presented following endotracheal intubation. Four of the cases (66.7%) resulting in failure had circumferential cicatricial scarring as opposed to 17 of the 31 total cases of subglottic stenosis (54.8%) and 12 of 25 successful cases (48%). Subglottic stenosis wider than 1 cm in vertical dimension was present in 3 cases of failure (50%), 15 of the total cases (48.4%) and 13 (52%) of the successfully managed cases. The incidence of preceding infection could not be adequately assessed to allow analysis. All cases resulting in failure had employed a stent (100%) while 21 of the 31 total cases of subglottic stenosis (71%) used stents. No prior cryosurgery was recorded at presentation in the 31 subglottic stenosis cases. No age relationship was evident as 5 of the failures (83.3%) and 22 of the successes (88%) were below 6 years of age.

Tracheal Stenosis. Two of the six cases of tracheal stenosis (33.3%) were successfully managed endoscopically. These two required an average of six endoscopic procedures to obtain a successful result. Both successful patients developed tracheal stenosis following intubation. One had undergone 4 previous operations elsewhere including tracheal resection of a 2 cm-wide stenotic ring with end-to-end anastomosis and 3 dilatations and required 4 further procedures: 2 laser excisions and 2 dilatations. The other patient had previously undergone 5 dilatations performed elsewhere and required 1 laser excision and 2 dilatations for a successful result. Neither case presented with tracheostomy and no stents were used. Both had narrow shelf-like noncircumferential stenosis.

Four of the six cases of tracheal stenosis (66.7%) resulted in failure. All 4 (100% of failures) had circumferential scarring wider than 1 cm, loss of tracheal cartilage and tracheomalacia, and tracheostomy present. Three of the failures (75%) had bacterial tracheal infection associated with tracheotomy prior to presentation. Three of the 4 failures were less than 6 years of age, while both successes were adults, and 3 of the total 6 (50%) were less than 6 years of age. Cryosurgery had been employed in one of the six total cases (16.7%) and this was a failure (25% of failures). Stents had been employed in all cases resulting in failure. Three failure patients were treated successfully with tracheal resection and end-to-end anastomosis. The other patient has a good voice with tracheostomy.

Combined Laryngeal and Tracheal Stenosis. Only one of the five patients having combined stenosis (20%) was treated successfully with endoscopic methods. This 2-year-old patient developed multiple fibrous bands in the larynx and proximal trachea after being intubated for croup. The bands were lysed with the laser and only one endoscopic procedure was necessary.

The remaining four cases of combined stenosis (80%) were failures. All had circumferential cicatricial scarring wider than 1 cm, significant loss of cricoid and tracheal cartilage and had preceding bacterial infections associated with their tracheostomies. One patient had elsewhere undergone more than 12 previous endoscopic surgeries including 6 cryosurgical applications. This patient was under ten years of age and represents 20% of the total number of combined stenosis patients and 25% of the failures. All four failures had stents employed.

DISCUSSION

Endoscopic management of laryngeal stenosis at all levels seems readily justified when the results are analyzed. Of all laryngeal stenosis cases 77.6%

were managed successfully, though 71.4% required multiple endoscopic procedures. Successful endoscopic management was possible in all parts of the larynx as shown by the success rates of 66.7% for supraglottic stenosis, 75% for glottic stenosis, and 80.6% for subglottic stenosis. These results also support the use of the carbon dioxide laser as a surgical instrument, as the laser was employed in all cases, whether or not a successful result ensued.

It is clearly apparent that purely endoscopic techniques are unsuccessful in most cases of severe tracheal stenosis and combined laryngeal and tracheal stenosis especially if the stenotic areas are wide, are circumferential, or if they are accompanied by significant loss of cartilage in the cricoid or trachea. Successfully managed cases in tracheal or combined stenosis showed more limited discrete lesions. Therefore, open operations should be employed in cases of extensive tracheal and combined stenosis. Endoscopic methods, however, may be justified in the initial management, if only to establish a lumen which later may be of help at open operations.

A major cause of failure at all levels was the reformation of the scar tissue following its excision. Abundant scar tissue of over 1 cm of vertical dimension, and/or if circumferential, was present in all failures at all levels except subglottic, where it was in the majority. Of special note is the observation that 2 cases of glottic stenosis involving fibrotic scar tissue in the interarytenoid area of the posterior commissure were failures to endoscopic management. This type of glottic stenosis seems best considered from the beginning for open surgical correction.

It would seem obvious that excessive application of laser energy should produce unnecessary necrosis in nearby tissue with resultant undesired scar-tissue formation. Such a factor in any failure proved difficult to analyze in this series as the cases resulting in failure did not seem to receive greater amounts of laser energy or longer periods of its application than did similar cases managed successfully. Experience with stenosis following widespread prolonged application of the laser, however, demands prudent caution. Extensive excision of severe subglottic stenosis proved successful if performed with brief (0.1 to 0.5 seconds), interrupted bursts of laser energy.

Superficially, tracheostomy would seem to be associated with failure, as a tracheostomy was present prior to endoscopic management attempts in all cases resulting in failure. It must be remembered, however, that tracheostomies existed in 75% of the total group on initial presentation, and were always necessary in the most severe cases of stenosis at any level. Furthermore, 93.5% of subglottic stenosis patients had tracheostomies present initially, yet 80.6% were successfully managed by endoscopic techniques alone, and 96% of the successful cases had tracheostomies.

A more significant factor in failure, and one associated with tracheostomy, is bacterial infection. While infection had not occurred in supraglottic and glottic stenosis cases, and could not be determined accurately in cases of subglottic stenosis, it represents a major pre-existent or predisposing factor in tracheal and combined stenosis. At these levels 87.5% of failures had sustained a severe bacterial infection of the trachea following tracheostomy and prior to any endoscopic management by our group. Such a history may predict the necessity of open surgery for management of tracheal stenosis alone or combined with other stenosis. The possibility of recurrent infection during endoscopic management with potential sequelae and failure may urge the endoscopic surgeon to employ antibiotics. Further data on patients in this series, now undergoing analysis, may support the use of prophylactic antibiotics in the endoscopic management of stenosis.

Of failing cases, 73.3% had a history of intubation prior to the diagnosis of stenosis, compared with 66.7% of the total series. A similar history was found in 72.5% of the cases managed endoscopically with success.

Soft Silastic stents were employed in all cases resulting in failure in subglottic, tracheal, and combined stenosis, but were associated with success in all cases where used in the supraglottis or glottis. Soft Silastic stents were used in 84% of the successful subglottic stenosis cases. As stents are obviously of benefit, especially in severe stenosis, and were so used, it appears that their use is not a factor in failure. Rather, the use of stents is associated with the most severe degrees of stenosis as it is here that they are most helpful.

Patient age was not associated with failure for endoscopic methods in any type of stenosis. In fact, in subglottic stenosis, 88% of the successful patients were less than 6 years of age, while 77.1% of all subglottic stenosis patients were in this age group. While three of the four failures in tracheal stenosis were patients under 6 years of age, they also were the patients with the most severe stenosis.

Cryosurgery had been previously employed elsewhere in one patient each with tracheal and combined stenosis who failed endoscopic management. Its prior use cannot be specifically indicted, however, as the relationship of the cryosurgery and the severe stenosis cannot be accurately determined. A history of previous cryosurgical techniques in a patient with severe stenosis may warn of future difficulties for endoscopic management methods.

Dilatation was not required at any time in virtually any patient in this series. It did prove helpful, however, in two patients with tracheal stenosis successfully managed endoscopically.

SUMMARY

Endoscopic management methods, including, as required, CO_2 laser excision, soft Silastic stents, and dilatations, are successful in most cases of laryngeal stenosis at all levels and of all etiologies. Endoscopic methods are successful only infrequently in major stenosis involving the trachea, either alone or in combination with laryngeal stenosis. To be managed endoscopically with success, stenosis involving the trachea must be limited in extent and without significant associated loss of cartilage, circumferential cicatricial stenosis or scarring wider than 1 cm in vertical width.

Major factors associated with failure of endoscopic management of stenosis at all levels of the larynx and trachea include preceding severe bacterial infection associated with tracheostomy, circumferential cicatricial scarring, scar tissue wider than 1 cm in vertical dimension and fibrotic scarring of the posterior laryngeal inlet with arytenoid fixation. Endoscopic management techniques should be considered with caution in the presence of a history of cryosurgery in the prior treatment of airway stenosis.

With consideration of these factors, the surgeon may choose either to proceed directly to open surgical methods, or to manage laryngeal and tracheal stenosis endoscopically with the expectation of a high likelihood of success.

ACKNOWLEDGMENT — We wish to express our gratitude to Mrs. Edna Joyner for the preparation of the manuscript.

REFERENCES

1. Kleinsasser O. Microlaryngoscopy and endolaryngeal microsurgery. Stuttgart: Schattauer-Verlag, 1976:156.
2. Evans JNG, Todd GB. Laryngotracheoplasty. J Laryngol Otol 1974; 88:589-97.

≈

PAN AMERICAN ASSOCIATION OF OTORHINOLARYNGOLOGY AND BRONCHOESOPHAGOLOGY

The XVIII Congress of the Pan American Association of Otorhinolaryngology and Bronchoesophagology will be held November 2-6, 1982, in San Juan, Puerto Rico. Dr. Hans von Leden has been elected President of the Association.

Ann Otol Rhinol Laryngol 91:1982

DIAGNOSIS AND CONSERVATIVE SURGICAL MANAGEMENT OF CHONDROSARCOMA OF THE LARYNX

JULIUS N. HICKS, MD

E. EARL WALKER, MD E. EUGENE MOOR, MD

BIRMINGHAM, ALABAMA

Tumors of cartilage rarely occur in the larynx. Most laryngologists see no more than one of these tumors. Therefore, information about the general knowledge, early diagnosis, and surgical treatment of these tumors accumulates slowly. In this paper we will discuss one type of cartilaginous tumor: chondrosarcoma of the cricoid cartilage. We will review general diagnostic information about this tumor, present a case report, and describe a method of conservative surgical excision.

INTRODUCTION

Cartilaginous tumors of the larynx occur as isolated cases in the practice of laryngology. Travers reported a case to the Medico-Chirurgical Society of London in 1816.[1]

Chondrosarcoma of the larynx is usually of low-grade malignancy and does not respond to treatment with irradiation and chemotherapy. Treatment is limited to surgical excision. The exact surgical procedure will vary from simple excision for a neoplasm of limited size and low-grade malignancy to total laryngectomy for a tumor of extensive size or high-grade malignancy.

Chondrosarcoma of the larynx is reviewed, with diagnostic factors outlined; the surgical treatment described; and a case reported. A conservative method of surgical excision of a chondrosarcoma arising in the cricoid region is described.

REVIEW

Incidence. The case reports of approximately 200 cartilaginous tumors of the larynx from 1816 to 1979 indicate 20% to be chondrosarcomas.[2] A review of 58 cases of chondrosarcoma of the larynx during a recent period of 80 years reveals an average patient age of 58 years, and there were 43 males and 15 females.[3]

Clinical Findings. The symptoms of chondroma of the larynx are those of any mass growing slowly inside the lumen of the larynx: hoarseness, dyspnea, and dysphagia. These symptoms are related to the location and size of the tumor. A lesion of the cricoid extending into the laryngeal lumen can cause decreased air flow and vocal cord mobility. Growth of a cricoid lesion posteriorly and laterally into the hypopharynx can cause dysphagia.

Location of Tumor in Larynx. Laryngeal chondrosarcomas usually arise from hyaline cartilage and show no evidence of elastic tissue. There is a striking predilection for the tumor to form in the region of the cricoid cartilage. A review of chondrosarcoma of the larynx has been done at the Armed Forces Institute of Pathology (AFIP).[4] This AFIP series notes 16 cases from 1929 to 1969 and shows that 11 (68%) of these tumors occurred in the cricoid region.

Etiology. The etiology of chondrosarcoma is unknown. Virchow wrote in 1863 that these tumors originate from the connective tissue stroma of the normal perichondrium, the body of the cartilaginous tissue, or the cartilaginous cell nests which serve as a matrix and then undergo ossification.[5] No scientist has offered a better explanation for the etiology of chondrosarcomas.

Clinical Diagnosis. The clinical diagnosis of chondrosarcoma is made on the basis of the history, physical examination, radiologic findings, and histopathologic findings. The patient presents with a history of hoarseness, dyspnea or dysphagia. Indirect laryngoscopy can reveal a smooth, rounded mass below the true vocal cords. Soft tissue x-ray films or xeroradiograms of the larynx can demonstrate the tumor. Mottled calcification is seen within the tumor in up to 75% of the soft tissue x-ray studies.[6] Planigrams can outline the tumor, but the CT scan can demonstrate the exact origin of the tumor.

The definitive diagnosis is made in the operating room with direct laryngoscopy and biopsy. Histopathological criteria which indicate a chondrosarcoma have been established by Lichtenstein and Jaffe:[7] 1) irregularity in the size of the cells and their nuclei; 2) increased numbers of cells; 3) hyper-

From the Division of Otolaryngology and Head and Neck Surgery, Department of Surgery, University of Alabama Hospitals and Clinics, Birmingham.

Presented at the meeting of the American Laryngological Association, Palm Beach, Florida, May 1-2, 1982.

REPRINTS — Julius N. Hicks, MD, Division of Otolaryngology and Head and Neck Surgery, Department of Surgery, University of Alabama in Birmingham Medical Center, University Station, Birmingham, AL 35294.

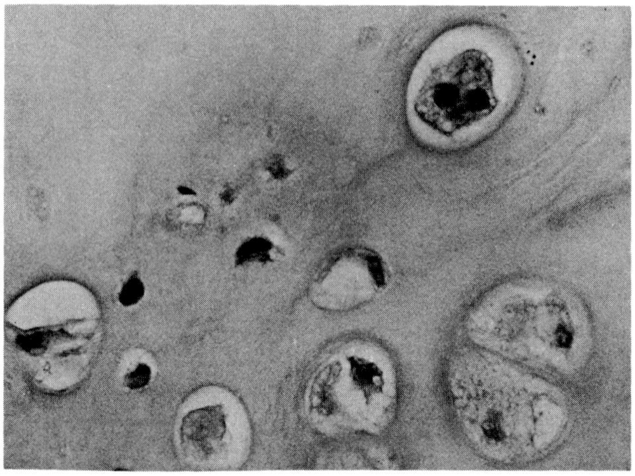

Fig. 1. Section of tumor showing at top a large binucleated cartilage cell which contributes to diagnosis of chondrosarcoma (H & E x600).

chromatic nuclei; 4) giant cartilage cells with single or multiple nuclei. These giant cartilage cells may be binucleated (Fig. 1).

Surgical Treatment. In most cases with significant airway obstruction a tracheotomy secures the airway and allows a direct laryngoscopy and biopsy to be done to establish the diagnosis. After the diagnosis is made, the grade of malignancy must be determined.

Since recurrences occur late and metastases are rare, surgical treatment should be as conservative as possible. Total laryngectomy may be required for a high-grade malignant tumor, a recurrent tumor, or a tumor which cannot be totally removed by a conservative surgical procedure. Adequate excision requires removal of the tumor with a margin of normal tissue. This can usually be done conservatively with a laryngofissure, thyrotomy, or partial laryngectomy. If adequate excision of the tumor requires removal of more than one half of the cricoid cartilage, a laryngectomy must be performed to avoid debilitating laryngeal and tracheal stenosis. In older patients the surgeon can sometimes remove the tumor with a curette and leave an adequate support of cricoid cartilage — the technique that was used in the case report following.

Since nodal metastases to the neck are rare, elective neck dissections are not indicated.

Although the tumor often recurs after conservative surgical treatment, most surgeons prefer laryngofissure exposure and total local excision, since the tumors recur many years later, grow slowly, and permit treatment by additional conservative surgical procedures.

CASE REPORT

A 67-year-old white female was referred to the University of Alabama in Birmingham Medical Center for definitive treatment. She had already been evaluated for periods of episodic shortness of breath. These episodes occurred at any time and had increased in frequency over the past year. A previous bronchoscopy revealed a subglottic mass. Her dyspnea increased and an emergency tracheotomy was performed on June 22, 1981, prior to transfer to the University of Alabama in Birmingham Medical Center for definitive treatment. At the time of the tracheotomy a biopsy was performed, and slides of the tissue were sent to the Armed Forces Institute of Pathology. The histopathological report by the AFIP revealed chondrosarcoma. Our pathology department confirmed this tissue diagnosis.

The patient's past history revealed that a surgeon performed a partial thyroidectomy in 1948, 31 years previously. An internist had ordered thyroid scans yearly for the previous five years.

Physical examination revealed an alert and cooperative female. The examination of the larynx revealed good true vocal cord movement. There was a large mass in the right subglottic region which completely filled the subglottic area except for a 1- to 2-mm space on the left side. The neck was supple, and the tracheostomy tube was in place. There was a 6-cm x 3-cm x 3-cm mass in the right thyroid lobe region. Admission laboratory studies revealed a normal hemogram, urinalysis, EKG and chest x-ray film. The electrolytes were normal. The GTT and alkaline phosphatase were slightly elevated.

A thyroid scan indicated an enlarged thyroid gland with increased uptake activity in the right upper lobe, consistent with multinodular goiter. The CT scan of the neck showed the large thyroid mass in the right neck and the smaller laryngeal mass in the lumen of the larynx and trachea. The laryngeal mass was attached to the right posterior lateral wall of the cricoid cartilage.

After completing the preoperative evaluation, the patient was taken to the operating room where laryngeal surgery was performed. The patient was given endotracheal anesthesia through the tracheotomy opening. The anatomic landmarks of the neck were identified. A skin mark was made with a marking pen for the horizontal skin incision over the midregion of the thyroid cartilage. The vertical limb of the incision was made through the previous vertical tracheotomy scar. After elevation of the skin flap, dissection was carried out to expose the thyroid cartilages. An incision was made through the midline and the superior margins of the perichondrium of the thyroid cartilages. Lateral extensions of the incisions on the superior margin were made to points medial to the superior laryngeal nerves and vessels.

The perichondrium was elevated on each side of all incisions. The larynx was transected in the midline of the thyroid cartrilages with scissors for a laryngofissure incisional approach. The lumen of the cricoid region was viewed by retracting each

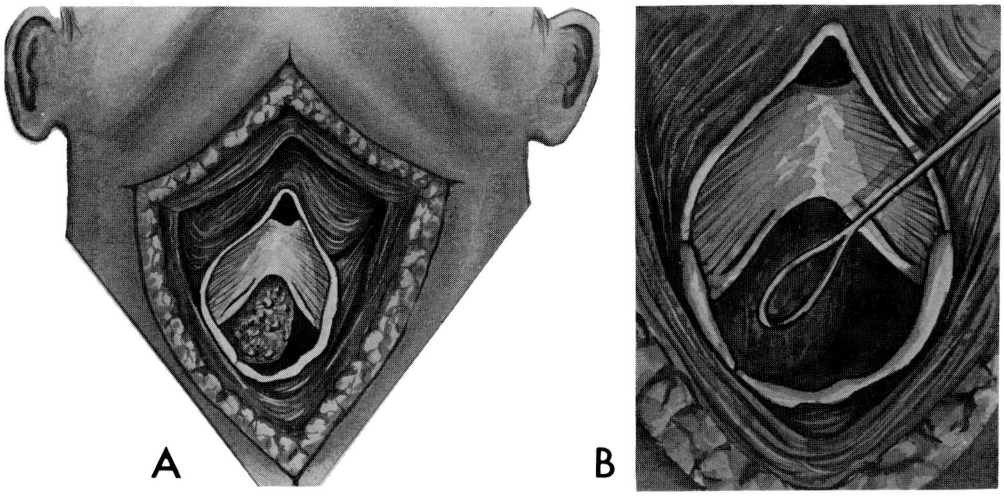

Fig. 2. Drawing showing A) subglottic mass and B) curette placed in raw surface after removal of tumor.

side of the thyroid cartilage with a skin hook. This maneuver exposed the site of attachment of the mass (Fig. 2A). The exact location of the attachment was determined by palpation with a small curette. The mucous membrane was incised so that there was a wide margin of normal mucous membrane around the mass. The mass was removed by curettage at its origin from the cricoid cartilage (Fig. 2B). The mass had a distinct difference in tissue density relative to normal cricoid cartilage. This tissue density could be appreciated during curettage and allowed complete excision of the tumor without taking an excessive amount of normal cricoid cartilage. The cricoid ring was not cut through and the integrity of the laryngeal airway was maintained.

The wound was irrigated with saline. The mucous membrane was cut so it would lie in the defect without tension. At this time the patient appeared to have a very satisfactory operative result.

The perichondrium was closed with 4-0 chromic catgut. A rubber drain was inserted. The muscles were approximated with 3-0 Vicryl sutures. Skin closure was performed with 5-0 nylon vertical mattress interrupted sutures. After the patient was breathing spontaneously, the Anode tube was removed and a No. 6 cuffed Shiley tracheostomy tube was inserted. The patient was awakened and taken to the recovery room in good condition.

The patient's postoperative course was uncomplicated. She was discharged on the third postoperative day to be followed by her referring physician. He decannulated her four weeks after her surgical procedure. It has been over nine months since excision of her tumor and there is no evidence of recurrence.

SUMMARY

The incidence, clinical findings, location, etiology, clinical diagnosis, and surgical treatment of chondrosarcoma of the larynx are discussed. Important features in the diagnosis and treatment of a chondrosarcomatous tumor of the larynx are demonstrated in a case report.

The patient's chief complaint was episodic shortness of breath occurring with increasing frequency over a period of 12 months. Her dyspnea progressed in severity until an emergency tracheotomy was required for airway control.

CT scan documented the attachment of the tumor to the right posterior lateral wall of the cricoid cartilage. Direct laryngoscopy and biopsy were done to obtain tissue for diagnosis. The histopathological examination revealed low-grade chondrosarcoma.

The tumor was removed totally with a wide-margin mucous membrane incision and careful curettement. A definite difference in the consistency of the tumor compared to normal cartilage allowed complete excision of the tumor with minimal sacrifice of healthy cricoid cartilage. This presentation emphasizes the conservative surgical removal of these tumors and notes how a curette can be used for this removal.

REFERENCES

1. Travers F. A case of ossification and bony growth of the cartilages of the larynx. Med Chir Trans 1816; 7:150.

2. Hellquist H, Olofsson J, Grontof T. Chondrosarcoma of the larynx. J Laryngol Otol 1979; 93:1037-47.

3. Cantrell RW, Jahrsdoerfer RA, Reibel JF, Johns ME. Conservative surgical treatment of chondrosarcoma of the larynx. Ann Otol Rhinol Laryngol 1980; 89:567-71.

4. Hyams VJ, Robuzzi DD. Cartilaginous tumors of the larynx. Laryngoscope 1970; 80:755-67.

5. Virchow R. Die Krankhaften Geschwulste. Vol. 1. Berlin: August Hirschwald Verlag 1863:442.

6. Zigmor J, Noyek AM, Lecois JS. Radiologic diagnosis of chondroma and chondrosarcoma of the larynx. Arch Otolaryngol 1975; 101:232-4.

7. Lichtenstein L, Jaffe H. Chondrosarcoma of bone. Am J Pathol 1943; 19:553-74.

CHONDROSARCOMA OF THE LARYNX: EXCISION OF MASSIVE RECURRENCE

FRANCIS E. LEJEUNE, JR, MD, FACS
HERBERT W. VAN HORN III, MD
GIST H. FARR, MD
NEW ORLEANS, LOUISIANA

Chondrosarcoma of the larynx is an uncommon, slow-growing malignant tumor of the larynx which tends to metastasize late. This paper adds to the literature a case which was followed for 18 years. During the first three years is was thought to be a benign chondroma. Conservative management by limiting surgical resection, at the patient's direction, allowed observation of the disease for this unusual length of time. Massive enlargement finally necessitated laryngectomy. The lesion, though unquestionably malignant, had not infiltrated adjacent neck structures and appears to have been totally excised, with the patient now being free of disease six months after surgery. This supports the view of conservative surgical management.

INTRODUCTION

Only approximately 200 cases of cartilaginous tumors of the larynx have been reported in the medical literature since 1822. Of these, approximately 20% have been malignant. In Cantrell et al's review,[1] 78% of the tumors arose from the cricoid, usually in the posterior or posterolateral areas. Another 15% arose from the thyroid cartilage. Males outnumbered females approximately 3 to 1. The ages of patients ranged from 33 to 91 years with the average being 58 years. No cases of documented chondroma transforming to malignant tumor have been reported, though one case was suspected.[2] In Ollier's disease, a familial syndrome characterized by multiple chondromatoses, approximately 10% of the cartilaginous tumors may be malignant.

CASE REPORT

In August 1981, a 72-year-old female with a tracheotomy was referred because of a large neck mass and purulent drainage (Fig. 1A). The history revealed that in 1963, at age 54, she had been evaluated by an otolaryngologist because of progressive dyspnea, hoarseness, and a slowly enlarging neck mass. A subglottic mass was noted and a biopsy indicated chondroma. In August 1966, progressive airway obstruction necessitated a tracheotomy. Biopsy again confirmed diagnosis of chondroma. She refused surgery at this time, electing to wear a tracheotomy tube for the next 12 years.

In 1978, she sought medical attention for progressive dysphagia and enlargement of the neck mass (Fig. 1B). In February 1979, she underwent a laryngofissure and partial excision of the mass. Pathologic diagnosis was chondrosarcoma. She refused definitive surgery but she changed her mind after noting drainage of purulent material from the large neck mass. In September 1981 a wide field laryngectomy was performed which appeared to completely excise all tumor. Healing was uneventful. The patient is now six months postsurgical treatment and is without evidence of disease (Fig. 1 C).

HISTOPATHOLOGY

Gross and Microscopic. The surgical specimen measured 12.5 x 9 x 8.5 cm. The cephalic aspect contained the epiglottis and the lower pharyngeal mucosa stretched over the submucosal tumor (Fig. 2 A, B). The caudal aspect of the specimen included the upper trachea, tracheostomy wound and surrounding skin. The anterior aspect of the specimen included portions of the thyroid gland and lymph nodes. The mass was unyielding to firm compression and a band saw was necessary to section the tumor. Contained within soft tissue was a roughly spherical mass having a rim of calcified tissue. The vast majority of the tumor was composed of semi-translucent, friable and focally mucoid material. Approximately midway into the specimen, a sinus tract was found, which extended from a 2-cm abscess cavity to the pinpoint lumen of the trachea (Fig. 2C). The latter was displaced laterally to the extreme left portion of the mass. At no point could tumor be found at a surgical margin. All lymph nodes and the thyroid were negative.

Microscopically, the tumor was a well-differentiated chondrosarcoma with areas of myxoid chondrosarcoma (Fig. 3A,B). Endochondral bone formation accounted for the incomplete bony rim. No areas of anaplastic tumor were identified. Some

From the Departments of Otolaryngology and Pathology, Ochsner Medical Institutions, New Orleans.
Presented at the meeting of the American Laryngological Association, Palm Beach, Florida, May 1-2, 1982.
REPRINTS — Francis E. LeJeune, Jr, MD, Ochsner Clinic, 1514 Jefferson Highway, New Orleans, LA 70121.

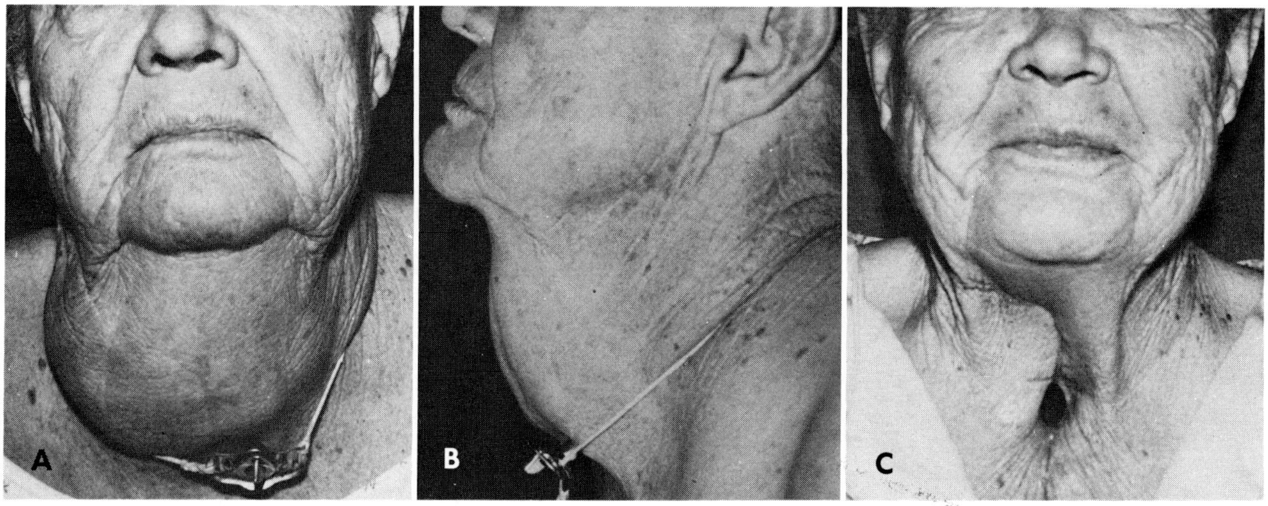

Fig. 1. A) Patient, 72-year-old female, with firm chondrosarcoma measuring approximately 15 x 18 cm, fixed to deep structures. B) Mass distorts neck contours, necessitating tracheotomy and causing progressive dysphagia. C) Six months postlaryngectomy, patient appears to be free of disease, and is being rehabilitated.

areas were very well-differentiated and adequate sampling was necessary to identify the various histologic pictures.

Only material from the 1979 excision was available for review. The tumor appeared no more aggressive in 1981 than in 1979.

DISCUSSION

The classic presentation of chondrosarcoma or of chondroma of the larynx includes hoarseness and dyspnea due to gradual expansion of the intraluminal tumor or dysphagia if the expansion extends toward the hypopharynx. A visible palpable mass will be present if the thyroid cartilage is involved.

At laryngoscopy, a smooth bulging contour is noted in the subglottic region. The mucosa overlying the mass is usually intact. Vocal cord motion may be limited if the mass encroaches. The firm nature of the mass makes the obtaining of an adequate biopsy specimen difficult.

Radiographic signs[3] include the location in the subglottis, often the posterior wall, of a mass which has a smooth surface but contains coarse, irregular scattered calcification; this does not provide a true distinction between benign and malignant masses.

Differential Diagnosis. Differential diagnosis should include the other primary lesions: neurilemoma, cylindroma, rhabdomyosarcoma, fibrosarcoma, calcified carotid artery, calcified thyroid adenoma, cysts, granular cell myoblastoma, amyloidosis, and tracheopathia osteoplastica. Metastatic lesions to the larynx are rare but prostatic and other primaries have been reported.

COMMENT

The slow growth of the lesion in the early years of this case seem to contrast with the more rapid expansion in the last several years. This apparent increase in rate of enlargement in its later states may be merely a function of its doubling time, a factor which can remain constant. To illustrate the exponential increase of this effect, if this page were

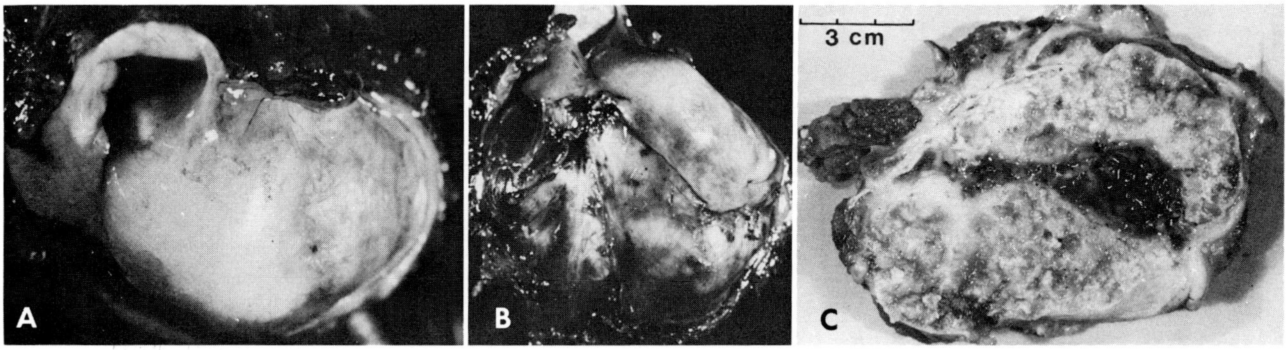

Fig. 2. A) Surgical specimen seen from above. Epiglottis and right arytenoid are seen in center. Mucosa covering right pyriform sinus is displaced by submucosal tumor, obliterating the sinus. B) Laryngectomy specimen viewed posteriorly. Chondrosarcoma mass and larynx measured 12.5 x 9 x 8.5 cm. C) Gross photograph of midsection of specimen, showing abscess cavity at right, with linear sinus tract to pinpoint trachea on the left.

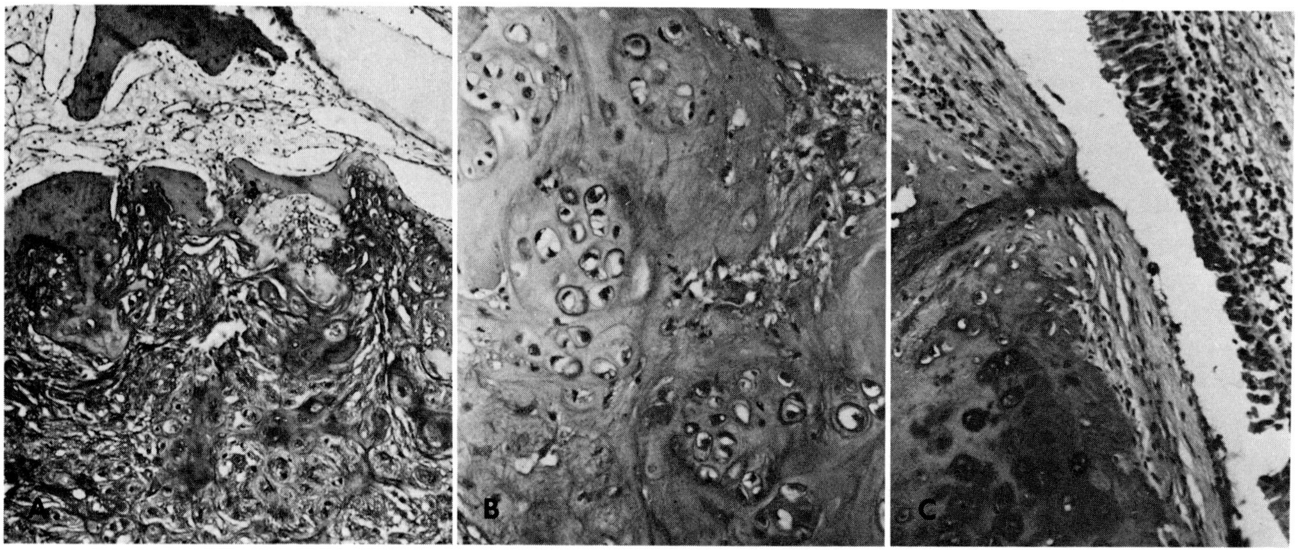

Fig. 3. A) Well-differentiated and myxoid chondrosarcoma, with areas of mature bone formation at periphery (H & E, x40). B) Well-differentiated chondrosarcoma, showing little myxoid change (H & E, x100). C) Pinpoint lumen of trachea, showing submucosal chronic inflammation at bottom and compressing chondrosarcoma at top (H & E, x 100).

torn in half and the two pieces of paper stacked and torn in half again and stacked and this were repeated for a total of 50 times, the stack of paper would reach far beyond the moon.

The apparent change in histologic pattern may represent a low-grade, well-differentiated chondrosarcoma with some areas closely resembling chondroma.

Management. The widely accepted rationale for treatment of cartilaginous tumor of the larynx by limited surgical resection[1,4-6] would appear to be supported by this case. Even though the initial surgical efforts were not successful in controlling the disease, the patient, by her strong rejection of greater surgical efforts, afforded an opportunity to see unaltered progression of the malignant disease. The eventual salvage of the patient in spite of the massive size of the lesion was possible because of its tendency to remain within the limits of the perichondrium of the larynx. No extension into adjacent tissues or structures was noted. Distant metastasis is an infrequent problem in the laryngeal chondrosarcoma cases studied, but is always a remote possibility.[7]

Conclusion. A case of chondrosarcoma of the larynx is reported in which the patient refused laryngectomy and survived 18 years before consenting to surgical extirpation. In spite of its long duration and massive size, the tumor appeared to be limited to the anatomical confines of the larynx at the time of wide field laryngectomy. She appears to be free of disease at this time, six months post-laryngectomy. Management by conservative excision of small lesions with laryngectomy reserved for large recurrent tumor is supported.

REFERENCES

1. Cantrell RW, Reibel JF, Jahrsdoerfer RA, Johns ME. Conservative surgical treatment of chondrosarcoma of the larynx. Ann Otol Rhinol Laryngol 1980; 89:567-71.

2. Busuttil A, Forbes J. Chondrosarcoma of the thyroid cartilage. J Laryngol Otol 1978; 92:633-8.

3. Zizmor J, Noyek AM, Lewis JS. Radiologic diagnosis of chondroma and chondrosarcoma of the larynx. Arch Otolaryngol 1975; 101:232-4.

4. Damiani KK, Tucker HM. Chondroma of the larynx. Arch Otolaryngol 1981; 107:399-402.

5. Hyams VJ, Rabuzzi DD. Cartilaginous tumors of the larynx. Laryngoscope 1970; 80:755-67.

6. Singh J, Black MJ, Fried I. Cartilaginous tumors of the larynx. Laryngoscope 1980; 90:1872-9.

7. Ross DE. Chondrosarcoma of the larynx invading thyroid gland. Laryngoscope 1971; 81:379-86.

EXTENDED TRANSANTRAL APPROACH TO PTERYGOMAXILLARY TUMORS

CHARLES J. KRAUSE, MD SHAN R. BAKER, MD

ANN ARBOR, MICHIGAN

A review of 14 patients treated between 1975 and 1979 is reported. The lesions were quite extensive in most of the patients, having extended beyond the nasopharynx in all but one. An extended transantral approach was utilized in nine of the patients to facilitate removal of lateral and superior extensions of tumor. Two of the patients (14%) developed recurrent tumor, one six months and one nine months following treatment. The extended transantral approach appears to be an effective method of approaching the pterygomaxillary extension of the tumor.

INTRODUCTION

The nasopharyngeal angiofibroma is an uncommon, highly vascular tumor which has a predilection for the nasopharynx of adolescent boys. Though only occasionally invasive, the tumor tends to spread anteriorly into the nasal cavity and ethmoid cells, and laterally through the sphenopalatine foramen and into the pterygomaxillary space (Fig. 1). From there the tumor may extend superiorly through the inferior orbital fissure, across the orbital apex, and through the superior orbital fissure into the middle cranial fossa (Fig. 2). Because of the predilection to lateral extension, preoperative evaluation with arteriography should always be done.

Many surgical approaches to these tumors have been advocated, including a vertical split of the soft palate, an anterior fishmouth approach through the palate, a transethmoid approach, a lateral rhinotomy and blunt dissection of the retromaxillary space. Selection of a preferred approach depends upon the extent of the tumor and the individual surgeon's experience and preference. Frequently more than one approach should be combined to offer optimum exposure.

When there is extensive involvement of the pterygomaxillary space, a transantral approach alone or in conjunction with other approaches offers access to the laterally extending tumor, to the internal maxillary artery for the purpose of ligation, and allows gentle dissection of tumor extending through the inferior orbital fissure. The technique employed and the results when utilized in a series of patients will be presented.

METHOD

An extended sublabial incision is made from the midline, laterally to the maxillary tuberosity, and carried down through the periosteum of the maxilla. The periosteum is elevated up to the infraorbital foramen and the face of the maxilla is widely excised using a Kerrison rongeur. The posterior wall of the sinus is then widely excised, allowing access to the pterygomaxillary portion of the tumor. Whenever possible, the internal maxillary artery should be ligated before beginning the tumor removal. By removing the medial wall of the sinus, the surgeon achieves access to the nose and nasopharynx (Fig. 3). When the tumor extends into the ethmoid cells, they may be opened from the antrum, and the tumor carefully dissected. When the tumor extends further laterally, the lateral wall of the sinus may be removed to improve exposure (Fig. 4). Finally, this approach allows excellent access to the inferior orbital fissure (Fig. 3) to allow gentle dissection of the tumor extending upward through the fissure.

The transantral approach may be combined with a transpalatal or external ethmoidectomy approach when tumor extension dictates. We prefer the fishmouth incision for the transpalatal approach, extending the incision behind the maxillary tuberosity on the side of greatest extension. The nasal mucoperiosteum is incised and sufficient bone is removed from the posterior edge of the hard palate to provide adequate access to the nasopharynx. An incision is then made through mucoperiosteum of the nasopharynx circumferentially around the tumor base. Using a periosteal elevator, dissection is carried all around the large feeding vessels which enter the pedicle at the base of the tumor. The vessels are then transected and the nasopharynx is packed for 5-7 days. Care must be taken to completely remove all tumor extensions.

RESULTS

Fourteen patients with nasopharyngeal angiofibroma who were treated at the University of Michigan between 1975 and 1979 were evaluated. A summary of their treatment and outcome is listed in the table. The age at onset ranged from 13 to 25, with the median being 15. Epistaxis and nasal obstruction were the most common symptoms noted at presentation, being present in all but one case. Four patients had been treated prior to undergoing surgical excision at the University of Michigan, including two who had received irradiation for extensive intracranial tumor. Arteriograms were performed in all patients preoperatively. In addition, computerized tomography (CT) scans were obtained in four patients. The extent of the tumor in each case is summarized in the table. All but two patients had lateral involvement of the pterygomaxillary space,

----

From the Department of Otorhinolaryngology, University of Michigan, Ann Arbor.

Presented at the meeting of the American Laryngological Association, Palm Beach, Florida, May 1-2, 1982.

REPRINTS — Charles J. Krause, MD, Department of Otorhinolaryngology, University of Michigan Hospitals, Ann Arbor, MI 48109.

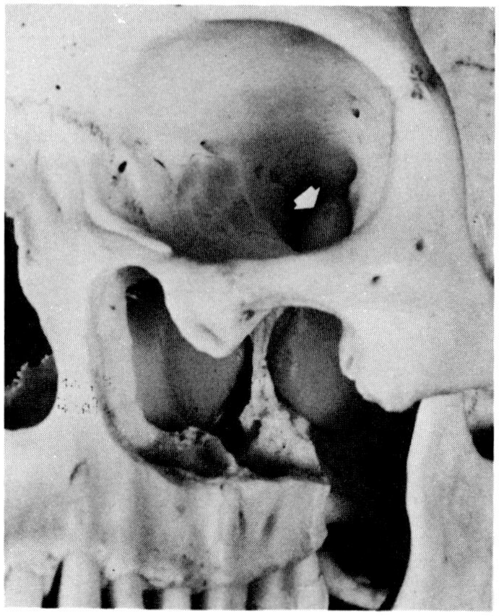

Fig. 1. Tumor extending through sphenopalatine foramen into pterygomaxillary space. Arrow indicates tumor crowding orbital apex.

and in five cases the tumor had extended intracranially as well. The extended transantral approach was utilized in 9 of the 14 patients, being combined with a transethmoid or transpalatal approach in 4 of them.

Five of the patients were found to have intracranial extension of their tumor; in 1 a craniotomy was performed to remove tumor, and 2 were successfully treated with radiation therapy. In the other two patients, the small amount of intracranial tumor was pulled downward through the inferior orbital fissure. Two of the patients developed recurrent tumor after treatment at the University of Michigan, one at nine months and one at six months. Both of these patients had been previously treated elsewhere, and had developed recurrent tumor prior to treatment at our institution. The remaining patients have been followed 18-60 months with no evidence of recurrence.

DISCUSSION

Angiofibromas appear to arise from fibrovascular

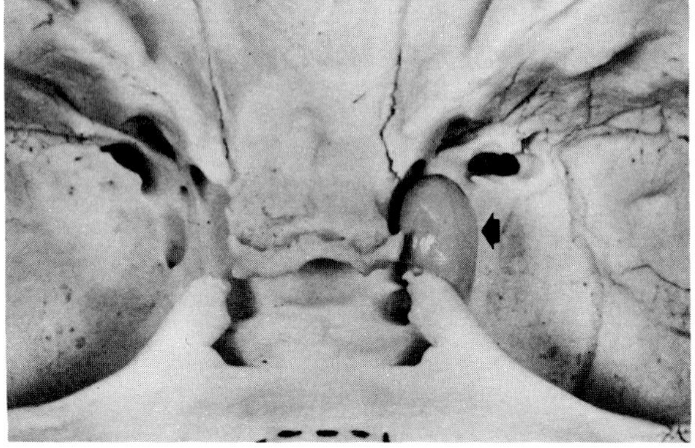

Fig. 2. Tumor extending through superior orbital fissure into middle cranial fossa.

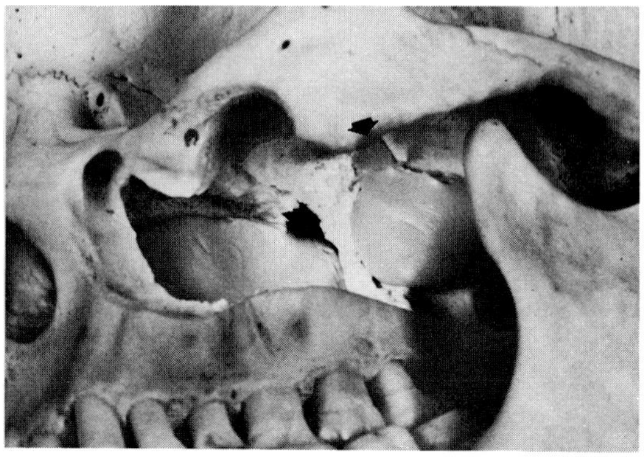

Fig. 3. Medial wall removed to provide access to nasopharynx and nasal cavity. Arrow indicates tumor extending upward through inferior orbital fissure.

stroma present in the nasopharynx,[1] most commonly from a broad base in the posterosuperior wall. The tumor, which consists of varying ratios of fibrous stroma and thin-walled vascular spaces, gradually enlarges and spreads, picking up blood supply as it goes.

The tumor tends to fill the nasopharynx and posterior choanae, then extends into the maxillary or ethmoid sinuses. Laterally it tends to extend through the sphenopalatine foramen into the pterygomaxillary space. From there the tumor extends upward through the inferior orbital fissure, and thence through the superior orbital fissure intracranially. Alternatively or additionally, the tumor may extend superiorly from the nasopharynx through the sphenoid sinus and into the sella turcica.[2]

Nasopharyngeal angiofibromas are nearly always found in males, with the onset of symptoms most commonly found during adolescence. More than a century ago, Gosselin suggested that angiofibromas spontaneously regress after adolescence.[3] It is of interest that one of our patients was more than 25 years of age when he began having symptoms, and

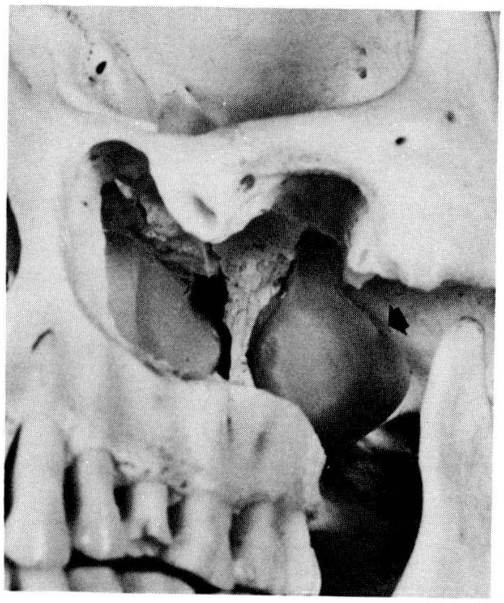

Fig. 4. Lateral wall of antrum has been removed along with posterior wall to provide access to lateral extension.

REVIEW OF PATIENTS TREATED FOR NASOPHARYNGEAL ANGIOFIBROMA

Pt. No.	Age at Onset	Symptoms	Duration of Symptoms (Mo)	Extent of Tumor	Procedure	EBL	Present Condition	Follow-up (Mo)	Comment
1	13	Epistaxis	12	Nasophar.	Transpalatal	500	NED	52	
2	13	Epistaxis Nasal obs.	12	Nasophar. P-M space Orbit	Transantral	1600	Recur	9	Had surgical excision prior to U of M Tx.
3	16	Nasal obs.	12-15	Nasophar. P-M space Orbit Intracran.	Transantral	1100	NED	18	
4	13	Epistaxis Nasal obs.	3	Nasophar. P-M space	Transantral	500	NED	20	
5	14	Epistaxis	4	Nasophar.	Transpalatal	250	Recur	6	2 previous surgical procedures
6	25	Nasal obs.	18	Nasophar. P-M space Ethmoid	Transpalatal Transethmoid	3000	NED	48	
7	18	Headache; proptosis	4	Nasophar. P-M space Orbit Intracran.	Transantral	7100	NED	24	
8	21	Nasal obs.	24	Nasophar. P-M space Orbit Intracran.	Transantral Craniotomy	2000	NED	23	
9	25	Nasal obs.	60	Nasophar.	Transantral	1100	NED	24	Radiation therapy for intracranial tumor
10	15	Nasal obs.	12	Nasophar. P-M space	Transantral Transethmoid	6000	NED	60	Treated with irradiation 1 yr earlier
11	14	Epistaxis Nasal obs.	12	Nasophar. P-M space	Transantral Transpalatal	—	NED	24	
12	13	Nasal obs. Mass R cheek	24	Nasophar. P-M space	Lat rhinotomy Blunt dissection of P-M space	1100	NED	24	
13	18	Epistaxis Nasal obs.	1	Nasophar. Ethmid	Transethmoid	600	NED	Lost to f/u	
14	14	Nasal obs.	12	Nasophar. P-M space	Transantral Transpalatal	—	NED	84	

EBL - Estimated blood loss; Nasal Obs. - Nasal obstruction; P-M - Pterygomaxillary space.

one other developed a recurrence of his tumor at 25 years of age, experiencing progressive nasal obstruction and epistaxis.

Most of these tumors were found to be quite extensive at the time of presentation here. The importance of including arteriography preoperatively to determine the extent of disease is illustrated by the fact that all but one of our patients were found to have extension of tumor beyond the nasopharynx, with lateral extension into the pterygomaxillary space in 12 of the 14 patients, and with tumor extending upward through the inferior orbital fissure in 4. In each of the latter patients it was possible to gently dissect the tumor downward out of the orbit.

Controversey exists regarding the use of hormone therapy preoperatively in an attempt to cause "maturation" of the angiofibroma. Martin et al[4] advocated testosterone, whereas Walike and MacKay[5] as well as Schiff[6] have reported beneficial effects from estrogen therapy. Only five of the patients in our study received estrogen therapy preoperatively, with no significant change in the size of the lesion noted.

Many different surgical approaches to nasopharyngeal angiofibromas have been advocated, ranging from a simple midline palatal split to craniotomy. The selection of an appropriate surgical approach is based primarily upon how extensive the tumor is, and which structures and spaces are involved. The extended transantral approach is primarily of benefit when there is extensive tumor in the pterygomaxillary space or evidence of extension upward through the inferior orbital fissure. The ability to safely dissect tumor from the orbit and even intracranially is primarily dependent upon having a limited amount of tumor to remove and the absence of feeding vessels of significant size located in these sites.

Only two of our patients (14%) developed a recurrence of their tumor; in both instances they had been treated earlier and had recurred prior to referral to this institution for treatment. These recurrences occurred nine and six months following completion of treatment here. This incidence of recurrence is somewhat lower than that of approximately 50% cited in many series.[2,7]

REFERENCES

1. Patterson CN. Juvenile nasopharyngeal angiofibroma. Otolaryngol Clin North Am 1973; 6:839-61.

2. Batsakis JF. Tumors of the head and neck. 2nd ed. Baltimore: Williams & Wilkins Inc, 1979.

3. Gosselin P. Clinique chirugicale de l'Hopital de la Charite. 2nd ed. Paris: JB Bailliere et Fils, 1876.

4. Martin H, Ehrlich HE, Abels JD. Juvenile nasopharyngeal angiofibroma. Ann Surg 1948; 127:513-36.

5. Walike JW, MacKay B. Nasopharyngeal angiofibroma light and electron microscopic changes after stilbesterol therapy. Laryngoscope 1970; 80:1109-21.

6. Schiff M. Juvenile nasopharyngeal angiofibroma. Laryngoscope 1959; 69:981-1016.

7. Smith MFW, Boles R, Work W. Cryosurgical technique in removal of angiofibroma. Laryngoscope 1964; 74:1071.

≈

THIRD INTERNATIONAL SYMPOSIUM ON RECENT ADVANCES IN OTITIS MEDIA WITH EFFUSION: CALL FOR PAPERS

Papers are being solicited for the Third International Symposium on Recent Advances in Otitis Media with Effusion, which will be held May 17-20, 1983, at the Bahia Mar Hotel, Fort Lauderdale, Florida. The deadline for submitting titles is November 15, 1982, and the deadline for submitting abstracts is January 15, 1983. For further information, write David J. Lim, MD, Program Chairman, 4331 University Hospitals Clinic, 456 Clinic Drive, Columbus, OH 43210.

PRIMARY MANAGEMENT OF LARYNGEAL TRAUMA

STEVEN D. SCHAEFER, MD
DALLAS, TEXAS

The management of 87 laryngeal trauma patients over the past 17 years is reported. During the last four years, 35 of these patients were prospectively studied by the author after drawing upon the treatment policies of the earlier experience. The results of this study demonstrate a successful program to preserve or restore the phonatory and airway function of the acutely injured larynx.

Laryngeal trauma threatens both the quality and preservation of life. Essential to the preservation of the phonatory and airway sphincter functions of the larynx is restoration of the skeletal framework and epithelium of this organ.[1] Various opinions exist regarding the extent of clinical evaluation and the indications, timing and form of surgical management.[1-4] With the exception of a few articles, most published reports are limited by the number of available patients to retrospective reviews of patients treated by several surgeons within a multiple-hospital institutional setting.[3,5]

Paralleling the experience of Harris and others over the past 17 years, the faculty of the University of Texas Health Science Center at Dallas adopted an aggressive and immediate management protocol for laryngeal trauma. A prior publication by the author reviewing results from the past 13 years permitted the identification of four treatment groups.[6] Utilizing the policies derived from this earlier work, a prospective study was begun four years ago to further clarify laryngeal injuries which might benefit from operative intervention and to test the rationale for various surgical procedures.

The purpose of this paper is to report a primary or immediate management protocol for blunt and penetrating trauma to the larynx that has yielded both predictable and successful results.

MATERIALS

Between 1965 and 1978, 52 laryngeal trauma patients were evaluated after treatment by the faculty of the University of Texas Health Science Center at Dallas Affiliated Hospitals (Parkland Memorial Hospital, Veterans Administration Medical Center, Presbyterian Hospital, and John Peter Smith Hospital). This retrospective report consisted of chart review and examination of available patients from one month to nine years after injury. After January 1978, 35 patients were prospectively managed by the author, primarily at Parkland Memorial Hospital (Table 1). Records were kept by the author beginning at the time of injury, and this information was supplemented by chart review. Follow-up in this population ranged from months to two years.

With the exception of two patients, diagnosis and treatment was performed within 24 hours after injury. Patients initially managed at other institutions or in whom a laryngeal injury was not immediately recognized have been excluded from this paper (one patient in the originally reported retrospective population has been eliminated for this reason).[6] This form of selection is intentional since the theme of the paper is the early management of acute laryngeal injuries, rather than secondary management of the late sequellae of laryngeal trauma.

MANAGEMENT

The diagnosis of laryngeal trauma was based on the history and physical examination (Table 2).[1] Emergent measures included preservation of the airway, cardiac resuscitation, control of hemorrhage, and stabilization of neural and spinal injuries, followed by a systemic search for other organ system trauma. The unstable airway was managed by tracheotomy, rather than endotracheal intubation. In the patient with a nondeteriorating airway, indirect laryngoscopy was considered an important part of the diagnostic evaluation.

Throughout the 17 years encompassed by this paper, lateral soft tissue x-ray examination of the neck was routinely performed, along with radiographic examination of the cervical spine. In the past two years, computerized tomographic scanning (CT) was selectively employed to identify patients who would benefit from surgery. Management in both the prospective and retrospective populations was divided into four groups.

Group 1. Findings included minor endolaryngeal hematomas or lacerations, and absence of a detectable laryngeal fracture. Computerized tomographic scanning was performed to confirm the clinical impression of the injury. Management consisted of close observation, head-of-bed elevation, and humidification of inspired air.

Group 2. Findings included edema, hematoma or minor mucosal disruption without exposed cartilage. Management consisted of tracheotomy, direct laryngoscopy and esophagoscopy. As was true of group 1, no further operative intervention was attempted because the potential for spontaneous resolution of the injured site was felt to be superior to surgery. Utilization of the CT scanner permitted examination of fracture sites. In the prospective group, nondisplaced fractures accompanied by hematoma or minor laceration and requiring tracheotomy were spared open exploration. Prior to CT application, such injuries might have undergone thyrotomy if the mucosal edema was massive enough to preclude an optimal direct endoscopic examination.

Groups 3 and 4. Findings included massive edema, mucosal tears, exposed cartilage and cord immobility. Following tracheotomy and endoscopy, the larynx was explored either through a midline thyrotomy or a laryngofissure in the case of a paramedian fracture. Computerized tomographic scanning was omitted

From the Department of Otolaryngology, The University of Texas Health Science Center at Dallas.

Presented at the meeting of the American Laryngological Association, Palm Beach, Florida, May 1-2, 1982.

REPRINTS — Steven D. Schaefer, MD, Department of Otolaryngology, The University of Texas Health Science Center at Dallas, 5323 Harry Hines Boulevard, Dallas, TX 75235.

TABLE 1. TREATMENT GROUPS (N = 87)

Group	*Retrospective* *1965-1977*	*Prospective* *1978-1982*	*Total*
1	7	7	14
2	5	17	22
3	14	4	18
4	26*	7	33
			87

*Excludes one patient in a previous report.

because these injuries were so significant that it was obvious that further surgery was needed. *All* mucosal injuries were carefully identified and approximated using 5-0 or 6-0 absorbable suture. The anterior free margin of each true vocal cord was sutured to the cartilage or external thyroid perichondrium at the thyrotomy site to reconstitute the anterior commissure. Particularly in the prospective group, this technique permitted one to avoid stenting if a mucosa-covered anterior commissure could be established. When the anterior half of the larynx (true and/or false vocal cords) were disrupted or the skeleton was likely to remain unstable, a lumen-keeping stent was employed. In group 4 patients, stability and mucosal injuries usually were of similarly severe magnitudes, with two or more fracture sites often accompanied by massive trauma to the laryngeal lining.

In the retrospective population, stenting was performed using either commercially available stents, a finger of a surgical glove filled with sponge rubber or a Portex endotracheal tube stent.[3,7] After 1975, the Portex stent was used exclusively. These "lumen keepers" were fixated with 2-0 Prolene suture passed externally through laryngeal ventricle and cricothyroid membrane. Further sutures were placed from the inferior stent to the chest skin via the tracheotomy and from the superior stent to the nose, to permit recovery of the stent if the fixation sutures failed. Prior to 1975, wire was used to fix these stents and was thereafter abandoned in three patients due to breakage. At no time during the entire 17 years covered by the study were skin or mucous membrane grafts utilized. Cartilage was repaired with either wire or nonabsorbable suture, with the latter method most often used in the prospective group. Removal or debridement of the laryngeal skeleton was limited to fragments which were totally avulsed from their perichondral blood supply. In both study populations, stents were removed by endoscopy under general anesthesia at four weeks.

RESULTS

The mechanism of injury for the prospective group is given in Table 2. The results by management group for both the retrospectively and prospectively treated patients are summarized in Table 3. Success was measured by the quality of the voice and airway. A good voice was one that was close to normal or comparable to the patient's preinjury voice. Moderate to marked hoarseness was described as a fair voice, and phonation just above a whisper was classified as poor. Airway quality was judged good if the patient denied restriction; fair with mild to moderate restriction; and poor if permanent tracheotomy was necessary.[6]

In groups 1 and 2 all 36 patients (12 retrospective and 24 prospective) obtained a good voice and airway. Within group 1, four patients were managed by observation only because CT examination showed nondisplaced fractures and hematomas which were likely to spontaneously resolve (Fig. 1). The CT scanner also proved useful in group 2 patients. In particular, one patient underwent an emergency tracheotomy in the emergency room. Computerized tomographic scanning revealed an intact laryngeal skeleton and massive edema was identified at direct laryngoscopy. Without CT examination and with edema that precluded adequate endolaryngeal assessment, open exploration would have been the next step in the care of this patient. Instead, further surgery was avoided and the patient was decannulated at five days with a good airway and voice. Nine prospectively managed patients in group 2 underwent concurrent open neck exploration without thyrotomy for vascular and pharyngeal injuries. Two of these patients had minor fracture dislocations which were repaired without entering the larynx.

Ten of the 18 group 3 patients were available for follow-up, ranging from one month to five years. One patient (prospective group) died from sepsis nine days after injury, following disruption of C-4 vertebrae, quadriplegia and CSF fistula secondary to a gunshot wound. With the exception of the one death, all patients were decannulated without complication within 14 to 35 days. Airway results were good in all patients, with nine having a good voice without further surgery. Another patient (retrospective group) suffered a thyroid-cricoid fracture and was explored at 48 hours. This patient developed a good airway and a fair voice. Six months after injury, one patient (prospective group) underwent left true vocal cord Teflon injection for recurrent laryngeal nerve paralysis. Following this procedure the patient achieved a good voice.

Thirty-three group 4 patients (26 retrospective and 7 prospective) were treated, and followed from two months to nine years postinjury. In this group, one patient died three days following injury from transection of the spinal cord and cerebral anoxia following carotid artery disruption from a missile wound. Another patient was assaulted and died three days after removal of the Portex stent. Stents consisted of soft sponge in 19 patients (retrospective group only) and Portex tube in 14 (7 retrospective and 7 prospective); both were removed four weeks

TABLE 2. PROSPECTIVE POPULATION PROFILE

	Presenting Symptoms							*Method of Injury*		
									Assault	
Group	*Hoarseness*	*Pain/ Tenderness*	*Hemoptysis*	*Dysphagia*	*Subcut Emphysema*	*Impaired Respiration*	*Hematoma*	*MVA*	*Blunt*	*Penetrating*
1	5	4						4	2	1
2	6	2	2	1	3	5	3	5	4	8
3	2	2	1	1		3		1		4
4	2	2		1	1	5		1	2	4

MVA - Motor vehicle accident.

TABLE 3. RESULTS OF TREATMENT OF EVALUABLE PATIENTS (N = 73)

Group	Voice Good	Voice Fair	Voice Poor	Airway Good	Airway Fair	Airway Poor
1	14	—	—	14	—	—
2	22	—	—	22	—	
3	9*	1	—	10	—	—
4†	18	8	—	25	—	2

*One patient achieved a good voice after Teflon injection of the true vocal cord following recurrent nerve injury.

†One patient not evaluated due to prolonged coma.

after injury. Decannulation varied from 35 to 100 days after injury, with two patients in the retrospective group requiring permanent tracheotomy. In one of these patients, cannulation was required for pulmonary toilet necessary for anoxic brain damage suffered following cardiac arrest. The other patient was an elderly woman who continued to use a small-diameter tracheotomy tube with a fair voice and a fair airway clinically (classified as poor for purposes of study) but refused decannulation.[6] Twenty-five other patients were available for evaluation, all of whom achieved a good airway. Eighteen (14 retrospective and 1 prospective) patients had a good voice and 7 (6 retrospective and 1 prospective) a fair voice. Complications in the group 4 patients included 1) avulsion of the entire mucosa of one side of the larynx following endotracheal intubation (Fig. 2), 2) slippage or expulsion of stent secondary to wire breakage in three patients (retrospective group), 3) total airway obstruction following attempted endotracheal intubation in four patients who were successfully rescued by tracheotomy, and 4) perichondritis nine years after injury necessitating temporary tracheotomy and hospitalization for antibiotic therapy.[6]

Antibiotics, usually a cephalosporin, were given for ten days or less to patients who underwent a surgical procedure. Infection was limited to those with massive pharyngeal and spinal column trauma following gunshot wounds. As stated earlier, such injuries accounted for the two deaths in this series. Steroids were used in a few of the group 1 patients, making their benefits difficult to assess.

DISCUSSION

The results following the prospective management of laryngeal trauma by the author for the past four years are considered along with the concepts established over the previous 13 years. A comparison of the two study populations shows an increase in the relative number of assaults and a decrease in automobile-related injuries. The intent of this paper is to draw upon this experience to improve airway and voice function following the various forms of laryngeal trauma.

Emergent Care. There is an unfortunate tendency for nonlaryngologists to regard all airway emergencies as best managed by endotracheal intubation. Following laryngeal trauma, intubation is hazardous. The few patients so managed (initial care conducted by nonotolaryngologist) developed serious iatrogenic complications. These findings lead the author to reinforce the statement of others recommending tracheotomy under local anesthesia for all suspected laryngeal trauma patients requiring airway support for either further diagnostic or surgical management.[1-3,5,6,8,9] In this series, stridor and difficulty breathing were the most consistent symptoms with severe airway trauma, and hence, the need for tracheotomy (Table 2).

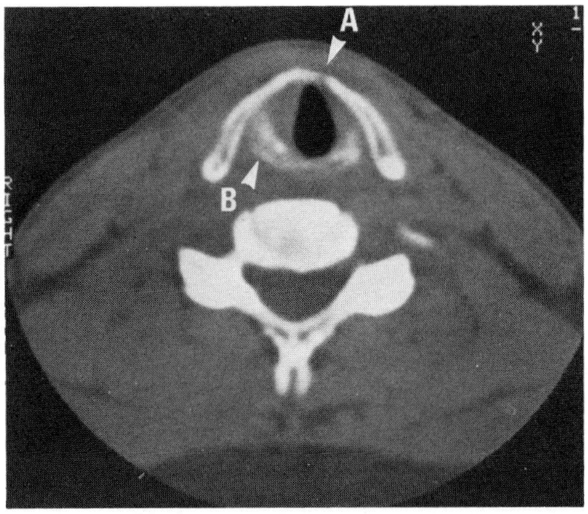

Fig. 1. Computed tomographic scan of patient with nondisplaced thyroid cartilage fracture (A). Right true vocal cord is enlarged due to hematoma, and right arytenoid (B) lies superior to left arytenoid, resulting from hematoma within cricoarytenoid joint.

Diagnostic Evaluation. In the stable airway, indirect laryngoscopy permits rapid assessment of the site and degree of injury. Computerized tomographic scanning has further refined this evaluation allowing one to visualize the skeleton and soft tissue of the larynx. However, as a costly radiographic procedure, the CT scan should be applied to those cases where the findings will influence a therapeutic decision, not to confirm a clinically obvious massive injury. Esophagoscopy was performed concurrently with direct laryngoscopy to exclude pharyngeal and esophageal injuries, and remains a valuable diagnostic adjunctive procedure.[10]

Operative Intervention. Beyond the need to establish an airway by tracheotomy, surgical therapy should be considered when spontaneous resolution of the laryngeal injury is unlikely. The results of this study and others suggest that a full recovery without operative treatment is likely with edema, hematomas without mucosal disruption, single nondisplaced thyroid cartilage fractures in the otherwise stable larynx and small lacerations (and moderate lacerations of the supraglottic larynx) not involving the anterior commissure.

The CT scan may complement the indirect laryngoscopy by evaluating the laryngeal skeleton and soft tissue, thereby either avoiding or supplementing direct laryngoscopy in *certain cases*. Open ex-

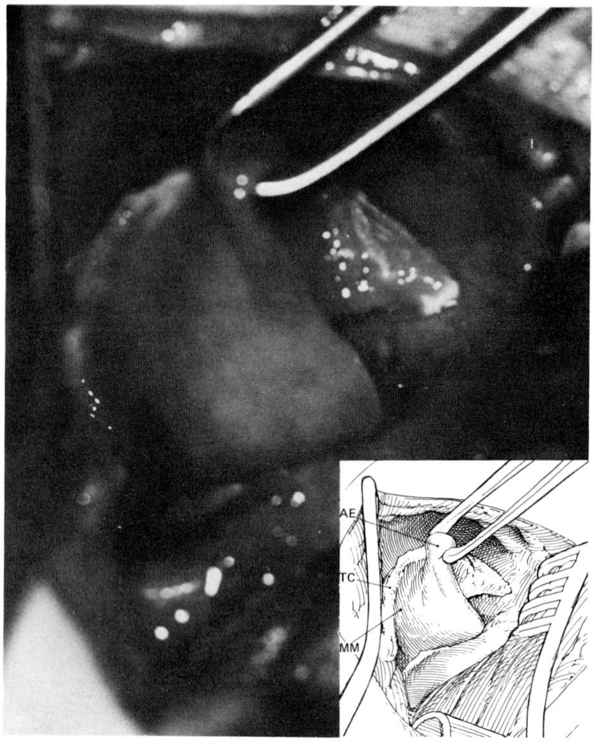

Fig. 2. Operative findings in patient with avulsion of right mucous membrane of larynx following false passage of endotracheal tube. Inset) Artist's drawing of same. AE -Avulsed epiglottis; TC - Thyroid cartilage; MM - Mucous membrane.

ploration of the larynx is felt to be indicated for large mucosal lacerations (particularly of the anterior commissure), displaced or comminuted cartilage fractures, avulsed mucosa and dislocated arytenoids.

Operative Timing. Acute operative management (within 24 hours) evolved as a policy at the University of Texas Health Science Center at Dallas in response to the large volume of trauma patients treated at Parkland Memorial Hospital and has been reinforced by other reports.[1-3,6,7] The results of the current study lend strong evidence to the efficacy of an early surgical management program, rather than waiting several days for edema to resolve.[11] Immediate surgical intervention aided identification of mucosal, muscular and cartilaginous injuries, permitting *primary* approximation of *all* involved tissues.

Laryngeal Stents. Internal stents or lumen keepers serve to splint unstable fractures and allow mucosal wounds to heal without leading to webs, adhesions or stenosis. Since many of the more severe injuries disrupt the anterior commissure and involve multiple cartilaginous fractures, stenting following thyrotomy is often indicated. In the present series, stenting was avoided when the laryngeal skeleton remained stable after open reduction and the mucous membrane of the anterior commissure was intact prior to open exploration. Stents were used when the anterior commissure had been traumatically disrupted despite primary repair of the mucous membrane to avoid the possible formation of a web. In choosing a stent, the surgeon should avoid rigid materials which might lead to further mucosal trauma. The stent should be fixed within the endolarynx in such a way that it moves with the larynx during swallowing and is consistently recoverable at endoscopy without further traumatizing the larynx.[2,7,11]

Grafts. In the present study (retrospective and prospective), skin or mucosal grafts were not utilized because in all 51 explored cases wounds were primarily closed. Grafts have been advocated as a supplement to primary closure to epithelialize areas of potential mucosal loss, and such a policy is certainly reasonable and well established.[1-3] The author would only comment that grafts *should not* be considered as a substitute for careful approximation of mucosa, muscle and cartilage necessary to preserve the dynamic function of the larynx.

The results presented in this paper represent an evolving process in diagnostic and surgical treatment of laryngeal trauma. From this work the term "primary management" has come to signify two meanings. In one sense, "primary" indicates immediate or acute surgical intervention. In another sense, "primary" refers to the tissue closure method which is possible in the early injury period. Following these concepts, it is possible to restore phonation and respiratory function to the acutely injured larynx.

REFERENCES

1. Cohn AM, Larson DL. Laryngeal injury: a critical review. Arch Otolaryngol 1976; 102:166-70.

2. Harris HH, Ainsworth JZ. Immediate management of laryngeal and tracheal injuries. Laryngoscope 1965; 75:1103-15.

3. Harris HH, Tobin HA. Acute injuries of the larynx and trachea in 49 patients. Laryngoscope 1970; 80:1376-84.

4. Chadwick DL. Closed injuries of the larynx and pharynx. J Laryngol Otol 1960; 74:306-24.

5. Downey WL, Owen RC, Ward PH. Traumatic laryngeal injury — its management and sequelae. South Med J 1967; 60:756-61.

6. Trone TH, Schaefer SD, Carder HM. Blunt and penetrating laryngeal trauma: a 13-year review. Otolaryngol Head Neck Surg 1980; 88:257-61.

7. Schaefer SD, Carder HM. Fabrication of a simple laryngeal stent. Laryngoscope 1980; 90:1561-3.

8. Bryce DP. The surgical management of laryngotracheal injury. J Laryngol Otol 1972; 86:547-87.

9. Curtin JW, Holinger PH, Greeley PW. Blunt trauma to the larynx and upper trachea. J Trauma 1966; 6:493-502.

10. Krekorian EA. Laryngopharyngeal injuries. Laryngoscope 1975; 85:2069-85.

11. Olson NR. Surgical treatment of acute blunt laryngeal injuries. Ann Otol Rhinol Laryngol 1978; 87:716-21.

ASSESSMENT OF INTUBATION IN CROUP AND EPIGLOTTITIS

JOHN J. ZULLIGER, MD
JOHN P. GARVIN, MD
DAVID E. SCHULLER, MD
HERBERT G. BIRCK, MD
THOMAS P. BEACH, MD
JOHN E. FRANK
COLUMBUS, OHIO

Nasotracheal intubation for the management of airway obstruction in acute epiglottitis has become a well-received practice. However, the same technique has not received widespread support in laryngotracheobronchitis. The purpose of this study was to update the series of nasotracheal intubations in croup and epiglottitis from Columbus Children's Hospital with the specific intent to evaluate its effectiveness. All patients were evaluated for any immediate and delayed complications. Delayed complications were evaluated using parent interviews and measuring expiratory flow rates. This study of 45 children intubated for epiglottitis and 83 intubations for croup reconfirms the earlier report from this institution about its safety in both conditions. However, it has identified a subset of the croup patients who are definitely at risk to develop complications of the technique. In those children under 1 year of age, a disturbingly high incidence of subglottic stenosis was identified and this appeared to be related to the patient's age, tube size, serial intubations (dilatations), and duration of intubation. Suggested guidelines for airway management in the light of the new information are presented.

INTRODUCTION

The treatment of laryngotracheobronchitis (croup) and acute epiglottitis has been gradually evolving over a number of years. Morgan and Wishart[1] cited a 75% mortality for these diseases in 1928. This rate improved dramatically as the importance of good airway management was appreciated. Although the use of endotracheal tubes for the relief of inflammatory upper airway obstruction was suggested as early as 1880 by MacEwan,[2] tracheotomy became the initial treatment of choice because of its effectiveness and supposed relative safety. The first modern use of nasotracheal intubation in the treatment of croup and epiglottitis patients was reported by Allen and Steven in 1965.[3] Since then there have been numerous reports in the literature demonstrating the safety of nasotracheal intubation in the airway management of epiglottitis patients.[4-9] However, there is little information available regarding the safety of intubation in croup cases.[4,10-14]

It is the purpose of this paper to expand the original series of intubated croup and epiglottitis patients from the Columbus Children's Hospital with particular attention being directed to the use of intubation in croup patients. The immediate and delayed complications directly attributable to nasotracheal intubation in croup and epiglottitis will be analyzed as well as technical factors felt to be responsible for them.

SUBJECTS AND METHODS

All patients admitted to Columbus Children's Hospital with either infectious croup or epiglottitis from January 1973 through December 1979, were included in the study (Table 1). However, three patients were admitted after tracheotomy had been performed at another institution and were subsequently excluded. The study population, therefore, included 626 cases of croup and 55 cases of epiglottitis. Eighty-three (13%) of the croup and 45 (82%) of the epiglottitis patients underwent endotracheal intubation.

Evidence of immediate intubation complications was collected from each patient's hospital record. The presence of delayed complications was investigated by three means: 1) the medical records were examined for records of subsequent hospital admissions related to upper airway obstruction, 2) the parents were contacted and carefully questioned regarding the persistence of any symptoms referrable to clinically significant upper airway damage, and 3) the peak expiratory flow rate was measured using the adult model Wright Peak Flowmeter, a pulmonary function test that has been found useful in assessing obstructive airway disease in children. This particular test was chosen because the normal values have been determined by testing over 4000 subjects and have shown close agreement among distinct, independent studies.[15,16]

RESULTS

Means of Intubation. The technique is the same as that described in an earlier paper from this institution.[4] Intubation is accomplished ideally in the operating room by a staff anesthesiologist, as performed in 76% of the epiglottitis intubations and 87% of the croup intubations. A greater percentage of the epiglottitis patients were intubated in the emergency room or at outlying hospitals than the croup patients, again revealing the fulminant nature of this disease.

It was not unusual for the first tube selected to be too large, requiring the selection of a smaller diameter tube. This was particularly true in the croup cases. Twenty-five percent of the croup patients had the initial tube replaced with a larger tube.

From the Department of Otolaryngology and the Department of Anesthesiology, The Ohio State University College of Medicine, and the Columbus Children's Hospital, Columbus. This research was supported in part by grant 1 K07 NS00417-04 from the National Institute of Neurological and Communicative Disorders and Stroke (Teacher-Investigator Award), and in part by grant 7430Z from the Columbus Children's Hospital Research Foundation.

Presented at the meeting of the American Laryngological Association, Palm Beach, Florida, May 1-2, 1982.

REPRINTS — David E. Schuller, MD, Department of Otolaryngology, The Ohio State University, 456 Clinic Drive, Columbus, OH 43210.

TABLE 1. PATIENTS ADMITTED WITH CROUP OR EPIGLOTTITIS

	No. Cases	Primary Tracheotomy	Population Studied	Nonintubated Cases	Intubated Cases No.	%
Croup	629	3	626	543	83	13
Epiglottitis	55	0	55	10	45	82
Totals	684		681		128	19

This was only necessary in seven percent of the epiglottitis patients. The tube changes occurred because of inadequate size for maintenance of the patient's airway. This often resulted in a dilatory effect on the edematous tissue. The critical factor with respect to tube size is that an *adequate* airway is established and *not a maximal* airway which would be more traumatic to the inflamed tissue. Uncuffed polyvinyl chloride tubes are used, and the tube is usually one or two sizes smaller than normal for the patient (Table 2). The tube is secured to a Logan bow which is taped to the face. Moderate to severe difficulty, as recorded on the anesthesia record, was encountered in intubating 29% of the epiglottitis patients and 35% of the croup patients. There have been no cases where an endotracheal tube could not be inserted.

Course of Intubation. The average duration of intubation was 60 hours in the epiglottitis and 144 hours in the croup patients (Table 3). Twenty-three (18%) of the patients extubated themselves accidentally and 14 of them required reintubation for continuing respiratory distress. In addition, seven (8%) of the croup patients required reintubation because of tube occlusion with thick secretions. The vital signs, especially temperature, and the patient's return to near-normal activity, were the parameters used to determine the optimal time for elective extubation. This was routinely done in the recovery room with a staff anesthesiologist in constant attendance. However, 19 (23%) of the intubated croup patients and one (2%) of the intubated epiglottitis patients continued to have respiratory distress following the tube removal and subsequently needed reintubation. Seven (8%) of the croup patients underwent tracheotomy because of inability to extubate after prolonged intubation. The intubated epiglottitis patients remained in the hospital an average of six days versus ten days for the croup patients.

Immediate Complication Rate. In the group of 45 intubated epiglottitis patients, there were no immediate complications. One patient had hypoxic brain injury before intubation at an outlying hospital.

In the group of 83 intubated croup patients, 73 (88%) had no immediate complications. One patient extubated himself the night of intubation and suffered hypoxic encephalopathy and a permanent neurologic deficit. Nine patients (11%) developed subglottic stenosis with seven of these patients requiring tracheotomy before discharge. One patient's tracheotomy tube became decannulated the night before discharge and he died.

Because of the disturbingly high incidence of subglottic stenosis in the patients intubated for croup, these patients were analyzed in greater detail in order to determine any similarities. Seven of these nine patients were under 1 year of age with the average being 11 months. Of the 20 intubated croup cases under 1 year of age, seven patients (35%) developed subglottic stenosis. Among the 7 of 9 stenosis patients in which nasotracheal tube sizes are reported, 6 had the inflamed subglottic larynx "dilated" with a larger tube which was felt to be a better size for airway maintenance. In addition, the tube sizes in the stenosis patients were usually larger and frequently approached the sizes generally used in children with normal airways (Table 2). The children who developed stenosis were intubated longer than those who did not develop stenosis (10.5 days vs 5.3 days). This longer duration reflects the

TABLE 2. SIZE OF ENDOTRACHEAL TUBE USED IN CROUP PATIENTS (N = 78)

	Age										
Tube Size (mm)	*0-6 mo*	*7-11 mo*	*1 yr*	*2 yr*	*3 yr*	*4 yr*	*5 yr*	*6 yr*	*7 yr*	*8 yr*	*9 yr*
3.0	6 (1)	1									
3.5	3	4	7 (1)	3							
4.0	3 (2)	4 (2)	14	7	1						
4.5			4	8	3	1		1			
5.0					2 (1)	1			1		
5.5							1			1	
6.0									1		1

( ) - Subglottic stenosis.
(hatched) - Tube size usually used in children with normal upper airways.
(shaded) - Recommended *maximal* tube size in croup patients.

TABLE 3. COURSE OF INTUBATION

	Croup (*n* = 83)	*Epiglottitis* (*n* = 45)
Self-extubation	18 (22%)	5 (11%)
Reintubation	12 (67%)	2 (40%)
Tube occluded and reintubated	7 (8%)	0
Total	25 (30%)	5 (11%)
Reintubation after elective extubation	19 (23%)	1 (2%)
Tracheotomy	7 (8%)	0
Average duration of intubation	144 hours	60 hours
Average hospital stay	10 days	6 days

difficulty encountered with extubation. An attempt was made to electively extubate all but one of the stenosis patients by the sixth day of intubation and two patients developed stenosis after being intubated for only three and four days respectively. All the stenosis patients underwent subsequent laryngoscopies with dilatations and/or steroid injection (range 1-23 procedures). Six of the seven patients requiring tracheotomy have been successfully decannulated with the one exception who is presently wearing a Silastic T-tube after laryngoplasty.

Delayed Complication Rate. A group of 43 croup patients (52%) were located for evaluation of any delayed complications. Inquiry regarding the existence of any postextubation symptoms revealed 100% to be asymptomatic. Measurements of peak expiratory flow rates were then attempted in 40 of these same patients. Due to the young age and resultant inability to comprehend the task in some cases, it was possible to obtain measurement in 36 of the patients, with 100% being normal. Of the 45 intubated epiglottitis patients, 26 (58%) were asymptomatic and 21 had normal peak flow rates.

DISCUSSION

Some guidelines for the management of acute upper airway obstruction in children have been formulated from the literature over the past decade. Several articles[4,6-9,17,18] have described the favorable use of nasotracheal intubation in the management of epiglottitis patients. The safety of this technique is reconfirmed in the present study. At the same time, other surgeons have reported large series of epiglottitis patients managed by tracheotomy with comparable morbidity and mortality.[5,19-23] Given the nearly equal morbidity and mortality for these two techniques, nasotracheal intubation appears to be preferable to tracheotomy because a surgical procedure is obviated and the duration of hospitalization is shortened, as reported in most series.[7,18,23]

Although there is now adequate guidance in the literature for the management of the airway in epiglottitis, a paucity of reports exists for croup. This is somewhat surprising as croup associated with respiratory failure is more frequently seen than epiglottitis. The few reports in the literature specifically addressing the use of nasotracheal intubation in croup patients have given mixed conclusions regarding its safety. Allen and Steven[24] concluded that nasotracheal intubation in croup patients was a safe technique as long as strict guidelines were followed. They reported three subglottic stenoses in 129 patients (2.3%) intubated for croup. Downes et al[10] reported three cases of subglottic stenosis and two cases of subglottic granuloma formation in 11 intubated patients. In a subsequent report,[11] they advised tracheotomy for croup patients suggesting that the nasotracheal tube acted as a foreign body which further irritated the inflamed, edematous mucosa. The previous report from our institution concluded that nasotracheal intubation for croup was a safe procedure. This report confirms that conclusion, but it also reveals some limitations of this technique for a particular group of children.

TABLE 4. RECOMMENDED MAXIMAL TUBE SIZE IN INTUBATED CROUP PATIENTS

Age	*Tube Size (ID mm)*
Neonate-1year	3.0
1-2 years	3.5
2-5 years	4.0
5-8 years	4.5
8 years- +	5.0

Management of the croup patient with respiratory failure is more difficult than that of the epiglottitis patient and this is probably related to the different histopathology. Unlike epiglottitis, croup is a diffuse inflammatory process involving the entire upper and lower airway. These patients are more difficult to intubate and the first tube selected will often not pass beyond the inflamed subglottic tissue. The younger age of children with croup compared with epiglottitis further exacerbates the problem. Thus, the clinician is caught between placing a tube large enough to adequately ventilate the patient, but not so large that it irritates the injured subglottic larynx.

The copious secretions seen in croup patients is a further complicating factor. These secretions, along with the smaller diameter tubes, account for the 8% incidence of tube occlusion. The higher incidence of self-extubation in croup (22%) compared to epiglottitis (11%) is probably related to the fact that the duration of intubation was twice as long with croup. Two thirds of the self-extubated croup children required emergency reintubation versus 40% for the self-extubated epiglottitis patients. Additionally, there is the high incidence of reintubation (23%) following elective extubation. When the patients who developed subglottic stenosis are analyzed for contributing factors, *young age, tube size, duration of intubation*, and *"dilating" the subglottic larynx* appear to be the most important. The infant larynx already injured by acute inflammation does not tolerate the additional insult of relentless pressure by an endotracheal tube.

Because of the unacceptably high incidence of subglottic stenosis in children with croup under 1 year of age, the following guidelines for airway management in children are currently being considered. When a croup patient develops signs of respiratory failure, he is taken to the operating room where nasotracheal intubation with general inhalational anesthesia is performed using the tube size listed in Table 4 (modified after Allen and Steven).[24] This table lists the *maximal* tube size utilized for each age group and does not correspond to the maximal tube size for normal children of a similar age. Gentle advancement of the tube beyond the edematous tissue is emphasized. If the first tube selected will not *gently* pass through the larynx, then a smaller size is attempted. After a tube is inserted, a larger tube should not be substituted. The edematous subglottic larynx should not be further stressed by dilating it. If the successfully passed tube seems too small in diameter to adequately sustain the patient's ventilation or is too small to permit effective suctioning, then an orderly tracheotomy should be performed.

After the tube is successfully passed, it is securely fixed to the patient's head and the patient is placed in the medical intensive care unit where he will receive continuous surveillance. All patients receive frequent suctioning and constant humidification to the tube. The use of restraints and/or sedation is important to hopefully avoid self-extubation. Techniques of objectively assessing the time for elective extubation are currently being developed. Those patients who require reintubation will undergo tracheotomy and subsequent laryngoscopy before tracheal decannulation.

Eighty-eight percent of the intubated croup patients in the present series and 92% in the total experience were successfully treated without serious complications. However, the percentage of patients less than 1 year old developing subglottic stenosis is too high. The above-mentioned recommendations will hopefully result in a dramatic improvement.

REFERENCES

1. Morgan EA, Wishart DES. Laryngotracheobronchitis — a statistical review of 549 cases. Can Med Assoc J 1947; 56:8-15.

2. MacEwan W. Clinical observations of introduction of tracheal tubes by mouth instead of a tracheotomy. Br Med J 1880; 2:122-65.

3. Allen TH, Steven IM. Prolonged endotracheal intubation in infants and children. Br J Anaesth 1965; 37:566-73.

4. Schuller DE, Birck HG. The safety of intubation in croup and epiglottitis: an eight year follow-up. Laryngoscope 1975; 85:33-46.

5. Cantrell RW, Bell RA, Morioka WF. Acute epiglottitis: intubation versus tracheotomy. Laryngoscope 1978; 88:994-1005.

6. Battaglia JD, Lockhart CH. Management of acute epiglottitis by nasotracheal intubation. Am J Dis Child 1975; 129: 334-6.

7. Oh TH, Motoyama EK. Comparison of nasotracheal intubation and tracheostomy in management of acute epiglottitis. Anesthesiology 1977; 46:214-6.

8. Blanc VF, Weber ML, Leduc C. Acute epiglottitis in children: management of 27 consecutive cases with nasotracheal intubation with special emphasis on anaesthetic considerations. Can Anaesth Soc J 1977; 24:1-11.

9. Tos M. Nasotracheal intubation in acute epiglottitis. Arch Otolaryngol 1973; 97:373-5.

10. Downes JJ, Striker TW, Stool S. Complications of nasotracheal intubation in children with croup. N Engl J Med 1966; 274: 226-7.

11. Striker TW, Stool S, Downes JJ. Prolonged nasotracheal intubation in infants and children. Arch Otolaryngol 1967; 85:210-3.

12. Thomson PD, Olinsky A. Nasotracheal intubation in acute laryngotracheobronchitis. S Afr Med J 1975; 49:785-8.

13. Wesley AG, Desai S, Holloway R. Nasotracheal intubation in the management of infective croup. S Afr Med J 1972; 46: 839-42.

14. Rahbar N, Krishnan V, Rapkin RH. Endotracheal intubation in laryngotracheobronchitis. J Med Soc NJ 1977; 74:771-3.

15. Nairn JR, Bennet AJ, Andrew JD, MacArthur P. A study of respiratory function in normal school children: the peak flow rate. Arch Dis Child 1961; 36:253-8.

16. Polgar G, Promadhat V. Pulmonary function testing in children: techniques and standards. Philadelphia: W. B. Saunders Company, 1971:188-94.

17. Milko DA, Marshuk G, Striker TW. Nasotracheal intubation in the treatment of acute epiglottitis. Pediatrics 1979; 53: 674-7.

18. Rowe LD. Advances and controversies in the management of supraglottitis and laryngotracheobronchitis. Am J Otolaryngol 1980; 1:235-44.

19. Baxter JD. Acute epiglottitis in children. Laryngoscope 1967; 77:1358-67.

20. Cohen SR, Chai J. Epiglottitis: twenty year study with tracheotomy. Ann Otol Rhinol Laryngol 1978; 87:461-7.

21. Mjeon S, Dahl T, Swenson T, Westheim A. Acute epiglottitis in children — an evaluation of the role of tracheotomy. J Laryngol Otol 1979; 93:995-1001.

22. Bjure J, Ejnell H, Jeppsson PH, Martinell S, Sixt R, Tornquist C. Tracheotomy — a satisfactory method in the treatment of acute epiglottitis. A clinical and functional follow-up. Int J Pediatr Otorhinolaryngol 1981; 3:37-43.

23. Crumley RL. Airway management of croup and epiglottitis. West J Med 1977; 126:184-9.

24. Allen TH, Steven IM. Prolonged nasotracheal intubation in infants and children. Br J Anaesth 1972; 44:835-40.

TREATMENT OF SEVERE SUBGLOTTIC STENOSIS WITHOUT TRACHEOTOMY

A PRELIMINARY REPORT

LAUREN D. HOLINGER, MD

CHICAGO, ILLINOIS

Subglottic stenosis in neonates, infants and children is one of the most challenging problems confronting the pediatric otolaryngologist today. Small patients with congenital or acquired stenosis severe enough to require tracheotomy must undergo repeated endoscopic procedures or laryngotracheal reconstruction; weeks, months, or years may be required to attain a lumen large enough to permit decannulation. During 1981, six infants and children with severe subglottic stenosis were managed without tracheotomy. The surgical technique employed involves endoscopic excision of the offending subglottic tissue using the CO_2 laser and suspension microlaryngoscopy. Intraoperative intubation is avoided by using an insufflation technique for general anesthesia which permits unobstructed visualization of the larynx, thereby avoiding laryngeal trauma and edema.

In 1974, Fearon and Cotton[1] startled the pediatric otolaryngologic community with their report of a 24% mortality rate in 25 infants and children with severe subglottic stenosis and tracheotomy who were managed conservatively. While the mortality in another series[2] (85 tracheotomy-dependent patients with subglottic stenosis) was considerably less (5.9%), the fact remains that the mortality among these small children is significant. Cotton and Evans,[3] among others, therefore began to advocate a more aggressive approach to the management of these patients; of 103 patients who underwent laryngotracheal reconstruction to treat mature, hard, fibrous, unresponsive scar in the subglottic larynx, they had only 1 surgical mortality: a mortality rate of less than 1%.

Ideally, severe subglottic stenosis would be treated without tracheotomy at all. Cotton and Seid[4] have been able to accomplish this in premature infants by using an anterior crocoid split as an alternative to tracheotomy when extubation attempts failed. Johnson and Stewart[5] and Downing and Johnson[6] have used the infant urethral resectoscope to treat three children with subglottic stenosis without tracheotomy. Koufman et al[7] reported endoscopic management of subglottic stenosis with the CO_2 surgical laser; tracheotomy was avoided in three children who had severe subglottic stenosis. The present report presents the preliminary results of six infants and children with severe subglottic stenosis managed endoscopically without tracheotomy using the CO_2 laser.

The indications for laser management of severe subglottic stenosis without tracheotomy are not yet well defined. It seems that any premature infant, full term infant, or child requiring tracheotomy who is stable and healthy enough to breathe spontaneously and undergo general anesthesia, would be a candidate for the procedure. The ideal application for the described technique is a discrete, short, soft tissue subglottic stenosis which does not involve the entire circumference of the subglottic larynx (Fig. 1). However, the technique has been used successfully in cases which have also had involvement of the supraglottic or glottic larynx, or upper trachea as well. A case report of the first child with severe subglottic stenosis managed without tracheotomy illustrates the indications and usefulness of the procedure.

CASE REPORT

Case 3. The patient was a 4½-month-old female who had been well until age 2 months, when she had begun to have typical symptoms of upper airway obstruction. Endoscopic evaluation by a pediatric surgeon yielded no specific diagnosis but the laryngeal aperture was felt to be slightly small. The patient was placed on steroids and her symptoms remained stable for one month. Increasing symptoms prompted the parents to seek the opinion of an otolaryngologist who observed a small larynx; severe respiratory distress following the laryngoscopy necessitated intubation. The patient extubated herself the night following the procedure; immediate reintubation was necessary.

When first seen by the author, the patient was resting comfortably with a 3.0# orotracheal tube securely in place. Chest x-ray films and barium esophagram had been normal; lateral xeroradiogram of the neck suggested airway compromise at the glottic or subglottic level. She was extubated 48 hours later. In spite of steroids and racemic epinephrine she developed progressive airway distress with increasing pCO_2 and therefore was taken to the operating room for laryngoscopy and bronchoscopy under general anesthesia. The larynx was erythematous and edematous throughout; the subglottic larynx had a fullness on the left covered with normal but traumatized mucosa. An eschar was present posterolaterally on the left where there was also early granulation tissue formation. Telescopic examination of the trachea and main bron-

From the Division of Otolaryngology and Communicative Disorders, Department of Surgery, The Children's Memorial Hospital, and the Department of Otolaryngology and Bronchoesophagology, Rush Medical College, Rush-Presbyterian-St. Luke's Medical Center, Chicago.

Presented at the meeting of the American Laryngological Association, Palm Beach, Florida, May 1-2, 1982.

REPRINTS — Lauren D. Holinger, MD, 155 North Michigan Avenue, Chicago, IL 60601.

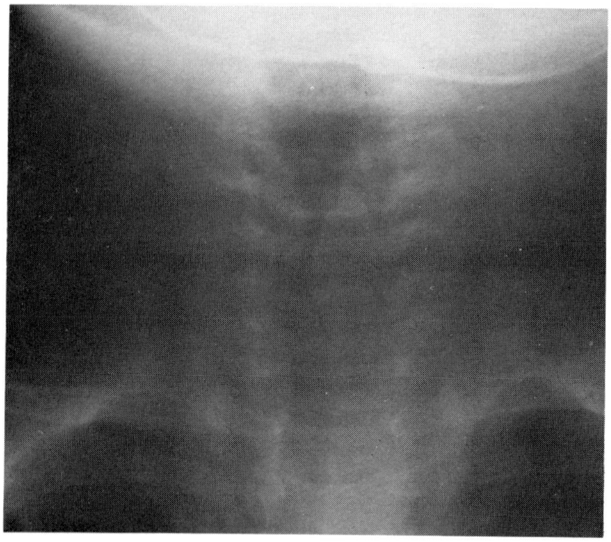

Fig. 1. (Case 4) Posteroanterior chest x-ray film demonstrating subglottic stenosis primarily involving left subglottic larynx.

chi was normal. Biopsies of the subglottic area showed fragments of columnar and squamous mucosa with inflammation and hyperplasia. The subglottic lumen was enlarged endoscopically with the CO_2 laser, removing tissue primarily from the left.

The patient had no respiratory symptoms for five days following the procedure. Over the next two days she developed intermittent stridor which responded dramatically to racemic epinephrine. At direct laryngoscopy seven days following the first laser procedure, an eschar was observed in the left subglottic larynx compromising the airway by 50%. It was removed with cupped forceps and the area was again biopsied. An 18 French brass laryngeal dilator was passed easily. The biopsy showed small fragments of squamous epithelium and fibrous tissue with acute and chronic inflammation and occasional foreign body giant cells.

Although she remained asymptomatic endoscopic re-evaluation was accomplished one week later. The mucosa in the left subglottic larynx was somewhat rough but the airway appeared normal; the 18 French dilator passed with ease through the larynx. She was discharged to be followed by her pediatrician.

Ten and one-half months later the parents were contacted to obtain follow-up information for the present study. Stridor and wheezing had recurred, which her pediatrician had diagnosed as asthma and was treating with bronchodilators. Shortly thereafter she developed acute, more severe respiratory distress which did not respond to subcutaneous epinephrine; racemic epinephrine and systemic steroids did relieve symptoms somewhat. A croup-like cough developed. Lateral xeroradiogram of the neck showed airway compromise at the glottic and subglottic larynx. The patient underwent endoscopic re-evaluation and laser excision of subglottic tissue on the left within one week (Fig. 2). Another similar procedure one week later relieved recurrent symptoms; she has had occasional mild stridor since.

METHODS AND MATERIALS

During 1981, 24 patients with subglottic stenosis were diagnosed by the author at The Children's Memorial Hospital and Rush-Presbyterian-St. Luke's Medical Center in Chicago. Follow-up is reported through May 1, 1982. A detailed review was made of the six patients whose subglottic stenosis was severe enough the require tracheotomy but in whom tracheotomy was avoided by enlarging the airway with the CO_2 laser (Table 1).

The diagnosis was confirmed endoscopically. Laryngoscopy and bronchoscopy were carried out in all patients to identify any other abnormalities of the larynx and tracheobronchial tree; usually this was not done at the initial procedure because of the extreme degree of airway obstruction. Any instrumentation of the subglottic larynx might have produced traumatic edema and precipitated tracheotomy. Examination of the tracheobronchial tree was accomplished without passing a bronchoscopic tube in three patients. They were examined with the Hopkins rod telescope (from a 3 mm x 20 cm Storz bronchoscope) which was passed carefully through the subglottic area into the trachea and each main bronchus, thus avoiding the additional trauma of the larger bronchoscopic tube.

The Cavitron CO_2 laser coupled to a Zeiss operating microscope was used for all patients. One to 1.5 mg/kg of dexamethazone (Decadron) was given intravenously prior to or during most endoscopic procedures to minimize postoperative edema. Postoperatively, patients were kept on high humidity oxygen or an ultrasonic nebulizer to minimize eschar formation. Build-up of fibrinous exudate and eschar formation often necessitated follow-up procedures to remove the eschar and re-establish an adequate airway. Typically, this occurred 3-6 days following a laser procedure. Racemic epinephrine (0.1-0.5 ml, 2.25% diluted in 2.5 cc normal saline) delivered with a nebulizer with 100% O_2 via face mask often provided temporary relief from respiratory distress.

Most patients were premedicated with atropine only (0.03 mg/kg). Pentazocine (Talwin), narcotics and barbituates were avoided because of their tendency to depress respiration. General

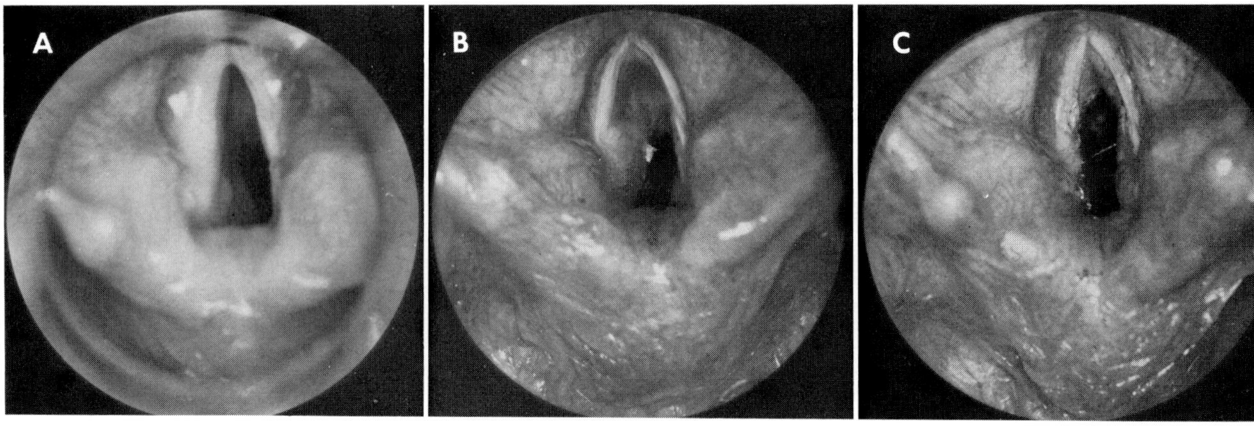

Fig. 2. (Case 3) A) Preoperative endoscopic view of recurrent soft subglottic stenosis at direct laryngoscopy. Lesion is primarily left-sided. Because laryngoscope is in right corner of mouth right vocal cord obscures right subglottic area. B) Intraoperative view. Laser excision of lower portion of stenosis has been accomplished. Trauma from laryngoscope has produced edema in anterior and superior portions of subglottic area. C) Immediate postoperative view. Endoscopic excision has been completed with enlargement of airway. Mucosa at the anterior commissure has been spared.

TABLE 1. SEVERE SUBGLOTTIC STENOSIS PATIENTS TREATED WITHOUT TRACHEOTOMY

Patient No.	Sex	Age at Onset of Symptoms	Age at Diagnosis (1st Endo.)	Nature of Airway Compromise	Clinical History	Duration of Intubation	No. of Procedures Laser	No. of Procedures Total Endo.	Etiology
1	M	18 mo	4½ yr	Subglottic: fibrous, circumferential (focal submucosal fibrosis, chronic inflammation) Glottic: bilateral cysts, posterior commissure synechia	Prematurity; RDS/BPD, croup 2/yr; 2 days severe progressive respiratory distress	2 mo	3	3	Acquired (following intubation)
2	F	14 mo	14½ mo	Subglottic: soft tissue; granulation tissue Glottic: anterior glottic web Supraglottic: bilateral ventricular protrusions; tracheal and bronchial compression	Aspiration and respiratory arrest 6 mo after division of vascular ring. Failed extubation	2 days x 2	3	10	Acquired (following intubation)
3	F	2 mo	4½ mo	Subglottic: soft tissue (acute and chronic inflammation, glandular hyperplasia, foreign body giant cells)	Progressive biphasic stridor; required intubation following diagnostic endo.	4 days	3	5	Congenital
4	F	3 wk	10 wk	Subglottic: soft tissue, left (glandular hyperplasia, chronic inflammation, foreign body giant cells)	Progressive stridor and barking cough; acute obstruction after diagnostic endo.	0	7	11	Congenital
5	F	Birth	8 wk	Subglottic: anterior, firm (not biopsied)	Progressive biphasic stridor; intubated and transferred following diagnostic endo. elsewhere	1 day	1	1	Congenital
6	F	5 mo	5 mo	Subglottic: soft tissue; edema, granuloma, exudate (necrosis, acute inflammation) Trachea: circumferential, high (7 mm below cords) fibrous stenosis; aberrant innominate artery	Failed extubation following meningitis, coma and seizures	0	2	9	Acquired (following intubation)
	Total						19	39	

Endo - Endoscopic or endoscopy; RDS - Respiratory distress syndrome; BPD - Bronchopulmonary dysplasia.

anesthesia was used in all cases. Routine induction was by mask using halothane (Fluothane), nitrous oxide and oxygen. Spontaneous respiration was maintained throughout, assisting the patient during induction only if necessary. Topical anesthesia using 1-2% lidocaine (Xylocaine) was administered to the trachea, larynx and hypopharynx with an atomizer. The dose of lidocaine did not exceed 3 mg/kg. After deepening anesthesia, a large bore suction catheter or a small (3-3.5 mm) endotracheal tube was placed through one nostril for delivery of anesthetic gases into the hypopharynx by insufflation. The position of the tip of the catheter in the pharynx was checked with a laryngoscope and the catheter carefully held or secured with a small piece of tape to the nose or cheek. The fraction of inspired oxygen (FiO_2) was limited to 50% (0.5).

A pediatric anterior commissure microlaryngoscope was used to visualize the larynx then stabilized with a Lewy laryngoscope holder supported on a Mayo stand brought across the patient's chest and abdomen (Fig. 3).

Biopsies were taken when the airway was adequate. The operating microscope and laser were positioned for removal of the offending subglottic tissue. If anesthesia lightened and the patient began to cough or if respiration became too shallow or ceased, intubation was easily accomplished through the laryngoscope. The endotracheal tube was removed when spontaneous respiration was restored, permitting an unobstructed view of the larynx for endoscopic surgery.

The laser may be used to remove tissue from the subglottic larynx and upper trachea, sometimes as far as 2 cm below the superior surface of the vocal cords. This is possible in some infants as well as children and adults. Trials with different pediatric microscopic laryngoscopes and various angles of alignment are necessary to determine which works best with each individual patient. Use of the left hand to manipulate the larynx and upper trachea while aiming the laser with the right obviates continual realignment of the laryngoscope and operating microscope (Fig. 4). One attempts to align the target area more perpendicular to the direction of the laser, giving a more precise burn rather than a tangential one. Removal of tissue from the entire circumference of the lumen at one procedure is avoided.

RESULTS

Six of seven infants and children with severe subglottic stenosis who were considered for (laser) treatment to avoid tracheotomy have indeed avoided tracheotomy. A total of 24 infants and children were diagnosed as having subglottic stenosis during 1981 (Table 2). Twelve of these had subglottic stenosis severe enough to require tracheotomy, only 6 of whom actually underwent tracheotomy; the other 6 were treated with endoscopic laser surgery and tracheotomy was avoided. For various reasons of logistics or timing, no attempt could be made to use the laser as an alternative to tracheotomy in five patients. In one patient, a laser procedure could not be initiated because of extreme respiratory distress, laryngospasm, and difficulty atttaining an adequate exposure for suspension microlaryngoscopy.

The clinical data of the six patients who were spared tracheotomy are presented in Table 1. These six patients underwent a total of 39 endoscopic procedures, an average of 6.5 procedures each. The

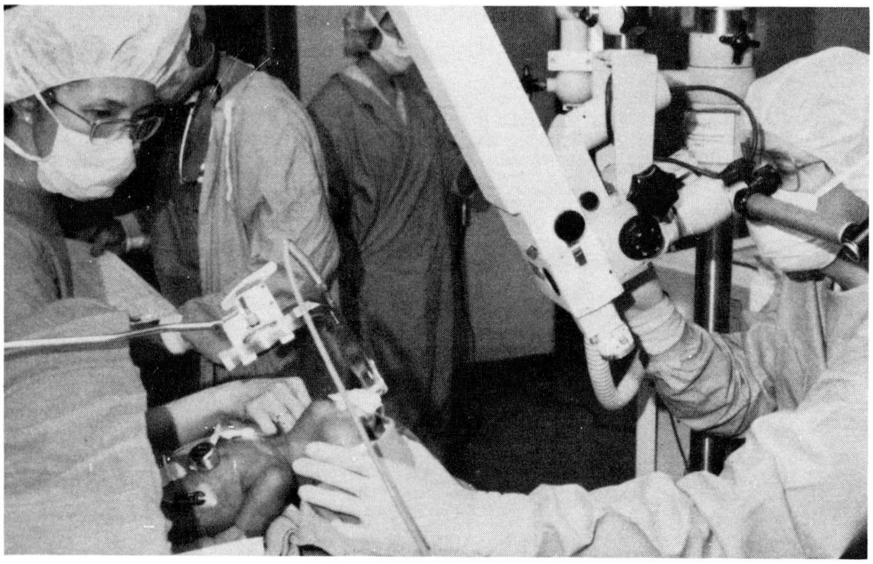

Fig. 3. Suspension microlaryngoscopy in a 3200 g infant undergoing laser removal of subglottic tissue. General anesthesia is maintained using insufflation technique.

laser was used in 19 (49%) of the procedures; the other 20 were done to remove eschar, to dilate or biopsy the larynx, or for diagnostic purposes only. Biopsies were taken when possible; the severity of the airway compromise precluded biopsy completely in one patient. Biopsies were sometimes taken at later procedures when a better airway had been established. Four of the six patients (cases 2, 3, 4, 6) exhibited a tendency for the soft tissue narrowing to recur; this tissue was quite soft and not a hard, fibrous, cicatricial or cartilaginous stenosis. Repeated biopsies showed no suggestion of hemangioma in any of these patients.

Of the 6 patients with severe subglottic stenosis treated without tracheotomy 5 were female, 1 male. The onset of symptoms occurred at age 14 months or younger in all except one patient; in four patients the onset of symptoms occurred under 6 months of age (Table 1). Three of the stenoses were congenital; three were acquired secondary to endotracheal intubation.

No deaths occurred in these patients, nor were any major complications encountered. One minor anesthetic complication occurred when the insufflation catheter was inadvertantly passed too far and entered the esophagus. The stomach was rapidly and massively distended with anesthetic gases. The problem was immediately recognized, the tube withdrawn and the stomach evacuated by passing a nasogastric tube. No long-term sequelae occurred.

DISCUSSION

Several authors have demonstrated the feasibility of treating subglottic stenosis without tracheotomy; anterior cricoid split,[4] the infant urethral resectoscope,[5,6] and the CO_2 laser[7] are the means by which this has been achieved. Of the many surgeons who have used the laser to treat subglottic stenosis, most have reported experience with patients in whom a tracheotomy was already in place and most report treatment exclusively or primarily of adult patients. Three children in the series of Koufman et al[7] had laser excision of subglottic tissue as an alternative to tracheotomy. Healy and his coauthors have used the laser in similar fashion in infants and children with subglottic hemangioma,[8] avoiding tracheotomy in many such patients. The use of the laser to treat severe subglottic stenosis without tracheotomy in infants and children is a logical application of these indications and techniques.

The use of the insufflation technique for administering general anesthesia to infants and small children is a most important technical aspect of the endoscopic treatment of severe subglottic stenosis without tracheotomy. It allows the surgeon unobstructed access to the subglottic space, since no tracheal tube of any type is used in the larynx. The technique is difficult and some anesthesiologists are reluctant to use it. Complete cooperation between the surgeon and the anesthesiologist is required; the anesthesiologist must allow the surgeon to accept full responsibility for the airway. Intermittent

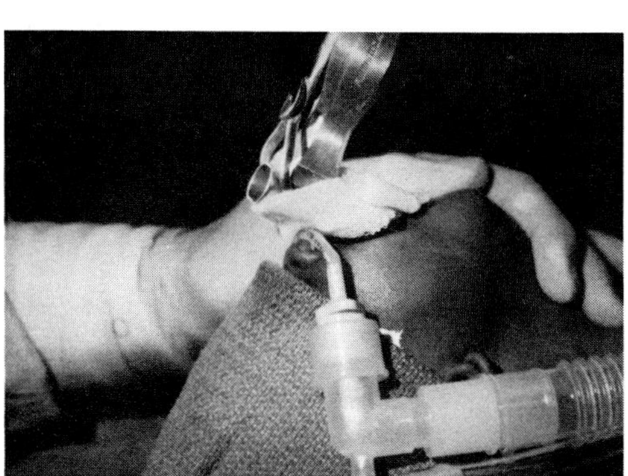

Fig. 4. Close-up of infant illustrated in Fig. 3 showing 3 mm endotracheal tube entering right nostril; tube tip rests in nasopharynx. A moist sponge protects the infant's gums and lips. Fingers of surgeon's left hand manipulate larynx and upper trachea.

TABLE 2. TRACHEOTOMY AND DEGREE OF SUBGLOTTIC STENOSIS

	No. of Patients
Mild or moderate subglottic stenosis	
Tracheotomy unnecessary	9
Tracheotomy for pulmonary pathology or pathology other than subglottic stenosis	3*
Severe subglottic stenosis	
No opportunity for laser	5*
Unable to use laser (laryngospasm and exposure problems)	1*
Tracheotomy avoided	6
Total	24

*Underwent tracheotomy.

laryngospasm and apnea occasionally complicate the procedure; another drawback is the exposure of operating room personnel to inhalation anesthetics. Scavenging of anesthetic vapors is performed whenever possible. For adequate protection, personnel in the immediate proximity (especially the surgeon and anesthesiologist) should wear an oxygen (or air) mask, or an activated charcoal absorbent mask.[9]

The term subglottic stenosis has been used with less precision recently, particularly by specialists in fields other than otolaryngology. By definition, the term applies to a narrowing or stricture of the subglottic larynx: the region extending from the insertion of the conus elasticus into the vocal cords to the inferior margin of the cricoid cartilage; the upper trachea is not included. The term should exclude all conditions such as neoplasms, extrinsic compression (such as vascular rings) and acute inflammatory conditions (such as croup).

Subglottic stenosis may be categorized in three ways: 1) etiology (congenital or acquired); 2) clinical/anatomic (hard or soft, degree [percent] of stenosis and precise anatomic location); 3) histopathology. The histopathologic classification is most helpful since knowledge of the precise histopathology of a lesion makes the treatment of choice almost self-evident. At present, however, it is possible to make this determination in two ways: 1) at the time of laryngotomy for a reconstructive procedure or 2) postmortem with whole-section organ mounts of the larynx. Continued advances in the technology of computer-assisted tomographic scanning will likely make earlier, more precise diagnosis possible in the future. At this time, however, the clinician is limited to the clinical/anatomic description of any particular lesion. This is correlated with the likely histopathologic diagnosis and therapy determined accordingly.

The more accurate the histopathologic diagnosis, the more precise and appropriate will be the treatment. Table 3 outlines the histopathologic classification of subglottic stenosis. Hard subglottic stenoses fall into two categories: fibrous (which can be dilated but tend to restenose shortly after each dilation) or cartilaginous (which cannot be dilated).

TABLE 3. HISTOPATHOLOGIC CLASSIFICATION OF SUBGLOTTIC STENOSIS

- Cartilaginous stenosis
  - Cricoid cartilage deformity (stenosis)
    - Normal shape
      - Small for infant's size
    - Abnormal shape
      - Large anterior lamina
      - Oval (elliptical) shape
      - Large posterior lamina
      - Generalized thickening
      - Submucous (occult) cleft
      - Other congenital cricoid stenoses
  - Trapped first tracheal ring
- Soft tissue stenosis
  - Submucosal fibrosis (fibrous connective tissue)
  - Submucosal mucinous gland hyperplasia
  - Granulation tissue

The clinical importance of diagnosing cartilaginous stenosis is that these stenoses are not responsive to dilation and must either be treated by a laryngotracheal reconstructive procedure or the child must wear a tracheotomy tube for an extended period of time (years) until the problem is outgrown. The prognosis for a hard, fibrous, cicatricial acquired subglottic stenosis is likely to be the same.

Soft subglottic stenoses usually represent granulation tissue, submucosal mucinous gland hyperplasia, or combinations in association with submucosal fibrosis. These stenoses dilate readily but collapse upon withdrawal of the dilator. Acquired subglottic or tracheal stenoses with loss of catilaginous support behave similarly. Soft tissue stenoses may be congenital (especially submucosal mucinous gland hyperplasia) or acquired (as with submucosal fibrosis and granulation tissue). The six cases reported here which were treated successfully without tracheotomy were soft stenoses; none were cartilaginous, nor had any of the acquired stenoses progressed to become the firm, circumferential, cicatricial type.

Many stenoses are not purely one histopathologic type or another. Often they are not confined exclusively to the supraglottic larynx but involve the glottic or supraglottic larynx or the upper trachea as well. Similarly, it is not unusual to find patients in whom an underlying congenital subglottic stenosis is complicated by submucosal fibrosis or granulation tissue acquired from endotracheal intubation. The ideal lesion for application of the technique described herein is a discrete, short, soft stenosis which does not involve the entire circumference of the subglottic larynx. However, it appears that the laser technique can be considered for any premature infant, full term infant, or child with adequate lungs who fails extubation or requires tracheotomy for congenital or acquired laryngeal (or high tracheal) chronic or subacute pathology.

The histopathologic classification of subglottic stenosis outlined in Table 3 incorporates recent contributions of Tucker et al[10] and a review by Morimitsu et al.[11] The latter article presents a case of congenital cricoid stenosis and contains an excellent illustrated diagrammatic summary of cartilaginous stenoses reported up to 1981. Tucker[10] has reported and detailed in a fine histopathologic study the trapped first tracheal ring and a small elliptical cricoid ring. He has also observed two cases of submucous (occult) clefts of the posterior cricoid lamina which probably represent incomplete laryngotracheoesophageal clefts (personal communication 1982).

In conclusion, six infants and children with severe subglottic stenosis have successfully undergone endoscopic laser surgery to avoid tracheotomy. All patients survived; no major complications occurred. The surgical technique employs suspension microlaryngoscopy and the CO_2 laser. An insufflation technique for administration of general anesthesia is used; spontaneous respiration is maintained and intubation avoided. The technique may be considered for any premature infant, full term infant, or child with adequate lungs who must undergo tracheotomy for severe subglottic stenosis.

ACKNOWLEDGMENTS — The author thanks Ms Carla Gaona for her assistance in the preparation of the tables and manuscript. Lucida Rita, MD, provided information for the description of the insufflation technique of general anesthesia. Gabriel F. Tucker, MD, contributed his expertise and advice for the histopathologic classification of subglottic stenosis.

REFERENCES

1. Fearon B, Cotton RT. Surgical correction of subglottic stenosis of the larynx in infants and children: progress report. Ann Otol Rhinol Laryngol 1974; 83:428-31.

2. Holinger PH, Kutnick SL, Schild JA, Holinger LD. Subglottic stenosis in infants and children. Ann Otol Rhinol Laryngol 1976; 85:591-600.

3. Cotton RT, Evans JNG. Laryngotracheal reconstruction in children: five year follow-up. Ann Otol Rhinol Laryngol 1981; 90:515-20.

4. Cotton RT, Seid AB. Management of the extubation problem in the premature child: anterior cricoid split as an alternative to tracheotomy. Ann Otol Rhinol Laryngol 1980; 89:508-11.

5. Johnson DG, Stewart DR. Management of acquired tracheal obstructions in infancy. J Pediatr Surg 1975; 10:709-17.

6. Downing TP, Johnson DG. Excision of subglottic stenosis with the urethral resectoscope. J Pediatr Surg 1979; 14:252-7.

7. Koufman JR, Thompson JN, Kohut RI. Endoscopic management of subglottic stenosis with the CO_2 surgical laser. Otolaryngol Head Neck Surg 1981; 89:215-20.

8. Healy GB, McGill T, Strong MS. Surgical advances in the treatment of lesions of the pediatric airway: the role of the carbon dioxide laser. Pediatrics 1978; 61:380-3.

9. Brummitt WM, Fearon B, Brama I. Anesthesia for laryngeal laser surgery in the infant and child. Ann Otol Rhinol Laryngol 1981; 90:475-7.

10. Tucker GF, Ossoff RH, Newman AN, Holinger LD. Histopathology of congenital subglottic stenosis. Laryngoscope 1979; 89:866-76.

11. Morimitsu T, Matsumoto I, Okada S, Takahashi M, Kosugi T. Congenital cricoid stenosis. Laryngoscope 1981; 91: 1356-64.

Ann Otol Rhinol Laryngol 91:1982

INFANT TRACHEOTOMY

CAROL ROBERTS GERSON, MD GABRIEL F. TUCKER, JR, MD

CHICAGO, ILLINOIS

The pediatric and neonatal tracheotomies done on our patients at Children's Memorial Hospital since 1975 have been reviewed. Patients' ages, birth weights, rates of complications, decannulations and deaths have been studied. As compared to previous studies, the proportion of procedures done on children in the first year of life has dramatically increased. A technique which has been modified for the small infant is described.

INTRODUCTION

Infant tracheotomy continues to evolve as the proportion of smaller patients increases. A number of modifications of operative technique for the neonate have seemed appropriate. These along with statistical analysis of our current experience are reported.

TECHNIQUE (Fig. 1)

Whenever possible, regardless of the age of the patient, all tracheotomies are performed under general anesthesia in the operating room with a controlled airway. Since many patients have an indwelling endotracheal tube and further need for prolonged ventilatory support, it is felt safest to perform the tracheotomies over the endotracheal tube and to defer definitive inspection of the larynx until the time of the initial tube change, usually one week. In all but three of these cases the tracheotomy was performed with an airway established and maintained easily with an endotracheal tube or bronchoscope. In these three cases attempts to pass either an endotracheal tube or a bronchoscope failed. One patient was a Pierre Robin child with an extremely small mandible, another was a case of massive maxillofacial and head trauma, and the third was a case of severe tongue swelling following a cleft palate repair in an infant.

A shoulder roll is placed and the patient is prepped and draped except for the face which is left visible both to the otolaryngologist and the anesthesiologist so that the patient's respiratory status and oxygenation can be easily monitored and the airway kept accessible. The hyoid bone and the cricoid cartilage are palpated (the neonatal thyroid cartilage is often difficult to palpate). The incision begins at the cricoid cartilage and extends 1-2 cm inferiorly, after injecting with a small amount of local anesthetic combined with 1:200,000 epinephrine. The soft tissues are dissected in the midline with sharp and blunt dissection and with the use of hemostats as retractors. When the thyroid isthmus is exposed a suture is placed in the trachea immediately below the cricoid cartilage and above the isthmus and thyroid. A suture is preferable to a hook since it will not disengage or tear the tracheal tissue as easily. Using the suture for traction, the trachea is elevated and a second suture is placed behind the thyroid isthmus. This suture can then be used to elevate the isthmus so that it is more easily dissected from the tracheal wall. The isthmus is double-clamped, divided, and oversewn with chromic suture, left long until the stay sutures are placed. The isthmus is always divided to prevent it from obscuring the tracheal incision in the event of an accidental decannulation. The isthmus divided, the initial suture can be laddered downward to provide traction slightly lower on the tracheal wall. The trachea is cleaned with cotton swabs and two black silk stay sutures are placed just to the right and left of the midline, circling tracheal rings 3 and 4. These sutures are tied several centimeters from the trachea and left long to be taped to the chest at the termination of the procedure. After the stay sutures are in place the thyroid sutures may then be cut and a vertical incision is made in the tracheal wall beginning inferiorly and proceeding superiorly to avoid traumatizing a high cupula or any mediastinal contents. An attempt is made to incise just the tracheal rings and then to complete the incision through the tracheal mucosa with a small hemostat to avoid any possibility of trauma to the posterior tracheal wall. A Shiley "neonatal" tracheotomy tube is placed in the incision under direct vision using the sutures as traction after the endotracheal tube has been withdrawn to just above the tracheal incision under our direct vision.

Once the tube is in place, the anesthesiologist then attaches to the tracheotomy tube and when adequate ventilation is assured, the endotracheal tube is fully withdrawn. Stay sutures are taped to the chest and kept in place for one week. At this

---

From the Division of Bronchoesophagology/Otolaryngology, Children's Memorial Hospital, Chicago. Support of the Edward Shedd Wells Fund is gratefully acknowledged.

Presented at the meeting of the American Laryngological Association, Palm Beach, Florida, May 1-2, 1982.

REPRINTS — Gabriel F. Tucker, Jr, MD, The Children's Memorial Hospital, 2300 Children's Plaza, Chicago, IL 60614.

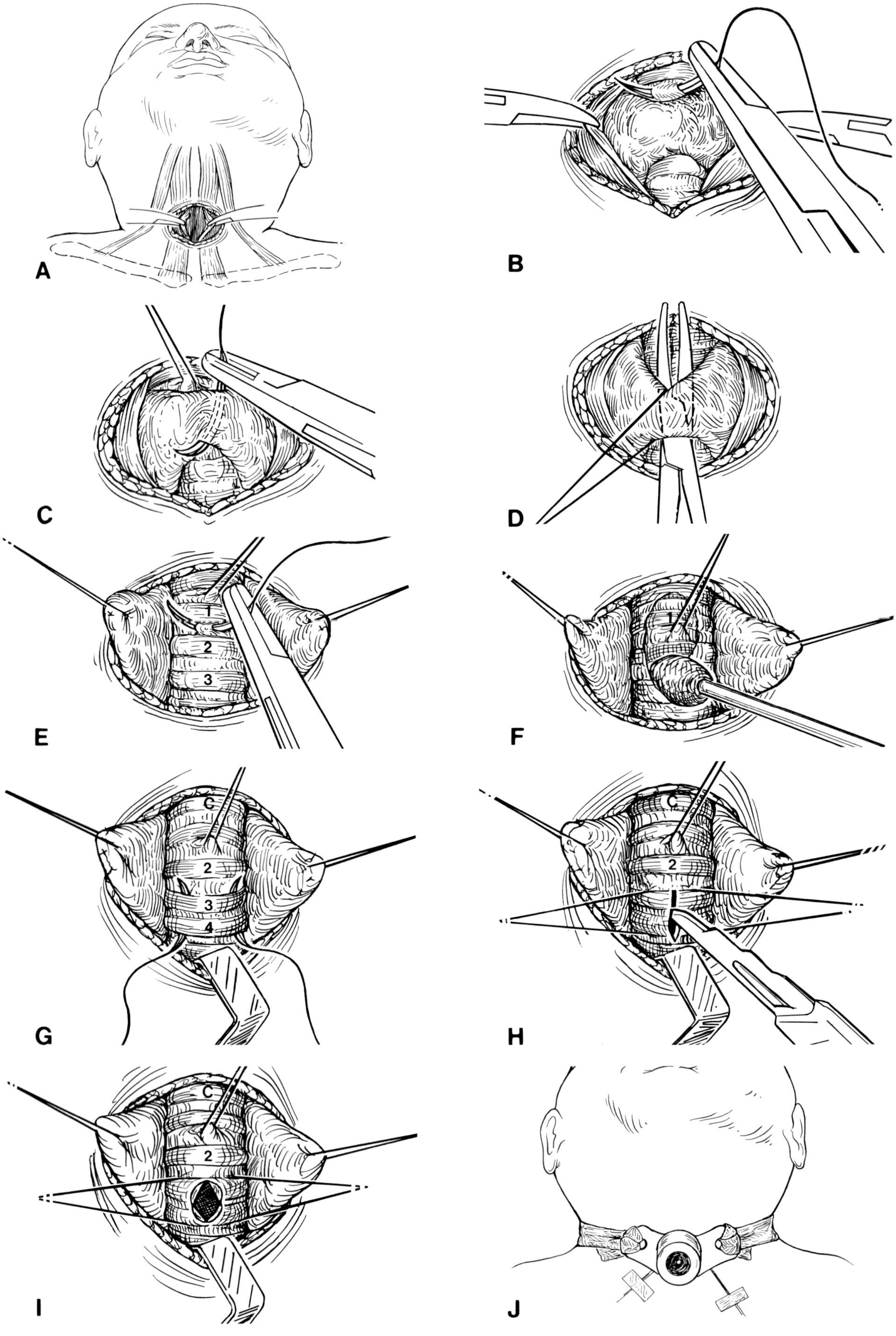
A
B
C
D
1
2
3
E
1
F
C
2
3
4
G
C
2
H
C
2
I
J

time it is hoped that the stoma will have begun to form. The initial tube change is done in the operating room under general anesthesia with the airway under endoscopic control, thus permitting a leisurely controlled inspection of the laryngeal pathology at a time when mucosal reaction, tube imprints, etc., have settled down. Further tracheotomy changes can be carried out by the resident or the nursing staff on a regular hospital floor. Daily tube changes, both in the hospital and at home, are advised to minimize stomal reaction, granulation tissue, etc; an antibiotic and/or steroid ointment is used to lubricate the replacement tube.

At this time it is worthwhile to note the introduction by Shiley of the neonatal tracheotomy tube. This is manufactured in the same sizes as the "pediatric" tube and has been modified to have a shorter cannula, more appropriate for the infant's trachea, and a smaller flange, more appropriate for the size of the infant's neck. This modifies the plastic pediatric tube to specifications similar to that of the silver Holinger tube.

Although developed for the neonate, the technical points just elaborated have been found applicable to the infant and child.

STATISTICS

Since 1975, 123 patients have undergone tracheotomy. Although previous studies have reported a consistent 2:1 male to female ratio, only 60% of the patients were male.[1-3] Over the last ten years there has been a significant change in the proportion of patients under one year of age who require tracheotomies. Sixty-four percent of the patients were less than 1 year of age, and 21% were between 1 and 5 years, only 11% being 5 years or older (Fig. 2).[1] This distribution is similar to that reported by Hawkins and Williams.[4] There were 18 premature infants included in this study. Their birth weights ranged from 600 to 2000 g, and gestational ages from 26 to 32 weeks. The age range of these patients at the time of tracheotomy was between 2 and 9 months. Most of the patients have been intubated for a significant portion of their lives prior to tracheotomy. A few who were intubated early in life were able to be extubated, but were found to have a subglottic stenosis and an inadequate airway after several months of extubation. There were seven full-term infants who were tracheotomized within the first 28 days of life.

The indications for tracheotomy were many and varied. There were a few patients, especially the neonates, who had primary upper airway insufficiency. These included bilateral cord paralysis, Pierre Robin syndrome, Treacher-Collins syndrome, arthrogryposis, and severe congenital subglottic stenosis. Most of the other patients were tracheotomized secondary to other medical problems, many of which were multisystem and complicated. There were numerous children with complex cardiac disease, significant neurological problems, and many with pulmonary disease related to prematurity. There were a few patients with tumors, several with head injuries and maxillofacial trauma, especially among those over five years of age. Only one patient was tracheotomized for upper airway respiratory infection.

There were few complications thought to be directly related to the procedure: two cases of pneumothorax, one case of which was secondary to displacement of the tube in the Neonatal Intensive Care Unit and attempts to ventilate through a tube in subcutaneous tissue. There were three cases of tube displacement within the first 24 hours after the procedure. There were two cases of postoperative bleeding, neither of which were directly related to the tracheostome; both appeared to be from dilated bronchial vessels traumatized by a suction catheter and to be coming from below the level of the tracheostome. A cardiac arrest occurred in one patient at the conclusion of the procedure, due to transient hypoxia when the tracheotomy tube replaced the endotracheal tube. The patient survived without sequelae. In one patient with a tracheoesophageal fistula the tip of the tracheotomy tube persistently fell into the fistula and rested in the esophagus. There were no operative deaths.

Thirty percent of our patients who are still alive have been decannulated. There are no patients at this time who are unable to be decannulated because of persistent stomal problems. Twenty percent of the original group of patients have died. In only one of these patients was there a suspicion that the death may have been caused by obstruction of the airway in a patient with an obligate tracheotomy. All other deaths were felt to be secondary to a progressive primary disease or multisystem failure. Because of the extreme fragility of our youngest babies, we have found a higher percentage of these patients do not survive; 36% of the premature babies died.[5]

DISCUSSION

There are several points which are of interest in reviewing these patients. As noted above, there is a higher proportion of females than in many of the previous studies. The significant preponderance of tracheotomy performed for infectious disease noted

Fig. 1. Technique used in infant tracheotomy. A) Incision in the midline with the use of hemostats as retractors. B) Traction suture above the thyroid isthmus. C) Suture behind the isthmus for easier dissection from the trachea. D) Elevation of the isthmus. E) Laddering downward of the traction suture. F) Cleaning of the trachea with cotton swabs. G) Stay sutures placed on either side of the midline between rings 3 and 4. H) Incision of the tracheal wall, to the mucosa, with a knife blade pointing superiorly. Mediastinum protected with a retractor. I) Use of the traction sutures to hold the incision open. J) Placement of the neonatal tube with a small flange; traction sutures taped to the chest. (Note: The thyroid isthmus reaches the second tracheal ring by the seventh week of fetal life.)

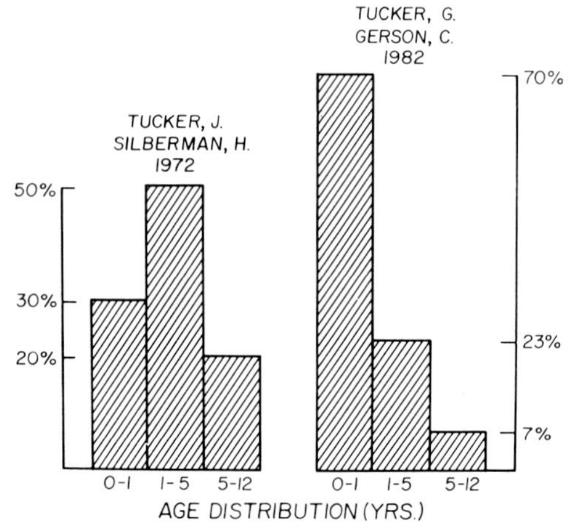

Fig. 2. Age incidence of tracheotomy under 12 years of age.

in previous studies has changed. Tracheotomies are not being performed for epiglottitis at The Children's Memorial Hospital today. We very rarely find it necessary to tracheotomize a patient secondary to laryngotracheobronchitis.[6] We are tracheotomizing many more very young and premature infants. It is possible that the change in emphasis on the indication for tracheotomy may relate to the change in sex distribution.

As our technology and skills in salvaging the premature and damaged child improves, the number of candidates in the youngest age group will, of course, increase. The youngest babies seemed to be carried for longer periods of time with endotracheal tubes in place than many of the older children. If our cardiac surgeons foresee a prolonged period of ventilation for a patient, they will request a tracheotomy after one or two weeks of intubation. The neonatologists, however, will frequently keep small infants intubated for a period of months. Only two of the premature infants have been successfully decannulated, whereas 13 of 21 children with congenital cardiac disease are decannulated. (Cardiac patients who have poor mucosal microcirculation might be expected to have more mucosal damage and a poorer chance for decannulation but this was not the case.) On the average, the patients with congenital cardiac disease were older, at least by gestational age, and larger in size than the premature infants. To begin with, the larynx in the older group is larger. This, and the fact that they were tracheotomized after a much shorter period of intubation, are the factors that may be significant. The prolonged need for a tracheotomy does not seem, to us, a complication of the tracheotomy procedure itself, but a complication of either the child's primary disease or of the prolonged period of intubation necessitated by that disease. If the smaller infants had been tracheotomized earlier it is possible that many of them would be decannulated at this point. In the home institution it is possible for the laryngologist to emphasize the need for the smallest endotracheal tube which can successfully ventilate the patient. It is not, however, possible to control this in patients transferred from multiple referring institutions. Many of these patients arrive with disproportionally large endotracheal tubes for the size of the child and significant laryngeal damage from those tubes.

The problem of tube displacement within the first 24 to 48 hours after the tracheotomy can be avoided by paying close attention to the tubes at the time the patient is moved from the operating table to the litter. If heavy ventilating equipment must be attached to the tracheotomy tube, it must be well supported externally so that it does not place torque on the tube itself. The pediatric tubes are quite flexible and the drag of heavy equipment can easily twist them out of the trachea. The division of the thyroid isthmus and the presence of stay sutures are important precautions to allow replacement of the tube with ease by whomever is present should an accidental decannulation occur. Keeping the dissection entirely in the midline and away from the mediastinum aids in preventing problems with pneumothoraces and pneumomediastina. Many of our patients have significant pulmonary disease and they have some hyperinflation of the lungs. It is not unusual to visualize the cupula of the lung in the lateral aspect of the operating field. In the three emergency tracheotomies there were no major complications of the procedure itself. It is, however, a procedure to be avoided whenever possible by prudent evaluation of any critical airway and placement of either an endotracheal tube or a bronchoscope.

SUMMARY

The records of 123 tracheotomized patients have been evaluated. The proportion of children treated in the first year of life is quite high. The use of techniques specifically designed for small infants can help avoid complications. The use of the neonatal tracheotomy tube allows a better fit for the small infant.

ACKNOWLEDGMENTS — We would like to thank Kathy Sisson and Robert Ossoff, DMD, MD, for their work on the illustration of technique.

REFERENCES

1. Tucker JA, Silberman HD. Tracheotomy in pediatrics. Ann Otol Rhinol Laryngol 1972; 81:818-24.

2. Oliver P, Richardson JR, Clubb RW, et al. Tracheotomy in children. N Engl J Med 1962; 267:631-7.

3. Holinger PH, Brown WT, Maurizi DG. Tracheostomy in the newborn. J Surg 1965; 109:771-9.

4. Hawkins DB, Williams EH. Tracheostomy in infants and young children. Laryngoscope 1976; 84:331-8.

5. Perrotta RJ, Schley WS. Pediatric tracheotomy. Arch Otolaryngol 1978; 104:318-21.

6. Bridges CP, Ryan RF, Longenecker CG. Tracheostomy in children: a 20-year study at Charity Hospital in New Orleans. Plast Reconstr Surg 1966; 37:117-20.

Ann Otol Rhinol Laryngol 91:1982

LARYNGEAL PARALYSIS IN CHILDREN
A LONG-TERM RETROSPECTIVE STUDY

SEYMOUR R. COHEN, MD
JEFFREY W. BIRNS, MD
KENNETH A. GELLER, MD
JEROME W. THOMPSON, MD
LOS ANGELES, CALIFORNIA

The charts of 100 children with laryngeal paralysis were reviewed. The patients in this study had either unilateral or bilateral abductor vocal cord paralysis. The literature and pathophysiology are reviewed. A statistical analysis of each group of patients according to etiology is reported. The follow-up, progress and recovery are detailed. The need for observation and conservative therapy is reinforced by the tendency for spontaneous recovery. Suggestions regarding treatment are given.

INTRODUCTION

The records of 100 infants and children with the diagnosis of laryngeal paralysis were reviewed.

Paralysis of the larynx is an important consideration in the differential diagnosis of airway obstruction, voice change and aspiration syndromes. The early recognition of this problem and the application of appropriate therapy will prevent potential life-threatening sequelae from hypoxia, anoxia or contamination of the lower respiratory tract.

This retrospective study reviews the literature and pathophysiology of laryngeal paralysis, summarizes the neuroanatomy, analyzes the historical data of these children, details the endoscopic findings in the larynx and studies the changes which occur over a period of months and years. The treatment of the child with a paralyzed larynx is analyzed and the details are reported. There is no similar study of long-term follow-up in the otolaryngological literature.

LITERATURE REVIEW

The otolaryngological and surgical literature is replete with papers on the subject of laryngeal paralysis in the adult patient. Fewer studies have been written on this problem in children and there are none which give an intensive long-term follow-up or detail the outcome of the infant and child with a paralyzed larynx. Clerf[1] in 1953 reported a series of 293 patients with unilateral vocal cord paralysis. Ten percent of the patients in this review had paralysis of congenital origin. The left recurrent nerve was involved two times more often than the right. Of the 19 patients with congenital paralysis, 13 had bilateral associated with various anomalies such as meningomyelocele, hydrocephalus, congenital heart disease and tracheoesophageal fistulae.

Cunning[2] in 1955 estimated that 10% of the unilateral cases of paralysis were caused by tumor, abscess, bulbar paralysis or by vascular accident and intracranial disease prior to the nerve leaving the skull. In his estimation 90% were caused by peripheral lesions along the course of the recurrent laryngeal nerve.

Holinger and Brown[3] in 1967, in a paper on congenital anomalies of the larynx, state that paralysis of one or both vocal cords in the newborn infant is usually a serious laryngeal manifestation of a gross anomaly of another organ system. These authors felt that bilateral vocal cord paralysis was rarely seen in an otherwise normal infant and that it was associated with cerebral agenesis, severe mental retardation, meningomyelocele and birth trauma.

Morse[4] in 1969 reported on paralysis of the larynx and gave the etiological factors as follows: 90% were due to trauma, neoplasms, cardiovascular disease, infections, toxins, heavy metals, and drugs; 10% were idiopathic.

Goff[5] in 1970 analyzed 229 cases of laryngeal paralysis and divided the etiology into congenital and acquired, unilateral or bilateral and sudden or gradual.

Bluestone et al[6] in 1972 reported 12 patients with vocal cord paralysis associated with hydrocephalus and meningomyelocele. Six of the 12 patients died during the first year and 2 died during the second year of life. Only 3 of these 8 patients had been tracheotomized. Paralysis of the larynx was described as being due to 1) compression of the vagus nerve, 2) traction of the cervical rootlets of the vagus nerve by caudal displacement of the brainstem and 3) brainstem dysgenesis.

Kirsch et al[7] in 1967 reported five patients with

From the Department of Surgery, Division of Otolaryngology, the Childrens Hospital of Los Angeles and the University of Southern California School of Medicine, Los Angeles.

Presented at the meeting of the American Laryngological Association, Palm Beach, Florida, May 1-2, 1982.

REPRINTS — Seymour E. Cohen, MD, 1300 North Vermont Avenue, Los Angeles, CA 90027.

abductor paralysis of the larynx in association with meningomyelocele with Arnold-Chiari malformation and hydrocephalus. These authors felt that a tracheotomy was necessary to relieve airway obstruction until the hydrocephalus could be controlled by ventricular taps and shunting procedures. Restitution of laryngeal function in their patients appeared to be dependent on reducing intracranial pressure.

Fearon and Ellis[8] in 1972 reported a series of 28 cases of vocal cord paralysis; 30% were bilateral, 70% were unilateral. Seventy-five percent had symptoms at birth and were diagnosed prior to 6 months of age. The etiology of the paralysis was neurogenic, meningomyelocele with hydrocephalus, birth trauma, cerebral agenesis and spastic paralysis. Thirty percent of the patients in this study required a tracheotomy.

Hengerer and Tucker[9] in 1973 described the use of a nerve pedicle graft using a motor branch with sternohyoid muscle to restore abduction in the paralyzed canine larynx.

Tucker[10] in 1975 described the use of the ansa hypoglossiomohyoid muscle pedicle graft to restore innervation of the paralyzed larynx in the human. He states that should this procedure fail, an arytenoidectomy may still be used.

Gacek[11] in 1976 reported a family in which the father and two sons had hereditary bilateral vocal cord paralysis; another 4 siblings, 1 male and 3 females, were normal. His patients also had other neurological findings later in life indicating possible association with the laryngeal defect.

Whitaker and Griffith[12] in 1977 reported three patients receiving vincristine and vinblastine, who developed hoarseness and were found to have recurrent laryngeal paralysis. In none of these patients was airway obstruction a problem. The incidence of side effects of these drugs in adults is three times greater than in children.

Holinger et al[13] in 1978 reviewed 21 infants and children with respiratory obstruction and apnea who had bilateral abductor vocal cord paralysis associated with meningomyelocele, hydrocephalus and Arnold-Chiari malformation. Tracheotomy, while relieving airway obstruction, did not stop the abnormal respiratory pattern or apnea and cyanosis. Fifteen of the 21 patients required a tracheotomy; 5 children died of significant apnea and all 5 had been tracheotomized. Ten patients had chronic aspiration from dysphagia. Autopsy on one patient revealed a paucity of neurons and degeneration of residual neurons in the nucleus ambiguus.

Ishak et al[14] in 1980 reported on the intraoperative dysfunction of the autonomic system in Arnold-Chiari malformation. Kinking and herniation of the brainstem is thought to cause impairment of its blood supply and the resultant ischemia leads to bilateral abductor vocal cord paralysis. Most of the signs of dysfunction are reversed with lowering of the intracranial pressure with ventriculoperitoneal shunting or decompression of the posterior fossa. Reduction of intracranial pressure by shunting or revision of a malfunctioning shunt may not relieve the apnea or bradycardia even with a tracheotomy.

Cohen et al[15] in 1977 reviewed 124 records of neonates requiring endoscopic procedures. Reported were 29 patients with vocal cord paralysis. The etiology of the paralysis was idiopathic in 25, 4 were associated with central nervous system (CNS) disease and 1 of these 4 had an associated meningomyelocele. Of the 4 patients born by breech delivery, 1 had a recurrent vocal cord paralysis. Of the 17 children born by cesarean section, 6 had vocal cord paralysis. Thirteen of the 29 patients with laryngeal paralysis required a tracheotomy.

Cohen[16] reported on the effectiveness of arytenoidectomy in children and performed this surgery in the preschool age period.

Pathophysiology. Dedo[17] in 1970 gave a detailed evaluation of laryngeal paralysis in humans and dogs. His work amply reinforces the following facts experimentally produced in dogs. 1) Section of the recurrent nerve causes momentary spasm with subsequent paralysis of the vocal cord in the paramedian position often with the arytenoid tilted forward. As the true cord becomes completely immobile, it lengthens and adducts slightly with each subsequent phonation. 2) Section of the superior laryngeal nerve with an intact ipsilateral recurrent laryngeal nerve always led to little or no visible change in the contracture of the vocal cords. However, the cricothyroideus muscle stopped contracting after spasm at the moment of dissection. 3) Section of the recurrent laryngeal nerve followed by ipsilateral section of the superior laryngeal nerve caused the essentially immobile cord in the paramedian position to become completely paralyzed in the more lateral position.

Gilmer et al[18] in 1970 reviewed the histological findings in two patients and confirm the modern concept of laryngeal paralysis.

Kirsch et al[7] gave a detailed study of laryngeal paralysis in association with meningomyelocele, hydrocephalus and Arnold-Chiari malformation in five patients. They gave an excellent review of the pathophysiology which follows in capsule form. Krause[19] in 1884 reported aphonia in dogs after bilateral extirpation of the gyrus precrucialis. Cushing[20] described coordinated laryngeal movements incidental to stimulating the human cortex at its caudal extremity adjacent to Broca's area. It was Foerster[21] who postulated the necessity of a bilateral lesion as a requisite to supranuclear laryngeal disturbances. Semon and Horsley[22] defined the topography of the medullary laryngeal centers in dogs by correlating regional stimulation along the floor of the fourth ventricle with direct laryngoscopy.

Furstenberg and Magielski[23] confirmed and extended these observations and defined the functional pattern of cerebral organization in the primate nucleus ambiguus. This nuclear group is considered a substrate for peripheral motor innervation for the ipsilateral branchiomerically derived skeletal muscle of the larynx, esophagus and pharynx in both primate and the human. The human nucleus ambiguus is an elongated structure approximately 2 cm in length and 0.3 cm in width and extends from the upper border of the medulla and stria medullosis caudalward to the level of the motor decussation. The small rostral segment of the nucleus is the somatomotor center for palate and pharynx, with a motor outflow via the glossopharyngeal and cephalad vagal rootlets. The larger caudal extent of the nucleus ambiguus subserves laryngeal function exclusively and mediates its effect via the vagus nerve. The four paired groups of muscles responsible for vocal cord movements and one unpaired interarytenoid muscle group have discreet regional representation within the nucleus ambiguus.

Pressman and Keleman[24] in 1955 presented evidence that laryngeal muscles were innervated by two branches of the vagus nerve, the recurrent and the external branch of the superior laryngeal nerve. The latter nerve, which supplies the cricothyroideus muscle, a cord tenser and adductor, originates from the cell bodies situated in the central portion of the laryngeal segment of the nucleus ambiguus. The posterior cricoarytenoideus which functions as a vocal cord abductor is innervated by the recurrent laryngeal nerve fibers derived from cells located immediately subjacent to the cricothyroid cell group. The remaining arytenoid muscles receive their nerve supply from the most caudally disposed cells within the nucleus ambiguus through the recurrent laryngeal nerve.

Murtagh and Campbell[25] observed that adductor fibers continue to propagate action potentials despite a chemical or thermal blockade sufficient to paralyze abductor function. In addition, the chronaxy of adductor fibers, one of the most rapid thus far identified (0.1 ms) is tenfold shorter than that found in fibers subserving abduction.

METHOD

This study is an analysis of the charts of 100 children with laryngeal paralysis treated at the Childrens Hospital of Los Angeles. The charts were chosen at random by the record room personnel and it is estimated that there is an equal number of children who had laryngeal paralysis who had been treated but are not included in this review.

All of the children were examined by the authors and two other senior endoscopists. The direct laryngoscopy was performed either awake or with the use of a light general anesthetic. The patient breathed spontaneously during the examination. The speculum of the laryngoscope was placed into the vallecula and the sensory and motor function of the larynx was evaluated. In children who had a tracheotomy, the tube was always occluded in order to observe laryngeal mobility. Bronchoscopy was performed in all children to evaluate the tracheobronchial tree and to perform the tracheotomy when it was necessary. The larynx was examined at monthly intervals whenever possible.

FINDINGS

The findings as a result of this study are related to the sex of the patient, etiological factors, the onset of the disease, the type of pregnancy of the mother and the type of delivery of the child, symptoms related to the disease, the type of paralysis and the vocal cord position, the need for a tracheotomy and the age of decannulation, the preoperative diagnosis, the neurological status of the patient, the congenital and associated anomalies, the course and progress of the disease with statistics on recovery and resolution.

The results of this study are divided into the above statistical analysis related to all children as a group and then are presented in detail according to each specific etiological factor.

Sex. In this study, 59 patients were male and 41 patients were female.

Etiological Factors. The causes of laryngeal paralysis were as follows. Central nervous system disease occurred in 18% of the patients. Meningomyelocele with Arnold-Chiari malformation and usually with an associated hydrocephalus occurred in 14% of the patients. Birth trauma accounted for 19% of the paralyses; surgical and blunt trauma to the neck caused 11% of the paralyses; idiopathic causes were noted in 36% of the patients; a tumor, ie, a neuroblastoma of the neck, was the cause for paralysis in one of the patients and a familial cause was found in one patient.

Onset of Paralysis. The mean age of onset of laryngeal paralysis in all etiological categories was 38 days. Fifty-eight percent of the paralyses occurred within the first 12 hours of life, 66% by the second day of life and 80% within the first 36 days of life.

Mother's Pregnancy. The mother's pregnancy was completely normal in 77% of the children in this study. The pregnancies were abnormal in 23%. The abnormalities were premature labor, abruptio placenta, placenta previa, abnormal bleeding, eclampsia, maternal diabetes, drug overdose and hepatitis.

Type of Delivery. The child's delivery was completely normal in 65% of the patients. Thirty-five percent of the children had complicated deliveries with cesarean section in 15 and forceps delivery in 20. The complicated deliveries were usually due to abnormal presentation of the infant. Of the children born by cesarean section, 43% presented with bilateral abductor vocal cord paralysis and 57%

with unilateral vocal cord paralysis. Of the 20 born by forceps delivery, two thirds had bilateral abductor vocal cord paralysis and one third had unilateral vocal cord paralysis.

Symptoms. Stridor was prominent in 71% of the children, obstruction occurred in 44%, dysphonia was seen in 35%, dysphagia occurred in 38% and aspiration was seen in 14% of the patients.

Type of Paralysis. In patients of all categories, unilateral paralysis occurred in 38%. In five patients the side was not specified. In 33 of the patients in which the side was recorded, the right side was involved in 21% and the left was involved in 79%. Bilateral abductor vocal cord paralysis occurred in 62% of the patients.

Vocal Cord Position. In the group of 100 patients, the vocal cords were in the median position in 43% of the patients, paramedian in 30%, lateral in 5% and 23% were normal.

Tracheotomy. A tracheotomy was not necessary in any patient with unilateral vocal cord paralysis except when another obstructive lesion or aspiration problem was present. In 62 patients with bilateral abductor vocal cord paralysis, 45 (73%) required a tracheotomy. The mean age at which tracheotomy was performed varied with the etiology of the paralysis. The mean age of performing a tracheotomy in children with laryngeal paralysis in all categories was 34 days. In 89% of the patients who required a tracheotomy, the procedure was performed at the time the diagnosis was confirmed.

Of the 45 patients with tracheotomy, only 43 charts had a statement regarding decannulation. Fifty-four percent of these patients were decannulated within a mean period of 33 months. The remaining patients were lost to follow-up. Decannulation was readily accomplished in all five patients who had an arytenoidectomy. In those patients who had either congenital or postintubation subglottic stenosis, decannulation was delayed by this complication although the paralysis had recovered.

Preoperative Diagnosis. The preoperative diagnosis as determined by otolaryngologists was as follows: laryngomalacia in 11%, subglottic stenosis in 10%, vocal cord paralysis in 48% and stridor of undetermined origin in 26%. A specific diagnosis was not made in 5% of the patients. A specific diagnosis could only be confirmed by direct laryngoscopy.

Neurological Abnormalities. Laryngeal paralysis was of neurological origin in 33% of the patients. The neurological abnormalities were as follows: hypotonia (floppy child), Möbius' syndrome, neurogenic arthrogryposis multiplex congenita, Charcot-Marie-Tooth disease, cerebral palsy, hypoxic encephalopathy, Arnold-Chiari malformation with meningomyelocele and one patient with neonatal meningitis who had an associated laryngeal paralysis.

Congenital Anomalies and Associated Abnormalities. The congenital anomalies associated with laryngeal paralysis were pulmonary in 12, cardiovascular in 10, esophageal in 10, cervical abnormalities in 6, bronchial anomalies in 4 and meningomyelocele in 14 patients. One patient with meningomyelocele in this group did not have hydrocephalus. Other associated abnormalities were congenital subglottic stenosis, Pierre-Robin syndrome, hemivertebrae and urinary tract abnormalities.

Course and Progress. The mean age of resolution of the paralyzed larynx in all categories was 21.4 months. One third of the patients were followed for a mean of 35.2 months. In 33% of the patients, observation showed that there was a gradual change from paralysis to paresis progressing to complete recovery.

Recovery occurred in 48% of all patients. Thirty-three percent of the bilateral abductor vocal cord paralysis patients (21) recovered completely. Forty-four patients were lost to follow-up, almost all of them unilateral paralysis patients and many of them having been endoscoped only on one occasion. Of the 38 patients with unilateral paralysis, 13 were known to have completely recovered.

DATA RELATED TO SPECIFIC ETIOLOGY

Central Nervous System Disease. There were 18 patients in this etiological category. The mean age of onset was ten days. A tracheotomy was required in 12 of the 18 patients. The mean duration of a tracheotomy in this group was 48 months. Bilateral abductor vocal cord paralysis was present in 14 patients, unilateral paralysis was present in 4 patients.

Sixty-six percent of all patients recovered. Three of 4 patients with unilateral paralysis recovered completely and 1 died of apnea due to CNS disease. Of the 14 patients with bilateral abductor vocal cord paralysis, 5 completely recovered, 4 partially recovered, 3 did not recover and 2 of the patients had no information regarding recovery. The mean follow-up period of this group was 64.4 months, the mean age of recovery was 26 months, the mean duration of a tracheotomy was 48 months. Seven of the 12 tracheotomized patients were decannulated.

Birth Trauma. There were 19 patients in this category. The mean and median age of onset of symptoms was 5.6 days. A tracheotomy was required in six (31%) of the patients. The mean duration of tracheotomy in 4 of the 6 patients was 49 months. In two patients there was no follow-up available. Paralysis in this group was bilateral in 12 (63%) and unilateral in 7 patients (37%).

Nine of the 19 patients are known to have recovered. In ten of the patients there was no information available regarding recovery. Of the seven patients with unilateral paralysis, one completely recovered. No information was available in six patients. There is no record of patients showing partial or no recovery in this group. Of the 12 patients with bilateral paralysis, 5 recovered completely, 3 recovered partially and 4 had no available information. The mean follow-up period was 25 months. The mean age of recovery was 29 months. The mean duration of a tracheotomy was 49 months.

In this group of 19 patients, 8 were delivered with forceps, 9 were delivered by cesarean section, 1 patient by breech delivery and 1 patient presented with shoulder dystocia. All of these patients had been the product of a normal pregnancy. Nine of these patients had respiratory problems at the time of the delivery and three had been intubated at the time of birth. When only partial recovery occurred in this group, it was usually on the left side. When recovery was complete, it was always on the right side.

Meningomyelocele. There were 14 patients in this group. The mean age of onset of symptoms was 47 days. A tracheotomy was required in 71% of the patients. The mean duration of the tracheotomy was 37.2 months. In 13 patients (93%) paralysis was bilateral and in 1 patient it was unilateral. Recovery was noted only in the bilateral vocal cord paralysis patients. No information regarding recovery was available in the one patient with a unilateral paralysis. Of the 13 patients with bilateral abductor vocal cord paralysis, 6 completely recovered, 2 partially recovered, 3 did not recover and 2 had no information available regarding recovery.

The mean follow-up period was 37.9 months. The mean age of recovery was 21.5 months; the mean duration of a tracheotomy was 37.2 months. Of the 14 patients, 7 were decannulated, 3 were not decannulated and 4 of the patients were lost to follow-up.

Idiopathic Category. There were 36 patients in this group. The mean age of onset of paralysis in this group was 53 days. A tracheotomy was performed in ten patients (28%). The mean age of decannulation of these patients who were followed was 33.5 months.

Paralysis in this group was bilateral in 19 patients (53%) and unilateral in 17 patients (47%).

Recovery of motion of the vocal cords was as follows. In the unilateral group of 17 patients, complete recovery was noted in 4. No information was available in 12, 0 had partial recovery and 1 did not recover. Of the 19 patients with bilateral abductor vocal cord paralysis, 4 completely recovered, 7 partially recovered, 3 did not recover. No information was available in five of these patients. The mean age of follow-up was 75.6 months and the mean age of recovery was 13 months.

Six of the ten patients who were tracheotomized were decannulated, 1 patient died of overwhelming sepsis. Two patients are still being followed and one patient was lost to follow-up.

Surgery. There were nine patients in this group. In eight patients the paralysis followed repair of a tracheoesophageal fistula and/or atresia. One patient developed paralysis following ligation of a patent ductus arteriosus. The mean age of onset of symptoms in this group was 42 days. A tracheotomy was required in three of the patients. The mean duration of a tracheotomy was 28 months.

The type of paralysis was bilateral in four and unilateral in five. Of the 5 children with unilateral paralysis, 1 completely recovered and 4 had no information available regarding recovery. Of the 4 patients with bilateral vocal cord paralysis, 2 completely recovered, 1 partially recovered and 1 had insufficient information regarding recovery.

The mean follow-up period in this group was 33.3 months. The mean age of decannulation was 28 months. Three of the nine patients had a tracheotomy. One child still has a tracheotomy and two have been decannulated.

Blunt Trauma. There were three patients in this group. One of the patients required a tracheotomy. In two of the patients, the paralysis was bilateral and in one it was unilateral. The tracheotomized child was lost to follow-up. In two patients in whom there was adequate follow-up, the mean duration of the paralysis was 6.5 months.

Familial Group. In this category of one patient, a female, the paralysis was bilateral. A tracheotomy was performed at the age of 14 months. An arytenoidectomy was performed at age 5 years and 1 month. The patient was decannulated three months later. The symptoms in this child were chiefly stridor with obstruction to the airway. This patient had the early diagnosis of arthrogryposis multiplex congenita which later, after further neurological developments, was diagnosed as Charcot-Marie-Tooth disease. This patient is still seen periodically almost 11 years after her arytenoidectomy and has had multiple orthopedic procedures requiring intubation.

Tumor. There was one patient in this group. His diagnosis was a primary neuroblastoma of the neck. The age of onset of symptoms in this child was 1 month. Two weeks following the diagnosis a tracheotomy was performed and was necessary for 17 months. The paralysis was unilateral and on the left side. This patient had been intubated prior to his tracheotomy and developed a laryngeal subglottic stenosis. He also had a mild form of laryngomalacia. The left vocal cord paralysis never recovered.

TREATMENT

The patients who have laryngeal paralysis require close observation. To prevent chronic hypoxia and brain damage a tracheotomy is mandatory in children with an inadequate airway. One should not await the development of cyanotic episodes before instituting an artificial airway. Isolated unilateral paralysis requires no treatment. Even when there is no recovery, compensation by the normal vocal cord gives adequate phonation except when the paralysis is in the lateral position.

In patients with bilateral abductor vocal cord paralysis due to meningomyelocele with Arnold-Chiari malformation, tracheotomy should not be performed until a shunt procedure has been done. The airway may be supported by a small endotracheal tube. If a functioning shunt tube does not clear the paralysis, a tracheotomy should be performed. This is especially necessary in children who display severe aspiration or apnea spells. The authors have seen a number of patients in whom shunt failure recreated bilateral abductor vocal cord paralysis. When the shunt tubes were revised and became functional, the vocal cord paralysis resolved.

In children who had arytenoidectomies performed, uniformly good results were obtained. The voice was excellent and an adequate airway was obtained so that decannulation was possible. Some exercise intolerance occurred in most of these patients.

A nerve pedicle reinnervation has not been done in any of the patients in this study. There has been no report of a large series of patients in the pediatric age group in which this procedure was performed successfully.

DISCUSSION AND CONCLUSIONS

The causes of laryngeal paralysis in the pediatric population are different from those in the adult. In the latter, unilateral vocal cord paralysis is the result of surgical procedures, trauma, neoplasia of the neck and chest, CNS disease, peripheral neuropathies and idiopathic causes. Bilateral abductor vocal cord paralysis in the adult may be the result of surgical injury, most often thyroidectomy, neurological disorders, malignancies of the neck and upper chest, in addition to other causes such as neuropathies.

In children, in contrast to the adult, the major causes of vocal cord paralysis, both unilateral and bilateral, are birth trauma, CNS disease, meningomyelocele with Arnold-Chiari malformation and hydrocephalus, idiopathic, surgical trauma and disease of the heart and great vessels.

A thorough examination of the larynx was performed in all children with care to evaluate both motor and sensory function. Cricoarytenoid fixation was excluded by direct palpation of the joint.

The sex distribution in this study tends to support the fact that the male is more often involved than the female.

The etiological factors as determined by this study were CNS disease, birth trauma, meningomyelocele with Arnold-Chiari malformation and hydrocephalus, idiopathic, surgical trauma, blunt trauma to the neck, familial and tumor of the neck. In this study, idiopathic laryngeal paralysis is so labeled when a specific etiological factor could not be elicited after extensive studies. The term familial paralysis is applied to the one child reported in this series because the mother and a sister of this patient also had bilateral abductor vocal cord paralysis associated with Charcot-Marie-Tooth disease.

The overall mean age of onset of symptoms of all categories was 38 days. The earliest evidence of laryngeal paralysis was in the group of children with birth trauma. Children with CNS disease showed evidence of laryngeal paralysis within the first ten days of life. However, in the group of patients with meningomyelocele with Arnold-Chiari malformation and hydrocephalus, the mean age of onset was 47 days. This delay in onset of symptoms may be related to the progressive development of hydrocephalus which followed the repair of the meningomyelocele. Uncomplicated hydrocephalus does not produce laryngeal paralysis. In the postoperative surgery and idiopathic groups, the mean age of onset of symptoms relates to the specific cause of the paralysis.

Complicated delivery with abnormal presentation or positioning of the infant and the need for cesarean section birth was associated with laryngeal paralysis in almost 20% of the patients. The relatively high incidence of bilateral abductor vocal cord paralysis in association with complicated deliveries should alert the physician to this group of high risk patients.

The symptoms of paralysis varied in degree of severity within the different etiological categories. Stridor was the most common presenting symptom; it was always inspiratory and crowing in character. The stridor was most pronounced in patients with CNS disease, surgical or birth trauma and meningomyelocele with Arnold-Chiari malformation. Severe obstruction to the airway, which required immediate intubation, was seen most commonly in patients with bilateral abductor vocal cord paralysis following surgical procedures and complicated deliveries. An endotracheal tube was usually inserted to insure the airway and to allow for possible recovery of the paralysis. In some of these patients, subglottic stenosis developed which prolonged the need for a tracheotomy even after the laryngeal paralysis had recovered. Dysphagia was more common in the CNS group of patients, frequently because of a poor suck reflex or associated cranial nerve deficiencies. Aspiration occurred in children with loss of laryngeal sensation, cranial nerve defects and lateral position of one or both vocal cords. This problem occurred in patients with CNS disease and meningomyelocele with Arnold-Chiari malformation which would indicate a defect of both superior and recurrent laryngeal nerves. Dysphonia was an uncommon symptom whether the paralysis was unilateral or bilateral. Apnea occurred in some patients with CNS disease and meningomyelocele with Arnold-Chiari malformation even after the hydrocephalus had been corrected by a shunt procedure or after a posterior fossa decompression had been performed. Patients with apnea required a tracheotomy for ventilation and in some patients a diaphragm pacemaker was necessary to control respirations.

The type of paralysis varied within each etiological category. Sixty-six percent of the patients in this study had bilateral abductor vocal cord paralysis. In the remaining patients with unilateral paralysis, the left side was involved in almost 80% of the children. It is significant that in the group with CNS disease, meningomyelocele and Arnold-Chiari malformation and birth trauma, that the right and left vocal cords were equally involved, whereas in the other categories the left vocal cord paralysis predominated. Although bilateral and unilateral vocal cord paralysis occurred in all etiological groups of patients, an overwhelming majority of the patients with meningomyelocele with Arnold-Chiari malformation and CNS disease had bilateral abductor vocal cord paralysis. Within the groups of birth and blunt trauma, bilateral vocal cord paralysis occurred in two thirds of the patients. In the other groups, the type of paralysis was almost equal in numbers.

In 5% of the patients, lateral position occurred in association with sensory paralysis and severe aspiration. This defect occurred in 2 patients within the meningomyelocele with Arnold-Chiari malformation group, 1 in the CNS group and 1 in the idiopathic group. The child with a unilateral vocal cord paralysis in the lateral position (idiopathic group) did not aspirate, but had an extremely poor voice.

A tracheotomy was not necessary in any patient with an isolated unilateral paralysis. In 73% of the patients with bilateral abductor vocal cord paralysis a tracheotomy was performed. The mean age of tracheotomy was 34 days.

Arytenoidectomy was performed in five patients who did not have spontaneous recovery from laryngeal paralysis. All of these patients were decannulated following surgery; they all had a good voice and adequate airway, but some had reduction in exercise tolerance.

Tracheotomy was necessary in patients with bilateral abductor vocal cord paralysis secondary to meningomyelocele with Arnold-Chiari malformation and hydrocephalus, CNS disease and in patients with surgical and birth trauma. In the patients with CNS disease and birth trauma, the tracheotomy was required for approximately four years. It should be noted that when a child with bilateral abductor vocal cord paralysis due to birth trauma did not require a tracheotomy, recovery was uniform within six months or less. Children with meningomyelocele with Arnold-Chiari malformation and hydrocephalus required a tracheotomy for almost three years. The presence of a subglottic stenotic lesion delayed decannulation.

When a neurological or congenital abnormality was associated with laryngeal paralysis, it was usually of a serious nature.

Some of the patients in this study were followed for a period of seven years or more. Almost all of the 14 patients who were lost to follow-up had unilateral paralysis. Of the patients with bilateral abductor vocal cord paralysis, one third recovered completely.

It must be emphasized that since recovery from paralysis of the larynx may occur in children, even after a period of a year or more from the time of its onset, observation rather than active surgical treatment must rule.

ACKNOWLEDGMENT — Gratitude is expressed to Rose Marie Lapicola for her dedication and help in the preparation of this manuscript. Gratitude is also expressed to Drs. Alden H. Miller and Max K. Pierce for allowing their patients to be included in this study.

REFERENCES

1. Clerf LH. Unilateral vocal cord paralysis. JAMA 1953; 151:900-3.

2. Cunning DS. Unilateral vocal cord paralysis. Ann Otol Rhinol Laryngol 1955; 64:487-93.

3. Holinger PH, Brown WT. Congenital webs, cysts, laryngoceles and other anomalies of the larynx. Ann Otol Rhinol Laryngol 1967; 55:744-52.

4. Morse HR. Vocal cord paralysis. Gen Pract 1969; 40: 79-84.

5. Goff WF. Vocal cord paralysis, analysis of 229 cases. JAMA 1970; 212:1378-9.

6. Bluestone CD, Delerme AN, Samuelson GH. Airway obstruction due to vocal cord paralysis in infants with hydrocephalus and meningomyelocele. Ann Otol Rhinol Laryngol 1972; 81: 778-83.

7. Kirsch WM. Duncan BR, Black FO, Stears JC. Laryngeal palsy in association with meningomyelocele, hydrocephalus and the Arnold-Chiari malformation. J Neurosurg 1968; 218:207-14.

8. Fearon B, Ellis D. The management of long-term airway problems in infants and children. Ann Otol Rhinol Laryngol 1971; 80:669-77.

9. Hengerer AS, Tucker HM. Restoration of abduction in the paralyzed canine vocal cord. Arch Otolaryngol 1973; 97:247-50.

10. Tucker HM. Human laryngeal reinnervation. Laryngoscope 1976; 86:769-79.

11. Gacek RR. Hereditary abductor vocal cord paralysis. Ann Otol Rhinol Laryngol 1976; 85:90-3.

12. Whittaker JA, Griffith IP. Recurrent laryngeal nerve paralysis in patients receiving vincristine and vinblastine. Br Med J 1977; 1:1251-2.

13. Holinger PC, Holinger LD, Reichert TJ, Holinger PH. Respiratory obstruction and apnea in infants with bilateral abductor vocal cord paralysis, meningomyelocele, hydrocephalus and Arnold-Chiari malformation. J Pediatr 1978; 92:368-73.

14. Ishak BA, McLone D, Seleny FL. Intraoperative autonomic dysfunction associated with Arnold-Chiari malformation. Childs Brain 1980; 7:146-9.

15. Cohen SR, Eavey RD, Desmond MS, May BC. Endoscopy and tracheotomy in the neonatal period. Ann Otol Rhinol Laryngol 1977; 86:577-83.

16. Cohen SR. Arytenoidectomy in children. Laryngoscope 1973; 83:1293-9.

17. Dedo HH. The paralyzed larynx: an electromyographic study in dogs and humans. Laryngoscope 1970; 80:1455-1517.

18. Gilmer WS, Arnold GE, Stephans CB. Vocal cord position in laryngeal paralysis. Two further neurohistologic studies. Arch Otolaryngol 1970; 91:575-80.

19. Krause H. Über die Beziehungen der Grosshirnrinke zu Kehlkeps und Rachen. Arch Physiol 1884; 8:203-10.

20. Cushing H. A note upon faradic stimulation of the postcentral gyrus in conscious patients. Brain 1909; 32:44-53.

21. Foerster O. Motorishe Felder un Bahnen. In: Bunke O, Foerster O, eds. Handbuch der Neurologie. Vol 6.; Berlin: Verlag von Julius Springler, 1936:1-357.

22. Semon F, Horsley H. On the relations of the larynx to the motor nervous system. DT Med Wschr 1890; 16:672-9.

23. Furstenberg AC, Magielski JE. A motor pattern in the nucleus ambiguus: clinical significance. Ann Otol Rhinol Laryngol 1955; 64:788-93.

24. Pressman JJ, Keleman G. Physiology of the larynx. Physiol Rev 1955; 35:506-54.

25. Murtagh JA, Campbell CJ. Physiology of the recurrent laryngeal nerve: report on progress. J Clin Endocrinol Metab 1952; 12:1395-1401.

≈

AMERICAN ACADEMY OF PEDIATRICS SECTION ON OTOLARYNGOLOGY AND BRONCHOESOPHAGOLOGY

The American Academy of Pediatrics Section on Otolaryngology and Bronchoesophagology Meeting will take place on Monday, October 25, 1982 (closed session), and Tuesday, October 26, 1982 (open session). The meeting will be held at the Sheraton-Center Hotel in New York City. For further information please contact Dr. Lyon Greenberg, Program Chairman, 980 Western Avenue, Albany, NY 12203.

LARYNGEAL PAPILLOMA: RESULTS OF TREATMENT WITH THE CO_2 LASER AND PODOPHYLLUM

HERBERT H. DEDO, MD ROBERT K. JACKLER, MD

SAN FRANCISCO, CALIFORNIA

From 1976 to 1982, 109 patients with recurrent laryngeal papillomas were treated with a total of 548 CO_2 laser excisions followed by podophyllum painting. There was high incidence of multiple sites of involvement, especially the tracheobronchial tree (18.3%) and palate (8.3%). Four patients had pulmonary parenchymal involvement. Patients were treated at 2-month intervals until they entered remission. Thereafter, microdirect laryngoscopies were advised at longer intervals. Remission was achieved in 41%; it occurred at all ages although it was most common during adolescence and rarest in the very young and very old. Many patients obtained remission with the CO_2 laser after multiple prior cup forceps removals had not achieved remission. Only two tracheotomies (1.8%) were required and no deaths occurred. When compared with mechanical methods of papilloma removal, CO_2 laser excision with podophyllum painting represents a clear advance in terms of preservation of laryngeal physiology and avoidance of life-threatening complications.

INTRODUCTION

Laryngeal papillomas (LP) were first described during the 17th century by Marcellus Donalus who wrote describing them as "warts in the throat."[1] A clear description did not emerge until the late 19th century when MacKensie differentiated papillomas from other benign lesions of the larynx.[2]

Squamous papillomas are the most common laryngeal tumor occurring in children. They are also among the most frequently encountered benign laryngeal growths at any age. Histologically, they are composed of multiple finger-like projections consisting of a central core of fibrous tissue covered by a fairly regular stratified squamous epithelium. On clinical rather than histological grounds they have been divided into two forms, adult and juvenile. In children, the disease often takes a more virulent course characterized by a rapid growth, formation of large exophytic clusters, and involvement of other areas of the upper aerodigestive tract in addition to the larynx. Adults, on the other hand, generally have a more quiet course with less frequent recurrences and better anatomic confinement. Malignant transformation has been reported to occur in a small percentage of cases most often following radiation therapy.[3]

ETIOLOGY

It is commonly held that LPs are caused by a virus of the papova group, although absolute proof has been elusive.[4] Recently, using an immunoperoxidase stain, human papilloma virus (HPV) has been identified in approximately 50% of LP.[5] Even more convincing is the work of Lancaster and Jenson who employed sophisticated DNA hybridization techniques to show the presence of papilloma virus genus-specific DNA sequences in LP tissue.[6] Unfortunately, reproducible tissue culture for HPV has yet to be achieved, and isolation of virus from LP has not yet been reported.

In a classical experiment Uhllman transplanted papilloma from a child with LP to his arm and then to the mucous membrane of a dog.[7] Others, more recently, have been unable to duplicate this work. Clinically, person-to-person transmission has long been suspected in neonates, but not in adults. The majority of young children with LP have a positive maternal history of genital warts (condyloma acuminata) during pregnancy.[8] The frequent association of LP and skin warts lends further circumstantial evidence of the viral etiology of this disease.

THERAPY

Although papillomas are histologically benign, they can potentially be life-threatening. As they grow within the larynx or tracheobronchial tree, they may compromise the airway, sometimes leading to asphyxiation. Goals of therapy are maintenance of airway patency, preservation of voice, and elimination of papillomas.

The plethora of real and purported therapies for LP testify to the frustration of the physicians who have dealt with this disease over the years (Table 1). Basically, three approaches have been used: 1) chemical inhibition of papilloma growth (eg, antimetabolites, hormones, podophyllum), 2) physical removal (eg, cup forceps removal, cryosurgery, ultrasound, laser), and 3) enhancement of the immune response (eg, vaccines, transfer factor, interferon). Standard care up to this time has consisted of repeated surgical removal with either cup forceps or the CO_2 laser. We believe this study clearly shows

From the Department of Otolaryngology-Head and Neck Surgery, University of California School of Medicine, San Francisco.

Presented at the meeting of the American Laryngological Association, Palm Beach, Florida, May 1-2, 1982.

REPRINTS — Herbert Dedo, MD, 727A, University of California School of Medicine, San Francisco, CA 94143.

TABLE 1. TREATMENT OF LARYNGEAL PAPILLOMA*

Medical
- Antibiotics (Aureomycin, chloramphenicol, etc)
- Chemotherapeutic agents (methotrexate, bleomycin, etc)
- Electrolytes (calcium, magnesium)

Immunologic
- Heterohemotherapy
- Interferon
- Lymphokines
- Transfer factor
- Vaccine (smallpox, bovine wart, inactivated autogenous)

Physical
- Cryosurgery
- Diathermy
- Electrocautery
- Laser
- Radiation
- Ultrasound

Surgical
- Cup forceps removal
- Thyrotomy with skin or vein graft
- Tracheotomy for "laryngeal rest"

*Partial list.

the advantage of the laser approach.

Although many techniques have been proposed to control the disease, a true cure most probably awaits elucidation of the host-virus immune interaction or the development of an effective antiviral agent. The latest enthusiasm is the use of interferon. Haglund et al[9] have reported seven patients treated with systemic leukocyte interferon with encouraging preliminary results. Unfortunately, papillomas had a tendency to recur following cessation of therapy.

MATERIALS AND METHODS

Patients who underwent laser excision of papillomas were admitted to the University of California Hospital, San Francisco (UCSF). Patients were usually discharged from the hospital on the morning following surgery, occasionally on the same day.

Most patients were referred to UCSF with the diagnosis of LP already having been made, but some were first diagnosed here. The diagnosis of pulmonary parenchymal extension presents a special problem. This was suspected in a patient with laryngeal or tracheal papillomas when radiographic evidence of bullous change, nodulation, or cavitation were present in the absence of an alternative explanation.[10]

For laser excision, patients were placed under general anesthesia via an endotracheal tube wrapped with aluminum tape. In children, a cuffless tube wrapped with 0.64 cm (¼ in) aluminum foil tape (Radio Shack Corp) was used. The wrap must begin at the very tip of the tube to protect against ignition. In adults, a 1.27 cm (½ in) tape (3M, Minnesota Mining & Manufacturing) was used, with the wrap commencing immediately above the endotracheal tube balloon. In both age groups, tape was carefully wound for 5.1 cm (2 in) up the tube. When a 5.1 cm wrap is used and the upper edge of the foil tape is set at the level of the tip of the epiglottis, the endotracheal tube tip will be at the correct level within the trachea. When necessary, for further protection, moist cottonoids attached to long strings were placed in the subglottic space. For best exposure, the smallest tube compatible with adequate ventilation was selected (Table 2). Laryngoscopy was performed with an adult, adolescent, or pediatric Dedo-Pilling laryngoscope using a tooth guard. For laser surgery this was held in a Lewy suspension arm supported by a Mayo stand over the patient's chest. While manipulating the laryngoscope, care was taken to avoid mucosal breaks which can lead to seeding of the papillomas. Following mapping of the papillomas and photography, biopsies were taken with cup forceps and sent for routine pathology. A model 400 or 450 Coherent CO_2 laser was then used to vaporize the papillomas. The laser was controlled by a micromanipulator attached to a Zeiss operating microscope when treating papillomas of the larynx, pharynx, nasopharynx, nose, or skin. A Coherent 450 CO_2 laser bronchoscope was used to remove tracheal or main stem bronchial disease.

TABLE 2. ENDOTRACHEAL TUBE SIZE FOR CO_2 LASER SURGERY

Patient's Age	*Tube Size (ID)*	*Type of Tube*
Infant-3 yr	2.5 mm	Cuffless plastic
3-7 yr	3.0 mm	Cuffless plastic
7-10 yr	3.5 mm	Cuffless plastic
10-16 yr	20 F (4.5 mm)	Cuffed red rubber or plastic
Adult female	22 F (5.0 mm)	Cuffed red rubber or plastic
Adult male	24 F (5.5 mm)	Cuffed red rubber or plastic

ID - Internal diameter; F - French.

Papillomas were excised with a 0.5 to 1 mm cuff of surrounding normal-appearing tissue. Excision was carried just past the base of the papillomas to the submucosal loose areolar tissue (Reinke's space). Vocalis muscle and perichondrium were carefully preserved. Slightly deeper excisions were required in areas where papillomas repeatedly recurred in the same anatomic location. We have observed trapped microcysts in the scar tissue under recurrent papillomas. Only when these microcysts were removed did these recalcitrant areas with papillomas finally clear. Care was taken not to denude both free edges of the anterior 3 mm of the true or false vocal cords to avoid web formation. Laryngoceles of the false cord will develop if the orifice of the ventricle is denuded circumferentially. This is avoided by excising the edge of the false cord and its papillomas with our ventricle protector (Pilling) in place to preserve the mucosa on the top of the true vocal cord. Occasionally, an existing web or adhesion had to be lysed in order to expose occult papillomas in the ventricle or subglottic region. The ventricle was exposed by cutting the false vocal cord back until its raw inferior edge rested upon intact mucosa on the ventricle floor. When anterior commissure webs were simply divided with the laser they virtually always recurred. Definitive treatment for extensive (20% or more) anterior commissure webbing at the false or true cord level was undertaken with the endoscopic Teflon keel technique.[11]

When skin papillomas were brought to our attention by the patient they were excised with the CO_2 laser along with a 1-mm cuff of normal skin. When excision was carried through the basal layer these seldom recurred. Papillomas of the pharynx and palate were exposed with a mouth gag and, when in the nasopharynx, required the use of metallic mirrors to direct the laser beam. Following papilloma excision, in all locations except the skin, the bed was treated wtih 25% podophyllum.[12] This caustic resin is used to discourage papilloma reimplantation on raw surfaces. After extensive experience no adverse effects have been found with its use.

Postoperative respiratory distress was uncommon except in patients with convex vocal cords or extensive tracheal disease. These patients were promptly treated with humidified oxygen, nebulized racemic epinephrine, and intravenous methylprednisolone, usually with good results. Reintubation was avoided, when possible, and tracheotomy was done only as a last resort. Some of the patients who developed postoperative respiratory distress were found to have convex vocal cords even after thorough papilloma removal. The bulging portion has been found to contain numerous trapped microcysts which expand the vocal cords thus impinging upon the airway. When the CO_2 laser was used to excise the convex portion back to a straight line from the anterior commissure to the arytenoid, postoperative distress did not recur.

Patients were scheduled for repeat treatments at 2-month intervals. Occasionally, a child with very rapidly growing disease required removal more often, even as frequently as once a week. When a patient became free of disease, he was re-examined under

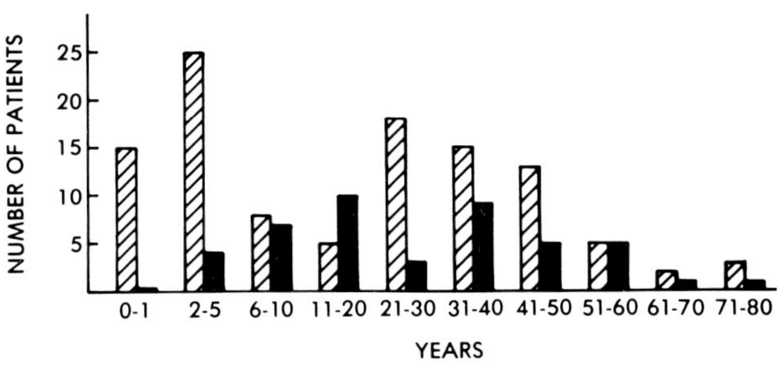

Fig. 1. Age at onset (▨ - 109 patients) compared with age at remission (■ - 45 patients).

anesthesia in approximately twice the preceding interval (4, 8, 16 months, etc), providing that papillomas had not recurred.

RESULTS

Over a 6-year period (1976 to 1982) a total of 109 patients underwent 548 laser removals of laryngeal papillomas. This averages just over five procedures per patient. Prior to commencing laser therapy, these same patients had undergone approximately 1050 conventional surgical removals, approximately 10 per patient, without eradication of their disease.

Sex Ratio. There were 66 male patients (60.6%) and 43 (39.4%) patients were female. This agrees with the slight male predominance often noted in the literature.

Race. A wide racial distribution was found: white — 81 (74.3%); black — 15 (13.7%); Hispanic — 8 (7.3%); oriental — 3 (2.8%); and Arab — 2 (1.8%). This is not substantially different from the distribution of patients within our referral population at large.

Geographic Location. The majority of our patients were from California with 44 (40.4%) residing in the San Francisco Bay area, and 46 (42.2%) from more distant parts of the state. Fifteen patients (13.8%) came from other states, and 4 (3.6%) from other countries.

Age at Onset. This was considered to be the age at which the patient first underwent a surgical procedure for papillomas (Fig. 1). Longer histories of hoarseness often existed, but accurate estimation of this period is difficult. Although no age is immune from LPs, they most often begin in childhood and are uncommon in old age. Forty-eight of our patients (44%) developed their disease in the first ten years of life, of these 40 (36.7%) in the first five years.

Sites of Involvement. We have confirmed the findings of others that this disease represents a diathesis of the entire upper aerodigestive tract, rather than a disease limited to the larynx (Table 3). Thirty-two of our 109 patients (29.4%) manifested extralaryngeal involvement. One half of these were under five years of age at the onset of their disease. Virtually all of the patients with widespread disease involving multiple sites were young children. Tracheobronchial disease was found in 20 patients (18.3%) making it the most common extralaryngeal site. Next common were the soft palate — 9 (8.3%), skin — 7 (6.4%), nasopharynx — 5 (4.6%), and tonsils — 5 (4.6%).

TABLE 3. SITES INVOLVED IN LARYNGEAL PAPILLOMATOSIS

Site	*No. of Patients*	*%*
Larynx	109	100.0
Trachea	17	15.6
Main stem bronchi	3	2.8
Lung parenchyma (suspected)	4	3.7
Pyriform sinus	2	1.8
Pharyngeal wall	4	3.7
Vallecula	4	3.7
Tongue	2	1.8
Tonsils	5	4.6
Palate	9	8.3
Oral mucosa	2	1.8
Nose	2	1.8
Nasopharynx	5	4.6
Skin	7	6.4

Pulmonary Papillomatosis. Four patients had suspected pulmonary parenchymal involvement. Only one patient (Case 2) developed this problem while undergoing laser therapy.

Case 1. A 29-year-old female whose disease began at age 2 years had a tracheotomy in infancy and has never been decannulated. She has lost count after more than 100 procedures including frequent removals from the tracheobronchial tree. Chest x-ray film reveals widespread scarring and chronic right upper lobe consolidation and abscess secondary to papillomas obstructing the right upper lobe bronchus.

Case 2. A 9-year-old male whose disease began at age 5 has had 17 procedures with frequent removals from the tracheobronchial tree, but no tracheotomy. His disease began on the tonsils and then spread sequentially to the larynx, trachea, and finally the lungs. At this time his only remaining disease is in the lung parenchyma. Chest x-ray film now reveals bilateral diffuse nodular disease.

Case 3. A 76-year-old male whose disease began at age 62 had a tracheotomy early in his disease course and was never decannulated. He has undergone 59 procedures with frequent removals from the trachea. Chest x-ray film reveals cavitary and bullous changes in both lungs.

Case 4. A 13-year-old male whose laryngeal disease began at age 9 has had neither trachoebronchial disease nor a tracheotomy. He has undergone 25 procedures to date. Chest x-ray film reveals severe bullous changes in both upper lobes.

Number of Procedures. The majority of patients, 66 (60.6%), had from 2 to more than 100 cup forceps removals prior to beginning laser therapy (Fig. 2). Another 24 patients (22%) had only a single diagnostic cup forceps removal prior to referral. Only 19 patients (17.4%) began their treatment with the laser. The average patient had a lifetime total of approximately 15 procedures, 5 of these being laser.

Remission Rate. Forty-five patients (41.3%) were free of disease at their last examination. In 80%, including all of the children, this was deter-

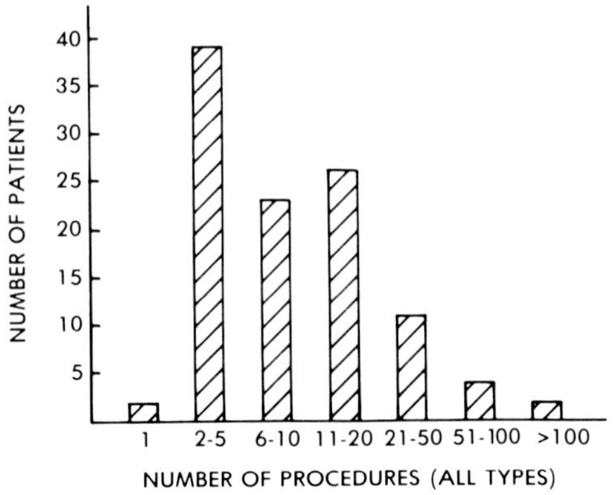

Fig. 2. All types of procedures (109 patients).

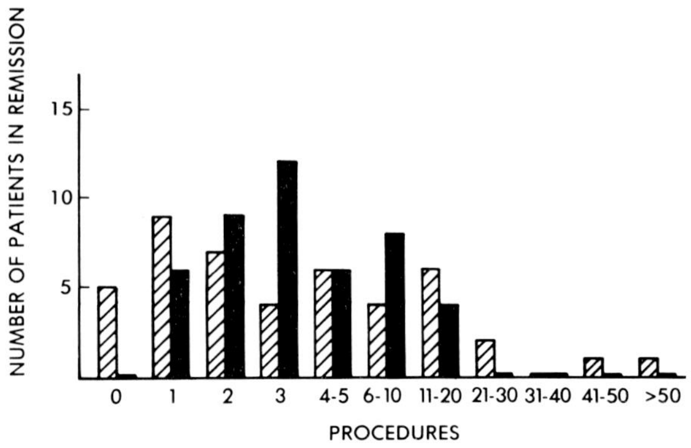

Fig. 3. Number of prior cup forceps removals without remission (▨ - 45 patients) compared with the number of laser removals required to achieve remission (■ - 45 patients).

mined at microdirect laryngoscopy. A few selected adults with easily visualized larynges were followed by indirect examination alone after no papillomas were evident at one microdirect laryngoscopy and symptoms were absent. However, it is preferable to use microdirect laryngoscopy for follow-up as indirect examination alone frequently misses subtle or anatomically hidden papillomas. We have had approximately ten patients in whom indirect laryngoscopy appeared clear while papillomas were found at microdirect laryngoscopy the very next day. Length of follow-up varied from two months to two years with the average being 8.5 months. There was a tendency for patients not to return for follow-up after two or three examinations revealed no papillomas.

Remissions occurred at all ages (Fig. 1), although it was most common in adolescence and rarest in the very young and very old. While 32.1% of patients developed their disease from birth to age 5, only 8.9% of remissions occurred in this age group. On the other hand, the 11- to 20-year-old group accounted for 22.2% of all remissions, while only 4.6% developed their disease during these years. We did not find the paucity of midlife remissions reported by Strong et al.[8]

The number of prior cup forceps removals bore little relation to the likelihood of achieving remission on laser therapy (Fig. 3). Fifty-two percent of patients who had undergone more than two previous mechanical removals entered remission on laser therapy. Twelve patients obtained remission despite more than ten previous cup forceps removals without remission. Two of these patients had more than 40 previous mechanical removals.

It has been our observation that most patients require several laser treatments before achieving remission (Fig. 3). This is because of the necessity of working on only one side of the anterior commissure at a time. Although our protocol calls for repeat excision at 2-month intervals, alternate sides of the anterior commissure are thus, in reality, treated only every four months. Occasionally, especially in children, this allows considerable regrowth during the interim. Patients not responding at all after ten laser treatments seldom enter remission. However, contrary to Strong et al,[8] we had four patients who remitted after more than 11 laser treatments.

Complications. Only two patients (1.8%) required tracheotomy while undergoing laser therapy. They were young, aged 1 and 2½ years. In each case, rapidly growing, circumferential, obstructing laryngeal papillomas resulted in acute upper airway obstruction. One patient was successfully decannulated three months post-tracheotomy and went on to have a clear larynx after 19 laser treatments over a 4-year period. The other remained cannulated despite multiple procedures and is now followed elsewhere. There were 12 patients who had undergone tracheotomy prior to beginning laser therapy. Decannulation was achieved in six of these.

Nine patients required endoscopic Teflon keel placement[11] for significant anterior glottic webbing; in seven of these the webbing was present upon referral. In two patients substantial webbing developed while undergoing laser therapy. These occurred early in our series before development of anterior commissure protectors (Pilling Co) which made it possible to remove papillomas precisely to the anterior midline.

No deaths have occurred to date, but there have been several close calls in patients with severe airway compromise.

Malignant Degeneration. Three adults, age 45, 72, and 78, developed squamous cell carcinoma of the larynx. All developed their papillomatous disease during adulthood at ages 43, 56, and 76 respectively. They had from 6 to 14 laser and cup forceps excisions prior to the diagnosis of malignancy. The final histology in each case was verrucous carcinoma. Earlier pathology specimens, when reviewed, still appeared to show benign squamous papillomas. In contrast to the literature, none of

TABLE 4. COMPLICATIONS — A REVIEW OF THE LITERATURE

Series	Year	No. Pts.	Tracheotomy (%)	Deaths (%)	No.
Mechanical removal					
Holinger[13]	1950	109	17.4	(?)	
Bjork[14]	1956	98	8.2	7.1	7
del Villar[15]	1956	112	52.7	7.1	8
Majoros[16]	1964	101	64.3	13.8	14
Dekelbaum[17]	1965	67	17.9	3.0	2
Klos[18]	1970	62	11.3	8.0	5
Cohen[19]	1980	90	4.4	3.3	3
Laser removal*					
Strong[8]	1976	110	2.7	0	
Dedo & Jackler	1982	109	1.8	0	

*Includes only tracheotomies performed while undergoing laser therapy.

our patients gave a history of prior irradiation therapy to the neck. All three are alive and well after laryngectomy, although one patient continues to form papillomas in the tracheostome.

DISCUSSION

Although laryngeal papillomatosis is a benign disease, it is traditionally associated with a substantial morbidity and mortality. The major sources of morbidity are 1) airway obstruction secondary to laryngeal stenosis or exophytic papilloma growth, 2) deterioration of voice, 3) pulmonary infections, and 4) loss of time from work or school. Mortality most often results from asphyxiation caused by exuberant papilloma growth, blockage of the tracheotomy tube, or postoperative edema. A high correlation between the presence of a tracheotomy and mortality exists. Death may also occur with malignant degeneration or where pulmonary papillomatosis results in extensive destruction of lung tissue.

A literature review (Table 4)[13-19] of seven major studies over the last 30 years reflects the high potential for complications in this disease. An average of 25% tracheotomies and 7% deaths was obtained with conventional therapy. Using CO_2 laser excision followed by podophyllum painting we had only 1.8% tracheotomies and no deaths in 109 patients. This agrees quite well with the only other large laser series in the literature, that of Strong et al.[8] They required only 2.7% tracheotomies and also were without deaths. We believe that these statistics demonstrate the clear-cut superiority of CO_2 laser therapy over traditional mechanical methods.

There are several factors contributing to the paucity of morbidity and mortality in this series. Most important is the combination of microdirect laryngoscopy and the surgical CO_2 laser which permits more precise, complete, and bloodless papilloma excision. The relatively minimal postoperative edema following laser surgery circumvents many of the acute airway problems encountered following mechanical avulsion. Also, the long-term effects of scarring, webbing, and stenosis are infrequent. Another important factor is the regular eradication of papillomas on a scheduled basis before extensive regrowth occurs. Formerly, many surgeons waited until symptoms of airway obstruction or severe vocal disturbance occurred before undertaking treatment. This only encourages complications and minimizes chances of remission. Also essential is skillful anesthesia performed by those experienced with using pediatric techniques and the smallest possible endotracheal tubes.

Another advantage of the CO_2 laser is the maintenance of vocal quality. In an earlier review of 67 papilloma patients treated with cup forceps at our own institution[17] 50% of patients had persistent hoarseness secondary to "thickened vocal cords, fibrotic changes, and recurrent papilloma." Although exact qualitative data are lacking, we have the strong clinical impression that vocal quality is better preserved with CO_2 laser therapy than with cup forceps removal.

The ultimate goal of papilloma therapy is a lasting cure. Unfortunately, this has been elusive, and papillomas may recur even after long periods of absence. The terms used in the literature to describe favorable results and duration of follow-up are highly variable. For future use we propose a nomenclature to classify the long-term follow-up of papilloma patients: 1) remission — no papillomas visible at the most recent examination; 2) clearance — no papillomas for three years; and 3) cure — no papillomas for five years. In this respect ours has been a preliminary study and we are in the process of collecting statistically significant data from 3- and 5-year follow-ups. Favorable immediate term results have been seen in those patients who have undergone first cup forceps removal and then laser excisions. These patients, who served as their own longitudinal controls, achieved a 52% remission rate on CO_2 laser therapy after repeated cup forceps removals had failed to control their disease. A few of these patients have now even gone four and five years without recurrence. Our hope is that meticulously done CO_2 laser excision, followed by podophyllum painting will achieve better long-term papilloma control than that obtainable with mechanical removal.

In summary, we have found that the treatment of LP with CO_2 laser followed by podophyllum painting represents a clear advance over traditional mechanical methods of papilloma removal when voice quality, remission rate, and especially incidence of complications, and occurrences of death are considered.

REFERENCES

1. Webb WW. Papillomata of the larynx. Laryngoscope 1956; 66:871-918.

2. MacKensie M. Essays on growth in the larynx with reports and an analysis of one hundred consecutive cases treated by the author. Philadelphia: Lindsay and Blakiston, 1871.

3. Batsakis JG. Tumors of the head and neck. Baltimore: Williams and Wilkins, 1979, 137-9.

4. Quick C, Faras A, Krzysek R. The etiology of laryngeal papillomatosis. Laryngoscope 1978; 88:1789-95.

5. Lack E, Jenson AB, Smith H, et al. Immunoperoxidase location of human papilloma virus in laryngeal papillomas. Intervirology 1980; 14:148-54.

6. Lancaster W, Jenson AB. Evidence for papillomavirus genus — specific antigens and DNA in laryngeal papillomas. Intervirology 1981; 15:204-12.

7. Uhllman EVL. On the etiology of laryngeal papillomatosis. Acta Otolaryngol (Stockh) 1923; 5:317.

8. Strong MS, Vaughn CW, Healy GB, Cooperband SR, Clemente MACP. Recurrent respiratory papillomatosis — management with the CO_2 laser. Ann Otol Rhinol Laryngol 1976; 85:508-16.

9. Haglund S, Lundquist P, Cantell K, et al. Interferon therapy in juvenile laryngeal papillomatosis. Arch Otolaryngol 1981; 107:327-32.

10. Rosenbaum HD, Alavi S, Bryant L. Pulmonary parenchymal spread of juvenile laryngeal papillomatosis. Radiology 1968; 90:654-60.

11. Dedo HH. Endoscopic Teflon keel for anterior glottic web. Ann Otol Rhinol Laryngol 1979; 88:467-73.

12. Hollingsworth J, Kohlmoos H, McNaught RL. Treatment of juvenile papilloma of the larynx with resin of podophyllum. Arch Otolaryngol 1950; 52:82-7.

13. Holinger P, Johnston K, Anison G. Papilloma of the larynx. A review of 109 cases with preliminary report of aureomycin therapy. Ann Otol Rhinol Laryngol 1950; 59:547-63.

14. Bjork H, Weber C, Papilloma of the larynx. Acta Otolaryngol (Stockh) 1956; 34:499-513.

15. del Villar R, Echeverria E, deAcosta V, et al. Laryngeal papillomatosis. Arch Otolaryngol 1956; 64:480-5.

16. Majoros M, Parkhill E. Devine K. Papilloma of the larynx in children. Am J Surg 1964; 108:470-5.

17. Dekelbaum A. Papillomas of the larynx. Arch Otolaryngol 1965; 81:390-7.

18. Klos J. Clinical course of laryngeal papillomatosis in children. Ann Otol Rhinol Laryngol 1970; 79:1132-8.

19. Cohen S, Seltzer S, Geller K, et al. Papilloma of the larynx and tracheobronchial tree in children. Ann Otol Rhinol Laryngol 1980; 89:497-503.

LEUKOCYTE INTERFERON IN PATIENTS WITH JUVENILE LARYNGEAL PAPILLOMATOSIS

HELMUTH GOEPFERT, MD
JORDAN U. GUTTERMAN, MD
WILLIAM J. DICHTEL, MD
ROY B. SESSIONS, MD
AYTEN CANGIR, MD
MARCELLE SULEK, MD

HOUSTON, TEXAS

Fourteen patients with aggressive juvenile laryngeal papillomatosis were treated with systemic administration of alpha-type interferon (IFN). The initial dosage of 2 million units alpha-interferon/m^2 was modified if a favorable response in the papilloma growth occurred, or if persistent drug-related side effects developed. Half of the patients showed a sustained response while on IFN, and two patients had a complete response. Persistent elevation in SGOT was the main dose-limiting toxicity, especially in infants below age seven years. All side effects subsided after the drug was discontinued. Further studies are recommended.

INTRODUCTION

Juvenile laryngeal papillomatosis (JLP) is the most common benign proliferative condition seen in the larynx of children,[1] has a relentless propensity for recurrence and a befuddling lack of behavioral predictability. The papillomas are consistently localized in the larynx and have an overall low incidence of growth in the tracheobronchial tree below the site of origin. Although the mortality from the disease is generally thought to be low, it has been reportedly high in several series.[2] Local aggressiveness can be a dominant feature and, in rare instances the disease has been associated with carcinoma of the larynx and cancer of the lung.[3,4]

The mainstay of treatment remains surgical ablation of all visible papillomas; however, recurrence in the majority of patients requires repeat surgery under general anesthesia. Cryosurgery, diathermy, electrofulguration, ultrasound, radiotherapy, topical application of podophyllin, steroid hormones, tetracycline, cytotoxic drugs, antimetabolites, and biologic response modifiers have also been utilized as treatment.[5-17] CO_2 laser vaporization has been the most popular method used in recent years.[18] The general philosophy of management is to control the growth of the papillomas with minimum danger to normal tissues in the hope that the aggressiveness of the tumor will diminish in time.

It seems that younger children are afflicted with more aggressive forms of the disease than are adolescents, and that in the adult, laryngeal papillomatosis tends to be even less active.[19] Contradictions in the disease's natural history and clinical behavior are plentiful. Puberty has been associated with spontaneous involution of disease and diminution of growth of papillomas in some patients; however, this finding has been inconsistent. It is uncertain at this time if pregnancy is associated with any significant change in growth pattern.[22] A spontaneous cessation of growth and even complete remission after periods of very active proliferation have been recognized. These variables make the evaluation of any therapeutic modality difficult.

Evidence of viral cause for JLP has not been conclusive. Indirect evidence of viral etiology is supported by the presence of tumorigenic intranuclear DNA virus belonging to the papovavirus group and by many past observations.[20,21] As early as 1890, Thost[22] described the concomitant occurrence of cutaneous and laryngeal papillomas in the same patient. Ullman[23] and Ishikawa[24] independently performed self-inoculation experiments with laryngeal papillomatosis. Meesen and Schutz,[25] Pinsker and Proud[26] and Timmel[27] made the initial cellular morphologic observations that suggested a viral etiology.

Papilloma viruses are a subgroup of the papova viridae family. These viruses are not only host- but tissue-specific and induce epithelial and fibroepithelial tumors in skin and mucosal epithelia.[28,29] Five different viruses have been identified in cutaneous papillomas in humans. It has been assumed that the human papilloma virus may not only be responsible for cutaneous lesions but may also be associated with mucosal papillomas such as laryngeal and anal genital warts. However, in vitro isolation has not yet been reproducibly accomplished. The data of Quick et al[29] suggests that the viruses that produce papillomas and cutaneous verrucae are of a similar family subgroup. Most cases of JLP would

---

From the University of Texas, M.D. Anderson Hospital and Tumor Institute at Houston, and the Departments of Otolaryngology and Communicative Sciences, Baylor College of Medicine, Houston. Supported by Grant CA 05831, National Cancer Institute, and Hoffman-La Roche, Inc. Research conducted in part by the Interferon Foundation and the Clayton Foundation for Research.

Presented at the meeting of the American Laryngological Association, Palm Beach, Florida, May 1-2, 1982.

REPRINTS — Helmuth Goepfert, MD, Department of Head and Neck Surgery, University of Texas, M.D. Anderson Hospital, 6723 Bertner, Houston, TX 77030.

be caused by one or more of the different serotypes of human papilloma viruses.

Because JLP seems to be a virally related disorder, there has been hope that interferon (IFN) may be helpful in its treatment. Interferon is a naturally occurring substance with clearly demonstrated antiviral and antiproliferative effects.[31-35] It has been used against myxovirus and herpes simplex virus infections by topical application to the respiratory mucosa and corneal epithelium, respectively. Haglund et al[36] recently reported the results using human leukocyte IFN (alpha-IFN) to treat seven patients with JLP. All seven patients showed some regression of papilloma growth. We report here the preliminary results of a study using alpha-IFN in patients with JLP.

INTERFERON — BACKGROUND

Interferons are potent antiviral, antiproliferative, and immunomodulating proteins. Since their discovery in 1957, a substantial body of knowledge on their biology and biochemistry has been promulgated.[37-44]

The IFN system itself is a complex defense mechanism involving the release of substances from cells infected with viruses. IFN is able to confer antiviral resistance on virus-susceptible cells. By itself, IFN has no direct antiviral action; however, it does induce synthesis of intracellular enzymes that act to control viral growth.[32]

Many cells are capable of producing IFN. In vivo, cells of the reticuloendothelial system are good producers; thus the lymphocyte, and probably the macrophage, are important sources of the substance. Fibroblasts are very productive of IFN. Transformed human lymphoid cells, such as those isolated from a Burkitt's lymphoma patient, can produce high levels of leukocyte IFN.[2,39,40]

The two major types of IFN are type I, which is induced by viruses, and type II, which is induced by antigens or mitogens. Type I IFNs include leukocyte (alpha) and fibroblast (beta); type II, or immune IFN, is called gamma. At present, alpha-IFN has been the main source for clinical trials, and most of the current knowledge of the pharmacokinetics, toxicity, and clinical efficacy is based on its study.

The IFNs are polypeptides and those that are produced in response to an antigenic challenge, ie, gamma-IFN, probably come from the T lymphocytes. Because IFN is a protein, it was originally anticipated that standard biochemical procedures would induce a pure, homogeneous material. This has not, in fact, been the case, and purification of the end-product has posed a major problem. Recently, however, progress has been made in this area, and homogeneous leukocyte IFN produced bacterially by recombinant DNA technology has been reported.[41]

IFN has an antiproliferative property that inhibits the division of tumor cells grown in culture, and the cell-multiplication-inhibition effects seem to influence inhibition of lymphocyte transformation as well as antibody synthesis.[42] In contrast, IFN enhances phagocytosis by increasing macrophage activation, increases sensitized cytotoxic lymphocyte activity, and activates the natural killer (NK) cell. Although little evidence exists regarding the in vivo role of NK cells in the antiviral activities of IFN, it is thought to be involved. It has been demonstrated that IFN has the capacity to induce certain tumor regressions;[42-44] however, the precise mechanism is unclear. A variety of immunopotentiating agents have been administered to cancer patients for the last decade, but tumor regression has rarely been observed. Thus, it is unlikely that the immune-enhancing properties of IFN are solely responsible for tumor regression. It may be that the direct effect of IFNs on the growth of tumor cells is important.[33]

METHODS

A randomized prospective study was conducted between March 1981 and February 1982 on 14 patients with aggressive laryngeal and/or laryngotracheobronchial (LTB) papillomatosis. Characteristics of the patient population are summarized in the table. Three patients had papillomatas in all three areas: larynx, trachea, and bronchi (patients 7,12,13). The adult patients had required two or more therapeutic endoscopies within the preceding year, and all children had four or more such procedures during that time. All patients required numerous endoscopies previously, with two patients requiring more than 60 procedures and one with over 300 endoscopies in his lifetime. Eight patients had previously required or were currently dependent on tracheostomy. Six patients had histories of at least one major crisis during their illnesses, such as acute airway obstruction or cardiopulmonary arrest. Eleven patients were male and 3 were female; there were 5 adults, 2 adolescents, and 7 were less than 10 years old. Ages ranged from 2 to 35 years. All patients were white.

Alpha-IFN was obtained from the Finnish Red Cross and Blood Transfusion Laboratories, Helsinki, Finland. Before the patients were admitted in the study, detailed histories were taken and physical examinations were performed. Complete blood counts, platelet count, liver function studies, serum urea nitrogen, creatinine determinations, and chest roentgenograms were obtained. Direct laryngoscopy and appropriate laser vaporization were performed on all patients prior to initiation of IFN treatment. Parents and patients received extensive counseling, and informed consent was obtained prior to each patient's enrollment in the study. Once treatment was initiated, patients underwent monthly laryngoscopies during the first three months, followed by laryngoscopies at 2 to 3-month intervals as dictated by clinical progress. Eleven of the 14 patients underwent laryngoscopies by the same surgeon (RBS). Papillomas were removed by endoscopic instrumentation as needed in the trachea and bronchi and by carbon dioxide laser vaporization in the larynx. The extent and distribution of papillomas were recorded diagrammatically in each case.

During each patient's treatment, complete blood differential and platelet counts were obtained weekly during the first month of treatment, twice a month during the second, and monthly during the remainder of the period of IFN administration. Liver and renal function studies were performed monthly for the first three months of treatment and subsequently on a bimonthly basis.

The initial dose of IFN was 2 million units/m^2 daily, intramuscularly. The frequency of administration was changed to three times weekly whenever the papilloma growth rate decreased or

SUMMARY OF CHARACTERISTICS OF PATIENT POPULATION

				Papilloma Natural History			*IFN Treatment*					
Patient	*Sex*	*Age (yr)*	*Onset Age (yr)*	*Location*	*Crisis**	*Endos*	*Months*	*Toxicity*	*Initial Response*	*Sustained Response*	*Dose Dependency*
1	M	3	1.5	Larynx	Yes	Many	7	Slight-liver	Slight	Yes	—
2	M	35	32	Larynx	No	Many	11	Slight-liver, WBC	Complete	Yes	Yes
3	M	3	1.5	Larynx/trachea (tracheostomy)	No	Many	11	Slight-liver, WBC	Complete	Yes	No
4	M	9	6	Larynx	No	Many	6	Marked-liver, WBC	None	—	—
5	M	30	25	Larynx (tracheostomy)	Yes	Many	10	None	Complete	No-grew at 7 mo	Yes
6	F	5	3	Larynx	No	Many	7	Marked-liver	Complete	LTF at 8 mo	No
7	F	2	1	Larynx, TBP (tracheostomy)	Yes	Many	12†	None	Moderate	No-grew at 6 mo	Yes
8	M	26	2	Larynx (tracheostomy)	No	60+	11	None	Complete	No-grew at 4 mo	No
9	M	27	2	Larynx (tracheostomy)	No	300+	9	None	Good	Yes	Yes
10	M	12	5	Larynx	Yes	60+	12	Moderate-liver, WBC	Good	No	Yes
11	F	8	5	Larynx (tracheostomy)	Yes	Many	11	Moderate-liver, WBC	Good	No-grew at 4 mo	Yes
12	M	14	4	Larynx, TBP (tracheostomy)	No	Many	7	Slight-WBC	Slight	Yes	No
13	M	4	2	Larynx, TBP (tracheostomy)	Yes	Many	12	None	Moderate	Yes	Yes
14	F	8	—	Larynx	No	Many	4	Marked-liver	Slight	No	—

TBP - Tracheobronchial pulmonary involvement; LTF - Lost to follow-up.
*History of either respiratory obstruction necessitating tracheostomy or cardiorespiratory arrest.
†Continuing.

remained stable over two successive endoscopies. Furthermore, changes in frequency and/or reduction in the individual dose (to 1 million units/m^2) was called for whenever the WBC count dropped below 2500/cu mm, or the level of SGOT rose above 100 units/ml. If toxicity persisted despite dosage changes, IFN was temporarily discontinued until blood test values returned to normal. Patients or family members were instructed in the technique of injection for at-home IFN administration. Withdrawal of the patients from IFN therapy was considered on an individual basis.

Response to treatment was graded by the evaluation of diagrammatic representation seen at the time of each endoscopy. A response was considered complete when no evidence of papilloma was present in the laryngotracheobronchial area; good response, an estimated 75% reduction of the overall papilloma volume relative to the disease at the time of entrance into the study; moderate response, 50 to 75% estimated reduction; and slight response, 25 to 50% reduction. If no discernible reduction in growth occurred or if growth increased, it was considered a negative response. Reductions in size were assumed to represent a response to IFN.

RESULTS

Twelve of the 14 patients completed a minimum of seven months of alpha-IFN therapy. Patient 4 was removed from the study because of continued toxicity (primarily SGOT elevation) despite dose modifications. Patient 14 was removed from the study at parental request after the first signs of significant liver toxicity. These two patients had shown no response or slight response while receiving the drug.

The responses were distributed as follows among the 12 evaluable patients: 5, complete response (2 of 5 having sustained responses); 3, good response (1 of 3 sustained); 2, moderate response (1 of 2 sustained); and 2, slight response (2 of 2 sustained).

Of the 5 complete responders, there were 3 adults and 2 children, ages 3 and 5 years. All the adults showed complete or good response. The two patients in whom slight responses were seen were 3 and 14 years of age. Six of the 12 patients who responded sustained the initial response throughout the entire period of IFN administration. One patient who showed a complete response was lost to follow-up after one month of observation (patient 6), and the remaining six patients had breakthrough of disease suppression and failed to sustain the initial tumor response. There was no apparent correlation between the degree of initial response and the predictability of sustaining such.

The response-dose relationship of individual responders cannot be judged on any patient with less than a moderate response. Of the ten complete, good, or moderate responses only four patients showed substantial changes in tumor response with alterations of the IFN dosage. Although there was a striking fluctuation of growth rate relative to dosage in very sensitive patients (2,5 and 9), it would appear that the sensitivity of response to this IFN is essentially an "all or none" phenomenon.

IFN has been discontinued in all but one patient (7). Nine patients were evaluated for periods longer than 7 months — three, 12 months; four, 11 months; one, 12 months; and one, 9 months. Eight patients have had at least one month's examination following cessation of IFN treatment. Two of these patients (1 and 12) had slight increase in growth relative to the volume of tumor noted at the time of IFN withdrawal. Two of these four patients (9 and 11) had marked and moderate increases in growth, respectively. Patient 13 showed a transient diminution of disease for approximately one month after cessation of treatment followed by renewed growth of papillomas. Patients 2,3, 5, and 6 have been followed for 1 to 3 months without any signs of increased growth. Patients 2 and 3 with complete responses remain free of disease until the present.

Toxicity was evaluated in 14 patients. Of the 9 patients who demonstrated signs of toxicity, 3 were in the group of complete responses, 2 had good responses, 3 had slight responses and 1 had no response. Neither of the two with moderate responses demonstrated any toxicity.

Temperature elevation was common during the first few injections of IFN but did not appear after the patients had received multiple doses. Malaise, fatigue, and a slight anorexia were not ignored but were usually thought to be of minor significance. As a matter of fact, the infants who showed marked regression of tumor usually became more active and had increased appetites. Toxicity was measured by WBC drop, and elevation in the SGOT level. The degrees of toxicity were classified as slight (1+) when the SGOT remained under 100 and returned to normal with the adjustment of the IFN dosage. It was considered moderate (2+) when the SGOT level was above 100 but returned to normal with proper dosage adjustment. Toxicity (3+) was considered marked when the SGOT level was progressive and forced discontinuation of the protocol. Two of the nine patients with toxicity were taken off the study because of persistent side effects. Depression of the WBC or elevation of the liver enzyme has been totally reversed by alteration of IFN level or cessation of the drug altogether.

No correlation between the response of papillomas and the susceptibility of the patient to IFN toxicity was seen. It is noticeable, though, that of the 8 patients who were under ten years of age, 6 demonstrated SGOT elevations and 4 of these 8 patients had myelosuppression as well. Only one of the five adult patients showed mild liver enzyme elevation and a slight bone marrow suppression. From these numbers, it appears that age of the patients is an important factor in tolerance to IFN.

DISCUSSION

Not only are there variations in the natural history of JLP from patient to patient, but in time different patterns of aggressiveness may be seen in the same patient. Several internal and external influences on the host, some of which escape our present knowledge, induce variations in the behavior of this benign tumor and add to the difficulty of evaluation of its treatment. More aggressive forms of the disease in the larynx, which is the site of most frequent involvement, or over the mucosa of the trachea and bronchi, have necessitated a variety of treatments other than surgical ablation of tumor. Chemotherapy, given systemically or applied topically, has enjoyed transient popularity, but, by and large, it has not given consistent results.[1-18,23]

The IFN system is described as a complex mechanism of cellular defense triggered or induced usually by the influence of viral antigen. The different types of IFN have species-specific antiviral, antiproliferative and antitumor effects.[32]

The majority of clinical studies have been carried out with leukocyte or alpha-IFN. This study was conducted using the product, originally developed by Cantell,[39] of the Finnish Red Cross Blood Transfusion Center and the Central Public Health Laboratory in Helsinki. The preparation obtained is approximately of 1% purity. Lymphoblastoid IFN and IFN obtained through the recombinant DNA technology are of 80-95% purity, respectively. Furthermore, it has been shown that the alpha-IFN obtained by the Cantell method is probably a mixture of several sub-types of IFN, each one with a specific activity.

This present study to a large extent duplicates what was reported by Haglund et al.[36] Although we administered a substantially higher dose of IFN on a daily basis to our patient population, neither the magnitude nor the rate of response could be judged to be very different, if we consider that the two patient populations are compatible. Most patients continued to receive IFN for over nine months without a substantial increase in the response rate. By and large, the beneficial effects of the drug were noticed within 6 to 12 weeks of therapy, and the dose-response relationship was only present in 4 of 10 patients. We did not find that severity of disease or amount of papillomas had any influence on the response rate of this drug. By study design, it was required that all patients have aggressive papillomatosis, and this may have had some influence on the relatively low response rate.

The most accurate possible documentation of any objective changes within the larynx and the tracheobronchial tree are mandatory. Photographic records of the laryngoscopic findings will only reflect the superficial and more proximal appearance of the papillomatosis and certainly fall short of any tumor volume determination. Graphic-pictorial documentation used in this study depends on the accuracy of the observer and is fraught with some margin of discrepancy. We believe that having one endoscopist (RBS) follow up the majority of the patients provided the most accurate, objective evaluation. Despite the method of recording disease some subtleties of change are difficult to describe. One finding that is difficult to document is the appearance of the epithelium of the papillomas during IFN treatment. Some studies have verified histologic changes of degeneration in the papilloma under the influence of treatment.[32,34] On repeated occasions, the observers noticed that under the influence of IFN, the florid, cauliflower-like raised, pinkish papillomas gradually changed to a flat, cobblestone-like pale mucosa, and that these changes reverted to the previous form when the disease process became more active. These visual findings require histologic and ultrastructural verification. Papilloma specimens were taken from all patients during their treatment, and these histologic and ultrastructural changes are under study and will be reported in the future.

Interferon acts as a biologic modifier; therefore, it is possible that when substantial numbers of papillomas are present, the benefits from treatment will be limited. For this reason, we believe that future studies should be designed in such a way that patients would, by conventional means, be rendered free of as much obvious papilloma as possible, prior to beginning IFN treatment. If we assume that papillomas are virally-induced, the best time to administer IFN is before the target cell is stricken by the virus. Furthermore, the antiproliferative and antitumor effects of IFN are most likely to be effective on a relatively small volume of papillomas.

An interesting observation was the increased papilloma proliferation and growth when IFN had to be reduced in dose or frequency of administration. This supports previous studies and places emphasis on the need to determine the optimal dose-time schedule to achieve the best results. A reverse rebound or delayed response effect was observed in patient 13 three weeks after the drug was discontinued when the endoscopist noted a striking improvement. Unfortunately, this was a short-lasting response. The exact mechanism of this rebound response is unknown, but similar effects have been noticed occasionally in patients with solid tumors treated with interferon.[42]

All patients experienced drug-related symptoms during treatment. Fever was present only following the first few injections, and malaise, fatigue, and anorexia were not considered significantly important. On the other hand, patients who had complete responses experienced a sensation of well-being and an increase in appetite.

The main dose-limiting side effect in our patient population has been an SGOT elevation. It is striking that this was particularly noticeable in the younger patients but, again, was not a consistent finding. In every instance, the laboratory values returned to normal within a week after IFN was discontinued and, in all, remained within normal range or slightly above normal when IFN was resumed at either lower dosage or a reduced frequency of administration (three times a week). All patients had slight decreases in WBC primarily due to a decrease in neutrophils. The myelosuppression was mild, with leukopenia below 3,000 in only a few instances. Opportunistic infections did not occur. At this time, the exact mechanism of the SGOT elevation is unclear, and it appears that it is not a manifestation of the IFN itself but may be due to the impurities of the preparation. From studies done in patients with solid tumors, this toxic effect is absent when the purified preparations are used.[43] The multiple anesthetics necessary for endoscopic surgery could be partially responsible for this enzyme elevation. None of the side effects nor the signs of toxicity have persisted after withdrawal from the drug.

Subsequent studies with IFN will have to be designed in such a way that maximum experience is gained to determine the exact dosage and route of administration. It is plausible that the drug could be used locally to the affected organ, which would lessen significant systemic side effects.[44] Whether daily treatment is necessary or an intermittent pulse schedule is more appropriate can only be answered by properly designed randomized studies. Pharmacologic data must be obtained and serum levels will, in part, reflect the degree of IFN-binding to the target tissues.

It is possible that the method of production of alpha-IFN influences its activity. The New York Blood Center has been producing IFN by methods similar to that used by Cantell and collaborators in Finland. Because of some methodologic differences in extraction, the final product may contain a different mixture of active substances. We are presently using this compound in all patients in whom disease continues to be active and who have failed to respond to previous treatment protocols.

The use of a biologic product in young organisms with a potential of a delayed sequela must be evaluated with care. In newborn animals, IFN may be toxic, not only to the hepatic, but also to the renal parenchyma.[38] Thus far, it has been confirmed in human studies.

Our data suggests the relatively impure preparations of alpha-IFN can lead to regression of papilloma. Our observations confirm that further studies and controlled trials in patients with laryngeal papillomas of a variety of clinical presentations are necessary.

REFERENCES

1. Quick CA, Foucan E, Dehner L. Frequency and significance of epithelial atypia in laryngeal papillomatosis. Laryngoscope 1979; 89:550-60.

2. Klos J. Clinical course of laryngeal papillomatosis in children. Ann Otol Rhinol Laryngol 1970; 79:1132-8.

3. Olofsson J, Bjelkenkrantz K. Grontoft O. Malignant degeneration of laryngeal papilloma. J Otolaryngol 1980; 9:329-33.

4. Brach B, Blein RC, Matthews AJ, Cook EW. Papillomatosis of the respiratory tract. Arch Otolaryngol 1978; 104:413-6.

5. Holinger PH, Schild JA, Mauriz DG. Laryngeal papilloma: a review of etiology and therapy. Laryngoscope 1968; 78: 1462-74.

6. Singleton GT, Adkins WY. Cryosurgical treatment of juvenile laryngeal papillomatosis. An eight year experience. Ann Otol Rhinol Laryngol 1972; 81:784-90.

7. Frookot NJ, Rogers JH. The treatment of juvenile multiple laryngeal papillomatosis by section and diathermy. J Laryngol Otol 1979; 93:373-81.

8. Birck HG, Mankart HE. Ultrasound for juvenile laryngeal papillomas. Arch Otolaryngol 1963; 77:603-8.

9. Land FT: Papillomata of the larynx. J Laryngol Otol 1950; 64:205-7.

10. Hollingsworth JB, Kohlmoos HW, McNaught RC. Treatment of juvenile papilloma of the larynx with resin of Podophyllum. Arch Otolaryngol 1950; 52:82-7.

11. Szpunner J. Laryngeal papillomatosis. Acta Otolaryngol (Stockh) 1967; 63:74-86.

12. Holinger PH, Johnson KC, Anison GC. Papillomas of the larynx: review of 109 cases with a preliminary report on aureomycin therapy. Ann Otol Rhinol Laryngol 1950; 59:547-64.

13. Sakurai S, Takahasi M, Nakajima Y, Ishizaka T. Juvenile papilloma of the larynx treated by bleomycin. Keio J Med 1975; 24:11-7.

14. Smith HG, Healy GB, Vaughan GW, Strong MS. Topical chemotherapy of recurrent respiratory papillomatosis. Ann Otol Rhinol Laryngol 1980; 89:472-8.

15. Holinger PH, Shipkowitz NL, Worland MC. Studies of etiology of laryngeal papilloma and an autogenous laryngeal papilloma vaccine. Acta Otolaryngol (Stockh) 1968; 65:63-9.

16. Stephens CB, Arnold GE, Butchko GM, Hardy CL. Autogenous vaccine treatment of juvenile laryngeal papillomatosis. Laryngoscope 1979; 89:1689-96.

17. Quick CA, Behrens HW, Bunton-Darnell M, Good RA. Treatment of papillomatosis of the larynx with transfer factor. Ann Otol Rhinol Laryngol 1975; 84:607-13.

18. Strong MS, Vaughan CW, Healy GB, Cooperband SR, Clemente MACP. Recurrent respiratory papillomatosis: management with the CO_2 surgical laser. Ann Otol Rhinol Laryngol 1976; 85:508-16.

19. Rubin JA. Papilloma of the larynx. Can Med Assoc 1954; 71:572-5.

20. Boyle WF, Riggs JL, Oshior LS, Lennette EH. Electromicroscopic identification of papova virus in laryngeal papillomatosis. Laryngoscope 1973; 83:1104-8.

21. Arnold W. Tubular forms of papova viruses in human laryngeal papilloma. Arch Otorhinolaryngol 1979; 225:15-9.

22. Thost A. Die gutartigen Neubildungen des Kehlkopfes. In: Denker A, Kahler O, eds. Handbuch der Hals-Nasen-Ohren-Heilkundemit Einschluss der Grenzgebiete. Band 5. Berlin: J Springer, 1926-29.

23. Ullman EV. On the etiology of the laryngeal papilloma. Acta Otolaryngol (Stockh) 1923; 5:317-34.

24. Ishikawa K. Klinische und Experimentelle untersuchungen über die Entstehungsursachen der Papilloma. Fukuoka Acta Med (abstr) 1936; 29:87-8.

25. Meesen H, Schutz H. Elektronenmikroskopisher Nachweis des Virus in Kehlkopfpapillom des Menschen. Klin Wochenschr 1957; 35:771-3.

26. Pinsker OT, Proud GO. Studies on the etiology of papilloma of the larynx. Arch Otolaryngol 1958; 56:268-70.

27. Timmel H. Zur Submicroskopischen Morphologie rezidivierender Larynxpapillome. Klin Wochenschr 1961; 39:307-8.

28. Faras AJ, Krzyzek RA, Ostrow RS, et al. Genetic variation among papilloma viruses. Ann NY Acad Sci 1980; 354:60-70.

29. Quick CA, Faras A, Krzyzek R. The etiology of laryngeal papillomatosis. Laryngoscope 1978; 88:1789-95.

30. Lack EE, Jenson AB, Smith HG, Healy GB, Pass F. Immunoperoxidase localization of human papilloma virus in laryngeal papilloma. Intervirology 1980; 14:148-54.

31. Krim M. Toward tumor therapy with interferons: part 2. Blood 1980; 55:875-84.

32. Gutterman JU. Clinical investigation of the interferons in human cancer. Cancer Bull 1981; 33:271-8.

33. Grossberg SE. The interferons and their inducers: molecular and therapeutic considerations. Part 3. N Engl J Med 1972; 287(3):122-8.

34 Strander H, Cantell K, Carlstrom G, Jakobsson PA. Clinical and laboratory investigations on man: systemic administration of potent interferon to man. JNCI 1973; 51:733

35. Strander H. Interferons: anti-neoplastic drugs? Blut 1977; 35:288-99.

36. Haglund S, Lundquist P, Cantell K, Strander H. Interferon therapy in juvenile laryngeal papillomatosis. Arch Otolaryngol 1981; 107:327-32.

37. Grossberg SE. The interferons and their inducers: molecular and therapeutic considerations. Part 1. N Engl J Med 1972; 287(1):13-9.

38. Strander H. Anti-tumor effects of interferon and its possible use as an anti-neoplastic agent in man. Tex Rep Biol Med 1977; 35:429-35.

39. Cantell K, Hirvones S, Mogensen KE, Pyhala L. Human leukocyte interferon: production, purification, stability and animal experiments. In Vitro 1974:35-8.

40. Berg K, Heron I. Production, purification and properties of human interferons. In: Stringfellow DA, ed. Interferon and interferon inducers. New York: Marcel Dekker, Inc, 1980.

41. Goeddel DV, Yelverton E, Ullrich A, et al. Human leukocyte interferon produced by E. coli is biologically active. Nature 1980; 287:411-6.

42. Gutterman JU, Blumenschein GR, Alexanian R, et al. Leukocyte interferon induced tumor regression in human metastatic breast cancer, multiple myeloma, and malignant lymphoma. Ann Intern Med 1980; 93:399-406.

43. Gutterman J, Fein S, Quesada J, et al. Recombinant leukocyte A interferon: pharmacokinetics, single dose tolerance and biologic effects in cancer patients. Ann Intern Med (in press).

44. Padovan I, Brodarec I, Ikic D, Kenzevic M, Soos E. Effect of interferon in therapy of skin and head and neck tumors. J Cancer Res Clin Oncol 1981; 100:295-310.

Ann Otol Rhinol Laryngol 91:1982

CRICOTHYROIDOTOMY: THE IMPACT OF ANTECEDENT ENDOTRACHEAL INTUBATION

ERNEST A. WEYMULLER, JR, MD CHARLES W. CUMMINGS, MD
SEATTLE, WASHINGTON

In light of the current debate regarding cricothyroidotomy, we elected to study the procedure at our institution. Cricothyroidotomy was instituted whenever tracheotomy was necessary for airway management. After a fairly short period of time, some significant complications of cricothyroidotomy were apparent and the study was aborted prior to achieving statistically significant results. The report reviews 15 consecutive cricothyroidotomies. Five (33%) developed significant complications requiring surgical intervention. Of the five, two had life-threatening airway obstruction. The major underlying factor in patients who developed complications was prolonged intubation prior to the institution of cricothyroidotomy. The study suggests that cricothyroidotomy should not be performed after prolonged intubation. The issue of primary cricothyroidotomy for short-term airway control remains unanswered.

INTRODUCTION

In 1976, Brantigan and Grow rekindled interest in cricothyroidotomy and initiated a debate marked by much emotional rhetoric.[1] Their study of 655 patients stands as the single largest accumulation of data on the subject of airway management. Their contention that cricothyroidotomy is an appropriate substitute for tracheotomy is resisted by traditionalists in otolaryngology who favor tracheotomy largely due to the influence and teachings of Chevalier Jackson.[2-5] Our study was initiated to attempt a further assessment of cricothyroidotomy with the intent of including careful laryngeal follow-up.

MATERIAL AND METHODS

Patients identified for the study were those who would have required tracheotomy for airway management. The patients fell into two major groups: 1) those intubated for prolonged periods and in need of further airway support, and 2) head and neck surgical cases without prior intubation who required cricothyroidotomy for airway management.

Patients requiring the procedure were taken to the operating room and, under sterile conditions, a standard cricothyroidotomy was accomplished and a No. 6 cuffed Shiley tracheotomy tube was inserted. Postoperative care included careful wound management using Betadine dressings and routine suctioning and humidification as normally applied to tracheotomy. None of the patients required mechanical ventilation for more than 24 hours.

The patients were registered in a follow-up system and carefully monitored by the authors. Each patient was followed after removal of the cricothyroidotomy tube (decannulation). When stridor or other airway symptoms developed, the patient was evaluated and treated with appropriate intervention.

Each patient in this series has been examined at least two months subsequent to decannulation or completion of therapy for complications of the cricothyroidotomy.

RESULTS

The study was aborted prior to accumulating a large group because significant complications became apparent in the patients who had prolonged intubation prior to cricothyroidotomy.

The total number of patients was 19; 3 died before removal of the cricothyroidotomy and were thus excluded, another patient disappeared one week after decannulation and is excluded. The study group consists of 15 patients, 10 of whom had prolonged intubation prior to cricothyroidotomy. In the group with prolonged endotracheal intubation, the average endotracheal intubation time was 14 days (range 11-21 days), and the average duration of cricothyroidotomy was 50 days (range 14-120 days). In the patients who had no antecedent endotracheal intubation, the average duration of cricothyroidotomy was 24 days (one patient 90 days, others 5-12 days).

There were no complications in ten patients (67%). Five patients (33%) developed significant complications. Two had progressive airway problems subsequent to the removal of the cricothyroidotomy. Each complication was relatively easy to manage with no permanent stenotic sequelae. All the complications occurred during the first month of decannulation.

Of the five patients with complications, four had prolonged endotracheal intubation, the fifth had a cricothyroidotomy performed for airway control (nonemergent) during management of a submandibular gland abscess.

The four patients with prolonged endotracheal intubation had anterior subglottic granulomata and fibrosis managed with endoscopic removal and steroid injection. The incidence of significant complications in this group was 4/10 (40%).

The fifth complication developed in a patient whose cricothyroidotomy became contaminated

---

From the University of Washington, School of Medicine, Seattle.

Presented at the meeting of the American Laryngological Association, Palm Beach, Florida, May 1-2, 1982.

after drainage of a submandibular abscess. The same bacterial organisms grew from the wound and the sputum on the seventh postoperative day and the same organisms were identified in subglottic granulation tissue one month later when stenosis was noted. The patient developed circumferential subglottic and tracheal edema. Successful therapy required four weeks of intravenous antibiotics. There was no vocal cord fixation and no irreversible stenosis as a complication of cricothyoidotomy in this series.

DISCUSSION

The detractors of elective cricothyroidotomy wax effusive but stumble over a lack of objective data. Two cases presented by Kennedy as complications of cricothyroidotomy have some limitations which must be mentioned.[3] The first patient had penetrating trauma of the neck and chest. The cricothyroidotomy is not clearly the source of the laryngeal pathology (fixed left vocal cord and anterior glottic and subglottic stenosis). The second patient had an endotracheal tube in place for four days after which she extubated herself with resultant airway obstruction requiring a cricothyroidotomy. It is clear in this instance that laryngeal pathology existed prior to the establishment of cricothyroidotomy. Mitchell cautions his readers against cricothyroidotomy without any case reports.[2] Carden responds emotionally to the subject without any objective substantiation.[5] Montagano and Passy mention seven cases of subglottic stenosis in a brief letter to the editor but fail to describe the cases and, therefore, leave much open to question.[4]

The champions of cricothyroidotomy on the other hand provide us with much clinical information (cumulatively numbering close to 1,000 patients).[1,6-9] Although their studies can be criticized for lack of patient follow-up, it is clear that the incidence of immediate and long-term complications of cricothyroidotomy in these authors' hands is notably low.

Experimental data from Nelson would suggest that cricothyroidotomy is unsafe.[10] He performed standard cricothyroidotomy on 3 dogs and noted moderate stenosis in 2, minimal stenosis in 1. This was a higher incidence of stenosis than in tracheotomized dogs. More recent studies using a total of 72 dogs have shown that cricothyroidotomy is safe in the experimental setting — even when some of the dogs had removal of cricoid mucosa at the time of cricothyroidotomy.[11,12]

It is important to note that even among the supporters of cricothyroidotomy, there are limitations to the procedure. Most importantly because of occasional complications, the authors are recommending that cricothyroidotomy is contraindicated subsequent to prolonged intubation.[8,13]

Although our series is limited in number, it seems appropriate to conclude that prolonged intubation is a contraindication to cricothyroidotomy. The presence of an endotracheal tube must be considered a source of acute laryngeal inflammation and mucosal ulceration and, therefore, a predisposing factor to complications from cricothyroidotomy.

It is interesting to note that even with a cricothyroidotomy in place for as long as 120 days, the subsequent granulation tissue and fibrosis were relatively easily managed with microscopic removal and instillation of steroids.

Two of the patients who developed complications did not give evidence of an airway problem until sometime after the removal of the cricothyroidotomy. All patients gave clear evidence of their complication within the first month after decannulation and two of them had acute evolution of obstruction, requiring urgent tracheotomy for airway control.

One patient from the series with complications was not examined by the authors after removal of her cricothyroidotomy. This patient had an urgent tracheotomy performed in another city after transfer from our hospital. The otolaryngologist who managed her subglottic stenosis reported that it responded readily to endoscopic dilitation and instillation of steroids. He has examined the patient and confirmed the return to a normal laryngeal status.

One patient had a cricothyroidotomy performed in the face of a rather severe upper airway infection, albeit nonlaryngeal. It would appear that this cricothyroidotomy was contaminated by the draining abscess and this would suggest the relative contraindication of cricothyroidotomy in the face of proximate soft tissue infection.

CONCLUSION

1. This series demonstrates the high probability of complication (40%) from cricothyroidotomy in the face of previous endotracheal intubation. It is the conclusion of the authors that prolonged intubation is a contraindication to routine cricothyroidotomy.

2. The few patients who had cricothyroidotomy without prolonged intubation had a totally benign course, but are too few in number to justify any conclusion.

3. The data in support of cricothyroidotomy as an elective procedure without antecedent intubation seem quite reasonable and the authors support the ongoing clinical research efforts to clarify the exact complication rate of primary cricothyroidotomy.

REFERENCES

1. Brantigan CO, Grow JB. Cricothyroidotomy: elective use in respiratory problems requiring tracheotomy. J Thorac Cardiovasc Surg 1976; 71:72-81.

2. Mitchell SA. Cricothyroidotomy revisited. Ear Nose Throat J 1979; 58:54-60.

3. Kennedy TL. Epiglottic reconstruction of laryngeal stenosis to cricothyroidotomy. Laryngoscope 1981; 90:1130-6.

4. Montagano J, Passy V. Letter to the editor. Plast Reconstr Surg 1981; 67:98.

5. Carden ET. Letter to the editor. Plast Reconstr Surg 1981; 67:99.

6. Boyd AD, Conlan AA. Emergency cricothyroidotomy: is its use justified? Surg Rds 1979; 2:19-23.

7. Brantigan CO, Grow JB. Cricothyroidotomy revisited again. Ear Nose Throat J 1980; 59:26-38.

8. Morain WD. Cricothyroidotomy in head and neck surgery. Plast Reconstr Surg 1980; 65:424.

9. Habel DW. Cricothyroidotomy as a site for elective tracheotomy. Trans Pac Coast Otophthalmol Soc 1977; 58:181.

10. Nelson TG. Tracheotomy: a clinical and experimental study. Am Surg 1957; 23:660-94, 750-83, 841-81.

11. Koopman CF, Feld RA, Coulthard SW. The effects of cricoid cartilage injury and antibiotics in cricothyroidotomy. Am J Otolaryngol 1981; 2:123-238.

12. Romita MC, Colvin SB, Boyd AD. Cricothyroidotomy — its healing and complications. Surg Forum 1977; 28:174-5.

13. Romita MC. Letter to the editor. Plast Reconstr Surg 1981; 67:98.

≈

WORLD CONGRESS OF OTORHINOLARYNGOLOGY

The XIIIth World Congress of Otorhinolaryngology will be held in Miami Beach May 26 — June 1, 1985. For further information please contact Anthony J. Maniglia, MD, Secretary-General, P.O. Box 016960 (D-48), Miami, FL 33101.

NERVE-MUSCLE PEDICLE REINNERVATION OF THE LARYNX: AVOIDING PITFALLS AND COMPLICATIONS

HARVEY M. TUCKER, MD

CLEVELAND, OHIO

The procedure for reinnervation of bilateral vocal cord paralysis using nerve-muscle pedicle technique has now been well established in the literature. Moreover, several other centers have reported success using this technique. Nevertheless, the author is aware that a significant number of well trained otolaryngology-head and neck surgery practitioners have found difficulty in making the procedure successful in their hands. It therefore seems appropriate to address those aspects of patient evaluation, technique and postoperative follow-up that have brought a satisfactory level of success in the author's hands. Preoperative evaluation of patients is the cornerstone of success in nerve-muscle pedicle reinnervation. It is imperative that the larynx be properly evaluated to be certain that there does not exist fixation or ankylosis of one or both arytenoids in addition to paralysis. Clearly if such fixation exists, nerve-muscle pedicle reinnervation cannot be successful. Several pertinent aspects of technique with special reference to the identification of the proper nerve-muscle pedicle, the design of the pedicle and proper identification of the posterior cricoarytenoid muscle will be discussed. Postoperative evaluation of patients may be difficult for inexperienced operators. The author has seen at least three patients who were operated on by other surgeons who were referred because of "failure" of the procedure only to find that all three of them were successfully reinnervated with satisfactory motion of the reinnervated cord for reasonable day-to-day activity. All aspects of postoperative evaluation and management will be discussed as well.

The procedure for reinnervation of bilateral vocal cord paralysis using nerve-muscle pedicle technique has now been well established in the literature.[1-3] Success with this technique has been reported from several centers.[4-6] Nevertheless, capable surgeons have informed the author of difficulty in achieving satisfactory results. This report is intended to address those aspects of patient evaluation, surgical technique and postoperative follow-up that have brought us success with the procedure and which may help to avoid complications or failure if adhered to closely.

PREOPERATIVE EVALUATION AND PATIENT SELECTION

Proper selection of patients and preoperative evaluation are the cornerstones of success in nerve-muscle pedicle reinnervation. In general, the procedure may be considered for any patient with unrecovered bilateral vocal cord paralysis which either has existed for one year from onset or in cases wherein it is known beyond any doubt that there can be no hope of recovery of either of the two recurrent nerves. The majority of patients that meet these criteria have suffered bilateral paralysis as the result of neck surgery, usually for carcinoma of the thyroid or other thyroid lesions.[7]

Analysis of over 200 cases of bilateral vocal cord paralysis that had existed for at least one year[7] shows that fully one third of the patients exhibited fixation or at least severe limitation of motion of one or both of the cricoarytenoid joints in addition to the recurrent nerve paralysis. Since it would be pointless to attempt to reinnervate a bilaterally paralyzed larynx which also exhibits significant fixation, it is imperative that patients be evaluated preoperatively to determine if the arytenoids are passively mobile. This should be accomplished under general anesthesia with paralysis either after performance of a tracheotomy or without intubation and by mask anesthesia only. With a hand-held anterior commissure laryngoscope in place and taking great care to position the laryngoscope so that it does not in any way affect or restrict movement of the vocal cords, a spatula or suction tip is introduced between the vocal cords to palpate them. It is important that the palpating instrument be placed as far posterior in the larynx as possible so that the body of the arytenoid will be displaced rather than the tip of the vocal process or the membranous vocal cord itself (Fig. 1). A normally mobile vocal cord will be easily displaced from its opposite neighbor and will produce a significant increase in the posterior glottic chink. If the arytenoid is ankylosed, it may be possible to displace it from its resting position, but in so doing the opposite arytenoid will be dragged along with it and there will be no significant increase in the posterior glottic chink (Fig. 2). On the other hand, if the palpating instrument is placed too far forward either on the vocal process or on the membranous cord itself, the observer can be easily misled, since the membranous vocal cord and vocal process can often be displaced even when the body of the arytenoid is fixed (Fig. 3). If the palpating instrument is placed too deeply into the larynx, it may impinge upon the cricoid itself and thus give a false impression of fixation of the arytenoid when in fact

From the Department of Otolaryngology and Communicative Disorders, The Cleveland Clinic Foundation.

Presented at the meeting of the American Laryngological Association, Palm Beach, Florida, May 1-2, 1982.

REPRINTS — H. M. Tucker, MD, Chairman, Department of Otolaryngology and Communicative Disorders, The Cleveland Clinic Foundation, 9500 Euclid Avenue, Cleveland, OH 44106.

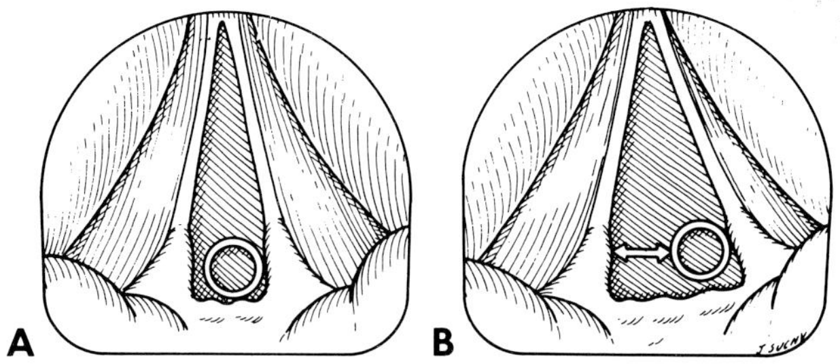

Fig. 1. A) Placement of palpating suction tip in posterior glottic chink. B) Note that lateral pressure is applied to body of arytenoid posterior to tip of vocal process, widening posterior glottic chink in mobile larynx.

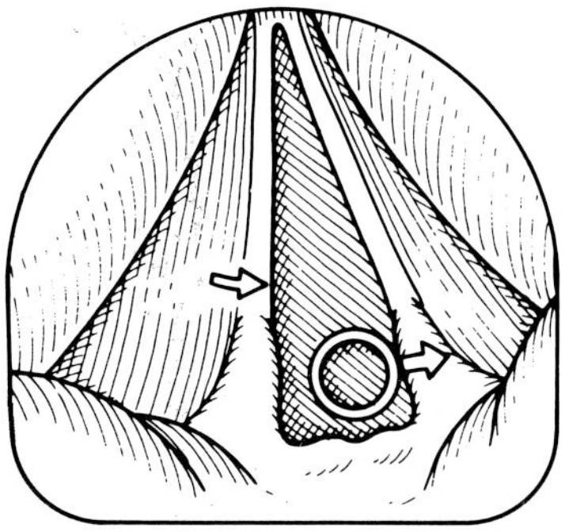

Fig. 2. Fixed arytenoid may still appear to be displaced by suction tip (right arrow). Arytenoid moves laterally, but opposite arytenoid is carried along with it (left arrow).

the joint is normally mobile.

Another factor to be considered in preoperative evaluation is that there must be no uncorrectable restriction of the airway other than the vocal cord paralysis itself. Clearly, if there is subglottic stenosis or other significant narrowing of the airway below the vocal cords, correction of the vocal cord paralysis will still not allow decannulation. As a general rule, such mechanical stenoses should be corrected before any attempt is made at reinnervation.

Another possible pitfall lies in the etiology of the paralysis. Only a 40-50% success rate has been achieved in reinnervating patients whose paralysis is the result of central nervous system problems such as Guillain-Barré syndrome or bulbar poliomyelitis. Any general neurologic disease process that might produce paralysis of the recurrent nerves also may interfere with the activity of the ansa hypoglossi which is necessary to reinnervation. Degeneration of the laryngeal muscles themselves, or direct damage to the nerves from surgery or radiation may interfere with development of the necessary nerve-muscle pedicle and thus prevent successful reinnervation.

SURGICAL TECHNIQUE

The details of surgical technique for nerve-muscle pedicle reinnervation have been described in several previous communications.[1-3] Discussions with several surgeons who have attempted the procedure indicate that the two major areas of potential technical difficulty are related to design of the pedicle and to proper identification of the posterior cricoarytenoid muscle. The pedicle is designed by identifying the branch of the ansa hypoglossi to the anterior belly of the omohyoid muscle. It is not essential that this particular branch be used since any of the strap muscles are suitable, but this nerve is fairly constant, is easily located in the surgical field, and is almost always of sufficient length and size to allow design of a good pedicle. The nerve is traced to the anterior belly of the omohyoid and the pedicle is designed about the actual point of entry of the nerve into the muscle. The nerve will often travel for 2-3 mm between muscle bundles before it actually arborizes into its terminal fibers (Fig. 4). It is essential, therefore, to gently separate these muscle fibers to observe the point of entry so that when the pedicle is designed, most of the terminal fibers and their subtended motor end-plates will be included. On the other hand, the pedicle should not be larger than 2 or 3 mm on a side. This small pedicle is quite adequate to include at least 80% of the subtended motor end-plates, provided it is placed at the very end of the nerve. More important, it avoids the possibility of excessive fibrosis that might occur if a larger pedicle were employed. Although it is true that free grafts of muscle measuring as much as 2 cm on a side can be readily transplanted and will survive, there will be significant loss of bulk and fibrous tissue replacement at the periphery of the graft if such a large piece of muscle is transposed. Since one of the mechanisms whereby nerve-muscle pedicle reinnervation occurs involves neurotization of the recipient muscle by invading nerve buds from the pedicle muscle, it is obviously important that fibrosis between the muscles should be minimized. Since the vasa nervora which are preserved in designing the pedicle will support the nerve but not the muscle, it is clear that the smaller the block of muscle used that will be adequate for preservation of a sufficient number of motor end-plates, the better. Excessively precise dissection of the soft tissue surrounding the nerve itself should be avoided. Since the vasa nervora are essential to the survival of the nerve, it is just as well to leave a fair amount of fat or areolar tissue intact on the surface of the nerve during its dissection to prevent unnecessary injury to these tiny vessels.

The other major potential area for error in the performance of nerve-muscle pedicle reinnervation is related to identification of the posterior cricoarytenoid muscle. After the pedicle has been prepared and laid aside, the lateral border of the thyroid cartilage is palpated and the retropharyngeal space is entered and is opened widely from the tip of the greater cornu of the thyroid cartilage to a point below the cricoid cartilage. If possible, the palpating finger should traverse this space and feel the posterior edge of the thyroid ala on the opposite side. This is relatively easy to do in children, young

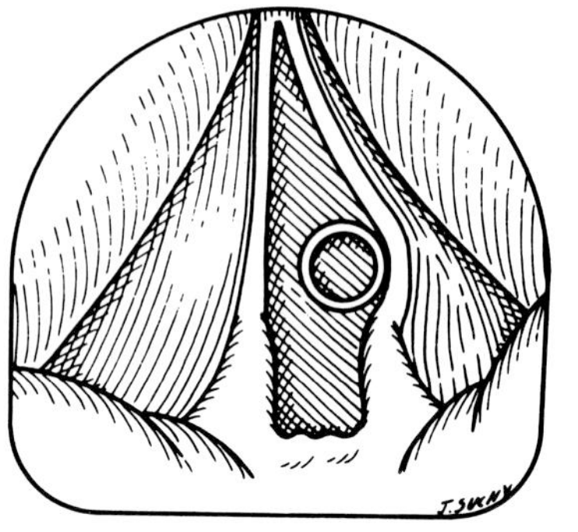

Fig. 3. Apparent displacement of arytenoid. Suction tip has been placed anterior to vocal process and therefore only membranous cord is being displaced.

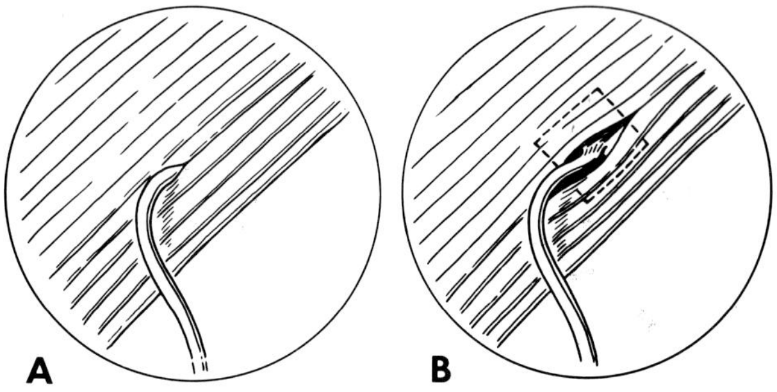

Fig. 4. Design of nerve-muscle pedicle. A) Apparent point of entry; B) actual point of entry. It is important to note point of aborization and entry of nerve into muscle by separating adjacent muscle bundles. (Reprinted with permission.[1])

people and patients who are fairly thin. The larynx can then be rotated almost 180°, which presents the posterolateral aspect of the cricoid and thyroid cartilages to the operator and fixes the larynx in position. The inferior cornu of the thyroid cartilage is then palpated and the approach through the inferior constrictor muscle is begun at a point 2 or 3 mm above the inferior cornu. Dissection is kept as close to the posterior edge of the thyroid cartilage as the anatomy will permit. The fascia is gently dissected free and the direction of the fibers of the inferior constrictor is noted. They travel from posterosuperior to anteroinferior. The fibers are separated along their long axes at the chosen point and widely retracted. In many patients, the inferior constrictor muscle is divided into two leaflets, an external one which inserts along the posterior edge and outer border of the thyroid cartilage and an internal one which inserts along the inner surface of the thyroid ala (Fig. 5). There will often be a plane of loose areolar tissue between these two leaflets. Therefore, having passed through what appears to be the entire inferior constrictor muscle and encountering such a fascial plane, it is easy to be misled into thinking that the next layer of muscle is the posterior cricoarytenoid muscle when it is actually the internal leaflet of the inferior constrictor muscle. It is important to note that the direction of the fibers of the posterior cricoarytenoid muscle is at right angles to those of the inferior constrictor. In most cases, having traversed both leaflets of the inferior constrictor, the reflection of the pyriform sinus mucosa will be encountered and this structure must be bluntly displaced from inferior to superior. In the majority of patients, an easily identifiable muscle structure will be encountered next, the fibers of which pass from posteroinferior to anterosuperior or at right angles to those of the inferior constrictor. This is the posterior cricoarytenoid muscle. If there remains any question as to its identity, the operator can simply pass through the muscle and will encounter the posterior aspect of the cricoid cartilage. When this has been done, if the operator "backs out" one muscle layer, he will have identified the posterior cricoarytenoid muscle. In the occasional patient, this muscle (although still present and capable of reinnervation) will have undergone sufficient wasting that it will be a fairly thin layer. If there is any question, a biopsy can be obtained to demonstrate that it represents striated muscle. Once the muscle has been identified, the nerve-muscle pedicle is sutured to it with one or two sutures of 5-0 nylon. These sutures are first placed through the muscle of the posterior cricoarytenoid and then carried through the muscle in the pedicle. It is only necessary to make contact between the raw surface of the transposed muscle block and the outer surface of the posterior cricoarytenoid muscle. The muscles of the larynx in this area have little or no fascia and in the process of dissecting the reflection of the pyriform sinus off the posterior cricoarytenoid muscle, the surface will be sufficiently denuded to allow good physiologic contact.

In some of the cases where the reinnervation procedure has failed, we have operated through the same incision in an effort to perform an arytenoidectomy and, in the process, have been able to inspect the nerve-muscle pedicle to try to determine reasons for failure. Lack of survival of the nerve-muscle pedicle and/or displacement of the pedicle from the recipient bed have been encountered only once, thus suggesting that these findings are not frequent reasons for failure.

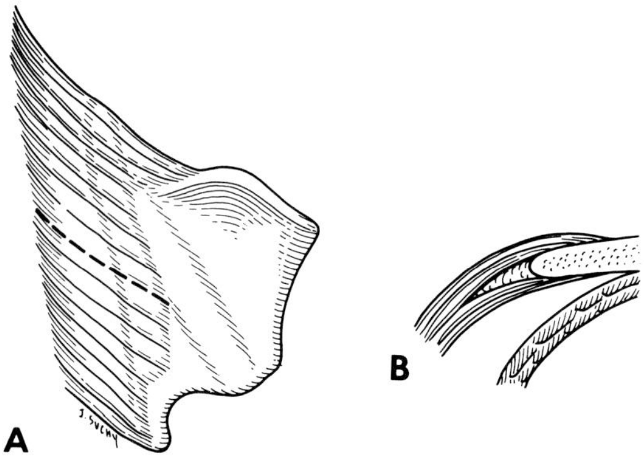

Fig. 5. A) Point of separation of fibers of inferior constrictor muscle (dotted line) to facilitate exposure of the pyriform sinus. B) Deepest muscle layer representing posterior cricoarytenoideus. Horizontal section of larynx at point of entry. External and internal leaflets of inferior constrictor muscle are visible as they insert on free edge of thyroid ala.

POSTOPERATIVE MANAGEMENT AND EVALUATION

There are three possible results of a properly done reinnervation procedure in a correctly chosen candidate: 1) there can be obvious improvement in the patient's airway and exercise capability without benefit of tracheotomy, accompanied by visible motion of the vocal cord during inspiratory effort; 2) there may be obvious improvement in the patient's airway and exercise capability without apparent movement of the vocal cord on inspiratory effort; and 3) there may be no appreciable improvement in the airway.

In the first situation, the success of the procedure is obvious and little need be said. These results will be obtained in approximately 40% of properly selected patients. In the third situation, postoperative evaluation is also fairly straightforward. If there is no visible motion in the cord, even with stress, and if the patient's airway with the tracheotomy tube occluded remains clinically inadequate six months after attempted reinnervation, the operation has failed and further improvement is not to be expected. Such a patient can be left with the tracheotomy tube as a more or less permanent solution to the bilateral cord paralysis problem or some type of vocal cord lateralization can be undertaken. In our current experience in over 200 cases, 20% of all patients subjected to reinnervation will have no improvement.

In the remaining 40%, the patient will have definite clinical improvement in airway and exercise capability with the tracheotomy tube occluded but there will be little or no visible motion of the vocal cord, even with inspiratory effort. These patients should be stressed by running in place with the tube occluded until they are panting and then observed again. In most of them, the reinnervated vocal cord will now be noted to have appropriate abduction with inspiratory effort (although not necessarily with each inspiratory effort) or there will be tonic abduction of the vocal cord. This phenomenon can be explained as follows. In many patients with bilateral vocal cord paralysis, the resting airway is at least adequate for resting ventilatory needs and even perhaps for a small amount of exertion. Since the nerve used to reinnervate abductor function of the vocal cord is derived from an accessory muscle of respiration which becomes highly active only under increased respiratory demand, there would be little or no motion expected unless the patient was stressed. In some patients there will be tonic contraction of the vocal cord because the strap muscles may increase activity under stress in either rhythmic or tonic fashion when respiratory effort is increased and thus the type of movement produced in the reinnervated cord will depend on which is true in the patient in question. The tonic type of contraction can be very subtle and it requires experience to really observe the increase in the cross-sectional area of the airway. This may amount to only 2 or 3 mm improvement at the posterior glottic chink over the resting state, but for many patients this is more than adequate. For this reason, the single most important factor in assessing whether or not a patient should be extubated after reinnervation is his ability to tolerate corking of the tracheotomy tube and still have satisfactory exertional capability. We have examined at least four patients who had successful reinnervation surgery by others, but the surgeon had been reluctant to remove the tube because of lack of apparent movement of the cord. In each of these cases, the patient reported definite improvement in exertional capability with the tracheotomy tube corked. In several of them it was possible to demonstrate subtle but definite lateralization of the reinnervated cord with appropriate exertional testing. All four of these patients were extubated and remained long-term successes.

In some patients a small improvement may be achieved by reinnervation surgery which perhaps is not sufficient for an optimal result. In such cases, if the opposite arytenoid was passively mobile and remained so, we have been able to perform reinnervation on the second side and achieve enough additional improvement that the patients could then be extubated with ability to exert themselves and with safety of the airway.

CONCLUSIONS

Nerve-muscle pedicle reinnervation for rehabilitation of bilateral vocal cord paralysis has been described in the literature and has been successful in the hands of its originator as well as in those of several other authors. Inability to reproduce these results may be related to pitfalls in at least three aspects of management of these patients, including preoperative assessment and selection of patients, design of the nerve-muscle pedicle, proper identification of the posterior cricoarytenoid muscle and postoperative evaluation. With further explanation and attention to these aspects of reinnervation surgery, we hope that other otolaryngologists will find that the procedure can be useful in their own practices.

REFERENCES

1. Tucker HM. Human laryngeal reinnervation: long-term experience with the nerve-muscle pedicle technique. Laryngoscope 1978; 88:598-604.

2. Tucker HM. Reinnervation of paralyzed larynx: a review. Head Neck Surg 1979; 1:235-42.

3. Tucker HM. Laryngeal paralysis: etiology and management. In: English GM, ed. Otolaryngology. Vol. 3. Hagerstown, MD: Harper and Rowe, 1981.

4. Applebaum EL, Alan GW, Sisson GA. Human laryngeal reinnervation: the Northwestern experience. Laryngoscope 1979; 89:1784-7.

5. May M, Lavorato AS, Bleyaert AL. Rehabilitation of the crippled larynx: application of the Tucker technique for muscle-nerve reinnervation. Laryngoscope 1980; 90:1-18.

6. Ward PH, Berci G. Observations on nerve-muscle preparation reinnervation of the paretic larynx — an evaluation of the Tucker procedure. Laryngoscope 1982 (in press).

7. Tucker HM. Vocal cord paralysis — 1979: etiology and management. Laryngoscope 1980; 90:585-90.

≈

INTERNATIONAL PIETRO CALICETI PRIZE

The International Pietro Caliceti Prize has been announced by the University of Bologna. This prize honors the memory of Professor Pietro Caliceti, former distinguished Professor of Clinical Otorhinolaryngology at Bologna University. The prize will be awarded to an Italian or foreign graduate in medicine and surgery, who during a four-year time span (November 1, 1976 to October 31, 1980) published a scientific work of unquestionable value and of recognized originality in the field of otorhinolaryngology. The prize consists of a gold medal, a cash prize of 3,000,000 Italian lire, and a diploma witnessing receipt of the prize. On or before December 31, 1982, interested individuals should send an application, a curriculum vitae, and six copies of the scientific work to the Secretary of the University of Bologna. For further information contact Il Rettore Prof. Carlo Rizzoli, the University of Bologna, Bologna, Italy.

SURGERY OF THE INFERIOR NASAL TURBINATES

William H. Saunders, MD
Columbus, Ohio

The inferior turbinates are responsible for nasal obstruction more often than commonly thought. When there is no other obvious cause for nasal obstruction, and when allergic disorder or other medical condition is not responsible, attention should be given to treatment of the inferior turbinates in many instances of nasal obstruction. Such treatment is usually surgical and may consist of submucous resection of the turbinate bone or excision of redundant hyperplastic turbinate tissue, or a combination of the two. Other treatments consist of electrocautery or cryotherapy. Injection of corticosteroids have produced blindness through embolism and, in general, this treatment is discouraged. The paper discusses in some detail which patients are best suited for submucous resection and which for excision of soft tissue. Techniques, which are simple, are also described.

Chronic nasal obstruction is one of the commonest complaints made by patients to their otolaryngologist. I look forward to seeing these patients with nasal obstruction, since there is virtually always something that can be done to improve their condition. Also, these patients, properly treated, tend to be grateful.

There are, of course, many causes of nasal obstruction. Some are medical causes, such as overuse of nosedrops producing rhinitis medicamentosa, and use of the rauwolfia drugs. An occasional patient has nasal obstruction because of overt hypothyroidism and others because of allergic conditions. All of these causes must be considered in the diagnosis and treated if possible. In this paper we assume none of these conditions to be present.

Surgically correctable conditions causing nasal obstruction include the deviated nasal septum, nasal polyposis, benign and malignant tumors, foreign bodies, and other conditions. One of the most common is disease or structural abnormality of the inferior turbinate. Often two or more causes of nasal obstruction exist together and should be treated simultaneously, but for the purpose of this paper we will consider only disorders of the inferior turbinate and make incidental references to other conditions.

INTRANASAL EXAMINATION

The first step is to establish an accurate diagnosis. To examine the intranasal chamber properly a system of bright lighting is needed. The head mirror reflecting light from a 150-W clear or bulls-eye bulb is the time-honored method because this permits an accurate focusing of light in the posterior aspects of the nose. I have found that the Zeiss operating microscope fitted with a straight head and a 250-mm objective lens offers brilliant illumination, magnification, and binocular vision. Proficiency in this technique is easy to acquire.

Also let me state in passing that while modern nasopharyngoscopes, such as the Machida and Olympus, are useful for special examination, they are not the primary tool for intranasal or postnasal examination.

Whenever the patient has nasal obstruction as a chief complaint, the intranasal examination should include the use of a vasoconstrictor, but not until after the nose has been inspected without the vasoconstrictor. I generally use 3% ephedrine applied on cotton pledgets, although other drugs will do. I do not use topical adrenalin because it produces too intense an effect. Occasionally I use small doses of topical anesthesia, such as Cetacaine spray (contains 2% tetracaine) to facilitate the examination.

An adequate examination must include a careful look at the postnasal space. Sometimes gagging or an inadequate space between the soft palate and posterior pharyngeal wall discourages observation. One must persist, however, since failure to see clearly in the epipharynx is one of the major pitfalls associated with accurate diagnosis. In my opinion the best method of examination is with the number zero nasopharyngeal mirror. Occasionally a palate retractor is needed. Also Valium, 10 mg intravenously, is useful to reduce gagging.

INFERIOR TURBINATE

Normally (Fig. 1A) the inferior turbinate does not obstruct breathing except occasionally when the patient is reclining. Then as blood and tissue fluids pool in the head he may find that one or the other side of his nose is blocked. By turning over in bed, the dependent, obstructive side becomes uppermost and the obstruction is relieved. Such alternating enlargement and diminishing of the soft tissue of the turbinates occurs several times daily regardless of posture, but usually does not cause symptoms. In

From the Department of Otolaryngology, The Ohio State University, Columbus.

Presented at the meeting of the American Laryngological Association, Palm Beach, Florida, May 1-2, 1982.

REPRINTS — William H. Saunders, MD, Dept. of Otolaryngology, The Ohio State University, 456 Clinic Drive, Columbus, OH 43210.

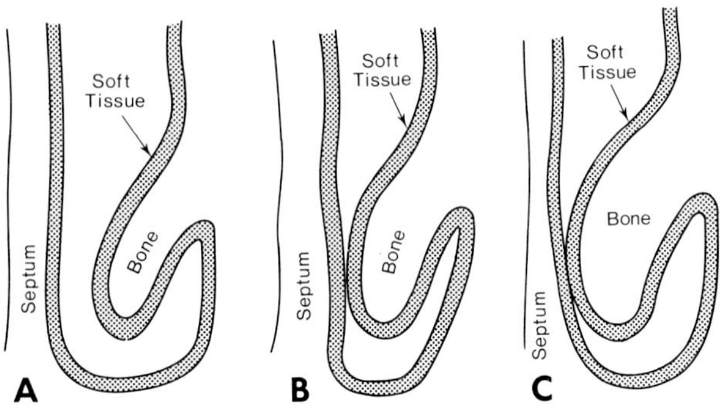

Fig. 1. Bone of inferior turbinate. A) Normal alignment. B) Bone approximates septum; small inferior meatus. C) Bone approximates septum; substantial inferior meatus.

short, the normal inferior turbinate should warm and moisten the air without producing symptoms.

Symptoms other than nasal obstruction such as headpain and postnasal discharge are not likely to be caused by deformity or disease of the turbinates and the patient should understand clearly, preoperatively, that the only symptom the surgeon is trying to relieve is nasal obstruction. Otherwise the operation, at least in the mind of the patient, fails before it starts.

There are, in general, three ways in which the inferior turbinate produces nasal obstruction. First, an undue prominence of the bony structure of the turbinate may cause it to touch or approximate the nasal septum (Fig. 1B). In this case application of vasoconstrictors reduces the size of the turbinate only minimally. When one palpates the turbinate it is apparent that the enlargement is bony and that the obstruction is not merely due to soft tissue engorgement or hyperplasia.

Treatment in this case consists of submucous resection of all or part of the turbinate bone so that the obstructive turbinate is reduced and no longer touches or nearly touches the nasal septum. This is best accomplished with the patient under local anesthesia. An incision is made down to the bone of the turbinate along most of its medial length. Then the soft tissue is elevated upward and downward and a substantial amount of bone exposed and removed. A chisel may be needed to fracture the bone, but often pieces can be broken off using a hemostat or submucous elevator. Gauze packing (preferably impregnated with Terramycin ointment) is applied and left in place at least 48 hours to prevent bleeding. The only complication of this procedure is postoperative hemorrhage, which is seen chiefly when packing is removed too soon. To be safe, I leave packs in place three to four days and remove them on an outpatient basis.

Sometimes it is worthwhile to crush an inferior turbinate laterally (toward the inferior meatus) when it is the bone of the turbinate that causes obstruction and not soft tissue. This procedure works best if the turbinate is first displaced toward the nasal septum and then pressed laterally. Even so, in most instances this procedure is not entirely effective since the fracture produced tends to be of the greenstick variety and later the turbinate tends to return to its original position. Lateral displacement works best in cases where there is a large inferior meatus to receive the newly displaced turbinate (Fig. 1C).

Second, there are patients with redundant hyperplastic turbinate mucosa (Fig. 2A). Their nasal obstruction may be severe unilaterally or bilaterally. The bony turbinate may or may not be enlarged, but certainly the soft tissue of the turbinates is excessive. Shrinkage with vasoconstrictors is incomplete and palpating the redundant lower and medial surfaces of the turbinate shows it to be flaccid and polypoid (Fig. 2B). The treatment here

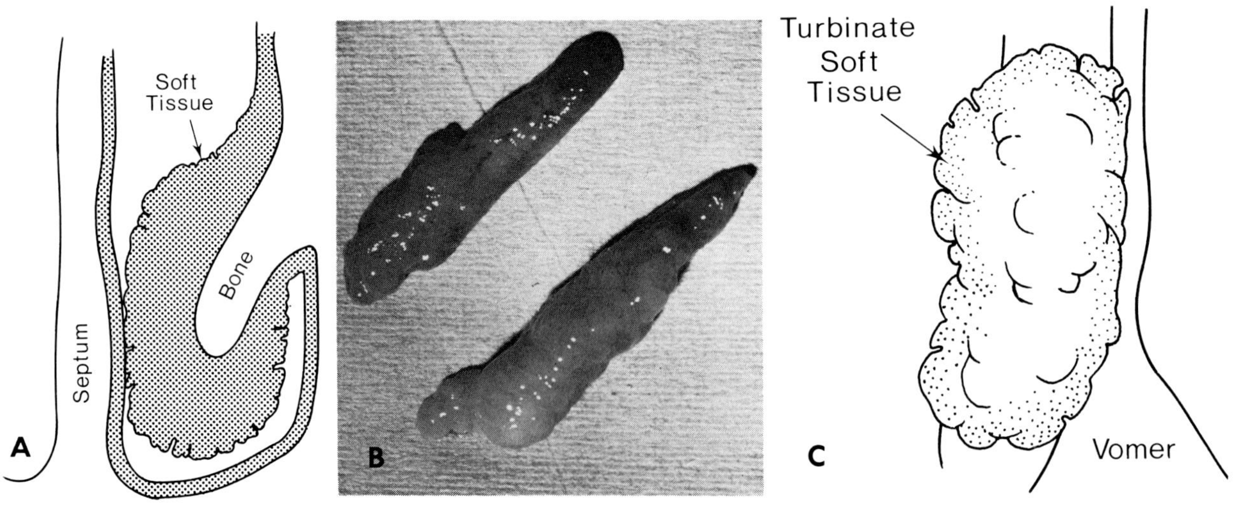

Fig. 2. A) Hyperplastic soft tissue of inferior turbinate with other relationships normal. B) Typical redundant, hyperplastic turbinate mucosa. This excision represents less than half of the entire turbinate tissue. C) Hyperplastic posterior tip of inferior turbinate.

(we assume no allergic condition) is to excise generously the redundant tissue with scissors. In addition, submucous resection of the bone may be required. In my opinion at least half of the soft tissue of the hyperplastic turbinate can be excised without danger of producing atrophic rhinitis.

Sometimes likened to a mulberry, the hyperplastic posterior end of the inferior turbinate may be so large as to fill one choana completely (Fig. 2C). The time to assess appearance of the posterior tip of the turbinate is preoperatively in the office using the postnasal mirror — not at the time of surgery. A snare passed around the posterior tip will cut it off, but there usually is need for additional work on the turbinate anteriorly. Even if only the posterior tip is snared away, be sure to pack the nose for three to four days or postoperative bleeding may be profuse.

Third, turbinates are often enlarged because of vasomotor changes. They seem simply engorged, and the mucosa is not particularly redundant or polypoid and the turbinate bone is not prominent. Vasoconstrictors should produce shrinkage. Again, it is assumed that there are no allergies identified.

Treatment may be with electrocautery by stripping the surface of the turbinate with the blade of the cautery instrument or inserting an electrode submucosally. In any case the result is tissue destruction and scarring so that there comes to be a reduction in the size of the turbinate. The treatment may have to be repeated. Local injectable anesthesia is adequate and the procedure may be done on an outpatient basis. Also, in patients of this type there is no reason that submucous resection of the turbinate should not be effective, and, as a matter of fact, I prefer it to cautery. Formerly, some doctors injected sclerosing solutions into the inferior turbinate to cause shrinkage, but now that there are reports of blindness from similar injections with steroids such injections are no longer done by most doctors.

MIDDLE TURBINATE

The middle turbinate also may contribute to nasal obstruction. When it does it is apt to be because of an ethmoidal air cell that dilates the turbinate. Also I have seen examples of mucoceles of the middle turbinate. In either case the treatment is easy: simply incise into the thin, shell-like structure and either crush it with a hemostat or other forceps, or resect some portion of the bone.

CORRECTION OF POSTERIOR GLOTTIC INCOMPETENCE FOLLOWING HORIZONTAL PARTIAL LARYNGECTOMY

HUGH F. BILLER, MD

WILLIAM LAWSON, MD, DDS

STEVEN SACKS, MD

NEW YORK, NEW YORK

Posterior glottic insufficiency following horizontal partial laryngectomy results in persistent aspiration. A new method of correction of this occurrence is described. The procedure is an extralaryngeal approach. A tracheotomy is not required. The procedure was successful in 4 of 6 patients.

Closure of the glottis on deglutition is essential for rehabilitation following horizontal partial laryngectomy or partial laryngopharyngectomy. Failure to achieve glottic closure in these cases is associated with chronic aspiration and recurrent or persistent pneumonitis. At the time of resection every effort is made to ensure adequate glottic closure postoperatively. Glottic insufficiency usually results from one of the following: 1) partial or total arytenoid removal; 2) partial resection of the true cord to obtain a tumor-free inferior margin; or 3) inadvertent injury of the recurrent laryngeal nerve during cricopharyngeal myotomy.

The first circumstance is the most common cause. Partial arytenoid resection with exposure of the residual cartilage frequently leads to arytenoid fixation in the abducted position. In these cases coverage of the exposed cartilage with a mucosal flap may avoid chondritis and, ultimately, fixation. Resection of the superior aspect of the arytenoid to the level of the vocal process will lead to fixation in most cases, even though mucosal coverage is performed. In these cases, even if the arytenoid moves when the anesthesia is lightened, the vocal cord should be fixed in the midline. This fixation is accomplished with a nonabsorbable submucosal suture extending from the vocal process to the perichondrium of the cricoid cartilage. This suture, when tightened, rotates the arytenoid internally, resulting in a vocal cord fixed in the midline. However, the defect created following complete arytenoid resection cannot be corrected by simply suturing the vocal process to the cricoid. Any attempt to do so will result in a defect in the posterior glottis postoperatively. In these cases, a free or pedicled cartilage graft is shaped to conform to the defect and is wired to the cricoid. The cut margin of the vocal process is then anchored, in the midline, to this piece of cartilage with a nonabsorbable suture. The entire reconstruction is now covered by a mucosal flap from the medial wall of the pyriform sinus.

Despite immediate reconstruction at the time of resection, a small number of patients will aspirate postoperatively because of incomplete glottic closure posteriorly. This failure may result from scarring, resorption of the cartilage graft, or inadequate reconstruction at the time of surgery.

This presentation introduces a technique for correction of postoperative posterior glottic deficiency. The diagnosis of postoperative posterior glottic incompetence is determined by indirect laryngoscopy in the patient with persistent aspiration. This circumstance is frequently, but not always, accompanied by a breathy voice. Indirect laryngoscopy confirms the diagnosis and also determines whether the defect is anterior in the membranous cord, or posterior at the arytenoid location. This determination is important for each area requires a different type of correction. Correction of deficiencies anteriorly along the membranous portion of the vocal cord has been adequately covered in previous papers[1-4] and will not be considered here.

TECHNIQUE AND MATERIALS

The approach entails an extralaryngeal exposure similar to the arytenoidectomy procedure as described by Woodman.[5] The operation is performed under general anesthesia utilizing endotracheal intubation with a 6.5 mm tube. If a neck dissection has been performed, a vertical incision is used so as to avoid exposure of the carotid. If a neck dissection has not been performed a horizontal incision (Fig. 1A-b) is made in the anterolateral neck. The remaining portion of the posterior border of the thyroid ala is identified. The attachment of the inferior constrictor muscle to the posterior border is divided. The cricothyroid articulation is separated and the posterior border of the thyroid cartilage is retracted anteriorly with a hook. The pyriform sinus mucosa is reflected superiorly and the posterior aspect of the cricoid cartilage is identified. A subperichondrial dissection is performed, if possible, exposing the posterior-superior cricoid border (Fig. 1B). The mucosa is elevated from the superior aspect of the cricoid laterally and to the midline. A piece of cartilage or bone is obtained, tailored and wired on to the cricoid at the arytenoid area (Fig. 1C). If a tear in the mucosa occurs, it is sutured. Direct laryngoscopy is then performed to evaluate whether the defect is adequately corrected (Fig. 2). Additional cartilage may be placed if necessary.

From the Department of Otolaryngology, The Mount Sinai Medical Center, New York.

Presented at the meeting of the American Laryngological Association, Palm Beach, Florida, May 1-2, 1982.

REPRINTS — Hugh F. Biller, MD, Dept. of Otolaryngology, Mount Sinai Hospital, 100th St. & 5th Ave., New York, NY 10029.

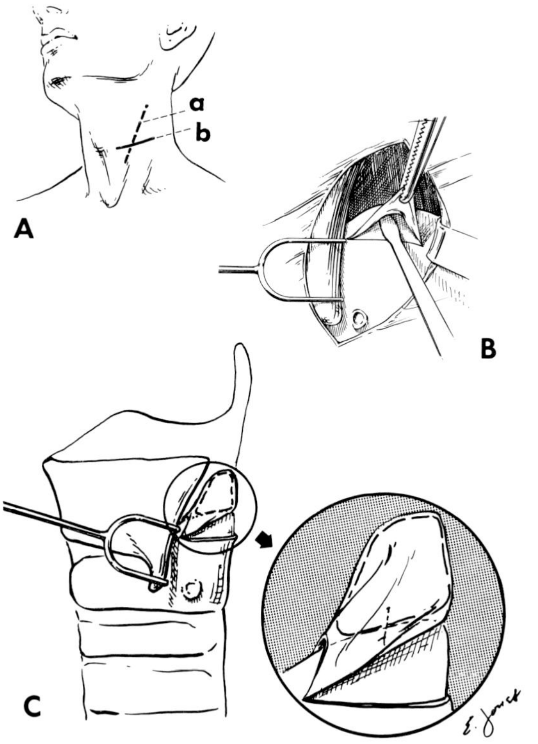

Fig. 1. A) Skin incision. a - Anterior border of sternocleidomastoid muscle; b - Horizontal incision in the anterolateral neck. B) Disarticulation of the cricothyroid articulation and subperichondrial dissection of arytenoid joint. C) Insertion and fixation of graft.

This procedure has been performed on six patients. The reconstructive effort occurred four months to two years following the initial extirpative surgery. Two of the six patients had partial laryngopharyngectomies performed for pyriform sinus cancers with complete excision of the arytenoid cartilage. Four patients had supraglottic carcinomas resected with partial or complete arytenoid removal. All patients aspirated sufficiently to require gastrostomy or nasogastric tube feedings. Three of the six patients had prior injection of Teflon without improvement.

RESULTS

Surgery was considered successful following the extralaryngeal cartilage implants in 4 of the 6 patients. These patients were able to feed orally without aspiration, gained weight, and had their nasogastric or gastrostomy tubes removed. These four patients have been followed for a minimum of 18 months. There has been no evidence of recurrence of the defect or aspiration.

One of the two patients who failed was noted to have extensive granuloma formation at the time of surgery, presumably secondary to the extravasation of Teflon. In this patient the anatomy was distorted and though a graft was inserted, minimal correction of the defect was obtained. The other failure had a graft which was small and only partially corrected the defect.

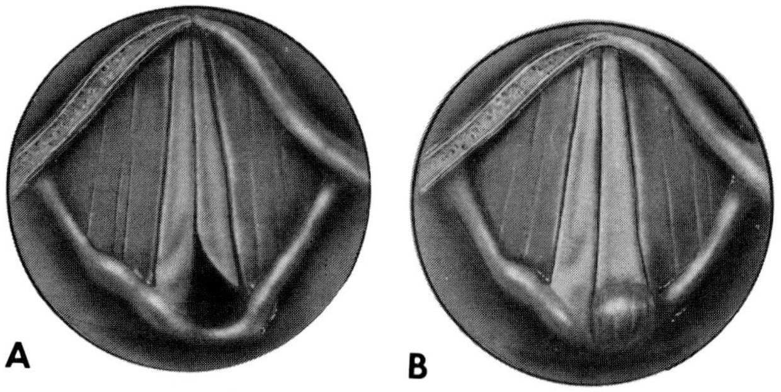

Fig. 2. A) Posterior defect and B) corrected.

DISCUSSION

The correction of late posterior glottic deficiency has received limited attention in the literature. Teflon injection, although successful in correcting the lateralized vocal cord secondary to paralysis or minimal scarring, is uniformly unsuccessful in the treatment of posterior glottic defects. The reason for this is that the dense adherence of the mucosa to the cricoid does not permit installation of this substance.

The only previous article addressing this problem is by Sessions et al.[3] These authors advocated correction of posterior defects by performing a thyrotomy and then dissecting a pocket between the vocal cord and the thyroid cartilage. This pocket was elevated posteriorly to the cricoid, following which a piece of cartilage was inserted. In our experience, this anterior approach is unsatisfactory because the cartilage graft is not fixed in position and, therefore, yields unpredictable results. A tracheotomy is also required. These deficiencies with correction through a thyrotomy led to the formulation of the present extralaryngeal approach. This extralaryngeal approach provides excellent exposure, wide mucosal undermining, permanent fixation of the graft, accurate assessment of the correction by direct laryngoscopy at the time of surgery and eliminates the requirement of a tracheotomy.

One of the failures in this series probably was due to prior extravasation of Teflon. It is apparent from our experience that Teflon installation should not be attempted for these posterior defects but rather cartilage grafting performed by the procedure described.

REFERENCES

1. Waltner J. Surgical rehabilitation of the voice following laryngo-fissure. Arch Otolaryngol 1958; 67:99-101.

2. Arnold G. Vocal rehabilitation of paralytic dysphonia IX. Technique of intracordal injection. Arch Otolaryngol 1962; 76:358-68.

3. Sessions D, Ogura J, Ciralsky R. Late glottic insufficiency. Laryngoscope 1975; 85:950-9.

4. Meurman Y. Operative medial fixation of the vocal cord in complete unilateral paralysis. Arch Otolaryngol 1952; 55:544-53.

5. Woodman D. A modification of the extralaryngeal approach to arytenoidectomy for bilateral abduction paralysis. Arch Otolaryngol 1946; 43:63.

Ann Otol Rhinol Laryngol 91:1982

TRACHEOSTOMAL STENOSIS FOLLOWING TOTAL LARYNGECTOMY

EUGENE N. MYERS, MD, FACS LOUIS J. GALLIA, DDS, MD

PITTSBURGH, PENNSYLVANIA

Stenosis of the tracheostoma after laryngectomy is an infrequent but often distressing postoperative complication. Recognition of possible predisposing factors will allow appropriate preventive measures in preoperative planning, surgical technique and postoperative care. We describe a surgical technique which can be utilized to correct tracheostomal stenosis or can be used at the time of initial stomal construction. Our method emphasizes mobilization of the tracheal stump, extensive excision of subcutaneous fat, excision of redundant skin and creation of a posterior-superior skin flap which is interdigitated into a vertical posterior tracheal incision. Our method is compared to other techniques described in the literature.

INTRODUCTION

Stenosis of the tracheostoma after laryngectomy is an infrequent but often distressing postoperative complication. It may occur in the immediate postoperative period or years later. Stomal stenosis will compromise not only optimum air exchange but also the ability to clear tracheobronchial secretions. The tracheal lumen may be reduced 50% in all diameters (resulting in a 75% reduction in luminal surface area) and a patient with normal lungs will maintain tolerance for normal exercise.[1] In a patient with emphysema or a chronic productive cough, the same defect may produce respiratory insufficiency. Stomal stenosis acts as a barrier to mucociliary transport resulting in a stagnation of mucus and a potential for recurrent pulmonary infection.[1] Severe stenosis, especially with the addition of crusting, may result in asphyxia.[2]

ETIOLOGICAL FACTORS

Factors contributing to stomal stenosis[2] include:

1. Radiation therapy
2. Excessive scar tissue formation
3. Wound dehiscence with healing by secondary intension
   a. Skin tension
   b. Infection
   c. Steroid usage
4. Keloid formation
5. Defective or absent tracheal rings
6. Inadequate excision of peristomal skin and fat at initial stomal construction
7. Recurrent tumor

PREVENTIVE MEASURES

The ideal method of dealing with tracheostomal stenosis is prevention. Preventive measures include careful preoperative planning, meticulous surgical technique and diligent postoperative care.

Planning. Subglottic extension of a laryngeal carcinoma will require resection of additional tracheal rings for adequate tumor clearance. In such cases, careful construction of the stoma, possibly with appropriate local flap design, will minimize tension-induced tracheocutaneous dehiscence and concentric scarring. There is a tendency for this dehiscence to occur in patients on chronic steroid administration; such cases should be constructed virtually tension-free.

If preliminary tracheostomy is required a few days or more prior to laryngectomy one may expect an extensive local inflammatory response which may predispose to stomal stenosis. A tracheal ring defect due to chondritis may predispose to stomal collapse.

In the grossly obese patient, the fat-laden peristomal tissues tend to bulge into the stoma resulting in a pseudostenosis. In the black patient, examination of previous wounds including surgical incisions will provide clues as to the potential for stomal keloid formation.

The stomal stenosis seen after radiation therapy presumably results from concentric scarring. Local flap transposition designed to enlarge the stoma and prevent formation of a circular scar may prevent the problem.

Surgical Technique. The primary objectives in the surgical prevention of tracheostoma stenosis are careful approximation of skin and mucous membrane, elimination of extensive compressive forces, active tension on the stoma margins, increased circumference, and redistribution of the forces of scar contraction.

From the Department of Otolaryngology, University of Pittsburgh School of Medicine, Eye and Ear Hospital.

Presented at the meeting of the American Laryngological Association, Palm Beach, Florida, May 1-2, 1982.

REPRINTS — Eugene N. Myers, MD, FACS, Professor and Chairman, Eye and Ear Hospital, 230 Lothrop Street, Pittsburgh, PA 15213.

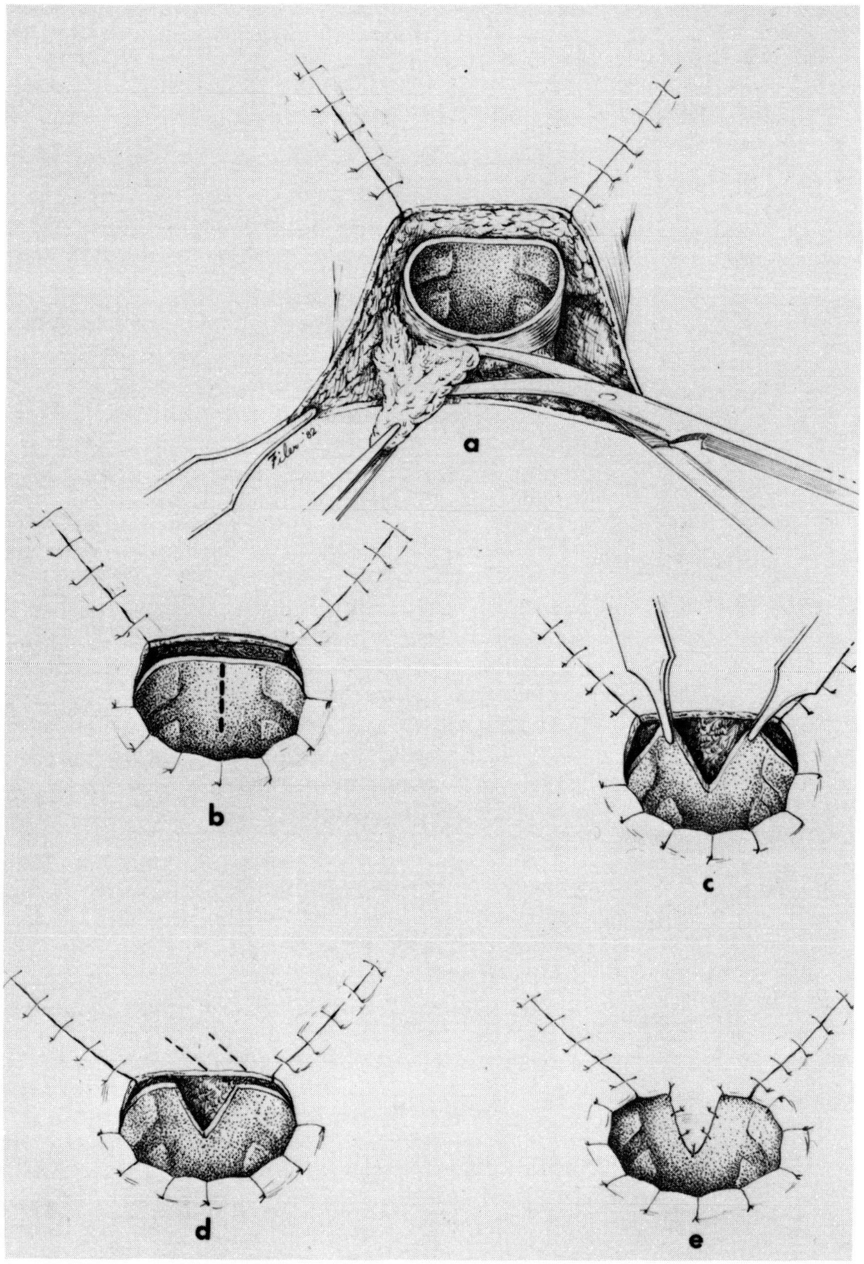

Fig. 1. a) Excision of peristomal adipose tissue. b, c) Incision in membranous posterior wall of trachea. d, e) Creation and transposition of local skin flap into tracheal incision with completion of stomal skin closure.

The most common techniques[2,3-5] to prevent stenosis include 1) oblique section of the tracheal stump (to increase stomal diameter); 2) semicircular or circular incision, to increase the circumference of the skin margin to adapt to the tracheal stump (to achieve tension radially on the stoma); 3) complete coverage of the cut edge of the tracheal cartilage with through and through or vertical mattress sutures.

In the obese patient, excision of excess adipose tissue will minimize the external compressive force of the adipose tissue.

Clairmont,[6] Jatho,[7] Isshiki and Tanabe,[8] Trail et al,[9] and Hartwell and Dykes[10] described a variety of similar techniques employing Z-plasty, double V and V-Y flap design methods of primary tracheostomal construction at the time of laryngectomy in order to prevent stenosis by enlarging the stoma and redirecting the forces of scar contraction.

Clairmont[6] created a "butterfly" or "bowtie" stoma by excising inferiorly based wedge-shaped triangles from the anterior and posterior tracheal stump. Superior and inferior skin flaps, created by lateral skin excision, are inset into the apex of the tracheal defects.

Trail et al[9] use a method of double rotation flap Z-plasty utilizing the skin posterior to the stoma transposed into an oblique incision in the posterior membranous tracheal wall. A small flap of mucosa of posterior tracheal wall is then transposed into the

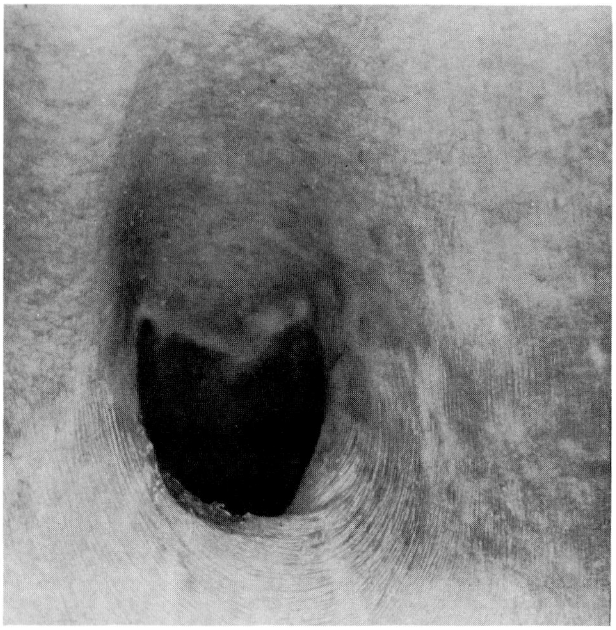

Fig. 2. Healed tracheal stoma in patient who had total laryngectomy and radical neck dissection one year following full course "curative" radiation therapy.

tumor site of the skin flap.

Isshiki and Tanabe[8] utilize superiorly based double skin flaps, created by a Y-shaped cutaneous incision, each of which is inserted into a separate oblique incision of the posterior tracheal wall.

Jatho[7] enlarges the stoma by a vertical anterior tracheal incision; edges created by this cut are pulled apart by permanent subcutaneous sutures which are affixed to the clavicle.

Hartwell and Dykes[10] created a triangular posterior-superior skin flap by excising a wedge of skin on each side of this flap. The flap is advanced and inset into a vertical incision of the posterior trachea. This technique differs from the technique we describe only in that this is an advancement flap which may tend to be redundant, whereas ours is a transposition flap.

Mumma and Pressman[11] described implantation of a subcutaneous tantalum ring around the stoma to prevent stenosis.

Postoperative care. Basic tenets of care which will minimize stomal stenosis include proper tube selection, meticulous local wound care and timely decannulation.

Some feel that an oversized tube may produce stenosis by producing mucosal inflammation and de-epithelization with subsequent concentric scarring. Removal of pericannular crusts and secretions, along with application of antibacterial agents such as Betadine, should minimize bacterial contamination and infection. Prolonged cannulation and especially prolonged mechanical ventilation provide the same type of provocative stimulation as an oversized tube. The patient should be decannulated as soon as possible.

MANAGEMENT OF TRACHEOSTOMAL STENOSIS

Once tracheostomal stenosis has developed, it is best managed by surgical correction. The many varieties of surgical procedures designed to correct stomal stenosis imply that the ideal solution to this problem has not yet been found.

An alternative nonsurgical technique of stenosis management involves dilation with progressively larger tracheostomy tubes and constant use of one of a variety of tracheostomy "buttons." This is usually unsatisfactory as a permanent solution since removal of the button even for a few hours often results in rapid restenosis.

Montgomery[2] reports that the method of tracheostoma repair will depend on the anatomical configuration of the stenosed stoma. He classifies the common types of stenosis as a) vertical slit, b) concentric, and c) "inferior shelf" stenosis. He demonstrates separate procedures for the correction of vertical stenosis. These techniques will effect lateral pull on the stomal margins by straight advancement and Z-plasty flaps or enlargement of the stoma with a double V-Y flap design.

For the correction of concentric stenosis, Montgomery recommends radial incisions made with an electrocautery knife followed by several weeks of cannulation with a large bore tracheostomy tube. He also presents a method of repair (the "donut" repair) where a 1 cm cuff of scar tissue is removed, the scarred edges undermined and the skin edges resutured to the tracheal margins.

For the correction of both concentric and "inferior shelf" stenosis, Montgomery recommends elevation of an inverted V skin flap with resection of a section of anterior tracheal wall and part of the skin flap to enlarge the stoma and supply an inferior traction on the stoma. Advancement of the lateral marginal incision supposedly applies additional pull on the stoma.

Converse[12] describes a swastika-shaped incision around the stenosed stoma; the stenosed skin is excised and the four created flaps are rotated, thus presumably creating a lateral tension to prevent recurrence.

Maruyama et al[13] utilized a 5 flap reconstruction consisting of two Z-plasties combined with a Y-V advancement which break up the superior of the stenosis and increase the circumference of the stoma.

TECHNIQUE

In the patient who has stomal stenosis following total laryngectomy, the most common problem is that there is a band of scar tissue present which concentrically narrows the stoma. Usually the caliber of the trachea is otherwise normal. The goal of this revision procedure is to excise this concentric scar and to prevent it from recurring.

The revision operation may be done under local or general anesthesia (Fig. 1). An incision is made around the periphery of the tracheostoma including the band of scar tissue. Clamps are applied to the scar tissue band and the trachea pulled up into the wound. The trachea is skeletonized for 1-2 rings thereby mobilizing the trachea for repositioning. The skin inferior to the tracheostoma is undermined for 2-3 cm, and the subcutaneous adipose tissue is removed. The excess skin in this area should be excised. The band of scar tissue is then excised from the tracheostoma and utilizing interrupted 3-0 chromic catgut sutures, the skin is sutured to the tracheostoma with a meticulous technique making certain that skin overlaps the raw edges of the cartilage and is in contact with the tracheal mucosa. This suturing is carried out to a level of 3 and 9 o'clock on the tracheostoma. The skin of the neck surrounding the posterior wall of the trachea is then undermined. Adipose tissue and redundant skin are excised. The membranous posterior tracheal wall is then incised vertically approximately 1 cm into the trachea itself. The suturing of the trachea to the skin inferior to the trachea is resumed. The circumference of the tracheostoma will now be considerably widened since the trachea has been split, thereby spreading open the tracheal lumen. A small incision is made in the redundant skin posterior to the trachea such that a small flap is developed. The flap is then transposed and sewn into the incision which has been made in the posterior wall of the trachea. The same 3-0 chromic suture material is utilized in this area. This breaks up the concentric circle of the tracheostoma thereby preventing the narrowing by scar tissue in the future.

Our technique emphasizes mobilization of the tracheal stump, the extensive excision of subcutaneous fat, excision of redundant skin, and creation of a posterior-superior skin flap which is interdigitated into a posterior tracheal vertical incision. The introduction of this flap breaks up the concentric circle of scar and prevents future stenosis. This is probably the single most important feature of this technique.

Our technique most closely resembles that of Hartwell and Dykes[10] in that a posterior-based skin flap is inserted into an incision in the posterior tracheal wall. Our technique seems to differ in that we advocate extensive subcutaneous fat excision and trimming the peristomal skin back as far as is necessary to provide slight tension on the closure. We also advocate a small transposition flap rather than an advancement flap.

Clairmont,[6] Isshiki and Tanabe,[8] Maruyama et al,[13] Converse,[12] and Montgomery[3] utilize the same principles of stomal enlargement and inhibition of circular scarring but are needlessly complex in design. We feel the simplest technique to accomplish the goal should be used. Our technique is adaptable to any type of stenosis, and the altering of the repair to the type of stenosis, as advocated by Montgomery, is probably unnecessary.

Implantation of foreign bodies as recommended by Mumma and Pressman[11] and Jatho[7] may result in infection, inflammation and actually accentuate scar formation and stenosis.

We have now begun to incorporate this exact same technique routinely in fashioning the tracheostoma in all patients undergoing total laryngectomy (Fig. 2). We believe that this is of particular importance to anticipate the potential for tracheostoma stenosis in patients who will receive postoperative radiation therapy particularly involving the tracheostoma.

DISCUSSION

In patients in which the tracheostoma area has been radiated postoperatively, extreme caution should be taken and minimal undermining should be carried out. Our three patients who have had complications from this type of tracheostomal revision all fall into this category. One patient had had several previous revision procedures. She lost considerable skin following our revision and restenosed. Two other patients lost some peristomal skin following revision, but did heal by secondary intention and fortunately did have correction of their tracheal stenosis.

SUMMARY

Stenosis of the tracheostoma after total laryngectomy is a distressing postoperative complication. Stomal stenosis can be prevented or minimized by careful preoperative planning, meticulous surgical technique and diligent postoperative care. Etiological factors, preventive measures, and a review of surgical corrective techniques have been described. The authors describe a technique which has provided a satisfactory solution to tracheostomal stenosis in most cases.

REFERENCES

1. Bain J. Late complications of tracheostomy and prolonged endotracheal intubation. Int Anesthesiol Clin 1972; 10:225-44.

2. Montgomery W. Stenosis of tracheostoma. Arch Otolaryngol 1962; 75:76-9.

3. Montgomery W. Surgery of the upper respiratory system. 2nd ed. Vol. 2. Philadelphia: Lea and Febiger, 1979.

4. Nauman HH. Kopf und Hals-chirurgie. Band 1. Stuttgart: Georg Thieme Verlag, 1972.

5. Barbosa JF. Surgical treatment of head and neck tumors. New York: Grune and Stratton, 1974.

6. Clairmont A. Tracheostoma construction during laryngectomy: techniques to prevent stenosis. J Laryngol Otol 1978; 92:75-8.

7. Jatho K. Das Kanul en Freie Tracheostoma Nack Kehlkopf Totol Extirpation. Laryngol Rhinol 1976; 55:631-6.

8. Isshiki N, Tanabe M. A simple technique to prevent stenosis of the tracheostoma after total laryngectomy. J Laryngol Otol 1980; 94:637-42.

9. Trail M, Chambers R, Leonard J. Z-Plasty of tracheal stoma at laryngectomy. Arch Otolaryngol 1968; 88:110-2.

10. Hartwell SW, Dykes ER. Construction and care of the end tracheostomy. Am J Surg 1967; 113:498-500.

11. Mumma C, Pressman J. A surgical technique to eliminate the tracheotomy tube after laryngectomy. Trans Am Acad Ophthalmol and Otolaryngol 1951; 55:418-23.

12. Converse JM. An operation for relief of stenosis of the stoma following total laryngectomy. Arch Otolaryngol 1950; 52: 950-1.

13. Maruyama Y, Kubota J, Nakajima H. A 5-flaps procedure for repair of stenosed tracheostoma. Acta Chir Plast (Prague) 1980; 22:107-10.

Ann Otol Rhinol Laryngol 91:1982

PREDICTING ESOPHAGEAL SPEECH

GEORGE A. GATES, MD

ERWIN M. HEARNE III, PHD

SAN ANTONIO, TEXAS

Patients undergoing laryngectomy in the 1980s have a low rate of acquisition of esophageal speech. The interaction of the factors of postoperative physical performance status, preoperative phonation duration, postoperative dysphagia, site of lesion, patient income, and postoperative radiation therapy correctly predict the acquisition of esophageal speech in 83% of cases and the failure to acquire esophageal speech in 96%. Such information may be helpful in selecting patients for alternative forms of postlaryngectomy speech rehabilitation.

INTRODUCTION

In spite of advances in diagnosis and therapy, about 7000 Americans lose their larynx to cancer every year. Most agree that the best method of postlaryngectomy rehabilitation for these patients is esophageal speech. In the past, the proportion of patients able to communicate effectively with esophageal speech was as high as 86%.[1] Subsequently this number has fallen to between 64-69%[2] and as low as 43%.[3] However, these reports[1-3] were based on retrospective studies. Using prospectively obtained data, we have determined that currently 26% of patients overall acquire esophageal speech and, if those who do not attempt to learn are excluded, the determinate success rate is 34%.[4]

The factors that influence esophageal speech are many and varied, but it appears to us that physical factors, ie, anatomical and physiologic, which affect esophageal speech acquisition directly, are the most difficult to overcome. In contrast, psychosocial factors, except for lack of motivation, are potentially susceptible to active intervention. In a previous communication[5] we identified and discussed individual factors that influence rehabilitation. In this paper we further analyze our data base to determine interactions among and combinations of multiple variables that might be useful to the physician in predicting which patients would be likely to fail to acquire esophageal speech. Such information would be of value in the early selection of patients for alternative methods of postlaryngectomy speech rehabilitation.

METHODS AND MATERIALS

The study records of 53 patients undergoing laryngectomy in the San Antonio area between 1975-1978 were analyzed. These records comprised all of the 103 patients with a clinical diagnosis of laryngeal cancer examined preoperatively during that time period who subsequently underwent laryngectomy. Of these, 47 patients were available for re-evaluation six months following the completion of their cancer therapy. The details of those examinations have been reported previously.[4]

The following variables were investigated as possible "discriminators" between esophageal speakers and nonspeakers in these 47 patients. They were chosen on the basis of logic, trial and error, and review of our data. For the first trial of the discriminant analysis, variables 1-6 were used. For the second trial all nine variables were used. These variables, along with brief definitions and their abbreviated symbol (in parentheses), are:

1. Tumor stage (STGE): 1 = T1N0M0, 2 = T2N0M0, 3 = T3N0M0, 4 - T3N1-3M0, 5 = T4N0M0, 6 = T4N1-3M0.
2. Postoperative radiation therapy (RADI): 1 = yes, 2 = no.
3. Physical status scale (PHYS): 5 = premorbid status, 1 = moribund.
4. Difficulty in swallowing (SWAL): 1 = yes, 2 = no.
5. Tumor site (SITE): 1 = glottic or supraglottic, 2 = pyriform sinus.
6. Preoperative phonation duration (DURA): the time, in seconds, that a subject could say /a/ on a single breath.
7. Education (ED): 1 = none, 2 = 1st-8th, 3 = 9th-12th, 4 = 1-2 college, 5 = 3-4 college, 6 = MA.
8. Number of homemates (HMATE).
9. Patient income (INC).

Of the 47 patients, eight nonspeakers were excluded from the first discriminant analysis because they were not able to participate in the preoperative phonation duration test (eg, because of a tracheostomy tube, or too ill) or because the data were missing. None of the eight subsequently acquired esophageal speech. For the second discriminant analysis one nonspeaker was excluded because no income information was available. Therefore, 39 patient records were included in the first analysis, 12 esophageal speakers and 27 nonspeakers, and 38 patients records in the second, 12 speakers and 26 nonspeakers.

The discriminant analysis was performed using forward stepwise selection of the variables. This technique chooses the variable with the largest F-statistic value, as long as the F is greater than or equal to 1. Then, the rest of the variables are chosen in a stepwise fashion, and the procedure is stopped when a variable has an F-statistic value of less than 1. Only the selected variables are used in the discriminant function.

RESULTS

The mean values of each variable for each group of subjects are displayed in Table 1. The results of the stepwise procedures are presented in Table 2. Notice that the only variables not selected as "significant" discriminators were tumor stage, education and number of homemates. The following

From the Division of Otorhinolaryngology, Department of Surgery, The University of Texas Health Science Center at San Antonio. This study was supported by a grant (RO1 CA 18629-02) from the National Institutes of Health.

Presented at the meeting of the American Laryngological Association, Palm Beach, Florida, May 1-2, 1982.

gives the standardized discriminant function for the first analysis.

$$Y = .28\ \frac{(X_{RADI} - 1.5)}{.51} + .37\ \frac{(X_{PHYS} - 2.5)}{1.14} + .61\ \frac{(X_{SWAL} - 1.6)}{.49} - .39\ \frac{(X_{SITE} - 1.3)}{.44} + .78\ \frac{(X_{DURA} - 10.1)}{7.09}$$

The general form of the equation is

$$Y = \frac{K_1(X_1 - \bar{X}_1)}{SD(X_1)} + \ldots + \frac{K_n(X_n - \bar{X}_n)}{SD(X_n)}$$

where Y = speaker score, ie, $Y = 1$ represents speaking and $Y = 0$ nonspeaking. The Xs are the data for a given patient. It should be noted that the absolute magnitude of the constants on the Xs show the relative importance of each discriminator, ie, preoperative phonation duration (DURA) was the most important variable.

The standardized discriminant function from the second analysis (9 variables) is as follows:

$$Y = .55\ \frac{(X_{RADI} - 1.5)}{.51} + .53\ \frac{(X_{PHYS} - 2.5)}{1.2} + .43\ \frac{(X_{SWAL} - 1.6)}{.49} - .41\ \frac{(X_{SITE} - 1.3)}{.45} + .85\ \frac{(X_{DURA} - 10.2)}{7.2} - .86\ \frac{(X_{INC} - 6981)}{5654}$$

The Ys for each patient can be used to "statistically" classify patients to the speaking or nonspeaking group. Table 3 presents the results of this classification. Notice that 66.7% of the speakers were correctly classified, and 85.2% of the nonspeakers were correctly classified, yielding an overall correct classification rate of 79.5% for the first trial. By adding the additional variables to the discriminant analysis the predictive ability increased to 92% overall with a correct classification score of 83% for speakers and 96% for nonspeakers.

DISCUSSION

Discriminant analysis is a powerful statistical method that allows inferences to be made about the relative weighting of multiple factors for purposes of predicting outcome. By applying the discriminant function to our patients we were able to "assign" them correctly to the appropriate category 80 to 92% of the time. Whether this predictive accuracy will hold up in other populations of laryngectomees remains to be seen; we hope it would be confirmed by other workers in the field.

We performed several trials of the discriminant analysis using a number of variables. We have chosen to include the two trials which most accurately reflect the interaction of the variables used in this study and our interpretation of their significance. This we did to indicate to those without an advanced background in statistics that there is an "art" as well as a "science" in this method of gleaning information about possible relationships from a large amount of data. Given this sample size and these subjects, it may be that these tests applied to different samples would give somewhat different results. The reader is urged to keep this in mind when applying this information to patient care. We do not suggest that this information will be 92% accurate when applied to any given group of patients.

It should also be stressed that statistical correlation does not imply causation. Even though factor A may be correlated strongly with factor B, both may be due to a third or more factors rather than the direct action of one on the other. For example, the mechanism whereby preoperative phonation duration influences the acquisition of esophageal speech is not readily apparent. Indeed, it might be a spurious coincidence or there may be a direct effect that should be studied further. One could postulate that patients with unimpaired phonation had smaller tumors, or that the patients in this category had better pulmonary function, or that they were not bashful about performing a phonatory test. In any event, this phenomenon carried too strong a statistical relationship to ignore even though the pathophysiology of this relationship is not obvious.

Logically, physical performance status would be expected to have a more direct effect upon acquiring esophageal speech. The physical rating scale we employed was relatively arbitrary. It varied from 1-5 with 5 being equivalent to the patients' preillness status and 1 indicating a bed-ridden preterminal condition. Common experience indicates that learning and using esophageal speech requires a fair amount of energy and vigor. Therefore, patients weakened by their disease, the effects of therapy, or depression would be expected to have difficulty speaking esophageally.

TABLE 1. MEANS ± STANDARD ERRORS OF THE MEANS (SEM) FOR EACH GROUP OF SUBJECTS

Group	*N*	*STAG**	*RADI*	*PHYS*	*SWAL*	*SITE*	*DURA*	*ED*	*HMATE*	*INC*
Speakers	12	3.3 ± .28	1.7 ± .14	3.3 ± .31	1.9 ± .08	1.1 ± .08	13.8 ± 2.2	2.8 ± .28	1.8 ± .55	4755 ± 1105
Nonspeakers	26	3.4 ± .25	1.4 ± .10	2.2 ± .21	1.5 ± .10	1.3 ± .10	8.5 ± 1.3	3.1 ± .20	1.1 ± .16	8008 ± 1199
Combined	38	3.4 ± .19	1.5 ± .08	2.5 ± .19	1.6 ± .08	1.3 ± .07	10.2 ± 1.2	3.0 ± .16	1.3 ± .20	6981 ± 917
Excluded nonspeakers	9	4.4 ± .48	1.2 ± 1.5	2.8 ± .47	1.5 ± .19†	1.4 ± .18	—	3.4 ± .24	1.8 ± .49	3457 ± 919§

* See text for definitions of variables.

† Based on N = 8.

‡ Based on N = 7.

TABLE 2. STEPWISE VARIABLE SELECTION RESULTS

	Step	Variable	F
First trial	1	PHYS	8.6
	2	DURA	6.3
	3	SWAL	4.8
	4	SITE	3.2
	5	RADI	1.2
Second trial	1	PHYS	8.2
	2	DURA	6.0
	3	INC	8.3
	4	RADI	6.8
	5	SITE	3.5
	6	SWAL	2.9

Similarly the effect of dysphagia would also appear to be direct. We categorized patients at their sixth month posttreatment examination into three groups on the basis of this variable: 1) those who had no difficulty swallowing, 2) those with mild to moderate difficulty but who did not require treatment, and 3) those who required dilations. None of the ten patients who needed dilations was able to make an esophageal voice. Only one of the esophageal speakers had dysphagia; 50% of the nonspeakers had dysphagia.

In the initial analysis of these patients the site of the cancer had no significant statistical relationship to esophageal speech acquisition. However, if the subjects were divided into two groups — 1) glottic and supraglottic vs 2) pyriform sinus — the success rate for group 1 was 33% and for 2 it was 7% (1/14) (Table 4). Thus one would conclude that patients with pyriform sinus cancer are less likely to develop esophageal speech than those with glottic or supraglottic primaries. Broken down according to tumor stage, the pyriform sinus group was staged: T_{1-2} –4, T_3 – 5, and T_4 – 6; one half had clinically evident cervical metastasis preoperatively. It is a common experience that the amount of pharyngeal mucosa available for closure of the pharynx is much less in patients with pyriform sinus cancer. The dysphagia rate (62%) for the pyriform sinus group differed ($p = .051$) from that of the glottic-supraglottic group of patients (30%). Therefore we may conclude that pharyngeal dysfunction leading to dysphagia is an important factor in mediating the deleterious effect of pyriform sinus cancer upon learning of esophageal speech.

The effect of radiation therapy appears to be confined to those who received postoperative therapy. In our previous report,[5] 4/12 esophageal speakers had postoperative radiation therapy in comparison to 23/35 nonspeakers. The statistical significance of this difference was $p = .06$. We postulate that postoperative radiation therapy has a direct effect upon learning esophageal speech because patients experience pharyngeal pain and dryness during the period in which they are attempting to learn esophageal speech. The majority of patients discontinue their speech lessons during radiation therapy; most do not resume. Therefore, we wonder about alternative rehabilitation plans, such as postponing the start of speech therapy until the effects of radiation therapy have subsided. We certainly do not advocate avoiding or postponing postoperative radiotherapy because of this effect but we do urge that it be considered in the rehabilitation planning.

TABLE 3. CLASSIFICATION RESULTS

	Actual Group	Predicted Group Membership: Speaking	Nonspeaking
First trial	Speaking	8 (66.7%)	4 (33.3%)
	Nonspeaking	4 (14.8%)	23 (85.2%)
		(79.5%)	
Second trial	Speaking	10 (88.3%)	2 (16.7%)
	Nonspeaking	1 (3.8%)	25 (96.2%)
		(92.1%)	

The importance of the patient income variable deserves comment. Contrary to previous reports which would indicate that the personal characteristics associated with affluence are important in motivating people toward learning esophageal speech, it is our opinion that socioeconomic status per se has a weak clinical relationship to esophageal speech. Even though our data would indicate statistically that low income predicts success, we interpret this finding to mean that high income does not influence success and that other factors, particularly physical factors, are far more important. We note that the mean income of the eight patients excluded from analysis because of missing data on phonation duration was much lower than the rest of the nonspeaker group. It is our impression that if these patients could have been included in the analysis, the predictive power of this variable would still be significant although statistically weaker.

We have not compared these data with the work of others in the literature for several reasons. First, our data were from a prospectively studied group, whereas all studies with which we are familiar were based on retrospectively obtained information. Second, our subject population was heterogeneous, coming from private, indigent clinic, military, and veterans' facilities, and cannot be compared to, for example, an all-male, veteran patient group. Third, this technique of analysis has not been applied previously to predicting outcome of postlaryngectomy rehabilitation. We look forward to the results of future studies of a similar nature.

It appears to us that substantive changes have occurred in the selection of patients for treatment of

TABLE 4. RELATIONSHIP OF SPEECH ACQUISITION TO SITE OF CANCER

	Glottic & Supraglottic	Pyriform Sinus
Speakers	11 (33%)	1 (7%)
Nonspeakers	22 (67%)	13 (93%)

(Corrected $X^2 = 2.3$, $p = .13$)

laryngeal cancer. Today's laryngectomee is more likely to be older, have more advanced disease, and receive multimodality therapy than was the case in the past. Thus, fewer patients are able to learn esophageal speech. Identification of patients who would be unlikely to be able to learn esophageal speech could result in the early use of alternative forms of speech rehabilitation for this high-risk group. Thus, months of delay and frustration could be replaced by early communication. For the 40% whose cancer therapy is not curative and whose lives are enriched by effective interpersonal communication, such early identification would greatly enhance the quality of their remaining days.

REFERENCES

1. Hunt RB. Rehabilitation of the laryngectomee. Laryngoscope 1964; 74:382-95.

2. Snidecor JC. Some scientific foundations for voice restoration. Laryngoscope 1975; 85:640-7.

3. King PS, Lowlles ES, Peirson GA. Rehabilitation and adaptation of laryngectomy patients. Am J Phys Med 1968; 97: 192-203.

4. Gates GA, Ryan W, Cooper Jr JC, et al. Current status of laryngectomee rehabilitation: I. Results of therapy. Am J Otolaryngol 1982; 3:1-7.

5. Gates GA, Ryan W, Cantu E, Hearne E. Current status of laryngectomee rehabilitation: II. Causes of failure. Am J Otolaryngol 1982; 3:7-14.

≈

PRIMARY VOCAL REHABILITATION USING THE BLOM-SINGER AND PANJE VOICE PROSTHESES

MICHAEL D. MAVES, MD RALEIGH E. LINGEMAN, MD

INDIANAPOLIS, INDIANA

Vocal rehabilitation by means of tracheoesophageal puncture and placement of either the Blom-Singer or Panje silicone prosthesis has become a standard method of speech production following total laryngectomy. The same technique has been employed primarily at the time of the laryngectomy by the Department of Otolaryngology-Head and Neck Surgery, Indiana University Medical Center, and our experience with 11 patients undergoing this technique forms the basis for this report. Of the ten patients available for evaluation, all have developed satisfactory prosthetic speech 2-12 weeks following total laryngectomy. Advantages of this technique include the utilization of standard laryngectomy without compromise of oncologic principles, elimination of a second procedure to place the tracheoesophageal puncture, elimination of the nasogastric tube, care in the pharyngeal closure to afford the maximum success of prosthetic speech production, and finally, the psychological boost. Limitations of the technique have been few but relate to limited voicing with postoperative radiotherapy and unrealistic patient expectations.

INTRODUCTION

Following total laryngectomy vocal rehabilitation by means of tracheoesophageal puncture and placement of either the Panje or Blom-Singer prosthesis has become a standard method of speech production with a high degree of success.[1-4] These two techniques, similar in concept and design, have offered new hope to many laryngectomees unable to use other means of communication and have found wide application. However, little has been written regarding the use of this technique primarily at the time of the ablative procedure. The purpose of this study was to evaluate the use of primary tracheoesophageal puncture as a means of vocal rehabilitation. A related phase of this investigation was to determine if alteration in the method of pharyngeal closure would have an effect on the incidence of pharyngoesophageal spasm in these prosthetic speakers.

SURGICAL TECHNIQUE

Primary tracheoesophageal puncture was performed following standard widefield laryngectomy or laryngopharyngectomy by creating a fistula in the superior midportion of the posterior tracheal wall. A finger is placed within the pharynx, exerting pressure on the party wall, while making an incision approximately 5 mm in length, 5-10 mm below the planned superior mucocutaneous junction of the stoma through the posterior tracheal wall into the esophagus. Once entrance into the esophagus has been made, the incision is gently dilated with a hemostat, and a 14 French Keofeed tube is introduced into the stomach and secured to the peristomal skin with an 0-silk suture.

Pharyngeal closure was altered in an attempt to decrease postoperative pharyngoesophageal spasm following the technique of Saunders.[5] A 36 or 38 French dilator was placed through the oral cavity into the pharynx for use as a "darner" or form to sew across. The mucosa and submucosa were then closed over this dilator in an interrupted fashion. The esophageal dilator, acting as a darner, allows the surgeon to detect gaps in the all-important first suture line. It also ensures that enough mucosa is present to prevent a tight pharynx. If one is unable to close the pharyngotomy defect with the 36 or 38 French dilator in place, then a myocutaneous flap or other augmentation should be used to reconstruct the pharynx. All closures were done in a T-shaped configuration. In no instance was an attempt made to close the pharyngeal musculature since it was suspected that traditional, tight, multilayered pharyngeal closures would increase the amount of scarring and lead to an increased incidence of pharyngoesophageal spasm.

In three preoperative irradiated cases, this same closure technique was used, but the suture line was reinforced with a pectoralis muscle flap in two cases and augmented with a pectoralis myocutaneous flap in another case.

Blenderized feedings were given through the fistula tube until the 10th to 14th postoperative day when oral alimentation was begun and the Keofeed tube was replaced with a 14 French silicone stent. Speech rehabilitation was initiated as early as the tenth postoperative day with voicing through the fistulous tract. Thereafter, fitting with either a Blom-Singer or Panje prosthesis was accomplished and standard instruction in the care of these appliances was begun.

RESULTS

Eleven patients undergoing total laryngectomy and primary tracheoesophageal puncture for T3 and T4 laryngeal and pyriform sinus neoplasms at the Indiana University Medical Center from July 1981 until April 1982 formed the basis for this report. Ten of these patients are available for evaluation. The unevaluable patient is currently still hospitalized and has been physically unable to begin voicing. Nine patients were male and all patients were in the sixth and seventh decades of life. Four patients underwent simultaneous radical neck dissection. Three patients received preoperative radiotherapy and the same number underwent postoperative irradiation.

All patients developed satisfactory, fluent, intelligible speech. The period of time from laryngectomy

From the Department of Otolaryngology-Head & Neck Surgery, Indiana University School of Medicine, Indianapolis.

Presented at the meeting of the American Laryngological Association, Palm Beach, Florida, May 1-2, 1982.

REPRINTS — Michael D. Maves, MD, Department of Otolaryngology-Head & Neck Surgery, 1100 W. Michigan Street, Indianapolis, IN 46223.

to the development of speech ranged from 2-12 weeks with an average of 5.2 weeks. If two patients requiring 12 weeks until voicing are eliminated, then the average time to voicing becomes 3.5 weeks.

Six patients were initially fitted with Panje prostheses and four with Blom-Singer. The choice of prosthesis type was based on the configuration of the stoma and final position of the tracheoesophageal fistula.

No difference in the eventual success of vocal rehabilitation was noted with patients undergoing either preoperative or postoperative radiotherapy. However, in two patients undergoing postoperative radiotherapy, voicing became limited because of peristomal reaction and pharyngeal edema.

Two patients, originally felt to be satisfactory prosthetic speakers, eventually used their prosthetic voice less. One of these individuals has a history of psychiatric illness and motivation tends to parallel his mood. Initial success was met with limited reception in another patient because of probable unrealistic preoperative expectations. There was one postoperative complication, a fistula in an unirradiated case. There was no evidence of pharyngoesophageal spasm.

DISCUSSION

Primary tracheoesophageal puncture has been found to be a procedure with favorable initial results. Standard wide-field laryngectomy or laryngopharyngectomy with no departure from established oncologic criteria may be performed. New techniques for approaching laryngeal neoplasms through subtotal laryngectomy have currently been under development and evaluation.[6] These techniques offer the hope of retention of limited laryngeal function and extension of traditional indications for conservation laryngeal surgery while maintaining the cure rates for laryngeal carcinoma now treated with total laryngectomy. However, further evaluation and follow-up are necessary before this can become a standard method of treatment. In the interim, primary tracheoesophageal puncture offers a single-stage method of prosthetic vocal rehabilitation with known cure rates.

Importantly, care can be given to the pharyngeal closure at the time of a laryngectomy. In our series, it was felt that by closing only the mucosa and submucosa we have allowed the wide myotomy of the pharyngeal constrictors which is present at the end of the laryngectomy to remain, and that this would result in a loose pharyngoesophageal segment less likely to spasm with air insufflation. In a large series of patients undergoing prosthetic vocal rehabilitation, Singer and Blom have noted an incidence of pharyngoesophageal spasm of 12% and postulate that it may even be higher.[7] Similar rates of pharyngoesophageal spasm have been noted by other investigators.[4,8,9] Although our initial results are encouraging, further investigation concerning variations of pharyngeal closure following laryngectomy and the role that such techniques play in the eventual production of pharyngoesophageal spasm merits further consideration.

By creating the tracheoesophageal fistula at the time of the ablative procedure, the puncture can be easily placed and a second operation, albeit a minor one, is avoided. The need for a nasogastric tube is also eliminated since feedings may begin via the tube in the fistula and this can be of considerable comfort to the patient who depends on central or enteral tube feeding for 10 to 14 days postoperatively.

Although vocal rehabilitation may begin as soon as 10 to 14 days postoperatively, this ideal was not always realized in our patient population. A patient with a postoperative fistula required a considerably longer interval to develop sustained effective voicing. In two of three patients undergoing postoperative radiotherapy some limited voicing was begun postoperatively only to decrease with radiotherapy because of pharyngeal edema and peristomal reaction. On the other hand, while postoperative radiation may limit voicing during radiotherapy, in no case was any long-term sequela apparent.

Finally, it must be emphasized that considerable psychological boost is given to both the patient and surgeon who realize that even in the face of total laryngectomy, efforts can be made at the time of the laryngectomy which will assist in postoperative vocalization. However, we have been careful to emphasize to our patients that the resultant voice will not be the same as their preoperative voice and that fluency will not come without diligent work and therapy. In one of our patients, unrealistic preoperative expectations led to disillusionment regarding tracheoesophageal speech and eventual decrease in the frequency of use, although he still wears his prosthesis. Considerable care in the selection of these patients is therefore required and one cannot yet advocate this as a universal standard technique to be applied to all laryngectomees. Lastly, it can be emphasized that in some of our patients initial efforts at esophageal speech were enhanced by the presence of the tracheoesophageal fistula. In fact, several patients have elected to proceed with education regarding esophageal speech and now use both methods of communication. One cannot regard this as a failure of tracheoesophageal speech; rather it reflects the interrelationship of these different modalities of postoperative vocal rehabilitation.

ACKNOWLEDGMENTS — The authors would like to recognize the invaluable assistance of James C. Shanks, PhD, and R. Edward Stone, PhD, who provided speech therapy for these patients, and Rhea Reynolds who typed the manuscript.

REFERENCES

1. Singer MI, Blom ED. An endoscopic technique for restoration of voice after laryngectomy. Ann Otol Rhinol Laryngol 1980; 89:529-33.

2. Panje WR. Prosthetic vocal rehabilitation following laryngectomy — the voice button. Ann Otol Rhinol Laryngol 1981; 90: 116-20.

3. Singer MI, Blom ED, Hamaker RC. Further experience with voice restoration after total laryngectomy. Ann Otol Rhinol Laryngol 1981; 90:498-502.

4. Panje WR, Van Demark D, McCabe BF. Voice button prosthesis rehabilitation of the laryngectomee — additional notes. Ann Otol Rhinol Laryngol 1981; 90:503-5.

5. Saunders WH. Techniques in laryngectomy to minimize postoperative complications and permit immediate feeding. Ann Otol Rhinol Laryngol 1963; 72:431-40.

6. Pearson BW. Subtotal laryngectomy. Laryngoscope 1981; 91:1904-11.

7. Singer MI, Blom ED. Selective myotomy for voice restoration after total laryngectomy. Arch Otolaryngol 1981; 107:670-3.

8. Donegan JO, Gluckman JL, Singh J. Limitations of the Blom-Singer technique for voice restoration. Ann Otol Rhinol Laryngol 1981; 90:495-7.

9. Wood BG, Rusnov MG, Tucker HM, Levine HL. Tracheoesophageal puncture for alaryngeal voice restoration. Ann Otol Rhinol Laryngol 1981; 90:492-4.

≈

THE SECOND INTERNATIONAL SYMPOSIUM ON AUDIOLOGICAL MEDICINE

The Second International Symposium on Audiological Medicine will be held April 10-13, 1983, in Verona, under the auspices of the International Association of Physicians in Audiology. For further information contact Dr. V. Colletti, Clinica ORL dell'Universita di Padova sede di Verona, Policlinico Borgo Roma, 37134 Verona, Italy.

CHEMICAL MODULATION OF THE HYPOXIC FRACTION IN THE TREATMENT OF HEAD AND NECK CANCER

RALPH R. WEICHSELBAUM, MD
THOMAS J. ERVIN, MD DANIEL MILLER, MD
BOSTON, MASSACHUSETTS

Treatment of large squamous carcinomas of the head and neck often requires intensive or multidisciplinary treatment. Despite such aggressive measures, local recurrence is common. Possible reasons for such local failure are numerous. Hypoxic but viable tumor cells may be one means of resistance to radiotherapy and chemotherapy. If surgical removal cannot eliminate these cells, tumor regrowth may occur. Modulation of the hypoxic fraction is one means of potentially altering resistance to radiotherapy. Misonidazole, a radiosensitizer, has been thought to increase free radical formation in hypoxic cells in vitro thus increasing the radiosensitivity. This observation is discussed with reference to advanced head and neck cancer.

Cancer therapists, regardless of discipline, have as their goal the elimination of the last clonogenic tumor cell or at least a reduction of the tumor cell burden so that the natural body defenses may eliminate any cell with malignant potential. In individuals with head and neck cancer, adequate local control may cure a large proportion of these patients. However, large tumors (T4) have considerably lower local control rates than smaller (T1) lesions.[1] Explanations frequently offered for this fact are 1) a larger tumor cell burden in T4 lesions, 2) greater efficiency of repair of x-ray and/or drug damage, 3) the presence of hypoxic cells which may reduce the efficacy of both drug and x-ray treatments, and 4) inherent or induced cellular resistance to drugs and x-rays.[2,3]

Survival curve analysis, whether involving x-rays or chemotherapeutic agents, has proven important in the conceptual design of cytotoxic cancer therapy. Figure 1 shows an x-ray survival curve. A logarithmic plot of the surviving fraction is shown on the ordinate and dose in rad on the abscissa. It should be noted that survival cures for chemotherapeutic agents are graphed in a similar fashion with concentration of drug on the abscissa instead of dose in rad. The inverse of the slope of the straight line portion of an x-ray or drug survival curve is known as the D_o (radiosensitivity or chemosensitivity). The back-extrapolation of the slope to the ordinate is known as the $\bar{n}$ or extrapolation number and represents the ability of cells to accumulate and repair sublethal damage. Survival enhancement after x-ray treatment, as reflected in a recapitulation of the extrapolation number, indicates that cells repair sublethal x-ray damage and any chemotherapeutic agent or host factor which influences this process is of great importance.

Thomlinson and Gray,[4] after histologic examination of lung tumors, noted that cells more than 150 μm from a capillary were necrotic and surrounded by a rim of hypoxic cells. This observation may be of great importance to the clinical cancer therapist, since the cytotoxic action of ionizing radiation and some chemotherapeutic agents such as adriamycin or cyclophosphamide in biological matter is mediated by production of free radicals. Free radicals contain unpaired electrons which create the chemical reactions that lead to molecular lesions which produce damage to DNA. The major forms of this damage are DNA strand breaks and/or base damage. Thus, when bacterial or mammalian cells are exposed to hypoxia (an environment less capable of free radical production), radioresistance or chemoresistance occurs (Fig. 2). A generalization is that in in vitro or in vivo treatment systems, absence of oxygen will result in a *decreased* cytotoxic effect. Conversely, it should be noted that radiosensitivity of virtually all hypoxic biological systems can be significantly *enhanced* in the presence of oxygen. Although the radiation dose necessary to produce a given degree of cell killing may be different under various conditions, the shape of the survival cures are identical when they are in aerated or hypoxic conditions. As Figure 2 shows, the ratio of the doses to reach the same biological end-point under oxic or hypoxic conditions is the same at each level of survival. This ratio is called the oxygen-enhancement ratio (OER) and can be calculated as the ratio of D_o values for hypoxic and aerated cells.[5] Tumors containing large fractions of hypoxic cells will be resistant, possibly as much as by a factor of three, to ionizing radiation. A clinical corollary to this phenomenon would be that tumors containing a population of hypoxic cells may require a dose of irradiation which exceeds normal (ie, oxic) tissue tolerance for local control.

From the Joint Center for Radiation Therapy and Sidney Farber Cancer Institute, Harvard Medical School, Boston.
Presented at the meeting of the American Laryngological Association, Palm Beach, Florida, May 1-2, 1982.
REPRINTS — Ralph R. Weichselbaum, MD, Joint Center for Radiation Therapy, 50 Binney Street, Boston, MA 02115.

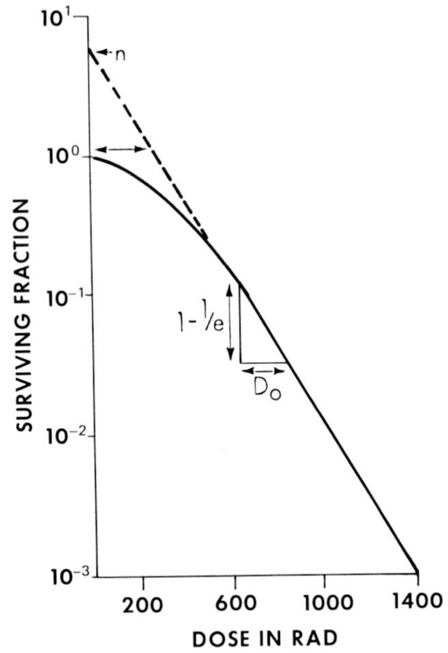

Fig. 1. Typical survival curve for mammalian tumor cells exposed to increasing doses of irradiation (or chemotherapy). Actual curve has initial "shoulder," and back-extrapolation of curve to ordinate (extrapolation number $\bar{n}$) is a measure of ability of treated cells to accumulate sublethal damage. Slope of curve (D_0) reflects sensitivity of cells to treatment.

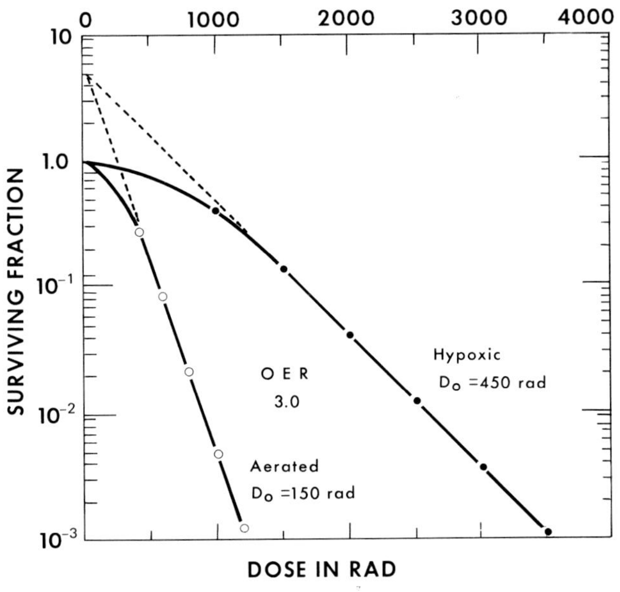

Fig. 2. Effect of hypoxia on cell survival following irradiation.

Several strategies have emerged by which hypoxia may be circumvented in radiotherapy. Although hyperbaric oxygen chambers have been employed with varying results, a more practical strategy has been the introduction into clinical radiotherapy of the nitroimidazoles as sensitizers of hypoxic cells.[6] These agents are electronic affinic compounds which have as their major mode of action the creation of free radicals in hypoxic cells. The prototype compound, metronidazole, a trichomonicide (Flagyl), was quickly followed by the development of misonidazole which is currently being investigated in clinical trials.[7] Figure 3 shows the effect of metronidazole in hypoxic cells in vitro. Note that the OER in the presence of metronidazole is decreased and the hypoxic cells are more like their well-oxygenated counterparts in their response to irradiation.[8] An increased cure rate in animals bearing tumors which contain a large hypoxic fraction of cells has been shown after the combined use of radiation and misonidazole.[9] Thus, it may be possible to enhance the therapeutic ratio in head and neck cancer with the employment of combinations of hypoxic cell, sensitizers and radiation therapy.

Rose and his colleagues[10] investigated the enhancement in tumor cell-kill which occurs when misonidazole is administered in combination with chemotherapeutic agents in animals bearing the Lewis lung carcinoma. Enhancement of melphalan cytotoxicity in tumors occurred when animals received misonidazole up to four hours before or one hour after melphalan. Enhancement was most marked with simultaneous administration (Fig. 4). Although misonidazole enhanced the response of intestine and bone marrow to melphalan treatment, enhancement ratios were considerably less than tumor enhancement ratios, resulting in a true therapeutic gain. Although the mechanism of potentiation of chemotherapeutic agents by the nitroimidazoles was unclear, Rose et al proposed that misonidazole might enhance melphalan activity by potentiating cytoxic action at the intracellular level by elaborating potentially toxic metabolites within the hypoxic tumor cells. These authors further suggested that these metabolites occur in concentrations insufficient to produce cytotoxicity by themselves, but which enhance the action of simultaneously delivered chemotherapy, perhaps through some electron affinic process.[10]

It is thus tempting to speculate that the nitroimidazoles originally investigated as radiation sensitizers may find use as chemosensitizers and that hypoxic cells originally thought to limit the effectiveness of radiation may alter the effectiveness of chemotherapy as well. Future clinical trials may include the employment of misonidazole with chemotherapy as well as during radiation itself.

In a previous study at the multidisciplinary Head and Neck Clinic at the Sidney Farber Cancer Institute and the Joint Center for Radiation Therapy, patients presenting with advanced stage III and stage IV squamous carcinoma of the head and neck were treated with high dose methotrexate (3-7 g/m^2 dose, with leucovorin rescue) given weekly for one month prior to definitive radiation and/or surgery. Six of 11 patients who showed a significant response (greater than 50% reduction of tumor to high-dose methotrexate) are alive and well at three years as opposed to 1 of 10 patients who showed less than a

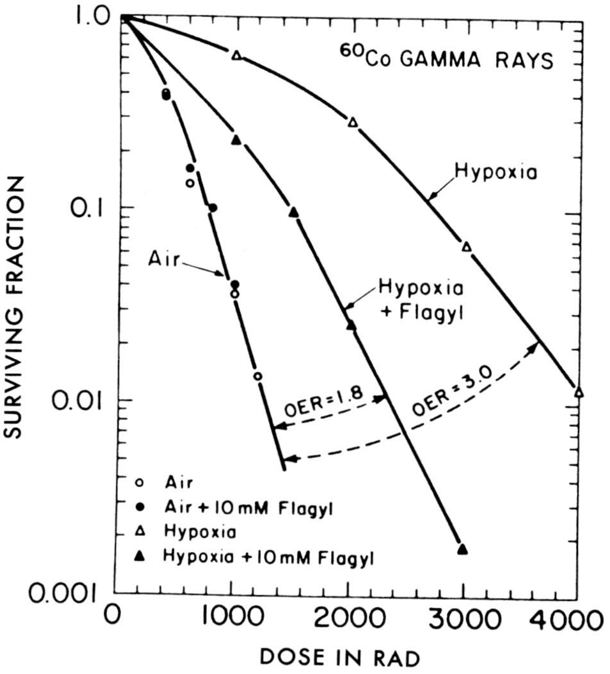

Fig. 3. Effect of misonidazole (Flagyl) on hypoxic inhibition of cell death following irradiation.

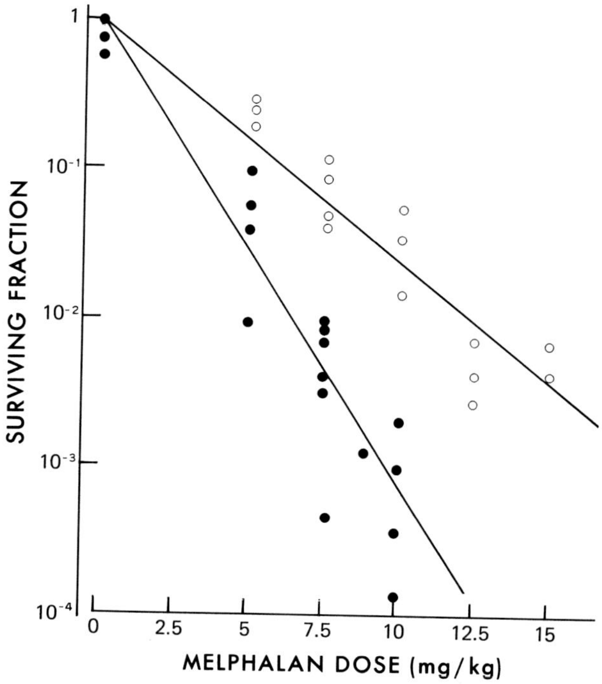

Fig. 4. Effect of misonidazole on cell survival after melphalan treatment.

50% reduction in tumor size.[11] An obvious interpretation is that an enhancement in cytoreduction was achieved by the chemotherapy and that the superiority in survival was solely due to a significant decrement in tumor cell burden. The fact that both the responding and nonresponding groups had the same incidence of distant metastases, however, suggests that the log-kill in the responding group might not have been significantly greater than in the nonresponding group. It is possible that the cytoreduction in the responding group was enough only to effect local control. This may have occurred by decreasing the local tumor burden or decreasing the local hypoxic cell population, thus making radiation surgery more effective. In explaining the effect of cytoreduction, several interesting experimental observations may be relevant. For example, several authors have shown experimentally that cells in small tumors are more sensitive to cytotoxic agents than those in large tumors. Also, in animals, pulmonary tumors as small as 20 mm in volume contain substantial numbers of hypoxic, presumably resistant, cells.[9,12] Thus, pre-definitive-treatment chemotherapy may have had the effect of reducing the hypoxic fraction by reducing the gross size of the tumor and rendered radiotherapy and presumably surgery more effective by size reduction as well.

The above principles have important implications for the surgical oncologist, since surgery may be curative by itself or in combination with chemotherapy and radiotherapy. Sound principles of oncologic management should be common to all disciplines involved in the care of head and neck cancer patients. For example, surgical debulking has been widely misinterpreted, but should take the form of complete excision of tumor deposits leaving only microscopic disease behind. Thus, cytoreductive surgery may be beneficial, not only because it reduces the total number of tumor cells, but may also reduce the number of hypoxic cells, leaving smaller numbers of well-oxygenated cells to be treated by chemotherapy and radiotherapy.

Tumor cell hypoxia is an example of only one problem which is common to all oncologic disciplines and demonstrates the necessity for combined clinical approaches to head and neck cancer. Other physiologic differences between tumors and normal tissues should be exploited. Potentiators of chemotherapy and radiotherapy and protectors of normal tissues which selectively take advantage of such differences should be explored. The nitroimidizoles and possibly hyperthermia are examples of such investigative efforts. With surgery, such interdigitation of disciplines might improve the therapeutic results for advanced squamous carcinoma of the head and neck.

REFERENCES

1. Fletcher G. Textbook of radiotherapy. Philadelphia: Lea & Febiger, 1980; 229-46.

2. Weichselbaum RR, Schmidt A, Little JB. Cellular factors influencing the radiocurability of human malignant tumors. Br J Cancer 1982; 45:10-6.

3. Ervin T, Karp D, Weichselbaum RR, Posner MR, Fabian RL, Miller D. The role of chemotherapy in the multidisciplinary approach to advanced head and neck cancer: potentials and prob-

lems. Ann Otol Rhinol Laryngol 1981; 90:506-11.

4. Thomlinson RH, Gray LH. The histiological structure of some human lung cancers and the possible implications of radiotherapy. Br J Cancer 1955; 9:539-49.

5. Hall E. Radiobiology for the radiologist. New York: Harper & Row, 1980.

6. Adams GE. Chemical radiosensitization of hypoxic cells. Br Med Bull 1973; 29:48-53.

7. Adams GE, Dische S, Fowler JF, Thomlinson RH. Hypoxic cell sensitizers and radiotherapy. Lancet 1976; 1:186-8.

8. Hall EJ, Roizin-Towle L, Theus RB, August LS. Radiobiological properties of high energy cyclotron produced neutrons used for radiotherapy. Radiology 1975; 117:173-8.

9. Denekamp J, Stewart FA. Sensitization of mouse tumors using fractionated irradiation. Br J Cancer 1978; 37 Suppl 3:259-63.

10. Rose C, Millar JL, Peacock JH, et al. Differential enhancement of melphalan cytotoxicity in tumor and normal tissue by mizonidazole. In: Brady LW, ed. Radiation-sensitizers. New York: Masson Publishers, 1980; 250-7.

11. Ervin TJ, Kirkwood J, Weichselbaum RR, Miller D, et al. Improved survival for patients with advanced carcinoma of the head and neck treated with methotrexate leucovorin prior to definitive radiotherapy or surgery. Laryngoscope 1981; 91:140-5.

12. Stanley JA, Peckham MJ, Steele G. Influence of tumor-size on radiosensitization by mizonidazole. Br J Cancer 1978; 37 Suppl 3:220-4.

PATHOLOGY CONSULTATION

METASTATIC PATTERNS OF SALIVARY GLAND NEOPLASMS

JOHN G. BATSAKIS, MD

PORTLAND, MAINE

Long-term follow-up of salivary gland carcinomas allows a better evaluation of their biologic malignancy than the traditional five-year period. Metastases (distant and local) are possible over the entire lifetime of a patient and are dependent upon histologic grade, persistence of neoplasm and clinical stage. Distant metastases to bone and lungs are manifested by nearly every carcinoma. Metastases to regional lymph nodes vary according to histologic type and it appears that the adenoid cystic carcinoma has the lowest incidence of that event.

An accurate assessment of the biologic activity of carcinomas of the salivary glands and the consequences of that activity on the host *cannot* be made on the basis of the traditional five-year "cure" or survival statistics. Metastases are events that occur over a protracted period, even in apparently disease-free subjects. Unfortunately the combination of the low incidence of salivary gland carcinomas and the often short follow-up periods in most of the publications thwart a circumspect analysis.

Malignancy (metastatic ability) of a salivary gland carcinoma is the result of a variety of interrelated factors; some are inherent in the neoplasm, others of more a facultative character; anatomic site of origin, clinical stage, adequacy of primary treatment and control or lack of control of the primary.

Histologic grade of the carcinoma by itself may be a determinant but in many instances the grade of the neoplasm is intimately related to clinical stage.[1] This appears to be true especially for mucoepidermoid and adenocarcinomas. Histologic grading of adenoid cystic carcinomas for the purpose of prognostication has had mixed "reviews."[2] For that neoplasm, it is unlikely that grade outweighs clinical stage in any instance. The same may be said for acinous cell carcinomas. Facial nerve paralysis (incorporated in clinical staging) is an ominous sign and frequently demonstrates a direct relationship to metastases.

Failure of local control, though it may have a protracted time period, with its repetitive surgery, irradiation and disruption of the tumor bed and vascular system, not only prolongs the chronological time of the neoplasm, it also provides opportunity for dissemination.

Anatomic site of origin definitely plays a role. Mucous gland carcinomas of the upper airway kill primarily through the ravages of local extension. Metastases, lymph node or distant, are less frequent than for comparable histologic types in the major salivary glands. Table 1 presents the percent frequency of metastases for adenoid cystic carcinomas, carcinomas in pleomorphic adenoma, and mucoepidermoid carcinomas. The data are derived from studies selected for long follow-up periods and identification of metastatic sites.[3-12] Except where indicated the neoplasms arose from *all* salivary sites.

As can be seen in Table 1, the three different carcinomas manifest different patterns of metastasis. Adenoid cystic carcinomas manifesting distant (hematogenous) dissemination outnumber those with lymph node involvement. For the latter, it is likely that the involvement of the regional lymph nodes is more often by contiguity than by lymphatic permeation. This should be kept in mind when

TABLE 1. SALIVARY GLAND CARCINOMAS: METASTATIC PATTERNS

Investigators	*No. Cases*	*Metastasis to Lymph Nodes (%)*	*Distant Metastasis (%)*
Adenoid Cystic Carcinoma			
Spiro et al[3]	242	15	42.0†
Conley and Dingman[4]	134	16	34.0
Zielke-Temme and Wannenmacher[5]	82	—	30.0
Eby et al[6]	54	15	24.0
Blanck et al[7]	35*	20	34.0
Grahne et al[8]	21	24	43.0
Carcinoma Ex Pleomorphic Adenoma			
Spiro et al[9]	150	25	32.0
Eneroth et al[10]	21	24	24.0
Mucoepidermoid Carcinoma (all grades)			
Spiro et al[11]	367 all patients	29	—
	342 with follow-up	—	15.0
	254*	28	—
Jakobsson et al[12]	63*	8	6.5

*Parotid only.
†70% assumed.

From the Department of Pathology and Laboratory Medicine, Maine Medical Center, Portland.

REPRINTS — John G. Batsakis, MD, Department of Pathology and Laboratory Medicine, Maine Medical Center, Portland, ME 04102.

planning treatment. It is also to be appreciated that adenoid cystic carcinomas of the paranasal sinuses and airway demonstrate approximately one half the frequency of lymph node involvement indicated in Table 1.[3]

Carcinomas ex pleomorphic adenoma (so-called malignant mixed tumors) involve regional nodes with a frequency nearly equal to their distant metastatic rate. This is to be expected since the carcinoma evolving from the pleomorphic adenoma is most often an adenocarcinoma of ductal type.

The statistics for mucoepidermoid carcinoma are skewed by inclusion of the more numerous low-grade carcinomas. These low-grade mucoepidermoid carcinomas manifest a biologic behavior not unlike a mixed tumor. Spiro and associates[11] have provided a more discriminating study. Forty-four percent (89 patients) of their patients with mucoepidermoid carcinoma of the parotid gland, other than grade 1, manifested cervical lymph node metastases at some time during their illness. Only primary squamous cell carcinoma (70%) and adenocarcinomas (36%) rivaled this metastatic rate. Once again signaling the apparent reluctance of adenoid cystic carcinomas to involve lymph nodes, Spiro et al[11] record a metastatic rate of only 10%.

Lack of long-term follow-up serves to give misconceptions over the potential lethality of acinous cell carcinomas. The study of 35 cases by Batsakis et al[13] and their accompanying review is a step in correcting this misconception. Metastases (local and distant) occurred in one third of the patients with hematogenous spread exceeding regional lymph node involvement by a 2:1 ratio.

SUMMARY

The frequency of lymph node and distant (hematogenous) metastases from salivary gland carcinomas is presented. Noteworthy findings are: 1) metastasis is often delayed beyond the traditional five-year surveillance period; 2) clinical stage and persistence of tumor are likely more important than histologic grade for metastasis; 3) hematogenous distant metastases, over the duration of the disease, is often more frequent than lymphatic metastases to regional lymph nodes.

REFERENCES

1. Spiro RH, Huvos AG, Strong EW. Cancer of the parotid gland: a clinicopathologic study of 288 primary cases. Am J Surg 1975; 130:452-9.

2. Batsakis JG. Tumors of the head and neck: clinical and pathological considerations. 2nd ed. Baltimore: Williams & Wilkins, 1979:33.

3. Spiro RH, Huvos AG, Strong EW. Adenoid cystic carcinoma of salivary origin: a clinicopathologic study of 242 cases. Am J Surg 1974; 128:512-20.

4. Conly J, Dingman DL. Adenoid cystic carcinoma in the head and neck (cylindroma). Arch Otolaryngol 1974; 100:81-90.

5. Zielke-Temme B, Wannenmacher M. Adenoid cystic carcinoma (cylindroma) in the head and neck. Acta Radiol Oncol Radiat Phys Biol 1978; 17:401-13.

6. Eby LS, Johnson DS, Baker HW. Adenoid cystic carcinoma of the head and neck. Cancer 1972; 29:1160-8.

7. Blanck C, Eneroth C-M, Jacobsson F, Jakobsson PA. Adenoid cystic carcinoma of the parotid gland. Acta Radiol [Ther] (Stockh) 1967; 6:177-96.

8. Grahne B, Lauren C, Holsti LR. Clinical and histological malignancy of adenoid cystic carcinoma. J Laryngol Otol 1977; 91:743-9.

9. Spiro RH, Huvos AG, Strong EW. Malignant mixed tumor of salivary origin: a clinicopathologic study of 146 cases. Cancer 1977; 39:388-96.

10. Eneroth C-M, Blanck C, Jakobsson PA. Carcinoma in pleomorphic adenoma of the parotid gland. Acta Otolaryngol (Stockh) 1968; 66:477-92.

11. Spiro RH, Huvos AG, Berk R, Strong EW. Mucoepidermoid carcinoma of salivary gland origin: a clinicopathologic study of 367 cases. Am J Surg 1976; 136:461-8.

12. Jakobsson PA, Blanck C, Eneroth C-M. Mucoepidermoid carcinoma of the parotid gland. Cancer 1968; 22:111-24.

13. Batsakis JG, Chinn EK, Weimert TA, Work WP, Krause CJ. Acinic cell carcinoma: a clinicopathologic study of thirty-five cases. J Laryngol Otol 1979; 93:325-40.

BOOK REVIEWS

Chronic Ear Diseases

By *Gordon D. L. Smyth*. Hard cover, black and white illustrations, indexed, 218 pages, 1980. Churchill Livingstone Inc., New York. Price $28.00.

Chronic Ear Diseases, a recent monograph by Dr. Gordon D. L. Smyth of Belfast in the "Clinical Otolaryngology" series published by Churchill Livingstone, is a valuable contribution to our knowledge of chronic otomastoiditis. His experiences with management and surgical reconstruction, namely tympanoplasty, will be of interest to otologists everywhere.

The pathology of chronic otitis media (CSOM) and mastoiditis is described with historical reviews and recent conceptions of etiology with appropriate attention to the increased incidence of middle ear effusion (MEE). As would be expected in a book on chronic ear disease, the subject of cholesteatoma is given detailed analysis. Smyth has summarized basic studies of the past and recent contributions. Theories for the genesis of cholesteatoma are well reviewed with discussions of histological characteristics and with considerations of "invasive" and "metaplastic" concepts. Smyth gives appropriate emphasis to the recent research and theoretical constructs of Sadé of Israel, whose publications have contributed greatly to concepts regarding cholesteatoma etiology.

In the section on "Eradication of Disease" there are special chapters on patient selection and management, surgical techniques in tympanoplasty and evaluations of tympanoplastic results. One may have differing opinions with the technical emphases of Smyth and his group, but his wide experiences have been meticulously analyzed and objectively reported.

Smyth, who pioneered in combined approach tympanoplasty (CAT) has presented dispassionate statistical analyses of results. When it was noted that CAT procedures were not always successful, Smyth and his colleagues began to emphasize the need for staging and for less emphasis on CAT procedures as "final answers." It is admirable that Smyth himself has led the soul searching in this surgical debate and presents reasoned and clearly presented objectivity in overall surgical approaches to chronic otomastoiditis. There are presentations of causes of graft failure, and critical studies contrasting "overlay" and "underlay" techniques, and discussions of such problems as anterior "blunting" which can complicate overlay techniques.

He emphasizes his preference for homologous preserved tissue in tympanoplastic procedures and although he mentions other tissues, including temporalis fascia and perichondrium, there is no mention of the use of gelfilm as an alternative to tissue grafts to allow spontaneous repair to occur in cases where tissue grafts are contraindicated. In those cases of keratoma (cholesteatoma) where recurrences are highly likely, any tissue grafts may be contraindicated. In such cases gelfilm can play a role in making possible "spontaneous" neotympanic membrane regrowth. He stresses the uses of banked tissues, specifically homologous dura, in preference to viable fresh tissues. This may be due in part to the fact that he and his colleagues are involved in a very large clinic with much surgery for chronic otomastoiditis. The convenience of banked material undoubtedly has played a role in this decision-making process.

Cholesterol granuloma with or without tympanosclerosis and/or keratoma is an important lesion within the rubric of "chronic ear disease." It is mentioned briefly in the introduction to cholesteatoma (Chapter 2). Cholesterol granuloma with or without cholesteatoma and/or tympanosclerosis is a fairly common cause of "chronic ear disease" in Southern California and as a definitive lesion can produce ossicular fixation, ossicular necrosis, and severe mucosal diseases in the tympanomastoid area. Although it can coexist with cholesteatoma and tympanosclerosis, it very frequently occurs by itself and requires consideration in any discussion of chronic ear disease.

In addition to stresses of etiology, surgical techniques and evaluations of postoperative results, there are useful chapters on simple tympanic membrane repair, ossiculoplasty, and on special problems such as postoperative sensorineural hearing loss, labyrinthine fistula, tympanosclerosis and facial nerve trauma.

This is a useful text, primarily of value to fellow otologic surgeons rather than to beginners. This excellent otologic monograph should be available in all otologic libraries.

Victor Goodhill, MD
Los Angeles, California

Tympanoplasty and Stapedectomy, a Manual of Techniques

By *Ugo Fisch*. Soft cover, black and white illustrations, indexed 79 pages. Thieme-Stratton, New York and Stuttgart. Price $24.00.

Dr. Fisch has compiled a manual of otologic surgical techniques for the treatment of middle ear and mastoid disease. This difficult book is written as a guide for the beginning ear surgeon with schematic illustrations presented in a stepwise fashion. The material is logically and graphically displayed and is the type of material that is missing in most comprehensive otology texts.

Dr. Fisch's experiences with the procedures are summarized at the end of each section. For the experienced surgeon, a discussion of various approaches is also included. The section on myringoplasty covers underlay and overlay techniques with specific indications for each. A large portion of the manual discusses the surgical treatment of cholesteatoma, illustrating open cavity and closed cavity techniques along with reconstructive measures. The final section discusses management of otosclerosis comparing stapedectomy and stapedotomy results, complications and revision techniques.

In summary the manual offers Dr. Fisch's approach to the surgical management of chronic middle ear and mastoid disease. The clear illustrations and variety of techniques displayed provide the beginning ear surgeon with an excellent laboratory guide. The experienced surgeon will be interested in the helpful hints and results sections. The manual sets a standard for technique tests that should be emulated in the future.

Bruce J. Gantz, MD
Iowa City, Iowa

LETTER TO THE EDITOR

Dear Editor,

In the May-June 1980 Supplement to the *Annals*,[1] my colleagues and I reported our results of a double-blind, placebo-controlled study which concluded that a short course of prednisone was an effective method in the treatment of persistent otitis media with effusion (OME). Recently I received a letter from an otolaryngologist which described two patients who developed serious complications while receiving corticosteroid therapy for OME. Both patients developed intracranial infections but only one patient received an antimicrobial agent plus the prednisone prior to the development of signs of meningeal inflammation. If another otolaryngologist is aware of additional cases of possible or definite intracranial complications of prednisone therapy for OME, I would appreciate information about such cases.

REFERENCES

1. Schwartz RH, Puglese J, Schwartz DM. Use of a short course of prednisone for treating middle ear effusion: a double-blind cross-over study. Ann Otol Rhinol Laryngol 1980; 89 Suppl 68:296-300.

Richard M. Schwartz, MD
4120 West Maple Avenue
Vienna, VA 21180

INFORMATION FOR AUTHORS

Send manuscripts by first-class mail to Editor Brian F. McCabe, MD, University of Iowa Hospitals, Iowa City, IA 52242, or to Co-editor Ben H. Senturia, MD, 4949 Forest Park Blvd., St. Louis, MO 63108. Original manuscripts which deal with clinical and scientific aspects of otolaryngology, bronchoesophagology, head and neck, maxillofacial and plastic surgery, audiology, speech pathology and related specialties will be considered for publication. It is understood that manuscripts will not have been published elsewhere.

MANUSCRIPTS. Papers should be limited to a maximum of 15 double-spaced typewritten pages including tables and references, so as not to exceed the permitted maximum of 6 typeset pages. This allows for one page of illustrations. If a manuscript of slightly greater length is approved by the Editorial Board all typeset pages in excess of 6 will be charged to the authors at the publisher's cost of $125 per page. An **original of the manuscript** and one set of **original illustrations** should be provided for reproduction. **Two clear copies** of the manuscript and illustrations should be submitted for review. Manuscripts should be typewritten on white bond paper ($8\frac{1}{2}$ x 11 in). Use double spacing throughout with margins of at least one inch. Each manuscript component should begin on a new page in the following sequence: title page, abstract and key words, text, acknowledgments, references, tables and legends for illustrations. Number pages consecutively in the upper right hand corner beginning with the title page.

COPYRIGHT. In compliance with the Copyright Revision Act of 1976, all manuscripts must be accompanied by a letter containing the following statement before they will be reviewed for publication: "In consideration of the *Annals of Otology, Rhinology & Laryngology* taking action in reviewing and editing my (our) submission the author(s) undersigned hereby transfers(s), assign(s) or otherwise convey(s) all copyright ownership to the Annals Publishing Company in the event such work is published in the *Annals of Otology, Rhinology & Laryngology.*" We regret that manuscripts not accompanied by such a letter will be returned.

TITLES of manuscripts should be concise and informative and worded to facilitate indexing.

RUNNING HEAD. An abbreviated form of the title, to be used at the top of each page, should be provided by the author.

GENERIC NAMES should be used in the text whenever possible.

REFERENCES should be numbered consecutively in the order in which they are first mentioned, and cited in the text in arabic numerals in superscript. The number of references should not exceed 30. Use the style of references given in *Uniform Requirements for Manuscripts Submitted to Biomedical Journals.* Include in the reference list manuscripts accepted but not yet published; designate the journal followed by "in press" in parentheses. Manuscripts submitted but not yet accepted should be referred to as "unpublished data" in parentheses in the text. Primary references only should be used and must be verified by the author(s) against the original documents. Examples of correct forms of references are given below.

Journal Article

(List all authors when six or fewer; when seven or more, list only first three and add "et al.")

Ketchum LD, Smith I, Robinson DW, et al. The treatment of hypertrophic scar, keloid and scar contracture by triamcinolone acetonide. Plast Reconstr Surg 1966; 38:209-18.

Books and Other Monographs

Personal Author(s)

Payne SW, Olson MA. The esophagus. Philadelphia: Lea and Febiger, 1974: 1-3.

Corporate Author

American Medical Association Department of Drugs. AMA drug evaluations. 3rd ed. Littleton: Publishing Sciences Group, 1977.

Chapter in Book

Belsey R. Diaphragmatic hernia. In: Jones FA, ed. Modern trends in gastroenterology. London: Butterworths: 1952:128-78.

ILLUSTRATIONS should be original drawings, glossy photographs or halftones. Line drawings should be in black on white paper. Letters, numbers and symbols should be clear and even throughout, and of sufficient size that when reduced for publication, each item is still legible. Titles and detailed explanations of illustrations must be listed on a separate sheet, not on the illustrations themselves. Each figure should have a label pasted on the reverse indicating the number of the figure, the names of the authors, title of the paper; the top of the figure should be indicated. Cite each figure in the text in consecutive order. If a figure has been published, acknowledge the original source and submit written permission from the copyright holder to reproduce the material. Actual publication cost of illustrations will be charged to the author. Color illustrations are acceptable for publication; cost estimates for color separations and printing will be provided upon request.

TABLES should be on separate sheets, numbered consecutively, each headed by a concise title. Place explanatory matter in footnotes. Cost of setting tables will be charged to the author.

MEASUREMENTS should be expressed in the metric system. Audiograms must be plotted according to ISO standards.

ABSTRACTS should contain not more than 150 words and should state the purposes of the study, primary procedures, main findings and the principal conclusions, emphasizing new and important aspects of the investigation.

PERMISSIONS. Materials taken from other sources must be accompanied by a written statement from both senior author and publisher giving permission to the *Annals* for republication. If permission for publication is required by the author's institution, such clearance should be provided. Written permission of subjects is required for identifiable photographs of individuals.

SUPPLEMENTS. A manuscript too long for inclusion in the *Annals* may be published as a supplement if approved by the Board of Editors. All costs must be borne by the author; estimates of cost will be provided upon request. Early publication of supplements is often possible since supplements are produced independently of the regular *Annals* issues.

PROOFS accompanied by prints of the illustrations will be sent to the first author and should be returned within 48 hours. Changes in galley proofs initiated by the author will be charged to the author.

AUTHOR RESPONSIBILITY. All accepted manuscripts are subject to copy editing. The author is responsible for all statements in his work, including changes made by the copy editor which were approved by the author on the proofs.

REPRINTS. Rates are quoted when the proofs are sent. Orders must be signed by the author and returned with the proofs.

These requirements are in accord with *Uniform Requirements for Manuscripts Submitted to Biomedical Journals* (Lancet 1979; 1: 428-30).

SINGULAR NEURECTOMY UPDATE

RICHARD R. GACEK, MD
SYRACUSE, NEW YORK

The results of a poll revealed that 96 singular neurectomies have been performed by ten surgeons in this country. Eighty-eight of these (91.7%) resulted in complete relief of benign paroxysmal positional vertigo (BPPV). In seven patients (7.3%) there was a sensorineural hearing loss as a result of this procedure. The average hospital stay for patients having this procedure ranged from 2-6 days, and the return to work time ranged from 1 to 3 weeks. These results indicate that singular neurectomy is an effective selective vestibular ablation procedure for BPPV and that the risks and disability are comparable to other routine middle ear procedures. The causes for failure of this procedure to relieve positional vertigo are a) misdiagnosis of BPPV and b) failure to recognize the singular nerve in the middle ear. Knowledge of the pathophysiology of the disorder and of the anatomical variation in the location of the singular canal will reduce these causes of failure.

INTRODUCTION

Benign paroxysmal positional vertigo (BPPV) is a unique clinical entity first described by Barany in 1921.[1] The accumulated clinical and histopathological observations of this disorder indicate[2-5] that 1) it is peripheral in origin, 2) one of the vertical semicircular canals is responsible for the symptomatology and 3) the ear positioned undermost in the provocative position is probably responsible for the positional vertigo. Schuknecht's description[6] of basophilic deposits embedded in the cupula of the posterior canal crista rendering it gravity-sensitive suggests that the posterior semicircular canal is the responsible sense organ in this condition (cupulolithiasis).

Most patients with BPPV experience spontaneous resolution over a period of months and many of those in whom resolution does not occur are able to live with the disorder by avoiding the provocative position. However, a small number of patients with this disorder are incapacitated sufficiently that surgical treatment is considered. In those patients who have a profound sensorineural hearing loss in the responsible labyrinth, surgical labyrinthectomy has proven effective in relieving the vestibular symptoms.[2,6] However, since most patients with this disorder have useful hearing in the involved ear, a method of selectively ablating function of the posterior semicircular canal is necessary.

In 1974, five patients with BPPV were described in whom the posterior ampullary nerve (singular nerve) was approached through a tympanotomy exposure under local anesthesia.[7] Transection of this nerve in the ear undermost in the positioning test provided complete and immediate relief of the positional vertigo in all five patients. Significant sensorineural hearing loss occurred in one patient. In 1978, an assessment of results in five more patients was added to the original series.[8] Transection of the singular nerve also provided complete relief of BPPV in this additional series with one patient experiencing a moderate sensorineural hearing loss.

At the present time, the author's series consists of 22 patients in whom singular neurectomy was performed for BPPV. This series includes the original ten patients reported in 1974 and 1978. Twenty-one of these 22 patients have experienced complete relief of the positional vertigo confirmed by a negative Hallpike maneuver. One patient has experienced almost complete relief of vertigo with a markedly reduced nystagmus response observed on Hallpike positional testing. Nevertheless, this patient noted a significant improvement in her vestibular symptoms following the procedure. In this series of 22 patients, 3 have suffered a significant sensorineural hearing loss postoperatively. The hearing loss was severe in one patient and moderate in two patients.

The results of other surgeons performing this procedure were collected by a mail poll so that a more significant assessment of the benefits and risks of this procedure could be formulated. The results of this poll are included in this report.

MATERIALS AND METHODS

In August 1981, a poll was conducted by mail to all members of the American Otological Society as well as to those nonmembers who had been known to perform this procedure for BPPV. The information requested in the questionnaire included 1) the number of singular neurectomies performed or attempted, 2) the type of anesthesia used for the procedure (local or general), 3) the average length of stay in the hospital of patients recovering from this procedure, 4) the average time of return to work, and 5) the effect of the procedure on the positional vertigo and on hearing.

From the Department of Otolaryngology and Communication Sciences, S.U.N.Y. Upstate Medical Center, Syracuse.

Presented at the meeting of the American Otological Society, Inc., Palm Beach, Florida, May 2-3, 1982.

REPRINTS — Richard R. Gacek, MD, Dept. of Otolaryngology and Communication Sciences, S.U.N.Y. Upstate Medical Center, 750 East Adams Street, Syracuse, NY 13210.

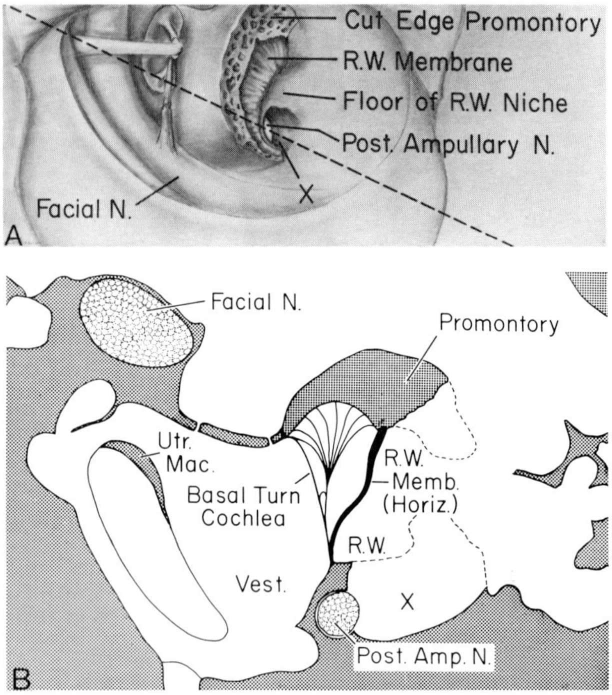

Fig. 1. Most common location of the posterior ampullary nerve (singular nerve). A) Surgical view. B) Outline of histological section which represents a vertical cut at the level of the dashed line in A. R.W. - Round window; N - Nerve; Utr. Mac. - Utricular macule; Vest. - Vestibule.

RESULTS

There were 73 respondents to the 120 questionnaires mailed out. Sixty-three of the respondents have not performed singular neurectomy, while 10 (including author) had performed the operation. Four of the surgeons had successfully transected the singular nerve in 15 or more patients while six had performed it on 5 or fewer patients. The highest number of procedures performed by a single surgeon was 27, while the lowest was 1.

The total number of singular neurectomies performed was 96. Eighty-eight (91.7%) of these procedures resulted in complete relief of the positional vertigo while in 8 patients (8.3%), incomplete or no relief was experienced. Seven (7.3%) patients experienced sensorineural hearing loss following the surgery. In five instances, the singular nerve could not be located in the middle ear. Three of these were recorded by the author. In one of the author's patients a middle cranial fossa vestibular nerve transection was subsequently carried out to relieve the BPPV with preservation of hearing. The remaining two patients continued to experience BPPV. General anesthesia was used routinely by six surgeons in performing singular neurectomy, while local anesthesia was preferred by four surgeons.

The average hospital stay for patients recovering from singular neurectomy ranged from 2 to 6 days. The six surgeons who had five or fewer cases indicated that their patients remained hospitalized $2^1/_2$ days. Those surgeons with the larger series (15 or more cases) indicated a longer hospital stay for their patients, averaging five days. The longer hospitalization probably reflects the fact that the surgeons performing more operations were treating patients referred from a larger geographic area and the hospitalization was longer in order to remove packing, evaluate hearing, etc, before discharge.

The average return to work time following this procedure ranged from 1 to 3 weeks for all but one surgeon. One surgeon who had performed 15 singular neurectomies indicated 6 to 12 months was required for patients to return to work and probably reflects a more conservative attitude of the surgeon.

DISCUSSION

The experience of ten surgeons who have performed singular neurectomy demonstrated the effectiveness and safety of this procedure for the relief of benign paroxysmal positional vertigo. A 92% chance for the relief of positional vertigo and a less than 8% risk of sensorineural hearing loss compares favorably with other established otologic procedures. As with any surgical procedure, the success and risks improve with increased experience of anatomical variations and modified surgical techniques. The hospital stay and the average time for returning to normal activities are also comparable to that required by patients recovering from routine middle ear surgery such as stapedectomy or tympanoplasty.

The success of this selective denervation procedure in relieving BPPV strongly supports the histopathology of this disorder.[6] The posterior semicircular canal sense organ of the downmost ear when placed in the provocative Hallpike position has been the target sense organ for this surgical procedure. The persistence of positional vertigo in those patients where a singular neurectomy could not be performed[8] strengthens the conclusion that denervation of the posterior canal crista relieves BPPV.

Singular neurectomy is not indicated for most patients with BPPV. Conservative management allowing sufficient time for spontaneous resolution and avoidance of the provocative position are effective, nonsurgical programs in the management of this disorder. However, a small number of patients having serious job or social limitations because of the positional vertigo for a sufficient duration to indicate permanency of the condition (at least one year) may be considered candidates for the operation. Selective transection of the singular nerve by a middle ear approach is indicated in those patients who have normal or very useful hearing in the involved (downmost) ear and who have sufficient disability that they are willing to risk a total hearing loss for the relief of the positional vertigo.

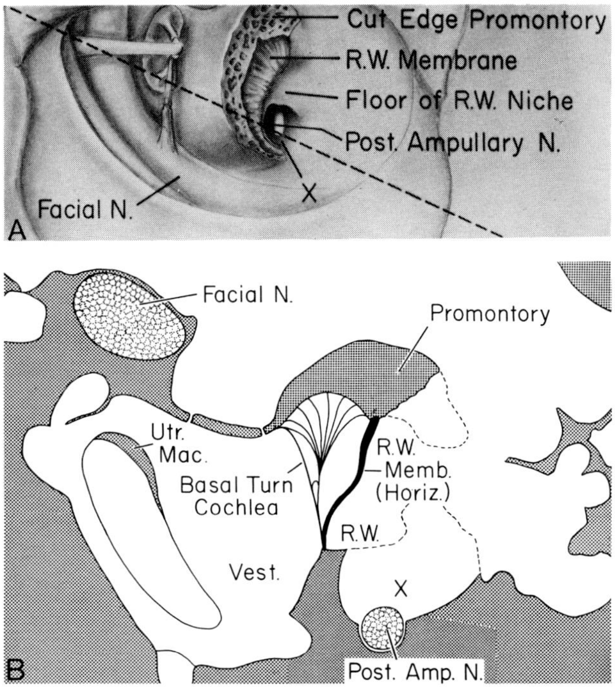

Fig. 2. Most favorable of other locations for singular nerve is illustrated in A) surgical and B) histological views.

Other procedures which ablate vestibular function can be used in the management of this disorder. 1) Transection of the vestibular nerve through a middle cranial fossa approach is an effective surgical technique which selectively ablates all vestibular function with preservation of hearing in the involved ear. However, it is a procedure which carries a greater potential for morbidity and mortality than singular neurectomy through a middle ear approach. Furthermore, all function in the involved ear is ablated by total vestibular neurectomy, requiring a longer period for central compensation; singular neurectomy ablates approximately one fifth of the function in an otherwise normal labyrinth, thereby providing the opportunity for compensation by the remaining sense organs of the involved labyrinth as well as the central vestibular system. In those patients where the singular nerve cannot be located safely in the middle ear, the middle cranial fossa vestibular nerve transection can be used to relieve the disorder. It is not practical to isolate and transect the singular nerve selectively in the internal auditory canal from the middle cranial fossa approach. The author relieved BPPV in one patient with a middle fossa vestibular nerve transection after an unsuccessful approach to the singular nerve in the middle ear. One respondent to the poll had relieved the BPPV in five patients by performing middle fossa vestibular nerve transection. 2) In the unusual circumstance where the BPPV is caused by pathology in an "only hearing" ear, the recommended procedure for selective vestibular ablation associated with the lowest risk of sensorineural hearing loss may be streptomycin sulfate delivered parenterally. 3) Labyrinthectomy performed by the transcanal route is an appropriate effective surgical approach in those patients where a profound or severe sensorineural hearing loss is present in the ear responsible for the BPPV.

Failure of singular neurectomy to relieve BPPV may be caused by 1) incorrect diagnosis or 2) failure to locate the singular nerve. An accurate diagnosis rests upon a careful history, properly performed positional test (Hallpike maneuver) and tests of hearing and balance function. The history usually reveals an antecedent event such as head trauma, viral infection, or surgical trauma which has produced an insult to the labyrinth (labyrinthitis). After a recovery period of several weeks, the syndrome of BPPV appears in which a head position to one side or straight back produces a brief period of violent vertigo. However, patients frequently give varying descriptions of their imbalance and often do not specifically describe the positional component. Therefore, the single most important test is the Hallpike positioning test where the examiner briskly places the patient's head in a dependent position either right or left and carefully observes eye movements unaided. Positioning nystagmus present only when recorded by eyes closed techniques (ENG) does not necessarily indicate pathology of the labyrinth (BPPV).[9] Only those patients in whom the positioning nystagmus can be observed unaided should be considered as candidates for singular neurectomy. A short (2-4 second) latency period followed by a rotatory nystagmus of 20 to 30 seconds duration is characteristic. The nystagmus is fatiguable on repeat positioning tests. Vertical components to the nystagmus may be seen sometimes. The nystagmus is directed upward (upbeat) in both eyes and is usually described as rotatory (clockwise when the left ear is dependent and counter-clockwise when the right ear is dependent).[10] These characteristics differentiate the peripheral (labyrinth) form of BPPV from the central (cerebellar vermis) type in which the nystagmus appears after a long latency (up to 50 seconds), is downbeat, and has a longer duration (30 to 180 seconds).[11]

Those forms of BPPV which are manifested by primarily vertical or horizontal nystagmus may not represent the syndrome caused by pathology of the posterior semicircular canal. Therefore, transection of the singular nerve may not be an appropriate form of vestibular ablation in those patients who exhibit a linear form of nystagmus. These nonrotatory forms of fatiguing positional nystagmus may represent pathology of other vestibular end-organs. If so, vestibular nerve section by the middle cranial fossa approach would be an appropriate form of ablation in these cases. Characteristically, caloric tests (ENG) are symmetrical and the hearing tests are normal both for pure tone thresholds and speech discrimination. A neurological evaluation per-

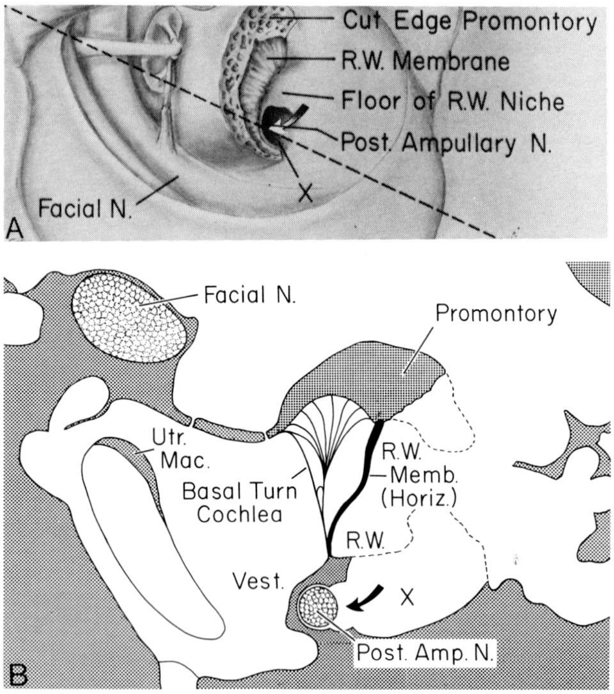

Fig. 3. Most unfavorable location of the singular nerve is shown in A) surgical and B) histological views.

formed to rule out any underlying central nervous system disease is normal.

Identification of the singular nerve in the middle ear depends upon thorough knowledge of microscopic and surgical round window anatomy, practice with the surgical approach and an awareness of the anatomical variations of the singular canal. It is frequently necessary to curette the posterior inferior bony wall of the ear canal in order to visualize the round window niche. Since the single most important surgical landmark is the round window membrane, it is essential that complete exposure of the membrane be accomplished by drilling away the bony overhang of the round window niche. This exposure must include the superior portion of the round window membrane which parallels the long diameter of the oval window as well as the surgeon's line of vision. Identification is confirmed by observing its displacement following depression of the stapes. The proper location for approaching the singular canal is just inferior to the attachment of this segment of the round window membrane in the floor of the round window niche. In order to protect against injury to the membrane and adjacent cochlea during the drilling procedure, it is advisable to leave a 1 mm margin of bone between the attachment of the round window membrane and the surgical defect in the floor of the niche.

The singular canal can be found in three positions (Figs. 1-3). 1) Usually only a small portion of the singular nerve can be exposed by drilling in the manner described (Fig. 1). Although only a portion of the nerve is visible, the nerve can be identified with certainty because of the patient's vestibular response to stimulation of the nerve under local anesthesia. 2) The most favorable but an infrequent (4 out of 22) position of the nerve is one where the nerve is located sufficiently inferior in the round window niche that its entire diameter can be seen (Fig. 2). Exposure and transection of the singular nerve in this location carries the least risk of cochlear trauma. 3) The other unusual position (3 out of 22) of the singular nerve is represented by its location under the attachment of the round window membrane (Fig. 3). This position should be suspected when the singular nerve is not seen after drilling to a depth of 2 to 3 mm in the appropriate location. If there has been no vestibular response noted by the patient, the nerve in this hidden position may be reached by directing a small (0.5 mm) burr in a superior direction from a starting point at the depth of the bony surgical defect in the floor of the round window niche. The maneuver resembles the use of a drill to enlarge a dental cavity; the location of the singular nerve is indicated by the patient's experience of vertigo. A small hook can then be used to palpate the lumen of the singular canal in order to transect the nerve. If the singular nerve cannot be found in any of these three locations, then it is advisable to cease the surgical approach through the middle ear and at a later date relieve the disorder by transection of the entire vestibular nerve through a middle cranial fossa approach.

Clinical signs following singular neurectomy are important to monitor not only as confirmation of successful denervation of the posterior semicircular canal sense organ but also to predict the patient's readiness to leave the hospital. Immediately following the surgical ablation a spontaneous vertical downbeat nystagmus can usually be observed unaided for a period of several hours. This spontaneous nystagmus is not usually visible on the first postoperative morning. When the Hallpike positioning test is performed on the first postoperative day, it does not provoke a transient rotatory nystagmus. Instead one observes a sustained vertical or horizontal nystagmus which appears without delay. This compensatory or "release" nystagmus is demonstrable for 3 to 4 days following the singular neurectomy. The patient does not have severe vertigo or nausea during this period and experiences only slight unsteadiness. Discharge from the hospital is usually possible after cessation of the release nystagmus produced in the positioning maneuver.

REFERENCES

1. Barany R. Diagnose von Krankheitserscheinungen im Bereiche des Otolithenapparates. Acta Otolaryngol (Stockh) 1921; 2:434-7.

2. Dix R, Hallpike CS. The pathology, symptomatology and diagnosis of certain common disorders of the vestibular system. Ann Otol Rhinol Laryngol 1952; 61:987-1016.

3. Cawthorne TE. Positional nystagmus. Ann Otol Rhinol Laryngol 1954; 63:481-90.

4. Lindsay JR, Hemenway WG. Postural vertigo due to unilateral sudden partial loss of vestibular function. Ann Otol Rhinol Laryngol 1956; 65:692-708.

5. Citron L, Hallpike CS. Observations upon the mechanism of positional nystagmus of the so-called "benign paroxysmal type." J Laryngol Otol 1956; 70:253-9.

6. Schuknecht HF. Cupulolithiasis. Arch Otolaryngol 1969; 90:765-78.

7. Gacek R. Transection of the posterior ampullary nerve for the relief of benign paroxysmal positional vertigo. Ann Otol Rhinol Laryngol 1974; 83:596-605.

8. Gacek R. Further observations on posterior ampullary nerve transection for positional vertigo. Ann Otol Rhinol Laryngol 1978; 87:300-5.

9. Barber HO. Positional nystagmus: testing and interpretation. Ann Otol Rhinol Laryngol 1964; 73:838-50.

10. Baloh RW, Sakala S, Honrubia V. The mechanism of benign paroxysmal positional nystagmus. In: Stahle J, ed. Frontiers in vestibular and oculo-motor research. Vol. 25. Adv Otol Rhinol Laryngol 1979; 161-6.

11. Fernandez C, Alzate R, Lindsay JR. Interrelations between flocculonodular lobe and vestibular system. In: Rasmussen GL, Windle WF. Neural mechanisms of the auditory and vestibular system. Springfield: C. Thomas, 1960:285-96.

≈

GUIDELINES FOR GRANTS
TRUSTEES OF THE RESERACH FUND OF THE AMERICAN OTOLOGICAL SOCIETY, INC.

The members of the Board of Trustees of the Research Fund of the American Otological Society have determined guidelines for making grants from the Fund. The following is the formulation of policy.

Grants will be given in the area of otosclerosis: its diagnosis and management, the possible causes and underlying conditions, and an understanding of the disorder that may lead eventually to its prevention or cure.

The present lack of understanding of the disorder and the absence of similar conditions in other animals makes research in this field difficult. A direct approach to the disease may or may not be feasible; therefore, a sound strategy would be to use other approaches, such as the investigation of bone development, growth and repair under various conditions and the study of other diseases that may be similar to otosclerosis. It is possible that investigations which may seem initially remote from otosclerosis may provide information which will eventually lead to a substantive further understanding of the disease process which underlies otosclerosis. The applicant should describe correlations between proposed research with the clinical pathological entity of otosclerosis.

The policy is to aid and encourage research in the immediate field of otosclerosis and also in adjoining fields, if, in the opinion of the Board, there is a substantial promise that results obtained will be of assistance in the ways indicated and may lead to the attainment of the objective of the further understanding of otosclerosis.

Applications for a research grant from the Research Fund of the American Otological Society may be obtained from the Office of the Secretary-Treasurer of the Research Fund of the American Otological Society. Write to Maxwell Abramson, MD, Secretary-Treasurer, Department of Otolaryngology, Columbia University, College of Physicians and Surgeons, 630 West 168th Street, New York, NY 10032; (212) 694-5820.

All grant requests must be submitted by January 31, 1983. All grants received after January 31 will not be considered.

INFRATEMPORAL FOSSA APPROACH FOR GLOMUS TUMORS OF THE TEMPORAL BONE

UGO FISCH, MD

ZURICH, SWITZERLAND

The surgical experience with 74 glomus tumors of the temporal bone is presented. The article proposes new refinements in the classification of types C and D tumors and describes in detail the technique of blind sack closure of the external auditory canal, double ligation of the sigmoid sinus and the use of a special infratemporal fossa retractor. The postoperative treatment and intraoperative management of the internal carotid artery, facial nerve and cranial nerves IX, X, XI and XII including the technique and results of a new type of V-VII anastomosis are discussed.

In the past years the surgical management of glomus tumors of the temporal bone has been influenced by two main factors. One is the introduction and refinement of computerized tomography, the other the development of the infratemporal fossa approach with permanent anterior transposition of the facial nerve.[1-3] High resolution computerized tomography permits the most accurate determination of tumor size and temporal bone invasion and has practically eliminated polytomography. The infratemporal fossa approach with permanent anterior rerouting of the facial nerve has opened the way for the radical removal of lesions situated in the infralabyrinthine and apical compartments of the temporal bone requiring exposure of the intratemporal course of the carotid artery. It is the purpose of this paper to review our experience with surgery of glomus tumors of the temporal bone in light of the above-mentioned developments.

CLASSIFICATION OF GLOMUS TUMORS

Accurate surgical planning and evaluation of the results require a precise classification of tumor size. In 1979[3] we proposed to classify the glomus tumors in four types: A — tumors limited to the middle ear cleft, B — tumors limited to the tympanomastoid area without destruction of bone in the infralabyrinthine compartment of the temporal bone, C — tumors extending and destroying bone of the infralabyrinthine and apical compartment of the temporal bone, and D — tumors with intracranial extension.

This classification based on the surgical approach required for tumor removal has remained valid. However, the following subdivision of types C and D has proven necessary in view of the different surgical problems encountered.

Type C

C_1 — tumors destroying the jugular foramen and jugular bulb and with limited involvement of the vertical portion of the carotid canal (Figs. 1 and 2A,B).

C_2 — tumors destroying the infralabyrinthine compartment of the temporal bone and invading the vertical portion of the carotid canal (Figs. 1 and 3A,B).

C_3 — tumors involving the infralabyrinthine and apical compartments of the temporal bone with invasion of the horizontal portion of the carotid canal (Figs. 1 and 4A,B).

Type D

D_1 — tumors with intracranial extension less than 2 cm in diameter; removal in one stage through the infratemporal fossa approach possible (Figs. 5A,B).

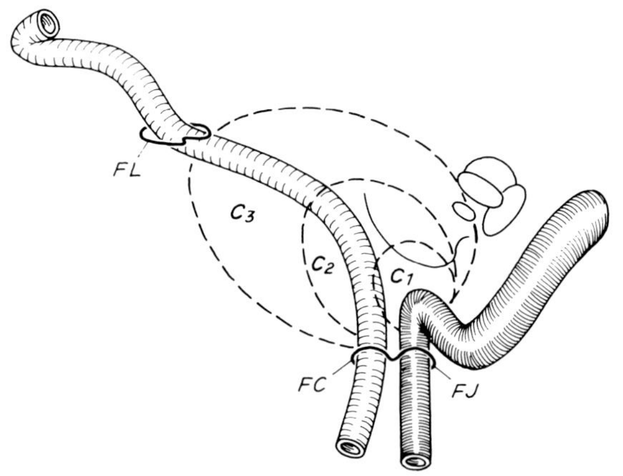

Fig. 1. Subdivision of type C glomus tumors of temporal bone according to their invasion of intratemporal carotid artery. FL - Foramen lacerum; FC - Foramen caroticum; FJ - Foramen jugulare.

From the ENT Department, University Hospital, Zurich.

Presented at the meeting of the American Otological Society, Inc., Palm Beach, Florida, May 2-3, 1982.

REPRINTS — Prof. Dr. Ugo Fisch, ENT Department, University Hospital, 8091 Zurich, Switzerland.

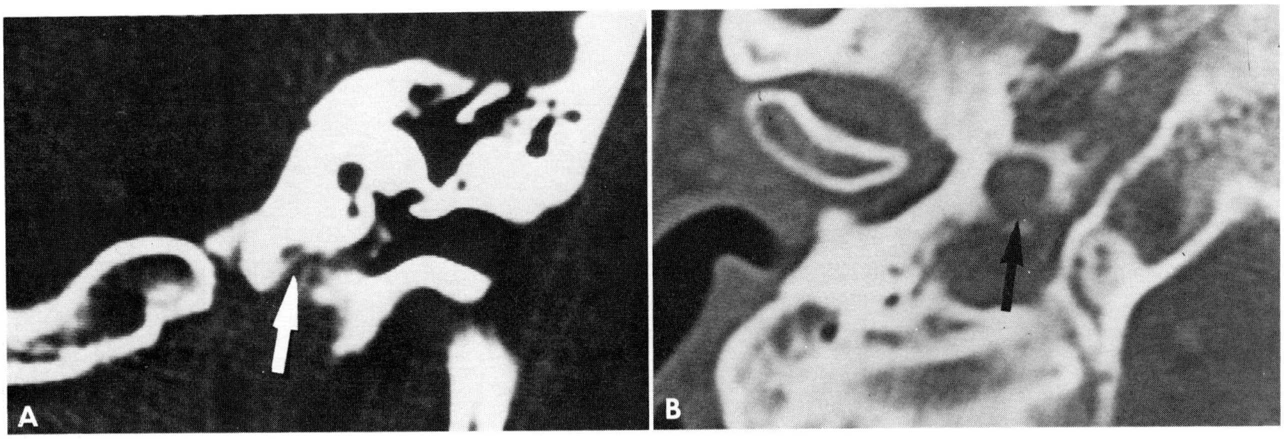

Fig. 2. (Patient 1, male, 37 yr) Type C_1 tumor destroying jugular foramen and jugular bulb with limited involvement of vertical portion of the carotid canal. A) CT, coronal section (arrow - jugular bulb). B) CT, horizontal section (arrow - vertical carotid canal).

D_2 — tumors with intracranial extension greater than 2 cm in diameter that require a combined two-stage otological and neurosurgical removal.

D_3 — tumors with inoperable intracranial invasion.

Table 1 shows the distribution of the tumors operated upon between 1970 and 1982 according to the above classification. The types A and B tumors were removed with conventional tympanoplastic techniques and preservation of the middle ear function. The radical removal of C_{1-3} tumors was only possible through the infratemporal fossa approach after permanent anterior rerouting of the facial nerve. Failure to do so in cases classified as B tumors before introduction of computerized tomography resulted in extensive recurrence after 4 to 5 years. D_1 tumors were all removed in one stage using the same approach as for C_{1-3} tumors. D_2 tumors require a two-stage, combined otological-neurosurgical removal. The extracranial portion of the D_3 tumors was removed using a similar approach as for D_1 lesions.

Selective external and internal carotid angiograms as well as vertebral angiography are still useful for determining vascularity, blood supply and relationship to involved major arteries. Embolization of the tumors is not carried out since it is fraught with risks, requires prolonged general anesthesia and does not present determinant advantages for subsequent surgery.

OPERATIVE TECHNIQUE

The main steps of the operative technique are described in previous papers,[2,3] and only a few details of technique will be mentioned here.

Blind Sack Closure of the External Canal. The external canal skin is transected at the level of the

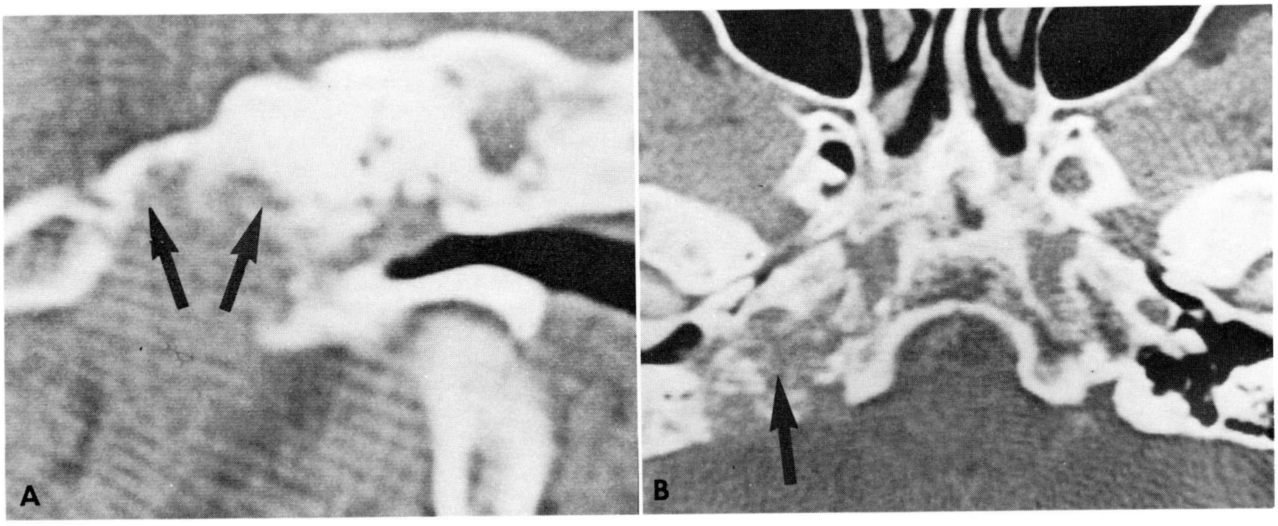

Fig. 3. (Patient 2, female, 69 yr) Type C_2 tumor destroying infralabyrinthine compartment of the temporal bone and invading vertical portion of carotid canal. A) CT, coronal section (arrows - infralabyrinthine compartment of temporal bone). B) CT, horizontal section (arrow - vertical carotid canal).

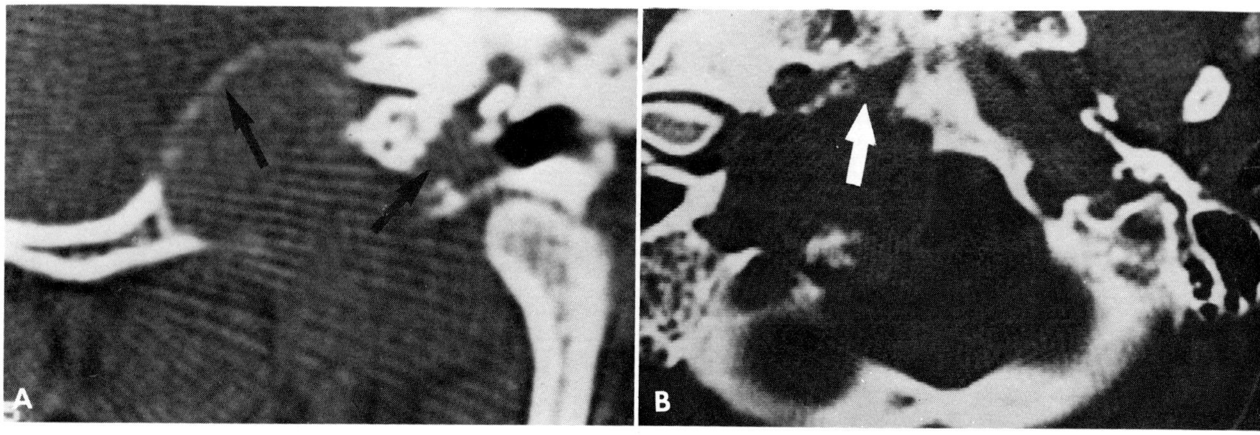

Fig. 4. (Patient 3, female, 27 yr) Type C_3 tumor involving infralabyrinthine and apical compartment of temporal bone. A) CT, coronal section (arrows - posterior fossa dura and hypotympanum). B) CT, horizontal section (arrow - vertical carotid canal).

bony cartilaginous junction. The skin of the external canal is elevated for approximately 1 cm and everted using temporary sutures pulled through the canal. The canal skin is closed with 4-0 vicryl sutures. The postauricular periosteal flap is sutured to the medial surface of the external canal forming a second layer closure.

Double Ligation of the Sigmoid Sinus. The bone covering the sigmoid sinus and the posterior fossa dura anteriorly and posteriorly to it is removed with the drill. Two incisions are carried out through the dura exposing the intact arachnoidal tissue anteriorly and posteriorly to the sinus. With the help of a special blunt, straight ligature needle (Fig. 6), a no. 2 silk suture is passed through the posterior dural opening along the medial wall of the sinus until the tip of the instrument has reached the anterior incision. The silk suture is pulled away from the tip of the instrument and cut leaving back two sutures across the sinus. These sutures are tied in order to block the venous circulation from the sinus in the jugular bulb. The double ligature of the sinus is performed if possible inferiorly to the mastoid emissary vein in order to maintain the venous blood flow superior to it. The sinus ligation according to the presented technique has been carried out to date in 52 cases without any complication.

Infratemporal Fossa Retractor for Displacement of the Ascending Mandibular Ramus. A special infratemporal fossa retractor has provided invaluable help in displacing the mandible for exposure of the intratemporal course of the carotid artery. The instrument has a long stump blade which is placed posteriorly to the ascending mandibular ramus and a short sharp blade which rests against the posterior margin of the wound (Fig. 7). With the help of the infratemporal fossa retractor the mandible is displaced anteriorly just as much as needed for correct exposure in the mandibular fossa avoiding undue traction on the displaced facial nerve. The use of the retractor has completely eliminated the need for resection of the mandibular condyle in glomus tumor surgery. Furthermore, the mechanical traction permits better control of the tension exerted on the transposed facial nerve, with correspondent reduction of risks of postoperative facial weakness, than manual retraction.

POSTOPERATIVE TREATMENT

Nasal intubation is left in place under sedation for 24 hours when cranial nerves IX and X were sacrificed. If in the course of radical removal of the tumor (types C_3, $D_{1,2}$) a large portion of the posterior fossa dura had to be resected, there is danger of a

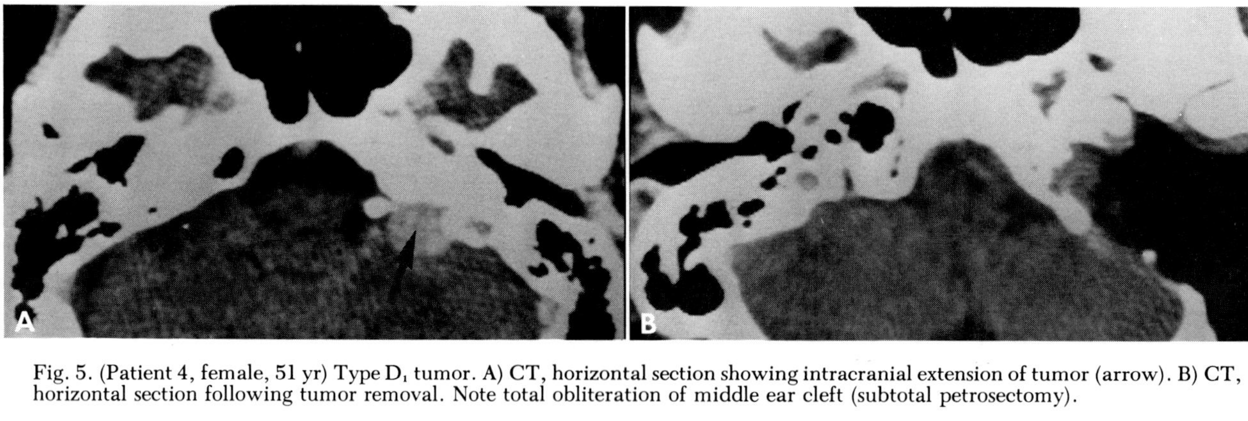

Fig. 5. (Patient 4, female, 51 yr) Type D_1 tumor. A) CT, horizontal section showing intracranial extension of tumor (arrow). B) CT, horizontal section following tumor removal. Note total obliteration of middle ear cleft (subtotal petrosectomy).

TABLE 1. DISTRIBUTION OF GLOMUS TUMORS OF TEMPORAL BONE OPERATED 1970-1982

Type	*No.*	%
A	6	8
B	16	22
C_{1-3}	35	47
D_{1-3}	17	23
Total	74	100

CSF leak through the wound, particularly when severe dysphagia and related continuous coughing have to be expected. In this situation an intralumbar drainage with a pressure-regulating system allowing a flow of 4 drops/min in horizontal position is introduced through a lumbar puncture and left in place for five days.

PRESERVATION OF STRUCTURES

Internal Carotid Artery. The infratemporal fossa approach with permanent transposition of the facial nerve permitted resection maintaining an intact carotid artery in 47 of 52 type C and type D glomus jugulare tumors. In three instances (one type C_2 and two type C_3 tumors), ie 6% of the cases, a perforation of the carotid wall occurred at the level of the caroticotympanic artery requiring repair with 5-0 vascular nylon suture. In two type C_3 tumors the internal carotid artery was found completely obliterated at surgery and was ligated and resected without any secondary effect (Table 2). The technique used for carotid artery manipulation has been reported recently in another paper.[4]

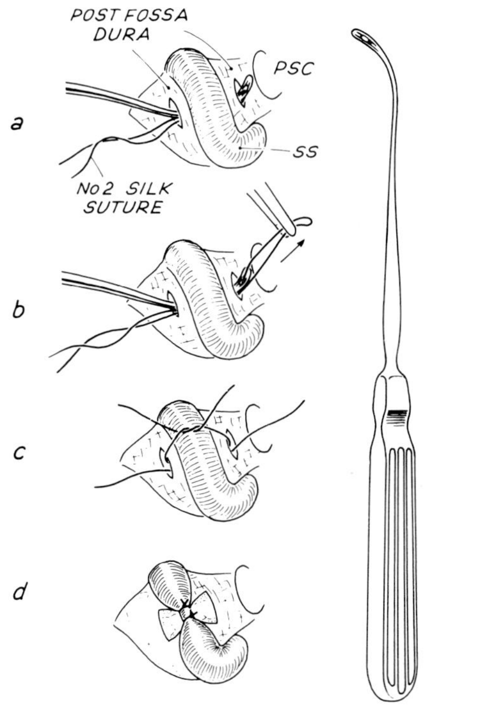

Fig. 6. Double ligation of sigmoid sinus. a) No. 2 silk ligature passed along medial wall of sinus with help of blunt, straight ligature needle. b) Silk suture is pulled away from ligature needle and cut, leaving back two sutures across the sinus. c,d) Sutures tied to block venous circulation from sinus in jugular bulb. PSC - Posterior semicircular canal, SS - Sigmoid sinus.

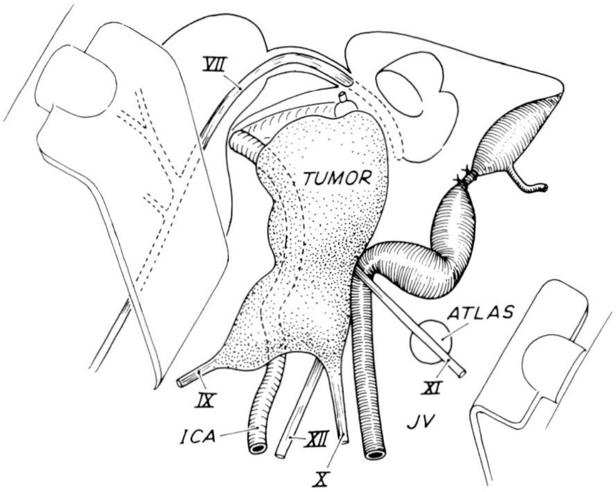

Fig. 7. Operative field after anterior rerouting of facial nerve. Anterior tumor pole is exposed with help of infratemporal fossa retractor. ICA - Internal carotid artery; JV - Jugular vein.

Facial Nerve. Table 3 shows the surgical manipulations carried out on the facial nerve and the corresponding results. The facial function was assessed at least two years after surgery by sending out questionnaires to 61 patients operated upon between 1970 and 1980. Forty-three useful answers (70%) were available for statistical evaluation. The types A and B tumors were removed without any deficit of facial function. The permanent anterior transposition of the facial nerve was followed on average by a recovery of 85% of facial function. No postoperative paralysis but only a facial weakness was observed when the epineurium of the transposed facial nerve remained intact. Complete, postoperative facial paralysis was the result of transposition of the nerve when a segment of the epineurium in the distal mastoid segment had to be left in place because of tumor invasion. Grafting combined with anterior transposition yielded results comparable to those obtained because of other pathologic changes along the original fallopian canal.[5] A 55% return of facial movements occurred after hypoglossal facial crossover. In two patients presenting with tumor invasion of cranial nerves VII, IX, X, XI and XII, the motor portion of the mandibular division of the trigeminal nerve was connected with the distal stump of the facial nerve in the parotid region via a graft from the sural nerve. The graft was routed in a bony groove drilled along the base and lateral

TABLE 2. MANAGEMENT OF INTERNAL CAROTID ARTERY IN TYPES C AND D TUMORS

Type Tumor	*No. Pt.*	*Intact*	*Suture*	*Resection + Ligature*
C_{1-3}	35	30	3	2
D_{1-3}	17	17	–	–
Total	52	47 (90%)	3 (6%)	2 (4%)

TABLE 3. FACIAL NERVE MANAGEMENT IN GLOMUS TUMORS OF THE TEMPORAL BONE (1970-1980, N = 43/61)

Type of Surgery	*No.*	*Result (SGE, $-\bar{X}$)*
Combined approach tympanoplasty	7	100%
Permanent anterior transposition (PAT)	23	85%
Grafting + PAT	6	65%
XII-VII	5	55%
V_3-VII	2	60%

SGE - Subjective global evaluation (assessed by questionnaire at least 2 years following surgery).

TABLE 4. MANAGEMENT OF CRANIAL NERVES IX, X, XI IN GLOMUS TUMORS OF THE TEMPORAL BONE

Tumor Type	*Lost*	*Preserved*
C_1	IX	X, XI
C_2	IX, X	XI
C_3	IX, X, XI	—
D_1	IX, X, XI	—
D_2	IX, X, XI	—

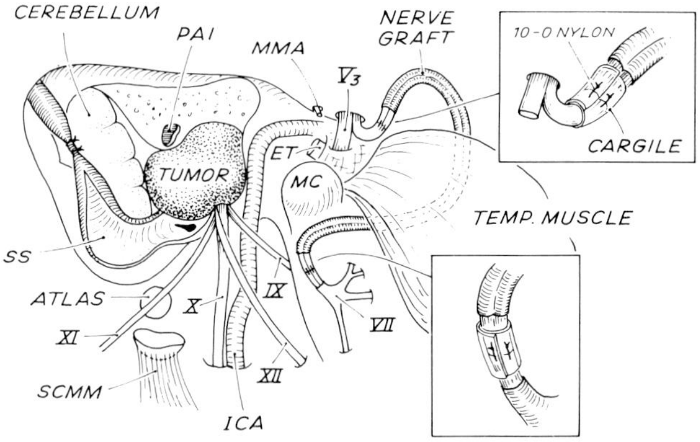

Fig. 8. Trigeminal-facial anastomosis in presence of D_2 glomus tumor. The intracranial portion of the tumor is left in situ for subsequent neurosurgical removal. In view of extensive infiltration of tumor into facial nerve, graft from sural nerve is interposed between motor portion of mandibular division of trigeminal nerve and stem of facial nerve in parotid region. PAI - Porus acusticus internus; MMA - Middle meningeal artery; ET - Eustachian tube; MC - Mandibular condyle; SCMM - Sternocleidomastoid muscle.

wall of the middle cranial fossa (Fig. 8). The anastomosis was performed as described previously.[6] Following placement of three 3-0 nylon sutures the anastomoses were covered with collagen membranes (Cargile Membrane, Ethicon, Inc., Somerville, NJ). The results obtained with this new trigeminal-facial anastomosis is shown in Figure 9. This type of repair can be a valuable addition in the management of extensive glomus tumors of the temporal bone.

Cranial Nerves IX, X, XI, XII. In spite of the introduction of microsurgical techniques, preservation of cranial nerves X-XI remains difficult to achieve and depends mainly on tumor size (Table 4). The close relationship between cranial nerve IX and the tumor makes separation of this nerve from the tumor impossible even in C_1 tumors. This loss is followed by a minimal dysphagia creating no problems to the patients. Sacrifice of cranial nerves IX and X is a regular feature when resecting types $C_{2,3}$ and $D_{1,2}$ tumors. When the function of these nerves was intact before surgery, severe aspiration of saliva accompanied by continuous cough is observed for at least one week. The resulting continuous increase of intracranial pressure leads to severe CSF leaks when the posterior cranial fossa dura had to be resected. This situation has led us to prefer a two-stage otological-neurosurgical resection in type D_2 tumors. The minimal morbidity and no mortality observed in our series is in contrast with one-stage procedures performed in type D_2 tumors by others.[7]

Cranial nerve XII had to be sacrificed at surgery in 13 (17%) of 74 patients. In these instances cranial nerves IX and X were also involved. In two patients nerve VII was resected because of tumor invasion together with nerve XII. In these instances the V_3-VII cross-over was performed as described above.

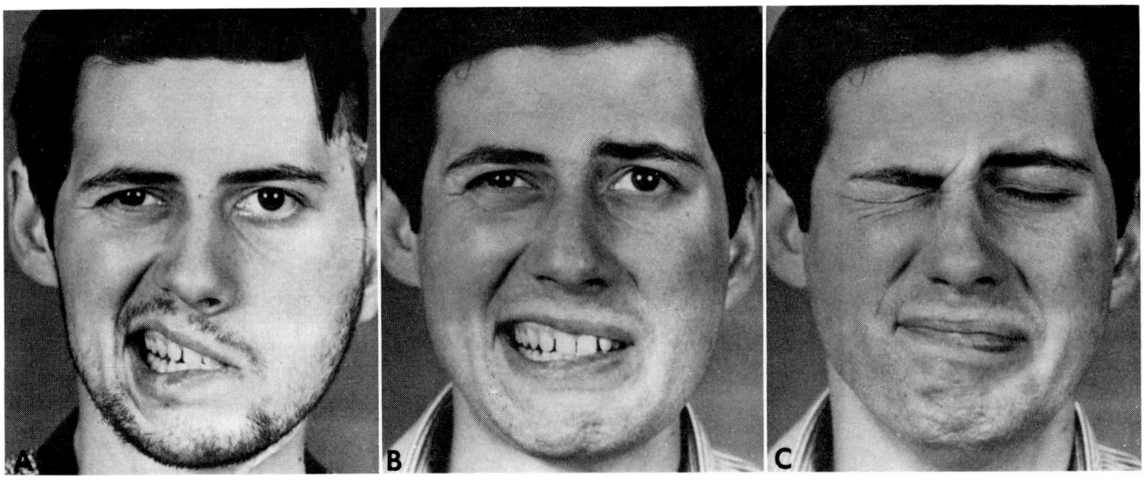

Fig. 9. Type D_2 glomus tumor of left temporal bone. A) Immediate result after removal of extracranial portion with trigeminal-facial anastomosis. B,C) Return of facial function after eight months.

CONCLUSIONS

The experience with 72 glomus tumors of the temporal bone has shown that the infratemporal fossa approach with permanent anterior rerouting of the facial nerve is necessary for removal of the tumor in 70% of the cases. For better surgical planning and evaluation of results a subdivision of type C and type D tumors is proposed. The development of a special infratemporal fossa retractor has facilitated the anterior displacement of the mandible eliminating the need for condyle resection. Using a straight blunt suture needle the double ligation of the sigmoid sinus was performed without complication in 52 patients. Next to the permanent anterior transposition of the facial nerve, the sacrifice of the middle ear function with complete obliteration of the middle ear cleft is the necessary prerequisite for total removal of type C and type D tumors. Grafting with anterior rerouting, XII-VII anastomosis or the V_3-VII anastomosis has been successfully employed. Preservation of cranial nerve X was only possible in C_1 tumors. The cranial nerve XI remained intact in C_1 and C_2 tumors. Since cranial nerves IX and X cannot be saved a two-stage otological-neurosurgical resection has to be preferred in D_2 tumors in order to reduce morbidity and mortality related to severe CSF leaks induced by dysphagia and continuous coughing.

REFERENCES

1. Fisch U. Infratemporal fossa approach for extensive tumors of the temporal bone and base of the skull. In: Silverstein H, Norell H, eds. Neurological surgery of the ear. Birmingham, Alabama: Aesculapius, 1977:34-53.

2. Jenkins HA, Fisch U. Glomus tumors of the temporal region. Arch Otolaryngol 1981; 107:209-13.

3. Oldring D, Fisch U. Glomus tumors of the temporal region: surgical therapy. Am J Otolaryngol 1979; 1:7-18.

4. Fisch U. Carotid lesions at the skull base. In: Brackmann DE, ed. Neurological Surgery of the Ear and Skull Base. New York: Raven Press, 1982.

5. Fisch U. Management of infratemporal facial palsy. Adv Tech Standards Neurosurg 1980; 7:215-38.

6. Fisch U. Facial nerve grafting. Otolaryngol Clin N Am 1974; 7:517-29.

7. Kempe LG. Glomus jugulare tumor. Neurol Surg 1982; 5: 3285-98.

≈

WORLD CONGRESS OF OTORHINOLARYNGOLOGY

The XIIIth World Congress of Otorhinolaryngology will be held in Miami Beach May 26 — June 1, 1985. For further information please contact Anthony J. Maniglia, MD, Secretary-General, P.O. Box 016960 (D-48), Miami, FL 33101.

POLYTOMOGRAPHY AND CONGENITAL ANOMALIES OF THE EAR

J. WILLIAM WRIGHT, JR, MD
J. WILLIAM WRIGHT III, MD
GEORGE HICKS, MD
INDIANAPOLIS, INDIANA

Conventional radiography and even high resolution computerized axial tomography leave much to be desired in demonstrating the minutiae of the anatomy of the temporal bone. Multidirectional tomography remains the examination of choice radiographically in cases of congenital anomalies of the temporal bone. Details of the inner, middle and even external ear in the presence of atresia are more clearly delineated by this method than any other to date. Such information is of inestimable value to the surgeon in the diagnosis and surgical correction of anomalies of the temporal bone. Important features of the vestibule, semicircular canals, cochlea, facial nerve, internal auditory canal, temporomandibular joint, pneumatization of the temporal bone, tegmen, tympanic cavity, ossicles, oval and round windows, jugular bulb and carotid artery and the external ear canal are discerned most clearly by multidirectional tomography.

INTRODUCTION

Visualization of the structures of the inner, middle and external ear canal is a great aid to the diagnosis and possible surgical therapy of congenital anomalies of the temporal bone. At this point in time, multidirectional tomography is the method of choice for roentgenographic examination of these patients. At times it may be definitive in determining both the etiology and the therapeutic course to be followed and always it is an indispensable roadmap for surgical exploration.

There are a great number of hereditary and congenital causes of hearing loss. Konigsmark[1] has estimated there are about 70 types of hereditary deafness in humans. He feels the differential diagnosis of these familial deafness syndromes is aided by examining 1) the mode of genetic transmission, 2) the characteristics of the deafness, 3) the age of onset, 4) the sonic frequencies involved and, 5) the associated abnormalities. He also pointed out what is well known, that hereditary deafness may be conductive, neural or mixed.

Ward[2] reminds us that "all cases of congenital deafness are not hereditary." He cites "the maternal ingestion of toxins, maternal rubella during the first trimester, Rh incompatibility, intrauterine accidents and birth injuries" which have "no genetic precursor."

Van Egmond[3] called attention to the fact that deafness may be hereditary but not congenital as in otosclerosis. Moreover, as Ward[2] recognizes, deafness can be both congenital and hereditary as exemplified in "sporadic recessive deafness."

Due to these and other considerations, classification of hereditary and congenital deafness has been most difficult and often confusing. In this paper, we are confining ourselves to those types of hereditary and congenital hearing loss, be they hereditary or congenital, which show demonstrable changes in the temporal bone by multidirectional tomography.

EMBRYOLOGY OF THE TEMPORAL BONE

According to Arey[4] the inner ear develops in the 3½-week-old human embryo as the otic placode, a thickening of the ectoderm on either side of the head. This area enfolds to become the otic pit and then pinches off to become the otocyst. By three months, it is differentiated into the endolymphatic duct and sac, the semicircular endolymphatic canals, the utricle, saccule and cochlear duct containing the organ of Corti. By the fifth month of fetal life, the sensory end-organ of the ear attains adult form and size as the cartilaginous otic capsule ossifies.[5]

The sound-conducting mechanism in the middle and external ear derives as follows:[6] the auricle, malleus and incus develop from the first branchial arch; the external auditory meatus develops from the first branchial groove; the tympanic cavity and eustachian tube develop from the first pharyngeal pouch; and the stapes develops from the second branchial arch.

By the third fetal month the pinna has been formed from the first and second branchial arches, but it is not until the seventh fetal month that the ectodermal chord of cells cannulizes to form the tympanic membrane and then the external auditory meatus. Pneumatization of the temporal bone also begins in the seventh fetal month and may continue into the petrous apex into adult life. Therefore, congenital anomalies of the inner ear occur during the second or third month of embryonic life, while congenital anomalies of the sound-conducting apparatus occur during the second to seventh month of fetal life.[5] It may be added that many, if not most, of the important developmental anomalies are initiated by changes occurring in normal development from the

Presented at the meeting of the American Otological Society, Inc., Palm Beach, Florida, May 2-3, 1982.
REPRINTS — J. William Wright, Jr, MD, Otologic Associates Inc., 5506 East 16th Street, Suite 22, Indianapolis, IN 46218.

seventh to ninth week of fetal life.

INNER EAR ANOMALIES VISUALIZED BY TOMOGRAPHY

The internal auditory canal (IAC) varies significantly in size both as to vertical height and also as to medial-lateral dimensions. It is, however, remarkably consistent in normal-hearing individuals when one side is compared to the other in the same person.

We have observed a narrow IAC in many individuals who have a sensorineural hearing loss which is not always progressive, although most of the time it is. It is extremely difficult to rule out other possibilities for the sensorineural hearing loss other than the size of the IAC itself. We have been impressed, however, that any IAC in which the vertical diameter of the canal is less than 3 mm in height may be of significance in sensorineural hearing loss. This is mentioned only because the association of such hearing losses with a narrow IAC seems to be greater than mere change would dictate. It is not, however, a proven correlation in our hands.

A frequent finding in congenital anomalies is what we have termed a "sloping tegmen." In the anterior-posterior (AP) view and somewhat less well-discerned in the lateral view, the floor of the midcranial fossa or tegmen may slope sharply from lateral to medial toward the foramen magnum. There is poorer, if any pneumatization, superior to the IAC and the effect of the deformity is to shorten the superior wall of the IAC and shorten the length of the entire canal. In extreme cases, this will cause the pors acousticus to open into the midcranial fossa rather than into the posterior cranial fossa. On occasion the IAC will be markedly short with a very poorly visualized crista falciformis.

Conversely, the tegmen may slope from medial to lateral in such a fashion as to descend to a level touching the horizontal semicircular canal. These deformities may coexist or be independent of each other.

The normal cochlea is well-delineated on multidirectional tomography and has a rather uniformly spherical appearance particularly in the AP view. In many of the named syndromes of congenital or hereditary hearing loss and also in some others not carrying an investigator's name but yet demonstrating neurosensory involvement, the cochlea appears to be somewhat "squashed" or "lopsided," as if it had been slightly squeezed between a thumb placed on the basilar turn and a forefinger on the apical. This leads to a slightly flattened appearance of the usual spherical form.

Probably the next most common inner ear pathology is seen with a dilation of the horizontal semicircular canal. This may present as a short and greatly enlarged horizontal semicircular canal in the AP view or may also be associated with an enlarged vestibule. Most often the superior and posterior canals are either normal or slightly underdeveloped. On rare occasions all three canals and the vestibule may be hugely dilated.

In Mondini's syndrome the basilar $1^{1}/_{5}$ coils of the cochlea usually appear normal, but there is a wide-open cavity above this with no separation between the second and the beginning of the third coil, so that there appears to be one coalescent cavity in the apical portion of the cochlea. Occasionally the vestibular aqueduct is dilated, becoming almost as broad in its lumen and as wide as the common crus. The vestibule itself may appear larger than normal.

The Michelle deformity is equal to an aplasia of the entire inner ear, wherein the vestibule, cochlea or semicircular canals are observed as not having any translucent lumen. The bony otic capsule is normally formed but without any fluid-containing spaces. In our experience, this is most often associated with a normal external ear canal and middle ear and, of course, presents a complete neurosensory hearing loss on the side or sides involved. Diagnosis is dependent entirely upon roentgenographic demonstration of the defect.

The normal facial nerve can be seen exiting from the lateral extremity of the internal auditory canal in both the AP and 20° oblique tomographic views. We have observed one case of Möbius syndrome with paralysis of the external rectus muscle and facial paralysis in which it was clear that no such exit existed in the tomographic examination.

Many of the named and unnamed syndromes of hereditary and congenital deafness show distortion of the normal architecture of the inner ear when examined tomographically. In our experience, these are found most often in Crouzon's, Apert's, Waardenburg's, Michelle's, Mondini's and Hurler's diseases. They are manifested by alterations in size, position and structure as well as possible obliteration or aplasia of the IAC, vestibule, cochlea, semicircular canals and tegmen. With the exception of the Michelle and Mondini syndromes, the tomographic findings are inconstant. Some patients demonstrate no significant changes in the inner ear, while others manifest severe alterations of normal anatomy.

There are many inconsistencies in the architecture of the temporal bone as observed in some instances of hereditary and congenital deafness. These inconsistencies initially give rise to great confusion in interpreting the tomogram. However, with experience one can begin to see what we like to call "consistent inconsistencies." Thus, it is observed that these deviations from normal tend to fall into a repetitive pattern making the analysis of the tomogram far easier.

EXTERNAL CANAL ANOMALIES SEEN IN TOMOGRAPHY

The external ear canal may have one of the three significant clinical abnormalities, ie, complete atresia, partial atresia, or abnormal angulation. Occasionally atresia, either partial or complete, may be confined to the lateral one third of the external ear canal which is its cartilaginous portion. Complete atresia of the canal, whether confined to the cartilaginous segment or involving the bony medial two thirds of the canal as well, is usually associated with deformities of the cartilaginous auricle.

When there is either incomplete or complete atresia of the bony external ear canal, it is most often due to either hypoplasia of the tympanic bone or failure of its cannulization.[7] Normally, through cannulization the tympanic bone contributes approximately two thirds to the substance of the external ear canal. It follows that hypoplasia or agenesis of the tympanic bone creates a much more difficult problem of surgical reconstruction.

Three things about the external canal are of importance to the surgeon. Agenesis or hypoplasia of the tympanic bone is of great importance since the larger and more normal this structure is, the more surgical room there is for reconstruction of an external canal. The surgeon is also interested in knowing the thickness and completeness of the bony atresia plate, since the thicker it is, the more drilling will have to be done in an area of few or little landmarks in order to reach the middle ear cavity. On the other hand, the smaller the tympanic bone, the more likely there is to be distortion of the normal relationships of the facial nerve and other important anatomical features.

If two surgeons are involved in the correction of an atresia with external ear deformity, one surgeon doing the former and the other surgeon doing the latter, consultation should be obtained to coordinate the position of the auricle and the external auditory canal. This is essential since the external canal can usually be placed in only one position, which is determined by the position of the middle ear and the amount of tympanic bone present for reconstruction of the external canal. The external ear must be moved to accommodate the position of the canal and not vice versa.

Partial atresia of the external ear canal can be well demonstrated in tomography and three important pieces of information gained. First is the important knowledge that there is indeed a track, no matter how small, which can lead the surgeon to the middle ear as opposed to his having to utilize other landmarks (which may in and of themselves be abnormally placed). Secondly, the demonstration of a patency regardless of size frequently assures that normal squamous epithelium is covering the outer surface of the eardrum. Thirdly, enlargement of the medial end of the external ear canal can be discerned. The latter situation is present on occasion when epithelial debris collects in the medial portion of the canal and is trapped by the partial atresia. Early correction can prevent this accumulation and the subsequent metamorphosis of fairly normal squamous epithelium into a cholesteatoma of the canal with pressure, necrosis and gross enlargement of the medial end of the canal. When marked enough, perforation of the drum can result with gross bone destruction of the medial end of the canal and the ossicles as well as facial paralysis.

ANOMALIES OF THE TYMPANIC CAVITY

The tympanic cavity, including the epitympanum and hypotympanum, varies from absent to larger-than-normal in size. Most consistently, when there is a diminution in size of the cavity, the attic area is usually best preserved. In studying the cavity by tomography, the AP view is more satisfactory for estimating the true size of the tympanic cavity than the lateral due to the frequent overlying atresia plate which obscures the details in the lateral view.

We have previously mentioned the medial-lateral slope of the tegmen in congenital cases which has a very deleterious effect upon the size of the tympanic cavity, and particularly the attic region. Should the tegmen slope so severely inferiorly that it comes to rest on the horizontal semicircular canal, this materially narrows the space available in the attic for surgical manipulation and reconstruction.

Within the tympanic cavity, the ossicles and oval and round windows all are subject to variation from normal.

The malleus quite frequently shows three minor deviations from normal, only one of which seems to have much clinical significance. The first variation is a hypertrophy or elongation superiorly of the head of the malleus. This appears in the lateral tomogram as if the malleus had a small peaked hat resting on the head and extending upward into the attic. The second alteration consists of a reduction in the posterior portion of the head of the malleus, which in turn is taken over by an extension of the body of the incus enlarging to fill this area. Sometimes this can cause some confusion in the AP view when the proper plane is cut, as it will appear to resemble a dislocation of the incus anteriorly over the malleus. We have observed no significant clinical effect from these two deformities.

The third and most common minor ossicular anomaly having any clinical significance is a right angle deformity of the long process of the malleus. This causes a right angulation of the long handle of the malleus, just beneath the neck of the malleus, to be pointed toward the cochlea, and sometimes, to be actually embedded in the mucosa of the medial wall of the middle ear. This fixation of the malleus limits its excursion and produces a significant conductive loss. Such a condition is best seen in the AP or oblique views.

Fusion of the malleus and incus into an inverted teardrop bony mass is the most common major deformity of the ossicular chain. Frequently this mass is fused to either the atretic plate or the attic. It is rarely seen without a marked conductive loss. It may be seen alone or in combination with stapedial malformation.

All ossicles, though appearing normal, may be congenitally fixed. A favorite spot for malleus fixation is immobilization of the head of the malleus by an anterior-superior fixation to the tegmen. On occasion, it may be immobilized by ossification and calcification of the anterior and posterior malleolar ligaments.

Hypertrophy, or failure of cannulization, of the posterior spine of the tympanic bone may result in lateral fixation of the incus.

Either the malleus or incus, or both, may rarely be fixed on their medial surfaces by a bony bridge. When the incus is involved this usually extends from the horizontal semicircular canal to the body of the incus and is best seen in the AP or oblique views. The malleus may have a medial fixation of the head to the medial wall of the attic, or may occasionally be fixed through the cochleariform process to the lower portion of the neck of the malleus. Again, the AP view best to delineates this situation.

The stapes suprastructure is not visualized well enough to estimate its condition. However, congenital footplate fixation can be demonstrated. The 20° oblique view is best for showing this condition. The tomograms show a bony barrier between the middle ear and the vestibule at the level of the oval window. The fixation is relatively sharp-appearing as opposed to the somewhat fuzzy appearance of otosclerosis. The oval window is quite often somewhat more shallow than normal and there is no vestibular extension of the footplate into the vestibule as is sometimes seen in otosclerosis.

The round window can fail to develop and may show complete absence. This can be discerned only by a series of tomographic cuts in the AP and oblique views usually placed slightly posterior to the level of the oval window.

ANOMALIES OF THE FACIAL NERVE

The facial nerve has a great tendency to be aberrant in hereditary and congenital anomalies. It is here that we see far more commonly the bifid or even tripartate nerves as well as the tortuous and circuitous route that the nerve may take. Here again, however, certain consistencies are helpful.

Probably due to the lack of development of the tympanic bone, the facial nerve tends to be found more anteriorly placed than usual. It can, on occasion, run through the middle ear cavity itself rather than its usual position posterior to the posterior wall of the tympanic cavity. In the normal temporal bone, the descending course or vertical portion of the facial nerve is on a vertical plane with the posterior limb of the horizontal semicircular canal. In congenital anomalies, a vertical line through this descending course tends to bisect the horizontal semicircular canal or lies even more anteriorly through the ampullary end of the canal.

Most congenitally aberrant facial nerves are short and relatively thick. Therefore, in searching for a difficult-to-locate facial nerve, one should always seek it more anteriorly than would be anticipated and search for a relatively short, wide translucency. The nerve is frequently somewhat more inferiorly placed in relationship to the horizontal semicircular canal than usual. It is not infrequently uncovered in its intratympanic course which is best seen in the 20° oblique view.

In following these tortuous nerves, it is necessary to take a series of views separated by 1 mm in both the lateral and AP positions in order to follow this abnormal pathway.

Commonly, a bifid nerve is one which is a single trunk just beneath the horizontal semicircular canal which then splits into two trunks throughout its descending vertical course and reunites either at or just outside the stylomastoid foramen into a single trunk. The most lateral of these trunks is usually the largest and is usually the one which receives the chorda tympani nerve. This condition is best seen in the AP view. One must not confuse the air cells of a coalescent-type sinus tympani with a medial branch of a bifid facial nerve. The clue to this distinction is that the medial branch of the facial nerve will exit through the stylomastoid foramen at some point, either with the lateral branch or apart from it. On the other hand, the sinus tympani does not exit from the base of the skull and no foramen can be visualized for its exit.

The vascular "bumps" which have been described elsewhere,[7] occur more frequently in congenital cases. These bumps can be distinguished from the true anomalous course of the facial nerve which tends to kink on occasion by the fact that the anterior wall of the facial nerve canal remains straight in the vascular bump while it also shows a deviation equal to the deflection of the posterior wall in the truly anomalous nerve. The vascular bump can also be distinguished from air cells immediately adjacent to the posterior portion of the descending course of the facial nerve by the fact that there is no intervening wall between the translucency of the vascular bump and the facial nerve itself, whereas air cells do have a bony wall or septum separating them from the integrity of the nerve itself.

A rare situation does occur wherein the facial

nerve passes inferior to the oval window rather than superior to it beneath the horizontal semicircular canal. AP and oblique views can demonstrate this situation by showing that there is a soft tissue opacity on the superior-lateral aspect of the promontory of the cochlea and no evidence of a bony canal for the facial nerve superior to the oval window and beneath the horizontal semicircular canal.

OTHER TOMOGRAPHIC FEATURES OF CONGENITAL AND HEREDITARY HEARING LOSSES

It is not unusual to see an alteration of the usual architecture of the temporomandibular joint principally because of the tendency for hypoplasia or agenesis of the tympanic bone. The glenoid fossa may be markedly flattened or even absent. Normally, the distance from the posterior aspect of the ramus of the mandible to the anterior surface of the tympanic bone is approximately 8 mm. In some congenital cases, depending upon the degree of hypoplasia or agenesis of the tympanic bone, this distance may reach as much as 40 mm.

The degree of pneumatization of the temporal bone and the size of the mastoid cells is important to observe in congenital anomalies. The more normal the cellular structure is the more likely other anomalies are not as severe. Conversely, the smaller and more sclerotic the mastoid, the more likely severe distortions of architecture are present, and consequently, the more difficult and hazardous the surgical correction.

The position and size of the jugular bulb and carotid artery are quite variable in congenital anomalies. Both lateral and AP views can reveal the presence of a high or uncovered jugular bulb, which may in some instances rise as high as the level of the oval window. The AP view in particular can reveal the position of a laterally-placed carotid or one that is not covered by bone.

CONCLUSION

Many of the deviations from normal in hereditary and congenital hearing losses may be clearly revealed by the use of multidirectional tomography, aiding both in the diagnosis of the condition and serving as a surgical roadmap for possible surgical intervention.

REFERENCES

1. Konigsmark, BW. Medical progress; hereditary deafness in man. N Engl J Med 1969; 281:713, 774, 827.
2. Ward PH, Kinne CE, Lindsay JR. Inner ear pathology in congenital deafness. Laryngoscope 1962; 72:435-55.
3. Van Egmond AAJ. Congenital deafness. J Laryngol Otol 1954; 68:429-43.
4. Arey LB. Developmental anatomy: a textbook and phonatory manual of embryology. 5th ed. Philadelphia: W. B. Saunders Co, 1946.
5. Shambaugh GE Jr. Developmental anomalies of the sound conduction apparatus and their surgical correction. Ann Otol Rhinol Laryngol 1952; 61:873-87.
6. Cliff MM, Lapayowker MS, Woloshin HJ. Congenital anomalies of the temporal bone. Semin Roentgenol 1969; 4:122-8.
7. Wright JW Jr. Polytomography and congenital external and middle ear anomalies. Laryngoscope 1981; 91:1806-11.

NORMAL NEONATAL BRAINSTEM AUDITORY EVOKED POTENTIALS

HOWARD H. ZUBICK, PHD

MARVIN P. FRIED, MD
MICHAEL F. EPSTEIN, MD

PETER FEUDO, JR, MA
MARSHALL STROME, MD

BOSTON, MASSACHUSETTS

Brainstem auditory evoked potentials present a unique opportunity to assess the neuronal and auditory status of the newborn. To date, sample data have been few in number, thereby limiting their interpretive value. The present study was undertaken in an effort to accrue data generated from a large sample size. One hundred fifty-five normal neonates were tested within the first 36 hours of life. No subjects qualified for inclusion in the High Risk Register for Hearing Loss established by the American Academy of Pediatrics. Each ear was tested independently, using click stimuli at a rate of 30.1 per second at 65 dB HTL. Test runs were replicated for purposes of reliability. A run consisted of 2,000 sweeps of data, each being 10 ms in length. Identification of wave forms were assessed by two or more observers. Total agreement was required from all observers for inclusion of wave peaks for analysis. Latencies of onset of stimulus to peak were obtained. Descriptive as well as inferential statistics were computed. Results provide standardized data for comparison.

Brainstem auditory evoked potential (BSAEP) assessment is an acceptable and facile method of measuring hearing and auditory maturation. One significant application is with individuals who are unable to participate in conventional behavioral testing. In the neonate, BSAEPs have been acquired from binaural stimulation at various stimulus intensity levels[1-4] and under various conditions of pulse rate and stimulus phase.[5]

The present investigation was performed to establish normative data for clinical use with BSAEPs in the assessment of hearing sensitivity and auditory maturation in normal birth neonates. As a result, each ear was to be assessed independently. Data were collected to describe frequency of occurrence of Jewett-Williston peaks,[6] the temporal relationships of each peak from the onset of the stimuli (latency), and to determine possible effects that may exist as a function of ear, trial replication, and intensity of stimuli.

METHODS AND MATERIALS.

During the period of data collection (20 days) there were 345 births of full-term infants who were admitted directly to regular nurseries of the Lying-In Division of the Brigham and Women's Hospital. None of these infants were at risk for hearing loss[7] as established by a joint committee of the American Academy of Pediatrics and the American Speech and Hearing Association. In addition, the five-minute Apgar score was greater than 7 in the study group (Table 1). Given time limitations, within 24 hours postpartum, 261 parents were contacted for participation of their newborns in this study in accordance with the guidelines of the hospital Human Subjects Committee. Of this number, 201 parents (77%) agreed to participate. Ultimately, 155 infants were tested, 79 males and 76 females.

Brainstem auditory evoked potentials were acquired on 155 infants within 36 hours of birth utilizing the Med-80 system (Nicolet Instrument Corporation). Following the placement of vertex and mastoid gold cup surface electrodes, each ear was stimulated independently in the following order: 1) right ear at 65 dB HTL; 2) replication at 65 dB HTL; 3) right ear at 45 dB HTL; 4) replication at 45 dB HTL; 5) left ear at 65 dB HTL; 6) replication at 65 dB HTL; 7) left ear at 45 dB HTL; 8) replication at 45 dB HTL. These particular stimulus levels were selected due to their relationship to normal and soft conversational speech, the attempt being made to rule out a loss significant enough to handicap the learning process. Presentation of stimuli below the 45-dB level were not utilized due to the need to accrue as many I-V peaks as possible for study.

Two thousand sweeps from a 10 ms window were collected for each stimulus series. Pulse duration was 100 μs delivered at a rate of 30.1 per second. A band-pass filter was set to limit collection of activity within the range of 150 Hz to 3,000 Hz. Artifact rejection level was set to 95%. Sensitivity of amplication was equal to 12.5 μV. By majority consent, three observers, all trained in brainstem evoked potential assessment, noted the presence or absence of peaks I-V. If a peak was present, the latency from onset of the stimuli to which the peak occurred was recorded. Figure 1 represents an example from one infant tested.

Although each infant was tested bilaterally with each ear stimulated independently, 10 of the 310 ears did not yield usable data. Consensus could not be reached among the observers for these ten infants. Thus, the initial data base included only the 145

TABLE 1. CRITERIA FOR IDENTIFICATION OF HIGH-RISK NEONATES[7]

History of hereditary childhood hearing impairment
History of rubella or other nonbacterial intrauterine fetal infections (eg, cytomegalovirus, herpes virus infections)
Defects of ear, nose or throat: malformed, low set, or absent pinnae; cleft lip or palate (including submucous cleft); any residual abnormality of the otorhinolaryngological system
Birth weight less than 1.5 kg
Bilirubin level greater than 20 mg/100 ml serum

From the Division of Speech & Hearing (Zubick, Feudo), the Department of Newborn Medicine (Epstein), Brigham & Women's Hospital, and The Joint Center for Otolaryngology (Fried, Strome), Harvard Medical School, Boston. The study was supported in part by a grant from the Brigham Surgical Group.

Presented at the meeting of the American Otological Society, Inc., Palm Beach, Florida, May 2-3, 1982.

REPRINTS — Howard H. Zubick, PhD, Chief, Division of Speech and Hearing, Brigham & Women's Hospital, 75 Francis Street, Boston, MA 02115.

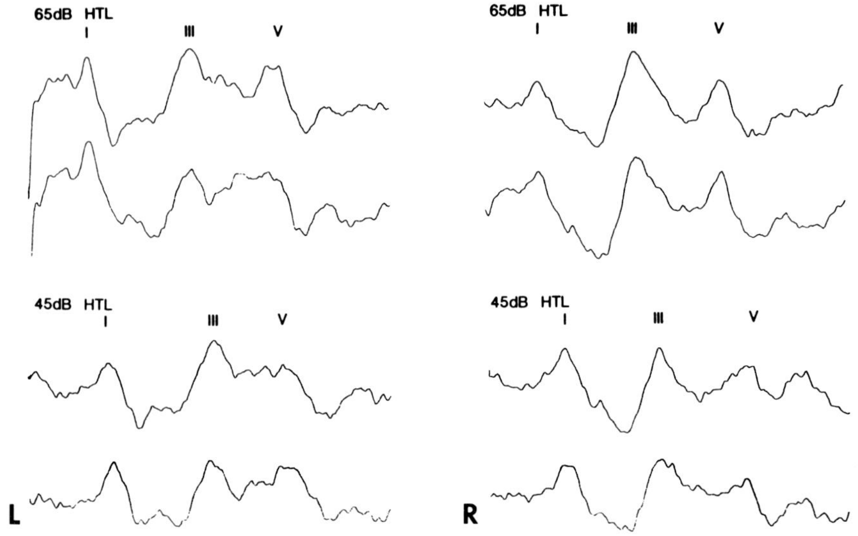

Fig. 1. BSAEP from one infant tested. L - Left ear; R - Right ear.

infants from whom data were acquired bilaterally. For these infants the binary endpoint of the presence or absence of each peak was calculated to reflect the effect of stimulus level (65 dB vs 45 dB), ear (right vs left), and replication (trial 1 vs trial 2). Following this, the mean latency of each peak was calculated for those infants. This was then performed for infants with observable peaks in both ears. These latency data were then treated using paired *t* tests to reveal the effects upon them by stimulus level, ear, and trial.

RESULTS

Figure 2A,B reveals the results of the rate of peak formation for each ear, for each replication, and for each of the five peaks at 65 dB HTL and 45 dB HTL respectively. A significantly greater incidence ($p < 0.05$) of peaks I, III, and V were observed compared to peaks II and IV. For peaks I, III, and V the difference between the number of peaks seen at 65 dB and at 45 dB is always statistically significant. A greater number of peaks were observed at the higher stimulus level. Further, peak V was observed most often. Peak III was observed more often than peak I. The effect of right ear vs left ear, and the effect of trial 1 vs trial 2 is not statistically significant. Thus, there was no difference in the number of peaks acquired per year or from the use of the replication.

Tables 2 and 3 represent the latencies of peaks observed in infants, with peaks recorded at both stimulus levels in the right ear and the left ear respectively. For each of the peaks, statistical tasks (paired *t* tests) performed reveal a consistent significance between the latencies of all peaks formed at 65 dB vs those at 45 dB. In moving from peaks I through V latencies are obviously longer. The absolute value of this comparison is presented within the tables. This value is termed the latency-intensity shift. A significant trial effect was not found in that a high replicability was noted.

Tables 4 and 5 present latency data for infants with peaks in both ears at 65 dB and 45 dB respectively. Paired *t* tests reveal a significant difference between the latencies of the peaks collected from

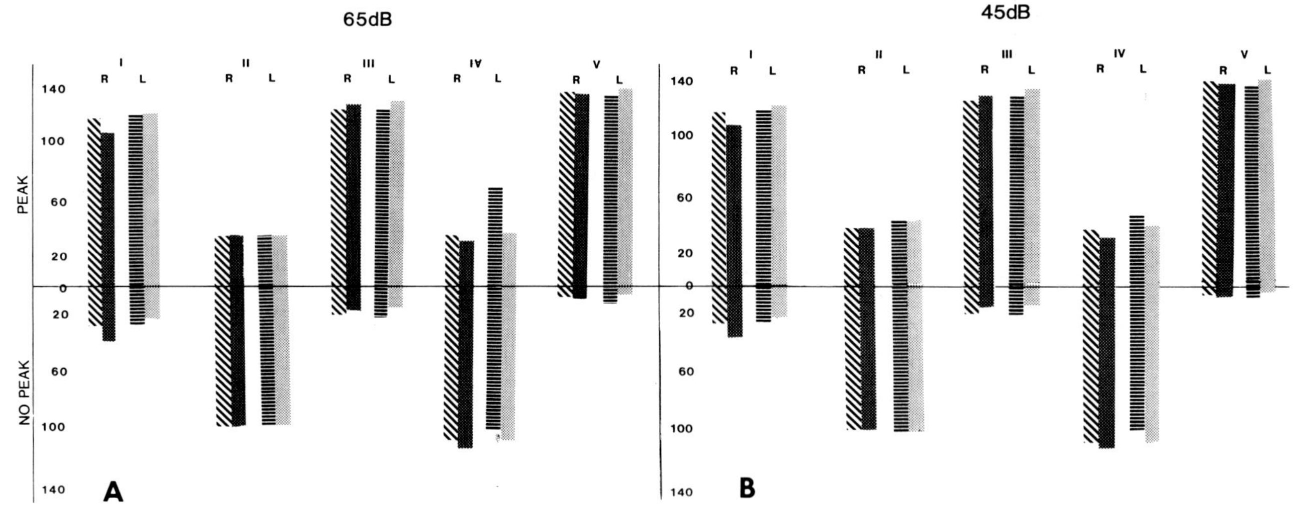

Fig. 2. Rate of peak formation for each ear and each replication. Frequency of occurrence A) 65 dB HTL; B) 45 dB HTL.

TABLE 2. LATENCY DATA FOR RIGHT EAR IN INFANTS WITH PEAKS AT BOTH LEVELS

			65 dB		45 dB		
Peak	Trial	N	X	SE	X	SE	Shift
I	1	80	2.26	0.05	2.72	0.05	0.46
	2	69	2.23	0.05	2.72	0.05	0.49
III	1	102	5.01	0.04	5.52	0.06	0.51
	2	101	5.00	0.03	5.52	0.06	0.52
V	1	113	7.18	0.05	7.78	0.05	0.69
	2	116	7.20	0.04	7.84	0.04	0.64

each ear. Although observed at both stimulus levels, this difference is somewhat greater at the 45-dB level (Table 5). It is interesting to note the very small standard error that exists in relation to all the mean data which are reported.

DISCUSSION

Based on this experience, BSAEP assessment has been found to be a reliable measure that is easily obtained. There were no present circumstances (eg, sedation, feedings) that must be met in order to acquire the data.

When peaks were observed at any intensity, at replication there was minimal latency variation. From this, the data suggests that trial replication may not be required. This may take on particular significance for those contemplating utilizing BSAEP techniques in screening a large number of newborns.

The evaluation of the neonatal BSAEP can be based on the latencies of peaks I, III, and V which are far more consistent in their presence than peaks II and IV. The same consistency existed for peaks which appeared following stimulation at 45 dB as well as 65 dB. For this reason, acquisition of data at 45 dB may preclude a 65 dB trial if hearing sensitivity is the issue to be resolved. If so, then trials at lower intensities may yield additional information regarding biologic threshold. The typical problem associated with stimulation below the 45-dB level is the diminution in the number of waveform data points available for analysis. The current study did not go below the 45-dB level in order to retain the wave I response for its relevance in determining the presence of a peripheral conductive loss in other than a normal test population.

Tables 4 and 5 depict a slight but statistically

TABLE 3. LATENCY DATA FOR LEFT EAR IN INFANTS WITH PEAKS AT BOTH LEVELS

			65 dB		45 dB		
Peak	Trial	N	X	SE	X	SE	Shift
I	1	79	2.20	0.04	2.79	0.04	0.59
	2	73	2.18	0.04	2.87	0.04	0.69
III	1	94	5.07	0.03	5.71	0.04	0.64
	2	94	5.09	0.04	5.66	0.03	0.57
V	1	114	7.29	0.04	7.95	0.04	0.66
	2	118	7.30	0.03	7.96	0.04	0.66

TABLE 4. LATENCY DATA AT 65 dB IN INFANTS WITH PEAKS IN BOTH EARS

			Right		Left		
Peak	Trial	N	X	SE	X	SE	Diff
I	1	96	2.26	0.05	2.19	0.03	0.07
	2	93	2.20	0.03	2.25	0.04	0.05
III	1	108	5.06	0.04	5.12	0.03	0.06
	2	117	5.07	0.04	5.16	0.04	0.09
V	1	127	7.24	0.05	7.32	0.03	0.08
	2	130	7.25	0.04	7.35	0.04	0.10

significant difference in latencies obtained from the right and left ears. This difference may be based in part on the design of the study. The study protocol used a systematic rather than a randomized order of presentations. All right ear trials were acquired prior to those from the left. The reliability of these data is such that even subtle differences between mean latencies were proven significant. In its extreme, the differences are less than 0.2 ms.

This issue was investigated through the additional testing of 20 normal infants for whom the order of presentation was randomized, since we found no similar study in the literature that compared interaural latencies. Each additional infant was selected according to the same criteria as the original group. Results of paired *t* tests for the data collected from the additional group were not significant for an interaural difference. In summary, the original minimal difference is resolved by randomizing order of presentation.

An analysis of the I-V conduction times that are shown in Tables 4 and 5 was performed. Trials 1 and 2 were averaged for waves I and V at both the 65-dB and 45-dB levels of stimulation. These times were then extrapolated by subtraction. The value for the right ear at 65 dB was 5.02 ms and 5.12 ms for the left. At 45 dB, the right ear I-V conduction time was 5.01 ms and 5.11 ms for the left. The resulting mean difference between conduction times for right and left ears is 0.10 ms for both levels of stimulation. The findings are consistent with the rigid protocol and statistical analysis.

The minor asymmetry between ears noted on the latency-intensity function appear to be of minimal, if any, significance. It is essentially eliminated through a randomized stimulus presentation. The authors, therefore, stress the need for this type of protocol design.

TABLE 5. LATENCY DATA AT 45 dB IN INFANTS WITH PEAKS IN BOTH EARS

			Right		Left		
Peak	Trial	N	X	SE	X	SE	Diff
I	1	60	2.76	0.05	2.79	0.04	0.03
	2	49	2.72	0.05	2.86	0.05	0.14
III	1	83	5.49	0.08	5.68	0.04	0.19
	2	82	5.57	0.04	5.63	0.04	0.06
V	1	98	7.76	0.05	7.95	0.04	0.19
	2	101	7.76	0.05	7.94	0.04	0.18

REFERENCES

1. Schulman-Galambos C, Galambos R. Brain stem evoked response audiometry in newborn hearing screening. Arch Otolaryngol 1979; 105:86-90.

2. Goldstein PJ, Krumholz AM, Felix JK, Shannon D, Carr, RF. Brain stem evoked responses in neonates. Am J Obst Gynecol 1979; 135:622-28.

3. Salamy A, Mendelson T, Tooley WH, Chaplin ER. Contrasts in brainstem function between normal and high-risk infants and in early postnatal life. Early Hum Devel 1980; 4:179-85.

4. Salamy A, Mendelson T, Tooley WH, Chaplin ER. Differential development of brainstem potentials in healthy and high-risk infants. Science 1980; 210:553-5.

5. Stockard JE, Stockard JJ, Westmoreland BF, Corfits JL. Brainstem auditory-evoked responses: normal variation as a function of stimulus and subject characteristics. Arch Neurol 1979; 36:823-31.

6. Jewett D, Williston JS. Auditory evoked far fields averaged from the scalp of humans. Brain 1971; 94:681-96.

7. Joint Committee of the American Academy of Pediatrics and the American Speech and Hearing Association. Proceedings of the Conference on Newborn Hearing Screening. Washington DC, AG Bell Association for the Deaf, 1971.

≈

≈

HARMONIC ACCELERATION TESTS AS A MEASURE OF VESTIBULAR COMPENSATION

WALLACE RUBIN, MD
METAIRIE, LOUISIANA

The material presented is excerpted from patient evaluations. The study was performed with the use of the Contraves rotary chair. This testing modality was used at each patient visit. All other conventional auditory and ENG tests were also performed. These patients have been selected to illustrate the value of the harmonic acceleration (HA) test as a modality for monitoring patient progress. The HA graphs produced were a result of the presence or absence of central vestibular compensation. The findings on these investigations further confirm that HA tests provide an objective monitor for vestibular abnormality.

Electronystagmographic recordings, rotation concepts, sinusoidal acceleration, graded low frequencies of rotation, sophisticated electronics and computer technology are not new. However, combining all these in the clinical area is new.

In 1972 Mathog stated in his treatise on testing of the vestibular system by sinusoidal angular acceleration[1] that ". . . it did provide a potential method for following a changing disease state."[1] Mathog was only able to conjecture that rotation testing would have monitor and other capabilities. He unfortunately did not have the advantage of sophisticated electronics and advanced computer technology. It took Wolfe et al[2] to put all of the pieces together so that we clinicians could finally "discover" it.

The clinical advantages of harmonic acceleration (HA) tests have been documented elsewhere.[3,4] The graphic advantages of the HA test have also been described in a number of other publications.[5,6] Suffice it to say here that there are two Bode plots which the XY plotter graphs for the clinician: phase lag and preponderance. The phase lag may be normal, describe a peripheral plot (low frequency abnormalities) or a central plot (all frequencies abnormal) (Fig. 1A-C). The preponderance plot may be normal, right preponderant or left preponderant (Fig. 1D-F).

Those with extensive ENG experience know that conventional ENGs (spontaneous, positional, gaze, optokinetic, tracking and thermic caloric tests) do not usually change as time elapses. Interval monitoring of a changing disease state or pathology, therefore, is not possible with conventional ENG. Of course, there are variations in ENG responses over time, as in some cases of hydrops. It is, however, impossible to follow and document the course of the majority of neurotologic patients with conventional ENG and relate the ENG findings to patient symptoms.

Conditioned by this prior prejudice as to the possibility of monitoring patient progress with ENG, I was surprised and utterly amazed to find that HA tests in fact could offer this monitoring capability. Patient progress can be classified according to the following format:

- I. Improvement (objective)
  - A. Sustained
    - 1. Subjective agreement (patient 1)
    - 2. Subjective disagreement (patient 2)
  - B. Not sustained (patient 4)
- II. No improvement (objective, patient 3)

CASE REPORTS

The following patient histories and test findings are illustrative of HA patient-monitoring advantages and capabilities.

Patient 1. A 34-year-old female was seen first on August 27, 1979, because of recurrent dizzy episodes accompanied by fullness, diplacusis and hearing loss in the right ear. There were no other general medical problems of significance. None of the medical regimens tried so far had been of benefit in controlling her rather obvious problem with endolymphatic hydrops. She was an intense, hard-working individual (both at home and in industry), and admitted to poor eating habits over a long period of time.

The evaluation revealed the following:

1. Physical examination: normal.
2. Hearing evaluation:
   - a. Conventional — right mild sensorineural hearing loss (low-tone primarily).
   - b. ABR-abnormal right.
3. Conventional ENG:
   - a. Right spontaneous nystagmus.
   - b. ABB — right reduced response.
   - c. SBB — peripheral right reduced response.

Presented at the meeting of the American Otological Society, Inc., Palm Beach, Florida, May 2-3, 1982.

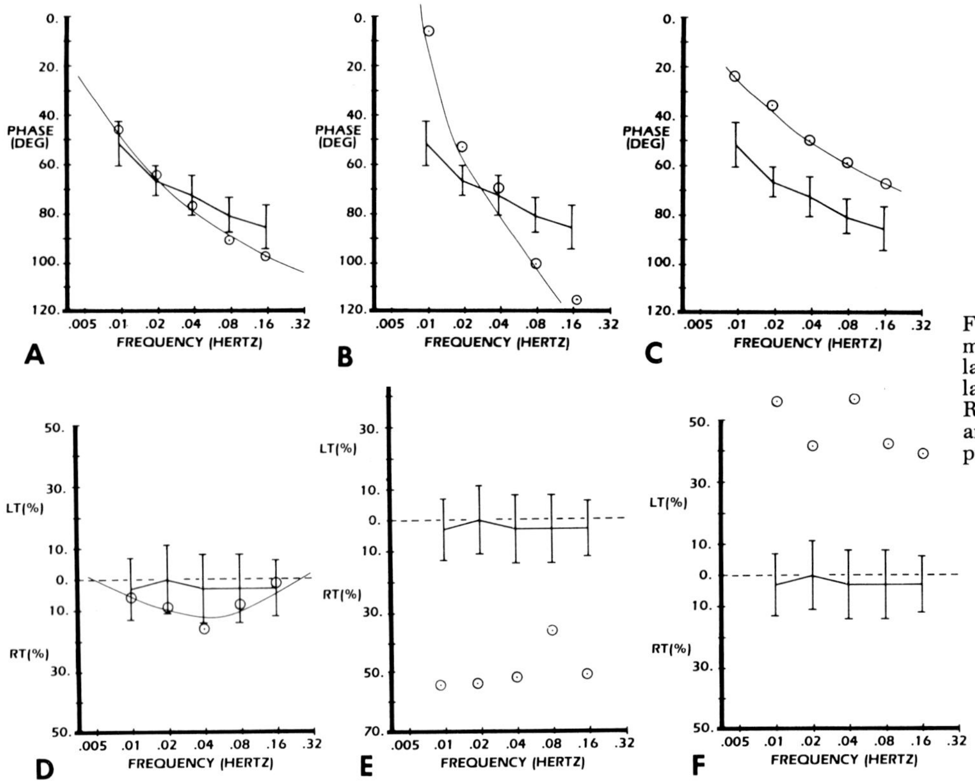

Fig. 1. HA tests showing A) Normal phase lag, B) Peripheral phase lag, C) Central phase lag, D) No labyrinthine preponderance, E) Right labyrinthine preponderance, and F) Left labyrinthine preponderance.

4. HA: Phase lag — peripheral abnormality; preponderance — right (marked) (Fig. 2).
5. Radiography: polytomes normal.
6. Biochemistry: normal except for flat glucose tolerance test.

The serial HAs correlated exactly with the remission and exacerbations of the symptoms related by the patient, but the hearing evaluations and the conventional ENGs from April 27, 1979, through July 21, 1980, did not correlate with the reported remission and exacerbations of the patient's symptoms.

Improvement was gradual but sustained, and there is complete agreement of HA tests with patient symptoms and progress.

Patient 2. A 31-year-old male industrial diver suffered caisson disease (bends) at 59 m (194 ft) on May 23 and 25, 1978. From that time until he was seen on November 8, 1978, he complained of irritability, forgetfulness, dizzy episodes, and hearing loss. He had been a commercial diver for ten years prior to the incident and had had caisson disease on at least two prior occasions, once in 1974 and once in January 1978. Both of these were episodes of bends involving the limbs. He was otherwise in excellent health.

Evaluation and findings on November 8, 1978, were as follows:

1. Physical examination: normal.
2. Hearing tests: high-tone sensorineural hearing loss (3,000, 4,000, 6,000 and 8,000 Hz); good discrimination bilaterally.
3. Conventional ENG:
   a. Left spontaneous nystagmus.
   b. Direction-changing positional nystagmus.
   c. ABB — left reduced response.
   d. SBB — normal.
4. HA: Phase lag — peripheral; preponderance — left (Fig. 3).
5. Radiography: polytomes normal.

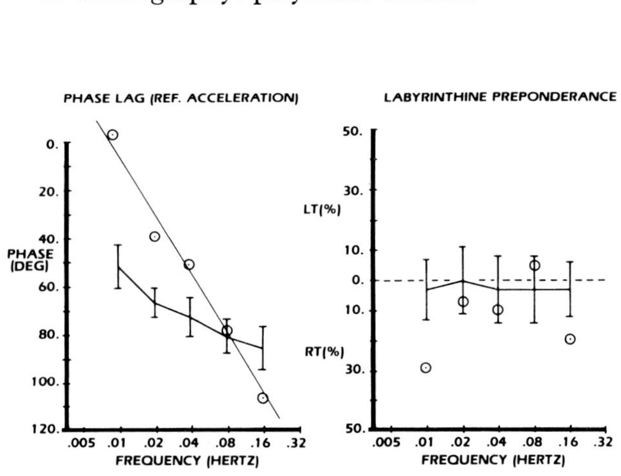

Fig. 2. (Patient 1) HA test showing peripheral phase lag and right labyrinthine preponderance.

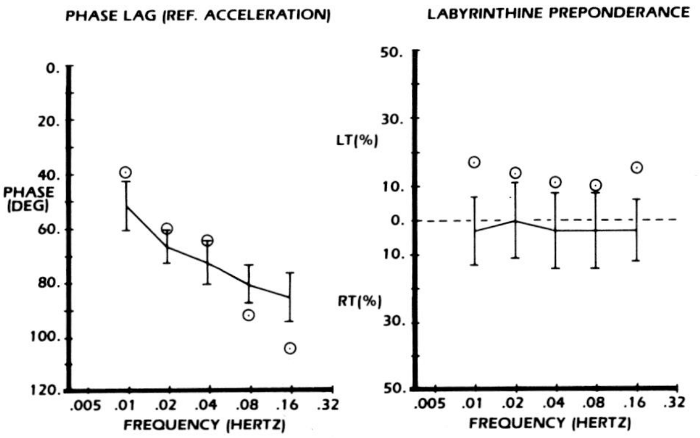

Fig. 3. (Patient 2) HA test showing peripheral phase lag and left labyrinthine preponderance.

6. Biochemistry: CBC — 7% eosinophilia; flat glucose tolerance test, otherwise normal.

The patient's HA findings improved gradually to complete recovery but he never quit complaining of dizziness and lightheadedness.

Patient 3. A 55-year-old male was first seen on May 14, 1979, because of complaints of staggering gait, wobbly posture, foggy head and dizziness since April 29, 1979. These symptoms followed a prostatectomy procedure done on April 25, 1979. He received 240 mg gentamicin per day for seven days starting April 5, 1979. Other than being a heavy smoker and drinker, his health was good.

Evaluation on May 14, 1979, revealed the following:

1. Physical examination: positive Romberg, abnormal gait and abnormal cerebellar function.
2. Hearing evaluation:
   a. Conventional — right sensorineural hearing loss, mild, flat.
   b. ABR — not done.

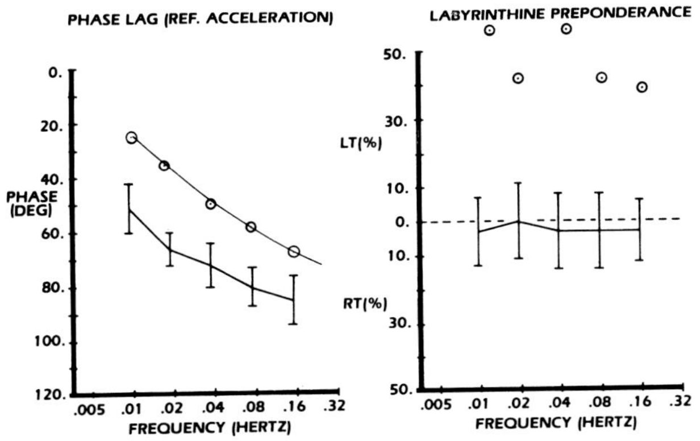

Fig. 4. (Patient 3) HA test showing central phase lag and left labyrinthine preponderance.

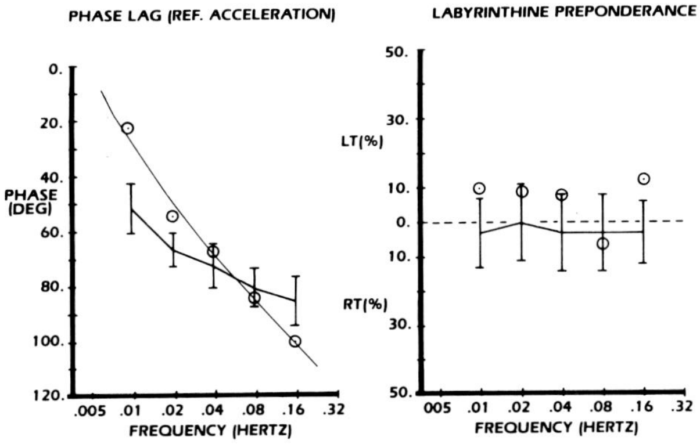

Fig. 5. (Patient 4) HA test showing peripheral phase lag and left labyrinthine preponderance.

3. Conventional ENG:
   a. Right spontaneous nystagmus.
   b. ABB — right reduced response.
   c. SBB — right preponderance.
4. HA: Phase lag — central abnormality; preponderance — left (Fig. 4).
5. Radiography: polytomes normal.
6. Biochemistry: normal.

An HA monitor over a 15-month period confirmed the negative progress for almost the first year after gentamicin therapy. The improvement which has now begun is confirmed by the correlation of the patient's symptoms and the HA tests.

Patient 4. A 59-year-old female was first seen on July 10, 1979, because of a week-long period of weakness, dizziness, vomiting, confusion and episodes of falling. She had been hospitalized for treatment of similar symptomatology on May 19, 1979. She had not improved on the previous treatment regimen (which she probably did not follow as prescribed).

Evaluation on July 10, 1979, revealed these significant findings:

1. Physical examination: obese female in obvious distress as a result of nausea and dizziness; abnormal Romberg, gait and cerebellar function.
2. Hearing evaluation:
   a. Conventional — normal except for bilateral high-tone loss (8,000 Hz).
   b. ABR — abnormal bilaterally.
3. Conventional ENG:
   a. Direction-changing positional nystagmus.
   b. ABB — left reduced response.
   c. SBB — left reduced response.
4. HA: Phase lag — peripheral abnormality; preponderance — left (Fig. 5).
5. Radiography: polytomes normal.

6. Biochemistry: elevated sugar (357), cholesterol (310), triglyceride (2030), type IV phenotype, HDL unreadable.

The patient improved markedly over the next 90 days but never did achieve the anticipated improvement because she followed instructions erratically. Her HA tests did, however, correlate completely with her biochemical surveys and her erratic performance.

CONCLUSION

These patients have been selected to illustrate the value of the harmonic acceleration test as a modality for monitoring patient progress. The harmonic acceleration test responses occurred as a result of the presence or absence of central vestibular compensation. Harmonic acceleration tests provide an objective and accurate monitor for vestibular abnormalities.

REFERENCES

1. Mathog RH. Testing of the vestibular system by sinusoidal angular acceleration. Acta Otolaryngol (Stockh) 1972; 74:96-103.

2. Wolfe JW, Engelken EJ, Kos CM. Low frequency harmonic acceleration as a test of labyrinthine function: basic methods and illustrative cases. Otolaryngology 1978; 86:130-42.

3. Rubin W. Symposium on low frequency harmonic acceleration, the rotary chair, SHA as a modality for monitoring patient progress. Laryngoscope 1981; 91:1282-4.

4. Rubin W. The SHA test in vestibular diagnosis. Laryngoscope 1981; 91:1702-4.

5. Wolfe JW, Engelken EJ, Olson JW, Kos CM. Vestibular responses to bithermal caloric and harmonic acceleration. Ann Otol Rhinol Laryngol 1978; 78:861-7.

6. Rubin W. Proceedings of the seminar on sinusoidal harmonic acceleration and computerized optokinetic tracking tests. Ann Otol Rhinol Laryngol 1981; 90 Suppl 86:18-24.

≈

INTERNATIONAL PIETRO CALICETI PRIZE

The International Pietro Caliceti Prize has been announced by the University of Bologna. This prize honors the memory of Professor Pietro Caliceti, former distinguished Professor of Clinical Otorhinolaryngology at Bologna University. The prize will be awarded to an Italian or foreign graduate in medicine and surgery, who during a four-year time span (November 1, 1976 to October 31, 1980) published a scientific work of unquestionable value and of recognized originality in the field of otorhinolaryngology. The prize consists of a gold medal, a cash prize of 3,000,000 Italian lire, and a diploma witnessing receipt of the prize. On or before December 31, 1982, interested individuals should send an application, a curriculum vitae, and six copies of the scientific work to the Secretary of the University of Bologna. For further information contact Il Rettore Prof. Carlo Rizzoli, the University of Bologna, Bologna, Italy.

COMPARISON OF VESTIBULAR SUBJECTIVE SENSATION AND NYSTAGMUS RESPONSES DURING COMPUTERIZED HARMONIC ACCELERATION TESTS

VICENTE HONRUBIA, MD
LOS ANGELES, CALIFORNIA

HERMAN A. JENKINS, MD
HOUSTON, TEXAS

ROBERT W. BALOH, MD
LOS ANGELES, CALIFORNIA

HORST R. KONRAD, MD
SPRINGFIELD, ILLINOIS

ROBERT D. YEE, MD
LOS ANGELES, CALIFORNIA

PAUL H. WARD, MD
LOS ANGELES, CALIFORNIA

A comparison was made between the phase of vestibulo-ocular reflex (VOR) responses to sinusoidal rotatory tests and the phase of the subjective sensation (SS) to rotation. A parallelism was found between the results of both sets of data such that they behaved in accordance with the prediction of the pendulum model of vestibular function. The time constant of the VOR (17.5 seconds) was longer, however, than that of the SS (13 seconds). Measurements in patients with unilateral labyrinthine pathology also showed comparable changes in both responses. One group of patients with complete unilateral labyrinthine paralysis showed an advance of the phase of the VOR and of the SS. However, phase measurements in the group of patients with only partial unilateral labyrinthine paralysis were not significantly different statistically from those of normal subjects.

Stimulation of the semicircular canals produces vestibulo-ocular reflexes (VOR) and the subjective sensation of rotation, both having similar characteristics. These responses follow qualitatively the predictions of the pendulum model of vestibular function.[1-4] During head movements of relatively high frequencies (0.1-0.5 Hz), the sensation of motion is in phase with the velocity of the head while the VOR response (the nystagmus slow component velocity) is compensatory, that is, eye velocity is 180° out of phase with the velocity of the head. At lower frequencies (0.05-0.01 Hz), there is a lead in phase angle between the two responses and head velocity. Recent studies of patients with peripheral unilateral labyrinthine paralysis have shown that the velocity of the slow component of the induced nystagmus demonstrates a permanent and forward shift of phase over the velocity of the head in comparison with that of normal subjects.[5-7] The change is most significant at frequencies of rotation between 0.025 and 0.05 Hz. Previous experiments have not addressed the question of whether changes occur in the phase of the subjective sensation to motion. To evaluate this question, angular sinusoidal acceleration was used to stimulate the horizontal semicircular canals. The characteristics of the VOR and of subjective sensations were compared in groups of normal subjects and in two groups of patients with peripheral labyrinthine lesions. The results indicate parallel changes in both reactions and suggest the possibility of conducting quantitative measurements of vestibular subjective sensation as an additional measurement for the clinical evaluation of patients with vestibular disorders.

PATIENTS AND METHODS

The data for this study were obtained from 9 normal subjects and 19 patients. A caloric examination was administered with water temperatures of 44 and 33°C. The patients' caloric responses fell into two groups. Ten patients had unilaterally decreased caloric responses with a maximum slow component eye velocity of the nystagmus produced from stimulation of one ear that was at least 27% smaller than that produced from stimulation of the other ear. This group is referred to as "partial" patients. A 22% difference in caloric response between each ear is the 95% confidence limit of our normal laboratory subject population. Nine patients had complete absence of caloric response in one ear. This group is referred to as the "total" patients. Eight of the latter had previously undergone eighth nerve sectioning for acoustic neuromas or Menière's disease. Three of these patients were in the acute postoperative period, having undergone surgery within one to two weeks before the test. One of the total patients was tested two times at one and two weeks after surgery.

The normal subjects underwent a series of sinusoidal rotations in the dark at a peak velocity of 60°/s and frequencies of 0.0125, 0.025, 0.05, and 0.2 Hz on an Inland Control Rate Table. The rotational platform was located inside a totally dark double-walled soundproof room. The subjects were asked to activate a switch located on the right armrest to indicate the perception of motion toward the right and the left-hand switch when they perceived motion toward the left. From a battery source the switch produced a constant voltage which was displayed as a step signal on the polygraph. The signal polarity depended on the switch that was activated; positive for clockwise-perceived motion and negative for counterclockwise.

Analysis of electronystagmographic (ENG) eye movement data was conducted with the aid of an LSI-11 minicomputer system. Details of the stimulating, recording, and on-line computer

From the Division of Head and Neck Surgery (Otolaryngology) (Honrubia, Ward), the Department of Neurology (Baloh) and the Department of Ophthalmology (Yee), UCLA School of Medicine, Los Angeles; the Department of Otolaryngology (Jenkins), Baylor College of Medicine, Houston; and the Department of Surgery (Konrad), University of Southern Illinois, Springfield. This research was supported by NINCDS grant NS 09823.

Presented at the meeting of the American Otological Society, Inc., Palm Beach, Florida, May 2-3, 1982.

REPRINTS — Vicente Honrubia, MD, Division of Head and Neck Surgery, UCLA School of Medicine, Los Angeles, CA 90024.

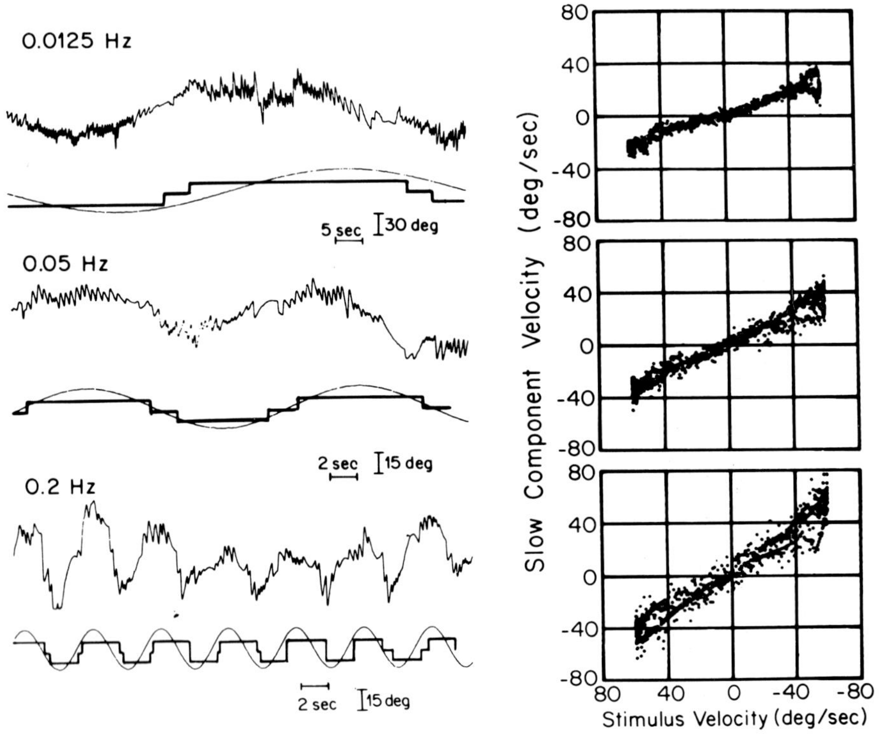

Fig. 1. Left — Electronystagmographic recordings obtained during stimulation of vestibulo-ocular reflex arc with three different frequencies with peak velocities of 60°/s. Underneath ENG tracings are records of sinusoidal trajectory of table velocity and steps of DC voltage indicating direction of motion as perceived by subject. Right — Computer-derived plots of velocity of slow component vs velocity of stimulus for each one of records reproduced on left.

analysis systems have been previously published.[8] The digitized eye position data were differentiated to obtain the instantaneous eye velocity. Data associated with the fast component of nystagmus were automatically removed and a Fourier analysis was performed on the remaining slow-component velocity.

Figure 1 shows a sample of the data as displayed on the polygraph obtained during stimulation at three different test frequencies. Below each record of the monitored ENG eye movement appears the sinusoidal trajectory of the stimulus velocity superimposed on a thicker trace which corresponds to the subjective perception record.

Figure 2 shows examples of computer outputs from programs used to evaluate the nystagmus data. The program performs a Fourier analysis of the slow-component eye velocity and the output provides the magnitude of the DC term, the gain (estimated as the ratio of the amplitude of the fundamental to that of the stimulus), the phase of the fundamental component, and the percentage of distortion (estimated as the ratio of the power of the first harmonic to that of the fundamental). In the normal subject (top) at this frequency (0.05 Hz), the amplitude of the response is very close to zero at the beginning, the middle and the end of each cycle. The phase angle difference is only 8°, equivalent to an advance of 0.4 second. In the patient, however, the response amplitude zero crossing takes place at a significant advance, 41°, equivalent to 2.3 seconds. Further details of methods used to evaluate gain and phase from the VOR have been described in an earlier publication.[9]

Subjective sensation was evaluated by recording the time at which switches were activated to indicate the beginning and the ending of rotational sensation. The phase angle of subjective sensation in relationship to the chair (or head) rotation was evaluated. In all cases, the data for the first settling cycle of rotation were disregarded. During stimulation with lower frequencies for a period of 80 seconds, measurements were made for one cycle only. For other frequencies, the second and third cycles of data were used.

RESULTS

Results of subjective sensation measurements in normal subjects are shown in Figure 3. The ordinate for each insert indicates the velocity of the chair whose trajectory is represented by a thin sinusoidal trace. Positive velocity corresponds to clockwise and negative velocity to counterclockwise motion. Stimulus peak velocity was always kept at 60°/s for each of the four different frequencies. Each circle corresponds to a measurement within a cycle and indicates the moment in the table trajectory when the subject indicated the perception of motion. The first column of data corresponds to sensation of movement toward the left and the second column to sensation toward the right. There are twice as many data points at the higher frequencies than at 0.0125 Hz. Filled circles indicate the beginning and empty circles the end of sensation. The abscissa shows the phase angle of the subjective sensation in relation to the stimulus. At the time subjects felt they were rotating to the left, during low frequency rotation, they were actually rotating to the right. The filled circle indicating starting movement to the left falls on the positive velocity trace. At the middle frequency (0.05 Hz), most subjects felt that they were rotating to the left at approximately the time the table started turning counterclockwise. At higher frequency (0.2 Hz), the subjective sensation of rotation was delayed relative to the chair rotation. The detection of sensation occurred after a significant delay of the table motion. Similar observations can be made during rotation to the right (second column).

In each subject, for every point indicating the end of a sensation of motion in one direction (eg, the left), there is a point indicating the beginning of sensation in the other direction (eg, to the right).

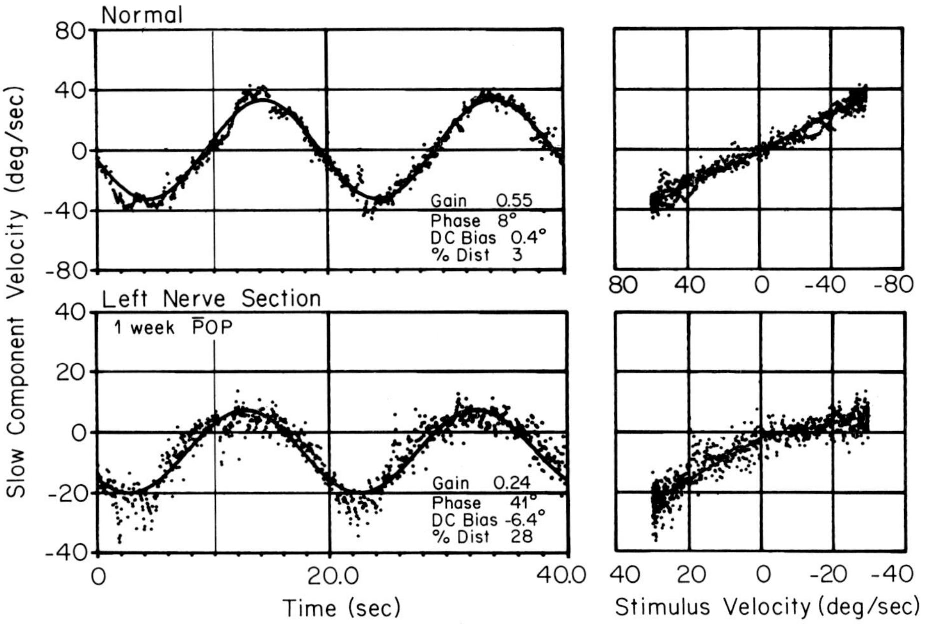

Fig. 2. Graphs illustrating method used to evaluate nystagmus responses in normal subjects and patients. Top — Response of normal subject; bottom — patient's response.

The time exactly midway between these values is indicated in the third column. The midpoints between the ending of sensation of turning to the right and beginning of sensation of turning to the left are shown as empty circles, the ending of sensation to the left and beginning to the right as filled circles. The midpoint values we interpret to represent the time when the sensation of motion should be minimal. (A simple physiological interpretation of this measurement, while not precisely correct, could be that the midpoint represents the time when ampullae of the horizontal semicircular canals were at the resting position on the crista.) Hence, this time has been used to estimate the phase angle relationship between the sensation and the platform motion.

Figure 4 shows the sensation detection phase angle at different peak velocities (as indicated on the right) for one frequency of stimulus (0.05 Hz) in five normal subjects. At 20°/s one subject did not respond. At 10°/s there was about a 50% failure to detect movement. The symbols used to describe the experimental results, ie, motion to the left and right and midpoint detection, are the same as in Figure 3.

The average duration of motion sensation for each half cycle of rotation for the data of Figures 3 and 4 is shown in Figures 5 and 6. The shaded rectangles indicate the time during the cycle when the subjects felt they were being rotated. The ends of the rectangles indicate the mean position of the platform (in degrees of angular deviation, abscissa) at the time of the switch activation. The variance associated with these measurements is represented by the lengths of the horizontal bars which indicate one standard deviation around the mean values. At 0.125 Hz the duration of the sensation is a fraction of the total movement. However, at high frequencies (0.2 and 0.05 Hz) the duration of the sensation is more than 90% of the total rotation cycle.

During stimulation with 0.05 Hz at different peak velocities (Fig. 6), the variability of the data increases with the diminution of the stimulus magnitude. The duration of motion sensation also decreases. Particularly during stimulation with 10°/s peak velocity the detection of motion in the clockwise direction lasts only two thirds of the cycle. This lower stimulus was subthreshold for approximately half of the subjects.

The phase of the subjective sensation response was evaluated as the mean value of the phase angle difference of the two clockwise and counterclockwise reactions. This value was compared with VOR data obtained from Fourier analysis of the slow-component velocity records (Fig. 7). Phase measurements for different frequencies could be conveniently included in the same graph and are indicated by different symbols. At the two lowest frequencies tested for both VOR and subjective sensation, the measurements show a lead in relation to the head velocity. The variability of data is greater for subjective sensation than for VOR measurements.

Phase eye velocity data lead the subjective sensation data (most of the data are below the isovalue line). However, if we assume that the measured phase of the subjective sensation represents two fractions — the actual phase angle and a fixed delay due to the reaction time — there is a logical explanation for the difference between the two sets of data. For example, if we assume a reaction time of 0.5 second, most of the high frequency measurements (0.2 Hz) will be shifted upward by a significant phase angle correction: 36°. The same reaction time, however, has little effect on very low frequencies of rotation. The correction will change the phase of 0.0125 Hz by only 2.25°. The average

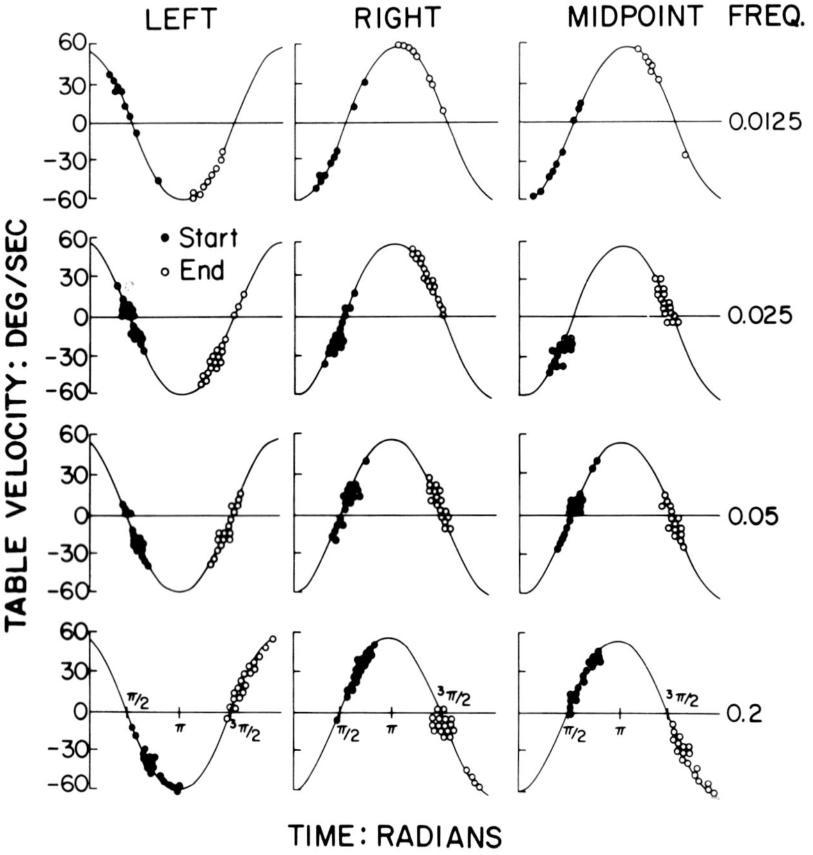

Fig. 3. Time during the rotation cycle when normal subject indicated beginning and ending of perception of motion to left or right. Sinusoidal traces indicate table velocity. Positive values correspond to clockwise motion and negative values to counterclockwise motion. Right-hand column shows phase measurement of response, referred to as midpoint between ending of sensation of motion to left and beginning of motion to right (filled circles) and ending of sensation of motion to right and beginning of motion to left (empty circles).

VOR phase lag at 0.2 Hz is $-4 \pm 2°$. The subjective sensation is $-33 \pm 20°$ which, if corrected by the presumed reaction time, will be similar to the phase of the VOR. At present, however, we do not have a procedure that will allow us to derive the vestibular reaction time with confidence, and these values are uncorrected in the graphs.

Another comparison of phase angle mean value measurements of VOR and subjective sensation is made in Figure 8. This is a Bode plot of the response amplitude and phase data for the VOR. In the ordinate of the top graph is shown the ratio of the eye velocity (°/s) to the head acceleration (°/s²) as a function of stimulus frequency (abscissa). The line indicates the prediction of the first-order model transfer function of the simplified pendulum model covering the range of frequencies used in this study ($T[f] = K/[1 + sT]$ with a gain value [K] of 6.5°/s of eye velocity for every °/s² of head acceleration and a time constant [T] of 17.5 seconds; this value of time constant [17.5 seconds] was selected because this was the derived value from mean VOR phase measurements at 0.125 Hz). Phase data (re: acceleration) for VOR and subjective sensation are shown in the bottom graph. The VOR phase data compare favorably to the first-order transfer function prediction. Subjective sensation phase data behave differently from VOR data. At lower frequencies (0.0125 Hz) the subjective sensation phase leads but, at higher frequencies, lags behind the VOR data. The difference at higher frequencies, however, as indicated before, has a more complex significance.

The results of VOR gain and phase measurements in a group of patients, including some from this study, have been reported in earlier publications.[6,9] Briefly, it was shown that phase measurements are a better discriminator of peripheral labyrinthine pathology than gain measurements. Among the patients, the phase angle at lower frequencies, 0.0125 and 0.05 Hz, is affected more than that of 0.2 Hz responses. Furthermore, the changes are greater in patients with complete absence of function than in those with partial paralysis. Is it possible that the data of subjective sensation can be used as a discriminator for identification of patients with peripheral vestibular lesions? To evaluate this possibility, measurements of subjective sensation were performed in patients. Individual measurements are displayed in Figure 9. The data have been separated to indicate whether the stimuli produced ampullopetal or ampullofugal flow of endolymph in the remaining or healthy semicircular canal organ. The displayed data were obtained with 0.0125 and 0.05 Hz stimuli. Both the total and partial groups of patients responded to 0.0125 Hz with a significant lead in relation to the platform velocity. During rotation with 0.05 Hz, the total patients responded earlier than the partial patients. This difference is reflected most clearly in the midpoint of phase

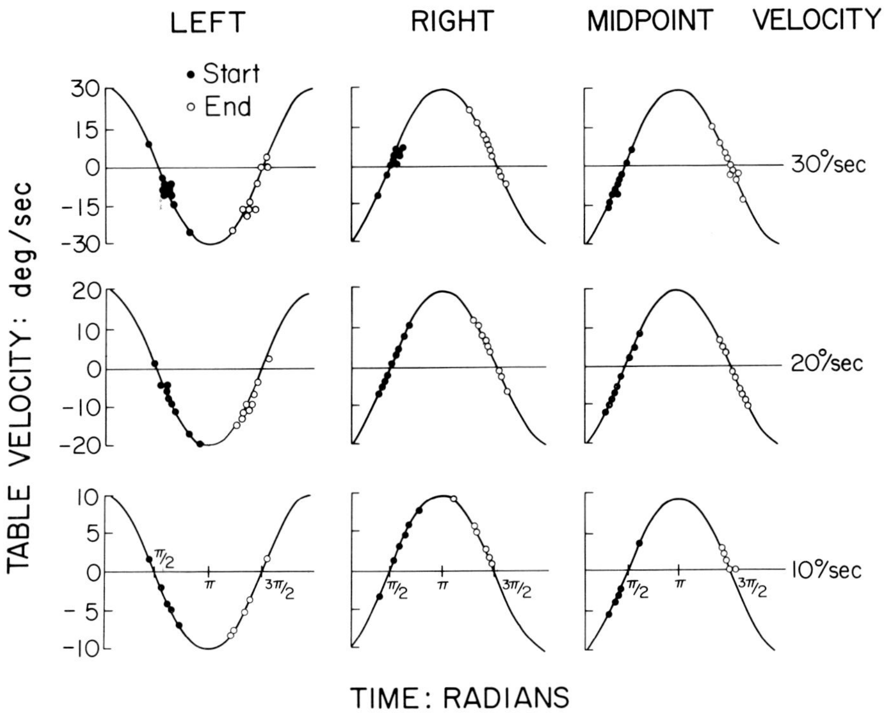

Fig. 4. Same measurements as those obtained in Fig. 3 in group of normal subjects using one frequency of rotation (0.05 Hz) but at three different peak velocities of stimulation.

angle measurements column. In the total patients most of the midpoint measurements fall on one side of the velocity trajectory.

In Figure 10, measurements of individual sensation (left) and VOR phase (right) are shown for each of the two stimulus frequencies (0.0125 and 0.05 Hz). Data have been separated to show the responses of total patients and partial patients. Also, comparison can be made between the individual patient measurements and the mean and standard deviation values for normal subjects. Especially with the 0.05 Hz stimulus, many total patients have significant phase leads. The same measurements of subjective sensations in patients show greater lead than with VOR measurements. The variability of the data on normal subject sensations, however, is greater than that of VOR measurements. Nevertheless, it is evident that not only do patients show abnormal VOR production but their perception of motion is different from that of normal subjects. The difference between the mean values of the subjective sensation phase measurements in normal subjects and those in total patients has a probability greater than 0.99 of being statistically significant for the two test frequencies of 0.0125 and 0.05 Hz. However, the difference between the normal subjects and the partial patients is not statistically significant.

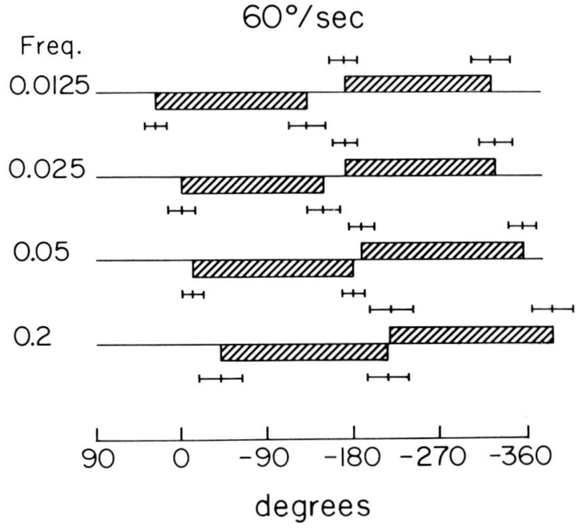

Fig. 5. Summary of results of rotation sensation measurements in normal subjects at four different frequencies of stimulation. Rectangles underneath baseline represent average duration of sensation of motion to left and, on top of baseline, to right. Bars indicate mean ± one standard deviation of measurements at beginning and ending of sensation.

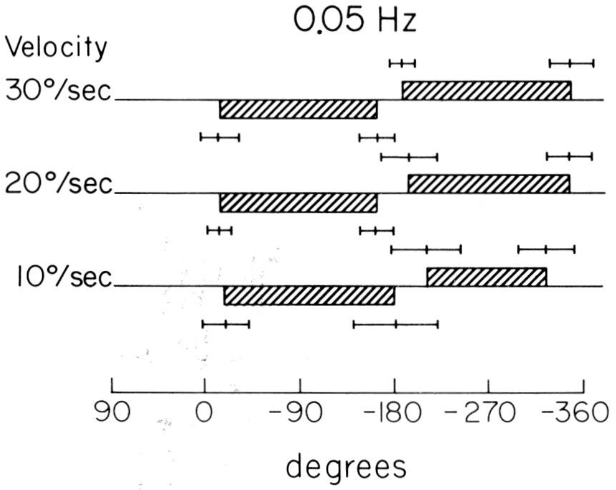

Fig. 6. Summary of results of rotation sensation measurements using one of frequencies in Fig. 5 (0.05 Hz) at three different magnitudes of stimulation.

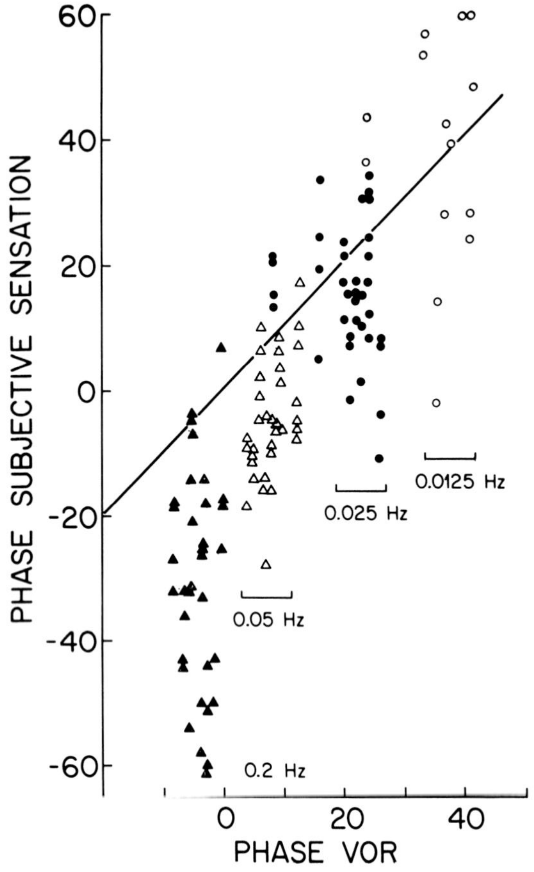

Fig. 7. Comparison of phase measurements during subjective sensation and vestibulo-ocular reflex (VOR) in group of normal subjects at four different frequencies of stimulation. Subjective sensation phase angle is shown in ordinate and VOR phase in abscissa. Positive number indicates phase lead and negative number phase lag of subjective response in relationship to stimulus velocity. Line through scatter plots is locus of equal values for each of measurements.

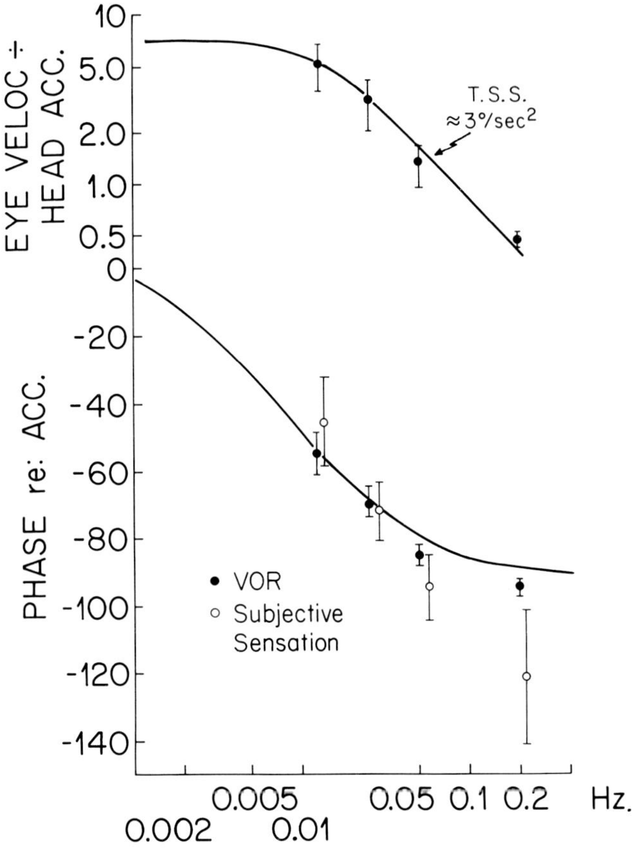

Fig. 8. Summary of gain and phase measurements in normal subjects. Bars indicate one standard deviation around mean values. Abscissa indicates frequency of stimulus and ordinate indicates ratio of eye velocity to head acceleration (top) or phase of responses in relation to head acceleration (bottom). In the latter, all values are negative, indicating lag of reflex reactions to stimuli.

DISCUSSION

Clinical tests of vestibular function are different from those of other sensory systems. Use is made of indirect methods such as measurements of VOR reactions instead of direct psychophysical evaluation such as in audition or visual system tests. Previous study of vestibular subjective sensation has focused mainly on threshold measurements or magnitude estimation of the rotational movement. Clinical application of measurement techniques based on subjective sensation and epitomized by cupulometry was not as successful as anticipated, and the use of vestibular sensation measurements for diagnostic purposes fell into disrepute.[10-14] The need for a method to evaluate the sensation of dysequilibrium suffered by patients or to quantify perception of motion as a clinical tool has persisted over the years. The motivation for this study arose from recent observations, made with the aid of rotatory devices, that the phase of the VOR in patients with peripheral labyrinthine deficits was a strong indicator of abnormal vestibular function. The use of this measurement for diagnostic purposes has been facilitated by new developments in quantitative measurements of VOR using precise stimulation and response evaluation. With such techniques, it has been shown that the VOR phase angle in normal subjects is the parameter with the least variance of all the routinely measured responses to rotatory tests. The standard deviation associated with phase measurements, in particular, is less than that with gain measurements.[5,6]

The results of this study indicate that the phase measurements of subjective sensation parallel the phase measurements of VOR in normal subjects and in patients, suggesting that the dynamics of the two reflexes are very similar. This must be because both reflexes use, at least in the initial segment, the same anatomical pathways: Scarpa's ganglion and the vestibular nuclei. A significant delay occurs at the level of the vestibular nuclei[15] but very little change must be introduced in the subsequent neural stations as the labyrinthine information is processed into the final VOR response of subjective sensation.

If it is accepted that the dynamics of the subjective sensation are adequately described by a model

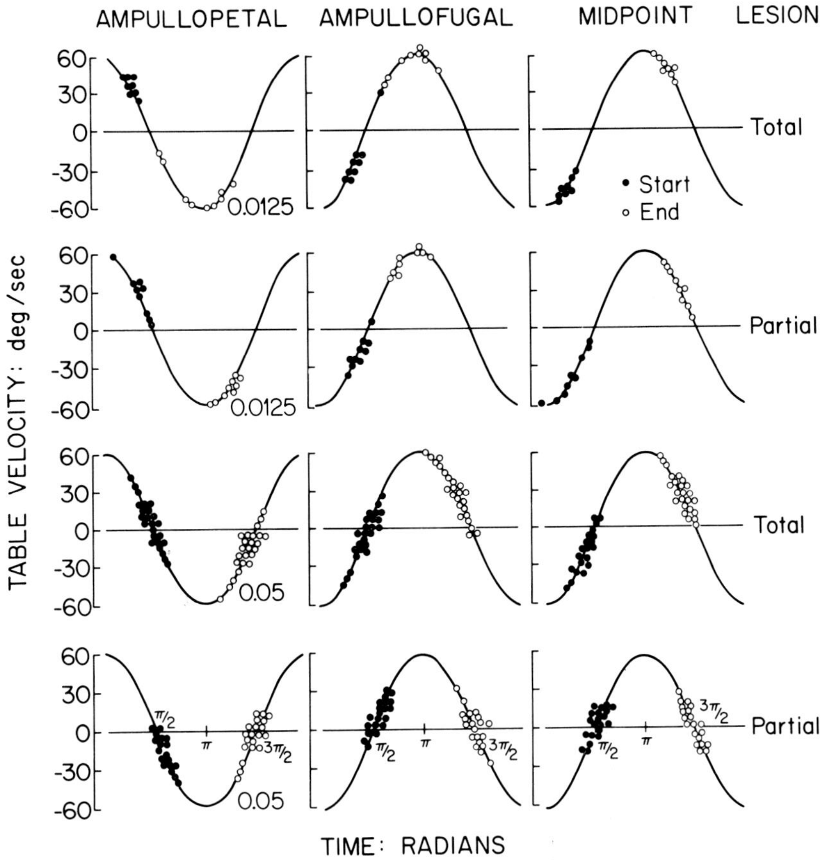

Fig. 9. Results of subjective sensation measurements in two groups of patients with either total unilateral labyrinthine paralysis or partial labyrinthine paralysis. Data points represent same measurements as those described in Figs. 3 and 4 in normal subjects.

similar to that for the VOR (as supported by the data in Fig. 7), it is possible to estimate the time constant of the transfer function of this system, as well as to estimate the threshold for constant acceleration sensation. For the phase angle measurements at 0.0125 Hz a time constant is derived of 13 seconds. This value is greater than that derived by Groen and Phil[16] but shorter than that derived by Rodenburg and Maas.[4] The differences are likely due to procedural causes since different stimuli were used in each study. Our results, however, are similar to those of Cramer[17] who used techniques similar to those used in this study.

Since the threshold of subjective sensation of 0.05

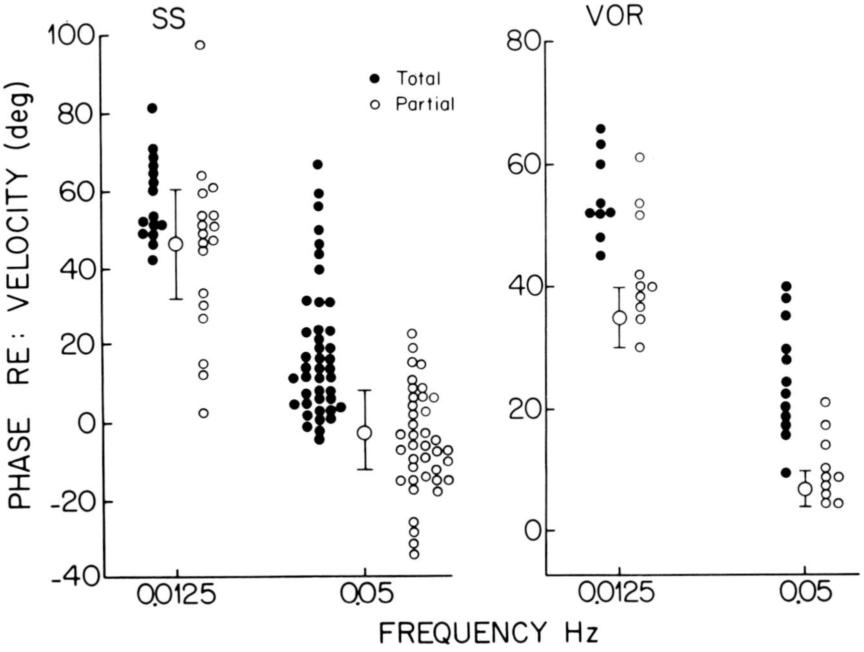

Fig. 10. Comparison of results of phase measurements of subjective sensation of motion and vestibulo-ocular reflex in normal subjects and in two groups of patients. Positive values indicate that reflex responses are ahead of stimulus velocity, and negative values that they lag behind. Data for all the normal subjects are indicated by large empty circles and vertical bars, representing one standard deviation around mean value. Data for individual patients with total unilateral labyrinthine paralysis are represented as filled circles and for those with partial unilateral labyrinthine paralysis as empty circles.

Hz is approximately 10°/s (which produced a 50% positive response in the subjects tested), an equal response (threshold) would be obtained with 0.3-0.5°/s² of constant angular acceleration. This value compares to those summarized by Clark[18] and Guedry et al[19] from studies using a variety of different methods.

The method used to detect phase in these experiments is rather simple. Perhaps with more sophisticated techniques than have been used for conducting psychophysical measurements in the study of other sensory modalities, such as a forced choice method, the variance could be reduced. Likewise, because of the singular characteristics of vestibular stimuli, it is possible to design new strategies that would be unique to the study of vestibular sensation. If this is the case, the probability of obtaining significant information about the perception of motion in patients with vestibular disorders is highly likely. The results of the present studies should encourage further development of tests of subjective sensation as clinical tools.

REFERENCES

1. Mayne R. A systems concept of the vestibular organ. In: Kornhuber HH, ed. Handbook of sensory physiology: vestibular system. Vol 6/2. Berlin: Springer Verlag, 1974:493-580.

2. Robinson DA. The use of control systems analysis in the neurophysiology of eye movements. Ann Rev Neurosci 1981; 4: 463-503.

3. Guedry FE. Psychophysics of vestibular sensation. In: Kornhuber HH, ed. Handbook of sensory physiology: vestibular system. Vol 6/2. Berlin: Springer Verlag, 1974:3-154.

4. Rodenburg M, Maas AJJ. Psychophysical determination of the phase characteristics of the vestibular system for sinusoidal oscillation in yaw. ORL 1977; 39:82-93.

5. Wolfe JW, Engelken EJ, Kos CM. Low-frequency harmonic acceleration as a test of labyrinthine function: basic methods and illustrative cases. Trans Am Acad Ophthalmol Otolaryngol 1978; 86:ORL 130-42.

6. Jenkins HA, Honrubia V, Baloh RW. Evaluation of multiple frequency rotatory testing in patients with peripheral labyrinthine weakness. Am J Otolaryngol 1982; 3:182-8.

7. Honrubia V, Kim YS, Jenkins HA, Lau CGY, Baloh RW. Ewald's second law of labyrinthine function and the vestibulo-ocular reflex. In: Gualtierotti T, ed. The vestibular system: function and morphology. New York: Springer Verlag, 1981:509-24.

8. Baloh RW, Langhofer L, Honrubia V, Yee RD. On-line analysis of eye movements using a digital computer. Aviat Space Environ Med 1980; 51:563-7.

9. Honrubia V, Jenkins H, Baloh RW, Lau CGY. Evaluation of rotatory vestibular tests in patients with labyrinthine lesions. In: Honrubia V, Brazier MAB, eds. Nystagmus and vertigo: clinical approaches to the patient with dizziness. New York: Academic Press, 1982:57-78.

10. Van Egmond AAJ, Groen JJ, Jongkees LBW. The mechanics of the semicircular canal. J Physiol (London) 1949; 110:1-17.

11. Hulk J, Jongkees LBW. The turning test with small regulable stimuli. II. The normal cupulogram. J Laryngol Otol 1948; 62:70-5.

12. Groen JJ, Jongkees LBW. The turning test with small regulable stimuli. III. The advantages of cupulometry over the classic technique of Barany. J Laryngol Otol 1948; 62:231-40.

13. Hallpike CS, Hood JD. The speed of the slow component of angular nystagmus induced by angular acceleration of the head: its experimental determination and application to the physical theory of the cupular mediarism. Proc R Soc London 1953; 141:216-30.

14. Bekesy G. Subjective cupulometry. Arch Otolaryngol 1955; 61:16-28.

15. Buettner UW, Buttner U, Henn V. Transfer characteristics of neurons in vestibular nuclei of the alert monkey. J Neurophysiol 1978; 41:1614-28.

16. Groen JJ, Phil M. Cupulometry. Laryngoscope 1957; 67: 894-905.

17. Cramer RL. Subjective responses to oscillation in yaw. Aerospace Med 1964; 38:457-8.

18. Clark B. Thresholds for perception of angular acceleration in man. Aerospace Med 1967; 38:443-50.

19. Guedry FE, Stockwell CW, Gilson RD. Comparison of subjective responses to semicircular canal stimulation produced by rotation about different axes. Acta Otolaryngol (Stockh) 1971; 72:101-6.

CT AIR-CONTRAST SCANNING OF THE INTERNAL AUDITORY CANAL

ROBERT ANDERSON, MD
DALLAS, TEXAS

JAMES OLSON, COL, USAF, MC
SAN ANTONIO, TEXAS

ROBERT DOWART, MAJ, USAF, MC
SAN ANTONIO, TEXAS

MARIE MERKLE, MD
DALLAS, TEXAS

STEVEN SCHAEFER, MD
DALLAS, TEXAS

Two hundred and four patients with audiometric and vestibular findings suggestive of a retrocochlear lesion were studied prospectively by computed tomographic scan with air contrast of the internal auditory canal. With this technique tumor limits are clearly defined. In the absence of disease the internal auditory canal has been completely air-filled in over 97% of cases. Soft tissue masses occluding the internal auditory canal were demonstrated in 11 patients. Four studies were inconclusive and there was one false positive. Headaches have been the only side effect and there have been no complications. In reporting their results the authors examine the indications, accuracy and limitations of this technique. This study demonstrates that computed tomographic scan with air contrast of the internal auditory canal should be considered as the radiologic procedure of choice for the evaluation of small acoustic tumors.

INTRODUCTION

Computed tomographic (CT) scanning has become a standard radiologic procedure in the evaluation of suspected retrocochlear tumors. Since 1979, CT scan with air contrast of the internal auditory canal (air cisternography) has been used to evaluate smaller tumors which are not consistently diagnosed on intravenous contrast-enhanced CT scans.[1] A preliminary study of 26 patients demonstrated the usefulness of this technique and a subsequent prospective study of an additional 178 cases forms the basis of this report.[2]

The purposes of this paper are to 1) present the results of CT air cisternography in 204 consecutive cases, 2) review the limitations of the various radiologic procedures currently used in the diagnosis of acoustic tumors, and 3) offer a protocol for the radiologic evaluation of the patient suspected of having an acoustic tumor.

METHODS

From January 1980 to March 1982 CT air cisternography was performed on 204 consecutive patients with suspected cerebellopontine angle (CPA) tumors. All studies were performed at The University of Texas Health Science Center at Dallas Affiliated Hospitals and Wilford Hall, USAF Medical Center, San Antonio, Texas. Patients were selected for this study on the basis of clinical history and audiometric or vestibular test results suggestive of a unilateral CPA tumor. All patients had a normal thin-section posterior fossa intravenous contrast-enhanced CT scan prior to the air-contrast study.

The technical aspects of patient positioning and CT beam angulation have been previously discussed.[2] Reference will be made only to specific techniques employed in the current investigation. Following normal (negative) intravenous contrast-enhanced CT scanning, lumbar puncture is performed and 3-5 ml of air are injected into the subarachnoid space. With the sagittal plane of the head remaining horizontal, the patient is brought to a near sitting position. This allows the air to flow to the appropriate (tumor suspect) CPA and internal auditory canal (IAC). After several minutes the patient is returned to the lateral decubitus position and the IAC is rescanned. The patient then rolls prone through 180° allowing air to enter the contralateral IAC which is also evaluated. The spinal needle may be left in position and the head rescanned to confirm entry of air into the CPA prior to removal of the needle, or the needle may be withdrawn prior to positioning the patient for rescan.

RESULTS

Two hundred and four patients (126 males and 78 females) ranging from 16-73 years of age were studied. Patients with the following symptoms and audiometric or vestibular test results were evaluated radiographically for a retrocochlear tumor: 1) unilateral or asymmetric sensorineural hearing loss, 2) audiometric test results suggestive of a retrocochlear hearing loss, 3) sudden sensorineural hearing loss, 4) unilateral tinnitus and 5) any unexplained dizziness, unsteadiness or sense of spatial disorientation in conjunction with a unilateral weakness on bithermal caloric electronystagmography. A total of 92% of the patients had either plain film radiographs or tomograms of the IACs prior to CT air cisternography (Table 1).

Only patients with a normal intravenous contrast-enhanced CT scan underwent evaluation with air contrast. The CPA and entire length of the IAC of the tumor suspect's side filled with air in 188 of 204 patients (Fig. 1). Partial air-fill of the IAC occurred in less than 3% of the cases. In these five pa-

From the Departments of Otolaryngology and Radiology, University of Texas Health Science Center and Veterans Administration Medical Center at Dallas, and the Departments of Otolaryngology and Radiology, Wilford Hall, USAF Medical Center, San Antonio.

Presented at the meeting of the American Otological Society, Inc., Palm Beach, Florida, May 2-3, 1982.

REPRINTS — Robert G. Anderson, MD, Department of Otolaryngology, University of Texas Health Science Center, 5323 Harry Hines Blvd, Dallas, TX 75235.

TABLE 1. RADIOGRAPHY OF INTERNAL AUDITORY CANALS

	No. of Cases
Plain film radiographs	177 (87%)
Tomography	10 (5%)
None	17 (8%)
Total	204

tients air filled only the medial 3-6 mm of the IAC, preventing adequate visualization of the entire length of the canal. One patient underwent small dose Pantopaque posterior fossa myelography which demonstrated a normal IAC. This was the one false positive case in this study. Another patient had a repeat CT air cisternogram which was equivocal for a small laterally situated tumor (Fig. 2). A middle cranial fossa vestibular nerve section was performed on this patient because of incapacitating unsteadiness and a 45% reduced vestibular response on electronystagmography in the tumor suspect ear. No tumor was found and the normal preoperative hearing was maintained postoperatively. Within two months the patient was symptom-free. The remaining three patients will have repeat CT air cisternography in the near future.

In 11 patients the IAC did not fill with air because of obstruction by a soft tissue mass (Fig. 3) All patients underwent translabyrinthine removal of the tumors because of nonfunctional hearing in the tumor ear. There were 9 acoustic neuromas, 1 hemangioma, and 1 calcified benign epithelial cyst. The largest tumor extended 1.5 cm into the CPA and the smallest was flush with the porus acousticus (Table 2).

The only side effect from CT air cisternography has been headaches. The majority of patients experience a mild postauricular stabbing or throbbing sensation when the air enters the CPA; however, this usually lasts less than 1-3 hours. Fewer than 20% of patients experience headaches lasting more than 6-8 hours postprocedure. Approximately 5% of patients had headaches longer than 24 hours and only five patients had headaches longer than 48 hours. Early in the study two patients suffered typical spinal headaches lasting up to seven days. One patient refused the blood patch procedure for closure of the cerebrospinal fluid leak and the other patient's attending physician did not advise her to have the blood patch procedure. Subsequently three patients have undergone the epidural blood patch procedure which is recommended at 48 hours for persistent headache. One patient experienced severe cervical muscle spasm for a period of eight days following CT air cisternography. The reason for this is not known. Depending upon the institution in which the x-ray study was performed, the patient was either directly admitted following the CT air cisternogram and remained flat at bed rest until discharge the following morning or stayed flat in bed in the otolaryngology clinic for 6-8 hours and was admitted overnight only if the headache persisted during that observation period. When a 22-gauge or smaller spinal needle was used and no more than 3-5 mL of air was injected, less than 20% of the patients required overnight hospitalization for analgesic control of headache pain.

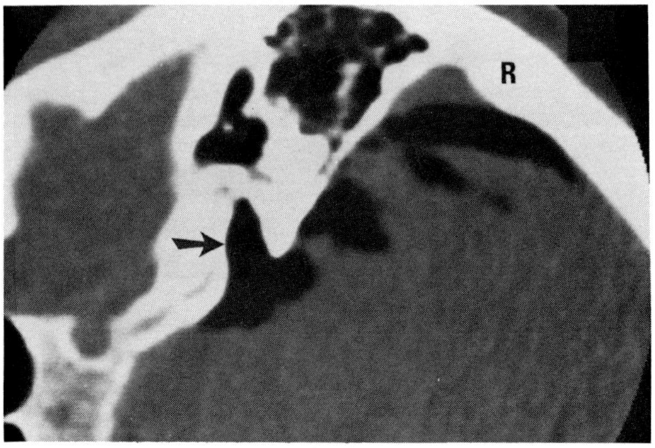

Fig. 1. Normal (negative) CT air cisternogram. Air completely fills the entire right IAC (arrow).

DISCUSSION

Acoustic tumor surgery has evolved dramatically since the introduction of the translabyrinthine and middle cranial fossa acoustic tumor procedures. At the present time operative mortality and morbidity are directly related to the size of the tumor. With small acoustic tumors operative mortality is uncommon and facial paralysis occurs less frequently than with removal of medium and larger tumors. If functional hearing exists in an ear in which the acoustic neuroma is confined to the IAC, preservation of hearing is possible through the middle cranial fossa approach. These facts make it imperative that earlier diagnosis of small tumors be attempted in any patient with signs and symptoms suggestive of a retrocochlear tumor.

Unilateral tinnitus is felt to be the initial symptom in 11% of acoustic tumor patients, and is present in 80% at the time of diagnosis. Virtually all patients will have a unilateral sensorineural hearing

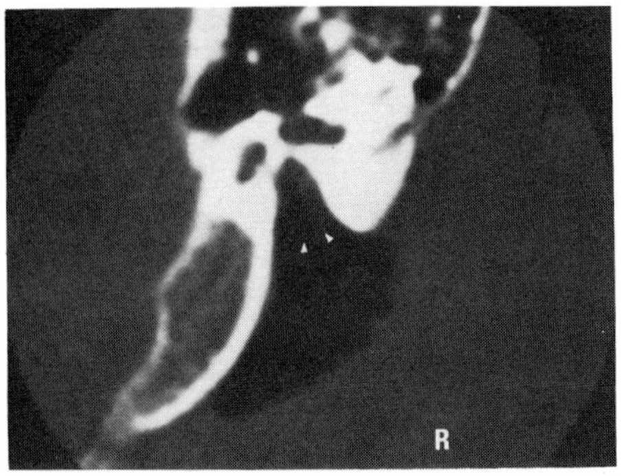

Fig. 2. Equivocal CT air cisternogram. At surgery (middle cranial fossa vestibular nerve section) the IAC was normal (arrows point to questionable laterally situated convex soft tissue mass).

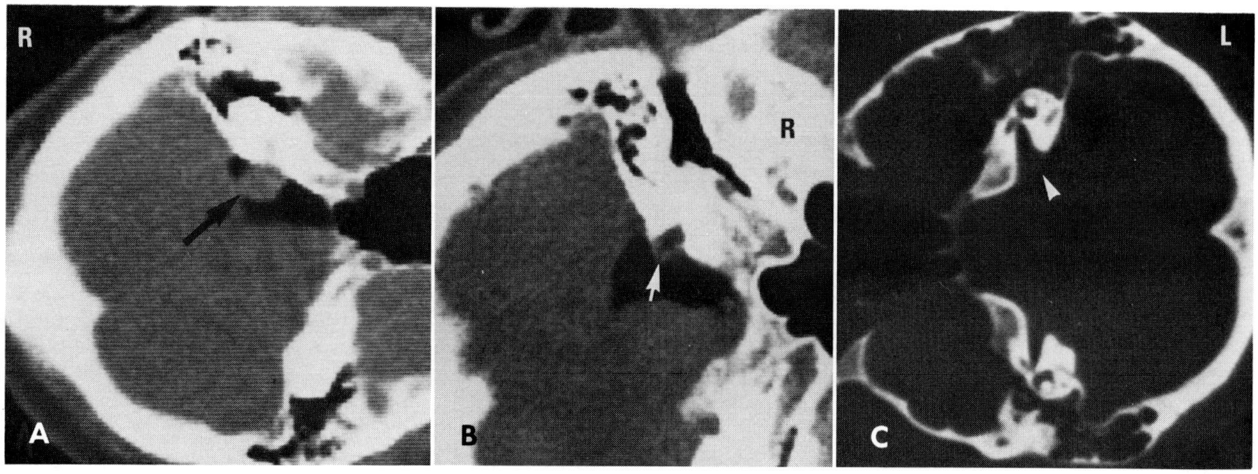

Fig. 3. CT air cisternogram. A) Right acoustic neuroma (arrow), 1.5 cm diameter, clearly outlined by air. B) Hemangioma (4 mm, arrow) outlined. C) Benign epithelial cyst (2 mm, arrow). Audiometric evaluation revealed a left 52% speech discrimination score and 60 dB pure tone average, and on ENG the patient had a 100% left unilateral weakness. Note the enlarged left IAC.

loss at the time of diagnosis with almost 1% of sudden sensorineural hearing loss due to acoustic tumors.[3,4] Vestibular dysfunction including any type of spatial disorientation is the presenting symptom in 11%, but is present in almost 70% of cases at the time of diagnosis.[3] It is these patients who are suspicious for having acoustic tumors and who were prospectively evaluated in this study.

Radiologic Evaluation. A number of radiographic procedures are available for evaluating the IACs and CPAs. These include plain film radiography, tomography, posterior fossa myelography, CT scan, and CT scan with contrast agents. The morbidity of the noninvasive procedures is limited to radiation exposure of vital structures in the head and neck region. Corneal radiation exposure with the potential for later cataract formation is a concern whenever x-ray films of the IACs are obtained. Although the cataractogenic dose in humans is not known, every effort should be made to obtain only those x-ray films of the IACs which are essential for the diagnosis of the acoustic tumor.

TABLE 2. POSITIVE CT AIR CISTERNOGRAMS

Case	*CT Measurement of Tumor Size (mm)*	*Histopathology*	*Radiography*
1	5	Acoustic neuroma	T Positive
2	15	Acoustic neuroma	PF Equivocal T Positive
3	15	Acoustic neuroma	T Positive
4	At porus acousticus	Acoustic neuroma	T Negative
5	4	Hemangioma	PF Positive T Negative
6	12	Acoustic neuroma	PF Positive
7	2	Benign epithelial cyst	Not done
8	5	Acoustic neuroma	PF Positive
9	5	Acoustic neuroma	PF Positive
10	12	Acoustic neuroma	PF Positive
11	10	Acoustic neuroma	PF Positive
			90% Positive

PF - Plain film; T - Tomography.

Morbidity of the invasive procedures includes local and central nervous system complications from Pantopaque, metrizamide, or gas installation into the subarachnoid space, in addition to corneal radiation exposure. Complications from Pantopaque are uncommon, but may be serious, resulting in pulmonary embolism, lipoid granulomatous pseudotumor, hydrocephalus, death from meningitis, and cranial nerve palsies from severe meningeal irritation.[5-10] The only serious metrizamide complication is the rare epileptic seizure which has been reported in only 17 cases out of more than 40,000 examinations.[11] Transient side effects from metrizamide include paresthesias, nausea, vomiting, and neck stiffness, among others. Recent animal studies have raised the question of metrizamide causing chronic arachnoiditis, but this has not been found on re-examination of patients having had metrizamide myelography.[12,13] The only side effect from air cisternography has been a headache which in the majority of patients lasted no more than several hours. One patient experienced severe cervical muscle spasm for eight days; however, this cannot easily be attributed to the subarachnoid installation of air.

Plain Film Radiographs, Tomograms, or Neither? Historically the initial radiographic procedure for evaluating an individual with audiometric or vestibular findings suggestive of a retrocochlear lesion has been either plain film radiographs or tomograms of the IACs. It is documented that for acoustic tumors these two procedures have about the same diagnostic potential (Table 3).[14-21] Of concern is the reported 10-25% incidence of normal x-ray films in surgically verified acoustic tumors. If audiometric studies suggest a retrocochlear site of hearing loss or vestibular evaluation indicates a

TABLE 3. ACCURACY OF PLAIN FILM RADIOGRAPHS AND TOMOGRAMS IN ACOUSTIC NEUROMA DIAGNOSIS

Author	Study Year	No. of Cases	% with Asymmetry/Abnormality of IACs: Plain Films (%)	% with Asymmetry/Abnormality of IACs: Tomograms (%)
Ebenius[14]	1934	34	80	—
Hodes et al[15]	1951	134	90	—
Crabtree and House[16]	1964	54	85	—
Reidy et al[17]	1975	156	75	—
Dubois et al[18]	1976	31	87	—
Crabtree and Gardner[19]	1979	500	90	—
Valvassori[20]	1969	78	—	78
Osborn[21]	1975	56	78.5	84
		Average	≈75-90	≈75-85

peripheral unilateral weakness, the possibility of an acoustic tumor cannot be excluded by negative (normal) plain film radiographs or tomograms of the IACs (10-25% false negative rate). In this situation CT air cisternography is obtained to definitely exclude the presence of, or define the limits of, a tumor. On the other hand if plain film radiographs or tomograms are positive (erosion or flaring of the IAC), tumor size must be determined to plan the operative approach (middle cranial fossa, translabyrinthine or suboccipital) and adequately counsel the patient regarding the morbidity and mortality of the planned procedure.

In the current study, patients who were suspected of having retrocochlear lesions by clinical history and audiometric or vestibular criteria underwent a CT scan regardless of the results of plain film radiographs or tomographs of the IACs. When the intravenous contrast-enhanced CT scan was positive for a CPA tumor, no further studies were required. If the CT scan was negative, as it is in 15-30% of all acoustic neuromas, the next step was CT air cisternography.[22-25]

Pantopaque, Metrizamide or Air. Pantopaque, metrizamide, and gas cisternography have all been used as contrast agents in the posterior fossa. The morbidity of Pantopaque has been discussed. Another distinct disadvantage of Pantopaque is that residual Pantopaque in the middle or posterior cranial fossa interferes with future CT scans which may be desired to evaluate tumor growth in patients who undergo a subtotal removal or to evaluate patients for hydrocephalus postoperatively. The rare serious morbidity of metrizamide, and the fact that the CT density of bone and metrizamide is so close that clear definition of small tumors is more difficult than with air contrast, has precluded its general acceptance as a contrast agent for the evaluation of the IAC. Air is an ideal contrast agent. It provides sufficient contrast and is stable at the pH of cerebrospinal fluid. It is nontoxic, nonsensitizing, resorbed and eliminated in a relatively short period of time and does not interfere with future radiological procedures.[10]

Protocol. In patients with a clinical history and audiometric or vestibular test results suggestive of a retrocochlear tumor, plain film radiographs and tomograms are no longer routinely performed. An intravenous contrast-enhanced CT scan is the initial radiologic procedure. CT air cisternography follows immediately if this is normal. In the absence of a retrocochlear tumor mass the IAC completely fills with air in over 97% of cases. In the presence of a tumor the limits of the soft tissue mass are clearly outlined by the air-contrast CT scan.

REFERENCES

1. Sortland O. Computed tomography combined with gas cisternography for the diagnosis and expanding lesions in the cerebellopontine angle. Laryngoscope 1979; 18:19-22.

2. Anderson R, Diehl J, Maravilla K, Fancher J, Schaefer S. Computerized axial tomography with air contrast of the cerebellopontine angle and internal auditory canal. Laryngoscope 1981; 91:1083-97.

3. Sheehy JL. Neuro-otologic evaluation. In: House W, Leutje C, eds. Acoustic tumors. Vol. 1: Diagnosis. Baltimore: University Park Press, 1979:199-208.

4. Shaia FT, Sheehy JL. Sudden sensori-neural hearing impairment: a report of 1220 cases. Laryngoscope 1976; 86:389-98.

5. Britton BH. Iophendylate examination of the posterior fossa in diagnosis of cerebellopontine angle tumors. In: House W, Leutje C, eds. Acoustic tumors. Vol. 1. Diagnosis. Baltimore: University Park Press, 1979:279-89.

6. Hinkel CL. Entrance of Pantopaque into the venous system during myelography. Am J Roentgenol 1945; 54:230-6.

7. Mason MS, Raaf J. Complications of Pantopaque myelography: a case report and review. J Neurosurg 1962; 19:302-11.

8. Sarkisian SS. Spinal cord pseudotumor: a complication of Pantopaque myelography. US Armed Forces Med J 1956; 7: 1683-6.

9. Hurteau EF, Baird WC, Sinclair E. Arachnoiditis following the use of iodized oil. J Bone Joint Surg 1954; 36-A:393-400.

10. DiChiro G, Fisher RL. Contrast radiography of the spinal cord. Arch Neurol 1964; 11:125-43.

11. Baker RA, Hillman BJ, McLennan JE, Strand RD, Kaufman SM. Sequelae of metrizamide myelography in 200 examinations. Am J Roentgenol 1978; 130:499-502.

12. Haughton VM, Ho KC, Larson SJ, Unger GF, Correa-Paz F. Experimental production of arachnoiditis with water-soluble myelographic media. Radiology 1977; 123:681-5.

13. Ahlgren P. Amipaque myelography: the side effects compared with Dumer X. Neuroradiology 1975; 9:197-202.

14. Ebenius B. The results of examination of the petrous bone in auditory nerve tumors. Acta Radiol 1934; 15:284-90.

15. Hodes PJ, Pendergrass EP, Dennis JM. Cerebellopontine angle tumors: their roentgenologic manifestations. Radiology 1951; 57:395-406.

16. Crabtree JA, House WF. X-ray diagnosis of acoustic neuromas. Arch Otolaryngol 1964; 80:695-7.

17. Reidy J, deLacey GJ, Wignall BK, Uttley D. The accuracy of plain radiographs in the diagnosis of acoustic neuromas. Neuroradiology 1975; 10:31-4.

18. Dubois PJ, Drayer BP, Bank WO, Ziad LD, Rosenbaum AE. An evaluation of current diagnostic radiologic modalities in the investigation of acoustic neurilemmonas. Radiology 1978; 126:173-9.

19. Crabtree JA, Gardner G. Radiographic findings in cerebellopontine angle tumors. In: House W, Leutje C, eds. Acoustic tumors. Vol. 1. Diagnosis. Baltimore: University Park Press, 1979: 241-52.

20. Valvassori GE. The abnormal internal auditory canal: the diagnosis of acoustic neuroma. Radiology 1969; 92:449-59.

21. Osborn JD. A comparative study of special petrous views and tomography in the diagnosis of acoustic neuromas. Br J Radiol 1975; 48:996-9.

22. Davis KR, Parker S, New P, et al. Computerized tomography of acoustic neuroma. Radiology 1977; 124:81-6.

23. Thomson JLG. Computerized axial tomography in posterior fossa lesions. Clin Radiol 1979; 29:1-8.

24. Wong ML, Brackmann DE. Computerized cranial tomography in acoustic tumor diagnosis. Presented at the American Neurotology Society, Los Angeles, California, March 3, 1979.

25. Tos M, Gyldensted G, Thomsen J, Lester J. Comparison of computer tomography and translabyrinthine surgery in the assessment of acoustic neuroma. Ann Otol Rhinol Laryngol 1980; 89: 117-20.

≈

INTERSPECIALTY FACIAL SURGERY CONGRESS FOR AESTHETIC, CANCER AND RECONSTRUCTIVE SURGERY

The IFSCACRS will be held at the Waldorf-Astoria in New York, April 27-30, 1983. This Congress is sponsored by the International Oculoplastic Society. For more information contact Pierre Guibor, MD, IFSC Secretary, 630 Park Avenue, New York, NY 10021; (212) 734-1010.

≈

FOURTH WORLD CONGRESS ON BRONCHOESOPHAGOLOGY

The Fourth World Congress on Bronchoesophagology will take place at the Foresta Conference Center in Stockholm, Sweden, June 20-23, 1983. This Congress is arranged by the International Bronchoesophagological Society, Swedish Otolaryngological Society and Swedish Society for Pulmonary Diseases. During the meeting, the Congress will update the knowledge within bronchology and esophagology. Further information may be obtained by writing IBES Congress 1983, c/o RESO Congress Service S-105, 24 Stockholm, Sweden, or Dr. Stig Haglund, Secretary of the Congress, Dept. of Otolaryngology, Karolinska Sjukuset, S-104 01 Stockholm 60, Sweden.

Ann Otol Rhinol Laryngol 91:1982

HINDBRAIN CIRCULATION AND ITS EVALUATION BY DYNAMIC COMPUTED TOMOGRAPHY

GALDINO E. VALVASSORI, MD GLEN D. DOBBEN, MD

CHICAGO, ILLINOIS

Permanent or transient reduction of blood flow to the end-organs and to the hindbrain is the single major cause of vestibular disorders and a common cause of sensorineural hearing loss. New imaging modalities have become available which allow the recognition of focal areas of hindbrain ischemia in the prestroke stage. The correlation between focal ischemic pathology and clinical findings opens a new approach to the mapping of central pathology. In addition a detailed knowledge of the vascular anatomy of the hindbrain is indispensible for the development of new microvascular surgical techniques aimed at the restoration of sufficient blood supply.

Permanent or transient reduction of blood flow to the end-organs and to the hindbrain is the single major cause of vestibular disorders and a common cause of sensorineural hearing loss. According to our statistics, vascular insufficiency is the etiopathogenic factor responsible for over 80% of central vestibular disturbances and for 20% of all sensorineural losses.

It is amazing that concentrated diagnostic and therapeutic efforts have been made to resolve far less common conditions; it is distressing that so little has been accomplished for the diagnosis and therapy of such a common problem as vascular insufficiency.

It is the purpose of this presentation to 1) review the vascular anatomy of the hindbrain with particular emphasis on the vascular supply of the territories containing the vestibular, auditory nuclei and their central pathways; 2) correlate anatomical pathology to physiologic changes; 3) emphasize new imaging modalities for the diagnosis of hindbrain ischemia; and 4) stimulate the otolaryngologist to become actively involved in the treatment of vascular pathology.

VASCULAR ANATOMY

The hindbrain is supplied by arteries arising from the vertebrobasilar system. The vertebral arteries enter the cranial cavity through the foramen magnum, course first laterally and then anteriorly to the medulla and join at the pontomedullary junction to form the basilar artery.

Branches of the vertebral arteries are 1) median perforating arteries penetrating the substance of the medulla oblongata and short circumferential branches. One of these branches, the artery of Foix and Hillemand, supplies the lateral aspect of the junction between the medulla and the pons and provides some blood supply to the vestibular nuclei (Fig. 1). 2) Posterior inferior cerebellar arteries supply the posteroinferior aspect of the cerebellum, tonsils, part of the inferior cerebellar peduncle and the lateral portion of the medulla including the nuclei from the 9th through the 12th cranial nerves.

The branches of the basilar artery are 1) median and circumferential pontine arteries which supply the pons, inferoposterior portion of the midbrain and ventrolateral aspect of the cerebellar cortex; 2) internal auditory or labyrinthine arteries which may arise either directly from the basilar artery or as a branch of the anterior inferior cerebellar artery; 3) anterior inferior cerebellar arteries which supply the anteroinferior aspect of the cerebellum, the middle cerebellar peduncles, the lateral part of the pons and adjacent portion of the medulla oblongata including the nuclei of the eighth cranial nerve (Fig. 1); 4) superior cerebellar arteries which supply the anterolateral portion of the superior half of the cerebellum, the superior cerebellar peduncles and the posterior portion of the midbrain; and 5) the posterior cerebral arteries which have predominantly a supratentorial distribution to the temporal and occipital lobes but also contributes to the blood supply of the upper portion of the midbrain.

Auditory Pathway. The cochlear nuclei, superior olivary, trapezoid body and lateral lemniscus nuclei[1] are supplied by branches of the anterior inferior cerebellar artery and circumferential branches of the vertebral artery. The inferior colliculus nuclei and its brachium receive blood from branches of the superior cerebellar artery. Finally the medial geniculate body receives branches from the posterior cerebral artery (Fig. 2).

Vestibular Pathway. The vestibular nuclei are supplied by branches of the vertebral and anterior inferior cerebellar arteries except for the inferior

From the Department of Radiology, Abraham Lincoln School of Medicine, University of Illinois, Chicago.
Presented at the meeting of the American Otological Society, Inc., Palm Beach, Florida, May 2-3, 1982.
REPRINTS — Galdino E. Valvassori, MD, 55 East Washington Street, Chicago, IL 60602.

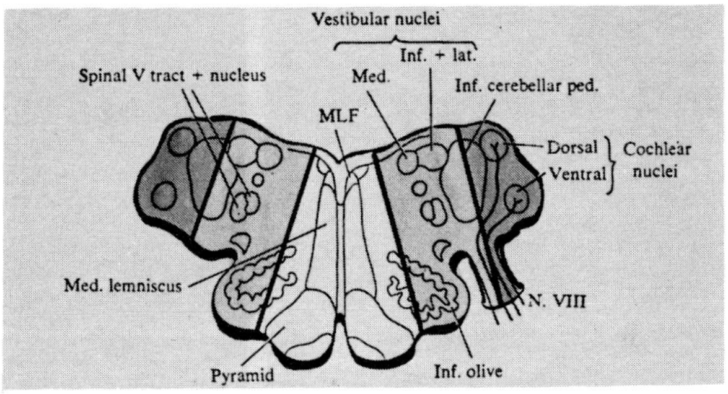

Fig. 1. Vascular supply of medulla oblongata at level of eighth cranial nerve. Light central area — Median perforating branches of vertebral artery; Grey middle area — Short circumferential branches of vertebral artery; Dark lateral area — Anterior inferior cerebellar artery.

spinal nucleus and the descending fibers which receive their blood supply also from the posterior inferior cerebellar artery. Branches of this artery supply the inferior cerebellar peduncle which contains fibers connecting the vestibular system to the cerebellum. Ascending fibers in the medial longitudinal fasciculus to the nuclei of the third, fourth and sixth cranial nerves are supplied by branches of the superior cerebellar artery and median pontine arteries.

CLINICAL CORRELATION

Variations in distribution of the cerebellar arteries and extensive anastomosis between their branches make it difficult to always correlate clinical symptoms to specific sites of vascular involvement.

It should also be emphasized that a decreased pressure in the carotid system due to stenosis or obstruction may cause a reversal of blood flow in the posterior communicating arteries with consequent stealing from the vertebrobasilar system. This will cause a reduction of blood flow in the hindbrain and hence symptoms of vascular insufficiency. Similar findings may also be present in patients with cardiac disorders and decreased output. The higher resistance in the vertebral arteries in comparison to the carotid, causes a disproportionate decrease of blood supply to the hindbrain.

In our series of 200 patients with vertebrobasilar insufficiency, the most common finding was dizziness which was present in almost 90% of the cases. Visual disturbances were observed in 45%, ataxia in 33%, spontaneous nystagmus in 27% and sensorineural hearing loss in 22% of the cases. Other less common findings were generalized or localized paresthesia, limb-weakness, tinnitus, Horner's syndrome and palsy of one or more cranial nerves.

As far as the auditory system, it should be pointed out that unilateral occlusion of the anterior inferior cerebellar artery or of the branches supplying the cochlear nuclei will produce ipsilateral total nerve deafness and slight impairment of the hearing of the opposite side. Unilateral occlusion of the vessels supplying the other nuclei of the auditory pathway, which are located after the decussation, will produce contralateral, severe, but not total, nerve deafness and mild ipsilateral hearing impairment.

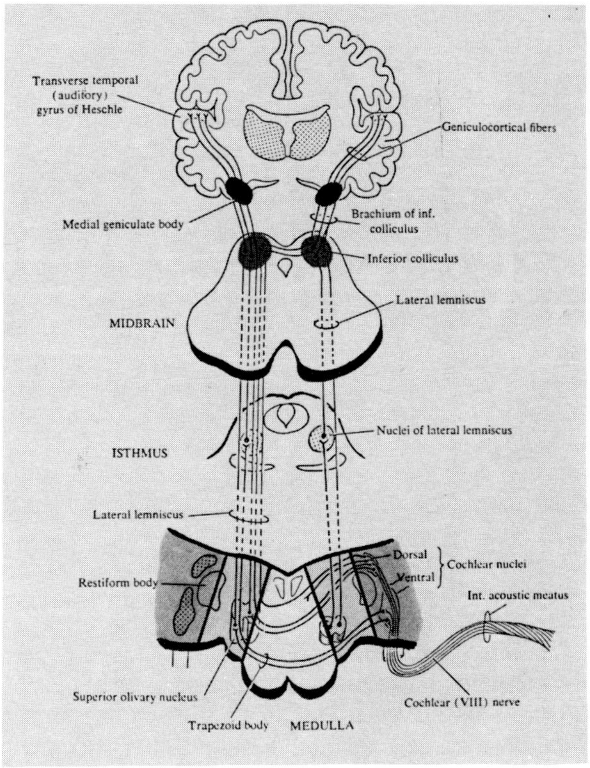

Fig. 2. Vascular supply of auditory pathway. Cochlear nuclei — Anterior inferior cerebellar artery; Superior olivary and trapezoid nuclei — Median and short circumferential branches of vertebral artery; Inferior colliculus — Superior cerebellar artery; Medial geniculate body — Posterior cerebral artery.

The vestibular system is by far more sensitive to vascular insufficiency than to auditory because of the extensive distribution and connections of its fibers in the brainstem and cerebellum.

Unilateral occlusion of the posterior inferior cerebellar artery will produce a classic Wallenberg's syndrome characterized by ipsilateral paralysis of the tongue, pharynx, larynx, ipsilateral loss of taste in the posterior third of the tongue, and loss of pain and sensation of feeling in the face, ipsilateral Horner's syndrome, asynergia and ataxia. Occlusion of the anterior inferior cerebellar artery or of its branches to the vestibular nuclei appears to cause partial ipsilateral vestibular paralysis. Incomplete or partial occlusion of the pontine arteries supplying the medial longitudinal fasciculus and of the superior cerebellar artery will cause findings which vary upon the site and extent of the injury.

IMAGING MODALITIES

Vertebral arteriography has been used in the past as the principal modality for the diagnosis of verte-

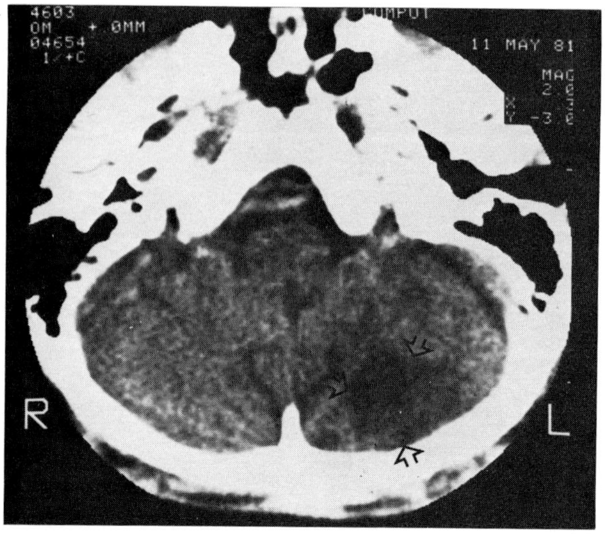

Fig. 3. Occlusion of left posterior inferior cerebellar artery with infarct. CT study reveals large area of decreased absorption in inferior aspect of cerebellum on left (arrows).

brobasilar insufficiency. There is, however, a justified reluctance to subject unselected patients to this invasive and risky procedure. More importantly, one should be aware that angiography may demonstrate signs of vascular pathology but not the presence of vascular insufficiency which is responsible for the patient's symptoms. Narrowing or obstruction of a vessel does not necessarily indicate cerebrovascular insufficiency since sufficient blood supply may be provided by collateral circulation. In addition arteriography does not demonstrate small vessels and parenchymal pathology.

Conventional CT studies performed before and after intravenous infusion of contrast material allow the study of the brain substance and the recognition of changes produced by vascular insufficiency such as infarcts, atrophy and encephalomalacia. The postinfusion examination may demonstrate the presence of luxury perfusion around the

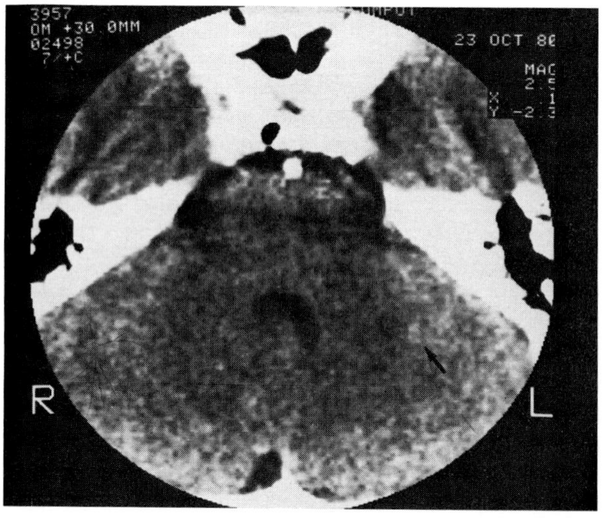

Fig. 4. Small infract (arrow) in left midcerebellum.

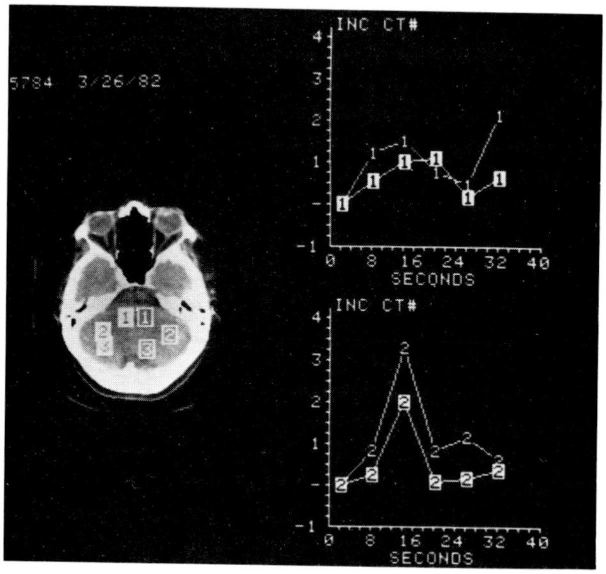

Fig. 5. Infratentorial dynamic study revealing focal area of abnormal circulation (peak time-22 s) in region of right vestibular nuclei (closed box 1). In other areas peak time is normal (16 s).

infarcted areas. The site of the brain damage can be correlated with a specific vascular territory and the size of the insult to the size of the involved vessel (Figs. 3 and 4).

A normal CT study does not, however, rule out the presence of vascular insufficiency which has not yet caused irreversible damage. This group of prestroke patients deserves particular attention because the early recognition of the territory of decreased blood flow, and if possible the surgical restoration of sufficient blood supply, can reverse the clinical course before permanent damage occurs.

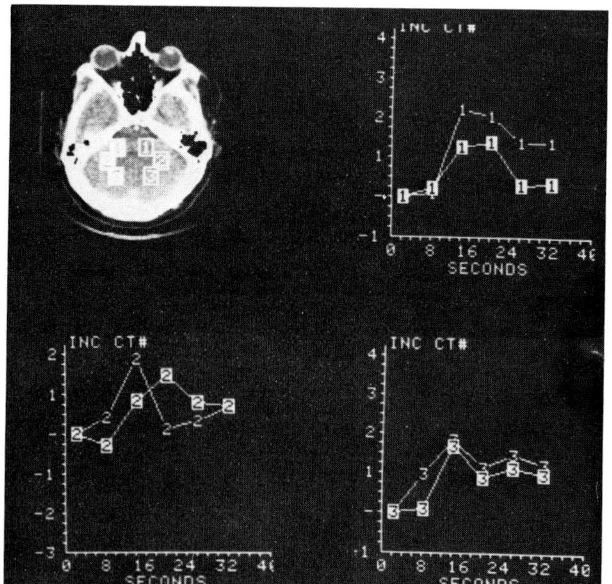

Fig. 6. Dynamic study demonstrating abnormal blood flow in right paraventricular region and midcerebellum (closed boxes 1 and 2). Conventional CT study was normal.

A new test is now available which allows the recognition of vascular insufficiency in the prestroke stage. The technique of dynamic CT has been described in previous reports.[2-6] Although this technique at present does not provide direct measurement of flow, the information obtained from CT dynamic images and CT numbers versus time curves provides several parameters which are directly related to blood flow and hence are a useful clinical index of brain circulation. Measurements are obtained in multiple areas of the hindbrain as small as 1 cc; therefore, specific territories of insufficient blood supply can be recognized (Figs. 5 and 6).

In our series of 200 patients referred with clinical diagnosis of vertebrobasilar insufficiency, we found that both conventional CT and dynamic studies were abnormal in 115 patients. In 49 patients or almost 25% of the cases, the conventional CT examination did not reveal parenchymal changes but the dynamic study demonstrated abnormal circulation patterns in the hindbrain.

Only after vertebrobasilar insufficiency is positively diagnosed by CT dynamic study should vertebral arteriography be performed in those selected cases where surgery is contemplated.[7] The arteriogram will demonstrate the site of vascular pathology and help the surgeon in planning the type of vascular bypass which could relieve the problem.

It should also be emphasized that the dynamic study should be repeated following surgery since this examination is the only available test which provides objective demonstration of any blood flow change in the ischemic areas.

A more precise and direct measurement of blood flow will hopefully be obtained in the near future by nuclear magnetic resonance (NMR). This technique allows the qualitative analysis of biologic structures or tissue samples. Proton determinations by NMR imaging can be used to evaluate pathological conditions related to water and blood content, distribution and movement.[8]

CONCLUSION

Since vestibular disturbances are usually the first sign of vertebrobasilar insufficiency, the otolaryngologist has a primary role and responsibility in the diagnosis and treatment of this common condition. He should become aware of the new sophisticated diagnostic tests now available for the recognition of hindbrain ischemia. In addition the unique expertise of the otolaryngologist in microsurgery provides him with the necessary knowledge and skill to extend into the field of microvascular surgery. It is a new challenge to your specialty, but a challenge which promises great rewards and the gratitude of a multitude of patients affected by this disabling, progressive, and often fatal condition.

REFERENCES

1. Pansky B, Allen DJ. Review of neuroscience. New York: Macmillan Publishing Co, 1980.

2. Valvassori GE, Dobben GD. Vertebrobasilar insufficiency. Ann Otol Rhinol Laryngol 1979; 88:689-92.

3. Dobben GD, Valvassori GE, Mafee MF, Berninger WH. Evaluation of brain circulation by rapid rotational computer tomography. Radiology 1979; 133:105-11.

4. Axel L. Cerebral blood flow determination by rapid-sequence computed tomography. Radiology 1980; 137:679-86.

5. Norman D, Axel L, Berninger WH, et al. Dynamic computed tomography of the brain: technique, data analysis and applications. Am J Neuroradiol 1981; 2:1-12.

6. Valvassori GE, Mafee MF, Dobben GD. Evaluation of the regional blood circulation of the hindbrain by dynamic computed tomography. Laryngoscope 1981; 92:1695-701.

7. Carney AL, Anderson EM. Diagnosis and treatment of brain ischemia. Adv Neurol 30:1981.

8. James AE, Price RR, Rollo FD, et al. Nuclear magnetic resonance imaging. JAMA 1982; 247:1331-4.

Ann Otol Rhinol Laryngol 91:1982

ANATOMIC SPECIFICITY OF CENTRAL VESTIBULAR SIGNS IN POSTERIOR FOSSA LESIONS

ARVIND KUMAR, MD, FRCS (ED)
MAHMOOD MAFEE, MD
NICHOLAS TOROK, MD
CHICAGO, ILLINOIS

The reliability of central vestibular signs such as decruitment in signifying retrolabyrinthine lesions has been well established. This study was initiated to determine if this and other central vestibular signs, individually or collectively, indicate involvement of specific anatomic structures in the posterior fossa. Forty-six patients with morphologic lesions defined by computerized tomography (CT), pneumo-CT or autopsy were studied. Oculomotor signs showed a statistically significant correlation with lesions of the archicerebellum. The other central vestibular signs did not show any correlations.

INTRODUCTION

When evaluating patients with complaints of disequilibrium and vertigo with or without hearing loss, our objectives are as follows:

1. To determine if there is an abnormality of the vestibular system responsible for the symptoms;
2. If so, to determine whether the lesion affects the labyrinth (peripheral lesion) or is central in origin (intracranial including the contents of the internal auditory canal);
3. If central, to determine the possible subtentorial location of the lesion; and finally,
4. To consider the pathologic nature of the abnormality.

A review of the patient's history of complaints is, in most instances, helpful in determining whether the vestibular system is affected or not. Differentiation of the site of the lesion, whether peripheral or central, can also be determined. This implies the application of a sensitive modality of recording eye movements and a neurotologic test protocol which is not exhausting for the patient and which provides accurate, reproducible and meaningful test results. Such a differentiation has been reported to be reliable and accurate[1-3] using the photoelectric principle[4] for oculography and a protocol of 1) calibration, 2) search for spontaneous nystagmus, 3) eye tracking, 4) optokinetic test, 5) Torok monothermal differential caloric test, 6) postural testing, 7) Wodak[5] past-pointing test, and 8) Romberg test. The predictive value of central vestibular signs in localizing subtentorial lesions, however, has not been studied in a substantive manner. The site of a lesion has been correlated with one or more central vestibular signs in several studies,[6,7] but the validity of the sign with a variety of lesions at the same location has not been confirmed.

With the availability of computerized axial tomography (CT) and CT dynamic flow studies (CT-rBBC), not only can very small lesions be identified but also their anatomic location can be accurately established. Because of this advantage, we assumed that the anatomic specificity of certain central vestibular signs could be substantiated. For example, a calibration overshoot[6] is believed to indicate a cerebellar lesion, while a downbeating spontaneous nystagmus is considered to indicate an involvement in the caudal brainstem. If central vestibular signs indicate a lesion in a specific area of the brain, then this will guide radiologists to investigate the corresponding area of the brain more intensively and help us understand basic pathophysiologic mechanisms of the vestibular system. This study was undertaken to investigate possible correlations between central vestibular signs and involvement of specific anatomic structures in the infratentorial region.

METHODS

In this study only those patients were selected in whom an identified morphologic lesion involving the subtentorial structures was detected either by a CT scan, pneumo-CT or autopsy. Forty-six patients were selected for this study. The extent of the lesion was determined at autopsy in only two patients. In the rest, the involvement and size of various neurologic abnormalities were obtained by CT scan or pneumo-CT. The latter contributed in the diagnosis of internal auditory canal lesions in six patients. Cuts (1.5 mm thick) for the CT scan were made in the axial plane, through the whole extent of the posterior fossa. In one patient coronal sections were also obtained. With a knowledge and understanding of the normal CT anatomy, the extent of a lesion could be mapped. Because the thickness of the sections was only 1.5 mm, the cephalocaudal dimension of a lesion could be mapped fairly accurately. Similarly the ventral-dorsal and lateral extensions of the lesion could be established. The neurologic structures involved by a particular lesion could thus be determined. Instead of including each subdivision of the cerebellum in the list of anatomic structures involved, the cerebellum was divided on an embryologic basis into the archicerebellum (vermis, flocculus,

From the Department of Otolaryngology-Head and Neck Surgery, College of Medicine, University of Illinois, and Illinois Eye and Ear Infirmary, Chicago.

Presented at the meeting of the American Otological Society, Inc., Palm Beach, Florida, May 2-3, 1982.

REPRINTS — Arvind Kumar, MD, Room B.45, 1855 W. Taylor St, Chicago, IL 60612.

nodule) and cerebellar hemispheres. The brainstem was divided into medulla, pons, and mesencephalon. The eighth nerve was categorized as a separate entity. The extent of each lesion was mapped on the basis of these six anatomic locations.

All 46 patients showed one or more central vestibular signs in their neurotologic examination. Table 1 summarizes the vestibular signs which indicate a posterior fossa lesion. Since oculographic calibration, sinusoidal eye tracking, and optokinetic responses all reflect oculomotor function, they were grouped as one. Spontaneous nystagmus, caloric abnormalities and postural signs are shown individually. In all, four signs and six anatomic locations were identified.

Data from 46 patients were classified according to absence (denoted by 0) or presence (denoted by 1) of four vestibular signs and corresponding lesions in six distinct anatomic locations. Our aim was to test associations between sign and location. The data were analyzed on an Amdahl V8 computer.

RESULTS

Grouping the central vestibular signs as described, their frequency of occurrence was as follows: spontaneous nystagmus, 36 times; caloric abnormalities, 26; oculomotor abnormalities, 15; and postural signs, 13. The frequency of involvement of the various anatomic sites was archicerebellum, 30; cerebellar hemispheres, 21; medulla, 18; pons, 21; nerve VIII, 17; and mesencephalon, 2. The varieties of pathologic lesions and their frequencies are shown in the figure. In the tumor category there were 10 acoustic neurinomas, 4 cerebellopontine angle meningiomas, 2 patients with von Hippel-Lindau disease, 2 astrocytomas, 1 hemangioblastoma, 1 glomus tumor, 1 metastatic tumor, and 1 lipoma.

Statistical evaluation indicated that individual neurotologic signs were not associated with any specific anatomic location of disease except oculomotor signs. These correlated with lesions in the archicerebellum. The chi square value was 4.57 for one degree of freedom. Combinations of pathologic signs could not be correlated with anatomic location.

TABLE 1. SUMMARY OF VESTIBULAR SIGNS INDICATING RETROLABYRINTHINE POSTERIOR FOSSA LESIONS

Test	*Central Vestibular Sign*
Calibration	Calibration overshoot or undershoot
Sinusoidal eye tracking	Saccadic eye tracking
Optokinetic responses	Optokinetic asymmetry Optokinetic fatigue
Spontaneous nystagmus and past-pointing	Horizontal unidirectional nystagmus with no drift Gaze nystagmus Vertical nystagmus Disconjugate nystagmus
Caloric responses	Vestibular decruitment Hyperactive responses
Postural study	Nystagmus unaccompanied by dizziness Nystagmus with dizziness, both persisting for as long as critical position is maintained and both being reproducible Vomiting unaccompanied by vertigo

DISCUSSION

In an effort to differentiate peripheral from central vestibular lesions, a variety of tests of vestibular and oculomotor function have been developed.[8,9] However, in routine clinical practice, the neurotologic test protocol usually consists of 1) tests of oculomotor function which include calibration, eye tracking, and horizontal optokinetic (OKN) stimulation; 2) search for spontaneous nystagmus (SN); 3) caloric stimulation; and 4) postural testing.

With respect to tests of oculomotor function there is general agreement about signs indicative of a central lesion (Table 1).

In 1954, Cogan[10] wrote that oculomotor dysmetria may be present when there is a consistent overshoot on changes of fixation from one target to another. It was his opinion that this sign occurs exclusively with diseases of the cerebellum or cerebellar pathways. In a retrospective study Haring and Simmons[6] found calibration overshoot in 40 patients. In 38 of these patients a neurologic lesion was confirmed involving the cerebellum. On the basis of their clinical observations in 38 patients with ocular dysmetria, Katsarkas and Younge[11] assumed that when this sign is found in association with certain other vestibular signs, a dysfunction of the flocculonodular lobe or its neural connections or both may be responsible. In the present study we had two patients in whom calibration overshoot was detected, and in both the archicerebellum was one of the anatomic locations involved. Conversely, the archicerebellum was involved by lesions in 30 patients, yet calibration overshoot was detected only in 2.

Saccadic eye tracking is a reliable sign of a posterior fossa lesion. This sign has been observed with both diffuse[12] and localized[13] lesions of the cerebellum. Abnormal ocular tracking patterns were reported by Benitez and Bouchard[13] in 9 of 10 patients

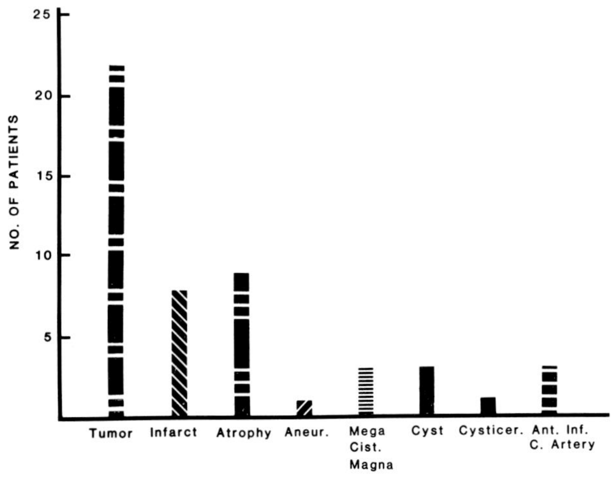

Pathologic findings in 46 patients with central neurotologic findings.

TABLE 2. DIAGNOSIS AND ANATOMIC LOCATION OF LESIONS ASSOCIATED WITH SACCADIC EYE TRACKING

Pt.	*Diagnosis*	*Anatomic Location of Lesion*
1	Cerebellar astrocytoma	Archicerebellum, medulla, pons
2	Cerebellar pseudotumor	Archicerebellum
3	Cerebellopontine angle meningioma	Archicerebellum, cerebellar hemisphere, pons, nerve VIII
4	Cerebellopontine angle meningioma	Archicerebellum, cerebellar hemisphere, pons, medulla, nerve VIII
5	Large acoustic neurinoma	Archicerebellum, cerebellar hemisphere, pons, medulla, nerve VIII
6	Acoustic neurinoma	Archicerebellum, cerebellar hemisphere, pons, nerve VIII
7	Large glomus tumor	Archicerebellum, cerebellar hemisphere, medulla, pons
8	Medullary, pontine and cerebellar atrophy	Archicerebellum, cerebellar hemisphere, medulla, pons
9	Cerebellar infarct and vermis atrophy	Archicerebellum, cerebellar hemisphere
10	Brainstem infarct	Archicerebellum, cerebellar hemisphere, medulla
11	Brainstem infarct	Medulla, pons

with cerebellopontine angle lesions. In the present series this sign was recorded in 11 patients, and 4 of them had large cerebellopontine angle lesions. With respect to diffuse cerebellar lesions resulting in saccadic eye tracking, the cerebellum as a whole was affected in 34 patients, yet saccadic eye tracking was recorded only 11 times (32%). The only structure in the posterior fossa not affected in all these patients showing saccadic eye tracking was the mesencephalon (Table 2).

The optokinetic test as an isolated abnormality in the neurotologic examination has no diagnostic importance. When it is found in association with other central signs it provides supportive evidence for a central lesion. In the present study eight patients demonstrated horizontal optokinetic asymmetry or fatigue. Four patients had large cerebellopontine angle lesions compressing the brainstem and cerebellum. Baloh et al[14] stated that when optokinetic responses are abnormal, the tumor is compressing the brainstem. In such a case, as previously stated, the abnormal optokinetic responses can serve as only supportive evidence. This was the finding in all four patients with neoplasms. In this series five other patients had large cerebellopontine angle tumors, but no optokinetic abnormalities were detected.

The localizing value of optokinetic asymmetry has been discussed. Coats[15] is of the opinion that when an optokinetic asymmetry is associated with gaze nystagmus the lesion is located in the pons or mesencephalon. Table 3 shows that the pons was one of the structures involved in one patient, but the mesencephalon was not affected in a single instance.

In our experience spontaneous nystagmus is considered of central origin when 1) horizontal nystagmus is recorded and the patient does not past-point; or 2) a gaze nystagmus is present, ie, the nystagmus beats in the direction of eye deviation (I° right and I° left); or 3) vertical upbeating or downbeating nystagmus or 4) disconjugate nystagmus is observed or recorded.

The literature dealing with SN resulting from chronic lesions in the posterior fossa is particularly conflicting. According to Hare et al[16] the representation of the eyes in the cerebellum exceeds that of any other anatomic structure. Lesions of the cerebellum could therefore be expected to result in nystagmus which is a form of disordered eye movement. Walsh and Hoyt[17] and Dow and Moruzzi[18] thought that SN in all cerebellar, spinocerebellar, and pontocerebellar atrophies is rare since the compensatory processes keep pace with the developing lesions. According to Bender,[19] patients with degenerative disease of the cerebellum per se rarely have nystagmus. He felt that when nystagmus is present, it is because of involvement of the brainstem or cerebellar peduncles. On the basis of clinical observations of circumscribed cerebellar lesions, Duke-Elder and Scott[20] believed that nystagmus can prob-

TABLE 3. DIAGNOSIS AND ANATOMIC LOCATION OF LESIONS ASSOCIATED WITH OPTOKINETIC ASYMMETRY

Patient	*Diagnosis*	*Spontaneous Nystagmus*	*Anatomic Location of Lesion*
1	Medullary pontine and cerebellar atrophy	Vertical downbeating nystagmus	Archicerebellum, cerebellar hemisphere, medulla, pons
2	Pseudotumor vermis	I°R and I°L	Archicerebellum
3	Cerebellopontine angle meningioma	Vertical upbeating nystagmus II°R I°R and I°L	Archicerebellum, cerebellar hemisphere, pons, medulla, nerve VIII
4	Von Hippel-Lindau disease	I°R and I°L	Archicerebellum
5	Cerebellopontine angle meningioma	None	Archicerebellum, cerebellar hemisphere, pons, nerve VIII
6	Cerebellopontine angle meningioma	None	Archicerebellum, cerebellar hemisphere, pons, nerve VIII
7	Infarct	II°L and I°L	Archicerebellum, medulla, pons
8	Acoustic neurinoma	II°R I°R I°L	Archicerebellum, medulla, pons, nerve VIII

TABLE 4. DIAGNOSIS AND ANATOMIC LOCATION OF LESIONS ASSOCIATED WITH VESTIBULAR DECRUITMENT

Pt.	*Diagnosis*	*Anatomic Location of Lesion*
1	Acoustic neurinoma	Nerve VIII
2	Acoustic neurinoma	Archicerebellum, cerebellar hemisphere, pons, nerve VIII
3	Acoustic neurinoma	Nerve VIII
4	Acoustic neurinoma	Archicerebellum, cerebellar hemisphere, nerve III, pons
5	Acoustic neurinoma	Archicerebellum, cerebellar hemisphere, nerve VIII, pons
6	Cerebellopontine angle meningioma	Archicerebellum, cerebellar hemisphere, pons, nerve VIII
7	Cerebellopontine angle meningioma	Archicerebellum, cerebellar hemisphere, medulla, pons, nerve VIII
8	Glomus tumor	Archicerebellum, cerebellar hemisphere, medulla, pons
9	Cerebellar metastatic tumor	Cerebellar hemisphere, medulla, pons
10	Dermoid cyst	Archicerebellum, medulla
11	Mega cisterna magna	Archicerebellum
12	Cerebellar atrophy and pontine infarct	Cerebellar hemisphere, pons
13	Cerebellar atrophy	Archicerebellum, cerebellar hemisphere
14	Cerebellar atrophy	Cerebellar hemisphere
15	Infarct brainstem	Pons, mesencephalon
16	Cerebellar and brainstem infarct	Archicerebellum, cerebellar hemisphere, medulla
17	Brainstem infarct	Medulla, pons
18	Lipoma of vermis	Archicerebellum
19	Medullary cyst	Medulla

ably be of direct cerebellar origin. Our findings agree with the view of Duke-Elder and Scott.[20] We had 12 patients with lesions affecting the cerebellum exclusively, and 9 of these showed spontaneous nystagmus. Table 4 shows that all patients except patient 1 had chronic lesions of the ceerebellum. However, in the case of patient 1, in addition to a cerebellar infarct there was evidence of marked cerebellar atrophy.

Similarly, brainstem lesions would be expected to result in SN. Six patients in our study had the lesions located exclusively in or adjacent to areas of the medulla, pons, or midbrain. Four patients showed SN.

Can SN (horizontal, gaze, vertical, or disconjugate) provide any clues as to specific areas of the brainstem or cerebellum affected by disease? Such correlations have been attempted both from results of animal experiments and clinically identified lesions. For example, downbeat nystagmus is believed to indicate damage to the caudal medulla. Of 27 cases of downbeat nystagmus reviewed by Cogan,[21] 8 proved to have abnormalities of the craniocervical junction, the most common being Arnold-Chiari malformation. Downbeat nystagmus has also been produced in monkeys by bilateral lesions in the median longitudinal fasciculus at the level of the brachium conjunctivum.[22] On the other hand, Gilman et al[23] in a clinicopathological study found that a primary position upbeat nystagmus can result from damage in the caudal brainstem. Thrush and Foster[24] felt that although nystagmus is a common finding in disorders of the brainstem and cerebellum, it has a poor localizing value and gives little indication of the underlying pathology. In this study we found three patients with vertical nystagmus. One showed a vertical upbeating nystagmus in addition to a horizontal nystagmus, and the lesion was a large cerebellopontine angle tumor. In the other two patients a strong downbeating nystagmus was the only SN recorded. In one patient an inferior cerebellar infarct was found on the CT scan, and in the second patient marked atrophy of the vermis and of the left cerebellar hemisphere was detected by CT scan. In four patients with lesions in the caudal brainstem-cerebellum area, no vertical nystagmus was detectable.

For the evaluation of vestibular function, the caloric test as described by Fitzgerald and Hallpike[25] has received the widest acceptance. Vestibular paresis and directional preponderance are the two abnormalities detectable with this technique of caloric stimulation. Umera and Cohen,[26] studying vestibular responses after creating lesions around the vestibular nuclear complex in monkeys, found vestibular paresis only when the lesions involved the nerve VIII root entry zone. According to Baloh and Honrubia[27] the lesion could be located anywhere from the end-organ to the nerve root entry zone when vestibular paresis is found. Directional preponderance, according to them, occurs with end-organ and nerve VIII lesions but also with lesions in the central nervous system from the brainstem to the cortex. The bithermal caloric test therefore does not contribute in differentiating end-organ from intracranial lesion. McCabe and Ryu,[28] testing normal subjects and experimental animals, concluded that directional preponderance is worthless in localizing vestibular disease. For these reasons we use the Torok monothermal differential caloric test, the diagnostic advantages of which have been described.[1] The two central vestibular signs obtained by this caloric test are vestibular decruitment and hyperactive responsiveness. The reliability of vestibular decruitment in detecting posterior fossa lesions has been reported as greater than 90%.[29] In the group of patients included in the present study, decruitment was detected 19 times. The anatomic locations of the lesions included all structures except the mesencephalon. In two patients (Table 4, patients 1 and 3) intracanalicular acoustic neurinomas were found.

TABLE 5. DIAGNOSIS AND ANATOMIC LOCATION OF LESION ASSOCIATED WITH POSTURAL TEST ABNORMALITIES

Pt.	*Diagnosis*	*Anatomic Location of Lesion*
1	Acoustic neurinoma	Nerve VIII
2	Acoustic neurinoma	Archicerebellum, cerebellar hemisphere, pons, nerve VIII
3	Cerebellopontine angle neurinoma	Archicerebellum, cerebellar hemisphere, pons, nerve VIII
4	Cerebellopontine angle neurinoma	Archicerebellum, cerebellar hemisphere, pons, nerve VIII
5	Cerebellopontine angle meningioma	Archicerebellum, cerebellar hemisphere, pons, nerve VIII
6	Cerebellar pseudotumor	Archicerebellum
7	Basilar artery aneurysm	Pons, mesencephalon
8	Mega cisterna magna	Archicerebellum
9	Mega cisterna magna	Archicerebellum
10	Dermoid cyst	Archicerebellum, medulla
11	Cysticercosis	Cerebellar hemisphere, medulla
12	Cerebellar and brainstem infarct	Archicerebellum, cerebellar hemisphere, medulla, pons
13	Cerebellar atrophy	Archicerebellum

Hyperactive caloric responses are indicative of defect of inhibition on the vestibulo-ocular reflex arc. Hyperactive caloric responses occurred in 8 patients in this study, and in 5 the lesion was located in the cerebellum. Of the 46 patients in this study 31 had lesions involving the cerebellum. Cerebellar lesions are also believed to be responsible for dysrhythmic postcaloric nystagmus.[30] This was not our observation in 31 patients who had confirmed cerebellar lesions.

The postural test is another reliable indicator of intracranial pathology. A central lesion is suspected when one of the signs listed under the postural test in Table 1 is detected. Thirteen patients showed such central postural signs. Table 5 summarizes the clinical diagnoses and the sites of the lesions in the posterior fossa in these cases. Again, no specific anatomic locations could be related to the central postural signs. Katsarkas[31] recently reported on 5 patients with positional nystagmus of the central type, and in 4 the lesions were located in the area of the fourth ventricle. He concluded that positional nystagmus of the central type is presumably due to pathology of the fourth ventricle. We had two patients with abnormalities around the fourth ventricle. In one patient the lesion was a dermoid cyst, and clear posturally-induced nystagmus was recorded without accompanying dizziness. In the other patient with hemangioblastoma no postural signs were present.

It is obvious that direct correlations between particular vestibular signs and specific neuroanatomic locations cannot be made with any certainty. It is clear from our study that while we may observe a particular central vestibular sign with a lesion in a specific area of the brain, it is also true that a lesion in the same area does not consistently create the same vestibular anomalies. The vestibular abnormality observed in a particular instance is probably due to more than just the neuroanatomic substrate involved.

This does not imply that attempts at making correlations should be abandoned. On the contrary, because clinical correlations can be made with much greater accuracy with the CT scan, we are encouraged to continue this study.

ACKNOWLEDGMENT — Glenn Krol assisted with the data collection and analysis. Edward Rackus and M. Patel helped with the statistical analysis.

REFERENCES

1. Kumar A. Diagnostic advantages of the Torok monothermal differential caloric test. Laryngoscope 1981; 91:1679-94.

2. Kumar A. Is spontaneous nystagmus a pathological sign? Laryngoscope 1982 (in press).

3. Kumar A, Torok N, Valvassori G. Central vestibular signs, posterior fossa pathology and computerized tomography-regional blood brain circulation. Ann Otol Rhinol Laryngol 1981; 90: 624-9.

4. Torok N, Guillemin V, Barnothy JM. Photoelectric nystagmography. Ann Otol Rhinol Laryngol 1951; 60:917-26.

5. Wodak R. Der Baranysche Zeigversuch. Berlin: Urban and Schwarzenberg, 1927.

6. Haring RD, Simmons FB. Cerebellar defects detectable by electronystagmography calibration. Arch Otolaryngol 1973; 98:14-7.

7. Tos M, Adser J, Rosborg J. Horizontal optokinetic nystagmus in cerebral diseases. Acta Neurol Scand 1972; 48:607-20.

8. Rubin W. The SHA test in vestibular diagnosis. Laryngoscope 1981; 91:1702-4.

9. Wennmo C. Eye movements in posterior fossa disorders. Doctoral dissertation, Lund University, Sweden, 1982.

10. Cogan DG. Ocular dysmetria, flutter-like oscillations of the eyes, and opsoclonus. Arch Ophthalmol 1945; 51: 318-35.

11. Katsarkas A, Younge BP. Electronystagmographic findings in cerebellar disease. J Otolaryngol 1976; 5:143-53.

12. Baloh RW, Konrad HR, Honrubia V. Vestibulo-ocular function in patients with cerebellar atrophy. Neurology 1975; 24:160-8.

13. Benitez JT, Bouchard KR. Electronystagmography: significant alterations in tumor of the cerebellopontine recess. Ann Otol Rhinol Laryngol 1974; 83:399-402.

14. Baloh RW, Konrad HR, Dirks D, Honrubia V. Cerebellar-pontine angle tumors: results of quantitative vestibulo-ocular testing. Arch Neurol 1976; 33:507-12.

15. Coats AC. Central electronystagmographic abnormalities. Arch Otolaryngol 1970; 92:43-53.

16. Hare WK, Magoun HW, Ranson SW. Localization within the cerebellum of reactions to faradic cerebellar stimulation. J Comp Neurol 1937; 67:145-82.

17. Walsh FB, Hoyt WF. Clinical neuro-ophthalmology. 3rd ed. Baltimore: Williams and Wilkins, 1969.

18. Dow RS, Moruzzi G. The physiology and pathology of the cerebellum. Minneapolis: University of Minnesota Press, 1958.

19. Bender MB. Disorders of eye movements. In: Vinken PV, Bruyn GW, eds. Handbook of clinical neurology. Vol. 1. Amsterdam: North Holland Publishing Co, 1969:574-630.

20. Duke-Elder S, Scott GI. Neuro-ophthalmology. In: Duke-Elder S, ed. System of opthalmology. Vol. 12. London: Kimpton, 1971.

21. Cogan DG. Down-beat nystagmus. Arch Ophthalmol 1968; 80:757-68.

22. Bender MB, Shanzer S. Oculomotor pathways defined by electric stimulation and lesions in the brainstem of monkeys. In: Bender MB, ed. The oculomotor system. New York: Paul B. Hoeber Inc, 1964:81-140.

23. Gilman N, Baloh RW, Tomiyasu U. Primary position upbeat nystagmus: a clinicopathologic study. Neurology 1977; 27: 294-8.

24. Thrush DC, Foster JB. An analysis of nystagmus in 100 consecutive patients with communicating syringiomyelia. J Neurol Sci 1973; 20:381-6.

25. Fitzgerald G, Hallpike CS. Studies in human vestibular function: 1. Observations on the directional preponderance ("Nystagmusbereitschaft") of the caloric nystagmus resulting from cerebral lesions. Brain 1942; 65:115-80.

26. Umera T, Cohen B. Effects of vestibular nuclei lesions on vestibulo-ocular reflexes and posture in monkeys. Acta Otolaryngol (Stockh) 1973; Suppl 315.

27. Baloh RW, Honrubia V. Clinical neurophysiology of the vestibular system. Philadelphia: F.A. Davis Company, 1979: 137-8.

28. McCabe B, Ryu J. Vestibular physiology in understanding the dizzy patient. Rochester, Minn.: American Academy of Otolaryngology, 1979:42.

29. Kumar A. Diagnostic reliability of vestibular decruitment. Presented at the XII World Congress of Oto-rhinolaryngology, Budapest, Hungary, June 1981.

30. Riesco-McClure J, Stroud M. Dysrhythmia in postcaloric nystagmus: its clinical significance. Laryngoscope 1960; 70: 697-721.

31. Katsarkas A. Vestibular and oculomotor disturbances in pathology of the fourth ventricle. Laryngoscope 1981; 91:71-7.

≈

STAPEDECTOMY — A LONG-TERM REPORT

JOHN J. SHEA, MD
MEMPHIS, TENNESSEE

The long-term results with large fenestra stapedectomy with vein graft and Teflon piston are compared with results with the small fenestra stapedectomy with Teflon piston directly into the vestibule. There were 1,943 operations in the former group and 2,155 in the latter when compared in 1970. One hundred consecutive patients from the beginning of each group with follow-up to present were compared. Results were generally the same with no great change in 15 and 20 years as compared to those at 5 years. The complication of perilymph fistula was caused by creating an opening in the footplate much larger than the prosthesis and was eliminated by interposing a living oval window seal if the opening was much larger than the prosthesis and a flap of lining membrane from the promontory when it was not. Other factors that influence a good result are discussed, including the type and the diameter of the piston used, the type of living oval window seal and the method of attachment to the incus. The small fenestra operation was found to be superior to the large, not only for the hearing gain achieved, but the ease of performance and the freedom from complications due to migration of the prosthesis and/or the oval window seal. At present we have done about all that can be done for the conductive components. What remains is the sensorineural component which our studies indicate may be due to an autoimmune response.

The question being debated now, a quarter century after the first successful stapedectomy, is not the wisdom of stapedectomy but the best way to reconstruct the sound-conducting mechanism of the middle ear. It is the purpose of this paper to re-examine the long-term results of large fenestra stapedectomy with vein graft and Teflon piston as compared to small fenestra stapedectomy with Teflon piston directly into the vestibule, and the other factors which influence a successful result.

In my 15-year report on stapedectomy to the American Academy of Otolaryngology in 1970,[1] I compared my results with these two groups of operations at that time. There were 1,943 operations in the large fenestra group and 2,155 operations in the small fenestra group. For the present analysis I went back and selected 100 consecutive operations from the beginning of each group with follow-up to the present.

In all of the large fenestra operations the same technique was followed meticulously. The stapedial tendon was cut, the arch of the stapes fractured away, the lining membrane of the middle ear elevated from around the circumference of the oval window, and the bleeding controlled. The footplate was fractured and as many of the fragments as would come away easily were removed. The oval window was covered with a compressed vein graft removed from the back of the patient's hand. A Teflon piston prosthesis 0.6 or 0.8 mm in diameter was then put into place on the vein graft projecting 0.25 mm below the inner rim of the oval window, and Gelfoam packed around to hold the prosthesis on the center of the vein graft (Fig. 1).

Results of the 1970 analysis are found in Figure 2. One hundred consecutive operations from this group operated upon in 1965 with follow-up to the present were selected so as to give a minimum of 15 years follow-up (Fig. 3).

It is interesting that 15 years after operation the percentage of closure of the air-bone gap and fur-

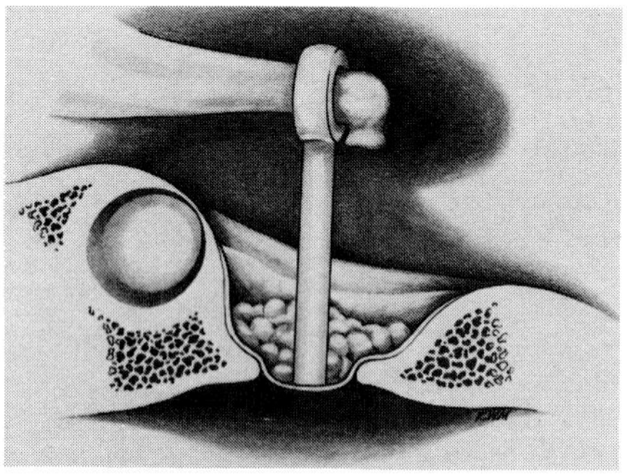

Fig. 1. Large fenestra stapedectomy with vein graft and Teflon piston prosthesis.

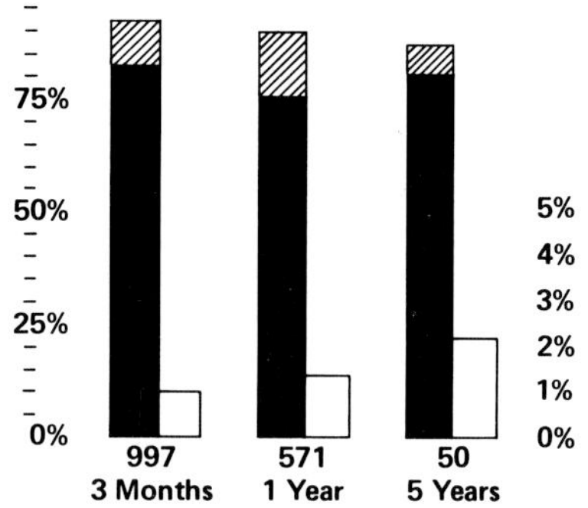

Fig. 2. Results of 1,943 large fenestra stapedectomies with vein graft and Teflon piston prosthesis. 1965-1970 analysis; no fistulas.

Presented at the meeting of the American Otological Society, Inc., Palm Beach, Florida, May 2-3, 1982.
REPRINTS — John J. Shea, MD, Shea Clinic, 1060 Madison Avenue, Memphis TN 38104.

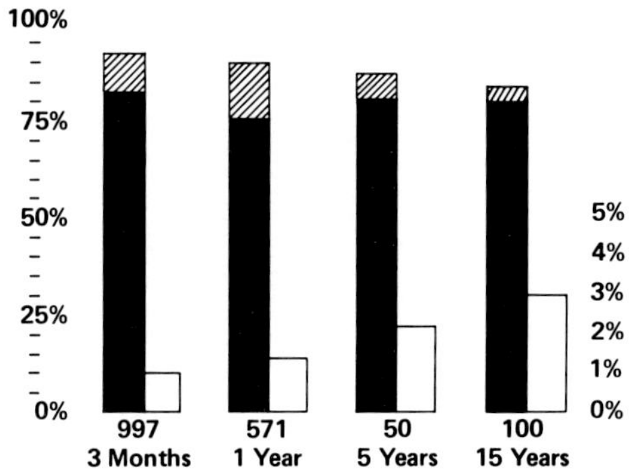

Fig. 3. Results of 1,943 large fenestra stapedectomies with vein graft and Teflon piston prosthesis. 1965-1982 analysis; no fistulas.

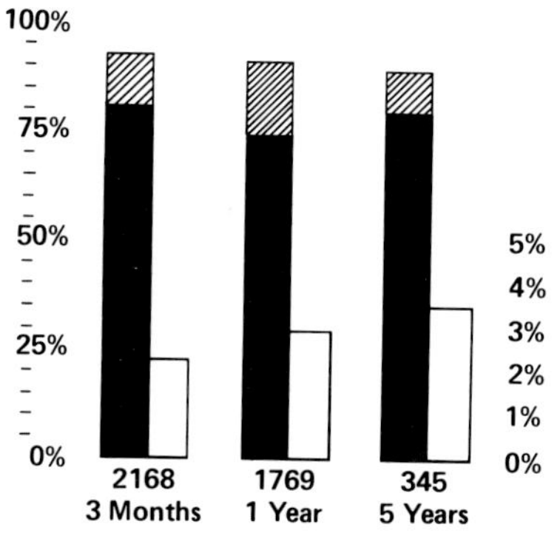

Fig. 5. Results of 2,155 small fenestra stapedectomies with Teflon piston directly into vestibule. 1960-1965 analysis; 2.4% fistulas.

ther cochlear loss had not changed much since the prior 5-year report. What this says is when the operation is successful after five years, it will usually remain successful for the rest of the patient's life.

In most of the small fenestra operations, the same technique was followed meticulously at first, but over time the technique was changed, which, unfortunately, caused the problem of perilymph fistula to develop.

The first such small fenestra operation was done in July 1960 on a young female with a congenital conductive hearing loss with a bifurcated facial nerve around the oval window (Fig. 4A). All I could do was remove the fragile arch of the stapes, which was not well attached to the footplate, drill a small opening in the footplate between the branches of the bifurcated facial nerve, and insert a 0.6 mm diameter Teflon piston prosthesis directly into the vestibule. Perivenous loose connective tissue was wrapped around the prosthesis as an oval window seal (Fig. 4B). The patient's hearing was improved at once, with eventual closure of the air-bone gap. With this good result it became apparent to me, for the first time, that total stapedectomy was not always necessary. I repeated this operation in this patient's other ear with the same good result the next year.

Because it was so successful and less traumatic and easier to perform, I gradually began to use this small fenestra operation on all patients with extensive otosclerosis, especially those with obliterative otosclerosis.[2] Results with this technique were very good, especially when compared to results with the large fenestra operation in ears with extensive and especially obliterative otosclerosis. Gradually, use of the technique was extended to those ears with less extensive otosclerosis. In some of these ears an opening much larger than the prosthesis was created, and in some as much as half the footplate was removed. Perivenous loose connective tissue and/or Gelfoam was always wrapped around the lower end of the Teflon piston to seal the oval window. Unfortunately, in some of these ears in which an opening much larger than the prosthesis was created perilymph fistula occurred, in 2.4% of the 2,155 operations in this group reported in 1970. Having discovered the problem and the cause, from 1970 onward a living oval window seal was always interposed unless the opening in the footplate was just larger than the prosthesis used. In 539 such operations since 1970 to date no more perilymph fistulas are known to have occurred. Even in these ears with an opening just larger than the prosthesis, whenever possible a flap of lining membrane from the promontory was elevated and turned over the fenestra to give a living oval window seal before the piston is inserted, penetrating no more than 0.25 mm below the inner rim of the oval window opening (Fig. 4C).

Results of the 1970 analysis are found in Figure 5. One hundred consecutive operations from this group with follow-up to the present were selected from those operated upon in 1960 so as to give a minimum of 20 years follow-up (Fig. 6). It is interesting that 20 years later the percentage of closure of the air-bone gap and further cochlear losses has not changed much since that prior analysis. Those patients who heard well at 1 year generally heard well at 10 and 20 years.

Fig. 4. A) Bifurcation of facial nerve around oval window. B) Small fenestra stapedectomy with Teflon piston directly into vestibule between bifurcated facial nerve. C) Small fenestra stapedectomy with Teflon piston prosthesis directly into vestibule, with flap of lining membrane from promontory over fenestra.

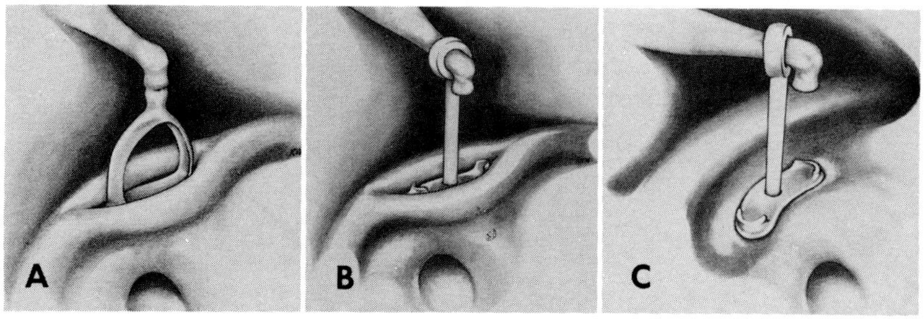

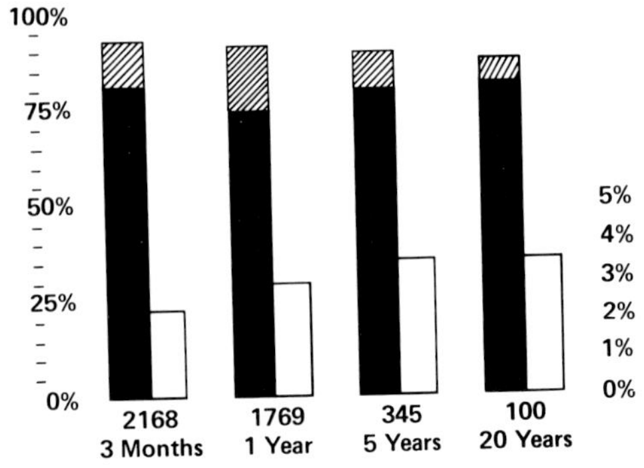

Fig. 6. Results of 2,155 small fenestra stapedectomies with Teflon piston directly into vestibule. 1960-1982 analysis; 2.4% fistulas.

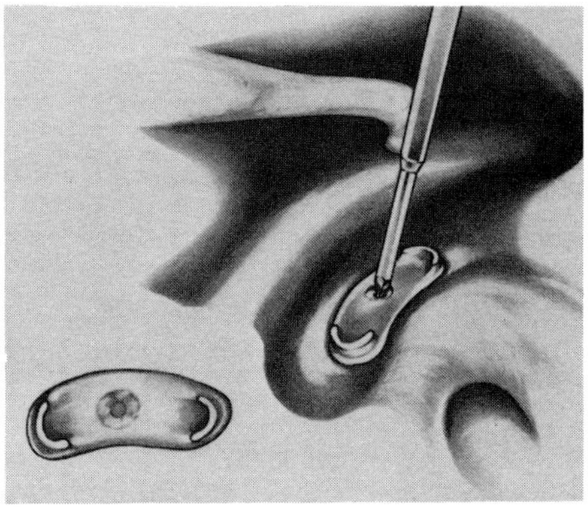

Fig. 8. Microdrill leaving cuff of footplate periosteum over oval window opening.

Our results indicate that if both operations are done properly, the hearing gain will be a little better, both at once and long-term, with the small fenestra operation than with the large. McGee came to the same conclusion comparing a small fenestra Teflon wire operation, very similar to this one, with a wire connective tissue-fat operation which is technically inferior to the vein graft and Teflon piston.[3]

If properly done the small fenestra operation is superior in several ways. It is certainly easier to do, especially with a drill which will create an opening in the footplate 0.65 mm in diameter that will just admit an 0.6 mm diameter piston (Fig. 7). The flap of lining membrane from the middle ear is easy to elevate. Sometimes the opening in the footplate can be created with this drill and a cuff of the footplate periosteum will remain over the opening to help seal the oval window (Fig. 8). The small fenestra operation is less traumatic to the inner ear because less of the lining membrane of the vestibule is disturbed and there is less chance of blood and the oval window seal to get into the perilymph.

I am not surprised that there was a fistula in the saccule in 3 of 8 cat ears in which a fenestra was created in the footplate with an argon laser in the experiment by Gantz et al.[4] It seems to me the argon laser is a difficult, potentially dangerous, and expensive way to create a fenestra in the footplate. Gardner et al (personal communication) have just concluded a similar experiment in our laboratory using a CO_2 laser to create a fenestra in the footplate of cats in which there was no injury to the saccule or other portions of the inner ear in seven ears. I am not in favor of using any type of laser at present to create an opening in the footplate, but of the two, the CO_2 laser is less expensive and, when used properly, would appear to be less potentially harmful to the inner ear.

If the opening is much larger than the piston and you must interpose a living oval window seal, it is best not to remove any more of the footplate than possible. That is, even in a large fenestra operation it is best to keep the opening as small as possible, but you must be sure to get the prosthesis into this small opening, projecting 0.25 mm below the inner rim of the oval window.

The complication of perilymph gusher, so disturbing in the early days of stapedectomy, can be managed by elevating the head to stop the leak, inserting a large living oval window seal and prosthesis, and keeping the head elevated for several days until the oval window seal heals into place. Most such patients will have large cochlear aqueducts as seen in polytome x-ray films.

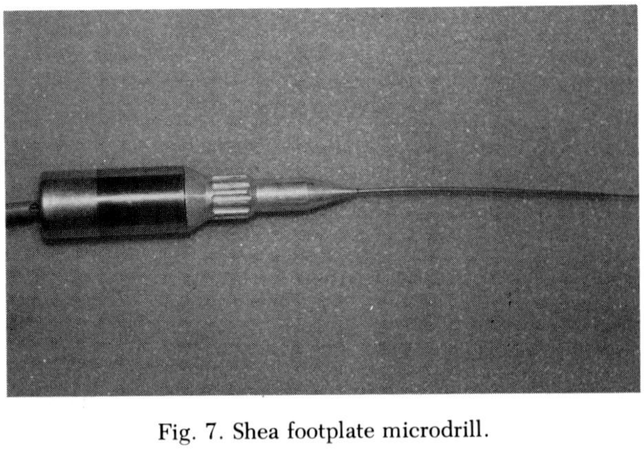

Fig. 7. Shea footplate microdrill.

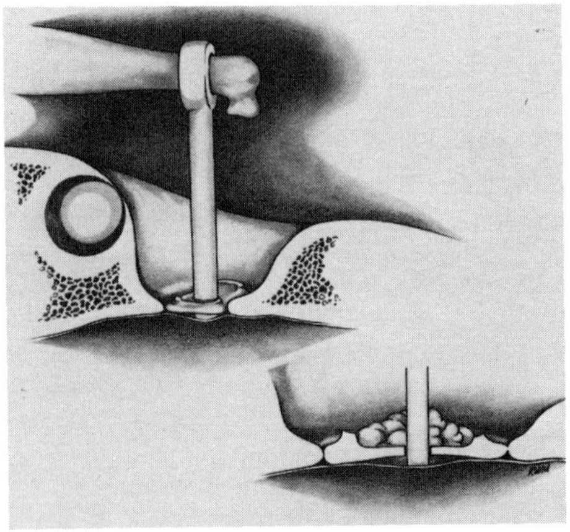

Fig. 9. Lining membrane of vestibule beneath piston driving fluid.

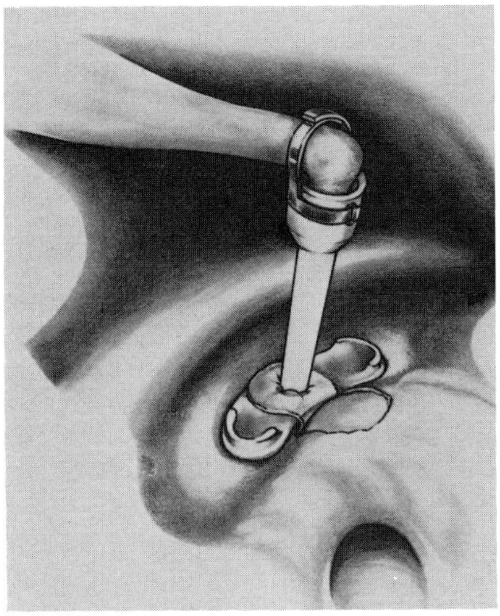

Fig. 10. Platinum Teflon cup prosthesis (0.6 mm) placed directly into vestibule with flap of lining membrane from promontory over fenestra.

From my analysis there was no statistical difference between the immediate or long-term hearing gain with a 0.6 or 0.8 mm diameter Teflon piston prosthesis, just as Schuknecht and Bentkover found,[5] which is not surprising, since, as Tonndorf (personal communication) has pointed out, the lining membrane of the vestibule heals beneath the piston in the vestibule to create a very efficient exponential cone-shaped membrane which moves the fluid (Fig. 9). My results with a small series of 0.3 mm diameter Teflon pistons were not good for low tones, closure and overclosure of the air-bone gap, so I stopped using this small diameter prosthesis. It is not usually possible to get an opening in the footplate to take a 1 mm diameter Teflon piston without getting into the oval window joint space, so the 1 mm diamter prosthesis is never used in the small fenestra operation.

The type of prosthesis used, and especially the

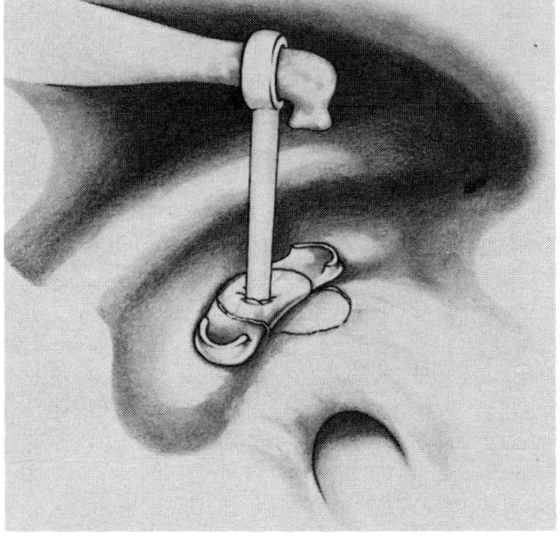

Fig. 11. Teflon piston on incus when lenticular process extends beyond oval window, with flap of lining membrane from promontory over fenestra.

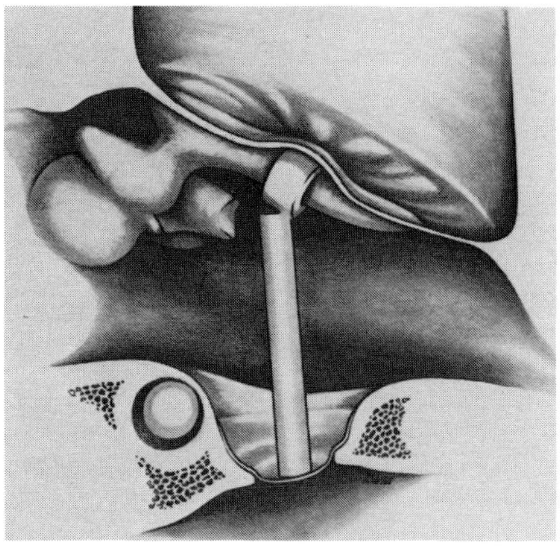

Fig. 12. Large-headed malleus Teflon piston in place.

method of attachment to the incus, are still very much in debate. My own experience from homograft cortical bone, to Teflon replica of the stapes, to pointed polyethylene tube, to Teflon piston to Teflon cup piston prosthesis with platinum loops has been one of gradual evaluation. At the present time, I use the 0.6 mm diameter platinum Teflon cup prosthesis with platinum loops (Fig. 10), except when the lenticular process extends beyond the center of the oval window and the 0.6 mm diameter Teflon piston on the lower incus will make a better fit into the oval window (Fig. 11).

When a large fenestra is created, a piston is less likely to become attached to the margins of the oval window than wire with a loop at its end. Attachment of a wire to the incus presents many immediate and long-term problems not present with a Teflon piston or cup piston prosthesis.

I prefer a Teflon cup piston to steel cup piston prosthesis, but I can see no great difference between the two.

If the incus is missing or defective, the long-headed malleus Teflon piston with a 30° angle between the loop at the end and the shaft of the prosthesis makes a good reconstruction of the sound-conducting mechanism of the middle ear (Fig. 12).

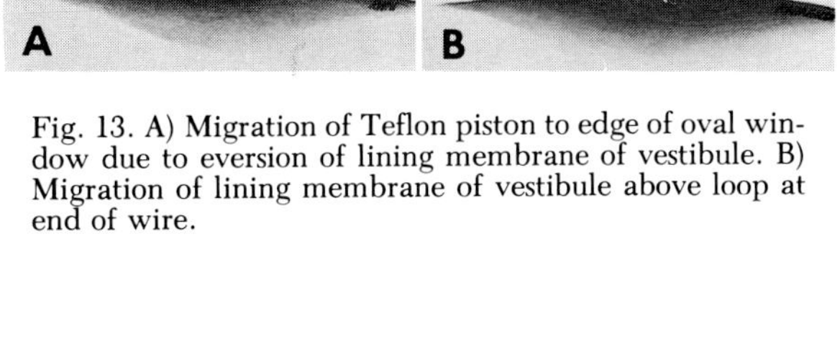

Fig. 13. A) Migration of Teflon piston to edge of oval window due to eversion of lining membrane of vestibule. B) Migration of lining membrane of vestibule above loop at end of wire.

The long debate about the value of Gelfoam as an oval window seal has just about ended with pretty general agreement that it should not be closed if a large opening is made in the footplate. While many ears will close with Gelfoam, enough will not, and granulomas, perilymph leaks, and other problems will occur, so that it should not be used.

The type of autogenous living oval window seal used is not as important as the prosthesis, since all of them thin down with time. My own preference for vein is due to the beautiful way it conforms to the oval window when compressed, which allows for a more accurate placement of the prosthesis.

The great long-term advantage of the small fenestra operation, besides its simplicity, is its stability, its freedom from delayed conductive hearing loss due to migration of the prosthesis and/or the oval window seal, from eversion of the lining membrane of the vestibule. The potential pressure gradient between the middle ear and perilymph is very great,[6] up to 950 mm water, and over time, in the large fenestra operation, can cause delayed conductive hearing loss due to migration of the prosthesis (Fig. 13A) and/or the lining membrane of the vestibule and incus necrosis (Fig. 13B), which just does not happen with the small fenestra operation.

We have come a long way from original attempts at mobilization of the stapes and stapedectomy by Kassel, Miot, Jack, and others, as resurrected by Rosen, and the multistage fenestration operation of Holmgren and Sourdille and others as perfected by Lempert, Shambaugh, House and others, to the small fenestra stapedectomy with Teflon piston of today. We have done about all that can be done for the conductive component. What remains is the sensorineural component, which continues, despite sodium fluoride, and is the challenge of the future. We have begun studies the preliminary results of which indicate that this sensorineural component is due to an autoimmune response, to the primitive cartilage in the fissula ante fenestrum and otic capsule in which the otosclerosis process begins. It may be that this research will lead to a method to prevent and/or treat this most distressing, and as yet, nearly untreatable sensorineural component of otosclerosis.

REFERENCES

1. Shea JJ Jr. A fifteen year report on fenestration of the oval window. Trans Am Acad Ophthalmol Otolaryngol 1971; 75: 31-47.

2. Shea JJ Jr. Teflon piston operation for otosclerosis. Arch Otolaryngol 1962; 76:516-21.

3. McGee TM. Comparison of small fenestra and total stapedectomy. Trans Am Otol Soc 1981; 69:633-9.

4. Gantz BJ, Jenkins HA, Kishimoto S, Fisch U. Argon laser stapedectomy. Ann Otol Rhinol Laryngol 1982; 91:25-6.

5. Schuknecht HF, Bentkover SH. Partial stapedectomy and piston prosthesis. In: Snow JB, ed. Controversy in otolaryngology. Philadelphia: WB Saunders Co, 1980:281-91.

6. Shea JJ Jr. Eversion of the lining membrane of the vestibule. Laryngoscope 1974; 84:1122-34.

WHAT CAN BE DONE FOR THE RECRUITING EAR?

MAURICE SCHIFF, MD
ROBERT E. SANDLIN, PHD
SAN DIEGO, CALIFORNIA

Probably one of the greatest problems in hearing aid fitting is to try to adapt hearing amplification to the recruiting ear. Sound is not loud enough, and then it is too loud. Microchips have permitted hearing aids to be smaller and smaller. However, they still remain either linear output- or input-compression types. Log-linear amplification permits the "smart aid" to automatically decrease the gain as the input power of speech or noise increases. This together with a patented low-frequency signal processor permits maximum discrimination with minimal violation of the patient's threshold of discomfort. This is a considerable step in ameliorating the major problem of the recruiting ear.

Probably one of the greatest problems in hearing aid fitting is to try to adapt hearing amplification to the recruiting ear. How often have we heard the patient narrate the sad lament, "What did you say?," and when the response is given back a little louder the patient's sharp reaction is "Don't shout, I can hear you!" These two phrases represent the discomfort and dilemma of the patient with the recruiting ear. At first it is not loud enough, and then with slight amplification it is suddenly too loud.

In recent years, hearing aids have been greatly improved. The electronics have been made smaller and more sophisticated, but the essential fundamental input/output gain relationship has not been changed. Several years ago a different approach was made electronically. This resulted in the application of log-linear amplification.[1-3] In brief, it can be stated that if the input increased, the gain would decrease logarithmically. And since the lag time was very short, the appreciation of the output would seem almost instantaneous. This type of aid is built so that an envelope made by the measurement of the threshold of discomfort (TD) and the threshold of detection is utilized. The aid's output is somewhere in the middle of this envelope and specifically is made never to violate the TD. At that level, the aid shuts itself down. Such a "smart" aid is almost totally self-regulating. This is not to be confused with output compression amplification.

Recruitment is a perplexing problem both for the physician and for the patient. This disproportionate growth in loudness, when compared to normal ear function, presents a most serious problem in the proper selection and fitting of hearing aid devices. In many instances, when the significantly recruiting ear is fitted with a hearing aid, sounds elevated only slightly above the most comfortable listening level (MCL) cannot be tolerated. Therefore, to avoid unpleasantness the patient will often turn down the acoustic gain of the hearing aid. By so doing, the overall efficiency of the amplification system is reduced.

It is true, unfortunately, that over the past several decades during which electronic hearing aid devices have been available to the acoustically impaired there has not been developed one single consensus on that amplification system best meeting the needs of the hearing-impaired patient.[4] Neither the otological, audiological, nor the hearing aid-dispensing community has presented a compelling hearing assessment procedure which, when applied to hearing losses, will provide unqualified parameters for hearing aid selection. In the medical community, for example, there is no consensus regarding candidacy for hearing aid amplification. There remains that vestige of the professional discipline which feels that patients presenting with confirmed sensorineural impairment are not candidates for hearing aid amplification, even in view of irrefutable evidence suggesting that the vast majority of patients who have a sensorineural deficit use hearing aids successfully.

Regardless of what the various philosophical approaches may be to resolving the acoustic needs of the hearing-impaired patients[5] who are not suitable subjects for medical or surgical intervention, there are problems which must be resolved if any hearing aid device is to be applied. In all instances of hearing loss, the patient has a reduced dynamic range (DR). DR may be best described as that range from the point of signal detection to the point of the TD level for a given acoustic stimulus. Diagrammatically, it may appear as shown in Figure 1. The solid line on the bottom portion of the chart suggests the normal threshold sensitivity for the best ears for frequencies from 125 to 8000 Hz. The dashed line shows the upper limits of normal threshold sensitivity. The solid line shown at the top suggests the TD for the frequency range indicated. The DR is quite broad and permits the processing of a host of inten-

From the Department of Otolaryngology-Head and Neck Surgery, University of California, San Diego.
Presented at the meeting of the American Otological Society, Inc., Palm Beach, Florida, May 2-3, 1982.
REPRINTS — Maurice Schiff, MD, 9834 Genesee Ave., Suite 128, La Jolla, CA 92037.

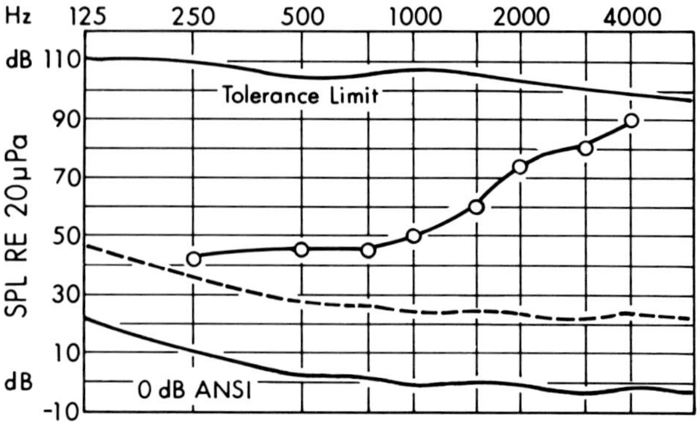

Fig. 1. Dynamics of hearing measurements. Threshold of normal hearing (bottom solid line); upper limit of threshold sensitivity (dashed line); normal tolerance limits (top solid line). Open circles — hearing loss showing reduced dynamic range.

sity/frequency inputs into the human auditory system.

The open circles on the graph indicate the elevation of threshold sensitivity for a hearing-impaired individual. It is apparent that there is a significant reduction in the DR and, therefore, a loss of information when the intensity/frequency input falls below the level of detection. There is always a loss of DR whether the loss is sensorineural, mixed, or conductive.

If one is aware that individual phonemes in the English phonologic system differ from one another as a function of their spectral distribution, some general statements can be made about problems of speech discrimination or the detection of information-bearing signals from nonspeech sources. One is aware, for example, that the identification of vowel and vowel-like sounds depends, for the most part, upon frequency content below 1500 Hz and that for much of the consonant discrimination frequency information above 1500 Hz is important. Further, it is well established that the energy present in the vowel components is significantly greater than is the acoustic energy for many of the consonant sounds.

Using the information suggested in Figure 1, one can predict that the vowel components can be detected with much greater facility than the consonant sounds when the DR is reduced, thus resulting in decreased discrimination. In short, the patient says, "I can hear what you are saying, but I can't understand it all."

From the standpoint of selecting the appropriate hearing aid with this in mind, the task is one of improving threshold sensitivity without violating the individual's tolerance threshold. Any hearing aid can improve threshold sensitivity and thus increase the probability of improved speech discrimination. However, if the task is that of reinstating normal threshold sensitivity as closely as possible then caution must be exercised in appropriate hearing aid selection practices. Again, the task remains that of

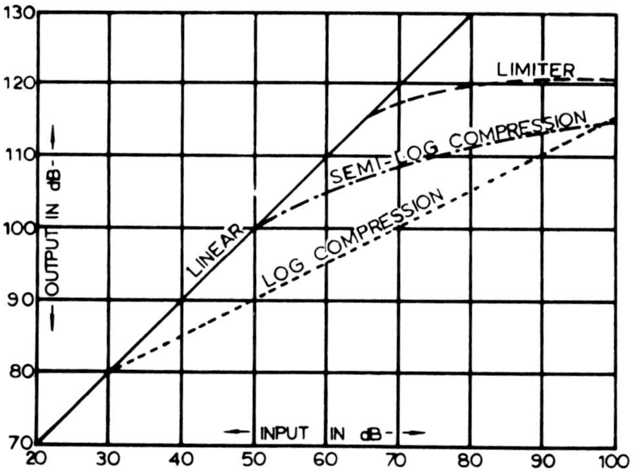

Fig. 2. Input-output functions of linear amplifier (solid line); output-compression amplifiers (dashed line labeled "limiter"); input-compression amplifiers ("semi-log" and "log" compression). Log-linear amplifier is linear to its knee and then becomes logarithmic.

improving threshold sensitivity without violating loudness tolerance. Parenthetically, it is the authors' view that in all cases of sensorineural impairment recruitment is present and serves to underscore the necessity of selecting hearing aid devices which will not compromise the TD.

The degree to which one succeeds in achieving this ideal goal of recapturing a normal DR depends, in large measure, upon the amplifier design of the hearing aid system selected by the individual physician or by the person to whom the patient is referred. To bring into a somewhat sharper focus the benefits accruing from increased threshold sensitivity, one should consider the following: assume that a patient wearing a hearing aid can just detect the presence of speech sounds when the talker is standing at 3 m (10 ft). Now, if the aided threshold could be improved by 6 dB that same talker could be heard at 6 m (20 ft). Suppose, then, one were able to improve threshold sensitivity for speech by 20 dB. The listener would then be able to detect speech at 30 m (100 ft). Therefore, when one considers the frequency/intensity distribution in the English sound system what may appear as a minor gain in threshold sensitivity may be a significant one for sound and speech intelligibility.[6]

In current use there are three basic types of amplifiers: linear, output-compression, and log-linear. Each amplifier has unique properties and treats the input/output function in a different manner. Figure 2 suggests the input/output functions of these amplifiers.

The linear amplifier has a 1:1 relationship between the input and output pressure of the hearing aid. For example, if there is a 10-dB increase in the input signal to the hearing aid there will be a 10-dB increase in the output signal. This linear relation will maintain until the maximum power output (MPO) of the hearing aid device is reached.

TABLE 1. INPUT-OUTPUT FUNCTIONS OF HEARING AID LINEAR AMPLIFIER

Assume 65 dB loss at 1000 Hz and threshold of discomfort at 115 dB MCL at 1000 Hz is 85 dB

	Input (dB)	Gain (dB)	Output (dB)
therefore —			
	65	20	85
	75	20	95
	85	20	105
	95	20	115
however —			
	55	20	75
	45	20	65

Signals less than 45 dB are not detected in aided mode.

In an output-compression amplifier the input/output function is linear up to a certain point, and then this relationship becomes nonlinear depending upon where the compression knee of the system is set. For example, all inputs into the hearing aid up to 70 dB will have a linear function. For each 10-dB increase in the input there will be a 10-dB increase in the output of the device. Above the 70-dB input level a 10-dB increase in signal strength may produce only a 6- or 7-dB increase in the output signal depending upon the specific design of the output-compression system. For rather high inputs the increase for each 10-dB input may be as little as 3 dB.

Input compression amplification is uniquely separate from other amplification systems in that all signal processing is accomplished before the volume control and the output amplifier. The slopes of the input/output function which are possible are limiting, semi-log, or log. The volume control will affect not only the gain of the hearing aid but also the final power output of the amplification system. In a log-linear aid, representative of input-compression devices, the input/output function is set at a fixed level, or ratio. That is, the log-linear design may be that which permits only a 5-dB increase in the output signal for each 10-dB increase in the input. The point at which the log-linear system is activated usually occurs at low input levels, perhaps around 35 dB sound pressure level (SPL) with the 0.5 ratio attaining at all inputs above this. The task is to examine each of the amplifiers and determine the efficiency with which each functions in a given DR.

It is the contention of the authors that one should strive to approximate the normal DR if instrument technology is available to do so. It is realized, of course, that some patients may reject hearing aids which provide normal approximation of threshold sensitivity for a number of reasons. To emphasize the practical advantages of one amplifier over another, let us assume the behavioral data indicated in Table 1 was obtained from a hearing-impaired patient using a complex speech input.

If one examines the function of a linear amplifier whose input/output is linear to the point of output saturation, one would observe something approximating the following: in order for a 65-dB speech input (normal conversation intensity) to achieve an 85-dB output pressure, an acoustic gain of 20 dB would be required. This acoustic gain is fixed and will be reflected in any change of the input signal. Therefore, a 65-dB input yields an 85-dB output pressure which approximates the listener's MCL. Increases of 10 dB in input continue to yield 10-dB increases in output until at 95 dB input the MPO of the amplification system is reached. However, as one reduces the intensity of the incoming signal, it is apparent that inputs less than 45 dB would not be detected as the outputs fall below the person's threshold of 65 dB.

TABLE 2. INPUT-OUTPUT FUNCTIONS OF COMPRESSION-OUTPUT LIMITING HEARING AID

Assume 65 dB loss at 1000 Hz and threshold of discomfort at 115 dB. Compression activated at 70 dB input MCL at 1000 Hz is 85 dB

	Input (dB)	Gain (dB)	Output (dB)
therefore —			
	65	20	85
	75	15	90
	85	9	94
	95	4	99
	105	3	102
	115	2	104
however —			
	55	20	75
	45	20	65

Signals less than 45 dB are not detected in aided mode.

Therefore, there would be a loss of information resulting in inappropriate processing of the intended message. In some instances, depending upon the input level, the patient may hear the vowel and vowel-like components but not the consonant sounds. Although an extremely useful amplification system, the linear amplifier cannot provide an approximation of normal threshold sensitivity in most hearing loss configurations.

When one examines the amplifier function of an output-compression amplifier as suggested in Table 2 and applies the same behavioral data as described for a linear amplifier, the following will obtain: assume that the compression system is activated for input signals 70 dB SPL or greater. A 65-dB input yields an 85-dB output pressure which is at the listener's MCL. Higher level inputs to the hearing aid are permitted without producing output pressures which violate the threshold of discomfort. This represents a significant advance in hearing aid function and has been a most useful advance for the acoustically-impaired hearing aid user. However, in that the compression function is activated only at input signals 70 dB or greater, input signals less than 70 dB produce a linear input/output function. Again, referring to Table 2, notice that acoustic signals into the system less than 45 dB will not be detected by the user of an output-compression device because the input/output

TABLE 3. INPUT-OUTPUT FUNCTIONS OF LOG-LINEAR INPUT-COMPRESSION HEARING AID

Assume 65 dB loss at 1000 Hz and threshold of discomfort at 115 dB. Compression activated at 35 dB.

	Input (dB)	*Gain (dB)*	*Output (dB)*
therefore —			
	30	3	65
	35	35	70
	45	30	75
	55	25	80
	65	20	85
	75	15	90
	85	10	95
	95	5	100
	105	0	105
	115	−5	110

Signal intensity ranging from 30 to 115 dB can be detected and/or tolerated.

function below 70 dB is identical in performance to the conventional linear amplifier. In essence, the output-compression device extends the acceptable range for the more intense signals but does not provide greater threshold sensitivity when compared to a hearing aid with linear amplification.

The reasonable question may be whether or not an amplification system is available which permits a wide range of input levels to enter the system and approximate normal threshold sensitivity without compromising the loudness discomfort of the patient. The answer is expressed in log-linear amplification. Using the same data suggested for linear and output-compression amplifier systems, a log-linear hearing aid having a 0.5 ratio for input/output function and the compression knee activated at 35 dB would provide the performance data given in Table 3. The gain of the aid is set to provide a 35-dB gain for input signals less than 35 dB SPL.

Immediately obvious is the broad range of signal intensities which can be processed by the user of the log-linear system. One will note that a 25-dB signal will be detected by the patient and that a signal of 115 dB can be easily tolerated. With the application of a log-linear hearing aid the aided DR is increased appreciably which enhances the hearing aid user's ability to process acoustic information presented to the auditory system. This results in improved control at high intensities and increased discrimination at high and low intensities.

Advances in amplifier design reflected in the log-linear amplifier are obviously advantageous to the hearing-impaired population, but there were some negative aspects of a log-linear device which present significant problems in the discrimination of speech in a noise background. The major disadvantage was the creation of foreground/background distortion.

In linear hearing aids all sounds amplified by the instrument maintain a constant foreground/background relationship until the output saturation of the hearing aid is reached. For example, when a speech signal (foreground) is at 65 dB SPL and the ambient noise (background) is 45 dB, this 20-dB difference in signal intensity is maintained when amplified by a linear system. The hearing-impaired person is not compromised relative to foreground/background separation.

However, in a log-linear system, and to some extent in other compression devices, foreground/background alteration can be considerable in that the compression function of the amplifier is intensity-specific. That is, all acoustic energies impinging upon the microphone of the amplification system alter the foreground/background separation depending upon the point at which the compression function is activated. This is especially apparent for a log-linear device which, in this instance, has its compression knee set at 35 dB SPL. Simply stated, input signals greater than 35 dB will activate the compression function and alter the foreground/background separation.

In rather high ambient noise environments such as restaurants, cocktail parties, sporting events, etc, the ability to discriminate speech is ordinarily a rather difficult task for the user of the log-linear device. Complaints of individuals in high ambient situations are often that they cannot understand the person seated across from them even though they can hear other noises or conversations generated at some distance. The reason is that the level of the ambient noise activates the compression function of the log-linear hearing aid thus creating a foreground/background distortion.

The limitation of this type of aid is that the initial adaptation takes much more time since the patient is now hearing all the sounds in the environment simultaneously. To an ear that has been unaccustomed to hearing for five to 20 years to suddenly hear the entire world with all its mixed signals can be a very serious rehabilitation problem.

Various attempts have been made to reduce problems associated with modifying the foreground/background separation. Of the several efforts made to resolve this problem those of Goldberg[1-3] have resulted in a log-linear hearing aid which incorporates an automatic low-frequency signal-processing function (Computer Hearing Aid, Dyn-Aura Engineering Laboratories, San Diego, Calif.). This particular application will suppress the low-frequency output of the hearing aid as a function of the frequency/intensity changes at the input to the log-linear system. In general, as the noise level in any given environment increases, the instrument automatically reduces the low-frequency output depending upon the overall intensity of the noise and its frequency distribution. The greater the noise level the more attenuation of the lower frequency range this instrument provides. In quiet there is no attenuation of the lower frequencies. This functional concept was derived in part from the equal loudness function of the human ear as well as the physiologic behavior of the tympanic membrane relative to its compliance as a function of the signal intensity impinging upon it.

It is assumed, generally, that the primary function of a hearing aid device is that of improving discrimination of acoustic events for the hearing-impaired individual. Such discrimination skills are improved if the aided DR of the user of the device is extended. The amplification system suggested by Goldberg[1-3] provides a means by which a greater DR can be accomplished. Others have made significant contributions to advances in hearing aid technology. Certainly, with the advent of sophisticated signal-processing devices capable of specific control of the input/output function of acoustic events, the probability for a more useful hearing aid is high. One's ability to control these input/output functions makes it possible to develop a "smart hearing aid" which will provide information at a restricted DR which heretofore has not been possible. Goldberg[1-3] has proposed that a log-linear hearing aid system with appropriate circuitry for specialized functions can, indeed, provide some of those desired features by incorporating existing technology into instrument design. His existing prototype device can exercise limited control over the low-frequency range. This absolute control of specific amplification functions should ultimately permit the physician and others to prescribe the acoustic performance of the hearing aid based upon the special acoustic needs of the acoustically-deficient person. It is in this area that the patient with recruitment problems is best helped.

CONCLUSION

The purpose of this paper has been to suggest that random, or unreasoned, selection of hearing aids does not result in the most efficient amplification system for the patient, especially the recruiting patient. It is to be repeated that all hearing-impaired patients present with a reduced DR. As such, informed attention should be given to the most effective amplification system which ameliorates the problem to the greatest extent possible.

Almost all patients having nontreatable hearing loss can benefit from appropriate hearing aid amplification. Obviously, all will not benefit equally in view of the several and diverse pathological conditions giving rise to hearing disorders.

It is not suggested that improving hearing sensitivity is commensurate with normal discrimination ability. Obviously, such is not true. Conversely, however, the potential for greater discrimination must lie with an appropriate amplification system when other avenues of intervention have not proven beneficial to the patient.

SUMMARY

1. The threshold of discomfort, or the uncomfortable loudness level, should not be violated.
2. All hearing aids strive to control the output.
3. Control of the input/output relationship permits a maximum control of the acoustical environment.
4. Suppression of the ambient noise level with a favorable signal-to-noise ratio improves the discrimination and intelligibility of sound and speech despite the ambient noise intrusion.
5. With particular reference to the patient with a recruitment problem it would appear that a log-linear device with an automatic low-frequency signal-processing circuit can best accomplish this in the present state of the art.

REFERENCES

1. Goldberg H. Electro-acoustic amplification, technical report. Dyn-Aura Engineering Laboratories, 1976.

2. Goldberg H. Hearing aid amplification, technical report. Dyn-Aura Engineering Laboratories, 1977.

3. Goldberg H. Hearing aid signal processes and their application to the hearing impaired. Hearing Aid J 1982; 35:23-8.

4. Byrne D, Tonisson W. Selecting the gain of hearing aids for persons with sensorineural hearing impairment. Scand Audiol 1976; 5:51-9.

5. Studebaker GR. Fifty years of hearing aid research: An evaluation of progress. Ear and Hearing 1980; 1:57-62.

6. Radio engineers. Electro-acoustics 37-21. New York: Howard W. Sams and Co, 1975.

Ann Otol Rhinol Laryngol 91:1982

EFFECT OF MASTOID CAVITY MODIFICATION ON MIDDLE EAR SOUND TRANSMISSION

JOHN T. MCELVEEN, MD
CHRIS MILLER, MS
RICHARD L. GOODE, MD
STEPHEN A. FALK, MD
PALO ALTO, CALIFORNIA

The modified radical mastoidectomy and intact canal wall mastoidectomy are the two most popular procedures used today for the treatment of chronic middle ear and mastoid disease. Their effects on the anatomy of the middle ear and mastoid cavity are quite different and it might also be expected that they would modify middle ear sound transmission in different ways. This paper describes experiments with human temporal bones and a middle ear computer analog model that attempt to define acoustic differences produced by cavity modifications in these two procedures. The temporal bone studies showed that blocking the aditus (as in modified radical mastoidectomy) produced improved sound transmission in the 1,500- to 4,000-Hz range and decreased transmission below 1,000 Hz when compared to the enlarged aditus and enlarged mastoid condition (as in intact canal wall mastoidectomy). The computer model showed better transmission at all frequencies with the intact canal wall mastoidectomy simulation.

INTRODUCTION

Despite widespread appreciation of the mechanics involved in middle ear sound transmission, the role of middle ear and mastoid cavity resonances is often overlooked by otologists and possibly underutilized in the design of otologic procedures. Tympanomastoid surgery modifies the middle ear cavities in various ways. These modifications may have important effects on middle ear sound transmission and, ultimately, the postsurgical hearing threshold. The acoustical effects of cavity modification produced by different types of tympanomastoidectomy are difficult to determine clinically by comparing preoperative and postoperative hearing thresholds because tympanic membrane (TM) and ossicular reconstruction often are performed as well. The combination of procedures obscures the significance of the cavity modifications in final hearing results.

Two of the most commonly performed mastoidectomy procedures — the modified radical mastoidectomy and the intact canal wall mastoidectomy — produce markedly different anatomic changes in the middle ear and mastoid cavities. The former operation closes off the aditus ad antrum, disconnecting the mastoid cavity from the middle ear, while the latter widely opens the aditus and enlarges the mastoid cavity. The acoustical effect of these two types of cavity changes would be expected to be quite different, all else being equal.

This paper discusses experiments using fresh human temporal bones and a middle ear analog circuit that attempt to define the effect on middle ear sound transmission of anatomical changes in the ear cavities similar to those produced by modified radical mastoidectomy and intact canal wall mastoidectomy.

BACKGROUND

Studies on human temporal bones[1,2] and in live subjects[3,4] have shown that ossicular vibration in response to a constant sound pressure level (SPL) begins to roll off above 2,000 Hz. Holographic measurements of the human TM[2,3] reveal this to be secondary to a breaking up of the TM into smaller, inefficient vibrating sections at higher frequencies. This roll-off in high-frequency efficiency of the middle ear is not always a gradually sloping curve; often there is a notch between 3,000 and 4,000 Hz with a great deal of individual variation above 1,500 Hz. This is shown in (Fig. 1) where umbo displacement in three fresh human temporal bones is measured with a constant SPL of 120 dB at the TM.

A similar middle ear transmission curve exists in the cat except that the roll-off begins at a higher frequency and the notch is present at around 4,500 Hz.[5,6] The notch is deep, averaging about 12 dB.

Modification of the ear cavities in the cat has significant effects on middle ear function. Experiments by Lynch[7] using admittance measurements at the TM have shown that blocking the foramen between the bulla and middle ear cavity eliminates the 4,500-Hz notch and decreases TM admittance by about 3 dB below 2,000 Hz. Removing the septum between the middle ear and bulla and opening the combined cavity to the outside also eliminates the 4,500-Hz notch and improves TM admittance below 2,000 Hz by 3 dB. Tympanic membrane admittance measurements correlate well with umbo

From the Division of Otolaryngology/Head and Neck Surgery, Stanford University Medical Center, and Palo Alto Veterans Hospital, California.
Presented at the meeting of the American Otological Society, Inc., Palm Beach, Florida, May 2-3, 1982.
REPRINTS — Richard L. Goode, MD, Division of Otolaryngology, Stanford Medical Center, 300 Pasteur Drive, Palo Alto, CA 94305.

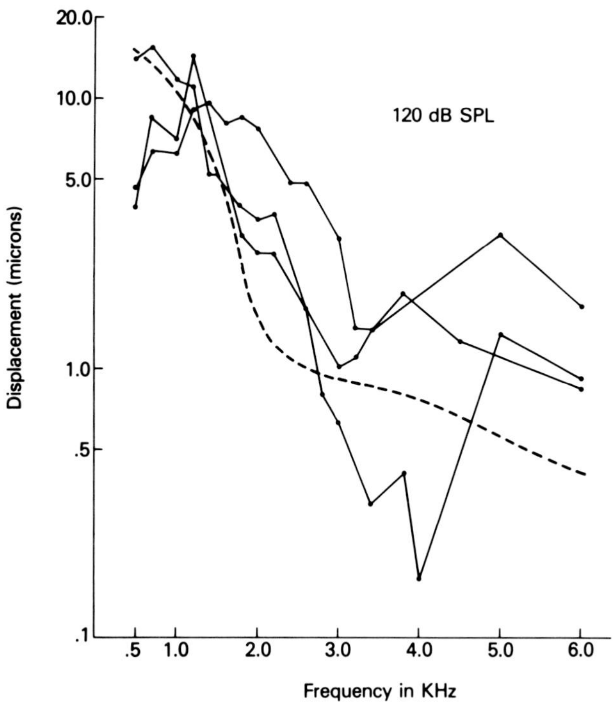

Fig. 1. Peak-to-peak umbo displacement measurements in three human temporal bones for constant sound pressure level of 120 dB at TM. Measurements were made at 200-Hz intervals for frequency range 500 to 6,000 Hz. Dotted line represents umbo displacement curve produced by Zwislocki middle ear analog. Reference point for this curve was arbitrarily set at 15 μm for 500 Hz.

velocity produced by a constant SPL at the TM and in the cat can be considered as an indirect measurement of sound transmission across the middle ear.[8]

The cat ear cavities appear to act acoustically as an impedance in series with the TM and ossicles. At low frequencies the impedance of the cavities is equivalent to the volume of the two cavities. At higher frequencies, the foramen acoustically closes and the impedance is that of the middle ear cavity alone. The notch at 4,500 Hz is thought to be due to the resonance of the cavities' compliance and inertance of the foramen. Blocking or widely opening the foramen would therefore be expected to eliminate the notch — the major acoustical effect of these anatomical manipulations. Blocking the foramen also eliminates the compliance of the larger bulla cavity thus stiffening the TM and decreasing low-frequency transmission, while enlarging the foramen and opening the bulla to the outside increases the cavity compliance, decreases TM stiffness and improves the low-frequency response.

Very little information is available on the effect of cavity modification in the human as compared to the cat. In man, the middle ear cavity averages 0.5 cc, while the mastoid cavity averages 8.6 cc with a wide range from 2.1 to 17.44 cc.[9] The human mastoid cavity consists almost entirely of pneumatic cells except for an antral cavity about 1 cc in volume. The cat middle ear has an average volume of 0.217 cc while the bulla averages 0.675 cc and is a single smooth-walled cavity. The foramen between the two is small and short, about 1 mm in diameter by 1 mm long, and is quite different from the human aditus ad antrum.[7,10] It is apparent that the anatomy of the cat ear cavities is less complex than that of humans; only the middle ear cavities are similar, except that the volume in the human is about twice that of the cat.

Onchi[11] studied middle ear sound transmission in three human temporal bones after aditus blockage and stated: "The antrum and mastoid cells increase the displacement of the tympanic membrane below 1,000 cps and decrease it in a frequency range of 1,000 to 3,000 cps. However, such an effect is within 10 dB." The temporal bones in his study had higher impedances than normal, raising the question of postmortem artifacts. To our knowledge, no data exist on the effect of enlarging the cavities on sound transmission in humans.

Since blocking the aditus mimics the middle ear cavity status after modified radical mastoidectomy, and enlarging the aditus and mastoid cavity simulates the cavity status following intact canal wall mastoidectomy, it would be of interest to the otologic surgeon to know the acoustical effect of these modifications.

The effect of cavity changes on sound transmis-

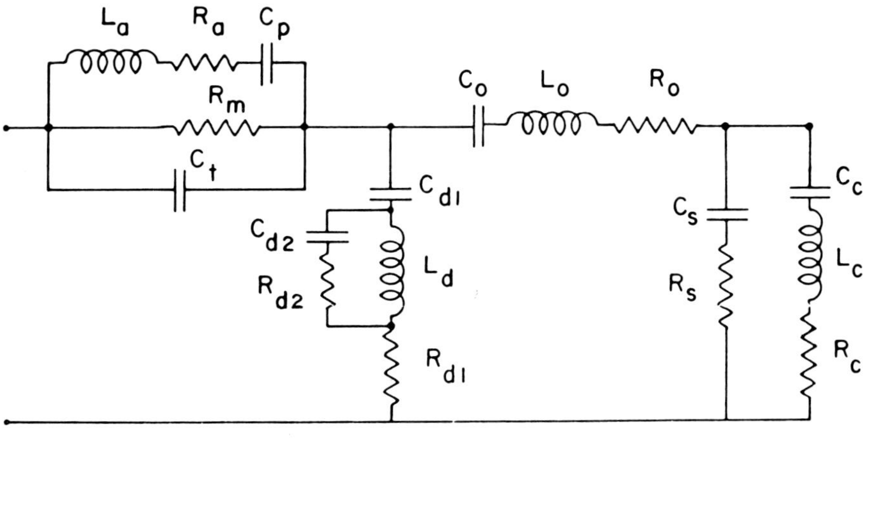

Fig. 2. Zwislocki electronic middle ear analog. Five-component section in upper left of figure represents middle ear and mastoid cavities. La - 14 mH, Ra - 10 Ω, Cp - 5.1 mF, Rm - 500 Ω, Ct - 0.35 mF.

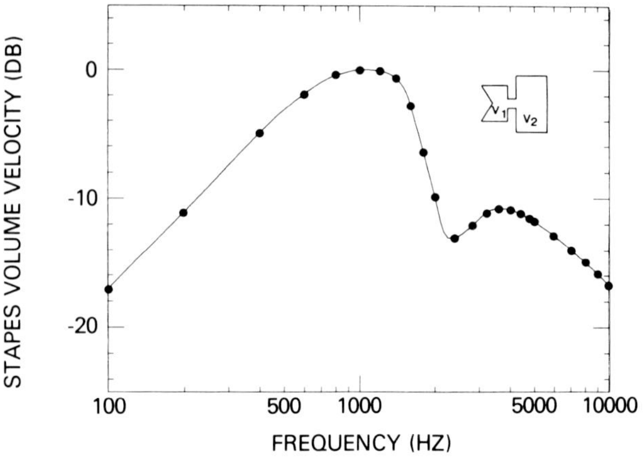

Fig. 3. Stapes volume velocity as predicted by Zwislocki analog for a constant SPL at TM in ear with normal cavities. Velocity at 1,000 Hz arbitrarily set as 0-dB reference. V_1 - Middle ear volume; V_2 - Mastoid volume.

sion in humans can also be studied using a middle ear electronic analog as described by Zwislocki[9] (Fig. 2). The middle ear and mastoid cavities are considered in the analog as two parallel capacitances. The smaller capacitance (Ct) represents the compliance of the middle ear volume (0.5 cc) while the larger (Cp) represents the compliance of an average mastoid cavity (8 cc). The aditus is represented as an inductance (La) and resistance (Ra) while sound absorption in the walls of the middle ear cavity and eustachian tube is represented by Rm.

In its usual form the analog circuit uses a constant voltage as the input, which represents a constant SPL at the TM. The output is the current through the cochlear portion of the circuit, which represents stapes velocity. Figure 3 shows a transmission curve produced by the circuit in Figure 2 for a normal middle ear with normal cavities. Output can also be converted to peak-to-peak umbo displacement so that it can be compared with measurements obtained in the temporal bones. (Measurement for the circuit in Figure 2 is shown as the dotted line in Figure 1). By modifying the values in the cavity section of the circuit, the effects of aditus blockage and cavity enlargement can be assessed.

METHODS

TEMPORAL BONE STUDIES

Umbo displacement in response to a constant SPL at the TM was the parameter used to measure middle ear sound transmission. In humans, umbo displacement is almost identical to stapes displacement[1] since the lever ratio between the umbo and lenticular process of the incus is low (1:3 to 1) and the ossicles move as a unit. Human cadaver temporal bones were obtained within 24 hours of death and tested within six days. The bones were inspected to rule out ear pathology and stored in 1:10,000 thimersal (Merthiolate) solution at 5°C as described by Onchi.[11] Using an American Electromedics model 83 impedance bridge, static compliance at 220 Hz was measured just prior to testing; bones that did not meet normal criteria were not used. Before testing, the bone's exterior was sealed with methylmethacrylate and a thin coat of safflower oil placed on the TM.

The bone was placed in a temporal bone holder attached to a heavy metal plate and a Mylar mirror (diameter 1.5 mm, weight 0.44 mg) glued to the umbo using cyanoacrylate adhesive. A 1-mm hole was drilled in the wall of the bony external auditory canal (EAC) 3 mm from the TM, and a 2.5 cm length of PE 60 tubing was placed through the hole and connected to a Brüel and Kjaer (B & K) model 4170 probe microphone. A separate 10-mm opening was made in the anterior wall of the bony EAC so that the displacement measuring probe could be directly focused on the umbo mirror in its usual plane of vibration.

The noncontacting optical measuring device used to measure umbo displacement was a KD100 Fotonic sensor with KD-1101 plug-in, a 109R fiberoptic probe and KD-LS-3 optical extender (Mechanical Technology Inc, Latham, NY).[12] The optical extender allowed umbo displacement measurements to be made at a distance of 3 cm from the TM when focused on the umbo mirror through the hole in the anterior wall of the EAC. The probe and optical extender were held in a Mitutoyo micromanipulator capable of 1-μm movements.

The Fotonic sensor's output passed through a narrow band (3 Hz) B & K model 2020 slave filter to a Princton applied research model 5204 lock-in analyzer which provided the readout. All readouts were converted to peak-to-peak umbo displacement.

The measuring device works in the following way: light produced by a source within the unit passes out sending fibers in the fiberoptic probe onto a reflective target attached to the object of interest. At a critical probe-target distance (focal point) a maximum amount of light is reflected back into light-receiving fibers within the probe. A photo-FET compares the reflected light with the transmitted light and produces a DC-voltage equivalent to the net amount of light. Thus, a null is produced at the focal point (maximum light reflected into receiving fibers) which is about 30 mm away when the optical extender is placed on the probe. Slight changes of probe-target distance produce a decrease in the amount of reflected light entering the probe and increase the voltage output until a peak is reached at about 30.7 mm. Halfway between these two points, 700 μm apart, is a linear, very sensitive measurement range which produces an output of about 1 mV for 0.1-μm changes under optimum conditions.

Before each measurement the system was calibrated with the micromanipulator as well as with a B & K model 4290 accelerometer calibrator; accuracy was within ± 2 dB in the 0.1- to 15-μm range using this method. Measurements of umbo displacement were made at 200-Hz intervals from 500 to 7,000 Hz at 110 and 120 dB SPL at the TM.

The sound source was a University ID-40T speaker driver with a 0.3-m long, 2-cm internal diameter rubber tube connected into the EAC via a speculum. The speaker was driven by a B & K model 1027 beat frequency oscillator (BFO) synchronized with the slave filter. The SPL at the TM was controlled by the probe microphone in the ear canal. Output was passed to a B & K model 2603 voltmeter and then back to the BFO. A second probe microphone connected to a B & K model 2606 voltmeter monitored middle ear cavity SPL. The probe microphones were calibrated in a B & K microphone calibrator. All tests were done in an IAC single-wall sound-treated room.

Two basic modifications of the mastoid and middle ear cavities were studied in the temporal bones:

Blocked Aditus (modified radical mastoidectomy experiment). Three temporal bones were studied. After initial baseline umbo displacement measurements the aditus ad antrum was blocked with a saline-filled balloon (Fogarty catheter) inserted through a hole in the tegmen made prior to the measurements and closed with clay. The balloon was inflated, the tegmen hole closed with clay and the measurements repeated. Measurements of the cavity volume were made with the impedance bridge through the tegmen hole after filling the EAC with clay.

Enlarged Aditus and Mastoid Cavity (intact canal wall experiment). In two temporal bones, the aditus ad antrum and facial recess were widely opened by the usual surgical approach. The mastoid cavity air cells were drilled out to provide a total cavity

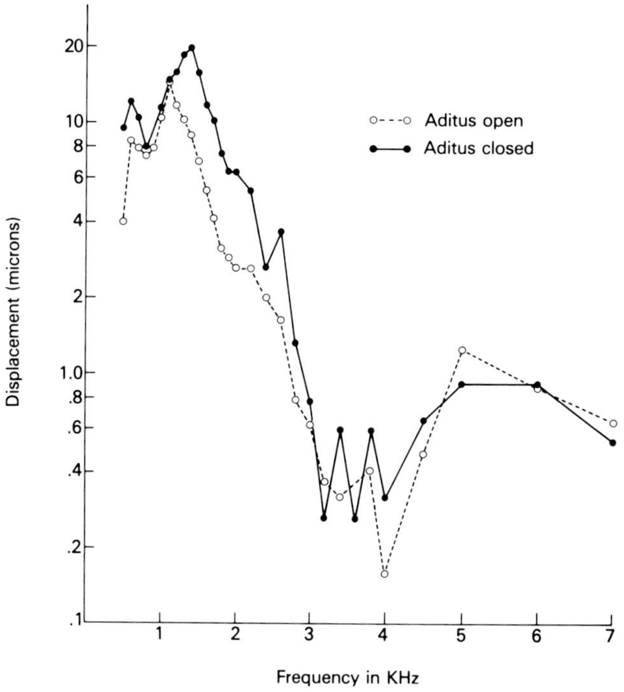

Fig. 4. Peak-to-peak umbo displacement, aditus opened v closed in human temporal bone 1, middle ear volume 0.6 cc. SPL at TM is 120 dB.

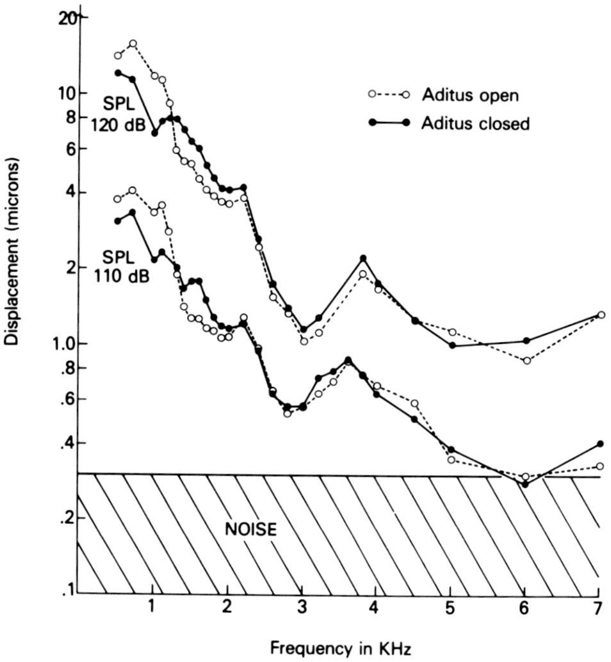

Fig. 6. Peak-to-peak umbo displacement, aditus open v closed in human temporal bone 3. Curves for 110 and 120 dB SPL at TM are shown. Noise floor was at 0.3 μm. Middle ear volume 0.7 cc.

volume of 6 cc and the external opening into the mastoid sealed with clay. The volume was determined with the impedance bridge as noted previously. Baseline measurements of umbo displacement were obtained, then the connection between the middle ear and mastoid cavity was blocked with clay and the measurements repeated. Clay was substituted for the balloon in these bones because it was found easier to use. The balloon and clay appeared to provide equally effective aditus blockage as determined in several temporal bones by mastoid cavity SPL measurements for known middle ear SPL. In one additional temporal bone, the mastoid cavity was widely opened to the outside without modifying the aditus and umbo displacement measured. The aditus was then blocked with clay and the measurements repeated.

Over 20 bones were used to perfect the measurement technique and an additional 20 bones were evaluted to obtain the 6 bones described in this study. Bones were unable to be used because of middle ear abnormalities, problems in performing the surgery or problems making the measurements.

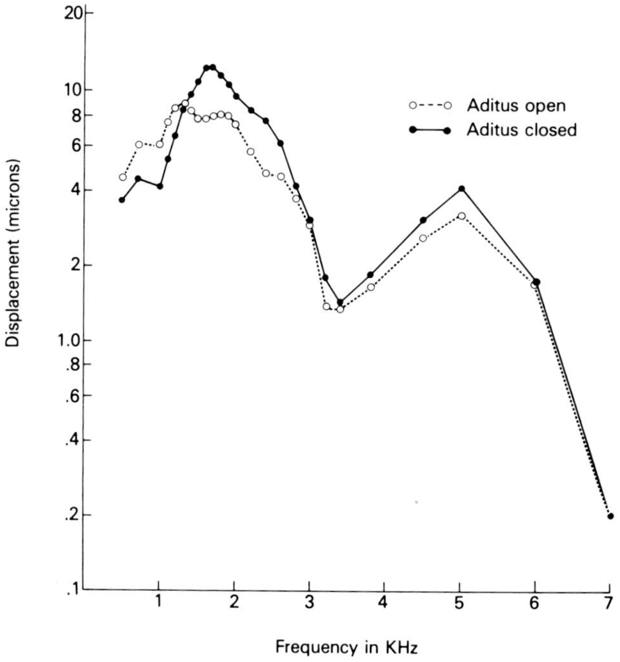

Fig. 5. Peak-to-peak umbo displacement, aditus open v closed in human temporal bone 2, middle ear volume 0.66 cc.

COMPUTER ANALOG SIMULATION

The cavity modifications performed on the temporal bones were also simulated on an IBM 3081 computer and a Versatec plotter using the circuit of Figure 2. For the blocked aditus (modified radical simulation), Ra was made infinitely high ($10^{12}\Omega$). For the enlarged cavity (intact canal wall simulation) Ra was raised to $10^{12}\Omega$ and Ct increased to 4.2 μF, equivalent to one large cavity of 6 cc.

RESULTS

TEMPORAL BONE STUDIES

The effect of blocking the aditus on umbo displacement, as compared to the normal state, is shown in Figures 4 to 6. Blocking the aditus decreased displacement in the lower frequencies below 1,500 Hz in two bones and increased it in one. Displacement in the midfrequencies was increased by aditus blockage with peak improvement found between 1,500 and 2,500 Hz. The notch at 3,000 to 4,000 Hz was not eliminated by blockage.

The effect of opening the aditus and facial recess widely, as in an intact canal wall mastoidectomy, is shown in Figures 7 and 8. The umbo displacement measurements for the widely open aditus and mastoid were compared with measurements made after

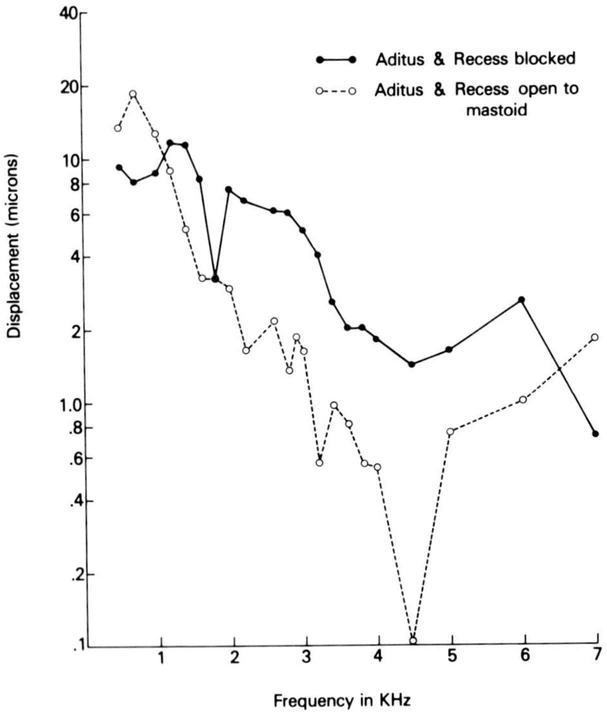

Fig. 7. Peak-to-peak umbo displacement, enlarged mastoid cavity, enlarged facial recess and aditus *v* blocked aditus and recess in human temporal bone 4. 120 dB SPL.

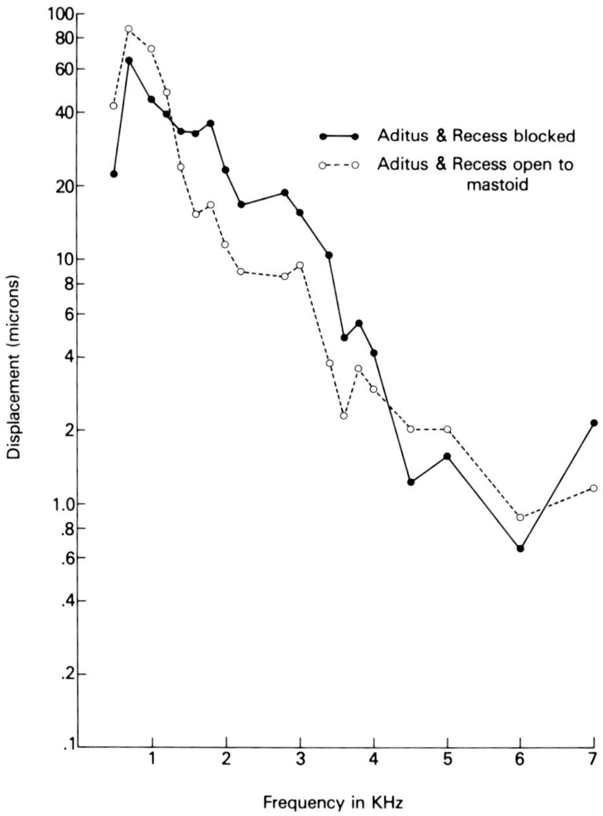

Fig. 8. Peak-to-peak umbo displacement, enlarged mastoid cavity, enlarged facial recess and aditus *v* blocked aditus and recess in human temporal bone 5. 120 dB SPL.

the opening was blocked with clay. The data obtained in these two bones allowed direct comparison of the aditus blocked *v* aditus widely open and mastoid cavity enlarged condition. Blockage of the enlarged aditus decreased umbo displacement in the lower frequencies, but in the mid-to-higher frequencies, displacement was increased by aditus closure. This was particularly marked in bone 4 Fig. 7).

The effect of widely opening the mastoid cavity to the outside in an otherwise normal bone, compared with the aditus blocked in the same bone, is shown in Figure 9. Opening the mastoid cavity produced a second notch in umbo displacement at 1,500 Hz but did not eliminate the 3,000 to 4,000-Hz notch. Blocking the aditus decreased low-frequency umbo displacement and eliminated the 1,500-Hz notch, but did not change the notch at 3,000 to 4,000 Hz.

COMPUTER ANALOG SIMULATION

The curves produced by the Zwislocki middle ear analog plot stapes volume velocity in decibels for a constant SPL at the TM from 100 to 10,000 Hz. The 0-dB reference was the volume velocity at 1,000 Hz in the normal cavity arrangement. Since the temporal bone measurements are of umbo displacement, the computer results must be converted into umbo displacement for comparison purposes. This has been done for the normal cavity arrangement and is shown as the dotted line in Figure 1.

Modified Radical Simulation. The effect of blocking the aditus ad antrum in the analog is shown in Figure 10. Compared with the normal cavity simulation (Fig. 3) there is a decrease in stapes volume velocity from 200 to 2,000 Hz, reaching 7 dB at around 1,000 Hz. The 2,500-Hz notch is eliminated with improvement between 2,000 to 5,000 Hz, reaching a maximum of 5 dB at 2,500 Hz.

Intact Canal Wall Simulation. The effect of enlarging the middle ear cavity to 6.0 cc so that it mimics the intact canal wall condition is shown in Figure 11. The curve is identical to the normal cavity arrangement up to 1,500 Hz. Between 1,500 and 5,000 Hz there is improved transmission reaching a peak of 9 dB at 2,500 Hz. The intact canal simulation is compared on the same graph with the modified radical in Figure 12, demonstrating the acoustical advantages of the former over the latter in the computer simulation.

In Figure 13, the output of the computer simulations have been converted from stapes volume velocity to peak-to-peak umbo displacement for easier comparison with the temporal bone experiments.

DISCUSSION

It appears from the temporal bone experiments that blocking the aditus improves middle ear sound transmission in the 1,500- to 3,000-Hz range when

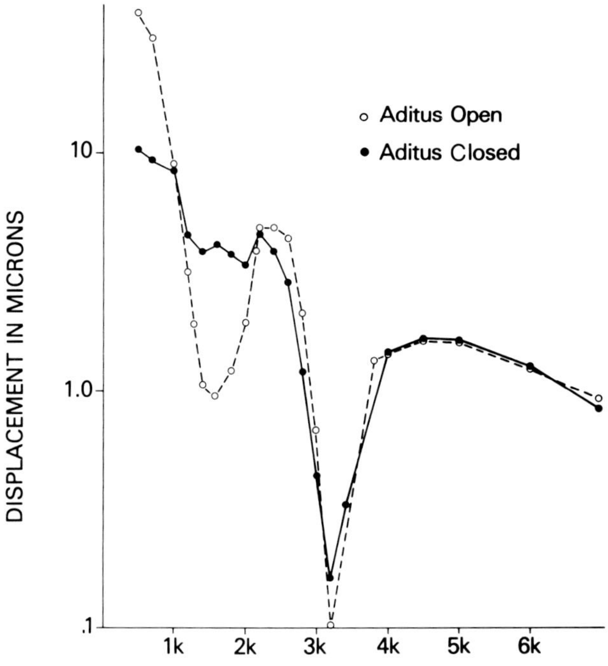

Fig. 9. Peak-to-peak umbo displacement in bone 6 with mastoid cavity widely opened to outside, aditus open *v* closed. 120 dB SPL at TM.

compared to the normal ear. Below 1,500 Hz, blocking the aditus decreased transmission in two bones and increased transmission in one bone. The effects were small, less than 10 dB. Interestingly, the 3,000- to 4,000-Hz notch, seen in many bones, was not affected by aditus blockage. In this respect the human appears different from the cat. As previously noted, there are significant anatomic differences between the ear cavities of man and cat, so that the transmission notch seen in both species may have different acoustical explanations.

The enlarged aditus and mastoid cavity condition provided better low-frequency sound transmission than the aditus closed situation, but in the important frequency range 1,500 to 4,000 Hz, transmission was better with the aditus closed.

Because of the small number of bones studied and the individual variations between bones, any conclusions regarding the clinical significance of the temporal bone results must be made cautiously. It does appear that blocking the aditus, such as occurs during modified radical mastoidectomy, is not acoustically detrimental and may actually be beneficial in the 1,500- to 4,000-Hz range when compared with the intact canal wall mastoidectomy, everything else being equal. For the low frequencies below 1,000 Hz, the latter procedure appears preferable.

The computer analog results did not correlate well with the temporal bone results. The analog

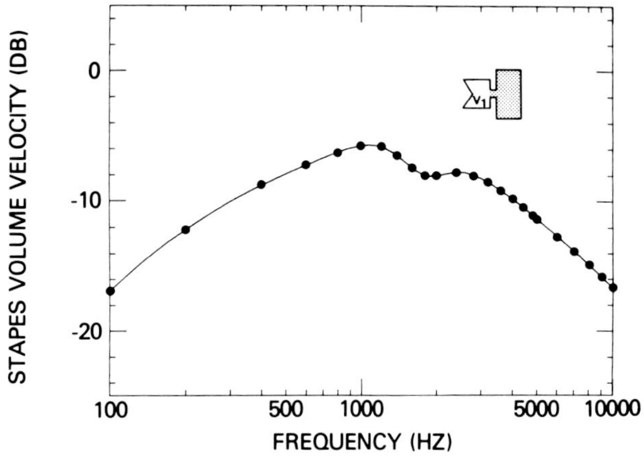

Fig. 10. Modified radical mastoidectomy. Effect of blocking aditus on stapes volume velocity as predicted by Zwislocki model. V_1 - Middle ear volume.

predicted optimal transmission with the intact canal wall mastoidectomy as well as elimination of the notch in both the intact canal wall and modified radical mastoidectomy simulation. There are several possible reasons for this. Zwislocki's model was primarily based on impedance measurements and he felt the data supporting the model was weak above 2,000 Hz.[9] The modeling of the mastoid cavity with a single capacitance (Cp) would be appropriate for the cat but not for man and the rationale for Rm is unclear; a better model is needed. Furthermore, the intact canal wall mastoidectomy was modeled as one large cavity of 6 cc while in the temporal bone; the situation was a normal middle ear cavity connected by an enlarged aditus and facial recess to a drilled-out mastoid with a total volume of 6 cc. The enlargement of the aditus and facial recess produced an opening between the two cavities about three times the normal diameter. Therefore, the computer simulation and temporal bone experiments may not be acoustically equivalent.

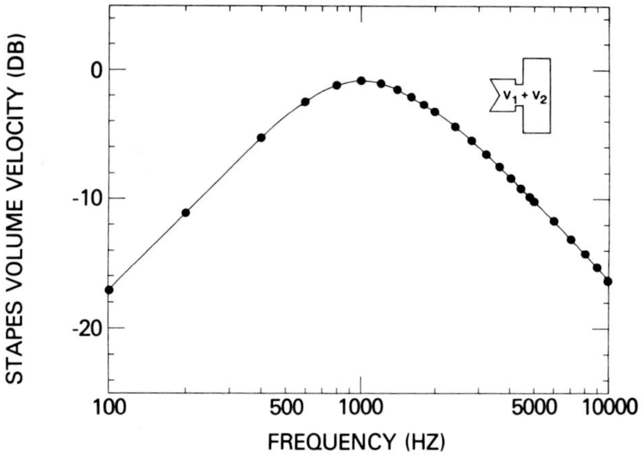

Fig. 11. Intact canal wall mastoidectomy. Effect of blocking aditus and enlarging middle ear cavity to 6 cc on stapes volume velocity as predicted by Zwislocki model. V_1 - Middle ear volume; V_2 - Mastoid volume.

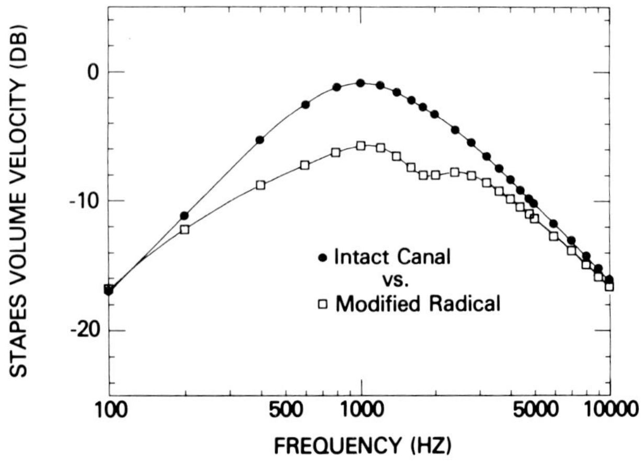

Fig. 12. Curves of Figs. 10 and 11 compared.

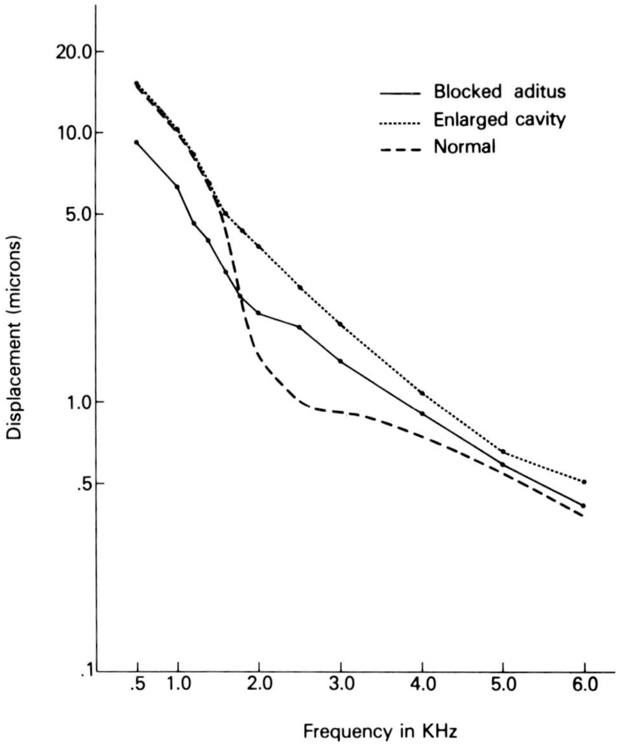

Fig. 13. Results of Zwislocki model simulations converted from stapes volume velocity to peak-to-peak umbo displacement. Reference point is 15 μm at 500 Hz for normal middle ear.

Accurate measurements of the modified anatomy of the two bones used in the intact canal wall mastoidectomy studies are currently being obtained with a CT scanner in order to better understand the exact changes produced and improve future modeling. In addition, the umbo displacement measurements are being compared with the middle ear SPL measurements to correlate TM displacement with the sound pressure difference across the TM. The results will be reported in a later paper.

When using human cadaver material, the question of postmortem artifacts must be addressed as a reason for the differences between the temporal bone, cat and model results. Onchi's[11] temporal bone impedance data showed an increase in reactance at low frequencies when compared to living subjects; no differences were present above 1,000 Hz. Postmortem changes have also been seen in cat experiments[12] and in situ temporal bone impedance measurements.[13] While the usual cause of these artifacts is drying, the in situ data of Zwislocki and Feldman[13] was undoubtedly influenced by postmortem negative middle ear pressures. We feel the use of careful microscopic inspection, impedance bridge screening and care in keeping the middle ear structures moist and lubricated minimized the likelihood of artifacts in these experiments. Furthermore, the umbo displacement curves obtained in our normal temporal bones are very similar to those obtained by Løkberg et al in live subjects.[4]

REFERENCES

1. Gundersen T. Prostheses in the ossicular chain — experimental and clinical studies. Baltimore: University Park Press, 1971.

2. Tonndorf J, Khanna SM. Tympanic-membrane vibrations in human cadaver ears studied by time-averaged holography. J Acoust Soc Am 1972; 52:1221.

3. von Bally G. Otological investigations in living man using holographic interferometry. In: von Bally G, ed. Proceedings of the International Workshop on Holography in Medicine and Biology. Berlin: Springer-Verlag, 1979:198.

4. Løkberg OJ, Høgmoen K, Gundersen T. Use of ESPI to measure the vibration of the human eardrum in vivo and other biological movements. In: von Bally G, ed. Proceedings of the International Workshop on Holography in Medicine and Biology. Berlin: Springer-Verlag, 1979:212.

5. Guinan JJ Jr, Peake WT. Middle ear characteristics of anesthetized cats. J Acoust Soc Am 1967; 41:1237-61.

6. Buunen TJF, Vlaming MSMG. Laser-doppler velocity meter applied to tympanic membrane vibrations in cat. J Acoust Soc Am 1981; 69:744-50.

7. Lynch TJ. Signal processing by the cat middle ear: admittance and transmission, measurements and models, thesis, Massachusetts Institute of Technology, Boston, Mass, 1981.

8. Möller AR. An experimental study of the acoustic impedance of the middle ear and its transmission properties. Acta Otolaryngol (Stockh) 1976; 60:129-49.

9. Zwislocki J. Analysis of the middle-ear function. Part I. Input impedance. J Acoust Soc Am 1962; 34:1514-23.

10. Silverstein H. Atlas of the human and cat temporal bone. Springfield, Ill: Charles C Thomas, 1972.

11. Onchi Y. Mechanism of the middle ear. J Acoust Soc Am 1961; 33:794-805.

12. Jako GJ, Hickman K, Adkins H. Use of a new photoelectric device (fotonic sensor) for vibration measurements in the ear. J Acoust Soc Am 1966: 40:1263.

13. Zwislocki J, Feldman AS. Post-mortem acoustic impedance of human ears. J Acoust Soc Am 1963; 35:104-7.

THE HOMOGRAFT TYMPANIC MEMBRANE AFTER 12 YEARS

ROGER E. WEHRS, MD
TULSA, OKLAHOMA

The homograft tympanic membrane has been utilized in reconstructive middle ear surgery since 1968. Previous reports describing its preservation and use were published in 1971, 1972, 1976 and 1978. Throughout this time the same preservative of 70% ethyl alcohol and the same surgical technique of covering the transplant with canal skin or fascia has been employed. These transplants have been used to supplement, not replace, other grafting tissues, and to improve the graft-take rate and hearing results. The graft-take rate has averaged over 90% for the past 12 years and 98% for the past 5 years. The hearing results have been satisfactory in 69 to 95% of the cases depending on the associated ossicular reconstruction. Furthermore these results have been consistent and have not deteriorated with the passage of time.

INTRODUCTION

Homograft tympanic membranes obtained from fresh unembalmed cadavers and preserved in 95% ethyl alcohol have been utilized routinely in reconstructive middle ear surgery since 1968. These transplants were not used as the primary grafting material but rather as a supporting matrix and have always been covered with living tissue in the form of canal skin or fascia. This technique which was first reported in detail in 1971 has changed very little over the years attesting to the durability of the method. In 1978 an extensive review of the hearing and anatomical results was reported.[1] This study reviews and compares those first seven years with the last five as well as looking at some long-term results.

The first homograft tympanic membrane was used in a 35-year-old male in October 1965. This patient had previously undergone bilateral radical mastoidectomies with several revisions and all ossicular tissue had been removed. In this case the homograft tympanic membrane was employed to support the homograft malleus in anatomical position, an indication that is still in use today. At this time in history the homograft incus had been successfully employed in several ears so there was no hesitancy in using another transplant bone; however, the fate and reaction of the homograft membranous eardrum was unknown. Therefore the fibrous annulus was removed from the homograft tympanic membrane in order that a minimum of foreign tissue would be introduced. (In subsequent years it has been discovered that the human body tolerates this dead tissue very well and replaces it with living tissue, therefore the fibrous annulus is now preserved and used over the patient's drum remnant.) The hearing mechanism was reconstructed with a homograft incus body with its short process on the stapedial footplate. These transplants were then covered with temporalis fascia. Fortunately the patient obtained a good result and still has serviceable hearing today (Fig. 1A, B).

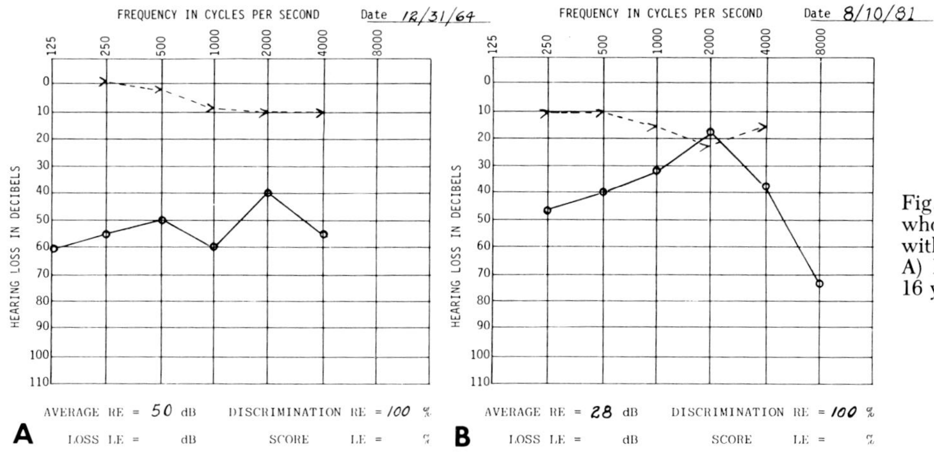

Fig. 1. Audiograms of first patient in whom homograft tympanic membrane with malleus was used in reconstruction. A) Preoperative. B) Postoperative, after 16 years.

From St. Francis Hospital, Tulsa.
Presented at the meeting of the American Otological Society, Inc., Palm Beach, Florida, May 2-3, 1982.
REPRINTS — Roger E. Wehrs, MD, 6465 S. Yale, Tulsa, OK 74177.

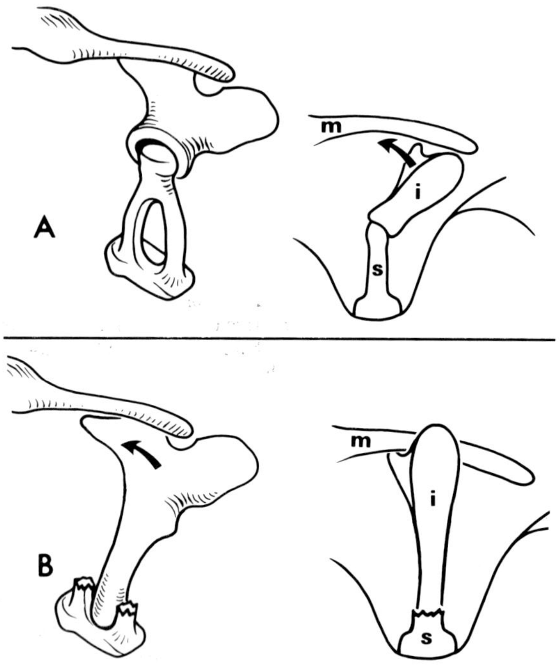

Fig. 2. Reconstruction of sound pressure mechanism. A) Stapes is intact. Homograft notched incus with short process is inserted flat under malleus (left) then moved upright to final position (right). B) Reconstruction directly to the stapedial footplate. Notched incus with long process is placed on promontory off tip of malleus (left), then raised to upright final position (right). m - Malleus; i - Incus; s - Stapes.

Although there was sporadic use of the homograft tympanic membrane in the next two years, it was not until the publication of a preliminary report by Glasscock and House[2] that interest was rekindled and its use became routine. The first report of 40 cases was published in 1971.[3] Subsequent reports were published in 1972,[4] 1976,[5] and 1977.[6] This study includes 300 ears and covers the years of 1976 through 1980, for a total of 920 ears to date.

Alcohol Preservation of Homografts. Homograft temporal bone cores are obtained from fresh unembalmed cadavers. These are placed in a plastic bag filled with water and frozen and they may be kept in the freezer for several months. At a convenient time the bones are thawed in cold running water and harvested. The epithelial layer is removed from the tympanic membrane and the fibrous annulus is removed from the bony annulus. The tensor tympani tendon is cut, the incudomallear joint separated, and the homograft tympanic membrane with attached malleus is removed. These structures are transferred to bottles containing 70% ethyl alcohol and stored until needed in surgery. The alcohol is changed every two weeks to compensate for evaporation.

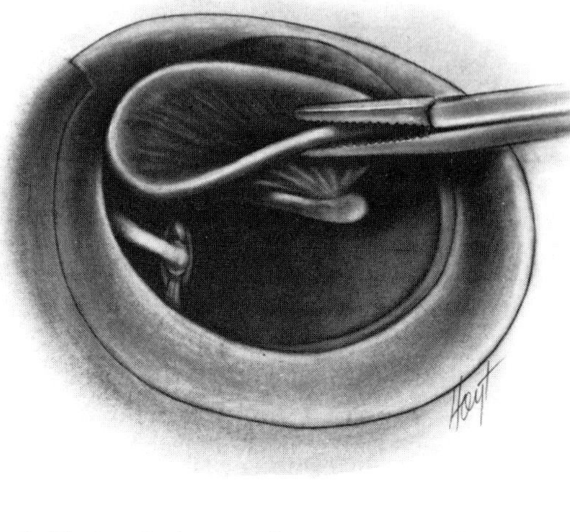

Fig. 3. Placing the homograft tympanic membrane. Note how cone shape of homograft drumhead contacts tip of patient's malleus.

No sterile technique is required until the homografts are needed in surgery. At that time the circulating nurse removes the lid from the bottle and the scrub nurse removes the homograft with a sterile instrument. It is immediately put through several rinsings of Ringer's lactate solution to remove the alcohol and it is then ready for use in the patient.

SURGICAL TECHNIQUE

This technique, published in detail previously,[1,3-5] differs from that described by others in that the homograft tympanic membrane is always covered with living tissue, usually the canal skin. Most procedures are performed entirely through the ear canal with the canal skin being reintroduced as a graft over the homograft drumhead. However, if the operation is combined with a mastoidectomy and carried out through a postauricular incision, then a fascial graft is placed over the homograft tympanic membrane. If the patient's malleus is usable, the homograft malleus is removed from the transplant drumhead and only the homograft tympanic membrane is utilized. However, if the malleus is

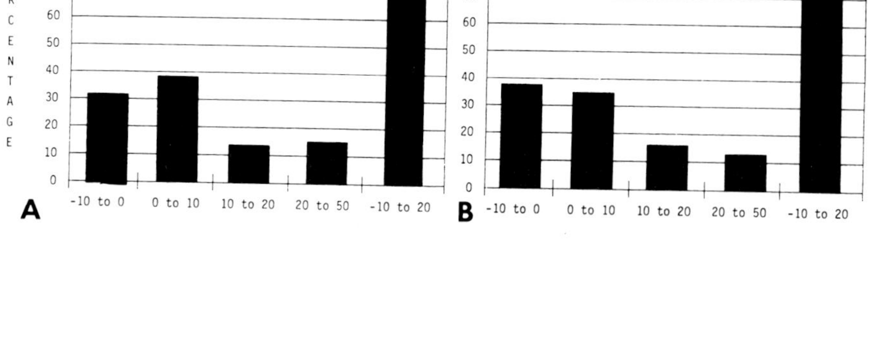

Fig. 4. Overall hearing results A) at six weeks and B) at six months with homograft tympanic membrane.

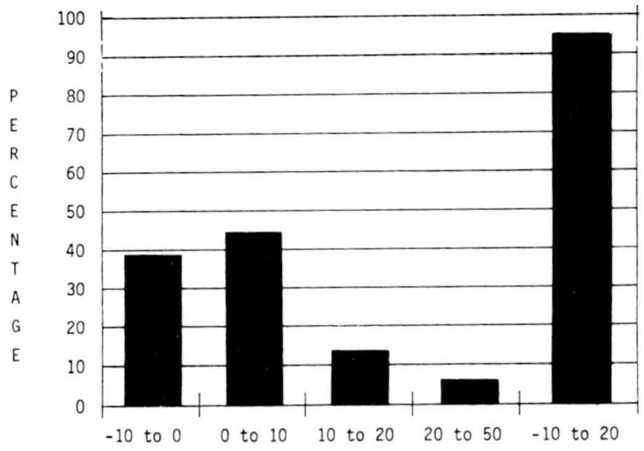

Fig. 5. Hearing results at six months when homograft tympanic membrane used over an intact and mobile ossicular chain.

eroded, involved in cholesteatoma or otherwise unsuitable, the homograft tympanic membrane and attached malleus become the main building block for the middle ear reconstruction.

When the patient's incus is also unfit for use, the middle ear is rebuilt with the homograft notched incus. If the stapes is intact the reconstruction is carried out with the homograft notched incus with short process. Here the cup created in the body of the incus fits over the stapedial head and the notch in the short process locks under the malleus (Fig. 2A). When the stapes superstructure is absent reconstruction is accomplished with the homograft notched incus with long process (Fig. 2B). In this instance the long process rests on the footplate and the prosthesis is stabilized by the malleus passing over the notch in the short process.

RESULTS

Anatomical. The new drumhead resulting from the above-described technique is thicker and more vascular than the normal tympanic membrane but this does not appear to affect its function. When the canal skin is placed over the homograft tympanic membrane it extends to but does not turn up on the anterior canal wall so as to preserve the acute angle so important to a good hearing result. Also if the ossicular chain is intact the umbo of the homograft contacts the tip of the patient's malleus thus reestablishing the cone shape of the normal tympanic membrane (Fig. 3).

The graft-take rate has averaged 98% over the past five years. When breakdown does occur it is usually due to infection within the first week or two following surgery. The graft has very little tendency to thin out and any late breakdown is due to a retained epithelial cyst.

CATEGORIES OF AUDIOMETRIC RESULTS OF TYMPANOPLASTY

Hearing	*Air-bone Gap (dB)*
Excellent	− 10 to 0
Good	0 to 10
Fair	10 to 20
Poor	20 to 50
Satisfactory	− 10 to 20

The audiometric results reported on the bar graphs correspond to these five categories.

Revision for a small perforation is usually carried out by raising a tympanomeatal flap and elevating just the epithelial layer of the remaining graft with the flap. When elevation has been obtained for a few millimeters around the perforation, a disc of homograft dura is placed over the drum remnant, and the flap and epithelial layer are then replaced. The dura can be seen shining through where the perforation had been. If the perforation is large and the canal skin which has regrown is of good character then the original procedure may be repeated. Another alternative is repair with a fascial graft.

Hearing. One of the most important criteria of a successful tympanoplasty is the hearing result obtained by the patient. These results therefore will be considered in detail (table).

The air-bone gap referred to in the text and graphs represents the difference between the postoperative air conduction and the preoperative bone conduction for the three speech frequencies. This format has for years been the one used for calculating the hearing results in otosclerosis as well as in tympanoplasty. One criticism of this method is that in some instances there is apparent overclosure of the air-bone gap. This is of course not possible. However, something has happened to produce this effect and it would seem to be that we have changed the dynamics of the conductive transformer mechanism of the operated ear. If this phenomenon can be shown to occur consistently and in a high percentage of postoperative cases, then that particular surgical technique may be changing the dynamics of the hearing mechanism in a beneficial way and should bear further investigation.

During the 5-year period of 1976 through 1980 a total of 300 ears were reconstructed with the homo-

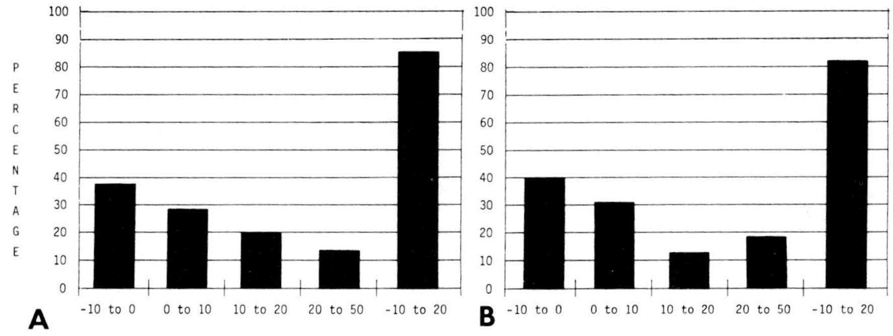

Fig. 6. Hearing results at six months with homograft tympanic membrane and homograft notched incus A) with short process; B) with long process.

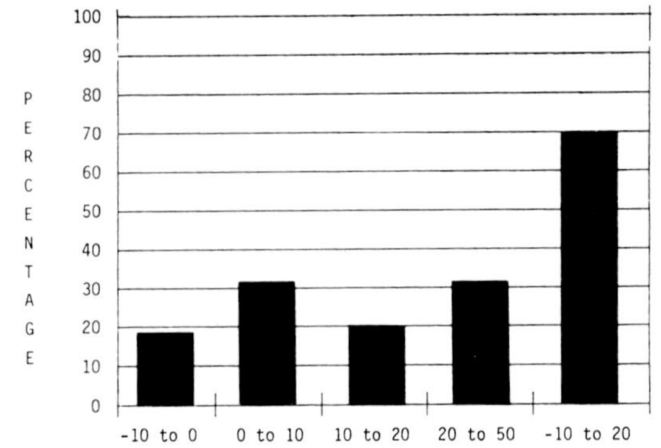

Fig. 7. Hearing results at six weeks with homograft tympanic membrane with homograft malleus and homograft notched incus.

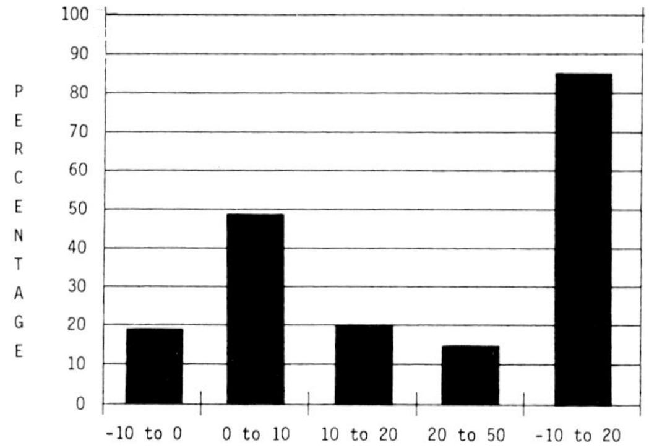

Fig. 9. Overall hearing results at five years with homograft tympanic membrane. Includes both past and present series.

graft tympanic membrane. This figure includes all cases in which a transplant drumhead was employed in the reconstruction regardless of the associated pathology.

The first postoperative hearing test six weeks following surgery demonstrates that 85% of those tested had closed the air-bone gap by 20 dB or less (Fig. 4A). Further breakdown of the graph shows that 31% fell in the *excellent* category. The *good* column was represented by 39% and the failure rate was 16%. At six months postoperatively the *satisfactory* column had improved slightly to 87% with only minor variations in the other categories (Fig. 4B).

Figure 5 represents those patients in whom the ossicular chain was intact and mobile. As might be suspected the results were satisfactory with 95% of the ears tested six months following surgery classified as satisfactory. The *excellent* category was 38% with the *good* column being 45% and the *fair* one totaling only 13%. The failure rate was 5%.

Reconstruction using the notched incus with short process is shown in Figure 6A. Here the first column representing the *excellent* results reached 37%. *Good* results were 28% and the most important column, *satisfactory*, was listed as 85% with 15% considered as failures.

Figure 6B depicts the hearing levels in those cases where the stapes superstructure was absent and the notched incus with long process was employed with the homograft tympanic membrane. Here the *excellent* category reached 40% but this was balanced out by a high failure rate of 18% so that the satisfactory column was only 83%.

The audiometric findings in the two preceding figures are probably tied more closely to the ossicular reconstruction than to the type of graft.

The homograft tympanic membrane with attached homograft malleus was also used to reconstruct 61 ears in which the patient's own malleus was missing or so extensively involved in disease that it could not be utilized. Reconstruction to the inner ear was carried out with the homograft notched incudi. The hearing results for these cases are given in Figure 7. Eleven ears or 18% of the total overclosed the air-bone gap by 0 to 10 dB. The percentage of patients reaching a satisfactory level stood at 69% with a failure column of 31%.

Now let us turn our attention once again to the overall long-term results of those cases in which a homograft drumhead was utilized regardless of the status of the ossicular chain or mastoid. Figure 8 tabulates the hearing results after one year in the present series. Of 129 patients who returned for au-

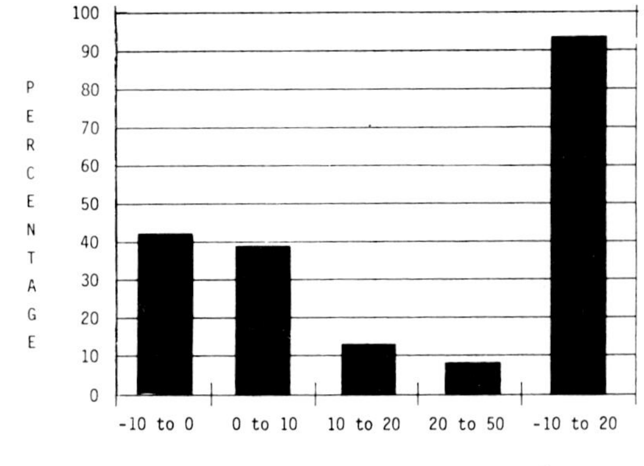

Fig. 8. Overall hearing results at one year in the present series with homograft tympanic membrane.

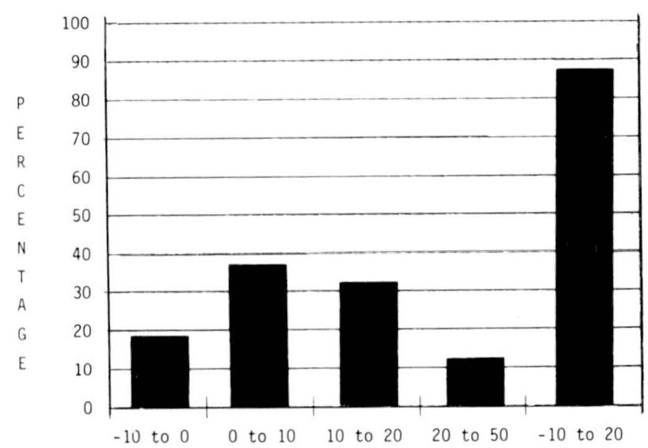

Fig. 10. Overall hearing results after ten years with homograft tympanic membrane. Includes both past and present series.

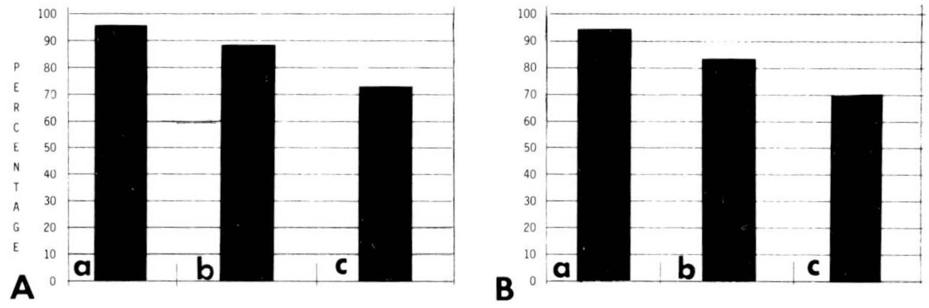

Fig. 11. Comparison of hearing results A) of past series (1970-1975) with B) present one (1976-1980). All cases met the *satisfactory* criteria of − 10 to 20 dB air-bone gap one year postoperatively. a - Intact chain; b - Patient's malleus; c - Homograft malleus.

diometric testing 10 patients (8%) exhibited an air-bone gap of greater than 20 dB and thus were considered failures. The satisfactory rate therefore represented 119 ears or 92% of the total. It was also gratifying to see more cases shifted to the *excellent* category with a reading of 42%.

The long-term hearing results are an important part of evaluating any grafting technique. Figures 9 and 10 list the audiometric findings for the 5-and 10-year intervals after the initial surgery. As noted in the graphs the improvement in hearing appears to be maintained with the *satisfactory* column being 86% at five years postoperatively and 87% after ten. The failure rates were 14% and 13% respectively.

Let us now compare the hearing results for the past series (1969-1975) with the present series (Fig. 11). These comparisons are for the intact ossicular chain, those cases in which the patient's malleus was used, and those utilizing the homograft malleus as well as the homograft tympanic membrane. As can be seen by the graphs they are almost identical. This would appear to indicate that even though progress had been made in shifting some of the *fair* and *good* results to the *excellent* category the overall failure rate remains unchanged.

CONCLUSIONS

The homograft tympanic membrane in conjunction with a tissue graft, usually canal skin, has proven to give satisfactory and consistent results in tympanoplasty. The graft-take rate has averaged over 90% for the past 12 years and 98% for the past 5 years.

The hearing results have been *satisfactory* in 69 to 95% of the cases depending on the associated ossicular reconstruction. Furthermore these results have been consistent and have not deteriorated over the longer term. Over the past five years progress has been made in that more of the *fair* and *good* results have been shifted to the *excellent* category, but the failure rate of 10-15% has not changed over the years even with modifications of technique. It is within this area that the greatest challenge exists for the future. However, at the present time the surgical technique herein described appears to yield equal if not superior results to contemporary procedures especially in the area of hearing improvement.

REFERENCES

1. Wehrs RE. Results of homografts in middle ear surgery. Laryngoscope 1978; 88:808-15.

2. Glasscock ME III, House WF. Homograft reconstruction of the middle ear: a preliminary report. Laryngoscope 1968; 78:1219-25.

3. Wehrs RE. Homograft tympanic membrane in tympanoplasty. Arch Otolaryngol 1971; 93:132-9.

4. Wehrs RE. Three years experience with the homograft tympanic membrane. Trans Am Acad Ophthalmol Otolaryngol 1972; 76:142-6.

5. Wehrs RE. Homograft tympanic membrane: a five year study. Trans Am Acad Ophthalmol Otolaryngol 1976; 82:34-9.

6. Wehrs RE. Hearing and anatomical results with homograft tympanoplasty. Otolaryngol Clin North Am 1977; 10:595-8.

Ann Otol Rhinol Laryngol 91:1982

LYOPHILIZED PARTIAL OSSICULAR REPLACEMENT ALLOGRAFTS

MANSFIELD F. W. SMITH, MD JOHN T. MCELVEEN, MD

STANFORD, CALIFORNIA

This report deals with the use of partial ossicular replacement allografts (PORAs) in the stable ear, ie, a middle ear free of any residual or recurrent disease process such as fluid, cholesteatoma or infection. PORAs have been used by Shinn and Smith at the Ear Medical Clinic of Santa Clara Valley between July 1978 and December 1981; they are used to span the distance between the malleus and the head of the stapes or tympanic membrane. Lyophilized ethylene oxide sterilized PORAs have been available through the Northern California Transplant Bank, San Francisco, since July 1978. Twenty-four of 32 PORAs (75%) used in stable ears closed the air-bone gap within 10 dB. Of the eight ears that did not have satisfactory functional hearing, it was evident within one year and there was no further deterioration noted up to four years. There was no evidence of PORA extrusion or erosion.

Since the 1901 report of Matte[1] of a myringostapediopexy, numerous methods have been employed to bridge the gap between the tympanic membrane and the labyrinthine fluids. Initial reconstructive efforts, such as those of Hall and Rytzner[2] focused on the use of autogenous materials. Jansen[3] and House et al[4] utilized homologous cartilage and ossicles, respectively, in the reconstruction of the ossicular chain.

Despite many excellent short- and long-term results[5,6] with autogenous and homologous prostheses, the success of polyethylene and Teflon pistons in stapes surgery focused attention on the potential role of synthetic biocompatible materials in ossicular chain reconstruction. The otologic literature of the early 1960s contains a number of case reports outlining the use of polyethylene prostheses of various shapes and sizes in the restoration of ossicular continuity.[7,8] Interspersed with these articles are reports of early and late extrusions, especially in cases requiring contact of the prosthesis with the tympanic membrane or graft.[9,10]

In 1974 Shea and Homsy introduced a polytetrafluroethylene-vitreous carbon prosthesis (Proplast) designed to present the tympanic membrane with a "soft gradual interphase of low modulus to overcome the problems of displacement, extrusion, and absorption."[11] Although one-year follow-up studies revealed only a 2% extrusion rate, this material was supplanted in 1978 by a high density polyethylene sponge prosthesis (Plastipore) which, according to Shea and Emmett, "was superior to the prosthesis made of Proplast."[12]

Despite encouraging short-term results, problems with extrusion persisted.[13] Placement of cartilage between the prosthesis and the tympanic membrane to prevent extrusion has been suggested by a number of surgeons including Sheehy, who has reported excellent results.[14] However, in a 1982 long-term study by Smyth,[15] a 57% failure rate in hearing restoration was noted with the use of PORPs (partial ossicular replacement prostheses) and further, the proportion of unsatisfactory results increased with the passage of time. Smyth also reported an 11% extrusion rate. Kerr[16] has recently reported electron microscope evidence of giant cell digestion of porous polyethylene when used as an ossicular replacement in the human middle ear.

There is a paucity of long-term reports with any type of ossicular chain reconstruction. It is evident that there have been a number of changes in techniques and materials in ossicular reconstruction but with few reports as to why. Figure 1 gives some indication of the changing trends in ossicular chain reconstruction. The analysis is based on the number of papers written about each type of ossicular reconstructive material in five-year blocks over 25 years. The materials considered are ossicles, bone, cartilage, and three synthetic materials — polyethylene, Proplast and Plastipore.

Freeze-dried otologic orthotopic allografts, with their superior mechanical design and minimal physiochemical alteration of donor tissue, offer an attractive alternative to the use of alloplasts and chemically-fixed or heat-processed ossicular grafts. The advantages of allograft bone over alloplastic materials (metals/plastics) depend upon host acceptance and viability of the implant. Controversy is evident in the variety of techniques which exist for processing ossicular grafts, including autoclaving, freezing, freeze-drying, organic mercurials, formalin and alcohol. Based on animal and clinical research, freeze-dried bone and fibrous tissue are stable transplants when stored in vacuum, function similarly to an autograft and retain their original molecular structure. Grafts can be stored at room temperature as long as the vacuum is retained.[17]

From the Division of Otolaryngology/Head and Neck Surgery, Stanford University Medical Center, Stanford, California.

Presented at the meeting of the American Otological Society, Inc., Palm Beach, Florida, May 2-3, 1982.

REPRINTS — Mansfield F. W. Smith, MD, Ear Medical Clinic of Santa Clara Valley, 2120 Forest Avenue, San Jose, CA 95128.

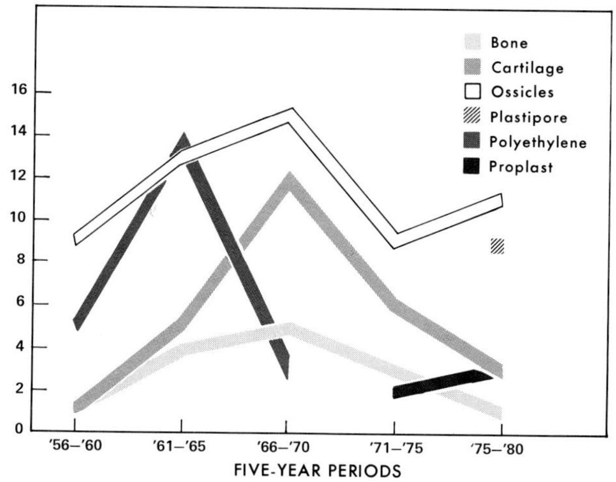

Fig. 1. Number of publications per 5-year period (1956-1980) for various types of ossicular reconstructive material.

PROCEDURES AND MATERIALS

PROCUREMENT

The process begins with procurement of the otologic allografts. The temporal bone cores are removed from the refrigerated cadaver within 24 hours of death. Only temporal bones uninvolved with neoplasm or infection are selected. There are no donor age limits.

The temporal bone cores are removed from the cadaver under clean, but not aseptic conditions. Cores are surface-decontaminated with an iodophor solution of providone-iodine (Betadine) and rinsed repeatedly with sterile 0.9% saline solution until the washings are clear; they are stored at 4°C for no longer than 14 days in normal saline.

PROCESSING

Ethylene-oxide sterilization and freeze-drying are carried out in the following manner:

1. The temporal bone is dissected, and the de-epithelialized tympanic membrane and periosteal cuff and attached malleus, incus and stapes are removed together or separately.
2. Graft tissue is placed in a container in which it is gas-sterilized. The 10% ethylene oxide/90% carbon dioxide gas sterilization is carried out in an ethylene oxide sterilizer (Steri-Vac, model 400, 3M Co, Minneapolis) at 29.4°C. The gas sterilization is performed under vacuum, which allows the gas to permeate the tissue thoroughly for a period of 4½ hours.
3. The graft is frozen to −70°C in a two-stage freezer for at least one hour. The graft may be stored indefinitively in this state.
4. The bottles containing grafts are transferred to the freeze-dryer (VerTis, model 25 SRC) using aseptic precautions. The grafts are freeze-dried for five days with the condenser temperature set at −56°C and the shelf temperature set at 20°C. This prolonged freeze-drying ensures a low water content and reduces dramatically the residual levels of ethylene oxide and its hydrolysis products left in the tissue.
5. The allograft containers are sealed. Test samples that underwent the same processing are cultured. The culture reports are available in 24 hours.

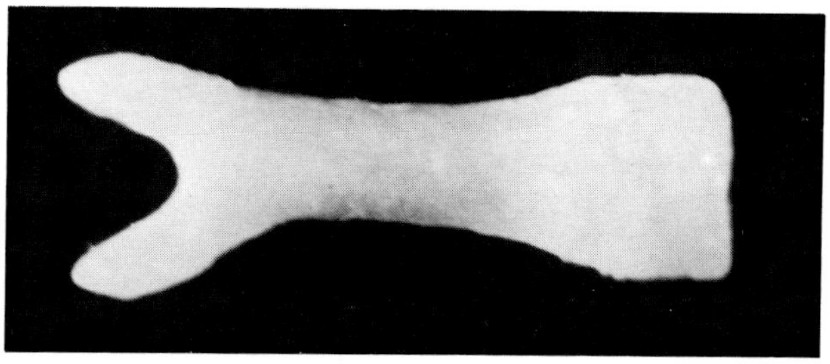

Fig. 2. Partial ossicular replacement allograft (PORA).

Ethylene oxide is used for sterilization because it is an effective agent against all microorganisms and causes no identifiable tissue alteration. Sterile, nontoxic implants are produced by this process. Ethylene oxide is a colorless gas at ordinary room temperatures; it liquefies readily at 10.9°C and freezes at −111.3°C. This chemical not only dissolves in ordinary solvents, including water, but also permeates solids from which unreacted ethylene oxide is slowly released. An inherent disadvantage of ethylene oxide is the fact that it, or its breakdown product, is retained.[18] Work at the Bone Transplant Unit of the Northern California Transplant Bank has demonstrated that residual concentrations of ethylene oxide and its toxic by-products are satisfactorily reduced following prolonged lyophilization. In addition, the depth of penetration of ethylene oxide necessary for sterilization of otologic transplants further reduces the potential for toxicity.

The PORA (Fig. 2) is positioned between the malleus neck and stapes head in stable ears. Reliable reconstruction of the middle ear transformer mechanism requires that the neck of the malleus be positioned over the oval window. Occasionally it is necessary to remove the entire tympanic membrane and malleus as an autograft and reposition the neck of the malleus over the oval window because of the poor angle or too much distance between the head of the stapes and the neck of the malleus. If the tympanic membrane and malleus are being reconstructed, an allograft de-epithelialized fibrous tympanic membrane with attached periosteal cuff is used to position the malleus neck over the oval window. Both of these procedures, the autograft and allograft repositioning of the tympanic membrane malleus unit, are done in two stages with a PORA placed between the neck of the malleus and stapes head approximately 4 to 6 months after the initial procedure.

The partial ossicular allografts come in various sizes and are measured from the end or central portion of the acetabulum to the center of the crutch. It is expected that these replacement allografts may need some modification by the otologic surgeon to adjust to the specific needs of each patient. These ossicular replacement allografts are homotropic in that they are fashioned from human ossicles. To fit between the malleus neck and stapes head, the PORAs are fabricated in sizes from 2 to 3 mm in 0.25 mm increments and from 3 to 5 mm in 0.5 mm increments.

Measuring Instruments. Measuring instruments are essential to accurately determine the distance between the neck of the malleus and head of the stapes or the mobile footplate. In addition, the measuring device (JedMed Instrument Co, St. Louis; Richards Manufacturing Co, Memphis) must serve as an instrument for lifting the malleus handle in order to obtain an accurate measurement, as the malleus handle may be slightly loose or need to be retracted laterally, in order to be in a more anatomically correct position.

RESULTS

Of 32 PORAs used in stable ears, 24 closed the air-bone gap to 10 dB, a 75% success rate. There was minimal deterioration after three months, and no evidence of extrusion. The maximum follow-up was $3^{1}/_{2}$ years; minimum follow-up was four months.

Of the eight ears that failed to close the air-bone gap to functional levels, there was either too great an angle between the neck of the malleus and stapes head or a distance in excess of 3.5 mm. Thus, it is essential that the surgeon determine accurately the distance between the head of the malleus and also calculate whether there is too much angle between the stapes head and malleus neck. At this point the surgeon must decide whether to reposition the tympanic membrane malleus unit which will require slightly more removal of the posterior osseous canal than is removed at a stapedectomy procedure to allow rotation of the malleus neck over the oval window. Then, at a second stage procedure, 4 to 6 months later, a PORA can be placed between the malleus neck and stapes head.

CONCLUSION

Use of alloplasts in middle ear reconstruction (other than stapes replacement in otosclerosis) are suspect for long-term foreign body extrusion and poor functional results. Otologic allografts (homografts), freeze-dried and ethylene-oxide-sterilized, offer an atractive alternative to the use of alloplasts and chemically fixed or heat-processed ossicular grafts for middle ear transformer reconstruction.

REFERENCES

1. Matte. Über Versuche mit Ainheilung des Trommelfells an das Kopfchen des Steigbügels nach operative Behandlung chronischer Mittelöhreiter-ungen. Arch Ohren Nasen Kehlkopfheilkd 1901; 53:96-9.
2. Hall A, Rytzner C. Stapedectomy and autotransplantation of ossicles. Acta Otolaryngol (Stockh) 1957: 47:318-25.
3. Jansen C. Über Radikaloperation und Tympanoplastik. Sitzungsber Fortbild. Ärztekamm. Ob V, Feb. 18, 1958.
4. House WF, Patterson ME, Linthicum FH Jr. Incus homografts in chronic ear surgery. Arch Otolaryngol 1966; 84: 148-53.
5. Guilford FR. Repositioning of the incus. Laryngoscope 1965; 75:236-41.
6. Smyth GD, Kerr AG. Homologous grafts for ossicular reconstruction in tympanoplasty. Laryngoscope 1967; 77:330-6.
7. De Sebastian G. The replacement of portions of the ear ossicles with artificial substances. Acta Oto-Rino-Laringol Ibero-Am 1960; 11:259-68.
8. Glaninger J. Zur operativen Wiederherstellung einer durch Schädeltrauma unterbrochenen Gehörknöchelchenkette. Z Laryngol Rhinol Otol 1964; 43:184-90.
9. Siedentop KH, Brown RC. Type 3. Polyethylene columella tympanoplasty. Long-range review of 28 cases. Arch Otolaryngol 1966; 83:560-5.
10. Sheehy JL. Ossicular problems in tympanoplasty. Arch Otolaryngol 1965; 81:115-22.
11. Shea JJ, Homsy CA. The use of Proplast TM in otologic surgery. Laryngoscope 1974; 84:1835-45.
12. Shea JJ, Emmett JR. Biocompatible ossicular implants. Arch Otolaryngol 1978; 104:191-6.
13. Strauss P. Vergleich von Ambossinterposition und Kunststoff-columella bei der Tympanoplastik. Laryngol Rhinol Otol (Stuttg) 1979; 58:15-22.
14. Sheehy JL. TORPs and PORPs in tympanoplasty. Clin Otolaryngol 1978; 3:451-4.
15. Smyth G. Five year report on PORPs and TORPs. Otolaryngol Head Neck Surg 1982; 90:343-6.
16. Kerr AG. Proplast and Plastipore. Clin Otolaryngol 1981; 6:187-92.
17. Smith MFW. Freeze-dried otologic implants. J Otolaryngol 1980; 9:222-7.
18. Rosomoff HL. Ethylene oxide sterilized, freeze-dried dura mater for the repair of pachymeningeal defects. J Neurosurg 1959; 16:197.

Pathology Consultation

MIDFACIAL NECROTIZING DISEASES

JOHN G. BATSAKIS, MD
HOUSTON, TEXAS

Necrotizing and apparently nonhealing disease of the upper aerodigestive tract can be the result of a host of underlying causes. Exclusion of specific agents and malignancy masquerading as so-called nonhealing granulomas is mandatory. This done, four disorders enter the differential diagnosis; Wegener's granulomatosis, non-Hodgkin's lymphoma, polymorphic reticulosis and idiopathic midline granuloma. Given representative biopsy material, the first three have sufficient specific diagnostic features that separation is possible. Such identification is important because of the varying responses to therapy.

Necrotizing lesions of the upper airway continue to frustrate pathologists, exasperate clinicians, and spawn a considerable literary effort. Vagueness in the literature, paucity of cases, and an inability to determine the causal basis of the lesions have led some to consider that clinical assessment of the patient is the only valid basis for making a diagnosis and treating the patient.[1]

For a pathologist there are three problem areas in the evaluation of a biopsy specimen from a necrotizing lesion of the nasal or oral cavities and the paranasal sinuses: 1) adequacy of the biopsy specimen, 2) elimination of specific infectious agents as the etiology, and 3) classification of the disorders.

Because surface necrosis and crusting are nearly obligatory with such lesions, the imposition of an inflammatory reaction may be so great that diagnostic features are obscured. Superficial biopsies will yield only a diagnosis of "nonspecific inflammation." Biopsy at the margins of the ulcers and/or deeper tissue representation will produce more representative tissue for examination.

The elimination by culture and special stains of specific etiologically determined diseases such as histoplasmosis and other fungal and microbial diseases is *mandatory*. This cannot be overstressed since these diseases account for a majority of such lesions on a worldwide basis.[2] Also to be eliminated are epithelial neoplasms that have provoked a localized necrotizing reaction.

The remaining patients, given representative biopsy specimens, fall into three disease categories; Wegener's granulomatosis, polymorphic reticulosis and idiopathic nonhealing (midline) granuloma. The number of synonyms and suggested "spectrum" array for these entities has served to confuse, rather than to clarify classification for pathologists and surgeons.

Owing to different responses to therapy, more precise definition of these clinicopathologic entities is required.[3] All have the common clinical feature of upper airway involvement, but their similarity largely ends there.

Wegener's granulomatosis is a systemic disease and the cardinal symptoms of the disease are related to a generalized hypersensitivity-like phenomenon involving the lungs and kidneys. Of the three disorders mentioned above, Wegener's granulomatosis is the *least* clinically destructive, an important differential diagnostic point.[2,3] It has a well-defined clinical course with development of a serious glomerulonephritis and involvement of the lungs and other organs. Given the symptom complex, it is certainly not reasonable to exclude the diagnosis when

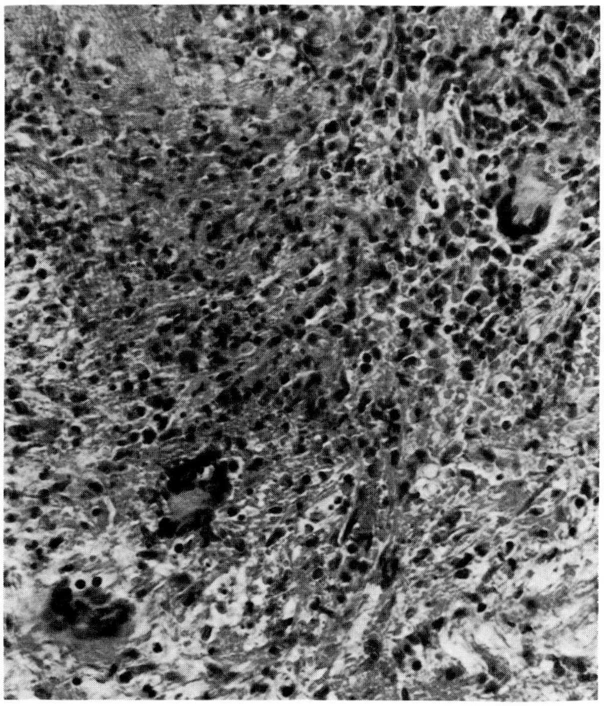

Fig. 1. Wegener's granulomatosis in maxillary sinus mucosa. Giant cells, fibrinoid necrosis and an inflammatory infiltrate are present in subepithelial tissue. (H & E, x85)

From the Department of Pathology and Laboratory Medicine, Maine Medical Center, Portland.
REPRINTS — John G. Batsakis, MD, Department of Pathology, M.D. Anderson Hospital, Texas Medical Center, Houston, TX 77030.

TABLE 1. MIDFACIAL NONHEALING LESIONS: DIFFERENTIAL FEATURES

	Wegener's Granulomatosis	*Polymorphic Reticulosis*	*Idiopathic Midline Granuloma*
Upper airway	Diffuse in upper airway, predominantly sinuses; erosion of facial bones and soft tissue is rare	Destructive localized or diffuse lesions; characteristic extension through palate and soft tissues	Most destructive of group; bone and soft tissue extension progressive and common
Systemic involvement	Classically a systemic disease; kidneys, lungs and small vessels	Localized *or* systemic; systemic manifestations are lymphoma-like	Localized to airway and upper aerodigestive tract
Association with malignancy	No known association	Very likely a form of lymphoma	May remain unspecific or evolve to polymorphic reticulosis
Histopathologic features	Necrotizing vasculitis, granulomas and giant cells, no atypical cells	Atypical and polymorphic cells, angiocentric and angioinfiltrative growth pattern, lymphoma or lymphoma-like	Nonspecific acute and chronic inflammation, usually no atypical cells
Treatment	Cyclophosphamide with or without steroids	Radiation therapy	Radiation therapy

a single biopsy specimen fails to demonstrate the histologic features.[3]

A triad of histologic findings characterize the microscopic appearance of Wegener's granulomatosis. These are a necrotizing *vasculitis*, *giant cell* granulomas, and a nonpleomorphic cellular infiltrate (Fig. 1).

Identification and elimination of Wegener's granulomatosis leave a collection of lesions that are more locally destructive and that also tend to exhibit a rather distinctive natural history. Within the group are the non-Hodgkin's extranodal lymphomas and a subset of lesions that behave clinically in a manner comparable to lymphomas. Ambiguity still exists over the exact nosologic status of this class of lesions. They are separable from those of Wegener's granulomatosis by an absence of necrotizing granulomas and giant cells; by a noticeable angiocentric and angioinfiltrative cellular growth pattern; and by an abundant, usually polymorphic and atypical lymphoreticular cellular component.[2-4]

The polymorphic infiltrate distinguishes the lesion from the typically monomorphic non-Hodgkin's lymphomas but only imperfectly from the mixed histiocytic-lymphocytic and histiocytic lymphomas. The terms polymorphic reticulosis and malignant midline reticulosis have been applied to these lesions. They clearly signify the pathologists' recognition of the atypical cellular infiltrate and also that the process is a lymphoreticular proliferative lesion rather than a vascular-based disorder (vasculitis).

Evidence is now accumulating that polymorphic reticulosis represents a form of lymphoma.[5] The local midfacial destructiveness, dissemination in the manner of lymphomas, and the cellular appearance certainly point to such an identity. Reluctance on the part of pathologists to cross the diagnostic "Rubicon" rests with a) their caution against making a diagnosis of lymphoma in such extranodal sites, b) difficulties inherent in histopathologic diagnosis of small-celled lesions from this area, and c) finding an acceptable position for the polymorphic lesion in existing classifications of lymphoma.

Idiopathic nonhealing (midline) granuloma is the most enigmatic of this group of lesions.[2,3] Not only is there no etiologic basis for the lesion, it presents with a completely nondescript, chronic, necrotizing inflammatory reaction. Clear-cut granuloma formation is found in about half of the cases and a vasculitis is seen on occasion. However, the vasculitis is not of a primary character but more of a endarteritis obliterans that is associated with tissue necrosis and infection. It is a localized disorder without systemic manifestations. Relentlessly progressive, idiopathic midline granuloma is likely the most mutilating of all of the midfacial disorders.[3]

The above is just a distillate of a rather extensive literature on these disorders. At the risk of reducing to dangerous simplicity, this brief report and Table 1 present contemporary thinking and allow a rather unencumbered, practical approach to diagnosis and treatment.

SUMMARY

Wegener's granulomatosis, a systemic disorder, manifests specific clinical and histopathologic findings that allow it to be separated from an unrelated group of upper airway lesions. Two of these, non-Hodgkin's lymphoma and polymorphic reticulosis, are related and may in fact be variable expressions of a lymphoma. A fourth, and fortunately rare, disorder presents as a severely destructive localized lesion without any specific histopathologic findings.

REFERENCES

1. Harrison DFN. Non-healing granuloma of the upper respiratory tract. Br Med J 1974; 4:205-9.

2. Batsakis JG. Wegener's granulomatosis and midline (nonhealing) "granuloma." Head Neck Surg 1979; 1:213-22.

3. Fauci AS, Wolff SM. Wegener's granulomatosis and related diseases. Dis Mon 1977; 23:1-35.

4. McDonald TJ, DeRemee RA, Harrison EG Jr, Facer GW, Devine KD. The protean clinical features of polymorphic reticulosis (lethal midline granuloma). Laryngoscope 1976; 86:936-45.

5. Michaels L, Gregory MM. Pathology of "non-healing (midline) granuloma." J Clin Pathol 1977; 30:317-27.

X-RAY STUDY OF THE MONTH

INTRACAVERNOUS INTERNAL CAROTID ARTERY ANEURYSM

A. L. WEBER, MD
BOSTON, MASSACHUSETTS

K. R. DAVIS, MD
BOSTON, MASSACHUSETTS

R. G. OJEMANN, MD
BOSTON, MASSACHUSETTS

M. NEGRI, MD
ROME, ITALY

PATIENT

Four months prior to admission this 45-year-old woman noted double vision when looking straight ahead or to the right. This improved after ten days, but recurred three weeks prior to admission. Neurological examination at the time of admission demonstrated a right 6th nerve paresis. The patient had experienced severe headaches for many years. At age 30, she had a meningeal syndrome with pleocytosis on spinal fluid examination. Her blood pressure at that time reached 160/100.

RADIOGRAPHIC FINDINGS

The tomographic section (Fig. 1A) reveals a sharply marginated hemispheric erosion of the right sphenoid bone at the level of the sella turcica (arrowheads). Coronal (Fig. 1B) and axial (Fig. 1C) CT scans demonstrate a contrast enhanced right parasellar mass lesion causing bony erosion (arrowheads).

DIAGNOSIS

An AP film of the carotid angiogram (Fig. 2A) following transfemoral catheterization confirmed the presence of a large intracavernous aneurysm of the right internal carotid artery (arrowheads). A Crutchfield clamp (Fig. 2B) was placed just above the origin of the right internal carotid artery and the vessel was totally occluded. A left vertebral angiogram following placement of the clamp revealed good collateral supply to the right hemisphere. (Fig. 2C), filling of the supraclinoid portion of the internal carotid artery (arrowhead), and nonfilling of the aneurysm.

DISCUSSION

Intracavernous carotid aneurysms occur in patients ranging in age from 22 to 71 years, chiefly in women over age 40.[1] The incidence of these aneurysms is from about 5% to 11% of cerebral aneurysms.[1,2] Bilateral aneurysms have been reported.[3] Rupture may occur when the aneurysm is small, causing a carotid-cavernous fistula with consequent pulsating exophthalmos, ocular palsy, and cephalic bruit.[4] Expansion of the aneurysmal sac causes com-

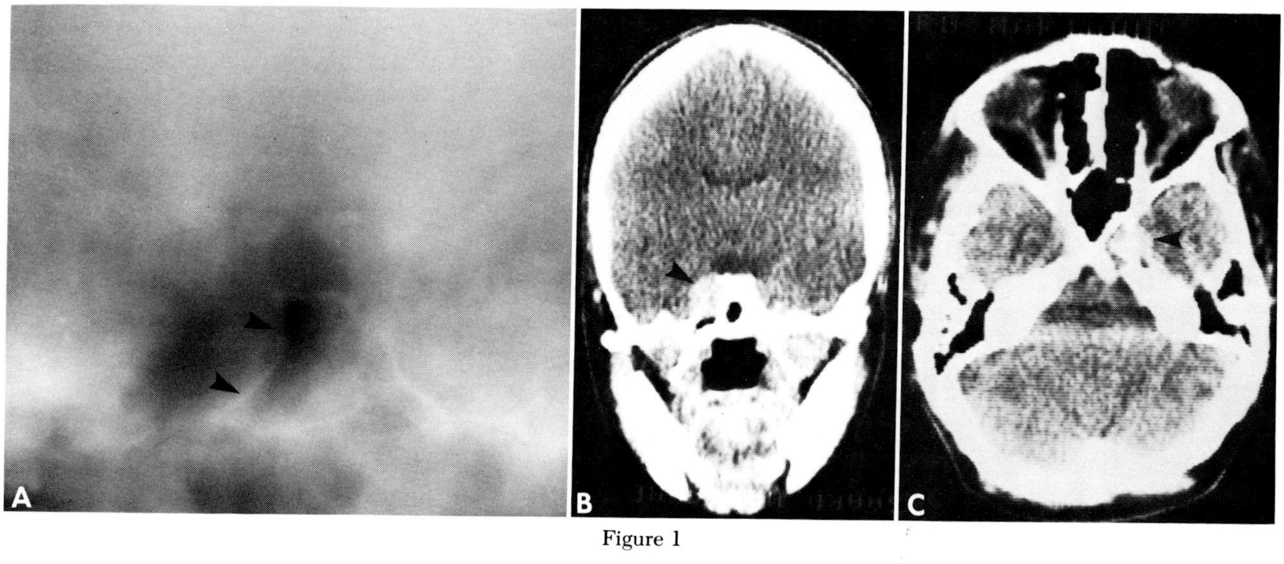

Figure 1

From the Department of Radiology, Massachusets Eye and Ear Infirmary, Boston.
REPRINTS — Alfred L. Weber, MD, Department of Radiology, Massachusetts Eye and Ear Infirmary, 243 Charles St., Boston, MA 02114.

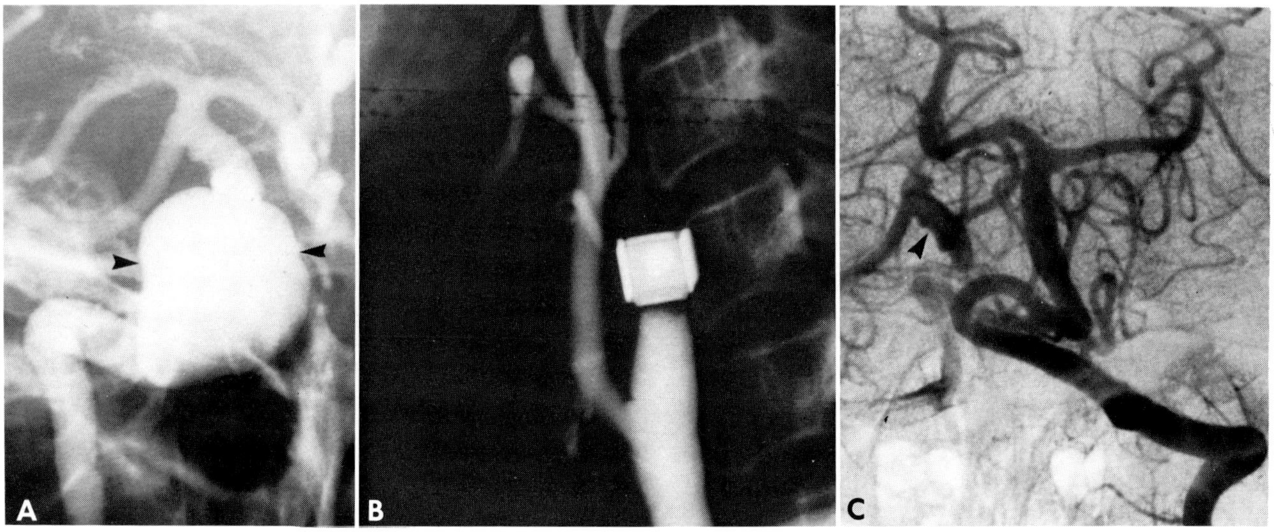

Figure 2

pression of the nerves in the cavernous sinus with paresis of the sixth, third, and fifth cranial nerves in that order of frequency. Disturbance of function of the sixth cranial nerve is almost always the first clinical feature and may be the only clinical sign for a considerable period of time as demonstrated in this case. Progressing visual failure, temporal defect of visual fields, exophthalmos, and loss of smell are other symptoms that may be encountered. The close relationship of these aneurysms to the base of the skull often produces osseous changes as demonstrated in our case. The roentgen findings[5] consist of undercutting of the anterior clinoid process, erosion of the lateral half of the sphenoid with or without erosion of the posterior clinoid process. If the aneurysm extends anteriorly there is enlargement of the superior orbital fissure and/or erosion of the inferolateral portion of the optic canal.[2] Posterior extension of the aneurysm may lead to erosion of the middle cranial fossa and in a large aneurysm erosion of the tip of the petrous pyramid. Complete or partial calcification of the wall of the aneurysm has been reported to occur in 33%, 38%, and 53% of cases.[1,2,6]

The plain CT scan may show elevated absorption values that are due to circulating blood within the unthrombosed aneurysmal sac.[7-9] The high values are a function of the protein content of the hemoglobin. Calcification of the wall of the aneurysmal sac or within areas of thrombosis may produce high values. Following infusion of contrast material, the circulating blood pool within the unthrombosed sac shows homogeneous enhancement (26 Hounsefield units per 100 mg% of iodine). The location of cerebral aneurysms is usually at the area of the circle of Willis, peripheral middle cerebral arteries from mycotic aneurysms and along the basilar artery or other large vessels for fusiform aneurysms. A meningioma has to be differentiated from a large aneurysm. The plain CT scan in meningiomas shows a high absorption coefficient due to psammomatous calcification in most cases, but there may occasionally be low absorption areas within an isodense or high absorption lesion.[10] Surrounding edema is often present as well as a mass effect. In meningiomas the contrast enhancement is uniform through the high absorption area. Aneurysms usually produce displacement of thin bony margins whereas meningiomas produce a hyperostotic bone reaction. The calcification in association with an aneurysm, if present, is usually along the sac wall whereas in meningioma may be scattered throughout the high absorption area. If the bone changes are not clear on CT scan, polytomes may provide additional information. Finally, angiography, which is necessary before surgery in either case, will show filling of the unthrombosed portion of an aneurysmal sac, and in case of a meningioma, dural feeders with a vascular blush. Excision of intracavernous carotid artery aneurysms is surgically not feasible and occlusion of the internal carotid artery on the side of the aneurysm by ligation or balloon placement, sometimes with prior superficial temporal-middle cerebral artery bypass, is the preferred treatment.

REFERENCES

1. Lombardi G, Passerini A, Migliavacca F. Intracavernous aneurysms of the internal carotid artery. AJR 1963; 89:361-71.

2. Rischbieth R, Bull J. Significance of enlargement of superior orbital (sphenoidal) fissure. Br J Radiol 1958; 31:125-35.

3. Noterman J, Warszawski M, Jeanmart L, Brihaye J. Bilateral aneurysm of the internal carotid artery in the cavernous sinus: case report. Neuroradiology 1972; 4:63-5.

4. Barr H, Blackwood W, Meadows S. Intracavernous carotid aneurysms. Brain 1971; 94:607-22.

5. Sosman M, Vogt E. Aneurysms of internal carotid artery and circle of Willis from a roentgenological viewpoint. AJR 1926; 15:122-34.

6. Meadows S. Intracavernous aneurysms of internal carotid artery. Arch Ophthalmol 1959; 62:566-74.

7. Laryne M, Kleefield J, Davis K, Ojemann R, Crowell R. Giant intracranial aneurysms of the anterior circulation. Clinical characteristics and diagnosis by computed tomography. Neurosurgery 1978; 3:356-63.

8. Pinto R, Kricheff I. Butler A, Murali R. Correlation of computed tomographic angiographic, and neuropathological changes in giant cerebral aneurysms. Radiology 1979; 132:85-92.

9. Schubiger O, Valavanis A, Hayek J. Computed tomography in cerebral aneurysms with special emphasis on giant intracranial aneurysms. J Comput Assist Tomogr 1980; 1:24-32.

10. Lee K, Lin S. Neuroradiology of sellar and juxtasellar lesions. Springfield, Ill.: Charles C Thomas, 1979.

≈

THIRD INTERNATIONAL SYMPOSIUM ON RECENT ADVANCES IN OTITIS MEDIA WITH EFFUSION: CALL FOR PAPERS

Papers are being solicited for the Third International Symposium on Recent Advances in Otitis Media with Effusion, which will be held May 17-20, 1983, at the Bahia Mar Hotel, Fort Lauderdale, Florida. The deadline for submitting titles is November 15, 1982, and the deadline for submitting abstracts is January 15, 1983. For further information, write David J. Lim, MD, Program Chairman, 4331 University Hospitals Clinic, 456 Clinic Drive, Columbus, OH 43210.

≈

CASSELBERRY AWARD

The American Laryngological Association announces that it will receive essays or theses relating to the art and science of laryngology and rhinology for consideration of the Casselberry Award for 1982-1983. The Award is open to physicians, interns, residents, and graduate students in laryngology and rhinology in the Americas and scientists in the field in laryngology and rhinology. For further information write to Eugene N. Myers, MD, Secretary, American Laryngological Association, Eye and Ear Hospital, 230 Lothrop St., Suite 1115, Pittsburgh, PA 15213.

BOOK REVIEWS

Oral Cancer and Precancer

By *Jens J. Pindborg*. Hard cover, black and white illustrations, indexed, referenced, 177 pages, 1980. John Wright and Sons Ltd, Bristol, Great Britain. Price $35.00.

In a unique approach to oral cancer and precancerous lesions of the mouth, Professor Pindborg's monograph explores these entities together in the same chapters. The first 11 chapters consider the epidemiology, clinical aspects, histopathology, etiology, and treatment of cancers and precancers of the lip, buccal mucosa, floor of mouth, tongue, palate, palatine arch, gingiva, and alveolar ridge. The remaining 12 chapters focus on etiology, treatment, histopathology, cellular and humoral immunity, and treatments of precancerous conditions. These chapters concentrate on the topognosis of precancer relating this complex entity to the clinical aspects of oral cancer. Pindborg documents his material with the most relevant, recent, and profound references from the world literature.

Pindborg defines and explains the histopathology of epithelial dysplasia, epithelial atypia, and dyskeratosis. His descriptions of lip cancer and precancer are exhaustive, divided equally between lesions of the vermilion border and labial commissures. The relationship between nodular leukoplakia and cancer is emphasized in the lips as well as buccal and floor of mouth areas. He establishes the erythroplakic lesion as a squamous carcinoma percursor and notes the seeming discrepancy between the relatively low numbers of oral leukoplakias found in certain high risk oral cancer populations. While his treatment of tongue cancer is limited, the epidemiologic features of this disease are thoroughly treated. Palate cancer is the rarest of all oral cancers in Europe and North America with a surprisingly high 37% of patients with soft palate carcinomas having regional lymph node metastasis. For otolaryngologists, Professor Pindborg's treatment of the palatine arch will be found superficial; it encompasses only one page of the monograph. In that brief encounter Pindborg points out that 17% to 19% of patients with palatine arch cancer have additional primary cancers elsewhere. His description of the serpiginous form of gingival cancer as "forme bourgeonnante" is memorable and precisely the description this lesion deserves; his review of the epidemiology of this disease is excellent.

It is unclear why Chapter 12, "Intraosseous Carcinoma of the Jaws," was included. Although a delightful little chapter describing both secondary carcinomatous invasion of the jaws along with primary carcinoma, it seems orphaned in the context of Pindborg's prior treatment of oral cancer and precancer. It serves as a transition, however, to the final 11 chapters devoted to general principles related to oral malignancies. The relationship of leukoplakia, carcinoma in situ, and epithelial dysplasia is considered in depth in Chapter 13. Again, Pindborg points out the danger of erythroplakic lesions. The discussion of etiology, topognostic considerations, and precancerous diseases includes complete discussions of syphilis, sideropenic dysphagia, lichen planus, submucous fibrosis, discoid lupus erythematosus, and dyskeratosis congenita.

The microscopic features of oral cancer are well-documented along with a schematic representation of McKinney and Singh's concept that "advanced dysplasia or carcinoma in situ lesions may produce excessive quantitites of collagenase or collagenase-like enzymes which are released into the intercellular spaces."

The final seven, quite brief chapters in this monograph include discussions of tobacco, alcohol, liver cirrhosis, diet, industrial hazards, social distribution and dental factors. Treatment of oral cancer is considered in a review of the literature of chemotherapy, surgery and radiation therapy. There is even a section on cryosurgery. Osteoradionecrosis is given a thorough treatment including histological characterization and the oral pathologist's plea for the conservation of teeth when radiation therapy is utilized.

The last four chapters include classification, histology, etiology, and treatment of oral leukoplakia. While the reader expects this section to be redundant, he is surprised and delighted to find microradiographic, cell kinetic, and electron microscopic studies to document Pindborg's thorough treatment of leukoplakia.

In summary, Pindborg has, in a stream of consciousness fashion, organized a huge volume of material relating to an area on which he is one of the world's great authorities. His documentation of precancerous oral lesions, their relationship to oral cancers, the etiologies, topognosis, treatment, and epidemiology of these conditions are included in a readable and condensed form. For the otolaryngologist, this monograph is a must read, invaluable addition to his library.

William H. Friedman, MD
St. Louis, Missouri

Acoustic Factors Affecting Hearing Aid Performance

By *Gerald A. Studebaker* and *Irving Hochberg*. Hard cover, black and white illustrations, indexed, referenced, 450 pages, 1980. University Park Press, Baltimore. Price $34.50.

The last decade has produced a vast amount of important, relevant and complex research in diverse areas related to hearing aids. An understanding of the overall importance of recent developments and their interaction requires considerable effort on the part of any professional who is concerned with electronic amplification. Consequently, a conference was held in June 1978 in which leading researchers presented some recent developments. This book is the proceedings of this conference and is intended to represent information on the current state-of-the-art in amplification for the hearing-impaired.

The title of the book implies that it is concerned only about acoustic factors of hearing aid performance; these include environmental acoustics, earmold acoustics, and transducer-related factors. A significant portion, however, is devoted to the effect of these acoustic factors on the hearing-impaired listener's performance. Thus, the book is more broadly based than its title implies.

The 18 chapters of this book are divided into four major sections. The first section deals with acoustics of the listening environment. Considerable emphasis is placed on signal changes due to reverberation and their effects on perception in both normal and hearing-impaired listeners. Also discussed are the effects of microphone location and the effects of acoustic environment on the effectiveness of directional hearing aids.

The second section deals mainly with acoustic factors related to the coupling of hearing aids to ears. The acoustics of the external ear and of the now much-used "Zwislocki" coupler are given in detail. On the application side, the acoustics of earmolds are given in sufficient detail to be used clinically. Important concepts which are discussed are the effects of commercial venting systems, open earmolds, and the "Killion" horn earmold.

The third section describes various quantitative modeling techniques which are capable of describing the acoustic coupling of hearing aids to ears. Sufficient detail is given for these models so that interested persons may implement them to make predictions about the signal reaching the eardrum.

Finally, the last section covers important issues related to frequency-selective hearing aid fitting techniques. Although no single method emerges as being optimal, the series of chapters clearly identifies some important concepts for frequency-specific amplification.

The overall quality of this book is excellent. It serves as an important reference book for researchers and clinicians interested in quantitative effects of amplification for the hearing-impaired.

Gerald R. Popelka, PhD
St. Louis, Missouri

Pocket Guide to Antimicrobial Therapy in Otolaryngology

By *David N. F. Fairbanks*. Soft cover, indexed, 57 pages, 1981. American Council of Otolaryngology — Head and Neck Surgery, Washington, D. C.

This publication is offered as a concise and practical guide to the practicing otolaryngologist caring for commonplace problems. The handbook begins with a section organized according to clinical diagnosis which is then followed by an overview of antimicrobials by category. A list of the "drugs of choice" according to infecting organism and clinical diagnosis is included in addition to a table of appropriate dosage schedules.

There are several points that can be commented upon. 1) The throat culture for group A β-hemolytic streptococci, although imperfect, is still a valuable guide to antimicrobial therapy when performed and interpreted properly. 2) In regard to exudative tonsillitis, Epstein-Barr virus, adenovirus, influenza A and herpes simplex are common causative agents of this syndrome. 3) The role of *Staphylococcus aureus* and *Hemophilus influenzae* as etiologic agents of pharyngitis is difficult to evaluate as these organisms are most often regarded as normal pharyngeal flora (carriage rates are approximately 40% and 15% respectively). 4) *H influenzae* does indeed cause mastoiditis and should be considered when prescribing for this entity. 5) The appropriateness of rifampin prophylaxis of family members of children with nonmeningitis *H influenzae* infections has not been established. 6) Several studies on the bacteriology of chronic sinusitis have reported different results. Only a single study, of a group of patients with very chronic infection (≥ 10 years), has reported a significant role for the staphylococcus (Frederick and Braude). The likelihood of anaerobic bacteria, *H influenzae* and viridans streptococci causing infection are noted but they are not provided for in the first "drug of choice" for chronic sinusitis. A cephalosporin might be a better first choice, with erythromycin/sulfasoxazole as an alternative agent for outpatient management. 7) Aminoglycosides are generally considered bactericidal rather than bacteriostatic, unless they are used in very small doses. 8) The drug of choice for diphtheria is penicillin or erythromycin. 9) Penicillin and chloramphenicol would be the drugs of choice for brain abscess secondary to an otic or a sinus focus. 10) The author notes that deep neck abscess is often a consequence of a mixed infection including anaerobes but neglects to provide antimicrobial coverage for these organisms in his recommended drug of choice.

The section on selection of drugs is a "nuts and bolts" approach which is both thoughtful and sensible. This publication will be useful to students, house officers and practitioners.

ELLEN R. WALD, MD
Pittsburgh, Pennsylvania

Manual of Electronystagmography, Second Edition

By *Hugh O. Barber* and *Charles W. Stockwell*. Hard cover, black and white illustrations, indexed, 224 pages, 1980. C. V. Mosby Co, St. Louis.

This book remains the standard textbook for otoneurologists and technicians who carry out electronystagmography. The text is complete and presents many theories concerning the integration of eye movement that is necessary for orientation in a space. The standard methods of otoneurological examination are well covered.

The chapter on physiology of eye movement contains a mass of information that is rather speculative. It may cause some difficulties of assimilation especially for technicians. A more general approach may be more appealing to many.

The clinical cases illustrated by electronystagmographic findings continue to be most helpful and instructive. All in all, the book is a "must" for otoneurological offices.

MALCOLM H. STROUD, MD
St. Louis, Missouri

Craniofacial and Upper Cervical Arteries: Functional, Clinical & Angiographic Aspects

By *Pierre L. LasJaunias* and *Alex Berenstein*. Hard cover, black and white and color illustrations, indexed, 195 pages, 1981. Williams and Wilkins Co, Baltimore. Price $57.00.

This book takes a novel and relevant approach to the anatomy of the external carotid artery and its craniofacial branches. Conventional texts have dealt with vascular anatomy by tracing arteries from origin to territory of supply discussing variations observed in dissected materials. With the advent of magnification and subtraction angiography, in vivo and thus functional anatomy can be deduced. Hypothesizing that the functional significance of a vessel depends more on its territorial distribution than its origin and proximal course, Dr. LasJaunias discusses the complicated anatomy of the external carotid system by proceeding from the angioarchitecture of the supplied tissue to variants of proximal supply expected within the constraints of development, hemodynamics, and osseus anatomy. The phylogeny and ontogeny of the major external carotid branches are also discussed at the beginning of their respective chapters.

After an introductory chapter on the branching pattern of the external carotid trunk and hemodynamics, the book is organized into sections covering major anatomic regions: the internal maxillary system, the pharyngo-occipital system, the upper cervical vertebral column and musculature and skin of the scalp, face and mouth. The final chapter covers the arterial supply of the transosseous peripheral nervous system discussing selected cranial and cervical spinal nerves.

The book contains many subtracted angiogram reproductions of very good quality and a large number of diagrams outlining vascular development and the subsequent variants of adult anatomy. Several color plates of injected cadaveric dissections are also included.

This text is of most value for angiographers, particularly those involved in embolization of vascular lesions of the head and neck, but it is a useful reference text for anyone whose practice includes arteriography of the external carotid system.

PATRICK J. DOYLE, MD
PHILIP HARRISON, MD
Vancouver, British Columbia, Canada

Vocal Fold Physiology

Edited by *Kenneth N. Stevens* and *Minoru Hirano*. Soft cover, black and white illustrations, 421 pages, 1981. University of Tokyo Press, Japan. Price $17.50.

This monograph represents a collection of papers delivered at a conference on Vocal Fold Physiology held January 15-19, 1980, at Kurume University in Japan. The conference was a collaborative effort among vocal physiologists to discuss and compare their work so that subsequent research could provide a more profitable means of understanding the mechanism of vocal fold vibration and control during speech and singing.

The book is divided into six sections. Section I discusses basic morphology and physiology of the larynx. In Section II various methods of observing vocal fold vibration are presented. Section III covers the control of physiologic parameters for speech and singing. Section IV develops models of vocal fold vibration. In Section V models of vibration are discussed with regard to voice quality. Section VI provides an overview of physical properties related to measurements from laryngeal models.

While the major strength of this monograph is its diverse approach to vocal physiology, its weakness, if one were to be identified, is its superficial treatment of complex and controversial issues in laryngeal research. Nevertheless, this document represents an important reference piece for the modern voice physiologist and is recommended for serious researchers in the field.

CLARENCE T. SASAKI, MD
New Haven, Connecticut

Physical Principles of Audiology

By *P. M. Haughton.* Hard cover, black and white illustrations, indexed, referenced, 183 pages, 1980. Adam Hilger Ltd., Bristol, England. Price $28.00.

As our knowledge of the auditory system increases, the technical information needed to understand and apply relevant concepts increases as well. Often there is a need to have a small summary reference book to fill the gap between the information provided by original research articles and that provided by comprehensive text books. *Physical Principles of Audiology* by P. M. Haughton fills this need very well.

This book is the third in a medical physics handbook series, which previously has dealt with ultrasonics and computer principles. The book is intended for use by medical physicists, engineers and audiologists. Organization of the book follows a format similar to that used in many hearing science textbooks which are now available. The beginning chapters deal with the physics of sound, anatomy and physiology of the auditory system, and psychoacoustic measures in the normal hearing ear. Two chapters outline important physiologic measures, namely evoked potentials and acoustic impedance, which are very useful clinically. Another chapter describes some common clinical entities and the routine audiologic measures which are relevant. Finally, a chapter is devoted to hearing aids.

The title of the book accurately describes its emphasis. For example, the acoustics chapter stresses the computational formulae and physical constants which are applicable to typical audiologic measures. The chapter on hearing disorders and the measurement of hearing only briefly describes the actual tests but goes into considerable detail on audiometric standards, calibration couplers and equipment. The acoustic impedance chapter goes into much more detail on measurement procedures and computations than on interpretation of test results.

I was particularly impressed with the precision of the book. The author concisely presents the basic relevant principles yet does not omit esoteric points such as the minutiae of acoustic impedance measurement terminology, small differences among calibration standards, and tabular notation of common sound pressure level meter weightings. Though no new information is presented, this book is a valuable reference which should be on the shelf of many professionals concerned with the auditory system.

GERALD R. POPELKA, PhD
St. Louis, Missouri

Cancer of the Head and Neck

Edited by *James Y. Suen* and *Eugene Myers.* Hard cover, black and white illustrations, indexed, 905 pages, 1981. Churchill Livingstone, Inc, New York. Price $89.00.

There is little doubt that this book represents a major contribution to the diagnosis, understanding, and treatment of head and neck malignancy. There are 32 chapters, each authored by an acknowledged expert in the field. Topics are inclusive of head and neck oncology, diagnosis, site of origin, natural history of disease, treatment, including surgery, radiation and chemotherapy, and pertinent adjunctive topics such as nutrition, dental considerations, and rehabilitation.

This book reflects the changing awareness of those who are committed to the management of head and neck malignancies away from the current dimensions of a therapist to the far more comprehensive role of the total physician. If one were to have at his command all of the information contained between the covers of this book, he would have undisputed expertise in the management of head and neck malignancies. It is quite impossible to single out one chapter over another in terms of excellence. Representative of the thoroughness of this book is the chapter on cancer of the nasal cavity and paranasal sinuses authored by George A. Sisson and Steven P. Becker. This is an exemplary chapter which accomplishes coverage of the topic from diagnosis to treatment, concisely, completely, and coherently.

The strength of the book is that it is complete and each topic is treated in a concise and comprehensive fashion. Every chapter is reflective of contemporary thought and the topics are all inclusive of head and neck oncology. The weakness of the book cannot be directed specifically toward this, but to any book that interrupts the continuum of evolution of a topic. Obviously, improvements and changes are occurring rapidly. The potential therefore exists for this book to drop out of date more rapidly than the text directed toward techniques alone. Regardless of this unavoidable weakness the thought reflected therein is contemporary.

In summary, this book is mandatory for all who are interested in head and neck oncology regardless of discipline. It must reside in the libraries of any department which professes to have interest in this field and should reside in the personal libraries of those in training as well as those on the clinical faculty.

CHARLES W. CUMMINGS, MD
Seattle, Washington

Pediatric Otolaryngology Case Studies

Edited by *W. Frederick McGuirt.* Soft cover, black and white illustrations, indexed, 484 pages, 1980. Medical Examination Publishing Co, Inc, Garden City, New York. Price $18.00.

This text represents a collection of 68 case studies encompassing common pediatric otolaryngology disorders, with occasional reference to the less common and controversial areas of the field. Topics covered include congenital head and neck anomalies; otologic, sinonasal, communicative, pharyngeal and airway disorders; head and neck oncology; trauma; and allergy and immunology. The format of each case study includes a patient history, pertinent physical findings, ancillary data and clinical course, followed by several multiple choice questions with detailed answers and an accompanying bibliography.

Although it does not represent a comprehensive text of pediatric otolaryngology, the book does cover the more common pediatric disorders seen by the otolaryngologist and is written in a very readable manner. The method of presentation is both stimulating and reinforcing. Moreover, the list of references accompanying each case study is complete and current. The only significant criticism is that some of the responses to the questions appear dogmatic and alternate viewpoints and therapeutic modalities are not covered adequately.

Although the book is primarily written and enthusiastically recommended for the otolaryngology or pediatric resident, the practicing otolaryngologist would also find it a useful, provocative review.

PETER G. SMITH, MD
St. Louis, Missouri

Diagnosis and Treatment of Palato Glossal Malfunction

Edited by *R. E. Ellis* and *F. C. Flack.* Soft cover, black and white illustrations, 89 pages, 1979. University Park Press, Baltimore. Price $9.95.

This small issue represents a state-of-the-art. Some of the authors are well-recognized authorities in the research aspect of cleft palate and in evaluation of clinical procedures. The individual papers have interesting material; however, since much of the conference was presented with video tape and cinematography, it has been difficult to include this material in the presentations. The text emphasizes the value of nasoendoscopy in the diagnosis of velopharyngeal abnormalities and this may be of interest to the otolaryngologist. However, few otolaryngologists are active in this field. The methods of speech evaluation and the research methods again are of interest to the speech therapist and prosthodontist and are not presented in a manner which may be of value to the otolaryngologist.

SYLVAN E. STOOL, MD
Pittsburgh, Pennsylvania

BOOKS RECEIVED

Proceedings of the Fourth International Symposium on Acoustic Impedance Measurements

Edited by Rui Penha and Paulo de Noronha Pizarro. Proceedings of Symposium held in Lisbon. Black and white line drawings, soft cover, 611 pages, 1981. Universidade Nova de Lisboa.

Sensorineural Hearing Loss, Vertigo and Tinnitus

Edited by M. M. Paparella and W. L. Meyerhoff. Black and white illustrations, indexed, hard cover, 170 pages, 1981. Williams and Wilkins Co., Baltimore, $26.

Respiratory Medicine

Edited by D. C. Flenley. Black and white illustrations, indexed, soft cover, 246 pages, 1981. Cassell Ltd., London (Macmillan Publishing Co. affiliate), $17.95.

New Perspectives on Noise-induced Hearing Loss

Edited by R. P. Hamernik, D. Henderson and R. Salvi. Papers presented at the National Institute of Occupational Safety and Health Symposium. Black and white illustrations, indexed, hard cover, 550 pages, 1981. Raven Press, New York, $63.

Surgery for Cancer of the Larynx and Related Structures

Carl E. Silver. Color and black and white illustrations, indexed, hard cover, 250 pages, 1981. Churchill Livingstone, Inc., New York, $65.

Surgery for Phonatory Disorders

Edited by Harvey M. Tucker. Volume 3, in *Monographs in Clinical Otolaryngology*. Black and white illustrations, indexed, hard cover, 130 pages, 1981. Churchill Livingstone, Inc., New York, $29.

Audiology and Audiological Medicine, 2 volumes

Edited by H. A. Beagley. Black and white illustrations, indexed with full chapter bibliographies, hard cover, 994 pages (total), 1981. Oxford University Press, London, $85 the set.

Physiological Acoustics

Edited by Juergen Tonndorf. Volume 15 in *Benchmark Papers in Acoustics*. Black and white illustrations, indexed, hard cover, 696 pages, 1981. Hutchinson Ross Publishing Co., Stroudsburg, Pennsylvania, $49.

Computed Tomography of the Head and Neck

Edited by Anthony A. Mancuso and William N. Hanafee. Black and white illustrations, indexed, 289 pages, hard cover, 1982. Williams & Wilkins Co., Baltimore, $55.

Textbook of Otolaryngology, 6th edition

Edited by David D. DeWeese and William H. Saunders. Black and white illustrations, indexed, hard cover, 474 pages, 1982. C. V. Mosby Co., St. Louis.

Benign Diseases of the Esophagus

Edited by R. H. Quinn, J. B. Gregg and C. Douglas Wood. Black and white illustrations, indexed, hard cover, 218 pages, 1982. Medical Examination Publishing Co., Inc., Garden City, $30.

Comprehensive Intervention with Hearing-Impaired Infants and Preschool Children

M. Suzanne Hasenstab and John S. Horner. Hard cover, indexed, 450 pages, 1982. Aspen Systems Corp., Gaithersburg, Md., $27.95.

Electronystagmography: A Systemic Approach

By Milind V. Kirtane. Black and white illustrations, subject index and bibliography, soft cover, 152 pages, 1982. Published by Dr. Kirtane, Bombay, India.

Disorders of the Facial Nerve: Anatomy, Diagnosis and Management

Edited by Malcolm D. Graham and William F. House. Black and white illustrations, indexed, hard cover, 576 pages, 1982. Raven Press, New York, $63.

Radiology of the Ear, Nose and Throat

By Galdino E. Valvassori, Guy D. Potter, William N. Hanafee, Barbara L. Carter and Richard A. Buckingham. Black and white illustrations, hard cover, 352 pages, 1982. W. B. Saunders, New York, $98.

Nystagmus and Vertigo: Clinical Approaches to the Patient with Dizziness

Edited by Vicente Honrubia, Black and white illustrations, author and subject indexes, hard cover, 296 pages, 1982. Academic Press, New York, $26.

The Nose: Upper Airway Physiology and the Atmospheric Environment

By Donald F. Proctor and Ib Anderson. Black and white illustrations, author and subject indexes, hard cover, 464 pages, 1982. Elsevier Biomedical Press, Amsterdam.

Central Auditory Assessment: The SSW Test, Development and Clinical Use

Edited by Dennis Arnst and Jack Katz. Black and white illustrations, chapter bibliographies, soft cover, 508 pages, 1982. College-Hill Press, Inc., San Diego, $32.50.

Advice to Parents of a Cleft Palate Child, 2nd edition

By Donna Konkel Wicka and Mervyn L. Falk. Black and white illustrations, bibliography, hard cover, 65 pages, 1982. Charles C. Thomas Co., Springfield, Illinois, $10.75.

Current Therapy in Otolaryngology — Head and Neck Surgery 1982-1983

Edited by George A. Gates. Black and white illustrations, subject index, hard cover textbook, 375 pages, 1982. B. C. Decker, Inc., Trenton, New Jersey, $44.50.

Vestibular Neurotology

Edited by P. Molina-Negro and R. A. Bertrand. Volume 28 in *Advances in Oto-Rhino-Laryngology*. C. R. Pfaltz, ed. Papers presented at the Symposium on Vestibular Neurotology, Montreal, September 9-12, 1980. Black and white illustrations, subject index, hard cover, 146 pages, 1982. S. Karger, Basel, Switzerland, $69.

HNO Praxis Heute, Volume 2

Edited by H. Ganz and W. Schatzle. Black and white illustrations, subject index, hard cover, 172 pages, 1982. Springer-Verlag, Berlin, $26.70.

Die Funktions-diagnostik der behinderten Nasenatmung. Einfuhrung in die Rhinomanometrie

By W. Bachmann. Black and white illustrations, subject index, reading list, hard cover, 143 pages, 1982. Springer-Verlag, Berlin, $39.10.

INFORMATION FOR AUTHORS

Send manuscripts by first-class mail to Editor Brian F. McCabe, MD, Department of Otolaryngology — Head & Neck Surgery, University of Iowa Hospitals and Clinics, Iowa City, IA 52242. Original manuscripts which deal with clinical and scientific aspects of otolaryngology, bronchoesophagology, head and neck, maxillofacial and plastic surgery, audiology, speech pathology and related specialties will be considered for publication. It is understood that manuscripts will not have been published elsewhere.

MANUSCRIPTS. Papers should be limited to a maximum of 15 double-spaced typewritten pages including tables and references, so as not to exceed the permitted maximum of 6 typeset pages. This allows for one page of illustrations. If a manuscript of slightly greater length is approved by the Editorial Board all typeset pages in excess of 6 will be charged to the authors at the publisher's cost of $125 per page. An **original of the manuscript** and one set of **original illustrations** should be provided for reproduction. **Two clear copies** of the manuscript and illustrations should be submitted for review. Manuscripts should be typewritten on white bond paper (8½ x 11 in). Use double spacing throughout with margins of at least one inch. Each manuscript component should begin on a new page in the following sequence: title page, abstract and key words, text, acknowledgments, references, tables and legends for illustrations. Number pages consecutively in the upper right hand corner beginning with the title page.

COPYRIGHT. In compliance with the Copyright Revision Act of 1976, all manuscripts must be accompanied by a letter containing the following statement before they will be reviewed for publication: "In consideration of the *Annals of Otology, Rhinology & Laryngology* taking action in reviewing and editing my (our) submission the author(s) undersigned hereby transfers(s), assign(s) or otherwise convey(s) all copyright ownership to the Annals Publishing Company in the event such work is published in the *Annals of Otology, Rhinology & Laryngology.*" We regret that manuscripts not accompanied by such a letter will be returned.

TITLES of manuscripts should be concise and informative and worded to facilitate indexing.

RUNNING HEAD. An abbreviated form of the title, to be used at the top of each page, should be provided by the author.

GENERIC NAMES should be used in the text whenever possible.

REFERENCES should be numbered consecutively in the order in which they are first mentioned, and cited in the text in arabic numerals in superscript. The number of references should not exceed 30. Use the style of references given in *Uniform Requirements for Manuscripts Submitted to Biomedical Journals.* Include in the reference list manuscripts accepted but not yet published; designate the journal followed by "in press" in parentheses. Manuscripts submitted but not yet accepted should be referred to as "unpublished data" in parentheses in the text. Primary references only should be used and must be verified by the author(s) against the original documents. Examples of correct forms of references are given below.

Journal Article

(List all authors when six or fewer; when seven or more, list only first three and add "et al.")

Ketchum LD, Smith I, Robinson DW, et al. The treatment of hypertrophic scar, keloid and scar contracture by triamcinolone acetonide. Plast Reconstr Surg 1966; 38:209-18.

Books and Other Monographs

Personal Author(s)

Payne SW, Olson MA. The esophagus. Philadelphia: Lea and Febiger, 1974: 1-3.

Corporate Author

American Medical Association Department of Drugs. AMA drug evaluations. 3rd ed. Littleton: Publishing Sciences Group, 1977.

Chapter in Book

Belsey R. Diaphragmatic hernia. In: Jones FA, ed. Modern trends in gastroenterology. London: Butterworths: 1952:128-78.

ILLUSTRATIONS should be original drawings, glossy photographs or halftones. Line drawings should be in black on white paper. Letters, numbers and symbols should be clear and even throughout, and of sufficient size that when reduced for publication, each item is still legible. Titles and detailed explanations of illustrations must be listed on a separate sheet, not on the illustrations themselves. Each figure should have a label pasted on the reverse indicating the number of the figure, the names of the authors, title of the paper; the top of the figure should be indicated. Cite each figure in the text in consecutive order. If a figure has been published, acknowledge the original source and submit written permission from the copyright holder to reproduce the material. Actual publication cost of illustrations will be charged to the author. Color illustrations are acceptable for publication; cost estimates for color separations and printing will be provided upon request.

TABLES should be on separate sheets, numbered consecutively, each headed by a concise title. Place explanatory matter in footnotes. Cost of setting tables will be charged to the author.

MEASUREMENTS should be expressed in the metric system. Audiograms must be plotted according to ISO standards.

ABSTRACTS should contain not more than 150 words and should state the purposes of the study, primary procedures, main findings and the principal conclusions, emphasizing new and important aspects of the investigation.

PERMISSIONS. Materials taken from other sources must be accompanied by a written statement from both senior author and publisher giving permission to the *Annals* for republication. If permission for publication is required by the author's institution, such clearance should be provided. Written permission of subjects is required for identifiable photographs of individuals.

SUPPLEMENTS. A manuscript too long for inclusion in the *Annals* may be published as a supplement if approved by the Board of Editors. All costs must be borne by the author; estimates of cost will be provided upon request. Early publication of supplements is often possible since supplements are produced independently of the regular *Annals* issues.

PROOFS accompanied by prints of the illustrations will be sent to the first author and should be returned within 48 hours. Changes in galley proofs initiated by the author will be charged to the author.

AUTHOR RESPONSIBILITY. All accepted manuscripts are subject to copy editing. The author is responsible for all statements in his work, including changes made by the copy editor which were approved by the author on the proofs.

REPRINTS. Rates are quoted when the proofs are sent. Orders must be signed by the author and returned with the proofs.

These requirements are in accord with *Uniform Requirements for Manuscripts Submitted to Biomedical Journals* (Lancet 1979; 1: 428-30).

CHEVALIER JACKSON LECTURE

ESOPHAGOLOGY: AN UPDATE

ARTHUR M. OLSEN, MD

ROCHESTER, MINNESOTA

Because of the great interest in the problem of gastroesophageal reflux, much emphasis has been placed on factors which control the competence of the lower esophageal sphincter (LES). Much study has been devoted to the effect of hormones and drugs on the LES. Of the various diagnostic methods available, 24-hour pH testing seems to offer the most information regarding reflux and its complications. Medical therapy should be given a careful trial before surgical procedures for reflux are considered. Diagnostic esophagoscopy is usually performed with fiberoptic instruments. Open-tube esophagoscopes are still preferable for most types of endoscopic therapy. However, flexible fiberscopes may be used for injection of esophageal varices and for laser coagulation of bleeding lesions or even tumors. Guide wires may be introduced through flexible scopes to aid in the dilation of esophageal strictures and also to aid in the placement of prosthetic tubes in patients with obstructing cancers. The performance of esophagoscopy by practitioners of several disciplines has resulted in fragmentation of the specialty. Ideally, all esophagoscopists should be competent with both open-tube and fiberoptic scopes and should be familiar with all of the newer knowledge of the physiology and pharmacology of the esophagus and its sphincters.

PHYSIOLOGY AND PHARMACOLOGY

In the past 30 years, much has been learned about the swallowing mechanisms.[1] With the help of manometry, the upper and lower sphincters have been well defined. The upper sphincter relaxes when swallowing begins, and the lower sphincter relaxes as the peristaltic wave passes into the stomach. Resting pressures at both sphincters normally prevent reflux from the stomach into the esophagus and airways. Except for some improvements in equipment and refinements in technique,[2] manometry has not changed appreciably in recent years. Motility studies are available in most hospitals and clinics, and manometry has taken its place as a diagnostic technique to supplement roentgen examination of the esophagus. Modifications of the pressure-detecting units permit a determination of potential difference[3] across the gastroesophageal mucosal junction, and pH electrodes can also be incorporated into the system.[3,4] All esophagologists should have some familiarity with these diagnostic techniques.

The lower esophageal sphincter (LES) is not anatomically identifiable. Its behavior is subject to the influence of a variety of neural, humeral, and mechanical stimuli.[5-7] Because maintenance of the pressure profile is so important in the prevention of reflux, the factors that increase or decrease the LES pressures are of considerable importance.

There is much evidence to suggest that intrinsic myogenic activity is chiefly responsible for the tone of the lower sphincter.[6,8] The normal LES pressure is reduced by esophagitis.[9] Reflux is favored by such factors as increased intra-abdominal pressure, impaired esophageal peristalsis,[7] and slow gastric emptying.[10]

Hormones have been implicated in the control of LES pressure. At one time, gastrin was thought to be of great importance,[11] but later studies have shown that serum gastric levels cannot be correlated with LES pressures or reflux.[12] However, estrogens (in pregnant women) apparently are responsible for incompetence of the LES.[13] Prostaglandins E_1 and E_2 cause a decrease in LES pressure.[14] A wide variety of other substances,[5] including foods and drugs, influence the pressure levels at the LES. Fats, chocolate, alcohol, and tobacco all cause a reduction in LES pressure. Anticholinergics reduce LES pressure, whereas drugs such as bethanechol, metoclopromide, domperidone,[15] carbenoxolone, and possibly antacids increase the sphincter pressures.[5]

ESOPHAGOSCOPY

There have been few advances in open-tube esophagoscopy in recent years. Fiberoptic illumination and improved magnifying telescopes have provided for better visualization and excellent photography. The *Atlas of Endoscopy* produced by Savary and Miller[16] is a testimonial to the Hopkins lighting system. Not only are the various diseases of the esophagus clearly shown but also the subtle changes of early esophagitis are demonstrated.

Flexible fiberoptic esophagoscopes have been with us for nearly 20 years. Constant improvements are being made in the optics and maneuverability of these instruments. Likewise, the channels for in-

From the Division of Thoracic Diseases and Internal Medicine, Mayo Clinic and Mayo Foundation, Rochester, Minnesota.

Presented at the meeting of the American Broncho-Esophagological Association, Palm Beach, Florida, May 3-4, 1982.

REPRINTS — A. M. Olsen, MD, Emeritus Office, Mayo Clinic, Rochester MN 55905.

strumentation have been enlarged. A variety of forceps for biopsy and foreign body removal are now available. Brushes for collection of material for cytologic study and snares for polypectomy may be passed through these channels. Also, these instruments will accommodate needles for injection of esophageal varices[17] and lasers for photocoagulation of bleeding lesions.[18]

Longer fiberoptic endoscopes are used to visualize the esophagus, stomach, and duodenum — all at one examination. Recently, sleeves, or "overtubes," have been passed over a 36-gauge rubber lavage tube or a small-caliber endoscope to permit repeated insertion and withdrawal of esophagoscopes.[19] The procedure is comparable to the use of an intratracheal tube for repeated passage of fiberbronchoscopes.

METHODS OF DILATING STRICTURES

The method described by Plummer in 1910[20] remains the safest and best way to dilate esophageal strictures. Bougies passed over a previously swallowed thread will dilate almost any type of esophageal stenosis. The only contraindications are gastroenterostomy and tracheoesophageal fistula, because the thread may drop back on itself after being swallowed. Admittedly, the method requires patience by both the patient and the endoscopist, but with time and effort, the thread will pass through the stricture and become anchored in the small intestine. This method is essential for multiple or tortuous strictures.[21]

In extreme stenosis, retrograde dilations with Tucker bougies are possible after gastrostomy and retrograde endoscopy with a cystoscope and passage of a ureteral catheter through the stricture into the hypopharynx.[21] After a few dilations, the gastrostomy can be closed and further dilations carried out over a swallowed thread.

When there is much retained food and secretion in the esophagus (as in achalasia), a mercury-weighted (0.5 ml) rubber or latex bag may be tied to the end of the thread to facilitate its passage. Otherwise, weights are neither necessary nor desirable.

Many endoscopists use Puestow or Rasmussen wires and bougies. Preferably, the wire should be passed through the stricture under direct vision and with the aid of fluoroscopy.[22] Recently, Savary developed a technique with a stainless steel wire and plastic, semiflexible bougies (Savary M, personal communication).

For "soft" strictures secondary to peptic esophagitis, the Hurst or Maloney mercury-filled, rubber bougies are adequate.[22] Often, the patient can dilate his own stricture with these bougies.

Open-tube esophagoscopes (or bronchoscopes) are often used to dilate short, soft strictures. The flexible fiberscope should not be used as a dilating instrument. However, guide wires can be passed through the fiberoptic esophagoscope and through the stricture under direct vision and preferably with fluoroscopic guidance.[22] Metal bougies and distensible balloons can be passed over the wires and very satisfactory dilation achieved (Hughes RW, personal communication). We can expect new advances in the techniques for dilating esophageal stenoses. However, it is important to emphasize that bougies and other dilators (except Maloney and Hurst dilators) must never be passed blindly.

MOTOR DISORDERS

Manometry has clearly shown that achalasia is a combination of motor failure of the esophagus and absence of relaxation of the lower sphincter.[23] If perfused polyvinyl tubing is used to record pressures, some patients with achalasia have increased pressures at the LES.[24]

The cause of achalasia (except in Chagas' disease) remains obscure. Methods of treating this disorder are designed to weaken the lower sphincter, either by forceful dilation or by myotomy. Both methods are effective, but they require considerable skill. In recent years, surgical treatment has been preferred because of more uniformly favorable results in a five-year-period of observation.

The myotomy should be esophageal, not gastric.[25] Extensive myotomies usually lead to reflux esophagitis and stricture. Our feeling is that antireflex surgical procedures are neither necessary nor desirable when myotomy is performed for achalasia.

Properly performed pneumatic dilations have a place in the management of achalasia. There is certainly a case for trying a pneumatic dilation before resorting to surgery.[26,27] However, surgical therapy is the treatment of choice in children, in patients with pain as the primary symptom, and in those who have manometric signs of vigorous achalasia. Obviously, surgical treatment should be used in patients who have not responded to dilation or who have had recurrent symptoms.

Diffuse spasm is a very different disorder.[23] Esophageal contractions are simultaneous, repetitive, and powerful in the smooth-muscle portion of the organ. The lower sphincter relaxes normally. Diffuse spasm is manifested clinically by substernal pain, tends to occur in nervous persons, and may be associated with peptic ulcer, biliary or pancreatic disease, and hiatal hernia.

The treatment of diffuse spasm is much less satisfactory than that of achalasia. Dilation is of very little value. Long myotomies extending up to the arch of the aorta may relieve symptoms in about 60% of patients.[23]

Some patients have clinical features and manometric characteristics of both achalasia and diffuse spasm.[28] Often, the roentgenographic appearance suggests diffuse spasm. Contractions are simultaneous, and there may be some relaxation of the lower sphincter, but premature contraction often takes place. Forceful dilation is not recommended for this syndrome. Results with esophagomyotomy are comparable with those obtained in classic achalasia. Recently, a patient with vigorous achalasia was reported to have had marked relief of pain and dysphagia[29] after administration of nifedipine. A European study suggested that the drug may be useful in diffuse spasm and achalasia.[30]

PULSION DIVERTICULA

Pharyngoesophageal diverticula arise in the hypopharynx just above the cricoid sphincter. Evidence suggests that malfunction of this sphincter is the probable cause of the diverticulum.[31] Manometric studies demonstrated that the sphincter contracts prematurely during swallowing and thus produces a physiologic obstruction.[32] The validity of this concept was recently challenged.[33] However, myotomy has been effective as a definitive treatment for small pharyngoesophageal diverticula. Relief of dysphagia may be obtained without resection of the diverticulum.[34]

Epiphrenic diverticula are usually asymptomatic unless they are associated with a motor disorder of the esophagus.[34] Motility studies are indicated whenever surgery is to be considered.[35] Achalasia or diffuse spasm is often present with symptomatic diverticula. Myotomy is essential, and an associated hiatal hernia should be repaired.[36] Diverticulectomy is optional unless the diverticulum is of good size.

GASTROESOPHAGEAL REFLUX

Reflux is one of the most common and distressing causes of dyspepsia. It is associated with incompetence (and usually hypotension) of the LES,[5] and it may or may not be associated with hiatal hernia. Reference has already been made to the factors that appear to influence the pressure elevation at the LES. It is likely that a combination of neural, humeral, and anatomic abnormalities cause incompetence of the sphincter.

When symptoms such as substernal burning or pain, sour regurgitation, and nocturnal choking or cough are present,[37] the fact that significant reflux is taking place should be established. Unfortunately, the patient's complaint of heartburn is poorly correlated with the actual amount of irritation or inflammation of the esophageal mucous membrane.[5] Roentgen examination and esophageal motility studies help demonstrate reflux, but they are not as valuable as pH measurements in the lower esophagus.[38] Esophagoscopy may reveal a normal-appearing membrane despite severe heartburn. Biopsy of the mucosa is often useful in demonstrating mild esophagitis.

Usually, pH studies of the lower esophagus are done by placement of a glass electrode (pH probe) in the lower esophagus about 5 cm above the esophagogastric junction.[39] After instillation of 300 ml of 0.1N hydrochloric acid into the stomach, the patient completes several maneuvers (such as deep breathing and Valsalva), and abdominal compression is also applied.[33] If reflux is present, the pH decreases to less than 4.

The standard pH study, just described, is not entirely reliable as an index of reflux. Twenty-four-hour pH monitoring gives much more accurate information about the exposure of the esophageal mucous membrane to gastric acid.[38] The patient's symptoms are correlated with the continuous pH recording. Documentation of this sort is desirable if surgery is being considered.

For most patients with symptoms of reflux, medical therapy is instituted. This consists of weight reduction, elevation of the head of the bed, avoidance of fat, chocolate, alcohol, tobacco, and particularly, refraining from eating for several hours before bedtime. Antacids are very helpful in alleviating symptoms and apparently strengthen the LES. As mentioned previously, drugs that increase sphincter pressure are bethanechol, metoclopromide, domperidone, and carbenoxolone.[5,15] Cimetidine, by inhibiting gastric acid secretion, may also be useful.

A further comment on nocturnal reflux is in order. Studies made during 24-hour pH monitoring have shown that reflux actually occurs more frequently during the daytime, when the person is upright, than during the night, when he is recumbent.[40] However, esophageal peristalsis occurs ten times more frequently during waking hours (72 times per hour) than when the person is asleep (seven times per hour). Thus, the total time of exposure of the esophageal mucosa to gastric acid is much greater at night. Hence, the frequency of peristalsis is of paramount importance in the clearing of acid secretions from the esophagus and is closely related to the incidence of reflux esophagitis.

Pulmonary aspiration associated with reflux may cause hoarseness, cough, wheezing, and pneumonitis.[38] Evidence suggests that the incidence of respiratory symptoms and complications may be related to the frequency of esophageal peristalsis and the integrity of the swallowing mechanism. It is well known that older persons and others with feeble peristalsis or other disturbances of esophageal motility are subject to aspiration pneumonitis. Hence, proper management of reflux in such patients is of particular importance.

Fundoplication procedures are widely used for the surgical management of reflux. The Belsey, Nissen, and Hill techniques appear to be equally effective in restoring the competence of the LES. However, surgery should be reserved for patients who cannot be managed successfully with medical measures.

ESOPHAGEAL VARICES

In 1939, Crafoord and Frenckner[41] reported the first successful injection of esophageal varices with a sclerosing solution through an esophagoscope. Using their technique, Moersch[42] began to inject esophageal varices with sodium morrhuate during the following year, and by 1947 he had treated 22 patients who had had bleeding from varices. Good results were obtained in 12 patients. Most of the patients with continued bleeding had associated gastric varices that could not be injected.

With the development of surgical techniques (especially portocaval shunts), interest in endoscopic treatment lagged, and little was written about sclerosing treatment for about 20 years. When it became apparent that surgical treatment left much to be desired, there was a renewal of interest in endoscopic sclerotherapy.[43,44] Recently, the needles used for injection have been passed through a fiberscope.[45,46]

Hughes and his colleagues[46] reported on a series of 75 patients with bleeding esophageal varices who were treated by sclerotherapy. Ethanolamine (5%) was the sclerosing agent. An average of six to eight treatments were required to obliterate the varices. About 10% of the patients had one or more complications, including esophageal ulcer, strictures, pneumonitis, mediastinitis, and febrile reactions.

For years, it has been known that balloon tamponade with Sengstaken-Blakemore, Linton-Nachlos, or Minnesota tubes temporarily controls bleeding from esophageal varices. Also, vasopressin (Pitressin) given intravenously may control bleeding for short periods. Recently, Lebrec and associates[47] reported that oral propranolol apparently reduces the incidence of recurrent hemorrhage from varices. Presumably, propranolol reduces portal pressure. Further studies are necessary to confirm the findings.

VOMITING AND THE ESOPHAGUS

Emesis is a common symptom of many disorders that affect mankind. It may occur with infectious diseases, various types of gastroenteritis, neurologic disturbances, and any disorder of the stomach or intestine that causes obstruction. Fortunately, vomiting usually is short-lived and causes little harm. Prolonged vomiting may not only cause serious nutritional disturbances but may also produce esophageal lesions. The esophageal problems are chiefly related to the regurgitation of gastric and intestinal secretions, especially gastric acids.

Violent vomiting, which may cause rupture of the lower esophagus (Boerhaave's syndrome), occurs most often in association with alcoholism. The clinical picture of severe chest pain, shock, and usually left hydropneumothorax is well known and should lead to an early diagnosis. Immediate surgical attention is essential, with thoracotomy and repair of the rent in the lower esophagus.[48]

Less violent and more prolonged vomiting may cause lacerations at the esophagogastric junction (Mallory-Weiss syndrome).[49] Like traumatic perforations, these lacerations are often related to increased esophageal and gastric pressure, and they are frequently associated with hiatal hernia. Hemorrhage is the most important symptom and may be manifested by hematemesis or melena or both. The lacerations are difficult to identify by radiologic techniques and often are not easy to demonstrate with open-tube esophagoscopy. With the flexible fiberesophagogastroscope, the lesions are easier to identify. Nevertheless, the Mallory-Weiss lacerations usually are seen for the first time at autopsy.

Bleeding from the Mallory-Weiss tears is difficult to control with tamponade, especially when hiatal hernia is associated. Recently, electrocoagulation[50] or laser photocoagulation[51] has been used with considerable success to control the bleeding.

Prolonged vomiting after surgical procedures or with pregnancy often produces long strictures that are difficult to dilate even when it is possible for the patient to swallow a thread. Such vomiting not only causes peptic stenosis but also results in shortening of the esophagus.[52] Because of continued reflux, a satisfactory esophageal lumen is difficult to maintain, and many of these patients require surgery. Interpositions of small or large bowel and Roux-en-Y gastric drainages may be necessary but are fraught with considerable hazard and frequent complications.

Much has been written about columnar-lined epithelium (Barrett) in the esophagus. It is likely that most patients with this disorder have had ulcerative esophagitis.[52] The high incidence of carcinoma associated with the Barrett esophagus is a matter of record.[53]

CANCER OF THE ESOPHAGUS AND CARDIA

The outlook for esophageal malignancies is still grim despite advances in surgical techniques and the use of roentgen therapy. Irradiation may provide temporary relief of symptoms, especially in the upper esophagus.[54]

From the endoscopist's point of view, improvements in technique for intubation of the patient who cannot be operated on are worthy of comment. Celestin[55] has modified his tube to prevent upward migration of the prosthesis. Recently, the Atkinson tube and Nottingham introducer have been used with considerable success (Hughes RW, personal communication).[56] Otherwise, periodic dilation is necessary to maintain an esophageal lumen.

FOREIGN BODIES

Endoscopists experienced with the flexible fiberscope continue to devise new instruments and methods of handling esophageal foreign bodies. Forceps, baskets, and snares that can be passed through the fiberscope are being improved, and there are many case reports of successful foreign body removal with the fiberscope. Meat impaction is being treated with meat tenderizers, with intravenous glucagon injections, or by "pushing" the bolus into the stomach with the endoscope. Also, by introduction of overtubes past the cricoid level, as previously mentioned,[19] the endoscope and forceps can be inserted into and removed from the esophagoscope repeatedly, and the "muzzle-loaded jumbo forceps" can be used for foreign body extraction.

COMPLICATIONS OF INSTRUMENTATION

The risks of perforation of the esophagus by passage of an open-tube esophagoscope are well known. Esophageal "splits" occur most frequently in the upper esophagus as the instrument is introduced. If hypertrophic changes in the cervical vertebrae are present, the chance of perforation is greater. Such accidents are less likely with the fiberscope,[57] but they may occur even if the operator is very skilled.

The incidence of perforation during dilation of benign strictures should be very low unless the procedure is carried out blindly. Complications after forceful dilation for achalasia occur in about 5% of cases.[23] Perforations are related to the number of dilations performed for each patient.[23]

The treatment of esophageal perforations is primarily surgical, but in small "leaks," antibiotics may control the infection. Certainly, if gross evidence of perforation is present in the upper esophagus (upper substernal pain, fever, tenderness in the neck, and subcutaneous emphysema), the superior mediastinum should be drained.[58] Obvious perforations of the midesophagus and esophagogastric junction should be treated by thoracotomy or extrapleural drainage.[58] Patients with cancer who have perforations after dilation can often be treated with antibiotics (Hughes RW, personal communication).

CHEST PAIN AND THE ESOPHAGUS

Various types of chest pain may be associated with esophageal disorders. The discomfort accompanying reflux esophagitis is characteristic and is unlikely to be confused with chest pain of cardiovascular origin. This is not the case, however, with esophageal dysfunction that produces both pain and manometric changes. Early or vigorous achalasia and diffuse spasm may cause pain that mimics angina pectoris. However, substernal chest pain also occurs when there are manometric abnormalities that are not typical of these entities. When associated with pain,[59] these nonspecific findings are likely to be peristaltic contractions of high amplitude, often repetitive and of considerable duration. Dysphagia may or may not be associated.

In most patients with atypical chest pain, coronary disease can be verified or excluded with electrocardiography or some type of stress test. In some instances, however, it would be helpful if chest pain of esophageal origin could be provoked (and supporting manometric evidence obtained) by injection of a pharmacologic agent. Ergonovine appears to be such a drug but is hazardous because it also can precipitate coronary artery spasm.[60] At present, edrophonium (Tensilon) appears to be the best drug available for provoking esophageal pain and compatible manometric changes.

INDICATIONS FOR FLEXIBLE AND RIGID ESOPHAGOSCOPES

In my opinion, the flexible fiberoptic endoscopes are primarily diagnostic instruments, and for this use they are vastly superior to the rigid tubes except in the upper esophagus. The length and flexibility of the fiberscope enables the examiner to inspect the esophagus, stomach, and duodenum. The fiberscope is certainly the instrument of choice in searching for the cause of unexplained hematemesis, particularly in the intervals between episodes of bleeding. The fiberscope is excellent for evaluation of esophagitis and gastritis, and it is very suitable for inspection of hiatal hernias and lesions near the esophagogastric junction. Biopsy specimens are smaller but usually adequate, and brushes can be passed for the collection of cytologic material.

The open-tube rigid esophagoscope is still the preferable instrument for inspection of lesions near the pharyngoesophageal junction. For most types of therapy, including foreign body removal, it is the preferable instrument. However, it is quite possible that esophageal varices can be injected just as well through the fiberscope, and instruments for electrotherapy or laser beams apparently can be passed as easily through the fiberscope. If an endoscope is to be used for dilating stenoses, the rigid instrument is obviously preferable. Once a diagnosis has been made and a thread passed into the small intestine, no endoscope is necessary. However, it may be desirable to perform dilations with fluoroscopic guidance. If difficulty is experienced in getting a thread past the obstruction, both an esophagoscope (either rigid or flexible) and fluoroscopy are necessary to pass a guide wire through the stenosis. Guide wires should not be passed blindly.

SUMMARY

Great progress has been made in the diagnosis and management of esophageal disorders. Esophagologists should be familiar with the newer knowledge of the physiology and pharmacology of the esophagus and its sphincters, and they should also be acquainted with the various techniques available for the study of esophageal disorders. Ideally, esophagologists should be proficient in the use of both rigid and fiberoptic endoscopes, and they should certainly be aware of the hazards of passing the tubes and all of the other equipment that can be inserted through the esophagoscope. Finally, they should be ever mindful of the basic principles of endoscopy enunciated by Chevalier Jackson many years ago.

REFERENCES

1. Olsen AM. Study of esophageal motility in health and disease. Ann Otol Rhinol Laryngol 1968; 77:892-905.

2. Arndorfer RC, Stef JJ, Dodds WJ, Linehan JH, Hogan WJ. Improved infusion system for intraluminal esophageal manometry. Gastroenterology 1977; 73:23-7.

3. Helm WJ, Schlegel JF, Code CF, Summerskill WHJ. Identification of the gastroesophageal mucosal junction by transmucosal potential in healthy subjects and patients with hiatal hernia. Gastroenterology 1965; 48:25-35.

4. Tuttle SG, Bettarello A, Grossman MI. Esophageal acid perfusion test and a gastroesophageal reflux test in patients with esophagitis. Gastroenterology 1960; 38:861-72.

5. Holloway RH, Winnan G, McCallum RW. Upper gastrointestinal motility. Part I. The pathophysiologic approach to the management of reflux esophagitis. Am J Gastroenterol 1981; 76: 280-90.

6. Behar J, Kerstein M, Biancani P. Neural control of the lower esophageal sphincter in the cat: studies on the excitatory pathways to the lower esophageal sphincter. Gastroenterology 1982; 82:680-8.

7. Stanciu C, Bennett JR. Oesophageal acid clearing: one factor in the production of reflux oesophagitis. Gut 1974; 15:852-7.

8. Christensen J, Freeman BW, Miller JK. Some physiological characteristics of the esophagogastric junction in the opossum. Gastroenterology 1973; 64:1119-25.

9. Eastwood GL, Castell DO, Higgs RH. Experimental esophagitis in cats impairs lower esophageal sphincter pressure. Gastroenterology 1975; 69:146-53.

10. McCallum RW, Berkowitz DM, Lerner E. Gastric emptying in patients with gastroesophageal reflux. Gastroenterology 1981; 80:285-91.

11. Cohen S, Lipshutz W. Hormonal regulation of human lower esophageal sphincter competence: interaction of gastrin and secretin. J Clin Invest 1971; 50:449-54.

12. McCallum RW, Callachan C, Avella J, Walsh JH. Normal antral gastrin concentration and endogenous release in gastroesophageal reflux (GER) patients [Abstract]. Gastroenterology 1979; 76:1197.

13. Fisher RS, Roberts GS, Grabowski CJ, Cohen S. Inhibition of lower esophageal sphincter circular muscle by female sex hormones. Am J Physiol 1978; 234:E243-7.

14. Rattan S, Goyal RK. Role of endogenous prostaglandins in the regulation of lower esophageal sphincter. In: Christensen J, ed. Gastrointestinal motility. New York: Raven Press, 1980: 29-36.

15. Goethals C. Domperidone in the treatment of post-prandial symptoms suggestive of gastroesophageal reflux. Curr Ther Res 1979; 26:874-80.

16. Savary M, Miller G. The esophagus: handbook and atlas of endoscopy. Colin-Jones D (trans). Solothurn, Switzerland: Verlag Gassmann AG, 1978.

17. Clark AW, MacDougall BRD, Westaby D, et al. Prospective controlled trial of injection sclerotherapy in patients with cirrhosis and recent variceal haemorrhage. Lancet 1980; 2:552-4.

18. Frühmorgen P, Bodem F, Reidenbach HD, Kaduk B, Demling L. Endoscopic laser coagulation of bleeding gastrointestinal lesions with report of the first therapeutic application in man. Gastrointest Endosc 1976; 23:73-5.

19. Cotton PE. An overtube concept in upper gastrointestinal endoscopy [Abstract]. Gastrointest Endosc 1981; 27:120.

20. Plummer HS. The value of a silk thread as a guide in esophageal technique. Surg Gynecol Obstet 1910; 10:519-23.

21. Rosenow EC III. Techniques of esophageal dilation. In: Payne WS, Olsen AM, eds. The esophagus. Philadelphia: Lea & Febiger, 1974:55-64.

22. Boyce HW Jr, Palmer ED. Techniques of clinical gastroenterology. Springfield, Ill: Charles C Thomas, 1975.

23. Ellis FH Jr, Olsen AM. Achalasia of the esophagus. Major Probl Clin Surg 1969; 9:1-221.

24. Cohen S, Lipshutz W. Lower esophageal sphincter dysfunction in achalasia. Gastroenterology 1971; 61:814-20.

25. Ellis FH Jr. The esophagus. In: Lewis' practice of surgery. Vol 5. Hagerstown, Md: Harper & Row, 1979:1-85.

26. Orringer MB. The treatment of achalasia: controversy resolved? [Editorial] Ann Thorac Surg 1979; 28:100-2.

27. Heimlich HJ, O'Connor TW, Flores DC. Case for pneumatic dilatation in achalasia. Ann Otol Rhinol Laryngol 1978; 87:519-22.

28. Sanderson DR, Ellis FH Jr, Schlegel JF, Olsen AM. Syndrome of vigorous achalasia: clinical and physiologic observations. Dis Chest 1967; 52:508-17.

29. Berger K, McCallum RW. Nifedipine in the treatment of achalasia. Ann Intern Med 1982; 96:61-2.

30. Weiser HF, Lepsien G, Golenhofen K, Siewert R. Clinical and experimental studies on the effect of nifedipine on smooth muscle of the oesophagus and LES. In: Duthie HL, ed. Gastrointestinal motility in health and disease. Lancaster, England: MTP Press, 1978:565-72.

31. Sutherland HD. Cricopharyngeal achalasia. J Thorac Cardiovasc Surg 1962; 43:114-26.

32. Ellis FH Jr, Schlegel JF, Lynch VP, Payne WS. Cricopharyngeal myotomy for pharyngo-esophageal diverticulum. Ann Surg 1969; 170:340-9.

33. Knuff TE, Benjamin SB, Castell DO. Pharyngoesophageal (Zenker's) diverticulum: a reappraisal. Gastroenterology 1982; 82:734-6.

34. Hiebert CA. Pulsion diverticula of the esophagus. In: Stipa S, Belsey RHR, Moraldi A, eds. Medical and surgical problems of the esophagus. Proceedings of the Serono Symposia. London: Academic Press, 1981; 43:248-51.

35. Olsen AM, Code CF, Clagett OT. Role of motility patterns in the diagnosis of esophageal disease. JAMA 1960; 172:319-24.

36. Allen TH, Clagett OT. Changing concepts in the surgical treatment of pulsion diverticula of the lower esophagus. J Thorac Cardiovasc Surg 1965; 50:455-62.

37. Olsen AM, Cameron AJ, Payne WS. Respiratory symptoms of gastroesophageal reflux. In: Stipa S, Belsey RHR, Moraldi A, eds. Medical and surgical problems of the esophagus. Proceedings of the Serono Symposia. London: Academic Press, 1981; 43: 130-7.

38. Pellegrini CA, DeMeester TR, Johnson LF, Skinner DB. Gastroesophageal reflux and pulmonary aspiration: incidence, functional abnormality, and results of surgical therapy. Surgery 1979; 86:110-8.

39. Kantrowitz PA, Corson JG, Fleischli DJ, Skinner DB. Measurement of gastroesophageal reflux. Gastroenterology 1969; 56:666-74.

40. Johnson LF. New concepts and methods in the study and treatment of gastroesophageal reflux disease. Med Clin North Am 1981; 65:1195-222.

41. Crafoord C, Frenckner P. New surgical treatment of varicose veins of the oesophagus. Acta Otolaryngol (Stockh) 1939; 27; 422-9.

42. Moersch HJ. Further studies on the treatment of esophageal varices by injection of a sclerosing solution. Ann Otol Rhinol Laryngol 1941; 50:1233-44.

43. Johnston GW, Rodgers HW. A review of 15 years' experience in the use of sclerotherapy in the control of acute haemorrhage from oesophageal varices. Br J Surg 1973; 60:797-800.

44. Terblanche J, Northover JMA, Bornman P, et al. A prospective controlled trial of sclerotherapy in the long term management of patients after esophageal variceal bleeding. Surg Gynecol Obstet 1979; 148:323-33.

45. Clark AW, Mitchell KJ, McDougall B, Silk DAB, Dawson JL, Williams R. Prospective controlled clinical trial of injection sclerotherapy in cirrhotic patients with recent variceal haemorrhage [Abstract]. Gut 1979; 20:A907.

46. Hughes RW Jr, Larson DE, Viggiano TR, Adson MA, van Heerden JA, Reeves CB. Endoscopic variceal sclerosis: a one-year experience. Gastrointest Endos 1982; 28:62-6.

47. Lebrec D, Poynard T, Hillon P, Benhamou J-P. Propranolol for prevention of recurrent gastrointestinal bleeding in patients with cirrhosis: a controlled study. N Engl J Med 1981; 305: 1371-4.

48. Olsen AM, Clagett OT, Spontaneous rupture of the esophagus: report on a case with immediate diagnosis and successful surgical repair. Postgrad Med 1947; 2:417-21.

49. Mallory GK, Weiss S. Hemorrhages from lacerations of the cardiac orifice of the stomach due to vomiting. Am J Med Sci 1929; 178:506-15.

50. Papp JP. Electrocoagulation of actively bleeding Mallory-Weiss tears. Gastrointest Endosc 1980; 26:128-30.

51. Geboes K, Rutgeerts P, Vantrappen G, Broeckaert L, Desmet V. A microscopic and ultrastructural study of hemostasis after laser photocoagulation. Gastrointest Endosc 1980; 26;131-3.

52. Andersen HA, Payne WS. Esophageal hiatal hernia, gastroesophageal reflux, and their complications. In: Payne WS, Olsen AM, eds. The esophagus. Philadelphia: Lea & Febiger, 1974: 107-37.

53. Hawe A, Payne WS, Weiland LH, Fontana RS. Adenocarcinoma in the columnar epithelial lined lower (Barrett) oesophagus. Thorax 1973; 28:511-4.

54. Pearson JG. The present status and future potential of radiotherapy in the management of esophageal cancer. Cancer 1977; 39:882-90.

55. Celestin LR. Palliation by internal tube. In: Stipa S, Belsey RHR, Moraldi A, eds. Medical and surgical problems of the esophagus. Proceedings of the Serono Symposia. London: Academic Press, 1981; 43:374-6.

56. Seifert E. Palliative treatment of inoperable patients with carcinoma of the cardia region [Abstract]. Gastrointest Endosc 1981; 27:128-9.

57. Tulman AB, Boyce HW Jr. Complications of esophageal dilation and guidelines for their prevention. Gastrointest Endosc 1981; 27:229-34.

58. Payne WS, Brown PW Jr, Fontana RS. Esophageal perforation, Mallory-Weiss syndrome, and acquired esophageal fistulas. In: Payne WS, Olsen AM, eds. The esophagus. Philadelphia: Lea & Febiger, 1974:171-89.

59. Benjamin SB, Gerhardt DC, Castell DO. High amplitude, peristaltic esophageal contractions associated with chest pain and/or dysphagia. Gastroenterology 1979; 77:478-83.

60. Eastwood GL, Weiner BH, Dickerson WJ II, et al. Use of ergonovine to identify esophageal spasm in patients with chest pain. Ann Intern Med 1981; 94:768-71.

≈

CORRECTION

In Part 2 of the September-October issue of the *Annals* (1982; 91 Suppl 97) an error appears in the article "Cochlear and Otoconial Abnormalities in Capsular Otosclerosis with Hydrops" by L-G. Johnsson, MD; J. E. Hawkins, Jr, DSc; R. C. Rouse, PhD; and F. H. Linthicum, Jr, MD. On page 14, column 2, paragraph 4, the second sentence reads *There appeared to be* no *relation between the amount of endosteum involved and the degree of sensorineural degeneration.* It should read *There appeared to be* a *relation between the amount of endosteum involved and the degree of sensorineural degeneration.*

Ann Otol Rhinol Laryngol 91:1982

OBSERVATIONS ON SO-CALLED IDIOPATHIC VOCAL CORD PARALYSIS

PAUL H. WARD, MD GEORGE BERCI, MD

LOS ANGELES, CALIFORNIA

A series of 238 patients with laryngeal paralysis seen during a six-year period (1976-1982) were studied with serial 16-mm motion picture filmstrips. There were 39 cases in which no etiological disease process could be found responsible for the paralysis; these were called "idiopathic." In all 39 cases, both the superior and recurrent laryngeal nerves were paralyzed indicating that the lesion involved the central (nuclear) lower motor neurons of the dorsal and ventral nucleus ambiguus. The high incidence of upper respiratory infections suggests a viral etiology in many cases. The ability to separate a pure recurrent from a combined superior and recurrent laryngeal paralysis on morphological indirect endoscopic appearance has significant diagnostic and therapeutic implications.

INTRODUCTION

Paralysis of one or both vocal cords is a sign, not a disease. This sign is most often related to a disease involving the vagus nerve or its branches somewhere along their courses in the brainstem, neck, or mediastinum. After extensive evaluation and work-up, there remain cases for which no etiological agent or disease can be found to be responsible for the paralysis or paresis. These cases have been labeled "idiopathic" laryngeal paralysis.[1-4] Major interest has centered around the known organic causes of vocal cord paralysis and relatively little has been written concerning the characteristics and behavior of the idiopathic group. This investigation is devoted to the study of a select group of cases: the incidence; the anatomical, pathophysiological characteristics of the paralysis; and the prognosis are discussed.

Of significant diagnostic and therapeutic importance is the striking finding of 39 cases of paralysis in which no organic etiology could be found and in all of which there was a paralysis or paresis of both the external branch of the superior and recurrent laryngeal nerves. Arthritis of the cricoarytenoid joint and intrinsic lesions (ie, tumors) of the larynx cause immobile vocal cords but will not be categorized with vocal cord paralysis.

The larynx is a remarkable and complex structure serving as the protective gate to the lower respiratory tract. Originally serving solely as a sphincteric organ, as is still the case in many lower animals, it has been adapted to produce sounds in many animals and speech in man. Interference with the nerve supply to the larynx in humans results in varying degrees of voice alteration, hoarseness, change in appearance of the larynx, dysfunction of swallowing, and aspiration. A better understanding of the physiological mechanisms of the larynx in health and disease can be facilitated by a brief anatomical review.

REVIEW OF ANATOMY

The cartilage structures of the larynx are held together by muscles and fibroelastic tissue covered and lined by mucosa. Two large cartilage masses, the cricoid and thyroid, along with the smaller paired arytenoids, make up the major superstructure of the larynx (Fig. 1). The epiglottis and the corniculate and cuneiform cartilages probably play less important roles in the function of the larynx. The intrinsic laryngeal muscles are divided for descriptive purposes into the abductors, adductors, and tensors of the vocal cords. The abductors of the vocal cords are the paired posterior cricoarytenoid muscles which, upon contracting, rotate the vocal process outward. The adductors include the paired lateral cricoarytenoid muscles, which turn the vocal process inward: the interarytenoid muscle extends between the two arytenoids which, upon contraction, pulls the arytenoids together; the internal and external thyroarytenoid muscles make up the bulk of the vocal cords and also serve as tensors. The externally located cricothyroid muscles, upon contraction, tilt the thyroid upon the cricoid cartilage, tensing and lengthening the vocal cords. Passive motion caused by flow of air and other motions induced by the extrinsic laryngeal muscles play less important roles in the position of the vocal cords.

The larynx is supplied by the paired superior and recurrent laryngeal nerves derived on each side from the vagus nerve trunks (Fig. 2). The lower motor neurons forming the vagus and, in turn, the superior and recurrent laryngeal nerves have their origin in the dorsal and ventral nucleus ambiguii.

From the Department of Surgery, Division of Head and Neck Surgery (Otolaryngology), UCLA School of Medicine, and the Department of Surgery, Cedars-Sinai Medical Center, Los Angeles.

Presented at the meeting of the American Broncho-Esophagological Association, Palm Beach, Florida, May 3-4, 1982.

REPRINTS — Paul H. Ward, MD, Chief, Department of Surgery, Division of Head and Neck Surgery (Otolaryngology), UCLA School of Medicine, 32-34 Rehabilitation Center, Los Angeles, CA 90024.

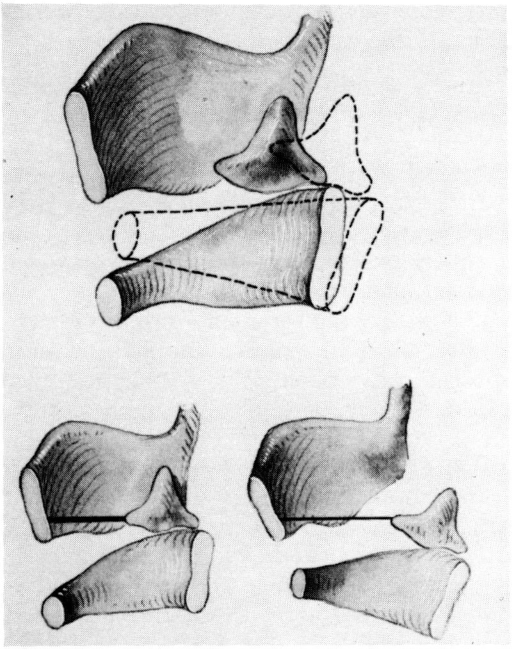

Fig. 1. Major suprastructure of larynx, showing contraction of cricothyroid muscle tilting thyroid cartilage on cricoid cartilage. Vocal cord is tensed and lengthened.

The two superior laryngeal nerves leave the vagus trunks on each side of the neck just below the nodose ganglion. They pass down and behind the carotid artery and curve forward toward the larynx. Each superior laryngeal nerve divides into the internal and external branches. The internal branches penetrate the thyrohyoid membrane and supply the supraglottic portion of the larynx with secretory and sensory fibers. The motor fibers of the superior laryngeal nerve are contained within the external branch which accompanies the superior thyroid artery moving caudally, inferiorly, and medially, to supply the cricothyroid muscle on each side.

The two recurrent nerves are the major motor nerves supplying the intrinsic muscles of the larynx. They also carry sensory and secretory fibers to the glottic, subglottic, and upper trachea. The right recurrent nerve initially pursues a different course from the left, leaving the vagus trunk at the level of the subclavian artery, passing backwards around the artery, and ascending medially and obliquely to the posterior lateral side of the trachea. The left recurrent nerve arises from the vagus trunk on the left side of the aorta, winds around the aorta at a point where the ligamentum arteriosum is attached, then ascends along the lateral wall of the trachea. Both nerves pass upward in their respective tracheoesophageal grooves, developing a close and variable relationship with the posterior aspect of the thyroid gland and the inferior thyroid artery. The close relationship and proximity of the recurrent and external branch of the superior laryngeal nerves to the thyroid gland invite frequent injury during thyroid surgery.[5]

During quiet respiration the vocal cords remain abducted and move minimally up and down with inspiration and expiration. Abduction is emphasized further during deep inspirations. During phonation the vocal cords are adducted, tensed, and lengthened (Fig. 1). Motor fibers passing within the recurrent nerves are responsible for supplying the intrinsic adductor muscles, while fibers initiating contraction of the cricothyroid muscles and thereby tensing and lengthening the vocal cords pass through the external branches of the superior laryngeal nerves. The midline position of the vocal cords pro-

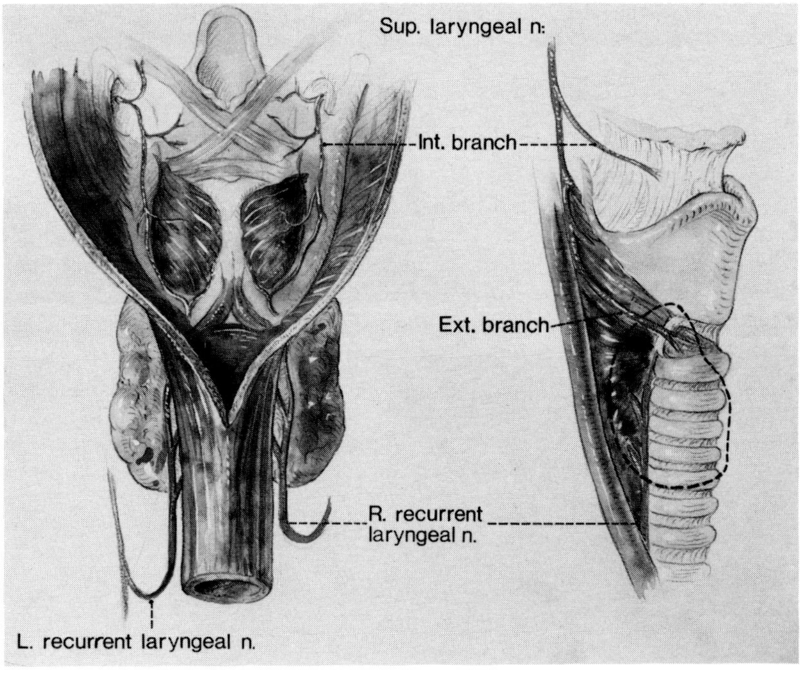

Fig. 2. Several pairs of laryngeal muscles are supplied by two pairs of motor nerves arising from vagus trunk. Relationships of recurrent laryngeal nerves to trachea and thyroid gland and entrance into larynx are shown in posterior view of laryngopharynx (left). Superior laryngeal nerve supplies motor fibers only to cricoid muscles on each side through its external branches. Internal branches contain secretory and sensory fibers supplying supraglottic portions of larynx on their respective sides.

CONVENTIONAL WORK-UP OF PARALYZED VOCAL CORD

History
Physical
Laboratory studies
Chest x-ray
Barium swallow
T3, T4, TSH scan and uptake
CBC, ESR, Hct,
FAT, FBS
Laryngoscopy
Bronchoscopy
Esophagoscopy
Mediastinoscopy (when indicated)

vides resistance to airflow until pressure builds up and then separates the cords. Separation of the cords reduces the pressure and allows them to return to the midline position. This process is repetitious, thus producing cordal oscillations and sound. The sounds are modified and speech is produced by the resonating qualities of the pharynx, nasopharynx, mouth, and other structures. Interference with delicate coordination of the intrinsic and extrinsic muscles of the larynx, or with the innervation and musculature of the pharynx, soft palate, tongue, or lips, alters phonation.

Secretory and afferent sensory fibers also are present in the superior and recurrent laryngeal nerves and play an important part in vocal reflexes and in reflex closure of the larynx to prevent aspiration.[6]

Paresis and paralysis of the larynx occurs with disease involvement anywhere along the pathway of the lower motor neurons from their origin in the medulla oblongata (dorsal and ventral nuclei ambiguii), through the vagus trunk, or the superior and recurrent laryngeal nerves. Disruption and interference with these neural pathways at various levels result in a variety of physical symptoms and alterations in appearance and function of the larynx.[7]

CRITICAL POINTS IN DIAGNOSIS

The importance of recognizing the dynamic positioning of the vocal cord and the lesion or combination of lesions responsible cannot be overemphasized. The literature is replete with poorly understood descriptions of various static cordal positions. The possible combinations of partial or complete paralysis of four nerves with reinnervation, contracture, and atrophy have made accurate assessment and correct understanding of these variable lesions almost impossible without cinematographic study. Documentation of the behavior and dynamic appearance of the larynx and correlation of this information with specific localized injury to the nerves has helped to clarify and provide a better understanding of some types of laryngeal paralysis.[7,8] The addition of electromyographic studies to further assess, confirm, and document the activity of the laryngeal musculature should add to our knowledge and diagnostic acumen.

An understanding of the appearance and behavior of the larynx in central and peripheral neural lesions is of great diagnostic significance.[9] The conventional work-up previously outlined by most authors for a paralyzed vocal cord can be modified for each patient if the examining physician can differentiate between a pure recurrent nerve paralysis and a combined superior and recurrent nerve paralysis. The history and physical examination (including indirect laryngoscopy) remain the mainstay in diagnosis for all patients.[10,11] Those patients having a pure recurrent nerve paralysis with an intact superior laryngeal nerve can have their evaluations modified to disregard central nervous system disease. Attention and investigation are devoted to the neck, mediastinum, and chest (Table). In this latter situation there is little need to search at the base of the skull or intracranially since, when the lesion or disease is central, the recurrent motor paralysis will be accompanied by a superior laryngeal motor paralysis. By contrast, when there is paralysis of both the superior and recurrent laryngeal motor nerves, the lesion (if a single lesion) has to be high in the neck, at the base of the skull, or located intracranially. Triple endoscopy, thyroid scans, and x-ray films of the chest and esophagus are not likely to produce information of value and are not cost-effective in the evaluation of central lesions.

This communication deals solely with recognition of unilateral paralytic and paretic, isolated and combined lesions. In analyzing the paresis or paralysis, it is critical to recognize the dynamic appearance of the larynx. As demonstrated in a film and exhibit presented to the American Academy of Ophthalmology and Otolaryngology in October 1976,[12] certain recognizable positions and motions of the larynx are predictable when specific surgical damage to the superior and recurrent laryngeal nerves is present.

Sectioning of a single recurrent nerve in the lower neck results in a cord resting in the paramedial (median) position (Fig. 3). During inspiration, it retains this position while the opposite and normally behaving cord abducts to provide a marginal to adequate airway. During phonation there is a tensing and lengthening of the paralyzed cord caused by the contraction of both cricothyroid muscles which tilt the thyroid on the cricoid cartilage. Since this tensing motion is present in both cords, it goes unnoticed unless looked for specifically. The intact cord moves toward the midline and approximates the paralyzed cord in its paramedial position. With forced expulsion of air, both cords vibrate and may appear grossly normal. The initially observed hoarseness readily disappears. After compensation, the speaking voice may be almost normal. Loss of the delicate coordination of the intrinsic muscles on

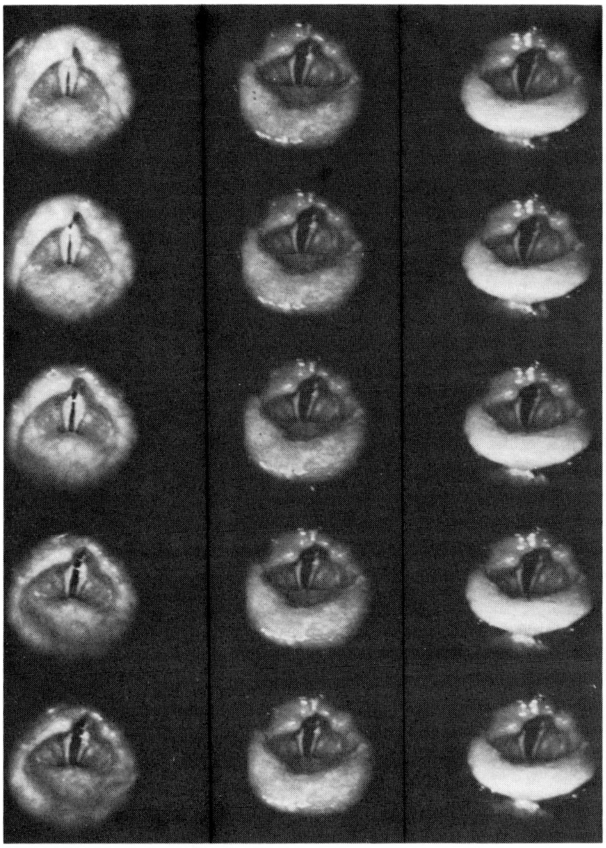

Fig. 3. Serial photographs from 16-mm motion picture film of patient with pure recurrent nerve paralysis secondary to surgical division of nerve. Vocal cord is in paramedial (median) position. During inspiration it retains this position while opposite cord abducts producing a marginally adequate airway. During phonation there is tensing and lengthening of both cords produced by contraction of both cricothyroid muscles tilting thyroid on cricoid cartilage. There is also a slight amount of adduction secondary to contractions of bilaterally innervated interarytenoid muscle.

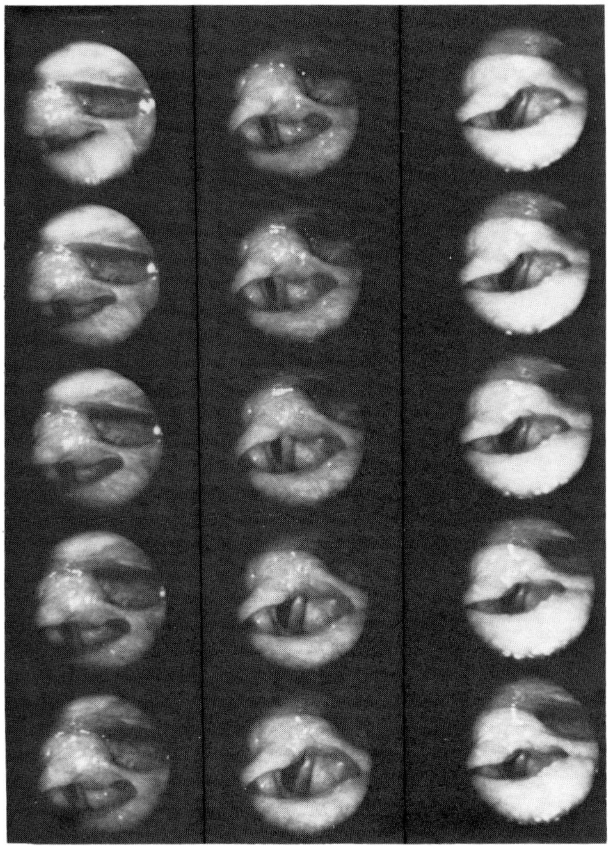

Fig. 4. Serial photographs from 16-mm motion picture film of patient with idiopathic vocal cord paralysis. Both superior and recurrent laryngeal nerves are paralyzed. During phonation contraction of opposite intact cricothyroid muscle produces an asymmetry of thyroid-cricoid cartilage tilt with lengthening and tensing of innervated cord. Tensed normal cord is thus at a different level than flaccid paralyzed cord, which may have an injected appearance due to hyperemia. There is an asymmetrical shift of posterior larynx toward paralyzed side during phonation.

one side of the larynx, however, severely impairs efforts to sing. Questioning the patient with recurrent laryngeal nerve paralysis concerning the onset of impairment of ability to sing may provide valuable medical data in identifying the onset of paralysis. In addition to the tensing and lengthening of the paralyzed cord during phonatory effort, there is also a slight amount of adduction secondary to contraction of the bilaterally innervated interarytenoid muscle.[13]

Complete unilateral superior and recurrent laryngeal nerve paralyses probably should be divided into two subgroups based upon current clinical and theoretical probabilities. The two subgroups consist of paralyses caused by those lesions involving 1) the external motor branch of the superior laryngeal nerve and the recurrent nerve, and 2) both internal and external branches of the superior laryngeal and recurrent nerves. The first subgroup is a central lower motor neuron paralysis in which the lesion or disease involves the dorsal and ventral nucleus ambiguus and can selectively spare the sensory and secretory pathways. When there is a complete absence of motor, sensory and secretory function of the superior and recurrent laryngeal nerves, the lesion is most likely an extracranial peripheral lesion. The known causes of unilateral complete sensory and motor paralysis studied in this investigation have been in cases of central nervous system disease (ie, Arnold-Chiari malformation and Wallenburg's medullary infarction) or resection of the vagus nerve during temporal bone resection for cancer. Some cases of resection of schwannomas of the vagus nerve and other tumors in the neck fell into both categories. In other words, when all sensory, secretory, and motor function is lost, the nerve trunks on both branches of the superior and recurrent nerves were involved. Lesions of the nuclei as seen in some CNS diseases and in all of the idiopathic cases may have only motor loss with sparing of secretory and sensory function.

In patients with a combination of superior and recurrent laryngeal nerve paralysis, phonation produces a breathy or whispery voice due to air leakage between the normal and the intermedial (lateral) position of the flaccid, nontensed paralyzed cord (Fig. 4). During respiration, the cord is motionless in the lateral position and provides a better airway than with simple recurrent nerve paralysis. During phonation, the paralyzed cord retains the intermedial (lateral) position, except that there is a faint adduction in the posterior commissure area due to contraction of the bilaterally innervated interarytenoideus muscle. The arytenoid portion of the aryepiglottic fold falls medially overlapping and partially obstructing visualization of the posterior portion of the flaccid cord. In only one case was there suggestive wrinkling of the flaccid cord. A bowed contour better describes its appearance. The contraction of the opposite intact cricothyroid muscle produces an asymmetry of thyroid-cricoid cartilage tilt with lengthening and tensing of the innervated cord. The tensed normal cord is thus at a different level than the flaccid paralyzed cord, which may have an injected appearance due to hyperemia. Recognition of these features and of the asymmetric shift of the posterior larynx of the intact side toward the paralyzed side, following contraction and tilt of the thyroid upon the cricoid cartilages by the intact contralateral cricothyroid muscle, assists in recognizing the superior laryngeal nerve component of the combined paralysis. There may be pooling of secretions in the pyriform sinus for some period of time. Aspiration is notably more severe in those cases in which there is known sensory denervation (ie, actual surgical division of the internal branch of the superior laryngeal nerve) of the ipsilateral supraglottic portion of the larynx.

When only the motor fibers of the external branches of the superior laryngeal nerve and the recurrent nerve are paralyzed, the appearance of the larynx and the voice changes are similar but the management of secretions and aspiration is less severely affected. In addition to some central lower motor neuron lesions, this situation also occurs when both the recurrent and external branches of the superior laryngeal nerve are sectioned during thyroid surgery or other surgery in the neck.

METHODS

During the past ten years, the authors have seen, examined, and photographed the larynges of 238 patients with laryngeal paresis and paralysis. The majority of the patients have had several serial 16-mm motion picture films made over a period of months. The recent application of the Hopkins rod lens optic system (Storz Endoscopy of America) has made photography of the larynx relatively simple.[8,9] Careful review, including stop-frame analysis, of 605 filmstrips of these 238 cases has provided us with a better understanding of the dynamic appearance and function of the larynx in the presence of various combinations of paresis and paralysis. Correlation with various injury and neurological diseases was achieved in many cases but was not possible in others. The latter group forms the so-called idiopathic paralysis, the central subject of this communication. Follow-up was available in all but seven of the idiopathic cases. The majority of these patients received the conventional work-up (previously outlined in the Table) unless the diagnosis was obvious. After becoming cognizant of the significance of a combined superior and recurrent laryngeal nerve paralysis, only the patients with pure recurrent nerve paralyses underwent the conventional work-up. In those patients with combined superior and recurrent laryngeal nerve paralysis attention focused upon a search for intracranial or base of the skull disease.

RESULTS

The most remarkable finding was that all 39 patients with 44 paralyzed cords had paralysis or paresis of both the superior and recurrent laryngeal nerves. One patient experienced paralysis and recovery of her left vocal cord three times. Two patients had bilateral paralysis of the superior and recurrent laryngeal nerves. One of these two patients sustained a paralysis of the right vocal cord followed by recovery, then a paralysis of the left cord which persisted, failed to compensate, and required Teflon injection. The patient with the second case of bilateral paralysis had a successful reinnervation followed by removal of her tracheostomy.

The sex distribution of this series consisted of 108 men and 132 women. The series reported in the literature are about equally divided between those with a majority of either sex. Those series with a predominance of women attribute the selection process to the higher incidence of thyroid disease in women. The series reporting a predominance of men suggested a higher exposure to cold in a manner similar to that suggested for Bell's palsy.[3,14] Of the idiopathic cases, there were 17 men and 22 women. Thus, it would appear that the sex of the patient is not a significant factor. In contrast to other series, in our group the right recurrent nerve was affected more often than the left (ie, left 17, right 25). Twenty-three of the 39 patients experienced adequate return of voice such that no operative procedure was required. Sixteen had partial or complete return of function of the cords. Seven patients showed little return of function but compensation by the other cord was such that the speaking voice was satisfactory. Sixteen patients failed to have any noticeable recovery. Twelve of these patients received Teflon injections of their vocal cords. All patients receiving Teflon injections had improvement in the strength of their voices; however, a raspy diplophonia developed in two patients. In 18 patients, a strong history was elicited of the paralysis or paresis accompanying an upper respiratory infection or bronchitis. Four patients had been driving with the window open shortly before the onset of the paralysis. No history of possible related factors could be elicited from the remaining 17 patients.

DISCUSSION

In previously published series of laryngeal paralysis approximately 30 to 50% were cases in which no etiological factor for the paralysis could be found.[1,3,4] However, Clerf[2] reported an incidence of 36 out of 293 cases as being idiopathic.

This is slightly lower than the 39 out of 238 cases of laryngeal paralysis in our series.

The prognosis for partial or complete recovery of vocal cord function is less than 50%; however, the return of voice was satisfactory in 59%. Of the 16 cases in which the voice was less than satisfactory and there was no return of function as well as inadequate compensation, 12 received Teflon injections of the paralyzed cord. Experience has shown that 80% to 90% of those patients sustaining a pure recurrent laryngeal nerve injury will get satisfactory return of voice through return of function or compensation. The patients with idiopathic paralysis (paralysis of both superior and recurrent laryngeal nerves) have less successful restoration of voice following Teflon injections. Only 6 of the 12 patients injected regained good speaking voices. Four were rather poor and breathy while two were unsatisfactory and developed a raspy diplophonia.

Several patients showed beginning recovery of their paralyses two to three weeks after the onset of their paralyses and several others had partial function when first seen, presumably at a similar period and after historical onset of the paralysis. The most common beginning of recovery was between five and six months. One patient was noted to begin recovery at 11 months. Clerf[2] appears to be correct when stating that absence of evidence of motion at six months carries a poor prognosis for recovery.

There were two additional cases classified as idiopathic laryngeal paralysis when initially seen. Both had a schwannoma of the vagus nerve detected three and five years after the initial idiopathic diagnosis was made.

In contrast to other series and to our own series of traumatic paralyses, there was a slightly higher incidence of paralysis in the right vocal cord than the left. This is not significant and, as would be expected of a central or nuclear paralysis, the incidence is probably the same for both sides. There are no major anatomical differences as there are in the peripheral recurrent laryngeal nerves.

Only 18 of the patients had the onset of the paralysis accompanied by an upper respiratory infection and four others had been exposed to cold and chilling weather. Nevertheless, idiopathic vocal cord paralysis unequivocally seems to be a CNS (nuclear) lesion. In all probability it is similar in origin to other idiopathic cranial nerve palsies such as facial paralysis, loss of olfaction, and sudden deafness. Viruses can cause a wide range of clinical manifestations. Different virus infections may also cause similar clinical pictures. For example, aseptic meningitis can be caused by a number of different viruses such as polio, Coxsackie, ECHO, and mumps. Many viral agents are known to infect man and not cause disease.[14] Evidence to support the viral etiology of isolated cranial nerve paralysis is scanty and primarily clinical but nevertheless at least some must be of viral etiology.

Improvement in our diagnostic abilities to detect and separate isolated recurrent nerve paralysis from central (nuclear) lower motor neuron paralysis (both superior and recurrent laryngeal), should result in a significant decrease in the number of so-called idiopathic paralyses. Recognition of the pure recurrent nerve paralysis allows concentration of the diagnostic studies to the neck, mediastinum, and larynx as the sites for the disease process responsible for the paralysis. If there is a complete superior and recurrent laryngeal nerve paralysis, attention can be directed to intracranial and immediate extracranial locations for the etiological process. Cinephotographic studies of the larynx that allow repeated viewing and stop-frame analysis of the dynamic pathophysiology of the vocal cords has contributed significantly to the localization of the lesions in laryngeal paralysis.

REFERENCES

1. New GB, Childrey JH. Paralysis of the vocal cords: a study of 217 medical cases. Arch Otolaryngol 1932; 16:143-59.

2. Clerf LH. Unilateral vocal cord paralysis. JAMA 1953; 151:900-3.

3. Williams RG. Idiopathic recurrent laryngeal paralysis. J Laryngol Otol 1959; 73:161-6.

4. Parnell FW, Brandenberg JH. Vocal cord paralysis: a review of 100 cases. Laryngoscope 1970; 80:1036-45.

5. Hollinshead WH. Anatomy for surgeons. II. The head and neck. New York: Harper and Row, 1954; 425-56.

6. Kirschner JH. Pressman and Kelemen's physiology of the larynx. 2nd ed. Rochester, Minnesota: American Academy of Ophthalmology and Otolaryngology, 1970.

7. Ward PH, Berci G, Calcaterra TC. Superior laryngeal nerve paralysis: an often overlooked entity. Trans Am Acad Ophthalmol Otolaryngol 1977; 84:78-89.

8. Ward PH, Berci G, Calcaterra TC. Advances in endoscopic examination of the respiratory system. Ann Otol Rhinol Laryngol 1974; 83:759-69.

9. Ward PH, Hanson DG, Berci G. Photographic studies of the larynx in central laryngeal paresis and paralysis. Acta Otolaryngol (Stockh) 1981; 91:353-67.

10. Ogura JH. Surgical decompression of the recurrent laryngeal nerve in idiopathic unilateral vocal cord paresis. Ann Otol Rhinol Laryngol 1961; 70:451-63.

11. Maisel RH, Ogura J. Evaluation and treatment of vocal cord paralysis. Laryngoscope 1974; 84:302-16.

12. Ward PH, Berci G, Calcaterra T. New insights into superior and recurrent laryngeal nerve paralysis. Film and exhibit presented at the meeting of the American Academy of Ophthalmology and Otolaryngology, Las Vegas, Nevada, October 6-10, 1976.

13. Dedo H. The paralyzed larynx: an electromyographic study in dogs and humans. Laryngoscope 1970; 80:1455-1519.

14. Saunders WH. Viral infections and cranial nerve paralysis. Arch Otolaryngol 1963; 78:85-90.

Ann Otol Rhinol Laryngol 91:1982

CONGENITAL HEREDITARY BILATERAL ABDUCTOR VOCAL CORD PARALYSIS

KENNETH M. GRUNDFAST, MD GREGORY MILMOE, MD

WASHINGTON, DC

Congenital hereditary bilateral abductor vocal cord paralysis has been found in a father, his son and daughter. Though the disorder was previously believed to be inherited in a sex-linked manner, it now appears that there is an autosomal dominant variant. The vocal cord paralysis was associated with swallowing difficulty during infancy in all three of the family members. Although both the son and daughter required tracheostomies during the neonatal period, both manifested improvement of vocal cord movement during infancy so that decannulation was possible before 14 months of age. Localized delay in neurologic maturation is suspected as the etiology.

GENERAL CONSIDERATIONS

Congenital bilateral abductor vocal cord paralysis can cause significant airway compromise in a neonate. Paralysis of one or both vocal cords can be the result of trauma during birth, or vocal cord paralysis can occur as part of a generalized neurologic disorder. Although evidence of vocal cord paralysis in a neonate traditionally has not been viewed as a finding warranting full neurologic evaluation, abnormal motion of the vocal cords may be the initial manifestation of a previously undetected neurologic disorder.

CASE REPORT

A father, then his son, and finally his daughter were born with breathing difficulty. The father, born Oct 17, 1951, had a weak cry and could not swallow properly during the first year of life. As an infant, he required gavage feedings to maintain adequate nutrition. The father did not undergo endoscopic evaluation and, therefore, the diagnosis made to explain his symptoms was "laryngeal stridor." At around 1 year of age, he began to breathe with less difficulty and was able to swallow normally.

The son was born March 9, 1977. He weighed 3,600 g and was delivered by cesarean section because of cephalopelvic disproportion after a 39-week gestation and uncomplicated pregnancy. The baby had stridor at birth. There was meconium in the amniotic fluid, the Apgar score was 7 at one minute, and the neonate was noted to be lethargic, had difficulty feeding and developed cyanotic episodes. Direct laryngoscopy on the third day of life revealed bilateral abductor vocal cord paralysis and a tracheostomy was performed. In the following days, additional observations during feeding and radiographic studies led to the diagnosis of velopharyngeal incompetence and cricopharyngeal achalasia. After direct laryngoscopy at age 4 months revealed normal vocal cord movement, the tracheostomy tube was removed and the boy subsequently had no severe respiratory distress.

The daughter was born Jan 23, 1980. She weighed 2,960 g and was born by repeat cesarean section. A high-pitched, low-volume cry was noted at birth. Stridor and substernal and intercostal retractions soon became evident. Cyanosis and bradycardia occurred with feedings. A barium swallow examination showed nasopharyngeal reflux. On the third day of life, direct laryngoscopy revealed right abductor vocal cord paralysis and left abductor vocal cord paresis. Tracheostomy was performed. At 2 weeks of age auditory brainstem response testing showed prolongation of central conduction time, more marked on the right than on the left. At age 14 months, direct laryngoscopy revealed normal vocal cord movement, the tracheotomy tube was removed and the girl has had no further difficulty breathing.

DISCUSSION

In a review of 389 cases of bilateral abductor vocal cord paralysis, including 149 infants and children, Holinger et al[1] reported only one family with an inherited vocal cord paralysis that was present at birth. In 1964, Plott[2] reported bilateral abductor vocal cord paralysis in three brothers. Dysgenesis of the nucleus ambiguus was suspected as the etiology. In 1973, Watters and Fitch[3] reported the occurrence of bilateral abductor vocal cord paralysis in three male infants, a proband and two maternal cousins. None of the children had tracheostomies but all had marked physical and mental retardation. Based on the cases reported, it had been assumed that hereditary abductor vocal cord paralysis is transmitted as a sex-linked recessive or an autosomal dominant gene with male sex limitation.[3] In the family presently reported a girl was born with abductor vocal cord paralysis. Thus, it appears

From the Department of Otorhinolaryngology, Children's Hospital National Medical Center, and Division of Otolaryngology, George Washington University School of Medicine, Washington, DC.

Presented at the meeting of the American Broncho-Esophagological Association, Palm Beach, Florida, May 3-4, 1982.

that there is also an autosomal dominant form of the disorder.

In 1976, Gacek[4] reported hereditary abductor vocal cord paralysis in a father and two sons who had required tracheostomy but did not have mental retardation. The disorder described in this report differs from "hereditary abductor vocal cord paralysis" described by Gacek.[4] Gacek described male family members who developed vocal cord paralysis from six months to nine years after birth. In contrast, stridor with vocal cord paralysis (assumed to be the cause of the father's stridor) was present at birth in the cases now reported. While the underlying etiology in the cases reported by Gacek apparently was an inherited neurodegenerative process, it seems that an isolated delay in neurologic maturation could explain the findings in the cases now being reported. Gacek described a progressive familial disorder while the distinctive characteristics in the cases now being reported are paralysis present at birth, autosomal dominant mode of inheritance, associated subtle neurologic abnormalities and improvement of vocal cord motion with lessening of airway obstruction throughout the first year of life.

In each of the three previous reports of hereditary abductor vocal cord paralysis, the site of lesion was considered. There seems to be general agreement among all authors that etiology of the vocal cord paralysis is dysgenesis of the abductor portion of the nucleus ambiguus.

Considering that abductor vocal cord paralysis could be the earliest manifestation of a localized neurologic disorder, the two children described in this report underwent objective and subjective assessment of neurologic function. The boy had a cine barium swallow examination and esophageal motility testing. Abnormal deglutition with nasal reflux was evident on the radiographic study and the pharyngoesophageal manometric study revealed abnormally low pharyngeal pressure. The girl also had nasal reflux and a manometric study revealed dyskinesis of the upper esophageal sphincter. Also, auditory brainstem response (ABR) testing in the girl at age 2 weeks revealed normal hearing sensation threshold with prolongation of wave I-V latency bilaterally. Repeat ABR at age 4 months showed more normal wave I-V latency in the right ear, while there was a more abnormal wave I-V latency in the left ear than had been evident at age 2 weeks. The findings are subtle, yet significant.

In a way, the ability to make a diagnosis and to determine the location and extent of related abnormalities depends upon the manner in which the infant's evaluation is approached. Many years ago, the neonate with stridor was usually diagnosed as having "congenital laryngeal stridor." As endoscopic methods improved, it became possible to assess laryngeal function more accurately. Consequently, infants with symptoms that once might have been collectively diagnosed as "laryngeal stridor" now can be examined in ways that enable more precise diagnoses. Further, with the advent of such methods of objective assessment as ABR testing and pharyngoesophageal manometric studies, it is possible to elicit quantifiable evidence of dysfunction that might otherwise not be apparent. Thus, at least in the father, son and daughter now reported, it appears that abductor vocal cord paralysis was not the result of an isolated dysgenesis in a minute area of the nucleus ambiguus. Rather, evidence of abnormalities of deglutition, esophageal motility and central auditory transmission seems to indicate a constellation of functionally and anatomically related abnormalities. This concept of related neurologic abnormalities was considered by Holinger et al[5] in a report on familial vocal cord paralysis occurring in association with peroneal muscular atrophy (Charcot-Marie-Tooth disease). Holinger used measurements of nerve conduction velocity and latency in the lower extremities to elicit objective evidence of neurologic dysfunction that otherwise might not have been apparent.

Further, a recent report by Finitzo-Hieber et al[6] revealed that 5 of 6 patients diagnosed as having adductor spasmodic dysphonia manifested abnormal latency parameters on ABR testing. This can be viewed as supporting the concept that a neonate with bilateral abductor vocal cord paralysis may be likely to manifest evidence of brainstem dysfunction in nuclei and tracts other than those specifically related to the vagus and recurrent laryngeal nerves.

SUMMARY

Three cases are presented involving infants who had stridor at birth. Direct laryngoscopy in the son and daughter revealed bilateral vocal cord paralysis; presumably, the father also had bilateral vocal cord paralysis. All had associated difficulties with swallowing. Difficulty breathing was most severe at birth; then, as vocal cord movement improved, ability to breathe through the larynx improved during the first year of life. In contrast to previous reports[3,4] of "hereditary" or "familial abductor vocal cord paralysis," this report describes a congenital condition. Apparently, there is an inherited tendency for delayed maturation in one neurologic subsystem. Most likely, the site of the abnormality is in the vicinity of the brainstem nuclei of the vagus nerve.

CONCLUSIONS

1. A rare disorder has been observed that can be termed congenital hereditary bilateral abductor vocal cord paralysis.
2. Tracheostomy during the neonatal period may be necessary to maintain an adequate airway.
3. Movement of the vocal cords slowly improves during the first year of life.
4. Feeding abnormalities and objective evidence of neurologic dysfunction within the brainstem may be associated with the disorder.

ACKNOWLEDGMENT — The authors wish to express their appreciation to Mrs. Carol Boyd and Ms. Joyce Johnson for assistance in preparation of the manuscript.

REFERENCES

1. Holinger LD, Holinger PC, Holinger PH. Etiology of bilateral vocal cord paralysis: a review of 389 cases. Ann Otol Rhinol Laryngol 1976; 85:428-36.

2. Plott D. Congenital laryngeal-abductor paralysis due to nucleus ambiguus dysgenesis in three brothers. N Engl J Med 1964; 271:593-7.

3. Watters GV, Fitch N. Familial laryngeal abductor paralysis and psychomotor retardation. Clin Genet 1973; 4:429-33.

4. Gacek RR. Hereditary abductor vocal cord paralysis. Ann Otol Rhinol Laryngol 1976; 85:90-3.

5. Holinger PC, Vuckovich DM, Holinger LD, Holinger PH. Bilateral abductor vocal cord paralysis in Charcot-Marie-Tooth disease. Ann Otol Rhinol Laryngol 1979; 88:205-9.

6. Finitzo-Hieber T, Freeman FJ, Gerling IJ, Dobson L, Schaefer SD. Auditory brainstem response abnormalities in adductor spasmodic dysphonia. Am J Otolaryngol 1982; 3:26-30.

≈

AMERICAN RADIUM SOCIETY

The 65th annual meeting of the American Radium Society will be held April 5-9, 1983, at the Hyatt Regency Hotel in Savannah, Georgia. For further information contact Mrs. Sally Polek, Office of the Secretariat, American Radium Society, 925 Chestnut Street, Philadelphia, PA 19107; (215) 574-3179.

≈

AMERICAN CLEFT PALATE ASSOCIATION/AMERICAN CLEFT PALATE EDUCATIONAL FOUNDATION

The ACPA/ACPEF annual convention will be held May 4-7, 1983, at the Hyatt Regency in Indianapolis, Indiana. For further information contact Jane Angelone Graminski, Administrative Secretary, American Cleft Palate Association, American Cleft Palate Educational Foundation, 331 Salk Hall, University of Pittsburgh, Pittsburgh, PA 15261; (412) 681-9620.

ATLANTOAXIAL INSTABILITY REVISITED

AN ALERT FOR ENDOSCOPISTS

MARTIN L. NORTON, MD, JD
ANN ARBOR, MICHIGAN

MANHAL A. GHANMA, MD
CLEVELAND, OHIO

Atlantoaxial instability in rheumatoid arthritis patients presents a particular hazard for endoscopists. The basic pathology, while well known to orthopedists, is not common knowledge among bronchoesophagologists or anesthesiologists. This paper describes the syndrome, potential complications and possible approaches to avoiding serious neurologic sequellae.

The endoscopist is routinely faced with the consequences of managing patients with multifaceted diseases. One of these, rheumatoid arthritis, has particularly serious aspects pertaining to endoscopy for diagnosis and therapy or endotracheal intubation.

Abnormalities of the atlantoaxial joint complex have been well documented in patients with rheumatoid arthritis. It is the purpose of this paper to alert not only anesthesiologists but all laryngobronchoesophagologists to this potentially disastrous situation. The precise definition of spinal instability has still not been agreed upon but certain general statements can be made. Clinical instability is defined as the loss of the capacity of the spine under physiologic loads to maintain relationships between vertebrae in such a way that there is neither damage nor subsequent irritation of the spinal cord or nerve roots and without development of incapacitating deformity or pain due to structural changes.[1]

DEMOGRAPHY

Atlantoaxial instability (AAI) is present in one fourth of all patients with rheumatoid arthritis. The condition is more frequent in males.[2] Its presence seems to be independent of the duration of the disease and of the patient's age. The finding of AAI is more likely in patients who have severe peripheral rheumatoid involvement. Subluxation is by far more common than dislocation and the clinical symptoms are indirectly related to the degree of instability of "slip." In one study,[3] 27 of 41 patients with subluxation, and 6 of 8 patients with dislocation, had central nervous system signs. Pain was present in 31 of 41 patients with subluxation and in 6 of 8 patients with dislocation. These findings are consistent with more recent reports in the literature.[4] From the above it is evident that several patients had radiographic evidence of instability but had no pain or signs.

ANATOMY

In the normal individual, integrity of the spine in the C-1 to C-2 area is maintained by the bony configuration as well as by ligamentous structures.

The first cervical vertebra (C-1) is named the atlas after Titan in Greek mythology because it supports the head. It is peculiar in that it has no body. It also has no spinous process, is ring-like and consists of an anterior and a posterior arch and two lateral masses.

The second cervical vertebra (C-2) is named the axis or epistropheus because it forms the pivot upon which the first vertebra rotates. The dens or odontoid process is an extension of the body of the second cervical vertebra which projects into the ring of C-1 just posterior to the anterior arch of C-1 (Fig. 1).

Of primary importance is the transverse ligament, which is a structure that attaches to both lateral masses behind the odontoid process of the axis, thereby preventing any posterior translocation or dislocation of the dens (odontoid process). This serves to protect the cord structures which lie immediately posterior. The second set of ligaments are the alar or wing ligaments. They are of questionable value in terms of providing mechanical stability but connect the odontoid process to the occipital condyles. The third set of ligaments are the cruciate ligaments which connect the axis to the border of the foramen magnum. The major motion at the C-1 to C-2 articulation is rotation. It is estimated that approximately 47% of axial rotation occurs at this point. There is no lateral bending at C-1 to C-2. In the normal individual there is also anteroposterior shift of the atlas on the axis or vice versa. Approximately 10° of flexion-extension normally occurs at C-1 to C-2.

In the patient with rheumatoid arthritis, the disease process affects the joints of the C-1 to C-2 ar-

From the Department of Anesthesiology, University of Michigan Hospitals, Ann Arbor, and the Department of Orthopedics, St. Luke's Hospital, Cleveland.

Presented at the meeting of the American Broncho-Esophagological Association, Palm Beach, Florida, May 3-4, 1982.

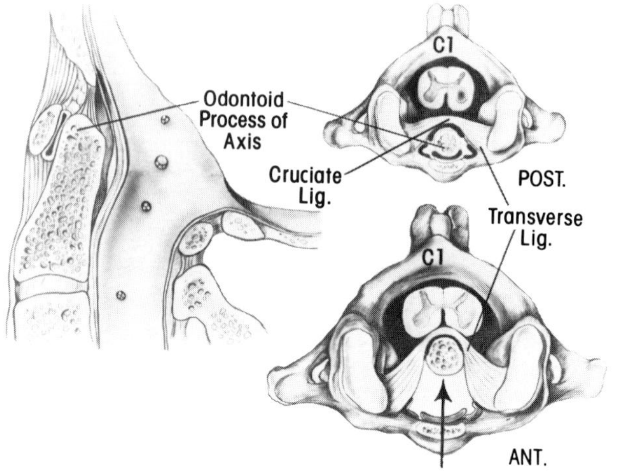

Fig. 1. Anatomy of atlantoaxial instabilty in severe peripheral rheumatoid arthritis.

ticulation (atlantodental, atlanto-occipital, and atlantoaxial joints). Subsequent to this, erosive changes occur in the odontoid process, along with weakening of the ligamentous structures there. The result is that neurological deficits or symptoms may ensue with definite instability of the spine.

Fielding et al[5] at Saint Luke's Hospital in New York have demonstrated that significant force is necessary to disrupt the transverse ligament. When this occurs, the odontoid process moves posteriorly, thereby producing a free space anteriorly. This space between the anterior arch of the atlas and the anterior cortex of the dens measured 5 mm when the transverse ligament was ruptured (Fig. 2). The remaining ligaments could then be disrupted easily. If all the other ligaments were disrupted and the transverse ligament was still *intact* the maximum displacement was 3 mm. Although the space anteriorly is a clue to the presence of instability, the true determinant of neurologic deficit is the space available for the cord (Fig. 3). This is measured between the posterior arch of the atlas and the odontoid process. The spinal cord itself measures approximately 1 cm in AP diameter at the C-1 level and approximately 2.2 cm in tranverse diameter. Damage to the cord can occur even if the available space is greater than 1 cm due to meningeal compression by the odontoid process.[6]

Symptoms of instability at C-1 to C-2 include upper neck pain, headaches, muscle weakness, incontinence, vertigo, nystagmus, dysphoria, and finally death. The finding of instability at C-1 to C-2 occurs in approximately 25% of rheumatoid arthritis patients and seems independent of duration of the disease (Figs. 2 and 3).

RADIOGRAPHY

In patients with suspected AAI a cervical spine radiographic series is recommended. This should include a lateral view of the cervical spine both in

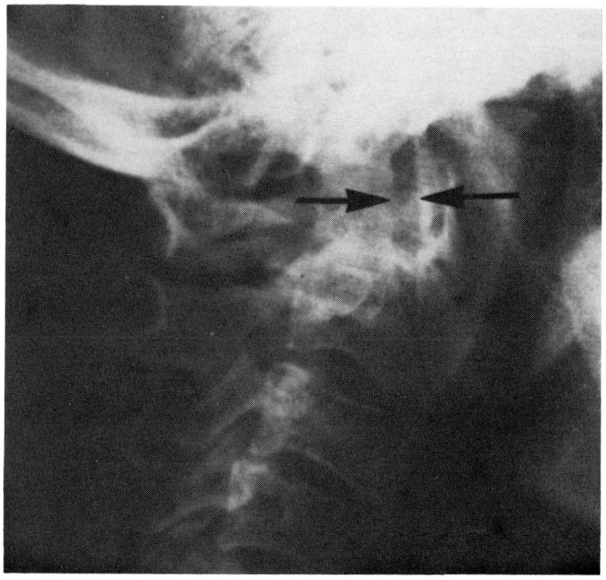

Fig. 2. Excessive mobility of odontoid process shown by space between anterior arch of atlas and anterior cortex of dens (arrows).

flexion and extension. It should also include an odontoid process view (open-mouth projection). If there is uncertainty as to the diagnosis, tomograms of the cervical spine should be done. The diagnosis is best made on a lateral view of the cervical spine in flexion, since the condition may not appear in extension.

Caution is necessary while obtaining flexion views of the spine. The patient himself should flex his neck as opposed to any forceful maneuver by the radiologist or radiology technician. If the patient has any untoward symptoms (increased pain, neurological deficits) from flexion of the spine, then his cervical spine should be immediately returned to the neutral position.

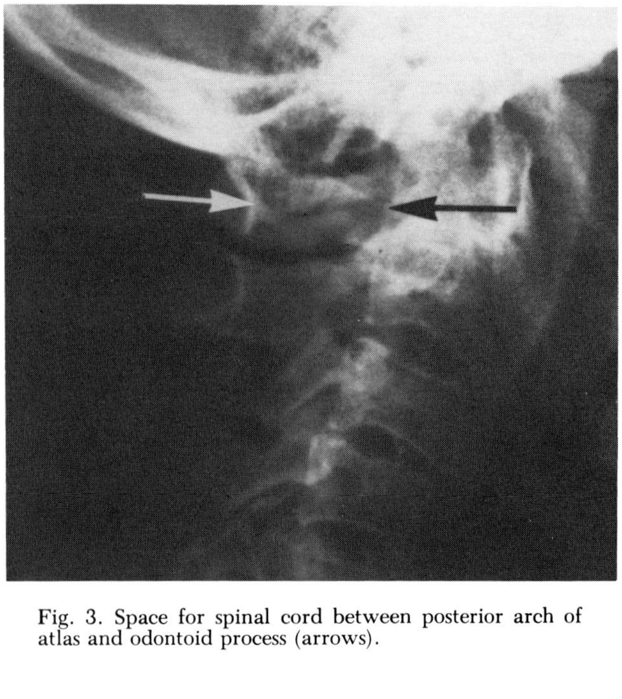

Fig. 3. Space for spinal cord between posterior arch of atlas and odontoid process (arrows).

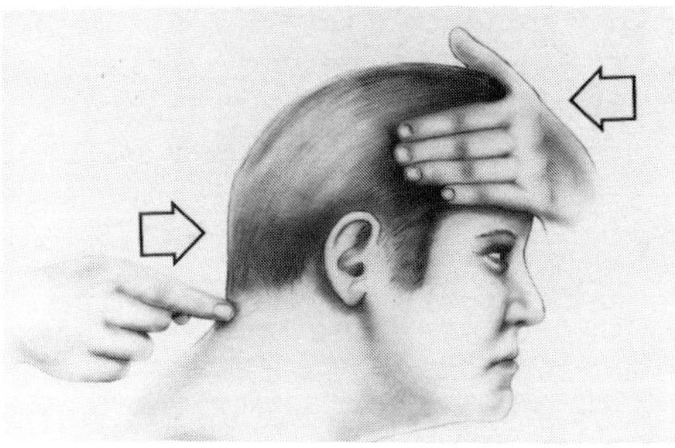

Fig. 4. Sharp and Purser test.

ENDOSCOPY AND ENDOTRACHEAL INTUBATION

Classic descriptions of endotracheal intubation techniques[7] describe many complications. Applebaum and Bruce[8] comment as follows:

> Traumatic mechanical injuries to the cervical spinal column and spinal cord may occur during positioning of the patient for intubation. These injuries are more likely in patients with preexisting spinal column trauma or weakness due to age, bone demineralization, malformation, or tumor. The person inexperienced at intubation further increases the possibility of injury by forceful hyperextension of the head (without flexing the neck) in a faulty attempt at improving laryngoscopic exposure of the larynx.

Katz and Kadis[9] primarily comment on the problems of corticosteroid therapy, but also refer to Edelist's admonition[10] that the neck and head should be manipulated with great care during positioning or intubation because cervical vertebral erosion and subluxation may occur especially at the atlantoaxial joint.

Dripps et al[11] stress flexion of cervical spine and extension at the atlanto-occipital joint according to the earlier advice of Chevalier Jackson[12] in contradistinction to the Rose position which stressed the anterior convexity positioning of the whole cervical spine.

Thus we see that the usual admonition of endoscopists[13] was and is for the "pecking position." Following this instruction in patients with potential atlantoaxial instability could cause cord compression by displacement of the odontoid process (dens) posteriorly. Flexion of the neck can produce a similar effect. While extension of the neck would appear to obviate the problem — this is *not* recommended. The biomechanics of extension should transfer the forces so that the atlas would tend to shift forward (ventrally) producing the feared subluxation and cord compression. We are therefore obligated to have the patient position the head while awake.

Althoff and Goldie[14] have recently studied the value of supportive collars for stabilization of C-1 to C-2 vertebrae. Their results indicate minimal effect on decreasing the instability in flexion even with the

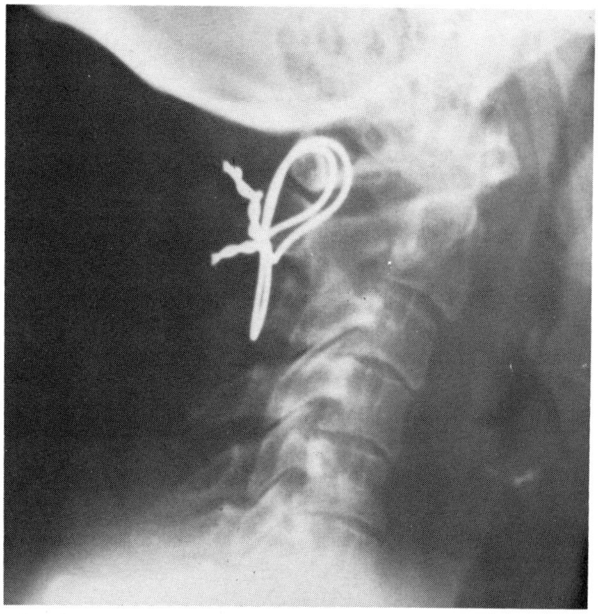

Fig. 5. Surgical repair wiring of atlas to dens.

Philadelphia or Guilford collars (38%-46% reduction). Unfortunately, these collars also impede the mechanics of endoscopy to some extent. A review of neurologic signs and symptoms relative to the upper cervical cord outflow should be completed. Then, and only then, should the patient be anesthetized. Endoscopy/intubation must be accomplished with no further change in position of the cervical spine. Access can be aided by intentional anterior dislocation of the temporomandibular joint (aided by general anesthesia and the use of nondepolarizing muscle relaxants). This will place the mandible in an anterior position with the mouth widely opened. After intubation we should return the mandible to the normal resting position as soon as possible before withdrawing the muscle relaxants.

Anesthetic management also requires muscle relaxant usage. Succinyldiacetylcholine causes marked neck muscle contraction with its potential for cervical vertebral slippage. The curare drugs do *not* manifest this effect, but do decrease the supportive muscle tension. On balance, we believe the hazards related to succinylcholine to be the greater risk.

In extreme cases, application of Crutchfield or Gardner-Wells tongs should be considered. The weights should not exceed 4.54 kg to avoid total destabilization of the atlantoaxial joint. The choice of this technique must be based on neurologic symptomatology in the awake patient. However, it is a useful approach even if temporarily applied.

What else can we do? First and foremost is awareness of the problems herein described. This responsibility is both ethical and legal. Secondly, there is the simple clinical test of Sharp and Purser[15] which can alert the endoscopist to the need for radiologic evaluation.

With the patient sitting upright, relaxed and with the neck flexed, the examiner places one hand on the forehead and the index finger of the other on the spinous process of the axis. Normally, pressure on the forehead produces no appreciable movement but when AAS is present a backward gliding motion of the head can be felt as the subluxation is reduced[16] (Fig. 4).

Similarly, because of the demography of this condition, another approach is to obtain a lateral radiograph of the neck in all patients over the age of 40 years with a history of either rheumatoid arthritis or ankylosing spondylitis, particularly if they have been medicated with steroids.

Perhaps most important is the obligation of the endoscopist to maintain his level of expertise in line with current knowledge.

TREATMENT

Although detailed descriptions of effective treatment of AAI are beyond the scope of this paper, it is important to mention that the treatment depends on the degree of instability. Patients who have minimal instability are advised to wear a collar and avoid activities that could possibly involve head injury. These patients should be cautioned about the increased risk of neurological deficits in car accidents producing whiplash-type injuries. As the degree of instability increases, the risk to the patient increases. In the acutely unstable spine, posterior cervical fusion or wiring of atlas to dens is indicated (Fig. 5).

CONCLUSION

We have presented a review of atlantoaxial instability in rheumatoid arthritis patients. These individuals represent an inordinate risk of cervical cord injury potentially leading to quadraplegia and even death. The ramifications of keeping informed about current medical knowledge obligates the physician to be alert to this syndrome.

REFERENCES

1. White AW, Panjabi MM. The clinical biomechanics of the occipitoatlantoaxial complex. Orthop Clin North Am 1978; 9:867-78.

2. Matthew JA. Atlantoaxial subluxation in rheumatoid arthritis. Ann Rheum Dis 1969; 33:260-6.

3. Rana NA, Hancock DD, Taylor AR, et al. Atlanto-axial subluxation and upward translocation of the odontoid process in rheumatoid arthritis. J Bone Joint Surg 1973; 55-A:1304.

4. Pellicii PM, Ranawat CS, Tsairis P, et al. A prospective study of the progression of rheumatoid arthritis of the cervical spine. J Bone Joint Surg 1981; 3:342-50.

5. Fielding JW, Cochran GVB, Lansing JF III, et al. Tears of the transverse ligament of the atlas. J Bone Joint Surg 1974; 55-A:1683-91.

6. Sherk HH. Atlantoaxial instability and acquired basilar invagination in rheumatoid arthritis. Orthop Clin North Am 1978; 19:1053-63.

7. Bannister FB, MacBeth RG. Direct laryngoscopy and tracheal intubation. Lancet 1944; 2:651.

8. Applebaum EL, Bruce DL. Tracheal intubation. Philadelphia: WB Saunders, 1976:80-1.

9. Katz J, Kadis BL. Anesthesia and uncommon diseases. Philadelphia: WB Saunders, 1973:408-12.

10. Edelist G. Principles of anesthetic management in rheumatoid arthritic patients. Anesth Analg 1964; 43:227.

11. Dripps RD, Eckenhoff JE, Vandam LD. Introduction to anesthesia. 5th ed. Philadelphia: WB Saunders, 1977; 15:216-30.

12. Jackson C, Jackson CL. Bronchoscopy, esophagoscopy and gastroscopy. 3rd ed. Philadelphia: WB Saunders, 1934:85-94.

13. Jackson C. Peroral endoscopy and laryngeal surgery. St. Louis: Laryngoscope Co, 1915.

14. Althoff B, Goldie IF. Cervical collars in rheumatoid atlanto-axial subluxation: a radiologic comparison. Ann Rheum Dis 1980; 39:485.

15. Sharp J, Purser DW. Ann Rheum Dis 1961; 20:47.

16. Stevens JC, Cartlidge NEF, Saundes M, et al. Atlantoaxial subluxation and cervical myelopathy in rheumatoid arthritis. Q J Med 1971; 159:391-408.

LARYNGEAL MALIGNANCIES AND COMPUTERIZED TOMOGRAPHY
A CORRELATION OF TOMOGRAPHIC AND HISTOPATHOLOGIC FINDINGS

JOYCE A. SCHILD, MD
MAHMOOD F. MAFEE, MD
GALDINO E. VALVASSORI, MD
WADI A. BARDAWIL, MD

CHICAGO, ILLINOIS

We compared the anatomic structures, computerized tomographic (CT) scan images and the histopathologic findings after surgery in 15 patients with laryngeal epidermoid carcinoma. We examined the horizontal whole-mount histologic sections along with the preoperative CT and verified the preoperative impression of the soft tissue changes of preepiglottic space involvement; true cord, false cord and aryepiglottic fold invasion; or subglottic extension in all 15 patients. It was impossible to judge reliably the microscopic invasion of bone or cartilage with this method. Preoperative CT evaluation of carcinoma of the larynx was a reliable method for judging gross tumor size, though decisions regarding conservation surgery cannot be based on CT evaluation alone.

INTRODUCTION

Until recently the specialized advanced radiographic procedures for diagnosis of laryngeal carcinoma included contrast laryngography, xeroradiography, tomography and arteriography. Each of these methods has failed to give an adequate view of deep invasion and early cartilage destruction because of the surface orientation of the technique or the indirect nature of the examination. Since 1973, when computerized tomography (CT) was first used clinically,[1] it has been effective in determining size, shape, location and tissue invasion of tumors in many anatomic locations.

To assess the accuracy of CT in laryngeal carcinoma, we compared the CT images with anatomic and pathologic structures. Removed whole or partial larynges with known epidermoid carcinoma were cut serially in the horizontal plane and studied alongside the preoperative CT scan done in the same horizontal plane.

METHODS AND MATERIALS

Fifteen patients with epidermoid carcinoma were examined preoperatively with CT scans of the neck from the base of the tongue to the upper trachea. The examination consisted of contiguous 5-mm horizontal (axial) sections with the infraorbitomeatal (Reid) line perpendicular to the table top. The patient was positioned supine, the head supported gently in position. Mobility of the vocal cords was studied with scanning during expiratory phonation. No patient required sedation. Equipment used was the GE CT/T 7800 for the early patients in the study, and the GE CT/T 8800 for the last eight patients.

The excised tissues were processed by the celloidin technique: fixed in 10% formalin for three to five days, decalcified in formic acid-sodium citrate solution for 3 weeks, washed, dehydrated in ascending concentrations of alcohol, cleared in ether/alcohol and imbedded in celloidin for 7 weeks. The last eight specimens were processed using a rapid method with staining properties equal to those of the longer processing technique. Following formalin fixation, washing and dehydration, specimens were decalcified for seven days in 1% nitric acid and neutralized in 5% sodium sulfate. All specimens were kept in a vacuum and placed in 1% celloidin for 24 hours, then in 4%, 8% and 12% celloidin for each successive 24-hour period. Finally, specimens were imbedded in 16% celloidin for 48 hours for improved cutting.

The sections of each whole or partial larynx were made in the horizontal plane and corresponded to the planes of the CT images. Early specimens were opened in the operating room by a vertical cut across the cricoid plate; however, better sections were obtained when the specimen was kept intact throughout the processing. Each section was 25 μm thick and stained with hematoxylin and eosin. The histologic sections of each larynx and the corresponding CT images were then examined simultaneously. Microscopic invasion was evaluated independently and compared to the preoperative CT evaluation.

RESULTS

In 1980 a preliminary report of the first four patients in this series was presented in poster form at the annual meeting of the American Academy of Otolaryngology (Schild et al, Computerized tomography of laryngeal malignancies: a correlation of tomographic and pathologic sections). Since that time 11 more larynges have been suitably processed for inclusion in the study, for a total of 15 patients. We continued to examine the horizontal whole-mount histologic sections along with the preoperative CT (Fig. 1) and verified the preoperative impression of the soft tissue changes of preepiglottic space involvement; true cord, false cord and aryepiglottic fold invasion (Fig. 2); or subglottic extension in all 15 patients.

The possibility of predicting cartilage or bone involvement was also studied (Table 1). In five patients neither CT nor histologic sections showed tumor invasion. Large defects of cartilage were recognized in two of the 15 patients both on CT and histologic sections (Fig. 3). In two more, erosion

From the Departments of Otolaryngology-Head and Neck Surgery (Schild, Valvassori), Radiology (Valvassori, Mafee) and Pathology (Bardawil), University of Illinois College of Medicine, University of Illinois Hospital and Eye and Ear Infirmary, Chicago.

Presented at the meeting of the American Broncho-Esophagological Association, Palm Beach, Florida, May 3-4, 1982.

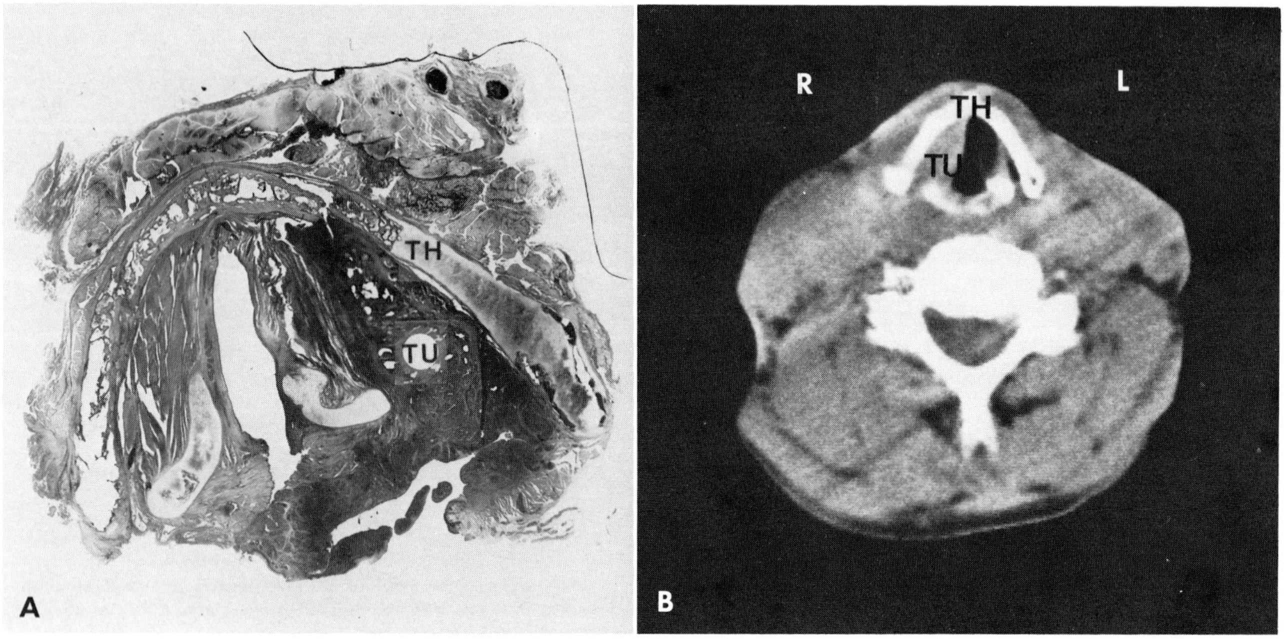

Fig. 1. A) Histologic section of larynx. B) CT scan of larynx in reversed orientation, right (R) to left (L). Tumor (TU) in right vocal cord appears on CT scan denser than left vocal cord and of different contour. Thyroid cartilage (TH) is intact.

was suspected on scan and was present histologically in one; in the other patient anatomic lack of ossification from tumor extension could not be differentiated by CT but histologically no tumor breakthrough was present. Tumor extended beyond the external surface of the thyroid cartilage in two additional patients, but had advanced via natural planes rather than through erosive action. The invasion of cartilage was seen microscopically in six larynges and was not predicted preoperatively by CT scan. These areas were less than the 4- to 6-mm size necessary to be visible by scan.

Vocal cord motility was specifically judged in only five patients on preoperative scans (Table 2). Patients were asked to phonate "E" on expiration, and the image was compared to that obtained during quiet breathing (Fig. 4). The CT image should show a difference in vocal cord position if the cords are mobile. While three of the five patients had decreased or absent motility on CT examination, two of the three had cartilage invasion histologically. Two of the five had good motility on CT; both had cartilage invasion. Thus, in only two of the five patients did radiologic findings regarding motility cor-

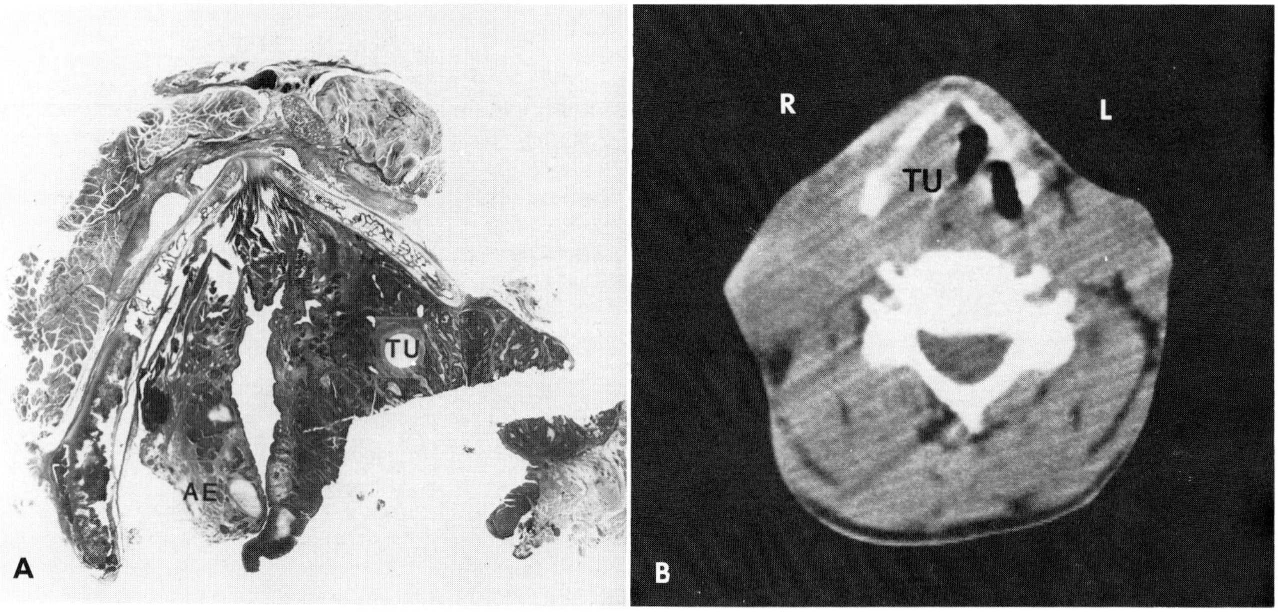

Fig. 2. A) Histologic section of larynx. B) CT scan (reversed orientation). Tumor (TU) obliterates right pyriform sinus, extending into false cord and aryepiglottic fold. Left aryepiglottic fold (AE) is normal. Separation artifact due to tissue processing is seen crossing tumor mass on right.

TABLE 1. CARTILAGE DEFECTS PREDICTED BY CT SCAN (N = 15 PATIENTS)

No. of Patients	*CT*	*Histology*
5	—	—
6	—	+
2	+	+
1	±	+
1	±	—

— - No defect predicted; + - Defect predicted; ± - Equivocal evidence for defect.

TABLE 2. EVALUATION OF VOCAL CORD MOTILITY

CT Motility	*Histologic Invasion*
Normal	+
Normal	+
Absent	+
Absent	+
Absent	—

+ - Invasion of cartilage; — - No invasion of cartilage.

relate with histologic findings of cartilage invasion.

Though nodal disease is sometimes predictable[2] and was recognized in some of our patients, it was not specifically evaluated in this study.

DISCUSSION

Radiographic demonstration of soft tissue abnormalities is hindered by the difficulty in defining differences in individual tissue densities. Xerography is an improvement because of so-called edge enhancement, but at the expense of increased radiation. Contrast laryngography yields surface information but may cause further obstruction in a patient with a diminished airway and requires local anesthetic for best results. Arteriography, while adding the possibility of tumor blush from intrinsic vascularity, often shows only deflection of vessels by the tumor in the larynx or neck and risks the patient's reaction to the dye or complications of arterial puncture.

In 1973 Hounsfield[3] and Ambrose[4] introduced clinical computerized transverse axial scanning (tomography) to evaluate lesions in the head. Subsequent improvements now allow CT scans of other body areas including the neck. Larynx lesions of all kinds are readily assessed visually by CT scanning.[5-7] Use of Hounsfield numbers defines tissue density differences precisely and is especially helpful for cystic lesions.[8]

Soft tissue abnormalities are particularly well displayed by CT of the larynx because of the cross-sectional view obtained.[9] This allows three-dimensional understanding of structural relationships of tissues of differing density when several CT levels are interpreted sequentially. In addition the effect of protruding tumor on airway size is startlingly visible. This was well demonstrated in this series when the CT scans were examined in conjunction with the tissue sections, as the tumor could be recognized easily in both methods at different levels. Furthermore, subtle asymmetry in the larynx is readily apparent on CT and indicates local pathology. Widening of the preepiglottic space, broadening of a normally delicate aryepiglottic fold, displacement of one arytenoid, or disturbance of motility are all important findings for identifying extension of tumor in various directions.

Invasion of cartilage can be a more difficult determination and may not be reliable. In our study, predicting cartilage or bone involvement was possible only with gross defects. Microscopically

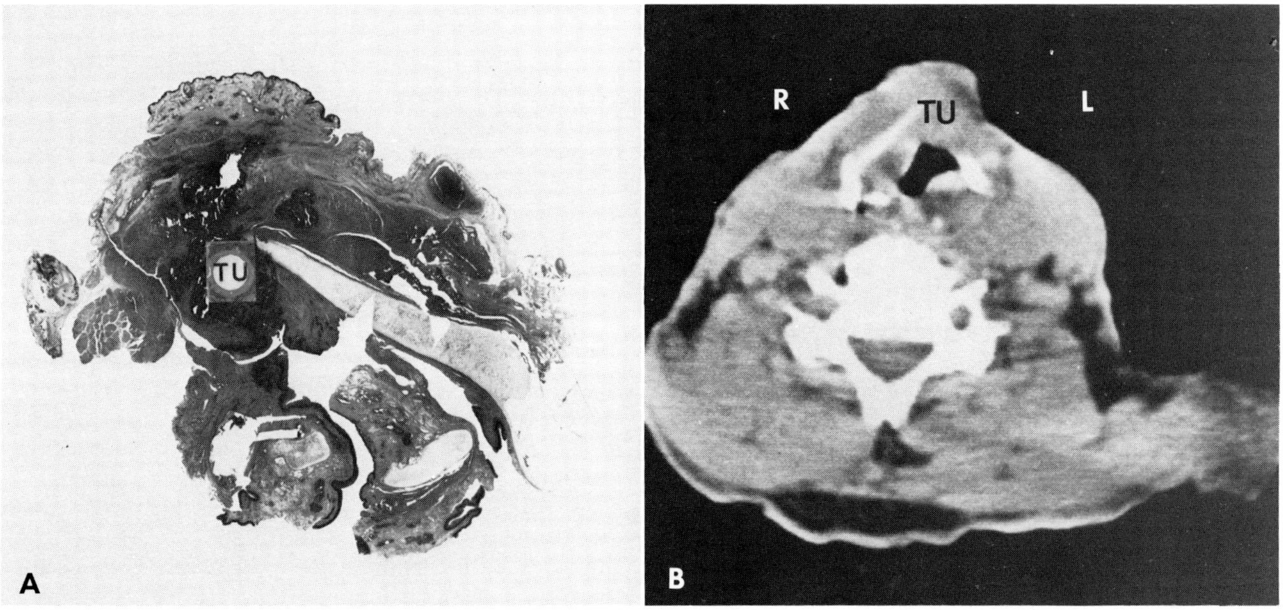

Fig. 3. A) Histologic section of left larynx. B) CT scan (reversed orientation). Previous left hemilaryngectomy with recurrent tumor (TU). Surgical absence of thyroid cartilage is shown on left.

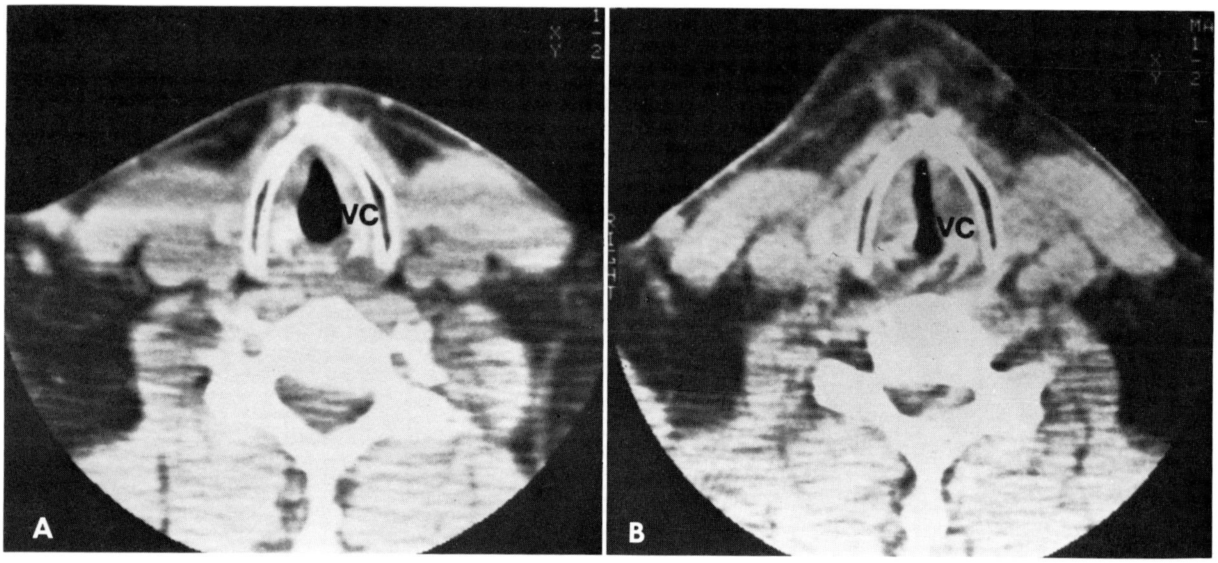

Fig. 4. CT scans of larynx comparing A) open vocal position in quiet breathing and B) phonation where glottis is smaller and both vocal cords have moved toward the midline. There is density difference in left vocal cord (VC) which is site of carcinoma.

identified invasion was not detectable on scan. Cartilage must be well calcified for good roentgenographic visibility, but calcification in laryngeal cartilages is highly variable. Irregular outlines and marked loss of symmetry, particularly when accompanied by surrounding tumor mass, become markers for judging the existence and extent of tumor erosion. In this series two patients had definite defects on CT, one by tumor invasion and one by previous surgery. The defects of both patients were confirmed on histologic sections. In two more patients cartilage defects were suspected which were confirmed on tissue examination in one. However, six patients were not suspected of having cartilage invasion on CT but did prove to have invasion microscopically. Because of the general size of the gross lesions, the inability to recognize microscopic invasion from CT did not affect the choice of therapy in these cases, although it might in patients with smaller lesions. It is our impression that cartilage erosion demonstrable on CT is significant prognostically, but that absence of recognizable erosion on CT is not a reliable guide in decisions regarding conservation surgical procedures. This is in agreement with the conclusions of others.[10]

Vocal cord motility can be evaluated by comparing the position of the cords during expiratory phonation and quiet breathing. Breath-holding and the Valsalva maneuver are alternatives to expiratory phonation because the glottis is obliterated during these maneuvers.[11] However, comparison must be made with quiet breathing in order to avoid confusion with a mass lesion. Though the number of patients reported here is small, this series suggests the reliability of CT scanning for evaluating vocal cord mobility; however it should not be solely depended upon for diagnosis.

CONCLUSIONS

We found that preoperative CT evaluation of carcinoma of the larynx is a reliable method for judging gross tumor size. Soft tissue swelling is well outlined and its extent can be correctly estimated medially into the airway and, more importantly, laterally into surrounding soft tissue because of the cross-sectional view obtained with this method. The superior-inferior extent of tumor is easily examined because multiple levels are obtained for viewing. Cartilage defects (surgical or neoplastic) can be visualized well only when they are macroscopic and when the underlying cartilage has no anatomic or calcification irregularity. Microscopic invasion of cartilage by tumor cannot be seen on CT scanning; therefore, decisions regarding conservation surgery cannot be based on CT evaluation alone. Vocal cord motility can be evaluated by comparing the cord position during quiet breathing with that during expiratory phonation, the Valsalva maneuver or breath-holding. However, observation of vocal cord immobility must be used with that of anatomic changes to estimate tumor size and invasiveness.

Overall, the cross-sectional view of the larynx obtained by CT scanning gives a three-dimensional image of the tumor not available by any other method. The patient can be positioned comfortably, no anesthetic is needed and no contrast materials are ingested or injected. We believe that the information gained from CT scanning is better than that from other available special radiologic procedures. It is, therefore, the preferred method for evaluation of tumors of the larynx.

REFERENCES

1. Ambrose J, Hounsfield G. Computerized transverse axial tomography. Br J Radiol 1973; 46:148-9.

2. Sagel SS, AufderHeide JF, Aronberg DJ, Stanley RJ, Archer CR. High resolution of computed tomography in the staging of carcinoma of the larynx. Laryngoscope 1981; 91:292-300.

3. Hounsfield GN. Computerized transverse axial scanning (tomography): 1. Description of system. Br J Radiol 1973; 46: 1016-22.

4. Ambrose J. Computerized transverse axial scanning (tomography): 2. Clinical application. Br J Radiol 1973 46:1023-47.

5. Pullen FW II. The use of computerized tomography in otolaryngology. Trans Am Acad Ophthalmol Otolaryngol 1977; 84:ORL 622-7.

6. Thawley SE, Gado M, Fuller TR. Computerized tomography in the evaluation of head and neck lesions. Laryngoscope 1978; 88:451-9.

7. Ward PH, Zwitman D, Hanson D, Berci G. Contact ulcers and granulomas of the larynx: new insights into their etiology as a basis for more rational treatment. Otolaryngol Head Neck Surg 1980; 88:262-9.

8. McCullough EC. Basic physics of x-ray computed tomography I. In: Norman D, Korobkin M, Newton TH, eds. Computed tomography 1977. St. Louis: CV Mosby, 1978.

9. Bergman AB, Neiman HL, Warpeha RL. Computed tomography of the larynx. Laryngoscope 1979; 89:812-17.

10. Nathan MD, El Gammal T, Hudson JH Jr. Computerized axial tomography in the assessment of thyroid cartilage invasion by laryngeal carcinoma: a prospective study. Otolaryngol Head Neck Surg 1980; 88:726-33.

11. Mafee MF, Schild JA, Valvassori GE. Computed tomography of the larynx: correlative anatomic and pathologic macrosection studies. Radiology (in press).

≈

CASSELBERRY AWARD

The American Laryngological Association announces that it will receive essays or theses relating to the art and science of laryngology and rhinology for consideration of the Casselberry Award for 1982-1983. The Award is open to physicians, interns, residents, and graduate students in laryngology and rhinology in the Americas and scientists in the field in laryngology and rhinology. For further information write to Eugene N. Myers, MD, Secretary, American Laryngological Association, Eye and Ear Hospital, 230 Lothrop St., Suite 1115, Pittsburgh, PA 15213.

Ann Otol Rhinol Laryngol 91:1982

TRACHEOSTOMA VALVE FOR POSTLARYNGECTOMY VOICE REHABILITATION

ERIC D. BLOM, PHD
MARK I. SINGER, MD
RONALD C. HAMAKER, MD, FACS
INDIANAPOLIS, INDIANA

Newer surgical techniques for postlaryngectomy voice rehabilitation provide a simple, effective method of communication but require manual occlusion of the tracheostoma during speech. We report the development of a unique tracheostoma valve that avoids the necessity for covering the stoma. This airflow-sensitive valve closes during speech and remains open with normal respiration. Results of a clinical trial with 50 patients over a ten-month period are encouraging. Our experience suggests that excessive vocal tract resistance to airflow is the principal limitation to effective valve use. Approaches to decreasing airflow resistance through the vocal tract to improve both voice production and tracheostoma valve use are discussed.

INTRODUCTION

With the introduction of the newer postlaryngectomy voice rehabilitation procedures, the need for intermittent occlusion of the tracheostoma during speech production is increasingly demanded.[1-3] Manual stoma occlusion is inconvenient, nonhygienic, and draws attention to the laryngectomized condition. This presentation describes a simple airflow-regulated tracheostoma valve that eliminates the need for manual diversion of pulmonary airflow for speech (Bivona Surgical Instruments, Inc, Hammond, Ind).

MATERIALS

The component parts of the tracheostoma valve include a flexible polyvinyl chloride housing that is convex to conform to a wide variety of stomal dimensions and configurations (Fig. 1-a). The housing is fixed to the peristomal skin with a disposable disc of double-faced hypoallergenic adhesive. A thin coating of clear liquid adhesive applied to the skin augments the seal around the stoma. This attachment design avoids an indwelling tracheal cannula and the potential problems of tracheitis, stoma dilatation, and air escape.

The inner rim of the housing is beveled to allow easy insertion of the valve assembly. A groove on the posterior aspect of the housing engages with a corresponding rib on the valve assembly (Fig. 1-b). This rib and groove design provides adequate retention of the assembly while permitting immediate removal for access to the airway. An arch-shaped crossbar prevents clothing from obstructing the valve inlet (Fig. 1-d). A precurved latex valve diaphragm is permanently attached to the shaft in the center of the valve assembly (Fig. 1-c). The diaphragm is airflow-sensitive and responds to variations in expiratory exchange. During normal respiration it remains in its fully open position (Fig. 2A). With the slight increase in expiratory flow for speech the diaphragm unfurls and seats circumferentially against the inner rim of the valve assembly, closing the tracheostoma (Fig. 2B). Decreasing expiratory airflow allows the diaphragm to return to the open position. During a cough, the valve may partially evert through the assembly to release excessive air pressure and is easily replaced (Fig. 2C).

Individual respiratory patterns are accommodated by selecting one of four available diaphragm thicknesses which determine valve sensitivity. The diaphragms are (0.055, 0.063, 0.073, and 0.083 cm (0.022, 0.025, 0.029, and 0.033 in, respectively) corresponding to the designations of ultralight, light, medium, and firm. The thicker diaphragms are less sensitive to airflow closure. During initial valve selection, the clinician matches the appropriate sensitivity to permit comfortable user respiration and phonation. Unimpeded respiration with routine physical activity is determined by having the user walk briskly for a distance as well as climb a flight of stairs. Closure or airway obstruction must not occur during these conditions. During physical exertion such as running, the valve can be temporarily withdrawn from the housing.

CLINICAL EVALUATION

The tracheostoma valve has been continuously used by 50 patients over a ten-month period. It has been accepted enthusiastically and has been free of complications. Patients rapidly accommodate to the aerodynamic principle of valve diaphragm function. They subjectively experience and report a more normal speech with the valve use.

The most frequent problem that patients identify is difficulty maintaining an airtight seal around the stoma for extended periods. Many found that the adhesive seal would loosen and require reapplica-

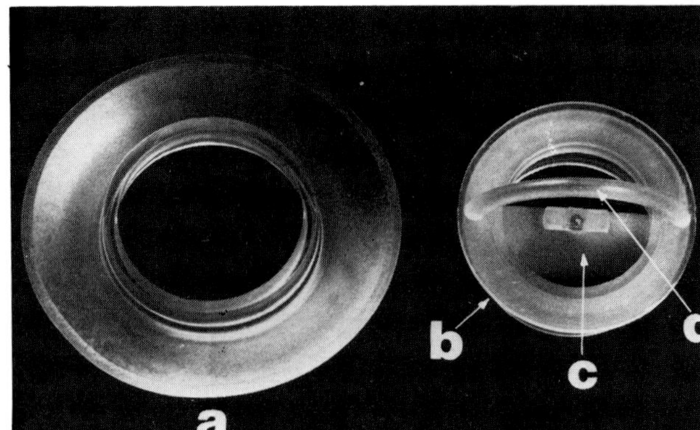

Fig. 1. Blom-Singer tracheostoma valve. a - Valve housing; b - Assembly; c - Latex valve diaphragm; d - Arched crossbar.

Presented at the meeting of the American Broncho-Esophagological Association, Palm Beach, Florida, May 3-4, 1982.

REPRINTS — Eric D. Blom, PhD, 1633 North Capitol Avenue, Medical Tower, Suite 780, Indianapolis, IN 46202.

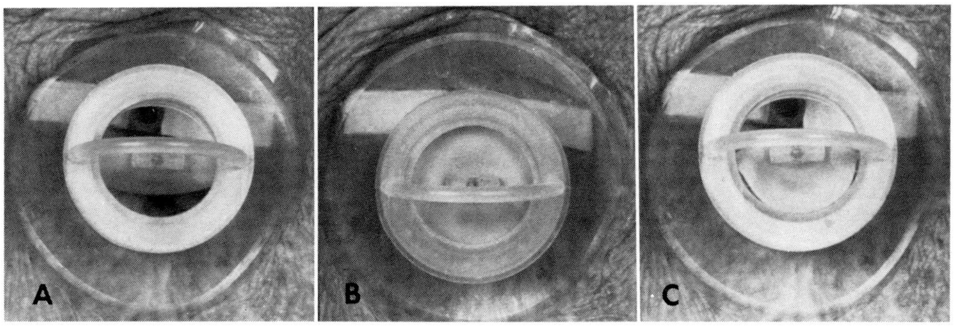

Fig. 2. Tracheostoma valve showing diaphragm A) open during normal respiration; B) closed diverting airflow for speech; and C) partially everted through assembly inlet to release cough pressure.

tion at least once during the day. Our assessment of this problem revealed that the main cause of this difficulty was related to airflow backpressure at the stoma during speech production. Backpressure that was formerly contained by the finger places a considerable stress against the adhesive seal, which eventually gives way to air leakage (Fig. 3).

We have noted that the two principal sources of vocal tract resistance are excessive pharyngeal constrictor tone and resistance offered by the voice prosthesis itself. In an earlier report, we concluded that selective division of the pharyngeal constrictor muscles enhances airflow through the upper esophageal sphincter and reduces the effort required to produce voice.[4]

Despite adequate pharyngoesophageal physiology for alaryngeal voice production, many patients in our tracheostoma valve series demonstrated an undesirable degree of airflow resistance revealed by backpressure at the tracheostoma. We speculated that residual opposition to airflow from the trachea to the esophagus was attributable to resistance offered by the duckbill (Blom-Singer) voice prosthesis. To test this hypothesis, we had each patient produce voice both with and without the prosthesis in place. In all instances, the patients reported that speech without the voice prosthesis was substantially easier and similar to the effort they formerly required for laryngeal voice.

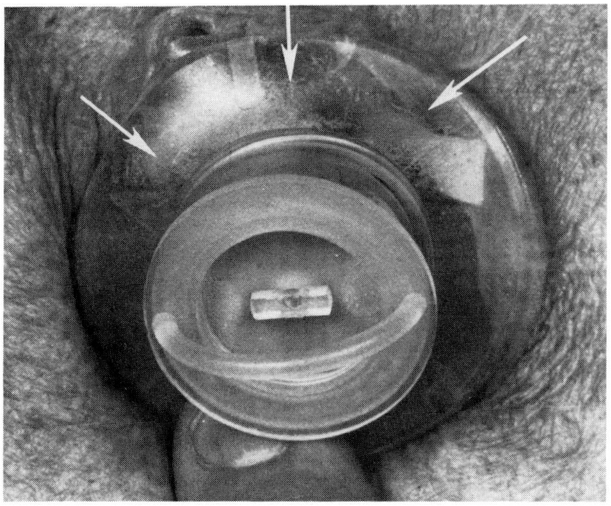

Fig. 3. Loosening of valve housing tape seal (arrows) caused by excessive airflow backpressure during speech.

Weinberg recently confirmed that in vitro airway resistances offered by the Blom-Singer voice prosthesis and the Panje voice button are considerably higher than the normal larynx.[5] Laboratory resistance calculations demonstrated that opposition to airflow through the Blom-Singer prosthesis ranged from 45 to 120 cm H_2O/ liters per second (LPS), while the Panje voice button was higher, ranging from 285 to 430 cm H_2O/LPS. These values compare to the resistance offered by the human larynx during voice production that range from 30 to 43 cm H_2O/LPS.[6]

LOW-PRESSURE VOICE PROSTHESIS

In an effort to decrease airflow resistance of the voice prosthesis to the range of the normal larynx, we have modified the valve design of the duckbill. The basic tubular design has been retained but increased in diameter from 5.3 to 6.6 mm to enhance airflow (Fig. 4-a). The slit valve has been replaced by a circular valve and recessed slightly into the distal end of the prosthesis. The beveled tip minimally protrudes into the esophageal lumen and provides a protective hood over the valve. A circular inner retention collar has been incorporated.

During speech, airflow diverted through the prosthesis opens the one-way valve (Fig. 4-b). With the

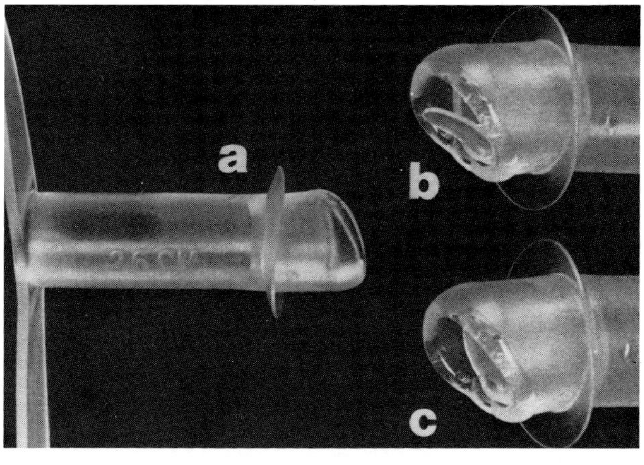

Fig. 4. a - Prototype voice prosthesis with inner retention collar and beveled distal tip. b - Hinged circular valve in open position during airflow for speech. c - Valve in closed position.

cessation of airflow, the hinged valve returns to its closed position and seats against a recessed circumferential ledge to provide a seal (Fig. 4-c). This design effectively eliminates regurgitation of fluids from the esophagus, and the positive pressure gradient generated within the esophagus during swallowing tends to assist valve closure. Calculations indicate the airflow resistance of this prototype low-pressure voice prosthesis is nearly within the range offered by the human larynx (Weinberg BW, personal communication). Thirty patients are using the prosthesis and no complications have been observed to date while substantial reduction in backpressure provided by the low-pressure voice prosthesis enables patients to maintain an airtight tracheostoma seal.

Our accumulated experience suggests that patients vary in their capacity to achieve a durable airtight seal enabling them to wear the tracheostoma valve. When vocal tract resistance is excessive, assessment of potential sources of resistance is indicated. As mentioned, prosthetic resistance is evaluated by tracheoesophageal airflow without the voice prosthesis. When substantial opposition to airflow is noted even without the voice prosthesis in place, assessment of pharyngoesophageal resistance is important. This can be achieved by a pharyngeal plexus nerve block under local anesthetic infiltration as previously described.[4] The contribution of the pharyngeal constrictor muscles after laryngectomy to excessive tone and diminished airflow is significant. This can be effectively reduced by selective constrictor myotomy with improved voice and diminished intratracheal pressures.

SUMMARY

The newer procedures for postlaryngectomy voice rehabilitation require manual occlusion of the stoma during speech. For many patients this is inconvenient, nonhygienic and draws attention to the laryngectomized condition. The tracheostoma valve described in this report provides an option for tracheoesophageal speakers without the necessity for finger occlusion of the stoma. Patients whose speech is characterized by low vocal effort and minimal resistance to tracheoesophageal airflow are candidates for this valve. Other patients will require adjustments of prosthetic or physiologic sources of airflow resistance to improve their capacity for extended tracheostoma valve use.

REFERENCES

1. Staffieri M, Serafini I. La riabilitazione chirurgica della voce e della respirazione dopo laringectomia totale. 29th National Congress of the Associazione Otologi Ospedalieri Italiana. Bologna: Associazione Otologi Ospedaliere Italiana, 1976:57-111.

2. Singer MI, Blom ED. An endoscopic technique for restoration of voice after laryngectomy. Ann Otol Rhinol Laryngol 1980; 89:529-33.

3. Pearson BW. Subtotal laryngectomy. Laryngoscope 1981; 91:1904-11.

4. Singer MI, Blom ED. A selective myotomy for voice restoration after total laryngectomy. Arch Otolaryngol 1981; 107:670-3.

5. Weinberg BW. Airway resistance of the voice button. Arch Otolaryngol (in press).

6. Smitheran JR, Hixon TJ. A clinical method for estimating laryngeal airway resistance during vowel production. J Speech Hear Disord 1981; 46:138-46.

FACTORS IN SUCCESSFUL DEGLUTITION FOLLOWING SUPRAGLOTTIC LARYNGEAL SURGERY

TORIBIO C. FLORES, MD
BENJAMIN G. WOOD, MD
HOWARD L. LEVINE, MD
LAWRENCE KOEGEL, JR, MD
HARVEY M. TUCKER, MD
CLEVELAND, OHIO

Aspiration is the major problem in deglutition associated with conservation laryngeal surgery. Closure of the glottic sphincter, depression of the epiglottis over the laryngeal inlet, elevation of the thyrohyoid complex under cover of the base of the tongue and appropriate relaxation of the cricopharyngeal muscle to permit unobstructed passage of food into the esophagus are important mechanisms that prevent food from entering the trachea. Partial laryngeal surgery can interfere with one or a combination of these mechanisms. Analysis of the records of all evaluable patients who underwent horizontal supraglottic resections from January 1976 to June 1981 was undertaken. The incidence of deglutition problems is reported. In addition, the effects of resection or preservation of the hyoid, arytenoid, base of tongue and branches of the vagus and the effect of cricopharyngeal myotomy upon ultimate swallowing function are analyzed.

INTRODUCTION

Over the past four decades, there has been gradual acceptance of conservation laryngeal surgery in the treatment of selected carcinomas of the intrinsic and extrinsic larynx. With partial laryngeal surgery, cure rates equivalent to those possible after total laryngectomy have been obtained[1] with the advantage of preservation of phonatory function and elimination of the need for a permanent tracheal stoma. Nevertheless, there remains some reluctance to perform partial laryngeal surgery because of concern regarding swallowing difficulties that may ensue. The literature has not been clear on the actual incidence of clinically significant dysphagia and aspiration following such procedures.

This paper attempts to analyze those factors which may be important in restoring swallowing function following horizontal supraglottic resection.

PHYSIOLOGIC AND SURGICAL CONSIDERATIONS

During the pharyngeal phase of swallowing, entrance of food into the upper airway is prevented by closure of the glottic sphincter, depression of the epiglottis over the laryngeal inlet, and anterior rotation and elevation of the larynx to appose the base of the tongue.[2-4] In addition, the cricopharyngeal sphincter must relax in time to facilitate the unobstructed passage of the food bolus into the esophagus.[5] Intact sensation in the pharynx is also important to maintain the integrity of this complex neuromuscular reflex. Partial laryngeal surgery may alter one or more of these mechanisms, depending on the specific areas resected and the type of reconstruction used.

With the exception of certain modifications by the individual surgeon, the technique of supraglottic laryngectomy used at the Cleveland Clinic is the same as that described by Ogura et al.[6] Standard supraglottic laryngectomy is an en bloc resection of the epiglottis, both aryepiglottic folds, the preepiglottic space, false cords and the upper third or half of the thyroid cartilage (Fig. 1A). Various extended operations may include the resection of one arytenoid, the pyriform sinus (partial laryngopharyngectomy, PLP) and/or base of the tongue. If one arytenoid is excised with the specimen, the vocal process of the remaining membranous cord is usually fixed to the cricoid in the midline so it can appose the other functioning cord and thus prevent aspiration. The closure of the supraglottic defect is accomplished by approximating the base of the tongue (or the hyoid if it has been preserved) to the preserved perichondrium of the larynx (Fig. 1B).[7] Regional flaps can be used to repair larger defects which result from more extensive resections of the base of the tongue or hypopharynx.[8]

In order to establish successful deglutition following horizontal supraglottic resection, the patient must accommodate to the alteration(s) in laryngopharyngeal anatomy. The epiglottis, which functions as a hood over the laryngeal vestibule, is eliminated and, more importantly, the relationship of the larynx to the base of the tongue is disrupted. Pharyngeal sensation may be altered when it is necessary to sacrifice one or both superior laryngeal nerves to accomplish an en bloc resection of the supraglottis. Such loss of sensation can be responsible for interference with cricopharyngeal sphincter function which has been reported following supraglottic laryngectomy.[5,9]

From the Department of Otolaryngology and Communicative Disorders, The Cleveland Clinic Foundation.
Presented at the meeting of the American Broncho-Esophagological Association, Palm Beach, Florida, May 3-4, 1982.
REPRINTS — Harvey M. Tucker, MD, The Cleveland Clinic Foundation, 9500 Euclid Avenue, Cleveland, OH 44106.

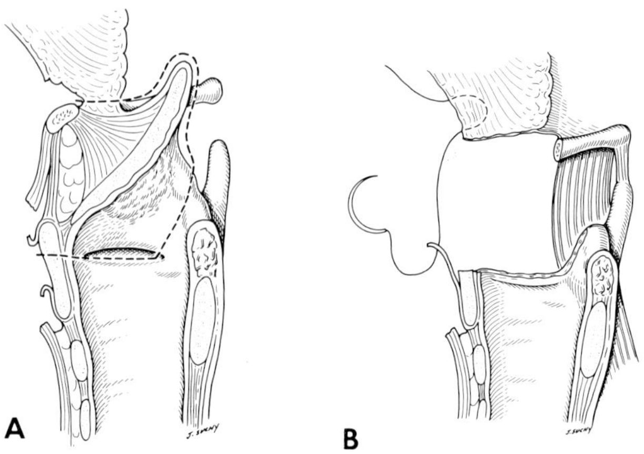

Fig. 1. Supraglottic laryngectomy. A) En bloc resection. B) Closure of supraglottic defect. (Reprinted with permission.[7])

Resection or preservation of the hyoid bone and the performance of cricopharyngeal myotomy have been performed routinely by some surgeons in our department but not by others. An analysis of these variables and the possible effects on successful deglutition is considered later in this report.

POSTOPERATIVE MANAGEMENT

Attempted deglutition is initiated after satisfactory healing has taken place. Because nearly all patients received high-dose radiation preoperatively, feeding is started no earlier than two weeks after surgery. The patient is first decannulated and 24 to 48 hours later, the nasogastric tube is removed and oral feedings are begun. Retraining for swallowing is done with the aid of a dietitian, a nurse and a speech pathologist. Swallowing difficulties are carefully monitored. Daily weights and intake and output are recorded. The patient may require intravenous supplements until oral intake is adequate. If the patient is still unable to swallow without significant aspiration within 1 week, the nasogastric tube is reinserted and the patient is discharged with tube feedings. He or she is readmitted for another attempt about 4 weeks later. Cineradiologic studies may be helpful at this point, although it is often difficult to identify the exact cause of dysphagia.

If the second attempt fails, a feeding gastrostomy may follow, providing the patient does not develop aspiration pneumonia from his or her own secretions. Completion laryngectomy is performed for the patient who develops severe pulmonary complications or who prefers to sacrifice voice in exchange for normal peroral deglutition.

MATERIALS AND METHODS

From January 1976 to June 1981,51 supraglottic laryngectomies (including PLPs) were performed at the Cleveland Clinic. At the time of the study, all living patients had been followed from 1 to 6 years. The effect of the following variables upon the success of deglutition was studied: age; resection of one arytenoid; preservation of the hyoid; sacrifice of the superior laryngeal nerve(s); resection of the base of the tongue and/or pyriform sinus; and the performance of cricopharyngeal myotomy.

The following were obtained from each record: date of surgery, date of first attempt to swallow, date of adequate swallowing and date of decannulation. The date of adequate swallowing was defined as the date on which the patient was able to rely solely on peroral nutrition, without the need for supplemental sources and without clinically significant aspiration. Retraining time, defined as the number of days between the first attempt to swallow and adequate swallowing, was used to compare all the independent variables.

RESULTS

Forty-six of the 51 patients were considered evaluable for this study. The five who were not evaluable never attempted to swallow after partial laryngectomy because of early postoperative mortality in three, residual carcinoma which required early completion laryngectomy in one and failure of fistula closure in another.

The distribution of patients according to success of deglutition is presented in Table 1. Of the 28 patients in the successful group, 27 swallowed adequately within three days and one in five days. None of these patients developed pneumonia and all were successfully decannulated.

Patients who were not successful in swallowing adequately within the first few days went through prolonged retraining. The nine patients in the delayed group eventually swallowed, but required retraining time from 4 weeks to 5 months. One of these patients developed pneumonia which was successfully treated medically. None required surgical intervention because of dysphagia. All were eventually decannulated.

The failed group consisted of the remaining nine patients who, at the time of this report, were still unable to swallow adequately. In this group, three are now fed via gastrostomy. Another three underwent gastrostomy, but required subsequent completion laryngectomy. Two patients were managed with completion laryngectomy alone. Recurrent tumor was found in one of the five patients who underwent completion laryngectomy. A single patient chose to retain the nasogastric tube indefinitely and has not been decannulated. In the failed group two deaths due to aspiration occurred and three patients developed pneumonia that responded to intensive medical treatment.

Age. The mean age for the successful group was

TABLE 1. DISTRIBUTION OF LARYNGECTOMY PATIENTS BY SUCCESS OF DEGLUTITION AND AGE (N = 46)

Adequate Swallowing	*No. of Patients*	*Mean Age (yr)*	*SD*	*Age Range (yr)*
Successful	28	54.9	9.8	27-73
Delayed	9	59.9	6.6	47-67
Failed	9	59.2	8.0	44-72

$F = 1.5$; $p = 0.24$.

TABLE 2. SUCCESS OF DEGLUTITION AND PRESERVATION OF HYOID BONE (N = 46)

	No. Patients with Adequate Swallowing			
	Successful	*Delayed*	*Failed*	*Total*
Hyoid preserved	6 (46%)	4 (31%)	3 (23%)	13
Hyoid partially preserved	11 (61%)	3 (17%)	4 (22%)	18
Hyoid completely resected	10 (72%)	2 (14%)	2 (14%)	14
Data not available	1 (100%)	—	—	1

$X^2_{(4)} = 2.1$; $p = 0.14$.

54.9 years and the range, 27 to 73 years. The mean ages for the delayed and the failed groups were 59.9 and 59.2 years respectively (Table 1). Analysis of the variance of age showed no statistically significant difference (p = 0.24).

Hyoid Bone. Table 2 shows the relationship between success of deglutition and preservation of the hyoid bone. Surprisingly, the highest success rate prevailed among those whose hyoid was completely resected. The failed and delayed percentages were lowest when the hyoid was totally resected. However, the differences were not statistically significant (p = 0.14).

Cricopharyngeal Myotomy. At the time of primary resection, 26 patients underwent cricopharyngeal myotomy and 20 did not (Table 3). The percentage of patients who failed to swallow was similar in the two groups, 19% when cricopharyngeal myotomy was performed and 20% when it was not. A higher immediate success rate (69%) resulted when the myotomy was done than when it was omitted (50%). As a result, there appeared to be more patients in the delayed category when the cricopharyngeal myotomy was omitted (30%) than when it was done (12%). However, the differences were not statistically significant (p = 0.26).

In an effort to improve deglutition for two patients in the failed group, cricopharyngeal myotomy was performed for one patient 1 year and for the other 3 years after primary resection. One was a repeat myotomy; the other was performed because it was not done at the time of primary resection. These late myotomies did not noticeably improve swallowing in either patient.

Superior Laryngeal Nerves. En bloc resection sacrificed at least one superior laryngeal nerve (at the side of most involvement) in 20 patients (Table 4). Twenty-six patients had more extensive resections in which both superior laryngeal nerves were sacrificed. Unexpectedly, deglutition was more successful when both nerves rather than one were resected. However, the difference was not statistically significant (p = 0.14).

TABLE 3. SUCCESS OF DEGLUTITION AND CRICOPHARYNGEAL MYOTOMY

Cricopharyngeal	*No. Patients with Adequate Swallowing*			
Myotomy	*Successful*	*Delayed*	*Failed*	*Total*
Performed	18 (69%)	3 (12%)	5 (19%)	26
Not performed	10 (50%)	6 (30%)	4 (20%)	20

$X^2_{(2)} = 2.7$; $p = 0.26$.

TABLE 4. SUCCESS OF DEGLUTITION AND RESECTION OF SUPERIOR LARYNGEAL NERVES

Superior	*No. Patients with Adequate Swallowing*			
Laryngeal Nerves	*Successful*	*Delayed*	*Failed*	*Total*
One sacrificed	9 (45%)	6 (30%)	5 (25%)	20
Both sacrificed	19 (73%)	3 (12%)	4 (15%)	26

$X^2_{(2)} = 4$; $p = 0.14$.

Arytenoid Excision. The impact of excision of one arytenoid upon the success of deglutition is shown in Table 5. In 15 patients an arytenoid had to be resected. A higher proportion of patients failed when one arytenoid was excised (47%) than when both were preserved (6%). Clearly, successful deglutition was more likely when both arytenoids were preserved (70%) than when one had to be sacrificed (40%). The difference was highly significant (p = 0.006).

Pyriform Sinus Resection or Partial Laryngopharyngectomy. Six patients underwent PLP (Table 6); 4 failed to swallow, 1 delayed and 1 was considered successful. Interestingly the successful patient was the only PLP case in which an arytenoid was not excised. However, the small numbers did not permit a valid chi square test.

Supraglottic Laryngectomy Extended to Base of the Tongue. Nine patients required extension of resection to the base of the tongue (Table 6). Six had extensive resections (up to the circumvallate papillae) with deltopectoral flap reconstruction; 5 of these patients swallowed successfully and 1 failed. Three patients had minimal base of tongue excision that could be closed primarily. Two of these swallowed successfully and one was delayed. Differences were not statistically significant.

DISCUSSION

Supraglottic laryngectomy is a well-established surgical procedure for treatment of selected carcinomas of the larynx. However, swallowing difficulties are frequent, especially with various extended modifications used to resect lesions adjacent to the laryngopharynx. The surgical effort to restore deglutition must begin with proper techniques at the time of resection.[10] Controversy remains as to whether cricopharyngeal myotomy[5,11] and hyoid preservation significantly affect deglutition following supraglottic laryngectomy.[6,12] This study suggests that failure rates were similar whether or not a myotomy was done. However, the possibility still exists

TABLE 5. SUCCESS OF DEGLUTITION AND ARYTENOID EXCISION

Excision of	*No. Patients with Adequate Swallowing*			
Arytenoid	*Successful*	*Delayed*	*Failed*	*Total*
One	6 (40%)	2 (13%)	7 (47%)	15
None	22 (71%)	7 (23%)	2 (6%)	31

$X^2_{(2)} = 10.4$; $p = 0.006$.

TABLE 6. SUCCESS OF DEGLUTITION AND RESECTION OF PYRIFORM SINUS AND BASE OF TONGUE

	No. Patients with Adequate Swallowing			
	Successful	*Delayed*	*Failed*	*Total*
Resection of pyriform sinus or PLP	1 (17%)	1 (17%)	4 (66%)	6
Resection of base of tongue.				
Extensive resection with DP flap reconstruction	5 (83%)	—	1 (17%)	6
Minimal resection with primary closure	2 (67%)	1 (33%)	—	3

PLP - Partial laryngopharyngectomy; DP - Deltopectoral.

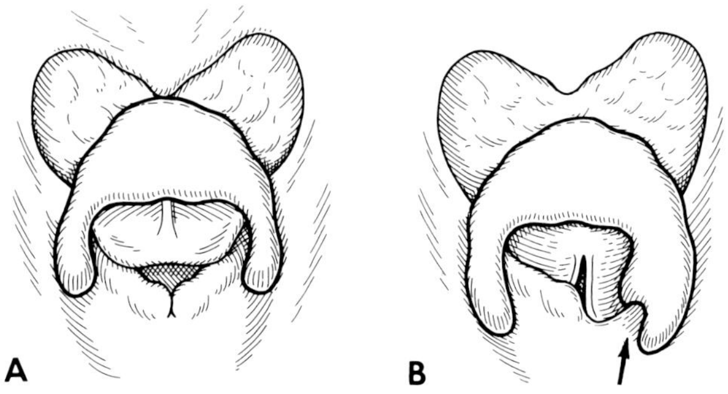

Fig. 2. Axial view of larynx before and after supraglottic laryngectomy with resection of one arytenoid and pyriform sinus. A) Preoperative; upper airway is well protected from aspiration. B) Postoperative; food bolus may be channeled into laryngeal aperture through pyriform funnel (arrow).

that the percentage with delayed swallowing, although not statistically significant, could be lowered and rehabilitation accelerated by performing a cricopharyngeal myotomy.

The notion that preservation of the hyoid may improve success in deglutition is purely anecdotal. Our data show no such difference and suggest that the patient who had the entire hyoid resected did better. Perhaps preservation of the hyoid bone which has been detached from the infrahyoid muscles interferes with the ability of the laryngeal remnant to rise toward the base of the tongue. Similarly, no significant difference was found between preservation of one superior laryngeal nerve and resection of both. This variable probably should not be considered separately since preservation of one superior laryngeal nerve is related to preservation of the hyoid bone.

This study suggests that the single most important factor measured in the success or failure of deglutition is the sacrifice of an arytenoid. Unfortunately, the decision to resect an arytenoid is determined by the extent of the tumor and is not the surgeon's discretionary choice.

Aspiration may be worse when resection must be extended to the pyriform sinus because extensive resection interferes with the three basic mechanisms providing protection to the larynx. In addition, resection of an arytenoid and the adjacent pyriform mucosa blunts the lateral food channel,[2] funneling the bolus on this side into the laryngeal aperture rather than into the introitus of the esophagus (Fig. 2A,B).

Yet judicious resection of the base of the tongue does not seem to affect the outcome of deglutition, provided proper reconstruction is done to fill in the gap and to insure that the movements of the base of the tongue and the remaining larynx are not limited.

Proper selection of the patient for conservation laryngeal surgery is important. Patients with chronic lung disease can be expected to have serious problems with aspiration. We do not quantify pulmonary function routinely unless there is an indication of significant deficit from history and physical examination. In addition, our data concur with previous studies[13] suggesting that advanced chronologic age alone is not a deterrent to the recovery of laryngeal function following horizontal supraglottic resection.

SUMMARY

Retrospective analysis of 46 patients who underwent horizontal supraglottic resections was undertaken. The occurrence of serious swallowing difficulties following the standard supraglottic laryngectomy was low (less than 10%). More swallowing difficulties occurred in the extended resections, notably in resections of the arytenoid and pyriform sinus. Resection of the base of the tongue did not preclude successful deglutition when suitable reconstruction was carried out. The effect of cricopharyngeal myotomy was equivocal. Superior laryngeal nerve preservation is ultimately associated with preservation of the hyoid bone. Neither of these could be shown to improve swallowing results.

ACKNOWLEDGMENT — The authors express their gratitude to Annie Polk and Marlene Goormastic for their help in gathering and analyzing the data presented in this study.

REFERENCES

1. Ogura JH, Biller HF. Conservation surgery in cancer of the head and neck. Otolaryngol Clin North Am 1969; 2:641-65.

2. Negus VE. The mechanism of the larynx. St. Louis: CV Mosby, 1929.

3. Adran GM, Kemp FH. The protection of the laryngeal airway during swallowing. Br J Radiol 1952; 25:406-16.

4. Litton WB, Leonard JR. Aspiration after partial laryngectomy: cineradiographic studies. Laryngoscope 1969; 79:887-908.

5. Staple TW, Ogura JH. Cineradiography of the swallowing mechanism following supraglottic subtotal laryngectomy. Radiology 1966; 87:226-30.

6. Ogura JH, Saltzstein SL, Spjut HJ. Experiences with conservation surgery in laryngeal and pharyngeal carcinoma. Laryngoscope 1961; 71:258-76.

7. Tucker HM. Surgery for phonatory disorders. New York: Churchill Livingstone, 1981.

8. Wood BG, Tucker HM, Levine HL. Regional flap reconstruction following "extended" partial horizontal laryngeal surgery. Laryngoscope (in press).

9. Lauerma KSL, Harvey JE, Ogura JH. Cricopharyngeal myotomy in subtotal supraglottic laryngectomy: an experimental study. Laryngoscope 1972; 82:447-53.

10. Sessions DG, Zill R. Deglutition after conservation surgery for cancer of the larynx and hypopharynx. Otolaryngol Head Neck Surg 1979; 87:779-96.

11. Dayal VS, Kane H. Supraglottic laryngectomy and swallowing: an experimental study. Can J Otolaryngol 1974; 3:581-5.

12. Bocca E. Supraglottic laryngectomy and functional neck dissection. J Laryngol Otol 1966; 80:831-8.

13. Tucker HM. Conservation laryngeal surgery in the elderly. Laryngoscope 1977; 87:1995-9.

≈

SATELLITE SYMPOSIUM ON PEDIATRIC OTOLARYNGOLOGY

A Satellite Symposium on Pediatric Otolaryngology will be held October 17, 1983, in Tokyo. For further information, contact Keijiro Koga, Department of Otolaryngology, National Children's Hospital, 3-35-31, Taishido Satagayaku, Tokyo, Japan.

≈

THE 16TH ANNUAL MEETING OF THE AMERICAN SOCIETY OF HEAD AND NECK RADIOLOGY

The 16th Annual Meeting of the American Society of Head and Neck Radiology will be held May 26-29, 1983, at the Boston Marriott Hotel. Inquiries should be directed to Barbara Carter, MD, North East Medical Center, 171 Harrison Avenue, Boston, MA 02111.

Ann Otol Rhinol Laryngol 91:1982

COMPLICATIONS OF INTUBATION

WILLIAM M. KEANE, MD
LEE D. ROWE, MD
JAMES C. DENNENY, MD
JOSEPH P. ATKINS, JR, MD
PHILADELPHIA, PENNSYLVANIA

Endotracheal intubation with current inert low-pressure, high-volume cuffed tubes is a safe procedure associated with few complications in the vast majority of patients. However, complications related to mechanical difficulties and mucosal injury can occur even under ideal circumstances. Immediate complications are primarily associated with problems during intubation and extubation while early and late complications represent the short- and long-term effects of epithelial trauma.

The intubation of the trachea is a commonly performed and safe act which enjoys a low complication rate. The procedure is not totally without risk, however, and complications with minor and major consequences are well described. In this paper, the complications relating to intubation are reviewed, drawing on the experience of the authors and that presented in the literature.

IMMEDIATE COMPLICATIONS

The complications of intubation can be classified as immediate, early and late. Blanc and Tremblay[1] have further divided the immediate complications as they relate to the process of intubation. Injuries may thereby be assigned to the act of intubation, the time of intubation and the act of extubation[1] (Table 1).

Act of Intubation. The act of intubation begins with the positioning of the patient with the head in the classic "sniffing" position (flexion of the cervical spine and extension of the atlanto-occipital joint). Overzealous attempts to achieve correct positioning may result in injury to the cervical spine and fractures with subluxation and spinal cord injury may result. Care must be taken with patients predisposed to such injuries in whom fragility of the cervical spine is the result of previous fracture or dislocation, congenital spinal malformation, osteoporosis, degenerative joint disease, connective tissue disorders or destructive bone tumors. The act of intubation can be particularly risky in patients with an acutely injured spine where cervical stabilization must be maintained during intubation.[1,2]

As the mouth is opened, unsuspected limitations to mandibular mobility may be encountered. Excessive force may dislocate or produce a pathologic fracture of the mandible. Dentition may be damaged with excessive digital prying and during laryngoscopy, instrumental dislodgment and aspiration can take place. The lip, tongue and buccal mucosa may become entrapped between the blade of the laryngoscope and the dentition, producing abrasions and lacerations. Careless manipulation of the laryngoscope has resulted in lacerations of the oropharynx, hypopharynx and larynx. Fragments of friable tumor mass and tonsillar tissue have been dislodged with subsequent aspiration. Excessive pressure on the tongue has resulted in paresis of the lingual and hypoglossal nerves.

The endotracheal tube itself or a protruding stylet may also produce direct injury. Lacerations of the oropharynx, hypopharynx, larynx, trachea and esophagus have been encountered. The area posterior to the cricopharyngeal muscle is particularly susceptible as is the pyriform sinus. Forcing the endotracheal tube or stylet into the endolarynx has produced lacerations, avulsions and dislocations of the vocal folds and arytenoids. These complications may be related to inadequate glottic paralysis, inappropriate tube or stylet selection or improper visualization and misdirection of the tube. With the safe passage of the endotracheal tube through the glottic chink, the subglottic space, trachea and bronchi become at risk, and injuries ranging from simple abrasion to severe laceration and rupture have been encountered as a result of the act of intubation. The esophagus may be similarly traumatized and endotracheal tubes have been swallowed during intubation.[1-5]

Blind nasotracheal intubation lends itself to a higher incidence of injury. The nasal septum may be dislocated, the nasopharynx abraded or deeply lacerated, and the hypopharynx and larynx subjected to risks similar in quality to those related to orotracheal techniques, but greater in frequency. Fragments of adenoid tissue have been dislodged and forced into the endobronchial tree. Intubations done in emergency situations, usually performed by less experienced personnel, are most likely to produce complications. In these less than optimal situ-

From the Departments of Otorhinolaryngology of the Pennsylvania Hospital and the University of Pennsylvania School of Medicine, Philadelphia.
Presented at the meeting of the American Broncho-Esophagological Association, Palm Beach, Florida, May 3-4, 1982.
REPRINTS — William M. Keane, MD, Pennsylvania Hospital, Eighth and Spruce Streets, Philadelphia, PA 19107.

TABLE 1. IMMEDIATE COMPLICATIONS

Nasal cavity	Trachea
Septal abrasion	Abrasion
Dislocation	Laceration
Alar rim abrasion	Rupture
Tearing	Main bronchus intubation
	Tube dislodgment
Nasopharynx	
Abrasion	Esophagus
Laceration	Abrasion
	Laceration
Oropharynx	Perforation
Lip abrasion	Intubation
Laceration	Swallowed tube
Mandibular dislocation	
Fracture	Equipment failure
Dental injury	Tube breakage
Aspiration of tooth	Obstruction
	Dislocation
Hypopharynx	Cuff obstruction
Abrasion	Fragmentation
Laceration	Tube ignition (laser)
Perforation	
	Neurogenic reflexes
Larynx	Pharmacotherapeutic side effects
Abrasion	
Laceration	
Dislocation	
Vocal cord paralysis	
Aspiration	

ations, the larynx may not be adequately visualized, inadequate muscle relaxation may be present and endotracheal tube selection may be limited.[1-7]

Blanc and Tremblay[1] describe three types of neurogenic reflex activity associated with the act of intubation. Laryngovagal reflexes produce laryngospasm and bronchospasm as well as bradycardia, arrhythmias and hypotension. Laryngosympathetic reflexes may be related to increased catecholamine levels and produce tachycardia, arrhythmias and hypertension. Laryngospinal reflexes produce coughing, vomiting and bucking.[1]

Transient sialadenopathy has been reported during intubation. The etiology is unclear, but neuromuscular blocking agents, belladonna drugs, succinylcholine and straining have been implicated.[8]

Time of Intubation. The most common complications during the time of intubation relate to improper ventilation. The tube position may be shifted during repositioning of the patient or by the operating surgeon. The tube may thus be advanced against the tracheal wall or into the main bronchi or withdrawn into the larynx or hypopharynx. Endoscopic equipment may interfere with proper ventilatory function and may shift tube position, produce kinking or lacerate the tube or cuff. Inappropriate cuff pressure may produce obstruction of the tube lumen by compression or by prolapse of the cuff over the tube tip. Rupture of the trachea has been reported during the time of intubation and may be related to excessive cuff pressure. This is especially true in elderly patients and in those emphysematous patients with a thin, friable posterior tracheal membrane. Rupture can lead to severe hemorrhage, pneumomediastinum and pneumothorax. The cuff also may burst or adhere to the tracheal wall, leaving fragments within the endobronchial tree. Vocal cord paralysis may result as a consequence of events during intubation. Excessive cuff pressure within the trachea may directly injure the recurrent laryngeal nerve. The diffusion of anesthetic gases into the cuff may increase the original pressure levels. Toxic neuritis may result from failure to clear agents used to cleanse the tubes. Ethylene oxide has been implicated most commonly.[4-9]

With the increased use of the CO_2 and argon lasers in surgery, the problem of incinerating endotracheal tubes with subsequent severe endobronchial injuries is well recognized. The use of metal endotracheal tubes and careful attention to detail has limited the incidence of that complication.[10]

Toxicity from products used to sterilize endotracheal tubes has been reported. Ethylene oxide and formaldehyde require periods of degassing before use or chemical burns of the trachea may result.[8]

Neurogenic reflex complications are also present at the time of intubation and are similar to those present during the act of intubation.[1]

Act of Extubation. Difficulty with extubation may result from failure or inability to deflate the cuff, with subsequent trauma to the larynx. Such trauma may range from simple abrasion to avulsion and dislocation injuries. Failure to deflate the cuff may produce recurrent laryngeal nerve injury by compressing the anterior branch of the nerve against the thyroid cartilage. The cuff or fragments of the endotracheal tube may become fixed to the tracheal wall and remain within the endobronchial tree. Tracheomalacia may be congenital or produced by prolonged internal cuff pressure or external pressure from paratracheal masses. This can result in tracheal collapse and respiratory obstruction. Occasionally, a patient may bite the tube and produce airway obstruction.[1,2,6,10]

Neurogenic reflex complications are present both during extubation and intubation. Laryngospasm and bronchospasm as well as cardiac arrhythmias are most common.[1]

EARLY COMPLICATIONS

Most complications of intubation are not apparent until extubation is accomplished and may present in the early or late postextubation period. The hazards associated with the process of placing and removing the endotracheal tube have been discussed and are relatively predictable. The residua produced by the presence of the endotracheal foreign body are particularly complex and insidious. Damage may result wherever the tube comes in contact with tissue, although the larynx and trachea are particularly at risk (Table 2).

Hilding[11] has shown that significant damage to the epithelium of the larynx and trachea occurs regularly with intubation. Injuries varied from desquamation and ulceration to separation of the epi-

TABLE 2. EARLY AND LATE COMPLICATIONS

Site	Early Complications	Late Complications
Nasal cavity	Edema Ulceration Epistaxis Infection	Alar rim erosion Septal perforation Synechiae Dysosmia
Nasopharynx	Edema Ulceration Infection	Ulceration Stenosis Eustachian tube dysfunction
Oropharynx	Edema Ulceration Infection	Tongue erosion Pharyngeal wall erosion
Larynx	Edema Ulceration Infection Vocal cord polyps	Granuloma Webs Synechiae Stenosis
Trachea	Edema Ulceration Infection	Stenosis Tracheomalacia Tracheoesophageal fistula
Hypopharynx	Edema Ulceration Infection	— — —

thelium from the basement membrane. The most serious injury occurred in the posterior larynx involving the cricoid cartilage and the vocal process of the arytenoids. The injury was related to the curvature of the endotracheal tube as it rested against the posterior larynx, which acts as a fulcrum forcing the distal end of the tube against the anterior tracheal wall. Hyperextension of the cervical spine and intraoral displacement of the tube further aggravate this mechanical advantage produced by the laryngeal fulcrum.[11]

Edema is frequently noted along the path of the endotracheal tube. Those areas most commonly involved are the epiglottis, aryepiglottic folds, and retroarytenoid and subglottic spaces where the presence of a loose submucosal attachment lends itself to the collection of edematous fluid. Although the degree of edema is typically of minor consequence, significant fluid can collect in these areas, pushing the epiglottis posteriorly or limiting vocal mobility with subsequent inspiratory obstruction. The most compromised area of postintubation edema is the subglottic space. Here the circumferential cricoid cartilage forces expansion of mucosal tissue into the airway lumen. The small diameter of the infant and child's airway is particularly at risk.[10-12]

As a result of edema, the patient may complain of hoarseness, sore throat, dysphagia, cough and, less commonly, dyspnea. The symptoms are typically of brief duration, clearing within 72 hours of extubation. Rarely does edema require reintubation or tracheotomy.

Intubation has also been linked to laryngeal incompetence and aspiration; this is related to a sensory and mechanical impairment of the glottis. The sphincteric function of the laryngeal folds is limited by the presence of edema and inflammation in the intrinsic musculature and cricoarytenoid space. The problem is typically a transient one, resolving within 12 to 24 hours following extubation.[13]

Injury beyond edema may result from brief periods of intubation. Donnelly[12] has shown that intubation as brief as one hour was associated with loss of mucosal epithelium. Prolonging intubation led to progressive injury and ischemic necrosis with bacterial infestation after 24 hours. Intubation beyond 48 hours is associated with perichondritis of the vocal process and cricoid laminae and after 96 hours severe damage can be found in these areas.[11,12,14]

Symptoms of ulcer formation are similar to those associated with edema. Pain is a more prominent complaint and the duration may be more prolonged. The most distressing aspect of these intubation injuries is their potential for developing into more severe late complications.

LATE COMPLICATIONS

Some mucosal damage is associated with every intubation. Most injuries are minor and heal without incident. More severe injuries result in mucosal erosion and chondritis. Granulation tissue often develops and wounds heal by secondary intention with an exuberant production of collagen. Because new collagen has a tendency to contract, a web or cicatrix develops and stenosis ensues. Although these changes may take place wherever the endotracheal tube rests, the vast majority are found in the larynx and trachea (Table 2).

A number of factors act alone or in concert in contributing to the frequency and severity of late complications. These include size of the tube relative to the size of the larynx and trachea, duration of intubation, shape and chemical composition of the cuff and tube, chemical irritants used in the cleansing of the tube, inflation pressure of the cuff, movement of the tube within the trachea, and intubation trauma. In addition, the biologic vulnerability of the mucosa resulting from infection, diabetes, hypotension, anemia and other underlying disease states has a clear influence.

The most common late complication is granuloma formation. It typically becomes apparent several weeks following extubation as symptoms of hoarseness, sore throat and dysphagia develop. The posterior aspect of the larynx, especially the area of the vocal process of the arytenoid, is most commonly involved. The thin mucosa and sparse submucosal space in this area make the cartilage susceptible to injury. The diameter of the endotracheal tube is maximal between the arytenoids, and repetitive stretching of tissue together with tube and laryngeal motion may produce significant repetitive insult. The posterior cricoid plate is subject to similar injury. The mechanical disadvantage of tube placement in this area has been discussed.[1,2,11,12,14]

Following the production of granulation tissue in this area, the reparative process may lead to the development of scar formation. Depending upon the pathogenicity of the process, simple narrowing of the posterior commissure and minor restriction of vocal cord mobility may result, synechiae and webs may develop or a circumferential cicatrix form. Fibrous tissue formation may cause ankylosis of the cricoarytenoid joints and narrow the subglottic space, resulting in severe laryngeal stenosis.

A similar sequence of events may occur in the trachea as a result of excessive cuff pressure or tube tip erosion. A minor area of insult may be followed by spontaneous resolution, or a devastating sequence of events may produce stenosis, tracheomalacia or even tracheoesophageal fistula. The same factors which influence the incidence and severity of laryngeal complication act within the trachea. The presence of the endotracheal cuff adds a new dimension, however. Cuff pressures in excess of 30 mm Hg produce a deficit in capillary perfusion, yet this level is often exceeded during intubation. Modern low-pressure, high-volume cuffs produce and maintain a compliant seal at safe pressures, but with overinflation even these cuffs become injurious.[11,12,14-16]

DISCUSSION

It is difficult to cite comparable statistical data on complications of intubation, although reports in the literature suggest that careful scrutiny of intubated patients would most likely show some injurious effect of the process. Hoarseness is the most common complaint and has been reported in 70% of patients.[2] Stauffer et al[2] found symptoms of sore throat, cough, sputum production and hemoptysis in descending frequencies ranging from 40% to 10% of patients studied. Dixon et al[17] reported a 5.5% incidence of postintubation stridor. Tonkin and Harrison[18] noted severe laryngeal damage in 4.2% of 166 long-term intubated patients.

The incidence of granuloma varies from 1:800 to 1:30 as reported in the literature. Most granulomas resolve spontaneously, although Lindholm removed seven postintubation granulomas in 312 patients studied.[4]

Stauffer et al[2] reported tracheal stenosis following intubation in 19% of patients studied with tomography. Although not clinically significant, this finding is in marked contrast to the 1% incidence reported by Lindholm[4] and illustrates the variability of statistical information on complications reported in the literature.

SUMMARY

In summary, endotracheal intubation with current, inert, low-pressure, high-volume cuffed tubes is a safe procedure associated with few complications in the vast majority of patients. However, complications related to mechanical difficulties and mucosal injury can occur even under ideal circumstances. Immediate complications are primarily associated with problems during intubation and extubation while early and late complications represent the short- and long-term effects of epithelial trauma.

REFERENCES

1. Blanc UF, Tremblay NAG. The complications of endotracheal intubation: a new classification with review of the literature. Anesth Analg (Cleve) 1974; 53:202-13.

2. Stauffer JL, Olson DE, Petty TL. Complications and consequences of endotracheal intubation and tracheotomy: a prospective study of 150 critically ill adult patients. Am J Med 1981; 70:65-76.

3. Levine PA. Hypopharyngeal perforation: an untoward complication of endotracheal intubation. Arch Otolaryngol 1980; 106: 578-80.

4. Lindholm CE. Prolonged endotracheal intubation. Acta Anaesthesiol Scand 1969; 33 Suppl 1:1-125.

5. Thompson DS, Read RC. Rupture of the trachea following endotracheal intubation. JAMA 1968; 204:995-7.

6. McGovern FH, Fitz-Hugh GS, Edgemon LJ. The hazards of endotracheal intubation. Ann Otol Rhinol Laryngol 1971; 80:556-64.

7. Wolf AP, Kuhn FA, Ogura JH. Pharyngo-esophageal perforations associated with rapid oral endotracheal intubation. Ann Otol Rhinol Laryngol 1972; 81:258-61.

8. Attas A, Sabawala PB, Keats AS. Acute transient sialadenopathy during induction of anesthesia. Anesthesiology 1968; 29:1050-2.

9. Nuntinen J, Karja J. Bilateral vocal cord paralysis following general anesthesia. Laryngoscope 1981; 91:83-6.

10. Schramm UL, Mattox DE, Stool SE. Acute management of laser ignited intratracheal explosions. Laryngoscope 1981; 91:1417-25.

11. Hilding AC. Laryngotracheal damage during intratracheal anesthesia: demonstration by staining the unfixed specimen with methylene blue. Ann Otol Rhinol Laryngol 1971; 80:565-81.

12. Donnelly WH. Histopathology of endotracheal intubation: an autopsy study of 99 cases. Arch Pathol 1969; 88:511-20.

13. Burgess GE, Cooper JR, Marino RJ, Peuler MJ, Warriner RA. Laryngeal competence after tracheal extubation. Anesthesiology 1979; 51:73-7.

14. Burns HP, Doyle VS, Scott A, Von Nostrand AWP, Bryce DP. Laryngotracheal trauma: observation on its pathogenesis and its prevention following prolonged orotracheal intubation in the adult. Laryngoscope 1979; 89:1316-25.

15. Cooper JD, Grillo HC. Analysis of problems related to cuffs on intratracheal tubes. Chest 1972; 62:21-7.

16. Conner GH, Bushet MJ, Maisels MJ. Prolonged orotracheal intubation in the newborn. Ann Otol Rhinol Laryngol 1980; 89:459-61.

17. Dixon TC, Sando MJW, Bolton JM, Gilligan JE. A report of 342 cases of prolonged intratracheal intubation. Med J Aust 1968; 2:529-33.

18. Tonkin JP, Harrison GA. The effect on the larynx of prolonged endotracheal intubation. Med J Aust 1966; 2:581-7.

WEGENER'S GRANULOMATOSIS OF THE SUBGLOTTIS AND THE UPPER PORTION OF THE TRACHEA

THOMAS J. MCDONALD, MD
H. BRYAN NEEL III, MD RICHARD A. DEREMEE, MD
ROCHESTER, MINNESOTA

A relatively little-known complication of Wegener's granulomatosis is involvement of the subglottis and upper part of the trachea, which is illustrated in this report on 17 patients. Each of the patients had biopsy-proved Wegener's granulomatosis of the nose and paranasal sinuses. Some had concomitant involvement of the eye, kidney, lung and skin. Nine of the 17 patients required tracheotomy; 5 still require a tracheotomy tube, and 4 have had decannulation (1 had successful reconstructive surgery of the trachea). Medical treatment consisted of cyclophosphamide, with or without corticosteroids. All 17 are currently alive, the average follow-up having been 81 months. The otolaryngologist plays a key role in the detection and management of patients with Wegener's granulomatosis, particularly when the onset is a sudden progressive upper tracheal obstruction with airway symptoms that may overshadow the sometimes more subtle nasal manifestations.

Wegener's granulomatosis is a specific granulomatous disease categorized with the respiratory vasculitides and characterized by necrotizing granulomas and vasculitis of the upper and lower respiratory tracts, systemic vasculitis and focal necrotizing glomerulitis. The concept of limited Wegener's granulomatosis, that is, lesions fulfilling the morphologic characteristics above and localized to certain areas or groups of sites, has already been widely accepted[1] and the nasal and paranasal manifestations, in particular, are recognized.[2]

Other sites in the upper airway, such as the mouth, notably the gingiva, and the oropharynx, can be involved but seldom are. Involvement of the nasopharynx is commonly associated with subsequent eustachian tube dysfunction, and otologic involvement with serous otitis media as the main manifestation has also been described.[3,4] In addition, vasculitis involving the cochlear artery, which may cause sensorineural deafness, has been described.[5] The third type of otologic involvement is chronic mastoiditis with chronic otitis media and destruction of the middle ear.[4]

Reports of Wegener's granulomatosis involving the glottis and supraglottic larynx have been conspicuously absent. What concerns us, therefore, is the following report on 17 patients with proved Wegener's granulomatosis in whom subglottic and tracheal stenosis developed during the course of the disease.

CLINICAL EXPERIENCE

Since 1964, 108 patients, 54 male and 54 female, with biopsy-proved Wegener's granulomatosis have been examined and treated at the Mayo Clinic. The ages ranged from 8 to 75 years. Each of the 17 patients with subglottic or tracheal involvement initially had nasal and paranasal manifestations of the disease, and in many patients, other organ systems were affected (Table). The nasal and paranasal findings, which have been described before,[2] consist mostly of nasal obstruction, bloody rhinorrhea, nasal crusting and bleeding, and, in many cases, perforation of the nasal septum and nasal dorsal saddling. Systemic symptoms that typically were out of proportion to the upper airway symptoms were observed in almost all patients. These symptoms consist of malaise, fatigue, night sweats and, usually, migratory arthralgias.[2,6]

Pulmonary involvement, ordinarily heralded by a cough, with or without hemoptysis, and demonstrated by roentgenographic changes of single or multiple cavitating lesions, was noted in 4 of the 17 patients. Concomitant renal involvement, characterized by abnormal urinary sediment, proteinuria and the presence of hyaline casts and red cells, was observed in 5 of the 17 patients, and in each of these patients an elevated serum creatinine level was found. The skin was involved in 3 of the 17 patients. Cutaneous lesions characteristically are small, red and slightly raised and are most commonly found on the lower limbs and occasionally on the upper extremities. They resemble tiny tick bites, and on biopsy, specimens show a vasculitis similar to the morphologic changes in other involved sites. In one patient, concomitant mononeuritis multiplex was found.

Involvement of the ear, generally serous otitis media, with or without chronic middle ear or mastoid changes, was noted in 5 of the 17 patients. Two of the five had associated sensorineural hearing loss.

Involvement of the orbit was seen in 8 patients, 5

From the Department of Otorhinolaryngology, Mayo Clinic and Mayo Foundation, Rochester, Minnesota.
Presented at the meeting of the American Broncho-Esophagological Association, Palm Beach, Florida, May 3-4, 1982.
REPRINTS — T. J. McDonald, MD, Mayo Clinic, 200 First Street SW, Rochester, MN 55905.

ORGAN SYSTEM INVOLVEMENT BY WEGENER'S GRANULOMATOSIS IN PATIENTS WITH TRACHEAL INVOLVEMENT (N = 17)

Organ	*No. of Patients*
Trachea	17
Nose	17
Eye	
Orbital mass	5
Cornea-sclera	3
Ear	5
Kidney	5
Lung	4
Skin	3
Central nervous system (mononeuritis multiplex)	1

of whom had an orbital mass. One patient with an orbital mass had extension of the disease from the nose to the orbit, with marked periorbital swelling and a tumefactive process that involved the entire orbit and resulted in marked proptosis. The remaining 4 patients with orbital masses had pseudotumor; in 1 the pseudotumor was not of the type associated with Wegener's granulomatosis, and in the 3 other patients with orbital involvement, the pseudotumors were of the histologic type ordinarily seen with Wegener's granulomatosis.[7]

The three remaining patients with ophthalmologic involvement had corneoscleral disease, generally a conjunctivitis, and one patient had a marginal corneal ulceration.

In 14 of the 17 patients, tracheal symptoms and signs, usually hoarseness with increasing stridor, were observed shortly after or concomitant with the nasal manifestations.

There was a different pattern, however, in three patients. In two, tracheal involvement developed that was characterized by hoarseness and stridor, $5^1/_2$ and nine years, respectively, after the initial nasal involvement was reported. The third patient, in whom tracheal symptoms developed concomitantly with involvement of the nose and orbit, did not require tracheotomy until 12 years later.

Tracheal Involvement. Each of the 17 patients had an identical type of tracheal lesion. On the average this was a 3- to 4-cm stricture of the upper portion of the trachea, usually a circumferential narrowing. The appearance of the lesion as observed on direct laryngoscopy was typical. Grossly, a reddish, friable, circumferential narrowing was seen just below the cords. In no instance was the distal part of the trachea involved. Tracheal tomograms clearly delineated the narrowed area.

Diagnosis. The investigation of each of the patients has been described before[6] and consisted of paranasal sinus and pulmonary roentgenography, urinalysis, complete blood count and determination of the serum creatinine level. Flow-volume loop studies (Fig. 1) and tracheal tomography (Figs. 2 and 3) were helpful in determining both the severity of the tracheal stricture and the success of treatment.

In each case, nasal biopsy was performed in the operating room with the patient under local anesthesia (cocaine anesthesia supplemented by intravenous sedative medication). Crusts had to be removed and then biopsy specimens of the friable mucosa underneath could be taken liberally. Cultures were done in each case to rule out specific fungal infections that can cause a granulomatous picture similar to Wegener's granulomatosis. In 3 of the 17 patients, tracheal biopsies were performed, revealing tissue consistent with Wegener's granulomatosis in each case.

Treatment. In nine patients, tracheotomy was necessary. Six of the 9 patients required tracheotomy shortly after the diagnosis was made, but in 3 others it was delayed.

Each of the patients was treated with cyclophosphamide, with or without corticosteroids. We ordinarily use both agents in patients who have a fulminating disease, especially in cases in which

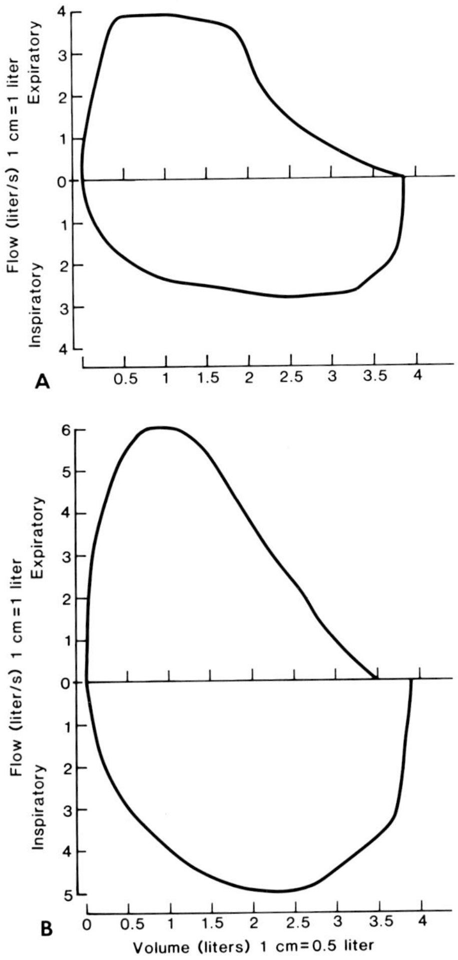

Fig. 1. Flow-volume loop study. A) Before treatment. Both inspiratory and expiratory peak flows are reduced. B) After treatment. Inspiratory and expiratory peak flows have increased.

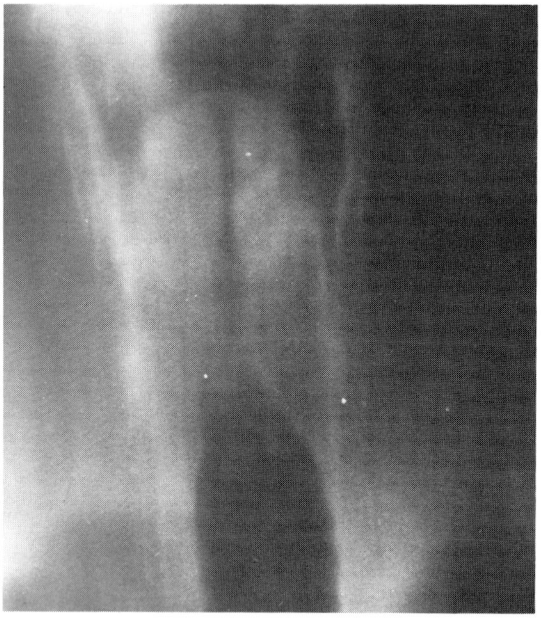

Fig. 2. Soft-tissue swelling associated with narrowing of subglottis due to Wegener's granulomatosis.

renal failure is present. In these instances, treatment with high doses of prednisone (60 to 80 mg a day) is begun immediately and is maintained until the disease is under control as indicated by an improved erythrocyte sedimentation rate and a more normal serum creatinine level. At that time, cyclophosphamide therapy (approximately 2 mg/kg per day as a single morning dose) is instituted. After 2 to 3 weeks, the prednisone dosage is reduced gradually and is ultimately tapered off completely. We continue cyclophosphamide therapy for 1 year beyond the last evidence of active disease and agree with Fauci et al[8] that there are dramatic responses to this agent in patients with Wegener's granulomatosis.

In patients with a more benign or indolent course but no renal involvement, glucocorticoids may not be necessary and cyclophosphamide may be used alone.

RESULTS

All patients are alive at the time of this writing, the average follow-up having been 81 months. Although five patients must still use tracheotomy tubes (later converted to a valved speaking tube), four others have undergone successful decannulation. One of these had successful tracheal reconstruction.

DISCUSSION

Sudden and progressive stridor due to upper tracheal narrowing is a challenging problem for the otolaryngologist. Specific nontraumatic and nonneoplastic causes have been reported[9] which include sarcoidosis, amyloidosis and relapsing polychondritis. Each of these conditions must be considered.

Sarcoidosis has certain manifestations that are not seen in patients with Wegener's granulomatosis: diffuse pulmonary infiltrates with or without bilateral hilar adenopathy, occasionally increased serum level, and hypercalciuria. In addition, even though nasal mucosal changes occur in sarcoidosis,[10,11] there are not the major ulcerative findings as seen in Wegener's granulomatosis. Moreover, sarcoidosis usually involves the supraglottic larynx rather than the trachea.[12]

Amyloidosis, when it does involve the trachea, is associated either with systemic amyloidosis or with multiple myeloma. When localized to the trachea,

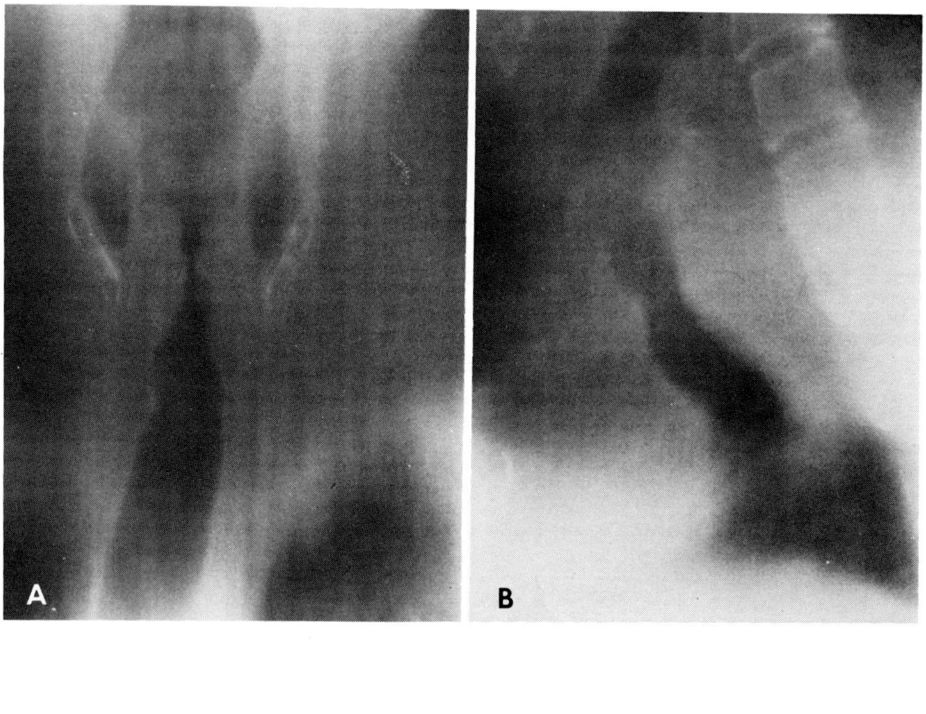

Fig. 3. A,B) Irregular narrowing of upper portion of trachea.

it usually occurs as a small, localized mass and not as a long, subglottic narrowing.[11]

Relapsing polychondritis remains to be differentiated from Wegener's granulomatosis when the patient presents with nasal and tracheal symptoms and signs. There is some help in making the distinction, however. First, patients with relapsing polychondritis do not have the nasal and nasopharyngeal mucosal destruction that we note in Wegener's granulomatosis. Moreover, the mucosal tissue in Wegener's disease usually yields the characteristic diagnostic findings. In relapsing polychondritis, the diagnosis is difficult to make by examining tissue from any site because the chondrolysis and other cartilaginous changes are relatively nonspecific and are seen only in the acute stage, at which time there is a certain appropriate reluctance to perform biopsy on an inflamed nose or pinna. In addition, other hallmarks of Wegener's granulomatosis, such as glomerulitis, skin changes and cavitating lesions on lung roentgenograms, are not characteristic of relapsing polychondritis. However, there are features — corneoscleral changes, nasal dorsal collapse and otologic manifestations (sensorineural deafness and serous otitis media) — that are similar to those observed in Wegener's granulomatosis.[13] On the other hand, the enlarged, reddened (and later deformed) pinna, classic in relapsing polychondritis, has been seen in only one of our patients with Wegener's granulomatosis. In addition to the nasal mucosal differences, the other differentiating feature between the two diseases seems to be the extent of tracheal involvement. In all patients in this series, the stricture was short (3 to 4 cm) and was directly below the glottis; the distal portion of the trachea was spared in all cases. Relapsing polychondritis, on the other hand, can involve the whole trachea and even extend into the adjacent bronchi.

We would again like to make a distinction between Wegener's granulomatosis and another disease so often confused with it, polymorphic reticulosis. The specific differences, notably morphologic contrasts, absence of otologic and renal involvement in polymorphic reticulosis, and differences in the response to treatment, have been referred to before.[14] We would like to add yet another differentiating feature in that we have observed tracheal involvement in only one of our patients with polymorphic reticulosis.[15] This is an interesting addition because the pulmonary involvement in both diseases is very similar.

In this context, we have continued to use the term "polymorphic reticulosis" in preference to "lymphomatoid granulomatosis." The latter term is inaccurate but is at least an improvement over the old name of "lethal midline granuloma," a wholly clinical and entirely nonspecific term under which Wegener's granulomatosis is still often discussed. Although polymorphic reticulosis is not necessarily the perfect term to describe a lymphomalike disease separate from Wegener's granulomatosis, it "stands at the watershed of the literature," links old and new reports and terms and consolidates them into a "sound, broad nosologic concept."[6]

The variations in behavior of the tracheal lesion in this group of patients and their response to treatment is noteworthy. The eight patients who did not need tracheotomy probably had a slightly less aggressive type of disease or were treated earlier (or both). These reasons probably explain the fact that in three of the patients decannulation was feasible. The other decannulated patient had resection of the stricture with successful tracheal repair.

The problems of any reconstructive surgery in patients with Wegener's granulomatosis are the same, whether the site of repair is nasal, orbital, otologic or tracheal. Most patients receive continuous immunosuppressive treatment; in addition, the disease does reactivate, as evidenced by the development of tracheal lesions in two patients some years after the initial upper airway lesions were controlled. This brings up the question of whether the disease behaves as a "continuum," being contained for a while in one part of the airway, only to skip and manifest itself later in another. These reasons, we believe, explain why surgical repair may not be attempted at all or, if performed, has poor results.

Finally, we find it difficult to explain the higher incidence of tracheal involvement in our female patients — 16 cases versus the single case in a male patient — especially when involvement of other parts of the airway is similar in the two sexes.

REFERENCES

1. Cassan SM, Coles DT, Harrison EG Jr. The concept of limited forms of Wegener's granulomatosis. Am J Med 1970; 49: 366-79.

2. McDonald TJ, DeRemee RA, Kern EB, Harrison EG Jr. Nasal manifestations of Wegener's granulomatosis. Laryngoscope 1974; 84:2101-12.

3. Karmody CS. Wegener's granulomatosis: presentation as an otologic problem. Otolaryngol Head Neck Surg 1978; 86: ORL573-84.

4. McCaffrey TV, McDonald TJ, Facer GW, DeRemee RA. Otologic manifestations of Wegener's granulomatosis. Otolaryngol Head Neck Surg 1980; 88:586-93.

5. Weaver M. Profound sensorineural hearing loss associated with collagen disease. Trans Pac Coast Otoophthalmol Soc Annu Meet 1972; 53:83-9.

6. DeRemee RA, Weiland LH, McDonald TJ. Polymorphic reticulosis, lymphomatoid granulomatosis: two diseases or one? Mayo Clin Proc 1978; 53:634-40.

7. Henderson JW, Orbital tumors. 2nd ed. New York: Thieme-Stratton, 1980.

8. Fauci AS, Haynes BF, Katz P. The spectrum of vasculitis: clinical, pathologic, immunologic, and therapeutic considerations. Ann Intern Med 1978; 89:660-76.

9. Djalilian M, McDonald TJ, Devine KD, Weiland LH. Nontraumatic, nonneoplastic subglottic stenosis. Ann Otol Rhinol Laryngol 1975; 84:757-63.

10. Miglets AW, Viall JH, Kataria YP. Sarcoidosis of the head and neck. Laryngoscope 1977; 87:2038-48.

11. McDonald TJ. Granulomatous diseases of the nose. In: Coates GM, Schenck HP, Miller MV, eds. Otolaryngology. Vol 2. Hagerstown: Harper & Row, 1979:1-13.

12. Devine KD. Sarcoidosis and sarcoidosis of the larynx. Laryngoscope 1965; 7:533-69.

13. McCaffrey TV, McDonald TJ, McCaffrey LA. Head and neck manifestations of relapsing polychondritis: a review of 29 cases. Otolaryngol Head Neck Surg 1978; 86:ORL473-8.

14. McDonald TJ, DeRemee RA, Weiland LH. Wegener's granulomatosis and polymorphic reticulosis — two diseases or one: experience with 90 patients. Arch Otolaryngol 1981; 107: 141-4.

15. McDonald TJ, DeRemee RA, Harrison EG Jr, Facer GW, Devine KD. The protean clinical features of polymorphic reticulosis (lethal midline granuloma). Laryngoscope 1976; 86:936-45.

≈

INTERSPECIALTY FACIAL SURGERY CONGRESS FOR AESTHETIC, CANCER AND RECONSTRUCTIVE SURGERY

The IFSCACRS will be held at the Waldorf-Astoria in New York, April 27-30, 1983. This Congress is sponsored by the International Oculoplastic Society. For more information contact Pierre Guibor, MD, IFSC Secretary, 630 Park Avenue, New York, NY 10021; (212) 734-1010.

≈

FOURTH WORLD CONGRESS ON BRONCHOESOPHAGOLOGY

The Fourth World Congress on Bronchoesophagology will take place at the Foresta Conference Center in Stockholm, Sweden, June 20-23, 1983. This Congress is arranged by the International Bronchoesophagological Society, Swedish Otolaryngological Society and Swedish Society for Pulmonary Diseases. During the meeting, the Congress will update the knowledge within bronchology and esophagology. Further information may be obtained by writing IBES Congress 1983, c/o RESO Congress Service S-105, 24 Stockholm, Sweden, or Dr. Stig Haglund, Secretary of the Congress, Dept. of Otolaryngology, Karolinska Sjukuset, S-104 01 Stockholm 60, Sweden.

WEGENER'S GRANULOMATOSIS APPEARING INITIALLY IN THE TRACHEA

J. CARLOS ARAUZ, MD ROLANDO FONSECA, MD

BUENOS AIRES, ARGENTINA

We treated ten patients with Wegener's granulomatosis whose clinical picture differed only in the stage of the disease at the time of the first visit. All patients were female with a mean age of 30 years and all presented with a picture of high tracheal obstruction. Three died and six have a permanent tracheostomy. Surgical treatment was unsuccessful; corticosteroids provided only transient improvement but cyclophosphamide induced remission. Removal of the stenosis either by open surgery or endoscopically by laser was not successful in accomplishing decannulation.

In 1936, Wegener[1] described the symptomatologic triad of necrotizing granulomatous processes in the upper and/or lower respiratory tract, necrotizing glomerulonephritis and generalized vasculitis of small arteries and veins.

In 1959, Atkins and Eisman[2] introduced this disease to laryngologists and reported that it was not always lethal and that incomplete forms could occur. They felt that the prognosis could be improved by immunosuppression.

Recently, De Remee et al[3] suggested the classification E, L and K be used for limited Wegener's granulomatosis. This classification is based on the anatomical regions involved. The classification E includes ears, nose and pharynx; L includes larynx, trachea and lungs; and K designates kidneys. The classic pathologic features are denoted as ELK, but also the combinations EL, EK and LK may occur.

Since 1959, we have treated ten patients with Wegener's granulomatosis who were first seen without a definite diagnosis. All were female and had respiratory obstruction due to subglottic involvement.

Illum and Thorling[4] reported 4 cases in a series of 17 who had a picture similar to that of our 10. At the time of diagnosis, we classified 3 as L, 4 as EL and 3 as ELK. In none of the cases was a biopsy helpful in establishing the diagnosis with certainty. This has been reported previously in other series. We believe that the diagnosis must be made on clinical grounds and, in some cases, according to the response to corticosteroids and cyclophosphamide.

The possibility of Wegener's granulomatosis must be kept in mind, particularly in patients with a history of chronic otitis or sinusitis.[5,6] In this series 4 patients had typical nasal deformity, 2 had lesions in the ear, and 1 had an ocular lesion. The findings on lateral x-ray films of the neck were similar in all cases. Seven of the 10 patients are alive and 6 required permanent tracheostomy.[7] Two patients were treated with surgical resection and end-to-end anastomosis, with transitory improvement. Corticosteroids provided only transient benefit, but cyclophosphamide induced remission and improved the prognosis.

CASE REPORTS.

Case 1. A 24-year-old woman (Figs. 1 and 2) complained chiefly of dyspnea of two months' duration. The medical history was noncontributory. Indirect laryngoscopy revealed subglottic infiltration and the biopsy specimen showed chronic inflammation. Chest x-ray films revealed pulmonary le-

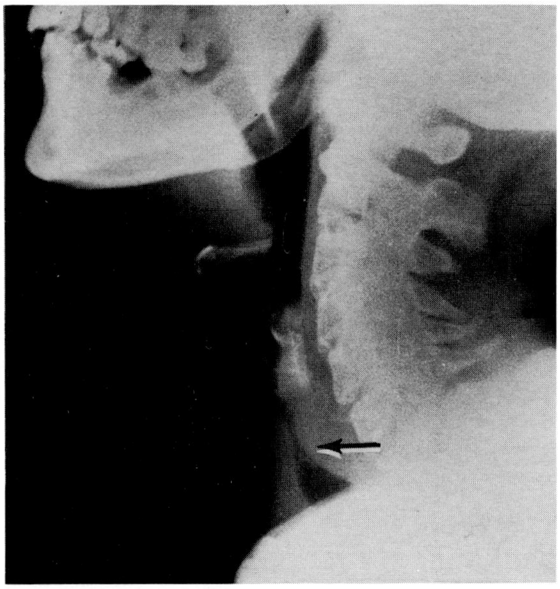

Fig. 1. (Case 1) Lateral neck x-ray film showing subglottic and upper tracheal stenosis (arrow).

From the Hospital de Clinicas, la. Catedra de O.R.L., Universidad de Medicine de Buenos Aires.

Presented at the meeting of the American Broncho-Esophagological Association, Palm Beach, Florida, May 3-4, 1982.

REPRINTS — J. Carlos Arauz, MD, Cangello 2150, 1040 Buenos Aires, Argentina.

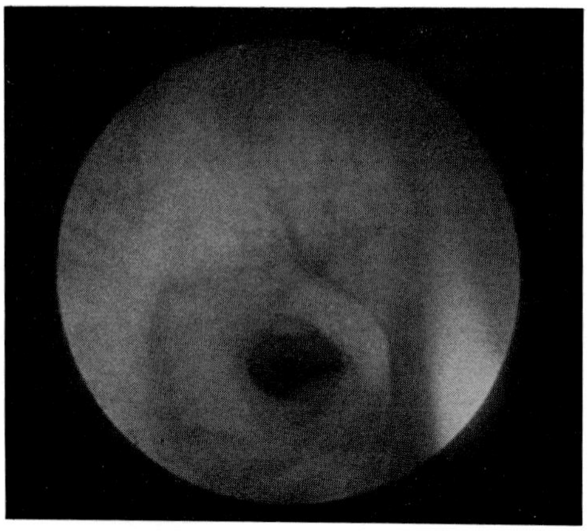

Fig. 2. (Case 1) Endoscopic view showing subglottic and upper tracheal stenosis.

sions, but tuberculosis was ruled out. Results of urinalysis were consistent with glomerulonephritis.

Treatment with cyclophosphamide resulted in marked improvement of the patient's renal status. The subglottic stenosis persisted and the lesion became cicatricial. After three years the attending internist agreed to perform surgery, and the lesion was removed, with end-to-end anastomosis of the trachea. Although the subglottic narrowing improved, it was impossible to remove the tracheostomy tube. The patient remains in good general health six years after the initial diagnosis.

Case 2. A 64-year-old woman presented with chief complaints of cough, nasal congestion and epistaxis of two months' duration. Recently she had developed dyspnea and hoarseness. On physical examination the vocal cords moved normally, but there was narrowing of the upper third of the trachea, particularly in the subglottic area, and the trachea collapsed on expiration. She had been admitted to another hospital two years previously with skin lesions and articular pains. A skin biopsy yielded results thought to be consistent with collagen vascular disease.

During the patient's final admission, respiratory function tests showed upper airway obstruction with the following values: pH, 7.34:P_{CO_2}, 46; P_{O_2}, 60. Her chest x-ray film showed a cavitary pulmonary lesion. She died after four days despite tracheostomy and medication. Autopsy revealed a granulomatous process in the trachea with fibrinoid necrosis and focal glomerulonephritis.

REFERENCES

1. Wegener F. Ueber generalisierte septiche Gefaesserkrankungen. Verh Dtsch Ges Pathol 1936; 29:2102-10.

2. Atkins J, Eisman S. Wegener's granulomatosis. Ann Otol Rhinol Laryngol 1959; 68:524-47.

3. De Remee RA, McDonald TJ, Harrison EG Jr, Coles DT. Wegener's granulomatosis: anatomic correlates, a proposed classification. Mayo Clin Proc 1976; 51:777-81.

4. Illum P, Thorling K. Wegener granulomatosis long term results of treatment. Ann Otol Rhinol Laryngol 1981; 90:231-5.

5. Reussi G, Arauz S, Yussem E, Vayo JM. Granulomatosis de Wegener. Rev Asoc Méd Argent 1973; 86: 23-31.

6. MacDonald TJ. Nasal manifestations of Wegener's granulomatosis. Laryngoscope 1974; 84:2101-11.

7. Arauz JC, Fonseca R. Granulomatosis de Wegener con manifestaciones iniciales en la laringe. Rev Asoc Méd Argent 1981; 94:127-8.

ANATOMIC ABNORMALITIES IN OBSTRUCTIVE SLEEP APNEA

DALE WILMS, MD

JOHN POPOVICH, MD
SHIRO FUJITA, MD

WILLIAM CONWAY, MD
FRANK ZORICK, MD

DETROIT, MICHIGAN

Both muscular hypotonia and anatomic abnormalities have been implicated in the pathogenesis of the obstructive sleep apnea syndrome (OSAS). The upper airways of 25 patients with OSAS were evaluated to determine potential sites of obstruction. Significant airway compromise was found in all patients with some patients having multiple sites of airway narrowing.

INTRODUCTION

Obstructive sleep apnea syndrome (OSAS) is due to intermittent collapse of the upper airway. Both muscular hypotonia and anatomic compromise of the airway have been implicated in its pathogenesis. Sleep apnea and upper airway obstruction have been demonstrated in patients with a variety of structural abnormalities of the upper airway and OSAS is commonly associated with obesity. To determine the contribution of structural abnormalities of the upper airway to OSAS we evaluated the upper airways of 25 patients with the disorder.

MATERIALS AND METHODS

The upper airways of 25 consecutive adult men with OSAS demonstrated by standard polysomnographic techniques were evaluated. The characteristics of these patients are shown in Table 1. All patients were somnulent and had typical manifestation of OSAS. The airway was evaluated by both direct inspection and fiberoptic visualization. The oropharynx and hypopharynx were evaluated for potential obstruction in the anteroposterior (AP) and lateral dimensions. The larynx was evaluated for its overall potential to obstruct the airway. Scoring of the airway abnormalities was performed by the examining physician and by two reviewers of video recordings of the airways, with the majority opinion of the appropriate score accepted. The structures were given a score of 1 to 3, a score of 1 being within the normal range and a score of 3 representing significant airway narrowing.

With the patient in the sitting position, the uvula, a potential source of obstruction in the AP dimension of the oropharynx, was given a relative size score. For the uvula scoring was as follows: 1 — normal in size; 2 — either elongated or widened to twice normal size; and 3 — both elongated and widened.

For evaluating the remainder of the airway nasopharyngolaryngoscopy was performed using an Olympus BF-3 bronchofiberscope. The patients were premedicated with intramuscular atropine and the nasal and oropharyngeal mucosa was anesthetized with topical 2% lidocaine. With the patient awake and supine, the bronchofiberscope was passed transnasally. The findings were recorded with still photography and the Circon color microvideo system. Still photographs were taken during inspiration.

The lateral dimension of the oropharynx was evaluated in terms of encroachment on the bronchoscopic visual field by the lateral walls of the oropharynx when the bronchoscope tip was positioned at the distal nasopharynx. The airway was scored as follows: 1 — lateral walls well beyond the bronchoscopic visual field; 2 — lateral walls approximately at the edge of the bronchoscopic visual field; and 3 — lateral walls within the bronchoscopic visual field.

The hypopharynx was also scored in the AP and lateral dimensions. The base of the tongue, which contributed to the AP narrowing, was evaluated in terms of obstruction of the bronchoscopic visual field when the tip of the bronchofiberscope was positioned halfway between the distal nasopharynx and the epiglottis. The relative degree of obstruction was scored as follows: 1 — one fourth of the visual field obstructed by the base of the tongue; 2 — half of the visual field obstructed; and 3 — three fourths or more of the visual field obstructed. The lateral dimension of the hypopharynx at the level of the epiglottis was scored relative to the outside diameter of the bronchoscope: thus, 1 — lateral dimension three or more bronchoscopic diameters; 2 — width approximately two bronchoscopic diameters; and 3 — width one or less bronchoscopic diameters.

The larynx was evaluated for narrowing by the lateral wall of the airway and redundancy of the aryepiglottic folds and was scored as follows: 1 — normal; 2 — appeared narrowed because of redundancy of the arytenoid mucosa and/or the aryepiglottic folds; and 3 — potential for airway obstruction by redundant aryepiglottic folds and/or arytenoid mucosa.

The oropharynx and hypopharynx were considered abnormal if the sum of the AP and lateral scores was 5 or 6; the larynx was considered abnormal if the score was 3.

RESULTS

Airway abnormalities were found in all patients evaluated. These included oropharyngeal obstruction in the AP dimension by the uvula and obstruction in the lateral dimension by bulging lateral walls. The hypopharynx was obstructed in the AP dimension by a large base of tongue and was also found to be narrowed laterally at the level of the

TABLE 1. CHARACTERISTICS OF PATIENTS IN STUDY

	Range	*Mean*
Age	33- 59	48
Percent ideal weight	101-197	153
Apneic episodes/hr	29- 87	62

From the Pulmonary Medicine Division (Wilms, Popovich, Conway), Otolaryngology Department (Fujita), and the Sleep Disorders Center (Zorick), Henry Ford Hospital, Detroit.

Presented at the meeting of the American Broncho-Esophagological Association, Palm Beach, Florida, May 3-4, 1982.

REPRINTS — Dale Wilms, MD, Loma Linda University Hospital, Division of Pulmonary and Critical Care Medicine, Loma Linda, CA 92354.

TABLE 2. SITES OF OBSTRUCTION IN UPPER AIRWAY (N = 25)

	No. of Patients	%
Oropharynx	19	76
Hypopharynx	11	44
Larynx	2	8
≥ 2 sites	9	36

epiglottis. Aryepiglottic abnormalities contributed most significantly to potential obstruction at the larynx.

A summary of the distribution of areas of abnormalities is shown in Table 2. The oropharynx was most commonly abnormal with the larynx being the least common abnormal site.

DISCUSSION

The sleep apnea syndrome with excessive daytime sleepiness, disturbed sleep, and loud snoring is a well-established entity. Polysomnography has demonstrated obstruction of the airway in patients with sleep apnea, but the pathogenesis of the obstruction remains unclear. A variety of anatomic abnormalities have been associated with the syndrome.[1-4] In many cases, particularly those associated with obesity, no anatomic abnormality has been described.[5]

Reports disagree regarding the site of obstruction with the oropharynx, epiglottis and larynx all being implicated.[6] Direct observation with fiberoptic instruments along with cinefluoroscopy and electromyography of the oropharyngeal muscles have aided in understanding the pathogenesis of upper airway obstruction.[7] While important in the respiratory cycle, it is not clear that oropharyngeal muscle dysfunction is the only pathologic mechanism in those patients previously felt to have no structural abnormalities.[5]

CONCLUSION

Significant airway compromise was found in all patients with OSAS. The abnormalities were frequent and often occurred at multiple sites. Our data suggest that structural abnormalities of the airway along with previously described neuromuscular dysfunction cause airway obstruction in OSAS.

REFERENCES

1. Orr WC, Martin RJ. Obstructive sleep apnea associated with tonsillar hypertrophy in adults. Arch Intern Med 1981; 141: 990-2.

2. Orr WC, Males JL, Imes NK. Myxedema and obstructive sleep apnea. Am J Med 1981; 70:1061-6.

3. Conway WA, Bower GC, Barnes ME. Hypersomnolence and intermittent upper airway obstruction. JAMA 1977; 237: 2740-2.

4. Baker SR, Ross J. Sleep apnea syndrome and supraglottic edema. Arch Otolaryngol 1980; 106:486-91.

5. Guilleminault C, Tilkian A, Dement WC. The sleep apnea syndromes. Annu Rev Med 1976; 27:465-84.

6. Remmers JE, DeGroot WJ, Sauerland EK, Arch AM. Pathogenesis of upper airway occlusion during sleep. J Appl Physiol 1978; 44:931-8.

7. Cirignotta F, Lugaresi E. Some cineradiographic aspects of snoring and obstructive apneas. Sleep 1980; 3:225-6.

BRAINSTEM EVOKED POTENTIALS IN ADULT SLEEP APNEA

NANCY L. SNYDERMAN, MD
JONAS T. JOHNSON, MD
MARGARETA MØLLER, MD, PHD
PATRICIA B. THEARLE, RN
PITTSBURGH, PENNSYLVANIA

Brainstem evoked potentials (BSEP) were recorded in 23 patients with adult sleep apnea (ASA). These patients were studied with all-night polysomnography prior to our testing. They were categorized as having obstructive, central, or mixed sleep apnea depending on the predominant sleep findings. All patients with central sleep apnea had abnormal BSEP with prolongation of wave V. A majority of the remaining patients with obstructive sleep apnea and mixed sleep apnea had abnormal BSEP, but without specific configurations. These findings substantiate our hypothesis that brainstem dysfunction may play a role in ASA.

INTRODUCTION

A population of people with sleep disturbance have sleep apnea. Apnea is the cessation of airflow past the nose and mouth for greater than 10s[1]. Episodes that occur more than 30 times per night may be considered to be sleep apnea. These patients can be further categorized as having apnea of either central or peripheral etiology. Those with obstructive sleep apnea (OSA) make persistent respiratory effort in spite of an anatomical obstruction to airflow. Patients with central sleep apnea (CSA) make no respiratory effort during the apneic periods. A mixed group (MSA) exists with both central and obstructive components.

At this time we do not understand the mechanism of sleep apnea of central origin. A theoretic consideration is that patients with the central disorder have an abnormality in the brainstem. A reliable method of distinguishing central from obstructive apnea would be clinically useful for diagnostic consideration and therapeutic decision-making. Brainstem evoked potentials (BSEP) might, therefore, provide information about brainstem abnormalities in patients with adult sleep apnea (ASA).

METHODS

Twenty-three patients with ASA underwent BSEP. These people had been diagnosed with all-night polysomnography (electroencephalogram, electrocardiogram, electromyogram, nasopharyngeal and oropharyngeal airflow monitors, and chest actograms) on two consecutive nights at the Western Psychiatric Institute and Clinic. Patients were then categorized as having CSA if respirations ceased during the apnea. Obstructive apnea was diagnosed when a respiratory effort was evident while the patient was apneic. Mixed apnea constituted a short CSA followed by a longer obstructive component. Pure-tone and speech audiometry were performed prior to BSEP. Two patients had a mild high-frequency sensorineural hearing loss, but no patients were excluded from the study because of hearing loss. The BSEP data was interpreted by an otologist who was unaware of any individual patient's diagnosis.

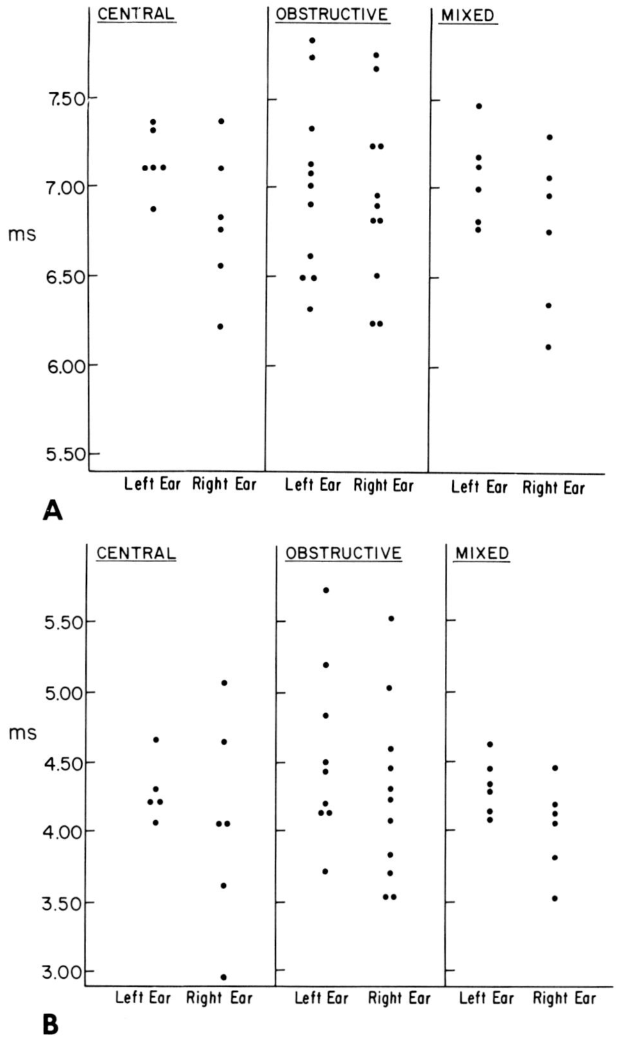

Brainstem evoked potentials. A) Absolute latencies of wave V. Normal range 4.90 to 6.80. B) Interpeak latency difference of peaks I-V. Normal range 2.90 to 3.90.

From the Department of Otolaryngology (Snyderman, Johnson, Thearle) and the Division of Audiology & Speech Pathology (Møller), University of Pittsburgh School of Medicine, Eye and Ear Hospital.

Presented at the meeting of the American Broncho-Esophagological Association, Palm Beach, Florida, May 3-4, 1982.

REPRINTS — Nancy L. Snyderman, MD, Department of Otolaryngology, 230 Lothrop Street, Pittsburgh, PA 15213.

Brainstem evoked potentials were recorded with the patient sitting in a sound-insulated room using the forehead and the mastoid.[2] The stimulation consisted of 2,000-Hz tone-bursts, 5 ms in duration, with a rise and fall time of 0.2 ms (to 90% and 10% of maximal amplitude, respectively). The hearing level corresponded to 85 dB. The tone-bursts were presented with an interstimulus interval of 150 ms and three tests were performed in each ear. Each test consisted of the averaged responses to 2,048 tone-bursts. Recordings were analyzed with regard to 1) the absolute latency of wave V and 2) the interpeak latency difference of peaks I-V.

RESULTS

Forty-seven percent of our patients had CSA. There were equal numbers of patients with OSA and MSA in the remaining 53%.

All patients with CSA had prolonged latencies of wave V, two of them had bilateral changes and the remaining four had a unilateral latency shift of wave V. The interpeak latency difference (ILD) I-V was abnormal in all cases with unilateral or bilateral abnormalities. Three subjects with OSA had a normal latency of wave V and normal ILD I-V. Seven patients had bilateral prolonged latencies of wave V with an increased ILD I-V except for one ear. One patient had a unilateral wave V shift, but with normal ILD I-V. The mixed group showed the same variations as the patients with OSA. Three patients had bilateral wave V abnormalities and two had unilateral changes. All of these had normal ILD I-V. Only one patient had normal latencies for wave V (the Figure).

DISCUSSION

The findings in this study support the assumption that a CNS component plays some role in CSA. A majority of patients with OSA and MSA also had abnormal tracings. It is unlikely that the mixed or obstructive patients have sleep apnea without a central component. The CNS control of pharyngeal musculature may be the important link between CSA and some patients in the other two groups. The underlying cause of the abnormality (ie, biochemical, histopathological, etc) is not known at this time.

Nodar et al[3] reported BSEP findings in six children at risk for sudden infant death syndrome (SIDS). The etiology of SIDS may be due to a breakdown in the central control of the breathing process. In this series, every BSEP was abnormal but no specific configuration could be delineated.

In 1981, Mosko et al[4] used BSEP to study five adults and one child with OSA. All were normal. Oxygen desaturation effect on brainstem neurons had neither an acute nor chronic effect as noted by the BSEP results.

In this series, all patients with CSA had prolonged absolute latencies of wave V. This differs from aforementioned studies in that the abnormality is specific. Seventy-six percent of patients with OSA and MSA had abnormal patterns, but the abnormalities were varied.

Multiple theories have been proposed to explain the underlying cause of ASA. The constant finding of increased latencies of wave V in CSA suggests a CNS role in the etiology. The fact that a single BSEP abnormality does not exist in MSA and OSA may indicate that there is more than one pathophysiologic mechanism involved in these groups.

ACKNOWLEDGMENT — The authors would like to thank Morris Z. Effron, MD, for his editorial assistance in the preparation of this manuscript.

REFERENCES

1. Guilleninault C, Tolkian A, Dement WC. The sleep apnea syndromes. Am Rev Med 1976; 27:465-84.

2. Møller AR, Janetta P, Møller, MB. Intracranially recorded auditory nerve response in man. Arch Otolaryngol 1982; 108: 77-82.

3. Nodar R, Lonsdale D, Orloski J. Abnormal brain stem potentials in infants with threatened sudden infant death syndrome. Otolaryngol Head Neck Surg 1980; 88:619-21.

4. Mosko SS, Pierce S, Holowach J, Sassin J. Normal brain stem auditory evoked potentials recorded in sleep apneics during waking as a function of arterial oxygen saturation during sleep. Electroencephalogr Clin Neurophysiol 1981; 51:477-82.

Ann Otol Rhinol Laryngol 91:1982

USE OF FOLEY CATHETER FOR REMOVAL OF ESOPHAGEAL FOREIGN BODIES

A SURVEY

W. FREDERICK MCGUIRT, MD

WINSTON-SALEM, NORTH CAROLINA

A survey was conducted among otolaryngologists, thoracic surgeons, pediatric surgeons and pediatric radiologists to determine the frequency of removal of esophageal foreign bodies with a Foley catheter. The 245 physicians responding reported 1,512 cases, 96% of which were treated with this technique by radiologists and pediatric surgeons. Although no deaths or serious complications were reported, the author warns that increasing use of this procedure by nonendoscopists carries the risk of serious complications unless certain safeguards are taken. These include trained personnel, use of fluoroscopy, a cooperative patient with a single, smooth, radiopaque foreign body lodged in the esophagus and a barium esophagogram with negative results for total obstruction and underlying esophageal disease.

INTRODUCTION

In 1966, Bilger[1] reported the removal of esophageal foreign bodies by use of a Foley catheter. Since that initial report, numerous articles have appeared[2-5] in the radiological, general surgical and pediatric literature endorsing the procedure. Few articles have been written by thoracic surgeons and bronchoesophagologists; those that have appeared have tended not to favor Foley catheter removal of esophageal foreign bodies.[6] Thus, the main advocates of the procedure are specialists who have not had specific training in the care of patients with foreign bodies in the upper aerodigestive tract. The lack of supportive articles by thoracic surgeons and bronchoesophagologists may imply an unfavorable attitude toward the technique and a preference for continued use of classical methods of extraction.

In an effort to obtain better documentation of the procedure and its results, the author sent a questionnaire to the directors of approved residency programs in otolaryngology and thoracic surgery and to members of the Society for Pediatric Radiology. Recipients were asked if they and other physicians in their departments used a Foley catheter for removal of esophageal foreign bodies and, if so, to describe the technique used and the number of cases treated. Information was also obtained on complications and indications and contraindications for the procedure. This report discusses the results of the survey.

RESULTS

Of the 540 questionnaires distributed, 245 were returned. A total of 1,512 cases were reported. As can be seen in Table 1, although radiologists and pediatric surgeons completed half of the returned questionnaires, they reported 96.2% of the procedures; otolaryngologists and thoracic surgeons completed almost half of the questionnaires, but accounted for only 3.8% of the procedures performed.

Only five of the 84 otolaryngologists stated that they had ever used the technique; of those five, two reported they no longer used it. Six of the 35 thoracic surgeons stated that they used the technique. In contrast, 57 of the 109 pediatric radiologists (52.3%) who responded had used the technique, as had six of the 15 pediatric surgeons. Surprisingly, otolaryngologists in 11 large teaching institutions stated that the procedure was not done in their institutions, while radiologists from the same institutions reported a series of cases and enthusiastically endorsed the procedure.

A large majority of users performed the procedure in a fluoroscopy suite, although nine respondents used the technique in a blind manner in the office, the emergency room or an operating suite. Only eight of the nonendoscopists who responded used the technique with the assistance of someone skilled in endoscopy, conventional extraction techniques and airway management. Another ten respondents reported a physician other than the radiologist in attendance in the fluoroscopic suite during the procedure, but did not describe resuscitative or intubation equipment.

No deaths were reported by the respondents, and only 25 complications were listed, none of long duration. Complications included 19 nosebleeds, four coins dislodged into the nose, one case of hyperpyrexia and one case of laryngospasm. These minor complications may have been more prevalent

From the Section on Otolaryngology, Department of Surgery, Bowman Gray School of Medicine of Wake Forest University, Winston-Salem, North Carolina.

Presented at the meeting of the American Broncho-Esophagological Association, Palm Beach, Florida, May 3-4, 1982.

REPRINTS — W. Frederick McGuirt, MD, Section on Otolaryngology, 300 S Hawthorne Road, Winston-Salem, NC 27103.

TABLE 1. SUMMARY OF RESPONSES

Specialty	Questionnaires Returned No.	Questionnaires Returned %	Respondents Using Procedure No.	Respondents Using Procedure % of Specialty Group	Reported Cases No.	Reported Cases %
Radiology	109	44.5	57	52.3	1,226	81.1
Otolaryngology	84	34.3	5	6.0 }		
					58	3.8
Thoracic surgery	35	14.3	6	17.1 }		
Pediatric surgery*	15	6.1	6	40.0	228	15.1
Miscellaneous*	2	0.8	1	50.0		
Total	245†		75		1,512	

*Recipients in the first three categories were asked to pass the questionnaire on to a more appropriate physician if they did not feel qualified to answer the questions.

†Of 540 questionnaires sent 45.4% were returned.

than reported, since almost all were reported in the smaller series of cases; only one respondent with a series of more than 25 cases reported a complication.

Failure to remove the foreign body by this technique was mentioned by some of the respondents reporting small series. Most reporters of large series did not cite a failure rate. The author's conclusion was that probably no more than 15% of attempts were unsuccessful. In five cases failure to detect underlying strictures was reported because the extraction was performed without concomitant barium esophagography.

Descriptions of the technique varied, but the majority of respondents reported using fluoroscopy and a No. 12 to No. 16 Foley catheter through the anesthetized nose. Most performed the procedure with the patient positioned head-down and on the side and restrained if struggling. The importance of using a symmetrically inflated balloon catheter was mentioned by several respondents.

Indications for the Foley catheter technique ranged from "coins only," noted by the majority of respondents, to "any foreign body," reported by one respondent. In general, respondents preferred the technique for removal of any smooth, radiopaque object and avoided using it for removal of sharp, rough or irregularly shaped objects.

The acceptable interval between time of lodgment and treatment varied, ranging from not over 12 hours to "no restrictions." Most respondents, however, stated that an interval of 48 to 72 hours was the maximum within which the technique should be used. Most respondents using the procedure did not recommend it for patients having known preexisting local disease or lesions identified by a barium esophagogram.

DISCUSSION

These data indicate that removal of esophageal foreign bodies with a Foley catheter has proved to be an uncomplicated and effective method. However, the procedure is being done by persons not trained in other methods of foreign-body extraction or airway maintenance, whereas persons who have the capability to perform all methods continue to prefer endoscopic removal.

The argument for the latter procedure is that it does not put the airway at risk. Compromise of the airway was not a reported complication but the possibility remains that obstruction can occur. The fact that physicians may perform it repeatedly without major complications does not make removal with a Foley catheter the safer procedure. While deaths have occurred relative to endoscopic esophageal foreign body removal, they are exceedingly rare and generally have been due to preexisting airway compromise and erosive esophagitis secondary to the foreign body and not to the procedure itself. Endoscopic removal is the method of choice by physicians capable of using all methods of extraction.

Those who argue against the use of a Foley catheter maintain that an underlying or associated disease may be missed; a second, unidentified foreign body may be left behind; blind manipulation of a rough foreign body or of a second, unsuspected foreign body may perforate the esophagus; radiation exposure may be prolonged if the procedure is done under fluoroscopic control; emotional trauma may be experienced by a patient, particularly a child, who has to be restrained forcibly; and that manipulation of the foreign body in the nonanesthetized esophagus may be painful.

Those who advocate the procedure maintain that it is cost-effective in that no admission and no operating room charges are incurred; it is less emotionally traumatic since no general anesthetic is required; and it can be performed in outlying areas not having adequate anesthesia and endoscopic facilities.

Based on the data it would seem that removal of an esophageal foreign body with a Foley catheter is a procedure that, while technically feasible and apparently safe, should be reserved for specific cases and used only when strict safety precautions are

TABLE 2. PREREQUISITES FOR FOLEY CATHETER EXTRACTION OF ESOPHAGEAL FOREIGN BODY

Cooperative patient
Smooth, inert, radiopaque foreign body
Duration of lodgment less than 48 to 72 hours
Barium esophagogram yielding negative results for total obstruction, multiple foreign bodies and underlying esophageal disease
Fluoroscopy available
Endoscopist standing by

followed (Table 2). In the patient with airway compromise the method is definitely contraindicated, as it is in the patient with total esophageal obstruction shown by preliminary barium esophagogram, and in the struggling, restrained, frightened child. Cooperation is needed from the patient with a foreign body in the pharynx if he or she is not to aspirate or reswallow the object as it is being removed. Even the patient who is willing to cooperate but who has a strong gag reflex may not be able to prevent aspiration or reswallowing.

The emotional trauma experienced by an uncooperative patient who must be restrained may be far greater than that which may occur during general anesthesia and endoscopic removal.

If the procedure is done, it should be performed under fluoroscopy and restricted to smooth, inert, radiopaque objects that have no risk of perforating the esophagus and can be watched as they are extracted (Table 2). If the object is inert, a time limitation of 48 to 72 hours seems reasonable. A barium esophagogram should always be done before removal is attempted to investigate the possibility of underlying disease, complete esophageal obstruction or a second, nonradiopaque foreign body.

During the procedure, the patient should be placed in a head-down, lateral position to minimize aspiration. In the fluoroscopy suite (or surgical suite with fluoroscopy) where the procedure is done, airway maintenance equipment, endoscopic grasping instruments and endoscopes must be available as well as trained personnel. If attempts to remove the foreign body with a Foley catheter are unsuccessful, the procedure should not be continued.

Because of the discrepancy in reports of otolaryngologists and radiologists from the same institutions, it is advised that endoscopists consult with their local radiology colleagues to see if Foley catheters are being used to remove esophageal foreign bodies. If so, the endoscopist should help establish strict criteria for use of the procedure and offer assistance when it is performed. Or, if an endoscopist has strong negative feelings about the procedure, the arguments must be made known to colleagues in the emergency department and in the community where he or she practices. Specific criticisms and suggestions must be made by the endoscopist since an increasing number of radiologists, emergency-medicine physicians and medical practitioners are using this technique for removing foreign bodies from the esophagus. If contraindications are not emphasized and complications not reported, the procedure may continue to be accepted and performed by an increasing number of physicians not specifically trained in airway management.

REFERENCES

1. Bilger FC. The use of a Foley catheter for removal of blunt foreign bodies from the esophagus. J Thorac Cardiovasc Surg 1966; 51:759-60.

2. Brown LP. Blind esophageal coin removal using a Foley catheter. Arch Surg 1968; 96:931-2.

3. Henry LM, Chamberlain JW. Removal of foreign bodies from esophagus and nose with the use of a Foley catheter. Surgery 1972; 71:918-21.

4. Chang JHT, Burrington JD. Removal of coins from the esophagus: nothing new under the sun. Pediatrics 1973; 51:313.

5. Davis RK. Management of infected foreign bodies in the esophagus in children. Mod Med 1980; 48:27-8.

6. Ritter F. Questionable methods of foreign body treatment. Ann Otol Rhinol Laryngol 1974; 83:729-33.

Ann Otol Rhinol Laryngol 91:1982

A SIMPLE ENDOSCOPIC INTUBATION TECHNIQUE IN ESOPHAGEAL OBSTRUCTION

ENJE TH. EDENS, MD JOS J. VAN OVERBEEK, MD

GRONINGEN, THE NETHERLANDS

Endoscopic intubation was effected in 42 cases of malignant esophageal stenosis during the period 1979-1981. The stenosis was dilated with the aid of thermoplastic probes passed through a rigid esophagoscope of sufficient length, whereupon a tube was introduced under endoscopic control and left in situ in the malignant stricture. This "rigid" technique is suitable for processes confined to the esophagus. Introduction of the tube requires adequate endoscopic skill and is not devoid of risk. Perforation, the gravest risk, occurred in two cases. Proximal tube migration was observed in five patients.

INTRODUCTION

Even before the turn of the century intubation was used in the treatment of malignant processes of the esophagus by Sir Charles Symonds,[1] who reported the first successful intubation in 1885. In his comprehensive textbook of laryngoesophagology the renowned London laryngologist Morell Mackenzie[2] also described an indwelling esophageal tube. Distal migration of this tube was prevented by means of sutures which were knotted via the nostrils around the ears or even to the moustaches. In France Guisez[3] developed a tube on the principle of the Pezzer catheter and in Germany Brünings and Albrecht[4] regularly treated patients with catheters of their own design. In the United States Mosher[5] and subsequently Holinger[6] designed an esophageal endoprosthesis. In 1924 the English surgeon Sir Henri Souttar[7] introduced a metal tube of silver alloy with a thin coating of gold. Its spiral shape was later modified by Amman and Collis.[8] In the course of the next 30 years, neither endoscopists nor surgeons took any interest in palliative intubation.

After 1954 it was felt that it might be better to pull a tube through a stenosis via a gastrostomy instead of pushing it through. The Mousseau-Barbin[9] and subsequently the Celestin[10] tubes were the first examples of this pull-through type.

Since 1970 the high incidence of immediate postoperative mortality revived the demand for a safe endoscopic technique.[11,12] Various endoprostheses designed and constructed in the course of the years are described in an excellent review by Earlam and Cunha-Melo[13] (Fig. 1).

Since Tytgat et al[12] published their description of an intubation technique with a flexible esophagoscope in 1976, we have become interested in this type of palliation, and have developed a similar technique using a rigid tube.

The construction of the Edens-Prins rigid insufflation esophagoscope (Fig. 2) has paved the way towards optimal localization of the tumor site.[14] In view of the risk of perforation we refrained from using the extension tubes developed in Haslinger's original design; instead, we have asked the instru-

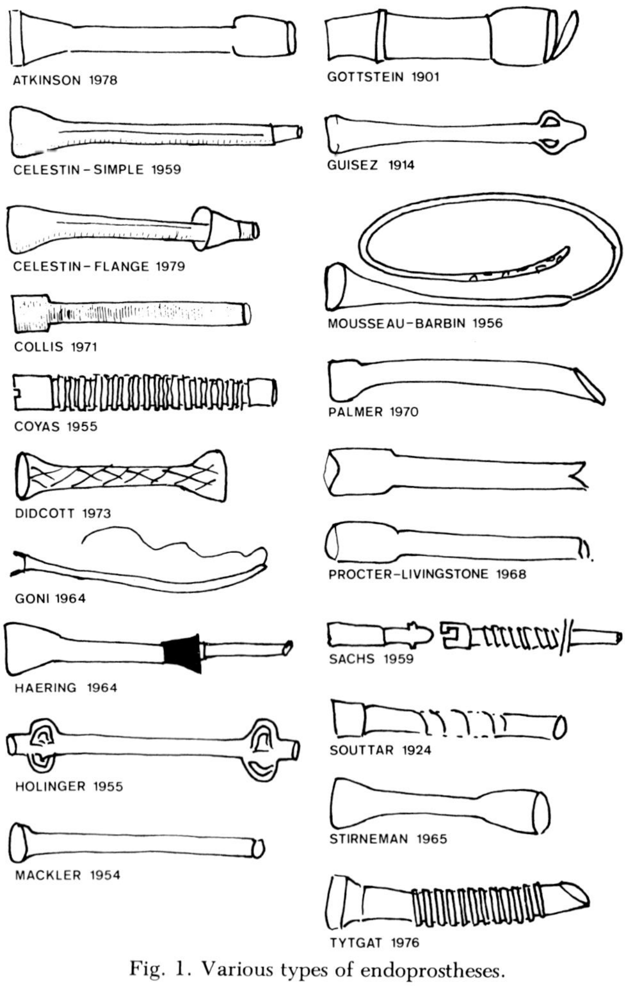

Fig. 1. Various types of endoprostheses.

From the Division of Endoscopy, ENT Department, University Hospital, Groningen, The Netherlands.

Presented at the meeting of the American Broncho-Esophagological Association, Palm Beach, Florida, May 3-4, 1982.

REPRINTS — E. Th. Edens, MD, Division of Endoscopy, ENT Department, University Hospital, PO Box 30.001, 9700 RB Groningen, The Netherlands.

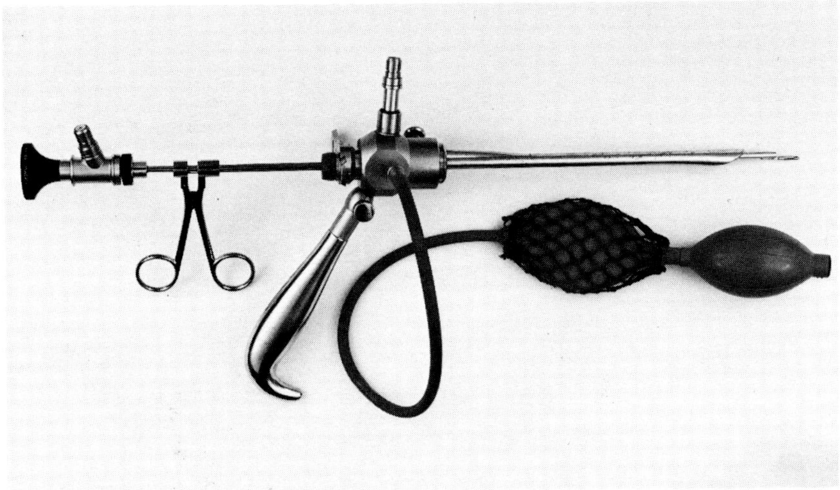

Fig. 2. Edens/Prins esophagoscope provided with optical forceps (Richard Wolf, Knittlingen, West Germany, and Medical Instruments Corp., Rosemont, Ill).

ment industry to provide tubes varying in length from 25- to 50-cm in 5-cm intervals. They enable the endoscopist to select the appropriate tube length on the basis of information obtained by barium swallow examinations. This rigid insufflation technique is not a necessary condition for successful therapeutic endoscopy, but it facilitates the search for the site of the stenosis.

TECHNIQUE

The procedure can be performed under local anesthesia, but we prefer general anesthesia. After tumor localization the esophageal lumen is dilated with the aid of thermoplastic bougies (Rüschelit esophageal bougie, Willy Rüsch Co, Rommelshausen [Stuttgart], West Germany, and Rusch Inc, New York, NY).

To ensure maximum flexibility, the most distal 5-cm length of these dilators is immersed in boiling water for at least five minutes.

Next, the stenosis is quickly dilated with the partially flaccid probes increasing in diameter from 10 to 34 French. Due to its maximum flexibility, the dilator tip seeks the path of least resistance. Rupture is usually avoided because dilation is effected very gradually.

The degree of dilation is determined by the external diameter of the tube. The maximum dilation effected with a flangeless Celestin tube (length, 18 cm; external diameter, 12 mm) is 34 French.

At the Groningen ENT Department we use several different tubes: Celestin-simple (Ambletin Ltd), Celestin-flange (Medoc Ltd) and Atkinson (Keymed), each of which is available in various diameters and lengths. We prefer the shortest Celestin tube without flange.

After dilation to a diameter slightly smaller than the external diameter of the tube to be introduced, a thin probe which fits snugly in the tube is left in situ in the stenotic part. The rigid endoscope (with the tumor distance marked) is removed, and the selected internally siliconized tube is slipped over the probe in situ and manually pushed as far distally as possible. An assistant is asked to keep the dilator fixed in position. The previously removed esophagoscope is reintroduced immediately alongside the probe in order to push the upper edge of the tube through the cricopharyngeal muscle into the esophagus. Exerting a little pressure, the endoscopist can leave the tube in situ in the stenosis (Fig. 3). After verification of the distance between maxilla and tumor, the dilator can be removed. Reflux of gastric juice is often visible when the lower rim of the tube lies in the stomach.

It is advisable to verify the intactness of the mucosa at the lower rim of the tube with the aid of a flexible endoscope of suitable size (Olympus BF-B3 or Gif P3). The rigid esophagoscope can then be removed. Immediately after this procedure an antiemetic, 10 mg (one ampoule) of metoclopramide (Primperan), is given intramuscularly and is repeated three times daily for three days. Chest x-ray films, anteroposterior and lateral, are made to control the position and to exclude perforation.

The first liquid food can be given six hours after the operation. One day later a barium swallow examination is done to verify the exact position and patency of the tube. When the end of the endoprosthesis lies in the stomach, the patient should be advised to assume a sitting position in order to prevent reflux.

RESULTS

Endoscopic intubation was requested for 45 patients during the period 1979-1981. In three cases the attempt was unsuccessful due to distal tumor localization. A carcinoma of the cardia region with extension to the stomach is not suitable for the technique described above. The Tytgat technique is indicated in such cases. Endoscopic intubation was successfully effected in 42 cases.

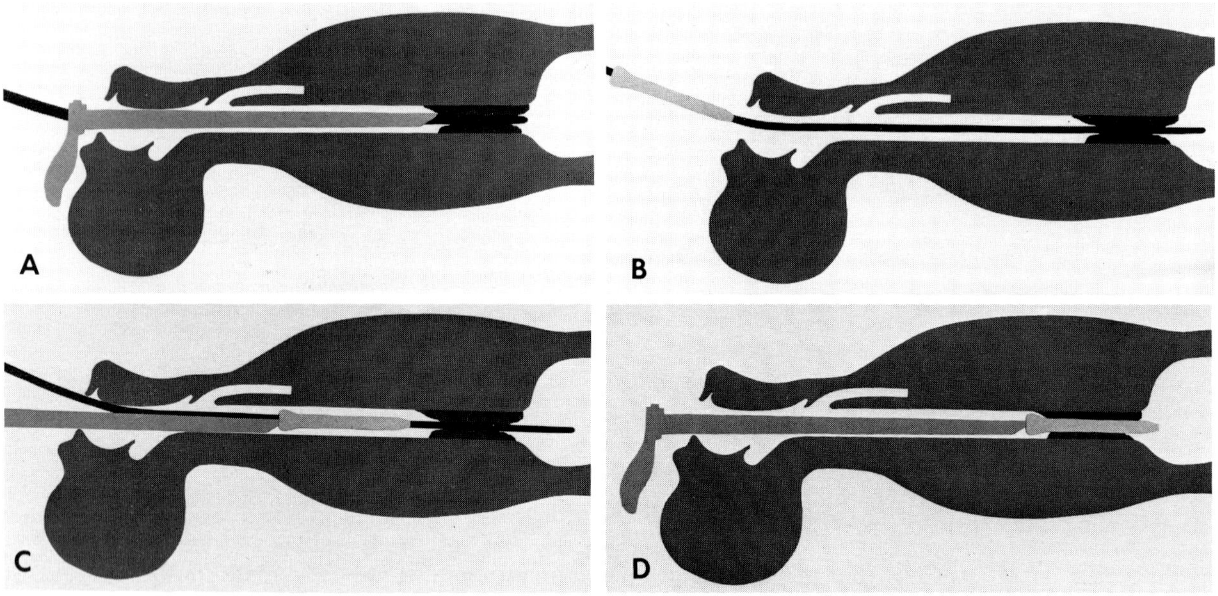

Fig. 3. Four important stages in endoscopic intubation. A) Tumor dilation till 34 French thermoplastic bougie. B) Endoprosthesis slipped over a thin 21 French probe. C) Esophagoscope placed immediately alongside probe to push down upper edge of endoprosthesis. D) Endoprosthesis in place after removal of 21 French bougie.

In two patients with an esophagobronchial fistula the coughing ceased immediately. Perforation due to rupture occurred in two cases. This complication was successfully treated conservatively by suction drainage of saliva, antibiotic medication and parenteral feeding. One patient died due to aspiration pneumonia. Tube migration occurred in five cases. Migration of the endoprosthesis can be prevented by using a flanged tube. The flange, however, makes introduction much more difficult due to the local increase in external diameter. The mean survival measured from time of intubation to death was 62 days.

CONCLUSIONS

When the passage of food is impeded by malignant processes in the esophagus or mediastinum, adequate palliation can be effected by endoscopic intubation. In the hands of experienced endoscopists, the procedure has complications which are acceptable. A careful follow-up is required for timely identification of problems of pain control, tumor overgrowth or pressure necroses. Thus monitored, the patient can look forward with confidence to an unmistakably improved quality of life.

ACKNOWLEDGMENT — We are indebted to Mr. A. de Jong and Mr. H. Leever, technicians, and Mr. M. Goslinga, photographer, for their valuable advice.

REFERENCES

1. Symonds CJ. A case of malignant stricture of the esophagus illustrating the use of the new form of oesophageal catheter. Trans Chir Soc Lond 1885; 18:155-8.

2. Mackenzie M. Die Krankheiten des Halses und die Nase. Berlin: Verlag August Hirschwald, 1884:35-6.

3. Guisez J. De l'intubation caoutchoutée oesophagienne. Presse Méd 1914; 22:85-7.

4. Brünings W, Albrecht W. Direkte Endoskopie der Luft- und Speisewege. Stuttgart: Verlag Ferdinand Enke, 1915:253.

5. Mosher HP. Some observations on esophageal cases and the presentation of two new instruments. Laryngoscope 1909; 19: 401.

6. Holinger PH. Self retaining esophageal intubation tube. Ann Otol Rhinol Laryngol 1955; 64:921.

7. Souttar HS. Method of intubating the oesophagus for malignant stricture. Br Med J 1924; 1:782-3.

8. Amman JR, Collis JL. Palliative intubation of the oesophagus: analysis of 59 cases. J Thoracic Cardiovasc Surg 1971; 61:863-9.

9. Mousseau M, le Forestier J, Barbin J, et al. Place de l'intubation à demeure dans le traitment palliative du cancer de l'oesophage. Arch Mal Appar Digest 1956; 45:208-16.

10. Etienne J, Celestin LR. La prothèse oesophagienne: passé et présent. Acta Endoscopica 1979; 9:235-43.

11. Atkinson M, Ferguson R. Fiberoptic endoscopic palliative intubation in inoperable oesophagogastric neoplasms. Br Med J 1977; 1:266-7.

12. Tytgat GN, de Hartog Jager FCA, Haverkamp HJ. Positioning of a plastic prosthesis under fiberendoscopic control in the palliative treatment of cardio-esophageal cancer. Endoscopy 1976; 8:180-5.

13. Earlam R, Cunha-Melo JR. Malignant oesophageal strictures: a review of techniques for palliative intubation. Br J Surg 1982; 69:61-8.

14. Edens ET. Insufflation esophagoscopy. Ann Otol Rhinol Laryngol 1978; 87:551-3.

INCENDIARY CHARACTERISTICS OF ENDOTRACHEAL TUBES WITH THE CARBON DIOXIDE LASER

SUPPLEMENTAL REPORT

C. THOMAS YARINGTON, JR, MD
GALE E. THOMPSON, MD
SEATTLE, WASHINGTON

In a previous report[1] we provided the results of experimental studies utilizing American Hospital, Portex, polyvinyl chloride and red rubber tracheal tubes in conjunction with a Cavitron carbon dioxide laser, indicating the levels of combustion with regard to time and watts for each tube. Subsequent to the publication of this report, a Silastic endotracheal tube which purports to have a threshold of combustion of approximately 700° or higher was brought to our attention by the Medical Engineering Corporation.

In reduplicating the experimental studies accomplished with the other tubes, we were unable to achieve combustion in this tube at the maximum power and time settings for our Cavitron laser in an environment of 20% oxygen. Using 5-s bursts of continuous application of the laser at the highest power setting achieved only a mild excoriation of the tube, without any evidence of combustion.

As a result of these studies, it would appear that the Silastic tube might offer a reasonably safe route for anesthesia when using the carbon dioxide laser and oxygen levels of approximately 20%.

REFERENCES

1. Treyve E, Yarington CT Jr, Thompson GE. The incendiary characteristics of endotracheal tubes with the carbon dioxide laser: an experimental study. Ann Otol Rhinol Laryngol 1981; 4:328-30.

Presented at the meeting of the American Broncho-Esophagological Association, Palm Beach, Florida, May 3-4, 1982.
REPRINTS — C. Thomas Yarington, Jr, MD, Mason Clinic, 1118 Ninth Avenue, Seattle, WA 98101.

Ann Otol Rhinol Laryngol 91:1982

HEAT SINK PROTECTION AGAINST LASERING ENDOTRACHEAL CUFFS

FRANCIS E. LEJEUNE, JR, MD, FACS
FRANCIS LETARD, MD, DABA
CHARLES GUICE, MD
HARVEY MARICE, MD

NEW ORLEANS, LOUISIANA

The ignition of an endotracheal cuff by CO_2 laser impaction has proved troublesome in several ignition sequences. Metal foil tape wrapped around the shaft of the tube will provide adequate protection for it, but the tape does not extend to the thin-walled cuff. When normal saline solution is used instead of air to fill the cuff, heat is rapidly conducted away from the wall and the cuff is prevented from reaching its kindling temperature. If penetration should occur, a fine jet of saline solution instantaneously sprays the field, extinguishing any early combustion. The reaction time of the surgeon or an assistant is not a factor in prevention of thermal injury, no new equipment is required and preparation time is minimal.

INTRODUCTION

As experience with the use of the CO_2 laser accumulates, a greater awareness of the hazards and their correction has followed.

Accidental ignition of the shaft of the endotracheal tube has been eliminated largely by wrapping the tube with self-adhering metal foil. This wrap is started immediately proximal to the thin-walled cuff and is continued in a spiral fashion toward the proximal end of the tube, usually stopping several centimeters short of the end. Flexion of the shaft of the tube may be done without exposing the combustible wall to a possible CO_2 laser strike because the overlapping spirals of tape tend to afford double-layered protection similar to the overlapping of shingles on a roof.

The inflatable cuff on the distal end of the shaft cannot be wrapped because of its need to expand. Should the cuffed portion of the tube migrate from the deeper portion of the trachea to the subglottic region, it approaches the range of the CO_2 laser beam. Moist cotton pads with or without flammable nylon tethers may become dry or drift aside, providing little protection from an errant laser beam. High oxygen concentrations of up to 99% are conducive to vigorous combustion. Should the laser beam or a fragment of carbonized tissue contact the thin-walled, air-filled cuff, immediate ignition could occur. Extubation of the patient within one second would probably avoid thermal injury to the subglottic and/or tracheobronchial areas, but a delay of two or more seconds could result in serious injury.

To avoid accidental ignition of the cuff, several factors are recognized. Silicone rubber has an ignition temperature of over 315°C while polyvinyl chloride plastic ignites at less than 149°C. Selection of a silicone cuff and tube will thus reduce combustibility. Latex rubber has an ignition temperature intermediate between silicone and polyvinyl chloride; therefore a red rubber endotracheal tube with a latex cuff is intermediate in combustibility.

Filling the cuff with an aqueous solution instead of air immediately reduces the combustibility of all three materials. The heat sink, or sump, is the heat-collecting property of the water which enables it to rapidly absorb and conduct localized heat away from the area of laser beam impact. The cuff wall does not reach ignition temperature and no combustion results. If, however, repeated pulses of the laser beam strike the cuff or if the beam is strong or continuous, the cuff wall will melt or become punctured. Instantly, a fine jet of solution will automatically spray the subglottic area, cooling and extinguishing any early combustion (Figs. 1 and 2). Normal saline solution is used rather than water in case any fluid finds its way into the alveoli of the lungs.

Filling the cuff with normal saline solution requires approximately five seconds more than filling it with air because of the increase in viscosity of the water. Approximately two minutes is required to prepare the cuff for intubation. Evacuation of air from the cuff is accomplished by filling and emptying the cuff with saline solution while digitally manipulating the air bubble to the orifice of the filling catheter inside the cuff as it is emptied. With some practice, this becomes a simple task and creates a built-in, automatic sprinkler system.

Special awareness of the flammability of small pediatric tubes which lack a cuff should be main-

From the Ochsner Medical Institutions, New Orleans.
Presented at the meeting of the American Broncho-Esophagological Association, Palm Beach, Florida, May 3-4, 1982.
REPRINTS — Francis E. LeJeune, MD, Ochsner Clinic, 1514 Jefferson Highway, New Orleans, LA 70121.

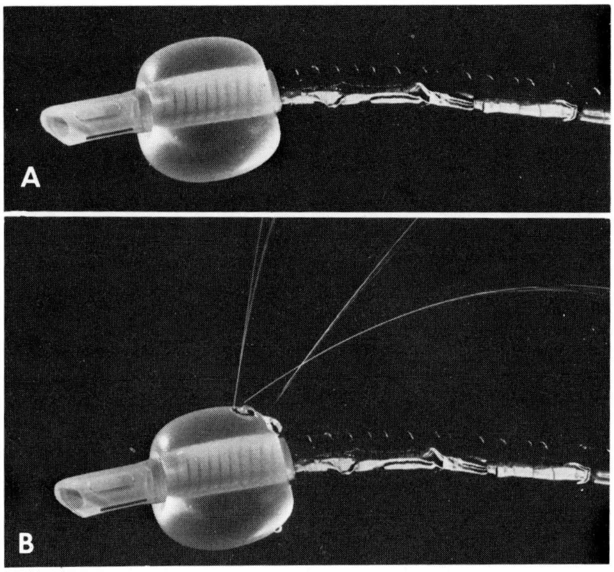

Fig. 1. A) Silicone rubber endotracheal tube with adhesive-backed aluminum tape wrapped around shaft and cuff filled with normal saline solution. B) After impact by two pulses of CO_2 laser beam, streams of saline solution spray environment of cuff.

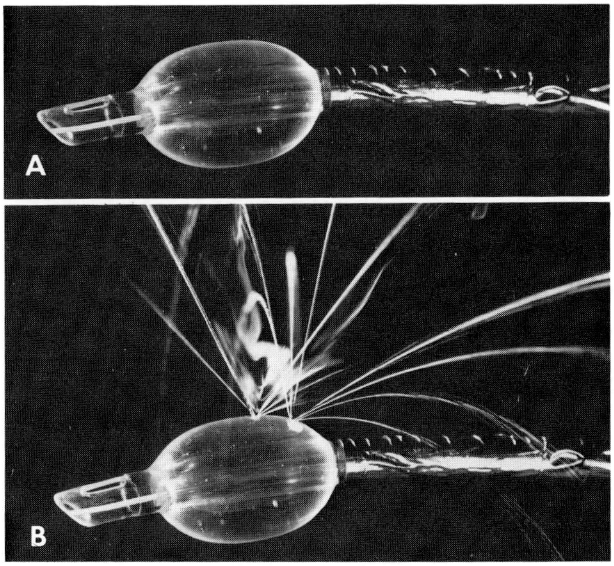

Fig. 2. A) Endotracheal tube and cuff constructed of polyvinyl chloride. Cuff is completely filled with normal saline solution; contains no air bubbles. Shaft is protected by metal tape. B) Moments after impact by two pulses of CO_2 laser, plume of smoke rises from cuff as streams of saline arch away from impact sites, creating automatic sprinkler system effect, extinguishing any early combustion.

tained. If a small tube is selected because of the reduced size of the glottic chink, remember that it is also shorter as well and that the unprotected beveled distal tip could be lying immediately beneath the cords where it is vulnerable to laser impact. Selection of a silicone rubber tube and the use of a pull cord for rapid extubation will help. Tracheotomy tape moistened and passed around the tube between the tip of the tongue and the lower central incisor teeth performs well as an emergency pull cord and can be held by the operator's left hand as the final stage of papilloma removal by laser is made. Extubation is readily accomplished in less than one second.

DISCUSSION

Studies on ignition potential of some of the commonly used endotracheal tubes have yielded varying results. Treyve et al[1] reported that polyvinyl chloride was less flammable, but Meyers,[2] Patel and Hicks[3] and Norton et al[4] described red rubber as less flammable. Wainwright and associates[5] believe that all rubber plastic materials burn in 100% oxygen and recognize the need for a nonflammable plastic tube which they hope to have available soon.

The cuff rather than the shaft of the tube seems to have been the kindling site of a certain number of endotracheal fires[6,7] as well as two of our own.[8] The prompt replacement of the deflated cuff tube with a tube having an intact cuff is supported by several authors.[2,7]

A desirable feature of a silicone rubber tube is that when there is continuous impact by a laser beam of 20W or more, an expanded ash forms which serves as a heat shield or insulator. Exposure of greater than one minute may be needed to penetrate the unprotected shaft.

CONCLUSION

The CO_2 laser operator can minimize the risk of troublesome ignitions by selecting materials of low combustion potential, using saline solution in place of air in cuffed endotracheal tubes, and exercising vigilance in the quick extubation of ignited tubes.

REFERENCES

1. Treyve E, Yarington CT Jr, Thompson GE. Incendiary characteristics of endotracheal tubes with the carbon dioxide laser: an experimental study. Ann Otol Rhinol Laryngol 1981; 90:328-30.

2. Meyers A. Complications of CO_2 laser surgery of the larynx. Ann Otol Rhinol Laryngol 1981; 90:132-4.

3. Patel KF, Hicks JN. Prevention of fire hazards associated with use of carbon dioxide lasers. Anesth Analg 1981; 60:885-8.

4. Norton ML, Strong MS, Vaughn CW, Snow JC, Kripke J. Endotracheal intubation and Venturi (jet) ventilation for laser microsurgery of the larynx. Ann Otol Rhinol Laryngol 1976; 656-63.

5. Wainwright AC, Moody RA, Carruth JA. Anaesthetic safety with the carbon dioxide laser. Anaesthesia 1981; 36:411-4.

6. Cozine K, Rosenbaum LM, Askanazi J, Rosenbaum SH. Laser-induced endotracheal tube fire. Anesthesiology 1981; 55:583-5.

7. Vourch G, Tannieres M, Freche G. Ignition of a tracheal tube during laryngeal laser surgery, letter. Anaesthesia 1979; 34:685.

8. Burgess GE, LeJeune FE Jr. Endotracheal tube ignition during laser surgery and laryngoscopy. Arch Otolaryngol 1979; 105:561-2.

Ann Otol Rhinol Laryngol 91:1982

UNIVERSAL ENDOSCOPIC COUPLER FOR CARBON DIOXIDE LASER SURGERY

ROBERT H. OSSOFF, DMD, MD

MARC S. KARLAN, MD

CHICAGO, ILLINOIS

A new set of endoscopic couplers has been designed by the authors for laparoscopic, arthroscopic and bronchoscopic carbon dioxide laser surgery. Certain safety features have been incorporated into this design which heretofore have been unavailable. The bronchoscopic coupler was designed with a gimbeled, partially reflective germanium window to facilitate direct, coaxial vision with the laser beam. A "joy stick" has been incorporated into the design to allow the surgeon to manipulate the helium-neon-aiming laser within the lumen of the bronchoscope. Bronchoscopes as small as 4 mm in diameter and 30 to 40 cm in length have been used with this coupler.

The carbon dioxide (CO_2) laser was coupled to a ventilating bronchoscope in 1973 by Strong and his colleagues[1] in Boston and was first presented[2] to our specialty at the 1974 annual meeting of the American Broncho-Esophagological Association in Palm Beach, Florida. Andrews and Horowitz[3] reviewed their experience with bronchoscopic CO_2 laser surgery in 1980.

These reports represented a logical extension of the clinical application of the CO_2 laser. Specifically, use of the CO_2 laser coupled to a ventilating bronchoscope allows the surgeon to perform hands-off endoscopic surgery through the relatively long and narrow operative field of a ventilating bronchoscope. The advantages of precision, hemostasis, decreased postoperative edema and decreased scarring facilitate visualization and control over the final result of the operation.

A new set of endoscopic couplers has been designed by the authors for laparoscopic, arthroscopic and bronchoscopic CO_2 laser surgery. Certain safety features have been incorporated into this design which heretofore have been unavailable.

Most laparoscopic and arthroscopic procedures are performed by a double-puncture technique. Therefore, the endoscopic coupler was designed with a gimbeled total reflector mirror; visualization and instrumentation are performed through a second endoscope. In cases where a single puncture technique is mandatory, the laparoscope or arthroscope can be attached directly to the endoscopic coupler.

Bronchoscopic CO_2 laser surgery must be performed utilizing only one endoscope. Therefore, the bronchoscopic coupler was designed with a gimbeled, partially reflective germanium window to facilitate direct, coaxial vision (Fig. 1A). The helium-neon-aiming laser beam is transmitted down the bronchoscope; this feature allows the surgeon to visualize the precise area of tissue to be impacted. In the past, centering of the laser beam within the lumen of the bronchoscope took place prior to introduction of the bronchoscope into the patient's tracheobronchial tree. Because standard bronchoscopes are slightly flexible, slight bending of the bronchoscope after insertion into the patient could cause the laser beam to reflect off of its inside wall with subsequent loss of power and possible heating of the bronchoscope itself. The "joy stick" allows the surgeon to manipulate the helium-neon-aiming laser within the lumen of the bronchoscope. Therefore, the laser beam can be centered within

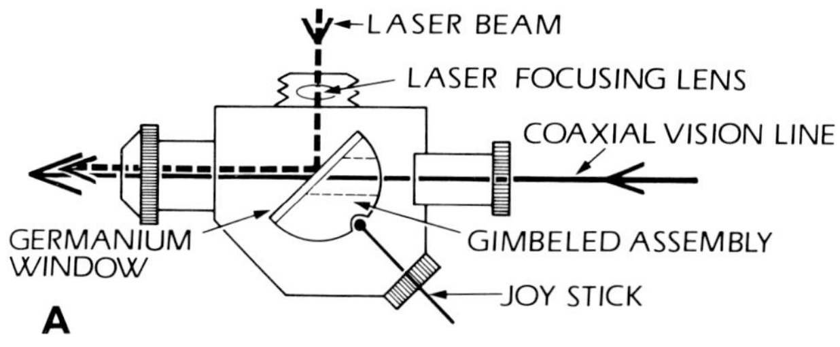

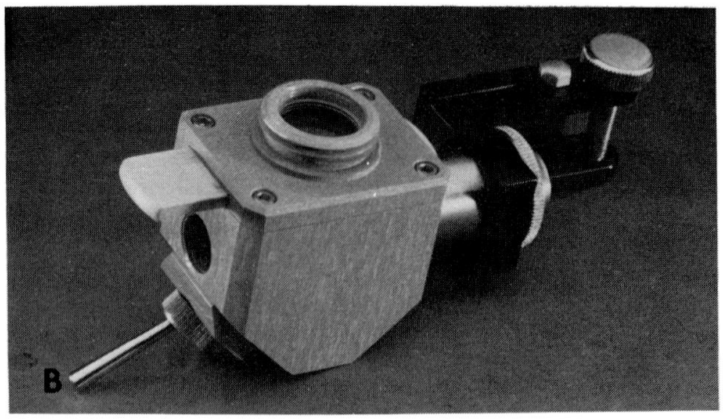

Fig. 1. A) Diagram of bronchoscopic coupler. B) Bronchoscopic coupler showing thumb screw attachment.

From the Department of Otolaryngology-Head and Neck Surgery, Northwestern University Medical School, and The Midwest Bio-Laser Institute, Chicago.

Presented at the meeting of the American Broncho-Esophagological Association, Palm Beach, Florida, May 3-4, 1982.

REPRINTS — Robert H. Ossoff, DMD, MD, Department of Otolaryngology and Maxillofacial Surgery, Northwestern University Medical School, 303 E. Chicago Avenue, Chicago, IL 60611.

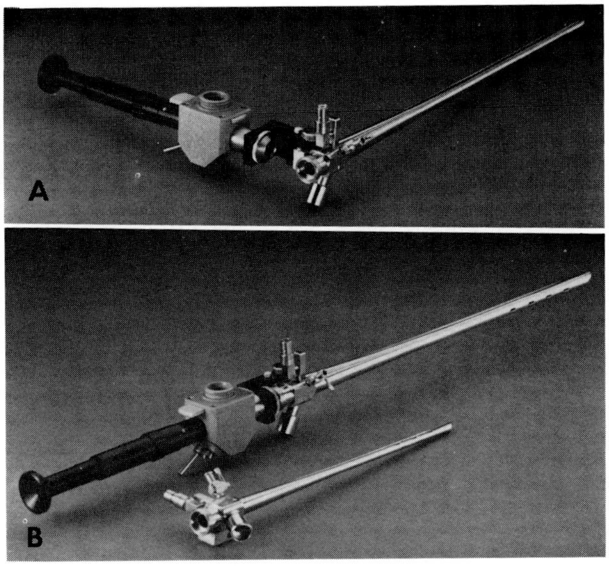

Fig. 2. A) Bronchoscope hinged on coupler by thumb screw. B) Bronchoscope (8 mm) attached to endoscopic coupler with 4-mm bronchoscope lying alongside.

the bronchoscope while in the patient's tracheobronchial tree. Additionally, the laser can be aimed to impact anywhere within the optical field of the bronchoscope should the clinical condition call for it.

The bronchoscope is attached to the endoscopic coupler by a thumb screw which passes through a mounting block on the side of the bronchoscope (Fig. 1B). The thumb screw acts as a hinge (Fig. 2A) to allow the coupler to swing away during insertion and instrumentation. An easy on/off adaptor has been designed to facilitate quick attachment and dislodgment of the bronchoscope to and from the coupler; the knurled thumb screw must be turned only 57° of the circle to accomplish this.

The endoscopic coupler itself weighs approximately 420 g; this allows the surgeon to easily grasp the coupler with attached bronchoscope in one hand.

Bronchoscopes as small as 4 mm in diameter and 30 to 40 cm in length have been used in conjunction with this coupler (Fig. 2B). Changes in the proximal end of existing bronchoscopes must be made to assure proper fit and coaxial alignment of the scope to the coupler. A new family of such bronchoscopes sized 4 mm through 10 mm with built-in distal steam evacuation ports will be the subject of a future report.

REFERENCES

1. Strong MS, Jako GJ, Polanyi T, Wallace RA. Laser surgery in the aerodigestive tract. Am J Surg 1973; 126:529-33.

2. Strong MS, Vaughan CW, Polanyi T, Wallace R. Bronchoscopic carbon dioxide laser surgery. Ann Otol Rhinol Laryngol 1974; 83:769-76.

3. Andrews AH, Horowitz SL. Bronchoscopic CO_2 laser surgery. Lasers in Surg Med 1980; 1:35-45.

Ann Otol Rhinol Laryngol 91:1982

ANESTHETIC GAS SCAVENGER FOR USE DURING OPEN RIGID BRONCHOSCOPY

DAVID J. STEWARD, MB, FRCP(C) BLAIR FEARON, MD, FRCS(C)

TORONTO, ONTARIO

A simple, effective method of scavenging waste anesthetic gases from an open-end bronchoscope by the use of a standard anesthesia t-piece is described.

Although closed-circuit anesthesia may be used for rigid bronchoscopy,[1] thus avoiding the dissemination of anesthetic gases into the atmosphere, it is sometimes essential to have the lumen of the bronchoscope open. At such times potent volatile agents escape from the proximal lumen of the bronchoscope and may be inhaled by the endoscopist. Such inhalation of modern, potent vapors may lead to impaired performance or even induce sleep.[2] On rare occasions repeated exposures may precipitate chronic diseases such as hepatic dysfunction.[3]

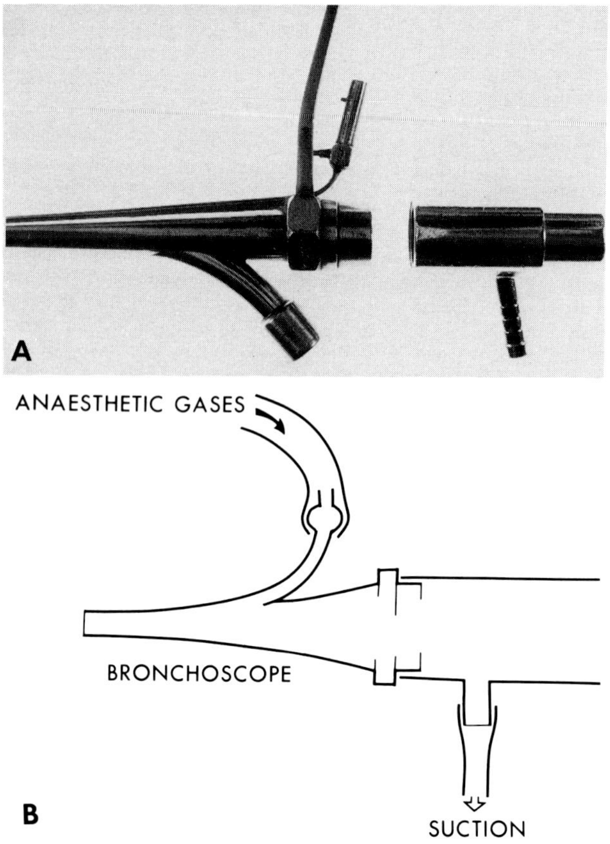

Fig. 1. A) Proximal end of Holinger bronchoscope with t-piece connector used to scavenge waste anesthetic gases. B) Bronchoscope with fresh anesthetic gases supplied as shown, and excess gases escaping from proximal lumen diverted into suction system.

Various methods have been used to protect the endoscopist and other operating room personnel from waste anesthetic gases. Masks provided with activated charcoal or a clean air supply may be worn. These methods are all cumbersome, however.

To prevent the escape of anesthetic vapors from the proximal end of the open bronchoscope we have devised a simple but effective scavenging technique which employs readily available standard equipment. A standard anesthesia t-piece connector (Medical & Industrial Equipment, Niagara Falls, Ontario) is attached to the proximal end of the appropriate Holinger bronchoscope (Fig. 1A). The side-arm of the t-piece is attached to the operating room suction systems. Anesthetic gases are supplied in the insufflation channel of the bronchoscope as usual, and excess gases escaping from the proximal lumen are diverted via the t-piece into the suction system (Fig. 1B). The anesthesia t-piece will fit a standard Holinger bronchoscope, is of similar internal diameter and does not obstruct the endoscopist's view.

In order to test the efficiency of this system we measured the concentration of nitrous oxide escaping from the proximal end of the bronchoscope after attaching the scavenging system (Fig. 2). Once suction is applied to the system there is no leak of anesthetic gases from the open end of the bronchoscope.

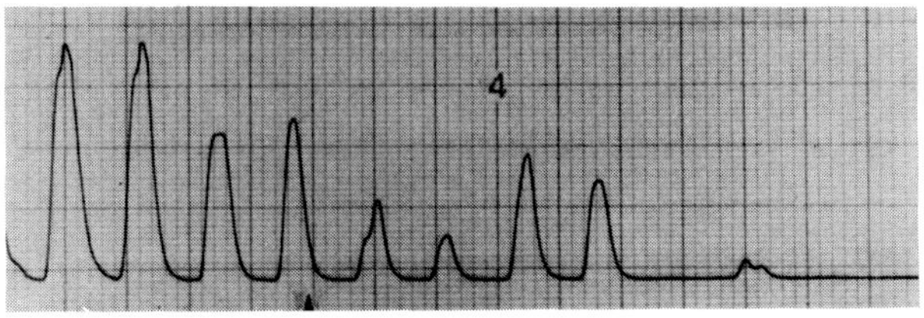

Fig. 2. Measurement of nitrous oxide escaping from proximal open end of bronchoscope, demonstrating effect of scavenging system. Suction is applied at arrow.

From the Departments of Anaesthesia and Otolaryngology of The Hospital for Sick Children and The University of Toronto.

Presented at the meeting of the American Broncho-Esophagological Association, Palm Beach, Florida, May 3-4, 1982.

REPRINTS — D. J. Steward, MB, FRCP(C), Department of Anaesthesia, The Hospital for Sick Children, 555 University Avenue, Toronto, Ontario, Canada M5G 1X8.

REFERENCES

1. Pelton DA, Conn AW. A bronchoscope adaptor for intermittent positive pressure breathing in children. Can Anaesth Soc J 1968; 15:628.

2. Bruce DL, Bach MJ. Effects of trace anesthetic gases on behavioural performance of volunteers. Br J Anesth 1976; 48: 871-6.

3. Klatskin G, Kimberg DV. Recurrent hepatitis attributable to halothane sensitization in an anesthetist. N Engl J Med 1969; 280:515-22.

≈

NINCDS NOTES*

NEW HEARING STUDY SECTION ESTABLISHED

The NIH Division of Research Grants is setting up a new Hearing Research Study Section for the peer review of applications in research and research training related to the structural and functional bases of ear disorders and the mechanisms of hearing. Fifteen authorities in the auditory system and hearing disorders, including otolaryngology, otology, psychoacoustics and bioengineering, will comprise the section. The new section originates from the former Communicative Sciences Study Section, which is now the Sensory Disorders and Language Study Section. Both sections review applications for several NIH institutes, but are primarily concerned with research of interest to NINCDS.

NINCDS REVISES EXTRAMURAL AND INTRAMURAL GUIDES

NINCDS has updated two booklets describing funding and training opportunities for basic and clinical research in neurological and communicative disorders. *NINCDS Extramural Research and Training Awards* lists NINCDS's research interests and explains how to apply for available grants, contracts and awards for research in the basic neurological and communicative sciences, stroke and nervous system trauma, neurological disorders and communicative disorders. *NINCDS Intramural Research Training Programs* briefly describes research at NINCDS branches, laboratories and special units in Bethesda, Maryland. Training opportunities exist for holders of PhD, MD and similar degrees as staff fellows. Qualified medical students can obtain training in genetics or medical/surgical neurology in the Clinical Elective Program. Foreign investigators may be eligible for a visiting fellow, associate, or scientist position. Copies of booklets are available without charge from the Office of Scientific and Health Reports, NINCDS, Building 31, Rm. 8A06, 9000 Rockville Pike, Bethesda, MD 20205.

----

*This information is prepared monthly by the Office of Scientific and Health Reports, National Institute of Neurological and Communicative Disorders and Stroke, National Institutes of Health, Building 31, Room A806, Bethesda, MD 20205; (301) 496-5751.

Ann Otol Rhinol Laryngol 91:1982

SCANNING ELECTRON MICROSCOPIC EXAMINATION OF NONBEATING CILIA

JAMES P. DUDLEY, MD

LANCE EISNER

JAMES D. CHERRY, MD

LOS ANGELES, CALIFORNIA

When cilia stop beating, their role in moving mucus ceases, but it is uncertain if nonmotile cilia preserve their external architecture and are thus capable of maintaining an additional role of retarding microbial access to the cell. Cilia of chicken embryo tracheal organ cultures were observed until their activity stopped. When examined with scanning electron microscopy, ciliary axonemes did not appear to differ significantly from normally functioning cilia when observed at lower magnifications. Since their density can remain essentially unchanged, nonbeating cilia may still have a role in protecting respiratory membrane from toxic microorganisms.

Cilia are cell organelles projecting from the surface of respiratory cells. Since normally functioning cilia have a beating pattern in which cilia shafts all move in the same direction, the tips of cilia act as an escalator for mucus and any bacteria or other foreign substances enmeshed in the mucus. This movement which they help to induce in the overlying mucus layer is probably the chief role which cilia have in respiratory membranes. We have demonstrated, however, that large portions of ciliated respiratory mucosa are not covered by mucus.[1] Cilia in those segments devoid of mucus may have an additional function of preventing access of microorganisms to the cell surface.[2] The density of 50 to 200 erect cilia per cell on healthy respiratory membrane must certainly act as an impediment to bacteria, mycoplasma and perhaps even viruses. On infected membrane we have demonstrated, however, that cilia do not maintain an erect position in relation to the surface of the cell.[3] The cilia shafts on these cells are bent in such a way that easy access to the cell surface may be provided to microorganisms. It has not been noted previously whether or not nonmotile cilia on uninfected membrane retain their density and external architecture, consequently providing a protective shield for respiratory cell membrane. Because ciliary activity in chicken embryo tracheal organ cultures does not continue unless the medium is changed frequently, cultures can be observed until no ciliary activity is noted. In order to determine whether alterations in the cilia occur, scanning electron microscopy (SEM) was used to examine nonmotile cilia.

MATERIALS AND METHODS

Tracheas were removed from 19- to 20-day-old chicken embryos, cut into ring sections 0.5 to 1 mm in thickness, and each ring placed in a 125- x 16-mm screw cap tube with 1 ml Eagles basal medium (BME) containing HEPES buffer and 1 mg/ml ampicillin trihydrate. Ciliary activity was observed daily using a lens with a magnification of ten and graded for vigor and extent of cilia distribution on the ring. Ten rings were used for each experiment, and the experiment was run in duplicate. In test cultures, the medium was not changed for the duration of the experiment. In cultures serving as controls, the medium was changed every four days, and 1 ml fresh medium was added. Representative rings were removed from test and control cultures every three days, fixed in 2% glutaraldehyde and processed for SEM by postfixing in 1% osmium tetroxide, rinsed with phosphate buffer (0.135 *M*, pH 7.4), dehydrated with the ethanol series, critical-point dried with liquid carbon dioxide and coated with palladium gold.

RESULTS

As noted previously by Cherry (unpublished observations), ciliary activity in control cultures was satisfactory even after 15 days of observation. On the 15th day ciliary activity was 82% and 67% in the control cultures in the first and second experiments, respectively (Table). In test cultures, ciliary activity dropped to 51% on the 9th and 12th days of observation in the first and second experiments, respectively. In some of these tracheal

COMPARISON OF CILIARY ACTIVITY IN CHICKEN EMBRYO TRACHEAL ORGAN CULTURES WITH MEDIUM CHANGE EVERY FOUR DAYS AND NO MEDIUM CHANGE

		Percent Ciliary Activity on Day					
Experiment	*Cultures*	*0*	*3*	*6*	*9*	*12*	*15*
1	Control (medium change)	94	93	90	78	82	82
	Test (no medium change)	86	89	89	71	51	50
2	Control (medium change)	87	87	80	73	70	67
	Test (no medium change)	87	75	76	51	47	38

From the Department of Surgery, Division of Head and Neck Surgery (Dudley), and the Department of Pediatrics, Division of Infectious Diseases (Cherry), UCLA School of Medicine, Los Angeles. This research was supported by grant CA 16042 from the Electron Microscopy Core Service of the UCLA Jonsson Comprehensive Cancer Center.

Presented at the meeting of the American Broncho-Esophagological Association, Palm Beach, Florida, May 3-4, 1982.

REPRINTS — James P. Dudley, MD, Division of Head and Neck Surgery, 62-158 CHS, UCLA Medical Center, Los Angeles, CA 90024.

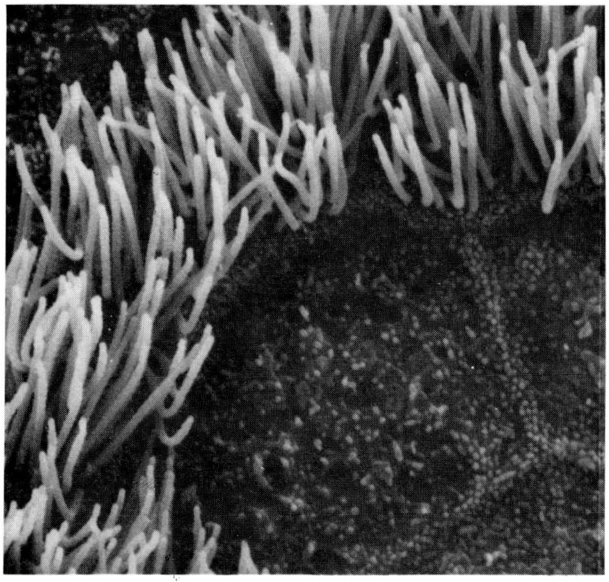

Fig. 1. Tracheal organ culture after three days of incubation. Most cilia shafts are erect. Tips of cilia are not bent. Adjacent epithelial cells without cilia are present. (x 8,000)

rings all ciliary activity had stopped. Those rings void of ciliary activity and other representative rings were processed for SEM.

As expected, cilia looked normal on the third day of incubation (Fig. 1). The shafts were upright, the tips were not bent and there did not appear to be any coalescence of cilia shafts. Cilia distribution also appeared normal (Fig. 2). Although some cells lacked cilia, there was a normal pattern of cilia. By the 15th day, cilia shafts had coalesced (Fig. 3). Although the coalescence was an alteration in the usual pattern of cilia, ciliary activity remained excellent in these cultures. Apparently, even when fused to a neighboring shaft, cilia were able to beat vigorously.

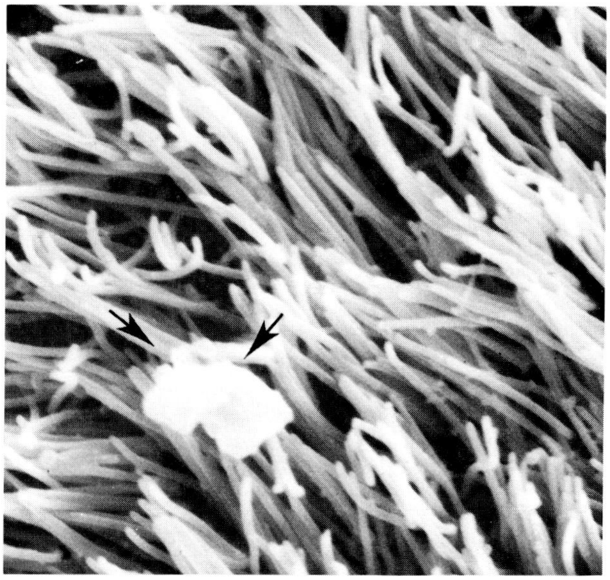

Fig. 3. Tracheal organ culture after 15 days of incubation with medium change every four days. Although some cilia shafts are fused, ciliary activity in this culture was almost normal. Piece of cellular debris is apparently being propelled across cilia tips (arrows). (x 8,000)

Nonmotile cilia shown in Figure 4 are from a 12-day-old tracheal culture in which no medium change occurred. Cilia were abundant, and except for a few nonciliated cells, there did not appear to be any gap or space between cilia shafts. Even though these cilia did not have visible movement, their appearance at a magnification of approximately 800 was not too dissimilar from cilia with normal movement. At higher magnification, however, cilia did not appear to be beating in the same direction (Fig. 5). Cilia having this appearance would not be capable of metachronal beating. This contrasted with normally beating cilia shown in Figure 6. These cilia all bend in the same direction

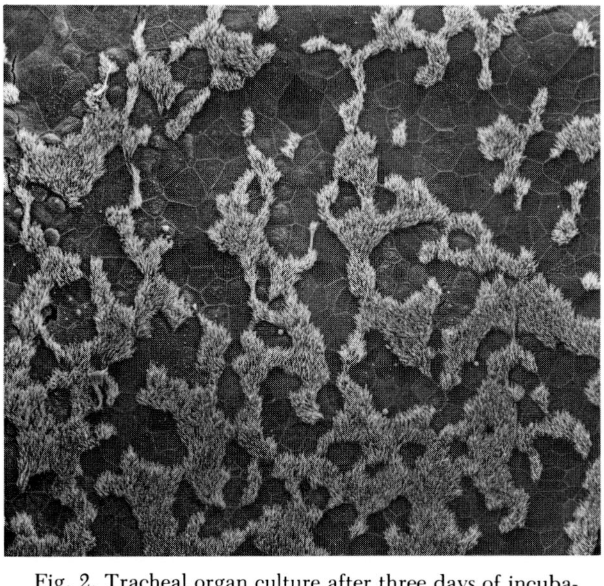

Fig. 2. Tracheal organ culture after three days of incubation. Some nonciliated respiratory cells are present. Large areas of cilia appear normal. (x 800)

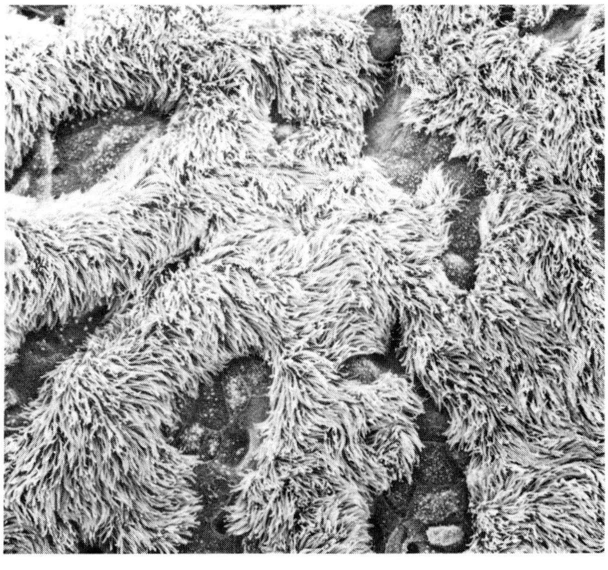

Fig. 4. Tracheal organ culture after 12 days of incubation with no medium change. Density of cilia appears normal with no gap bertween cilia shafts. (x 800)

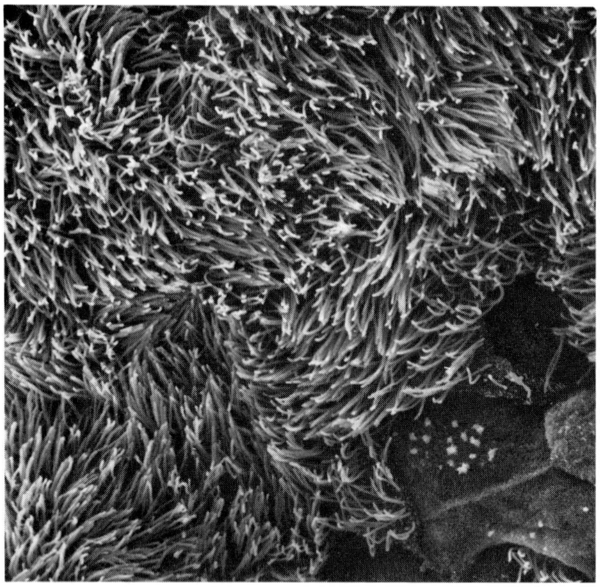

Fig. 5. Tracheal organ culture after 12 days of incubation with no medium change. Although cilia are present in normal numbers, they appear slightly irregular and are not beating in same direction. (x 2,000)

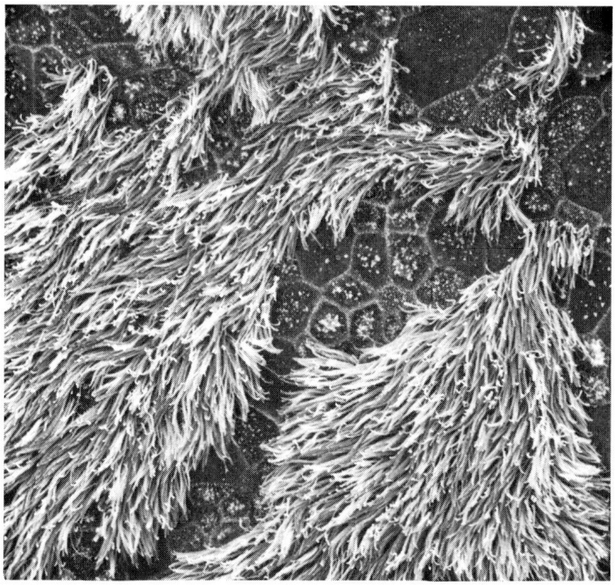

Fig. 6. Tracheal organ culture after 15 days of incubation with medium change every four days. These normally beating cilia have a regular appearance and are all inclined in one direction. Even after 15 days these cilia appear capable of metachronal beating. (x 1,200)

and are from a 15-day-old tracheal culture treated with medium change.

DISCUSSION

Although there is a disparity in the alignment of cilia shafts in tracheal cultures with beating and nonbeating cilia, their density remains similar. This barrier to the cell surface, which both beating and nonbeating cilia provide, may give cilia a second role in defending the host. A "Maginot Line" of dense organelles would appear to make it difficult for bacteria, mycoplasmas and perhaps viruses to reach the cell membrane. Since it is the contact microorganisms make with the cell surface which is toxic for that cell, retarding access to the cell may help to prevent cell death. Although the outer limiting membrane of a cilium is really an extension of the cell membrane, the toxicity produced by microbial proximity to these cell organelles may possibly be diluted. Since the role of microbial attachment is of importance in this toxicity, the effect of the presence of these cell organelles may be to prevent or to prolong the time required for microbial pathogens to produce disease. Although evidence of this is lacking in vivo, there is evidence that this occurs in vitro. In *Mycoplasma gallisepticum*-infected chicken embryo tracheal organ cultures, attachment to nonciliated surfaces occurs during the first day of incubation.[3] Adherence to ciliated cells, however, does not begin until the third or fourth day of incubation. The presence of cilia appears to be a reason for this delay. Since a mass of healthy, erect cilia occupy most of the space adjacent to the cell surface, adherence to ciliated respiratory cells is delayed until cilia become scrambled and lose their erect posture. This irregularity in cilia shafts is no doubt a toxic effect of microorganisms which become enmeshed in the tips of cilia. This "opening up" of the cell surface by the loss of ciliary regularity is probably an early step in microbial attachment to that surface.

Although cilia do not have a life independent of the cell from which they arise, there are some environmental influences responsible for loss of ciliary movement. Reduced temperatures can induce decreased ciliary movement and sometimes cilia stasis.[4] Alterations in pH apparently can do the same.[5] Since there are times when normal cilia do not beat and perform their primary function of propelling mucus, a secondary function as a protector of respiratory membrane may still be intact.

REFERENCES

1. Dudley JP, Cherry JD. Scanning electron microscopic demonstration of goblet cell discharge and mucous layer on nasal ciliated respiratory epithelium. Otolaryngol Head Neck Surg 1980; 88:439-41.

2. Dudley JP, Cherry JD. Cilia coalescence demonstrated by scanning electron microscopy in *Mycoplasma gallisepticum*-infected chicken embryo tracheal organ cultures: relation to pathogenesis of infection. Surg Forum 1980; 31:539-41.

3. Dudley JP, Cherry JD. Demonstration of adherence of *Mycoplasma gallisepticum* to chicken tracheal organ cultures using scanning electron microscopy. Read before the American Lung Association Annual Meeting, Las Vegas, May 15, 1979.

4. Rylander R. Current techniques to measure alterations in the ciliary activity of intact respiratory epithelium. Am Rev Respir Dis 1966; 93:67-85.

5. Sleigh MA. The biology of cilia and flagella. Oxford: Pergamon Press, 1962:96-8.

DYNAMICS OF VENTURI JET VENTILATION THROUGH THE OPERATING LARYNGOSCOPE

PEAK WOO, MD

STEPHEN EURENIUS, BS

BOSTON, MASSACHUSETTS

Venturi jet ventilation with the oxygen injector needle placed within the lumen of the laryngoscope was studied systematically in two dogs undergoing repeated general anesthesia suspension laryngoscopy. Using a total body plethysmograph, the effect of changes of needle angle, position and its effect on tidal volume delivery were measured. The changes of pressure regulator, flow rate and needle size were correlated with the volume delivery. Intratracheal pressure during Venturi ventilation was measured. Correlation of arterial blood gases and minute ventilation with the system was done. While ventilatory capacity is able to be achieved predictably, there are many variables. Optimal placement of the needle tip for maximum safety and efficiency appears to be at the midthird or lower third of the laryngoscope. It is important to center the needle axis to the laryngoscope axis. Other parameters subject to choice are the selection of needle size, regulator pressure setting and flow rate setting. By first selecting the correct needle size that will hyperinflate the subject, the pressure regulator can then be reduced to achieve ventilatory volumes similar to spontaneous tidal volumes. In prolonged use, the Venturi system was able to provide excellent ventilation safely and predictably.

INTRODUCTION

The advantages of ventilation during microlaryngoscopy with an oxygen injector system has been appreciated for a number of years. Several techniques have been described in the literature.[1-4] These techniques include placement of an oxygen-bearing catheter within the trachea, transtracheal stylet placement, high frequency positive pressure ventilation and Venturi jet ventilation.

Venturi jet ventilation with the oxygen injector needle placed within the lumen of the laryngoscope has been in use for several years.[4,5] The advantages during laser microlaryngoscopy are 1) the excellent unobstructed view of the larynx during surgery and 2) the absence of a potentially combustible endotracheal tube.

Because of the "open" nature of ventilation, accuracy of volume delivery to the patient during ventilation with the Venturi jet apparatus has been difficult. This has meant that accurate volume delivery to the patient has not been correlated with arterial blood gas values. The placement and position of the needle is believed to influence volume delivery but has not been tested. In man, the choice of needle size, the selection of oxygen driving pressure and oxygen flow rate has not been systematically studied. In the clinical situation, the anesthesiologist and otolaryngologist have been guided by empirical observation for adequacy of chest expansion and by random arterial blood gas determinations.[6,7] The method has not achieved wide popularity because of doubt concerning the adequacy of the ventilation provided and the fear of causing cervical and mediastinal emphysema. Recent investigators have developed lung models to test this system.[8] For the varying compliances and different lung volumes encountered in clinical work, criteria and limits for ventilation with the Venturi jet method must be established. This is necessary to provide for optimal ventilation and to minimize possible hazards.

The purpose of this study is to investigate the Venturi jet ventilation system in an animal model. In the animal model, we will determine the optimal needle size, needle tip position, gas pressure and gas flow rate needed to provide adequate ventilation. Long-volume delivery and arterial blood gases will be measured in the dog to assess various parameters subject to change during Venturi jet ventilation. These parameters are 1) needle size, 2) needle placement, 3) pressure regulator setting, and 4) oxygen flow rate selection. In addition, measurements will be made to assess 1) the pressure in the trachea during Venturi jet ventilation and 2) the prolonged effect of Venturi jet ventilation on blood gas and lung volume delivery.

MATERIALS AND METHODS

The conventional instrumentation consisting of a 7.5 cm, 14 or 16 gauge needle placed on a clamp attached to the wall of a large bore operating laryngoscope was used in this experiment. An intravenous (IV) connector tubing from the needle is connected to a toggle switch placed in line with an H tank of medically pure oxygen. A two-stage reducing valve with adjustable pound per square inch (PSI) and liters per minute (L/min) oxygen is placed to complete the circuit.

The manual toggle switch was modified by replacing the manual switch with a solenoid valve triggered by an adjustable timer circuit. The duty cycle is set to deliver one-second long bursts of gas injection. This was defined as the inspiratory cycle. The off-duty cycle is adjustable from 1 to 5 seconds and is defined as the expiratory cycle. Thus the timer allows us to adjust total cycles per minute in a repeatable manner from 10 to 30 respiratory cycles per minute.

From the Department of Otolaryngology, University Hospital, Boston University School of Medicine.

Presented at the meeting of the American Broncho-Esophagological Association, Palm Beach, Florida, May 3-4, 1982.

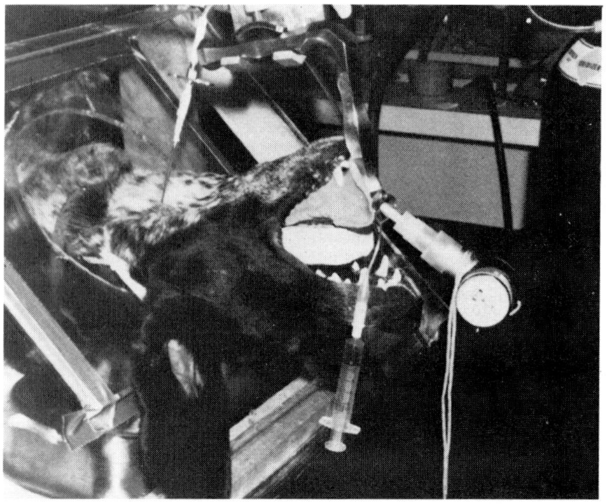

Fig. 1. Animal sealed in plethysmograph with suspension laryngoscopy instruments in place. Spontaneous ventilation measured via Wright's spirometer fitted on end of endotracheal tube.

Needle sizes 12G, 15G, 19G (spinal) were fitted onto an adult Jako-Pilling laryngoscope. The fixation to the laryngoscope allowed no moving parts.

A Wright spirometer was used to measure dog tidal volumes and minute ventilation in the spontaneously ventilating dog.

A total body plethysmograph was built and used to house the animal for the purpose of measuring volume delivery during Venturi jet ventilation.

Arterial blood gases were measured in the standard manner by arterial puncture or via an indwelling arterial catheter line. Two adult mongrel dogs were used repeatedly. Their weights were 12.3 and 16 kg. Anesthesia was obtained by giving 10 mg/kg of Nembutol IV. After anesthesia was obtained, the dog was placed into the plethysmograph. An IV and arterial (A)-line were started. The plethysmograph was then sealed. A 6-mm endotracheal tube was inserted. Spontaneous ventilation was maintained and the tidal volume and minute ventilation recorded (Fig. 1). Appropriate plethysmograph correction factors were calculated. A baseline blood gas was drawn.

The endotracheal tube was then withdrawn and the laryngoscope placed in position. The anterior tip of the laryngoscope was placed immediately above the level of the glottis. The laryngoscope was centered over the glottic aperture and was fixed in position by a Lewy holder. The Venturi jet apparatus was then placed in position.

Succinylcholine (Anectine, 20 mg) was given. After full paralysis, the Venturi jet system was activated and the experiment was initiated. An Anectine drip was used to insure full muscle paralysis (0.1 mg/kg/min). A Nembutol IV was given as needed to maintain anesthesia.

Upon completion of the experiment, the dogs were given physostigmine as needed to reverse the paralysis. When they could respond to pain stimuli and maintain spontaneous ventilation, they were returned to the animal shelter. Postoperative checks were done the next day. A maximum of two anesthesias per week were done to allow for adequate anesthetic recovery. The usual length of anesthesia was 6-8 hours.

RESULTS

Volume Delivery and Needle Placement along the Length of the Laryngoscope. Figure 2 summarizes the effect of placement of the Venturi jet needle along the length of the laryngoscope on delivery of tidal volume. The spontaneous preparalysis tidal

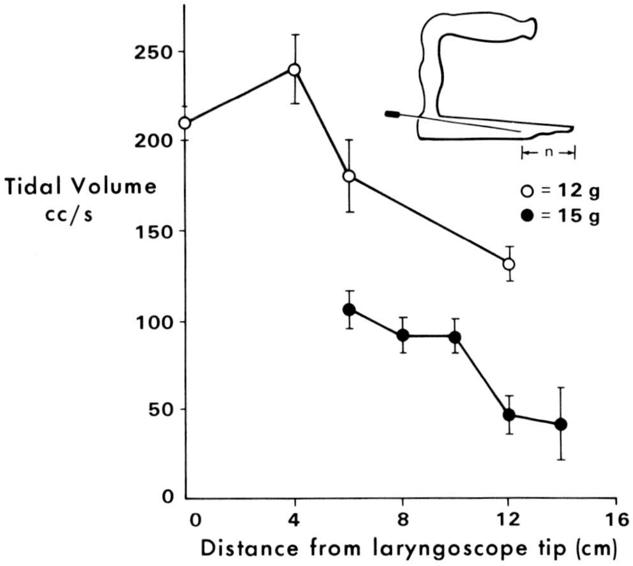

Fig. 2. Change of needle tip-to-glottis distance and its effect on tidal volume delivered to paralyzed dog (12.15 kg female) ventilated with Venturi jet apparatus at 40 PSI and 10L/min. n - Centimeters.

volume was 150 cc per cycle. The needle was centered between the vocal folds with all other parameters being equal. Regulator settings were 40 PSI and a flow rate meter reading set at 10 L/min. The figure represents graphically the fall-off of volume delivery as the needle is placed further from the vocal cords. The two graphs are for the nos. 12 and 15 gauge needles. From a strictly volume delivery capability point of view, the best volume delivery is achieved at or slightly above the level of the vocal fold. With the no. 12 needle, ventilatory volumes similar to spontaneous tidal volume can be achieved even with the needle placed further away from the vocal fold level. The no. 15 needle could not sustain volume delivery similar to spontaneous tidal volume when the needle is withdrawn further into the laryngoscope lumen. We did not measure volume delivery with the needle placed subglottically

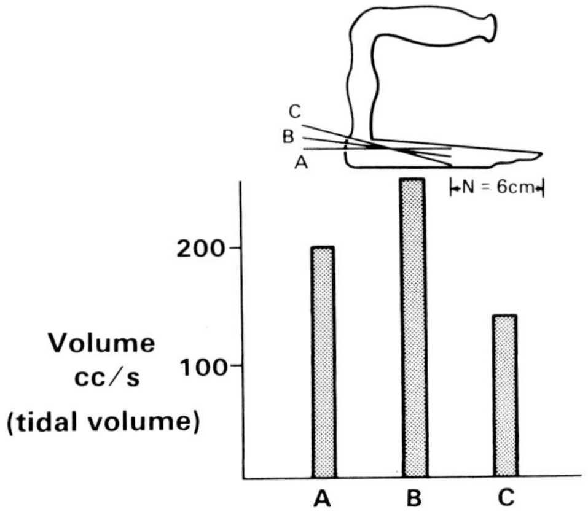

Fig. 3. Angle of Venturi jet needle placement within laryngoscope and tidal volume measured.

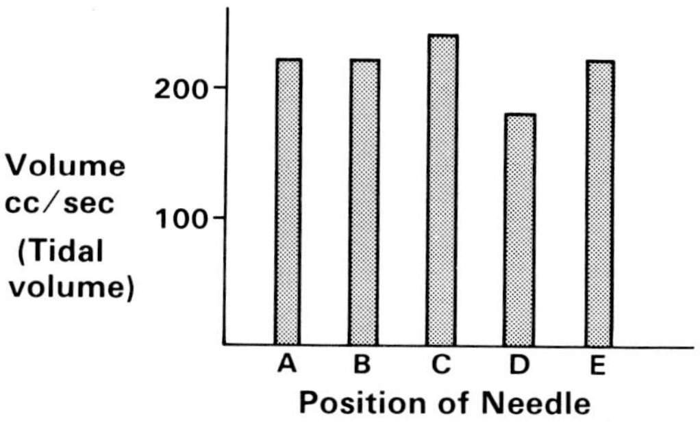

Fig. 4. Tidal volume and needle placement fixation on different walls of the laryngoscope (16.7 kg male).

because of the known hazard of producing mediastinal emphysema.

Volume Delivery and Change in Angle of Needle Placement. Figure 3 depicts the volume delivery in one second as the needle angle is changed. The regulator setting was set at 40 PSI and 10 L/min using a 15 gauge needle. The needle tip is at a distance of 6 cm from the vocal folds, spontaneous tidal volume is 200 cc. In column A, the length of the needle is placed against the laryngoscope wall. In column B, the needle axis is centered down the laryngoscope. In column C, the needle axis is aimed at the posterior lip of the laryngoscope. The volume delivery with each burst in the designated position is represented graphically. The greatest volume is delivered to the dog through the laryngoscope when the Venturi jet needle is aimed in the center of the laryngoscope. A 20% volume loss is noted when the needle is placed along the laryngoscope wall, a full 50% volume loss is noted when the tip of the needle is not directed in line with the laryngoscope.

In Figure 4 the needle is placed in various positions of the laryngoscope wall along the axis of the laryngoscope. Position A is with the needle in the left light carrier port. Position B is with the needle placed in the left light port with the needle aimed in the center of the scope. Position C is with the needle placed through the right light port, the needle being aimed in the center of the laryngoscope. Position D is with the needle placed through the right light carrier port with the needle along the laryngoscope wall. Position E is with the needle placed on a screw clamp fixed onto the inferior scope wall. Within the error of measurement, no significant difference in volume delivery was seen provided the needle was aligned with the axis of the laryngoscope.

Volume Delivery with Different Needle Sizes, Pressure and Oxygen Flow Regulator Setting. The Table indicates the volume delivery in one second to a paralyzed dog whose spontaneous tidal volume was 150 to 170 cc per cycle. The needle size, pressure regulator valve, oxygen flow indicator on the two-stage reducing valve was varied. The resultant tidal volume was measured. Representative data is tabulated for the nos. 19, 15, and 12 gauge needles.

TIDAL VOLUME AT VARIOUS VENTURI APPARATUS SETTINGS

		Flow Rate in L/Min		
Needle No.	*Pressure (PSI)*	*5L*	*10L*	*15L*
19	20	0	10	10
	40	—	20	30
	60	—	40	40
15	20	35	50	30
	40	—	90	100
	60	—	100	130
12	20	40	90	150
	40	—	160	180
	60	—	200	220

Female dog (12.2 kg) spontaneous tidal volume - 150 cc. All tidal volumes with Venturi are cubic centimeters per one second inspiration. All needles placed 6 cm from glottis, between vocal cords.

The position of the needle was fixed at 6 cm from the true cord and the needle aimed along the axis of the laryngoscope. With the needle position fixed, three variables were seen to affect the tidal volume delivery in the same test animal undergoing Venturi ventilation. These were 1) needle size, 2) reducing pressure gauge value and 3) oxygen flow regulator setting.

The volume delivery was quite variable. Little lung expansion and volume delivery were recorded during the use of Venturi with low pressure settings and no. 19 gauge needles. A volume 150% that of spontaneous tidal volume was consistently delivered when the no. 12 needle was used with the higher pressure setting with the oxygen regulator flow at 15 L/min. This large volume delivery in one second often resulted in a jerking type of motion as the dog lung was expanded to a hyperinflated state. The other intermediate valves of tidal volume delivery and the different needle size, pressure settings and oxygen regulator settings are tabulated in the Table.

It was noted that with a smaller size no. 19 needle, a maximal pressure of 60 PSI was not able to deliver adequate volume to mimic spontaneous tidal volume. As the pressure regulator was increased from 20 to 60 PSI using a no. 19 needle the increased volume delivery was small; it could not deliver adequate ventilatory volume for the test animal. The no. 12 needle was the largest needle tested and afforded the best volume delivery of the three needle sizes tested. This was true for all the pressure reducing valve settings and for all the oxygen flow rate settings. The pressure regulator was seen to have a more profound effect on volume delivery when used for the no. 12 needle. As the driving pressure was reduced from 60 to 20 PSI the fall-off of volume delivery to the lung was marked. Using the no. 12 needle, tidal volume similar to tidal volume prior to paralysis could be easily achieved even with a reduced pressure regulator setting; when the volume delivered was approximately that of the spontaneous tidal volume, the jerking type of chest motion observed with hyperventilatory tidal volume delivery was minimized.

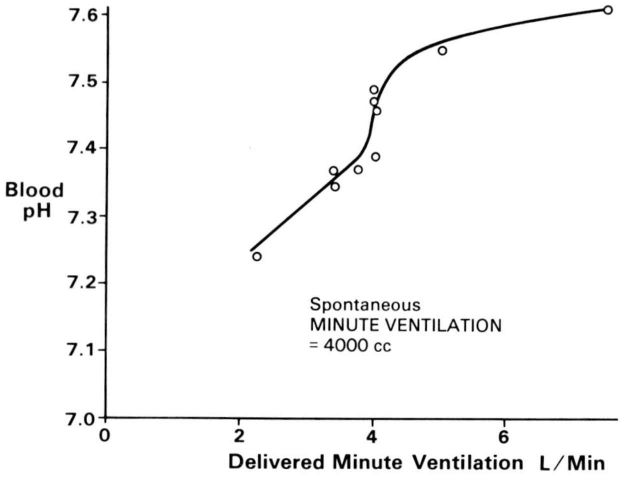

Fig. 5. Change in minute ventilation with Venturi jet ventilation and its effect on blood pH.

Venturi Jet Ventilation and Blood Gas Measurements. Using the total body plethysmograph, the tidal volume could be accurately measured while the test animal is being ventilated with the Venturi apparatus. By varying the expiration time, the cycles per minute of ventilation were manipulated. Using the equation: minute ventilation = tidal volume times cycles per minute, the minute ventilation was measured. This was made to equal the spontaneous ventilation of the test animal prior to paralysis. This technique also allowed us to deliver minute ventilation greater than or less than the volume of spontaneous minute ventilation. These ventilatory values correlated with blood gases.

Figure 5 shows graphically the effect on blood pH. Similarly the effect on oxygenation is presented in Figure 6. When the measured Venturi minute ventilation matched that of the spontaneously breathing animals' minute ventilation, adequate oxygenation was observed. When Venturi jet minute ventilation exceeded that of the spontaneous minute ventilation, the effect on blood gas was hypocapnia and respiratory alkalosis. When the minute ventilation via the Venturi was less than that of the spontaneous minute ventilation, the effect observed was hypercapnia and respiratory acidosis. In all blood gas measurements hypoxia (PO_2 less than 80 torr) was not measured. PO_2 values all stayed above 150 torr and increased slightly with increased minute ventilation. Even at levels of respiratory acidosis, the oxygenation remained excellent.

Serial Blood Gas Study in Dogs Ventilated with Venturi Apparatus. The long-term effects of Venturi ventilation on blood gases were evaluated. A Venturi apparatus was set up to deliver an effective tidal volume to the dog similar to that of tidal volume preparalysis. Cycles per minute on the timer were adjusted to simulate the dogs preparalysis respiratory rate. Serial blood gases were obtained. Two representative studies are shown in Figures 7 and 8. The longest time ventilated was 90 minutes. All experiments were terminated voluntarily. In each figure the values recorded are for one dog, ventilated at minute ventilations slightly greater than spontaneous tidal volume and for another dog ventilated at a value slightly less than spontaneous minute ventilation. pH and oxygen remained stable through both studies.

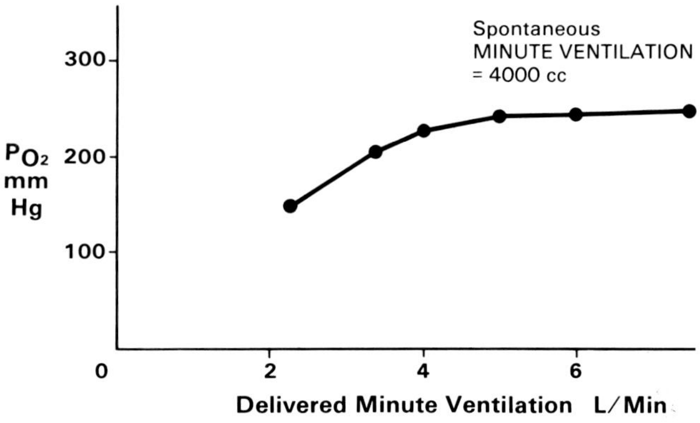

Fig. 6. Change in PO_2 with increasing minute ventilation using Venturi jet apparatus.

Intratracheal Pressure Changes. Pressure in the trachea caused by the Venturi apparatus was measured. Tidal volumes delivered by Venturi injection similar to that of spontaneous tidal volumes were used. The needle was placed at the level of the glottis. The trachea was then surgically exposed for 10 cm. Pressure along the path of the Venturi needle

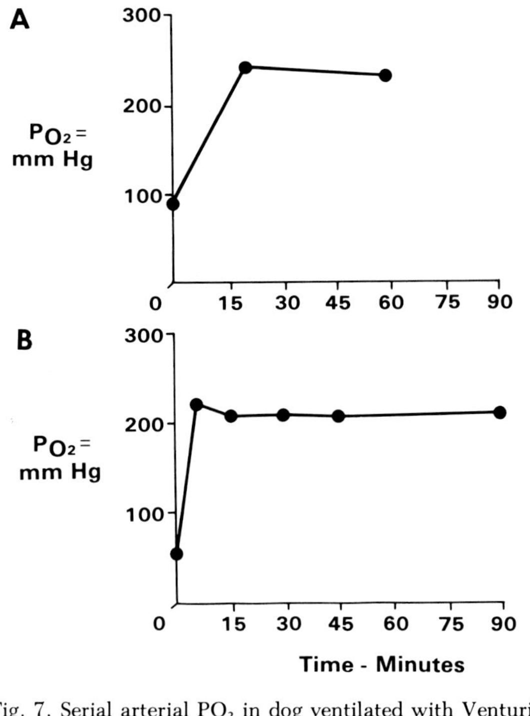

Fig. 7. Serial arterial PO_2 in dog ventilated with Venturi jet apparatus. A) Dog spontaneous tidal volume - 210 cc; Dog minute ventilation - 4000 cc; Venturi minute ventilation - 4200 cc. B) Dog minute ventilation - 4000 cc; Venturi minute ventilation - 3750 cc.

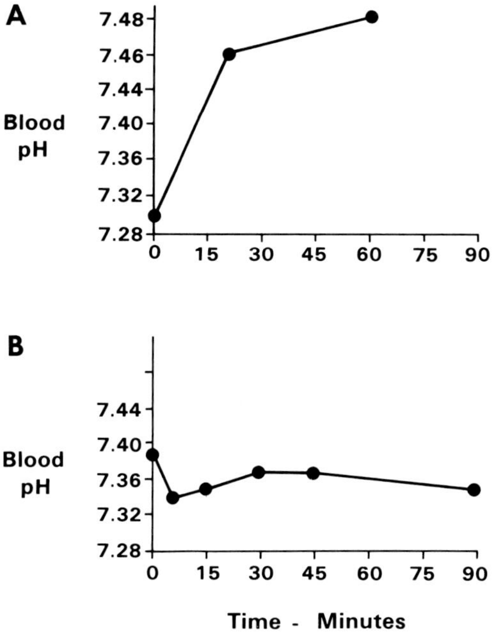

Fig. 8. Serial arterial pH in dog ventilated with Venturi jet apparatus. A) Dog spontaneous tidal volume - 210 cc; Dog minute ventilation - 4000 cc; Venturi minute ventilation -4200 cc. B) Dog spontaneous tidal volume - 210 cc; Dog spontaneous minute ventilation - 4000 cc/min; Venturi minute ventilation - 3750 cc/min.

and the pressure exerted against the tracheal wall was measured. A no. 10 needle attached to a manometer was used to cannulate the dog trachea and the peak pressures recorded. These pressures were measured in increasing increments of distance from the needle tip. Graphically it is presented in Figure 9. A large difference in the pressure between that at the path of the oxygen jet and that exerted against the trachea was found. The tip pressure along the axis of the needle was very high. The fall-off of the pressure from the needle tip was also very rapid. In the lower trachea the difference between the tracheal wall pressure and the tracheal lumen pressure was less and the two values approached one another. There was little difference between the two at 5 cm. The initial negative tracheal wall pressure at the level of the needle tip represents the Venturi effect. The differential between the pressure at 1 mm from the needle tip to that at 5 cm from the needle tip was 150 cm to 11 cm of water.

We have no data on the effect of placing the needle tip closer than 1 mm from the tracheal mucosa and the pressures generated.

DISCUSSION

This study was done on a test animal model to approximate the situation in man. However, several limitations must be noted. These study animals had no intrinsic laryngeal abnormality. Their pulmonary and thoracic compliances were not measured and were assumed to be normal.[9] The dog compliance measurements may not correlate with that of man. These lung volume delivery measurements would probably not be applicable in disease states such as outlet obstruction from, eg, laryngeal papilloma. Obstructive and restrictive lung disease states and their effects on the use of the system have not been addressed.

In the test animal model, we have shown that ventilation through the laryngoscope can offer a wide range of ventilatory capability. Volume delivered can be varied from 10 cc per second to a value one and a half times the value of spontaneous tidal

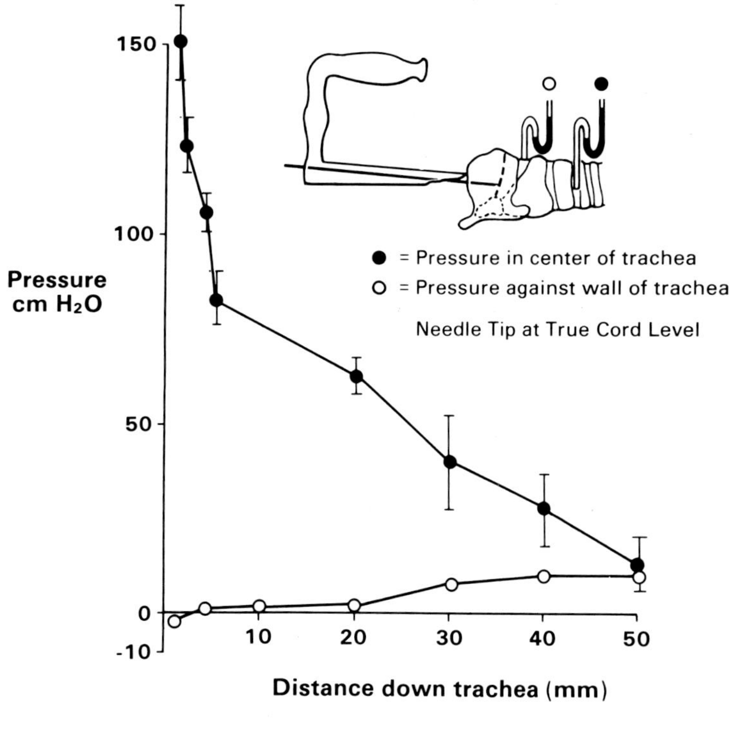

Fig. 9. Peak intratracheal pressures and tracheal wall pressures generated with Venturi jet ventilation measured at different distances down trachea.

volume in a similar one-second period. As shown, the parameters which will affect the volume delivered depend on needle size, needle position, regulator pressure, regulator flow rate. When tidal volume can be accurately measured, accurate minute ventilation can be delivered with the Venturi system to simulate that of spontaneous minute ventilation. Furthermore, we have shown that it is correlated with excellent blood gas values indicating adequate ventilation and oxygenation. In our study there is a direct correlation between volume delivery and its effect on blood gas values. Hyperventilation is associated with clinical alkalosis, hypoventilation with acidosis. In the clinical application of Venturi jet ventilation, volume measurements are not possible because of the open nature of the ventilatory circuit. At present, the best predictor of adequate ventilation in the endoscopy suite is the observation of chest expansion similar to that of tidal volume.[10,11] Needless to say, a more accurate predicator of volume delivery is needed. The use of multiple normograms depending on patient size may be one possible solution to predict which needle size and pressure values to use when the patient is paralyzed.

There exists situations in the study where adequate volume delivery could not be achieved. Using the no. 19 needle, adequate ventilation could not be done because of the low volumes delivered. The no. 15 needle could achieve adequate ventilation at 60 PSI and 30 cycles per minute. The no. 12 needle could achieve hyperventilation easily and can afford a range of volume delivery necessary to allow for regulation of minute ventilation. There appears to be a limiting factor exerted on volume delivery by the needle size. The smaller the needle size, the less the maximum volume achievable at any pressure up to 60 PSI. The pressure regulator further adjusts to volume delivery capabilities in more discrete steps allowing for more controlled volume delivery.

The above information may be applicable in the clinical usage of the Venturi ventilation apparatus. When an infant is being ventilated, its high compliance and the low volume needed coupled with the need to avoid hyperinflation would point toward the usage of a smaller sized needle. Similarly, in an obese and muscular individual with intrinsic lung disease, a small gauge needle would be quite unsatisfactory. A large needle size coupled with high regulator pressures may be needed to achieve lung expansion. In the experience from this study, a needle size is chosen to perform ventilation at 60 PSI which is greater than normal chest expansion, the pressure regulator is then lowered to a level where the chest is seen to move to approximate tidal volume. Although cycle length can also be varied, the frequencies have been between 20 to 30 per minute. These measurements usually gave blood gases indicating adequate ventilation.

With regard to the needle placement and volume delivery, several observations are valid. The needle axis should be placed in line with the laryngoscope, the larynx and the trachea. This provides for optimal volume delivery. The oxygen flow should not be aimed at any part of the laryngoscope except the lumen. Because of the fall-off of the volume delivery capability as the needle is withdrawn from the scope, the needle should be kept as nearly to the glottic level as is safe.

Because of the high pressure at the needle tip and the reported cases of mucosal tear and mediastinal emphysema associated with use of the oxygen injector system,[12,13] the needle tip was placed further back from the laryngoscope tip.[14] This protected the needle tip from inadvertently coming in contact with respiratory mucosa. However, from Figure 3 it can be seen that there is a drop in volume delivery efficiency as the needle is pulled back from the vocal fold level. A compromise distance of 6 cm from the vocal fold was made. From Figure 8B the maximal pressure in the tracheal lumen at a distance of 5 cm from the needle tip is 10 to 15 cm H_2O. This is similar to peak pressures achieved while using manual ventilation with a face mask. The apparatus therefore allowed for delivery of tidal volume, adjustable minute ventilation and excellent blood gases without risk of trauma with the high pressure needle. Further withdrawal of the needle tip from the vocal cord level will result in worsening volume delivery capability without the advantage of increased protection from the high pressure experienced at the needle tip. Because of the rapid fall-off of the tip pressure, the positioning of the Venturi needle tip within the laryngoscope should eliminate the reported complications of mucosal tear, subcutaneous emphysema, pneumomediastinum. From the study on dogs, a distance of 6 cm in the adult laryngoscope appeared to be most suitable. In our continued use of these dogs we did not see any of the above complications.

The initial negative pressure across the larynx at the level of the needle tip is the Venturi effect. There is some entrainment of air within the laryngoscope into the trachea with this system. The actual entrained volume and its effect on dilution of the delivered oxygen in various clinical situations is not addressed in this study. The effect of entrainment is seen clinically when the vocal fold is observed to move inward slightly with each oxygen injection. We are in the process of measuring the volume delivered from the needle tip and correlating it with the chest expansion volume to assess the importance of entrainment in this system.

Laryngeal pressure and lung volume measurements support the concept that Venturi jet ventilation is similar to conventional ventilation with a volume ventilator. Peak tracheal pressure of 8 cm H_2O is needed to inflate the normally compliant lung and chest wall in our animal model. This is similar to that of ventilation in man. Volume delivery and blood gas measurements indicate that when minute ventilation was adjusted to that of preparalysis minute ventilation, excellent ventilation can be achieved.

The stability of the system has been tested over 90 minutes of ventilation with the Venturi jet system. Blood gases remained within acceptable limits and was stable without evidence of deterioration. The excellent pH and PO_2 achieved over time would imply that there is no adverse effect on the pulmonary circulation or alveolar exchange over the time tested. Complications which were observed in the prolonged use of the Venturi system for ventilation included the excessive mucosal drying. This is from use of the dry oxygen. The effect is to be seen greatest at the vocal cords and subglottically. Tongue edema was seen when suspension on the laryngoscope was maintained for more than 60 minutes. When there was blood or mucus in the larynx, the jet had a tendency to blow the blood further into the tracheobronchial tree. These should be watched for and corrected. In addition, adequate anesthesia coupled with complete muscular relaxation must be achieved prior to use of the Venturi apparatus. In prolonged clinical usage, blood gases and cardiac activity should be monitored continuously.

The use of Venturi jet ventilation has advantages in certain aspects of laryngeal surgery. There are several distinct disadvantages associated with ventilation and operation without an endotracheal tube in place. The most prominant difference is the movement of the vocal cords while the Venturi jet is being used. The vocal cords will move in with inspiration and move out with expiration. The vocal aperture will change in diameter depending on the respiratory cycle. This can be of concern when using the laser in critical microlaryngeal work. The movement may be very small but must be compensated for. The effect of drying is reduced by frequent spraying with saline from a nebulizer. The necessity for complete paralysis may require longer anesthesia time for reversal. When working in the anterior commissure area of the vocal cords it is difficult to obtain wide abduction without the use of the endotracheal tube to stent the glottic aperture. The importance of alignment of the needle down the laryngoscope and the trachea necessitates careful positioning of the patient. Finally, while the endolaryngeal surgery is being performed, care must be exercised not to move the needle tip and not to obstruct the laryngeal opening for prolonged periods of time with the microlaryngoscopic instruments.

In summary, the introduction of suspension microlaryngoscopy coupled to the laser offers new challenges in patient management. The Venturi jet ventilation apparatus is one method devised to offer optimal anesthesia while allowing the otolaryngologist the time and room to perform the necessary surgery. This is particularly helpful in the region of the vocal processes of the arytenoids. The anesthesiologist must be concerned with muscle relaxation, adequate ventilation, and cardiopulmonary stability. The technique used must be sufficient to allow the team to feel that proper ventilation is being delivered with confidence throughout surgery. While the technique has a definite place in laryngology, it is limited in part by how safe this can be made to the type of endolaryngeal surgery being performed. This study indicates that if the guidelines outlined here are adhered to and if there is a high degree of cooperation between the surgeon and the anesthesiologist that adequate ventilation can be confidently provided.

REFERENCES

1. Spoerel WE, Narayanan PS, Singh NP. Transtracheal ventilation. Br J Anaesthes 1971; 43:932-9.

2. Borg U, Eriksson I, Sjøstrand U. High frequency positive-pressure ventilation: a review based upon its use during bronchoscopy and for laryngoscopy and microlaryngeal surgery under general anesthesia. Anesth Analg (Cleve) 1980; 59:594-603.

3. Carden E, Becker G, Hamood H. Percutaneous jet ventilation. Ann Otol Rhinol Laryngol 1976; 85:652-5.

4. Norton ML, Strong MS, Snow JC, et al. Endotracheal intubation and Venturi (jet) ventilation for laser microsurgery of the larynx. Ann Otol Rhinol Laryngol 1976; 85:656-63.

5. Carden E, Ferguson GB. A new technique for microlaryngeal surgery in infants. Laryngoscope 1973; 83:691-9.

6. Sander RD. Two ventilating attachments for bronchoscopes. Del Med J 1967; 30:170-6.

7. Albert SN, Shibuya J, Albert CA. Ventilation with an oxygen injector for suspension laryngoscopy under general anesthesia. Anesth Analg (Cleve) 1972; 51:866-70.

8. Lyons D, Stenzler A, Steinberg H, Abramson A, Ruder C. The airway mechanics of jet ventilation. Otolaryngol Head Neck Surg 1981; 89:364-9.

9. Schroter RC. Quantitative comparisons of mammalian lung pressure volume curves. Respir Physiol 1980; 42:101-7.

10. Snow JC, Kripke BJ, Strong MF. Anesthesia for carbon dioxide laser microsurgery on the larynx and trachea. Anesth Analg (Cleve) 1974; 53:407-12.

11. Rontal M, Rontal E, Wenokur M. Jet insufflation anesthesia for endolaryngeal surgery. Laryngoscope 1980; 90: 1162-8.

12. Oliverio R, Ruder CB, Fermon C, Cura A. Pneumothorax secondary to ball-valve obstruction during jet ventilation. Anesthesiology 1979; 51:255-6.

13. Chang JL, Meeuwis H, Bleyaert A, Babinski M, Petruscak J. Severe abdominal distention following jet ventilation during general anesthesia. Anesthesiology 1978; 49:216.

14. Tobias MA, Nassar WY, Richards DC. Naso-tracheal jet ventilation for micro-laryngeal procedures. Anesthesia 1977; 32:359-62.

FOREGUT CYSTS IN INFANTS AND CHILDREN

DIAGNOSIS AND MANAGEMENT

Seymour R. Cohen, MD Kenneth A. Geller, MD Jeffrey W. Birns, MD
Jerome W. Thompson, MD Bert W. Meyer, MD George G. Lindesmith, MD
Los Angeles, California

The charts of 15 patients with foregut cysts were reviewed. The lesions were intrathoracic in 14 patients and in the cervical area in one child. The importance of early diagnosis and surgical management is stressed. In untreated infants with foregut cysts, severe progressive and life-threatening airway obstruction may develop. Since the symptoms of this congenital lesion may simulate other more common diseases of the tracheobronchial tree and esophagus, the physician should become familiar with this disease entity so that proper diagnosis and surgical treatment will not be delayed. The study includes symptomatology, methods of diagnosis, pathologic findings and classification of the cysts.

INTRODUCTION

Duplication cysts of the esophagus, a term used synonymously with enteric cysts, bronchogenic cysts and foregut cysts, constitute 10% of all mediastinal tumors.[1,2] Few detailed reports regarding this rare congenital defect appear in the otolaryngological literature. A thorough review has failed to reveal any reports of the occurrence of cervical duplication cysts, and rarely is it mentioned in the differential diagnosis of neck masses in children.

A retrospective study of 15 children with cysts of foregut origin is presented. It includes one patient in which the cyst occurred in the cervical area. Four patients with cervical foregut cysts were not included in the study and will be reported at another time.

This unusual lesion was first described by Blasius in 1711,[3] but its earliest clinical recognition was by Hare[4] in 1899. Since then well over 100 cases have been reported.

Duplication of the foregut must be included in a differential diagnosis of stridor, respiratory distress and neck masses in infants and children. This anomaly most commonly occurs in the thorax and abdomen, but may be located anywhere from the mouth to the anus.[5] The removal of the mass is usually successful in relieving obstructive symptoms.

REVIEW OF LITERATURE

Gans et al[6] in 1968 reported two children with duplications of the esophagus in the cervical area. One patient had a neck mass associated with respiratory distress; the other had no clinical evidence of respiratory obstruction. After exhaustive research of the literature, the authors found two case reports in which the foregut cysts arose in the neck, with one originating in the upper thorax.

Grosfeld et al[5] in 1970 reported an 18-year review of the literature of enteric duplications in infants and children. The review included a series of 23 patients, 16 females and 7 males. The duplications included a variety of cysts, diverticula and tubular malformations, all believed to have a similar embryonic origin. The exact mechanism of production remains unknown. The authors considered the lesions to be thoracic, thoracicoabdominal and abdominal. In 15 of the 23 patients, the lesion was diagnosed within the first week of life and in 8 patients, by the third month. Only four patients became symptomatic after the first year of life. Respiratory distress was the most common symptom. Others included a palpable mass and intestinal obstruction with vomiting. Respiratory obstruction is common in thoracic and thoracolumbar duplications. Occasionally, perforations occurred when ectopic gastric mucosal activity was present, which may lead to pulmonary hemorrhage. In abdominal lesions, intestinal obstruction may be prominent.

Fallazadeh and Harderer[7] reported a 21-year-old man who had an esophageal duplication cyst and symptoms of chest pain. The lesion resembled stomach radiologically and filled the entire apical portion of the left side of the chest.

Kirwan et al[8] in 1973 suggested that foregut cysts be classified into three categories based on embryology: bronchogenic, a result of defective lung budding; intramural esophageal, a true duplication cyst; and enteric, resulting from a split notochord syndrome. They reported 41 patients examined between 1948 and 1971 and stressed the need for surgical removal of all foregut derivatives in order to

From the Department of Surgery, Divisions of Otolaryngology and Thoracic Surgery, Childrens Hospital of Los Angeles and the University of Southern California School of Medicine, Los Angeles.

Presented at the meeting of the American Broncho-Esophagological Association, Palm Beach, Florida, May 3-4, 1982.

REPRINTS — Seymour R. Cohen, MD, 1300 N. Vermont Ave., Los Angeles, CA 90027.

prevent complications. All patients had foregut cysts in the intrathoracic area.

Sethi et al[2] in 1974 reported a case of duplication cyst of the esophagus in a 5-month-old infant. The cyst occurred on the right side. In their experience, cysts of this type constituted 10% of all mediastinal tumors. Sixty percent occurred in the lower third of the esophagus; others were divided equally among the upper and middle third. Symptoms of dysphagia, regurgitation, failure to thrive, recurrent pneumonia and airway obstruction are described.

Graves et al[9] in 1974 reported a 5-month-old boy with a congenital bronchopulmonary foregut malformation with a pulmonary artery blood supply and pulmonary venous drainage.

Haller et al[1] in 1975 reported life-threatening respiratory distress from mediastinal masses in five infants. Two had intramural bronchial cysts; 1 had a giant esophageal duplication; and of the remaining 2, 1 had a benign teratoma and 1 had a highly malignant neuroblastoma.

Bower and Kiesewetter[10] in 1977 reported 11 duplication cysts and 6 bronchogenic cysts in 93 infants and children with mediastinal masses.

Sherman et al[11] in 1978 reported a 6-week-old infant with three distinct duplications occurring in the esophagus, duodenum and ilium. The infant, who was treated surgically, also had hemivertebrae and mild bilateral hydronephrosis.

EMBRYOLOGY AND HISTOPATHOLOGY

The respiratory system develops as a median ventral diverticulum of the cranial portion of the primitive foregut. The tracheobronchial tree and respiratory epithelium of the alveoli arise from the diverticulum. When abnormal budding of the bronchial tree occurs, abnormal cystic structures, or bronchogenic cysts, may develop which may or may not communicate with the bronchial tree. About the fourth embryonic week, the esophagus arises from the caudal portion of the foregut and elongates. The lining epithelium proliferates and converts the esophagus into a solid tube. About the sixth week of embryonic life, vacuoles develop within the solid esophagus, eventually coalescing to form the esophageal lumen. When a vacuole persists, an intramural esophageal cyst may develop and form a true duplication.[8]

Gray and Skandalakis[12] classify foregut cysts as bronchogenic, tracheobronchial, esophageal, gastric and enterogenous duplications. Confusion arises because some authors use classifications based on anatomic site and/or embryology, while others use classifications based on epithelial lining. Gray and Skandalakis believe that classification should be based on anatomic location and embryologic origin. They describe three categories of intrathoracic foregut derivatives: bronchogenic cysts, intramural esophageal cysts and enteric cysts.

Bronchogenic cysts result from abnormal budding of the bronchial tree. A part of the lung bud becomes separated and develops independently. Bronchogenic cysts are never associated with vertebral anomalies and are distinct from ciliated intramural esophageal cysts. Histologically, the bronchogenic cyst is related to the bronchial tree and is lined with ciliated columnar epithelium often having cartilage within the walls.

Intramural esophageal cysts are less common than bronchogenic cysts. The intramural cyst lies in close proximity to the wall of the esophagus and is lined with ciliated columnar epithelium. Some have nonciliated columnar or squamous epithelium. These are true duplications and result from defects in the vacuolation process. Intramural esophageal cysts are never associated with vertebral anomalies.

Enteric cysts are usually separate from the esophagus and lie in the posterior mediastinum. They have variable types of epithelium and a muscular wall which resembles that of the intestine. Enteric cysts are commonly associated with vertebral abnormalities. Embryologically, they are part of the split notochord syndrome and are usually attached firmly to the body of the vertebra by fibrous tissue which results from degeneration of that part of the fistula which penetrates the spine. The position of the cyst is usually caudal to that of the vertebral defect because of the difference in elongation between the spine and the foregut. Radiographs may demonstrate the vertebral anomaly.[12]

As previously stated, classification of congenital cysts may also be based on anatomic position.

Duplications of the trachea, or paratracheal cysts, are usually attached to the right lateral wall of the trachea just above the carina. However, they may be much more craniad as demonstrated in a case report by Brosnan[13] in 1959, in which the cyst extended from the level of the glottis to the sixth tracheal ring. These cysts are usually asymptomatic, but one death from tracheal compression has been reported.[14]

Hilar and carinal cysts are referred to as duplications of the bronchi. They are usually in proximity and distal to the bifurcation of the trachea, and are most often attached to the trachea or a bronchus by a strand of tissue. Histologically, the cyst wall is bronchial in structure.

Esophageal or paraesophageal cysts of Maier's classification,[15] although lined with ciliated epithelium, are attached to or embedded in the wall of the esophagus. These cysts are true derivatives of the primitive foregut which differentiates into the trachea and esophagus. They represent earlier sequestration than the paratracheal, carinal or hilar cysts.[12]

SUMMARY OF PATIENT POPULATION

The charts of 15 patients with the diagnosis of foregut cysts were reviewed. Four cases diagnosed postoperatively but not preoperatively as foregut cysts were not included in this study.

Nine patients (60%) were male and six were female. A familial tendency for foregut cysts could not be discerned from these records.

Presenting Symptoms. Ten patients had symptoms of chest pain or cough (6, cough alone; 2, chest pain; and 2, both). Stridor was a symptom in one patient. Five patients with severe pneumonia associated with cyanosis had major respiratory distress and required oxygen. Forty-seven percent of the patients had wheezing and five patients (33%) had gastroesophageal complaints consisting of epigastric pain, vomiting and gagging. There were no patients with cardiac symptoms or cardiac failure. One patient complained of severe sore throat.

Age. The mean age of onset of symptoms was 49.4 months; the mode was 1 month and the median was 3 months (range, 1 month to 18 years). The mean age at which a diagnosis was made was 65 months and the median was 48 months.

Initial Diagnosis. In five patients, the initial diagnosis of a foregut cyst was made from an x-ray film of the chest. Various diagnoses were made for other children, including bronchial asthma, vascular ring, foreign body in the tracheobronchial tree, mediastinal tumor and pneumonia. A foregut cyst was found incidentally at surgical exploration in one patient who had a thyroid nodule. When removed, the mass was found to be an esophageal duplication cyst. In the three patients who were treated for asthma, a routine x-ray film of the chest showed the mediastinal mass. In one patient with a diagnosis of a possible foreign body, who had hyperaeration of the left lung and persistent pneumonia, bronchoscopy revealed a compressive lesion at the carina. A barium esophagram showed the posterior deviation of the esophagus consistent with a bronchogenic cyst. The diagnosis was either a mediastinal tumor or a bronchogenic cyst for nearly two thirds of the patients. Many patients had previous chest x-ray films that had been read as normal.

Radiographic Findings. The plain x-ray studies showed a mass outside of the mediastinum in two patients. A neck mass was seen on the x-ray film of one patient, and the tumor was found on physical examination. Ten patients had mass lesions identified within the mediastinum on a roentgen study of the chest. In six patients, pneumonia was diagnosed also. Three patients had obstructive emphysema; one had pleural effusion. Thirteen patients had mass lesions within the chest: on the left side in 9, on the right side in 4 and in the midline in 2 patients. Nine patients (60%) had a barium esophagram which confirmed a compressive lesion deviating the esophagus within the mediastinum. In two patients the barium esophagram was essential to the diagnosis. Compression of the left upper lobe was noted in two patients.

Pathology. In 11 patients the cyst was lined with a pseudostratified columnar ciliated epithelium. Of the remaining cysts, 1 had a squamous epithelial lining, 1 a gastric mucosal lining, 1 a combination of squamous and respiratory epithelium and 1 a combination of squamous and gastric epithelium. Smooth muscle was found in 73% of the cystic lesions. One cyst, a duplication of the esophagus, had skeletal muscle. Many secretory glands were found, and 40% of the cysts had cartilage. All cysts were ovoid; the contents were usually of a mucoid character. Cyst size, which ranged from 1 cm^3 to 5 cm^3, was not related to the age of the patient.

Site of Origin of Cysts. The cysts were attached to the trachea by a fibrous band in 3 of the 15 patients (20%). The cysts of three patients were attached to a bronchus. One of the 15 patients had a mass involving the neck, mediastinum and abdomen. In one patient, the cyst had an attachment to the trachea by a fibrous strand and was attached firmly to the wall of the esophagus. Six of the cysts were intramural esophageal duplications. One of the bronchogenic cysts was intrapulmonary and was surrounded by lung parenchyma (Fig. 1). All cysts were extraluminal.

Associated Anomalies. Most of the children had no other abnormalities of foregut origin. Associated defects were laryngomalacia, sickle cell trait, nephrotic syndrome, cystic adenomatoid disease of the lung and patent foramen ovale.

Endoscopic Findings. Direct laryngoscopy in 5 of the 15 patients showed the larynx to be normal, except in the child with laryngomalacia. One of the 5 patients had a normal tracheobronchial tree; 3 had compression of the left main stem bronchus; and 1 had severe blunting and splaying of the carina, indicative of compression by a peritracheal and peribronchial mass lesion. The child with a normal tracheobronchial tree had an intramural esophageal

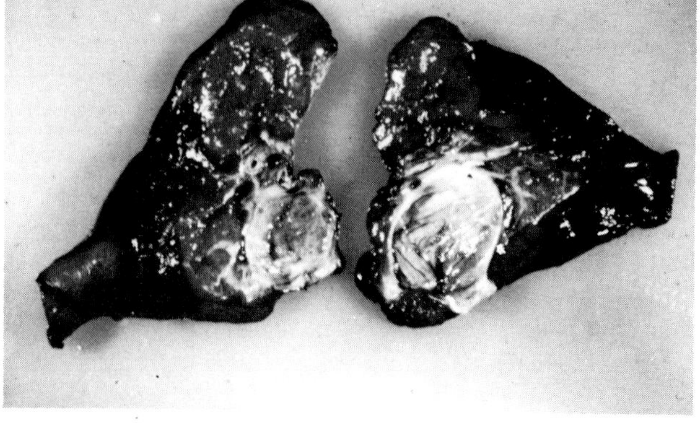

Fig. 1. Unusual bronchogenic cyst lying within normal lung parenchyma.

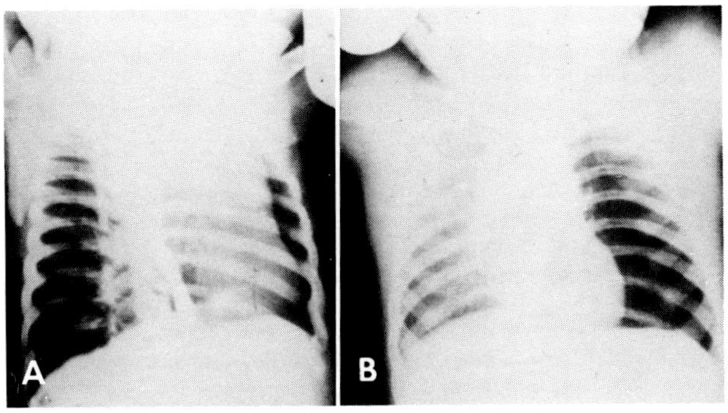

Fig. 2. (Case 1) X-ray films showing obstructive emphysema of left lung and posterior displacement of esophagus by cystic mass. A) Right anterior oblique view; B) P-A view.

duplication. Esophagoscopy in one patient revealed a posterior compression of the esophagus which was later confirmed by a barium esophagram. Only one bronchogram was performed to confirm compression of the left main stem bronchus.

TREATMENT AND RESULTS

All 15 children were treated surgically. A mass was found and successfully removed from 14 patients (93%). Three patients had postoperative complications (one developed a pleural effusion). One, who did not recover, had surgery performed at another institution and was transferred to Childrens Hospital for follow-up care. The cyst in this case was a gastric duplication extending from the neck to the abdomen and had never been removed. Death was ascribed to sepsis. Another child whose cystic mass could not be found at surgery and who had postoperative difficulties died approximately two months later from severe respiratory obstructive disease.

CASE REPORTS

Case 1. A 7-month-old girl was admitted on Nov 2, 1948, with a history of expiratory wheezing since 6 weeks of age. Her pediatrician, after noting the wheeze, had followed her with serial roentgenograms. Two months prior to admission a barium esophagram (Fig. 2) showed a compressive lesion suggestive of a mediastinal tumor. The child had increased wheezing with crying or stress and her symptoms became markedly pronounced with respiratory infections. There was no cough or cyanosis. Family and past history were noncontributory.

The admission examination revealed a normocephalic chubby girl with normal findings except those within the chest. The chest was symmetrical with no retractions or splinting. The left side of the chest was dull to percussion and had markedly diminished breath sounds. The heart was not displaced.

An x-ray film showed marked emphysema of the left lung with a shift of the mediastinum to the right. Posterior displacement of the esophagus was noted. Hemoglobin level (Hb) was 13.6 g with a WBC count of 11,500. The day after admission, the infant was taken to surgery and an exploratory thoracotomy was performed. The left lung was markedly emphysematous and would not collapse, which created severe difficulty in palpation of the mediastinum. The thymus was thought to be enlarged and a mediastinal or hilar mass was not found. Postoperatively, the patient developed marked stridor. Radiation therapy was given to the thymus.

The patient was readmitted on Dec 29, 1948. Apparently she had done well at home until the day before readmission. She developed a cold with marked respiratory distress and stridor, fever and vomiting. Examination showed moderate to marked cyanosis, labored respirations with a loud expiratory stridor and marked retractions. Both lungs were dull to percussion, more so on the left than on the right, with extremely poor air exchange. An x-ray film showed marked emphysema of both lungs with a shift of the heart to the left. The child was given oxygen, appeared to be doing well, then developed respiratory arrest. Artificial respiration was futile and the child died.

At autopsy, a mass lesion could not be palpated in the mediastinum. However, when dissecting the mediastinum, it was noted that the trachea was pushed to the right. Lying posterior to the carina and extending 2.5 cm down the left main stem bronchus was a soft cystic mass. The main portion of the cyst was to the left of the trachea and a small protrusion was seen posterior to the right main stem bronchus. The mass measured 5.5 x 3.5 x 3 cm and weighed 19 g. The mass lesion was connected by a fibrous band to the trachea at a point 2 cm above the bifurcation. It was also connected to the esophagus by a small band of connective tissue 1 mm thick. There was no dimpling of either the tracheal or esophageal mucosa. The cyst was filled with clear fluid, and was lobulated but not multiloculated (Fig. 3A). The esophagus was markedly deviated to the right by pressure of the cyst. The cyst wall consisted of loose, fibrous connective tissue, smooth muscle and ciliated columnar epithelium. Cartilage and acinar structures were also seen, with ducts leading to the surface. Several small septa were noted to be covered with ciliated columnar epithelium (Fig. 3B).

Case 2. A 5-month-old boy was admitted on Aug. 10, 1954. The chief complaint was wheezing that had persisted for a number of weeks following an upper respiratory infection and had partially cleared with antibiotic therapy. The family history was noncontributory. The clinical history showed that wheezing was first noted in this child at 5 weeks of age. He had periodic wheezing which cleared with antibiotics. He was the product of a normal pregnancy and a normal, full-term delivery.

Upon admission, examination showed a well-developed, well-nourished male infant with marked wheezing. The chest was symmetrical, but high-pitched wheezes were heard throughout the lung fields bilaterally. Coarse rales were heard at the base, especially anteriorly. His heart was normal. Fluoroscopic examination showed a shift of the mediastinum to the right. A radiopaque foreign body was not identified. He was admitted for endoscopic examination which revealed tracheobronchial obstruction either by a vascular ring, mediastinal tumor or tracheal anomaly. A barium esophagram performed three days after admission showed a mediastinal mass compressing the left bronchus with displacement of the esophagus (Fig. 4).

A left thoracotomy was performed on Aug 18, 1954, and a

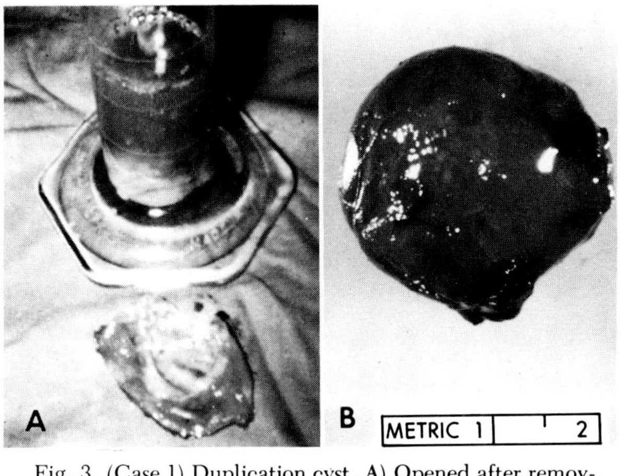

Fig. 3. (Case 1) Duplication cyst. A) Opened after removal. Fluid was aspirated from cyst. B) Intact showing ovoid shape.

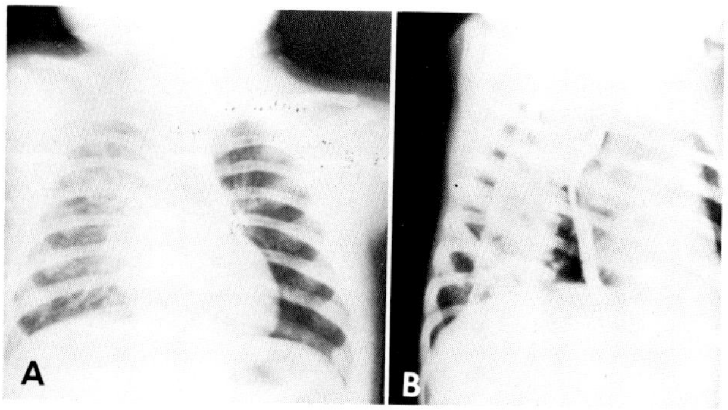

Fig. 4. (Case 2) X-ray films showing hyperaeration of both lungs and cystic shadow within mediastinum displacing esophagus posteriorly. A) P-A view; B) Right anterior oblique view.

bronchogenic cyst was removed. The child was discharged six days after surgery, after an uneventful postoperative course. The findings at thoracotomy showed the left lung to be markedly emphysematous. The thin-walled cyst contained clear fluid. It was located in the left mediastinum between the aorta and the left main stem bronchus and compressed the posterior wall of the bronchus. The esophagus was displaced to the right. The cyst arose from the left main stem bronchus 1 cm from the bifurcation of the trachea and there was a narrow pedicle attachment to the cartilaginous portion of the left bronchus.

Laboratory findings prior to the surgery were Hb level, 13.7 g; WBC count, 26,300 and normal urine. The cyst was 2 x 1 x 1 cm, multilocular and contained cartilage at the line of excision. The structure was lined with pseudocolumnar ciliated epithelium and contained amorphous noncellular material. The wall was fibrous between multilocular areas and no alveolar components were seen. Follow-up examination of this patient indicated complete recovery and cure.

Case 3. A 5½-month-old male infant was admitted June 12, 1981, with a history of numerous respiratory infections since birth. At 2 months of age he was admitted to another hospital with bronchiolitis and pneumonia. He was treated with numerous antibiotics, but at the time of his discharge, he continued to have wheezing. The wheezing respirations progressed rapidly, accompanied by fever of 39°C with cough. The child was treated for asthma and pneumonitis without response. Vital signs were normal. Positive findings were those noted in the chest. The lungs were symmetrical but wheezing was heard at both bases, more on the left than on the right. There were decreased breath sounds in the right upper lobe area. Hematologic studies showed an Hb level of 12.7 g, 14,800 WBC, with a normal differential. Urine was also normal. An x-ray film of the chest showed the bony thorax to be intact and the size of the heart to be normal. There was a density along the right side of the heart and an area of atelectasis in the right middle lobe. No specific masses were identified on this film. A barium esophagram revealed an indentation just below the left main stem bronchus. Direct laryngoscopy revealed a mild form of laryngomalacia. Both the trachea and the right bronchial tree were normal. The left main stem bronchus was severely compressed distal to the mouth of the left main bronchial orifice. The child tolerated the endoscopic procedure well. The findings were reported as severe compression of the left bronchial orifice due to an external mass in the mediastinum. The child was discharged on June 18, 1981, with persistence of the wheezing respirations. He was to be readmitted for surgery.

On June 24, 1981, the infant developed nausea, vomiting and diarrhea and was readmitted with increased respiratory distress and wheezing. Cyanosis was not present. An x-ray film of the chest revealed increased atelectasis in the right middle lobe. A rounded circumferential edge of a bronchogenic cyst could be seen in the mediastinum. On June 29, 1981, a right thoracotomy was performed and an esophageal duplication cyst was removed. His postoperative course was uneventful and he was discharged July 3, 1981.

A CT scan of the chest performed prior to surgery showed the presence of a cystic mass between the esophagus and the trachea in the subcarinal area. Upon entering the right side of the chest, a cystic structure was found bulging through the mediastinal pleura. The mass was overlying the midesophagus just below the area of the tracheal bifurcation in the subcarinal area. There was no intimate attachment to the trachea or bronchial tree. Surgeons were unable to determine the extent to which the respiratory tract was compressed. The mass arose from the wall of the esophagus with an area of esophageal muscularis coming up over the cyst wall. There was no apparent communication with the upper gastrointestinal tract or the tracheobronchial tree. The cyst was 1.3 x 1 x 0.7 cm. Microscopically, sections of the cyst showed a ciliated pseudostratified columnar epithelium thrown into folds. The cyst wall was composed of an inner circular and an outer longitudinal smooth muscle layer. Cartilage was not present in the mass. The postoperative pathological diagnosis was esophageal duplication.

The patient did well for two months, then developed asthmatic symptoms and recurrent pneumonia. Because of wheezing, endoscopic examination was again performed and the left main stem bronchial stenosis was shown to be resolved.

DISCUSSION AND CONCLUSIONS

Foregut cysts within the thoracic cavity can be classified according to embryogenesis as bronchogenic, intramural esophageal and enteric cysts. Of the 15 cases reported in this study, 14 foregut cysts were intrathoracic and 1 was in the cervical region.

The most prominent symptoms were cough, chest pain, wheezing and respiratory distress. Respiratory distress was of major proportion at times and was most likely to occur in small infants. Symptoms such as epigastric pain, vomiting and gagging were most likely to occur in children with esophageal and gastric duplications. The foregut cyst sometimes remained asymptomatic for months or years. However, when symptoms developed in early infancy, they were most likely to progress rapidly and produce major, even dramatic, airway obstruction. Complete surgical extirpation was mandatory.

Foregut cysts may simulate asthma, a vascular ring (or sling), tracheal or severe bronchial stenosis, foreign body aspiration and bronchiolitis.

Six patients developed symptoms prior to 6 months of age (40%) and 7 patients (46%) developed symptoms within the first year of life.

The diagnosis was established in 10 of the 15 patients by an x-ray study of the chest. However, a barium esophagram was necessary for the diagnosis in two patients. It is important that a barium esophagram be performed in children with persistent wheezing, intermittent stridor, a brassy cough, chronic or recurring pneumonia or when endoscopic examination reveals a compression of the trachea or bronchial tree.

Endoscopic examination was performed only when the diagnosis was not confirmed by an x-ray film of the chest or when a foreign body or intrinsic tracheobronchial abnormality was suspected.

As has been suggested by others,[8,12] the authors believe that foregut cysts should be classified on the basis of embryogenesis and not on location or type of epithelial lining. Foregut cysts may be bronchogenic, esophageal duplication or enteric cysts. The first type arises from abnormal budding of the precursor of the larynx, trachea and bronchial tree. Esophageal duplication cysts arise from defects of vacuolization during the development of the lumen of the esophagus and therefore are truly duplication cysts. Enteric cysts arise from the split notochord syndrome and are associated with defects of the spine. The cysts do not communicate with the lumen of the organ from which they arise.

Of the foregut cysts in the 15 children studied, 8 were bronchogenic, 6 were esophageal and 1 was intralobar bronchogenic. No enteric cysts were found. Associated anomalies were not serious.

Thirteen patients (93%) were cured by surgical extirpation of the lesion. Two deaths occurred; one was associated with severe postoperative sepsis and the other with sudden obstruction of the airway.

Excision of the lesion was accomplished with minimal loss of normal tissue and postoperative morbidity was minimal. Most patients were discharged by the fifth or sixth postoperative day.

The tendency for intrathoracic foregut cysts to enlarge and produce airway obstruction is sufficient reason for early diagnosis and surgical removal.

ACKNOWLEDGMENT — Gratitude is expressed to Rose Marie Lapicola for her help in the preparation of this manuscript, and to Hart Isaacs, MD, for supplying photographs of the gross pathology.

REFERENCES

1. Haller JA, Shermeta DW, Donahoo JS, White JJ. Life threatening respiratory distress from mediastinal masses in infants. Ann Thorac Surg 1975; 19:364-70.

2. Sethi GK, Marsden J, Johnson D. Duplication cysts of the esophagus. South Med J 1974; 67:616-8.

3. Blasius G. Observationes medicae, anatomicae, variores. 3rd ed. Leyden:1711.

4. Hare HA. The pathology, clinical history and diagnosis of affections of the mediastinum other than those of the heart and aorta. Philadelphia: Blakiston's, 1899.

5. Grosfeld JL, O'Neill JA Jr, Clatworthy HW Jr. Enteric duplications in infancy and childhood: an 18-year review. Ann Surg 1970; 172:83-90.

6. Gans SL, Lackey DA, Zuckerbraun L. Duplications of the cervical esophagus in infants and children. Surgery 1968; 63: 849-52.

7. Fallazadeh H, Harderer O. Esophageal duplication cyst with unusual manifestations. Chest 1973; 63:827-8.

8. Kirwan WO, Walbaum PR, McCormick RJM. Cystic intrathoracic derivatives of the foregut and their complications. Thorax 1973; 28:424-8.

9. Graves VB, Dahl DD, Power HW. Congenital bronchopulmonary foregut malformation with anomalous pulmonary artery. Pediatr Radiol 1974; 114:423-4.

10. Bower RJ, Kiesewetter WB. Mediastinal masses in infants and children. Arch Surg 1977; 112;1003-9.

11. Sherman NJ, Morrow D, Asch M. A triple duplication of the alimentary tract. J Pediatr Surg 1978; 13:187-8.

12. Gray SW, Skandalakis JE. Embryology for the surgeons. Philadelphia: Saunders, 1972.

13. Brosnan ML. Report of a case of double trachea. J Laryngol Otol 1959; 73:853-5.

14. Blackader AD, Evans DN. A case of mediastinal cyst producing compression of the trachea ending fatally in an infant of 9 months. Arch Pediatr 1911; 28:194.

15. Maier HC. Bronchogenic cysts of the mediastinum. Ann Surg 1948; 127:476-502.

PEDIATRIC TRACHEOSTOMY

EXPERIENCE DURING THE PAST DECADE

RALPH F. WETMORE, MD

STEVEN D. HANDLER, MD   WILLIAM P. POTSIC, MD

PHILADELPHIA, PENNSYLVANIA

A retrospective review of a decade of experience with pediatric tracheostomy encompassed 420 children. Analysis was performed with respect to primary diagnosis, age, duration of tracheostomy and hospitalization, early and late complications and mortality. While the incidence of tracheostomy per hospital admission decreased over the period of review, there was substantial increase in duration of tracheostomy. Approximately half of the patients sustained complications. While overall mortality approached 28%, tracheostomy-related deaths occurred in only eight patients (2%). Almost one fifth of children with tracheostomies were discharged to home care, and 3% were involved in our home ventilator program.

INTRODUCTION

A review of the medical literature shows pediatric tracheostomy to be a surgical procedure with significant morbidity and mortality.[1-9] Complication rates are greater in children than in adults. This difference in complications is a reflection of the primary disease process, the age of the child and the duration of the tracheostomy.

Chew and Cantrell[10] reviewed 1,928 tracheostomies in adults and found an overall complication rate of 15.8% and an overall mortality rate of 1.6%. By comparison, tracheostomy-related mortality in children ranges from 3.2% to 8.5%. Mortality from all causes approximates 25% but may reach 50% or more in selected groups under 1 year of age.[1-9]

A recent 10-year review of pediatric tracheostomy was performed to identify trends in airway management in children and to recognize those groups of patients who are at greater risk for complication and mortality.

METHODS

All tracheostomies performed in the operating room between January 1971 and December 1980 were reviewed retrospectively. A list was compiled initially from the operative log and included procedures done by otolaryngology, general surgical and cardiothoracic services. A total of 441 charts were identified and 420 were located and analyzed with respect to the following variables: age, diagnosis, indication for procedure, duration of tracheostomy, early and late complications and mortality. Early complications were defined as those occurring in the operating room or during the first postoperative week. At one week, the tracheostomy stoma has usually matured, and the first tube change is performed. Late complications were defined as those occurring after the first week.

RESULTS

While the absolute number of tracheostomies has remained constant each year, the incidence per hospital admission has shown a slight decrease (Table 1). There was a slight male predominance (1.4:1.0). The racial incidence appeared to reflect the racial pattern of the referral region for Children's Hospital. The age range spanned one day to 21 years; 244 patients (58%) were 2 years of age or younger; 197 (47%) were under 1 year of age. Over the 10-year period, there was a relative increase in the number of children under the age of 2 (Fig. 1).

Table 2 illustrates the distribution of primary diagnoses in patients who underwent tracheostomy. Along with CNS disorders, diseases of the upper airway were the most common primary diagnoses. Further breakdown of the upper airway obstruction category is shown in Table 3. Over the review period there was an increase in tracheostomies in elective craniofacial procedures, CNS disorders and respiratory distress syndrome (RDS) and a decrease in patients with congenital heart disease (CHD).

Prolonged ventilation was the most common indication for tracheostomy in our series (53%). Other major indications included upper airway obstruction (39%) and pulmonary toilet (4%). One infant required a tracheostomy because of recurrent apnea and bradycardic episodes. Another child had bleeding of the upper aerodigestive tract which required a controlled airway. A third child could not be adequately ventilated through an endotracheal tube. An additional 4% of patients had multiple indications for tracheostomy.

With the exception of six cases which were done

From the Division of Otorhinolaryngology and Human Communication, Children's Hospital of Philadelphia and the University of Pennsylvania School of Medicine.

Presented at the meeting of the American Broncho-Esophagological Association, Palm Beach, Florida, May 3-4, 1982.

REPRINTS — Ralph F. Wetmore, MD, Children's Hospital of Philadelphia, 34th Street and Civic Center Boulevard, Philadelphia, PA 19104.

TABLE 1. INCIDENCE OF TRACHEOSTOMIES IN 420 PATIENTS

Year	*No. of Tracheostomies*	*% of Hospital Admissions*
1971	55	0.9
1972	38	0.6
1973	35	0.5
1974	47	0.6
1975	32	0.3
1976	36	0.3
1977	50	0.5
1978	39	0.4
1979	46	0.4
1980	42	0.4

using either local anesthesia or mask inhalation, the vast majority of cases were performed with an endotracheal tube or, rarely, an open bronchoscope controlling the airway.

The duration of tracheostomy ranged from one day to more than 10 years and averaged approximately 180 days (Fig. 2). Since long-term tracheostomies tended to skew the yearly averages, omission of those in place longer than 1 year provided a better indication of a trend — a doubling of the duration of tracheostomy over the 10-year period. This finding is supported by an almost threefold increase in the length of hospital stay over the period of review.

There were 341 complications in 204 children (49%). Early complications, those which occurred intraoperatively or within the first postoperative week, numbered 119 (Table 4). Two complications occurred intraoperatively. In one patient, the esophagus was entered inadvertently when the rigid esophageal stethoscope was mistaken for the trachea. The other occurred when a tracheostomy tube was acutely obstructed during the procedure. Accidental decannulation and pneumonia were most commonly encountered.

Late complications, those which occurred after the first postoperative week, totaled 222 (Table 5). Persistent tracheocutaneous fistula and accidental decannulation were seen most frequently.

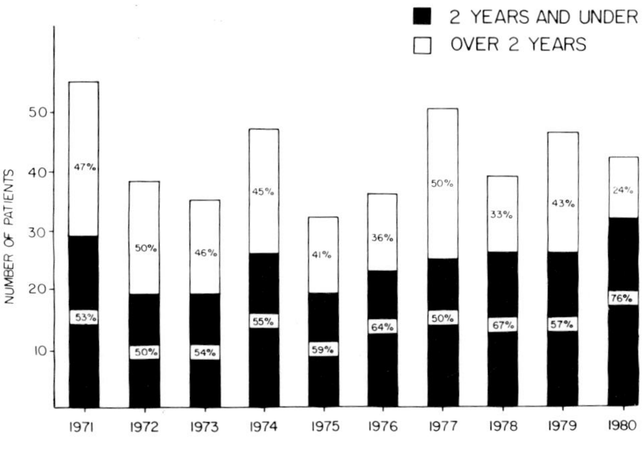

Fig. 1. Pediatric tracheostomy patients (n = 420).

TABLE 2. PRIMARY DIAGNOSES IN 442 TRACHEOSTOMY PATIENTS

Upper airway obstruction	105	(24%)
CNS disorders	105	(24%)
Miscellaneous disorders	81	(18%)
Congenital heart disease	73	(17%)
Respiratory distress syndrome	51	(12%)
Craniofacial disorders	27	(6%)

*20 patients with two or more diagnoses.

Table 6 lists the primary diagnoses of patients who sustained one or more complications. When compared to the overall frequency of primary diagnoses, there appeared to be a higher incidence of complications in patients with upper airway obstruction and RDS. Children with CHD or elective craniofacial surgery requiring tracheostomy appeared to sustain relatively fewer complications.

Of the 204 children with complications, 116 suffered one, 56 developed two and 32 had three or more. The average duration of tracheostomy in those patients with complications was significantly longer (305 days) than the overall average of 180 days.

Early complications occurred in 61% of children 2 years of age or younger, a frequency similar to the overall distribution of patients by age. More late complications (79%) were seen in the age group 2 years and under. The ratio of early to late complications remained relatively constant during the review period (Fig. 3).

Overall mortality for the period of review was 116 patients (28%). In eight children (2%), death was attributed to the tracheostomy: obstructed tube (4), accidental decannulation (2), massive tracheal hemorrhage (1) and sepsis due to erosion by the tube (1). Primary diagnoses in those patients with tracheostomy-related deaths included CNS disorders (3), RDS (2), miscellaneous disorders (2) and craniofacial disorders (1). Four of these deaths occurred at home, two at Children's Hospital and two at other institutions.

Nontracheostomy-related deaths numbered 108, and the primary diagnoses are listed in Table 7. One operative mortality occurred in a patient

TABLE 3. CAUSES OF UPPER AIRWAY OBSTRUCTION IN 105 PATIENTS

Laryngotracheobronchitis	32	(30%)
Subglottic stenosis (congenital or acquired)	22	(21%)
Acute epiglottitis	16	(15%)
Pierre-Robin syndrome	7	(7%)
Head and neck neoplasms	7	(7%)
Multifactorial causes	7	(7%)
Adenotonsillar hypertrophy	5	(5%)
Respiratory papillomatosis	3	(3%)
Laryngeal cysts	2	(2%)
Tracheal stenosis	2	(2%)
Laryngeal trauma	1	(1%)
Vocal cord paralysis	1	(1%)

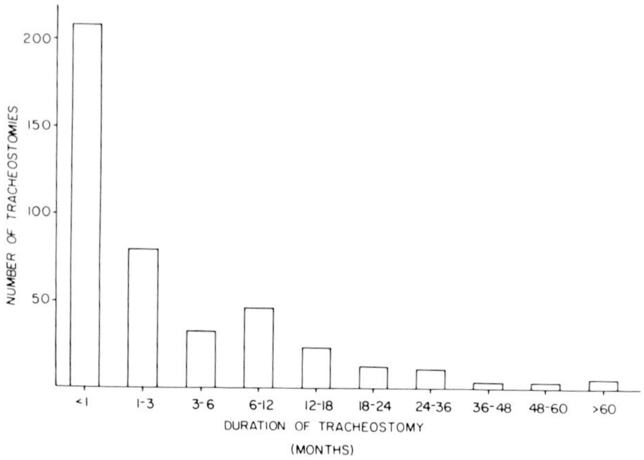

Fig. 2. Duration of tracheostomies (n = 420).

undergoing cardiac surgery for CHD. A tracheostomy was performed at the onset of the procedure, and the death was unrelated to the tracheostomy.

Seventy-two patients (17%) were discharged directly from the hospital to home after an intensive period of training family members in tracheostomy care. Eleven patients (3%) required home ventilators for continued respiratory support. Sixty-three patients were transferred to other institutions for further care. The remaining patients were either decannulated during initial hospitalization or succumbed with an indwelling tracheostomy while still hospitalized.

DISCUSSION

With 106,298 pediatric admissions from 1971 to 1980, the average incidence in our study was 3.9 tracheostomies per 1,000 admissions. The gradual decrease over the decade (Table 1) is probably a reflection of the increasing acceptance of prolonged intubation for croup, epiglottitis and some cardiac and CNS disorders.

The higher incidence of tracheostomy in male patients has been cited by both Tucker and Silberman[5] and Oliver et al[1] and is felt to represent an increased male susceptibility to congenital and acquired disorders.

The relative increase in tracheostomy in children under 2 years of age appears to parallel the increase in survival in children with bronchopulmonary dysplasia and other congenital disorders over the past decade.[11]

Along with CNS diseases, obstruction of the upper airway comprised the most frequent primary diagnosis. The incidence of tracheostomy in cases of upper airway obstruction, however, remained relatively constant over the 10 years of review, while CNS disorders have shown a steady increase — a reflection of prolonged survival of children with these diseases.[12,13] Elective craniofacial procedures have been performed more frequently and often require tracheostomy.[14] Prolonged ventilation has been associated with improved survival in premature infants with RDS and often necessitates tracheostomy. Only in patients with CHD has there been a substantial decline in tracheostomies, a factor which reflects changes in the philosophy of our cardiothoracic surgeons.

Over the 10-year span, both length of hospitalization and duration of tracheostomy have shown substantial increases. Again this indicates the prolonged survival of critically ill children who probably would have succumbed in the past. Children with RDS and CNS disorders frequently fall into this category. Many of these children require a tracheostomy for months for prolonged ventilation or access for pulmonary toilet.

The complication rate of 49% is similar to that reported by Tucker and Silberman[5] (46.5%) but higher than that reported by Hawkins and Williams[6] (36%), Gaudet et al[9] (33%) and Palva et al[8] (19%). Some series have included delayed decannulation as a complication. Delayed decannulation may be due to tracheostomy but is more often a result of the primary disease. This difference may be difficult to distinguish and is rarely well documented. Likewise persistent tracheocutaneous fistula is often not included as a complication since it occurs after successful decannulation. We have

TABLE 4. EARLY COMPLICATIONS (N = 119)

Accidental decannulation	29	(24%)
Pneumonia	24	(20%)
Pneumothorax	11	(9%)
Subcutaneous emphysema	11	(9%)
Obstructed tube	8	(7%)
Hemorrhage	8	(7%)
Stomal infection	7	(6%)
Tracheitis	7	(6%)
Pneumomediastinum	5	(4%)
Other	9	(8%)

TABLE 5. LATE COMPLICATIONS IN 222 PATIENTS

Tracheocutanous fistula	42	(19%)
Accidental decannulation	40	(18%)
Tracheal granuloma	30	(14%)
Excessive stomal granulation	24	(11%)
Obstructed tube	23	(10%)
Hemorrhage	22	(10%)
Stomal infection	18	(8%)
Tracheomalacia	12	(5%)
Other	11	(5%)

TABLE 6. PRIMARY DIAGNOSES IN PATIENTS WITH COMPLICATIONS (N = 218)

Upper airway obstruction	71	(33%)
CNS disorders	47	(22%)
Miscellaneous disorders	40	(18%)
Respiratory distress syndrome	39	(18%)
Congenital heart disease	20	(9%)
Craniofacial disorders	1	(1%)

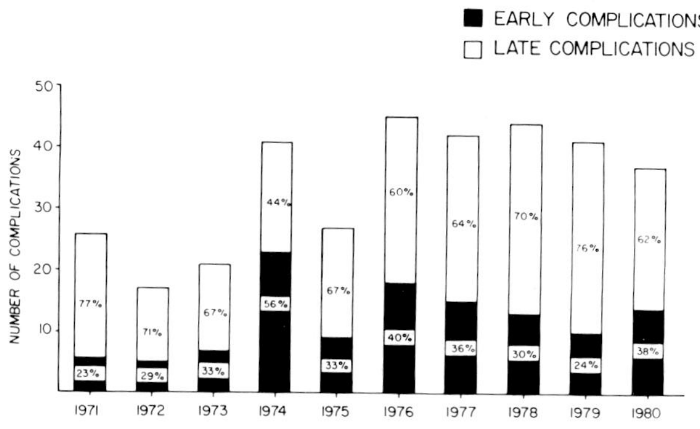

Fig. 3. Early and late complications of pediatric tracheostomies (n = 341).

considered it a complication since a secondary closure procedure is often required.

Tracheostomy in adults has generally been associated with a lower complication rate than in children. The low incidence of intraoperative complications in our series (0.5%) is most likely a result of almost all tracheostomies being performed by or under the direction of a few pediatric surgeons who are otolaryngologic, general or cardiothoracic surgeons. Almost all were performed with a controlled airway, usually an endotracheal tube. This permits a safe general anesthetic and is helpful in identifying the trachea, which tends to be less rigid in children than in adults. Meticulous attention is paid to hemostasis, and careful dissection in the midline can avoid such complications as pneumothorax. Once the trachea is identified, stay sutures are placed on either side of the midline to provide easy access to the trachea postoperatively if decannulation or tube obstruction should occur. A vertical incision through one or two tracheal rings is made between the stay sutures. In older children, particularly adolescents, an inferiorly based flap is frequently employed. After the endotracheal tube is withdrawn to a level just above the operative site, the tracheostomy is placed and secured. The skin incision is closed only partially to prevent pneumomediastinum or subcutaneous emphysema. The endotracheal tube is not completely removed until the tracheostomy tube is well secured and bilateral auscultation of the lungs reveals good breath sounds. A postoperative chest radiograph is obtained either in the operating room or in the intensive care unit. The tracheostomy tube is changed routinely at the end of the first week by a member of the operative team. The patient remains in the intensive care unit

TABLE 7. PRIMARY DIAGNOSES IN NONTRACHESTOMY-RELATED DEATHS (N = 115)*

Congenital heart disease	33	(29%)
Miscellaneous disorders	29	(25%)
CNS disorders	27	(23%)
Respiratory distress syndrome	18	(16%)
Upper airway obstruction	8	(7%)

*Five patients with two or more diagnoses.

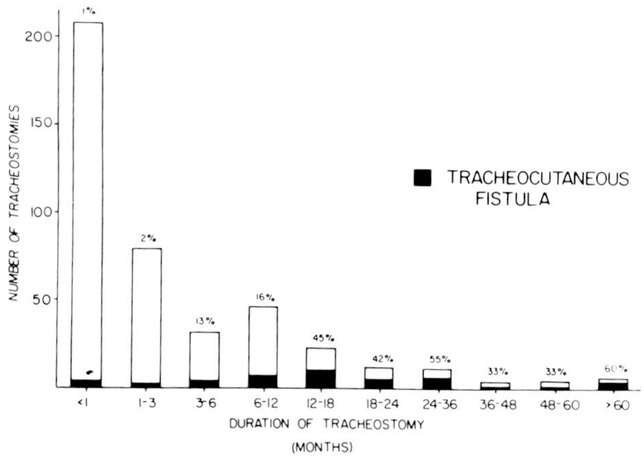

Fig. 4. Incidence of tracheocutaneous fistulas and duration of trachestomies (n = 420).

for monitoring at least through the first tube change or longer if indicated by the general medical condition.

Contrary to most other series[1,5,7,9] in which pneumothorax and pneumomediastinum were the most frequent early complications, our most common early complication was accidental decannulation followed by pneumonia. Pneumothorax is reported to occur more often in infants and younger children; our results paralleled those of Bridges et al[3] which showed a slightly higher incidence in older children. Inclusion of pneumonia as an early complication is controversial since the process may have preceded the tracheostomy. We included only those postoperative cases of pneumonia that were not clinically or radiographically evident prior to the tracheostomy as early complications.

The most frequent late complication, persistent tracheocutaneous fistula, occurred in a direct relationship to the duration of tracheostomy; approximately half of the tracheostomies of more than 1 year's duration developed a fistula (Fig. 4). Oliver et al[1] also reported a significant incidence of tracheocutaneous fistula after decannulation. Accidental decannulation was the second most common late complication and the most common overall complication. In most cases of tracheal hemorrhage, the etiology was uncertain. Several cases accompanied abnormal clotting, usually in the presence of overwhelming sepsis. In only one case was postoperative bleeding a result of operative technique, ie, a vein which required ligation. There was one occurrence of massive hemorrhage, presumably an innominate artery rupture, which resulted in the death of a patient.

As noted by Gaudet et al,[9] infants with RDS had a higher incidence of complications. Children with upper airway disease also sustained more morbidity, while there appeared to be fewer problems in cardiothoracic patients, contrary to other series.[9] The higher incidence of late complications in younger age groups has also been noted by other authors.[1,9]

Our overall mortality rate is comparable to those of other series,[1,6] while tracheostomy-related deaths are slightly fewer than most other series. As noted by Tucker and Silberman,[5] accidental decannulation and tube obstruction are the most common causes of tracheostomy-related deaths. Recently, all children, either hospitalized or at home and with critical airways, have been provided with airway occlusion or cardiac monitors to prevent asphyxia in the event of accidental decannulation or tube obstruction.

In nontracheostomy-related deaths, mortality is a function of the severity of the underlying illness. Patients with cardiac and CNS disorders and congenital anomalies (miscellaneous disorders) demonstrated high rates while craniofacial patients and those with upper airway obstruction had significantly lower rates.

Children with long-term tracheostomies, especially those associated with prolonged ventilation, present difficult management problems. There are currently several children who have spent most, if not all, of their lives hospitalized for prolonged ventilation or tracheostomy care. With intensive instruction, monitoring, and humidification and suctioning equipment, home care of children with tracheostomy can be successful. While half (four) of the tracheostomy-related deaths occurred at home and were due to accidental decannulation or tube obstruction, most occurred prior to the increased availability of airway occlusion monitors. Our home ventilator program has also provided an alternative to continuous hospitalization in patients who require only respiratory support.[15]

In addition to the complications previously described, speech and swallowing difficulties in children with tracheostomies have also been recognized as significant long-term problems. Our experience has revealed that speech therapy is beneficial in assisting the child's normal language development.[16] A communication disorders clinic has been established at Children's Hospital of Philadelphia to help monitor and treat these problems.

CONCLUSION

Pediatric tracheostomy during the past decade has been subject to changes brought on by improvements within pediatric medicine. The decrease in incidence of tracheostomy reflects an increase in the use of endotracheal intubation. The increase in duration of tracheostomy and decrease in age are a result of improvements in survival of infants with RDS and other children with chronic and complicated primary disease. With good operative technique, operative complications can be minimal. Postoperative complications frequently mirror the complexity of the child's overall medical care. While these complications have a significant incidence, related mortality can be limited both in the hospital and at home with good training and the proper equipment, especially humidification and monitoring.

ACKNOWLEDGMENT — We would like to acknowledge the assistance of Vera Rogers in the collection of medical records and Dottie Archer in the preparation of the manuscript.

REFERENCES

1. Oliver P, Richardson JR, Clubb RW, Flake CG. Tracheostomy in children. N Engl J Med 1962; 267:631-7.

2. Holinger PH, Brown WT, Maurizi DG. Tracheostomy in the newborn. Am J Surg 1965; 109:771-9.

3. Bridges CP, Ryan RF, Longenecker CG, Vincent RW. Tracheostomy in children: a twenty-year study at Charity Hospital in New Orleans. Plast Reconstr Surg 1966; 37:117-20.

4. Hatcher CR, Abbott OA, Logan WD, Patterson JH. Tracheostomy in infancy and childhood. South Med J 1967; 60:411-5.

5. Tucker JA, Silberman HD. Tracheotomy in pediatrics. Ann Otol Rhinol Laryngol 1972; 81:818-24.

6. Hawkins DB, Williams EH. Trachoestomy in infants and young children. Laryngoscope 1976; 86:331-40.

7. Perrotta RJ, Schley WS. Pediatric tracheotomy: a five-year comparison study. Arch Otolaryngol 1978; 104:318-21.

8. Palva A, Jokinen K, Niemela T. Tracheostomy in children. Arch Otolaryngol 1975; 101:536-9.

9. Gaudet PT, Peerless A, Sasaki CT, Kirchner JA. Pediatric tracheostomy and associated complications. Laryngoscope 1978; 88:1633-41.

10. Chew JY, Cantrell RW. Tracheostomy: complications and management. Arch Otolaryngol 1972; 96:538-45.

11. Sarasohn C. Care of the very small premature infant. Pediatr Clin North Am 1977; 24:619-32.

12. Bruce DA, Schut L, Bruno LA, Wood JH, Sutton LN. Outcome following severe head injuries in children. J Neurosurg 1978; 48:679-88.

13. Bruce DA. Current management of pediatric brain tumors. Curr Concepts Oncol 1982; 4:21-7.

14. Handler SD, Beaugard ME, Whitaker LA, Potsic WP. Airway management in the repair of craniofacial defects. Cleft Palate J 1979; 16:16-23.

15. Ziegler MM, Shaw S, Goldberg AI, Kettrick R, Koop CE. Sequlae of prolonged ventilatory support for pediatric surgical patients. J Pediatr Surg 1979; 14:768-72.

16. Simon B, Handler SD. The speech pathologist and management of children with tracheostomy. J Otolaryngol 1981; 10:440-8.

HOME CARE OF THE PEDIATRIC PATIENT WITH A TRACHEOTOMY

R. J. RUBEN, MD
L. NEWTON, MD
D. JORNSAY, RN, PNP
R. STEIN, MD
H. CHAMBERS, MD
J. LIQUORI, CSW
C. LAWRENCE, MA, RN
BRONX, NEW YORK

Forty-seven infants and children with tracheotomies were cared for at home for a follow-up period of 1,581 months. There were two relevant fatalities which gave a death rate of 0.13 deaths per 100 months. The average age at the time of tracheotomy was 13 months and the tracheotomy was in place for an average of 33 months per patient. The ability to care for these children was provided through coordinated, intensive training and a home-care program in which the inpatient nurse, nurse practitioner, social worker, pediatrician, and otorhinolaryngologist worked as a team.

INTRODUCTION

The care of infants and children with tracheotomies presents a special problem to the family and the clinician. There are large numbers of infants and children who undergo tracheotomies and who have no other deficits which would require their continued hospitalization. The safety and feasibility of discharging these infants to their homes, or to other care institutions, is a subject upon which there are few reports.[1-4] The present report is a retrospective study of all of the infants and children discharged from The Hospital of the Albert Einstein College of Medicine (HAECOM) with tracheotomies in place between January 1, 1970, and December 31, 1981. It presents information concerning epidemiology, mortality, home-care management and the implications of long-term tracheotomy.

The management of these infants and children requires the coordination of a number of health providers including the pediatric otorhinolaryngologist, pediatrician, inpatient and outpatient nursing services and social workers. The relationship of the health-care providers and the family is felt to be a most important factor in the successful care of these patients. There have been a few reports on the social and medical support service needs for the home care of infants and children with tracheotomies.[3,5]

METHOD

All the patients under the age of 12 discharged from HAECOM with tracheotomies from Jan 1, 1970, to Dec 31, 1981, were reviewed. Information was obtained from chart analysis. In addition, parents of children who had not been seen within the preceding 12 months were contacted for further follow-up information. The records of the monthly reviews of home care of infants and children with tracheotomies were also utilized in obtaining the information presented in this report. All statistics include the total time during the study when the children had their tracheotomies in place.

The children were cared for at home in two different programs. Approximately half of the children resided within the geographic confines of the pediatric home care (PHC) program previously described[6,7] as an ambulatory special care unit. The remaining children resided outside the geographic area of the PHC program and were cared for by local pediatricians, visiting home nurses and, in some instances, services of the regional Departments of Health.

RESULTS

For the period studied, 47 infants and children were identified who had tracheotomies in place and were cared for at home or in residential institutions. The average number of months with tracheotomies in place as of Dec 31, 1981, was 33 months. There were 12 cases in which tracheotomies were in place from 0 to 12 months, 16 cases from 13 to 24 months, 4 cases from 25 to 36 months, and 15 cases which had the tracheotomies in place for greater than 37 months. The average time for follow-up, as of Dec 31, 1981, with or without tracheotomies was 38 months. There were 11 cases followed for 1 to 12 months, 11 cases from 13 to 24 months, 8 cases from 25 to 36 months, and 17 cases that were followed for greater than 36 months. The total time with tracheotomies in place was 1,581 months or 132 years; and with or without tracheotomy tubes in place there were 1,826 months or 152 years of follow-up. The average age at which the child received the tracheotomy was three months. There were 37 children who had their tracheotomies done from 0 to 12 months of age; 4 children from 13 to 24 months of age; 2 children from 25 to 36 months of age; and 4 children who had tracheotomies put in place at ages greater than 36 months of age. There were 35 boys and 12 girls. The etiologies for the

From the Departments of Otorhinolaryngology (Ruben, Newton), Pediatrics (Stein, Chambers), Nursing (Lawrence), and Social Service (Liquori), Albert Einstein College of Medicine of Yeshiva University and Montefiore Hospital and Medical Center; and the Department of Nursing, Bronx Municipal Hospital Center (Jornsay).

Presented at the meeting of the American Broncho-Esophagological Association, Palm Beach, Florida, May 3-4, 1982.

REPRINTS — R. J. Ruben, MD, Department of Otolaryngology, Albert Einstein College of Medicine, 1300 Morris Park Avenue, Bronx, NY 10461.

TABLE 1. ETIOLOGY

Acquired subglottic stenosis	18
Congenital subglottis stenosis	8
Subglottic stenosis*	3
Hemangioma	8
Papillomata	3
Other	7
Tracheomalacia & granuloma	
Vocal cord paralysis	
Cricoarytenoid fixation	
Laryngeal cleft	
Cystic hygroma	
Unknown	
Total	47

*Insufficient information to determine whether stenosis was congenital or acquired.

TABLE 2. DAYS IN HOSPITAL AFTER TRACHEOTOMY

No. of Days	*No. of Cases*
7-14	4
15-21	8
22-28	3
29-35	2
36-42	1
>42	4
Total	22

Average no. of days — 30.

Tracheotomies (22) performed at HAECOM; data not available on those performed at other institutions.

tracheotomies are detailed in Table 1. Over one half (29 of 47) of the children had their tracheotomies for either acquired or congenital subglottic stenosis. The average length of hospital stay for those children who had tracheotomies performed at HAECOM was 30 days (Table 2). Several of these children had prolonged hospital stays because of either medical or social problems that prevented their discharges within three weeks of the placement of the tracheotomy tubes. The mean age at discharge for these 22 patients was five months (Table 3), and 21 out of 22 were less than 12 months of age at the time of discharge.

At the time of this survey (Dec 31, 1981), 27 had the tracheotomies in place, 14 were decannulated, 3 were dead and the status of 3 of the children was unknown. The cause of death in one child was neurological disease, the other two deaths occurred at home one to three days after an endoscopic procedure was performed. Autopsies were obtained in both cases and did not show any occlusion of the airways below the tracheotomies. The autopsy revealed neurological disease in both children. One child had a total occlusion of the subglottis and the other had a 2-mm opening in the subglottic space. In this study both of these deaths are considered to be airway-related.

Five of the patients had total occlusion of their airways proximal to the tracheotomy tubes for various periods of time; 2 for one month; 1 for one year; 1 for two years and 1 for more than three years. One child died having had total occlusion for one month.

Repeat tracheotomies were needed in 3 of the 47 children (all statistics include the total time during the study when the children had their tracheotomies in place). These three children developed severe respiratory distress after upper respiratory infections and needed to have their tracheotomy tubes put back in place. The underlying pathology was acquired subglottic stenosis (one case), congenital subglottic stenosis (one case), and supraglottic hemangioma (one case). One of these children was accidently decannulated at home, another was decannulated early because of social problems and the third was decannulated as the hemangioma appeared to have regressed and was no longer impinging on the airway.

Data was available concerning the living status of 44 of the 47 children, as 3 children were lost to follow-up: 3 were dead; 38 of the remaining 41 children were at home; and 3 were in institutions, 2 because of severe central neurological diseases and 1 was a quadriplegic.

All of the six children who had tracheotomies in place and were born before June 1, 1975, that is, who were older than $6^1/_2$ years and who should have been in school, and for whom information was available, were in school. Five of the 6 were in regular schools and 1 was in a special school because of mental retardation.

DISCUSSION

The information presented reveals that it is possible to care at home successfully for infants and children with tracheotomies. The mortality reported in this study is compared with a previously published study in which data was collected from a number of different institutions[4] (Table 4). The present study differs in a number of ways from the previous studies and shows a significant decrease in the death rate, from 1.81/100 months of tracheot-

TABLE 3. AGE AT DISCHARGE FROM HAECOM AFTER TRACHEOTOMY

Age (mo)	*No. of Cases*
1	1
2	3
3	5
4	1
5	4
6	2
7	3
8	1
9	0
10	1
11	0
12	0
13	0
14	1
Total	22

Average no. of months — 5.

TABLE 4. MORTALITY RATE

	Present Study	*Previous Study*[4]
Children	47	38
Months tracheotomy in place	1581	332
Tracheotomy deaths	0	2
Unknown deaths	2	4
Deaths (%)	4	16
Death rate per 100 tracheotomy months	0.13	1.81

omy home care to 0.13/100 months of tracheotomy home care. The data in the present study shows that the patients were able to be discharged from the hospital an average of 30 days after the tracheotomies were performed. In cases without other medical and social problems, the children could be discharged within 2 to 3 weeks.

The two deaths, which were considered for this study to be due to airway failure, occurred in children with neurological disease, total or almost total subglottic occlusion, shortly after an endoscopic procedure. These three factors should be assessed in the future care of these children. It may have been possible to prevent these deaths by retaining these children in the hospital with monitoring for a few days after the procedure or by instituting a more rigorous monitoring system at home for the first few days after the procedure.

The ability to discharge children from the hospital and care for them at home, to integrate them into the family, to arrange attendance at regular school, and to provide for their continued care is based upon a program of home care which begins in the hospital. This program of home care is dependent upon the management by and coordination of a number of health providers including the pediatric otorhinolaryngologist, the pediatrician, inpatient and outpatient nursing services and social workers. The relationship between the health care providers and the family is a most important factor for the successful care of these patients.

The experience of 11 years of home management of children with tracheotomies shows that the situation in which the child is hospitalized in the intensive care unit or is placed close to the nurse's station for necessary observation intensifies the difficulty of hospital-to-home care transition for the family. Unfortunately, this required level of hospital care reinforces fears regarding the parents' abilities to care for the child at home. The large majority of parents are able to overcome these fears; however, there are some children for whom the possibility of home management does not exist, either because of the social situation or overwhelming fear on the part of the parents. For these children, placement in a chronic care facility may be the only reasonable alternative. Only one child of our group who could have been at home was placed in a chronic care facility. This child remained in the chronic care facility for two years and was then accepted into the home.

Due to the difficulty of transition from hospital to home, work begins with the child and the family on an inpatient service in which parents are helped to understand why the tracheotomy was needed, and instruction is begun on how to care for the child with a tracheotomy. When parents understand the reason for the tracheotomy, they are better able to learn how to care for the child.[8] Lengthy discussions and explanations, usually augmented with diagrams, are needed. Explaining the etiology of the problem to the parents is the responsibility of the pediatric otorhinolaryngologist and pediatrician. The social worker assesses the family's needs and resources, works out the mechanisms to obtain necessary equipment at home and provides psychological support for the family. Initial instruction on tracheotomy site care, postural drainage, suctioning and then tracheotomy tube changes is given by the inpatient nursing and medical staff and is coordinated with the nurse who will follow the child after discharge. A teaching check-list is used which documents when a procedure was taught, when it was reinforced, when the parents or caretakers were able to demonstrate that they had gained proficiency in the care. This check-list includes basic knowledge of the anatomy and physiology appropriate to the patient, use of humidification, the parts of the tracheotomy tube, the cleaning of the inner cannula, peristomal care, the use of the suction, the change of the tracheotomy ribbon, the change of the tracheotomy tube, emergency procedures, the availability of contacting community support, including the Visiting Nurse Service, Home Care, Public Health Nurse and the local utilities and local ambulance, the use of the portable suction and saline instillation. Cardiopulmonary resuscitation from mouth to tracheotomy stoma is taught. If the child is old enough and has appropriate social maturity (between 5 and 6 years), he or she is involved in the instruction.

At least two family members are taught tracheotomy care. These are usually both parents, and whenever possible a third person with whom the child is familiar and comfortable and with whom the parents can leave the child, is also instructed.

Prior to discharge, supplies are ordered. These supplies consist of a portable suction machine, a de Lee trap for emergency suction, Kelly clamps, a spare tracheotomy tube, tracheotomy care kits, tracheotomy suction kits, hydrogen peroxide, sterile saline in liter bottles and syringes for saline instillation. The parents are advised to keep a list of where these materials can be ordered and to keep at least a two-week supply on hand. A home visit is made by the Visiting Nurse Service or the Home Care Service to help the parents set up the equipment. Equipment is arranged in the room where the child will sleep

TABLE 5. THE CHILD WITH A TRACHEOTOMY MANAGEMENT HINTS A GUIDE FOR PARENTS

Home Environment
1. Keep all tracheotomy care equipment in one place.
2. Keep dusty items away from the child.
3. Humidify the room if you use an air-conditioner.
4. Instruct a "sitter" in tracheotomy care.

Bathing and Hair Washing
1. Do not leave the child alone in the tub.
2. For hair washing — place the child on his or her back on the vanity or kitchen counter, his or her head hanging over the sink.

Clothing
1. No turtleneck shirts.
2. No fabric that sheds.

Feeding
1. Prevent food or liquids from entering the tracheotomy.
2. Suction the child and do tracheotomy cleaning before feeding the child.

Traveling
1. Bring a deLee suction with you for short trips (store, doctor's office). For long trips take your battery-powered suction, replacement tube, suction and cleaning equipment.

Report the Following to the Otolaryngologist:
1. Change in color or consistency or odor of mucus.
2. Skin breakdown around the stoma.
3. Child's admittance to the hospital.

Emergency Telephone Numbers
1. Otolaryngologist
2. Pediatrician
3. Local hospital
4. Local police, fire, or rescue squad, depending on which has the equipment and personnel to aid with resuscitation
5. Utility company
6. Neighbor

within easy reach of the child's bed or crib. Several electrical outlets and sufficient current to support two appliances concurrently are needed. The suction pump should be plugged in at all times and a humidifier kept in the room in which the child spends the main part of his or her time. A sterile tracheotomy tube and scissors are taped at the head of the child's bed; for a toddler, these are taped on the outside of the crib out of the child's reach. The safety of the child at home with a tracheotomy is paramount, so families are always taught to keep an extra tracheotomy tube available.

It is desirable for parents to stay in the hospital with the child and to participate in and ultimately to provide the child's tracheotomy care there, especially a few days before the child is ready to be discharged. After the equipment is in place at home, arrangements are made so the child may spend a few hours there. Passes home have been found to relieve anxiety a great deal and are useful in helping all involved to anticipate and raise questions and concerns. In some institutions the child is allowed to go home on an overnight pass prior to actual discharge. When this is not possible arrangements are made for the mother to sleep-in and care for the child in the hospital overnight if she has not already done so.

Usually children are discharged at the beginning of the week so families are somewhat comfortable by their first weekend. The parents are given the home phone numbers of the nurse, pediatrician, pediatric otorhinolaryngologist, and nearest hospital emergency room. These phone numbers, along with the numbers of the ambulance service and fire department, are permanently posted adjacent to the phone for easy accessibility in an emergency. The local power company and fire department are notified that a child with life-sustaining equipment is living in the area so that provisions can be made in the event of a power failure. Some centers recommend sending children home with an Ambu bag, but this has not been our policy. It is important, however, for the family to have and to know how to use deLee suctioning traps. The parents are given a short guide for home care of the patient (Table 5) and a copy of *A Guide to Pediatric Tracheostomy Care.*[5]

At the time of discharge, several family members are competent in giving tracheotomy stoma care and suctioning. Although they have all been taught to change the tracheotomy tube, parents tend to be much more fearful of this procedure when they are outside the protected environment of the hospital. An initial home visit is made on the day of discharge, and daily if needed, until the family is comfortable with the procedure. At these visits, the parents demonstrate their suctioning techniques. Emphasis is placed on hand washing before beginning care of the tracheotomy. While in the hospital parents are taught sterile technique; in the home, clean technique has been found sufficient for preventing infection.

When teaching or reviewing suctioning procedure the importance of positioning the child with the neck hyperextended is emphasized. The inner cannula is removed prior to suctioning. Suction catheters are always tested with a small amount of normal saline prior to being inserted. Depending on the moisture of the secretions, instillation of sterile water may be required. Generally 0.5 to 1 cc of sterile water is sufficient. If the child has difficulty coughing or bringing up secretions, deeper suctioning may be needed. The suction catheter is inserted until it meets resistance. The child is suctioned with the head turned first to one side and then to the other. No suction is applied until the catheter is being withdrawn. The catheter is rotated as it is withdrawn. The amount of time for each aspiration should not exceed five seconds. The child should be suctioned until the catheter return is clear; the child will need a rest period between aspirations. The suction catheter should be cleared of mucus between aspirations. After the child appears comfortable and free of mucus, the suction catheter should be cleared of mucus. Catheters can be cleaned with soap and hot water and stored for reuse in a clean jar. During the entire procedure the child must be observed closely for any signs of respiratory distress.

Cardiopulmonary resuscitation and the emergency phone numbers are reviewed on the initial home visit.

Ideally the tracheotomy tube should be changed daily to minimize granulation tissue. The absolute frequency, however, will be dependent on the parents' level of expertise and comfort with the procedure. This procedure may require two people, one to position and hold the child and the other to change the tube. Initially, tracheotomy site care should be performed, the inner cannula removed, and the child suctioned. The new sterile tracheotomy tube with clean ties should be ready with the obturator in place. With the child held with the head hyperextended, the tracheotomy ties are cut and the tube is held in place. One hand removes the dirty tracheotomy tube, while the other hands holds the clean one ready for insertion. The obturator is removed immediately once the clean tube is inserted and the clean inner cannula is replaced. To tie the tracheotomy, the child's head should be flexed forward onto the chest. There should be room for one adult finger between the ties and the neck. Finally the ties are tied with at least a triple knot.

If the child is sent home with parents who have been taught and know the procedure for changing the tracheotomy tube but are too fearful to do this alone, the home care nurse works toward a gradual increase in parental independence. Initially she helps the mother, then stands next to her while she does it, then in the next room. This gradual increase of parental responsibility enables even the most fearful parent, within a few weeks, to change the tracheotomy tube independently.

When the inner cannula is removed prior to suctioning, it should be placed in a solution of one-half strength hydrogen peroxide and water. It should not be left in the solution for longer than three minutes or it will blacken. The lumen of the inner cannula should be well cleaned with either pipe cleaners or gauze prior to being sterilized.

Tracheotomy tubes are sterilized by placing them in boiling water and being boiled for 15 minutes. They are then removed and stored in a clean towel. If the suction bottle itself develops an odor, it can be cleaned with alcohol in addition to the usual soap and water. There is no need to purchase sterile water and normal saline. These solutions are easily made at home. Normal saline is made by mixing 2 tsp of table salt with 0.95 L (1 qt) of sterile water which is then labeled and stored.

When traveling outside the home the child should wear a bib made from a triangularly folded handkerchief to protect the open tracheotomy, and the parent should carry an emergency kit which contains several portable deLee mucus traps, a scissors, an extra tracheotomy tube, and forceps to keep the stoma open.

Other factors in home safety include making sure the nebulizer gives cold rather than a hot mist to prevent the possibility of scalding, screening the environment of the infant or toddler for any small objects which could be inserted into the tracheotomy tube, and watching young siblings for "trach play." Powders, aerosols, fine animal hair and cigarette smoke are all irritating to the tracheotomy and should be avoided. When bathing the child or washing his or her hair, parents must be careful to keep water from entering the tracheotomy tube. If any water gets directly into the tracheotomy tube, the child should be suctioned immediately. Restrictive clothing such as turtlenecks should not be worn.

The most common complication encountered by parents is partial or complete obstruction of the tracheotomy site with symptoms of fright, restlessness, clammy skin, tachypnea, nasal flaring, and, if allowed to progress, frank cyanosis. Parents should be taught how to handle this situation initially by suctioning and then removing the inner cannula. This will frequently remove the mucus plug. If the parents are unable to dislodge the plug by suctioning, they should make sure the child's neck is hyperextended, and stimulate a cough by instilling up to 1 cc of sterile water into the tracheotomy tube. They must continue to suction and stimulate coughing and never leave the child alone. If unsuccessful, they should change the tracheotomy tube and be prepared to call the ambulance should this fail to alleviate the problem.

Another complication is displacement of the tracheotomy tube. If the tracheotomy tube is displaced or comes out partially, it should be reinserted and tightened. When it comes out completely, a new sterile tracheotomy tube should be reinserted when available; if unavailable, the old one should be reinserted. This situation is likely to be frightening both to the parent and child, making tracheotomy tube insertion difficult, but if the parent can remain calm, the child will relax and reinsertion of the tube will be easier. In the event that the parent is unable to reinsert the tube, someone should stay with the child while an ambulance is called. Speaking to parents about this specific problem in advance, and even role-playing the situation, can be helpful to parents in preparing them to remain calm should the actual problem arise.

Respiratory distress may occur secondary to a number of causes. The parents should be taught to observe for dyspnea, orthopnea, retractions, nasal flaring, tachypnea, and cyanosis. When tachypnea occurs parents should observe level of activity and the presence of any fever. True tachypnea or any of the other signs of respiratory distress warrant immediate investigation by the doctor or nurse.

Children with tracheotomies appear to be more susceptible to respiratory infections than the average child. Parents should be told that when the child has an infection, the secretions may become thicker and change in color. The secretions may also develop an odor. The child is also more likely to require suctioning more often than usual. Postural drainage is also an important aspect of treatment of the children with upper and lower respiratory infections. Children with tracheotomies also contract other common episodic illnesses of childhood. Parents need to learn fever control, the importance of suctioning after any vomiting episode, and postural drainage. The parents are instructed to call the nurse or the doctor for any temperature greater than 38.3°C (101°F) or any change in the nature of tracheal secretions.

Bleeding is another complication that is very frightening to parents. If the "bleeding" is pink-tinged mucus without any other symptoms of illness, anxiety may be reduced if parents are informed that this may result from increased frequency or vigor of suctioning. When irritation of the trachea is suspected, review of suctioning procedures and especially catheter rotation during suctioning is undertaken with the parent. Any bright red mucus or prolonged bleeding warrants immediate medical attention.

A common parental concern regarding a child with a tracheotomy is the issue of speech. Most children with tracheotomies have a sufficient airway to allow some air to pass through the vocal cords and thereby to produce sound. Parents may initially hear babies produce some sound with crying, then babbling and eventually talking. Toddlers quickly learn to cover the hole in their tracheotomies with their chins or fingers to make a noise. Unless the child has an associated hearing loss, he will develop some speech. Children with complete upper airway obstruction and hence without the ability to transmit air through their larynges must be handled with special techniques.[9,10]

Although parents are concerned about speaking, the more major problem in the area of communication is the fear that the child will be unable to summon help. This is especially true of the infant or young child. For this reason, parents are advised to tie a bell around the child's ankle. A child in respiratory distress will not lie quietly, but rather will thrash about, thereby "ringing" for help. The older child can be given a squeeze horn, squeeze toy or a bell.

The fear of the child's inability to call for help and the increased risk of infection causes the parents of children with tracheotomies to live with nearly constant reminders of their child's vulnerability. Even when they understand the medical cause, parents often cannot understand why or how this particular misfortune has happened to their child, so they review all the events of the pregnancy, and/or the child's birth and infancy looking for any possible cause. In the two-parent family, they may accuse one another and it is the role of the primary care provider to help the family maintain a realistic medical appraisal of the situation. It is very important, therefore, to give new information regarding prognosis or outcome of procedures to both parents together whenever possible, so that one parent is not put in the role of being the messenger of bad news.

Parents fear that such things as smoking or not taking vitamins during pregnancy caused or contributed to their child's problem. This almost universal guilt, plus the feeling of responsibility for the child's airway, exacerbate any pre-existing family problems to the point that they may require intervention. It is helpful for medical providers to understand that this is a potential effect of having a tracheotomy in a family.

The fear of their child's inability to communicate is perhaps the single most disruptive force in the family. Parents anticipate their child having respiratory distress at night and being unable to call for help, and will therefore sleep in shifts or not at all. In addition to the changes in sleeping patterns, there is frequently also a change in sleeping arrangements and physical reorganization of space. Many times the child who was previously sleeping in his or her own crib or bed in another room is moved into the parents' room. Commonly, the father is displaced from the bed, or the room, and the child may begin sleeping with the mother. As one might well imagine, this is all very disruptive to the parents' sexual relationship.

Although we have not done a statistical survey, we feel we should note that during our 11 years' experience of home management of children with tracheotomies, we have observed a relatively high incidence of fathers leaving the home at least temporarily after the child with the tracheotomy returned home from the hospital.

Many working mothers leave their job to care for the child with a tracheotomy; this exacerbates the financial burdens imposed upon the family. In addition to the direct medical expenses, there are the expenses of days lost from work for the parent who continues to work. There are also numerous direct and indirect medical expenses, such as transportation to and from the hospital, meals while in the hospital, and babysitters for the children at home.

Another source of parental anxiety and guilt is the risk of anesthesia to which their child is repeatedly subjected for endoscopic procedures. This situation is compounded if these treatments involve an overnight admission, rather than a stay in the one-day unit. Parents also must handle the problem of the child's fear concerning his or her repeated hospitalization.

The child with a tracheotomy will usually decrease the mobility of the members of the family. This will also serve to create a realignment of the family. There is less available time for self, spouse and siblings and an overinvestment in and overprotectiveness of the one "sick" child. The entire family starts to expect all the attention to be focused on the child with the tracheotomy and family members may resent the lack of available time. The child with the tracheotomy becomes cast in his or her "sick" role, exempted from normal social responsibilities and expectations. The school-age child, for example, does not do the dishes or go to camp, or the younger child can't go to preschool because he or she is "sick." If this is allowed to continue, the child is put into a dilemma. The child knows that he or she should want to get well, but sees the advantages and secondary gains of being sick, and also bears tremendous guilt. He or she is the reason why the family can't have a pet or must move closer to the hospital. The child also feels the burden of the responsibility placed on the siblings. One school-age child with a tracheotomy related that his father would not allow his year-older sister to hit him because if he cried he would produce more mucus. The child was most distressed by the fact that he could hit his sister and get away with it, but the same rules did not apply to his older sister. He perceived this as more responsibility than he wanted.

While the sick role has implications for the child with the tracheotomy, there are also overwhelming implications of the tracheotomy on the child's well siblings. The siblings feel anger and jealousy at their "sick" sibling and guilt for their anger, for being healthy, and for their fantasies in which they are certain they caused their sibling to need a tracheotomy. Many manifest fears about "catching" the disease that necessitated the tracheotomy. They are often unable to talk about these fears or frustrations or anger. When people within the family are unable to speak about their feelings or concerns about the tracheotomy, an enlarging circle of dangerous subjects develops which cannot be spoken about because it is feared that they will trigger a discussion about the dreaded topic. This is especially true regarding sibling and parental fears that the child will die.

In any family there is a great amount of competition among siblings for parental attention. Siblings of children with tracheotomies usually try to win back some parental attention by initially being the best child or best sibling to the sick child. Some as young as three years old have learned to help their mothers with tracheotomy-site care and suctioning. If the siblings are unsuccessful at being the best child, they may attempt to gain parental attention by having something worse, being more sick, having frequent accidents, etc. Older siblings experience the increased burdens of babysitting and, in bilingual families, of translating for their non-English-speaking parents. Frequently, the older sibling is responsible for the management of the household while the parents are in the hospital with the child with a tracheotomy and are thus prematurely forced into adult roles.

Babysitting also presents a problem. The babysitter must be someone with whom the child is comfortable as well as someone who is able to suction, knows cardiopulmonary resuscitation and is able to respond to an emergency. Unfortunately, many families deal with this problem by never going out or leaving the child with a babysitter. In order to avert this problem, parents should be encouraged to teach other family members or close friends. Another resolution is the use of a homemaker or skilled nurse to relieve the parents for short periods of time. The most viable solution to this problem, however, seems to come from alliances between parents of children with tracheotomies who can exchange babysitting services and feel comfortable that their child is being left with someone competent to provide the necessary care.

The lack of available school programs for children with tracheotomies has presented a problem to almost all parents. Generally, schools will not permit a child with a tracheotomy in the classroom unless there is a full-time registered nurse in attendance. This nursing situation exists in New York City only in programs for multihandicapped children. For nonmentally handicapped school-age children there are several other alternatives: 1) home tutoring, which is definitely inadequate for purposes of socialization and generally inadequate educationally because the time is so limited; 2) parent or guardian accompaniment in the classroom, which is not a feasible alternative for families with younger children and a questionable alternative from the perspective of socialization as well; or 3) special arrangements whereby the parent assumes responsibility for the tracheotomy by being "on call" to the school in case of an emergency. This seems to be the most workable solution although it is only feasible for the child who can cough up secretions easily, is able to remove his or her own inner cannula if needed, and lives relatively near the school. In this situation, the child should carry a clean inner cannula with him or her at all times.

The child with a tracheotomy is as much in need of recreational services as his or her normal peers. A camp experience is a particularly good way of meeting this need and giving the child an opportunity to be independent of the parents' usual overprotectiveness. Some sleep-away camps for children with a chronic disease exist that are properly staffed and are willing to take a child with a tracheotomy. Here the child may have the opportunity to experience some independence and take part in normal camp activities without the stigma of being the only one with a health condition or other chronic disease, and thereby may gain a different perspective of himself or herself.

The stress imposed on the family by the tracheotomy often requires the intervention of social work services for counseling and assistance obtaining financial support. The availability of these services on an outpatient basis is quite limited.

Although many aspects of the home management of the child with a tracheotomy are problematic, they are outweighed by the benefits to the child and family. The primary benefit of involvement of family members in the treatment plan is that it minimizes the inherent impact of the tracheotomy by preserving the basic family structure and by providing the child with a supportive environment which fosters acceptance of the child and his or her condition by the family.

CONCLUSION

Infants and children with tracheotomies in this home care program have a low mortality rate. The most important element in the maintenance of a safe and effective home-care program is the availability of otolaryngic, nursing, pediatric and social service support for the training of the parents, and continued monitoring and care of the child. An intensive, planned, coordinated parental training and home-care program is felt to be a major factor in the low mortality reported in this series.

REFERENCES

1. Foster S, Hoskins D. Home care of a child with a tracheotomy tube. Pediatr Clin North Am 1981; 28:855-7.

2. Funel AE, Putnam JS. Patients with tracheostomies: goals of management. Primary Care 1978; 5:557.

3. Kaler J, Kaler H. Michael had a tracheotomy. Am J Nurs 1974; 74:852-5.

4. Okamoto E, Fee WE Jr, Boles R, et al. Safety of hospitals vs. home care of infant tracheotomies. Trans Am Acad Ophthal mol Otolaryngol 1977; 84:92-9.

5. Amado P. A guide to pediatric tracheostomy care. Springfield, Ill: Charles C Thomas, 1981.

6 Stein REK. Pediatric home care: an ambulatory special care unit. J Pediatr 1978; 92:495-9.

7. Stein REK. A special home care unit for care of chronically ill children. In: Bryce M, Lloyd JC, eds. Treating families in the home: an alternative to placement. Springfield, Ill: Charles C Thomas, 1981:313-26.

8. McCormick RM, Gelson-Parkavich TJ. Patient and family education, tools, techniques and theory. New York: John Wiley & Sons, Inc, 1979.

9. Kaslon K, Grabo D, Ruben RJ. Voice speech and language habilitation in young children without laryngeal function. Arch Otolaryngol 1978; 104:737-9.

10. Tucker HM, Rusnov M, Cohen L. Speech development in aphonic children. Laryngoscope 1982 (in press).

BRONCHOSCOPIC LIMITED LAVAGE FOR CYSTIC FIBROSIS PATIENTS

AN ADJUNCT TO THERAPY

BRUCE F. ROTHMANN, MD
ROBERT T. STONE, MD
LEWIS H. WALKER, MD
FRANCOIS W. SEGUIN, MD

AKRON, OHIO

Bronchoscopic aspiration of the tracheobronchial tree in patients with cystic fibrosis is a controversial procedure. Results of therapy are difficult to evaluate. Many different techniques have been described, adding to the confusion. Our experience using limited lavage with 4% acetylcysteine and saline have been most gratifying in 114 procedures at the Children's Hospital Medical Center of Akron, Ohio. Each was performed under general anesthesia using the rigid bronchoscope. There were no deaths. Timing of the procedure and patient selection are partially subjective. The most impressive results have been improved pulmonary compliance and improved quality of life in the patient. Details of the procedure, techniques of anesthesia, and results of therapy are presented.

Management of the thick, viscous, partially obstructing secretions in the tracheobronchial tree of the patient with cystic fibrosis remains a continuing challenge. This problem is more pronounced during periods of acute exacerbation of pulmonary infection. It is manifested by marked decrease in pulmonary function, increased P_{CO_2}, and decreased P_{O_2}, to the extent that conventional cystic fibrosis pulmonary therapy loses its effectiveness. Endoscopic removal of tracheobronchial secretions has been performed in recent years in an attempt to improve the clinical condition of the patient. This has included volume-controlled lung lavage as reported by Kylstra and coworkers[1-3] and bronchoscopy and bronchial lavage as reported by Altman and coworkers.[4,5] Both the rigid[4] and flexible bronchoscopes[6,7] have been used with general or local anesthesia. At Children's Hospital Medical Center of Akron, 114 procedures have been performed on 35 patients (20 men, 15 women) since 1970. The youngest patient was three months old and the oldest 31 years. Each procedure was performed under general anesthesia using the rigid bronchoscope. There were no operative deaths.

METHODS

Bronchoscopy with limited lavage has been performed most commonly after the patient is admitted to the hospital and placed on intensive medical therapy including intravenous antibiotics for 72 hours, postural drainage and vigorous nutritional support. Occasionally, bronchoscopy has been performed on an emergency basis due to the marked secretions and, on clinical judgment, if the patients were drowning in their own secretions. Early in our experience, several patients developed elevation of temperature after minimal preoperative preparation. It was for this reason that we arbitrarily initiated, as part of the "tune-up," a minimum of a 72-hour preparation with intensive intravenous antibiotic therapy. Cultures are obtained on all patients with cystic fibrosis on a monthly basis, so we generally have an excellent idea of both the bacteria and the sensitivity.

The patient is induced with thiopentone 4 mg/kg intravenously followed by succinylcholine 1.5 mg/kg. During induction, a rigid bronchoscope of the largest size which can be comfortably introduced is passed into the trachea. The thick, tenacious secretions are aspirated by suction, and the specimen collected for bacteriologic, fungal, and cytologic studies. Ventilation is accomplished by bag injection of 100% oxygen through the sidearm of the bronchoscope. Relaxation is maintained by 0.2% succinylcholine drip. A 4% solution of acetylcysteine (Mucomyst, Mead Johnson Labs, Evanston, Ind) is injected forcibly through the bronchoscope in 8-ml increments. After positive pressure ventilation, the secretions are aspirated by suction. Usually a large volume of secretions including bronchial casts is obtained. The injection is repeated on each side selectively as indicated. Brevital (Eli Lilly Co, Indianapolis, Ind) 1 mg/kg is given intravenously. Normal saline 10 ml is injected and aspirated from each main stem bronchus. The succinylcholine drip is discontinued, and the patient is allowed to react with the bronchoscope in place. Once coughing and spontaneous ventilation are effective, the bronchoscope is withdrawn. We have not had complaints of awareness, and the patient is awake on leaving the surgical suite. The volume of lavage fluid is usually 50 to 60 ml. The procedure requires approximately 20 minutes.

RESULTS

The only difficulty related to anesthesia occurred early in the study. Curare was used for relaxation and reversal was difficult. Most cystic fibrosis patients are in a state of chronic acidosis which may impede the reversal of curare. This problem has not existed since the administration of succinylcholine as the relaxing agent. Extreme cooperation between the anesthetist and bronchoscopist is essential. Occasionally, ventilation is improved by forcibly blowing through the open end of the bronchoscope.

Successful lavage induces effective cough with massive production of mucus in the next 24 hours.

From the Surgical Service and Cystic Fibrosis Clinic, Children's Hospital Medical Center of Akron, Ohio.

Presented at the meeting of the American Broncho-Esophagological Association, Palm Beach, Florida, May 3-4, 1982.

REPRINTS — Bruce F. Rothmann, MD, Surgical Service, Children's Hospital Medical Center of Akron, OH 44308.

Bronchial casts may be expectorated for a period up to 72 hours. Hemoptysis is rarely a problem.

Improvement in clinical status following bronchoscopy and limited lavage has been most gratifying. Objective assessment is difficult; however, several physiological factors have been identified. There is a marked improvement in lung compliance noted by the anesthesiologist and the bronchoscopist. The patient immediately recognizes that it is easier to breathe and that the secretions are more liquid and easily eliminated. Pulmonary function studies performed preoperatively and postoperatively on six patients showed an increase in vital capacity in each patient with an average increase of 19.5%.

Exercise tolerance, school and work attendance are improved. Most striking in our group of patients is their request for periodic washouts as part of their inpatient tune-ups. Radiologic evidence of improvement is not consistent, although it has been extremely dramatic in some patients. Improvement in chest films seems to be maintained for a period of three to six months. Stabilization of weight loss and weight gain has been noted in patients in the months following washout.

DISCUSSION

We have found that the overall improvement in patients with cystic fibrosis following bronchoscopy and limited lavage is of sufficient benefit to continue its integration as part of the therapeutic regimen. There is little doubt that the progressive disease process is not altered. However, an improved quality of life can be achieved. The sense of well-being and improvement in the quality of life expressed by our patients has been most impressive. A large number of patients, particularly in the adolescent and adult age groups, have requested the procedure, noting the benefit of a previous lavage. We have not used this procedure on a routine or prophylactic basis. It has not replaced pulmonary physiotherapy or antibiotic therapy but is viewed as an adjunct to vigorous medical treatment of this most difficult disease.

The use of 4% acetylcysteine as shown by Shaw[8] is an effective mucolytic and has not presented the problem of bronchial irritation or spasm. Most patients are discharged within one week of the procedure. Following the lavage, the intravenous antibiotics are maintained for a minimum of 72 hours before being switched over to appropriate oral antibiotics. It is our impression that patients have been able to enjoy a more productive life as a result of integrating this procedure with the overall medical tune-up that we offer.

CONCLUSIONS

1. Bronchoscopy and limited bronchial lavage have been performed safely under general anesthesia 114 times in 35 patients at Children's Hospital Medical Center of Akron.

2. Stabilization of weight loss and, in many patients, an actual weight gain has occurred in the four- to eight-week period following medical tune-up and lavage.

3. It is imperative that intravenous antibiotics be used for a minimum of 72 hours prior to the procedure and for a period of at least 72 hours following the procedure in order to avoid bacteremia and febrile responses.

4. As an emergency procedure, bronchial lavage in patients who are literally drowning in their own secretions is an effective adjunct to medical therapy.

5. Bronchoscopy and limited lavage is an adjunct not a substitute for conventional cystic fibrosis pulmonary therapy.

ACKNOWLEDGMENTS — We are indebted to Mary O'Neil RN, PNA; Donald S. Nelson, MD; and Jeanette Kilgo for their assistance in the preparation of this manuscript.

REFERENCES

1. Kylstra JA, Rausch DC, Hall KD, Spock A. Volume controlled lung lavage in the treatment of asthma, bronchiectasis, mucoviscidosis. Am Rev Respir Dis 1971; 103:651-65.

2. Lober CW, Saltzman HA, Kylstra JA. Volume controlled lung lavage in a woman with cystic fibrosis. Chest 1975; 68:382-3.

3. Blenkarn GD, Lanning CF, Kylstra JA. Anesthetic management of volume controlled unilateral lung lavage. Can Anaesth Soc J 1975; 22:154-63.

4. Altman RP, Kulczycki LL, Randolph JG, McClenathan JE. Bronchoscopy and bronchial lavage (BBC) in children with cystic fibrosis. J Pediatr Surg 1973; 8:809-14.

5. Millis RM, Young RC Jr, Kulczycki LL. Validation of therapeutic bronchoscopic bronchial washing in cystic fibrosis. Chest 1977; 71:508-13.

6. Dahm LS, Ewing CW, Harrison GM, Rucker RW. Comparison of three techniques of lung lavage in patients with cystic fibrosis. Chest 1977; 72:593-6.

7. Quick CA, Warwick W. Bronchoscopy and lavage in management of pulmonary complications of cystic fibrosis. Chest 1978; 73:755-8.

8. Shaw A. Safety of n-acetylcysteine in treatment of meconium obstruction of the newborn. J Pediatr Surg 1969; 4:119-25.

RESPIRATORY REHABILITATION WITH TRANSTRACHEAL OXYGEN SYSTEM

HENRY J. HEIMLICH, MD
CINCINNATI, OHIO

A system of transtracheal oxygen administration has been developed which is more effective for rehabilitating chronic obstructive pulmonary disease (COPD) patients than traditional systems for providing continuous oxygen therapy. The procedure involves administering oxygen continuously through a No. 16 intravenous catheter inserted transtracheally. Therapeutic PaO_2 levels are attained with an oxygen flow of 0.25 to 1 liter per minute. Transtracheal oxygen administration has numerous advantages over nasal cannula or Venturi mask devices. With this system, the patient requires 3 to 4 times less oxygen; therefore, a 2.7-kg (6-lb) portable tank will last most of one day. Oxygen-enriched air via transtracheal catheter reaches the lungs directly with less respiratory effort. Delivery of oxygen is not impaired by sinusitis, mouth-breathing, displacement of nasal cannula or loss of oxygen into the room. Patients experience an immediate sensation of being able to breathe more easily, begin ambulating the day of the procedure, have improved nutrition and return to many normal activities.

As emphysema, black or brown lung and other chronic lung diseases advance in severity, patients become dependent upon oxygen inhalation therapy for comfort and survival. Hypoxemia ravages all organ systems of the body, causing functional and psychological incompetence. Oxygen therapy alleviates hypoxemia for patients with chronic obstructive pulmonary disease (COPD) while decreasing the actual work of breathing. Clinical studies indicate that patients experience increased exercise tolerance as well as general physical and mental improvement with supplemental oxygen.

Traditional systems for providing continuous oxygen therapy delivered by a nasal cannula or mask have several disadvantages. Due to the high flow necessary to attain therapeutic levels, large quantities of oxygen are required; therefore, oxygen containers are heavy and cumbersome and limit ambulation. In addition, oxygen irritates the nasopharynx, diminishing patient acceptability. To overcome these problems, a system of transtracheal oxygen administration has been developed which is effective for rehabilitating COPD patients. The technique consists of inserting No. 16 gauge plastic tubing through the lower neck into the trachea and delivering oxygen directly into the tracheobronchial tree (Figure). The nasopharynx is bypassed, eliminating irritation, and therapeutic blood oxygen levels are attained with considerably lower flow than was possible with previous oxygen delivery equipment. As a result, smaller, lightweight containers can be used, permitting ambulation for patients dependent upon a continuous oxygen supply.

RATIONALE

Oxygen administered by nasal cannula or face mask is largely wasted because much of it dissipates into the atmosphere through the nose and mouth before it can reach the lungs. In addition, the oxygen introduced into the nasopharyngeal and laryngotracheal dead space is not utilized for respiratory exchange. Consequently, high flows, at least 2 to 4 liters per minute (LPM), are required for adequate therapy. Small portable containers provide oxygen for only a short time and larger units must be rolled on wheels. Mobility generally is limited by 15 m of tubing connected to a stationary concentrator or cylinder.

Oxygen delivered through the nose or mouth dries the nasopharyngeal mucosa, resulting in irritation that may not be relieved by humidification. Nasal cannulas cause bleeding at the orifices of the nose. An oxygen mask is uncomfortable and often produces pressure sores. These devices are also cosmetically unsightly. Patients resist continuous oxygen therapy by these methods. The result is decreased functional capacity of internal organs and generalized deterioration attributable to hypoxemia and immobility.

It was conceived that direct intrabronchial oxygen delivery would require less oxygen flow to provide adequate therapy by bypassing the dead space and eliminating oxygen waste associated with nasal cannulas and masks. Furthermore, providing oxygen transtracheally eliminates nasopharyngeal irritation.

Prompt improvement in respiratory exchange by eliminating the effect of dead space has been well established as demonstrated when tracheotomy is performed to relieve respiratory distress. Tracheostomy is not acceptable to COPD patients, how-

From Xavier University, Cincinnati.
Presented at the meeting of the American Broncho-Esophagological Association, Palm Beach, Florida, May 3-4, 1982.
REPRINTS — Henry J. Heimlich, MD, Professor of Advanced Clinical Sciences, Xavier University, Cincinnati, OH 45207.

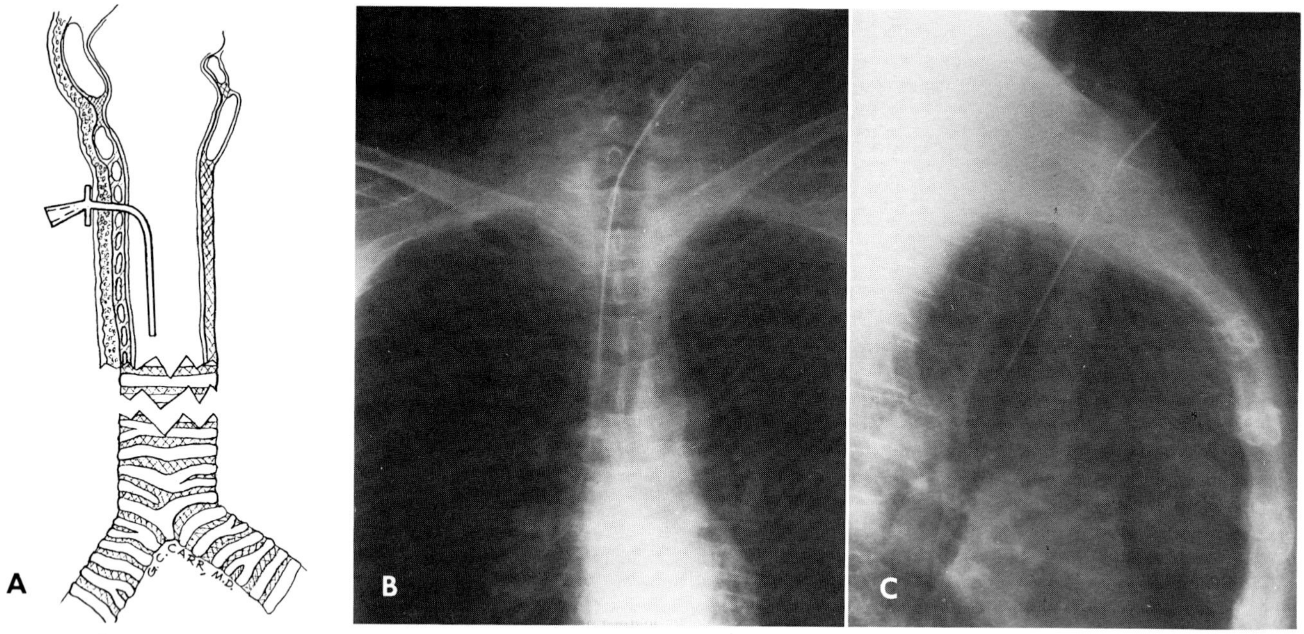

Radiopaque catheter extending from outside neck into trachea. A) Diagram; B) PA and C) lateral cervical roentgenograms.

ever, due to loss of voice and complicated care of the operative site.

To overcome the disadvantages of the usual tracheostomy, while retaining the benefits of intratracheal oxygen delivery, the possibility of inserting a permanent small plastic tube transtracheally was considered. Transtracheal insertion of plastic tubes, such as those used for intravenous therapy, is a common practice. The tubes are left in place several days for introduction of saline to induce cough and to thin secretions in postoperative and comatose patients.[1] Pratter and Irwin[2] report transtracheal aspiration to be highly successful with minimal risk when routinely performed for aspiration biopsies. It was felt that transtracheal catheters would be well tolerated on a permanent basis when constructed of inert plastics since standard large tracheostomy tubes have been left in place for many years without adverse effect.

LABORATORY STUDIES

Four beagle dogs were anesthetized and intubated with a No. 36 endotracheal tube. Baseline PaO_2 was taken. Pure (100%) oxygen was delivered through either a No. 8 or a No. 16 catheter inserted into the endotracheal tube and studies performed with flows from 1 to 5 LPM. Blood samples were taken every 15 minutes. The catheters were placed in the following positions: just inside the endotracheal tube, halfway down the tube, at the inside tip of the tube, 5 cm past the tip of the tube and in the left lung main bronchus. Blood gases were also analyzed with the catheters in these same positions as they were withdrawn.

Results. Tests with compressed air rather than oxygen demonstrated no change in PaO_2 regardless of the catheter level. Using 100% oxygen at a constant flow, there was a marked increase in PaO_2 the deeper the catheter location. The arterial oxygen pressure dropped slightly, however, as the catheter was passed into the left main bronchus, then increased when it was pulled back to 5 cm below the tip of the tube, just above the carina. It was determined that PaO_2 in normal dogs could be maintained with four times less oxygen when it was delivered directly into the distal trachea, rather than at higher levels of the endotracheal tube.

Subsequently, a No. 8 Teflon catheter was inserted through the trachea of one dog and a No. 16 in another; the external end of each tube was implanted under the skin for long-term observation. An initial increase in cough rate decreased after a few days; temperature and white blood cell counts remained within the normal range. Intratracheal visualization of the catheter was performed through a fiberoptic bronchoscope after five and seven months. The tracheal mucosa appeared normal without irritation or infection. The tubes were tolerated up to one year with no evidence of infection or adverse reaction.

CLINICAL EXPERIENCE

Case Selection. Criteria for patient selection were based on indications for long-term oxygen therapy included in the Standards of the American Thoracic Society.[3] Eleven men and three women, aged 40 to 77 years (mean age, 61.7 years), underwent insertion of the transtracheal ambulatory oxygen system and were followed from 2 to 22 months. All 14 patients had a history of chronic pulmonary disease and respiratory disability, one with restrictive pulmonary function, one with obstructive pulmonary function and 12 with both. Nine had emphysema and five had coal pneumoconiosis (black lung disease). Seven patients had one or more myocardial infarctions and seven had cor pulmonale.

All patients were unable to ambulate without supplemental oxygen despite use of medications, but were able to ambulate with a minimum of 1 LPM oxygen via nasal cannula. They were unable to work or pursue hobbies and had severe restriction in daily activities. All had a history of respiratory disability longer than eight years, had been on home oxygen therapy for 1½ to 2½ years and showed an increasing dependency on oxygen. Three patients were considered "last resort" cases, one of them terminal.

CLINICAL AND LABORATORY DATA* (N = 14)

Case No.	Age/Sex	Pretranstracheal Data Arterial Blood Gases† PCO₂	PO₂	Sat.(%)	Posttranstracheal Data Arterial Blood Gases (0.5 LPM) PCO₂	PO₂	Sat.(%)	Course
1	61/M	35	56	89	40	74	95	Working part-time; full independence
2	51/M	45	66	93	47	84	96	Full activity
3	65/M	40	64	93	80	49	87	Limited outdoor activity
4	68/M	35	83	96	40	99	98	Died 8/27/81; CVA & CHF
5	64/M	36	58	92	33	86	97	Full independence
6	67/M	44	34	67	41§	78	95	Died 1/12/82; CVA
7	43/F	58	37	69	63§	60	87	Outdoor activity 3-4 times weekly
8	74/M	36	43	85	40	64	94	Outdoor activity 3-4 times weekly
9	61/M	46	48	87	39	69	95	Died 3/2/82; CVA
10	69/M	64	32	60	51	70	96	Died 2/12/82; CHF & ASHD
11	55/M	44	55	89	44	60	90	Outdoor activity 5-6 times weekly
12	69/F	55	31	56	75§	44	75	Full home activity
13	40/F	35	63	94	38§	104	97	Employed as account executive
14	77/M	48	53	87	49§	65	93	Full independence

LPM - Liters per minute; PCO_2 - Carbon dioxide pressure; PO_2 - Oxygen pressure; Sat. - Saturation; M - Male; F - Female; CVA - Cerebrovascular accident; CHF - Congestive heart failure; ASHD -Arteriosclerotic heart disease.

*Complete data available from author.

†Room air.

§1 LPM.

Preplacement tests included arterial blood gases on room air, 0.5, 1 and 2 LPM oxygen per nasal cannula and, in some, 28% oxygen per Venturi mask; pulmonary function tests; exercise tolerance and treadmill tests (when possible); chest x-ray studies; ECG; alpha$_1$-antitrypsin level; urinalysis; complete blood cell count; electrolyte studies; and clotting time.

Procedure. The procedure was performed under local anesthesia in the intensive care unit. Through a specially designed needle that was subsequently extracted, a modified No. 16 Teflon catheter (Erie Medical, Milwaukee) was inserted between the second and third tracheal rings, then sutured to the skin, and secured around the neck with umbilical tape. Tubing connected the catheter to a 2.7-kg oxygen tank fitted with a valve and meter that could be accurately regulated by the patient in increments of 0.25 LPM.

Oxygen was delivered through the transtracheal catheter at a flow of 0.25 to 1.5 LPM based on PaO_2, clinical response and amount of exercise. Three patients showed mild local subcutaneous emphysema which disappeared in a few hours. In such instances, nasal cannulas were used for the first 24 hours. Initially, cannulas also were used at night and when patients were not being observed to avoid inadvertent displacement of the transtracheal catheter.

Ambulation was begun on the day of the procedure. The length of hospital stay was evaluated individually and ranged from 1 to 2 weeks.

Results. The Table lists pertinent clinical and laboratory data for the patients who underwent transtracheal ambulatory oxygen insertion. Thirteen patients were ambulatory the day of the procedure and were improved. The terminal patient had limited ambulation.

There was an average 57% reduction in oxygen requirement, while maintaining therapeutic arterial blood gases, using transtracheal oxygen as compared with nasal cannulas. Before placement of the catheter average PaO_2 was 52 mm Hg with average O_2 saturation of 83%. With 2 LPM per nasal cannula of oxygen, average PaO_2 was 77 mm Hg with average O_2 saturation of 94%. The average PaO_2 with 0.5 LPM per transtracheal catheter was 73 mm Hg with average O_2 saturation of 94%. An average PaO_2 of 82 mm Hg resulted from 1 LPM per transtracheal catheter with average O_2 saturation of 92%. (The average arterial blood gas studies do not include case No. 10, in which the patient was terminally ill and required 1.5 LPM oxygen for therapeutic response.)

Complications included mild site irritation and occasional initial purulent drainage. Catheters were easily removed and reinserted by patients after 2 to 3 months when a tract had developed.

No deaths were related to the procedure. One patient died of a cerebrovascular accident 8 months following catheter insertion. Of the three patients considered last-resort cases, one died two months and two died 4 months postplacement due to cerebrovascular accidents or preexisting arteriosclerotic heart disease and congestive heart failure.

CASE REPORTS

Case 1. A 61-year-old man with emphysema suffered a crushing chest injury in 1973. He experienced increased shortness of breath, with marked dyspnea on exertion becoming increasingly severe in the year prior to placement. Hospitalization was required nine times for acute exacerbation, totaling 19 weeks in the year prior to conversion to transtracheal catheter. In 1979, continuous oxygen therapy was begun at home at 2 LPM per nasal cannula. Chronic bronchitis resulted in expectoration of large amounts of mucus. Sleep was brief and intermittent and he complained of weakness and fatigue. Occasional rectal bleeding occurred, and steroid dependency was diagnosed in March 1980.

Blood gas studies yielded the following results: pH, 7.46; PCO_2, 35 mm Hg; PaO_2, 56 mm Hg with average O_2 saturation of 89%. Pulmonary function tests showed severe obstructive airway disease with slight but significant improvement with bronchodilators. The ratio of residual volume (RV) to total lung capacity (TLC) was 77%. Chest x-ray films indicated hyperaeration of the lungs. Electrocardiogram changes were consistent with COPD.

A transtracheal catheter was inserted in July 1980. Arterial blood gases with 0.5 LPM oxygen per transtracheal catheter were pH, 7.45; PCO_2, 40 mm Hg; PaO_2, 74 mm Hg with average O_2 saturation of 95%. The patient was discharged from the hospital on 0.5 to 1 LPM oxygen via transtracheal catheter. His symptoms subsided and medications were decreased by 70%. He resumed work four months after insertion of the catheter.

Case 2. A 51-year-old man was diagnosed in 1970 as having COPD which gradually worsened until he was forced to retire from his occupation as a paper mill worker. Following hospitalization in 1979, home oxygen therapy was prescribed. He was hospitalized again in 1980 for 19 days. The patient had extreme dyspnea when walking 3 to 30 m. Oxygen by nasal cannula was prescribed for 1 to 2 hours at 2 to 2.5 LPM in the evening but was often skipped to avoid discomfort and a feeling of dependence.

Results of blood gas studies were pH, 7.40; PCO_2, 45 mm Hg; PaO_2, 66 mm Hg and average O_2 saturation of 93%. Results with nasal oxygen at 2 LPM were pH, 7.39; PCO_2, 47 mm Hg; PaO_2, 102 mm Hg and average O_2 saturation of 98%. Pulmonary function tests indicated severe COPD with decreased diffusing capacity. The ratio of RV to TLC was 77% with no change after bronchodilators. Chest x-ray films revealed bilateral bullous emphysema.

A transtracheal catheter was inserted in June 1981 without incident. Blood gases on 0.5 LPM oxygen via transtracheal catheter were pH, 7.41; PCO_2, 47 mm Hg; PaO_2, 84 mm Hg and average O_2 saturation of 96%. The patient ambulated within 48 hours and has been maintained on 0.5 LPM oxygen flow since discharge from the hospital. Four months after insertion of the catheter he walked several hours a day.

DISCUSSION

Home oxygen therapy is essential in treating advanced COPD. It provides immediate functional competence and mobility, preventing the otherwise rapid physical deterioration. Such treatment has become increasingly practical in recent years and is considerably less expensive than hospitalization. Petty[4] states that COPD patients given controlled oxygen "were markedly improved in terms of functional capability and facility in coping with advanced disease while living at home," a finding which confirmed earlier studies by Levine et al.[5]

Continuous oxygen therapy has proven to be more beneficial than 12-hour nocturnal oxygen therapy for patients suffering from severe respiratory impairment. In a recent study, overall mortality in the nocturnal oxygen therapy group was nearly twice that of the continuous oxygen therapy group.[6]

With transtracheal administration, oxygen-enriched air enters the lungs directly. Subjectively, patients experienced an immediate sensation of being able to breathe more easily. Delivering oxygen-enriched air directly into the lungs relieved patients of the constant respiratory effort required to draw oxygen from the nasopharynx into the trachea when traditional masks or nasal cannulas were used. Furthermore, oxygen delivery was not impaired by sinusitis, mouth breathing, displacement of the cannula or loss of oxygen into the room. Nutrition improved because the oxygen supply was not interrupted while eating.

Early evidence indicates an increased mental alertness as hypoxemia is relieved. The patient's general physical status benefits from ambulation and continuous relief of hypoxemia, and the quality of life is significantly enhanced. When wearing a shirt and tie or dress with a collar, neither the catheter nor connective tubing, which runs under the clothes, is visible.

Most patients formerly had been housebound and required a wheelchair for mobility. They have returned to normal functioning including fishing, hunting, vacationing, shopping, driving and family-related activities. All patients carry the 2.7-kg tank with ease.

With transtracheal oxygen, patients require three to four times less oxygen than with nasal or oropharyngeal methods. Portable 2.7-kg tanks maintain patients 6 to 10 hours. When intermittent flows of 0.25 to 0.5 LPM are used during the day and a large tank or concentrator at night, the 2.7-kg tank lasts up to 20 hours.

Analysis of oxygen consumption and related costs before and after placement of the transtracheal catheter shows a substantial decrease in the amount of oxygen used. One patient's oxygen consumption had averaged 164 kg costing $408.74 per month for the five months prior to placement of the catheter. During the first five months with the transtracheal ambulatory oxygen system, the patient used an average of 61 kg oxygen per month costing $145.92, a 64% reduction.

The same patient was hospitalized 19 weeks for severe respiratory failure at a cost of approximately $33,250 in the year preceding placement of the transtracheal oxygen system. In the first 1½ years after placement, the patient was not hospitalized for the pulmonary condition.

The need for medications such as bronchodilators has diminished. Lanoxin, digoxin, furosemide (Lasix), and prednisone dosages prescribed for the effects of deterioration caused by hypoxemia have gradually decreased for some patients. One reported that for the months immediately following insertion, his medication costs dropped from a previous monthly average of $50 to $25.

As of August 1982, 23 additional patients underwent transtracheal ambulatory oxygen insertion and results are promising.

ACKNOWLEDGMENTS — Research and clinical studies were supported by The Joseph and Helen Regenstein and the Claude Worthington Benedum Foundations. Professor Neil A. Armstrong, Edward A. Patrick, MD, PhD and George Rieveschl, PhD, participated in preclinical studies. Patients with black lung disease and other conditions in Beckley, West Virginia, were cared for by John M. Daniel, MD, under sponsorship of Beckley College, John W. Saunders, EdD, President. Karon R. Mazzaro provided editorial assistance.

REFERENCES

1. Bartlett RH, Gazzaniga AB, Geraghty TR. Respiratory maneuvers to prevent postoperative pulmonary complications: a critical review. JAMA 1973; 224:1017-21.

2. Pratter MR, Irwin RS. Transtracheal aspiration: guidelines for safety. Chest 1979; 76:518-20.

3. Oxygen Therapy Committee of the American Thoracic Society. Oxygen administration in the home. Am Rev Respir Dis 1977; 115:897-9.

4. Petty TL. Home oxygen in advanced chronic obstructive pulmonary disease. Med Clin North Am 1981; 65:615-27.

5. Levine BE, Bigelow DB, Hamstra RD. The role of long-term continuous oxygen administration in patients with chronic airway obstruction with hypoxemia. Ann Intern Med 1967; 66:639-50.

6. Nocturnal Oxygen Therapy Trial Group. Continuous or nocturnal oxygen therapy in hypoxemic chronic obstructive lung disease: a clinical trial. Ann Intern Med 1980; 93:391-8.

≈

THE SECOND INTERNATIONAL SYMPOSIUM ON AUDIOLOGICAL MEDICINE

The Second International Symposium on Audiological Medicine will be held April 10-13, 1983, in Verona, under the auspices of the International Association of Physicians in Audiology. For further information contact Dr. V. Colletti, Clinica ORL dell'Universita di Padova sede di Verona, Policlinico Borgo Roma, 37134 Verona, Italy.

≈

ASSOCIATION FOR RESEARCH IN OTOLARYNGOLOGY

The Association for Research in Otolaryngology will hold its annual midwinter research meeting on January 24-26, 1983, in St. Petersburg Beach, Florida. To register, contact Donald W. Nielsen, PhD, Secretary-Treasurer, Association for Research in Otolaryngology, Otological Research Laboratories, 7036 E&R Building, Henry Ford Hospital, Detroit, MI 48202.

TRACHEOBRONCHIAL OBSTRUCTION FROM METASTATIC DISTANT MALIGNANCIES

STANLEY M. SHAPSHAY, MD
BURLINGTON, MASSACHUSETTS

M. STUART STRONG, MD
BOSTON, MASSACHUSETTS

Tracheal or endobronchial metastases from distant primary malignancies are rare. Hemoptysis, dyspnea and cough are common nonspecific presenting symptoms. Renal, breast, thyroid and colon cancers are the most common malignancies associated with tracheobronchial metastases. Since 1979, five patients with tracheobronchial metastases from distant sites have been treated by the otolaryngology service at the Boston University Medical Center. Patients with advanced tumors previously treated by conventional modalities were referred for palliation of airway obstruction. Satisfactory palliation without significant morbidity was achieved in four out of five patients utilizing a CO_2 surgical laser through a rigid bronchoscope system. Four patients died from advanced cancer, 1 to 18 months after laser surgery. Although tracheobronchial metastasis from extrathoracic malignancy is associated with a poor prognosis, palliation of airway obstruction can be achieved in most patients with endobronchial or tracheal tumor.

Extrathoracic malignancies commonly metastasize to the lung parenchyma, pleura and mediastinal lymph nodes. The trachea and bronchi are, however, rare sites of metastasis from distant cancers.[1] A misdiagnosis of bronchogenic carcinoma is often made by the clinician because of a "low index of suspicion" for endobronchial metastasis.

Since 1979, five patients with tracheal or endobronchial metastases have been treated by the otolaryngology department at the Boston University Medical Center. These patients were referred specifically for palliation of their tracheobronchial obstruction utilizing a rigid CO_2 laser bronchoscope system. This unusual series of patients prompted a literature review of the incidence, treatment and prognosis of endobronchial or tracheal metastasis. The otolaryngologist should consider this diagnosis when dealing with tracheobronchial obstruction and be aware of therapeutic options. A cancer patient with symptoms of persistent cough, hemoptysis, wheezing and increasing dyspnea should alert the clinician to the possibility of metastases to the tracheobronchial tree. This paper will present our experience with this group of patients and review selected literature on this topic.

METHODS AND MATERIALS

Since 1979, five patients with severe tracheobronchial airway obstruction from endobronchial or tracheal metastases were referred to our otolaryngology service. These patients had previously been treated both at the primary and metastatic site with conventional modalities for their tumors. Only one patient (Table, patient 4) was referred for both histological diagnosis and treatment; diagnosis of distant metastasis was otherwise previously established. Two patients had renal cell carcinoma and the others were thyroid, colon and uterus carcinoma.

A 50-W CO_2 laser coupled to a rigid ventilating bronchoscope was used in all cases. This instrumentation has been previously described.[2,3] General anesthesia utilizing nonflammable anesthetics was delivered through the ventilating channel on the bronchoscope and also cleared the smoke from tumor vaporization. Standard bronchoscopic cup biopsy forceps was often used to remove carbonized tumor particles. Occasionally epinephrine-soaked sponges (1:1000) were applied to facilitate hemostasis.

PATIENT SUMMARIES

Patient 1. A 50-year-old man had a nephrectomy and partial hepatectomy for an extensive renal cell carcinoma in 1977. A solitary metastasis was removed from the left humerus a year later. Pulmonary metastases were removed by multiple lobar resections (both lungs) in 1979. A year after the lung metastases were removed, the patient noted increasing dyspnea and hemoptysis. A flexible bronchoscopy revealed endobronchial metastases obstructing the right bronchus intermedius and left posterior basal segment. Radiation therapy and subsequent endobronchial insertion of radioactive gold seeds failed to alleviate the obstructive symptoms (Fig. 1). He was then referred for laser bronchoscopic removal of tumor (Figs. 2 and 3). Successful palliation of dyspnea and hemoptysis was achieved over an 18-month period (nine laser bronchoscopies) before his death. An autopsy was not done.

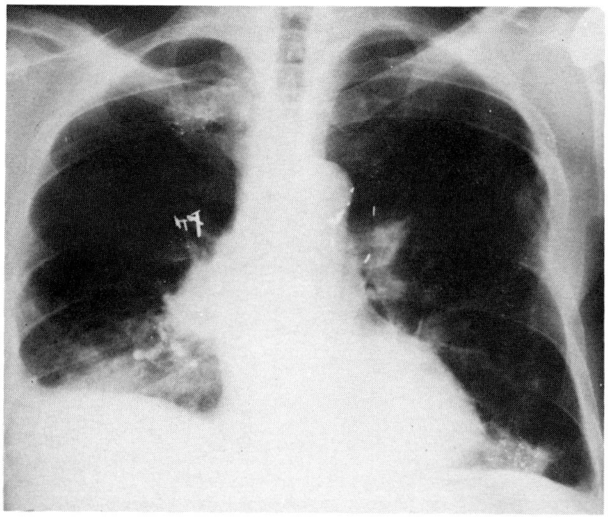

Fig. 1. (Patient 1) Chest radiograph showing bilateral pulmonary metastases treated with radioactive gold seed implants and lobar resections.

From the Department of Otolaryngology, University Hospital, Boston University School of Medicine.
Presented at the meeting of the American Broncho-Esophagological Association, Palm Beach, Florida, May 3-4, 1982.

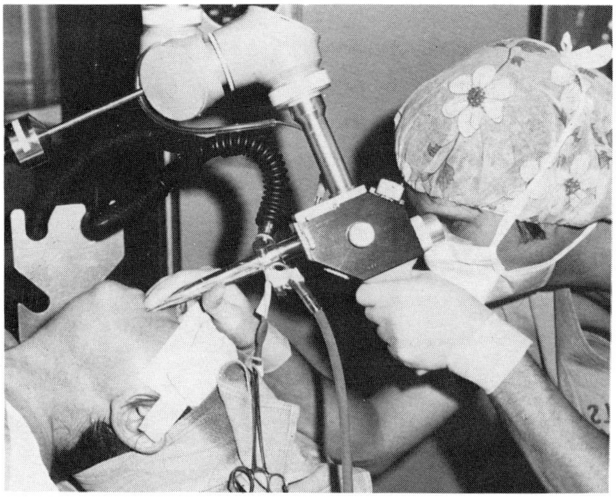

Fig. 2. Ventilating laser bronchoscope system in use. Note protective covering over patient's eyes to prevent inadvertent laser deflection-injury.

Patient 2. A 49-year-old man with renal cell carcinoma metastatic to the carina was referred with symptoms of severe airway distress. He had a nephrectomy in 1969 without recurrence at the primary site. Pulmonary and bone metastases were removed in 1977. Radiotherapy was used to treat cerebral metastasis in 1979. A year later severe dyspnea and hemoptysis were noted. A fungating carinal metastasis partially obstructing both main bronchi (approximately 80%) was discovered. Successful palliation was achieved with one laser bronchoscopy without morbidity. The patient died without airway obstruction three weeks later.

Patient 3. A 61-year-old woman had a colon resection in 1974 for a colonic adenocarcinoma. Liver metastasis was discovered in 1979 and distal tracheal spread noted in 1980. Radiation therapy failed to control the tracheal metastases and she was referred for palliative laser surgery. Bilateral main stem bronchial obstruction (90%) was removed with the CO_2 laser bronchoscope. The patient died from liver failure two months later.

Patient 4. A 61-year-old woman with a history of adenocarcinoma of the uterus was referred for diagnosis and treatment of a large carinal mass. Her uterine carcinoma was successfully treated with radiotherapy in 1975 with no evidence of recurrence over five years. Flexible bronchoscopy showed a friable tumor mass partially (approximately 50%) obstructing both main bronchi. A biopsy was taken and the rigid laser bronchoscope system used to remove the obstructing mass. There was histologic confirmation of metastatic adenocarcinoma consistent with the uterus primary. She is presently free of tumor (six months follow-up) and asymptomatic after a course of radiotherapy.

Patient 5. A 46-year-old man with thyroid follicular adenocarcinoma was referred for alleviation of airway distress. A thyroidectomy and left radical neck dissection were done in 1975 and mediastinal metastasis was treated with radiotherapy in 1978. Distal tracheal metastases were partially removed elsewhere with cup forceps through a rigid bronchoscope on several occasions, moderate hemorrhage occurring with these procedures. Increasing dyspnea was noted in 1980 due to bilateral main stem bronchi obstruction. Laser bronchoscopic removal of distal tumor obstruction (both lower lobes) could not be done. The patient died of respiratory insufficiency a month later.

RESULTS

Successful palliation of airway obstruction was achieved in four out of five patients. The patient with endobronchial thyroid cancer (Table, patient 5) had extensive proximal and distal endobronchial tumor which could not be entirely removed. Best palliation thus far was achieved in patient 1 (Table) with endobronchial renal cell carcinoma. He was able to work and function well for 1½ years, requiring nine laser bronchoscopies. Progression of pulmonary parenchymal metastases eventually led to his death. Pulmonary edema, the only complication in this series, occurred immediately after laser surgery. There were no hemorrhage, tracheobronchial perforation or burns in this series.

DISCUSSION

Possible routes for endobronchial or tracheal metastases from distant sites are 1) a parenchymal mass with direct extension into the bronchus, 2) mediastinal lymph node metastasis with secondary bronchial extension and 3) direct metastasis to the trachea or bronchus. The first two possibilities should be evident because of associated roentgenographic changes. Direct endobronchial metastases was most probable in all but patient 5.

The incidence of direct endobronchial metastases from distant sites was reported to be 2% in a large autopsy series of extrathoracic tumors.[1] Another autopsy series reported an incidence of 18% but also included invasion of bronchi by direct extension.[4] If histologic evidence of bronchial involvement was included, then a 25% incidence of endobronchial metastases was noted.[5]

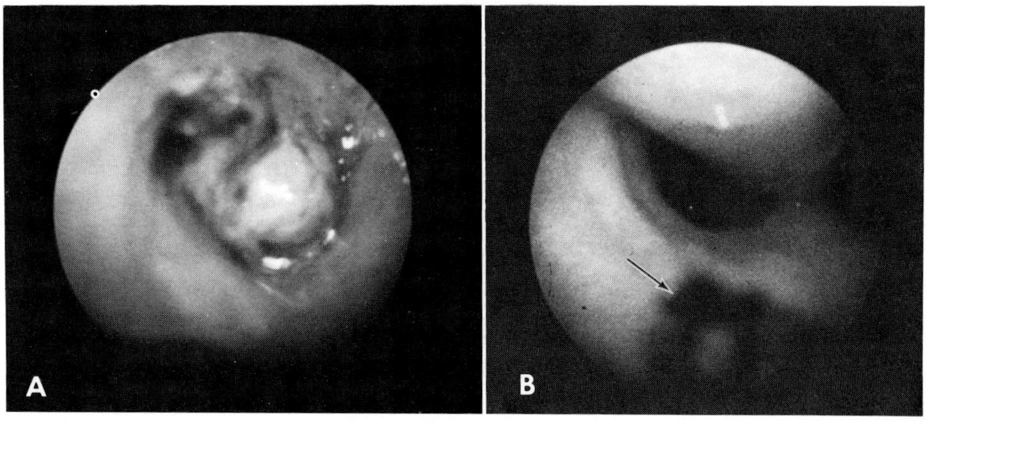

Fig. 3. (Patient 1) Endobronchial photographs of right bronchus intermedius. A) Obstructing renal cell carcinoma metastasis; B) Immediately after laser removal of tumor. Note lack of edema in bronchus and presence of carbonized particles (arrow).

DIAGNOSIS, TREATMENT AND FOLLOW-UP IN PATIENT SERIES

Pt. No.	Age	Sex	Diagnosis	Endobronchial/Tracheal Site of Metastasis	Previous Treatment	No. of Laser Operations	Survival After Laser Surgery
1	50	M	Renal cell carcinoma	Right bronchus intermedius, left postbasal segment	Nephrectomy 1977 Resection of humerus, metastasis 1978 Bilateral pulmonary metastases, surgery 1979 Endobronchial metastases, radiotherapy and implant with radioactive gold seeds 1979	9	18 mo*
2	49	M	Renal cell carcinoma	Carina — both main stem bronchi	Nephrectomy 1969 Right lower lobectomy 1977 Bone metastases, radiotherapy 1977 Brain metastases, radiotherapy 1979	1	3 wk*
3	61	F	Colon adenocarcinoma	Carina — both main stem bronchi	Colon resection 1974 Liver metastases, chemotherapy 1976 Tracheal metastases, radiotherapy 1979	1	2 mo*
4	61	F	Uterus adenocarcinoma	Carina — both main stem bronchi	Uterus carcinoma, radiotherapy 1975	1	Alive — 6 mo follow-up
5	46	M	Thyroid follicular adenocarcinoma	Carina — both main stem & distal lower lobe bronchi	Thyroidectomy 1975 Neck and mediastinum metastases, radiotherapy	1	1 mo*

*Died.

The most common extrathoracic tumors associated with endobronchial or tracheal metastases were carcinomas of the kidney, breast, colon and thyroid in order of decreasing incidence.[1,6-9] Gerle and Felson presented and reviewed 17 cases of metastatic endobronchial renal carcinoma and concluded that endobronchial metastasis was a terminal event in most patients.[6] Seldom did their patients survive more than 1 year from the time of diagnosis. Malignant melanoma and lymphoma have also been reported to metastasize to the tracheobronchial airway.[10-12]

Treatment of endobronchial or tracheal metastases is usually for palliation of airway obstruction and occasionally for control of hemoptysis. Bronchoscopic electrocoagulation and forceps removal of tumor particles may restore airway patency but carry the risk of hemorrhage and scarring (particularly with repeated coagulations). Endoscopic cryosurgery has been utilized but the depth of tissue destruction is not easily predictable.[13]

We have had 8 years' experience with a rigid CO_2 laser bronchoscope system in over 400 cases. Previous reports have documented the safety, indications and contraindictions for this technique.[2,3,14,15] Good hemostasis due to laser heat coagulation of small blood vessels and excellent wound healing have been noted. Disadvantages have been the limitations associated with a rigid system and relatively poor optics when compared to a flexible fiberoptic system. Newer systems such as a ND-YAG laser and phototherapy with laser — hematoporphyrin deviative may prove to be useful.[16-18]

Palliation of tracheobronchial obstruction in this small series of patients was generally short-term; three patients died one month or less after laser surgery. Only one patient, however, died of airway distress (Table, patient 5). There were two long-term survivors, 1 which required nine laser bronchoscopic tumor removals over an 18-month period. The other long-term survivor (uterine carcinoma) is still alive without recurrence six months after radiation therapy. Since airway obstruction and ultimate suffocation is a particularly dreaded event, palliation of this symptom certainly seems worthwhile if the patient can tolerate general anesthesia.

CONCLUSION

1. Metastasis to the tracheobronchial tree from extrapulmonary sites are uncommon but should be considered when symptoms of airway obstruction, cough and hemoptysis occur in a cancer patient.

2. Carcinomas of the kidney, breast, thyroid and colon appear to be the most common malignancies associated with tracheobronchial metastases.

3. Palliation of airway obstruction without significant morbidity can be achieved utilizing endoscopic laser surgery. Laser surgery is usually hemostatic, associated with minimal swelling and can be used repeatedly.

REFERENCES

1. Braman SS, Whitcomb ME. Endobronchial metastasis. Arch Intern Med 1975; 135:543-7.

2. Strong MS, Vaughan CW, Polanyi T, Wallace R. Bronchoscopic carbon dioxide laser surgery. Ann Otol Rhinol Laryngol

1974; 83:769-76.

3. Andrews AH Jr, Horowitz SL. Bronchoscopic CO_2 laser surgery. Lasers Surg Med 1980; 1:35-45.

4. King DS, Castleman B. Bronchial involvement in metastatic pulmonary malignancy. J Thorac Cardiovasc Surg 1943; 12:305-15.

5. Rosenblatt MB, Lisa JR, Trinidad S. Pitfalls in the clinical and histologic diagnosis of bronchogenic carcinoma. Dis Chest 1966; 49:396-404.

6. Gerle R, Felson B. Metastatic endobronchial hypernephroma. Dis Chest 1963; 44:225-33.

7. Fitzgerald RH Jr. Endobronchial metastases. South Med J 1977; 70:440-1.

8. Baumgartner WA, Mark JBD. Metastatic malignancies from distant sites to the tracheobronchial tree. J Thorac Cardiovasc Surg 1980; 79:499-503.

9. Schnur MJ, Austin JHM. Radiopaque hemithorax in an elderly woman. Chest 1979; 76:209-11.

10. Webb WR, Gamsu G. Thoracic metastasis in malignant melanoma. A radiographic survey of 65 patients. Chest 1977; 71:176-81.

11. Andrews AH Jr, Caldarelli DD. Carbon dioxide laser treatment of metastatic melanoma of the trachea and bronchi. Ann Otol Rhinol Laryngol 1981; 90:310-1.

12. Samuels ML, Howe CD, Dodd GD Jr, Fuller LM, Shullenberger CC, Leary WL. Endobronchial malignant lymphoma. Am J Roentgenol 1961; 85:87-95.

13. Carpenter RJ, Neel BH, Sanderson DR. Comparison of endoscopic cryosurgery and electrocoagulation of bronchi. Trans Am Acad Ophthalmol Otolaryngol 1977; 84:313-23.

14. Laforet EG, Berger RL, Vaughan CW. Carcinoma obstructing the trachea. Treatment by laser resection. N Eng J Med 1976; 294:941.

15. Shapshay SM, Davis RK, Vaughan CW, Norton M, Strong MS. Endoscopic management of airway obstruction from tracheobronchial neoplasia, abstracted. Chest 1980; 78:3.

16. Toty L, Personne C, Colchen A, Vourc'h G. Bronchoscopic management of tracheal lesions using the neodynium yttrium aluminum garnet laser. Thorax 1981; 36:175-8.

17. Dumon JF, Reboud E, Garbe L, Aucomte F, Meric B. Treatment of tracheobronchial lesions by laser photoresection. Chest 1982; 81:278-84.

18. Hayata Y, Kato H, Konaka C, Ono J, Takizawa N. Hemotoporphyrin derivative and laser photoradiation in the treatment of lung cancer. Chest 1982; 81:269-77.

≈

WORLD CONGRESS OF OTORHINOLARYNGOLOGY

The XIIIth World Congress of Otorhinolaryngology will be held in Miami Beach May 26 — June 1, 1985. For further information please contact Anthony J. Maniglia, MD, Secretary-General, P.O. Box 016960 (D-48), Miami, FL 33101.

Ann Otol Rhinol Laryngol 91:1982

HEMATOPORPHYRIN-DERIVATIVE PHOTOTHERAPY FOR LOCAL TREATMENT OF CANCER OF THE TRACHEOBRONCHIAL TREE

DENIS A. CORTESE, MD

JAMES H. KINSEY, PHD

ROCHESTER, MINNESOTA

In this paper the potential use of hematoporphyrin-derivative (HpD) phototherapy in the local treatment of bronchogenic carcinoma is discussed. Ten patients with cancer involving the tracheobronchial tree have completed at least one course of HpD-mediated laser phototherapy administered by means of the flexible fiberbronchoscope. Complete response was obtained in four cases, and in each case the tumor was small and superficial. Larger tumors with greater degrees of invasion showed only a partial response. Two patients with tumors eroding through the bronchial wall died following treatment. It appears that HpD phototherapy may be useful for control of only small, superficial squamous cell carcinomas of the tracheobronchial tree and only those within the range of the flexible fiberbronchoscope.

Hematoporphyrin derivative (HpD) has been used for localizing cancer for at least 20 years. During the past seven years this chemical has also been useful in the phototherapy of cancer. A summary of the current knowledge about HpD will help in understanding its mechanism of action and the rationale for its use in the local treatment of certain types of human cancers.

Hematoporphyrin is an iron-free porphyrin. It can be prepared in vitro from protoporphyrin, a naturally occurring, iron-free porphyrin, or from the iron protoporphyrin complex hemin, which is a breakdown product of hemoglobin. Several years ago, crude hematoporphyrin was shown to localize in rat tumors, transplanted mouse tumors, several types of sarcomas, carcinomas, lymph node tissue, traumatized tissue, and embryonic tissue.[1,2] Subsequently, a specialized, prepared derivative of crude hematoporphyrin, which is now the substance called HpD, was shown to have better tumor-localizing ability than the crude hematoporphyrin.[3,4] The original technique for the preparation of HpD is still followed today. This involves dissolving crude hematoporphyrin in a mixture of glacial acetic acid and concentrated sulfuric acid in a ratio of 19:1, followed by subsequent steps of filtration, precipitation, washing, and lyophilization. The resultant dried powder is then dissolved in normal saline solution, and a final adjustment to physiologic pH is made with sodium hydroxide.[3] The product HpD is not a pure compound but is known to be a complex mixture of vinyl porphyrins, hematoporphyrin monoacetate, hematoporphyrin diacetate, protoporphyrin, deuteroporphyrin, and several additional porphyrin compounds.[5]

HpD has been successfully used as an aid in the localization of human cancer. This is possible because HpD is preferentially concentrated by cancer cells, and it produces a characteristic salmon-red fluorescence when irradiated with blue light at a wavelength of approximately 405 nm.[3,6-10] With the use of appropriate optics and filters, one can see the fluorescence emanating from cancer tissue containing HpD. Until recently, however, HpD fluorescence from early bronchogenic carcinoma could not be seen because of the technical limitations of the rigid and the standard flexible bronchoscopes. Development of a photoelectric hematoporphyrin fluorescence detector has allowed detection of hematoporphyrin fluorescence during flexible bronchoscopy performed with white light illumination. This device has been used successfully as an aid in the localization of radiologically and endoscopically occult in situ and early invasive bronchogenic squamous cell carcinoma of the lung.[11-14]

In animals and humans, photochemically significant quantities of HpD remain in the skin for several weeks after intravenous administration. HpD photosensitizes the skin to a point that after even mild exposure to direct and indirect sunlight, a severe sunburnlike reaction can occur.[3,4,6-9] The skin photosensitivity reaction suggested a possible role for HpD in the treatment of cancer.

Pursuing this observation, many investigators have successfully shown in cell culture and in animal experiments that the photodynamic effect of the combination of HpD and light irradiation is capable of destroying cancer cells.[15-26]

Phototherapy with HpD in the case of a human carcinoma was first reported in a patient with bladder cancer.[17] Subsequently, work by Dougherty and associates[20,21] has shown the potential of this technique for treatment of a variety of solid malignant tumors of the skin and subcutaneous tissues.

From the Division of Thoracic Diseases and Internal Medicine and Department of Physiology and Biophysics, Mayo Clinic and Mayo Foundation, Rochester, Minnesota. This investigation was supported in part by Research Grant CA-28923 from the National Institutes of Health, Public Health Service.

Presented at the meeting of the American Broncho-Esophagological Association, Palm Beach, Florida, May 3-4, 1982.

REPRINTS — D. A. Cortese, MD, Mayo Clinic, 200 First Street SW, Rochester, MN 55905.

The literature indicates that after an intravenous injection, HpD is concentrated in the cytoplasm of normal and cancer cells within three hours. However, after 24 hours, HpD begins to wash out of normal cells, while being retained in the cytoplasm of cancer and reticuloendothelial cells.[27,28] Why HpD is retained in cells is unknown; however, there are indications that HpD binds to cell membranes (Moses HL, personal communication).[29-32] Moreover, photochemical reactions mediated by porphyrins have an effect on cell membrane properties, and it is likely that damage to this membrane plays an important role in the cytotoxicity produced by HpD phototherapy.[30,31]

The cellular mechanism responsible for the cytotoxic effect after HpD phototherapy is thought to involve the production of singlet oxygen and toxic oxygen radicals. The major cytotoxic agent responsible for ultimate cell destruction appears to be singlet oxygen, an excited molecular species that is formed by the transfer of energy from the excited sensitizer, the hematoporphyrin.[19-22,33,34] In addition, superoxide and hydroxyl radicals are generated after HpD phototherapy.[35,36] Production of singlet oxygen and the free oxygen radicals leads to disruption of the cell membrane by lipid oxidation and protein sulfhydryl oxidation. The radicals apparently can also produce single-strand breaks in DNA that are structurally similar to DNA breaks seen after ionizing radiation.[37] Singlet oxygen has been demonstrated to form lipid peroxides in the lysosome membrane, and this results in the breakdown of the lysosome.[32]

With the foregoing information as background, we report now the use of a bronchoscopic laser system to assess HpD phototherapy in patients with lung cancer. Early results are presented for ten patients who completed one course of HpD phototherapy administered by means of the flexible fiberbronchoscope.

METHODS

All patients had biopsy-proved malignancy involving the tracheobronchial tree. All had had previous pulmonary resections or were considered to have inoperable conditions for medical or technical reasons. Furthermore, they were considered ineligible for, or had failed to respond to, conventional radiation therapy and chemotherapy. Before HpD phototherapy was administered, each patient's condition was evaluated by a team of physicians, including a pulmonologist, a thoracic surgeon, and an oncologist. Each patient was repeatedly warned to avoid exposure to intense sunlight up to four weeks after intravenous administration of HpD, and informed consent was obtained. HpD was prepared by a modification of the method of Lipson et al.[3]

A continuous-wave argon ion laser with a maximum power output of 20 W was used to pump a dye laser. Rhodamine B dye was circulated in the dye laser to produce an output wavelength of 630 nm. Adjustments were made so that the dye laser beam was focused directly into an optical fiber. The proximal end of this fiber was coupled to the dye laser by a specially designed positioning device. Almost all of the dye laser output could be transmitted through the fiber because the optical losses were minimal. The optical guide was a medical-grade quartz optical fiber, 5 m in length with a core diameter of 400 μm (Quartz et Silice, Paris). The exit beam divergence was approximately 20°.

The fiber was passed through the open channel of a flexible fiberbronchoscope so that the distal end protruded from the tip of the bronchoscope. The distal end of the fiber was positioned 1 to 1.5 cm from the surface of the tumor when the light was directed onto its external surface during treatment. In this case the beam diameter was approximately 10 mm with a central intense spot of 4 to 5 mm. To increase the diameter of the intense spot, we rounded the distal tip of the fiber by heating it in a flame. In essence, a small microlens was produced, and light could be more evenly distributed over a diameter of 10 to 12 mm when the fiber was held 1 to 1.5 cm from the surface of the tumor. In some patients the distal tip of the fiber was inserted directly into the body of the tumor for intralesional therapy. The output from the optical fiber was measured in a calibrated, flat-response, continuous-wave power meter.

Procedure. The protocol for treatment of our patients followed the procedures reported by Dougherty et al.[20,21] All patients received between 2.5 and 5 mg of HpD per kilogram of body weight, intravenously, from three to five days before light irradiation. General anesthesia was used for most of the procedures. Topical anesthesia was used at the request of a few patients.

The small, superficial mucosal tumors were treated with light irradiation directed onto the external surface of the tumors. Even though the superficial tumors were no more than 3 cm^2 in surface area, the diameter of the spot of light irradiation was often too small to cover the entire tumor when the probe was held in one position. However, all the tumors seemed to be adequately covered by administration of irradiation in two overlapping locations. The larger cancers were treated by inserting the probe into the mass of the tumor.

Photographs were taken before treatment and at each subsequent bronchoscopy. Biopsies and brushings were performed either several days before the administration of HpD or immediately after the laser irradiation in order to prevent interference with the absorption of the light by traumatic bleeding. Doses of light ranged from 180 to 480 J for each treatment session. The spot size ranged from 5 to 10 mm when irradiation was directed onto the external surface of the cancer.

Follow-up and Interpretation of Results. All patients understood the need for close follow-up, which included multiple bronchoscopies. The first six patients underwent bronchoscopy at least once, and in most cases twice, within the first seven days of treatment. A characteristic exudative reaction develops within several days of treatment. It takes at least four weeks for the initial edema and the exudative reaction to subside before it is possible to obtain adequate revisualization, photographic documentation, and biopsy proof of the therapeutic result. Accordingly, the last four patients had bronchoscopy repeated between four and eight weeks after phototherapy. Photographs were taken at each bronchoscopy to determine tumor response and size. Bronchoscopic brushings and biopsy specimens were obtained on each examination to determine the histologic changes.

Results were analyzed according to the following definitions: complete response — no tumor demonstrable in biopsy and brushing specimens; partial response — a greater than 50% reduction in tumor size but cancer still present in biopsy or brushing specimen; regression — a less than 50% reduction in tumor size and cancer still present in biopsy or brushing specimen; stable — no change in tumor size and cancer still present in biopsy or brushing specimen; and progression — visible enlargement of the tumor.

RESULTS

All ten patients completed one course of therapy and follow-up. The longest follow-up interval was 14 months. The results reflect the outcome of a single course of HpD phototherapy. There were a total of 11 cancers; 10 were squamous cell carcinomas and 1 was a tracheal cylindroma.

Complete response was obtained in four cancers and a partial response was obtained in five cancers. Two patients, each with a single cancer, died.

The cancers for which complete response was obtained were all small, superficial squamous cell carcinomas. Two of the four cancers were occult but were localized by the technique of HpD-fluorescence bronchoscopy. The third cancer was also occult but was localized by random brushings at routine bronchoscopy. The fourth cancer was endoscopically visible and showed subtle mucosal changes. Although the extent of the invasion of these four cancers cannot be proved without histologic section of resected tissue, our experience with small superficial cancers of this sort would indicate that these were most likely in situ with microinvasion to a depth of less than 5 mm.

The cancers in which a partial response was demonstrated included a tracheal cylindroma and four endoscopically visible squamous cell carcinomas. All the cancers were exophytic to some extent, protruding into and narrowing the normal lumen of the trachea or the bronchus. The smallest cancer in this group involved the lateral wall of the trachea in such a position that only tangential light irradiation was possible. Patients in this group will soon complete a second course of HpD phototherapy and follow-up.

None of the squamous cell carcinomas reported above were visible on chest radiographs and computed tomographic scans. In the case of the tracheal cylindroma, extratracheal involvement of the mediastinum was demonstrated on computed tomography of the chest. The eight patients in the two groups are still alive as of this writing.

The remaining two patients died within two weeks of HpD phototherapy. Both patients had squamous cell carcinomas involving a main stem bronchus. In each case the tumor measured at least 4 cm and was visible on a radiograph. Bronchoscopically, the tumors were seen to be eroding through the bronchial wall. The major portion of each tumor was extrabronchial. Both patients had experienced significant hemoptysis before HpD phototherapy. Each received 5 mg/kg of HpD intravenously. The light dose was 630 J in the first case and 480 J in the second case. Death was caused by bleeding, aspiration, and subsequent cardiac arrest six days after treatment in the first case and 11 days after treatment in the second case. Postmortem examination was not performed in either patient. It is probable that the HpD phototherapy produced extensive tumor necrosis in an already necrotic carcinoma, which resulted in further hemorrhage.

Hyperthermia seems to be an important factor in this form of phototherapy if the dye laser power output is 300 mW or greater. This is particularly true with intralesional therapy. Smoke emanating from the site of the fiber insertion was seen with treatment at the higher power levels. Bronchoscopy within a few days of treatment demonstrated a black central eschar where the probe had been inserted.

Edema and necrosis developed after treatment in four patients. In one patient, rehospitalization was required for shortness of breath and wheezing localized to the area of treatment. The patient responded to therapy with bronchodilators and corticosteroids and was able to leave the hospital in three days. Three other patients specifically complained of a cough lasting from three days to two weeks. They each noted that the cough promptly disappeared after the expectoration of a gray plug of tissue. Histologic examination of one of the tissue plugs revealed squamous cell carcinoma.

Three patients had mild first-degree sunburnlike reactions that responded promptly to antihistamine therapy.

DISCUSSION

Phototherapy with HpD is new, experimental, and unproved in the local treatment of lung cancer. It has the potential for becoming a successful modality in the treatment of in situ and early invasive bronchogenic carcinoma. With the combination of HpD-fluorescence bronchoscopy and HpD phototherapy, it is now possible to localize early occult bronchogenic carcinoma and to proceed with local bronchoscopic treatment. Local treatment is particularly appealing in patients with lung cancer because they are at high risk for surgical resection and for the development of a subsequent primary lung cancer.

It is not clear whether HpD phototherapy will prove successful in curing or even in controlling solid tumors of the tracheobronchial tree. HpD phototherapy for palliation of large endobronchial and extrabronchial cancers seems of limited use because of the potential for producing a bronchopleural fistula or hemorrhage from the necrotic tumor. Furthermore, the edema produced during the treatment could result in temporary worsening of bronchial obstruction. HpD therapy is therefore not suited for urgent treatment of an obstructed major airway.

Current requirements for HpD phototherapy include that the lesion be within the range of the flexible fiberbronchoscope, that the lesion be less than 2 to 3 cm, and that there be no evidence of erosion through the bronchial or tracheal wall. Definite indications for treatment include 1) a recurrent carcinoma in a patient in whom chemotherapy or radiation therapy (or both) failed and 2) a second primary in a patient who is ineligible for additional chemotherapy or radiation therapy. Possible indications for this therapy include 1) a second primary in a patient who is not a surgical candidate and 2) simultaneous primaries not resectable or treatable with radiation therapy. The decision to treat an individual patient should be made in concert with a pulmonologist, an oncologist, and a thoracic surgeon.

REFERENCES

1. Auler H, Banzer G. Untersuchungen über die Rolle der Porphyrine bei geschwulstkranken Menschen und Tieren. Z Krebsforsch 1942; 53:65-8.

2. Figge FHJ, Weiland GS, Manganiello LOJ. Cancer detection and therapy. Affinity of neoplastic, embryonic, and traumatized tissues for porphyrins and metalloporphyrins. Proc Soc Exp Biol Med 1948; 68:640-1.

3. Lipson RL, Baldes EJ, Olsen AM. The use of a derivative of hematoporphyrin in tumor detection. J Natl Cancer Inst 1961; 26:1-11.

4. Lipson RL, Baldes EJ. The photodynamic properties of a particular hematoporphyrin derivative. Arch Dermatol 1960; 82: 508-16.

5. Clezy PS, Hai TT, Henderson RW, van Thuc L. The chemistry of pyrrolic compounds. XLV. Haematoporphyrin derivative: haematoporphyrin diacetate as the main product of the reaction of haematoporphyrin with a mixture of acetic and sulfuric acids. Aust J Chem 1980; 33:585-97.

6. Lipson RL, Baldes EJ, Gray MJ. Hematoporphyrin derivative for detection and management of cancer. Cancer 1967; 20:2255-7.

7. Gregorie HB Jr, Horger EO, Ward JL, et al. Hematoporphyrin-derivative fluorescence in malignant neoplasms. Ann Surg 1968; 167:820-8.

8. Leonard JR, Beck WL. Hematoporphyrin fluorescence: an aid in diagnosis of malignant neoplasms. Laryngoscope 1971; 81:365-72.

9. Kyriazis GA, Balin H, Lipson RL. Hematoporphyrin-derivative-fluorescence test colposcopy and colpophotography in the diagnosis of atypical metaplasia, dysplasia, and carcinoma in situ of the cervix uteri. Am J Obstet Gynecol 1973; 117:375-80.

10. Carpenter RJ III, Neel HB III, Ryan RJ, Sanderson DR. Tumor fluorescence with hematoporphyrin derivative. Ann Otol Rhinol Laryngol 1977; 86:661-6.

11. Kinsey JH, Cortese DA, Sanderson DR. Detection of hematoporphyrin fluorescence during fiberoptic bronchoscopy to localize early bronchogenic carcinoma. Mayo Clin Proc 1978; 53:594-9.

12. Cortese DA, Kinsey JH, Woolner LB, Payne WS, Sanderson DR, Fontana RS. Clinical application of a new endoscopic technique for detection of in situ bronchial carcinoma. Mayo Clin Proc 1979; 54:635-41.

13. Kinsey JH, Cortese DA. Endoscopic system for simultaneous visual examination and electronic detection of fluorescence. Rev Sci Instrum 1980; 51:1403-6.

14. Cortese DA, Kinsey JH. Hematoporphyrin-derivative fluorescence for lung cancer localization. Semin Respir Med 1981; 3:37-41.

15. Diamond I, Granelli SG, McDonagh AF, Nielsen S, Wilson CB, Jaenicke R. Photodynamic therapy of malignant tumours. Lancet 1972; 2:1175-7.

16. Granelli SG, Diamond I, McDonagh AF, Wilson CB, Nielsen SL. Photochemotherapy of glioma cells by visible light and hematoporphyrin. Cancer Res 1975; 35:2567-70.

17. Kelly JF, Snell ME. Hematoporphyrin derivative: a possible aid in the diagnosis and therapy of carcinoma of the bladder. J Urol 1976; 115:150-1.

18. Dougherty TJ, Grindey GB, Fiel R, Weishaupt KR, Boyle DG. Photoradiation therapy. II. Cure of animal tumors with hematoporphyrin and light. J Natl Cancer Inst 1975; 55:115-21.

19. Dougherty TJ, Gomer CJ, Weishaupt KR. Energetics and efficiency of photoinactivation of murine tumor cells containing hematoporphyrin. Cancer Res 1976; 36:2330-3.

20. Dougherty TJ, Kaufman JE, Goldfarb A, Weishaupt KR, Boyle D, Mittleman A. Photoradiation therapy for the treatment of malignant tumors. Cancer Res 1978; 38:2628-35.

21. Dougherty TJ, Lawrence G, Kaufman JH, Boyle D, Weishaupt KR, Goldfarb A. Photoradiation in the treatment of recurrent breast carcinoma. J Natl Cancer Inst 1979; 62:231-7.

22. Weishaupt KR, Gomer CJ, Dougherty TJ. Identification of singlet oxygen as the cytotoxic agent in photo-inactivation of a murine tumor. Cancer Res 1976; 36:2326-9.

23. Signorelli CD, Ammirati M, Tajana G. Photochemotherapy of human glioma cells in culture by hematoporphyrin and visible light (preliminary experiment). Acta Neurol (Napoli) 1978; 33:105-12.

24. Sery TW. Photodynamic killing of retinoblastoma cells with hematoporphyrin and light. Cancer Res 1979; 39:96-100.

25. Christensen T, Moan J. Photodynamic inactivation of synchronized human cells in vitro in the presence of hematoporphyrin. Cancer Res 1979; 39:3735-7.

26. Kinsey JH, Cortese DA, Moses HL, Ryan RJ, Branum EL. Photodynamic effect of hematoporphyrin derivative as a function of optical spectrum and incident energy density. Cancer Res 1981; 41:5020-6.

27. Bugelski PJ, Porter CW, Dougherty TJ. Autoradiographic distribution of hematoporphyrin derivative in normal and tumor tissue of the mouse. Cancer Res 1981; 41:4606-12.

28. Chang CT, Dougherty TJ. Photoradiation therapy: kinetics and thermodynamics of porphyrin uptake and loss in normal and malignant cells in culture, abstracted. Radiat Res 1978; 74:498.

29. Kessel D. Transport and binding of hematoporphyrin derivative and related porphyrins by murine leukemia L1210 cells. Cancer Res 1981; 41:1318-23.

30. Kessel D. Effects of photo-activated porphyrins on cell-surface properties. Biochem Soc Trans 1977; 5:139-40.

31. Kohn K, Kessel D. On the mode of cytotoxic action of photo-activated porphyrins. Biochem Pharmacol 1979; 28: 2465-70.

32. Torinuki W, Miura T, Seiji M. Lysosome destruction and lipoperoxide formation due to active oxygen generated from haematoporphyrin and UV irradiation. Br J Dermatol 1980; 102: 17-27.

33. Bodaness RS, Chan PC. Singlet oxygen as a mediator in the hematoporphyrin-catalyzed photooxidation of NADPH to $NADP^+$ in deuterium oxide. J Biol Chem 1977; 252:8554-60.

34. Moan J, Pettersen EO, Christensen T. The mechanism of photodynamic inactivation of human cells in vitro in the presence of haematoporphyrin. Br J Cancer 1979; 39:398-407.

35. Buettner GR, Oberley LW. The apparent production of superoxide and hydroxyl radicals by hematoporphyrin and light as seen by spin-trapping. FEBS Lett 1980; 121:161-4.

36. Hariharan PV, Courtney J, Eleczko S. Production of hydroxyl radicals in cell systems exposed to haematoporphyrin and red light. Int J Radiat Biol 1980; 37:691-4.

37. Gomer CJ. DNA damage and repair in CHO cells following hematoporphyrin photoradiation. Cancer Lett 1980; 11: 161-7.

Ann Otol Rhinol Laryngol 91:1982

PEDIATRIC CAUSTIC INGESTION

JEFFREY S. ADAM, MD HERBERT G. BIRCK, MD

COLUMBUS, OHIO

Accidental caustic ingestion in the pediatric age group continues to be a controversial and difficult problem. This retrospective study gives clinical support to treating this problem with early esophagoscopy, steroids, antibiotics and dilatation. Four hundred two patients were evaluated for possible caustic burn of the esophagus. Of the 70 patients who had esophageal burns demonstrated at esophagoscopy and who were treated with steroids, antibiotics and dilatation, none developed strictures. The two patients not treated in this fashion developed strictures.

INTRODUCTION

Accidental caustic ingestion in the pediatric age group remains a major challenge to the practicing otolaryngologist. Estimates show that over 5,000 accidental caustic ingestions occur in the United States yearly in the 5-and-under age group.[1] The late 1960s saw a sharp increase in the number of burns with the introduction of strong alkaline drainpipe cleaners. When Liquid-plumr first came on the market, it consisted of a 30% sodium hydroxide solution, which is very caustic. The potentiation for ingestion of caustic material, coupled with the inherent difficulty of surgically dealing with the esophagus, makes the possible adverse consequences of caustic ingestion quite protean. This study reviews the experience of the Columbus Children's Hospital with accidental caustic ingestion and assesses the efficacy of our present treatment protocol. A review is presented of the pathophysiology of caustic burns of the esophagus, which is important to the development of a rational treatment regime.

A distinction should be made between alkali and acid ingestion. Because acid causes a coagulation-type necrosis, it does not penetrate the esophageal lining deeply; hence, gastric ulceration, perforation or pyloric stenosis are the more likely consequences. In contrast, alkalis cause a liquefaction-type necrosis that allows penetration to the deep muscular layers of the esophagus, occasionally resulting in perforations. The esophageal changes caused by alkaline burns are divided into three phases. The first is the acute necrotic phase in which cell death occurs due to coagulation of intracellular protein. An intense inflammatory reaction develops in the viable tissues surrounding the overlying area of necrosis and vessel thrombosis occurs. The phase ends with the sloughing of the superficial necrotic layer two to four days after injury.

MATERIAL AND METHODS

This study represents the retrospective review of 402 consecutive cases. It includes actual as well as possible accidental caustic ingestion in a pediatric group seen during the period from Jan 1, 1970, to Dec 31, 1979. There were no suicidal attempts in this series. The study also excludes transfers from other hospitals if the patient was not started on steroids and antibiotics less than 48 hours after ingestion.

All children who underwent esophagoscopy had a strong history pointing to accidental caustic ingestion, ie, a responsible adult either witnessed the ingestion or discovered the child crying near an open container of a caustic agent. Thus, in the presence of strongly implicating circumstantial evidence, a child was a candidate for esophagoscopy, even though caustic burns in or about the oral cavity were not obvious.

The 402 patients were managed by a treatment protocol in use since the early 1960s. First, an esophagoscopy under general anesthesia is performed 24-36 hours after ingestion. This is usually done on an outpatient basis. The esophagoscope is passed up to but not past the point of injury. Done in this manner, early esophagoscopy has proven to be a totally safe procedure. The gross mucosal changes seen in the early acute necrotic phase include erythema, edema, ulceration and fibrinous exudate. If there are no changes the patient is discharged. If there are positive findings, steroids are administered, 2 mg/lb/day prednisone, and the patient remains hospitalized. When the esophagus is moderately or severely burned, steroids are administered for 2 weeks with tapering during the third and fourth week. Antibiotics, specifically ampicillin or amoxicillin, 50 mg/kg/day by mouth, are given simultaneously, as the major reported infections are usually due to gram-positive cocci. Steroids are empirically administered to patients whose esophagoscopy is scheduled later than 36 hours after ingestion. (Such delays are practiced to prevent the expense of mobilizing the operating room team in the middle of the night.) Dilatation is started on the second day and, to be effective, should be continued until a No. 34 Maloney dilator can be accommodated to prevent later foreign body complications. All patients are given a full diet by the third day as we feel that the food bolus itself acts as a dilator. A barium swallow x-ray examination is done on an outpatient basis 3-4 weeks after ingestion to rule out the possibility of early stricture formation.

RESULTS

At the time of endoscopy, 330 (82%) of the patients had normal esophageal examinations; 72 (18%) had positive findings. The Figure demonstrates that the 22- to 24-month age group appears to be the most commonly involved. These data are in agreement with the studies of others.[2,3] At this age the toddler demonstrates an active curiosity for

From the Department of Otolaryngology, Children's Hospital and Ohio State University, Columbus.

Presented at the meeting of the American Broncho-Esophagological Association, Palm Beach, Florida, May 3-4, 1982.

REPRINTS — Herbert G. Birck, MD, Children's Hospital, Columbus, OH 43205.

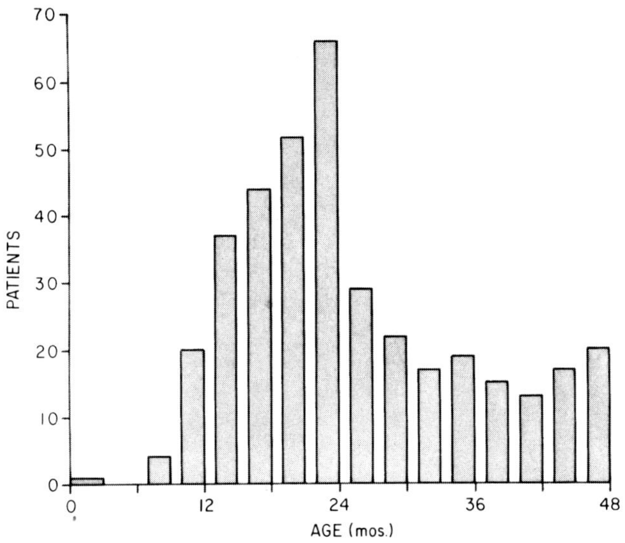

Caustic ingestion in pediatric patients by age.

the environment and is physically able to explore the surroundings. The commonly encountered caustic agents in our patients are listed in the Table along with the total number of patients ingesting each agent and the number of positive and negative esophagoscopies performed. Liquid Drano, a 20% sodium hydroxide solution, was the most commonly ingested agent. Hawkins et al[3] feel that solid caustic agents have a higher incidence of esophageal burns than liquid agents. He reasons that a solid bolus of caustic material is more likely than a liquid agent to have prolonged contact with the esophageal mucosal lining since the solid agent is quickly swallowed while the liquid agent is expelled from the mouth immediately after the oral mucosa is burned. This observation was not borne out in our study. A lower rate of positive findings resulted from solid Drano crystals than from liquid Drano (15% versus 20%) or the Clin-O-Test tablets.

Reports on the physical examination of the positive extraesophageal burns ranged from mild hyperemia on the dorsum of the tongue to ulceration of the oral mucosa or skin. The extraesophageal burns are classified as significant or minor on the basis of how they were described. Thirty-six of the 72 patients with positive esophagoscopies had significant extraesophageal burns while three with positive esophagoscopies had no extraesophageal burns. Thus the status of the esophagus cannot be related to the presence or absence of an extraesophageal burn.

Analysis of our management of these cases indicates that of eight patients who received no treatment, two developed strictures. In six cases it was the feeling of the attending physician that the positive findings at esophagoscopy were so minimal that further treatment was not warranted. The two patients in the untreated group who eventually developed severe strictures were judged normal at the time of their initial esophagoscopies. Obviously the

CAUSTIC AGENTS INGESTED (N = 402)

Agent	*+ Esoph.*	*− Esoph.*	*Total*
Drano			
Liquid	21	86	107
Solid	7	41	48
Lye	14	40	54
Toilet bowl cleaner (Vanish, Saniflush, Vansol)	7	45	52
Ammonia cleanser	7	29	36
Ammonia ampules	0	18	18
Plunge	3	15	10
Clin-O-Test tablets	0	10	10
HTH (pool cleaner)	0	10	8
Oven cleaner	0	8	8
Dry cleaning fluid	0	2	2
Unknown, miscellaneous	13	26	39

+ - Esophageal burns; − - No esophageal burns.

burns were missed at that time. The remaining 64 patients were treated with ampicillin or amoxicillin, prednisone and dilatation. There was no stricture formation in this group. In an attempt to quantitate the severity of the esophageal burns, we classified them as mild, moderate and severe on the basis of the following criteria. Burns were classified as mild if only erythema and/or edema of the mucosa was observed. Burns were classified as moderate if erythema, blister formation, superficial ulceration and fibrinous exudate were seen at the time of the esophagoscopy. Severe burns were diagnosed if erythema, deep ulceration and eschar formation were observed at esophagoscopy. The information needed to classify each burn was obtained from the description in the operative report. Of the eight patients in the untreated group, six had mild burns; of the 64 patients receiving treatment, 26 had mild burns, 21 had moderate burns and 17 had severe burns.

DISCUSSION

The protean complications of caustic esophageal burns in the pediatric age group can be devastating to patient and family. This fact is readily demonstrated by one of our patients who progressed to a severe stricture after an esophagoscopy described as normal. This 2-year-old child was readmitted 1 month after ingestion with increasing difficulty swallowing. She had another esophagoscopy at this time which resulted in an esophageal perforation. A thoracic surgeon drained her cervical esophagus, performed a gastrostomy and placed a string inside the esophagus for future retrograde dilatation. She was subsequently readmitted for division of her cervical esophagus and creation of a cervical esophagostomy. She was admitted 8 months later and had a colon interposition with takedown of her cervical esophagostomy and pyloroplasty. Subsequently, she was admitted six times over a 10-month period and had six endoscopic procedures for dilatation of her esophagus and esophago-colonic anastomosis. To date, a total hospital bill of $69,780 has been incurred for this child.

Prior to the work of Spain et al in 1950[4] which

demonstrated the anti-inflammatory properties of steroids, treatment plans were aimed at dealing with stricture formation. The Salzer method[5] recommended early dilatation beginning just two to three days after burn. The Jackson method, however, recommended delaying dilatation until 2-3 weeks after burn.[6] Various stenting techniques, such as the one described by Reyes and Hill,[7] were also employed.

After the work of Spain et al in 1950, many investigators used steroids both in experimental and clinical settings.[8-14] Since Spain et al did the basic research on which steroid management of caustic ingestion is based, a closer look at their work seems warranted.

Spain et al also emphasized the importance of early steroid usage. In another group the same dose of steroids was given but administration began 48 hours after wounding. No difference in quality or quantity of granulation tissue was found when compared to the control groups. Antibiotics were also shown to be effective in the treatment of alkaline burns of the esophagus. Haller et al[10] described the risk of pulmonary infection from aspiration secondary to dysphagia and obstruction due to inflammatory edema at the site of injury. He also pointed to the possibility of bacterial invasion of the mediastinum through the wall of the injured esophagus even though gross perforation was not present. He therefore recommended the use of antibiotics. Krey[11] showed that experimentally antibiotics control inflammation and hasten the injury-repair process, thereby helping to decrease stricture formation. It should be remembered that these patients are usually treated concomitantly with steroids and, therefore, are immunosuppressed; antibiotics are a necessity in preventing infection. Many authors have reported the benefits of early esophagoscopy.[2,3,10,14,15] The presence or absence of an esophageal burn can be established immediately and should a burn be present, appropriate treatment can be started. It is cost effective; the total cost of an esophagoscopy in our institution is approximately $658, compared to the total cost of $69,780 for the patient described above. Three hundred thirty of our patients were discharged the day of surgery, resulting in obvious savings of time and resources. We feel that an esophagoscopy as described in the early stages of the acute necrotic phase is a safe procedure. Esophagoscopy can provide knowledge of the severity and extent of the injury not obtainable from a barium swallow examination. Lastly, as our results and the results of others have demonstrated, the presence or absence of extraesophageal burns may not be an accurate indicator of esophageal status. An esophagoscopy is necessary. Our treatment protocol represents an aggressive approach to the problem of caustic ingestion in children, which we believe is preferable from the outset to more conservative treatment.

CONCLUSION

This review of 402 patients provides strong clinical support for the use of steroids, antibiotics and early dilatation in the treatment of caustic burns of the esophagus. We feel that early esophagoscopy is the best method of evaluating the esophagus for caustic burn. In addition to its effectiveness in treating caustic esophageal burns, the protocol described above has proved to be cost effective.

REFERENCES

1. Reyes HM, Lin CY, Schlunk FF, Replogle RL. Experimental treatment of corrosive esophageal burns. J Pediatr Surg 1974; 9:317-27.

2. Tewfik TL, Schloss MD. Ingestion of lye and other corrosive agents — a study of 86 infant and child cases. J Otolaryngol 1980; 9:72-7.

3. Hawkins DB, Demeter MJ, Barnett TE. Caustic ingestion: controversies in management. A review of 214 cases. Laryngoscope 1980; 90:98-109.

4. Spain DM, Molomut N, Haber A. The effect of cortisone on the formation of granulation tissue in mice [Abstract]. Am J Pathol 1950; 26:710.

5. Bosher LH. The pathology of experimentally produced lye burns and strictures of the esophagus. J Thorac Cardiovasc Surg 1954; 24: 483-9.

6. Tucker JA, Yarington CT. The treatment of caustic ingestion. Otolaryngol Clin North Am 1970; 12:343-9.

7. Reyes HM, Hill JL. Modification of the experimental stent technique for esophageal burns. J Surg Res 1976; 20:65-70.

8. Lund-Iverson L. Cortisone treatment of corrosive lesions of the oesophagus. Acta Otolaryngol (Stockh) 1978; 92:364-9.

9. Weisskopf A. Effects of cortisone on experimental lye burns of the esophagus. Ann Otol Rhinol Laryngol 1952; 64:681-9.

10. Haller JA, Andrews HG, White JJ, Tamer MA, Cleveland WW. Pathophysiology and management of acute corrosive burns of the esophagus: results of treatment in 285 children. J Pediatr Surg 1971; 6:578-83.

11. Krey H. On the treatment of corrosive lesions in the esophagus. Acta Otolaryngol (Stockh) 1952; 102 Suppl:1-49.

12. Webb WR, Koutras P, Ecker RR, Sugg WL. An evaluation of steroids and antibiotics in caustic burns of the esophagus. Ann Thorac Surg 1970; 9:95-102.

13. Haller JA, Bachman K. The comparative effect of current therapy on experimental caustic burns of the esophagus. Pediatrics 1964; 34:236-45.

14. Middelkamp JN, Ferguson TB, Roper CL, Hoffman FD. The management and problems of caustic burns in children. J Thorac Cardiovasc Surg 1969; 57:341-7.

15. Viscomi GJ, Beekhuis GJ, Whitten CF. An evaluation of early esophagoscopy and corticosteroid therapy in the management of corrosive injury of the esophagus. Pediatrics 1961; 59:356-60.

MEDIASTINOSCOPY FOR EXTRATHORACIC MALIGNANCIES

LOUIS W. WELSH, MD
JENKINTOWN, PENNSYLVANIA

JOHN J. WELSH, MD
JENKINTOWN, PENNSYLVANIA

J. C. CHINNICI, DO, MS
PHILADELPHIA, PENNSYLVANIA

GEORGE F. HUCK, JR, MD
ABINGTON, PENNSYLVANIA

Metastatic tumors from extrathoracic sources appear in the mediastinum infrequently and from a variety of locations. In this series of approximately 350 malignancies of the mediastinum, 20 (6%) originated from the breast, prostate, kidney, pelvis, and gastrointestinal tract. A radiologic review of these cases does not identify a unique pattern, although paratracheal masses present most often, while unilateral hilar adenopathy occurs somewhat less frequently. The history of previous surgery for malignancy suggests metastatic disease into the mediastinum. However, other entities of second primaries, lymphoma, Hodgkin's disease, and benign processes warrant consideration. Mediastinoscopy is reemphasized as a valuable diagnostic technique for the solution of these problems.

Metastatic neoplasms appearing in the mediastinum from extrathoracic sources are relatively uncommon. Consequently, awareness of this remote possibility is essential from a diagnostic and therapeutic standpoint. In the investigation of the mediastinal mass, mediastinoscopy plays an important role in procuring the tissue essential for the ultimate confirmation of the pathologic process.

There are several goals of this presentation, namely, 1) an overview of the many types of space-taking lesions appearing in the mediastinum through an analysis of our experience, 2) a consideration of metastases from extrathoracic or intrathoracic malignancies, and 3) the radiologic and endoscopic investigation of such entities.

A number of historical and clinical points should be considered as background material for the evaluation of mediastinal disease. For many years we have been aware of the diagnostic and therapeutic value of mediastinoscopy following the report by Carlens.[1] The surgical and medical literature abounds with application, diagnostic value, and therapeutic gain. The present authors' personal advocacy can be summarized in two areas, namely, the diagnosis and staging of lung cancer,[2] and the procurement of tissue for histologic confirmation in the disease entities of lymphoma, Hodgkin's disease, and sarcoidosis.[3,4] Prognosis and survival time can be predicted for carcinoma of the lung via positive endoscopic biopsy of the mediastinum.[2] Furthermore, a differentiation of similarly appearing inflammatory and neoplastic disorders may be readily solved by endoscopic biopsy.

From the radiologic standpoint, pulmonary abnormalities illustrating the classic presentation of a peripheral or a central density and with associated mediastinal adenopathy suggest the the diagnosis of lung cancer. By contrast, a mediastinal lesion described as either solitary or multiple nodular masses without a pulmonary parenchymal infiltrate relates to a wide spectrum of disease. As our data suggest, the most likely tissue of origin is based upon statistical probability. Viewed as a radiologic challenge, it is this group of mediastinal masses that is the most difficult to consider from a secure diagnostic standpoint. We should also comment that a significant number of highly anaplastic or undifferentiated tumors cannot be identified with regard to the cell of origin. Further, the experienced clinician realizes that radiologic interpretation of mediastinal space-taking lesions is often more descriptive than diagnostic, identifying in turn the location, size, density and configuration of the lesion. Although specific chambers within the mediastinum contain a number of tumors unique to that location (eg, neural tumors in the posterior compartment), nonetheless, the variety of neoplastic entities is sufficiently broad that the presumptive diagnosis necessarily falls within a group of several or more possibilities.

The composite clinical and radiologic evaluation may not suggest a specific diagnosis, yet some findings such as neural interruption and venous obstruction would infer a more ominous entity such as malignancy rather than inflammatory response. The nonspecific vague history is often of minimal diagnostic assistance. Finally, curative surgery in the mediastinum is severely limited by the invasive behavior of many neoplasms into essential structures, precluding total removal.

The authors, having outlined the major goals of this paper, suggest that the most important role of mediastinoscopy for metastatic disease is identification of the cellular origin of the neoplasm. Conclusions are derived from the evaluation of 20 cases from seven extrathoracic sources. The pertinent

Presented at the meeting of the American Broncho-Esophagological Association, Palm Beach, Florida, May 3-4, 1982.
REPRINTS — Louis W. Welsh, MD, 179 Washington Lane, Jenkintown, PA 19046.

anatomy of the mediastinal lymphatics plus the associated peripheral connections and the modes of spread are discussed as appears relevant to the understanding of these cases.

ANATOMY OF DISSECTION

Metastatic disease extending into the mediastinal chambers for the most part spares the anterior region. This is surgically fortunate due to the relative inaccessibility of this region for endoscopic exploration. The middle compartment which contains the bulk of lymphatic connections permits satisfactory dissection with relative ease. The posterior segment is a secondary area of concern with relatively infrequent first- or second-level metastatic activity. The superior mediastinum which is related to the paratracheal and visceral lymphatics (ie, thyroid gland) is accessible, easily explored and provides a high yield in advanced head and neck neoplasms.

LYMPHATIC NETWORK

The anatomy of the lymphatic system concerned with the cases in this presentation will be reviewed. We draw attention to the fact that an occasional site of metastasis is apart from the anticipated pattern of lymphatic spread. This devious development can be explained as secondary lymphatic streaming into minor channels still within the normal anatomic pattern.

The lymphatic system[5] may be considered regionally with significant channels terminating in the mediastinum from the head and neck, breast, cutaneous areas of the trunk and the abdominal and pelvic viscera.

The upper body drains into the bronchomediastinal trunk by way of the peripheral smaller ducts and trunks.

In the head and neck region, integration of the cervical visceral channels is through the jugular and bronchomediastinal trunks. The thoracic cutaneous lymphatics relate to the posterior intercostal nodes or anteriorly to the internal mammary nodes. The breast associates by quadrants ultimately into the mediastinal nodes from channels along the internal mammary vessels and axillary system.

The major abdominal trunk is the cisterna chyli and is ultimately confluent with the thoracic duct.

The gastrointestinal lymphatic system flows through subsidiary nodes along the regional arteries, subsequently into an intestinal trunk entering the cisterna chyli and terminating in the thoracic mediastinal region. The kidney drains via channels into the lateral lumbar nodes, sequentially thereafter into the lumbar trunk and the cisterna chyli.

It is apparent in the regions under discussion that while the immediate lymphatic connections may not be mediastinal (eg, the lateral breast and the abdominal viscera), the ultimate fate of lymph-flow bearing neoplastic cells is through the mediastinum into the venous terminals of the jugular and subclavian veins. Surgical, radiotherapeutic, inflammatory, or neoplastic conditions may further alter lymphatic flow resulting in unusual or relatively aberrant metastases. This is the condition of most of the cases under review in this paper.

LITERATURE REVIEW

An informative paper by Winterbauer et al[6] discussed the interpretation of bilateral hilar adenopathy and clinical correlation with established diagnosis. A wide experience with sarcoidosis and other diseases which produce mediastinal adenopathy was presented. The spectrum included 99 patients with sarcoidosis, 212 with lymphoma, 500 with bronchogenic carcinoma and 354 instances of pulmonary metastases from extrathoracic tumors. In addition to a clinical evaluation, important radiologic correlates were drawn with each disease class. In this series, 74 of 99 patients with sarcoidosis presented with symmetrical hilar adenopathy at the time of diagnosis. Of this group, hilar adenopathy was the only radiographic abnormality in 29 patients, and in addition, peritracheal nodes (usually right side and unilateral) were an associated finding in 30 of 74 patients with hilar adenopathy. The important observation made by these authors is that peritracheal without hilar adenopathy was not seen in any patient with sarcoidosis. Evaluation of the 212 patients with lymphoma was subdivided into 96 with Hodgkin's disease, 62 with reticulum cell sarcoma, 27 with lymphoblastic lymphoma, 18 with lymphocytic lymphoma and 9 with unclassified lymphoma. Of these confirmed 212 with the various subgroups of lymphoma, 63 presented with abnormal chest x-ray studies. These authors indicate that bilateral hilar adenopathy does not relate to any specific form of lymphoma. The chest film, by contrast with sarcoidosis, demonstrated peritracheal masses without hilar adenopathy and was the most common abnormality. Forty-three percent of the total had unilateral hilar enlargement, pleural effusion, an anterior mediastinal mass and parenchymal nodules. Delayed bilateral adenopathy appeared at a mean of 24 months after confirmation of the diagnosis in 12 patients while 8 of 63 presented with bilateral densities. Clinically, systemic and thoracic symptoms were associated with lymphoma and mimicked sarcoidosis. Peripheral nodes were identified and biopsied in a small group of this series and were diagnostic for lymphoma. It is interesting that in the 500 cases with bronchogenic carcinoma (confirmed by extrathoracic tumor biopsy), two cases presented with bilateral adenopathy. The group with extrathoracic tumors included 354 cases with evidence of intrathoracic metastases, but only two cases presented with bilateral hilar node enlargement.

The authors[3] cite a number of cases in which the histologic report "consistent with" sarcoidosis conflicts with the clinical course and ultimate diagnosis of malignancy. Three cases were eventually categorized as one generalized form of malignant melanoma with reactive change in the mediastinal nodes, and two instances of Hodgkin's disease. Three cases were considered to have the epithelioid reaction as a response to regional malignancy. The radiologic appearance in each instance was atypical and not consistent with sarcoidosis, such as unilateral hilar disease, or symmetrical bilateral mediastinal widening due to peritracheal adenopathy.

Mediastinoscopy has not been employed extensively for the evaluation of metastatic carcinoma of the breast. A report by Neifeld et al[7] cites their experience with mediastinoscopy as a diagnostic aid in six patients to obtain tissue for estrogen receptor analysis. The authors limit the procedure to those individuals with evidence of mediastinal disease by chest roentgenography, tomography, or gallium scintigraphy, where more easily accessible sites were not apparent.

The natural course of renal carcinoma with extension by metastases into lymph nodes is discussed by Arkless.[8] In his series of 152 patients, 12 developed obvious supradiaphragmatic nodal disease 11 of which were located in the carinal, hilar, or paratracheal areas. Five patients in the same group had anterior cervical or supraclavicular adenopathy. An unusual case presentation by Khan and Khan[9] cited a 52-year-old man with minimal symptoms and radiographic findings of bilateral hilar adenopathy resembling sarcoidosis. A scalene node biopsy established the site of origin, later confirmed by diagnostic studies, to be the left kidney. The authors suggest tissue confirmation for the diagnosis of sarcoidosis as a consequence of this case. Subsequent to this report another case was cited by Ahmad and Zevallos[10] describing a similar pattern of bilateral hilar adenopathy consistent with sarcoidosis but confirmed via mediastinoscopy as renal in origin. Robson et al[11] commented upon the value of mediastinoscopy in determining the presence of lymphatic metastasis from renal cell carcinoma and wrote that "it is used routinely to determine the need for extensive subdiaphragmatic lymphatic dissection."

Feldman and Kricun[12] discussed a malignant melanoma presenting as a mediastinal mass. Confirmation was by mediastinoscopy though the primary site of origin was not determined.

Webb[13] surveyed 65 patients with intrathoracic metastases from melanoma of which 35 patients had metastases to hilar or mediastinal nodes. Five of the 28 patients with pulmonary nodules demonstrated symmetrical hilar adenopathy resembling sarcoidosis, and seven individuals had unilateral involvement of lung, hilar and mediastinal nodes.

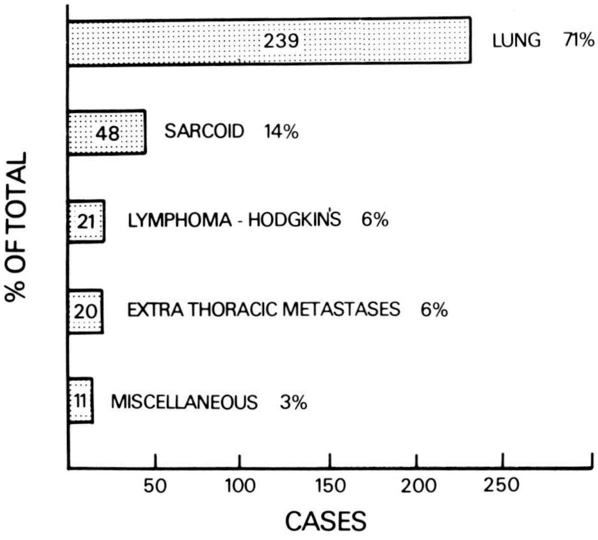

Fig. 1. Analysis by tissue of 339 cases of mediastinal metastases.

The inferolateral lymphatic channels emanating from the thyroid gland empty into the pretracheal, paratracheal, and infraglandular nodes.[14] As described by Sisson and Feldman,[15] extension and spread of malignancy into the anterior mediastinum is through this system and warrants surgical removal.

DATA

The authors have reviewed 339 cases in which mediastinoscopy and biposy furnished a positive tissue diagnosis. Surgery has been limited, with a few exceptions, to the cases in which standard roentgenographs or planigrams clearly demonstrated adenopathy or widening of the compartment compatible with diffuse neoplastic expansion. This policy was adopted to minimize the cases in which the surgical yield was low (ie, below 10%) or in which the metastatic potential was similarly insignificant or established by bronchoscopic biopsy.

Figure 1 identifies the relative importance of malignant and inflammatory disease in the mediastinal lymph nodes. Cancer of the lung is the most significant component of the five major headings, encompassing 71% of the total series. This preponderance reflects the relative importance and high incidence of pulmonary neoplasms in a general hospital census. Sarcoidosis is less frequent in this review, but still comprises 14% of the series. Hodgkin's disease, non-Hodgkin's lymphoma, and leukemic infiltrate diminish in quantity, appearing in approximately 6% of the total.

Miscellaneous diagnoses include tuberculosis and fungal infections of lymph nodes, thymic diseases (cyst and thymoma), substernal thyroid, and developmental cysts. Finally the metastatic group, although statistically small, is 6% of the series.

When the lung cancers are excluded, there are approximately 100 diagnostic problems of mediastinal masses. The presence of asymptomatic hilar adenopathy particularly associated with uveitis or cutaneous nodules is classic for sarcoidosis and these individuals may be withdrawn from further consideration. This exclusion reduces the diagnostic census to approximately 50 individuals.

SITE OF ORIGIN

There were 20 cases of mediastinal metastases from extrathoracic primary malignancies with seven sites of origin. Consequently the data are diluted, almost anecdotal, and not statistically significant for any site of origin. The sex ratio is seven men to 13 women, skewed by the eight cases of female breast malignancy; the next largest group (4) originated in the prostate. Six patients conclude the group with sites of origin being kidney (2), gastrointestinal tract (2), thyroid gland (1), and uterus (1). The ages range from 35 to 78 years with a mean of 59 years; the melanoma patients are in their 30s (35 and 36 years) and the most senior patient (78 years) is in the group with prostatic carcinoma. These 20 cases will be detailed briefly and some of the appropriate films presented.

BREAST CANCER

Breast malignancies, as the most common in this series, will be considered first. The patients, but for one, have been followed in the breast tumor clinic undergoing periodic chest x-ray studies. Films are taken for new pulmonary complaints in addition to a routine screening plan. Shortness of breath and cough were the most common presenting complaint (5/8); other symptoms were a pathologic fracture of the hip, headache due to intracerebral metastases, and posterior fossa spread with cerebellar and brainstem disorders. Only one individual was symptom-free at the time of the abnormal chest film.

While the bronchoscopic evaluation as a preliminary investigation is quite valuable, only one of this group exhibited endoscopic evidence of neoplasm which was reported initially as poorly differentiated epidermoid carcinoma, probably of pulmonary origin. Later, the diagnosis was corrected to adenocarcinoma of the breast after reception of more adequate tissue from mediastinoscopy.

The radiologic appearance presented a broad spectrum of abnormality. The most common form of presentation is parenchymal nodules due to pulmonary showering of neoplasm. Hilar adenopathy is associated less frequently with peripheral nodules and rarely with a pleural effusion.

The onset of clinically evident metastases ranged from as brief as three months postmastectomy, to 13 years of apparent tumor freedom.

Case 1. The chest radiograph of a 61-year-old woman with generalized spread through the parenchyma and with mediastinal metastases is presented. This individual had previously undergone radical mastectomy two years before the current investigation and positive axillary nodes were identified (Fig. 2A,B).

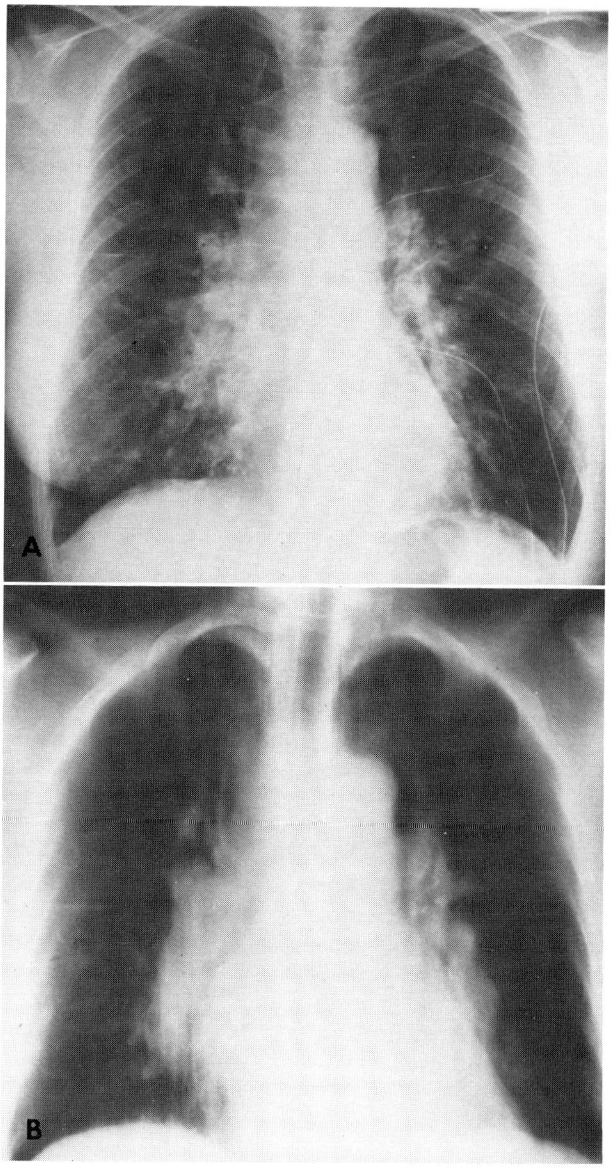

Fig. 2. (Case 1) A) Bilateral hilar and suprahilar adenopathy with scattered densities in pulmonary parenchyma. Note absent left breast. B) Tomogram more clearly illustrates diffuse nodular mediastinal disease than standard chest film.

The endoscopic examination was unremarkable and randomized transbronchoscopic biopsies showed only bronchitis and essentially normal alveolar tissue. Exploration by mediastinoscopy revealed a number of tumor-bearing nodes in the paratracheal region and tracheobronchial groove.

PROSTATIC CANCER

Malignancy of the prostate gland with mediastinal metastases is considered in four cases. The out-

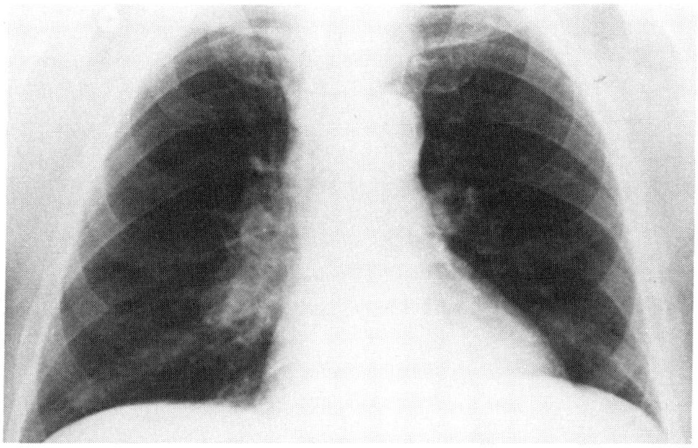

Fig. 3. (Case 2) Patient demonstrated right hilar and infrahilar masses confirmed as metastatic neoplasm from primary prostate cancer.

standing symptoms related to bone pain from metastases into the pelvis and lumbar spine in two cases, hoarseness due to interruption of the left recurrent laryngeal nerve in one case, and one symptom-free individual with an abnormal chest x-ray study. The significant x-ray studies identified pulmonary nodules (one patient) and abnormal mediastinal configuration (three patients). Bronchoscopy identified compression of the trachea in one patient but was otherwise unrewarding in the three remaining cases. The history of relatively recent prostate surgery was obtained in each case with a maximum period of three years intervening before distant symptoms appeared.

Case 2. A 69-year-old man was symptom-free and therefore the chest x-ray study was routine, demonstrating right hilar and infrahilar adenopathy (Fig. 3). Though this patient was asymptomatic, metastatic neoplasm was identified and confirmed in the right hilar region.

CANCER OF THE KIDNEY

Two cases of renal carcinoma underwent mediastinoscopy and biopsy for adenopathy in the paratracheal and tracheobronchial areas. One individual was asymptomatic; the initial complaint of the second individual was hip pain. Nonetheless, in the latter case, metastatic disease was confirmed from a primary renal lesion seven years before the current evaluation.

Case 3. This 69-year-old man presented with a painful hip. During the investigation, chest films disclosed an abnormality in the right infrahilar region confirmed by tomography. The film of the pelvis identified a large lytic lesion destroying most of the ilium. Subsequent radiologic investigation by renal angiography depicted the vascular pattern of neoplasm (Fig. 4A,B).

MALIGNANT MELANOMA

The unpredictable behavior pattern of malignant melanoma is exemplified by the following two cases. Two young women, ages 36 and 35 respectively, underwent wide excision of primary neoplasm from the back and flank, 4 and 11 years before their current problems developed. Mediastinoscopy was positive in each instance.

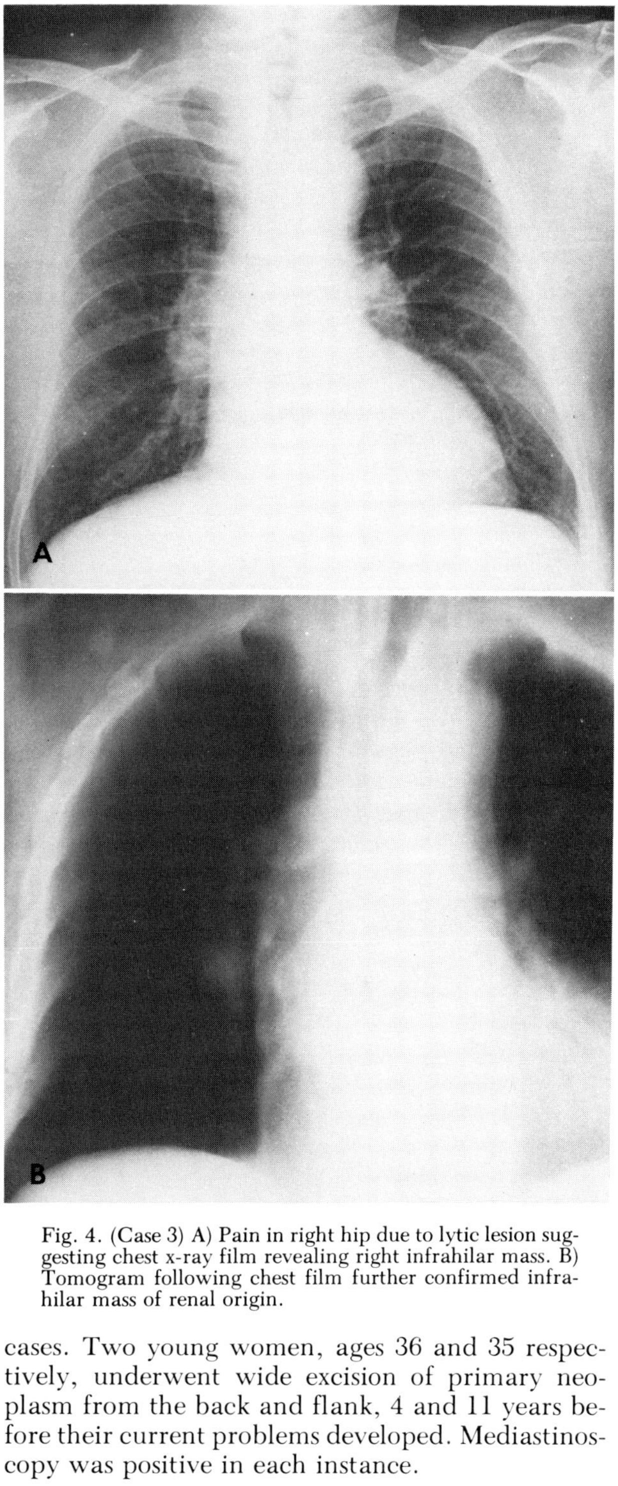

Fig. 4. (Case 3) A) Pain in right hip due to lytic lesion suggesting chest x-ray film revealing right infrahilar mass. B) Tomogram following chest film further confirmed infrahilar mass of renal origin.

GASTROINTESTINAL MALIGNANCIES

There are two representative cases; one case with primary carcinoma originating in the stomach and in the second case originating in the pancreas. The patients were a 55-year-old man and a 49-year-old woman. In each instance, the presenting complaint was intractable, excruciating back pain. Radiographs indicated large right paratracheal masses with no evidence of bone erosion in the rib cage or

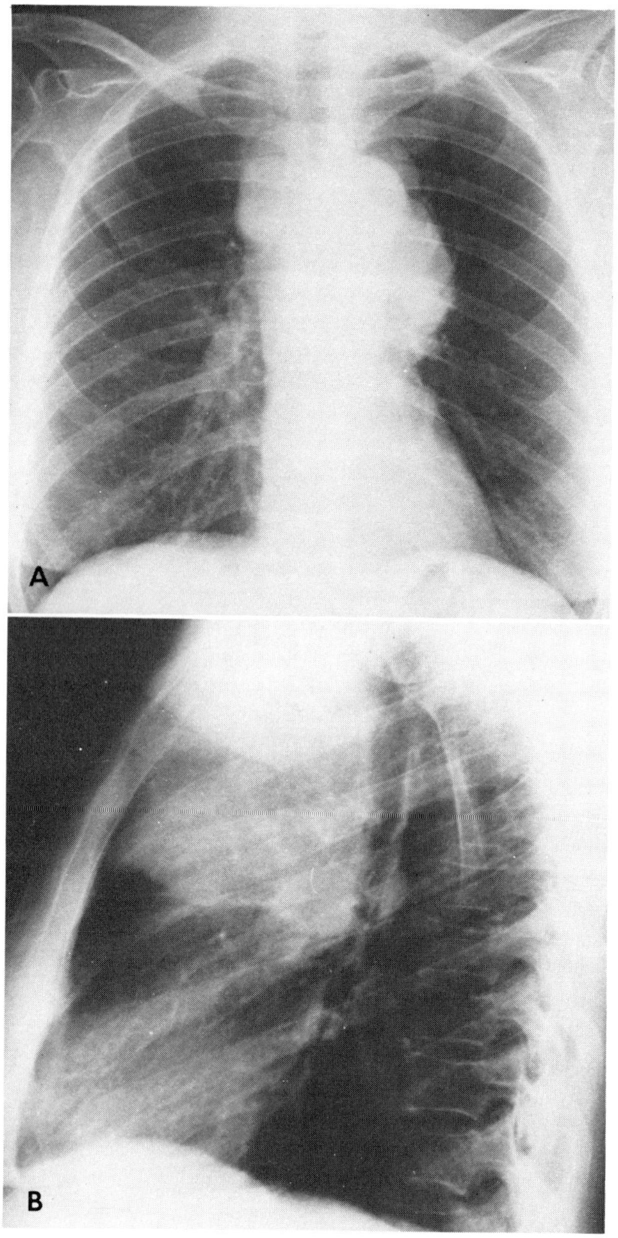

Fig. 5. (Case 4) A) Large lobulated mass in right and left paratracheal area in this 50-year-old woman originated from stromal cell sarcoma of uterus. B) Lateral projection indicates mass anterior to trachea extending anteriorly to sternum.

thoracic spine. Mediastinoscopy identified tumor in the superior and middle compartment in one patient, and adherence of a tumor mass to the thoracic spine in the second patient. Tissue investigations confirmed adenocarcinoma suggesting gastrointestinal tract origins. Retrospective investigations revealed a previous bowel malignancy in one patient, and the subsequent course of the second patient confirmed the site of origin as the pancreas.

THYROID CARCINOMA

A 58-year-old man was investigated for progressively increasing right paravertebral pain between T-4 and T-7. A chest x-ray study revealed a large mass filling the right paratracheal region with posterior projection to the thoracic spine and was documented by tomography. At mediastinoscopy, the right paratracheal region was filled by a large tumor mass extending to the spine; tissue analysis was reported as papillary thyroid carcinoma.

PELVIC CANCER

Case 4. A 51-year-old woman previously in only fair health due to a neurologic disorder classified as a dystonia, had a chest x-ray study for a variety of vague symptoms described as "chest spasm" associated with a cough of four-weeks duration. The chest radiograph suggested a large superior mediastinal tumor, lobulated and irregular, with compression of the tracheal lumen. The radiologic diagnosis, based upon the tumor size and location, suggested lymphoma as the primary consideration with thymoma as the secondary diagnosis. (Fig. 5A,B).

At mediastinoscopy, the right paratracheal area contained a firm mass which on dissection proved to be a collection of individual lymph nodes. Multiple biopsies were taken. After numerous pathologic consultations, the tissue was considered to be a large-cell anaplastic carcinoma of unknown origin. This interpretation suggested a reevaluation of the patient for an occult primary; following reappraisal, a pelvic neoplasm was identified. Subsequent intravenous pyelogram and examination suggested an extrinsic tumor distorting the ureter and bladder. Laparotomy and pelvic exploration revealed a large ovarian mass which was removed. The histopathologic report from this mass was stromal cell sarcoma. The mediastinal tumor was reviewed and found to be consistent with metastases from the pelvis.

DISCUSSION

Comparison of chest x-ray studies and, when necessary, tomographs of the mediastinum does not indicate a common denominator of neoplastic appearance suggestive of intrathoracic or extrathoracic origin. However, malignancy is suggested by the location of isolated masses in the paratracheal region or unilateral hilar nodularity.

The authors consider the negative aspects of bronchoscopy in relation to the radiological findings. Our experience indicates that when metastases are confined to the regional lymphatic system and spare the pulmonary tissue, the yield from bronchoscopic biopsy is negligible. Additionally, the endoscopic appearance of tracheobronchial distortion is absent until late tumor expansion and compression becomes evident. The exception to this general observation is breast cancer with relatively early peritracheal and submucosal infiltration.

Nine of the described 20 cases originated from

tumors above the diaphragm (8 breast and 1 thyroid); 9 cases were infradiaphragmatic in location, either abdominal or pelvic in origin, and the remaining 2 cases originated from cutaneous areas on the trunk.

In this series of metastatic disease and in other cases in our files, a major problem has been identified with regard to origin of the cell line of the biopsied tumor. There is sufficient characterization in the well and moderately differentiated carcinoma, whether of cutaneous or glandular origin, to establish the probable and in most instances accurate organ source. By contrast, when the cell pattern is described as highly undifferentiated, anaplastic, or primitive-cell type, and other similarly general terms, the question of primary *v* metastatic neoplasm may not be answered. In our series, thoracotomy for additional tissue, once representative material has been derived by mediastinoscopy, yields relatively little additional information. Furthermore, when external irradiation has been applied to the mediastinum for shrinkage of a neoplasm, the cellular morphology identified thereafter is distorted or modified further impeding a definitive diagnosis.

From a historical standpoint, the background of previous cancer surgery is most significant, irrespective of the interval before the primary neoplasm and on the onset of symptoms or radiologic findings. This fact is documented by the breast malignancies with occasional long periods of tumor control. Second primaries or neoplasms of lymphatic origins may intervene as the immunosurveillance system is depressed or modified. Consequently, the newly discovered abnormalities require evaluation for current therapeutic programming.

There are some applications of mediastinoscopy to specific regions of neoplasm that warrant discussion. The use of staging of head and neck cancer has been reported;[16,17] the obvious goal is determination of substernal spread. The authors counter that head and neck cancer usually, though not always, spreads via the cervical chain with the primary relationship to specific regional nodes. When spread occurs due to elaboration of tumor emboli from an involved node or as a secondary area of deposit in the neck, it is usually within the immediate vicinity and therefore clinically palpable. An isolated substernal metastasis, skipping the intervening lymphatic system is a relatively unusual event, and therefore the authors do not suggest routine mediastinal exploration.

With improving chemotherapeutic techniques of tumor suppression, it is essential that tissue diagnosis of mediastinal disease be established. Temporary or prolonged regression of breast cancer dissemination can be achieved; less successful is the control of other forms of malignancy. The areas in which adjuvant therapy is minimally or at best moderately effective, such as bowel malignancies and malignant melanoma, still warrant diagnostic evaluation to apply the modality most effective at this time.

REFERENCES

1. Carlens E. Mediastinoscopy: a method for inspection and tissue biopsy in the superior mediastinum. Dis Chest 1959; 36: 343-52.

2. Welsh LW, Welsh JJ. Mediastinoscopy: the predictive survival value in staging carcinoma of the lung. Ann Otol Rhinol Laryngol 1978; 78:544-52.

3. Welsh LW, Welsh JJ. Mediastinoscopy: application for hilar adenopathy. Laryngoscope 1974; 84:848-56.

4. Welsh LW, Welsh JJ. Problems of diagnosis in the evaluation of mediastinal sarcoidosis. Laryngoscope 1977; 87:1635-44.

5. Lockhart RD, Hamilton GP, Fyfe RN. Anatomy of the human body. Philadelphia: Lippincott Company, 1972.

6. Winterbauer RH, Belic N, Moores KD. A clinical interpretation of bilateral hilar adenopathy. Ann Intern Med 1973; 78:65-77.

7. Neifeld JP, Ingle JN, Tormey DC, Lippman ME, Richman SD, Michaelis LL. Mediastinoscopy, a diagnostic aid in metastatic carcinoma of the breast. Cancer 1976; 137:1973-7.

8. Arkless R. Renal carcinoma: how it metastasizes. Radiology 1965; 84:496-502.

9. Khan A, Khan FA. Hypernephroma: a rare cause of bilateral adenopathy, and an example of the importance of tissue diagnosis in suspected cases of sarcoidosis. Chest 1974; 66:722-4.

10. Ahmad M, Zevallos P. Metastatic hypernephroma presenting as bilateral hilar adenopathy. Chest 1975; 68:849-50.

11. Robson CJ, Churchill BM, Anderson W. The results of radical nephrectomy for renal cell carcinoma. Urology 1969; 101: 297-302.

12. Feldman L, Kricun ME. Malignant melanoma presenting as a mediastinal mass. JAMA 1979; 241:396-7.

13. Webb WR. Hilar and mediastinal lymph node metastases in malignant melanoma. AJR 1979; 133:805-10.

14. Block MA, Miller JM, Horn RC. Significance of mediastinal lymph node metastases in carcinoma of thyroid. Am J Surg 1972; 123:702-5.

15. Sisson GA, Feldman DE. The management of thyroid carcinoma metastasis to the neck and mediastinum. Otolaryngol Clin North Am 1980; 13:119-27.

16. Suzuki B, Kreutzer E. Mediastinoscopy for cancer of the head and neck. Ear Nose Throat J 1981; 60:191-6.

17. Tucker JA. Application of mediastinoscopy to carcinoma of the larynx, a preliminary report. Laryngoscope 1969; 79: 118-24.

X-RAY STUDY OF THE MONTH

CHEMODECTOMAS (NONCHROMAFFIN PARAGANGLIOMAS) OF THE GLOMUS JUGULARE, GLOMUS VAGALE AND CAROTID BODY

ALFRED L. WEBER, MD
KENNETH R. DAVIS, MD
JOSEPH B. NADOL, JR, MD
BOSTON, MASSACHUSETTS

PATIENT

This 20-year-old woman complained of fluctuating hearing in the left ear for approximately three months. Otoscopic examination revealed a bulging erythematous left drum. A diagnosis of acute suppurative otitis media was made, and the patient was treated with oral antibiotics. A myringotomy was performed one week later because the appearance was unchanged and serous fluid was aspirated. A second week later an exploratory tympanotomy was done and profuse bleeding encountered. When referred to the Massachusetts Eye and Ear Infirmary three weeks later a bilobed mass was seen in the posteroinferior quadrant of the mesotympanum. Other than a moderate conductive hearing loss on the left, the remainder of the head and neck examination was normal.

The patient's father was said to have had a chemodectoma removed from each side of the neck and a paternal uncle was said to have had a solitary chemodectoma in the neck.

A combined exploration of the left mastoid and neck was performed and a carotid body tumor was encountered at the carotid bifurcation and totally removed. A second tumor was found in the area of the inferior ganglion of the vagus nerve. Exploration of the middle ear and mastoid revealed a large glomus tumor at the jugular foramen which was incompletely removed because of extension of the tumor into the carotid canal.

RADIOGRAPHIC FINDINGS

Towne's view (Fig. 1) of the temporal bones show a diffuse nonspecific increase in density in the left middle ear cavity and adjacent mastoid (arrowheads). Semiaxial polytome study of the base of the skull (Fig. 2) shows a normal right jugular fossa with a sharp cortical outline (asterisk). There is erosion of the lateral superior portion of the left jugular fossa with loss of the jugular spine (arrowhead). There is also destruction of the floor of the left tympanic cavity (arrow) together with increased density in the left tympanic cavity. A lateral polytomographic study (Fig. 3) reveals destruction of the caroticojugular spine (arrowhead). There is also erosion of the bony outline of the jugular fossa (arrow).

A lateral subtraction view of the inferior tympanic branch of ascending pharyngeal artery angio-

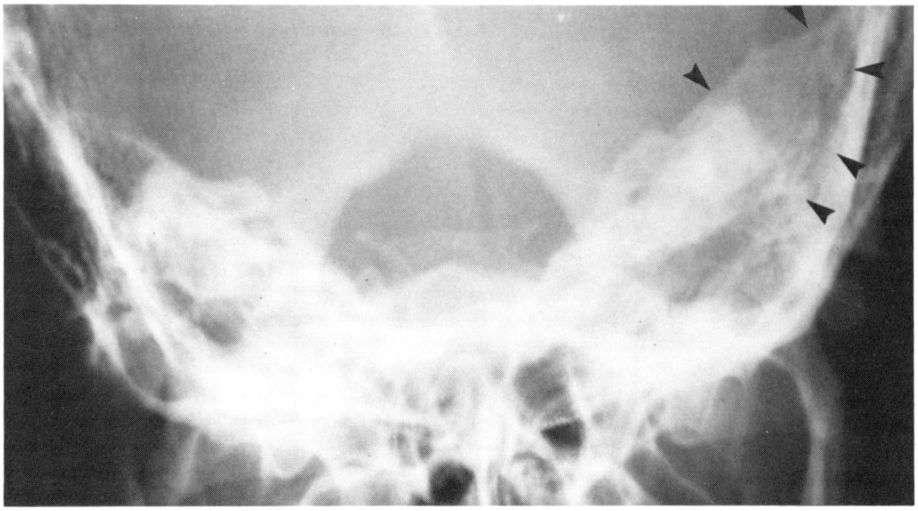

Figure 1

From the Department of Radiology, Massachusetts Eye and Ear Infirmary, Boston.
REPRINTS — Alfred L. Weber, MD, Department of Radiology, Massachusetts Eye and Ear Infirmary, 243 Charles St., Boston, MA 02114.

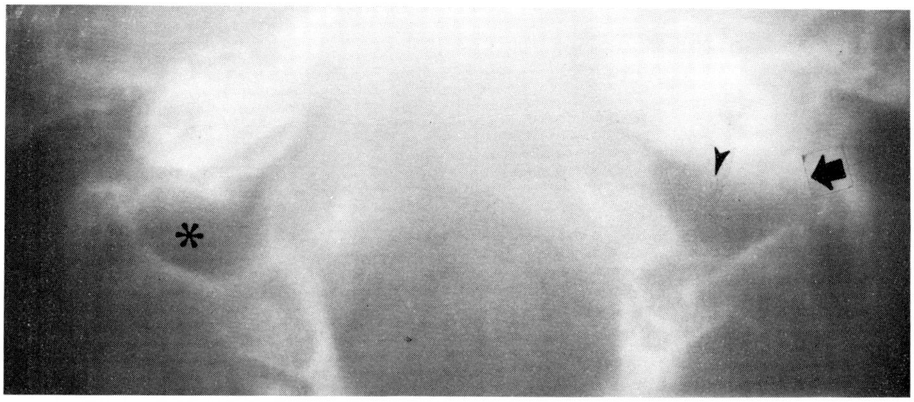

Figure 2

gram demonstrates a dense vascular stain of a glomus jugulare tumor in the jugular fossa (arrowheads). Early venous shunting is evident (Fig. 4). A lateral subtraction view of the more proximal ascending pharyngeal artery angiogram reveals retrograde filling of a very vascular nodule (arrowheads) at the level of the second cervical (C-2) vertebra along the vagus nerve (Fig. 5). The lateral subtraction view following injection near the origin of the superior thyroidal artery (arrowhead) demonstrates branches producing hypervascularity at the common carotid bifurcation (arrow) and antegrade filling of the nodule at the level of C-2 (Fig. 6).

DISCUSSION

Chemodectomas (nonchromaffin paragangliomas) are slow-growing tumors ranging in size from a few millimeters to ten or more centimeters. They are more common in females, particularly the intratympanic and glomus jugulare tumors. The majority of these lesions are unilateral, but bilateral tumors or glomus jugulare tumors associated with vagal tumors and carotid body tumors are encountered.[1] A rare feature is a heredofamilial tendency.[2] These tumors are usually encapsulated and the vast majority of chemodectomas are histologically benign. They are composed of many small capillaries surrounded by epithelial cells[3] and may invade locally, recur and metastasize in 2% to 6% of cases.[4]

Glomus jugulare tumors arise from the adventitia of the internal jugular vein within the jugular fossa. The most frequently encountered symptoms are conductive hearing loss, fullness in the ear, tinnitus, discoloration of the tympanic membrane caused by the tumor, facial nerve or 9th through 12th nerve palsy, aural bleeding or discharge, and a mass within the bony external canal or behind the tympanic membrane. The radiographic findings of glomus jugulare tumors depend on the size and extension of the lesion.[5] Initially there is erosion of the cortical outline followed by enlargement of the jugular fossa. A large jugular fossa without erosion of the cortical outline is not of diagnostic significance since asymmetry of the two fossae of the same patient is common with the right side often larger than the left side. There may be erosion of the bony septum (caroticojugular spine) between the jugular foramen and the intrapetrous portion of the carotid canal. Erosion of the floor of the middle ear cavity is commonly seen with extension of a soft tissue mass of variable size into the middle ear cavity. If the mass is extensive, involvement of the mastoid and bony external canal may occur. Anterior extension may cause destruction of the inferior aspect of the petrous pyramid. Extension posteriorly causes erosion of the occipital bone and enlargement or de-

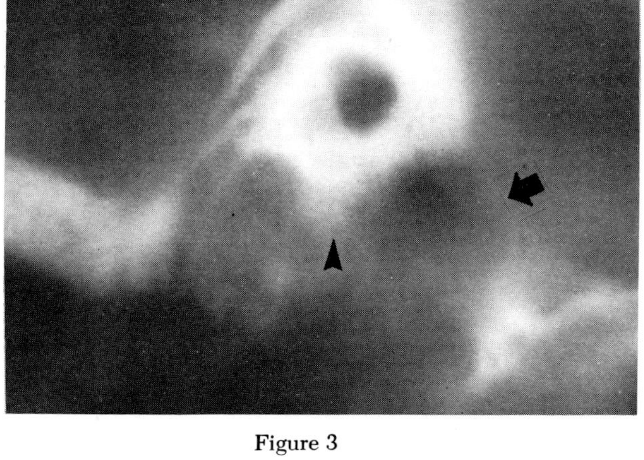

Figure 3

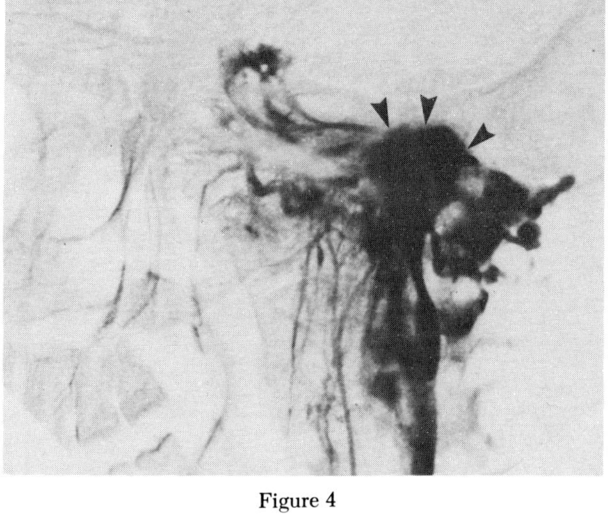

Figure 4

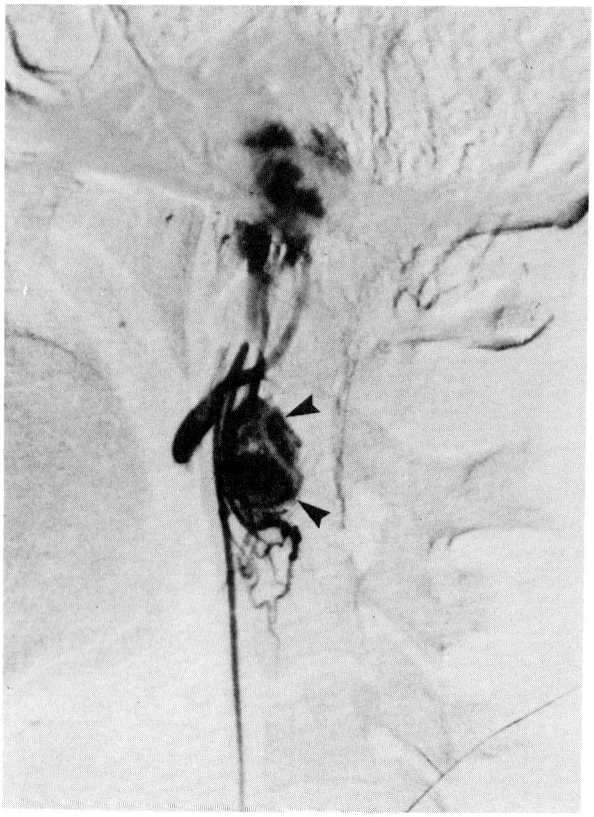

Figure 5

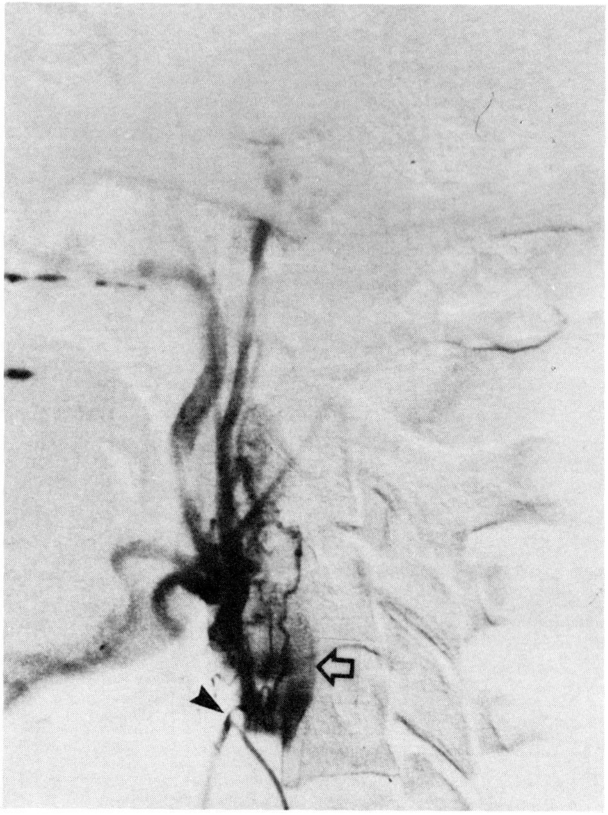

Figure 6

struction of the hypoglossal canal.[6] Angiography yields important information regarding the size of the lesion and extension. The blood supply of these tumors frequently arises from the tympanic branch of the ascending pharyngeal artery. Therefore, selective angiography of the external as well as the internal carotid arteries and vertebral artery is necessary for complete evaluation of the tumor. Contrast medium accumulates within a network of small irregular vessels and the late angiographic phase demonstrates a uniform tumor blush. Jugular venography helps to outline the inferior extent of the tumor. The jugular bulb may be indented extrinsically by the tumor or there may be actual invasion of the vein over a variable distance inferiorly. Computerized axial tomography following infusion of contrast material may demonstrate intracranial extension of the tumor. Chemodectomas in the neck enhance following infusion of contrast material and thus can be differentiated from avascular tumors and cysts. In the tympanic cavity glomus tumors should be differentiated from an ectopic carotid artery and vein, cholesterol granuloma and hemangioma.[7]

Chemodectomas arising from the inferior ganglion of the vagal nerve (ganglion nodosum) are manifested by a painless mass behind the angle of the mandible which frequently bulges into the pharyngeal wall in the peritonsillar area producing dysphagia. Simultaneous occurrence with other chemodectomas, as presented in this case, has been previously reported.[8] Metastases have been reported in 19% of 37 reported cases.[9]

Carotid body tumors manifest as a painless mass in the lateral aspect of the neck. The duration of growth may range from a month to many years before detection. When the lesion is large, pressure on surrounding structures causes dysphagia, hoarseness, and coughing. Physical examination reveals a tumor mass at the carotid bifurcation usually movable laterally, but not vertically. The mass may be pulsatile and associated with a thrill or bruit making its differentiation from an aneurysm difficult. Angiography outlines the size of the lesion and its relationship to the internal and external carotid arteries. The opposite side should also be assessed by angiography to rule out a possible second lesion which occurs in 2.8% of cases but increases to 26% in patients showing a familial tendency.[10] The cerebral flow from the opposite side of the lesion should be assessed either by performing carotid angiography on the unaffected side or by compression of the uninvolved carotid artery during injection of contrast medium in the affected side. The study of cross-flow intracerebrally is important in case the internal carotid artery has to be sacrificed during the excision of the lesion. The angiographic findings consist of a dense tumor blush along with separation and/or displacement of the internal and external carotid vessels. The vessels may also be narrowed, but are almost never occluded.

REFERENCES

1. Spector GJ, Ciralsky R, Maisel RH, Ogura JH. IV. Multiple glomus tumors in the head and neck. Laryngoscope 1975; 85: 1066-75.

2. Hayes HM Jr, Fraumeni JF Jr. Chemodectomas in dogs: epidemiologic comparison with man. J Natl Cancer Inst 1974; 52:1455-8.

3. Batsakis JG. Tumors of the head and neck: clinical and pathological consideration. 2nd ed. Baltimore: Williams & Wilkins Co, 1979.

4. Irons GB, Weiland LH, Brown WL. Paragangliomas of the neck: clinical and pathologic analysis of 116 cases. Surg Clin North Am 1977; 57:575-83.

5. Rice RP, Holman CB. Roentgenographic manifestations of tumors of the glomus jugulare (chemodectoma). AJR 1963; 89: 1201-8.

6. Handel SF, Miller MH, Miller LS, Goepfert H. Angiographic changes of head and neck chemodectomas following radiotherapy. Arch Otolaryngol 1977: 103:87-9.

7. Valvassori GE, Buckingham RA. Middle ear masses mimicking glomus tumors: radiologic and otoscopic recognition. Ann Otol Rhinol Laryngol 1975; 83:606-12.

8. Someren A, Karcioglu Z. Malignant vagal paraganglioma. Report of a case and review of literature. Am J Clin Pathol 1977: 68:400-8.

9. Druck NS, Spector GJ, Ciralsky RH, Ogura JH. Malignant glomus vagale. Report of a case and review of the literature. Arch Otolaryngol 1976; 102:634-6.

10. Cook RL. Bilateral chemodectomas in the neck. J Laryngol 1977; 91:611-8.

≈

GUIDELINES FOR GRANTS
TRUSTEES OF THE RESERACH FUND OF THE AMERICAN OTOLOGICAL SOCIETY, INC.

The members of the Board of Trustees of the Research Fund of the American Otological Society have determined guidelines for making grants from the Fund. The following is the formulation of policy.

Grants will be given in the area of otosclerosis: its diagnosis and management, the possible causes and underlying conditions, and an understanding of the disorder that may lead eventually to its prevention or cure.

The present lack of understanding of the disorder and the absence of similar conditions in other animals makes research in this field difficult. A direct approach to the disease may or may not be feasible; therefore, a sound strategy would be to use other approaches, such as the investigation of bone development, growth and repair under various conditions and the study of other diseases that may be similar to otosclerosis. It is possible that investigations which may seem initially remote from otosclerosis may provide information which will eventually lead to a substantive further understanding of the disease process which underlies otosclerosis. The applicant should describe correlations between proposed research with the clinical pathological entity of otosclerosis.

The policy is to aid and encourage research in the immediate field of otosclerosis and also in adjoining fields, if, in the opinion of the Board, there is a substantial promise that results obtained will be of assistance in the ways indicated and may lead to the attainment of the objective of the further understanding of otosclerosis.

Applications for a research grant from the Research Fund of the American Otological Society may be obtained from the Office of the Secretary-Treasurer of the Research Fund of the American Otological Society. Write to Maxwell Abramson, MD, Secretary-Treasurer, Department of Otolaryngology, Columbia University, College of Physicians and Surgeons, 630 West 168th Street, New York, NY 10032; (212) 694-5820.

All grant requests must be submitted by January 31, 1983. All grants received after January 31 will not be considered.

LETTERS TO THE EDITOR

Dear Editor,

I have mixed feelings about the article by Dr. Ernest A. Weymuller, Jr, and Dr. Charles W. Cummings, "Cricothyroidotomy: The Impact of Antecedent Endotracheal Intubation" (*Ann Otol Rhinol Laryngol* 1982; 91:437-9). This article does little more than add more confusion to an already heated issue. It was an attempt to prove or disprove the value of cricothyroidotomy, but the study as designed could hardly be considered a scientific project. The authors, complaining of other articles and the lack of objective data, should certainly review their own article and data. I never contended that my article, "Epiglottic Reconstruction of Laryngeal Stenosis Secondary to Cricothyroidostomy," (*Laryngoscope* 1980; 90:1130-6) was a scientific paper, but only cautioned against outright acceptance of the procedure. I disagree with their comments on my two cases and only ask readers to review it for themselves. I find their comments cautioning readers against articles without any case reports rather ironic, since they present none themselves. I also find their third concluding point recommending cricothyroidotomy as an elective procedure without antecedent intubation *quite unreasonable* and without support in their article or any other that I have read. Furthermore, one gets rather disturbed in reading an allegedly objective report, like this one, which calls those against this operation the "detractors" and the advocates for the procedure "champions."

I find the subject cricothyroidotomy perplexing to say the least. As an otolaryngologist, I can find no support for a procedure which involves trauma to an organ (the larynx) that otherwise could be handled by a classic tracheotomy. The limited number of cases that would probably be candidates, such as those without prior intubation and those not requiring mechanical ventilation, would be so infrequent as to not warrant popularizing this procedure for fear of its indiscriminate use. Articles written in support of cricothyroidotomy stress time as a major advantage over a tracheotomy. If the time difference is substantial between a classical tracheotomy and a cricothyroidotomy by a particular surgeon, that surgeon should not be doing either of the procedures.

Yes, more clinical research rather than laboratory research will most likely be continued as this article encouraged; and no doubt we will see more complications as a result.

Thomas L. Kennedy, MD
Associate, Otolaryngology
Geisinger Medical Center
Danville, PA 17822

Dear Editor,

To respond to the comments made by Dr. Kennedy regarding our article discussing cricothyroidotomy:

1. Our study is certainly not a prospective randomized trial of cricothyroidotomy and cannot be considered totally "scientific." We felt it imperative to abort the use of cricothyroidotomy after seeing significant complications related to prolonged intubation.

2. We presented in cumulative form the objective data regarding our patients. Specific case reports are not essential to our main point.

3. We concluded that cricothyroidotomy as an elective procedure is indeed reasonable. This was supported by our limited personal experience and by massive experience cited in the literature (references 6-9). I would suggest that Dr. Kennedy and others who question the appropriate use of cricothyroidotomy familiarize themselves with the large body of information available on elective cricothyroidotomy.

4. The major benefits to be gained by cricothyroidotomy are not only the time factor, but more specifically as pointed out by Boyd and Conlan, cricothyroidotomy removes the incision from proximity to a median sternotomy making it popular with thoracic surgeons. As mentioned by Morain, cricothyroidotomy is attractive to the head and neck surgeon because it can be done through a limited incision and is easier to separate from a radical neck dissection field thus preventing the sometimes bothersome air leak that complicates the establishment of suction drainage in the presence of a tracheotomy.

It seems that cricothyroidotomy continues to strike an emotional response which we regret. It should remain our responsibility to accumulate objective data and recognize the information made available by nonotolaryngologists (Boyd and Conlan, Brantigan and Grow, Morain).

Ernest A. Weymuller, Jr, MD
Associate Professor
Charles W. Cummings, MD
Professor and Chairman
Department of Otolaryngology
University of Washington
Seattle, WA 98195

BOOK REVIEW

Larynx: Microlaryngoscopy and Histopathology

Edited by *Willy Lehmann*, *Jean-Marie Pidoux* and *Jean-Jacques Widmann*. Hard cover, color illustrations, indexed, bibliography, bilingual text (French/English), 135 pages, 1981. International Pharmaceuticals, Zambon, Switzerland.

This photographic atlas of laryngeal pathology is unique for two reasons. First, it provides a pictorial correlation between macroscopic identification of mucosal lesions matched to their histologic descriptions. Second, it offers some of the most vivid photographs of endolaryngeal pathology ever published. The endolaryngeal photographs are of uniformly high quality characterized by surprising color accuracy and vivid clarity. Color illustrations used in the Introduction provide helpful anatomic references and are especially useful to the student beginning the study of laryngology.

There are a few minor deficiencies in this atlas. Since the text was originally written in French, at times the English translation suffers from awkward medical terminology with which the American physician may be unfamiliar. I was also somewhat disappointed not to see photographic descriptions of tuberculosis, sarcoidosis and fungal infections included among the granulomatous diseases. Examples of cleft larynx and laryngoceles would also have been of interest.

Nevertheless, this atlas is a magnificent attempt to bring together gross and microscopic descriptions of laryngeal pathology. Photographic quality is outstanding. This compendium represents a very worthwhile addition to the otolaryngologist's library.

Clarence T. Sasaki, MD
New Haven, Connecticut

INDEX

AUTHORS

Abramson M, 156
Abbs JH, Suppl 100:15
Adam JS, 656
Alatorre G, 220
Anderson DJ, Suppl 100:9
Anderson R, 501
Arab M, 363
Arauz JC, 593
Atkins JP, Jr, 584

Bailey BJ, Suppl 100:21
Baker BM, 277
Baker CD, 277
Baker SR, 395
Baloh RW, 493
Bardawil WA, 571
Barrett KA, 82
Bartal A, 261
Batsakis JG, 342, 465, 541
Beach TP, 403
Bean SF, 142
Berci G, 558
Berlin CI, Suppl 100:15
Berliner KI, Suppl 91:11, 55, 59, 90
Berlinger FG, 363
Bhatnagar KP, Suppl 89
Biller HF, 246, 448
Birck HG, 403, 656
Birns JW, 417, 622
Black FO, Suppl 100:17
Blalock PD, 372
Blanks RHI, 185
Blitzer A, 156
Blom ED, 576
Bluestone CD, 179, Suppl 100:10
Bordley JW, Suppl 100:10
Bosma MM, 285
Breipohl W, Suppl 89
Bretlau P, 131
Briggs BR, Suppl 93, part I
Brimacombe JA, Suppl 91:27
Brinn JE, 82
Brook I, 41
Brookes GB, 299
Brookhouser PE, Suppl 100:19
Bumsted RM, 115
Burnett PA, 169
Bustamante-Balcárcel A, 166

Callier J, 175
Canalis RF, 27, 160
Cangir A, 431
Cantekin EI, 179, 256
Carlborg B, 209
Carlsson B, 76
Carniol PJ, 152
Catanzaro A, 70
Chambers H, 633
Cherry JD, 612
Chinnici JC, 659
Chung CT, 94
Clemis JD, 304
Cleveland PH, 70
Clopton BM, 285, Suppl 98
Cohen SR, 417, 622
Collard ME, 330
Conway W, 595
Cooper B, 310
Corral-Romero MA, 166
Cortese DA, 652
Costa F, 323
Crary WG, Suppl 91:55, 59
Cummings CW, 94, 370, 437, 670, Suppl 100:7
Curthoys IS, 185

Dabelsteen E, 131
Daniel HJ, III, 82
Danley MJ, Suppl 91:21
Daroff RB, 316
Davis KR, 543, 666
Davis LE, 90
Dayal VS, Suppl 95
Dedo HH, 425
Dee A, Suppl 97:62
Degreef F, 175
Dell'Osso LF, 316
DeLozier HL, 336
DeMaria TF, Suppl 93, part II
Denneny JC, 584
Dent LJ, Suppl 91:41
Densert B, 209
Densert O, 209
De Proost W, 175
DeRemee RA, 588
Deviri E, 261
Diamond SG, 225
Dichtel WJ, 431
Dobben GD, 506
Dobie RA, Suppl 100:15
Doslak MJ, 316
Dowart R, 501
Doyle KJ, Suppl 91:100
Doyle WJ, 150, 179, 256
Duckert LG, 33
Dudley JP, 612
Duncan RB, 200, 281

Eavey R, 230
Edens ET, 602
Edgerton BJ, Suppl 91:35, 100, 104, 117
Eisenberg LS, Suppl 91:27, 47, 62, 67
Eisner L, 612
Eliachar I, 261
Elkins E, Suppl 100:17
Emery PJ, 234
Epstein MF, 485
Ervin TJ, 461
Escajadillo JR, 220
Eurenius S, 615
Eylan E, 163

Falk SA, 526
Farr GH, 392
Fearon B, 610
Fee WE, Jr, Suppl 100:17
Fenton E, 119
Fermin CD, 44
Feudo P, Jr, 485
Fisch U, 25, 474
Flores TC, 579
Fonseca R, 593
Frank JE, 403
Fredrickson JM, Suppl 100:15
Fretz RJ, Suppl 91:21
Fried MP, 152, 485
Friedman EM, 41
Friedman M, 363
Frye-Osier HA, 272
Fryksmark U, 268
Fujita S, 595
Fulghum RS, 82
Furuya N, 225

Gacek RR, 469, Suppl 100:15
Gallia LJ, 450
Gantz BJ, 25
Garvin JP, 403
Gates GA, 454, Suppl 100:7, 19, 23
Gayler BW, Suppl 99
Geller KA, 417, 622
Gerson CR, 413
Ghanma MA, 567
Giebink GS, 20
Goepfert H, 431
Goldsher M, 261
Goldstein R, 272
Goode RL, 526
Goodhill V, 351
Grundfast KM, 564
Guice C, 606
Gussen R, 27
Gutterman JU, 431

Hamaker RC, 576
Hamaya M, 101
Hamilton LH, 106
Handler SD, 628
Harford ER, 20
Hasegawa M, 112
Hartman MT, 70
Hawkins JE, Jr, Suppl 97:3, Suppl 100: 11
Healy M, 310

Healy GB, 230, 384
Hearne EM III, 454
Heaton SL, 292
Heimlich HJ, 643
Heller KA, 20
Helmerich LF, Suppl 91:35
Hicks G, 480
Hicks JN, 389
Hirano K, 101
Hirsch JE, 272
Hitselberger WE, Suppl 91:117
Holinger LD, 407
Honrubia V, 493
House HP, Suppl 100:10
House WF, Suppl 91:11, 15, 47, 67, 74, 100, 104, 117
Huang C-C, 156
Hubbard DG, 193
Huck GF, Jr, 659
Hürzeler D, 57

Igarashi M, 44, Suppl 100:17

Jackler RK, 425
Jackson RT, 216
Jafek BW, 136, Suppl 100:7
Jares A, Suppl 95
Jenkins HA, 25, 493
Johns ME, Suppl 100:9
Johnson JT, 94, 597, Suppl 100:9
Johnsson L-G, 193, Suppl 91:74, Suppl 97:3
Jørgensen MB, 131
Jornsay D, 633
Joy MLG, Suppl 95

Karlan MS, 608, Suppl 100:10
Kashima H, Suppl 99
Keane WM, 584
Kennedy DW, Suppl 92
Kennedy, TL, 670
Khan WN, 328
Kileny P, 61
Kimmelman CP, 339
Kimura RS, 5
Kinsey JH, 652
Kirchner FR, 382
Kishimoto S, 25
Kitamura K, 5
Kleinsasser O, 378
Kodama A, Suppl 96
Koegel L, Jr, 579
Kohut RI, Suppl 100:9
Konrad HR, 493
Kopstein E, Suppl 92
Kosugi T, 101
Koufman JA, 372
Kraus EM, 237
Krause CJ, 395, Suppl 100:11
Krueger LJ, 115
Kumar A, 510

Lawrence C, 633
Lawson W, 448
Le HT, 277
Lechago J, 160
Leipzig B, 94
LeJeune FE, Jr, 392, 606
LeTard F, 606
Lewis DM, Suppl 93, part II
Levine HL, 579
Lim DJ, Suppl 93, parts I, II, Suppl 100:11
Lindeman RC, 169
Lindesmith GG, 622
Lingeman RE, 458
Linthicum FH Jr, Suppl 91:74, Suppl 97:3
Liquori J, 633
Liston SL, 98
Lloyd GAS, 234
Lo A, Suppl 95
Lundberg C, 76

Maeda S, Suppl 94
Mafee MF, 510, 571
Maisel RH, 98
Malmgren LT, Suppl 100:15
Mangham CA, Jr, 169
Marice H, 606
Markham CH, 185, 225
Marshak G, 256
Mathog RA, Suppl 100:19
Martinez CR, Suppl 99
Matsuo O, 101
Mattox DE, Suppl 100:11
Matulionis DH, Suppl 89
Maves MD, 458
McCabe BF, 1, 237, 350
McDonald TJ, 359, 588
McElveen JT, 526, 538
McGee TJ, 304
McGuirt WF, 599
Merkle M, 501
Mesolella C, 323
Meyer BW, 622
Mihara H, 101
Millen SJ, 122
Miller C, 526
Miller D, 461
Miller JM, 33, Suppl 100:17
Miller LW, Suppl 91:55, 59
Milmoe G, 564
Mogi G, Suppl 93, part II; Suppl 94
Møller M, 597
Montgomery WW, 65, 344
Moon RE, Suppl 95
Moor EE, 389
Moore EJ, Suppl 100:15
Morelli G, 323
Mori S, 250
Morris HL, 115
Myers EN, 450

Nadol J, Jr, 666
Nager GT, Suppl 92, Suppl 97:33
Naunton RF, Suppl 100:19
Needleman SW, 145
Neel HB, III, 359, 588
Neely JG, Suppl 100:9
Negri M, 543
Nelson JR, Suppl 91:47
Newton L, 633
Niimi S, 119
Nomura Y, 250
Norton ML, 567

Obiako MN, 325
Ogawa A, 14, 136
Oh M, Suppl 94
Ohlsson K, 76, 268
Ojemann RG, 543
Olsen AM, 551
Olson J, 501
Ossoff RH, 608

Panje WR, 53, Suppl 100:7
Paparella MM, Suppl 100:10
Pashley NRT, 204, 332
Pfingst BE, Suppl 98
Phelps PD, 234
Polling Å, 268
Popovich J, 595
Potsic WP, 339, 628
Proctor B, Suppl 97:33
Proctor L, Suppl 100:7
Pulec JL, 122

Rapin I, Suppl 97:62
Reardon EJ, 65
Redianu C, 163
Reed GF, 352
Robinson E, 261
Rodriguez WJ, 328
Rohn D, 150
Rothmann BF, 641
Rouse RC, 193, Suppl 97:3
Rowe LD, 584
Rubel EW, Suppl 100:17
Ruben RJ, 633, Suppl 97:62, Suppl 100:21
Rubin W, 489
Rubinstein A, 205
Ryan AF, 70

Sacks S, 448
Sagerman RH, 94
Sakurai T, 250
Sandlin RE, 521
Sando I, 14, 136, Suppl 96
Santulli B, 323
Sasaki CT, 670
Saunders WH, 445
Schaefer SD, 292, 399, 501
Schiff M, 521
Schild JA, 571
Schley WS, 119
Schuknecht HF, 5, Suppl 97:16
Schuller DE, 403, Suppl 100:9
Schwartz RH, 328
Schwartz RM, 467
Schut L, 339
Seguin FW, 641
Senturia BH, 2, 4, 126
Sergeant R, 53
Sessions RB, 142, 431
Shanon E, 163
Shapiro ED, 150
Shapshay SM, 384, 648
Shea JJ, 516
Shelton VK, 363
Shugar JMA, 246
Shugar MA, 65
Siegelman SS, Suppl 99
Simmons FB, 266, Suppl 100:10
Simpson GT, 384
Singer MI, 576
Skolnik EM, 363

Smith LE, 266
Smith MFW, 538
Smith RJH, 142
Snow JB, Jr, Suppl 100:21
Snyderman NL, 597
Sohmer H, 205
Som PM, 246
Sørensen CH, 131
Spelman FA, Suppl 98
Stearns MP, 370
Stebbins WB, Suppl 100:19
Stein R, 633
Steinitz R, 261
Steward DJ, 610
Stone RT, 641
Strome M, 485
Strong MS, 384, 648
Sulek M, 431
Supance JS, 256

Tegner H, 268
Testa B, 323
Thearle PB, 597
Thielemeier MA, Suppl 91:27
Thompson GE, 605
Thompson JW, 417, 622
Thomsen J, 240
Tingwald FR, 330
Torok N, 510
Tos M, 240
Tucker HM, 440
Tsuchida M, 250
Tucker GF, Jr, 413
Tucker HM, 440, 579
Tung M-S, 297
Valvassori GE, 506, 571
Van Horn HW, III, 392
Vannieuwenhuyse E, 175
Van Overbeek JJ, 602
Vaughan CW, 384
Ventruto V, 323
Wagner CA, 330
Wald ER, 150
Walker EE, 389
Walker LH, 641
Ward PH, 493, 558, Suppl 100:11
Watanabe N, Suppl 93, parts I, II
Weber AL, 230, 344, 543, 666
Weber K, 272
Wehrs RE, 533
Weichselbaum RR, 461
Weinberg AG, 193
Welsh JJ, 310, 659
Welsh LW, 310, 659
Wessberg GA, 292
Wetmore RF, 628
Wexler M, Suppl 91:55, 59
Weymuller EA, Jr, 437, 670
Wiederhold ML, Suppl 100:7
Wilms D, 595
Wilson WR, 344
Windle-Taylor PC, 234
Wolf G, Suppl 100:15
Woo P, 615
Wood BG, 579
Work WP, Suppl 90
Wright CG, 193
Wright JW, Jr, 480
Wright JW, III, 480

Yanagisawa E, 354
Yarington CT, Jr, 605
Yee RD, 493

Zárate A, 220
Zikk D, 163
Zorick F, 595
Zubick HH, 485
Zulliger JJ, 403

SUBJECTS

Abductor vocal cord paralysis, congenital hereditary bilateral, 564
Abscess, periapical, in children, and intracranial complications of sinusitis, 41
Acoustic reflex latency, standardization of in humans and nonhuman primates, 169
Adult sleep apnea, brainstem evoked potentials in, 597
Alexander's law, model and study of, 316
Allergies; vocal quality, articulation and audiological characteristics in children and young adults with, 277
Allografts, ossicular replacement, lyophilized partial, 538
American Board of Otolaryngology: 1950-1979, Suppl 90
Ampicillin, use in treatment of pneumococcal otitis media (chinchilla model), 256
Ampicillin-resistant *Hemophilus influenzae*, otitis media secondary to, 328
Anesthetic gas scavenger, use during open rigid bronchoscopy, 610
Aneurysm, intracavernous internal carotid artery (X-ray study of the month), 543
Annals, history of, 1892-1982, 2
Anomalies, congenital, and polytomography of ear, 480
Antigen, introduction into middle ear, humoral and cell-mediated immunity in peripheral blood, 70
Antileukoprotease, distribution in upper respiratory mucosa, 268
Apnea, adult sleep, brainstem evoked potentials in, 597
Obstructive sleep, anatomic abnormalities in, 595
Argon laser and stapedotomy, 25
Artery, labyrinthine, and eighth cranial nerve, inner ear pathology following injury to, 136
Artificial larynx, endotracheal, Suppl 95
Artificial stapes, hair-clip type piston, and safety auger, 297
Atlantoaxial instability, alert for endoscopists, 567
Auditory brainstem evoked response, accuracy with unknown hearing level, 266
Auditory brainstem response and effects of conductive hearing loss, 304
Auditory brainstem responses, indicators of hearing aid performance, 61
Auditory canal, internal, computed tomographic air-contrast scanning of, 501
Auditory evoked potentials, normal neonatal brainstem, 485
Auditory nerve response, latency in neonates one to eight hours old, 205
Auditory prosthesis, neural mechanisms relevant to design: location and electrical characteristics, Suppl 98
Autosomal dominant inheritance, presumed, and familial laryngeal abductor paralysis, 323
Binocular counterrolling during sustained body tilt, and unilateral vestibular nerve section, 225
Biofeedback rehabilitation, use in seventh nerve paralysis, 166
Blom-Singer and Panje voice prostheses, primary vocal rehabilitation using, 458
Blood, peripheral, humoral and cell-mediated immunity following introduction of antigen in middle ear, 70
Blood vessels, nasal, evidence for presynaptic parasympathetic receptors on, 216
Bone cyst, aneurysmal, of sphenoid in child, 339
Bone labeling, tetracycline, improved technique using incident fluorescence, 160
Bone resorption in human cholesteatomas, 131
Bony auditory tube and otitis media with effusion, 200
Book Reviews
Barber HO, Stockwell CW, *Manual of electronystagmography*, 547
Bess FH, McConnell FE, *Audiology, education and the hearing-impaired child*, 346
Dayal, VS, *Clinical otolaryngology*, 233
Desmedt JE, *Spinal and supraspinal mechanisms of voluntary motor control and locomotion*, 347
Ellis RE, Flack FC, *Diagnosis and treatment of palatoglossal malfunction*, 548
Fairbanks DNF, *Pocket guide to antimicrobial therapy in otolaryngology*, 547
Fisch U, *Tympanoplasty and stapedectomy, a manual of techniques*, 467
Greene MCL, *The voice and its disorders*, 346
Haughton PM, *Physical principles of audiology*, 548
Hill B, *Verbal dyspraxia in clinical practice*, 347

LasJaunias PL, Berenstein A, *Craniofacial and upper cervical-arteries: functional, clinical & angiographic aspects*, 547
Lehmann W, Pidoux J-M, Widmann J-J, *Larynx: Microlaryngoscopy and Histopathology*, 670.
Lesavoy MA, *Reconstruction of the head and neck*, 347
McGuirt WF, *Pediatric otology case studies*, 548
Pindborg JJ, *Oral cancer and precancer*, 546
Proctor DF, *Breathing, speech, and song*, 347
Ramwell P, *Prostaglandin synthetase inhibitors: new clinical applications*, 346
Smythe GDL, *Chronic ear diseases*, 467
Snow JB, Jr, *Controversy in otolaryngology*, 233
Stevens KN, Hirano M, *Vocal fold physiology*, 547
Studebaker GA, Hochberg I, *Acoustic factors affecting hearing aid performance*, 546
Suen JY, Myers E, *Cancer of the head and neck*, 548
Van den Brink G, Bilsen FA, *Psychophysical, physiological and behavioural studies in hearing*, 233

Brainstem auditory evoked potentials, normal neonatal, 485
Brainstem dysfunction, cortical, subcortical and, in dyslexic children, 310
Brainstem evoked potentials in adult sleep apnea, 597
Brainstem responses, auditory, as indicators of hearing aid performance, 61
Bronchoscopic lavage, limited, adjunct to therapy for cystic fibrosis patients, 641
Bronchoscopy, fluorescence, new techniques and results, 57
Open rigid, anesthetic gas scavenger for use during, 610

Canal, facial, anatomy; variations and anomalies of, Suppl 97:33
Cancer, metastatic head and neck, basic principles of chemotherapy in treatment of, 145
Cancer of head and neck, chemical modulation of hypoxic fraction in treatment of, 461
Cancer of tracheobronchial tree, hematoporphyrin-derivative phototherapy for local treatment of, 652
Capsular otosclerosis with hydrops, cochlear and otoconial abnormalities in, Suppl 97:3
Carbon dioxide laser, heat sink protection against lasering endotracheal cuffs, 606
Incendiary characteristics of endotracheal tubes with (supplemental report), 605
Carbon dioxide laser and podophyllum in treatment of laryngeal papilloma, 425
Carbon dioxide laser surgery, universal endoscopic coupler for, 608
Carcinoma, anterior tongue, 94
Head and neck, in patients under 40 years old, 152
Laryngeal, in Israel (1960-1976), occurrence of primary additional neoplasms in patients with, 261
Squamous cell, of human parotid gland, collagenase activity in, 156
Thyroid, laryngotracheal invasion by, 363
Carcinomas, middle ear, bilateral, and Waldenström's macroglobulinemia, 299
Carotid artery, intracavernous internal aneurysms of (X-ray study of the month), 543
Catheter, Foley, use for removal of esophageal foreign bodies, 599
Caustic ingestion, pediatric, 656
Chemotherapy, basic principles of treatment of metastatic head and neck cancer, 145
Cholesteatomas, human, bone resorption in, 131
Chondrosarcoma of larynx, diagnosis and conservative surgical management of, 392
Excision of massive recurrence of, 392
Cilia, nonbeating, scanning electron microscopic examination of, 612
Circulation, hindbrain, evaluation by dynamic computed tomography, 506
Cochlea (guinea pig), acute morphological changes following electrical stimulation, 33
Cochlear abnormalities, otoconial abnormalities, and in capsular otosclerosis in hydrops, Suppl 97:3
Cochlear aqueduct, functional patency of, 209
Cochlear hydrops, collapsed saccule and ductus reuniens, 5
Cochlear implants. *See* Implants, cochlear
Cochlear prosthesis, tissue impedance and current flow in implanted ear, Suppl 98
Cochleovestibular lesions and typhoid fever, 220
Collagenase activity in squamous cell carcinoma of human parotid gland, 156
Computed tomography, dynamic, evaluation of hindbrain circulation by, 506
Computed tomography of neck, Suppl 99
Computerized tomography, laryngeal malignancies and, correlation of tomographic and histopathologic findings, 571
Congenital palatal incompetence, indications before diagnosis, 115
Cortical dysfunction, subcortical, brainstem and, in dyslexic children, 310
Cranial nerve, eighth, and labyrinthine artery, inner ear pathology following injury to, 136
Cricothyroidotomy, antedecent endotracheal intubation and, 437
Croup and epiglottitis, assessment of intubation in, 403
Cryoglobulinemia, deafness in, 250
Cryoprobe for palliative care, 204
Crypts, tonsillar, microcrypt extensions of, Suppl 94
Cuffs, endotracheal, heat sink protection against lasering, 606
Cyst, aneurysmal bone, of sphenoid in child, 339
Cystic fibrosis patients, bronchoscopic limited lavage as adjunct to therapy for, 641
Cysticercosis cerebri, neurotologic implications of, 122
Cysts, foregut, diagnosis and management in infants and children, 622

Deafness, sudden, resulting from infection by *Mycoplasma pneumoniae*, 163
Deafness in cryoglobulinemia, 250
Deglutition, successful, following supraglottic laryngeal surgery, factors in 579
Deltopectoral flap, and combined pectoralis major myocutaneous flap for closure of large pharyngocutaneous fistulas, 98
Diseases, midfacial necrotizing (Pathology consultation), 541
Ductus reuniens, collapsed saccule and cochlear hydrops, 5
Dyslexic children, cortical, subcortical, and brainstem dysfunction in, 310
Dysplasia, fibrous, review and manifestations in temporal bone, Suppl 92
Otoconial membrane, vaterite otoconia in, 193

Ear, inner, experimental viral infections (in hamster) and viremic spread of reovirus to eighth nerve ganglion cells, 90
Middle, bilateral carcinomas of, Waldenström's macroglobulinemia, 299
Middle, cavity, comparative anatomy of eustachian tube for otitis media (animal models), 82
Middle, electrical stimulation for activating central auditory pathways, 285
Middle, findings and tympanic configurations in otitis media, 20
Middle, sound transmission, effect of mastoid cavity modification on, 526
Polytomography and congenital anomalies of, 480
Recruiting, 521
Editorial, 4
Effusions, middle ear, granulocyte proteases in, 76
Electrical stimulation of middle ear for activating central auditory pathways, 285
Electroencephalic response components to clicks, early- and middle-AER, indices for neonatal hearing screening, 272
Electron microscope, scanning, in examination of nonbeating cilia, 612

Endolymphatic sac and vestibular aqueduct, postnatal development of, Suppl 96
Endolymphatic sac (rugose portion) and vestibular aqueduct in human temporal bones, dimensional anatomy and statistical analysis of, Suppl 96
Endoscopic coupler, universal, for carbon dioxide laser surgery, 608
Endotracheal artificial larynx, Suppl 95
Endotracheal cuffs, heat sink protection against lasering, 606
Endotracheal intubation, antecedent, and cricothyroidotomy, 437
Endotracheal tubes, incendiary characteristics with carbon dioxide laser (supplemental report), 605
Epiglottitis and croup, assessment of intubation in, 403
Epithelium, olfactory (in mouse), degeneration and regeneration of, Suppl 89
Epithelium of monkey larynx, age-related changes in, 370
Esophageal obstruction, simple endoscopic intubation technique in, 602
Esophageal speech, predicting, 454
Esophagology, update on, 551
Eustachian tube, middle ear cavity and comparative anatomy for otitis media (animal models), 82
  Normal function of, comparison in rhesus monkey and man, 179
Evoked potentials, brainstem, in adult sleep apnea, 597
  Normal neonatal brainstem auditory, 485
Evoked response, auditory brainstem, and unknown hearing level, 266
Extraskeletal mandibular fixation, monophasic, head and neck surgery and, 292

Facial canal, anatomy, variations, anomalies, Suppl 97:33
  Spatial occupancy of vessel and facial nerve, 14
Familial laryngeal abductor paralysis, presumed autosomal dominant inheritance, 323
Fever, typhoid, and cochleovestibular lesions, 220
Fibrous dysplasia, review and manifestations of disease in temporal bone, Suppl 92
Fistula, pharyngocutaneous, large, pectoralis major myocutaneous flap with medially based deltopectoral flap for closure of, 98
  Simultaneous round and oval window, in child, 332
  Tracheoesophageal, complication of foreign body, 325
Flap, deltopectoral, and combined pectoralis major myocutaneous flap for closure of large pharyngocutaneous fistulas, 98
  Pectoralis major myocutaneous, combined, and deltopectoral flap for closure of large pharyngocutaneous fistulas, 98
Foley catheter, use for removal of esophageal foreign bodies, 599
Foregut cysts, diagnosis and management in infants and children, 622
Foreign bodies, esophageal, use of Foley catheter in removal of, 599
Fossa, infratemporal, approach for glomus tumors of temporal bone, 474
Fossa lesions, posterior, anatomic specificity of central vestibular signs in, 510

Ganglion, eighth nerve, and viremic spread of reovirus in experimental viral infections of inner ear (hamster), 90
Giant apical air cell syndrome, 237
Glottic incompetence, posterior, correction following horizontal partial laryngectomy, 448
Granulomatosis, Wegener's, appearing initially in trachea, 593
  Of subglottis and upper portion of trachea, 588

Hair-clip type piston artificial stapes and safety auger, 297
Harmonic acceleration tests, computerized, vestibular subjective sensation and nystagmus responses during, 493
Harmonic acceleration tests as measure of vestibular compensation, 489
Hearing, preservation and acoustic neuroma surgery, 240
Hearing loss, conductive, effects on auditory brainstem response, 304
Hearing screening, neonatal, early- and middle-AER components to clicks as response indices in, 272
Hematoporphyrin-derivative phototherapy for local treatment of cancer of tracheobronchial tree, 652
Hemophilus influenzae, ampicillin-resistant, secondary to otitis media, 328
History, *Annals*, 1892-1982, 2
Home care of pediatric tracheotomy patient, 633
Homograft tympanic membrane after 12 years, 533
Hypertelorism in nasal and paranasal sinus polyposis (X-ray study of the month), 344
Hypoxic fraction, chemical modulation in treatment of head and neck cancer, 461

Idiopathic vocal cord paralysis, so-called, observations on, 558
Implants, cochlear, progress and perspectives, Suppl 91
  Audiological results, 27
  Bilateral; otopathological findings, 74
  Cochlear nucleus stimulation in humans, 117
  Comparison in promontory and cochlear implants in single subject, 100
  Initial experience with children, 67
  Multiple-electrode, 104
  Overview, 11
  Psychoelectric measurements and results from patients, 35
  Psychological effects: patient and "index relative" perceptions, 59
  Psychometric studies and clinical interviews, 55
  Risks and benefits of, 90
  Single electrode; design and functioning of units, 21
    Effects on vestibular system of profoundly deaf, 47
    Vowel discrimination, 41
  Surgical considerations, 15
  Use by prelingually deaf, 62
Incident fluorescence, use in tetracycline bone labeling, 160
Infant tracheotomy, 413
Ingestion, pediatric caustic, 656
Instability, atlantoaxial, alert for endoscopists, 567
Interferon, leukocyte, and juvenile laryngeal papillomatosis, 431
Internal auditory canal, computed tomographic air-contrast scanning of, 501
Intubation, antecedent endotracheal, and cricothyroidotomy, 437
  Assessment in croup and epiglottitis, 403
  Complications of, 584
Intubation technique, simple endoscopic, in esophageal obstruction, 602
Invasion, laryngotracheal, by thyroid carcinoma, 363

Labyrinthectomy, behavior of vestibular nerve following, Suppl 97:16
Labyrinthine artery and eighth cranial nerve, inner ear pathology following injury to, 136
Language development, speech development and, in parent-infant total communication program, Suppl 97:62
Laryngeal papilloma, treatment with carbon dioxide laser and podophyllum, 425
Laryngeal papillomatosis, juvenile, and leukocyte interferon, 431
Laryngeal paralysis, endoscopic rehabiliation of airway in, 382
Laryngeal paralysis in children, 417
Laryngeal sarcoidosis, 359
Laryngeal stenosis and tracheal stenosis, endoscopic management and predictive factors of success or failure, 384
Laryngeal surgery, supraglottic, factors in successful deglutition following, 579
Laryngeal trauma, primary management of, 399
Laryngectomy, horizontal partial, correction of posterior glottic incompetence following, 448
  Total, tracheostomal stenosis following, 450

Laryngoscope, operating, dynamics of Venturi jet ventilation through, 615
Larynx, age-related changes in epithelium of monkeys, 370
Chondrosarcoma of, diagnosis and conservative surgical management of, 389
Excision of massive recurrence in, 392
Endoscopic rehabilitation of airway in laryngeal paralysis, 382
Endotracheal artificial, Suppl 95
Intrinsic malignant schwannoma of, 336
Nerve-muscle pedicle reinnervation of, 440
Office telescopic photography of, 354
Laser, argon, and stapedotomy, 25
Carbon dioxide, heat sink protection against lasering endotracheal cuffs, 606
Incendiary characteristics of endotracheal tubes with (supplemental report), 605
Surgery, universal endoscopic coupler for, 608
Latency, acoustic reflex, standardization in humans and non-human primates, 169
Lavage, bronchoscopic limited, adjunct to therapy for cystic fibrosis patients 641
Lesions, cochleovestibular, and typhoid fever, 220
Posterior fossa, anatomic specificity of central vestibular signs in, 510
Letters to the Editor, 234, 467, 670
Leukocyte interferon, juvenile laryngeal papillomatosis with, 431
Levodopa-treated Parkinson's disease, vocal symptoms in, 119

Macroglobulinemia, Waldenström's, and bilateral middle ear carcinomas, 299
Malignancies, extrathoracic, mediastinoscopy for, 659
Laryngeal, and computerized tomography, correlation of tomographic and histopathologic findings, 571
Metastatic distant, tracheobronchial obstruction from, 648
Malleus handle probe, middle ear and, 281
Mandibular fixation, monophasic extraskeletal, head and neck surgery and, 292
Mastoid cavity, effect of modification on middle ear sound transmission, 526
Mediastinoscopy, use in extrathoracic malignancies, 659
Membrane, otoconial, dysplasia and vaterite otoconia in, 193
Middle ear, electrical stimulation for activating central auditory pathways, 285
Findings and tympanic configurations in otitis media, 20
Humoral and cell-mediated immunity in peripheral blood following introduction of antigen, 70
Middle ear carcinomas, bilateral, and Waldenström's macroglobulinemia, 299
Middle ear cavity, comparative anatomy of eustachian tube for otitis media (animal models), 82
Middle ear muscle tinnitus, conditioned, 330
Middle ear sound transmission, effect of mastoid cavity modification on, 526
Mixed tumor, malignant (Pathology consultation), 342
Mucormycosis, temporal bone, 27
Mucosa, upper respiratory, distribution of antileukoprotease in, 268
Mucous membrane, paranasal, characteristics of tissue plasminogen activator in chronic sinusitis, 101
Mycoplasma pneumoniae, infection and sudden deafness resulting from, 163
Myocutaneous flap, free, and revascularization of skin using myovascular pedicle (animal model), 53
Pectoralis major, and deltopectoral flap for closure of large pharyngocutaneous fistulas, 98
Myovascular pedicle, and revascularization of skin using animal model, 53

Nasal cycle, postural variations in nasal resistance and, 112
Nasal resistance, nasal cycle and postural variations in, 112
Nasal turbinates, inferior, surgery of, 445
Nasopharynx, rhabdomyosarcoma of (X-ray study of the month), 230
Neck, computed tomography of, Suppl 99
Neonates one to eight hours old, latency of auditory nerve response in, 205
Neoplasms, additional primary, occurrence in patients with laryngeal carcinoma in Israel (1960-1976), 261
Salivary gland, metastatic patterns of, 465
Nerve, auditory, latency of response in neonates one to eight hours old, 205
Eighth cranial, and labyrinthine artery, inner ear pathology following injury to, 136
Facial, and spatial occupancy of vessels in facial canal, 14
Nerve-muscle pedicle reinneration of larynx, 440
Nerve section, unilateral vestibular, and binocular counter-rolling during sustained body tilt, 225
Neurectomy, singular, update, 469
Neuroma, acoustic, surgery and preservation of hearing, 240
Nonbeating cilia, scanning electron microscopic examination of, 612
Nystagmus responses and vestibular subjective sensation during computerized harmonic acceleration tests, 493

Obituary, French K. Hansel, 232
Samuel Rosen, 126
Ben H. Senturia, 351
Obstruction, esophageal, simple endoscopic intubation technique in, 602
Tracheobronchial, from metastatic distant malignancies, 648
Obstructive sleep apnea, anatomic abnormalities in, 595
Olfactory epithelium (in mouse), degeneration and regeneration of, Supp 89
Open rigid bronchoscopy, anesthetic gas scavenger for use during, 610
Operating laryngoscope, dynamics of Venturi jet ventilation through, 615
Ossicular replacement allografts, lyophilized partial, 538
Otitis media, comparative anatomy of eustachian tube and middle ear cavity (animal models), 82
Experimental, tympanic configurations and middle ear findings, 20
Experimental (in chinchillas), Suppl 93: baseline immunological investigation, part 1; middle ear immune response to *S Pneumoniae* types 3 and 23, part 2
Pneumococcal, ampicillin in treatment (chinchilla model), 256
Secondary to ampicillin-resistant *Hemophilus influenzae*, 328
Otitis media with effusion and bony auditory tube, 200
Otoconial abnormalities, cochlear abnormalities and, in capsular otosclerosis with hydrops, Suppl 97:3
Otoconial membrane dysplasia, vaterite otoconia in, 193
Otolaryngology, American Board of, 1950-1979, Suppl 90
First National Conference on Research Goals and Methods in, Suppl 100
Otolaryngology-head and neck surgery, dilemma of subcertification in, 352
Otosclerosis, capsular, with hydrops, cochlear and otoconial abnormalities in, Suppl 97:3
Oval window fistula and round fistula, simultaneous, in child, 332
Oxatomide, use in treatment of chronic allergic rhinitis, 175

Palatal incompetence, congenital indications before diagnosis, 115
Palliative care, use of inexpensive effective cryoprobe for, 204
Panje and Blom-Singer voice prostheses, primary vocal rehabilitation using, 458
Papilloma, laryngeal, treatment with carbon dioxide laser and podophyllum, 425

Papillomatosis, juvenile laryngeal, leukocyte interferon use in, 431
Paralysis, abductor vocal cord, congenital hereditary bilateral, 564
Familial laryngeal abductor, and presumed autosomal dominant inheritance, 323
Laryngeal, endoscopic rehabilitation of airway in, 382
In children, 417
Seventh nerve, biofeedback rehabilitation in, 166
Vocal cord, observations on so-called idiopathic, 558
Parkinson's disease, vocal symptoms in levodopa-treated, 119
Parotid gland, human, collagenase activity in squamous cell carcinoma of, 156
Patency, functional, and cochlear aqueduct, 209
Pathology consultation: malignant mixed tumor, 342
Metastatic patterns of salivary gland neoplasms, 465
Midfacial necrotizing diseases, 541
Pediatric tracheostomy, 628
Pedicle, myovascular, and revascularization of skin (animal model), 53
Nerve-muscle, reinnervation in larynx, 440
Pemphigoid, benign mucous membrane, 142
Periapical abscess, and intracranial complications of sinusitis in children, 41
Peripheral blood, humoral and cell-mediated immunity following introduction of antigen into middle ear, 70
Photography, telescopic, of larynx in office, 354
Phototherapy, hematoporphyrin-derivative, for treatment of cancer of tracheobronchial tree, 652
Podophyllum and carbon dioxide laser, treatment of laryngeal papilloma with, 425
Polyposis, nasal and paranasal sinus, hypertelorism in (X-ray study of the month), 344
Polyps, vocal cord, pathogenesis of, 378
Polytomography, and congenital anomalies of ear, 480
Probe, malleus handle, middle ear and, 281
Propylhexedrine, nasal decongestant effect of, 106
Prosthesis, auditory, neural mechanisms relevant to design: location and electrical characteristics, Suppl 98
Cochlear, tissue impedance and current flow in implanted ear, Suppl 98
Proteases, granulocyte, and middle ear effusions, 76
Pterygomaxillary tumors, extended transantral approach to, 395

Receptors, presynaptic parasympathetic, evidence on nasal blood vessels, 216
Reovirus, viremic spread (in hamster) to eighth nerve ganglion cells and experimental viral infections in middle ear, 90
Research goals and methods in otolaryngology, first national conference on, Suppl 100
Resorption, bone, in human cholesteatomas, 131
Respiratory rehabilitation with transtracheal oxygen system, 643
Rhabdomyosarcoma of nasopharynx (X-ray study of the month), 230
Rhinitis, chronic allergic, oxatomide in treatment of, 175
Round fistula and oval window fistula, simultaneous, in child, 332

Saccule, collapsed, ductus reuniens and cochlear hydrops, 5
Salivary gland neoplasms, metastatic patterns of, 465
Sarcoidosis, laryngeal, 359
Schwannoma of larynx, intrinsic malignant, 336
Schwannomas, paranasal sinus, management of, 65
Semicircular canal structure, postnatal development in cat and guinea pig, 185
Senturia, Ben H. Dedication, 1; In Memoriam, 349; Tribute, 350
Seventh nerve paralysis, use of biofeedback rehabilitation in, 166
Sleep apnea, adult, brainstem evoked potentials in, 597
Obstructive, anatomic abnormalities in, 595
Sinus, maxillary, bacteriology in rhesus monkeys, 150
Paranasal, schwannommas of, 65
Sinusitis, chronic and tissue plasminogen activator from paranasal mucous membrane, 101
Intracranial complications in children with periapical abscess, 41
Speech and language development in parent-infant total communication program, Suppl 97:62
Sphenoid, aneurysmal bone cyst of, in child, 339
Squamous cell carcinoma of human parotid gland, collagenase activity in, 156
Squirrel monkey, vestibular ganglion of, 44
Stapedectomy, long-term report, 516
Stapedotomy, argon laser, 25
Stapes, artificial, hair-clip type piston and safety auger, 297
Stenosis, laryngeal and tracheal, success or failure in endoscopic management of, 384
Severe subglottic, treatment without tracheotomy, 407
Tracheostomal, following total laryngectomy, 450
Subcertification in otolaryngology-head and neck surgery, 352
Subcortical dysfunction, and brainstem and cortical dysfunction, in dyslexic children, 310
Subglottic stenosis, severe, treatment without tracheotomy, 407
Subglottis and upper portion of trachea, Wegener's granulomatosis of, 588
Supraglottic laryngeal surgery, factors in successful deglutition following, 579
Syndrome, giant apical air cell, 237

Telescopic photography of larynx in office, 354
Temporal bone, infratemporal fossa approach for glomus tumors of, 474
Mucormycosis, 27
Review and manifestations of fibrous dysplasia in, Suppl 92
Tetracycline bone labeling using incident fluorescence, 160
Thyroid carcinoma, laryngotracheal invasion by, 363
Tinnitus, conditioned middle ear muscle, 330
Tissue plasminogen activator and paranasal mucous membrane, characteristics in chronic sinusitis, 101
Tomography, computed, air-contrast scanning of internal auditory canal, 501
Computed, of neck, Suppl 99
Computerized, laryngeal malignancies and, correlation of tomographic and histopathologic findings, 571
Dynamic computed, evaluation of hindbrain circulation by, 506
Tongue, anterior, carcinoma of, 94
Tonsillar crypts, microcrypt extensions of, Suppl 94
Total communication program, parent-infant, speech and language development in, Suppl 97:62
Trachea, upper portion, and subglottis, Wegener's granulomatosis of, 588
Wegener's granulomatosis appearing initially in, 593
Tracheal and laryngeal stenosis, endoscopic management and predictive factors of success or failure in, 384
Tracheobronchial obstruction from metastatic distant malignancies, 648
Tracheobronchial tree, cancer of, hematoporphyrin-derivative phototherapy for local treatment, 652
Tracheoesophageal fistula, a complication of foreign body, 325
Tracheostoma valve, postlaryngectomy voice rehabilitation with, 576
Tracheostomal stenosis following total laryngectomy, 450
Tracheostomy, pediatric, experience during past decade, 628
Tracheotomy, infant, 413
Treatment of severe subglottic stenosis without, 407
Tracheotomy patient, pediatric, home care of, 633
Transtracheal oxygen system, respiratory rehabilitation with, 643
Trauma, laryngeal, primary management of, 399
Tumor, malignant mixed (Pathology consultation), 342
Warthin's, 246

Tumors, glomus, of temporal bone, infratemporal fossa approach for, 474
Pterygomaxillary, extended transantral approach to, 395
Turbinates, inferior nasal, surgery of, 445
Typhoid fever and cochleovestibular lesions, 220

Valve, tracheostoma, for postlaryngectomy voice rehabilitation, 576
Vaterite otoconia in otoconial membrane dysplasia, 193
Ventilation, Venturi jet, dynamics through operating laryngoscope, 615
Venturi jet ventilation, dynamics through operating laryngoscope, 615
Vestibular aqueduct and endolymphatic sac, postnatal development of, Suppl 96
Vestibular aqueduct and endolymphatic sac (rugose portion) in human temporal bones, dimensional anatomy and statistical analysis of, Suppl 96
Vestibular compensation, harmonic acceleration tests as measure of, 489
Vestibular ganglion in squirrel monkey, 44
Vestibular nerve, behavior following labyrinthectomy, Suppl 97:16
Vestibular nerve section, unilateral, and binocular counter-rolling during sustained body tilt, 225
Vestibular signs, central, anatomic specificity in posterior fossa lesions, 510
Vestibular subjective sensation and nystagmus responses during computerized harmonic acceleration tests, 493
Vocal cord paralysis, congenital hereditary bilateral abductor, 564
So-called idiopathic, observations on, 558
Vocal cord polyps, pathogenesis of, 378
Vocal rehabilitation, primary, use of Blom-Singer and Panje voice prostheses in, 458
Voice disorders, functional, classification and approach to patients with, 372
Voice rehabilitation, postlaryngectomy, tracheostoma valve for, 576

Waldenström's macroglobulinemia and bilateral middle ear carcinomas, 299
Warthin's tumor, 246
Wegener's granulomatosis appearing initially in trachea, 593
Wegener's granulomatosis of subglottis and upper portion of trachea, 588

X-ray study of the month: hypertelorism in nasal and paranasal sinus polyposis, 344
Intracavernous internal carotid artery aneurysm, 543
Rhabdomyosarcoma of nasopharynx, 230

DEGENERATION AND REGENERATION OF OLFACTORY EPITHELIUM IN THE MOUSE

A Scanning Electron Microscopic Study

Daniel H. Matulionis, PhD

W. Breipohl, MD

Kunwar P. Bhatnagar, PhD

This publication was supported in part by Parke-Davis
Division of Warner-Lambert Company.

DEGENERATION AND REGENERATION OF OLFACTORY EPITHELIUM IN THE MOUSE

A Scanning Electron Microscopic Study

Daniel H. Matulionis, PhD
Lexington, Kentucky

W. Breipohl, MD
Essen, West Germany

Kunwar P. Bhatnagar, PhD
Louisville, Kentucky

Surface morphological events which occur during degeneration and regeneration of mouse olfactory epithelium following nasal irrigation with 1% aqueous zinc sulfate solution are described at the scanning electron microscope level. Degeneration of olfactory epithelium occurred over extensive areas during the first 24 hours after treatment. Degenerative conditions ranged from a slightly altered surface to a surface revealing the underlying basal lamina. Onset of regeneration was suggested by the appearance of squamous cells two days post-treatment and occurred simultaneously over large surface areas. At this time the surface was perforated by numerous pore-like openings from which protruded cells as though in a process of migration. It is suggested that the presumed migrating cells contribute cellular elements to olfactory epithelium during early regeneration. Regrowth of the epithelium was uniform over the entire regenerating epithelium. Neural elements first appeared 14 days after treatment. The surface of olfactory epithelium appeared nearly normal 28 to 42 days after the zinc sulfate treatment. The distinctive degenerative and regenerative surface manifestations extend and confirm previous observations made at the transmission electron microscopic level.

INTRODUCTION

A relatively large number of studies deals with the effects of zinc sulfate ($ZnSO_4$) on olfactory epithelium.[1-10] These studies reveal that irrigation of the nasal cavity with aqueous $ZnSO_4$ solution causes a selective destruction of olfactory epithelium. Nasal respiratory epithelium is affected by the same treatment to a lesser degree.[11] This treatment allows the assessment of neuronal regeneration which occurs uniquely in the olfactory epithelium.

The most important region of olfactory epithelium is its surface since it is here that receptor sites for olfaction are located. Investigators have described the degenerative and regenerative episodes at the light and/or transmission electron microscopic (TEM) levels which occur below the surface. A clear idea of events manifested at the surface of this epithelium during such drastic alteration and reorganization of the tissue is lacking. For example, surface manifestations that occur during de-epithelization and regrowth of the epithelium have not been described prior to the present study. The extent of epithelial areas affected by the $ZnSO_4$ treatment, the surface morphology of the bare basal lamina, and the events occurring during the reconstitution of the surface brush border lack documentation. Further, the origin and surface morphology of cells which initially contribute to the reformation of the epithelium are unclear. In addition, the degree to which cell migration, from edges of epithelium which escaped the $ZnSO_4$ solution, contributes to the new epithelium is unknown.[9,10] The present scanning electron microscope (SEM) study documents the morphological events that occur at the surface during degeneration and regeneration of olfactory epithelium and provides information in regard to the above points.

METHODS

A total of 54 adult male C57BL/6J mice were used for the SEM assessment of olfactory epithelium. The nasal cavities of 45 mice were irrigated with 1% $ZnSO_4$ solution according to a method described previously.[10] Five sham-treated and four untreated animals served as controls. Sham treatment consisted of irrigating the nasal chambers with distilled water. Olfactory epithelium from the posterior nasal vault, the posterior portion of the nasal septum, and the medial surface of the endoturbinate bones of both nasal chambers was examined from five $ZnSO_4$-treated animals at 0.5, 1, 2, 3, 4, 8, 14, 28 and 42 days after the treatment. Before the tissues were dissected free from the nasal cavities, the animals were anesthetized by intraperitoneal injections of Nembutal (Abbott Laboratories, North Chicago, Ill.). After careful dissection of the olfactory mucosa, the samples were washed by gently pipetting Hank's balanced salt solution over the surface of the tissue. This washing removed surface mucus and cellular debris, allowing the visualization of the epithelium surface. The initial fixation was carried out in cacodylate buffered 3% glutaraldehyde (pH 7.35) for 16-18 hours at 4°C. After several washings in the cacodylate buffer, the samples were postfixed in 1% osmium tetroxide[12] for two hours. Following another brief buffer rinse, the samples were dehydrated in graded methanol and passed through graded methanol-amyl acetate to a final concentration of 100% amyl acetate. Critical point drying was carried out with liquid CO_2 in a Polaron critical point drying apparatus. The dried samples were mounted on aluminum stubs affixed with colloidal silver, gold-sputtered (4 cm from the anode) on a water-cooled stub holder (in an argon atmosphere) in a vacuum of 10^{-1} torrs twice for one minute and examined in a Cambridge SEM 180 at

From the Department of Anatomy, University of Kentucky Medical Center and the Kentucky Tobacco Health and Research Institute, Lexington; Institut für Anatomie, Universitätsklinikum, Essen, West Germany; and the Department of Anatomy, University of Louisville School of Medicine. This study was supported by the University of Kentucky Anatomy Department, the University of Kentucky Research Committee Grant and Deutsche Forschungsgemeinschaft (SFB 114).

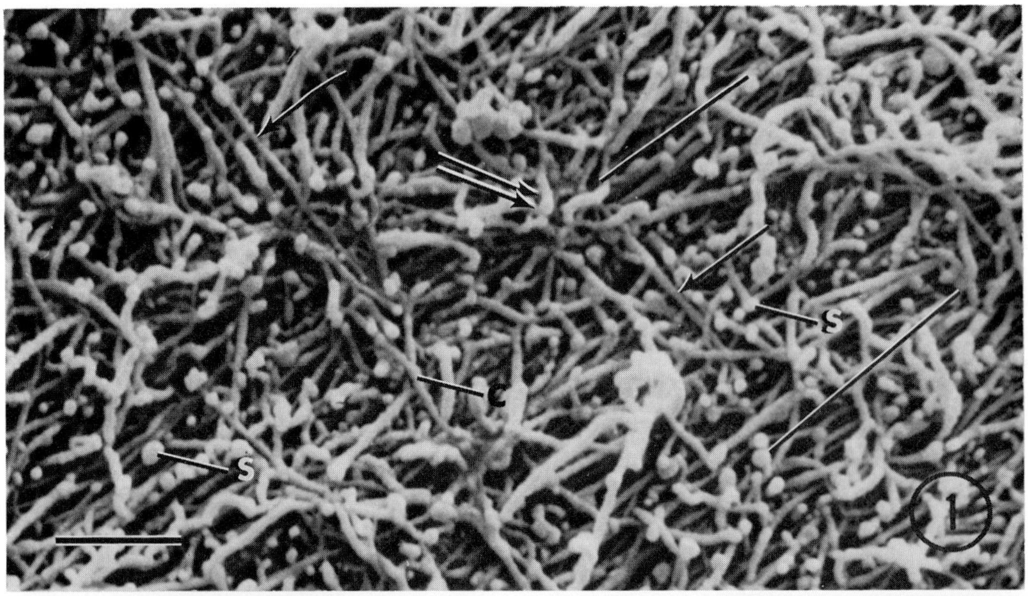

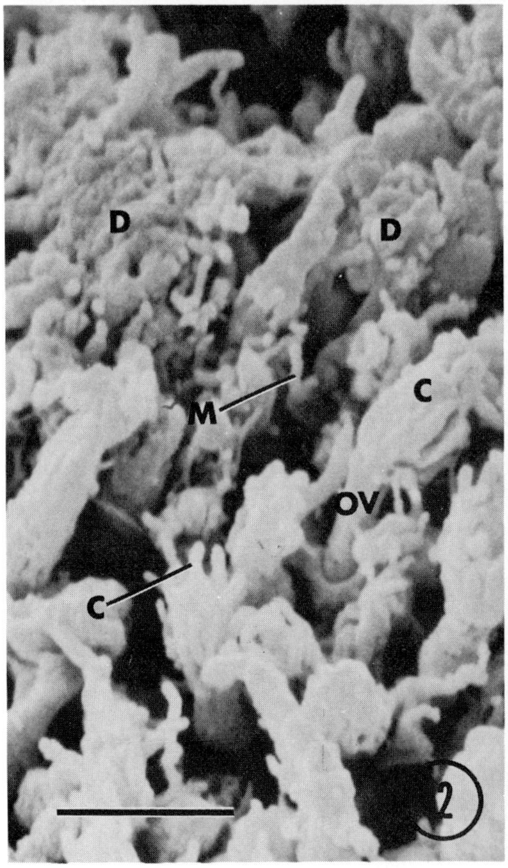

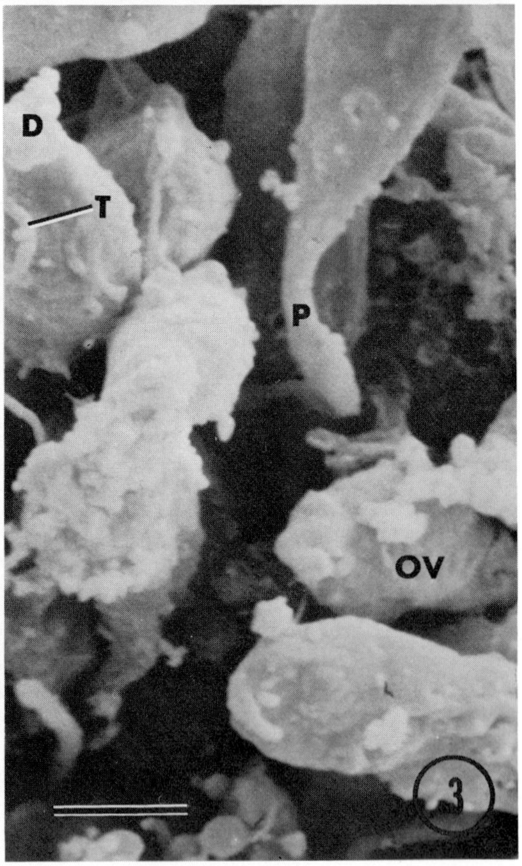

Fig. 1. Olfactory epithelial surface of a control mouse. In several regions cilia (C) appear to be radiating from central points of origin (double arrows). The thin distal portion of many cilia, somewhat removed from their origin, appear to be in parallel arrangement (lines). Other cilia orient themselves perpendicularly to those arranged in a parallel fashion (arrow). S - Terminal swellings. (Bar 3 μm unless otherwise noted in all figures.)

Fig. 2. Surface of olfactory epithelium one-half day after treatment showing the least severely altered degenerative condition. Olfactory vesicles (OV) are covered with short segments of cilia (C). Cellular debris (D) represents remnants of severely altered supporting cells. M - Microvilli.

Fig. 3. Olfactory epithelial surface one-half day after treatment depicting the "more severely altered degenerative condition" which contained swollen vesicles (OV) devoid of cilia. T - Tubular structures; D - Cellular debris; P - Tapering processes.

20 kV. The tilt angle of the specimen in the SEM ranged from 15-30°.

Olfactory mucosa of nine additional C57BL/6J mice treated with $ZnSO_4$ were also available for TEM assessment. These tissues were prepared using methods reported earlier[10] with one modification: the dissected olfactory mucosa was washed in a fashion similar to that used in preparing the tissue for SEM. Tissues from three animals were available at each of the 1-, 2- and 3-day sampling periods after the $ZnSO_4$ treatment. These tissues were examined in a TEM (Philips 200) at 60kV.

RESULTS

The surface of untreated and sham-treated olfactory epithelium was similar in appearance, consisting of presumed olfactory cilia which measured about 0.1-0.4 μm in diameter (Fig. 1). The cilia appeared to originate from numerous central points, radiated in all directions and often terminated with spherical swellings. The terminal enlargements (swellings) are characteristic of normal cilia (Matulionis DH, unpublished data). Somewhat removed from the point of origin, the orientation of cilia was more or less parallel to each other and to the free surface. Few cilia were seen oriented perpendicular to the majority. Orientation of the cilia was confirmed by TEM observation (Matulionis DH, unpublished data). Terminal enlarged dendritic endings (olfactory vesicles) of sensory cells were hidden due to the large number of the cilia at the surface, as were the apical surfaces of supporting cells.

Half Day after $ZnSO_4$ Treatment. Twelve hours after the nasal cavities were irrigated with $ZnSO_4$ the surface morphology was highly altered when compared to the control tissue. Although quantitative measurements were not made, the altered areas were extensive. Three general conditions were prominent, each suggesting a different progressive stage of degeneration. The least severe condition revealed numerous olfactory vesicles (1.2 μm in diameter) devoid of the long olfactory sensory cilia (Fig. 2) which normally are so numerous that they conceal the olfactory vesicles and the components of the epithelial surface. Instead, short cylindrical surface structures (approximately 0.93 μm long, 0.25 μm in diameter), presumed to be altered cilia, emanated from these vesicles.

The more severe degenerative condition was characterized by swollen olfactory vesicles (about 3.6 μm in diameter) with occasional cylindrical structures (altered cilia) emerging from their surface (Fig. 3). The vesicles appeared free in the nasal chamber but were attached to the epithelium by elongated tapering processes which were most likely the dendritic components of the olfactory neurons. Small particles of cellular debris were noted on the vesicles and tapering processes.

The most marked state of degeneration at 12 hours after $ZnSO_4$ treatment was characterized by a relatively uniform noncellular surface littered with considerable debris consisting of strands and irregularly shaped material and occasionally groups of small spherical cells (Fig. 4). Occasionally irregular tears and holes were noted, indicating a fragile surface. The morphology of the surface suggested that it was the bare basal lamina of the epithelium. Of the three degenerative conditions noted at this time, the most severely altered condition was least frequently observed.

One Day after $ZnSO_4$ Treatment. The prevailing condition noted at this time resembled the most severely altered condition of the previous stage and was observed over large areas of the mucosa. The surface morphology was different from that of the previous stage. The sensory olfactory vesicles were completely absent and the amount of cellular debris on the surface was reduced (Fig. 5). TEM assessment of tissue at this time revealed a bare basal lamina also free of debris (Fig. 12). Irregular, well-demonstrated openings were seen on the surface (Fig. 5). In some cases, the orifices of these openings appeared to be congested with cells which were studded with short microvilli. The cells within the openings were located below the basal lamina in the subjacent lamina propria. These were cellular components of Bowman's glands. This type of surface morphology marks the terminal stage of degeneration after the epithelial cells have completely sloughed off. Normally basal lamina is covered by basal, receptor and supporting cells (cells of olfactory epithelium).

Two and Three Days after $ZnSO_4$ Treatment. The surface of the olfactory mucosa was almost uniformly covered with squamous cells, suggesting onset of epithelial regeneration (Fig. 6). The area populated by the squamous cells was extensive and corresponded with the area of the bare basal lamina seen in the previous stage. Surface cells were irregular, stellate, or fusiform in shape, and were covered with short microvilli (Figs. 6, 7). Certain areas, however, were devoid of cells demonstrating the naked basal lamina (Fig. 7). Such areas were perforated with small holes that occurred randomly over the surface of the tissue. In addition, many larger openings were present at the surface (Figs. 6, 7). These larger openings were congested with cells which in turn were covered with numerous microvilli. On many occasions cells covered with microvilli were noted protruding through these larger openings as though in the process of migration onto the surface (Fig. 8). Such protruding cells were uniformly distributed over the surface of the regenerating olfactory epithelium. TEM assessment revealed these cells to be covered with microvilli and glandular in nature (Fig. 13).

Four and Eight Days after $ZnSO_4$ Treatment. The surface of regenerating epithelium at four and eight days after treatment with $ZnSO_4$ was similar. The most common surface manifestation at these times appeared as extensive areas composed of rela-

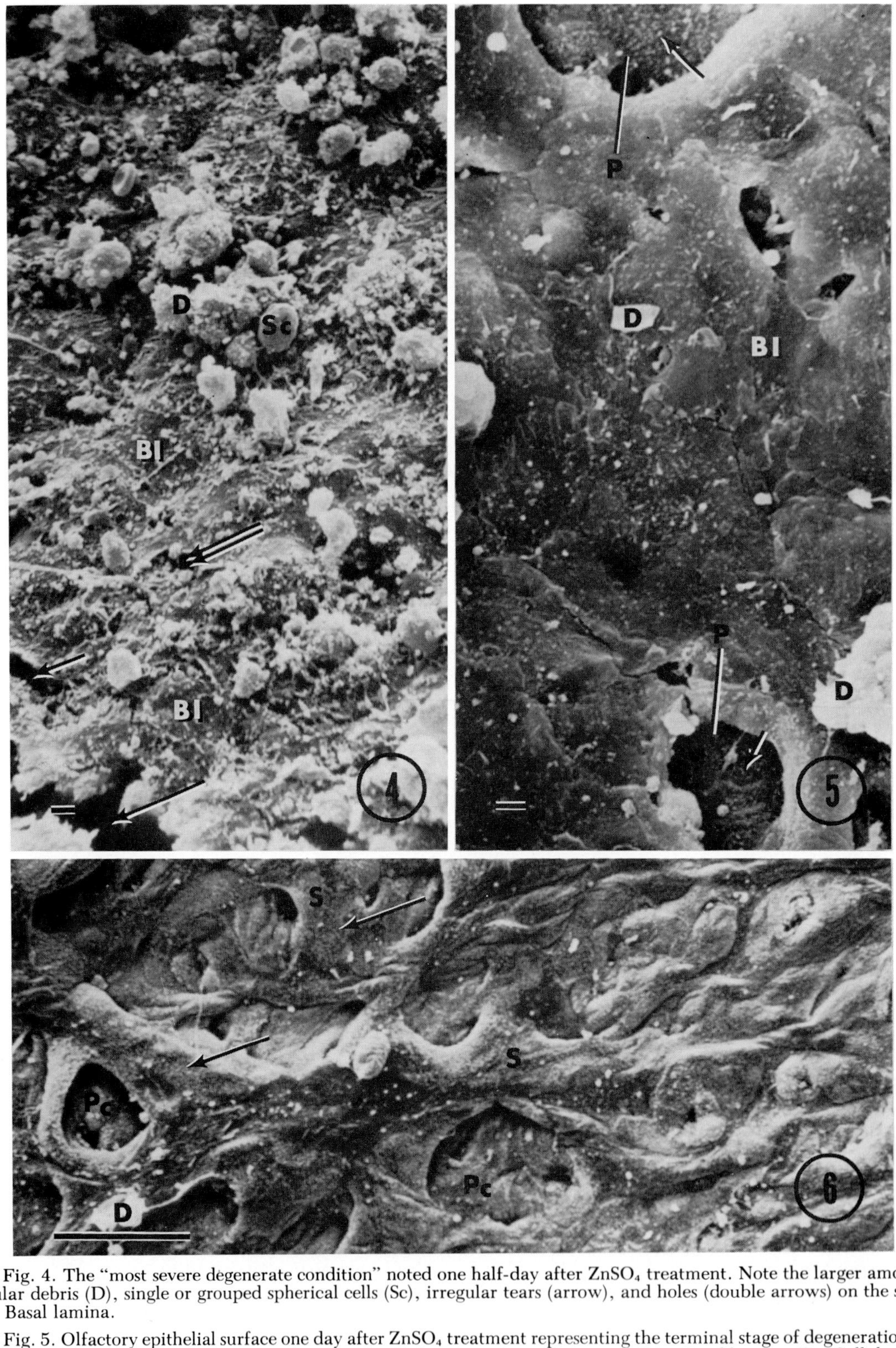

Fig. 4. The "most severe degenerate condition" noted one half-day after $ZnSO_4$ treatment. Note the larger amounts of cellular debris (D), single or grouped spherical cells (Sc), irregular tears (arrow), and holes (double arrows) on the surface. B1 - Basal lamina.

Fig. 5. Olfactory epithelial surface one day after $ZnSO_4$ treatment representing the terminal stage of degeneration. Note the pore-like openings (P) which are congested with cells bearing microvilli (arrow). B1 - Basal lamina; D - Cellular debris.

Fig. 6. Regenerating olfactory epithelial surface two days after treatment. The surface is no longer flat but composed of irregularly shaped squamous cells (S) which are covered with short microvilli (arrow). The bar in the lower left corner represents 30 μm. Pc - Cells in the opening of pores; D - Debris.

tively uniform elongate cells (Fig. 9). These cells were covered with numerous microvilli, the length and diameter of which seemed to be slightly variable on different cells. Surface outlines of individual cells were evident. In one animal, four days after treatment, normal epithelium was observed adjacent to regenerating tissue. The regenerating epithelium next to the normal epithelium was

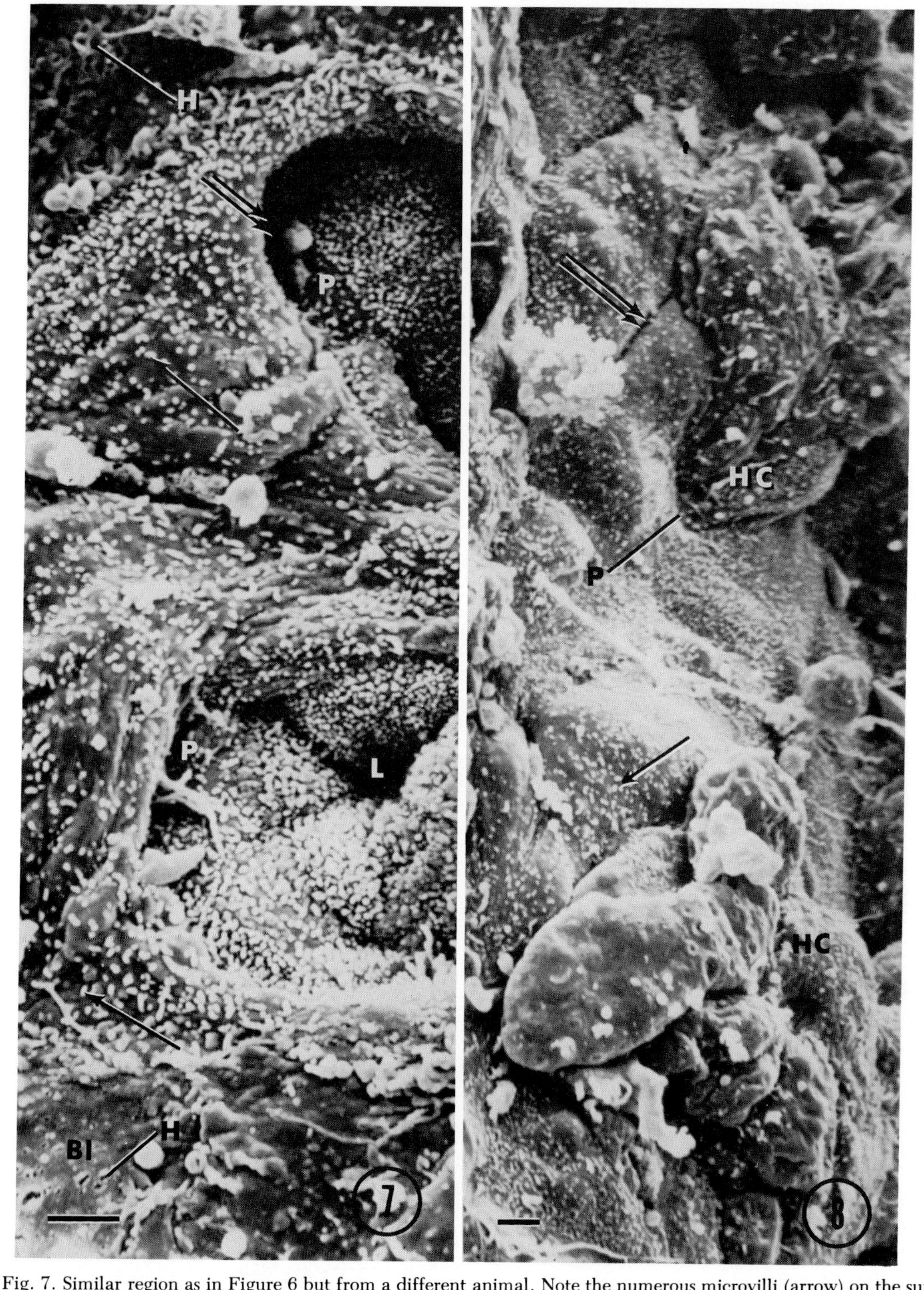

Fig. 7. Similar region as in Figure 6 but from a different animal. Note the numerous microvilli (arrow) on the surface cells. Areas which represent the basal lamina (Bl) contain holes (H). L - Lumen of Bowman's glands; P - Pores; Double arrow - Cells in the opening of pores.

Fig. 8. Similar region as in Figure 6 but from a different animal which shows cells migrating (HC) through pores (P). Arrow - Microvilli. Double arrow - Breaks between cells.

similar in every respect to that farther removed from the unaffected normal tissue.

Fourteen Days after $ZnSO_4$ Treatment. Surface morphology 14 days after treatment was considerably different when compared to the previous stages. Large numbers of microvilli, now elongated, obstructed the visualization of epithelial cell surfaces (Fig. 10). Individual cell boundaries were no longer discernible. Clusters of projecting microvilli-like structures (approximately 2.2 μm in diameter) seemingly originating from a common

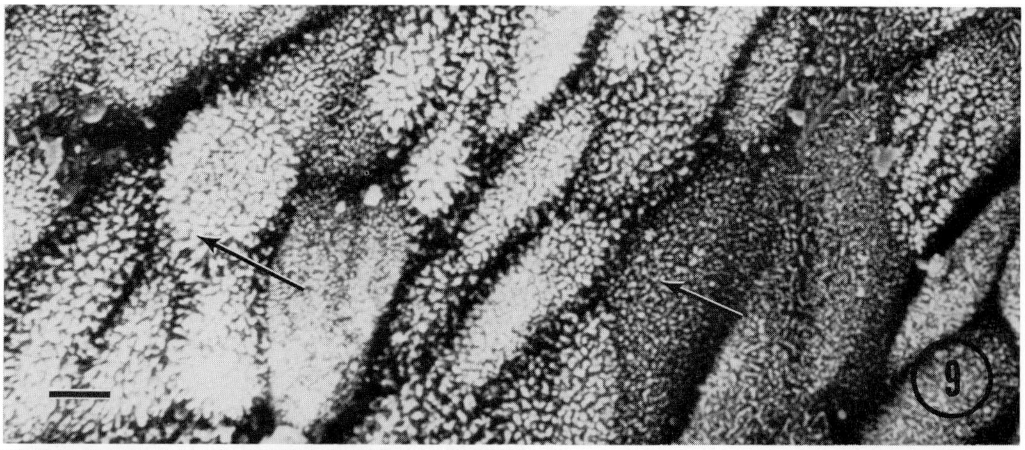

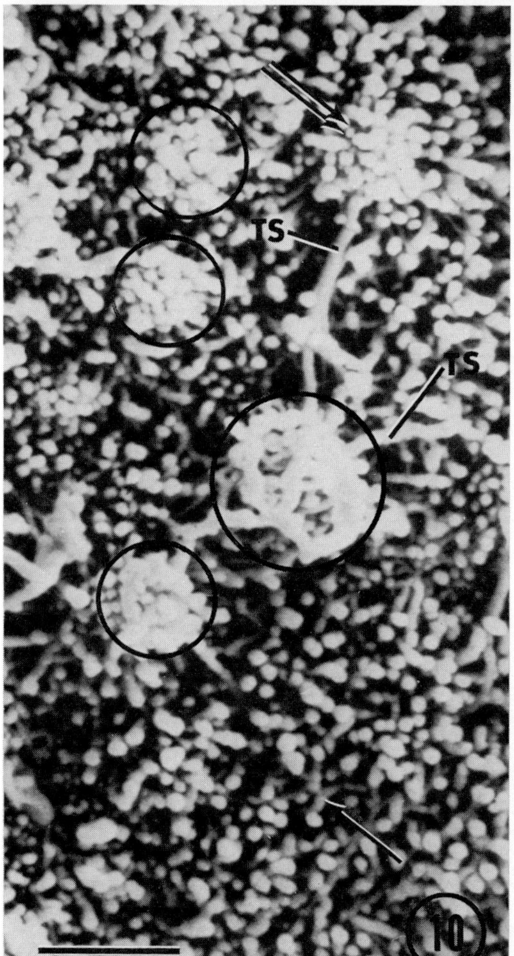

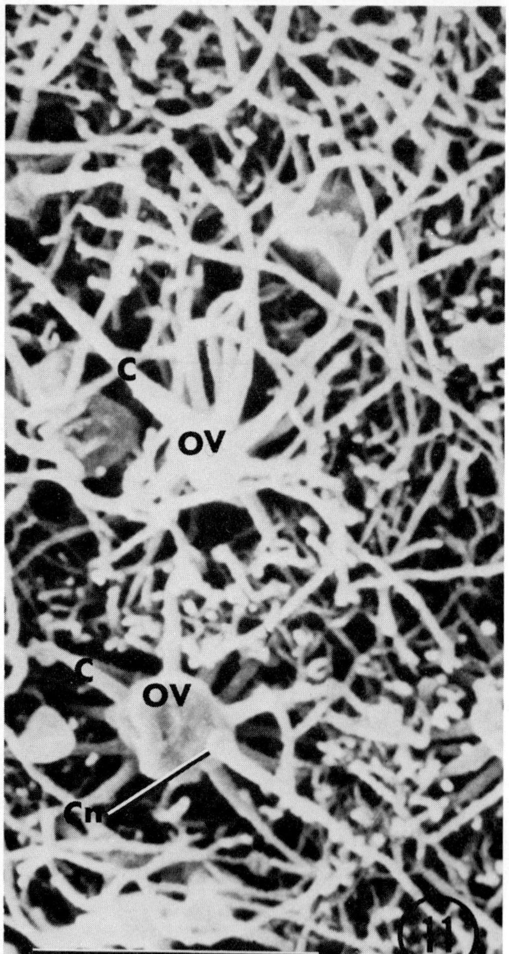

Fig. 9. Regenerating olfactory epithelial surface four days after $ZnSO_4$ treatment depicting relatively uniform cells covered with microvilli of different sizes (arrow).

Fig. 10. Regenerating olfactory epithelium 14 days after treatment. Note the large numbers of microvilli (arrow) and developing olfactory vesicles (circle). The vesicle, covered with microvilli (double arrows), possesses outgrowing longer tubular ciliary structures (TS).

Fig. 11. Nearly normal olfactory epithelium 28 days after treatment depicting several olfactory vesicles (OV) with well-developed cilia (C). A ciliary neck (Cn) is seen at the base of a cilium.

source, were noted in certain areas of the epithelial surface. Longer rounded elongate projections were noted emanating from the clusters and occasionally formed entanglements. The longer projections were interpreted as developing olfactory sensory cilia of the olfactory vesicles.

Twenty-eight and Forty-two Days after $ZnSO_4$ Treatment. Surfaces of regenerating epithelium at

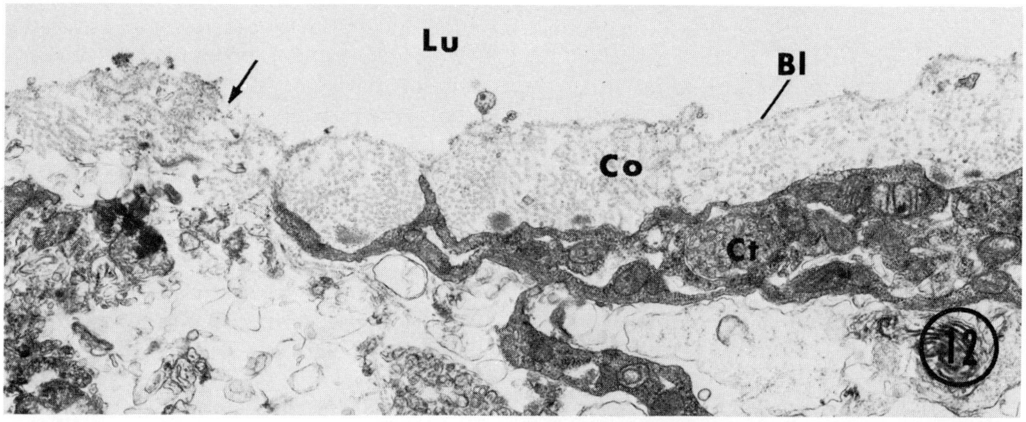

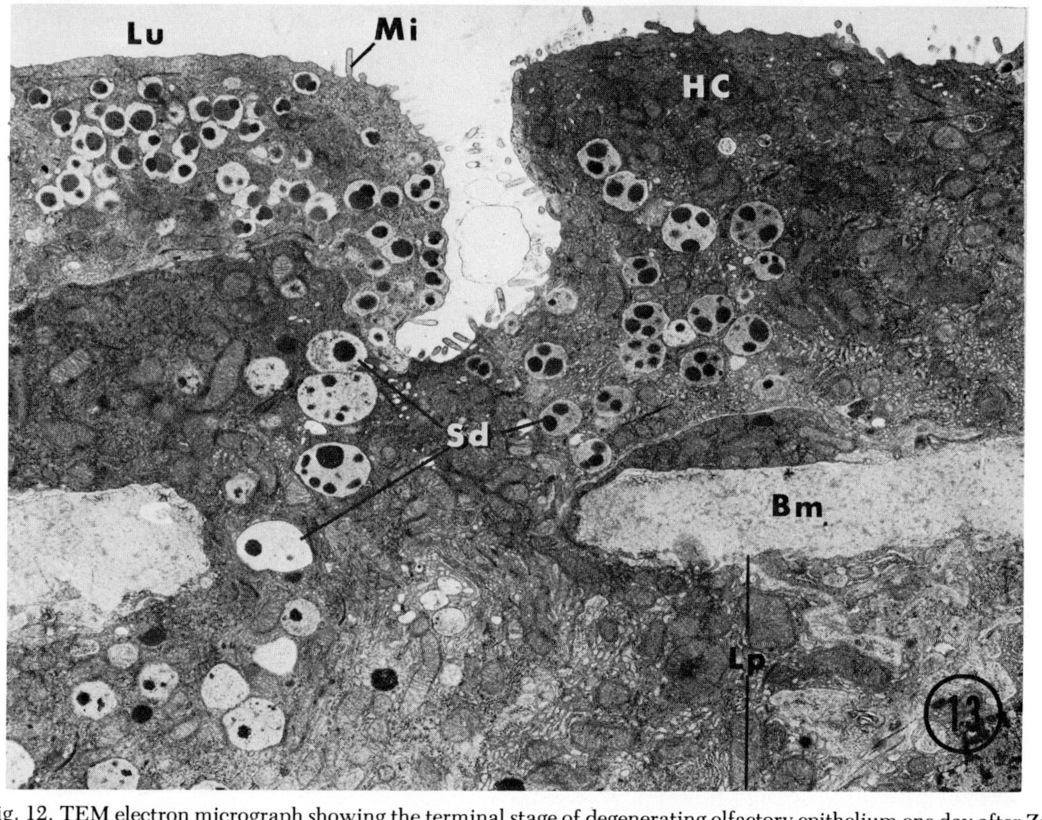

Fig. 12. TEM electron micrograph showing the terminal stage of degenerating olfactory epithelium one day after $ZnSO_4$ treatment. Note the bare basal lamina (Bl) with small breaks (arrow). Lu - Lumen of the nasal cavity; Ct - Connective tissue cell; Co - Collagen in the basement membrane. (x 9180)

Fig. 13. TEM electron micrograph showing glandular cells (HC) migrating from the lamina propria (Lp) onto the surface of the basement membrane (Bm) two days after $ZnSO_4$ treatment. Mi - Microvilli; Lu - Lumen of the nasal cavity; Sd - Secretory droplets. (x 7150)

28 and 42 days past $ZnSO_4$ treatment were similar and appeared normal (Fig. 11). The dendritic swellings of the olfactory neurons, the thick proximal (ciliary neck) segment (approximately 0.18 μm in diameter) and the thin distal segment (about 0.1 μm in diameter) of the olfactory sensory cilia were clearly evident. The density of the cilia was, however, lower than that of control tissue (compare Figs. 1 and 11). The lower density of these structures could be a reflection of their shorter length rather than fewer numbers. Also, the parallel arrangement of the cilia was not evident at this stage of degeneration. The epithelium appeared immature but almost totally renewed.

DISCUSSION

The present SEM study describes the degenerative and regenerative events that are seen at the surface of the olfactory mucosa following irrigation of the nasal chambers with 1% aqueous $ZnSO_4$ solution. The following points, pertinent to the regenerative capacity of olfactory neurons, are discussed: 1) visual assessment of the extent of olfactory mucosal surface affected by the treatment, 2) events that occur during early regeneration, focusing on the cells which initially colonize the mucosal surface, and 3) the reconstitution of the epithelial border, a region containing sites for olfactory reception.

Degeneration of the olfactory epithelium occurred rapidly over the first 24 hours after the $ZnSO_4$ treatment. During this time, the epithelial surface was conspicuously free of sloughing cells and cellular debris, a prominent feature of degenerating epithelium seen previously with the TEM.[10] The debris-free surface was undoubtedly a result of the method used to prepare the tissue for SEM. Numerous washings of the epithelial surface were necessary to remove the mucous film which would normally obscure surface features. Tissues which were similarly washed for TEM also revealed a debris-free surface. SEM observation of the initial changes seen at the washed surface revealed olfactory vesicles devoid of the normal complement of olfactory cilia. It appears that the cilia are markedly and rapidly affected by the $ZnSO_4$ treatment rather than tissue processing procedures since the cilia of the control and sham-treated animals were intact. The fragile nature of these structures has been previously observed by other investigators.[13,14] The deleterious effects of $ZnSO_4$ appears to rapidly disrupt those structures (cilia) which have been purported to contain chemoreceptor sites.[15-18]

The altered or degenerating areas of epithelium were extensive and no normal (unaffected by the treatment) olfactory epithelium was seen 24 hours after treatment. However, four days after $ZnSO_4$ application, a region of normal-appearing tissue adjacent to regenerating tissue was noted. Wide expanses of altered tissue in mice, as seen with SEM, correlate well with the 78 to 97% of olfactory epithelial destruction produced by $ZnSO_4$ in hamsters.[19] Present observations indicate that irrigation of the nasal cavities with $ZnSO_4$ is an effective means of destroying large areas of olfactory epithelium. Such a treatment provides an opportunity to study the dynamics and plasticity of this tissue.

The degenerative process culminated in a surface totally devoid of epithelial cells (24 hours posttreatment) revealing a bare basal lamina. Presence of irregular randomly-oriented artifactual tears and holes in the surface of the basal lamina suggested a thin fragile surface. Previous and present TEM observations of the terminal degenerating phase of mouse olfactory epithelium revealed regions of basal lamina devoid of cells one day after $ZnSO_4$ treatment.[10] However, it was difficult to assess with TEM the extent of the naked basal lamina present after such a treatment. SEM analysis, on the other hand, clearly demonstrated large regions of exposed basal lamina, comparable to those of degenerating epithelium present over the mucosa one day after $ZnSO_4$ irrigation.

Initial signs of regeneration appeared approximately two days after treatment. At this time the surface was covered with squamous cells which were studded with short microvilli. The squamous nature of the surface cells at the onset of regeneration has been reported[10] and confirms the present observations. The borders of these cells were clearly visible with occasional separations between them. This observation supports the notion that the tissue surface at one day after treatment represents a fragile bare basal lamina, rather than a cellular surface since the breaks on the surface at that time were randomly oriented.

At two and three days after $ZnSO_4$ treatment, cells were often noted protruding through openings of the basal lamina. The morphological configuration of these cells suggested that they were in a migratory process. TEM assessment of the migrating cells revealed them to be glandular in nature. Similarly, migrating cells were noted previously and suggested as originating from Bowman's glands.[8,10] The observation of such migrating cells lends itself to speculation in regard to their role in the regenerating epithelium. Could these cells be the progenitor cells for olfactory epithelium? It has recently been proposed that basal cells give rise to stem cells for regeneration (after transection of the olfactory nerve) and normal replacement (during adult life) of olfactory neurons.[20-23] These studies, however, do not address themselves to the origin of the basal cells. It is unlikely that the migrating cells are basal cell precursors since their cytoplasmic ultrastructure is similar to that of supporting cells.[10] However, similar morphology of migrating and supporting cells suggests that the former cells are precursors of the latter. Such an interpretation would agree with data reported by Graziadei and Graziadei.[21] They stated that "in adult mice basal cells generate only neurons," which suggests a different cell lineage for supporting cells. The origin of new epithelial cells from glandular elements may reflect their common embryonic source; both the neural epithelium and glands develop from the olfactory placode.[24]

One may speculate that squamous cells could also originate from edges of unaffected areas and migrate over the naked basal lamina. If this were true, it would seem logical to expect that regions of regrowing epithelium near the unaltered tissue (which presumably escaped the $ZnSO_4$ treatment[10]) would exhibit more advanced stages of regeneration than those areas farther removed from the normal (unaltered) tissue. Such conditions were not observed in the present study. On the contrary, degeneration and regeneration in individual samples occurred uniformly over the surface of the mucosa. For example, the protruding (migrating) cells were evenly distributed over the surface of the basal lamina, new squamous surface cells covered the regenerating area uniformly and the reconstitution of the sensory structures (cilia) at the border occurred, for the most part, simultaneously over the affected regions. Thus, the present observations suggest that migration of cells from the edges of unaffected epithelium, if occurring at all, is not the principal mechanism for epithelial reconstitution. Further, it appears that the migrating cells contribute cells to the formation of olfactory epithelium during early regeneration. However, the fate of these cells and the degree of their contribution to the definite epithelium remains uncertain.

Olfactory neural elements appeared at the surface 14 days after treatment in the form of surface protrusions covered with short microvilli. The latter originated from olfactory vesicles. Longer cilia-like structures of uniform diameter were often noted emanating from the microvillus-covered olfactory vesicles. The presence of microvilli and cilia on mammalian olfactory vesicles is not surprising since a similar condition has been observed by Breipohl and Fernandez[25] in developing chick olfactory epithelium. Also, developing regions of bovine olfactory epithelium appear to have both cilia and microvilli on presumably newly formed neural elements.[26] As regeneration and maturation of the olfactory mucosa progress over the next 14 days, the microvilli disappear from the surface of the vesicles. The surface of the epithelium, 28 to 42 days after $ZnSO_4$ treatment, is formed by a loose entanglement of olfactory cilia. It appears that these structures have not yet reached their normal length and thus produce a less dense olfactory border. Also the cilia have not attained their mature parallel arrangement to each other. In contrast, normal olfactory epithelium is covered with many cilia which obscure the vesicles.[27,28] The sparsity of the cilia at this time of regeneration has also been reported previously.[9]

A final comment appears necessary in reference to the variation of morphological alterations during regeneration at the various times the tissue was examined. The morphological surface manifestations noted were the most common and prominent conditions observed. However, it should be pointed out that some morphological variations occurred among individual animals. For example, in two animals sampled 12 hours after treatment, the predominant condition of degenerating epithelia was the "least severely altered state." In the remaining three animals all of the degenerating stages were equally present. Further, the terminal stage of degeneration (naked basal lamina) was noted in several areas of one animal as late as four days after treatment and the initial regenerative stage (surface covered with squamous cells) was observed in a few regions of two animals one day after treatment. Such variations were similar to those observed earlier,[9,10] and undoubtedly result from the multiple irrigation approach used to insult the tissue.[9] Although some variations in the degree of morphological alterations were found among individual animals and among experimental groups, they appeared uniform in each animal and the distinctive pattern of degeneration and regeneration of olfactory epithelial surface described above was always evident.

ACKNOWLEDGMENTS — The authors wish to express their gratitude to Linda Simmerman, Marion Ummels, and Renate Kerschek for their expert technical assistance.

REFERENCES

1. Smith CG. Changes in the olfactory mucosa and the olfactory nerves following intranasal treatment with one percent zinc sulfate. Can Med Assoc J 1938; 39:138-40.

2. Stuart-Harris CH, Francis T. Studies on the nasal histology of epidemic influenza virus infection in the ferret: resistance of regenerating respiratory epithelium to reinfection and to physicochemical injury. J Exp Med 1938; 68:803-12.

3. Hunnicutt LG. The effect of zinc sulfate on the olfactory mucus membrane in dogs and monkeys. Trans Pac Coast Otoophthalmol Soc 1939; 24:72-80.

4. Schultz EW. Regeneration of olfactory cells. Proc Soc Exp Biol Med 1941; 46:41-3.

5. Schultz EW. Repair of olfactory mucosa. Am J Pathol 1960; 37:1-19.

6. Moulton DG, Beidler LM. Structure and function in the peripheral olfactory system. Physiol Rev 1967; 47:1-52.

7. Mulvaney BD, Heist HE. Regeneration of rabbit olfactory epithelium. Am J Anat 1971; 131:241-51.

8. Takagi SF. Degeneration and regeneration of olfactory epithelium. In: Beidler L, ed. Handbook of sensory physiology. Vol. 4. New York, Springer Verlag, 1971:75-94.

9. Matulionis DH. Ultrastructural study of mouse olfactory epithelium following destruction by $ZnSO_4$ and its subsequent regeneration. Am J Anat 1975; 142:67-89.

10. Matulionis DH. Light and electron microscopic study of the degeneration and early regeneration of olfactory epithelium in the mouse. Am J Anat 1976; 145:79-99.

11. Matulionis DH. Light and electron microscopic study of the effects of $ZnSO_4$ on mouse nasal respiratory epithelium and subsequent responses. Anat Rec 1975; 183:63-81.

12. Dalton AJ. A chrome-osmium fixative for electron microscopy. Anat Rec 1955; 121:281.

13. Reese TS. Olfactory cilia in the frog. J Cell Biol 1965; 25:209-30.

14. Tucker D. Olfactory cilia are not required for receptor function. Fed Proc 1967; 26:544.

15. Ottoson D. Sustained potentials evoked by olfactory stimulation. Acta Physiol Scand 1954; 32:384-86.

16. Ottoson D. The slow electrical response of the olfactory end organs. Exp Cell Res Suppl 1958; 5:451-59.

17. Koyama N, Sawada K, Kurihra K. Isolation on some properties of plasma membranes from bovine olfactory epithelium. Biochim Biophys Acta 1971; 241:42-8.

18. Parker GH. Smell, taste and allied senses in the vertebrates. Philadelphia: JB Lippincott Co, 1922.

19. Winans SS, Powers JB. Olfactory and vomeronasal deafferentation of male hamsters: histology and behavioral analysis. Brain Res 1977; 126:325-44.

20. Kiyohara S, Tucker D. Activity of new receptors after transection of the primary olfactory nerve in pigeons. Physiol Behav 1978; 21:987-94.

21. Graziadei PPC, Graziadei GAM. Neurogenesis and neuron regeneration in the olfactory system of mammals. I. Morphological aspects of differentiation and structural organization of the olfactory sensory neurons. J Neurocytol 1979a; 8:1-18.

22. Graziadei PPC, Graziadei GAM. Neurogenesis and neuron

regeneration in the olfactory system of mammals. II. Degeneration and reconstitution of the olfactory sensory neurons after axotomy. J Neurocytol 1979 b; 8:197-213.

23. Graziadei PPC, Okano M. Neuronal degeneration and regeneration in the olfactory epithelium of pigeon following transection of the first cranial nerve. Acta Anat 1979; 104:220-36.

24. Laugwitz H. Morphologische Untersuchungen zur Ausreigung des Riechepithels beim Haushuhn. Inaugural dissertation: Essen, West Germany, 1980.

25. Breipohl W, Fernandez M. Scanning electron microscopic investigations of olfactory epithelium in the chick embryo. Cell Tissue Res 1977; 183:105-14.

26. Menco BPM. A qualitative and quantitative investigation of olfactory and nasal respiratory mucosal surfaces of cow and sheep based on various ultrastructural and biochemical methods. Wageningen: Veeman H and Zonen BV, 1977.

27. Greenwood MF, Holland P. The mammalian respiratory tract surface. A scanning electron microscopic study. Lab Invest 1972; 27:296-304.

28. Menco BPM, Leunissen JLM, Bannister LH, Dodd GH. Bovine olfactory and nasal respiratory epithelium surfaces. Cell Tissue Res 1978; 193:503-24.

THE AMERICAN BOARD OF OTOLARYNGOLOGY: 1950-1979

WALTER P. WORK, MD

GREEN VALLEY, ARIZONA

This report concerns historical aspects of the American Board of Otolaryngology during the period 1950 to 1979. There has been gradual evolution from a partially structured clinical didactic and clinical oral examination to a highly standardized and uniform type of examination with broad modern content. The use of patients in the clinical oral part of the examination was discontinued in 1970. In the 1950s the American Board of Otolaryngology sought ways and means for the specialty to redirect its goals following the introduction of antibiotic drug therapy. As a result of the gradual shift of its objectives, the Board initiated many changes in the examination during the 1960s which helped to define the future of the specialty. In the 1970s multiple choice written and oral simulated patient examinations were developed. Many hundreds of hours were spent by Directors of the Board, task force members, guest examiners and educational consultants in preparing, administering and grading the examinations. However, the Directors have always retained the perogatives as to the selection of candidates, final evaluation of candidates and the issuance of certificates. The advanced format has allowed the American Board of Otolaryngology to test 400, plus or minus, candidates during each examination session. Prior to 1970, in order to test increasing numbers of candidates, two and occasionally three examinations were given each year. The whole broadened field of otolaryngology was included in the content of the examinations so that modern otolaryngology was represented. In addition, the Board continued to uphold standards for otolaryngologists who desired certification and encouraged development and maintenance of highest standards in the teaching and training of otolaryngologists. Liaison with otolaryngologists was maintained through specialty societies and the Residency Review Committee in Otolaryngology. In organized medicine as a whole, otolaryngology has been and is represented through its membership in the American Board of Medical Specialties.

INTRODUCTION

Nineteen hundred seventy-nine marks the 55th year of the existence of the American Board of Otolaryngology. In 1950, Proetz[1] published an historical account of the Board's first 25 years. The only board established prior to 1924 was the American Board of Ophthalmology, which was organized in 1917. Since these two boards were established, 21 other boards in medicine and surgery have been formed.

The American Board of Otolaryngology was planned as a private organization in 1924 and incorporated in the State of Missouri. The objectives of the Board are to establish standards of qualifications for otolaryngologists who desire and request Board certification, to determine which candidates fulfill these standards of qualification, to examine such candidates and issue certificates upon satisfactory completion of requirements, and to encourage development and maintenance of the highest standards in teaching and training of otolaryngologists.[2]

The certificate of the American Board of Otolaryngology, like the certificate of the 22 other medical and surgical boards, carries no licensure to practice medicine. This is frequently not understood by American and foreign graduates alike. Proetz[1] gave a vivid picture of the American Board of Otolaryngology's activities and summarized in the final paragraph of his report: "These are crucial times for American medicine. What more can one say for a body such as this, on its Silver Jubilee, than that it has always been and always will be dedicated to the highest ideals and a tireless devotion to the public weal?"

THE 1950s

December 1949 marked the 25th year of incorporation of the American Board of Otolaryngology.

EXAMINATIONS ADMINISTERED BY THE AMERICAN BOARD OF OTOLARYNGOLOGY 1950-1979.

YEAR	*CITY*	*YEAR*	*CITY*	*YEAR*	*CITY*
1950	New Orleans	1957	Chicago	1968	New Orleans
	San Francisco	1958	Chicago		Chicago
	Chicago	1959	Chicago	1969	Los Angeles
1951	New York	1960	Chicago		Chicago
	Richmond, Va.	1961	Chicago	1970	New Orleans
	Chicago	1962	Chicago		Toronto
1952	Toronto	1963	Chicago		Chicago
	Chicago		New York	1971	Chicago
1953	New Orleans	1964	New Orleans	1972	Chicago
	Chicago		Chicago	1973	Chicago
1954	Boston	1965	Chicago	1974	Chicago
	New York	1966	New Orleans	1975	Chicago
1955	Chicago		Chicago	1976	Chicago
1956	Montreal	1967	Toronto	1977	Chicago
	Chicago		Chicago	1978	Chicago
				1979	Chicago

Dr. Work is Emeritus Professor and Chairman, Department of Otorhinolaryngology, University of Michigan; and Lecturer, Surgery, Section of Otolaryngology, University of Arizona.

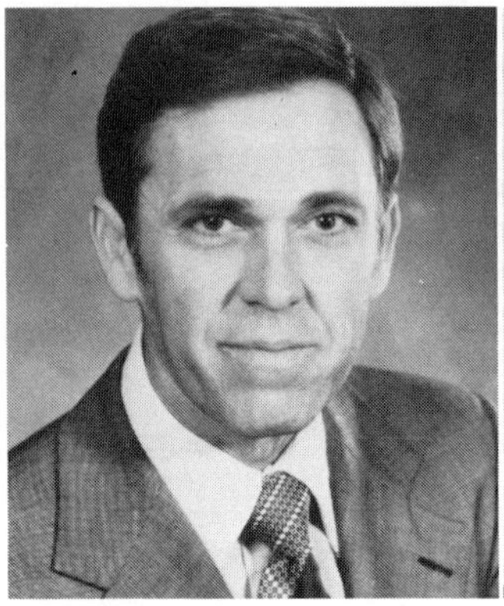
Bobby R. Alford, MD

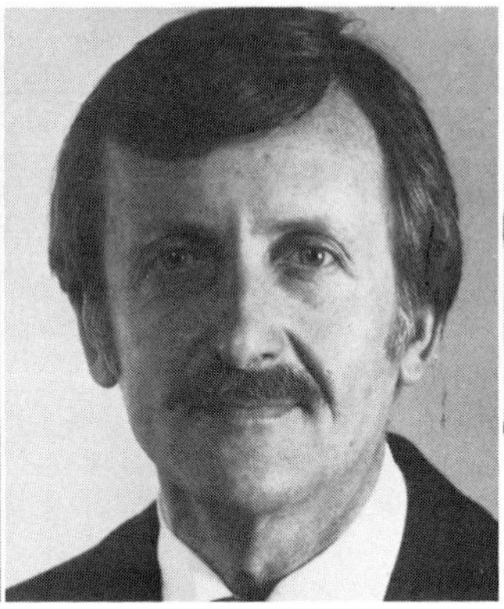
Byron J. Bailey, MD

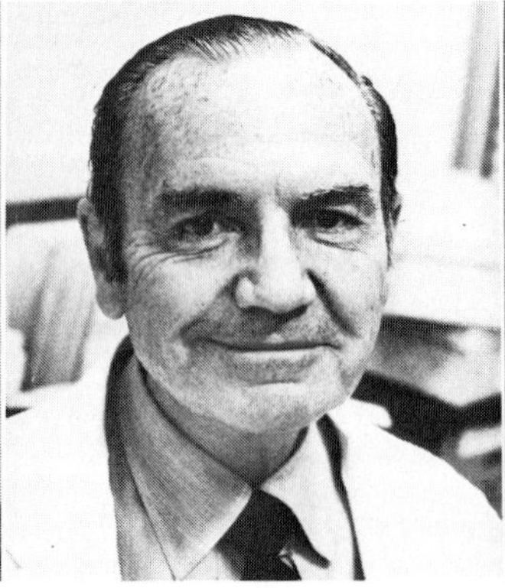
Daniel C. Baker, Jr, MD

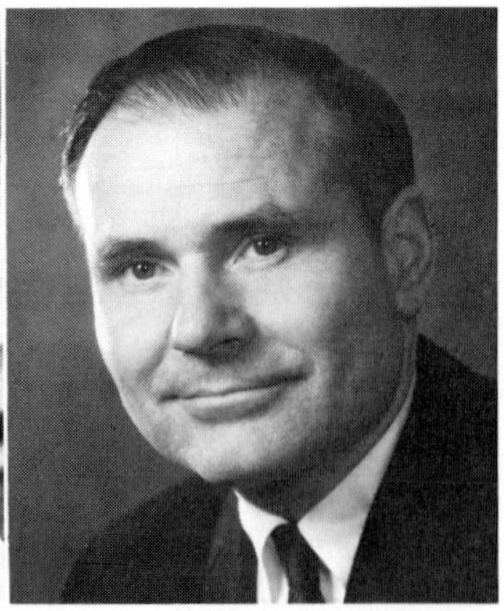
Roger Boles, MD

The present report deals with the 30 years of the Board's existence starting at the conclusion of Proetz' report of 1950 through 1979. Otolaryngology experienced difficult times as a specialty in the 1950s. The introduction of antibiotic drugs seemed to affect otolaryngology adversely at the time, but as events proved later, their introduction proved to be a benefaction in disguise. These adverse effects upon otolaryngology during the 1950s were compensated in part by advances in otolaryngology and Lempert's introduction of the one-stage fenestration operation for hearing loss in patients with clinical otosclerosis. Many other otolaryngologists were contributing heavily of their time and efforts during these years.

Resident teaching and education suffered; many resident programs in otolaryngology had great difficulty in attracting qualified physicians to fill positions. Records of the business meetings of the Directors of the Board during this period are replete with discussions of ways and means to improve teaching at all levels so that young doctors would be attracted to residencies in otolaryngology. Some said the best way to do this was to eliminate excessive numbers of resident education programs. In actuality, through the Board's initiative, resident programs were visited by its Directors not for accrediting purposes, but to act as consultants and counselors to program directors. The Society of University Otolaryngologists and the American Academy of Otolaryngology (American Academy of Ophthalmology and Otolaryngology at that time) acted as advisors in these efforts. The National Institutes of Health supplied funds through the Society of University Otolaryngologists for the survey visits. It was realized early that the more effective resident programs were departments which functioned independently as to budget, space, equipment, research and teaching. Many resident education and medical student teaching programs benefitted from these efforts.

An internship as well as three years in resident education in otolaryngology was required at this time. Formal structuring of residencies allowed for development of a broader content base in otolaryngology. The Board had anticipated this broadening and structured its certification examination accordingly.

Medical and surgical aspects of the specialty were stressed in the examination. In addition to otology, audiology, communicative disorders, laryngology, rhinology and bronchoesophagology, surgery of the head and neck evolved to include regional oncology and regional plastic surgery. Another broad development took place in the fields of allergy and immunology. Clinical and basic research was also stressed and developed into an integral part of the

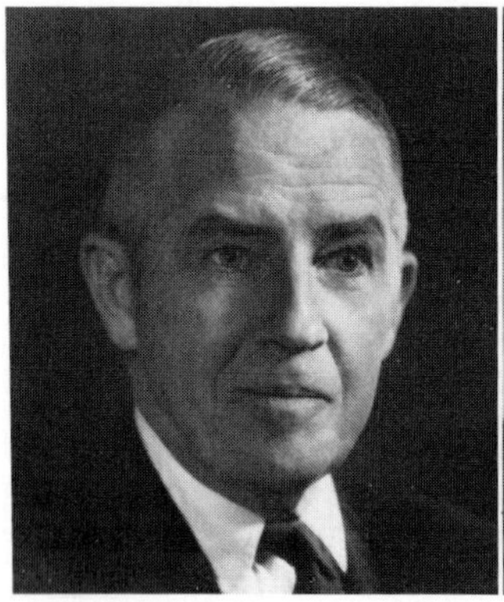
John E. Bordley, MD

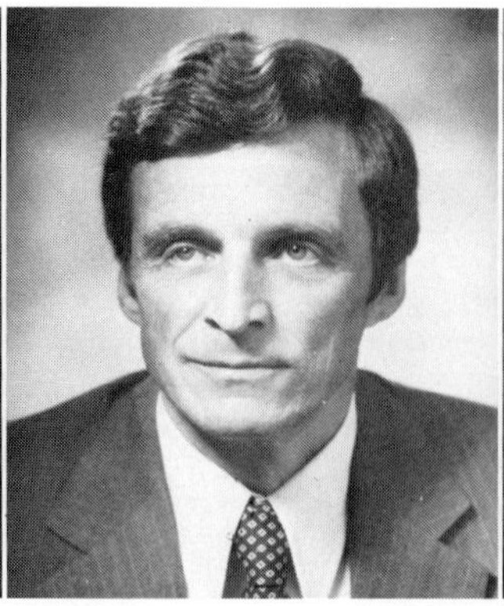
Wesley H. Bradley, MD

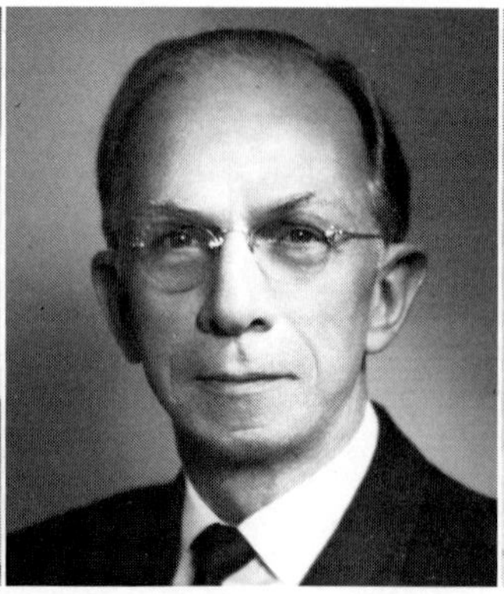
Lester A. Brown, MD

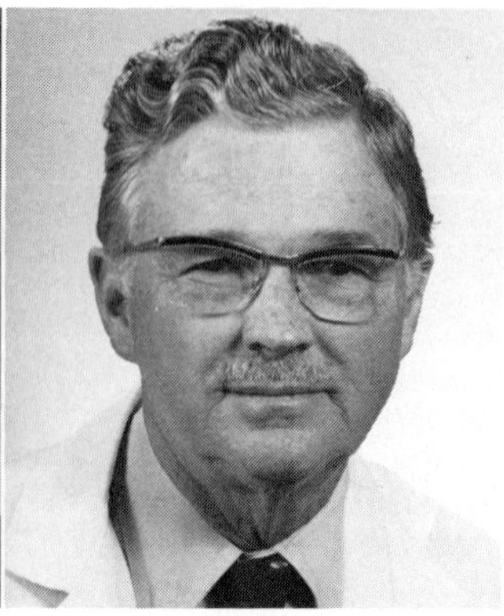
Douglas P. Bryce, MD

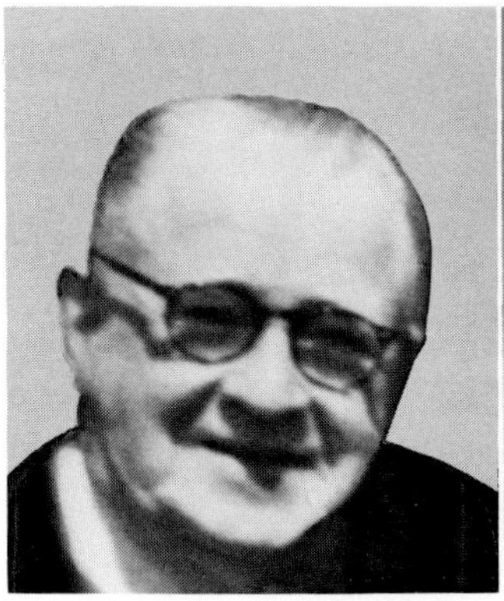
Daniel S. Cunning, MD

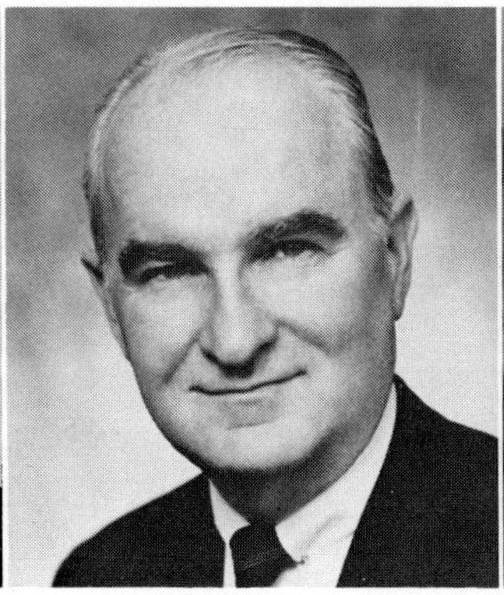
John F. Daly, MD

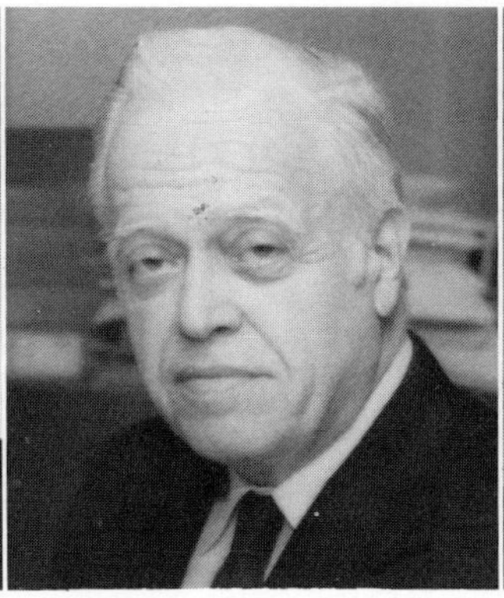
David D. DeWeese, MD

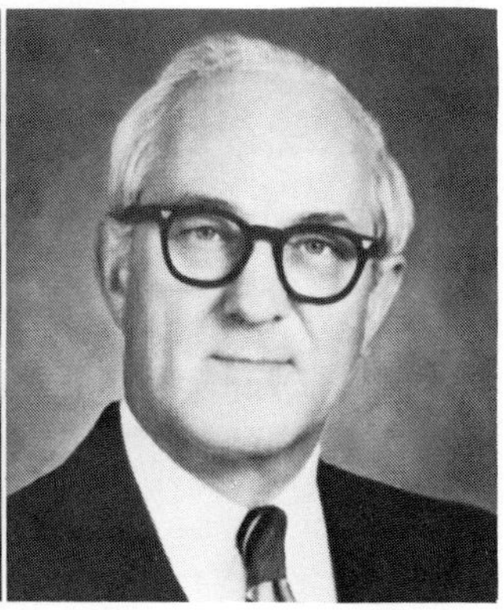
John T. Dickinson, MD

resident programs in many centers. The certifying examination during these years was clinically oriented and patients were still examined by candidates. In this manner, the examiner was able to evaluate the candidate in an "office set-up."

An attempt was made to structure both the oral didactic and the oral clinical examination and to standardize them as much as possible. The oral clinical examination included otology, audiology and speech, rhinology, laryngology, throat disorders and bronchoesophagological diseases. The oral didactic examination included pathology, physiology, embryology, pharmacology, microbiology, anatomy and biochemistry. At one point, the Board was so concerned about the content and structuring of the examination that an ad hoc committee was appointed to prepare that part of the oral didactic examination which dealt only with audiology.

During the 1950s, an average of 111 candidates were certified annually. A backlog of candidates developed in 1950 and 1951 (see table), and the examination was given three times; 195 and 210 candidates were certified in these two years, respectively. The high number of examinations per year proved to be prohibitive due to the expenses involved. However at one point in the mid-1950s, only one examination was given and only 48 candidates were certified. This decline continued during the last years of the decade and was truly the low ebb of the specialty.[3] During this 1950 decade only 1115 certificates were issued.

Another function of the American Board of Otolaryngology during the early 1950s was to accredit resident education programs. This effort proved to be extremely time-consuming and expensive. In 1950, 185 residencies in otolaryngology were available and only 135 were filled.[4]

The Residency Review Committee in Otolaryngology became a functioning body in 1954 and its parent sponsors were the American Board of Otolaryngology, the American Medical Association and the American College of Surgeons. This committee assumed the duties of accreditation of resident training programs for otolaryngology and thus eased some of the pressure on the Board.

In addition to the site surveys conducted by the Board of Directors, two questionnaires were sent to program directors in the latter part of the decade. The first questionnaire was aimed at determining the best way to improve resident training and medical student teaching so that candidates could be attracted to resident programs in otolaryngology. The second questionnaire was designed to determine whether general surgical resident education should be included as a requirement in the training of an otolaryngologist. Replies to the first questionnaire unanimously agreed that quality of education was the key to success, that the specialty should be

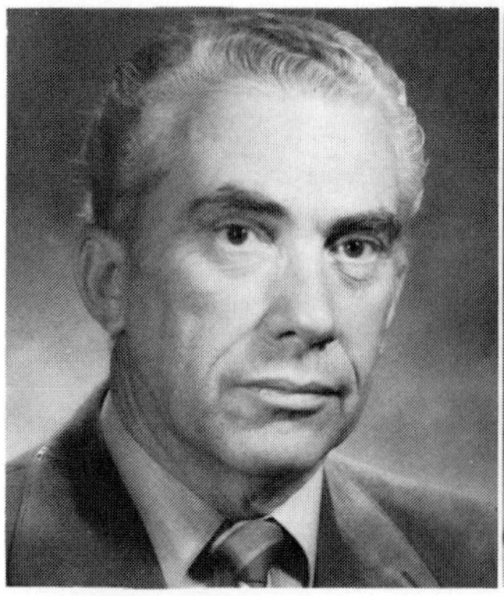
Patrick J. Doyle, MD

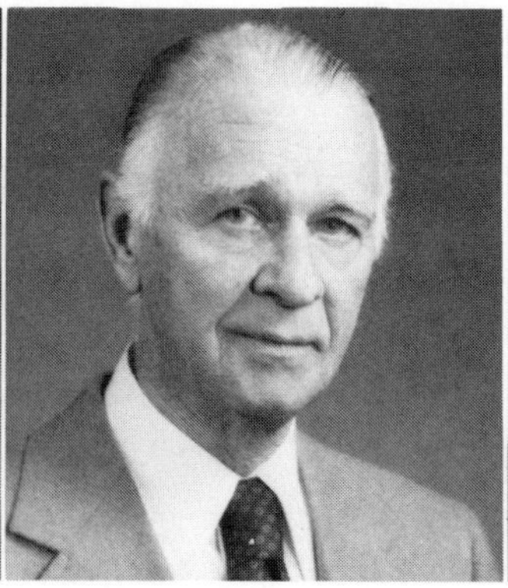
James A. Harrill, MD

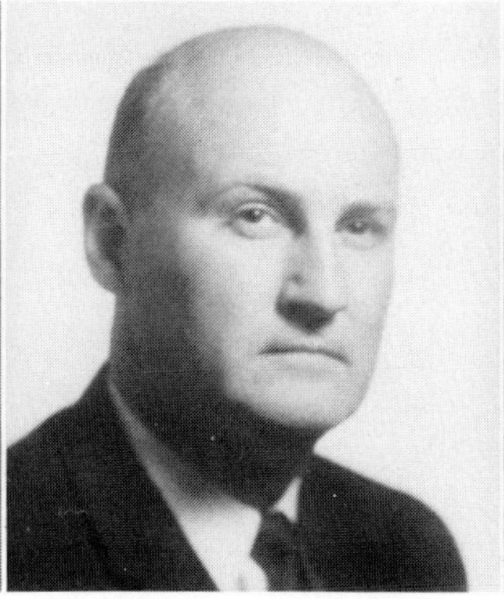
Jerome A. Hilger, MD

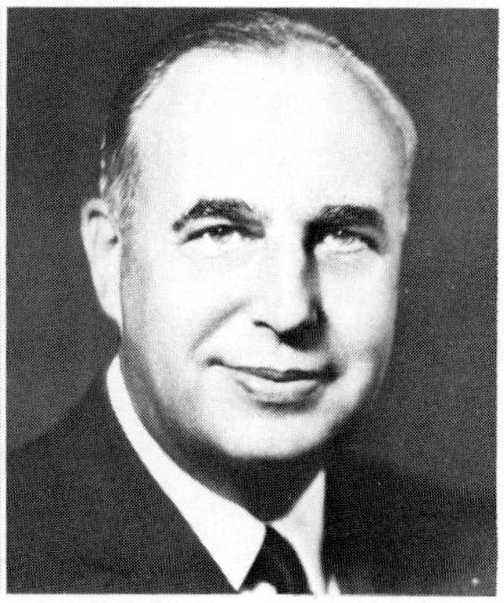
Paul H. Holinger, MD

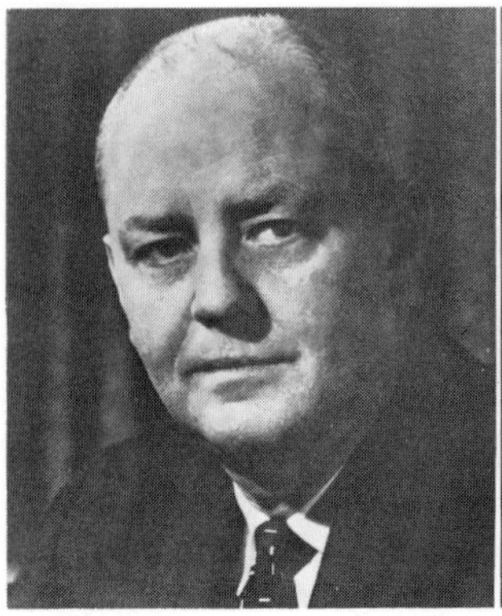

William C. Huffman, MD

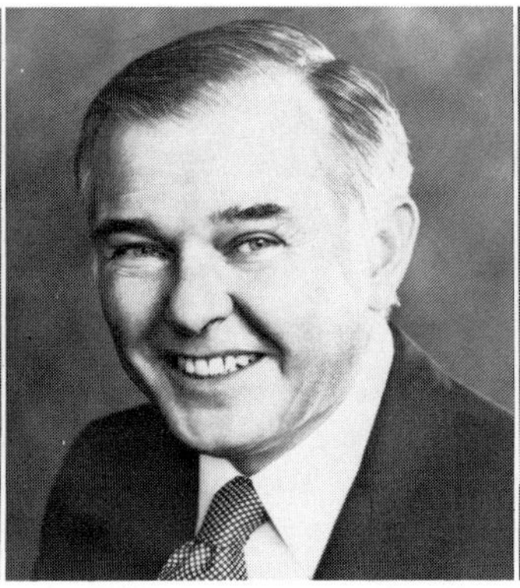

Robert I. Kohut, MD

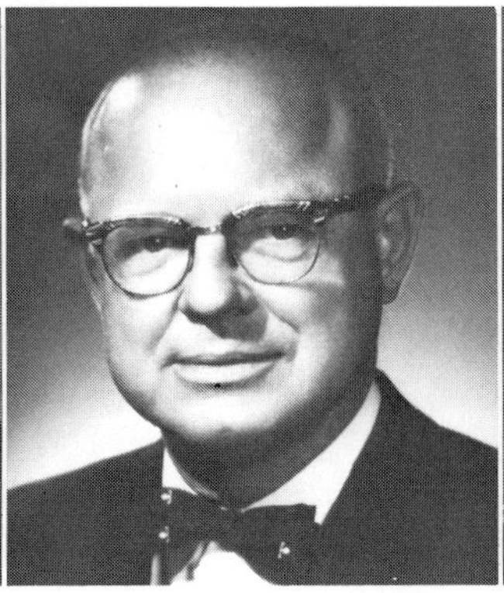

Clair M. Kos, MD

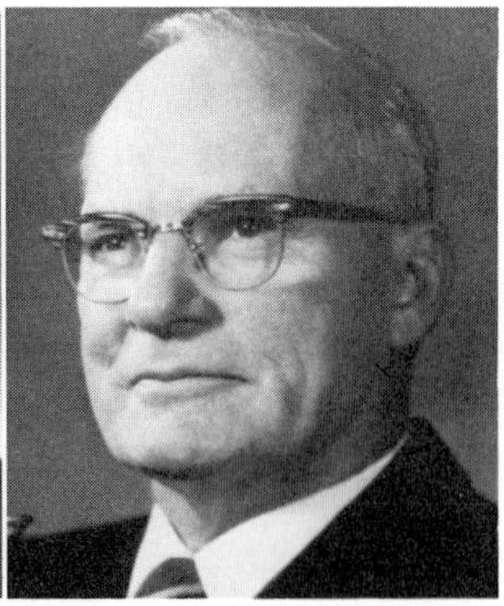

Frank D. Lathrop, MD

broadened, and that the program directors should spend more time and effort in teaching, administration, clinical activities and research. Only 25% of those answering the second questionnaire indicated that they required otolaryngology residents to supplement their otolaryngology training by general surgical resident education. However, 100% of the respondents indicated that general surgery should be required for residents. As circumstances developed, this extra year evolved into the required year of general surgery, and surgical services in this country and Canada soon made surgical training possible for all residents entering otolaryngology. Thus, during the 1950s, resident education in otolaryngology developed into a well-organized, broad-based experience.

By mid-decade the American Board of Otolaryngology described the following paths a candidate could pursue to meet requirements for voluntary application toward certification:

1. One year of internship (approved by AMA).

2. Proficiency in the applied basic sciences, including the anatomy of the ear, nose and throat, neck, chest, esophagus and nervous system, gross pathology and histopathology, bacteriology, physiology, didactic otolaryngology and the general fundamentals of surgery.

3. In addition to a general internship, the required clinical training in otolaryngology may be acquired in any of the following ways:

a) A 3-year residency or fellowship in otolaryngology.

b) A 2-year approved residency or fellowship in otolaryngology or a 3-year approved combined residency or fellowship in otolaryngology and ophthalmology, provided two years have been in otolaryngology and have been preceded by at least one year of approved residency training in surgery or medicine or by an additional year in an approved internship.

4. In exceptional circumstances, certain candidates who do not meet all the above Board requirements may be accepted for examination.

5. At least one year must be spent in private, group or institutional practice in otolaryngology after the period of special training. This requirement may be waived for candidates from foreign countries.

6. A candidate may be qualified for examination at the discretion of the American Board of Otolaryngology . . . "if" he has limited his practice to otolaryngology for seven years in association with a hospital staff approved by the AMA.

7. A physician who limits himself exclusively to the practice of peroral endoscopy may be granted limited certification in this field.[5]

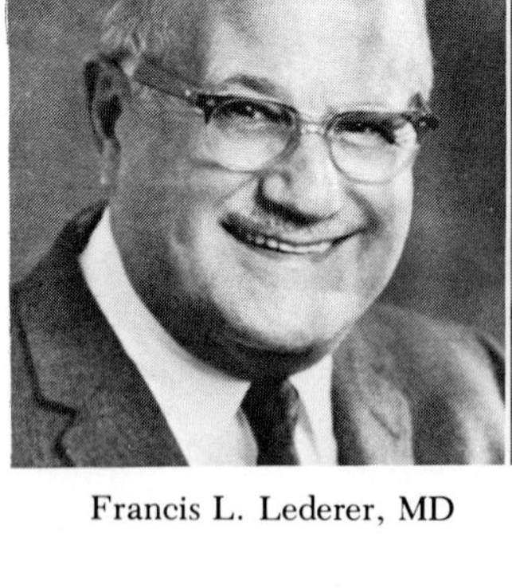

Francis L. Lederer, MD

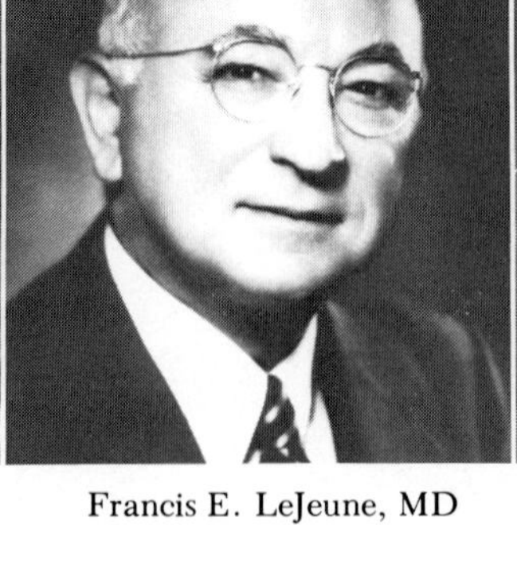

Francis E. LeJeune, MD

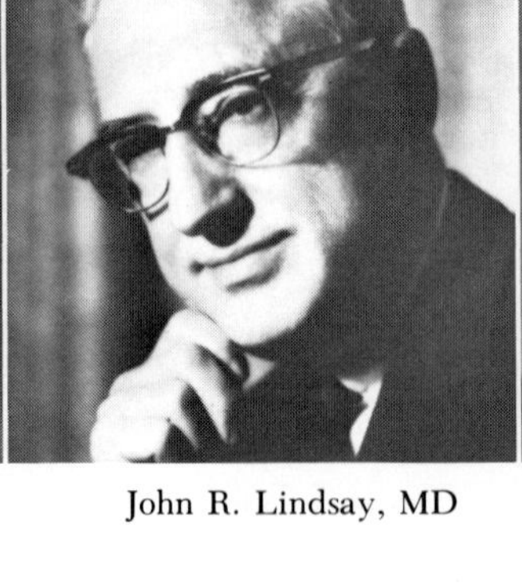

John R. Lindsay, MD

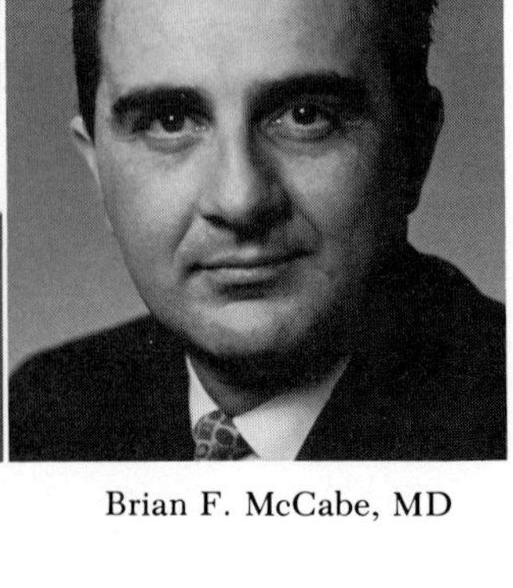

Brian F. McCabe, MD

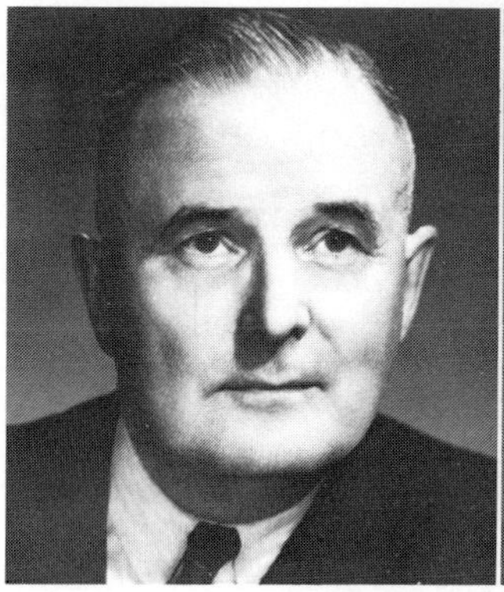
William J. McNally, MD

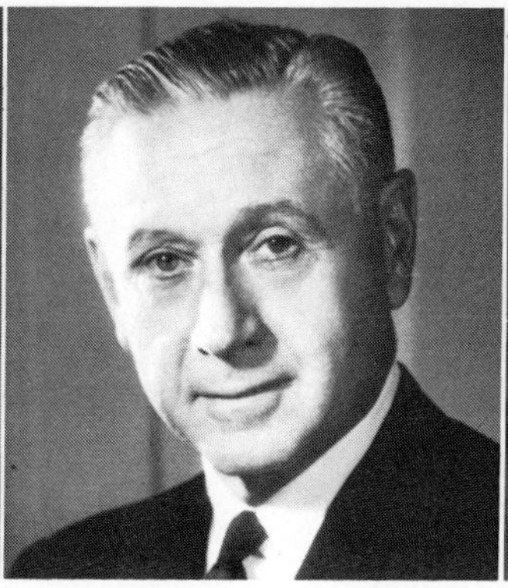
Alden H. Miller, MD

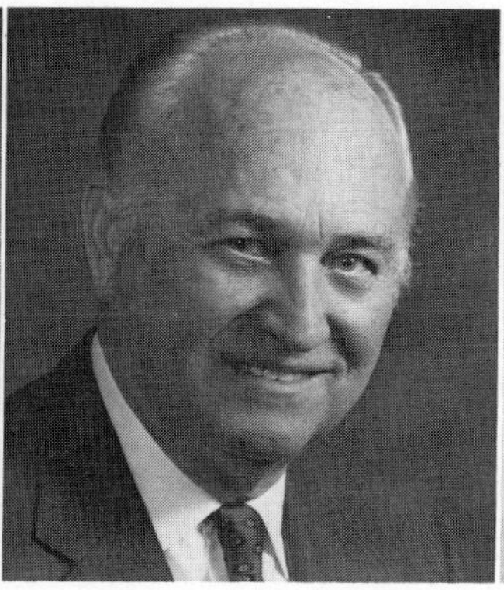
James A. Moore, MD

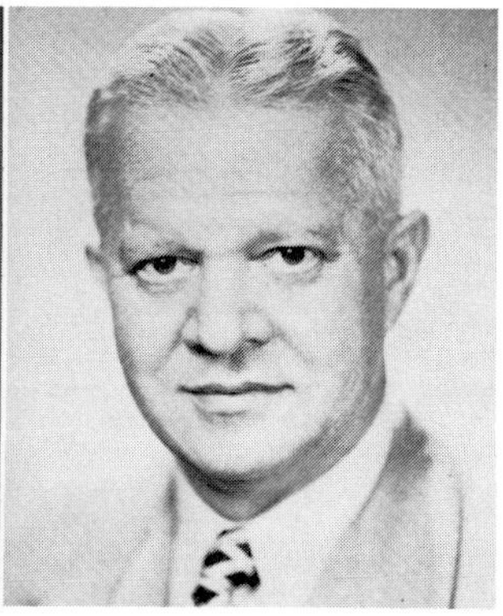
Lewis F. Morrison, MD

The special requirements quoted above reflect the Board's exploratory years. For example, in the latter part of the 1950s the combined residency requirement in ophthalmology and otolaryngology was dropped, as was the seven years of practice requirement. In 1959, the Board revised its special resident education requirements to include more concisely:

1. One year of internship (approved program AMA).

2. One year of general surgery resident education (approved program).

3. Three years of otolaryngology (approved program).

4. A candidate may be examined at the conclusion of his training.[6]

As in other changes in resident education planned by the Board, "lead time" for initiation of the proposed changes was and is usually from two to three years so such was the case in 1959 regarding general surgery.

All in all, otolaryngologists who were active in the 1950s planned well for the future. During this decade, the Board was constantly aware of the importance of revitalization of otolaryngology and made every effort to plan for the future. Cooperative efforts among otolaryngologists were the key-notes during these years.

THE 1960s

The 1960s were marked by many changes in the teaching of medical students and residents in the field of otolaryngology. Quality patient care continued to be the overall goal. Basic and clinical research efforts were introduced into many resident programs. The National Institutes of Health awarded research contracts to institutions so that research efforts could be enhanced by the hiring of necessary personnel and the acquisition of space and equipment. Other funds were granted to help program directors train young specialists so that they might be encouraged to enter academic careers. Site visits to resident programs by Directors of the Board continued mainly for counseling purposes. The certifying examination was reevaluated and slowly modified to include the areas being taught in medical schools, medical centers and resident programs. The Board finalized its concepts regarding the one year of general surgical resident education by making it a special requirement in 1961.

The Residency Review Committee for Otolaryngology was becoming increasingly active in accrediting those institutional programs in which the broad concept of otolaryngology was being taught. Resident education consisted of one year of surgical and three years of otolaryngology resident education in approved programs in the United States or Canada in addition to the internship year. This was the pattern of resident education throughout the decade.

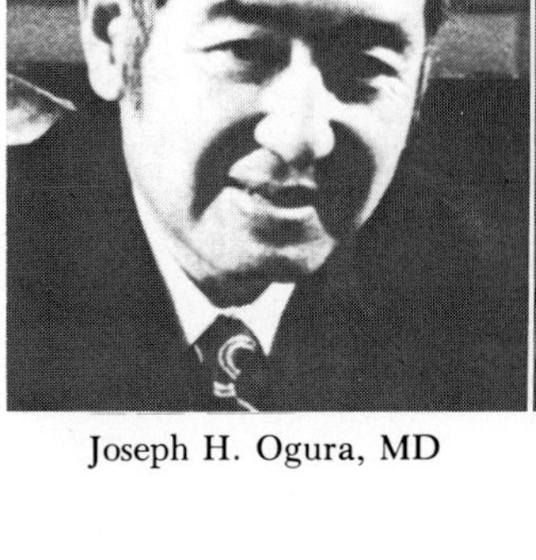
Joseph H. Ogura, MD

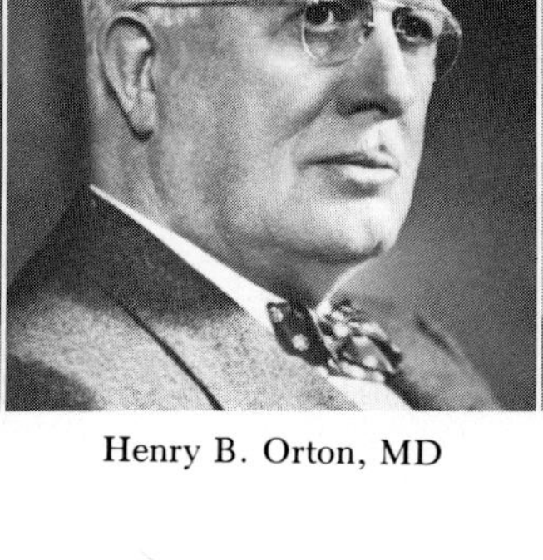
Henry B. Orton, MD

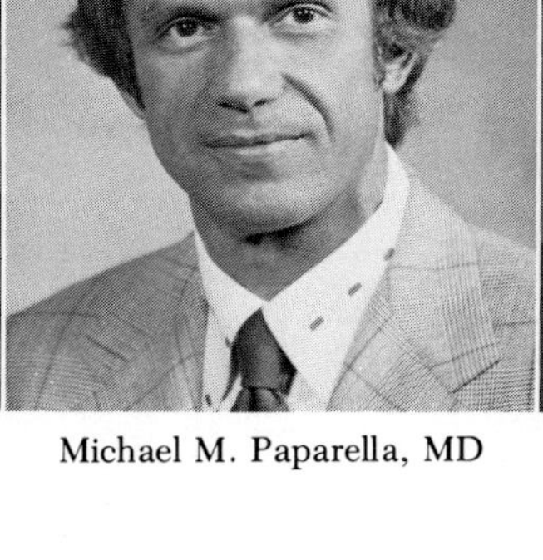
Michael M. Paparella, MD

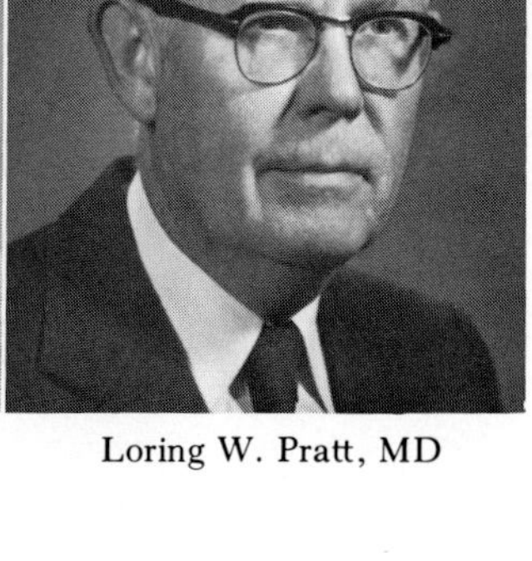
Loring W. Pratt, MD

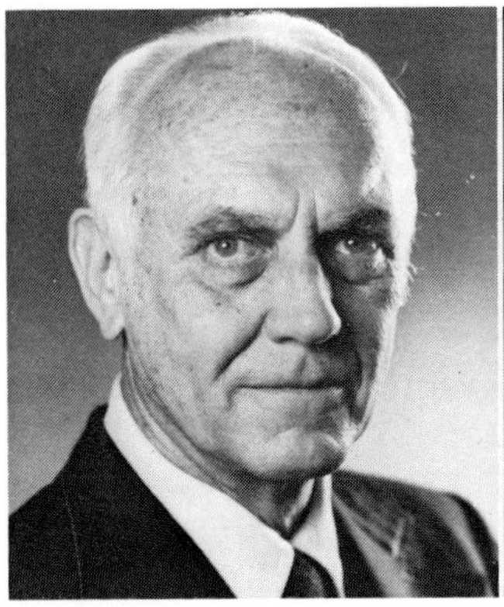

G. O. Proud, MD

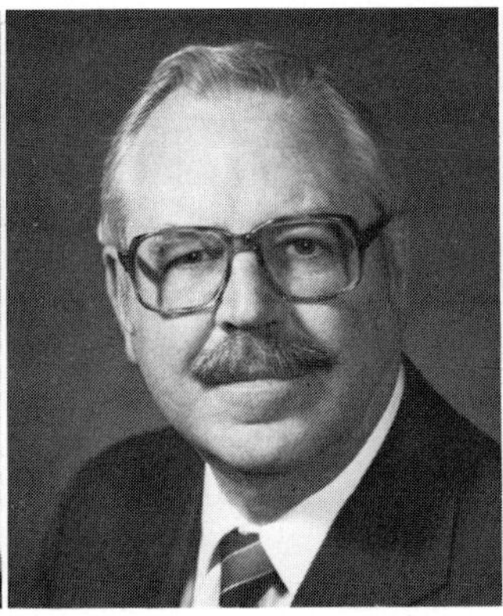

George F. Reed, MD

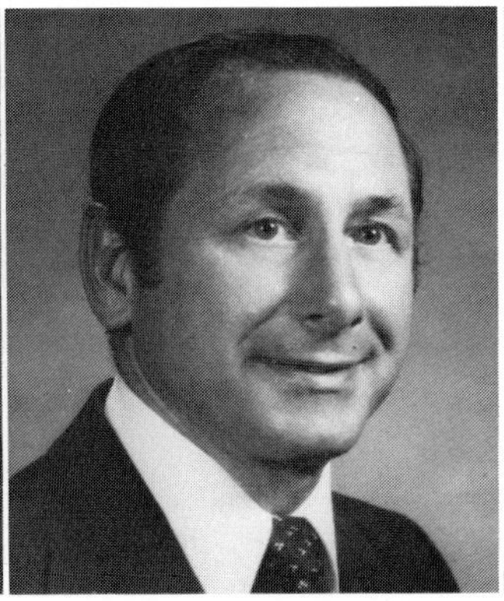

Frank N. Ritter, MD

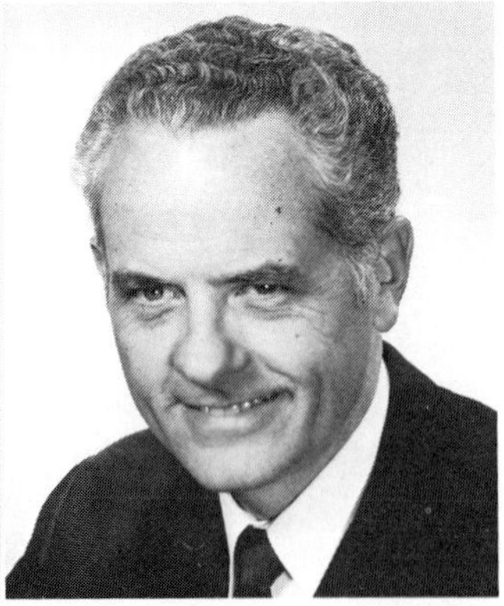

William H. Saunders, MD

Oral didactic and oral clinical examinations were used exclusively. The content of the oral didactic examination was broadened to include wider areas of basic science and research. The clinical oral examination was becoming expensive and complicated. Cooperating hospitals which participated simply could not furnish patients for the examination due to rising cost of travel, insurance and administration. However, by close cooperation with host institutions, the Board was able to keep the clinical oral examination intact during the whole of the decade. The examination process during this time was organized so that increased number of candidates could be examined in a uniform and standard manner.

New concepts in medical education and its evaluation were developing under physicians' guidance. An educational consultant was employed and members of the Board were utilized in an advisory capacity. Constant liaison was maintained with the Resident Review Committee, and in addition, a great spirit of cooperation existed among all otolaryngologists during the 1960s. With the cooperation of all parties a new certifying examination was formulated for the 1970s.

The American Board of Otolaryngology also played a role in organized medicine through its activities in the Advisory Board for Medical Specialties. Although the latter was strictly advisory at this time, it was influential in keeping each medical and surgical specialty board up-to-date on evaluation activities throughout the whole of medicine and surgery. As events unfolded in the latter part of the 1960s, plans were made by all boards to change the Advisory Board for Medical Specialties to the American Board of Medical Specialties.

In the 1960s, a total of 1,206 candidates were certified for an average of 120 candidates per year, a slight increase over the previous decade. This was a decade of revitalization. It was a period in which resident education was further improved and formalized so that the foundation was laid for further broadening the specialty. The year of required general surgery resident education, introduced in the early 1960s, gave a resident an opportunity to be trained along surgical principles that allowed for diversified surgical activities in caring for patients. The Board considered this surgical education a milestone in the specialty's development.

THE 1970s

In 1970 three examinations were given; the first in February (in New Orleans), when 78 certificates were issued; the second in May (in Toronto), when 77 certificates were issued, and the third in September (in Chicago), when 84 certificates were issued; a total of 239 for the year. All three examinations followed the older design of oral didactic and oral clinical types, while the third also included written multiple choice and oral-simulated patient sections.

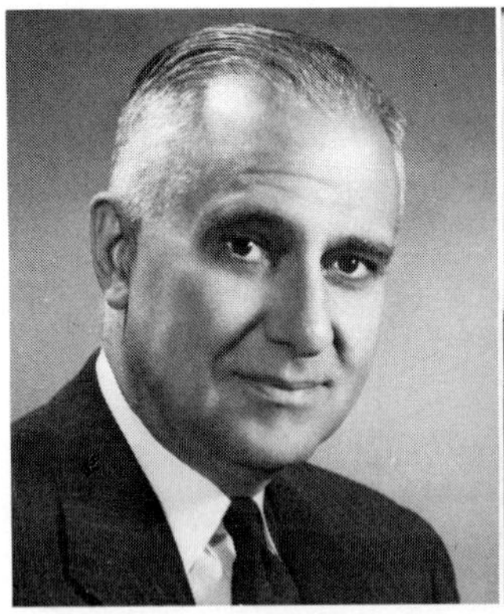

Harry P. Schenck, MD

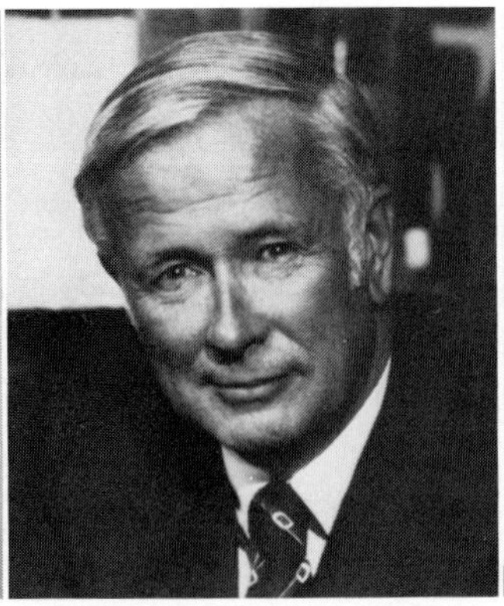

George A. Sisson, MD

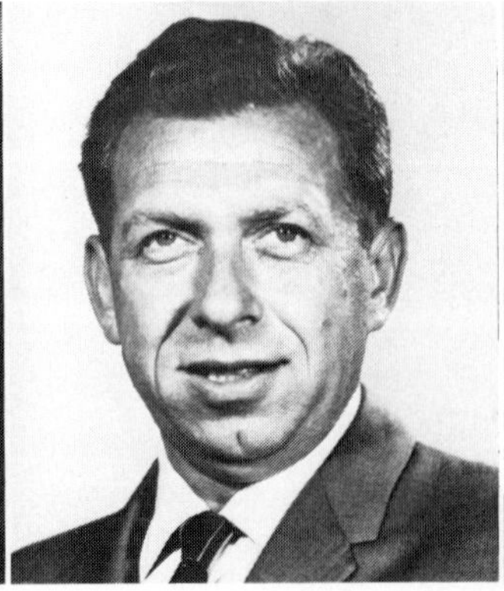

Emanuel M. Skolnik, MD

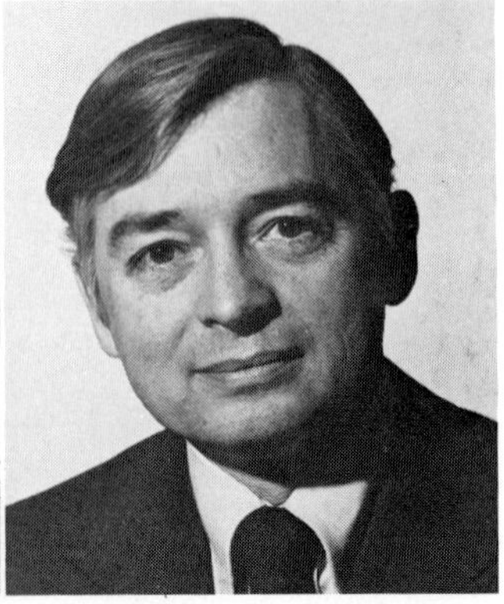

James B. Snow, Jr, MD

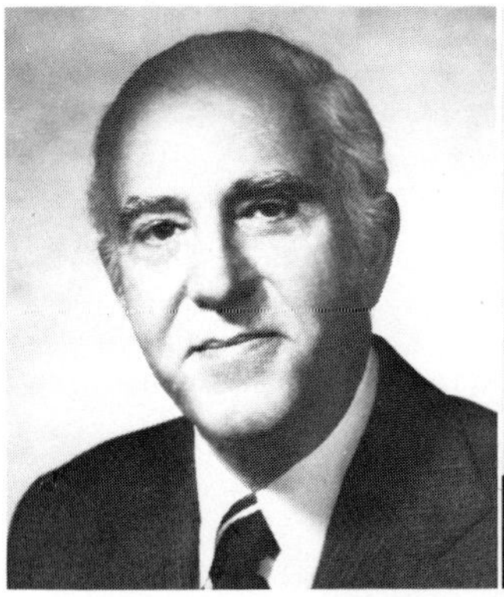
Burton J. Soboroff, MD

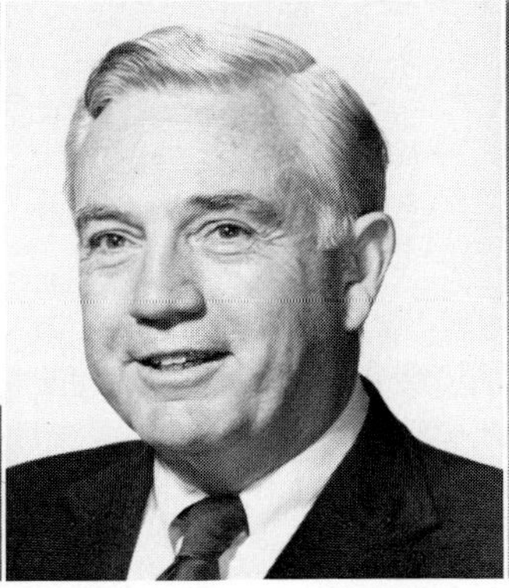
Francis A. Sooy, MD

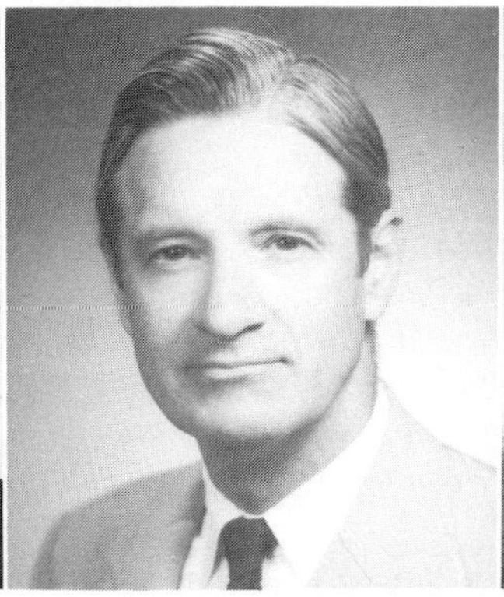
M. Stuart Strong, MD

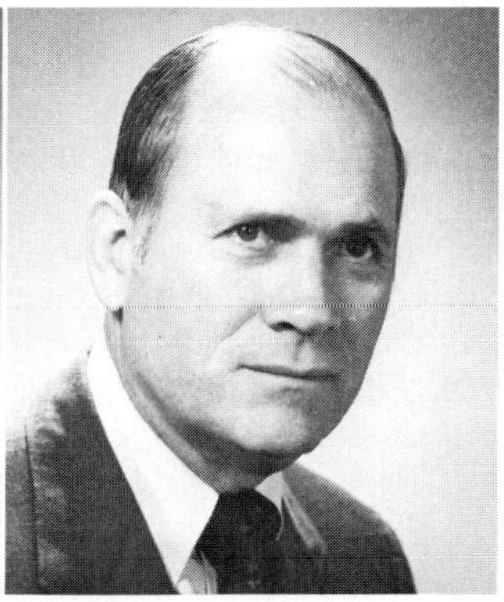
Harold G. Tabb, MD

These added features were an attempt by the Board to introduce a wholly new examination so that the shift from the "old to the new" would be a gradual one.

In November 1971, an entirely new certifying examination was offered to 329 candidates. This was the greatest number of candidates the Board has been able to accommodate at any one time. This examination[7] consisted of written multiple choice and oral patient-simulated parts. For the first time in many years patients were not used. The first evidence of "the third wave"[8] in evaluation techniques was truly upon us. Task forces made up of otolaryngologists from the United States and Canada were now organized to prepare examination materials that represented current otolaryngology. The new examination format was costly to prepare and administer; the number of guest examiners increased seven-fold. This meant that special orientation and instructional sessions had to be prepared for the guest group as well as for participating Board members so that uniformity in the examination would be maintained. Final evaluation continued to be the responsibility of the Directors of the Board since they participated fully in directing all phases of the examining and evaluating processes.

The format of the new examination lasted through 1979. During the 1970s there were constant refinements of the examination in an effort to increase its reliability and validity. An educational consulting firm continued to work with the Directors. Despite the large numbers of candidates, security of examination materials and anonymity of candidates were maintained so that fairness prevailed.

The year of required internship was dropped in 1972. Resident education stabilized to include one year of general surgery and three years of otolaryngology, to be served successfully in the United States or Canada in approved programs.

In order to meet the demands of the expanded and diverse fields of modern otolaryngology, new special requirements for resident education were approved by the parent sponsors of the Residency Review Committee for Otolaryngology (American Medical Association, American College of Surgeons and the American Board of Otolaryngology). This meant that organized medicine was aware of and endorsed a much broader concept of otolaryngology than ever before. The American Board of Otolaryngology had already anticipated this endorsement and modified the certifying examination content during the time when otolaryngology program directors were making broad changes in resident education.

Items such as recertification and subcertification were discussed by the American Board of Otolaryngology on numerous occasions during this period. In fact, ad hoc committees of the Board have contin-

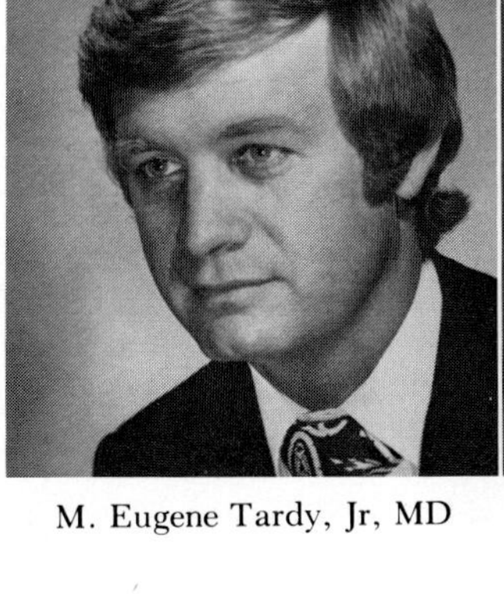
M. Eugene Tardy, Jr, MD

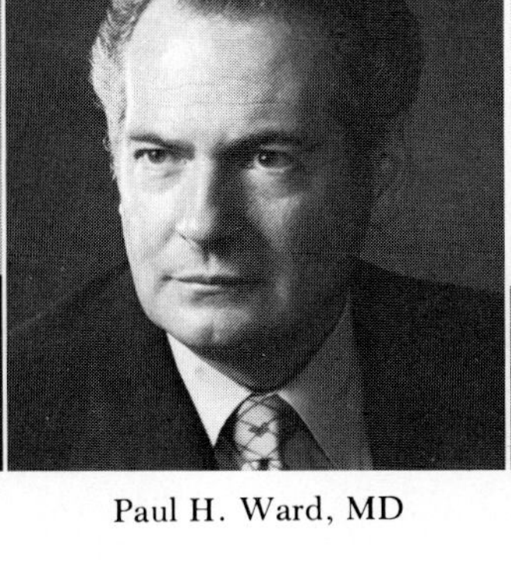
Paul H. Ward, MD

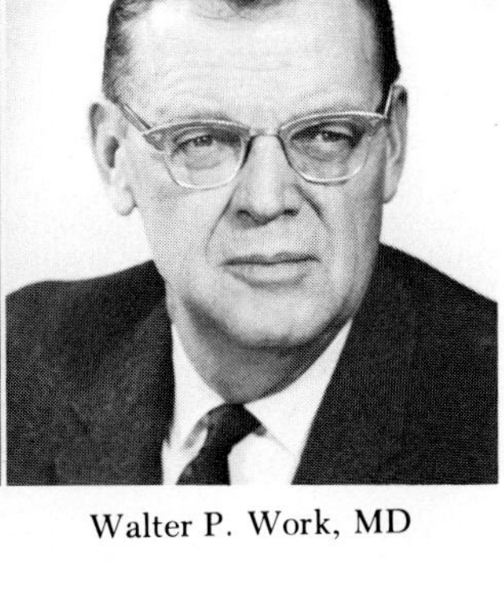
Walter P. Work, MD

ued to study these items over the years. The American Board of Medical Specialties, (established in 1970 and formerly the Advisory Board for Medical Specialties) has been the forum for open discussions of these and other items by all the boards. During this same period the American Board of Otolaryngology was greatly concerned with upward spiraling costs, increasing numbers of serious legal matters, the ongoing relationship of otolaryngology diplomates to the Board and the regulatory mechanisms contemplated by government in the certification process.

The American Board of Medical Specialties is a sponsor parent of the Accreditation Council on Graduate Medical Education, the Accreditation Council on Continuing Medical Education and the Liaison Council on Medical Education. Since the American Board of Otolaryngology is a member of the American Board of Medical Specialties it was and is represented throughout the hierarchy of organized medicine via this channel.

Toward the latter part of this decade, the American Board of Otolaryngology and the Residency Review Committee announced that on July 1, 1981, resident education would be lengthened to five years to meet requirements for primary certification. In preliminary studies, it had been discovered that two thirds of resident education programs were already requiring a fifth year and a few, six years. One year of surgery and three years of otolaryngology in resident education is to be served in programs approved by the Accreditation Council of Graduate Medical Education in the United States or the appropriate medical authority in Canada. The additional year can be flexible and must be served in an approved resident program also in the United States or Canada, and cannot be served as the fifth year of residency since this fifth year must be spent as a senior or chief resident in otolaryngology.

The five years of resident education to meet requirements for primary certification will go far toward clarifying the issue of subcertification in head and neck oncology, regional plastic and reconstructive surgery and allergy and immunology. Trends in organized medicine indicate cooperation among medical and surgical specialty groups which will lead to combined efforts of various interested parties to subcertify jointly in areas of mutual interest.

During the 1970s, 2,896 certificates were issued by the Board, an average of 289 per year. In this 10-year period, 575 more certificates were issued than in the previous 20 years (2,321 certificates were issued from 1950 to 1969). It was only in the early years after incorporation that the Board issued relatively large numbers of certificates in a short period of time due to the existing "grandfather clause" then in effect. As of December 31, 1979, 9,615 certificates had been issued by the Board: 4,398 in its first 25 years and 5,217 in the next 30 years. Since its incorporation 90 Directors served on the Board through 1979.

In closing, it would be well to recall the 50th Anniversary of the Board which was celebrated in November 1974.[9-12] On this occasion it was pointed out that otolaryngology had become a dynamic force among the medical and surgical specialties as well as throughout medicine. The lean earlier years were over.

During the 55 years in which the American Board of Otolaryngology has issued certificates, it made every effort to improve the validity of the certifying examination. The examination more than ever reflects the broad content of otolaryngology and evaluates all candidates in a uniform and standard manner.

REFERENCES

1. Proetz AW. Backstage with the board. Ann Otol Rhinol Laryngol 1950; 59:231-41.

2. American Board of Otolaryngology booklet of information 1979; 3-4.

3. Lierle DM. The present status and future of otolaryngology. Ann Otol Rhinol Laryngol 1950; 59:496-506.

4. American Board of Otolaryngology business meeting record. New York: January 8, 1951:2.

5. American Board of Otolaryngology booklet of information 1956; 5-7.

6. American Board of Otolaryngology booklet of information 1959; 7-8.

7. Lierle DM. American Board of Otolaryngology 1971 certification examination. Arch Otolaryngol 1971; 93:547-8.

8. Toffler A. The third wave. New York: Bantam, 1980.

9. Bradley WH. The American Board of Otolaryngology — a 50th birthday, editorial. JAMA 1974; 6:880.

10. McNally WJ. Fiftieth anniversary of the American Board of Otolaryngology 1924-1974, editorial. Arch Otolaryngol 1974; 99:249.

11. McCabe BF. 50th anniversary of the American Board of Otolaryngology, editorial. Ann Otol Rhinol Laryngol 1974; 83:563.

12. McCabe BF. Remarks on the 50th anniversary of the American Board of Otolaryngology, editorial. Laryngoscope 1974; 84:1729.

REPRINTS — Walter P. Work, MD, 172 Paseo de Golf, Green Valley, AZ 85614.

COCHLEAR IMPLANTS: PROGRESS AND PERSPECTIVES

Editors
William F. House, MD
Karen I. Berliner, PhD

CONTENTS

Contributors 5
Dedication 7
Acknowledgments 8
Preface 9

PART 1: THE SINGLE-ELECTRODE COCHLEAR IMPLANT

The Cochlear Implant Program: An Overview. K.I. Berliner, PhD; W.F. House, MD 11
Surgical Considerations in Cochlear Implantation. W.F. House, MD 15
Design and Functioning of the Single-Electrode Cochlear Implant. M.J. Danley; R.J. Fretz, MSEE, MSBME 21
Audiological Results with the Cochlear Implant. M.A. Thielemeir, MA; J.A. Brimacombe, MA; L.S. Eisenberg, MA 27
Psychoelectric Measurements and Results from Cochlear Implant Patients. L.F. Helmerich; B.J. Edgerton, PhD 35
Vowel Discrimination with the Single-Electrode Cochlear Implant: A Pilot Study. L.J. Dent, PhD 41
Effects of the Single-Electrode Cochlear Implant on the Vestibular System of the Profoundly Deaf Adult. L.S. Eisenberg, MA; J.R. Nelson, MD; W.F. House, MD 47
Psychometric Studies and Clinical Interviews with Cochlear Implant Patients. W.G. Crary, PhD; M. Wexler, PhD; K. I. Berliner, PhD; L.W. Miller, PhD 55
Psychological Effects of Cochlear Implant: Patient and "Index Relative" Perceptions. M. Wexler, PhD; L.W. Miller, PhD; K.I. Berliner, PhD; W.G. Crary, PhD 59
Use of the Cochlear Implant by the Prelingually Deaf. L.S. Eisenberg, MA 62
Initial Experience with the Cochlear Implant in Children. L.S. Eisenberg, MA; W.F. House, MD 67
Otopathological Findings in a Patient with Bilateral Cochlear Implants. L-G. Johnsson, MD; W.F. House, MD; F.H. Linthicum Jr, MD 74
Risk Versus Benefit in Cochlear Implantation. K.I. Berliner, PhD 90

PART 2: EXPERIMENTAL SYSTEMS

Comparison of Promontory and Cochlear Implants Within a Single Subject. B.J. Edgerton, PhD; W.F. House, MD; K.J. Doyle, MS 100
A Multiple-Electrode Cochlear Implant. W.F. House, MD; B.J. Edgerton, PhD 104
Hearing by Cochlear Nucleus Stimulation in Humans. B.J. Edgerton, PhD; W.F. House, MD; W.E. Hitselberger, MD 117

CONTRIBUTORS

House Ear Institute
Los Angeles, California

Karen I. Berliner, PhD
Director of Clinical Trials
Assistant Clinical Professor of Psychiatry (Psychology)
University of Southern California School of Medicine

Judy A. Brimacombe, MA
Research Associate, Audiology

William G. Crary, PhD
Consultant in Psychology
Associate Professor of Psychiatry (Psychology)
University of Southern California School of Medicine

Michael J. Danley
Senior Electronic Technician

Laurel J. Dent, PhD
Research Associate, Linguistics
(October 1979-September 1980)
Division of Otolaryngology
Stanford University School of Medicine
Palo Alto, California

Karen J. Doyle, MS
Research Associate, Audiology

Bradly J. Edgerton, PhD
Director of Auditory Research

Laurie S. Eisenberg, MA
Senior Research Associate, Audiology

Robert J. Fretz, MSEE, MSBME
Consultant in Engineering

Lawrence F. Helmerich
Research Associate, Audiology

William E. Hitselberger, MD
Professional Associate in Neurosurgery

William F. House, MD
Director of Research
Clinical Professor of Otolaryngology
University of Southern California School of Medicine
Otologic Medical Group, Los Angeles

Lars-Göran Johnsson, MD
Consultant to House Ear Institute on
cochlear implant study
Kresge Hearing Research Institute (1966-1981)
Department of Otorhinolaryngology
University of Michigan Medical School
Ann Arbor
Department of Otorhinolaryngology
University of Helsinki
Helsinki, Finland

Fred H. Linthicum, Jr, MD
Director of Histopathology
Clinical Professor of Otolaryngology
University of Southern California School of Medicine
Otologic Medical Group, Los Angeles

Linda W. Miller, PhD
Senior Research Associate, Psychology
Clinical Instructor of Psychiatry (Psychology)
University of Southern California School of Medicine

James R. Nelson, MD
Consultant in Neurology
Department of Neurosciences
School of Medicine
University of California at San Diego
La Jolla

Margaret A. Thielemeir, MA
Research Associate, Audiology

Murray Wexler, PhD
Consultant in Psychology
Professor of Psychiatry (Psychology)
University of Southern California School of Medicine

DEDICATION

Jack Urban, PE, 1902-1981

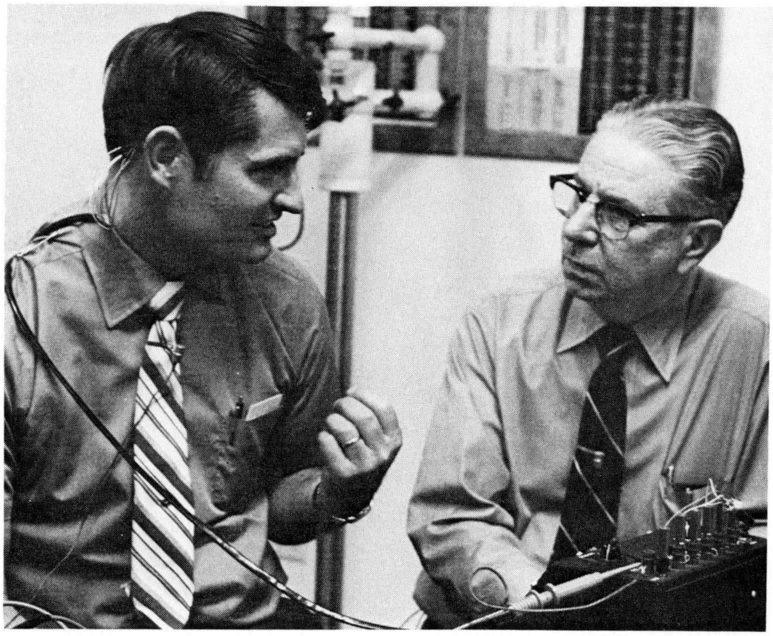

Jack Urban worked on the cochlear implant almost from its inception, and remained active as a consultant until his death last year.

The implant project started slowly in the early 1960s with electrical stimulation of the inner ear during stapes and chronic ear surgery being performed under local anesthetic. A few deaf patients were then tested with electrical stimulation of the promontory through the stapes approach. Jack and I were both excited by what we learned, and Jack began producing electrode configurations for insertion in temporal bones through different approaches. This was followed by construction of hard-wire buttons that Jack ingeniously designed and fabricated in his shop.

Finally, we implanted three patients with hard-wire multiple-electrode systems. This started a series of trials and disappointments that required building and rebuilding. We spent endless hours trying various electrical inputs. We would try some sophisticated device, only to have the patient tell us it was just so much noise. Jack never seemed discouraged. He only talked of what was learned and what we would try next. After two years of many evening sessions, a wearable device was constructed. Over these past ten years, the device was not fundamentally changed from Jack's original design.

In the early years, funding for the project was very sparse, and Jack Urban devoted his time and the facilities of his company at no charge. Through all of this, I came to appreciate Jack's deep religious feelings, his orientation toward the vast unknowns of biology and medicine, and his devotion to helping his fellow man. It is my sincere hope that his contributions will never be forgotten.

William F. House, MD
March 1982

ACKNOWLEDGMENTS

Preparation of this supplement was supported by the Commonwealth Foundation, New York, and assistance in the publication was provided by Union Pacific Foundation, New York.

Significant gifts in direct support of the research came from Mrs. Thurmond Clarke, Newport Beach, Calif.; Mrs. Lillian Disney, Los Angeles; and Mr. George Eccles, Salt Lake City. Major grants were provided by the following: The Ahmanson Foundation, Los Angeles; The Albertson Foundation, Los Angeles; C.H.E.A.R., Inc., Yonkers, NY; Charles E. Culpepper Foundation, Inc., New York; The Fluor Foundation, Irvine, Calif.; The Daniel and Florence Guggenheim Foundation, New York; Hollywood Turf Club Associated Charities, Inc., Inglewood, Calif.; W.M. Keck Foundation, Los Angeles; The Robert J. Kleberg, Jr, and Helen C. Kleberg Foundation, San Antonio, Tex.; and Harry G. Steele Foundation, Newport Beach, Calif.

The following otologists and audiologists are coinvestigators with the House Ear Institute who have implanted one or more patients each. They have spent many hours in their own right collecting data and filling out data forms. Much of the data presented in this supplement comes from these coinvestigators: Pedro Albernaz, MD; Marlene Albernaz; H.A. Ted Bailey, Jr, MD; James Pappas, MD; Sharon Graham, MS; Michael E. Glasscock III, MD; Susan Logan, MA; Anne Forest Josey, MS; J.V.D. Hough, MD; Kathy Waterfall, MS; Larry Englemann, MS; Tomokazu Kamio, MD; Sam E. Kinney, MD; Denise Caferelli, MS; Charles M. Luetje, MD; Donald Lawrence, PhD; H. Edward Maddox III, MD; Todd Porter, MA; Michelle Lynn, MS; Charles Mangham, Jr, MD; Patricia Burnett, MS; Brian McCabe, MD; Bruce Gantz, MD; Mary Lowder, MA; G. Tom McMurry, MD; Barbara Eisenmenger, MA; William L. Meyerhoff, MD; Christine Painter, MA; Robert Mischke, MD; Tim Campos, MA; Richard T. Miyamoto, MD; Jon Shallop, PhD; Molly Pope, MAT; Marjorie Kienle, M Ed; Fred Owens, MD; Asher Wolfe, PhD; Jorge A. Schwartzman, MD; Viviana Wilkinson, PhD; Fred T. Shaia, MD; Nancy Lambdin, MA; James B. Snow, Jr., MD; James Hall, PhD.

We would also like to thank Linda Dal Soglio, MA; Nancy Ogulnick, MS; and Bonnie Baehr, MA; audiologists at the Otologic Medical Group who performed the preoperative evaluations on many of our patients; and Kenneth Brookler, MD, and his staff who have provided follow-up care and data for several of our patients.

Additionally, we would like to acknowledge Bonnie Gill, Julia Graham, Leticia Rodriguez, and Ron Charbonneau, who spent many hours typing manuscripts or helping with the preparation of this supplement in other ways. Ed Zilberts, MA, did an outstanding job in preparing the medical illustrations and figures.

PREFACE

The articles in this supplement are summaries of the vast amounts of data collected over many years and uncountable hours of staff and patient time. One of the papers was completed nearly two years ago, and another more than a year ago. They were held for publication with this supplement because we wanted to present a comprehensive view of our cochlear implant research in a manner easily accessible to the reader.

The articles have been divided into two sections, one dealing with the single-electrode cochlear implant currently undergoing clinical trials, and a second presenting research with experimental systems. Papers in this supplement include a brief overview of the implant program, a detailed discussion of the surgical technique, engineering aspects of the device, results of audiological and psychological studies, a vestibular study, clinical results with special patient populations, risks and benefits in cochlear implantation, and studies of three different experimental systems for electrical stimulation of the auditory pathways.

The reader will find that a variety of terms have been employed when referring to the cochlear implant system we use at the House Ear Institute. Single-electrode induction coil cochlear implant, single-channel implant, House-Urban implant, House implant, and 16 kHz AM system all refer to the same device.

In this supplement, acoustic sound intensity has been expressed in decibels sound pressure level (re: .0002 dyne/cm^2). This method of data presentation was selected since at the present time there is no general agreement as to the values that should be used to convert minimal audible field data to equivalent earphone hearing threshold levels (HTLs). Factors such as the orientation of the measuring microphone, the azimuth of the ear relative to the speaker, the acoustic characteristics of the test environment, the type of stimulus used, and monaural versus binaural stimulation must be considered before a standard can be provided. However, for those readers who desire a general indication of the relationship between the minimal audible field warbled tone thresholds and earphone thresholds, we present the clinical standard for warbled tone thresholds proposed by Morgan, Dirks, and Bower:[1]

Test Frequency (Hz)	250	500	1000	2000	4000
dB correction*	15.0	11.5	8.0	2.5	2.5

*Subtract from sound field warbled tone thresholds to estimate equivalent hearing threshold levels.

The correction factor for speech signals delivered at a 0° azimuth is approximately 16.5 dB.[2] Thus, subtraction of 16.5 dB from the sound field speech thresholds should yield an approximation to the earphone HTL.

The House Ear Institute cochlear implant program has been an ongoing endeavor for over 20 years. The implant must now be considered a practical clinical alternative for the profoundly deaf patient. However, we are still in the pioneering phase, and much work remains to maximize the potential of implantable auditory prostheses.

REFERENCES

1. Morgan DE, Dirks DD, Bower DR. Speech audiometry: earphone and sound field. J Speech Hear Dis 1979; 44:37-54.

2. Dirks DD, Stream RW, Wilson RH. Suggested threshold sound pressure levels for frequency-modulated (warble) tones in the sound field. J Speech Hear Dis 1972; 37:162-76.

PART 1

THE SINGLE-ELECTRODE COCHLEAR IMPLANT

THE COCHLEAR IMPLANT PROGRAM: AN OVERVIEW

Karen I. Berliner, PhD

William F. House, MD

The single-electrode cochlear implant used at the House Ear Institute is undergoing clinical trials under Food and Drug Administration regulations governing medical devices. The program involves selection and evaluation of suitable subjects, surgery, basic guidance or training in implant use, and regular follow-up. As of November 1, 1981, 199 deaf subjects have had cochlear implant surgery. They range in age from 3.5 to 75 years old. Subjects with a wide variety of etiologies have been successfully implanted. The vast majority use their device on a daily basis, and subjects as a group have received more than 800,000 hours of electrical stimulation. Fifteen other otologists in the United States have implanted one or more subjects as coinvestigators in this clinical trials program. The otologists and their implant teams are trained by the House Ear Institute. Results indicate that the implant program can be performed adequately in a variety of clinical settings.

It is now more than two decades since the first reports that a deaf subject had been implanted with a coil and electrodes for the purpose of electrically stimulating the auditory nerve.[1] Auditory sensation through electrical stimulation seemed to promise hope for those with a profound sensorineural hearing loss.

In recent years, the amount of research on cochlear implants has increased dramatically. Although work at the House Ear Institute (HEI) on implants began as early as 1961, the bulk of research has occurred just since 1973. In that year, a comprehensive, multidisciplinary program was launched to study the single-electrode induction coil cochlear implant.

A monograph supplement detailing the work at HEI through 1975 has been published previously.[2] Most aspects of the implant program, including the selection and evaluation of subjects, surgery, rehabilitation, and follow-up evaluations have not changed greatly, nor have the basic electronic concepts of the implanted device and external stimulator. However, in all of these areas there has been continued development, modification, and refinement. Changes have been made in evaluation batteries, and new research areas have been approached.

Other papers in this supplement present specific information from each of the disciplines involved in the program, including otology, audiology, psychology, and engineering. An overview of the program is presented here, followed by an update on the current status of subjects who have received the single-electrode cochlear implant.

DESCRIPTION OF IMPLANT

The implant system is pictured in the figure. A microphone, usually mounted at ear level, picks up acoustic stimuli and transmits them to a stimulator unit. The stimulator processes the signal and then transmits it to an induction coil worn externally and placed directly over an implanted coil. The signal is magnetically induced across the skin barrier to the internal coil where it flows down an electrode that has been placed through the round window and into the scala tympani. Current flows between the active electrode and a second or ground electrode placed into the eustachian tube, stimulating remaining nerve fibers and producing a sensation of sound. Details of the design and functioning of the implant can be found in Danley and Fretz.[3]

SELECTION AND EVALUATION OF SUBJECTS

Subjects are selected for the implant procedure on the basis of medical, audiological, and psychological criteria. Many of the evaluative procedures are repeated at specified intervals to measure changes that may occur with use of the implant.

Medical. The medical evaluation includes history and physical examination, electronystagmography, x-ray films, and promontory response to electrical stimulation. The Promontory Response to Electrical Stimulation test is used to determine whether the candidate has a sensory loss with at least some neural elements intact.[4] In the past, only subjects who responded to electrical stimulation at the promontory of the cochlea with a sensation of sound and at voltages below the threshold of pain were further considered as candidates for an implant. However, experience has shown that the promontory test is highly variable, depending on placement of the electrode and other factors. Further, some subjects who do not stimulate at the promontory may, in fact, have a response to an intracochlear electrode. The vast majority of subjects with profound sensorineural deafness do have a positive promontory test. A subject who does not stimulate would be counseled appropriately and given the option to proceed with the implant.

X-ray films are studied with attention to the basal coil. Bone formation in the scala does not necessarily exclude a subject from having the implant surgery. However, such a case may require drilling as far as possible and then placing a shortened electrode into the cochlea. In these cases, results may be

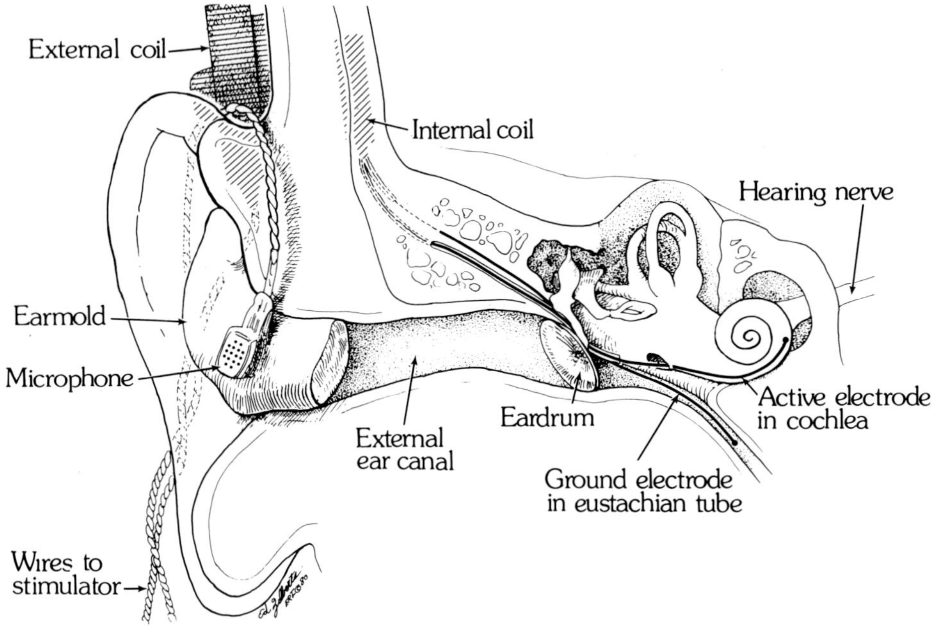

Single-electrode cochlear implant showing placement of internal coil and electrodes.

successful for one subject, and yet not for another. Again, the subject is counseled regarding this situation. X-ray studies are repeated after surgery to document placement of the electrodes, the presence of kinks in the electrodes, and so on.

Hearing and Speech. Subjects being evaluated for the implant program undergo audiological testing, and speechreading and voice production assessments. Audiological testing is used to select subjects who are profoundly deaf. More than 50% of the subjects who have received the implant had no unaided responses to the limit of the audiometer for the speech frequencies.[5,6]

In addition, performance with a hearing aid is evaluated on a number of discrimination tasks that include speech stimuli and environmental sounds. The subject's performance on these tests is compared to that achieved by subjects using a cochlear implant. If the prospective candidate scores as well with a hearing aid as implant users score, it is strongly recommended that he or she forego the implant and use a hearing aid. The audiologically poorer of the two ears is always chosen for implantation, so that the ear that uses an aid the best or is most preferred by the subject for hearing aid use is not implanted (even if no aid is currently being used).

SINGLE-ELECTRODE COCHLEAR IMPLANT PATIENTS*

	Late Loss	*Early Loss*	*Total*
Users	120	28	148
Nonusers	12	5	17
In process	19	1	20
Device failure	8	1	9
Deceased	5	0	5
	164	35	199

*November 1, 1981.

Speechreading and voice production assessments as well as further audiological testing may be performed prior to implant surgery. Testing is carried out both unaided and with an appropriate hearing aid. Test procedures are repeated at follow-up intervals with the implant. See Thielemeir et al[6] for a detailed discussion of the audiological procedures and results.

Psychology. As part of the selection and evaluation process, prospective implant candidates are psychologically assessed using interviews, tests, and questionnaires to measure cognitive, neuropsychological and personality functions. They should demonstrate no evidence of severe organic brain impairment, no evidence of psychosis, no mental retardation, no unremitting unrealistic expectations, and no personality traits that would markedly decrease their probability of completing the program.

The psychological battery is also repeated at regular follow-up intervals in order to monitor the subject and measure any changes in psychological functioning that may occur with use of the implant. Psychological test results and clinical findings are detailed in Crary et al[7] and Wexler et al.[8]

Subject Counseling. The decision to implant a particular subject goes beyond test results. The subject must decide that he or she wants to have this surgical procedure, to wear a rather large and bulky instrument, and to spend time learning how to use what will not be normal hearing. To this end every effort is made to insure that the subject understands the benefits and the limitations of the single-electrode cochlear implant, and that the expectations for the implant are realistic. The subject is given written materials answering commonly asked questions about the implant, meets with implant staff to discuss the pros and cons in relation to his or her own needs, and, finally, meets with a previously implanted subject to ask questions of an experienced implant user.

SURGERY

With the subject under general anesthesia, an incision is made behind the ear and a mastoidectomy is performed. A circular seat is drilled in the temporal bone above and behind the ear to secure the magnetic induction coil in place. The ground electrode is placed into the attic and down into the opening of the eustachian tube. The active electrode is led down through the facial recess. The round window lip is removed, the membrane lifted out of its sulcus, and the active electrode inserted into the scala tympani for a distance of about 14 mm. This places the ball tip of the electrode a little less than half-way around the basal turn with the uninsulated portion of the electrode lying along the higher frequency regions. Following insertion of the electrode, the round window membrane is replaced and fibrous tissue is placed around the electrode to promote sealing. The postauricular opening is sutured. About two months are allowed for healing before beginning electrical stimulation. A detailed description of the surgical procedure can be found in House.[9]

REHABILITATION

After the healing period the subject is ready to begin the rehabilitation program. Primary emphasis initially is on "basic guidance": teaching the subject how to handle the stimulator, fitting the coil holder so that the transmission between external and internal coils is strong, adjusting the electronic settings of the stimulator for the individual, and beginning training in critical listening with the implant. Subjects receive approximately 25-30 hours of training in implant use during individual sessions at HEI as well as having home lessons and assignments to complete.

Intensive therapy for development of specific skills may be offered on an individual basis according to each subject's need. Continuing guidance and support after the primary training period is provided by regular mail contact for the first few months, and occasional mail contact and visits to HEI thereafter. Long-term follow-up care continues as necessary. (Subjects are seen on an annual basis for retesting.)

SUBJECTS

Description. As of November 1, 1981, 199 deaf subjects have undergone surgery to receive a single-electrode cochlear implant. The surgeries were performed by William F. House, MD, and other otologists working as coinvestigators with the HEI cochlear implant program.

The subjects ranged in age at time of implant from 3.5 to 75 years old, with a mean of approximately 45 years. There are 108 males and 91 females. The age at onset of a profound hearing loss varied from birth to 64 years old, with a mean age of onset of 30 years. The subjects had experienced profound deafness for an average of 15 years prior to receiving the implant. One subject had had a profound loss for only six months prior to receiving the implant, while another had been profoundly deaf for almost 50 years.

A wide variety of etiologies have been found suitable for cochlear implantation. The most commonly occurring causes of deafness in the subjects who have had the cochlear implant are otosclerosis (20%), meningitis (15%), unknown (14%) and ototoxic (11%). The remaining cases included Menière's disease, congenital lues, trauma, rubella, and Usher syndrome, among others.

Little relationship has been found between years of deafness and auditory performance with the implant.[6] Etiology also does not appear to be a major factor, although statistical analyses do show some relationship of etiology to implant performance. For example, the otosclerosis patients tend to have better auditory thresholds with the implant at 1000 and 2000 Hz than other etiologies. This difference led to a statistically significant analysis of variance effect of etiology on threshold for those two frequencies ($p \leq .0025$ and $p \leq .001$, respectively). There was also a tendency for patients with meningitis and deafness of unknown etiology to perform more poorly than ototoxic and otosclerotic patients on discrimination tasks. However, there was considerable overlap in the distributions, and minimum and maximum scores were similar for all groups. Thus, etiology does not seem to be a major predictor of implant performance.

Status. The current status of subjects with an HEI single-electrode cochlear implant is presented in the table. HEI's own series of cases, implanted by House, includes 98 subjects. Coinvestigators working in conjunction with HEI have implanted an additional 101 subjects. Subjects have been grouped according to age of onset of their profound hearing loss. Subjects suffering a profound loss at or prior to age 5 have been listed as "early childhood" losses. Some of these may have congenital or prelingual losses. The majority of subjects for an implant have postlingual losses that occurred in at least late childhood and more often in adulthood.

The implant subjects have been classified with respect to how much they use their implants. Those who use their device on a regular basis, usually every day, are considered "users." Those who have chosen to use their implants only sporadically or not at all are termed "nonusers." Some subjects cannot use their implant because the internal device has failed due to a wire breakage, leakage of fluid into the coil, etc. These failures can be corrected by replacing the failed coil and electrodes with a new system, under a local anesthetic. Also classified as "device failure" would be cases that do not stimulate well for physiological reasons. For example, two recent HEI subjects were found on x-ray studies to have bone growth in the lower basal turn of the cochlea. They were informed that placement of the implant electrode could be attempted but might or might not yield satisfactory results. Both chose to have the procedure. In one, electrical stimulation was successful. In the other, the bone was apparently too dense to allow flow of the electric current, and this subject could not be stimulated within acceptable voltage limits.

Subjects are categorized as "in process" if they are within the 2-month period following completion of the basic guidance rehabilitation program. It is felt that classification prior to that time is premature. A subject may be wearing the stimulator every day during the rehabilitation period because he or she is being seen at HEI every day but might go home and discontinue daily use. On the other hand, a subject may require a period of experience before deciding to use the implant regularly. Thus, judgment on the subject's status as an implant user is delayed until after an interval of experience. Five implanted subjects are now deceased. One died before receiving an external stimulator and therefore had never used the implant.

As shown in the table, the vast majority of cochlear implant subjects use their prostheses regularly. Most use them all day long, every day. In total, subjects have received approximately 800,000 hours of electrical stimulation. The longest-term user has been wearing an implant daily for nine years. There have been almost no measurable adverse effects, and the implant has clearly been of significant benefit to these subjects. The risks and benefits of cochlear implantation are discussed fully in Berliner.[10]

CLINICAL TRIALS PROGRAM

The single-electrode cochlear implant used by HEI is undergoing clinical trials under the FDA regulations governing investigational medical devices. Fifteen other otologists in the United States have implanted one or more subjects as coinvestigators with HEI in the clinical trials program. These otologists and their implant teams are trained by HEI and provided with detailed manuals on all aspects of the program.[11-14]

Each coinvestigator is required to bring his or her first patient to Los Angeles, where the surgery is performed under the supervision of House. The coinvestigator's audiologist must come to HEI to observe the preoperative audiological evaluation procedures and be trained in the use of the implant equipment. After the healing period, the basic guidance program is performed with the subject by one of the HEI staff, and the coinvestigator staff observes the process. Thereafter, each coinvestigator team evaluates, implants, and trains subjects using the procedures specified by HEI.

Data forms are provided by HEI, and all coinvestigators are required to report subject data using these forms. In this way, all coinvestigators perform the same test procedures and report results in a standardized fashion. HEI has developed interactive data entry programs for entering all cochlear implant data into a computer for storage, retrieval, and analysis.

The clinical trials program is directed toward gathering safety and efficacy information on the single-electrode cochlear implant. The coinvestigators enlarge the data pool as well as making the implant available closer to home for those patients who might be suitable candidates. An important result of this program is the finding that the implant procedure is clinically feasible and can be performed adequately in a variety of clinical settings. Although it is not a cost effective procedure for the otologist in clinical practice, the implant program allows the clinician to offer something to patients he or she has not been able to help in the past.

REFERENCES

1. Djourno A, Eyries C. Prothese auditive par excitation electrique a distance du nerf sensoriel a l'aide d'un bobinage inclus a demeure. Presse Med 1957; 35:14-7.

2. House WF, Berliner K, Crary W, et al. Cochlear implants. Ann Otol Rhinol Laryngol 1976; 85 Suppl 27:1-93.

3. Danley MJ, Fretz RJ. Design and functioning of the single-electrode cochlear implant. Ann Otol Rhinol Laryngol 1982; 91 Suppl 91:21-6.

4. House WF, Brackmann DE. Electrical promontory testing in differential diagnosis of sensorineural hearing impairment. Laryngoscope 1974; 84:2163-71.

5. House WF, Bode DL, Berliner KI. The cochlear implant: performance of deaf patients. Hear Instr 1981; 32:13-8.

6. Thielemeir MA, Brimacombe JA, Eisenberg LS. Audiological results with the cochlear implant. Ann Otol Rhinol Laryngol 1982; 91 Suppl 91:27-34.

7. Crary WG, Wexler M, Berliner KI, Miller LW. Psychometric studies and clinical interviews with cochlear implant patients. Ann Otol Rhinol Laryngol 1982; 91 Suppl 91:55-8.

8. Wexler M, Miller LW, Berliner KI, Crary WG. Psychological effects of cochlear implant: patient and "index relative" perceptions. Ann Otol Rhinol Laryngol 1982; 91 Suppl 91:59-61.

9. House WF. Surgical considerations in cochlear implantation. Ann Otol Rhinol Laryngol 1982; 91 Suppl 91:15-20.

10. Berliner KI. Risk versus benefit in cochlear implantation. Ann Otol Rhinol Laryngol 1982; 91 Suppl 91:90-8.

11. House WF. Cochlear implant clinical trials manual. Los Angeles: Hearing Rehabilitation Research Center, 1980.

12. Norton NB, Eisenberg LS, Berliner KI, Thielemeir MA. Cochlear implant rehabilitation manual. Los Angeles: Hearing Rehabilitation Research Center, 1980.

13. Thielemeir MA. Cochlear implant equipment manual. Los Angeles: Hearing Rehabilitation Research Center, 1980.

14. Eisenberg LS. Introduction to sound: a therapy program developed for the prelingually deafened adult using a cochlear implant. Los Angeles: Hearing Rehabilitation Research Center, 1980.

SURGICAL CONSIDERATIONS IN COCHLEAR IMPLANTATION

WILLIAM F. HOUSE, MD

A detailed description of the surgical technique for the single-electrode cochlear implant is presented. Principles of implant surgery, techniques for revision of failed devices, and postoperative complications are also discussed.

Twenty years of experience with cochlear implants has taught us a number of principles regarding surgery and long-term use and tolerance of these devices. This paper is a summary of my present thinking regarding cochlear implant surgery.

PRINCIPLES OF IMPLANT SURGERY

The surgical problem simply stated is how do we implant a device capable of introducing electrical fields close enough to remaining cochlear nerve fibers so that they will discharge in complex enough patterns to result in meaningful sound? In this paper I will not discuss the questions relating to numbers of electrodes and types of electrical stimulation, but confine the discussion to surgical methods of introducing electrodes and passing electrical potentials through these electrodes.

Electrodes capable of introducing electrical fields that discharge cochlear nerve fibers can be placed outside the otic capsule in the middle ear, in the cochlear fluids, in the modiolus (Rosenthal canal), the eighth nerve trunk, and at the ventral cochlear nucleus where the eighth nerve fibers synapse with the nuclear cells on a one-to-one basis.

All of these placements except electrodes along the eighth nerve in the internal auditory canal or cerebellopontine angle have been tried and reported clinically.[1-3] So far, the most successful electrode placements have been the electrodes in the intracochlear fluids. If the cochlea or eighth nerve has been destroyed, then ventral cochlear nucleus electrodes are possible.[4]

Electrodes have been introduced into the cochlear fluids by pushing them into the scala tympani through the round window area, or through holes drilled through the otic capsule into the various turns of the cochlea. In general, the larger the area of exposed electrode surface in the fluids, the lower the electrode impedance and the less the current density adjacent to the electrode. The higher the current density, the greater the likelihood of local tissue damage.

Electrode arrays have been inserted as far as 24 mm into the scala tympani through the round window. This is the length of the basal turn of the cochlea (24 mm out of a total of 35 mm length of the scala) and includes the frequency areas from 1500 to 20,000 Hz.

Multiple holes can be drilled through the otic capsule and electrodes inserted into the various scalae. At House Ear Institute (HEI) we have presently a patient with a 14 mm electrode inserted into the scala tympani, an electrode inserted into the second turn of the cochlea, and an electrode inserted into the helicotrema. The details of this surgical procedure and the results of the multiple-electrode stimulation are reported elsewhere.[5]

In addition to the electrode placement considerations there is the problem of how best to introduce the electrical potentials to the electrodes.

Hard-wired methods refer to bringing the wires through the skin to various types of plugs that can be attached to external potential sources. At HEI, whenever any new electrode system has been tried, hard-wire systems have been used so that the variables of across-the-skin transmission of the electric signals are eliminated. Experience with these hard-wire systems has shown remarkable tolerance in some cases. Our first hard-wire patient in 1969 used such a system in one ear for seven years. However, another patient developed loosening of the button and infection that required removal after six weeks of experimentation. Hard-wire systems, therefore, are not stable for long-term use in large numbers of patients.

There are a number of possible ways to transmit electrical potentials across the skin. Among these are electromagnetic induction, radio frequency transmission, and infrared transmission. At HEI we have experimented with each of these. Each has its advantages and disadvantages. The system that has proven the most practical to date has been electromagnetic transmission.

The principal problems have been the approximately 10 to 1 loss of power in transfer across the skin and the problem of keeping the internal coil and the external coil aligned for adequate power transmission. The greater the distance between internal and external coil the more the power loss. Therefore, surgically we have attempted to keep the scalp over the internal coil as thin as possible, yet with adequate blood supply. The alignment problem has been greatly helped by the use of magnets to keep the internal and external coil aligned and by well-designed brackets to fit the external coil to glasses frames. Various head bands, tapes and skin glues have not proven satisfactory except in a few cases.

In general, a cochlear implant consists of a system for transmission of electrical potential across the skin, wires to lead the potentials to the inner ear, and electrodes to create electrical fields that stimulate cochlear nerve discharges.

The basic surgical problem is to introduce this hardware into the temporal bone and have it function over a lifetime without rejection.

Our long-term clinical experience to date indicates that this is possible. A basic principle in this surgical tolerance has emerged. This is simply that all hardware must be kept as far away from skin surfaces as possible, consistent with function.

In the case of the imbedded electromagnetic coil we want it as close to the skin surface as possible in order to increase electrical efficiency. However, if the blood supply to the dermis of the scalp is interfered with by thinning the skin too much during surgical placement or placing the incision too close to the coil, rejection and infection could result. Also, too much pressure of the external coil on the internal coil could collapse the vessels in the interposed dermis between the coils and skin with resulting necrosis. To date, these potential problems have been satisfactorily avoided. In two cases the internal coils have become exposed, apparently due to the coil edge being too close to the incision. In each case surgical revision has corrected the problem.

The wires leading from the internal coil to the cochlear electrodes should be placed through the mastoid and facial recess to keep them as far away from skin surfaces as possible. Putting a groove down the posterior aspect of the external auditory canal and running the wires in the groove is very likely to result in infection and rejection. The problem is that the thin skin of the external auditory canal retracts onto the wire and the slightest trauma or crusting abrades the skin and allows infection to start. This infection cannot be controlled in the presence of the foreign body wires. Likewise, techniques that create a mastoid cavity are unstable since the skin lining the bowl is likely to retract over the wires passing through the cavity and become eroded and infected.

I have implanted several patients who have presented with radical mastoid cavities. To get the wires as far away from the skin as possible I have put bone pate over the wires and under the skin lining. This has proved satisfactory so far, but clinical experience with mastoid obliteration techniques has taught me that 5-year follow-up will be required to eventually assess the success of this technique.

COCHLEAR IMPLANTS IN CHILDREN.

At HEI our youngest implant patient to date is 3½ years old. The surgical result with this child has indicated that cochlear implants during the third year of life (24-36 months) are feasible. It is well documented that the cochlea is adult size at birth and, in general, the middle ear, eardrum, and ossicles are also adult size. Surgical dissection of skulls from newborn through age 48 months indicate that by 24 months the facial recess is adult size and the mastoid antrum and air cells are well developed. The squamous part of the mastoid bone, however, is small and only 2-3 mm thick. The scalp is still thin, but small internal coils have been tolerated well over this area. The electrode and wire placement is similar to adult surgery. The electrode wires have enough length that they can tolerate the increase in height and width of the skull without pulling the active electrode out of the scala tympani.

SURGICAL TECHNIQUE OF THE SINGLE-ELECTRODE COCHLEAR IMPLANT

The surgical technique of the cochlear implant relies on the techniques developed for intact canal wall facial recess approaches that I developed during the late 1950s and early 1960s for chronic ear surgery.

Continuous irrigation suction and diamond stone drills are essential. Surgeons who have mastered these techniques need, in addition, to study the relationships of the round window niche and basal coil (especially the hook area) to the facial recess. This must be done in the temporal bone dissection laboratory, and at the same time practice electrodes can be inserted into the scala tympani of the basal coil.

The procedure starts with locating the position of the external coil above and behind the pinna. A dummy coil of the size and shape of the external coil is placed on the skin before distortion of the tissues with local anesthetic. The placement of the external coil should be as close to the pinna as possible without touching it. Postoperatively, if the external coil touches the pinna it will cause a pressure sore. The position of the internal coil must then be established so that it will be directly under the external coil. This is accomplished by pushing a slender sharp drill through the center of the dummy external coil, and a small hole is drilled in the squamous part of the temporal bone (Fig. 1).

The postauricular scalp is infiltrated with Xylocaine and 1/100,000 adrenalin and a large postauricular incision is made. The incision should be 1 cm wide of the external-internal coil edge (Fig. 2). Making this large incision outside the position of the internal coil minimizes any damage to the superficial temporal vessel supply to the skin of the area. The lower pole of the incision likewise should not be brought in too close to the postauricular crease since

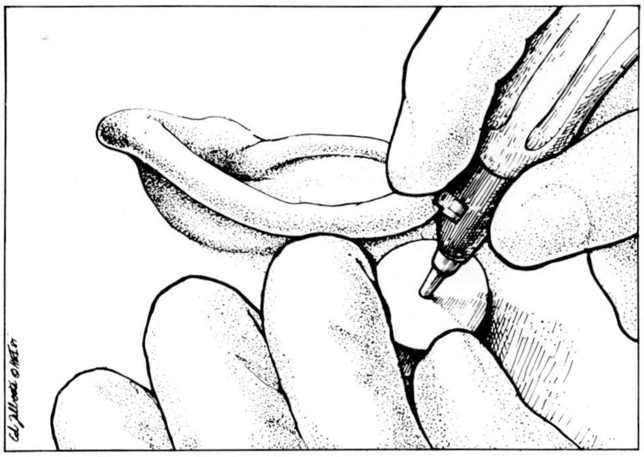

Fig. 1. Marking position for placement of internal coil by use of dummy external coil.

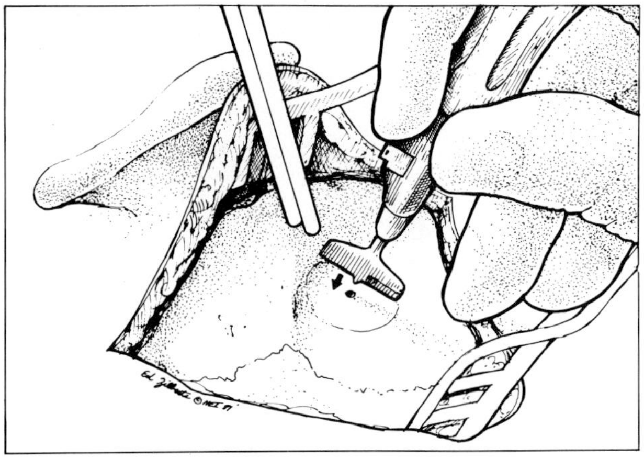

Fig. 3. Butterfly burr (reamer) forming seat for internal coil.

it is not desirable to cut across the branches of the occipital artery that also suppy the postauricular scalp.

The postauricular flap is then elevated forward. The avascular plane between the scalp and the temporalis muscle is developed and the periosteum over the mastoid below the linia temporalis is elevated using a Lempert periosteal elevator. The flap is developed forward to the spine of Henle. One should not cut between the periosteum and the scalp as this only diminishes the blood supply and does not increase access.

Retractors are placed and a large piece of temporalis muscle is removed over the squamous part of the temporal bone. Removing this muscle allows a better seating of the internal coil; postoperatively the scalp heals down against the bone around the internal coil, thus making it easy to palpate and minimizing the thickness of the scalp over the internal coil.

Removing the temporalis muscle also brings into view the small drill hole that was made through the center of the dummy external coil at the beginning

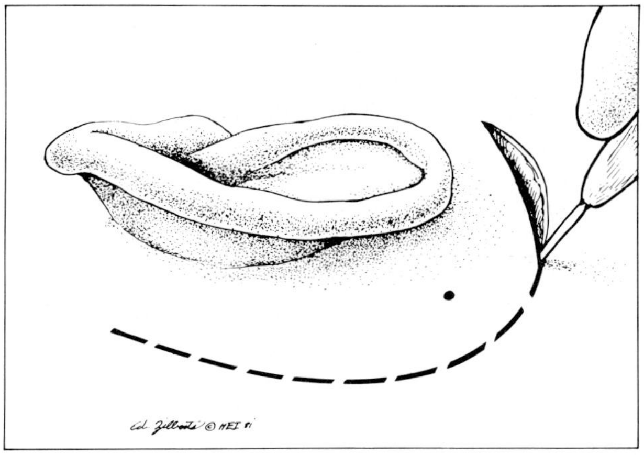

Fig. 2. Large postauricular incision 1 cm wide of the edge of the internal coil.

of the operation. This hole is enlarged and deepened to 4 mm (in adults) with a special drill that has a guard on it to prevent plunging through the bone into the underlying dura and brain. Using a reamer that is the same size as the internal coil (I call this a butterfly burr) a seat is made in the bone to accept the internal coil (Fig. 3). This seat accepts the internal coil, locates it properly on the bone and keeps the coil from shifting out of place during the healing period. The seat must be made at the proper plane so the internal coil will be parallel to the scalp surface.

A mastoidectomy is now done using conventional burrs and irrigation suction techniques. The bone removal extends back to the sigmoid, but collapse of the sigmoid is not required unless it is very far forward. The middle fossa plate is skeletonized, and the antrum and horizontal canal are located. The bone in the attic is removed enough so that the top of the incus can be clearly seen. I do not dislocate or remove the incus or other ossicles. The posterior bony canal wall is thinned as much as possible without exposing the overlying vascular strip skin. This is necessary because in viewing the round window area the direction of vision is parallel to the external auditory canal bone.

The facial recess is now opened. The facial nerve is skeletonized at the mastoid genu, but effort is made to avoid exposing the nerve sheath. Drill forward to the chorda tympani. This is a good landmark to the eardrum annulus since the chorda enters the middle ear at the annulus level. If the facial recess is very restricted, it is occasionally necessary to remove the chorda, but usually this is not necessary for adequate visualization of the round window niche.

Once the facial recess is opened, the lip of the round window niche is usually visible just inferior to the stapedius tendon and head of the stapes. Using a small diamond stone and intermittent irrigation, the lip of the niche is removed, and the round window membrane comes into clear view.

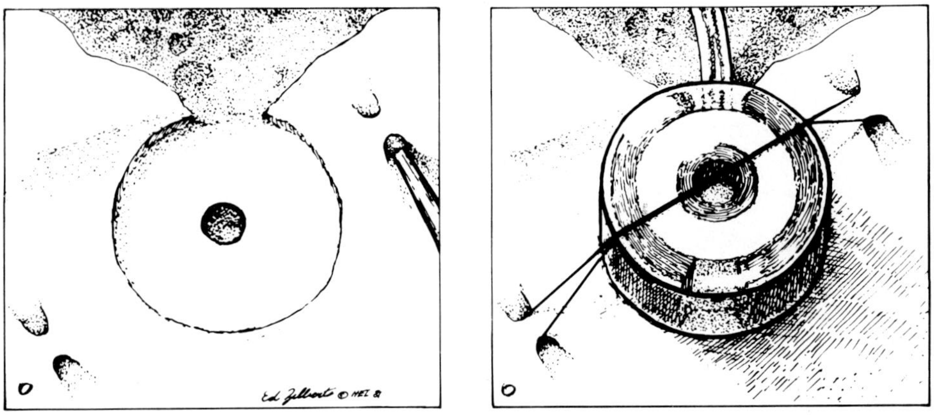

A B

Fig. 4. A) Making a tunnel hole for suture retention of internal coil. B) Placement of retention suture to hold internal coil in place.

With a smaller diamond stone and small hooks an opening large enough to accept the ball of the active electrode is made just anterior to the annulus of the round window membrane. The surgeon must be extremely careful not to have the diamond stone rotating when passing through the facial recess to the round window area. On one occasion, I had the rotating burr hit the anterior bone edge of the facial recess and bounce against the facial nerve. Fortunately, the facial nerve had not been exposed so no harm was done; but it scared me and warned me to be more careful.

Occasionally the round window niche will be almost hidden under the pyramidal process. In this case, one must drill forward thinning the promontory until the scala tympani is entered. This is not difficult provided you have done your homework with temporal bone dissection and thoroughly understand how the basal coil curves from the round window forward along the base of the promontory.

In 30 or 40% of cases, the round window niche and membrane will be replaced with new bone growth. This is especially true in otosclerosis and meningitis cases. Careful preoperative study of polytome x-ray films, properly made to show the basal coil and round window areas, will usually warn of this problem. From these x-ray films the surgeon can usually determine how far forward along the basal coil he or she will have to drill. In some cases, this may be as much as 5 or 6 mm. Usually the new bone is white and can be demarcated from the surrounding otic capsule. Following this white plug of bone with the drill will eventually lead to the patent scala and an opening made to accept the active electrode.

In one case, x-ray films showed almost total obliteration of the cochlea (except the apical turn) by bone following meningitis. As a trial I drilled forward 7 mm through the soft bone of the scala tympani. No true opening was made into a patent scala, but there seemed to be some perilymph moisture seeping through the porous bone. An electrode was placed in this 7 mm hole, and the patient does get sound from stimulation. He wears the implant device on a full-time basis.

The next step is the coil and electrode placement. On each side of the internal coil seat a small tunnel hole is made to accept a 4-0 silk suture (Fig. 4A).

The internal coil, which comes packaged sterile, is placed in the bony seat and sutured into place (Fig. 4B). Once the coil is secured in place, the ground electrode, which is an exposed platinum wire, is placed into the attic superior to the tensor tendon and down into the protympanum (eustachian tube) (Fig. 5).

The active electrode, which has a 0.5 mm ball on the end and wire exposed 14 mm to the silicone rubber insulation is inserted into the opening in the scala tympani. To minimize damage to the basilar membrane, it is pushed in so that it follows the outer curve of the scala tympani. To do this the surgeon imagines he or she is directing the electrode in the direction of the patient's nose (downward and forward). The electrode is inserted so that the edge of the insulation is at the round window membrane and the entire exposed metal electrode is in the scala tympani (Fig. 5). When first starting with the single-electrode, we inserted it 24 mm, but we found it would occasionally kink and cause damage to the basilar membrane.[6] We gradually have shortened the electrode to the present 14 mm. Experience has shown that probably even this length is not critical so we are considering further shortening to about 10 mm. Fascia is packed around the active electrode at the round window.

The operation is now complete except for skin closure. A word of caution: once the electrodes are placed, we feel it could be hazardous to use conventional cautery where the current flows from the active electrode through the body (path of least electrical resistance) to the large ground electrode under the patient. With this type of cautery, it is conceivable that part of this path of least electrical resistance could be the active or ground electrode.

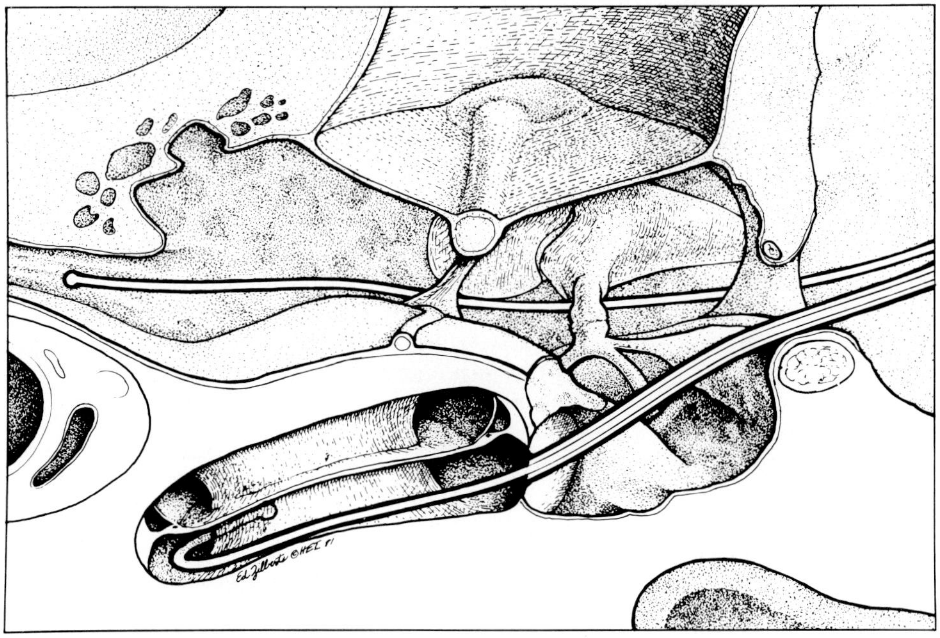

Fig. 5. Active electrode in the basal coil scala tympani. Insulation ends at the round window. Ground electrode (bare) placed in attic and eustachian tube.

For this reason, once the electrode is in place we use only bipolar cautery to control skin bleeders.

Each surgeon has his own preference for skin suturing of postauricular incisions. Mine is subcuticular 2-0 chronic catgut. Care is taken not to allow the needle to penetrate the silicone rubber covering of the internal coil.

REVISION IMPLANT SURGERY

Cochlear implant failures have occurred due to shorting of the internal coil. In this situation, usually the patient noted complete loss of stimulation or intermittent stimulation followed by complete failure. In these cases a promontory test showed that the inner ear still was capable of being stimulated and tests of the external stimulator showed it to be functioning. The only possibility, therefore, was internal unit failure. Most of these failures occurred anywhere from 2 to 7 years after the original placement of the internal coil and electrodes.

Patients with internal coil failures have undergone revision surgery under local anesthesia. The postauricular incision was again made and the entire electrode and internal coil system removed. A new coil and electrode system was placed. Fortunately there did not seem to be calcification of the scala tympani, so the new active electrode slipped in easily.

Analysis of these removed units revealed that water vapor had penetrated the silicone rubber insulation, and shorts had developed, usually at solder joints or occasionally between the copper wire turns in the internal coil. Due to these findings, design changes such as sealing the internal coil with epoxy before silicone rubber encapsulation were made. This has definitely reduced the failure rate. However, silicone rubber will transmit water vapor (no other ions are apparently allowed to pass). As long as we cannot prevent water vapor transfer through the silicone rubber covering, failure will always be a possibility with this type of system. Use of a hermetically sealed container and of platinum rather than copper coils are being explored as a means to further reduce coil failures.

Since internal coil failures may never be completely eliminated, I began looking at better methods of internal device replacement. The electrodes removed from temporal bones after several years of use were studied with electron microscopy to see if the surfaces were pitted, indicating loss of metal due to electrolysis. No difference in surface appearance between control unimplanted electrode wires and those stimulated over long periods of time were noted.[7] This finding indicated that once the electrodes were in the cochlea and middle ear, they would probably be stable for a lifetime.

The surgical problem then became: how can the internal coil be replaced without replacing the electrodes that had become stabilized in the inner ear? Two possibilities were evident: 1) develop a disconnect system that could be implanted, or 2) develop a way of connecting cut electrodes to new coil leads and reinsulating them in surgery. The technology for disconnect-reconnect pacemakers was looked at and found to be too bulky for temporal bone operations. Smaller systems developed by FB Simmons (personal communication, 1977) and by ITT Cannon Company also proved bulky and difficult to manipulate in the surgical situation.

It was found that the platinum electrode wire could be connected to the internal coil lead by slipping a platinum tube over the end of each and crimping the tube on the wire. The problem remained, however, of how to insulate this connection from the surrounding tissue. This seems to have been solved by the use of bone wax. Bone wax is very impervious to transmission of water vapor.[8] For this reason, then, at surgery bone wax is melted and flowed around the exposed connection. We now have two cases where this technique has been used to replace the internal coils that have been functioning for more than one year. Improved instrumentation for this technique is now being developed by Spire Medical under the direction of S. Waldron.

POSTOPERATIVE COMPLICATIONS

Fortunately, complications following implant surgery have been remarkably low. Specifically, there have been no cases of meningitis, cerebrospinal fluid leak, middle ear infection, persistent unsteadiness, vertigo, facial nerve spasm, or facial paralysis. There have been no adverse neurological or psychological effects.[9] This includes the entire HEI and coinvestigator cases numbering 199.

In this series there have been two cases of failure of primary healing over the implanted coil. One of these was corrected by a secondary skin flap procedure. In the other case, the coil was disconnected and removed, leaving the electrodes in place for later placement of a new coil. Another case was noted to have persistent perilymph leak around the active electrode at the round window. The electrode was removed, and the leak closed. The patient has subsequently had a successful implant in the other ear.

SUMMARY

Cochlear implants and cochlear implant surgery will continue to evolve. Principles and do's and do not's are beginning to emerge, and the next 20 years will undoubtedly see greater changes than the past 20 years.

REFERENCES

1. Douek E, Fourcin AJ, Moore BCJ, Clark GP. A new approach to the cochlear implant. Proc R Soc Med 1979; 70:379-83.

2. House WF, Berliner K, Crary W, et al. Cochlear implants. Ann Otol Rhinol Laryngol 1976; 85 Suppl 27:1-93.

3. Simmons FB. Electrical stimulation of the auditory nerve in man. Arch Otolaryngol 1966; 84:2-54.

4. Edgerton BJ, House WF, Hitselberger WE. Hearing by cochlear nucleus stimulation in humans. Ann Otol Rhinol Laryngol 1982; 91 Suppl 91:117-24.

5. House WF, Edgerton BJ. A multiple-electrode cochlear implant. Ann Otol Rhinol Laryngol 1982; 91 Suppl 91:104-16.

6. Johnsson L-G, House WF, Linthicum FH. Bilateral cochlear implants: histological findings in a pair of temporal bones. Laryngoscope 1979; 89:759-62.

7. Graham MD. Long term intracochlear electrode implantation in man: scanning electron microscopic observations. Ann Otol Rhinol Laryngol 1976; 85 Suppl 27:58-61.

8. Enger CC, Rhinelander FW. Implantable impermeable flexible encapsulants for artificial organs. J Biomed Mater Res Symposium 1971; 1:149-68.

9. Crary WG, Wexler M, Berliner KI, Miller LW. Psychometric studies and clinical interviews with cochlear implant patients. Ann Otol Rhinol Laryngol 1982; 91 Suppl 91:55-8.

DESIGN AND FUNCTIONING OF THE SINGLE-ELECTRODE COCHLEAR IMPLANT

MICHAEL J. DANLEY

ROBERT J. FRETZ, MSEE, MSBME

The single-electrode cochlear implant used by the House Ear Institute was first implanted in a patient in 1972; it is essentially this same device that is in use today. This paper presents a physical description of the major components of the device, as well as a discussion of the signal processing that occurs.

In the early 1960s, an electrical system capable of stimulating the auditory nerve in profoundly deaf patients seemed feasible. At the House Ear Institute (then the Los Angeles Foundation of Otology), a major engineering thrust in this direction began when William F. House, MD, teamed up with an engineer, Jack Urban. They designed a multiple-electrode cochlear implant with a percutaneous plug that was first implanted in a human subject in 1969. The hard-wire multiple-electrode system contained five active electrodes in the scala tympani and an extracochlear ground. Three subjects were implanted in 1969-1970, and extensive testing on one of these subjects led ultimately to the design of the current single-electrode system.

Special equipment was built to stimulate the electrodes with analog signals; square, triangle, or sine waves; or an amplitude modulated carrier wave. The square wave could be changed to a pulse with a delay time of up to 7.5 ms from first to last electrode. A dual trace oscilloscope was used to monitor the signal, and enabled exact measurement and control of the stimulus to be fed to the implanted electrodes. Bandpass filters that could be adjusted for each electrode independently were used for some of the testing. During this early testing, no clear advantage was found for the use of multiple electrodes rather than a single active electrode. This finding simplified considerably the task of developing a wearable stimulator unit.

Thus, the development began on a single-electrode device that would not protrude through the skin and for which a take-home stimulator would be available. It was decided that a passive system which required neither a power source for the internal components nor demodulation of the signal would be the simplest and most clinically efficient system. The single-electrode magnetic induction coil was designed. The system included the internal induction coil, a matching external coil for transmission through the skin, and the external electronics package. The idea of amplitude modulating a "carrier" had been explored earlier, and 16 kHz was chosen for three reasons: 1) it was high enough to prevent foldover of the lower side band into an audio range already limited by the tuned circuitry to frequencies below approximately 3 kHz, 2) it allowed economical energy transfer, and 3) experience indicated that subjects preferred the region above 12 kHz.

The House-Urban single-electrode induction coil cochlear implant was implanted in a patient in 1972. Although numerous minor modifications have occurred over time, it is essentially this same system that is in use today. Following is a physical description of the major components of the current device and a discussion of the signal processing that occurs.

PHYSICAL DESCRIPTION

Internal Coil. The implanted device consists primarily of three parts, the electromagnetic coil and two platinum electrodes (Fig. 1). The electrodes are used in a monopolar configuration with the active implanted in the scala tympani and the ground placed in the eustachian tube. The electrodes are 99.9% pure platinum wire with a diameter of 0.008 inches (0.2 mm) and an 0.5 mm ball formed at the end. The total length of the active lead is 78 mm from the edge of the coil body to the ball end, with 15 mm left uninsulated to form the electrode. For the ground lead, the total length is 68 mm with 53 mm left uninsulated to form the electrode. The platinum electrode wires are insulated with silicone rubber tubing.

The implanted coil is wound on a Delrin plastic bobbin (EI du Pont de Nemours and Co, Wilmington, Del) with 450 turns of 42 gauge copper wire insulated with a heavy Isonel coating (Schenectady Chemical, Inc, Schenectady, NY). A ferrite pot core is used in conjunction with the coil to direct and concentrate the magnetic field from the external stimulator coil. The platinum electrode leads are connected to the coil wires by way of a solder joint, and the coil windings are impregnated with Epoxylite (Epoxylite Corp, Anaheim, Cal) to fill the voids between the coil turns and increase long-term reliability. A silicone rubber coating is used to cover the outside of the coil and the ferrite core so that the implantable device is totally encapsulated. The sili-

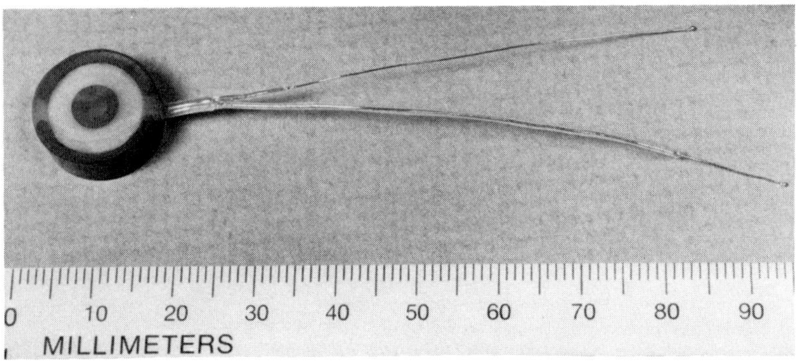

Fig. 1. Internal electromagnetic coil with active and ground platinum electrodes.

cone coating on the outside of the ferrite core is approximately 0.64 mm thick which allows a total device dimension of 15.5 mm diameter and 6.1 mm thickness. The electrical properties of the coil exhibit an inductance of 6.7 millihenrys (mH) and a DC resistance of 73 Ω.

External Coil. The external stimulator coil (Fig. 2) is constructed from 600 turns of 40 gauge copper wire with heavy Isonel insulation wound on a Delrin plastic bobbin. A ferrite pot core of slightly larger size than the implanted coil is used to make the coupling of the coils less sensitive to misalignment. There is a 2-pin female connector which is affixed to the ferrite core that allows easy electrical connection to the coil. The entire external coil assembly is encapsulated by a polyester resin to increase its reliability. The total dimension of the external coil is 19 mm diameter and 8.9 mm thick. The electrical characteristics of the coil are an inductance of 14 mH and a DC resistance of 76 Ω.

In the past there have been many ideas on how to place the external stimulator coil over the internal implanted coil with reliable alignment. This placement must be comfortable and convenient for the patient who will in many cases use the stimulator for 8 to 15 hours a day. These ideas have included a holder mounted on glasses, double-back adhesive tape, special toupee glue, and a headband. The most effective method has been a special coil holder which is attached to a glasses temple piece (Fig. 3). The device is made with Delrin plastic material in the form of a cup to hold the coil in position over the implant. On the back of the cup a small ball and socket system is used that allows the coil to align itself with the surface of the skin above the internal implanted coil. The coil holder must be custom-fitted to each glasses temple piece and positioned for each implant. When the holder is properly fitted, the coil exerts a force of approximately 40 g onto the surface of the skin.

Microphone. The microphone used with the stimulator is a subminiature electret type which has a flat response within the audio range. A miniature 3-pin female connector is affixed to the back side of the microphone which allows easy electrical connection (Fig. 4). The microphone with connector can be attached to a glasses temple piece, an earmold, or clipped onto clothing with a special adaptor.

External Stimulator. The external electronic stimulator is composed of three sections, a printed circuit board with all of its associated components, the battery compartment and contact strip, and the metal case which is used to house the stimulator package (Fig. 5). The electronic circuit is powered by two 9 V alkaline batteries which supply a nominal power of 70 to 100 mW depending on the output voltage needed for the patient. The battery life is on the order of 40 to 80 hours. The printed circuit board contains three integrated circuit packages and three internal variable adjustments which are the carrier, symmetry, and clipping controls. These controls are set so that the proper output voltage levels do not exceed the patient's uncomfortable

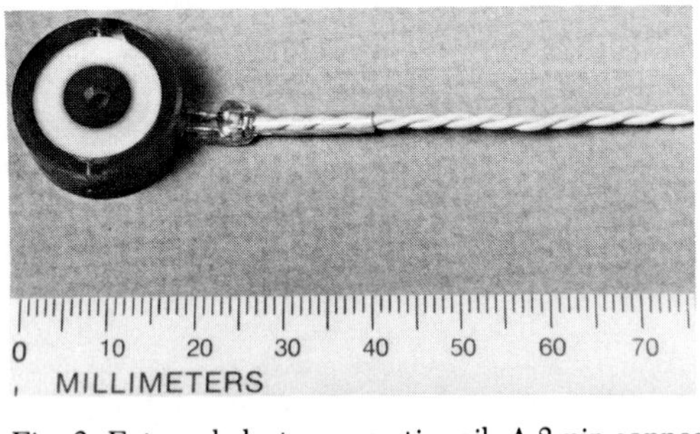

Fig. 2. External electromagnetic coil. A 2-pin connector is affixed to the core for easy electrical connection to the coil.

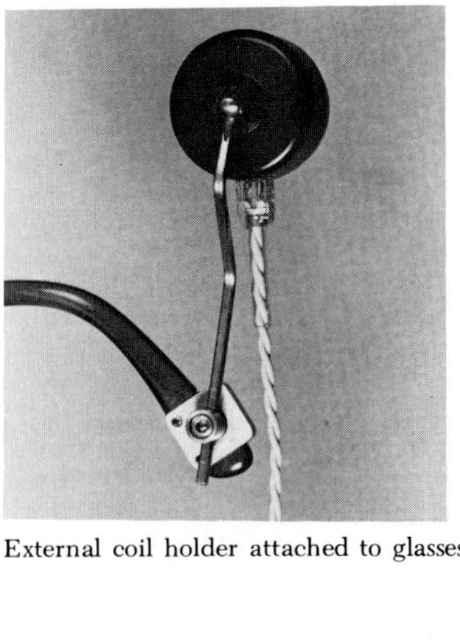

Fig. 3. External coil holder attached to glasses temple piece.

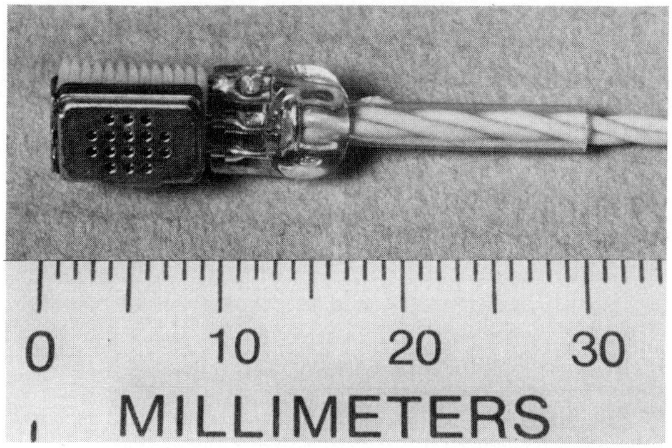

Fig. 4. Subminiature electret type microphone. A miniature 3-pin connector is affixed to the back of the microphone for easy electrical connection.

loudness level. There are also two external controls which may be adjusted by the patient. The "V" or volume control is used to adjust the output level up to an internally preset maximum, and the "M" or modulation control is used to adjust the sensitivity of the modulation level. There is a miniphone plug used for the external stimulator coil and a 3-prong female plug for the microphone input. These connectors allow easy replacement of the wire cords in case of damage or normal wear. The dimensions of the metal case are 12.7 cm x 6.35 cm x 2.54 cm, and it is made of aluminum. The construction is in two parts. One is a shallow drawn case which houses the circuit board and batteries, and the other is a protective lid which covers the entire top opening. The stimulator weighs 150 g by itself and with alkaline batteries weighs approximately 240 g.

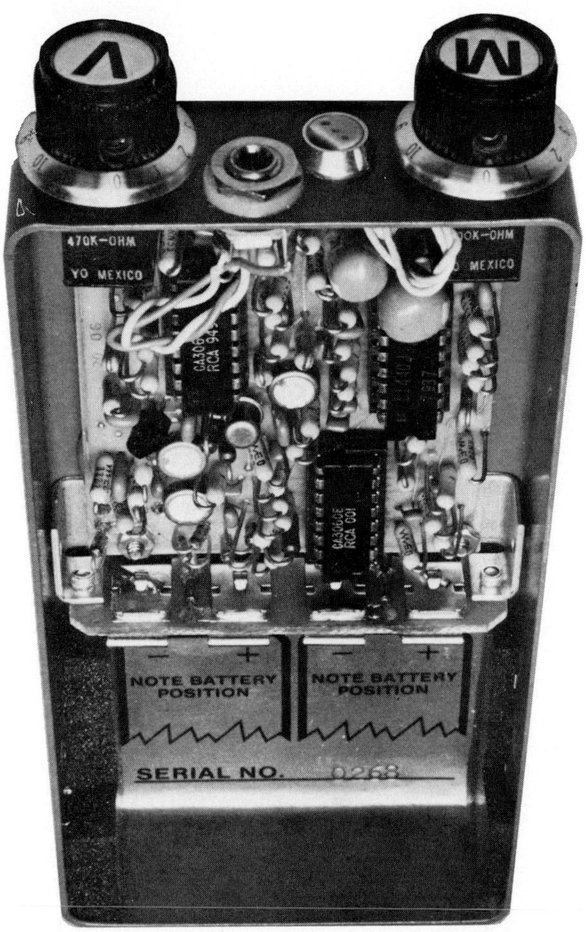

Fig. 5. Cochlear implant stimulator. Back has been removed to show printed circuit board and battery compartment.

SIGNAL FLOW

The following discussion will trace the signal as it moves from the microphone to the cochlear electrode, describing the signal processes and transformations that occur along the way. Figure 6 is a block diagram of various sections of the signal path that will be addressed. The microphone, preamplifier and filter, 16 kHz oscillator, AM modulator and the output buffer are all part of the external electronic package where the majority of the signal transformation occurs. The external and implanted coils will be considered together as a loosely coupled transformer. Finally, some data on the electrode characteristics will be given.

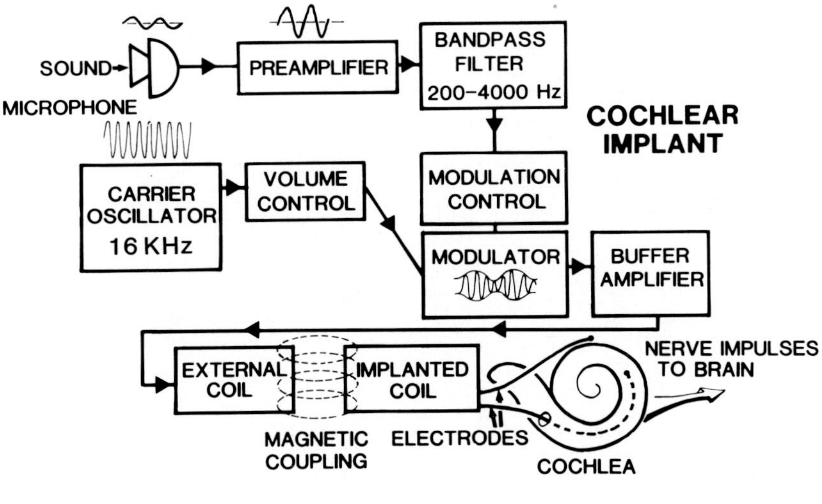

Fig. 6. Block diagram of cochlear implant signal processing scheme.

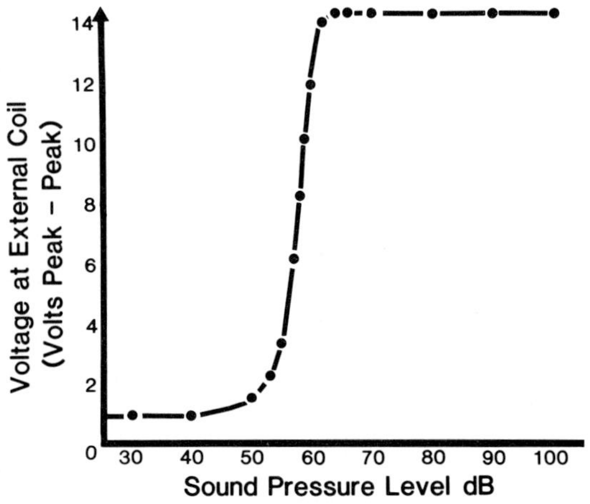

Fig. 7. Output of stimulator to external coil in relation to sound pressure level input at the microphone, for sine-wave signals. Stimulator was set for a threshold of 1 V peak-to-peak and a clipping level at 14.3 V peak-to-peak.

The microphone, preamplifier and filter are straightforward systems and need little description. The electret microphone with standard operational amplifier circuitry provides more than adequate fidelity. Following the preamplification is a bandpass filter. It has approximately 15 dB per octave high and low frequency rolloffs and 3 dB cut-off frequencies of about 200 and 4000 Hz. The filter is included to remove some of the sounds that might annoy and confuse the user. The total gain from the microphone to the modulator is controlled by the "modulation control." This primarily varies the sensitivity of the device. Increasing the gain allows lower intensity sound to be heard at the cost of increased background noise and distortion.

Unlike the preamplifier and filter, the 16 kHz AM modulator has unusual characteristics. The circuitry itself, however, is not complicated. A 16 kHz signal is generated by a free running multivibrator, while the modulation is accomplished by a voltage divider network with a field effect transistor (FET). The audio signal changes the resistance of the FET, in turn varying the amplitude of the 16 kHz signal. The unusual feature is the highly nonlinear nature of this modulator. The modulator is the only section of the signal pathway up to the electrode that is nonlinear. Figure 7 is a graph of a typical voltage amplitude at the output of the external unit versus the sound pressure level at the microphone. The external unit was set to the threshold of 1 V peak-to-peak and a clipping level of 14.3 V peak-to-peak. This input-output characteristic holds for all input frequencies within the bandpass of the filters.

The modulator function may be viewed as three separate regions. The first region is at very low input levels. In Figures 7 and 8 this region is for inputs less than about 45 dB SPL. At these input levels the 16 kHz signal is held at a low level, referred to as the "carrier level." Typically the carrier level is 10% of the maximum level. Input level changes in this region have little effect on the output.

The second region is for input acoustical levels between about 45 and 65 dB SPL. In this region the output to the external coil increases relatively greatly with small increases in the input level.

The third region is for input acoustic amplitudes of about 65 dB SPL or greater. In this region the output is a series of bursts of the 16 kHz signal, synchronized with the input signal. The amplitude of the signal is at a fixed level referred to as the "clipping level." In between the bursts of 16 kHz, the signal is near zero. For acoustic levels greater than 75 dB, increasing input amplitude increases the fraction of the period during which the 16 kHz is on, in other words the duty cycle is increased, but the maximum amplitude stays constant.

The nonlinearity characteristic of the modulator leads to a predictable perceived loudness to the patient; signal levels lying within the first region are below the patient's threshold. As signal levels in-

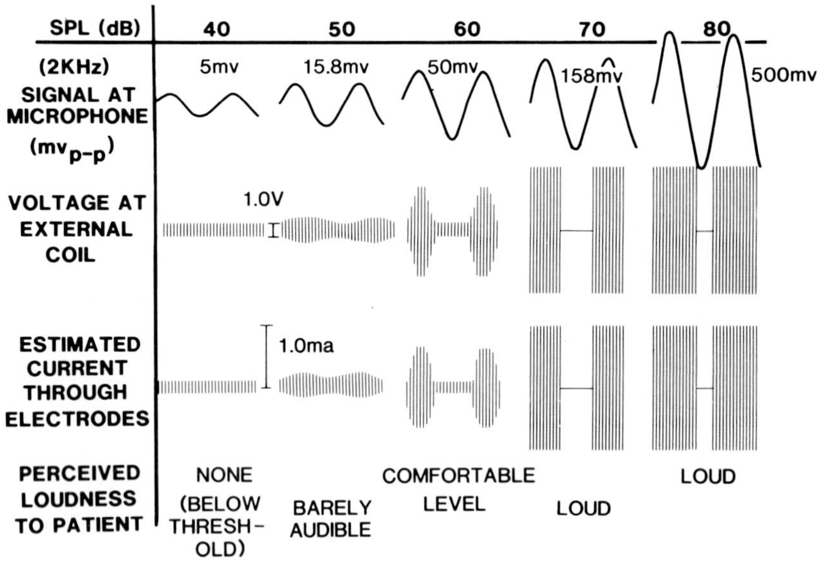

Fig. 8. Relationship of signal intensity at the microphone to voltage at external coil, current at the electrodes, and perceived loudness for a 2000 Hz signal.

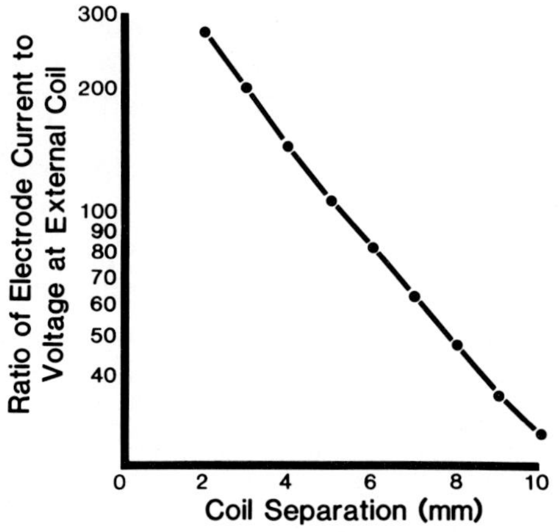

Fig. 9. In vitro estimate of the ratio of electrode current to voltage at the external coil for a 16 kHz sinusoid, as a function of the distance between the internal and the external coils.

crease through the second region, the patient perceives a rapid loudness growth. After the signal level passes into the third region, the patient perceives only minimal loudness increases. It is possible that another mapping from input amplitude to perceived loudness might prove superior for discrimination and this is a current area of research.

Following the modulator is a buffer amplifier. Constructed of operational amplifiers and emitter follower circuitry, the buffer drives the external coil with an amplified version of the modulator output. The buffer drives the coil differentially. For example, as one terminal of the coil goes up to 1 V, the other terminal goes down 1 V. Since the power source is two 9 V batteries, theoretically a maximum of 36 V peak-to-peak voltage could be applied to the coil. Actually, because of variations in battery voltage and voltage drops in the buffer, about 23-36 V is the maximum peak-to-peak voltage that can be consistently applied to the external coil.

The volume control functionally works to vary the gain of the buffer amplifier. In the circuit, the volume control is accomplished by varying the amplitude of the oscillator output. In series with the volume control is an internal control making it possible to set the full on volume equal to the patient's maximum comfortable level.

The external coil and the internal implanted coil are, of course, physically distinct and different, but electrically they can be treated as parts of one transformer. The coupling coefficient between the coils is quite low over the normal range of skin thicknesses. This results in the impedance of the external coil as seen by the buffer amplifier being equal to the impedance of the coil alone. Likewise the internal impedance driving the electrode is that of the internal coil. The coupling coefficient, and hence internal voltage and current, drops off as the coil separation increases or the two coils are misaligned. Using a model for the electrode impedance (to be discussed below) and the assumption that the skin is transparent at these frequencies of magnetic fields, the ratio of the internal current to external voltage can be experimentally determined. This ratio is shown as a function of coil separation in Figure 9. The range of coil separation is a function of skin thickness and internal coil encapsulated thickness, and has been estimated to range from 3.2 to 6 mm in most implanted patients.

The coil system in use, unlike more sophisticated transmission designs such as FM transmitters, has some disadvantage in its sensitivity to misalignment and separation and perhaps power transfer efficiency. However, the simplicity of having only a single coil with no other electronic component as the implanted part is a strong case for continuing to use it. Work is underway on new coil designs that have improved efficiency and less sensitivity to misalignment.

The last item in the signal flow path to the scala tympani is the electrode itself. Actually, of course, there is a pair of electrodes, the larger one in the eustachian tube serving as a "ground" for the scala tympani electrode. Because the electrodes are connected directly to the implanted coil, the long-term average potential applied across the electrode is zero. The surface area of the electrode is quite large so that the charge and current densities are much smaller than many other functional nerve stimulating electrodes in use. Estimates of the actual charge density are discussed in detail in Berliner.[1]

The electrode impedance was measured on one patient who had the electrodes directly accessible via a percutaneous plug. The measured impedance is shown in Figure 10 (Edgerton BJ, Spelman F, personal communication). Measurements were ob-

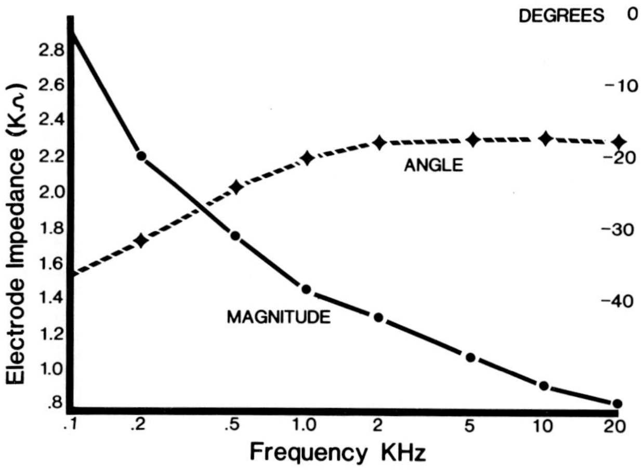

Fig. 10. Electrode impedance, magnitude and phase as a function of frequency obtained on one patient by direct measurement via a percutaneous plug.

tained using sinusoidal signals at voltage levels of 10 to 70 mV rms.

Using the data on electrode impedance and a measurement of the coil separation, the current in the electrode can be roughly estimated. The coil separation is determined by measuring the change in the inductance of the external coil caused by its proximity to the internal coil. This inductance change can then be correlated empirically to coil separation. Using these techniques, the data of Figure 8, showing current levels in the electrode for a representative patient, have been calculated.

FUTURE DIRECTIONS

There are many engineering improvements that are being pursued. Several aspects of the signal processing are being explored. For example, systems using differently shaped nonlinear compressors are being tried and evaluated using audiologic and psychoacoustic measures. Also, experiments are being conducted on the possibility of giving an analog signal to the electrode in place of the 16 kHz amplitude modulated signal. Many convenience engineering features are being addressed. Several new coil designs have been constructed that show better transmission efficiency. Work at House Ear Institute and elsewhere[2] has shown the feasibility of incorporating permanent magnets in the coils to provide for holding the external coil in place. The other major convenience feature in progress is to simply reduce the size of the external unit. This will require major redesign of the package and redesign of the circuitry to reduce the complexity and power required.

REFERENCES

1. Berliner KI. Risk versus benefit in cochlear implantation. Ann Otol Rhinol Laryngol 1982; 91 Suppl 91:90-8.

2. Dormer KJ, Richard GL, Hough JVD, Nordquist R. The use of rare-earth magnet couplers in cochlear implants. Laryngoscope 1981; 91:1812-20.

AUDIOLOGICAL RESULTS WITH THE COCHLEAR IMPLANT

MARGARET A. THIELEMEIR, MA
JUDY A. BRIMACOMBE, MA
LAURIE S. EISENBERG, MA

Audiological test results from 135 adult, profoundly deaf, single-electrode cochlear implant subjects are presented. Unaided, aided, and cochlear implant warble-tone and speech detection thresholds have been analyzed, as well as word, word stress, and environmental sound discrimination scores. Results indicate that implant thresholds are significantly better than aided thresholds at all frequencies tested and for speech detection. Also, word, word stress, and environmental sound discrimination scores are all significantly better with the implant than with a hearing aid. Although the implant does not provide speech discrimination, subjects report that it does provide valuable speech and sound awareness, which aids in speechreading and voice monitoring. A small group of subjects has shown that an implant in the poorer ear can also be successfully combined with a hearing aid in the better ear. The audiological test results clearly show that the implant is a viable alternative for the profoundly deaf.

The single-electrode cochlear implant has been used successfully by profoundly deaf adults at the House Ear Institute since 1972. This paper describes the audiologic tests that have been used to assess auditory performance of these profoundly deaf subjects. Current test results are presented, and the benefits and limitations of the implant from the subject's perspective are discussed.

Initial testing and observation revealed that cochlear implant subjects could recognize some environmental sounds but scored at zero or chance level on standard speech discrimination measures. For example, a speech detection threshold could be obtained at 50 to 60 dB SPL (approximately 35-45 dB HL, re ANSI 1969[1]); but a speech (spondee) reception threshold (SRT) could not be obtained with an open list of familiar spondees regardless of the presentation level. Implant users could discriminate speech stimuli if a small, closed list was used, or if stimuli varied in durational or intensity cues rather than pitch cues. Subjects could differentiate between two or three consonant-vowel-consonant words (CVCs) that differed in voicing or manner of articulation, eg, "shake" vs "shame" (unvoiced plosive vs voiced continuant) or "pass" vs "lass" vs "sass" (unvoiced plosive vs glide vs unvoiced sibilant). A few implant users were able to achieve an SRT using a 10-spondee list and the method advocated by Wilson et al.[2]

The task facing the cochlear implant team was to develop tests to objectively measure what implant users subjectively reported. Tests were needed to 1) select candidates for the implant project, 2) compare performance across different groups of implant users, and 3) monitor performance over time to assess long-term effects of electrical stimulation in the cochlea. Such clinical research tests were developed and tried in two areas: speech perception and environmental sounds recognition. In addition, a protocol was established for measuring speech and warble tone thresholds and uncomfortable loudness levels (ULLs) as well as direct electrical thresholds and ULLs. The tests described here were developed for postlingually deafened adults who have a clear memory of speech and environmental sounds. Test development for prelingually and congenitally deafened adults and children will be discussed later.

TEST MATERIALS

SPEECH PERCEPTION TESTS

A variety of speech discrimination tasks have been tried, including a 6-item closed-list spondee recognition test, a conversational sentence differentiation task, a monosyllable-trochee-spondee discrimination test and a CVC rhyme discrimination test. The rhyme test is a 50-item task in a 4-item forced-choice format that allows limited feature analysis. The test is described in Eisenberg et al[3] and Norton and Edgerton (unpublished). Rhyme test and spondee recognition test results show significantly better performance with an implant than with a hearing aid for both independent and matched groups.[4,5] The rhyme test is currently being revised and is not part of the current clinical trials test battery.

Monosyllable-Trochee-Spondee (MTS) Test. This test was developed by Erber and Alencewicz[6] and consists of four simple words in each of three stress categories: monosyllable, trochee (a 2-syllable word with stress on the first syllable, eg, "butter") and spondee (a 2-syllable word with both syllables equally stressed). We refer to this test as the MTS Test (Table 1).

The test utilizes a forced-choice format, with the subject referring to an instruction sheet which lists the 12 answer choices. Prior to test administration, the subject hears each test item once in the order printed on the instruction sheet. Following this familiarization process, each word occurs twice, in random order, for a total of 24 items. Each test item may be repeated once if necessary. A ready light is flashed to alert the subject to each stimulus presentation. There are six randomizations of the original recorded stimuli.

The subject's responses are recorded on an error matrix and analyzed in two ways: number of words correctly identified, and number of stress categories correctly identified (ie, the number of monosyllables identified as monosyllables plus the number of trochees identified as trochees plus the number of spondees identified as spondees).

ENVIRONMENTAL SOUNDS TESTS

The original Hearing Rehabilitation Research Center (HRRC) Environmental Sounds (ES) Test[7] consisted of 30 sounds derived

TABLE 1.
MONOSYLLABLE-TROCHEE-SPONDEE (MTS) TEST

Monosyllables	*Trochees*	*Spondees*
Bed	Button	Baseball
Cat	Chicken	Birdhouse
Duck	Doctor	Popcorn
Pig	Turtle	Toothpaste

from commercially available records or recorded especially for this test. It was a 5-choice forced-choice task. Answer choices were randomly selected from seven sound categories such that each foil came from a different category. All sounds used were readily identified by a group of ten normal-hearing listeners. There were two forms of the test and two randomizations of each form.

In 1979, one form of the test was reduced to a 20-item task. The five test items most commonly chosen correctly in the 30-item test were removed, as were the five sounds that were most commonly missed. Sounds were rerecorded to be more equal in overall intensity and, where possible, in length. Four randomizations of the 20-item test were taped. The ES Test scores reported in this paper are for the revised 20-item form of the test.

Subjects are instructed to read the five answer choices and circle the one they hear. Sounds are presented once, and may be repeated once if necessary. Guessing is encouraged. A ready light is flashed while each sound is presented, and the tester shows numbered cards to the subject to indicate the test item number. These visual cues are used to augment the subjects' minimal auditory capabilities, particularly during preoperative testing.

EVALUATION PROTOCOL

PREOPERATIVE TEST PROCEDURES

Subjects being evaluated for the cochlear implant undergo an extensive audiological assessment. Unaided speech detection and warble tone thresholds and ULLs for octaves and interoctaves of 250-4000 Hz are measured binaurally under headphones. An ascending method is used to measure thresholds, and all data are recorded in decibels SPL (re 20 μPa). A most comfortable loudness level (MCL) is established, if possible, and the MTS Test is administered binaurally at MCL. Warble tone thresholds and ULLs are used to select the gain and maximum power output characteristics of hearing aids to be used in this evaluation. Aids are selected to give the greatest amount of gain without exceeding an individual's discomfort level. If no ULLs are measured, testing is done with the aid adjusted to not exceed a 130 dB SPL output at any frequency.

At least two aids are tested on each side. The volume control of the aid is adjusted until spondees presented at 70 dB SPL, an average speech level, are judged to be comfortable. Once the gain of the prosthesis is set, the test battery is given. The battery consists of a spondee detection threshold (SDT); warble tone thresholds at 250, 500, 1000, 2000, and 3000 Hz; the MTS Test; and the ES Test. The MTS and ES Tests are presented at 70 dB SPL. If the output of the aid is at the allowable limit (130 dB SPL) and the subject does not detect spondees at 70 dB SPL or below, the MTS and ES Tests are not given. Warble tone thresholds are assessed, and a second aid is tried.

Subjects selected for implantation are profoundly deaf and demonstrate poorer performance with a hearing aid than implanted subjects can demonstrate. They must also meet medical and psychological criteria and express realistic expectations for the implant.

POSTIMPLANT TEST PROCEDURES

Audiometric Test Battery. The same audiometric test battery that was given preoperatively is readministered postoperatively with the subject using the cochlear implant. It is given during basic guidance (the initial rehabilitation period approximately 2-3 months after surgery), six months after basic guidance, and annually thereafter. Tests are presented at 70 dB SPL and subjects adjust their units until speech at 70 dB SPL is heard comfortably.

Electrical Measurements. In addition to audiometric testing, the performance of the implanted coil is assessed directly without going through the stimulator device. Two measurements are made: electrical threshold, and electrical ULL. These measurements are used to 1) initially set the stimulator unit, and 2) to monitor the performance of the internal coil/auditory system over time.

Test stimuli are produced by the HRRC Threshold Tester, a battery-operated, portable waveform generator. The output of the Tester goes directly to the subject's external coil, which is held in place over the implanted coil. Electrical threshold is measured using an ascending technique with a pulsing (500 ms repetition rate) 16 kHz sine wave, similar to the carrier wave in the current stimulator units. The stimulus used for ULL measurements is a pulsing 16 kHz sine wave modulated by a 1 kHz sine wave, similar to the stimulus produced when a 1 kHz sine wave is picked up by the stimulator unit microphone. Measurements are read on an oscilloscope and reported in peak-to-peak voltage across the external coil.

RESULTS

Audiological test results from 135 adult House Ear Institute and coinvestigator cochlear implant subjects have been analyzed. For this group, the mean age at time of implantation was 46 years (range = 18 to 75 years). The mean age at time of profound bilateral deafness was 31 years (range = birth to 64 years). The cause of deafness for this population was ototoxic drugs (11%), otosclerosis (20%), meningitis (15%), unknown (14%), and other (40%; including Menière's disease, congenital lues, trauma, rubella, and Usher syndrome). Characteristic onset of hearing loss was classified as progressive (48%), sudden (36%), fluctuant (4%), and congenital (12%).

TABLE 2. MEAN, STANDARD DEVIATION. MEDIAN, AND RANGE OF PREOPERATIVE, UNAIDED WARBLE TONE AND SPEECH DETECTION THRESHOLDS FOR COCHLEAR IMPLANT PATIENTS (N = 135)

	Frequency (Hz)					
	250	*500*	*1000*	*2000*	*3000*	*SDT*
Mean* (SD)	123 (12.2)	122 (10.9)	125 (9.0)	127 (7.0)	129 (5.5)	120 (13.2)
Median	NR	NR	NR	NR	NR	NR
Range	(76-NR)	(87-NR)	(97-NR)	(104-NR)	(100-NR)	(70-NR)
%NR	71	57	76	84	94	56

In dB SPL re: 20 μPa.

SDT - Spondee detection threshold; NR - No response.

*Mean thresholds were calculated using 130 dB SPL when no response was obtained.

TABLE 3. MEAN, STANDARD DEVIATION, MEDIAN, AND RANGE OF PREOPERATIVE WARBLE TONE (N = 73) AND SPEECH DETECTION (N = 91) THRESHOLDS FOR THE IMPLANTED EAR, WITH A HEARING AID

	Frequency (Hz)					
	250	*500*	*1000*	*2000*	*3000*	*SDT*
Mean* (SD)	86 (22.8)	83 (25.2)	84 (28.0)	99 (26.2)	108 (23.4)	68 (22.3)
Median	81	80	75	NR	NR	64
Range†	(45-NR)	(40-NR)	(39-NR)	(42-NR)	(36-NR)	(35-NR)
% NR	25	23	40	62	78	14

In dB SPL re: 20 μPa.

*Mean thresholds were calculated using 120 dB SPL when no response was obtained.

†The minimum values presented here reflect the inability of several patients to benefit from conventional amplification for reasons other than threshold responses (eg, recruitment, poor discrimination).

AUDIOMETRIC TEST FINDINGS

Table 2 presents the mean and median unaided, preoperative auditory thresholds for this profoundly deaf population, in the ear that was implanted. A large percentage of these subjects had no measurable hearing at the frequencies tested (250, 500, 1000, 2000, 3000 Hz).

Subject selection for cochlear implant surgery is dependent, in part, upon auditory thresholds and performance with a powerful hearing aid (eg, Unitron 960P, Widex S20). Table 3 displays the mean and median preoperative, aided warble tone thresholds for 73 patients, in the ear to be implanted. Mean aided auditory thresholds ranged from 83 to 108 dB SPL across the frequencies tested, with a large percentage of "no responses" (NR) at the limit of the audiometer at 2000 and 3000 Hz. Due to the difficulty of finding an appropriate value to substitute for NR, median values were also calculated for the aided warble tone and speech detection thresholds. These values, which are not affected by the substitution of an arbitrary value (in this case, 120 dB SPL) for NR, are similar to the mean values obtained, but better reflect the large percentage of NRs at 2000 and 3000 Hz.

Mean audiometric thresholds with the cochlear implant are shown in Table 4. They ranged from 53-64 dB SPL across the frequencies tested. It can be seen that these thresholds are consistent from the subjects' basic guidance period to their most recent audiological testing. It is also interesting to note the lack of NRs to auditory input with the cochlear implant activated. This is in direct contrast to the high percentage of NRs obtained from these same subjects with conventional amplification. An analysis of subjects' auditory thresholds with hearing aids and with the cochlear implant reveals that implant thresholds are significantly better at all frequencies and for speech detection ($p \leq .001$).

The figure presents unaided, hearing aid, and cochlear implant auditory thresholds in relation to both the average speech spectrum and to normal hearing. It can be seen that for the majority of these subjects, auditory thresholds with a hearing aid do not permit detection of speech, while implant thresholds are within the speech range.

SPEECH AND ENVIRONMENTAL SOUNDS DISCRIMINATION

Speech and environmental sounds discrimination scores have been obtained for 86 subjects with the

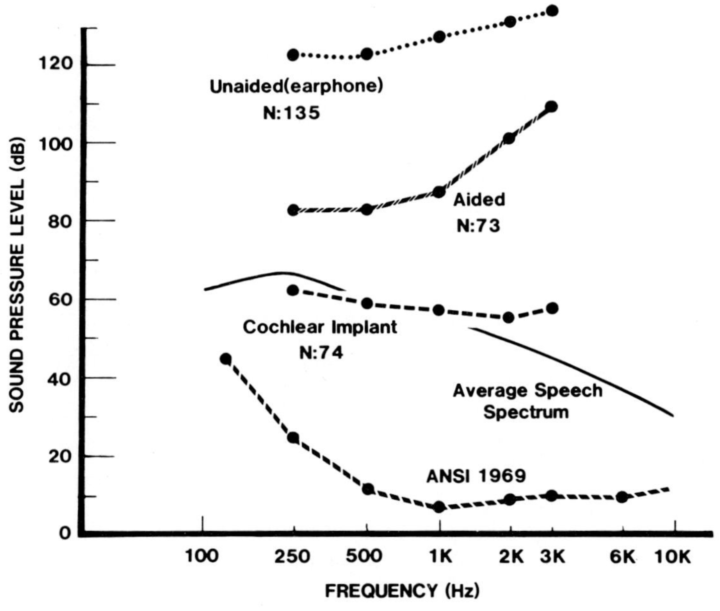

Mean unaided, hearing aid, and cochlear implant warble tone thresholds in decibels SPL. Also shown are SPL values for the average speech spectrum at about 1 m (from Davis[8]) and for normal hearing thresholds as defined by the American National Standards Institute (ANSI-1969). Unaided and ANSI-1969 values are measured under earphones; aided and implant thresholds are for sound-field conditions.

TABLE 4. MEAN, STANDARD DEVIATION, AND RANGE OF WARBLE TONE AND SPEECH DETECTION THRESHOLDS WITH COCHLEAR IMPLANT AT BASIC GUIDANCE TRAINING (N = 74) AND MOST RECENT AUDIOLOGICAL TESTING (N = 65)

	Frequency (Hz)					
	250	*500*	*1000*	*2000*	*3000*	*SDT*
Basic Guidance						
Mean	64	60	58	57	60	56
(SD)	(7.9)	(7.7)	(7.5)	(7.7)	(7.2)	(6.8)
Range	(43-87)	(40-75)	(39-72)	(38-73)	(42-75)	(40-72)
% NR	0	0	0	0	0	0
Recent*						
Mean	61	56	56	57	59	53
(SD)	(9.2)	(8.1)	(6.8)	(7.5)	(8.9)	(5.6)
Range	(36-79)	(40-80)	(39-78)	(40-76)	(35-85)	(40-65)
% NR	0	0	0	0	0	0

In dB SPL re: 20 μPa.

*Most recent test was an average of two years postimplant.

cochlear implant. Mean MTS scores were 34.5% and 73.9% for word and stress discrimination, respectively. The mean ES Test score was 55.1%. A comparison was made of the MTS and ES discrimination scores obtained from a select subgroup of 37 subjects who were tested both preoperatively with hearing aids in the ear to be implanted and postoperatively with the cochlear implant. This subgroup included only those subjects who were able to detect speech with a hearing aid at levels better than 70 dB SPL. Since the majority of the subjects tested had SDTs poorer than 70 dB SPL, this subgroup represents those subjects with the best preoperative aided thresholds. Despite this, Table 5 shows that MTS word and stress scores, as well as ES Test scores, were all significantly better with the cochlear implant than with a hearing aid ($p \leq .001$).

A paired comparison of 28 subjects' basic guidance and most recent MTS and ES Test scores indicated that discrimination with the implant improved over time (Table 6). Both speech and environmental sound discrimination scores were higher after at least six months experience with the implant.

ELECTRICAL MEASUREMENTS

Mean electrical thresholds and ULLs with the cochlear implant are presented in Table 7. Over time, mean thresholds were very consistent, despite the large intersubject variance. The large range in subjects' thresholds can be attributed to several factors. First, skin thickness varies between subjects and affects the efficient transduction of the electrical signal from the external to the internal coil. Appropriate coil alignment is a second factor affecting subjects' thresholds over time. Slight misalignment of the external coil increases the amount of power required for threshold perception. The composition of the induction coil system is a third factor which accounts for a great deal of the variance in electrical measurement data. Some coils are now being used that contain a magnet. These magnet systems increase the impedance of the induction coil system, thus requiring more power to achieve a percept of hearing.

As shown in Table 7, mean ULLs tend to vary to a greater degree than mean thresholds as a function of time. Also, the range of subjects' ULL measurements is larger. The variability in ULL measurement is also attributable to patient skin thickness, coil alignment, and type of coil used (ie, magnet). Additionally, there is a psychological element to the ULL measurement which increases intersubject variability. For example, congenitally deaf subjects tend to describe sound as being uncomfortable at lower voltage levels than the postlingually deafened.[9]

CORRELATIONAL ANALYSES

Auditory Thresholds. Statistically, it was found that cochlear implant auditory thresholds and electrical measurements did not correlate with any of the following: 1) age at onset of profound deafness, 2) years of profound deafness, or 3) age at time of cochlear implant. In addition, unaided warble tone thresholds and thresholds with a powerful hearing aid were not predictive of cochlear implant auditory thresholds.

TABLE 5. PAIRED COMPARISON OF DISCRIMINATION SCORES WITH HEARING AID AND COCHLEAR IMPLANT

			Mean Percent Correct		
Test	*N*	*Chance*	*Hearing Aid*	*Cochlear Implant*	*t test*
MTS Word	37	8	18.0	33.8	$p \leq .001$
MTS Stress	37	33	50.6	72.4	$p \leq .001$
Environmental Sounds	32	20	34.1	53.3	$p \leq .001$

TABLE 6. PAIRED COMPARISON OF DISCRIMINATION SCORES WITH COCHLEAR IMPLANT AT BASIC GUIDANCE AND AT MOST RECENT AUDIOLOGICAL TESTING

		Mean Percent Correct		
Test	*N*	*Basic Guidance*	*Recent**	*t test*
MTS Word	28	27.5	35.4	$p \leq .02$
MTS Stress	28	70.8	79.8	$p \leq .004$
Environmental Sounds	29	54.3	63.3	$p \leq .004$

*Most recent test was an average of two years postimplant.

TABLE 7. MEAN ELECTRICAL THRESHOLDS AND UNCOMFORTABLE LOUDNESS LEVELS IN VOLTS PEAK-TO-PEAK, WITH COCHLEAR IMPLANT, OVER TIME

	Threshold			ULL		
	N	Mean	Range	N	Mean*	Range
Basic guidance	87	3.0	(0.5-17.0)	50	14.0	(2.2-33.0)
Six months	42	2.6	(0.7-13.0)	23	13.7	(5.2-31.0)
One year	27	2.4	(0.5-8.0)	24	12.6	(3.3-31.0)
Most recent†	28	2.7	(1.0-8.8)	27	15.0	(4.0-31.0)

*Mean uncomfortable loudness levels (ULLs) were calculated by substituting 33 V when ULL could not be measured using equipment with a maximum output of 32 V (p-p).

†Most recent test was an average of two years postimplant.

Speech and Sound Discrimination. A moderate correlation (r = .44, p≤.05) was found between MTS stress discrimination scores with a hearing aid preoperatively in the ear to be implanted and with the cochlear implant. The same was found for ES discrimination. That is, those subjects who scored higher on these measures with a hearing aid were also the highest scoring cochlear implant subjects. This relationship may reflect the ability of certain subjects to use minimal auditory cues (eg, rhythm and intensity) better than others to discriminate word stress and environmental sound patterns. No relationship was found between MTS word discrimination with a hearing aid and with the cochlear implant.

MTS word and stress scores and ES discrimination scores were found to correlate negatively with years of profound deafness (r = −.40 to −.54, p≤.01). That is, discrimination scores were found to be poorer as years of profound deafness increased. This inverse relationship suggests that both experience with sound and auditory memory may play an important role in cochlear implant subjects' ability to effectively discriminate different elements of speech and environmental sounds. Physiological differences in the state of the remaining auditory system may also play a role in these statistically significant, though small, relationships.

WHAT THE SUBJECT HEARS: SUBJECTS' PERSPECTIVE

Postlingually deaf subjects have provided a vast amount of information regarding what the implant sounds like and how that sound can be used. Subjects are amazingly consistent in their reports. They generally describe the sensation received from the implant as sound perceived deep within the ear, as sound should be. In contrast, these same subjects typically describe the sensation they received from hearing aids as sound coming toward or being "forced" into the ear.

Sound, as it is perceived by implant users, is not described as normal, but rather as having a "mechanical" or "static-like" quality. Subjects consistently report that initially everything sounds the same; "scratchy," "tinny," "crackling," or "metallic." Patients have likened the sound to "the buzz of an electric drill," "humming on a comb covered with waxed paper," or "the speech of Donald Duck." All voices initially sound the same, and the subject may find his or her own voice particularly foreign and disturbing.

It is at this point that guidance from a rehabilitation staff member is essential. By demonstrating how to make use of the simple timing and intensity cues provided by the implant, the subject is given a basis for interpreting different sounds. In time, a maturation or learning occurs. Voices and speech patterns begin to sound different from other environmental sounds. As early as the second day, subjects begin noticing differences between men's and women's voices, and their own voice becomes more acceptable. With experience, subjects are able to recognize many sounds occurring within the environment, without visual clues.

The quality of sound also changes over time. Subjects report that the initially monotone signal becomes more tonal in quality, with some pitch variation. Sound is still not described as "normal," but rather as "more natural." Subjects describe speech as "muffled," "like talking into a hanky," or like a radio tuned slightly off station. For example, the subject may know someone is talking, but he or she can't quite understand the words. Some environmental sounds are described as sounding very natural. These sounds include running water, footsteps, knocking on a door, clapping, hitting or banging on metal, shuffling cards, and crumpling paper.

Many subjects find competing noise, such as background traffic, particularly troublesome during the early stages of implant use. However, as different sounds take on specific qualities, it becomes easier to focus on the signal. Background sounds seem less dominant.

Subjects report that sometimes when speechreading family or friends, they feel as if they were hearing normal speech. But when the speaker turns away, the speech "changes" dramatically to become unintelligible. Subjects also report that once in a while an occasional word or words may come through very clearly even when the subject does not see the speaker's face. This can happen over the telephone, when the speaker is in another room, while watching television, or when someone is speaking from behind the subject. Subjects report the very strong feeling that the word sounded exactly like it used to before they lost their hearing.

Although the implant does not provide speech discrimination, it does enhance communication. Subjects consistently report that their speechreading abilities are improved when the implant is activated. Families and friends confirm the subjects' reports. Further, implant users know when people are speaking, and do not inappropriately interrupt others' conversations. The volume and pitch of the subjects' voices tend to be more appropriate, and this adds to their increased confidence in social situations.

Implant subjects report hearing many sounds within the environment. From the warble tone threshold data it is clear why so many sounds can be detected. Most moderate and loud sounds, as well as some soft sounds, can be heard. Conversational speech, for example, can be detected in a quiet room at distances of 15 to 20 ft (4.5 to 6 m). Subjects subjectively report hearing sounds from outside the house such as trucks and cars coming from down the street and airplanes and helicopters flying overhead. Sounds from other rooms in the house are also typically reported. Experienced implant users report being able to detect two and three sounds occurring simultaneously, such as clock chime and cooking fan and water running; boss talking and traffic (outside) and radio; conversation and television and newspaper rustling; vacuum cleaner and dog barking in another room.

Many subjects enthusiastically praise the implant. However, they also report disappointments and dislikes. The major disappointment is in not being able to understand speech. Every subject is counseled prior to surgery regarding the limitations of the implant. Most, however, maintain some hope that they will be able to understand at least some speech. Also frustrating is the feeling that speech is on the verge of being understandable. Another common disappointment is music. One subject described it as "jumbled, like someone talking real fast in a lot of background noise . . . no tune to it." It has also been described as a "low rumble" or "clanking." On the other hand, subjects have reported being able to dance again because they hear the beat, or sing because they can hear themselves. Some subjects have even resumed playing musical instruments.

There are a number of sounds that are commonly disliked. These include such sounds as motorcycles, noisy cars, vacuum cleaners, and banging or hitting of metal. There are also situations where the implant is typically not helpful. These include watching television, following conversation in a group, and very noisy situations.

In spite of the limitations of the cochlear implant, most of the implanted subjects use the device all day long, every day. They frequently liken deafness to death and say that the implant makes them feel "alive" again. It brings them out of isolation and back into contact with a living world.

BINAURAL PROSTHESES: HEARING AID AND IMPLANT

During the selection evaluation, a candidate's aided thresholds and test scores are compared with those of implant users. The audiological criteria for implantation are met if the aided scores are equal to or poorer than the average implant user's scores.

What if a subject meets the criteria in one ear, but scores slightly better than implant users in the other ear? Can a cochlear prosthesis on the poorer side combine with the aided sound in the better ear to provide greater benefit than the aid alone? Will sound from the implant and aid in opposite ears merge or conflict?

Six postlingually deafened adult subjects (three male, three female; age range 35 to 51) successfully combine aid and implant in opposite ears and use both prostheses 12 to 16 hours per day. All subjects met audiological criteria for implantation in the poorer ear, but varied in aided performance in the better ear. Three subjects demonstrated aided MTS scores between the average and top implant user results, but scored zero on phonetically-balanced (PB) monosyllabic word discrimination lists (W-22s) presented under headphones at the most comfortable loudness level (MCL) or the limit of the audiometer. The remaining three subjects demonstrated more usable hearing in the nonimplanted ear. These subjects demonstrated aided MTS scores equal to or better than the best implant user score. One subject scored perfectly on the MTS test. These three subjects also demonstrated PB word discrimination scores under headphones of 50 to 65%.

TABLE 8. PERCENT CORRECT DISCRIMINATION SCORES FOR SUBJECTS USING HEARING AID IN BETTER EAR AND IMPLANT IN POORER EAR*

	MTS Word			*MTS Stress*			*Environmental Sounds*		
Patient	*CI*	*HA*	*CI + HA*	*CI*	*HA*	*CI + HA*	*CI*	*HA*	*CI + HA*
A	75	71	71	92	96	92	71	63	75
B	63	79	79	88	96	96	50	50	50
C	79	63	92	100	92	100	79	79	75
D	50	100	DNT†	96	100	DNT†	75	75	DNT
E	50	92	88	96	92	92	54	71	79
F	25	100	DNT†	83	100	DNT†	79	79	DNT

*Testing was done after six months of implant use in three conditions: implant alone (CI); hearing aid alone (HA); and implant and aid together (CI + HA).

†Did not test in CI + HA condition because HA alone scores were 100%.

TABLE 9. COMPARISON OF DISCRIMINATION SCORES IN THE IMPLANT-ONLY CONDITION FOR SUBJECTS WITH IMPLANT ONLY, AND SUBJECTS WITH IMPLANT AND HEARING AID

	Mean Percent Correct		
Subjects	*MTS Word*	*MTS Stress*	*Environmental Sounds*
Implant only (N = 37)	33.8	72.4	53.3
Implant and hearing aid (Testing done with implant only) (N = 6)	61.3	88.3	67.5

Subjects were tested in three conditions: aid alone, implant alone, and aid and implant together. Test results reveal that performance on the MTS and ES Tests is neither improved nor decreased for these subjects when sound from the implant is added to sound through the hearing aid (Table 8). Subjects report that addition of the implant does not necessarily make speech more understandable, but it does make sound "fuller," "sharper," and "adds depth." All report that soft sounds are easier to detect with the implant and aid than aid alone. Sound from the implant is described as "filling in the blanks" of frequencies not perceived through the aid. Subjects receiving primarily low-frequency signals through the aid are able to detect high-frequency sounds (up to 4000 Hz) through the implant. One subject receives high frequencies better than low frequencies through the hearing aid, and reports that the implant adds low-frequency perception. Most subjects reduce hearing aid volume when adding the implant. Most report that loud sounds are bothersome or uncomfortable through the aid but not through the implant.

Subjects that use aid and implant tend to perform better on discrimination measures with the implant alone than typical implant users. Table 9 reveals that aid and implant users perform better than implant-only users on MTS and ES Tests when both groups are tested in the implant-only condition. Preoperative unaided and aided scores for the implanted ear do not appear to be different between the two groups; and implant alone, warble tone and speech thresholds are within 2 dB at all frequencies. Therefore, it remains unclear what might account for this difference. Perhaps the continuing experience with minimal cues in the aided ear improves the ability of these patients to make use of the auditory information from the implant. Alternatively, it may be that these subjects do exceptionally well with hearing aids because they possess greater ability to use minimal cue information, and this ability serves them equally well for making use of the implant.

Pilot work with six cases reveals that the cochlear implant in the poorer ear can be successfully combined with a hearing aid in the better ear. The benefits and limitations of this binaural fitting need to be investigated more fully. However, the subjects seem to feel that there is enough added benefit to warrant wearing the hardware for two devices.

SUMMARY

Audiological results gathered on a large number of profoundly deaf adults clearly show that this select population can benefit significantly from the cochlear implant. Audiometric thresholds, environmental sounds discrimination, and speech and stress discrimination on a closed-list task are significantly better with the implant compared to the preoperative aided scores in the same ear.

Implant users report that sound through the implant allows identification of many environmental sounds, enhances speechreading and voice monitoring, and provides contact with sound that was unavailable through hearing aids. The implant does not allow speech discrimination on open-list tasks, and does not provide many benefits in noise. Despite the limitations of the cochlear implant, and the large size of the external device, the vast majority of the subjects are using it daily, many for all waking hours. A small group of subjects who could gain limited benefit from a hearing aid are successfully combining an aid in the better ear with an implant in the poorer, unaidable ear.

A number of speech and environmental sounds recognition measures were developed for the profoundly deaf population because standard speech discrimination tests were too difficult. The present results indicate that these tests are clinically useful for differentiating performance of profoundly deaf subjects, both in comparing hearing aids to implant and in comparing different aids. Many profoundly deaf subjects were found to be able to score above chance with conventional aids. These tests, however, were developed for postlingually deafened adult subjects who had an auditory memory of speech and sound, and are not appropriate for subjects with early childhood or congenital losses who do not have an extensive auditory memory. Test development for this population is continuing in two areas: 1) psychophysical tests which do not require extensive auditory memory, and 2) speech and sound differentiation tests which require training prior to administration. Tests are also being modified or developed for children.

The cochlear implant has shown itself to be a feasible prosthetic alternative for the profoundly deaf. Audiologic results demonstrate the ability of these subjects to perform significantly above chance on discrimination tasks and to detect sound at moderate to soft levels of intensity. This must be considered a substantial improvement over a world of total silence.

REFERENCES

1. American National Standards Institute Specification for Audiometers. ANSI 53.6-1969. New York: American National Standards Institute, Inc, 1970.

2. Wilson R, Morgan D, Dirks D. A proposed SRT procedure and its statistical precedent. J Speech Hear Dis 1973; 38:184-91.

3. Eisenberg LS, Luckey R, Norton NB, Berliner KI. A discrimination task for profoundly deafened adults: HRRC rhyme test. Presented at American Speech and Hearing Association, Chicago, 1977.

4. House WF, Berliner KI, Crary WG, et al. Cochlear implants. Ann Otol Rhinol Laryngol 1976; 85 Suppl 27:1-93.

5. House WF, Berliner KI, Eisenberg LS. Present status and future directions of the Ear Research Institute cochlear implant program. Acta Otolaryngol (Stockh) 1979; 87:176-84.

6. Erber N, Alencewicz C. Audiologic evaluation of deaf children. J Speech Hear Dis 1976; 41:256-67.

7. Norton NB, Berliner KI. Environmental sounds: test and training program for the hearing impaired. Presented at American Speech and Hearing Association, Chicago, 1977.

8. Davis H. Acoustics and psychoacoustics. In: Davis H, Silverman SR, eds. Hearing and deafness. New York: Holt, Rinehart, and Winston, 1970: 28.

9. Eisenberg LS. Use of the cochlear implant by the prelingually deaf. Ann Otol Rhinol Laryngol 1982; 91 Suppl 91:62-6.

PSYCHOELECTRIC MEASUREMENTS AND RESULTS FROM COCHLEAR IMPLANT PATIENTS

LAWRENCE F. HELMERICH BRADLY J. EDGERTON, PhD

Psychoelectric experiments, including threshold, uncomfortable loudness level, loudness growth and frequency discrimination were performed with six cochlear implant patients. All subjects used a single-channel transdermal induction coil implant system. Stimuli were presented directly to the external induction coil and not through a signal processing device. A method is reported in which current at the electrode is derived from voltage measures at the external coil. The derived thresholds were on the order of 1 to 120 μA peak-to-peak and are similar to those reported by other investigators. Loudness growth was more rapid for implant patients, being over twice that of normal listeners. Frequency difference limens were determined using both analog and 16 kHz amplitude modulated signals. Frequency discrimination was better with the analog system than with the 16 kHz amplitude modulated system. In general, below 100 Hz the patients' difference limens were essentially normal, but rapidly deteriorated until at approximately 600 Hz there was little frequency discrimination.

The cochlear implant (CI) research program at the House Ear Institute was developed to meet needs in two major areas: 1) clinical evaluation protocols which can be used in the selection and monitoring of patients, and 2) basic science studies which provide information for designing new or refined systems for neural stimulation. In this chapter, psychoelectric data are presented which have been collected to begin defining the limits and variability in perception among patients receiving single-channel cochlear stimulation. Basic experiments in the areas of intensity and frequency are reviewed, and a new method of estimating stimulus current levels at the implanted electrode site from voltages applied across the House-Urban transdermal magnetic induction system is described. In the following series of experiments, stimulation was achieved by routing sinusoids directly to the external induction coil without processing by the standard CI stimulator.

ELECTRICAL THRESHOLDS

Voltage, current, and charge or charge density have all been used by researchers to express threshold results. The use of different referents has made difficult the direct comparison of data across laboratories. Different stimulus referents have been used due to limitations imposed by the CI systems of some researchers, and by a lack of unanimity of opinion regarding the expression which best describes the stimulus characteristics eliciting the neural response. In general, when induction coil systems have been used to couple signals from external equipment to the implanted electrodes, voltage has been the unit of measure since coil characteristics and separation and alignment affect the signal transmitted to the implanted electrodes. In cases where direct connections exist between test equipment and implanted electrodes, current measurement is usually the method of choice. Charge levels, expressed in coulombs, can be calculated from a knowledge of current levels and stimulating frequency.

Electric threshold levels may vary as a result of stimulus waveform, electrode configuration and placement, or neural density and distribution. Merzenich et al[1] reported threshold data obtained for two patients with an intracochlear multiple bipolar electrode array. Trapezoidal stimuli were introduced directly and thresholds were expressed in volts. Thresholds varied from about 141 mV peak-to-peak (p-p) at about 25 Hz to about 42 mV at 100 Hz and then increased to slightly less than 1400 mV p-p at 10,000 Hz. House et al[2] reported thresholds for 12 patients for a 16 kHz sinusoid which ranged from 1.3 to 10 V p-p with a median of 3.2 V p-p. These values are consistent with the voltages reported in this monograph for our present CI system. Tong et al[3] have reported thresholds for pulsatile stimuli at rates of 200 and 1000 pulses per second (pps) for nine different intracochlear electrode sites. Thresholds were in the range of 60 to 70 μA across all electrodes but showed considerable variability among the sites of stimulation. At all electrodes, thresholds were higher for 200 pps than for 1000 pps.

Eddington et al[4] reported thresholds obtained from two patients (direct stimulation) with 6-electrode intracochlear arrays. Patients were stimulated with sinusoids and biphasic pulses. Thresholds for sinusoidal and pulsatile stimuli were similar across all electrodes. For sinusoids, thresholds ranged from 5-10 μA p-p at frequencies below 100 Hz. When pulsatile stimuli were used, thresholds were higher than for sinusoids (70-115 μA p-p at 25 pps and 40-90 μA p-p at 10,000 pps) and decreased as frequency increased. The difference between thresholds as a function of frequency for the sinusoidal and pulsatile stimuli is related to the amount of charge transferred per unit time with fixed pulse width stimuli versus sinusoids. Note that the find-

TABLE 1. ACTUAL AND ESTIMATED THRESHOLDS IN MICROAMPERES AT STIMULUS FREQUENCIES OF 0.2, 1, AND 16 kHz

Frequency (kHz)	*Actual Threshold (μA)*	*Estimated Threshold (μA)*
0.2	12	9
1.0	18	24
16.0	87	72

ings of Eddington et al do agree with those reported by Tong et al.

Procedure. Thresholds measured at the external induction coil reflect both the coil transduction properties and the actual electrical thresholds. The present induction coil system acts as a high pass filter with a 3 dB down point at about 1000 Hz. In addition to the filter characteristics, the power transmission across the coils drops as the square of the distance between them increases. Thus no definitive statements can be made regarding true thresholds unless an alternative procedure for estimating current at the electrodes is used.

In order to determine the thresholds in current at the internal electrodes, the coil separation, transfer function, and electrode impedance function must be established. Determination of the distance between the external and internal coils has been the major obstacle to estimating current levels at the electrodes in the House-Urban CI. Measurements of coil separation were achieved as follows. 1) The inductance of the external coil separated from the internal coil at distances ranging from 1 to 10 mm in 0.5 mm steps (L) was measured. 2) The inductance of the external coil alone (L2) was measured. 3) The ratio of L-L2/L was calculated. This ratio reflects the percentage of change in inductance as a function of coil proximity. Thus, by measuring inductance changes, the coil separation due to skin and tissue interposed (transparent to electromagnetic fields) can be estimated. Measurements were made with an HP 4274A multifrequency Inductance/Capacitance/Resistance meter at a frequency of 1 kHz and voltage setting of 0.5 V rms to determine the effects of the coil transfer function and electrode impedance characteristics. Model loads were built which fit the magnitude and phase angle of the impedance measured at the internal coil of a directly coupled patient for the frequency range from 50 to 20,000 Hz. For each coil separation from 1 to 10 mm (0.5 mm steps) a constant voltage was applied to the external coil and the current at the electrodes (under load) was measured.

Results. Recently the direct coupled patient whose impedance data formed the basis of our model loads was reimplanted with an induction coil system due to a failed percutaneous plug/electrode interface. Thresholds in voltage were measured at the external induction coil of our standard system. The procedures for estimating electrode current levels were applied and then compared to the pre-

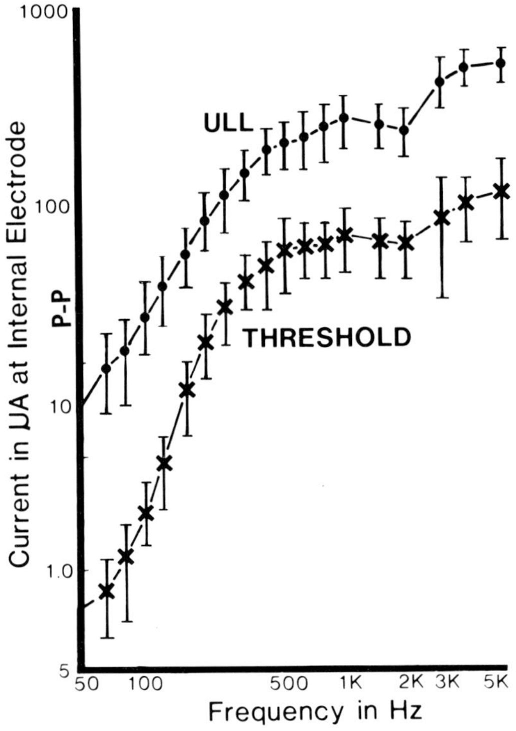

Fig. 1. Mean current (p-p) needed to obtain threshold and ULL as a function of frequency, for six implant patients.

viously obtained direct coupled thresholds. Table 1 presents the actual threshold current levels measured in a direct coupled condition and those estimated using the above procedure at 0.2, 1, and 16 kHz. Table 1 reveals that there was exceptionally good agreement between the actual and estimated thresholds.

Figure 1 presents the mean threshold current levels estimated at the internal electrodes for six patients. Test frequencies ranged from 50 to 6000 Hz. The current at the electrode was lowest at low frequencies and rose continuously as frequency increased until about 500 Hz, at which point the current remained steady out to 2000 Hz. From 2000 to 6000 Hz, the current increased rapidly. The current was lowest at 50 Hz averaging 0.9 μA p-p, and greatest at 6000 Hz averaging 118 μA p-p. The range of thresholds varied considerably depending on the stimulus frequency. The lower frequencies yielded ranges on the order of 2 to 5 μA p-p while the highest frequencies yielded ranges on the order of 70 to 100 μA p-p.

Comparison of the threshold data obtained in this study with the data reported by Eddington et al[4] reveals very similar results. For example, at 100 and 1000 Hz there were differences of only about 5 and 20 μA respectively between the results of Eddington et al and ours. This is noteworthy since the data obtained in the present investigation represent estimates of current levels and not actual direct-coupled measurements, and differences exist between the

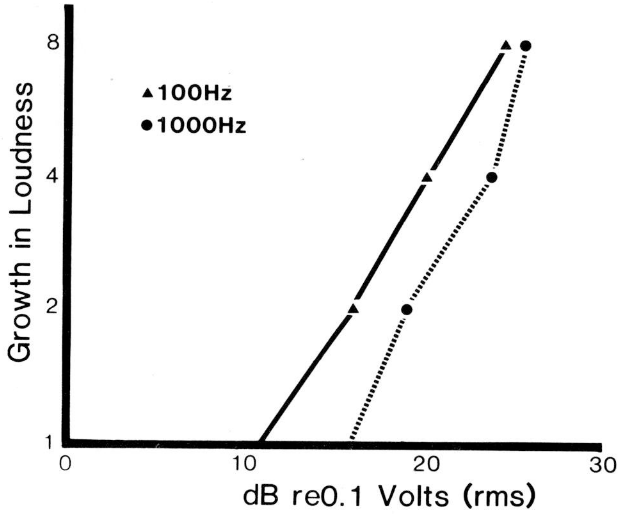

Fig. 2. Loudness growth functions for a single subject using 100 and 1000 Hz standards.

electrode configurations for the two studies. Thresholds are lower at all frequencies than have been reported for pulsatile stimuli.[3,4]

DYNAMIC RANGE

It has been hypothesized by Simmons[5] that the dynamic range, ie, the stimulus intensity range from threshold to discomfort level, may be an indicator of the number or distribution of the neurons excited by electrical stimulation. Researchers have reported dynamic ranges of 4 to 30 dB for sinusoidal and pulsatile stimuli.[2,4,6,7] Eddington et al[4] reported that with one patient the dynamic range was only about half as large for pulsatile stimuli (5-7 dB) as for sinusoids (12-15 dB). In addition, they found that dynamic ranges were "constant with stimulus frequency and remained so over the long term."

Procedures and Results. Threshold measurement procedures were previously described; only sinusoidal stimuli were used. Uncomfortable loudness level (ULL) was defined as the level that the patient "would not want to listen to for more than five minutes." The ULL was approached from threshold in approximately 100 mV (p-p) steps. The ULL was taken as the average of at least five ascending trials.

Figure 1 provides the averages and standard deviations for the ULLs at the frequencies from 50 to 6000 Hz. From the figure it can be seen that the ULL curve runs roughly parallel to the electric threshold curve across the frequency range. Comparison of the dynamic range across frequency reveals that it is about 20 dB for the low frequencies, decreases to about 11 dB by 250 Hz, remains constant up to about 4000 Hz at which point it gradually begins to increase. The standard deviations of the dynamic ranges were about 4 dB at the low frequencies, 2 to 3 dB over the middle frequencies and 3 to 4 dB at the highest frequencies. These results are in agreement with the findings of previous researchers.

LOUDNESS GROWTH

Michelson et al[8] determined the relationship between loudness and stimulus intensity for three cochlear implant patients. The patients were asked to rate the loudness of the stimuli on a scale ranging from 1 to 100. Michelson et al found that loudness increased logarithmically from threshold to ULL. This growth was much more rapid than the growth of loudness for normal listeners.

Procedures and Results. The loudness growth was obtained by asking a patient to determine when the loudness of a comparison tone was twice and half that of a standard tone. All results are an average of ten trials at each loudness level. The stimuli consisted of 500 ms sinusoids with 25 ms rise/fall time presented serially. The loudness functions for 100 and 1000 Hz are shown in Figure 2, and the loudness functions of other frequencies tested are similar to those in Figure 2. Loudness grows rapidly as the intensity of the stimuli increases. There is approximately a 2-fold increase in loudness for a 4 dB increase in intensity. It should be noted that the growth of loudness function for both low and high frequencies is essentially the same. Although it is difficult to compare the results of Michelson et al[8] to the present study, this study similarly found that loudness function increases logarithmically with increases in intensity, and that both functions increase more rapidly than for normal-hearing listeners. It should be noted that although the loudness growth function is not normal for CI patients, the

TABLE 2. MEAN AND STANDARD DEVIATIONS FOR FREQUENCY LIMENS (△f) at 125, 250, 500, 750, 1000, AND 2000 Hz STANDARDS FOR PULSED AND SINUSOIDAL STIMULI*

	Frequency (Hz)					
Waveform	*125*	*250*	*500*	*750*	*1000*	*2000*
Pulse						
△f (Hz)	9.35	71.70	100.50	96.30	285.20	224.30
SD	8.48	152.80	91.50	115.90	326.00	287.10
(N)	(19)	(16)	(11)	(7)	(10)	(14)
Sinusoid						
△f (Hz)	9.56	36.40	106.90	75.70	283.80	306.90
SD	12.80	48.10	137.50	—	456.00	496.40
(N)	(14)	(16)	(16)	(1)	(13)	(9)

*This table summarizes results which were obtained and reported for seven different sensation levels. Data were pooled for 12 patients. However, patients may be present in categories more than once, and all patients are not represented in each category. (From Bilger et al[11].)

intensity difference limen is on the order of 0.5 to 1 dB at comfortable loudness levels, ie, it is within the normal range.

FREQUENCY STUDIES

Frequency discrimination is requisite to high levels of performance on speech recognition tasks and therefore of considerable importance in the design of limited-channel auditory prostheses. In single-electrode neural stimulation, frequency resolution is limited by the ability of the nerve to follow or volley at high frequencies. It is not clear at this time, however, what the range of maximum volley rates is across CI patients, or what effects different stimulus waveforms have in maintaining neural synchrony at high repetition rates.

To access frequency perception among CI patients, both frequency difference limen and pitch scaling techniques have been used. Eddington et al[4] used biphasic pulses to determine difference limens for two subjects, one being postlingually deaf and the other prelingually deaf. The postlingually deaf subject obtained frequency DLs of approximately 25 Hz for frequencies from 25 to 400 Hz. The prelingually deaf patient, however, required changes of 50 to 80% of the test frequency to detect differences. Both patients were capable of correctly ranking (scaling) the pitch of 100, 175, and 300 Hz pulses across six intracochlear electrodes.

Herndon[9] reported frequency DLs for one subject implanted with a modiolar electrode. Using rectangular pulses, DLs of 3.5 to 23.5 pps at 100 pps, 9.5 to 45.5 pps at 200 pps, and 63 pps at 300 pps were found. These results were similar to the findings of Simmons,[10] who obtained DLs of 30 pps for stimuli from 50 to 300 pps. Herndon also reported that his patient could scale pitch, ie, increasing pitch with increasing frequency, up to a pulse repetition rate of approximately 300 Hz.

Using sinusoids, Merzenich et al[1] found discriminable hearing in implant patients up to 500 Hz. Difference limens in this study for one patient were 1 to 2 Hz at 100 Hz, 5 Hz at 300 Hz and 7 to 10 Hz at 500 Hz. A second patient revealed DLs of 30 Hz at 500 Hz. Pitch scaling experiments revealed that pitch increased as frequency increased rapidly up to about 400 Hz and then more slowly up to 1000 Hz. Beyond 1000 Hz pitch did not change with corresponding frequency increases.

Bilger et al[11] provided the most comprehensive report of CI patient frequency discrimination. Twelve patients with single-electrode devices were tested, 2 with analog systems and 10 with standard House-Urban CI systems. The stimuli included both pulses and sinusoids and were administered at seven different sensation levels. Unfortunately, the same patients were not evaluated under all conditions at specific test frequencies. Thus the variability of the data was very great. Table 2 presents data from the Bilger et al study on frequency difference limens for pulses and sinusoids with the sensation levels pooled. The test stimuli were 125, 250, 500, 750, 1000, and 2000 Hz. There was a wide range of variability for all stimuli. Performance got poorer as frequency increased for sinusoids and pulses, and in general both yielded similar frequency discrimination. Bilger et al noted that patients using the House-Urban CI systems performed better than the patients using the analog system.

Results reported by the above investigators reveal that below approximately 300 Hz, patients can discriminate frequency differences very well. However, from about 300 to 1000 Hz implant patients' frequency discrimination becomes markedly poorer, and above 1000 Hz there is little frequency discrimination. The pitch scaling experiments confirm the results of the frequency difference limen test and also reveal that above 1000 Hz virtually all signals have the same pitch although there may be some qualitative differences.

Procedure. Frequency difference limens were studied using analog and 16 kHz amplitude modulated and clipped stimuli. Six patients were studied. All testing was done at a "comfortable listening level" and the standard and comparison tones were adjusted to equal loudness prior to the frequency limen measurement. Loudness was controlled, since previous experience has demonstrated that pitch changes can occur with relatively small changes in signal intensity.[12]

Stimuli were presented in pairs with the standard tone at a fixed frequency and the comparison tone

TABLE 3. MEAN DIFFERENCE LIMENS IN HERTZ FOR FREQUENCY (△f), AND NUMBER OF PATIENTS SUCCESSFULLY COMPLETING THE TASK (N), FOR BOTH THE ANALOG AND 16 kHz AM SYSTEM

	Frequency (Hz)					
	50	*100*	*200*	*315*	*500*	*630*
Analog						
Ascending △f	1.5	4.8	19.5	46.2	105.0	70.0
(N)	(6)	(6)	(6)	(4)	(3)	(1)
Descending △f	2.0	4.6	12.7	29.2	88.3	115.0
(N)	(6)	(6)	(6)	(6)	(3)	(3)
16 kHz AM						
Ascending △f	6.7	11.0	25.0	50.0	260.0	—
(N)	(6)	(6)	(3)	(2)	(1)	—
Descending △f	2.5	6.2	25.0	20.0	55.0	—
(N)	(4)	(6)	(5)	(2)	(1)	—

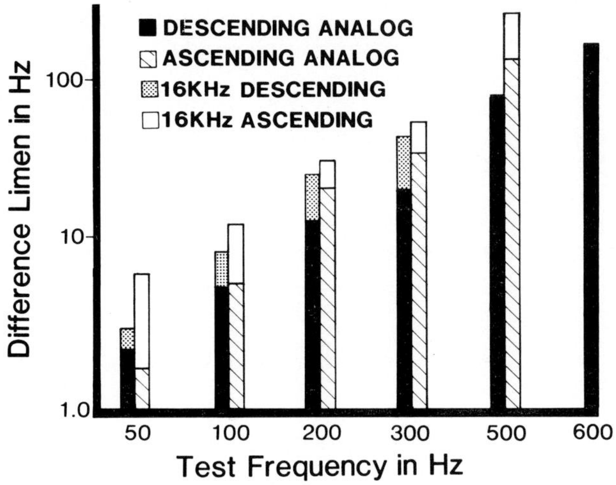

Fig. 3. Mean ascending and descending frequency limens (Hz) for analog and AM carrier stimuli at 50, 100, 200, 300, 500, and 600 Hz, for six subjects.

varied. Ascending and descending trials were used. For the standard tones 50, 100, 200, and 315 Hz, steps of 1 Hz were used. For the standard tones at 500 and 630 Hz, steps of 5 Hz were used. If the distance between the comparison tone and the standard tone exceeded one octave, the test was terminated.

Patients were instructed to determine whether the pitch of the comparison was lower or higher than the pitch of the standard. This procedure was used instead of same/different or 4-interval forced choice methods since some patients could discriminate differences at high frequencies, but could not specify the correct direction. The frequency limen was taken as the point at which the patients correctly responded to at least 75% of the comparison stimuli.

Results. Figure 3 presents the mean ascending and descending frequency limens for the analog and 16 kHz AM stimuli. In the figure, both ascending and descending frequency limens are presented since large differences existed between them, particularly at high frequencies. In addition to the asymmetry of ascending and descending frequency limens for CI patients, the frequency limens may not be obtainable at high frequencies. For example, in Table 3 the frequency limens are presented along with the number of patients from whom they were obtainable. As the standard frequency increased, the number of patients successfully completing the task decreased. Thus, presenting frequency discrimination results requires careful description of the ranges of patient performance, the technique of measurement, and the proportion of patients capable of completing the task.

When both the average of the frequency limens and the number of patients successfully completing the task are considered, the analog frequency limens were better at all frequencies than the 16 kHz AM frequency limens. The analog stimuli frequency limens were within normal limits at 100 Hz and below; at 200 Hz frequency limens were obtained from all patients although they were larger than normal (>5 Hz), and above 200 Hz the frequency limens increased rapidly, and not all patients could complete the task. For the 16 kHz AM system, the frequency limens were generally slightly poorer than normal even at the very low frequencies. At 200 Hz and above not all patients could complete the task. It should be noted that all of the preceding data are pooled across subjects. For one patient, frequency limens were consistently better for the 16 kHz AM system than for the analog, and for another patient, there was no appreciable difference in frequency limens between the two stimuli. It was also found that two patients could distinguish 1000 from 2000 Hz stimuli but that differences were qualitative, ie, no frequency limens could be obtained.

The results obtained for the analog and 16 kHz stimuli in this study are not congruent with the findings of Bilger et al[11] of better performance for the 16 kHz AM stimuli. However, it should be noted that the data from Bilger et al were obtained with patients using the House-Urban 16 kHz AM wearable stimulator while this study used stimuli direct from a wave generator to the external coil. In addition, the two analog patients studied by Bilger et al were using stimulators which were not described and different implanted electrode systems than were used in this experiment.

CONCLUSION

The present studies confirm that substantial limitations in frequency and intensity discrimination exist for single-channel CI users. However, clinical

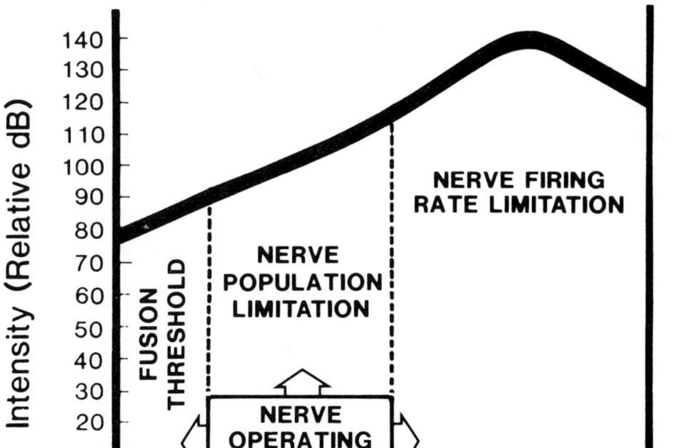

Fig. 4. Approximate discrimination limits and limiting factors for single-channel cochlear implant wearers superimposed on normal auditory perceptual space for frequency and intensity.

and experimental data generally indicate that temporal cues are perceived normally by CI patients. Figure 4 shows the normal auditory perceptual space for frequency and intensity as well as the approximate discriminable space for the single-channel CI user. It is clear that at the present time single-channel devices probably will not allow normal second and third formant tracking since frequencies are not easily discriminable above about 500 Hz. Since CI patients do have relatively normal gross temporal perception, and intensity distortion alone probably does not account for the limited speech recognition, poor frequency discrimination is considered the most limiting single factor.

A great deal of research has yet to be done to define alternative methods of increasing frequency discrimination using single-channels of stimulation. However, as our data have revealed, waveform may be an important consideration as well as electrical configuration. It remains to be seen if slight improvements in psychoelectric performance will result in improved performance in the real world context for single-channel CI users.

REFERENCES

1. Merzenich MM, Michelson RP, Pettit CR, Schindler RA, Reid M. Neural encoding of sound sensation evoked by electrical stimulation of the acoustic nerve. Ann Otol Rhinol Laryngol 1973; 82:486-503.

2. House WF, Berliner KI, Crary WG, et al. Cochlear implants. Ann Otol Rhinol Laryngol 1976; 85 Suppl 27:1-93.

3. Tong YC, Black RC, Clark GM, et al. A preliminary report on a multiple-channel cochlear implant operation. J Laryngol Otol 1979; 93:679-95.

4. Eddington DR, Dobelle DH, Brackmann DE, Mladejovsky MG, Parkin JL. Auditory prostheses research with multiple channel intracochlear stimulation in man. Ann Otol Rhinol Laryngol 1978; 87 Suppl 53:1-39.

5. Simmons FB, Walker MG, Mathews RG, White RL. Percepts and discrimination by auditory nerve stimulation: a summary of results and some proposals for nerve viability evaluation. In: McPherson DL, ed. Advances in prosthetic devices for the deaf: a technical workshop. Rochester, NY: National Institute for the Deaf, 1978; 271-4.

6. Michelson RP. Electrical stimulation of the human cochlea. Arch Otolaryngol 1971; 93:317-23.

7. Michelson RP, Merzenich MM, Schindler RA, Schindler DN. Present status and future development of the cochlear prosthesis. Ann Otol Rhinol Laryngol 1975; 84:494-8.

8. Michelson RP, Merzenich MM, Petit CR, Schindler RA. A cochlear prosthesis: further clinical observations; preliminary results of physiological studies. Laryngoscope 1973; 83:1116-22.

9. Herndon MK. Psychoacoustics and speech processing for a modiolar auditory prosthesis. Technical Report No. G906-5. Stanford Electronics Laboratories, Stanford University.

10. Simmons FB. Electrical stimulation of the auditory nerve in man. Arch Otolaryngol 1966; 84:24-76.

11. Bilger RC, Black FO, Hopkinson NT, et al. Evaluation of subjects presently fitted with implanted auditory prostheses. Ann Otol Rhinol Laryngol 1977; 86 Suppl 38:1-176.

12. House WF, Edgerton BJ. A multiple-electrode cochlear implant: preliminary test results. Paper presented at West Coast Cochlear Prosthesis Conference, Seattle, 1980.

VOWEL DISCRIMINATION WITH THE SINGLE-ELECTRODE COCHLEAR IMPLANT: A PILOT STUDY

LAUREL J. DENT, PhD

Eight normal-hearing individuals and six single-electrode cochlear implant users were asked to discriminate tape recorded pairs of spoken monosyllables consisting of 11 English syllabic nuclei /i, ɪ, e, ɛ, æ, a, ɔ, ʌ, o, ʊ, u/ bounded by the consonant frame. A same-different paradigm was used. Most normal-hearing subjects discriminated all pairs intended by the talker as different; two normal listeners confused monosyllables containing /a/ and /ɔ/. Cochlear implant users showed some intersubject variation, but for 4 of the 6 subjects, discriminations were consistent enough to allow the data to be pooled for analysis. The pooled data for these four subjects indicated that high front and high back vowels were discriminable from low vowels. The basis for the discriminations is difficult to evaluate, since the naturally spoken stimuli varied with respect to formant frequencies, fundamental frequency, intensity, and duration.

The single-channel cochlear implant has been demonstrated to be highly successful in reuniting the profoundly deafened adult with the world of sound.[1,2] Not only does the implant permit the user to reestablish auditory contact with the environment, but it greatly facilitates participation in spoken communication. With the implant, the user can monitor and hence better regulate his or her own voice, and speech reception is improved in several respects. First, lowered audiometric thresholds (relative to those measured prior to implantation) result in the cochlear implant user's ability to follow the voice of someone speaking at a comfortable conversational level. This reduces the amount of effort required on the part of both the talker and the listener to communicate and receive messages. Secondly, the implant provides the user with useful information to supplement what he or she obtains through speechreading. Thirdly, cochlear implant users do better with the implant than with a hearing aid on a task requiring the listener to identify which of four words he or she has heard, where the words differ only with respect to the initial or final consonant.[3]

In the present discussion we ask to what extent the single-electrode cochlear implant user can distinguish between spoken pairs of English monosyllables that differ from each other only with respect to the vowel nuclei. The ability to recognize the vowels of one's language is an important prerequisite for speech understanding. (The word "prerequisite" is appropriate because the identity of consonants is signalled in part by the formant transitions contained in the adjacent vocalic portions of the speech wave.[4,5]) For example, a spondee recognition test for the assessment of speech reception ability on the part of hearing-impaired listeners developed by Erber[6] has been asserted by Risberg and his associates[7] to be largely a test of vowel recognition.

To our knowledge, the present study represents the first report of cochlear implant user's ability to discriminate English syllable nuclei produced in a consonantal context by a human talker. (The "Vowel Test" of the Minimal Auditory Capabilities Test Battery is a closed set vowel identification test, rather than a discrimination test. Most recent results of cochlear implant subjects' performance on the Vowel Test are reported by Owens and Telleen[8] and by Herndon.[9]) Other investigators have reported the performance of cochlear implant users in discriminating synthetically generated vowels and vowel-like sounds. Bilger et al's results[10] show that cochlear implant users can distinguish between single-formant vowels having center frequencies characteristic of the high back vowel /u/ and of the low vowel /a/. Eddington[11] used two synthetically generated high vowels /i, u/ and one low vowel /a/ and reported that /i/ and /u/ were each discriminable from /a/ and from each other. (Subjects' best performance on this task was obtained with the use of a particular signal processing scheme for a multiple-channel electrode system.[11]) Clark and his associates[12] have reported that different "vowel-like sensations" have been induced by different parameters of electrical stimulation of the implanted electrodes in their subject, although no vowel discrimination tests have been administered.

Vowels produced by human talkers vary with respect to their spectral characteristics[13-16] and secondary characteristics.[16,17] Spectral characteristics include the frequencies of the first three formants, which correspond to the first three resonances of the vocal tract, spectral balance, and, in a consonant-vowel-consonant (CVC) context, the first-, second-, and third-formant transitions. That vowel quality is determined by the frequencies of the first three formants is amply documented.[13-15] High vowels are characterized by a low first formant, for example, while low vowels have a relatively high first formant. Spectral balance refers to the distribution of energy throughout the amplitude spectrum. For high front vowels energy is concentrated in the high-frequency region of the spectrum, for low central vowels in the middle-frequency range, and for high back vowels in the low-frequency region.[16] In a single consonantal context, different vowels show different formant transitions to the adjacent consonants.[18,19] These three properties of vowels are considered to be primary because they are crucial for identification of vowels by normal listeners. That is, changing one of these characteristics by a sufficient amount will cause the listener to perceive a change in vowel quality.

The secondary characteristics of vowels are the voice fundamental frequency, duration, and intensity of the vowels. These three parameters are observed to vary systematically with changes in vowel quality.[16,17] For instance, low vowels produced by a human talker tend to be characterized by lower fundamental frequency, greater intensity, and greater duration than high vowels. This generalization seems to hold for vowels of many languages,[17] and therefore these secondary attributes are considered intrinsic to the vowels they characterize (although it is certainly possible for humans to produce vowels with secondary characteristics other than the values considered to be "intrinsic" to each vowel). As such, they constitute potential contributors to the identities of these vowels.[20-22]

Synthetic approximations to English vowels can be produced with or without appropriate values of secondary characteristics. It might be argued that, when presented with two synthetic vowels of the same duration, intensity, and fundamental frequency, regardless of any spectral differences between the vowels, a listener is not being given a fair chance to identify the sounds as speech sounds, ie, as sounds emanating from a human vocal tract, because the vowels are not produced in the way that they would be in nature (Lea W, personal observations).

A certain amount of confusion between spoken vowels adjacent in the vowel triangle (as defined by, say, an F1-F2 plot) is expected on the part of normal listeners, and most normal listeners seem to be able to identify certain vowels with greater accuracy than others.[13] It has been shown that synthetically produced vowels are more accurately identified by normal listeners if they are embedded in a CVC context than if they are presented in isolation.[23]

The two foregoing considerations suggest that a test of the ability to distinguish vowels as it is applied to the perception of human speech should be based on stimuli that provide the listener with all of the cues which are naturally available to a human listener when he or she decodes speech produced by a human talker. (We recognize that in order to answer certain types of questions definitively, tests of discrimination of synthetic stimuli may be more appropriate.) Equipped with these assumptions, we constructed a test requiring a subject to discriminate between tape recorded pairs of spoken monosyllables that consisted of 11 English syllable nuclei bounded by a single consonantal frame.

METHODS

Two groups of listeners participated. Eight normal-hearing native speakers of English, four males and four females, comprised one group. Six cochlear implant users, all profoundly hearing-impaired native English-speaking listeners, made up the second group. Three were female and three were male. Normal-hearing listeners ranged in age from 24 to 52 years with a mean of 33 years. The hearing-impaired listeners' ages ranged from 39 to 63 years with a mean of 51 years. Tables 1 and 2 list some of the characteristics of the six cochlear implant users. All subjects have bilateral profound hearing loss. It can be seen that there was no attempt made to match these subjects for etiology of deafness, age of profound loss, or length of experience with the implant (Table 1). Four of the six subjects had had their right ear implanted (Table 2), and of these, two had some residual hearing in the left ear, in which they customarily used a hearing aid (although the tests reported here were administered via the implant only). All of the hearing-impaired subjects were right-handed. They also had in common the fact that they were all postlingually deafened adults who used their implants virtually all day every day (Table 2).

The instrumentation and calibration procedures differed for presentation of stimuli to normals and cochlear implant users. For presentation to normal listeners, the output of a tape deck (Ampex ATR-700) was routed to an amplifier (Crown D75) and then fed to a speaker (Allison 2043) in a double-walled sound suite (IAC-400 series). To calibrate the level of stimulus presentation on different testing occasions, we recorded a 1000 Hz tone on a section of the audio test tape preceding the recorded speech materials. The experimenter adjusted the amplification level to one the normal subject identified to be a comfortable listening level. The level of the calibration tone was registered by a sound level meter (General Radio 1933 Precision Sound Level Meter). Readings for the eight normal subjects in the pilot study varied from 57-76 dB SPL.

For presentation to the cochlear implant users, the output of a tape recorder (Ampex ATR-700) was amplified (Crown D75 Am-

TABLE 1. COCHLEAR IMPLANT SUBJECTS FOR PILOT STUDY

Subject	*Age*	*Sex*	*Age at Profound Loss*	*No. Years Deaf*	*Etiology*
1	53	F	29	24	Ototoxic drugs
2	63	M	52	11	Meningitis
3	39	M	**	—	Cochlear otosclerosis
4	53	F	44*	—	Cochlear otosclerosis
5	46	F	**	—	Cochlear otosclerosis
6	51	M	30	21	Ototoxic drugs

*Gradual loss becoming profound at the age listed.

**Subjects 3 and 5 both have progressive hearing losses that have become worse very recently. They still have some residual hearing, so age at profound loss is not applicable.

TABLE 2. COCHLEAR IMPLANT SUBJECTS FOR PILOT STUDY

Subject	*Implanted Ear*	*Length of Experience With Implant*	*No. Hours Daily Implant Use*	*Hearing Aid in Unimplanted Ear*
1	R	7 yr	14-16	No
2	L	1 yr	14-16	No
3	R	4 mo	14-16	Yes
4	L	2 yr	14-16	No
5	R	1 mo	10-14	Yes
6	R	7.5 yr	12	No

TABLE 3. COCHLEAR IMPLANT DISCRIMINATION PERFORMANCE

Subject	*Same Items*	*% Correct Same*	*Different Items*	*% Correct Different*
1	55	93	550	50
4	55	78	550	46
5	55	89	550	50
6	55	90	550	62
2	44	70	440	47
3	44	18	440	89

plifier) and routed to the input of a standard hearing aid test box (Bruel and Kjaer 4212). A microphone (Knowles miniature) was placed in the test box, and the output of the microphone (Bruel and Kjaer 2.5 cm [1 in] condenser microphone 4133) adjacent to the first allowed monitoring of the sound pressure in the test box on a measuring amplifier (Bruel and Kjaer type 2609). All stimuli were delivered at a level of 70 dB SPL as measured for the 1000 Hz calibration tone.

The speech materials for the pilot study consisted of 9 English words and 2 nonsense words, for a total of 11 stimulus types. These are composed of the following 11 English vowels in a /b_t/ context: /i, ɪ, e, ɛ, æ, a, ʌ, ɔ, o, ʊ, u/. Of course, /bat/ and /but/ do not constitute lexical items of English. Each stimulus was combined with other stimuli including itself, for a total of 12 stimulus frames. The order of the 121 stimulus frames was randomized, and a list of the pairs was drawn up.

The list was read by a male talker who sat in a double-walled sound suite (IAC-400 series). A microphone (Electrovoice RE-15) was positioned approximately 30 cm from the talker's mouth. The signal was recorded on a tape recorder (Ampex ATR-700) at 7.5 inches (19 cm)/s. An intrastimulus interval of approximately 200 ms was used, and the interstimulus interval was approximately three seconds. There was a pause of approximately 20 seconds after every 20 items. The talker uttered the individual tokens as naturally as possible. Therefore there was variation in duration and intensity of the tokens. There was some effort, however, to utter the words on a consistent pitch, in order to avoid the possible signaling effect of falling intonation at the ends of the groups of 20 pairs. Still, the fundamental frequency of the talker's voice did vary to some degree, often providing an additional cue for discriminability between items in a stimulus pair. The plosive at the end of each stimulus was exploded.

Each subject was tested individually. The subject was seated in the sound booth. For the normal subjects, a comfortable listening level was determined by the method of limits, and for the cochlear implant users, by the method of adjustment, ie, the user adjusted the controls on his or her own stimulator unit. The normal subjects took the test without practice, while the cochlear implant users were given one presentation of the test list as practice. The normal subjects were given the following instructions:

> You will hear a list of word pairs. For each pair of words that you hear, please decide whether the words are the same or different, and indicate your decision by putting an X through the S for "same" or through the D for "different" on your answer sheet. After 20 pairs there will be a long pause. There are 121 pairs in all.

The cochlear implant users were given these instructions:

> You will hear a list of word pairs. For each pair of words that you hear, please decide whether the two words sound the same or different to you, and tell the person running the test either "same" or "different." Each word is a one-syllable word. Do not be concerned with *what* the words are. We just want you to say whether they are the same or different. If you are not sure, please make a guess. After each 20 pairs there will be a long pause.
>
> Don't worry about making mistakes. Even normal-hearing people have made mistakes on this test. Besides, we learn from your mistakes. They tell us what has to be done to improve the implant. So sit back, relax, and just do the best you can. First we will do a *practice* test. If there is time today, we will do another test. If it is too late, we will repeat the test another day.

Each normal subject took the test once. The test was administered at least four times to each cochlear implant user. The normal subjects recorded their own judgments on a response sheet. The cochlear implant subject communicated his or her response for each pair either by signing or mouthing the words "same" or "different." The subject's responses were recorded on an answer sheet by the experimenter, who sat outside the booth watching the subject through the window.

RESULTS AND DISCUSSION*

The results take the form of matrices with 11 rows and 11 columns, or 121 cells. Since each of 11 vowels was combined with each other vowel including itself, 11 of the pairs (on the diagonal) are the same, and there are 110 different pairs. On each occasion that a subject took the test, he or she had one chance to judge each same pair and two chances to judge each different pair (if the ordering of the members of each pair is disregarded).

The lexical items are arranged along the matrix in the following fashion: high front vowels are at the top, proceeding to low front vowels, then low back vowels, and finally to high back vowels at the bottom (as if we were to go around the periphery of the vowel triangle from high front to high back vowels). Across the tip, the same order is followed from left to right, so that high front vowels are on the left, low (front and back) vowels in the middle, and high back vowels on the right. This means that in the upper left corner of the matrix are the pairs consisting exclusively of high front vowels. The lower left corner contains the pairs of syllable nuclei that each consists of a high front vowel and a high back vowel, while the lower right corner contains the set of pairs of high back vowels. The pairs containing high front vowels and low vowels are along the bottom of the matrix. Low vowel pairs are to be found near the center of the diagonal.

The results for the eight normal subjects were pooled into an 11 x 11 confusion matrix. Every subject correctly labelled every pair intended as the same by the talker, with one exception (/bʌt bʌt/). Every pair intended by the talker as different was judged as such by every normal listener except two, who confused the items /bat/ and *bought*. This is not surprising, as there are several dialect areas in the country where no distinction is made between the vowels in *cot* and *caught*.[25]

There was some intersubject variation among the cochlear implant users' patterns of discrimination (Table 3). Four subjects took the test five times, had 55 chances to judge same pairs, and scored between 75-95% correct on these pairs. On the average they correctly identified about half of the different pairs

*These results have been discussed with a different emphasis in a presentation by Dent and Edgerton.[24]

as different. Two subjects took the test four times each and had 44 chances to judge pairs that were the same. Subject 2's performance resembles that of the other four subjects, but subject 3 clearly had some response bias toward the judgment "different." He correctly identified 89% of the different pairs as such, but only 18% of the same pairs did he correctly label as the same.

In spite of the fact that most cochlear implant users judged only about half of the different pairs correctly, the patterns of discrimination that they were able to accomplish were not random. Subject 1 took the test five times and so had ten chances to judge each pair of different monosyllables. This subject had little trouble discriminating monosyllables containing high and middle back vowels from those containing low vowels /æ/ and /a/, and was able to discriminate the words with high front vowels from the words with the low front vowel at a level better than chance.

Subject 2 took the test four times and hence had eight chances to judge each of the different pairs. Like subject 1, subject 2 was able to discriminate the monosyllables containing back vowels from those having low and middle front vowels, with a couple of exceptions. Also like subject 1, he discriminated the monosyllables with high front vowels from one with a low central vowel. In addition, subject 2 was able to discriminate the word containing the high front vowel /i/ from those containing high and middle back vowels. Furthermore there is some indication that *bought* (low back vowel) was distinguishable from syllables containing two higher back vowels. Finally there are two pairs *beat-bait* and */bʊt/-boot* which this subject was able to discriminate at a level higher than chance.

Subject 3 also took the test four times, so he had four chances to judge each same pair and eight chances to judge each different pair. As noted above, subject 3 seemed to have a response bias toward "different," as indeed practically every pair sounded different to him, including many of the pairs that the talker intended as the same.

Subject 4 took the test five times. (For the first two test trials, subject 4 used the stimulator unit to which she was accustomed, while for the last three trials she had been given another stimulator unit. The pattern of pooled results for the first two trials are slightly different from those for the last three.) This subject's discriminations patterned slightly differently from those of subjects 1 and 2 in that monosyllables containing the high back vowel /u/ seemed discriminable from virtually everything else. This subject was also able to discriminate the syllables containing the high front vowel /i/ from those with the back vowels. In addition, subject 4 discriminated between words containing back vowels and front vowels, between those with high front vowels and low vowels, and between high and middle back vowels and low vowels.

The last two subjects, 5 and 6, were the best subjects in terms of their ability to apply consistently the same label, same or different, to a given pair. Subject 5 accurately judged more same pairs as same than any other subject, followed by subject 6. At the same time, these two subjects also led the others in numbers of pairs consistently discriminated, subject 6 with the highest number of matrix cells representing pairs judged different each time they occurred in the test. Subjects 5 and 6 each took the test five times.

For subject 5, monosyllables containing high front vowels were discriminable from those containing low vowels. The word *bought* was distinguishable from nearly everything except *but* and *bat*. Syllables with back vowels were discriminable from those containing /æ/ and /a/, both low vowels. The syllable containing the middle front nucleus /e/ was distinguishable from those containing high back nuclei. There is some evidence that tense and lax syllable nuclei were distinguishable, as *bet* and *but* (lax nuclei) were discriminated from *bat* and */bat/* (tense nuclei) at a level higher than chance.

Subject 6 discriminated high front vowels and high back vowels from low vowels. Again there was evidence that tense/lax syllable nuclei could be discriminated by subject 6 (as by subject 5). Other

	beat	bit	bait	bet	bat	/bat/	/bʌt/	bought	boat	/bʊt/	boot
beat											
bit	18										
bait	32										
bet											
bat	47	68		63							
/bat/	82	82		68							
/bʌt/	42		58		63	76					
bought	60	74	55	55	42	37	47				
boat	29	60	47	66	95	92	55	79			
/bʊt/	50		63	42	89	97		71	26		
boot	39	66	79	58	97	97	68	89		34	

Fig. 1. Percentage of stimuli pairs judged different by cochlear implant (CI) subjects at a level higher than chance. Numbers have been entered in every cell that represents a pair that was discriminated at a level higher than chance by at least one of the four subjects. A blank cell indicates that no subject discriminated the pair in question at a level higher than chance. Dotted lines enclose those pairs that were discriminated at a level higher than chance by the aggregate of subjects. Circles represent those pairs that every one of the four subjects discriminated at a level above chance.

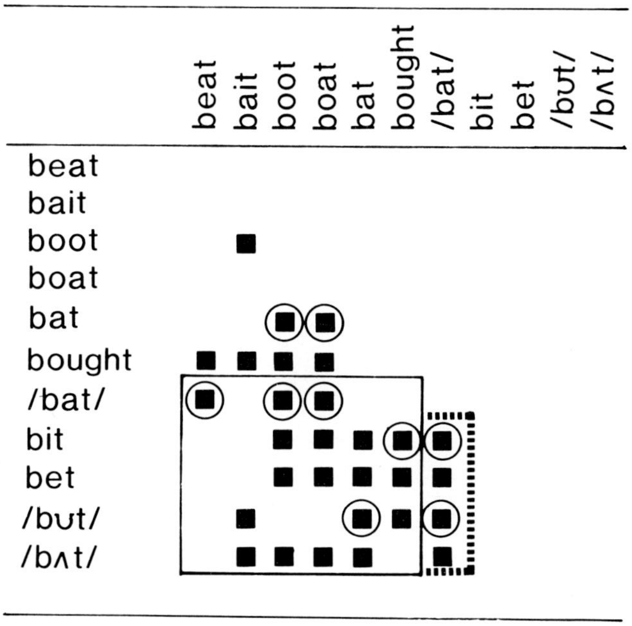

Fig. 2. Stimuli regrouped into tense and lax syllable nucleus classes. The pairs of monosyllables containing only tense vowels are represented in the upper left-hand corner, while the lax/lax syllable nucleus pairs are in the lower right. A line is drawn around all of the pairs in which one word contains a tense syllable nucleus, and the other a lax syllable nucleus. Squares represent syllable pairs that were discriminated at a level higher than chance by the aggregate of subjects. Circles represent pairs that were discriminated by every subject at a level higher than chance.

highly discriminable tense/lax pairs are *beat-bit, beat-/b ʊ t/, boot-bit,* and *boot-/b ʊ t/.* Subject 6 was able to distinguish the low back syllable nucleus *(bought)* from all other back syllable nuclei.

Four of the subjects' judgments seemed to pattern in a similar fashion, so the results for these four subjects are pooled in Figure 1. The number in each cell represents the percentage of pairs judged different by the four subjects. Looking at the cells containing circled numbers, we see that words with high and middle back vowels /u, ʊ, o/ are distinguishable from those with front and central low vowels. The class of back vowels are those with the first and second formants closely approximated to each other and located below the region of about 700-800 Hz (for a male talker). For the low vowels /æ/ and /a/, the first two formants are also relatively closely approximated, but the center of spectral gravity is higher for these two vowels. This observation is in agreement with the results reported by Bilger,[10] ie, cochlear implant users can distinguish between single-formant vowel-like stimuli with center frequencies approximating those of high back vowels and low vowels.

A second group of highly discriminable syllable nuclei are those composed of high front vowels and low vowels. The rest of the monosyllables that were discriminated at a level above chance by the aggregate are distributed around these two cores of highly discriminable words.

Finally, there is evidence that cochlear implant users can distinguish tense and lax syllable nuclei. Tense vowels, according to Jakobson et al,[26] are produced with "a longer sound interval" than their lax counterparts and with "a greater sum of the deviation of their formants from the neutral position." Thus tense vowels tend to be considerably longer than their lax counterparts. (In English, tense syllable nuclei are distinguished from lax ones on the basis of their distribution in syllables as well. Tense vowels can occur both in open syllables and closed syllables, whereas lax vowels can occur only in closed syllables. Thus words exist that end in /i, e, o, u/ but not in /ɪ, ɛ, æ, ʊ/.)

In Figure 2 we have regrouped the lexical items into tense and lax syllable nucleus classes. A line is drawn around all of the pairs in which one word contains a tense syllable nucleus, and the other a lax syllable nucleus. The rationale for including / ɔ / as a tense vowel[27] is that sound changes in English have had the effect of expanding the occurrence privileges of the phoneme / ɔ / so that it can now occur in word-final position, eg, *law, saw.* As a "phonologically tense" vowel, then, / ɔ / has been lengthened.[25] Similarly /æ/ has become long and tense in many dialects,[25] although it is still barred from occurring in open syllables. The case of /a/ is also special. This vowel can occur in open syllables of certain borrowings (eg, *Shah, spa*) but not in native English words. It happens, however, to be a longer vowel than the other vowels of English, in accordance with the universally observed tendency for low vowels to be longer than high vowels (all else being equal).[17] Therefore although /a/ is "phonologically lax," it is phonetically long in comparison to the other lax vowels of English. Pairs of monosyllables containing /a/ have been set off by a dotted line in Figure 2.

Every square shown in Figure 2 represents a syllable pair that was discriminated at a level higher than chance by the aggregate of subjects. Most of the squares fall within the boundaries of the demarcated class of tense/lax pairs.

From the data presented here we can say that monosyllables containing high back syllable nuclei, and, to a lesser extent, those containing high front syllable nuclei, can be distinguished from monosyllables containing low syllable nuclei by single-electrode cochlear implant users. In addition, cochlear implant users are able to distinguish words containing tense nuclei from those containing lax nuclei. In order to determine the basis for these discriminations, controlled studies with synthetic vowel stimuli are indicated.

ACKNOWLEDGMENTS — The author would like to thank Lori L. Eberle, Bradly J. Edgerton, PhD, and Laurie S. Eisenberg, MA, for their assistance in data collection, and Karen I. Berliner, PhD, Wayne A. Lea, PhD, and Hisashi Wakita, PhD, for helpful discussion during the course of the work.

REFERENCES

1. House WF, Berliner K, Crary W, et al. Cochlear implants. Ann Otol Rhinol Laryngol 1976; 85 Suppl 27:1-93.

2. House WF. Continued implantation of cochlear prostheses in a limited number of postlingually deaf subjects is appropriate. In: Snow B, ed. Controversy in otolaryngology. Philadelphia: WB Saunders, 1980:423-32.

3. Eisenberg LS, Norton NB. Consonant discrimination with the cochlear implant. Presented at 14th International Congress of Audiology, Acapulco, Mexico, 1978.

4. Delattre PC, Liberman AC, Cooper FS. Acoustic loci and transitional cues for consonants. J Acoust Soc Am 1955; 27:769-73.

5. Delattre P. From acoustic cues to distinctive features. Phonetica 1968; 18:198-230.

6. Erber NP. Pure-tone thresholds and word-recognition abilities of hearing-impaired children. J Speech Hear Res 1977; 17:194-202.

7. Risberg A, Agelfors E, Boberg G. Measurement of frequency discrimination ability of severely and profoundly hearing-impaired children. Stockholm Speech Transmission Laboratory, Quarterly Progress and Status Report 1975; 2:40-8.

8. Owens E, Telleen CC. Speech perception with hearing aids and cochlear implants. Arch Otolaryngol 1981; 107:160-3.

9. Herndon MK. Psychoacoustics and speech processing for a modiolar auditory prosthesis. Stanford University: unpublished doctoral dissertation, 1981.

10. Bilger RC, Black FO, Hopkinson NT, et al. Evaluation of subjects presently fitted with implanted auditory prostheses. Ann Otol Rhinol Laryngol 1977; 86 Suppl 38:1-176.

11. Eddington DK. Speech discrimination in deaf subjects with cochlear implants. J Acoust Soc Am 1980; 68 Suppl 1:885-91.

12. Clark GM, Tong YC, Bailey QR, et al. A multiple electrode cochlear implant. J Otolaryngol Soc Austral 1978; 4:208-12.

13. Peterson GE, Barney HL. Control methods used in a study of the vowels. J Acoust Soc Am 1952; 24:175-84.

14. Fant G. Acoustic theory of speech production, with calculations based on x-ray studies of Russian articulations. s'Gravenhage: Mouton, 1960.

15. Ladefoged P. Three areas of experimental phonetics: stress and respiratory activity, the nature of vowel quality, units in the perception and production of speech. London: Oxford University Press, 1967: 50-142.

16. Lea WA. Prosodic correlates of linguistic structures. In: Broad OJ, ed. Topics in speech science. Los Angeles: Speech Communications Research Laboratory, 1977: 394-564.

17. Lehiste I. Suprasegmentals. Cambridge, Mass: MIT Press, 1970.

18. Potter RK, Kopp GA, Green HC. Visible speech. New York: Van Nostrand, 1947.

19. Stevens KN, House AS. Perturbations of vowel articulations by consonantal context. J Speech Hear Res 1968; 6:111-28.

20. Ainsworth WA. Perception of synthesized vowels and h_d words as a function of fundamental frequency. J Acoust Soc Am 1971; 49:1323-4.

21. Ainsworth WA. Duration as a cue in the recognition of synthetic vowels. J Acoust Soc Am 1972; 51:648-51.

22. Stevens KN. Effect of vowel duration upon vowel identification. J Acoust Soc Am 1959; 31:109[A2].

23. Strange W, Verbrugge R, Shankweiler DP, Edman TR. Consonant environment specifies vowel identity. J Acoust Soc Am 1976; 60:213-24.

24. Dent LJ, Edgerton BJ. Cochlear implant users discrimination of vowels in /b_t/context. Presented at West Coast Phonetics Forum UCLA, March 1980.

25. Labov W, Yeager M, Steiner R. A quantitative study of sound change in progress. Philadelphia: US Regional Survey, 1972.

26. Jakobson R, Fant CGM, Halle M. Preliminaries to speech analysis: the distinctive features and their correlates. Cambridge, Mass: MIT Press, 1952.

27. Chomsky N, Halle M. The sound pattern of English. New York: Harper & Row, 1968.

EFFECTS OF THE SINGLE-ELECTRODE COCHLEAR IMPLANT ON THE VESTIBULAR SYSTEM OF THE PROFOUNDLY DEAF ADULT

LAURIE S. EISENBERG, MA
JAMES R. NELSON, MD
WILLIAM F. HOUSE, MD

Twenty-two profoundly deafened adults, implanted with the single-electrode cochlear implant, were involved in a study to observe the effects of cochlear electrical stimulation on the vestibular system. Previous investigators had found evidence that the implant might disrupt postural stability. As there had been no general complaints of dizziness or dysequilibrium by the implant subjects, a study was undertaken to replicate the earlier study and to compare the results to more standardized procedures. A Sono-Postural Test was devised from the Ataxia Test Battery for the testing of balance with and without an auditory prosthesis. Electronystagmography was also performed on the subjects before and after surgery as a means of monitoring vestibular status over time. Results from these tests indicate that the single-electrode implant does not disrupt the balance system to any significant degree. In fact, evidence indicates that postural stability may actually improve with the cochlear implant activated.

Because of the close proximity of the vestibular apparatus to the cochlea any deliverance of an electrical stimulus to the hearing mechanism may also activate the balance system. As early as the beginning of the 19th century, Ritter[1] and Augustin[2] independently published reports of vertigo being evoked as a result of an electric current sent through the head. Purkinje[3] additionally noted nystagmus being elicited and equilibrium disrupted due to galvanic stimuli delivered to the labyrinth. The issue must therefore be of concern to those involved in the study of implanting electronic prosthetic devices as an aid to the profoundly deaf.

The House Ear Institute (HEI) in Los Angeles has been involved in the development and evaluation of such a device.[4-6] Under the direction of William F. House, MD, profoundly deaf adults have been implanted in the scala tympani with a single-electrode, induction coil device. The implanted coil is electrically stimulated by an external induction coil via magnetic field induction through intact skin. This external coil is connected to the battery-driven stimulator unit, which delivers to the internal coil a 16 kHz carrier wave that is amplitude modulated by the electrical analog of the auditory signal.

In 1976, a group of independent investigators from Pittsburgh evaluated 13 subjects fitted with single-electrode cochlear implants in order to observe the benefits and side effects of electrically stimulating the cochlea.[7] Eleven of those subjects had been implanted by House. One aspect of the Pittsburgh study involved evaluating the effects of cochlear electrical stimulation on the vestibular system. Computerized Posturography was the method employed.[8] This recording of the Classic and Sharpened Romberg Test on a computerized platform allowed for quantifying vestibular status with and without the implant activated. The investigators reported the following results: "All 13 subjects demonstrated evidence of additional instability by one or more of the posturography test measures employed when tested with their unit on and the gain set for use in usual circumstances."[8(p143)] This was particularly noted in testing with eyes closed. It was, therefore, suggested that the cochlear implant had a galvanic effect on the vestibular system. A closer look at the individual subject data, however, shows that there was also some *improvement* in postural stability on 1 or more of the 16 measures for most of the subjects. In addition, postural stability seemed to show some improvement when the implant was activated and a broadband noise stimulus was delivered simultaneously.

Subjectively, the HEI implant subjects do not report any specific balance problems or dizziness complaints when using the stimulator. Some subjects do experience some vestibular symptoms such as oscillopsia or problems when walking in the dark. This, however, is a result of absent vestibular function secondary to the etiology of their inner ear problem, and was experienced prior to implant surgery. Most subjects do report slight dysequilibrium immediately postsurgery. (As a clinical observation, House reports this immediate postoperative unsteadiness seems to be less than seen in patients undergoing stapes surgery.) This disappears within a week or two following surgery. The subjects are not given the stimulator unit until two months postsurgery.

Several subjects at the beginning of implant use did report some lightheadedness. These subjects are currently using the implant 12-14 hours a day and have not had these complaints since initial stimulation. If anything, subjects have reported either no change, or that equilibrium seems somewhat more stable with the implant activated.

As there are no general complaints of balance problems by the subjects when using the implant,

TABLE 1. SUBJECT SUMMARY

Subject No.	*CI No.**	*Age*	*Etiology*	*Age at Onset of Profound Loss*	*Date(s) of Cochlear Implant Surgery*
Long-term group					
1	4	50	Ototoxicity	30	Rt 6/70, Lt 10/72
2	5	50	Ototoxicity	39	Rt 5/72
3	7	47	Unknown	Birth	Lt 6/73
4	8	66	Otosclerosis	45	Lt 11/73
5	9	57	Unknown	35	Rt 1/74
6	11	41	Renal infection/ototoxicity	23	Lt 6/74
7	12	60	Meningitis	53	Lt 7/74, Rt 1/77
8	13	61	Otosclerosis	44	Lt 7/74
9	15	67	Otosclerosis	55	Rt 7/74
Short-term group					
10	20	53	Otosclerosis	40	Rt 4/77
11	21	54	Scarlet fever	37	Rt 4/77
12	22	25	Meningitis/ototoxicity	7	Rt 8/77
13	23	51	Otosclerosis	45	Lt 8/77
14	24	58	Otosclerosis	37	Rt 2/78
15	25	64	Menière's/ototoxicity	61	Lt 3/78, Rt 6/78
16	27	63	Ototoxicity	51	Lt 4/78
17	28	57	Meningitis	13	Rt 4/78
18	29	37	Cogan syndrome	32	Lt 4/78
Group with hearing aid data only					
19	26	39	Unknown	34	Rt 4/78
20	30	61	Ototoxicity	57	Lt 5/78
21	31	52	Bilateral basilar skull fracture	23	Lt 6/78
22	41	34	Malaria/ototoxicity	5	Rt 1/79

*Subjects in order of entry into the cochlear implant program at HEI.

and the posturography data appear somewhat inconsistent, a test protocol was devised to further investigate the Pittsburgh conclusions and determine if electrical stimulation of the cochlea disrupts the balance system to any significant degree.

METHODS

SUBJECTS

Twenty-two profoundly deaf adults implanted by House participated in this study. All subjects met the following criteria for implantation set by HEI:

1. 100+ dB HL bilateral, audiometric pure-tone responses averaged for the speech frequencies.
2. No speech reception threshold with a hearing aid, using a closed set of ten spondees.
3. Neural responses from electrical promontory testing.[5,9]

The implant subjects were divided into two groups. Long-term implant users were those subjects receiving electrical stimulation for over a year. Nine subjects were in this group. Short-term implant users were those subjects with less than one year of usage. Nine subjects were in this group. On four subjects, only preoperative data was collected as the study ended prior to their availability for posttesting. It should be noted that due to subject availability (ie, illness, out-of-town, etc) not all subjects were able to participate in all test measures.

Subjects ranged in age from 25 to 67 years, with a mean age of 50.9 years. All but one subject were postlingually deafened. Etiology for the subject group included the following: ototoxicity, cochlear otosclerosis, meningitis, trauma, scarlet fever, and Cogan syndrome. In several subjects the diagnosis was unknown.

Most of the subjects had received implant surgery on one side only. Three subjects, however, had received bilateral implants, with only one (subject 15) currently receiving binaural stimulation. For a summary on the individual subjects, refer to Table 1.

MATERIALS AND PROCEDURES

Electronystagmography (ENG). All prospective implant candidates were tested by electronystagmography as part of the initial evaluation. The ENG results do not affect the subject's selection for the program, but rather aid in further defining the subject's status. Horizontal eye movements were tested on a single channel Instrument and Control Systems nystagmographic recorder. The testing included the following procedures:

1. Spontaneous nystagmus — eyes open and eyes closed.
2. Positional nystagmus — eyes open and eyes closed: supine, left, supine right, supine left, postural right, postural left, head hang right, head hang left.
3. Pendular tracking to observe smooth pursuit movements of the ocular system: both eyes together, right eye only, left eye only.
4. Fitzgerald-Hallpike Bithermal Caloric Test to determine status of vestibulo-ocular function: 30°C, right and left; 44°C, right and left; observation for fixation suppression; ice water testing and positional inversion if indicated.

For those subjects involved in this special vestibular study, ENG data was collected postoperatively after a period of stimulation in order to observe any changes over time.

A more expanded test battery was devised for a small group of subjects to seek any possible central vestibular findings. This evaluation involved testing for disconjugate eye movements.[10] Seven electrodes were employed for monocular recordings, and the subjects were tested on the Beckman 4-channel Dynagraph. In addition to the standard screening procedure, optokinetic nystagmus (6 and 13 rpm) and torsion swing testing were included. A small group of subjects were additionally tested postoperatively but prior to receiving their stimulator units, for the purpose of observing the direct effects of surgery.

Ataxia Test Battery. The Ataxia Test Battery of Graybiel and Fregly[11] and Fregly et al[12-16] is a measure devised for assessing vestibular ataxia. According to Fregly,[16(p 321)] vestibular ataxia is defined as "a person's limited ability to coordinate voluntary muscular movements while walking or standing due to the

TABLE 2. STATUS OF VESTIBULAR FUNCTIONING

Subject No.	Ear Implanted	Electronystagmography Presurgery	Electronystagmography Postcochlear Implant	Ataxia Test Battery Results
1*	Rt, Lt	Bilateral hypoactive caloric response Rt beating spontaneous nystagmus	No response to calorics bilaterally No spontaneous nystagmus	Positive
2*	Rt	Rt beating spontaneous nystagmus Direction changing positional nystagmus	Normal ENG	Negative
3	Lt	Response to ice calorics with eyes open only Lt beating positional nystagmus	Inappropriate direction of beating to ice water, eyes open No positional nystagmus	Positive
4	Lt	No response to calorics bilaterally Direction changing positional nystagmus	No response to calorics bilaterally No positional nystagmus	Positive
5	Rt	Bilateral hypoactive caloric responses	No response to calorics on lt ear Response on rt only to ice	Positive
7	Rt, Lt	Borderline bilateral hypoactive caloric response Rt beating positional nystagmus	Bilateral hypoactive caloric response Lt beating positional nystagmus	Borderline
8	Lt	Bilateral hypoactive caloric response Lt beating positional nystagmus	No response to calorics bilaterally No positional nystagmus	Negative
10	Rt	Normal ENG	Normal ENG	Negative
11	Rt	RVR† on rt ear	RVR on rt ear Slight lt beating spontaneous nystagmus	Negative
12	Rt	No response to calorics bilaterally Lt beating spontaneous and positional nystagmus	No response to calorics bilaterally No spontaneous or positional nystagmus	Positive Positive
13	Lt	RVR on rt ear	RVR on rt ear	Negative
14	Rt	Normal ENG	Bilateral hypoactive calorics Slight rt beating spontaneous nystagmus	Negative
15	Rt, Lt	RVR on lt ear	RVR on lt ear	Positive
16	Lt	Rt beating directional preponderance	Normal ENG	Negative
17	Rt	No response to calorics bilaterally	No response to calorics bilaterally	Positive
18	Lt	No response to calorics bilaterally	No response to calorics bilaterally	Positive

*Tested prior to second surgery.
†RVR - Reduced vestibular response.
Significant positive relation between ENG and the Ataxia Test Battery (Fisher's test, $p < .05$).

absence, disturbance or loss of function of the vestibular apparatus." This test measure was chosen for the purpose of gathering baseline information as a means of defining vestibulospinal function. Because this test battery had been standardized and applied to groups with varying degrees of vestibular function loss,[13,17] it was believed to be an adequate index for classifying the subject with respect to postural performance, and as an alternative measure to compare with the results of Computerized Posturography.

The battery includes the following seven different subtests:

1. SR = Sharpened (Tandem) Romberg.
   a. Feet heel-to-toe; arms folded; eyes closed.
   b. Four trials; one point per second of holding stance.
2. Walk E/O = walk on 2 cm (3/4 in)-wide rail, eyes open.
   a. Feet heel-to-toe; arms folded.
   b. Five trials; one point per step taken.
3. Stand E/O = stand on 2 cm (3/4 in)-wide rail, eyes open.
   a. Feet heel-to-toe; arms folded.
   b. Five trials; one point per second of holding stance.
4. Stand E/C = Stand on 5.6 cm (2 1/4 in)-wide rail, eyes closed.
   a. Feet heel-to-toe; arms folded.
   b. Five trials; one point per second of holding stance.
5. SOLEC-R = Stand on one leg (right), eyes closed.
   a. Arms folded.
   b. Five trials; one point per second of holding stance.
6. SOLEC-L = Stand on one leg (left), eyes closed.
   a. Arms folded.
   b. Five trials; one point per second of holding stance.
7. WOFEC = Walk on floor, eyes closed.
   a. Feet heel-to-toe; arms folded.
   b. Five trials; one point per step taken.

Subjects were given the specified number of trials per test, and score was determined according to the number of steps or seconds the subject was able to perform for that task. Vestibular ataxia was arbitrarily defined by the developers of the test as performance below the fifth percentile (fourth for "walk on floor" test) for all the floor tests and the "stand on 5.6 cm (2 1/4 in) rail" test.[14]

The subjects in the long-term group (more than one year of implant use) were tested postoperatively, as these subjects had all been implanted prior to the initiation of the study. The short-term subjects were all tested prior to surgery. No auditory prosthetic device was used during this test.

Sono-Postural Test. The Sono-Postural Test was devised for comparison testing with and without the prosthesis activated. This test is based on the four maneuvers of the floor battery of the Ataxia Test Battery:[12] SR, SOLEC-R, SOLEC-L, WOFEC. Each maneuver was performed with eyes open and eyes closed, thus making up eight subtests.

Originally, the Ataxia Test Battery (which includes the rail tests) was to be used for comparison testing. However, the rail tests were found to be extremely difficult for the HEI subjects, the majority of whom exhibited partial or total loss of vestibular function. Fregly et al[14(p398)] state:

> In our experience the use of the "floor battery" alone appears sufficient for clinical, or even laboratory purposes. It has proved consistently to be equal, or better, in sensitivity to the "rail battery" in the detection and charting of spontaneous and induced vestibular and related disturbances. In combination, however, the full test battery offers the advantages of greater sampling of multidimensional ataxia test behavior. . .

The rail battery was therefore utilized one time only to classify the subject according to vestibulospinal functioning by way of ataxic behavior, whereas the floor battery (eyes open and eyes closed) was repeated over time for comparison purposes.

The long-term subjects were tested first without activation of the implant and then with the implant activated. The short-term group was tested prior to surgery first with no prosthetic device, and then with a high-powered hearing aid. They were again tested after surgery, first with the implant turned off and then with the implant activated. The test environment was not soundproof.

Computerized Posturography. A computerized posture platform* was installed at the House Ear Institute in 1977, and a protocol was devised to replicate the Pittsburgh study.[8] Paralleling the Pittsburgh study, the Classic Romberg (feet together) and Sharpened Romberg (heel-to-toe) tests were used. Each maneuver was 15 seconds in duration. The subjects were tested in the following conditions: implant turned off, implant activated, and implant activated plus noise. The noise utilized was a 90 dB HL continuous, broad-band signal delivered via a headphone placed approximately 2.5 cm over the microphone of the stimulator unit. During all implant-activated trials, the volume was set for comfortable listening in usual circumstances.

The HEI protocol included an additional condition which required the use of a galvanic stimulus as a control. A bipolar, mastoid-to-mastoid technique was employed whereby the positive electrode was placed over the mastoid contralateral to the ear implanted. A current of 2 mA to 2.5 mA was delivered for ten seconds in duration.

The Pittsburgh protocol required that all of the subjects perform the two Romberg maneuvers with eyes open and eyes closed. The subjects had difficulty standing alone, especially with eyes closed, due to their vestibular deficits. "All subjects required support during some portion of the posture test series."[8(p141)] It is assumed that this support was manually provided, as no descriptions were given of the method of support. In the HEI study, if a subject could not perform a maneuver with eyes closed for the entire 15-second trial, then that maneuver was only performed with eyes open throughout the test.

The subjects were tested on the two Romberg maneuvers with shoes off and arms folded in each of the four test conditions (no prosthesis, implant activated, implant and noise, and galvanic stimulus), for a total of eight tests. Each test was performed twice in a random order determined by using a standard table of random numbers.

RESULTS

ELECTRONYSTAGMOGRAPHY

The ENG was performed on 16 subjects before and after cochlear implantation to observe any changes with regard to status of vestibular functioning. The long-term group was composed of seven subjects who had been using the implant for a period ranging from 4 to $8^1/_2$ years, and averaging $5^1/_2$ years. The short-term group was composed of nine subjects who had only received stimulation within a 1-year period ranging from 4 to 9 months, with an average of 6 months.

Preoperative data on the 16 subjects revealed that three subjects demonstrated normal test results, one had normal responses on calorics with spontaneous and direction changing positional nystagmus, three had a unilateral reduced vestibular response and four subjects demonstrated bilateral hypoactive responses on calorics. Five subjects showed no response to caloric testing (including ice water tests), except for one subject who demonstrated strong nystagmus only with eyes open on ice water calorics. For individual subject data refer to Table 2.

Six of these 16 subjects (subjects 10-15) were tested with the expanded ENG protocol, which included separate eye recordings, optokinetics, and torsion swing. No significant findings were revealed from the additional testing.

Four subjects (subjects 10-13) had ENGs postoperatively, but prior to receiving their stimulating units, in order to determine any vestibular changes as a direct result of the implant surgery. No changes in these four subjects were detected.

On postoperative testing, after a period of time with implant use, it was revealed that for the short-term group 8 of the 9 subjects demonstrated essentially no change from the preoperative ENGs. It must be mentioned that of the 8 subjects, 3 showed no response to calorics bilaterally on pretesting. One of the 9 subjects (subject 14), however, did show a bilateral reduction in calorics on posttesting. No symptoms were noted by this subject.

Long-term group data revealed that 3 of the 7 subjects showed no significant change from pretest to posttest, with 1 of those subjects having no response to calorics on preoperative tests. One of the 3 subjects had spontaneous and positional nystagmus on pretests, but showed a normal recording on posttesting. Three of the 7 subjects revealed a decrease in calorics when comparing predata and postdata. However, in all three cases the decrease was bilateral, rather than being localized to the ear receiving stimulation. Two of these subjects (5, 8) had surgery on only one side, but one subject (1) had had multiple surgeries on both sides. This decrease may or may not be attributed to the bilateral implant surgeries, as other subjects (6, 15) with bilateral surgeries showed no changes in calorics. Again, no symptoms were reported by the subjects.

The one subject (3) who demonstrated "central" findings (caloric induced nystagmus with eyes open only) on pretesting showed a change in direction of nystagmus on posttesting. The six subjects who were given the expanded test battery revealed no significant abnormalities on posttesting.

ATAXIA TEST BATTERY

The Ataxia Test Battery was performed on 19 subjects. Seven were long-term implant users (average of 4.9 years) while the other 12 were short-term subjects and were therefore tested prior to surgery.

*Contraves Automatic Postural Stability Test System (Contraves Goerz Corp, Pittsburgh). Technical description: The posture platform senses the forces caused by gravity acting on the mass of the test subject. Measurement of the forces enables the location of the center of gravity to be accurately determined with respect to the platform surface. Data presentation: x-y coordinates, polar coordinates, phase plane and power density spectra plots.

TABLE 3. SONO-POSTURAL TEST TOTAL SCORES ON EYES-CLOSED MEASURES FOR SHORT-TERM SUBJECTS*

Subject	*No Prosthesis Preoperative*	*No Prosthesis Postoperative*	*Implant Activated Postoperative*
10	333	329	356
12	57	41	52
13	73	69	79
14	267	284	305
15	36	38	45
16	58	80	96
17	94	63	50
18	48	56	52
N = 8	996	960	1035
Mean	120.75	120	129.375
SD	113.3	116.55	126.07

*The higher score indicates the better performance.

According to the normative criteria established by Fregly and Graybiel,[11-16] the HEI results revealed that 9 subjects did not demonstrate vestibular ataxia, while 10 did. To further validate the results on the Ataxia Test Battery, a small sample size nonparametric statistical test was utilized in order to compare the test with ENG results. There was a significant positive relation found between the two tests (Fisher's test, $p<.05$, Table 2).

SONO-POSTURAL TEST

The Sono-Postural Test (based on the floor battery of the Ataxia Test Battery) was given to 20 subjects. Eight subjects were long-term implant users, with an average of 4.8 years of stimulation, and eight were short-term implant users, with an average of 5.3 months of stimulation. An additional four unimplanted subjects together with three of the short-term implanted subjects were used to obtain hearing aid data.

The eight short-term subjects were tested without any prosthesis preoperatively and postoperatively, and with the cochlear implant activated postoperatively. The eyes-closed maneuvers of the floor battery were combined to give one score for comparison purposes. These scores can be found in Table 3. Analysis revealed that there were no significant differences between any of the three conditions (no prosthesis preoperatively, no prosthesis postoperatively, and implant activated).

TABLE 4. SONO-POSTURAL TEST MEAN SCORES ON INDIVIDUAL TEST MANEUVERS (N = 16)

	Postoperative Mean Scores		
Maneuver	*Implant On*	*Implant Off*	*Difference*
SREO	186.375	144.06	+ 42.315
SREC	43.75	45.125	− 1.375
SOLEO-R	86.562	74.25	+ 12.312
SOLEC-R	17.875	14.187	+ 3.688
SOLEO-L	84.937	83.06	+ 1.877
SOLEC-L	18.062	14.5	+ 3.562
WOFEO	25.25	24.56	+ 0.69
WOFEC	10.937	10.437	+ 0.5

+ Direction of better performance with the cochlear implant activated.
− Direction of better performance with the cochlear implant turned off.

TABLE 5. SONO-POSTURAL TEST MEAN TOTAL SCORE AND STANDARD DEVIATION OF 8 MANEUVERS*

	CI (N = 16)		*HA* (N = 7)	
	Off	*On*	*Off*	*On*
Mean	409.6	449.3	625.4	613.6
SD	259.7	255.0	223.6	246.6

*The higher score indicates the better performance.
CI - Cochlear implant; HA - Hearing aid.

The Sono-Postural Test was given postoperatively to eight long-term subjects as well as to the eight short-term subjects. All 16 subjects were first tested with the implant off and then with the implant activated in order to determine if there were any significant quantitative changes as a direct result of electrical stimulation. Analysis on individual subtests revealed no significant differences, although total mean differences were generally in the direction of better performance with the implant activated (Table 4). This difference does reach statistical significance for the total score of the eight subtests, which was significantly better for the implant-activated condition than the implant-off condition ($t = 1.94$, $p<.05$). (Due to the high variability exhibited as a result of combining subjects with varying vestibular function, a nonparametric analysis was additionally performed. The Wilcoxon Matched-Pairs Signed-Ranks Test revealed a significant difference in the direction of better performance with the implant activated [$T = +25$, $p<.05$].) It is interesting that for the hearing aid subjects ($n = 7$), the mean difference on total score was in the direction of better performance in the unaided condition. This difference, however, was not significant (Table 5).

Total scores for the 16 implant subjects were also analyzed to assess the role of duration of implant use (long-term vs short-term), ataxic behavior (presence or absence), and combinations of the four. These data are presented in Table 6. In subjects with or without vestibular function as measured by the Ataxia Test Battery, activation of the implant evoked very similar improvements. On the duration of use comparison, both long-term and short-term groups showed better performance with the implant activated as opposed to the implant-off condition. However, the short-term group demonstrated much larger mean differences than the long-term group for both the ataxia present and ataxia absent comparisons.

COMPUTERIZED POSTUROGRAPHY

Fourteen subjects were evaluated by Computerized Posturography. Eight subjects were long-term implant users (average of 4.8 years), and six were short-term (average of 6.3 months). On the Classic Romberg test, all subjects were able to perform the maneuver with eyes closed. On the Sharpened Romberg test, two of the subjects could not perform the maneuver for the entire 15-second trial

TABLE 6. SONO-POSTURAL TEST SCORES COMPARING VARIABLES OF PROSTHESIS ACTIVATION, ATAXIC BEHAVIOR AND DURATION OF IMPLANT USE

	Subjects	No.	Implant On	Mean of Total Score Implant Off	Difference
	Long-term	5	231.4	221.8	+ 9.6
Ataxia demonstrated	Short-term	4	388.25	313.5	+ 74.75
	Total	9	301.11	262.56	+ 38.6
	Long-term	3	462.67	449.33	+ 13.34
Ataxia not demonstrated	Short-term	4	772.5	710.75	+ 61.75
	Total	7	639.7	598.7	+ 41

+ Direction of better performance with cochlear implant activated.

(even with eyes open), and were therefore not tested on this task. Of the remaining 12 subjects who could perform the maneuver, 4 were tested with eyes closed, and 8 with eyes open. Differences as a direct result of electrical stimulation were evaluated using paired *t* tests. The measure looked at was "total energy." This was the sum of the energy of the x and y displacements; cartesian coordinates of the center of mass. It is a measure of the amount of "sway" of the subject. If the subject has disturbed vestibular function he or she sways more and uses more energy to maintain posture. In other words, that individual's center of gravity (or mass) moves more and at greater speed.

Quantitative analysis revealed that subjects' scores were so variable for the same two maneuvers per test condition that the data had to be looked at in two ways: the best of the two scores and the average of the two scores. Even then, extreme variability was shown on total group scores for each condition. For a summary of total group data, refer to the figure.

Data analysis on the Classic Romberg maneuver revealed that the subjects as a group tended, though not significantly so, to exert less energy with the implant activated than with the implant turned off.

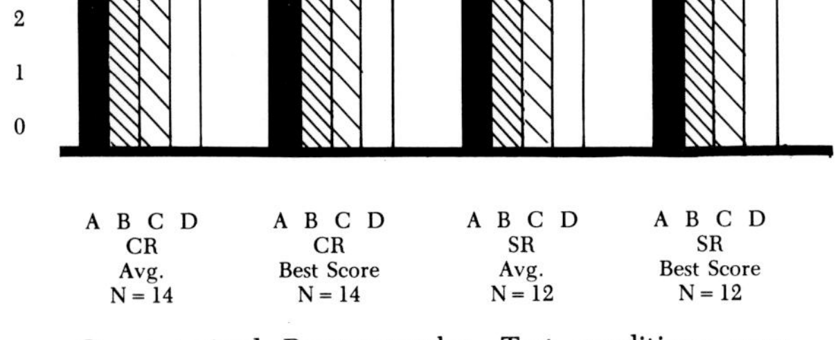

Computerized Posturography. Test conditions were A - No prosthetic device; B - Implant activated; C - Implant noise; D - Galvanic stimulus; CR - Classic Romberg (feet together); SR - Sharpened Romberg (heel-to-toe). The higher score indicates more difficulty in maintaining balance, ie, more energy exerted.

There was a further slight decrease in energy with the implant-plus-noise condition, which bordered on significance when compared to the implant-off condition (for best score, $t = 1.96$, $p < .08$). This general pattern was also demonstrated on the Sharpened Romberg maneuver for the averaged-scores analysis. On the best-scores analysis for the Sharpened Romberg, however, the opposite pattern was shown. There was slightly more energy exerted with the implant activated. For 3 of the 4 analyzed measures, the subjects as a group demonstrated increased energy scores with the galvanic stimulus control when compared to the implant-off condition. This suggests that it was possible to activate vestibular structures by at least a strong level of electrical stimulation.

Data were additionally analyzed with subjects divided into smaller categories with regard to duration of implant use (long-term or short-term), status of vestibular functioning (either absent or present), and combinations of the four. The purpose was to observe any consistent patterns as a result of these variables. It was revealed that those subjects who tended to demonstrate less energy exerted with the implant activated (compared to implant off), while showing increased energy exerted with the galvanic stimulus, were those subjects who were long-term implant users, particularly with some residual vestibular functioning. Subjects who tended to show further improvement with noise input were those who demonstrated absent vestibular function, particularly long-term users. A rather interesting finding was the trend of the short-term implant users, who tended to show less energy exerted not only in the implant-activated condition but with the galvanic stimulus as well, when compared to the unaided condition. Finally, for those subjects who tended to demonstrate poorer scores for the implant-activated condition when compared to inactivated, this pattern was scattered over all subject categories with a slight trend for long-term subjects with absent vestibular function to predominate.

A final analysis was performed to compare the Computerized Posturography with the Sono-Postural Test results. Using nonparametric procedures, no significant relation was found between the two tests.

DISCUSSION

In summary, vestibular function tests performed as a means of detecting the possible effect of cochlear electrical stimulation on the balance system indicate that equilbrium is not disrupted to any significant degree. Predata and postdata comparisons, as shown by ENG records, reveal essentially no change in vestibular sensitivity. For those subjects, however, who demonstrated a significant decreased response in caloric testing after a period of time with implant use, the decrease was bilateral rather than localizing to the ear being electrically stimulated. This suggests either a further spontaneous deterioration in vestibular function from the inner ear pathology, or central compensation. The subjects who did reveal this decrease did not report any subjective changes.

The Ataxia Test Battery, Sono-Postural Test and Computerized Posturography were administered to determine if there were any quantitative changes in vestibulospinal function as a direct result of electrical stimulation. The Ataxia Test Battery, in defining vestibulospinal status, showed a significant positive relation to vestibulo-ocular data. Results on the Sono-Postural test (based on the floor maneuvers of the Ataxia Test Battery) revealed no significant difference between any of the test conditions (preoperatively and postoperatively unaided, and postoperatively with implant activated) for short-term subjects ($n = 8$). However, with the implant activated, improved postural stability was demonstrated as compared to the postoperative implant-off condition for long-term and short-term subjects combined ($n = 16$).

On Computerized Posturography, analysis of the total energy measure showed that most implant subjects tended to exert more energy in attempting to maintain stability during a strong transtemporal galvanic stimulation than in the implant-off condition. On the other hand, with the implant activated, subjects tended to exert less energy than with the implant off. These findings are not consonant with Black's[8] suggestion that the cochlear implant delivers a sufficient galvanic stimulus to the vestibular system to produce increased postural instability.

In addition to the present findings on human implanted subjects, animal studies undertaken by Kimm et al[18] provide evidence indicating that electrical stimulation can be directed to the auditory nerve without any significant activation of the vestibular system.

Electrical stimulation of the cochlea, by creating an electrical field through the cochlear fluids, certainly has the potential for affecting the balance system especially as a byproduct of fitting an electrical prosthetic device for such a sensory deficit as profound deafness. What must particularly be noted is the wide variety of vestibular functioning exhibited in the deaf population, ranging from normal sensitivity to unilateral weakness, hypoactive functioning and total loss of function. This variability might well confound any attempts to study galvanic vestibular effects. It is difficult to determine whether test results represent a direct effect of the electrical stimulation or some interactive effect dependent upon vestibular status secondary to etiology.

The Pittsburgh report bases its conclusions on a relatively new measurement from which standardized data were gathered only on a population of normals. The varying degrees of vestibular deficits and accompanying central compensatory mechanisms may be of importance to subject performance. The fact that all of the subjects evaluated by Pittsburgh were tested with eyes closed and required support to prevent them from falling may have biased performance data. Since this support apparently was provided manually by the experimenter, it would be difficult to insure consistency from subject to subject. Of even more importance was the incidence of extreme variability exhibited between and within tests, both by subjects evaluated at HEI and those evaluated in Pittsburgh. Interpretation based solely on posturographic records must, therefore, be treated conservatively and regarded with some reservation.

The fact that human studies undertaken at HEI do not support the hypothesis that electrical stimulation as produced by the implant disrupts equilibrium, but rather point to the contrary, suggests that sound itself can be a factor in the maintenance of balance. It is speculated that this phenomenon may be a result of cochlear-induced CNS effects that somehow sharpen postural equilibrium. To our knowledge, the hypothesis that sound has a positive effect on equilibrium has not been studied. There is, however, some anecdotal clinical data that support this. Many subjects in an anechoic chamber report a feeling of unsure stability in complete silence. Certainly posturography and other postural tests with normal subjects in such a chamber would be most interesting.

On the other hand, intense sound can stimulate the vestibular system.[19-23] This tendency was shown in our own deaf subjects who tended to show deterioration in their Sono-Postural scores with high-powered hearing aids on, which deliver sound pressure levels up to 130 dB. Indeed, most normal persons in these sound levels become unsteady or faintly dizzy. To us this indicates the possibility of direct stimulation of the vestibular system by sound.

CONCLUSIONS

The hypothesis that electrical stimulation of the cochlea will affect any neurons surviving in the vestibular nerve is certainly reasonable. However, results from vestibular test measures recorded on human implanted deaf adults at HEI indicate the following:

1. There is no evidence that the electrical current delivered to the cochlea via the cochlear implant disrupts the balance system by stimulating vestibular neurons.

2. On subjects with total or partial loss of vestibular function in association with profound deafness, postural stability appears to improve with the implant activated.

ACKNOWLEDGMENTS — Diane Churchill, formerly Head Technician of the Vestibular Test Laboratory at the Otologic Medical Group in Los Angeles, performed the Computerized Posturography and the Electronystagmography tests for this study. Karen Berliner, PhD, Cognitive Psychologist and Director of Clinical Trials at the House Ear Institute, assisted in the statistical analysis for this study.

REFERENCES

1. Ritter J. Ueber die Anwendung der Voltaischen Säule. Hufeland's J Pract Heilk 1803; 7:30-53.

2. Augustin FL. Versuch einer Vollständigen systematischen Geschichte der galvanischen Electricität und ihrer medicinischen Anwendung. Berlin: Felisch, 1803.

3. Purkinje J. Beitrage zahnaheren Kenntniss des Schwindels aus heautognostichen Daten. Wich Med Jahrb 1820; 6:79-125.

4. House WF, Urban J. Long term results of electrode implantation and electronic stimulation of the cochlea in man. Ann Otol Rhinol Laryngol 1973; 82:504-17.

5. House WF, Berliner K, Crary W, et al. Cochlear implants. Ann Otol Rhinol Laryngol 1976; 85 Suppl 27:1-93.

6. House WF, Berliner KI, Eisenberg LS. Present status and future directions of the Ear Research Institute cochlear implant program. Acta Otolaryngol (Stockh) 1979; 87:176-84.

7. Bilger RC, Black FO, Hopkinson NT, et al. Evaluation of subjects presently fitted with implanted auditory prostheses. Ann Otol Rhinol Laryngol 1977; 86 Suppl 38:1-176.

8. Black FO. Effects of the auditory prosthesis on postural stability. In: Bilger RC, Black FO, Hopkinson NT, et al. Evaluation of subjects presently fitted with implanted auditory prostheses. Ann Otol Rhinol Laryngol 1977; 86 Suppl 38:141-64.

9. House WF, Brackmann DE. Electrical promontory testing in differential diagnosis of sensori-neural hearing impairment. Laryngoscope 1974; 84:2163-71.

10. Kimm J, MacLean JB. Disconjugate eye movements during electronystagmographic testing in patients with known central nervous system lesions. Ann Otol Rhinol Laryngol 1975; 84:368-73.

11. Graybiel A, Fregly AR. A new quantitative ataxia test battery. Acta Otolaryngol (Stockh) 1966; 61:292-312.

12. Fregly AR, Graybiel A. An ataxia test battery not requiring rails. Aerospace Med 1968; 39:277-82.

13. Fregly AR, Graybiel A. Labyrinthine defects as shown by ataxia and caloric tests. Acta Otolaryngol (Stockh) 1970; 69:216-22.

14. Fregly AR, Graybiel A, Smith MJ. Walk on floor eyes closed (WOFEC): a new addition to an ataxia test battery. Aerospace Med 1972; 43:395-9.

15. Fregly AR, Smith MJ, Graybiel A. Revised normative standards of performance of men on a quantitative ataxia test battery. Acta Otolaryngol (Stockh) 1973; 75:10-6.

16. Fregly AR. Vestibular ataxia and its measurement in man. In: Kornhuber HH, ed. Handbook of sensory physiology, vol VI. Vestibular system part 2: psychophysics, applied aspects and general interpretations. Berlin: Springer-Verlag, 1974:321-60.

17. Nelson JR. Long-term effects of acoustic neuroma surgery. Arch Otolaryngol 1968; 88:675-86.

18. Kimm J, Winfield JA, Sutton D, et al. Vestibular effects of electrical stimulation of the cochlea: monitored in the awake primate. Arch Otolaryngol 1979; 105:175-9.

19. Ades HW, Graybiel A, Morill SN, et al. Nystagmus elicited by high intensity sound. Research Project NM 13-01-99. sk 2, rept. 6. Pensacola Fla: US Navy Research Laboratory, 1957.

20. McCabe BF, Lawrence M. The effects of intense sound on the non-auditory labyrinth. Acta Otolaryngol (Stockh) 1958; 49:147-57.

21. Kryter KD. Effects of noise on man. New York: Academic Press, 1970.

22. Harris CS. Effects of acoustical stimuli on the vestibular system. Technical report 71-58. Aerospace Medical Research Laboratory, Wright-Patterson Air Force Base, Ohio, 1971.

23. Parker DE, Ritz LA, Tubbs RL, et al. Effects of sound on the vestibular system. AMRL-TR-75-89. Aerospace Medical Research Laboratory, Wright-Patterson Air Force Base, Ohio, 1976.

PSYCHOMETRIC STUDIES AND CLINICAL INTERVIEWS WITH COCHLEAR IMPLANT PATIENTS

WILLIAM G. CRARY, PhD
KAREN I. BERLINER, PhD
MURRAY WEXLER, PhD
LINDA W. MILLER, PhD

Selection of suitable candidates for an implant was a central issue in planning clinical trials. Psychological techniques were included, the purpose being to screen out individuals who, on an a priori basis, we considered cognitively and/or emotionally inappropriate. Psychological measures were further used to assess the effect of the implant on those candidates who did undergo the surgical procedure. The present paper describes the preimplant and postimplant interviews and psychometric assessment. Based on the data developed from the interviews, we concluded that the recipients of implants are in almost unanimous agreement that the implant is a very positive contribution to their lives. Tests of cognitive functioning conducted over time indicate that the implant does not impair cognitive or neuropsychological functions. Personality tests were also administered, and no significant changes in these dimensions were found.

Once the cochlear prosthesis was ready for human trials, it was necessary to develop a set of criteria for selecting candidates. It was clear from the outset that psychological factors should be included since the implant's effects on human cognition and personality were unknown. In order to evaluate these issues, two courses of action were decided upon. Any individual who displayed significant signs of psychopathology would be eliminated as a candidate and those who were implanted would be studied over time to determine what effects, if any, the implant had on human behavior. Clinical interviews and psychological tests were utilized to screen candidates, and those who were selected were reinterviewed and retested at periodic intervals in order to track any changes which may have occurred since the prosthesis was implanted.

PSYCHOMETRIC STUDIES

Psychometric studies were included in our procedures in order to provide objective measures of cognitive and emotional functioning. We wanted to assess change over time which might presumably be due to the implant. In particular, we were concerned about organic effects. "Since the issue of brain damage from cochlear implants is a matter of potential significance, periodic monitoring of intellectual deficits referable to cerebral dysfunction will play a major role."[1]

The data presented are those obtained on 46 English-speaking, postlingually deafened adults. There were 29 males and 17 females. The mean age was 48 years and ranged from 19 to 75 years. Patients were tested prior to receiving the implant, at approximately one year postimplant, and annually thereafter. One year and most recent follow-up tests are reported here. Some patients have had as many as five annual retests, while others are not beyond the first year. The data reported were obtained from 23 of the patients at one year postimplant and from 16 patients at two years or more postimplant. For the group as a whole, the final test period reported here averaged three years and eight months from the point the patients were first stimulated, ranging from two years to almost seven years.

COGNITIVE STUDIES

Tests Used. Wechsler Adult Intelligence Scale (WAIS)[2] yields a verbal, performance and full IQ as well as other significant data concerning intellectual functions. Graham-Kendall Memory For Designs (MFD)[3] measures the capacity for immediate recall. Trail Making Test (Trlmk)[4] reflects the ability to maintain a cognitive set and pursue a task sequentially. Bender Visual Motor Gestalt (BNDR)[5] and Bender Visual Motor Interference Test (BIP)[6] are designed to assess visual motor functions at two levels of difficulty. All have normative data available for assessing presence of organic brain dysfunction.

Results. Table 1 describes the cognitive test findings preimplant and for the two follow-up periods. As a group, these patients can be classified in the lower range of bright-normal intelligence. Other scores do not indicate difficulties in immediate recall, set and sequencing, or visual-motor coordination. Follow-up studies indicate that the scores remained stable through time. That is, they show very little change from testing to testing. Slight improvements in IQ postimplant are probably attributable to practice effects.

Tests of significance (paired t tests) were computed for each variable between the three testing periods, ie, 1 vs 2; 1 vs 3; 2 vs 3. In each instance, no significant differences appeared.

When we began the cochlear implant project, we could not predict with certainty what effects, if any, the implant would have on cognitive func-

TABLE 1. MEANS AND STANDARD DEVIATIONS OF COGNITIVE TEST SCORES

	Preimplant I		Postimplant II		Postimplant III	
	Mean	SD	Mean	SD	Mean	SD
WAIS						
Verbal IQ	110.8	16.7	112.5	19.3	113.0	23.4
Performance IQ	110.4	11.5	113.9	11.0	113.9	14.1
Full IQ	111.6	13.8	112.9	15.7	113.3	19.8
MFD (no. of errors)	1.8	2.6	1.7	1.9	1.1	1.5
Trlmk (credits)	13.3	3.6	13.6	3.9	14.6	3.6
BNDR (no. of errors)	1.8	1.5	1.8	1.4	1.6	1.2
BIP (no. of errors)	1.8	1.3	1.7	1.1	2.1	1.1

tions. Although we felt it would not impair these processes, we could not be sure.

The results are in and our original optimism has been confirmed. There is no evidence from the sample studied that there is any damage to cognitive function. At least from this perspective, we can conclude that the implant does not produce cerebral impairment. Clinical evidence also supports this conclusion in that our patients have continued to pursue their daily activities with the same efficiency as they did prior to the implant. Indeed, there are several individuals whose performance has improved which we feel is a direct contribution of the implant.

PERSONALITY STUDIES

A variety of personality tests and measures of emotional status were used at the inception of our research. These have been described[5] and include measures of anxiety, stress, self-esteem, depression, and other personality and behavioral characteristics. Due to a consistent finding that patients' scores did not change significantly over time, and given the substantial effort required to answer so many questionnaires, it was decided to drop these from the research plan. Currently, patients are required to complete the Minnesota Multiphasic Personality Inventory (MMPI).[7] (Early patients received the "Mini-Mult,"[8] a shorter version of the MMPI which is considered valid for group data. Mini-Mult and MMPI scores have been intermingled in this analysis. Each patient received the same test preimplant and postimplant.) However, for the purposes of monitoring individual patients, those who initally responded to the original tests have continued to answer them at follow-up intervals. Data are therefore available from 14 patients on these measures, both at one year postimplant and at most recent testing.

Results. Cochlear implant patients score in the normal range on all personality and affective measures. Mean scores on the MMPI for the three test intervals can be found in Table 2. The normative mean for all MMPI scales is 50, with a standard deviation of 10. Scores above 70 would be considered evidence for pathology. Paired t tests done for those patients having postimplant data at one year and at two years or more indicate no significant changes on any of the MMPI scales from preimplant to postimplant. As in the past, the other measures employed showed few significant changes. There was a decrease on one measure of anxiety and an increase in energy level, but the majority of scores remained unchanged.

As with the cognitive studies, we conclude that since there are no significant shifts, particularly in a negative direction, the implant appears to have no adverse psychological effects.

CLINICAL INTERVIEWS

The interview has a long and significant history in the practice of medicine. It has always served as a major source of data upon which clinical decisions could be based. In clinical psychiatry and psychology it is the primary screening device in the evaluation of psychopathology. Since the nature and degree of emotional disturbance was incorporated in our selection criteria, the open-ended interview became a routine part of our procedures for identifying acceptable candidates for implants.

The technical details of the clinical interview we use have been described and discussed elsewhere.[9-12] The objective, preimplant, is to obtain a history, the purpose being to identify signposts pointing to psychological stability or instability, and to evaluate the patient's current mental status.

Postimplant follow-up interviews are scheduled a year after beginning implant use, and annually thereafter. The purpose here is to evaluate the impact of the cochlear implant, problems related to

TABLE 2. MEANS AND STANDARD DEVIATIONS ON THE MINNESOTA MULTIPHASIC PERSONALITY INVENTORY

	Preimplant I		Postimplant II		Postimplant III	
Scale	Mean	SD	Mean	SD	Mean	SD
L	52.5	7.1	52.5	8.0	52.9	8.0
F	53.2	7.4	53.3	6.1	54.9	8.6
K	56.1	8.4	50.4	6.2	59.1	6.9
1 Hs	59.1	12.1	56.9	12.1	62.1	8.7
2 D	58.0	10.3	62.6	10.3	57.1	10.2
3 Hy	60.9	8.3	60.8	7.6	60.4	7.6
4 Pd	58.9	10.7	54.6	9.0	62.1	9.0
6 Pa	60.7	9.7	59.8	6.6	58.7	10.0
7 Pt	52.8	12.7	51.6	13.7	50.3	9.9
8 Sc	54.8	11.0	49.6	13.9	55.6	10.6
9 Ma	49.0	9.6	48.3	8.9	48.7	6.9

implant use, and so on. In our study population, we found most patients have been constant users. A few are nonusers (less than 10% of the total implant population have been classified as nonusers). After a brief period of trying to adjust the unit many patients experienced a sense of disappointment. It is as though each had secretly hoped that he or she would be the first to experience speech discrimination. At this point they may begin to "fiddle" with the unit, seeking to adjust it because "with a little change here or there, I just know I could understand what people say." The postlingually deafened patient is no different from any other chronically impaired individual: there is always the desire to return to the predeficit level of functioning. Most patients come to terms with this unrealistic fantasy, as evidenced by their continued use of the device over many years, their enthusiasm for the other benefits obtained from the implant, and their self-reports regarding this topic. However, all patients report this to be a variably frustrating reality with which to cope.

On a few occasions individuals experienced failure of the internal coil. In all cases the patients responded with understandable disappointment but without profound anger or depression. They had been apprised of the investigative nature of the implant and were informed that replacement would be much simpler than the original surgical procedure. Unit failure is realistically frustrating, but not devastating, to implant recipients.

The common themes encountered in the interviews are 1) the implant reduces the sense of isolation, of being "cut off from the world"; 2) it helps restore the patients' confidence that they can function interpersonally; 3) many patients feel the cochlear implant helps them in speechreading; 4) for many, hearing warning sounds is valued. The most common frustrations encountered revolve around not being able to discriminate speech and, to a lesser degree, with keeping the external coil properly aligned with the internal coil.

Our overall impression from the clinical interviews is that, to date, the patients report no significant intellectual, emotional, occupational or interpersonal problems with the implant. The majority "like" their units, use them daily, and feel comfortable wearing them. For these individuals, the implant is not perceived as being crucial to their survival. They are willing to accept the current limitations of the implant because they find it improves the quality of their lives.

DISCUSSION

Psychometric data show no evidence of any deficits in cognitive functioning following electrical stimulation. Other tests do not show any changes in the patient's personality status. Since negative effects were not observed in either sphere, the cochlear implant appears safe from the psychological perspective.

On the other hand, the psychometric data provide little evidence of positive changes related to implant use. There are three probable explanations for this. First, it is unlikely that cognitive abilities and long-standing personality characteristics in an individual would change greatly, particularly over the short term. Second, population norms indicate that this sample of patients performed in the normal range on all measures, preoperatively and postoperatively. It would not be reasonable to expect the implant to make deaf individuals significantly more effective than their normal counterparts in the hearing population. Finally, the selection process screened out individuals with obvious pathology. We do not know what effects, positive or negative, the implant might have had on a population of deafened adults who were more emotionally disturbed.

It is clear, however, from the clinical interviews that both patients and their relatives feel that the cochlear implant has improved the quality of their lives. They report specific ways in which the implant makes a difference. Since our current batteries of tests do not reflect these changes, we have recently designed a questionnaire using a 5-point ordinal scale to more specifically define the psychosocial and interpersonal changes that may occur with use of the implant. This questionnaire and the results obtained with it are discussed elsewhere in this supplement.[13]

Identifying variables which predict the outcome of rehabilitation would be highly desirable. In particular, we were interested in spotting those who might turn out to be nonusers. In order to determine whether our psychological measures had predictive value, a multiple-regression analysis was performed using hours of daily use of the implant as the dependent variable and the cognitive tests and MMPI scales as the independent (predictor) variables. Although all of these variables taken together accounted for approximately 50% of the variance in hours of use, only two were weighted heavily enough to be worth noting. These were the Trail Making Test which accounted for 15% of the variance, and MMPI Scale 3 (Hysteria) which accounted for another 23%. These tests, therefore, have little predictive value, at least in terms of the rehabilitation variable studied, ie, hours of implant use.

One of the authors recently completed a study in which hours of use was studied in relation to the presence or absence of the character trait of compulsive self-reliance.[14] Some evidence was adduced that patients who have this character trait may be nonusers of the implant. Further studies along these lines are planned in order to cross validate these findings.

One difficulty encountered in both of the studies noted here is the small number of nonusers. There are only 12 postlingually deaf nonusers, fewer at the time of these studies. In one respect, it appears that the selection process may have been highly successful in identifying those patients who will use the prosthesis, and who find it of significant benefit in their lives.

It is difficult to quantify the effect that the cochlear implant may have on an individual's quality of life. The psychometric studies have shown no evidence that the implant is harmful to the patient. Clinical interviews yield extremely consistent responses across a large number of patients regarding the benefits of the implant. These data must not be discounted in evaluating the worth of the cochlear implant as an auditory prosthesis for the deaf.

ACKNOWLEDGMENT — Sheryl Duvall, MS, performed the multiple-regression analysis regarding prognostic indices of rehabilitative success.

REFERENCES

1. House WF, Berliner KI, Crary WG, et al. Cochlear implants. Ann Otol Rhinol Laryngol 1976; 85 Suppl 27:1-93.

2. Matarazzo JD. Wechsler's measurement and appraisal of adult intelligence. 5th ed. Baltimore: Williams and Wilkins, 1973.

3. Graham FK, Kendall BS. Performance of brain-damaged cases on a Memory-for-Designs test. J Abn Soc Psychol 1946; 41:303-14.

4. Reitan RM. Validity of the Trail Making Test as an indicator of organic brain damage. Percept Mot Skills 1958; 8:271-6.

5. Hutt ML, Briskin I. The clinical use of the revised Bender Gestalt Test. New York: Grune and Stratton, 1960.

6. Canter A. A background interference procedure to increase sensitivity of the Bender Gestalt Test to organic brain disorder. J Consult Clin Psychol 1966; 30:91-7.

7. Dahlstrom WG, Welsh GS, Dahlstrom LE. An MMPI handbook, rev ed. Minneapolis: University of Minnesota Press, 1972.

8. Kincannon JC. Prediction of the standard MMPI scale scores from 71 items: the Minimult. J Consult Clin Psychol 1968; 32:319-25.

9. Crary WG, Johnson CW. The mental status exam. In: Johnson CW, Snibbe J, Evans L, eds. Basic psychopathology. 2nd ed. Jamaica, NY: Spectrum Publications, 1980.

10. Enelow A, Wexler M. Psychiatry in the practice of medicine. New York: Oxford University Press, 1960.

11. Strimmel G, Crary WG. Techniques for successful patient interaction. California Pharmacist 1980; 27:26-8.

12. Wexler M, Adler LM. Help the patient tell his story. Oradell, NJ: Medical Economics Book Division, 1970.

13. Wexler M, Miller LW, Berliner KI, Crary WG. Psychological effects of cochlear implant: patient and "index relative" perceptions. Ann Otol Rhinol Laryngol 1982; 91 Suppl 91:59-61.

14. Miller LW. Individual differences in rehabilitation as a function of attachment behavior. Unpublished doctoral dissertation. California School of Professional Psychology, Los Angeles, 1981.

PSYCHOLOGICAL EFFECTS OF COCHLEAR IMPLANT: PATIENT AND "INDEX RELATIVE" PERCEPTIONS

Murray Wexler, PhD
Karen I. Berliner, PhD
Linda W. Miller, PhD
William G. Crary, PhD

The ultimate judge of the value of a technological advance is the patient. The patient's evaluation of the cochlear implant is one way of judging its effects. A second method is from observations of the patient made by an individual in close relationship, ie, an "index relative." In order to determine implant effects as experienced by both patient and observer, we devised preimplant and postimplant questionnaires. We found that patients feel the implant gives them a greater sense of safety; self-sufficiency is considerably enhanced; emotionally negative episodes are significantly reduced; the feeling of being a burden to others is diminished; communication with others is much smoother; and, while engaging in group activities is still difficult, participation is less threatening than before the implant. The index relatives agree with these perceptions. They also are emotionally relieved because they feel the patients have a device which extends their range of mastery. In turn, the index relatives feel less burdened and responsible.

The ultimate arbiter of the value of medical advances is the consumer. While science requires objective measures of the efficacy of a therapeutic procedure, phenomenological (that is, experiential) evidence is often ignored. Since recipients of treatment are exclusively concerned with how it will alter or improve their lives, their perception of therapeutic effects cannot be excluded from the pool of data used in the final assessment of the worth of a technological development. Although the patient is the primary informant, a secondary but nonetheless vital source of information comes from individuals who live in close proximity.

Illness is a social event as well as a biological one. Its impact extends beyond the victim, in adversely affecting the lives of people with close ties to the patient. When the disaster of profound deafness strikes, those closest to the patient feel helpless. Anxiety, panic, depression and anger are the common emotional accompaniments of this state of affairs. Fears for the welfare of the victim predominate. As the inevitability of the deafness fully sinks into awareness, a second, often equally profound fear surfaces. Deafness in the patient also means that new and heavy burdens will fall upon the shoulders of those closest to the victim. Since the individual is now profoundly handicapped, the "index relative" in one way or another must try to help the patient compensate for the deficit. New tasks are imposed upon them which, in turn, further disrupt their lives. In addition, since patterns of communication are at the heart of all human relationships, deafness is devastating since it is so disruptive to this process. Restoring some semblance of communication is a long and arduous course. The results are rarely, if ever, really satisfactory to the people involved. As a consequence of these events there are now, in fact, two or more patients: the victim and one or more individuals with whom he or she is closely allied.

Since the cochlear implant influences both informational input and patterns of communication, it frequently has a significant impact on the lives of the patient's close associates. The investigation described in the following pages provides substantial evidence that the implant patient and the index relative perceive that their lives are modified, often for the better, in a variety of ways.

METHOD

From the inception of the cochlear implant project, careful attention was given to the behavior of both the recipients of the prosthesis and the index relatives. The primary method of observation was through extensive interviews, and the design of the questionnaires used in the present study was based on the data obtained from several hundred interviews.

Our interviews elicited eight major themes which were incorporated into the questionnaires: 1) sense of safety, 2) emotional reactions, 3) nature of interpersonal relationships, 4) social activities, 5) sense of isolation, 6) communication problems, 7) employment, and 8) involvement with hobbies/recreational activities. Parallel questionnaires were constructed for the implantee and the index relative. There was a preoperative and postoperative questionnaire for both, which contained 38 questions for patients, and 23 questions for index relatives.

The questionnaires consisted of questions which were to be answered by circling one of five choices. The statements were the same except for brief changes of wording depending on the informant, ie, patient or index relative. For example:

To what degree are you concerned about your
(your relative's) safety or welfare because of deafness?

not concerned	somewhat concerned	moderately concerned	quite concerned	extremely concerned

Most of the questions appeared in both the preoperative and postoperative forms, although there were additional questions in the latter concerning the observed effects of the prosthesis. An example from the postoperative questionnaire for the patient is:

About how long would you say
it took for you to adapt to the implant?

no time	hardly any time	moderate amount of time	quite some time	a very long time

For the index relative:

Have you noted many changes in the patient's
emotional state since he/she began using the implant?

no change	hardly any change	moderate amount of change	quite a lot of change	a great deal of change

Both preoperative and postoperative forms of this questionnaire were mailed to postlingually deafened cochlear implant patients and their index relatives. Results are based upon data returned by 22 patients (13 men and 9 women) and 13 index relatives (7 men and 6 women). Patients in this sample were highly variable on dimensions of age and etiology as well as how long the cochlear implant had been used. The latter variable ranged from six months to ten years.

The response scale ranged from 0 to 4. The higher the score, the more the patient endorsed a given situation (eg, comfort at social events). The Wilcoxon Matched-Pairs Signed-Ranks Test was used to determine significance between comparable questions, ie, preimplant and postimplant surgery. For qualitative evidence concerning implant effects, we used material from interviews with index relatives and patients.

In one important respect the present design is weakened since our patients had implants at the time of testing. In effect, we instructed the index relatives to recall what they thought and how they felt before the patient had an implant. Obviously, several factors can contaminate "after the fact" memories. It is conceivable that our results are skewed because uncontrolled factors unduly influenced recall. However, our statistical findings do dovetail nicely with our qualitative assessment of interviews which were done preoperatively. In this respect, at least, we feel more confident in the validity of our findings. Nevertheless, the results should be read with the caveat in mind.

RESULTS (PATIENTS)

Thirty-eight questions were asked of each patient, preimplant and postimplant. Results for all questions indicated change in the direction of improvement and increased adaptation with the implant. The mean change for all responses was 0.5 on the 5-point scale. Mean change scores ranged from 0.07 to 1.22 across the different questions.

Twenty-four questions met the criteria for statistical significance of the difference between preimplant and postimplant ($p \leq .05$). Of these, questions that demonstrated the greatest improvement were those concerned with the following: feelings of isolation, issues of safety, comfort at social events, difficulty and frustration in communication, participation in solitary activities (eg, going to a store or restaurant alone), feelings of being a burden. Table 1 presents the mean ratings for these items preimplant and postimplant.

TABLE 1. MEAN PATIENT RATINGS PREIMPLANT AND POSTIMPLANT FOR THOSE ITEMS SHOWING GREATEST IMPROVEMENT (N = 22)

	Preimplant	*Postimplant*	*T**	*p*
Feelings of isolation	2.8	1.6	3	.0006
Concern for safety	2.0	1.0	0	.0005
Comfort at social events	1.1	2.2	0	.0005
Difficulty in communication	2.0	1.0	2.5	.0013
Frustration in communication	2.1	1.1	0	.0007
Difficulty in solitary activities	1.3	0.4	8	.0026
Feelings of burden	1.4	0.6	5	.0023

**T* is the smaller sum of like-signed ranks of the Wilcoxon Matched-Pairs Signed-Ranks Test.

Of the 14 questions that did not reach statistical significance, most were close. For example, questions 29 and 30 were concerned with interest and degree of comfort in employment. The significance levels were $p \leq .0899$ and .1125 respectively. Although these values did not meet the statistical criteria, nevertheless many patients indicated that both interest and comfort in employment were better than prior to the implant.

The questions demonstrating less improvement were primarily those concerned with hobbies and recreational activities. In general, the quality and quantity of those experiences did not appear to be affected by the implant to any significant degree whether or not the activity required sound.

Lastly, patients reported the least change in reference to the number and quality of their friendships. This remained unchanged despite the wearing of an implant.

DISCUSSION (PATIENTS)

The patients report that they feel much safer since they have an implant. Since they are able to encode a wide variety of environmental sounds such as warning signals, they can detect and evaluate potential dangers more effectively. They note that they are more secure in going shopping, to the library, driving a car, and the like, and do not need to be accompanied by others. They appear to have fewer episodes of depression and/or anxiety than prior to the implant. An increased sense of mastery is also evidenced by the fact that they report feeling generally less upset. Emotional well-being has been significantly improved. One major contribution to the sense of increased independence and emotional security is the finding that they feel they are less of a burden to their families. This undoubtedly diminishes guilt and anger, and bolsters self-esteem.

Communication is a much smoother process. Extreme feelings of frustration about difficulties in communication appear to have been modulated. The implant provides a larger number of verbal cues which can lead to improved communication, particularly with people with whom the patient is frequently in contact. They are almost in unanimous agreement that one of the effects of the implant in relation to communication is that it promotes their capacity for lip reading. One outcome of improved communication is that the patients sense a greater ability to express ideas and make their needs more directly known to others.

While participation in group activities is difficult, the patients tend to be much more comfortable in such situations than prior to the acquisition of the prosthesis. They are somewhat more facile in picking up the drift of conversations. They report that in family settings, and to some degree in other groups, they feel less isolated because their under-

TABLE 2. MEAN INDEX RELATIVE RATINGS PREIMPLANT AND POSTIMPLANT FOR THOSE ITEMS SHOWING GREATEST IMPROVEMENT (N = 13)

	Preim-plant	*Postim-plant*	*T*	*p*
Concern for patient's safety	2.8	1.8	0	.0038
Patient's negative emotional reactions	2.7	1.2	0	.0017
Frustration in communication	1.9	0.8	0	.009
Quality of patient's voice	2.4	3.2	3.5	.012

standing about what is transpiring has improved. While they continue to favor more isolated activities, as they did when they were profoundly deafened (eg, reading), they nevertheless have an enhanced feeling of belonging to a social group and can make use of such situations more frequently. This reduces the number of episodes in which they feel extremely lonely.

The patients report that the implant has a decided effect on their lifestyle because it has extended their sensory capacities which, in turn, permits them to engage in human activities formerly denied them.

RESULTS (INDEX RELATIVE)

There were 23 questions where the index relative responded to preimplant and postimplant. As was the case with the patients, *all* comparisons elicited change in the direction which supported the view that the index relative perceived a positive change in the patient and a personal sense of relief because the latter seemed to be functioning more satisfactorily. The mean change for this sample for all questions was 0.47; mean change scores for individual questions ranged from 0.07 to 1.16.

Twelve questions met the criteria for statistical significance ($p \leq 0.05$). Of these, the greatest improvement was demonstrated in the following areas: concern for patient's safety, patient's negative emotional reactions, frustration in communication, and the quality of the patient's voice. Table 2 presents mean index relative ratings for those items.

The areas that showed the least improvement were all related to the quality of the index relative's relationship with the patient. Not surprisingly, this relationship appeared to remain unchanged despite the other positive lifestyle changes reported as related to the wearing of an implant.

DISCUSSION (INDEX RELATIVE)

The index relative tends to perceive events in a manner similar to that of the patient. Now that the patient has the implant, the index relative is relieved about matters of safety. The patient is perceived to have fewer episodes of emotional distress. By the same token, the index relative is less upset and this is attributed to the contribution of the implant toward the patient's well-being. Communication is perceived to be smoother in that the patient seems to understand more, is a better speechreader and can modulate his or her voice more successfully. Because of these factors, the index relative is less frustrated when communicating with the patient. This factor is doubtless a significant contribution to the reduction in emotional tension in both the patient and the index relative. In addition, they noted there has been some increase in the number of social situations they have attended with the implantee.

There were some contradictions in the way the index relatives responded to questions. For example, many index relatives noted that, prior to the implants, they did not consider the deafened individual with whom they were involved to be a burden or that they harbored negative feelings toward him or her. This can only be ascribed to denial and guilt since fears for the patient's safety, heightened levels of frustration due to severe impediments in communication, and the like, must have made them feel that their profoundly deafened relative was indeed a burden.

SUMMARY

The ultimate value of any invention is its effect on human experience. The cochlear implant provides the profoundly deafened with a limited range of sound, although discriminated speech is beyond its grasp. Does it make a difference to the recipient's lifestyle? The answer derived from our data is clearly in the affirmative. For the profoundly deafened, the implant increases the sense of security, diminishes dependence on others, reduces the frequency and intensity of emotional distress, promotes communication, particularly through more efficient speechreading, and there is a significant decrease in dread when social situations are encountered. These events are confirmed by outside observers, namely the index relatives. These improvements in the patient's experience have a secondary but highly salutary effect in the index relatives. In short, the latter also feel more secure and optimistic that the deafened relative or friend has a new resource which extends his or her coping abilities.

The questionnaire used for this study was based on information gathered from many patient and index relative interviews. It provides a means for quantifying an individual's perceptions of the effect of the cochlear implant on his or her life. That effect is the primary concern that dictates the value of a prosthetic device for the consumer/patient.

USE OF THE COCHLEAR IMPLANT BY THE PRELINGUALLY DEAF

LAURIE S. EISENBERG, MA

Introducing sound to the prelingually deaf adult presents a special challenge to those concerned with the rehabilitation of the deaf utilizing the cochlear implant. Twelve subjects with an early loss have undergone implant surgery and have been fitted with external stimulator devices. Eight of the 12 subjects are considered successful users. Electrical thresholds are comparable to those for the postlingually deaf. However, the prelingual subjects initially have a reduced tolerance for sound and often react differently than the postlinguals. The prelinguals do not always respond to the sensation as sound, but rather as a feeling or vibration in the head. However, like the postlinguals, the prelingually deaf report being able to respond to attention-getting sounds, such as horn-honks and their names being called; and voice quality changes have been noted. These subjects find music particularly enjoyable through the implant. In addition, they have reported feeling more independent, more social, and even less lonely.

To most people the term deafness often evokes an image of an individual who attended special schools for the deaf, uses sign language to communicate, and primarily associates with other deaf people. This, in fact, is often an accurate description of the individual who was born deaf or lost his or her hearing early in life. The congenitally or prelingually deaf, in most cases, are individuals who have devoted their entire childhood to trying to overcome this profound sensory impairment, an impairment which potentially can retard linguistic, cognitive, and social development, as well as alienate the child from family members due to an inability to communicate wants and needs.

With the exception of a small percentage, most deaf children are born to hearing parents.[1] As hearing loss is detected, parents attempt to seek out all of the educational options available. Often they are told that the learning of sign language may seriously limit the child's chance for being successful in a hearing world. So the child begins the laborious process of learning language and speech through an oral/aural approach. Some of those children are successful, depending on such factors as severity of loss, early detection, and ability to make use of residual hearing through effective amplication. But often there is minimal or no progress, and then manual communication is reconsidered. Of those children who continue in oral education, many eventually learn sign language as the easiest way to communicate with their deaf friends and schoolmates. By the time adolescence is reached, most deaf children have made the decision to either join the deaf world or attempt to live in the hearing world; the majority choose the deaf world.

There is another group of deaf individuals — those who acquired a profound hearing loss after having developed speech and language. In most cases, these are people who attended normal schools, come from a hearing family, work and socialize with hearing people. In other words, sound had at one time been an integral part of their lives. Onset of deafness affects every aspect of life; job, family and friend relationships, etc. There is a tendency to withdraw from most social situations. In addition, absence of sound results in an extreme sense of isolation. The postlingually deaf do not fit into either the hearing or the deaf world.

The cochlear implant has been studied primarily with the postlingually deafened adult. These subjects were originally chosen as a source for comparing normal hearing (auditory memory) with hearing from the implant. But even more, these subjects had a strong need to be back in an auditory environment. While we know that the implant does not provide even near normal speech discrimination, it does give enough clues from timing and intensity information to aid in lipreading. Additionally, it allows the deaf individual to hear his or her own voice for purposes of monitoring volume and pitch. Thus, communication is enhanced, giving more confidence and less tendency to withdraw from social settings.[2,3]

With the implant the majority of the profoundly deaf subjects attain thresholds for warble tones from about 50-70 dB SPL through the speech frequencies.[4,5] This enables the individual to come into contact with many sounds within the environment. It likewise gives a greater sense of security and independence in the ability to perceive and recognize warning signals, and to use the telephone for emergency situations.

The findings to date indicate that the cochlear implant can be of significant benefit for the postlingually deafened individual. But the majority of congenital or prelingually deaf have accommodated to a life without hearing and have learned to rely on alternate sensory modalities as a substitute. Can the benefits provided by the cochlear implant be of significance for the prelingually deaf?

Human and animal studies indicate that extensive sensory hair cell damage results in some further, but not total, retrograde degeneration of spiral ganglion cells, cochlear nerve fibers, and cells within the cochlear nucleus. This is found in both adventitious and congenital hearing loss.[6-10] Findings of Webster and Webster[11,12] suggest that congenital deafness (or any early deprivation of sound) causes an incomplete maturation of cells in the cochlear nucleus; this development takes place postnatally and apparently requires auditory stimulation. Ruben and Rapin[13] cite a number of animal studies which show behavioral effects of early auditory deprivation.

The House Ear Institute (HEI) has recently devoted considerable effort to the study of those adults either born deaf or deafened in early childhood. The electrical stimulation of the auditory system in these subjects poses two questions: 1) can an individual who has reached maturity without normal development of auditory pathways now receive and make use of an auditory signal; and 2) if so, can these subjects learn to make use of this sound to improve their quality of life?

A therapy plan was developed at HEI which teaches the concepts of sound to the prelingually deaf adult using the cochlear implant.[14] The program takes a multisensory approach whereby auditory input is integrated with visual and tactile information as a means of developing auditory perceptual skills. The lessons progress in a hierarchy of difficulty which begins with the production of sound. Many deaf individuals do not realize that most objects are capable of producing sound, even if only by actions (eg, fork hitting plate).[15] Instruction regarding more abstract conceptualization, such as viewing of sound being produced on film, progressing to listening to sound on audiotape, is gradually introduced. Music and environmental sounds form the basis of the program. Music in particular has been found to be a successful therapeutic tool in helping to facilitate a carryover from vibrotactile experience to auditory experience. The basic parameters of sound (such as timing and intensity) are taught using music, and reinforced through a series of familiar associations (environmental sounds) which serve to convey the meaning and usefulness of sound.

PRELIMINARY FINDINGS

Prelingually Deaf Adult. Experimentation with a small group of subjects suggests that electrical stimulation of the residual auditory neurons in the prelingually deaf adult does provide useful information. Currently, 12 adult subjects evaluated at HEI with early childhood hearing losses (prelingual — arbitrarily defined by HEI as any subject deafened before age 5 — and congenital) have undergone implant surgery and been fitted with external stimulator devices. Table 1 provides a description of the subjects. Their ages at time of implant range from 19 to 41 years with a mean age of 26 years. The majority of the subjects had some experience with hearing aids at some time in their lives. It should, however, be pointed out that only two subjects were using amplification at the time of receiving the implant. Eight of the 12 subjects are considered successful users in that they use the implant on a daily basis. Of these 8, 6 are congenitally deaf. With respect to mode of communication, it is interesting that all four subjects who come from an oral/aural (speech- and lipreading) background are successful users. Subjects from either a manual (sign language) or total (oral/manual) background are evenly distributed between the users and nonusers. Two successful users are from essentially a manual background. Both of these subjects had etiologies of Usher syndrome, and were in need of a back-up system should their vision completely fail. One additional trend was that the most successful users tended to be those subjects with strong family support during the rehabilitation process. With regard to those subjects classified as nonusers, the only consistent pattern appeared to be that 3 of the 4 subjects had concurrent emotional and/or personality traits which seemed to interfere with their lives.

Table 2 presents test results which indicate that electrical thresholds for the prelingually deaf subjects are comparable to those for the postlingually

TABLE 1. COCHLEAR IMPLANT ADULT SUBJECTS WITH EARLY CHILDHOOD HEARING LOSS

Subject	*Implant Use on a Daily Basis*	*Date of Beginning Stimulation*	*Onset of Deafness*	*Age at Time of Receiving Implant*	*Use of Hearing Aid At Time of Receiving Implant*	*Mode of Communication*
A	Nonuser	10/73	Birth	23	No	Manual
B	User	10/73	Birth	41	No	Manual/oral
C	User	8/74	6 mo*	37	No	Oral
D	Nonuser	9/78	2 yr	19	No	Manual
E	User	1/79	Birth	32	No	Manual
F	User	2/79	4 yr	34	No	Oral
G	Nonuser	7/79	4 yr	19	No	Manual/oral
H	User	1/80	Birth	19	No	Manual
I	Nonuser	3/80	Birth*	26	No	Manual/oral
J	User	4/80	Birth	19	No	Oral
K	User	6/80	Birth	22	Yes	Oral
L	User	8/80	Birth	26	Yes	Manual/oral

*Not profound at onset.

TABLE 2. ELECTRICAL TEST RESULTS IN VOLTS* AT THE EXTERNAL COIL (PRELINGUAL VS TOTAL SUBJECTS)

	Threshold		Uncomfortable Loudness Levels	
	No.	*Mean(V)*	*No.*	*Mean(V)*
Prelinguals	9	2	4	5.9
Pre- & postlinguals combined	87	3	50	14.0

*Peak-to-peak.

TABLE 3. MEAN WARBLE TONE THRESHOLDS WITH THE COCHLEAR IMPLANT IN THE SOUND FIELD (PRELINGUAL VS TOTAL SUBJECTS)

	Mean Warble Tone Thresholds (dB SPL*) Frequency in Hertz				
	250	*500*	*1000*	*2000*	*3000*
Prelinguals (N = 5)	74	64	61	64	63
Pre- & postlinguals combined (N = 74)	64	60	58	57	60

*Re: 20 μ Pascal.

deaf subjects. However, the prelingual subjects take quite a bit longer to acclimate to sound. They initially can only tolerate stimulation for short periods of time such as 1 to 2 hours a day. This tolerance increases with time. The prelinguals are varied in their daily usage, ranging from 7 or 8 hours per day for some subjects to 14-16 hours per day for others. The prelingual subjects also tend to have a reduced tolerance for the intensity of the stimulus. The mean uncomfortable loudness level (ULL) for four prelingual subjects is 5.9 V (p-p) when measured at the external coil. (The majority of the subjects were not tested for ULL; this is a very difficult measure for subjects with little or no previous sound experience.) This contrasts with the mean ULL for 50 implant subjects (combined early and late losses) which is twice as high at 14 V. Therefore, the implant stimulator units for the prelinguals are set rather conservatively. This results in slightly higher warble-tone thresholds in the sound field (Table 3). With time, the subjects can generally tolerate higher voltage settings.

Initial reactions to sound for the prelinguals have been varied. Most of the subjects (congenitals even more so than those who lost their hearing in early childhood) have described such sensations as dizziness, spinning in the head, pulsation of the eyes deep inside the head, and bodily reactions such as feelings in the chest or throat. Hearing is predominantly described as feeling or vibration in the head, either in the forehead or all over the head, but not in the region of the ear. This contrasts with the postlingually deaf subjects who have described it as an auditory sensation usually deep within the ear. (One subject totally deaf for 48 years — commencing at age 6 as a result of trauma to the head — also described the stimulus from the implant as a sensation in the center of the forehead.)

Two congenitally deaf subjects who had early and continuous exposure to sound through hearing aids (and were planning to continue using them on the ear opposite the implant) likewise reacted to the sound with descriptions of bodily sensations and vibrations in the head. Using both prostheses together, these subjects were eventually able to merge the two different sensations (hearing and feeling), and were less aware of "vibrations." As one of these subjects described:

When I wore the implant for the first time, I felt vibrations in my head and didn't hear anything through my ear. I had a terrible headache caused by a lot of vibration for a couple of weeks. A few months later, the vibration in my head stopped. Then I felt sounds going through my ear with the implant, as same as with my hearing aid.

The other subject noted that after approximately three months of using the implant the vibrations in the head were still present, but that sounds in the ear were also being experienced. Nevertheless, rehabilitation for these two subjects required a comprehensive program of introducing the basic parameters of sound and auditory training techniques — the program specially developed for those with little or no previous auditory experience.

The fact that the congenital subjects relate to this sensation as vibration or feeling in the head is reasonable when one considers that the deaf have always been able to perceive sound (if intense enough) in the form of vibrations on the skin. However, we recently had the opportunity to observe two very unusual cases. One case, reported by our coinvestigator team from Houston (Porter T, Maddox HE, personal communication), was a woman prelingually deafened in one ear and postlingually deafened (onset during teens) in the other ear. This enabled her to develop normal language and speech, in addition to retaining a memory for sound. Cochlear implant surgery was performed on the ear which was prelingually deafened. Initial testing with the implant evoked similar reactions to those of the congenital subjects, that is, "pressure" or "vibration in the head." By making the signal stronger in intensity, she was able to perceive it as auditory.

Of even more interest is a case seen at HEI of a 34-year-old male who lost his hearing in the right ear in childhood reportedly due to measles. An acoustic tumor later developed on the left side, and hearing had been slowly deteriorating over the last 13 years. This resulted in a severe sensorineural loss, which was aided with a BICROS system. The subject was investigating various medical/surgical treatments for the tumor, and decided to have an implant on the right ear as a precaution, should removal of the tumor result in total deafness.

This subject reacted to electrical stimulation as the congenitals did; initial reaction was dizziness, and as the intensity was increased a "pounding" in the forehead was experienced. He was able to give us some very interesting descriptions.

> . . . I felt a sudden sensation. This sensation came from the middle of my head almost directly above the bridge of my nose about four inches up, and seemed to be emanating from where my hairline begins. It felt like a pounding sensation, like a rush of air coming across from my eyes and protruding from my eyes up through the back of my nose and pushing towards the top of my skull . . .

His description of the second day was:

> It's like a search beacon swimming in my head, swirling around and affecting my eyes, and the left and right side of my head from the eye level straight up and over, and then down over the other right eye level, and across over the bridge of the nose almost like a rectangle. It's almost as if it makes my hair stand on end. It's discomforting, but it does not hurt.

After one week of stimulation the sensation changed to a "horizontal-like feeling" from ear to ear, about eye level. He perceived it as being a bit stronger on the right. After approximately six months of stimulation, the sensation moved to the locale of the right ear, and was definitely perceived as hearing.

Unlike the Houston subject, this subject did not perceive sound with increases in intensity, but rather experienced only an increase in discomfort. These reactions lead us to believe that his implanted ear was very possibly a congenital loss, as primarily only the congenitals have responded this way. The subject indicates that this is indeed a possibility. Thus this case may have provided us with an ear that has never received any acoustic stimulation before in a patient who is postlingually deafened and has years of sound experience from the other ear. We had assumed that the reactions of the congenitally deaf were of a cognitive nature. That is, that the congenitally deaf did not have the experience or the vocabulary to describe sound. The fact that this subject also did not interpret the stimulus as auditory raises the issue that such perception of sound may additionally have a developmental or physiological basis.

Another major difference between the postlinguals and the prelinguals is in response to music. The postlingual subjects are quite disappointed when hearing music through the implant. This is understandable in that the signal they receive lacks the tonal/harmonic structure which comes to be representative of music for the hearing person. The prelingual subjects, in contrast, find music particularly enjoyable with the implant. In some cases music has been the major motivating factor behind acceptance of the implant. This may be attributed to the fact that the prelingual deaf also have a defined representation of what music is. By using primarily the tactile sensory mode, the deaf pick up vibrations of varying duration, intensity and tempo, and give an aesthetic interpretation to this code. The implant, likewise, provides the temporal/intensity cues of music. In this way music, via the newly acquired hearing modality, maintains its structural integrity within a defined construct. In fact, the implant provides the prelingually deaf with more sensations from music than they could otherwise obtain.

The benefits derived from the implant by a postlingually deafened adult were discussed early in the paper. The prelingual subjects, likewise, report similar advantages. As with the postlinguals, the prelingually deaf subjects report being able to respond to attention-getting sounds such as horn-honks and their names being called. Voice quality changes (toward a more habitual pitch) have been noted in these subjects. In addition, subjects have reported feeling more independent, more social, and even less lonely.

The subjects generally report that the implant brings in more sounds than had ever been experienced through hearing aids. One subject, who had worn an aid all her life, stated that this was the first time she had ever heard such sounds as water flowing, paper crackling, a kiss on the hand, chalk on a board, and even hands hitting while using sign language. The knowledge that most objects are capable of producing sound through action, and that sounds can be experienced from a distance has been a revelation to these subjects.

Contact with sounds in the environment has been of extreme importance to man from an evolutionary standpoint. As Berliner[16] states:

> It seems reasonable that the continual awareness of or sensing of the environment through the auditory modality has had survival value for humans in their evolutionary history. They come equipped with adult size cochleas at birth, the only organ of the body that is adult size at birth, and hearing provides some of the first contacts with the world . . . The infant uses his sense of hearing in a number of ways before he has acquired speech perception ability, and prehistoric man undoubtedly used audition to advantage before development of a spoken language.

Man has an innate need for sound. For our prelingually deaf implant subjects there seems no doubt that the ability to hear sound adds a new dimension of sensory awareness for interacting with the environment.

The cochlear implant does not take the prelingually deaf adult out of the world of deafness, nor does it significantly alter any style of living, as these patterns have been long established. However, the fact that these subjects have accepted sound and find it useful and enjoyable, has encouraged us to begin looking at the deaf child.

Subjects under Age Eighteen. To date, 12 profoundly deaf children have undergone implant surgery and been fitted with external stimulator devices. The results on these subjects can be found in this monograph as a separate chapter devoted just to children.[17] However, with our knowledge of how the congenitally deaf adults initially describe the sensations, we were concerned about how the congenitally deaf children would respond, particularly the first child, a 10-year-old male. His first reaction to sound through the implant was similar to that of the prelingual adults, a sensation experienced in the head. This was understandably quite disturbing to him, and he began to exhibit symptoms of anxiety. Rather than run the risk of conditioning him to sound as an aversive stimulus, a behavior-shaping approach using techniques of desensitization was initiated. The stimulator device was fit on him, but set below his level of awareness. We had him participating in sound-producing activities which were pleasurable for him. Gradually the volume was increased. With each increment he was positively reinforced with some reward. By the end of two weeks he was able to make simple discriminations such as a door knock from a doorbell ring from his name being called. He was using the implant 10-11 hours a day.

The ultimate goal for this project is to be able to implant the very young deaf child who cannot benefit from traditional amplification. In this way, residual cochlear nerve fibers can receive some benefit of auditory stimulation during those critical years when sensory pathways are being integrated into the central nervous system and the development of speech and language is at an optimum. Experience with the prelingually deaf adult has been one more step toward this goal. From this very special group we have learned that an auditory signal can be perceived at the adult stage, and become an integral part of the life experience.

REFERENCES

1. Schein JD, Delk MT. The deaf population of the United States. Silver Spring: National Association of the Deaf, 1974.

2. House WF, Berliner KI, Eisenberg LS. Present status and future directions of the Ear Research Institute cochlear implant program. Acta Otolaryngol (Stockh) 1979; 87:176-84.

3. House WF. Continued implantation of cochlear prostheses in a limited number of postlingually deaf subjects is appropriate. In: Snow JB, ed. Controversy in otolaryngology. Philadelphia: Saunders, 1980: 423-32.

4. House WF, Berliner KI, Eisenberg LS, Edgerton BJ, Thielemeir MA. The cochlear implant: 1980 update. Acta Otolaryngol (Stockh) 1981; 91:457-62.

5. Thielemeir MA, Brimacombe JA, Eisenberg LS. Audiological results with the single-electrode cochlear implant. Ann Otol Rhinol Laryngol 1982; 91 Suppl 91:27-34.

6. Kerr A, Schuknecht HF. The spiral ganglion in profound deafness. Acta Otolaryngol (Stockh) 1968; 65:586-98.

7. Otte J, Schuknecht HF, Kerr AG. Ganglion cell populations in normal and pathological human cochleae: implications for cochlear implantation. Laryngoscope 1978; 88:1231-46.

8. Webster DB, Webster M. Cochlear nerve projections following organ of Corti destruction. Otolaryngology 1978; 86: ORL 342-53.

9. Ylikoski J, Collan Y, Palva T. Pathologic features of the cochlear nerve in profound deafness. Arch Otolaryngol 1978; 104:202-7.

10. Ghorayeb B, Sarwat A, Linthicum FH. Viable spiral ganglion cells in congenital and acquired profound hearing loss. J Laryngol Otol 1980; 94:367-76.

11. Webster DB, Webster M. Neonatal sound deprivation affects brain stem auditory nuclei. Arch Otolaryngol 1977; 103:392-6.

12. Webster DB, Webster M. Effects of neonatal conductive hearing loss on brain stem auditory nuclei. Ann Otol Rhinol Laryngol 1979; 88:684-8.

13. Ruben RJ, Rapin I. Plasticity of the developing auditory system. Ann Otol Rhinol Laryngol 1980; 89:303-11.

14. Eisenberg LS. Introduction to sound: a therapy program developed for the prelingually deaf adult using a cochlear implant. Los Angeles: Hearing Rehabilitation Research Center, 1980.

15. Liben LS. Developmental perspectives on the experiential deficiencies of deaf children. In: Liben LS. Deaf children: developmental perspectives. New York: Academic Press, 1978: 195-215.

16. Berliner KI. Human contact with the environment: environmental sounds. Master's Thesis. California State University, Los Angeles, 1975: 1-2.

17. Eisenberg LS, House WF. Initial experience with the cochlear implant in children. Ann Otol Rhinol Laryngol 1982; 91 Suppl 91:67-73.

INITIAL EXPERIENCE WITH THE COCHLEAR IMPLANT IN CHILDREN

LAURIE S. EISENBERG, MA WILLIAM F. HOUSE, MD

The decision to implant cochlear prostheses in children came after positive findings with deaf adults and the belief that the benefits of receiving sound far outweigh the potential risks involved. As of December 1981, 12 profoundly deaf children have received the single-electrode cochlear implant. Their ages range from 3.5 to 17 years. Test results are consistent with those of adults. Mean thresholds across the frequency range fall between 59-64 dB SPL. With the implant, these children can perform specific timing and intensity differentiations which could not be done with hearing aids. Their voices are quieter and more modulated, and the children are not quite as noisy with objects in the environment (eg, do not slam doors any more). This preliminary data demonstrates that implanting subjects under the age of 18 years is feasible.

Most educators of the deaf advocate the need to fit young deaf children with amplification as early as possible. Traditionally, high-powered hearing aids have been the prosthesis of choice, even though there existed a potential risk of doing further damage to inner ear structures.[1] The rationale supporting this view maintains that children need auditory input most particularly during those critical early years when language development is at an optimum.

Often, however, children with total or profound hearing loss have not been able to benefit from hearing aids. In recent years, the single-electrode cochlear implant has been proven a clinically feasible alternative for profoundly deaf adults. The decision to implant children came as a result of the belief that the benefit of sound to a profoundly deaf child far outweighs the potential risks involved.[2] Extensive experience with a large number of implanted deaf adults gives us objective evidence that the implant provides significant benefit. Warble tone thresholds across the frequency range show detection between 55-70 dB SPL.[3] This allows for contact with a great many sounds within the environment. Psychoacoustic measurements reveal near normal durational and intensity information, with measurable frequency difference limens to 500 Hz.[4,5] While this does not provide enough cues to understand speech, it does provide prosodic elements of speech (such as stress and syllabication) which can supplement lipreading. The subjects, likewise, are able to spontaneously monitor their voices toward a more appropriate volume and pitch.

The majority of subjects implanted have been postlingually deafened. The postlingual adults have demonstrated an ability to make reasonable judgments regarding the sound, and thus are good test subjects. However, congenitally (or prelingually) deaf adults had to be investigated as a prelude to considering children. From a physiological point of view, there was a need to know if one either born deaf, or deafened in early childhood, had an auditory system that was capable of being stimulated. Additionally, it was necessary to know whether the prelingually deaf could receive benefit from the implant similar to that of the postlinguals.

A small sample of 12 prelingually deaf adults was implanted and put through a rehabilitation program developed at the House Ear Institute. From these subjects it was learned that even with long-term auditory deprivation from birth or early childhood, the auditory system is still capable of being stimulated. It was also shown that these subjects receive and can make use of the timing/intensity patterns used by the postlingual adults. They, likewise, report similar benefit such as contact with the auditory environment; feeling more independent, more social, less lonely; and improvement in voice quality.[6]

Yet, while the postlingual subjects consistently report significant improvement in quality of life, the prelingual subjects indicate that the addition of an auditory channel has limited effect on their lives, as patterns and habits for living in a deaf world (a world without need for sound) have been long established.

Thus, from these results it was hypothesized that the younger that one can be implanted, the greater the chance for effecting a change, particularly if hearing can be integrated into the central nervous system during those critical developmental years, and before reliance on alternate sensory modalities becomes habitual. It is to be expected that the young subjects will receive the same information from the implant as the adults. Yet the potential for benefit is perhaps even greater. Timing and intensity information cannot be underestimated with respect to speech reception and production. Simmons[7] reports three cases with no hearing above 750 Hz, but normal hearing below that frequency. All three of the cases developed the losses prior to age 2, yet are able to communicate quite effectively. He at-

TABLE 1. SUBJECTS UNDER AGE 18 RECEIVING COCHLEAR IMPLANT

Subject	*Sex*	*Age At Onset of Deafness*	*Etiology*	*Age in Years at Time of Receiving Implant (Beginning Stimulation)*	*Use of Hearing Aids at Time of Receiving Implant*	*Mode of Communication*
A	M	Birth	Unknown	10.8	No	Manual
B	M	7.5 yr	Trauma	12.3	No	Oral/aural
C	F	Birth	Unknown	17.1	No	Manual
D	F	3 yr	Meningitis	3.5	Yes	Oral/aural
E	M	Birth	Unknown	11.8	Yes	Manual
F	M	1 yr	Meningitis	8.7	Yes	Manual
G	F	Birth	Maternal rubella	4.0	Yes	Manual
H	M	Birth	Unknown	13.5	Yes	Oral/aural
I	F	1.3 yr	Meningitis	9.0	Yes	Manual
J	M	Birth	Unknown	17.0	No	Manual
K	F	5 yr	Meningitis	10.5	Yes	Oral/aural
L	M	2.8 yr	Meningitis	6.8	Yes	Manual

tributes this to an ability to make use of rate-pitch coding during the early years. This is the kind of information the implant can provide.

Animal and human studies on auditory deprivation indicate that absence of acoustic stimulation in early developmental years can result in the inability of the auditory neural network to reach full maturity.[8-10] Giving the young deaf child some auditory stimulation now may make that child better able to use more sophisticated systems available in years to come.

The ultimate measure of success with deaf children has to lie in how the implant can influence the receptive and productive elements of speech. The most appropriate way to determine the potential effect of the implant on speech and language is a controlled study which can directly compare profoundly deaf children using an implant to those using a hearing aid and those with no prosthesis at all. Such an investigation will take much planning and will necessarily be a long-term endeavor. However, prior to undertaking such an investigation a pilot study is necessary. Such issues as ability to wear equipment, assessment procedures, and development of a habilitation program all require studying a select group of profoundly deaf children of varying ages on which to base the development of a protocol for a controlled study.

The most immediate concern prior to initiating even a pilot study is the issue of surgery in the young deaf child. It has been well documented that the cochlea and middle ear structures are adult size at birth. At approximately two years, the facial recess reaches adult size. However, the squamous portion of the mastoid bone is small and the skull thin. Small internal coils have been tolerated well, and the electrodes have enough length to compensate for growth of the skull. Thus from a surgical standpoint it is feasible to implant at two years of age.[11]

Another issue is a medical concern. With the occurrence of otitis media, the risk of infection invading the cochlea cannot be ruled out. The fact that no insulating material enters the scala significantly reduces the risk. One adult implant subject developed an otitis media that resolved with no complications. However, the children must be watched carefully in this regard.

A further consideration is that of equipment. The adult subjects are required to wear a pair of glasses as a means of holding the external coil to the head. Prior to the actual implanting of children, internal magnet/coil systems were implanted in animals[12] and then adults. These were found to be a successful replacement for the glasses. They also make alignment between the two coils much easier.

SUBJECTS

The children chosen for the pilot study were tested under headphones, with hearing aids, impedance audiometry, and brainstem evoked response tests (subjects under age 5) to confirm bilateral profound deafness. The ear chosen for the implant was the poorest of the two ears with respect to hearing aid performance. Educators of deaf preschoolers have remarked on the importance of allowing a trial period with hearing aids (especially prior to the age of three years) before making a decision as to benefit. Thus, the children under five years had at least six months' prior experience with aids.

All previous audiological and academic records were required from each child. Contacts were set up with the schools the children attended. As important as it is for us to learn about the child, it is equally important that the schools begin to learn about the implant.

To date, 12 profoundly deaf subjects under the age of 18 have been selected to undergo cochlear implant surgery.

Table 1 provides a description of the 12 subjects. The ages of these subjects range from 3.5 to 17 years, with a mean age of 10.3 years. Five of the subjects are female and seven are male. Six of the subjects were born deaf, while the other six were deafened due to either meningitis or trauma. Eight

TABLE 2. PREOPERATIVE WARBLE TONE THRESHOLDS (dB SPL*) UNDER HEADPHONES IN EAR RECEIVING IMPLANT ON SUBJECTS UNDER AGE 18

	Frequency (Hz)				
Subject	*250*	*500*	*1000*	*2000*	*3000*
A	120.5	96.5	117	NLA	NLA
B	NLA	NLA	NLA	NLA	NLA
C	90.5	91.5	107	NLA	NLA
D	NLA	NLA	NLA	NLA	NLA
E	NLA	NLA	NLA	NLA	NLA
F	130	NLA	NLA	NLA	NLA
G	NLA	NLA	NLA	NLA	NLA
H	115.5	121.5	NLA	114	NLA
I	110.5	NLA	NLA	NLA	NLA
J	NLA	100	110	110	105
K	NLA	NLA	NLA	NLA	NLA
L	115.5	121.5	NLA	NLA	NLA

*re: 20 μ Pa.

NLA - Not to the limit of the audiometer.

of the 12 subjects utilize manual communication (sign language) as their primary means of communication while the other 4 use oral modes. Subjects B, D and K had developed language prior to onset of deafness, and were using speech and lipreading (oral/aural) to communicate. Subject H, while born deaf, had enough usable residual hearing with aids to develop oral skills. All of the children have had some experience with hearing aids. Eight of the children were still wearing aids at the time of receiving the implant.

Table 2 demonstrates the profoundness of the hearing loss in the ear undergoing implantation. Table 3 shows hearing aid performance in the ear receiving the implant. Subjects C, H and J show responses out to 3000 Hz. However, these subjects had extremely small dynamic ranges and could not tolerate any aid of enough gain to provide adequate sound awareness for general use.

RESULTS

All 12 of the subjects have successfully undergone cochlear implant surgery. Four of the subjects were implanted in the right ear, and eight were implanted in the left ear. The dates of stimulation commence with subject A, who began stimulation in August 1980, to the most current subject, who started in December 1981. All of the children have been implanted with magnet/coil systems. The figure shows how the implant is worn by a young subject. The two youngest subjects wear the

TABLE 3. PREOPERATIVE WARBLE TONE THRESHOLDS WITH HEARING AIDS IN SOUND FIELD (dB SPL*) IN EAR RECEIVING IMPLANT

	Frequency (Hz)				
*Subject***	*250*	*500*	*1000*	*2000*	*3000*
B	NR	90.0	NR	NR	NR
C	65.5	36.5	47	74	85
D	NR	NR	NR	NR	NR
E	80.0	NR	NR	NR	NR
F	85.0	90.0	NR	NR	NR
G	NR	NR	NR	NR	NR
H	80	75	60	80	80
I	80	60	90	NR	NR
J	80	66.5	78	82.5	82.5
K	90	90	NR	NR	NR
L	80	70	80	NR	NR

*re: 20 μ Pa.

**Subject A did not test with hearing aid; aided speech threshold -75 dB SPL.

NR - No response at 90 dB SPL.

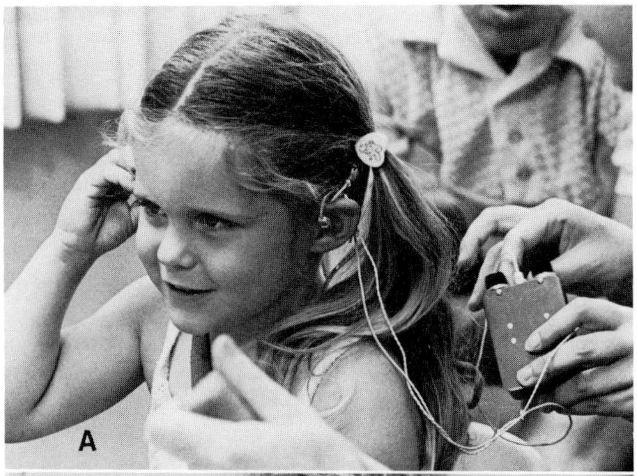

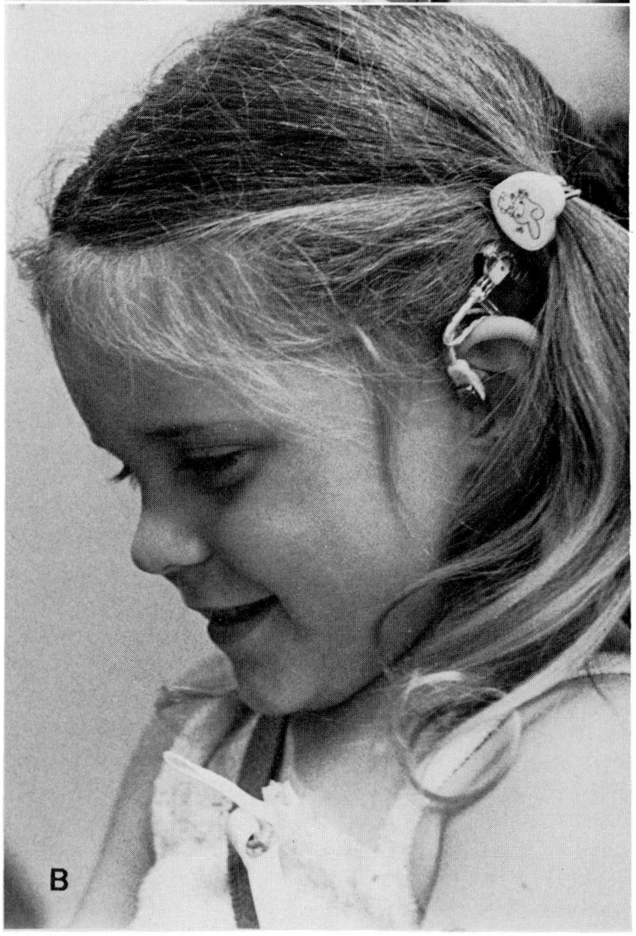

A) External coil, microphone, and stimulator unit as shown on young implant subject. B) Closeup of center magnet coil and microphone worn by young implant subject.

TABLE 4. MEAN WARBLE TONE THRESHOLDS (dB SPL*) WITH COCHLEAR IMPLANT: CHILDREN VERSUS ADULTS

	Frequency (Hz)				
Subjects	250	500	1000	2000	3000
Children	65	61	59	61	62
Adults (n = 74)	64	60	58	57	60

*re: 20 μ Pa.

TABLE 5. WARBLE TONE THRESHOLDS (dB SPL) WITH COCHLEAR IMPLANT FOR SUBJECTS UNDER AGE 18

	Warble Tone Thresholds (dB SPL*) Frequency (Hz)				
Subjects**	250	500	1000	2000	3000
A	58	53	54	64	60
B	59	53	56	50	60
C	58	55	56	63	62
D	78	67	65	61	56
E	66	65	55	56	62
F	73	69	65	69	64
H	65	64	62	61	64
I	66	60	57	63	64
J	51	56	53	55	57
K	66	66	62	60	66
L	62	62	60	67	75

*re: 20 μ Pa.
**Subject G could not be conditioned to respond to sound.

stimulator unit in a very small backpack on their backs. Worn in this manner it doesn't get in the way when they are very physically active. The older children wear the device in the same manner as adults.

Initial Reactions to Stimulation. From the experience we have had with congenitally deaf adults, we know that initial reaction to the implant can be disturbing. The sensation is often first perceived as "dizziness" and feelings in the chest or throat. As the signal is made a little stronger, the sensation is perceived as a feeling or vibration in the center of the forehead. This, understandably, is somewhat discomforting. With time, the strangeness wears off, and subjects report that the vibration disappears and the sensation is perceived in the ear. Knowing this, a primary concern was how the children would initially react, as many would be congenitally impaired.

Initial reactions to electrical stimulation were varied. Subject A was visibly distressed. He began to cry and then pull the coil away. A process of desensitization was initiated whereby hearing was paired with sound-producing activities which were enjoyable to the subject. On the other hand, subject E (who was of a similar age to subject A) was literally enthralled by sound. His eyes would widen at every sound heard. From the very first days he was using the implant up to 13 hours a day.

Subjects F and I, while not having quite as enthusiastic a reaction as subject E, did accept the implant very well. Subject G, our youngest congenital, experienced a reaction similar to subject A. She was visibly confused and startled by the sound. Her response was to take the coil off and go to her mother for comfort. Subject L, likewise, was frightened by the sensation and began to cry. Our goals with these two subjects were to build a tolerance to sound (as with subject A), while at the same time teaching what the sensation is and how to relate to it. This involved a very controlled situation, where the child was either producing the sound or watching it being produced.

Subject D, the youngest subject (and most recently deafened) had a completely different reaction from any other subject (child or adult). She showed no real response to sound for the first three days. Her case is extremely unusual, and will be discussed later in this paper.

The four oldest subjects (B, C, H and J) and subject K reacted like the adult subjects, and were able to be put through the therapy programs developed for the adult implant subjects. In contrast, the two youngest subjects could not even give us the feedback required to know if the stimulator unit was set adequately. Therefore, means for establishing optimum unit settings have been devised that involve techniques of operant conditioning, judgments on voice changes, and ability of the subject to respond to sound while asleep.

Finally, it should be noted that most of the young congenital subjects indicated that the sensation was perceived as a feeling in the forehead. Subject C reported that after approximately six months of using the implant, the sensation localized to her ear, and the "vibration" sensation had disappeared. Subject E reported that after six months hearing was perceived in both the ear and the forehead. The children with acquired deafness indicated that the sound was perceived in the ear, the same as reported by the postlingually deaf implanted adults.

Subject Performance. Test results on these subjects as a group are consistent with those found on the adult subjects. Table 4 shows the mean warble tone thresholds for the children versus adult subjects. Mean warble tone thresholds (in the sound field) across the frequency range fall between 59 and 64 dB SPL for the children (n = 11). This is comparable to the adults, who range from 57 to 64 dB SPL.

Table 5 shows individual test results for the 12 young subjects. These were obtained during the first few weeks of stimulation. The younger children had higher warble tone responses than the older children. We expect to see lower thresholds in time as listening skills are further developed. Subject G could not be taught to respond during this initial period, even with conditioning. She did, however, show definite changes in vocalizing when the implant was activated. After approximately five weeks with stimulation, she did start showing consistent awareness to sound.

With the implant, these subjects are able to perform specific timing and intensity differentiations, none of which could be done with hearing aids. With the exception of the two youngest subjects, the children were able to make judgments between loud and soft sounds the very first session with stimulation. They were also able to count and tell differences in numbers of sounds the first or second day. By the second week they were able to transfer this to numbers of syllables in words and sentences. Additional abilities have included differentiating continuous versus interrupted, long versus short, and fast versus slow. As with the adult subjects, the children can easily discriminate between two and three sounds within the environment, such as a doorknock versus a siren versus their name being called.

Parents' and Teachers' Reactions. From the parents' reports we were able to make better judgments as to appropriate unit setting and effective use. It also enabled us to better modify and tailor therapy for each child's individual needs.

In general, all of the parents have observed that their children have become much quieter when the implant is activated. Their vocalizations become softer in intensity and, thus, more appropriate. The pitch tends to be less shrill and piercing. Objects in the environment are treated with more gentleness. For example, doors are no longer slammed shut and toys are treated less roughly. Some of the parents have remarked that their children seem to focus more on the faces when conversation is going on, and seem very curious about speech. Almost all of the children use their voices when turning the implant on to test the loudness of the setting.

Teachers and speech therapists of the children have remarked that the voices have become more relaxed and natural sounding with the implant activated. Practicing with speech is easier and more progressive now that the children are able to auditorily monitor their voices. One child's teacher, speech therapist, and program coordinator all came to observe him undergoing therapy at the Institute. They commented that he was performing tasks he had never been able to do with the hearing aids. They additionally noted his increased attentiveness for the auditory training activities.

Current Status. Eleven of the 12 children are considered to be successful implant users in that they use the implant on a daily basis. Hours of usage range from 5 to 13 hours a day, with the majority using it 8 to 10 hours. The one subject not using the implant is subject A. This subject initially had a difficult adjustment to the implant. He also had a history of rejecting hearing aids. Prognosis with the implant was believed to be good because after two weeks he was using the implant up to 11 hours a day, and performing simple discrimination tasks. After leaving the Institute he had great difficulty in adjusting to sound, particularly in the school setting. From his reactions to both the implant and to hearing aids in school, there is evidence that the addition of an auditory stimulus somehow interferes with his processing of other information.

To date, no measurable adverse effects have been observed. Surgery and the postoperative period have been unremarkable. One subject developed a slight infection over the incision. This was treated in the early stages and resolved. Two other subjects developed otitis media in the ears having received the implant. Both were treated with antibiotics. The problem resolved without any further complication.

Summary. To summarize, test results as a group are consistent with those of adult subjects. With the implant, the children are able to perform specific timing and intensity differentiation tasks, none of which could be done with hearing aids. Subjects have exhibited a variety of reactions to initial stimulation. The majority of the congenitally deaf children indicate that the sensation is perceived in the forehead, the same as reported by the congenital adults. The children with acquired deafness are similar to the postlingual adults in perceiving the sensation in the ear. Parents and teachers have reported that voices sound modulated and less piercing. It has also been noted that the children are not quite as noisy with objects in the environment. To date, 11 of the 12 subjects use the implant on a daily basis. No adverse effects have been measured.

DISCUSSION

Experience with 12 implanted children has given us the opportunity to evaluate performance in comparison with adult implant subjects. Results indicate that the majority of the children are able to perform specific discrimination tasks within a 2-week period after having received stimulation. The children of age 13 years and older were able to be put through the adult rehabilitation programs, as they were intrinsically motivated to succeed with the implant. The children between the ages of 6 and 12 years required techniques of behavior modification, as motivations were more reward-oriented. The two preschool-age children (subjects D and G) were the most difficult to work with from a therapeutic standpoint. The case of subject D is of major interest in that she is the youngest subject (aged 3.5 years) to have undergone cochlear implant surgery.

This subject became suddenly and profoundly deaf around the time of her third birthday as a result of meningitis. Within a month following the illness, her speech began to deteriorate at an extremely rapid rate. She became completely unintelligible.

Conrad has noted that onset of deafness in early childhood has profound consequences: "...the effects of normal exposure to auditory language for a period of three years appear to become totally erased."[13 p 264] She was fit with hearing aids and put in a preschool deaf classroom. This class advocated the oral/aural method of communication, which relies heavily on usable residual hearing. As the subject was showing no progress, a program of manual communication was recommended by her school audiologist. The cochlear implant was considered as a last resort for providing an auditory feedback mechanism in an effort to facilitate the relearning of speech.

The subject underwent surgery for a cochlear implant in April 1981. She began electrical stimulation the following June. The first week of electrical stimulation, the subject gave very inconsistent responses to sound or even vibration. The stimulator unit was gradually set up to maximum voltage. Yet she showed no conscious awareness to sound either in a play activity or in a therapy/test situation. She did, however, respond consistently to sound while asleep with such responses as body reflexes, eye blinks, and even arousal. Her parents reported that she seemed to lipread them better. That is, they were repeating much less when conversing with her.

During the second week, the subject was using the implant six hours a day. At this point her voice became very quiet. The voltage of the unit was decreased, and her voice became stronger. It was also noted that with the implant activated her voice was less shrill or piercing. At this time we were able to elicit an awareness to sound during audiometric testing. She, likewise, started showing an awareness to loud sounds in the environment (eg, truck passing by).

By the third week she was talking much more, even going up to strangers and talking. Her parents were understanding her a little more. This reduced some of her frustration in trying to communicate her needs. Other people were commenting on the improvement in her speech. She began responding to music on television by getting up and dancing to it. She started to imitate sounds by vocalizing in a similar rhythmic pattern.

In the fourth week the subject was using the implant approximately seven hours per day. She was reciting the songs and nursery rhymes she used to know prior to becoming deaf. During this week we were able to determine auditory thresholds using techniques of behavioral conditioning. She was also able to differentiate between one and two sounds (nonsense syllables). Her awareness to sound in the environment continued to expand. At this point, however, her voice again became very quiet. The voltage of the unit was lowered. This brought the voice back up. The same phenomenon again occurred in the fifth week, so the voltage was again lowered, resulting in a return of the voice.

By the sixth week, the subject was using the implant 10 to 11 hours a day. She was beginning to enunciate syllables in words, where prior to this the words were all slurred together. By this time she was responding to her name being called about 70% of the time (primarily in a quiet environment).

In summary, the case just reviewed is that of the youngest child to have received the cochlear implant. This child could not give us the information needed to know if the implant was set appropriately or even being activated as there was no immediate awareness to the sound. We were able to approximate unit settings based on her voice. With the unit set too low, her voice would go into a very high-pitched shrill tone when screaming to get attention. With the unit set too high, her voice would drop to almost nothing. Over time we were able to lower the unit setting more and more, as she seemed to become more sensitized to sound.

The case of subject D is interesting in that her responses have been atypical for an implant subject, adult or child. Specifically, she differs in the fact that she did not show an immediate awareness to sound. Several explanations are offered. One possibility is that she was perceiving the sound as tinnitus, and was just ignoring it. Another explanation could be that having had normal hearing until recently, this sound was different and she could not immediately relate to it. A third possibility is that this is a result of the meningitis, and of such recent onset of hearing loss, for as disturbing as her initial responses to sound were to us, it was just as disturbing that she had such very inconsistent responses to vibration also, almost as if there had been an anesthetizing effect on the system. Teachers of the deaf are continually baffled by meningitic children's total lack of response. The fact that subject D is becoming more sensitized to sound (as evidenced by decreased unit settings and increased awareness) tends to lend some support to this possibility.

In contrast to this, the other very young child, subject G, (aged 4 years) showed an immediate reaction to sound, yet could not be conditioned to it. Nor did she show any awareness for several weeks after acclimating to the sensation, even though there was a definite change in vocalization. A possible explanation for this is that subject G, being congenitally deaf, may have received a sensation similar to that received initially by the adult congenitals, that is, "dizziness," bodily sensations, and feelings in the forehead. As the discomfort of these symptoms diminished with implant use, she might have become less consciously aware of the sensation. Again, it must be repeated that very young deaf children often require a long trial with acoustic stimulation before showing awareness to it. After about one month of consistent stimulation, subject G not only began to show a conscious awareness to sound in the test situation, but also started responding to sound from her hearing aid in the other ear (for the first time). After five weeks, she could differentiate between four different sounds.

Although reasons are only speculative as to both these subjects' initial reactions, it should be brought to mind that the auditory neural system is still developing at these ages in normal-hearing children.[14] Time and experience with deaf subjects under the age of five years should give us greater insight into what may be occurring to an auditory system just going through the process of maturation.

CONCLUSION

Initial results on 12 implanted children indicate that children receive sound field thresholds and timing/intensity information similar to that received by adult implant subjects. All of the subjects but one are considered successful implant users, and use the implant daily. To date, no measurable adverse effects have been observed. How the processing of auditory information provided by the cochlear implant can influence speech and language development will become the main thrust of a long-term investigation.

REFERENCES

1. Ross M, Lerman J. Hearing-aid usage and its effect upon residual hearing: a review of the literature and an investigation. Arch Otolaryngol 1967; 86:639-44.

2. Berliner KI. Risk versus benefit in cochlear implantation. Ann Otol Rhinol Laryngol 1982; 91 Suppl 91:90-8.

3. Thielemeir MA, Brimacombe JA, Eisenberg LS. Audiological results with the cochlear implant. Ann Otol Rhinol Laryngol 1982; 91 Suppl 91:27-34.

4. Helmerich L, Edgerton BJ. Psychoelectric measurements and results from cochlear implant patients. Ann Otol Rhinol Laryngol 1982; 91 Suppl 91:35-40.

5. Bilger RC, Black FO, Hopkinson NT, et al. Evaluation of subjects presently fitted with implanted auditory prostheses. Ann Otol Rhinol Laryngol 1977; 86 Suppl 38:1-176.

6. Eisenberg LS. Use of the cochlear implant by the prelingually deaf. Ann Otol Rhinol Laryngol 1982; 91 Suppl 91:62-6.

7. Simmons FB. The electrical stimulation of the acoustic nerve. In: Merzenich MM, Schindler RA, Sooy FA, eds. Proceedings of First International Conference on Electrical Stimulation of the Acoustic Nerve as a Treatment of Profound Sensorineural Deafness in Man, San Francisco 1973. San Francisco: University of California, 1974; 123-5.

8. Webster DB, Webster M. Neonatal sound deprivation affects brain stem auditory nuclei. Arch Otolaryngol 1977; 103:392-6.

9. Webster DB, Webster M. Effects of neonatal conductive hearing loss on brain stem auditory nuclei. Ann Otol Rhinol Laryngol 1979; 88:684-8.

10. Ruben RJ, Rapin I. Plasticity of the developing auditory system. Ann Otol Rhinol Laryngol 1980; 89:303-11.

11. House WF. Surgical considerations in cochlear implantation. Ann Otol Rhinol Laryngol 1982; 91 Suppl 91:15-20.

12. Dormer KJ, Richard G, Hough JVD, Hewett T. The cochlear implant (auditory prosthesis) utilizing rare earth magnets. Am J Otol 1980; 2:22-7.

13. Conrad R. The deaf school child: language and cognitive function. London: Harper & Row, 1979.

14. Eggermont JJ. Physiology of the developing auditory system. Presented at the symposium Auditory Development in Infancy, University of Toronto, June 1981.

OTOPATHOLOGICAL FINDINGS IN A PATIENT WITH BILATERAL COCHLEAR IMPLANTS

LARS-GÖRAN JOHNSSON, MD

WILLIAM F. HOUSE, MD

FRED H. LINTHICUM, JR, MD

The death in 1976 of a patient who had a multiple-electrode cochlear implant in one cochlea and a single-electrode cochlear implant in the other provided a unique opportunity for both clinical and histological study of the effects of such implants in a human subject. The patient was 68 years old at the time of his death. In 1969, at the age of 61, and after 11 years of profound deafness, apparently as a result of lues, the patient was implanted on the left side with a hard-wired 5-wire multiple-electrode cochlear implant. Five years later, his right side was implanted with a single-electrode induction coil cochlear implant. Audiological and psychoacoustic studies were performed by a number of investigators. The results are reviewed. Following the patient's death, his temporal bones were obtained and examined using microdissection techniques followed by serial sectioning. The histological findings are described.

This paper presents the clinical findings and the postmortem labyrinthine pathology in a patient who had received bilateral cochlear implants. The temporal bones were examined by microdissection of the inner ear tissues followed by serial sectioning of the modiolus. It is the first complete report of labyrinthine pathology in such a patient.

CLINICAL FINDINGS

HISTORY

The temporal bones were obtained at autopsy from a 68-year-old male who was first seen at the Otologic Medical Group in 1961. He is referred to as "CR" in House et al,[1] as "M" in Bilger et al,[2] and by both initials in Johnsson et al.[3] The patient experienced sudden profound deafness on the left side 18 years prior to death and a similar loss on the right side 3 years later. He complained of bilateral tinnitus and unsteadiness.

By the time of death he had carried a single-electrode induction coil implant of platinum-iridium in the right ear for two years and a multiple (5) hard-wired silver electrode implant in the left ear for seven years.

The patient had a history of luetic infection at the age of 18 and his VDRL test had remained positive despite a full course treatment with antibiotics. It was assumed that the patient's deafness was related to vascular changes secondary to lues.

In 1963, a myringotomy was made in the left ear and an electrode placed as close as possible to the round window membrane. Stimulation with square waves resulted in a sensation of sound when the frequency was below 50 Hz. Following this test, six years elapsed before a permanent electrode system was developed.

IMPLANTATION OF A MULTIPLE-ELECTRODE PROSTHESIS

In September 1969 a 2½-hour procedure was performed for insertion of cochlear electrodes. The operative record reads as follows:

> Under general anesthesia supplemented by a local, a postauricular incision was made. The mastoid cortex and air cells were removed with a drill. The facial recess was opened. The stapes and the round window niche were visualized through the facial recess. The round window niche was drilled off with a diamond stone to completely visualize the round window membrane. A metal stud was then placed in the mastoid process bone and attached to this was a button with five wire insertion sockets; these five wires were then let down to the round window and the electrodes were placed into the basal coil of the cochlea through the round window membrane. The incision was then closed with No. 2-0 gut . . .

The five silver wire electrodes were inserted into the scala tympani so that the apical-most electrode was about 20 mm around the basal coil, with the other four electrodes spaced at approximately 4 mm intervals between the round window and the first electrode. The connecting button and its sockets were covered with a screw-on water-tight cap to prevent moisture from entering.

By 1974, the button had begun to disintegrate with some possibility that the implant might fail. Therefore, a single-wire induction coil cochlear implant was considered for the patient's right ear.

IMPLANTATION OF A SINGLE-ELECTRODE PROSTHESIS

Promontory testing with electrical stimulation indicated that the patient did have responses in his right ear. In October 1974 surgery was performed for placement of an induction coil implant. The operative record reads as follows:

> Under general anesthesia a postauricular incision was made and the position of the induction coil was located. A seat was made for the induction coil using a drill and tre-

The histological investigation was supported by USPHS Research Grants NS 05065 and NS 12706 and Programs Project Grant NS 05785.

phine. Mastoidectomy was done and the facial recess was opened. A round window niche was exposed and the edge of the round window drilled back to expose the round window membrane. It was found then on placing the electrode coil and the electrodes and coil assembly that the place for the seat was too far from the round window and therefore a new seat was made for the induction coil. The induction coil was then placed in the seat and it was anchored in place with a 4-0 Mersilene suture, tied to the bone, and the ground wire was placed in the attic; the active wire was then slipped into the cochlea, and the fascia was placed around the active electrode. The postauricular incision was closed with subcuticular 2-0 gut . . .

In December 1974, the patient suffered a congestive heart failure. He had continuing, though intermittent, problems and in August 1976, at the age of 68, he died. He had activated the implant in his left ear for a total of approximately 27 months of electrical stimulation, using the implant 6 to 8 hours a day, six days a week once a wearable stimulator was available. Due to his illness, fitting of a wearable stimulator for his right ear induction coil implant was delayed, and such a unit was worn off and on for only about three months of total time of usage. Unless otherwise stated, the audiological results presented are for the multiple-electrode implant.

AUDIOLOGIC FINDINGS

Hearing without a Prosthesis. Prior to implantation in 1969, the patient demonstrated unaided pure tone responses in the right ear of 90 dB HL at 500 Hz and 100 dB at 1000 Hz. Response in the left ear was found for 105 dB at 500 Hz. All other frequencies tested (250 to 4000 Hz) for both ears showed no response to the limit of the audiometer. There was no response to bone conduction and no understanding of speech discrimination tests.

Bilger et al [2] tested this patient's unaided auditory response again in 1975 as part of a study of implanted patients by the Eye and Ear Hospital of Pittsburgh. They report no response for either ear at any frequency (125 to 4000 Hz) to full-range Bekesy audiometry for interrupted and continuous tones. Other tests using narrow-band noise indicated what were probably vibrotactile thresholds.

Implant Activated. Until the end of 1970, this patient was tested in the laboratory for the purpose of developing an external stimulator for the multiple-electrode implant. During these sessions it was found that applying a sine wave of one frequency to an electrode elicited a different hearing sensation than did another frequency applied to the same electrode. Similarly, if the same signal was applied singly into each of the five electrodes, the patient reported a different sound sensation at each one. However, before a wearable unit was developed the patient moved away from the city. Therefore, he did not have use of his cochlear implant until 1974 when he returned and was fitted with a wearable external stimulator like that being used for single-electrode induction coil implants. It was modified

LIST OF ENVIRONMENTAL SOUNDS HEARD BY PATIENT

Jigsaw	Shopping carts
Sander	Organ and piano
Cars	Dishes and pans banging
Trucks	Voices (own and others)
Motorcycles	Cracking eggs
Dog bark	Children talking
Lawnmower (hand)	Turning pages of newspapers and books
Grandson's laugh	Screen door closing
Bell on toy telephone	"Riffle" of playing cards
Rubber duck squeak	Voices on TV and radio
Footsteps	Vacuum cleaner
Crunching of paper	Hammer
Cupboard door shut	Slamming doors
Running water	Rattling of silverware
Cash registers	

to be used with his hard-wired system. Stimulation was accomplished by using the most apical and most basal electrodes as active and ground, thus producing a single-electrode type of functioning.

The rehabilitation records at the House Ear Institute, including daily diaries kept by the patient and rehabilitation report forms filled out by the rehabilitation audiologist, indicate that this patient could hear a wide variety of environmental sounds with his implant. The table presents a list of some of the sounds the patient reported hearing. He reported knowing the difference in whether a passing vehicle was a car, a truck, or a motorcycle. His wife reported he could distinguish music from speaking on the radio approximately 75% of the time. During auditory training, the patient could discriminate between /m/ and /b/ as presented in "man" and "ban."

In November 1975, the patient reported that when he played the bass notes of the piano they "came in at different frequencies." A final written report from the patient in March 1976, five months before his death, indicated that his implant was still working, apparently as well as previously.

Utah Studies. After having worn his stimulator for several months, the patient participated in a cooperative program with the University of Utah, Division of Artificial Organs. Results have been reported in Mladejovsky et al[4] and Eddington et al[5] and are summarized below. Electrode impedances, electrical thresholds, and frequency and loudness discrimination were explored for the multiple-electrode implant.

Mean impedances for a biphasic pulsatile stimulus at each of the five electrodes varied from 5.6 kΩ at electrode 5 (basal-most electrode) to 10 kΩ at electrode 2. No significant day to day variations in impedances were observed. Amplitude thresholds in microamps peak-to-peak were also measured for each electrode. The mean threshold ranged from 68.6 μA for electrode 4 to 118 μA for electrode 3.

Place and periodicity-pitch perception tasks were performed to determine to what extent these mechanisms of pitch perception were provided by the multiple electrode implant. Place-pitch was examined by stimulating two different electrodes in rapid succession and asking the patient to judge the relative pitch of the two sounds. The stimuli at both electrodes were identical, and a response was correct if it matched the response expected based on the tonotopic organization of the cochlea. The pitch produced at the most apical electrode was always perceived as lower than that produced at any of the other electrodes. Adjacent electrodes elicited the lowest percentage of correct responses, while those separated by two or more inactive electrodes were judged correctly 100% of the time.

Periodicity-pitch was also investigated. Two different frequencies were presented in succession at one electrode and relative pitch judgments were reported. An attempt was made to determine the smallest change in stimulation frequency that the patient could reliably report as being in the same direction as the stimulus frequency change. An average frequency change of 25 Hz could reliably be detected, at all five electrodes, over the range from 25 to 400 Hz. Between 400 and 1000 Hz, stimulation did not result in perceivable differences in pitch.

In addition to frequency discrimination, the minimum change in current amplitude which resulted in a discernible change in loudness was investigated. For pulsatile and sinusoidal stimulation, the average minimum discernible changes were 8 and 19 μA, respectively.

The patient is reported to have been consistent in describing the pitch of the sound as "high" or "low" and the loudness as "loud" or "soft." The sounds he heard seemed to be more complex than "pure" tones but had enough tonal quality to allow pitch comparison.

Pittsburgh Studies. In late 1975 and early 1976, the University of Pittsburgh School of Medicine, through the Eye and Ear Hospital of Pittsburgh, evaluated the patient as part of a study of subjects with implanted auditory prostheses.[2] His left ear was tested using a stimulation pattern that produced a "single-electrode" type of stimulation. Unfortunately, the patient's external stimulator failed before testing was completed. It is difficult to determine from the published results which results may have been obtained with an adequately functioning unit and which were not. (Even those results obtained with a nonfunctioning unit were included in the tables). However, results can be found in which the patient's scores were better than chance on at least some discrimination tasks. For example, he scored better than chance on a vowel-discrimination task for discriminations of /a/ versus /i/, /e/, and /ɛ/. He also could discriminate between a narrow band of noise (259±50 Hz), an amplitude-modulated tone (250 modulated by 50 Hz), and a sine wave (250 Hz). His results on these tasks were similar to those of subjects using a single-electrode induction coil cochlear implant. Few other psychoacoustic results were obtained on this patient.

Upon the patient's death, his temporal bones were obtained, fixed in buffered formalin, and hand-delivered to the histopathologist.

HISTOLOGICAL FINDINGS

It is absolutely essential that the temporal bones from all patients with cochlear implants be properly examined postmortem. Such examination will provide useful information for improving both implant design and surgical techniques. Not only should the patient be persuaded to sign a temporal bone pledge, but the next-of-kin should be fully informed about the importance of this examination for otologic research and progress.

Microdissection is employed in this study as a means for examining the temporal bones from these particular patients. Because the cochlea contains a hard implant the bones cannot be sectioned. Sectioning a celloidin-embedded specimen close to the implant and observing the implant through the translucent celloidin would be possible. It would, however, be necessary to remove the prosthesis to allow further sectioning and that would, in all probability, cause extensive damage to the cochlear structures, and the position of the implant in relation to surrounding structures could no longer be determined. It would also be difficult to evaluate the tissue reaction around the implant. Furthermore, the combination of studying the first order neuron in surface preparations of osseous spiral lamina as well as in celloidin sections of the modiolus gives a much more reliable picture of the condition and distribution of the remaining neurons than examination of sections alone. The microdissection technique also allows the usage of transmission and scanning electron microscopy, plus microanalysis of tissue with the electron probe.

METHODS

The external ear canal was removed and the middle ear was inspected under the Zeiss operating microscope. Both windows were exposed. There was no active inflammation in either middle ear and no gross pathology was observed that would warrant discussion here.

A complete microdissection of the labyrinth was performed according to the method that we and others have outlined elsewhere.[3,6-8] The inner ear was stained with a perilymphatic perfusion of a 1% solution of osmium tetroxide through the oval window. Because the implants occupied the round window, a small hole was drilled in scala tympani in the basal turn as an outlet for the fluid. The otic capsule was reduced to a thin shell by means of dental burrs and then carefully removed.

The microdissections were photographed under the Wild-Heerbrugg M-5 Stereo-microscope, with the specimen immersed in 70% alcohol. The membranous labyrinth was dissected into surface preparations and studied with the phase-contrast micro-

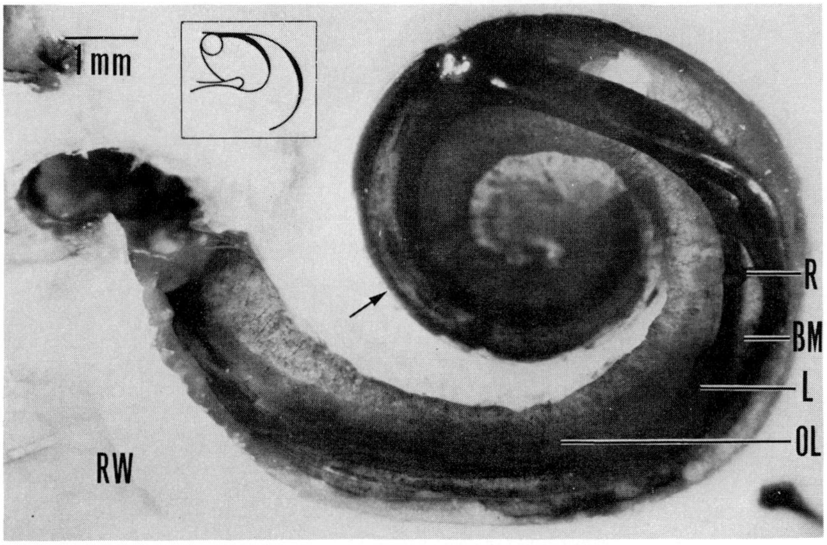

Fig. 1. Right cochlea showing single electrode entering scala media along bony wall c 12 mm from opening of niche. Most of the spiral ligament has been dissected away except in upper basal turn, where implant has pulled away the stria vascularis and the basilar membrane from the spiral ligament which is left in situ. A small hole cut in the ligament opens a view into scala tympani. Insert) Schematic drawing showing the position of the implant as if seen in a cross section. Arrow - Two patches of Corti organ with inner hair cells supplied by darkly stained bundles of nerve fibers. RW - Site of round window niche. The tip of the electrode cut at the former opening of the niche is seen. R - Remnants of Reissner membrane left in situ; BM - Basilar membrane covered only by a flat epithelium; L - Spiral limbus; OL - Osseous spiral lamina, void of myelinated nerve fibers. (OsO_4)

scope. Portions of the osseous spiral lamina from both ears were embedded in Araldite, and "thick" (c 1 μm) cross sections were cut for examination in light microscopy and ultrathin sections were prepared for transmission electron microscopy. Portions of the osseous lamina were viewed with the scanning electron microscope. The sensory cell population in the vestibular organs was also evaluated with the scanning electron microscope. The abnormal saccular otoconia were analyzed by powder x-ray diffraction. The electron probe was used for identifying the presence of silver. After the dissection was completed the temporal bones were decalcified and the modiolus sectioned using conventional techniques for temporal bone histology.

The cochlear nerve was dissected out from the internal meatus and embedded in paraffin. The sections were stained with hematoxylin and eosin plus Holmes silver stain. Unfortunately, it was not possible to obtain good vertical sections of the nerve samples available. The sections obtained showed nerve degeneration, but were in general not very informative.

We recommend that in future specimens from implantation cases the cochlear nerve and the vestibular nerves as well be carefully dissected out in their entire length from the internal auditory canal. This requires time and care. The posterior wall of the canal should be drilled away and each nerve should be identified with certainty and separated from the others. After this the nerves can be cut at the fundus of the internal meatus. The length of the nerve samples can be increased if at autopsy the eighth nerve is cut as close as possible to the brainstem. The nerves should then be stained with osmium tetroxide and embedded in Araldite so that the long axis as well as the proximal and distal ends of the nerve fiber can be determined. From these blocks vertical sections can be cut for study by light as well as by electron microscopy.

COCHLEAR PATHOLOGY

STATE OF THE IMPLANTS

The right ear had a single-electrode and the left ear a multipolar implant. Both round windows were well sealed by extensive formation of soft tissue around the implant in the niche. The implants were lying in scala tympani in the lower portion of the basal turn, but at the first curvature about 12 mm from the original opening of the niche and c 12-13 mm from the basal end of the cochlea each implant deviated from its intended spiral course in scala tympani (Figs. 1 and 2). They took a lateral direction toward the basilar membrane and the spiral ligament, following the bony wall closely, and entered the scala media. The right electrode (Fig. 1), which was inserted more deeply, was bent at that point and took a straight, more or less posterior course, mostly inside the cochlear duct, until it was stopped by coming into contact with the

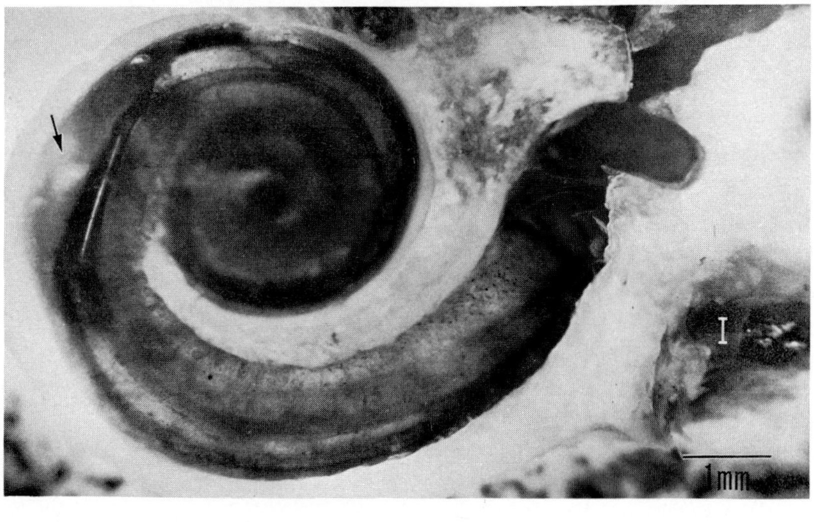

Fig. 2. The left cochlea showing the distal end of the multipolar electrode entering the scala media and scala tympani (cf Fig. 1). There is a partial ossification of the spiral ligament next to the exposed electrode (arrow). The proximal end of the electrodes surrounded by a cuff of connective tissue cut at the opening of the round window niche is seen at the right (I). There is a complete degeneration of Corti organ and of nerve fibers in osseous spiral lamina. (OsO_4)

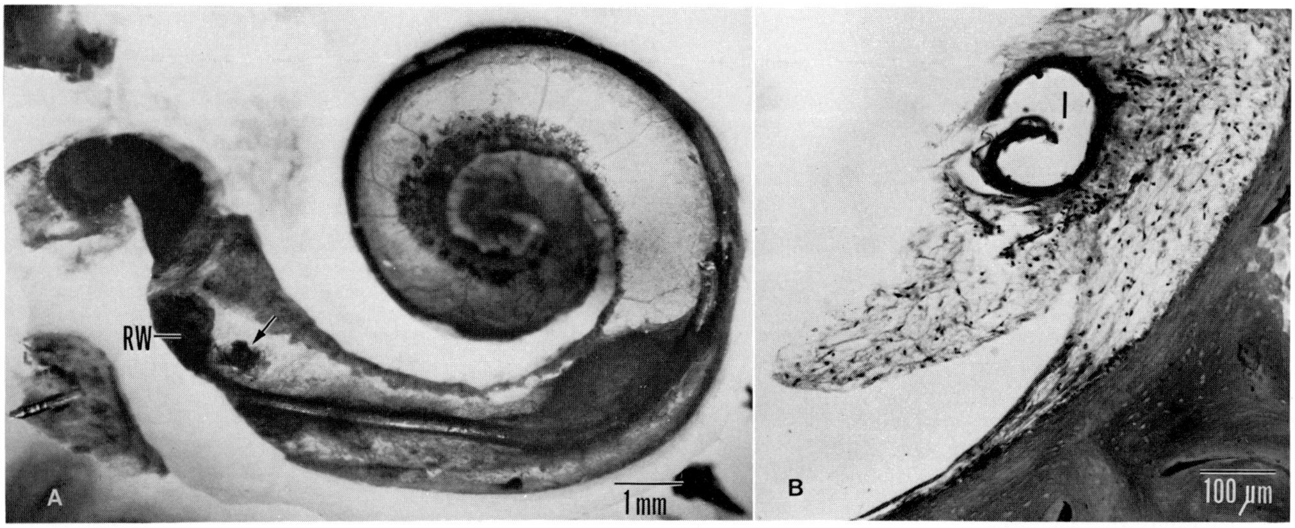

Fig. 3. A) Right ear, view of scala tympani with several radiating venules descending along the bony wall toward the modiolus. The electrode is clearly seen bending along the bony wall toward scala media at the first curvature. The implant was cut just above the basilar membrane. Note the formation of loose connective tissue around the implant in the first curvature. Along the rest of its course the implant was surrounded by a dense but thin layer of connective tissue. No bone formation is present. RW - Round window membrane. Arrow - Opening of cochlear aqueduct. (OsO_4) B) Detail of a celloidin section showing the connective tissue formation seen in A. It is sparse and poorly vascularized, but forms a dense sleeve of fibroblasts around the implant (I), which has been removed. (H & E stain after initial OsO_4 staining, bright-field.)

bony wall of scala vestibuli in the upper basal turn, c 17 mm from the basal end of the cochlea. The implant in the left ear (Fig. 2) was deflected less and did not reach as deep as on the right side.

Both implants appeared otherwise intact. There was no visible erosion of their surfaces. The single electrode on the right side was surrounded by a thin irregular layer of soft tissue. The electrode on the left side had a shiny brownish surface and the Pyre-ML varnish layer[1] covering it seemed undamaged.

RIGHT COCHLEA

Implant-Related Pathology. There was relatively limited tissue reaction visible in the right ear, especially compared to the opposite side. No osteoneogenesis was observed. In the scala tympani next to the implant and around it a thin layer of darkly stained loose irregular tissue was present. At the first curvature of the cochlea, there was a circumscribed mass of loose tissue which in the stereo-microscope had the appearance of an accumulation of cobweb or cotton (Fig. 3A). Some of the tissue in the scala tympani was adherent to the outer margin of the basilar membrane.

Conventional sections of the dissected bone showed that the meshwork in the scala tympani was formed by poorly vascularized connective tissue. No lymphocytes were present. There was a stromal con-

Fig. 4. Right ear, the entire basilar membrane (BM) with osseous spiral lamina (OL) and the distal end of implant dissected out. Two stretches of Corti organ in the upper half of the basal turn and in the upper middle and apical turns (insert), respectively, each with their separate bundles of nerve fibers. L - Limbus; SL - Spiral ligament; S - Site of atrophic stria vascularis; DR - Ductus reuniens. (OsO_4)

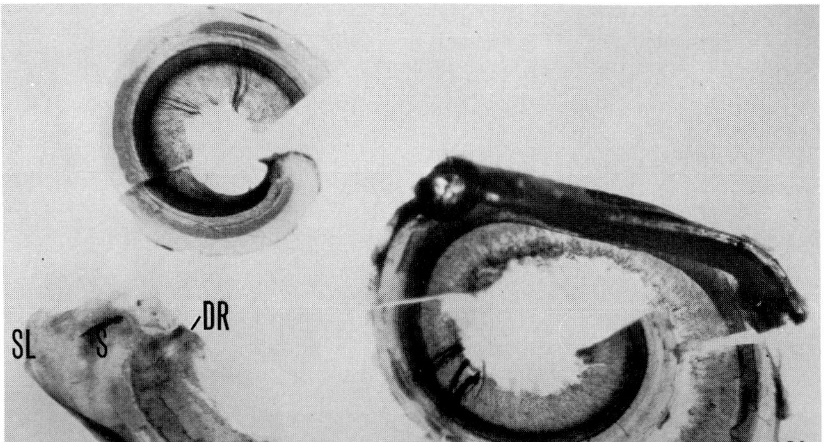

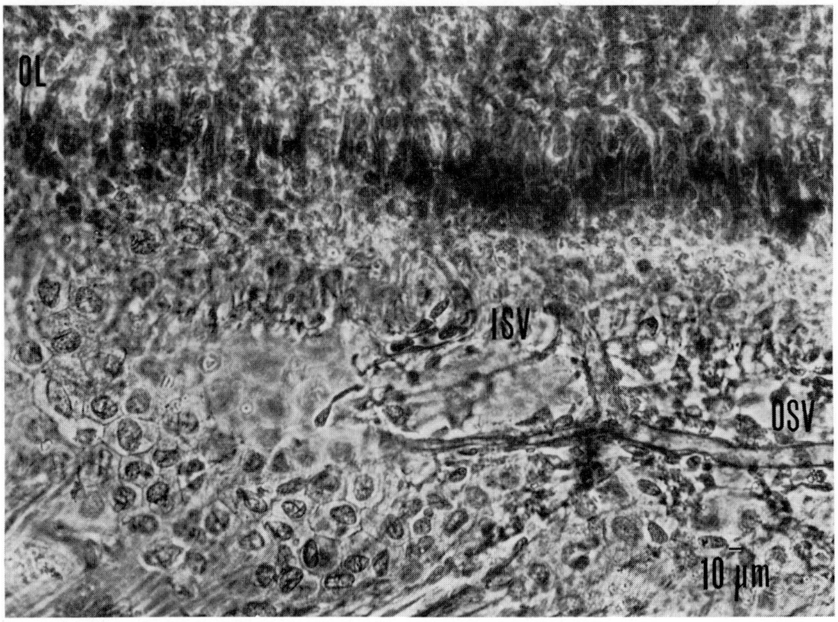

Fig. 5. Right ear, higher magnification of the displaced basilar membrane (see Fig. 1) showing the epithelium covering the basilar membrane. The T-junction of the outer spiral vessel (OSV) is seen to the right. The left hand arm was apparently interrupted during implantation and ends blindly. So does branch of the inner spiral vessel (ISV). OL - Osseous spiral lamina. (Phase-Contrast, OsO_4)

densation around the implant which was formed by a dense envelope of fibroblasts. It appeared that the tissue in the scala tympani was derived from the endosteum (Fig. 3B).

It is remarkable that at the time of dissection the walls of the cochlear duct in spite of being displaced showed no obvious ruptures or defects. The part of the implant which had deviated from the scala tympani was lying within the displaced scala media (Fig. 1). The basilar membrane and Reissner membrane were intact. It appeared as if the stria vascularis had been pulled off the spiral ligament during implantation and had then been replaced by osmiophilic scar tissue which formed the outer wall of the displaced scala media in the upper basal turn.

Reissner membrane was inserted at the upper margin of the strip of scar tissue which was adherent to the spiral ligament. The spiral ligament itself remained in normal position attached to the bony wall. Localized changes in the spiral ligament at this site of apparent maximal damage were remarkably small. The spiral ligament was fibrotic and somewhat thicker than elsewhere. Radiating arterioles and capillaries were present, however, and no marked localized devascularization could be observed.

In areas where Corti organ was absent the basilar membrane was transparent and covered only with a flat epithelium of polygonal cells which almost invariably pave the membrane after complete degeneration (Figs. 4 and 5). In this instance, however, the cells in some areas were smaller, and more numerous and osmiophilic than usual. The outer spiral vessel was interrupted for a long stretch where the implant had entered the scala media and tapered off to form a pointed end (Fig. 5). Several vessels were seen crossing the basilar membrane toward the former site of the stria in the upper basal turn. Vessels traversing the basilar membrane are not common[9,10] and in this instance their presence probably was the result of vasculoneogenesis.

The shape and arrangement of the epithelial cells in Reissner membrane were more regular than usually seen in adults, with fewer spindle-shaped cells forming the characteristic "whorls" usually present in the mature membrane. The membrane was covered by numerous radially arranged melanocytes; this has been observed in our material previously, and was presumably related to the fact that the patient had dark hair and brown eyes.[11]

Sensorineural Degeneration. Widespread complete sensorineural degeneration was present along

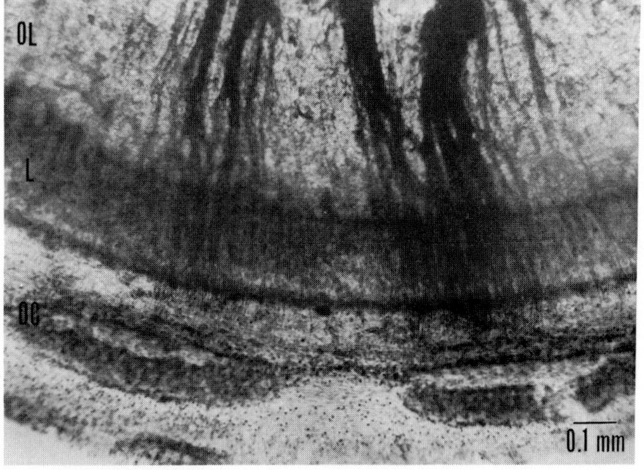

Fig. 6. Right ear, higher magnification of the two patches of Corti organ (OC) (see Figs. 1 and 4), each with their bundles of myelinated nerve fibers. OL - Osseous spiral lamina; L - Spiral limbus. (OsO_4, bright-field)

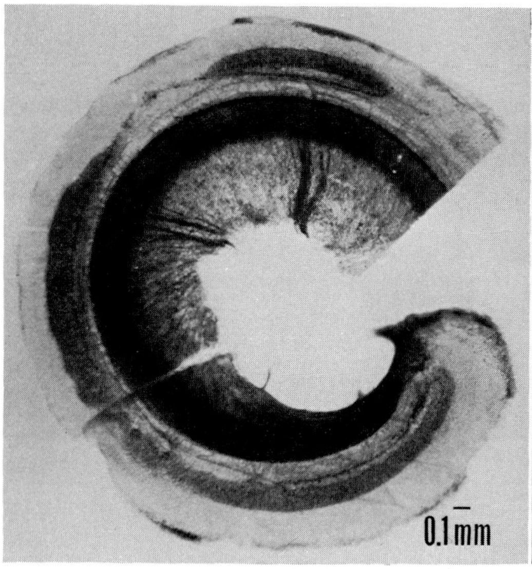

Fig. 7. Right ear, higher magnification of the upper half of the middle and the apical turn in Fig. 4 displaying two stretches of supporting cells and myelinated nerve fibers.

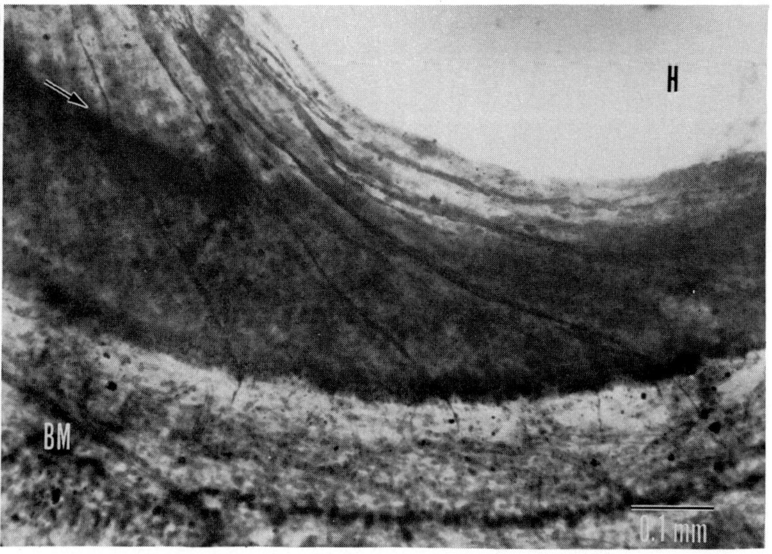

Fig. 8. Right ear, higher magnification of the very apical end in Fig. 3A showing the arrangement of the few myelinated nerve fibers remaining in osseous spiral lamina. Arrow pointing at the boundary between the osseous (upper) and nonosseous (lower) portion of the spiral lamina. BM - Basilar membrane; H - Helicotrema. (OsO_4, bright-field)

most of the cochlea. Two small islands of Corti organ were seen in the vicinity of the tip of the electrode c 20 mm from the basal end (Figs. 4 and 6). They were supplied by two narrow but relatively dense bundles of nerve fibers, 0.19 and 0.41 mm in width, respectively (as measured at the level of habenula perforata). The more apically located patch contained Deiters cells, pillar cells, and 12 inner hair cells. The other similar patch with fewer nerve fibers had only four inner hair cells.

In the apical turn (Figs. 7 and 8) the distal 4.8 mm of the basilar membrane was covered with supporting elements, with the exception of a small 0.5 mm gap. Two dark, very narrow bundles of nerve fibers were going to each patch. In addition, numerous thin, lightly stained nerve fibers were seen in the apical end of the cochlea, corresponding to the longer stretch of supporting elements (Fig. 9).

The cochlea was 28.7 mm long. Since the entire spiral at one time must have been populated with nerve fibers and 1.11 mm of its length was still supplied with fairly dense bundles of nerve fibers at the time of death, in addition to a thin network present in the apical turn, it appeared that c 4% of the original number of ganglion cells had distal processes and thus remained reasonably viable in this ear. (The "dendritic" fibers with their main portion located in the osseous spiral lamina will be referred to as *distal processes* and the "axonal" fibers with their main portion in the internal auditory canal as *proximal processes*.)

The faint outlines of thin myelinated radial fibers in the osseous spiral lamina which were seen in all three turns in both specimens (Fig. 4) did not represent nerve fibers. Cross sections of samples of the spiral lamina from the right ear studied in light and transmission electron microscopy revealed a series of holes enclosing only tiny dark strands of tissue which appeared to be remnants of the myelin sheaths of degenerated nerve fibers in their canals (Fig. 9). In a scanning electron micrograph of one of the samples a single nerve fiber taking a spiral course was seen.

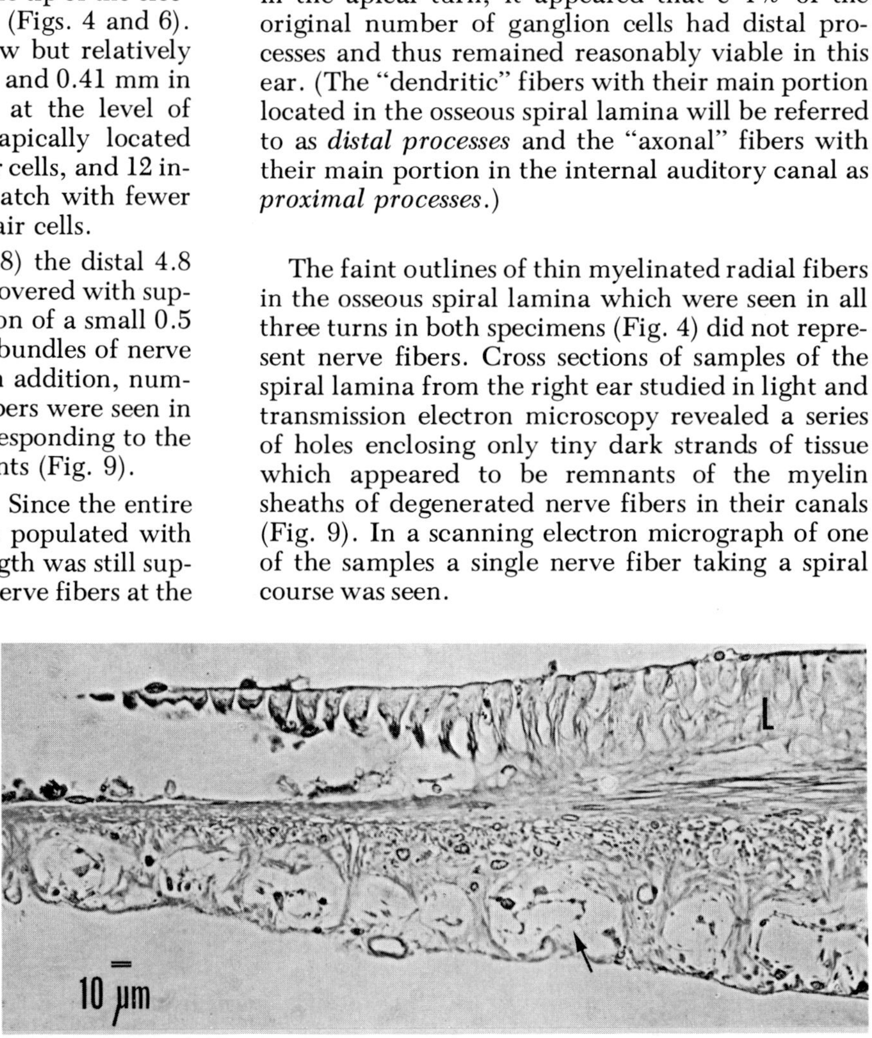

Fig. 9. Right ear, semitangential cross section of the osseous spiral lamina, basal turn, including the limbus (L) showing the empty channels remaining after nerve degeneration. Arrow pointing at thin dark strands probably representing remnants of a myelin sheath.

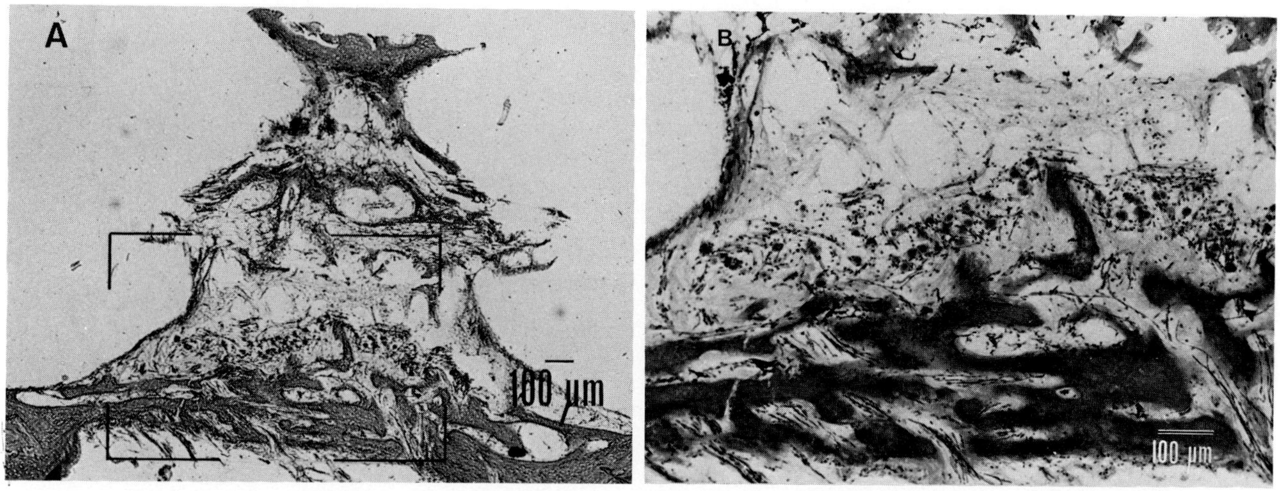

Fig. 10. A) Right ear, horizontal midmodiolar section after dissection. The lower half of the basal turn is to the right, the upper half to the left. Several ganglion cells with their proximal processes seen above the fundus of the internal meatus; nerve has been evulsed. (OsO_4, H & E) B) Right ear, higher power magnification of the area corresponding to the upper half of the basal turn indicated by lines in A.

These and subsequent photomicrographs of sections through the modiolus and the floor of scala tympani are printed so that their orientation is the same as that of the corresponding photomicrographs of the cochlear spiral.

Horizontal sections (Fig. 10A, B) of the temporal bone showed two small clusters of ganglion cells in the apical and basal portion of the modiolus, respectively. The cells obviously corresponded to the sectors of the osseous lamina which had nerve fibers (Fig. 4). From the latter group of cells a small dark fascicle of distal processes could be observed in one of the slides, apparently going to one of the two nerve bundles seen in the upper basal turn. Numerous proximal processes were present in the base of the modiolus (Fig. 10A, B).

Spiral Ligament and Stria Vascularis. Both of these structures, and especially the stria vascularis, showed severe atrophy. The atrophy was complete in the basal turn. In the middle and apical turns, five small islands of atrophic stria remained interspersed between areas of complete atrophy. The spiral ligament in the lower half of the basal turn showed an uneven, patchy atrophy, which we have not seen in our material before.

LEFT COCHLEA

Implant-Related Pathology. In this ear the multipolar implant was completely buried in bone along its entire course in the scala tympani (Fig. 11A, B). The extensive formations of new bone occluded the scala in the lower half of the basal turn, covering the round window and the opening of the cochlear aqueduct. Large masses of the new bone were fused with the osseous spiral lamina. Grossly, the condition was somewhat reminiscent of what is seen in temporal bones with bone formation in the scala tympani secondary to extensive capsular otosclerosis.[12] The implant was lying in a narrow tunnel inside the new bone, surrounded by an irregular loose layer of connective tissue. Examination of conventional sections (Fig. 12A-C) showed that this was new immature trabecular bone in the scala tympani. Just apical to the area of ossification there was loose connective tissue, which was more or less identical with the connective tissue we observed in the scala tympani of the right ear, except that it contained a few small islands of new trabecular bone. Little or no bone formation was found in the connective tissue in the second and the third turns, where the tissue layer was for the most part relatively thin, just covering the bony wall of the scala tympani. As in the opposite ear, no lymphocytic infiltration was observed. Since the tissue formation in the middle and apical turn was separated from similar changes in the basal turn by an intact stretch of smooth bony wall apical to the tip of the implant (Fig. 11A), it may well have been caused by factors unrelated to surgery.

There was circumscribed ossification of the spiral ligament along the uncovered distal end of the electrode in the scala media and scala vestibuli (Fig. 2). In this region there was also a marked blackening of the spiral ligament. The discoloration was clearly seen through the translucent bone when some of the otic capsule was being removed prior to staining in the initial phase of preparation. This particular implant was made of silver, and despite its varnish covering it had caused local argyrosis. The presence of silver was confirmed using the electron probe. (Electrodes of silver were used only in the early multiple-electrode system. Since 1970, platinum or platinum-iridium has been used for all electrodes.)

The tectorial membrane in the upper half of the basal turn was displaced from its normal position and was atrophic and shortened. It rested on the osseous spiral lamina, making two straight lines which converged at the basilar membrane forming an angle of approximately 90° at about 12 o'clock of

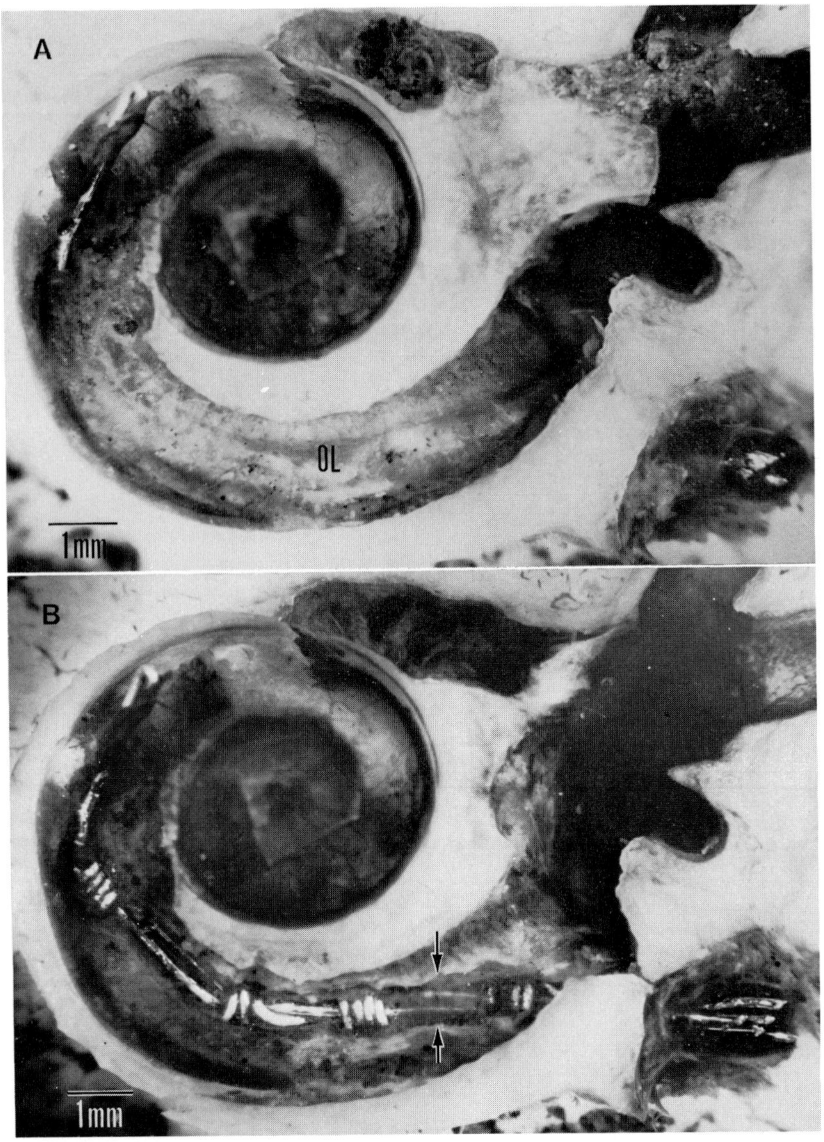

Fig. 11. Left ear (see Fig. 2). A) Massive new bone formation around the implant during its course in scala tympani occluding the scala in the lower half of the basal turn where most of osseous spiral lamina (OL) was fused to the new bone. There is also connective tissue covering the floor of the scala in the middle and apical turn, which probably was caused by factors unrelated to surgery. (OsO_4, H & E) B) Multipolar electrode uncovered from bone. Implant was lying in a narrow tunnel inside the bone (arrows) surrounded by loose connective tissue.

the cochlea. Such a severe displacement of the tectorial membrane has not been observed in any of our specimens before, including the hydropic ones and the finding is therefore likely to be the result of surgical trauma. Furthermore, the tectorial membrane was more or less abnormal along the entire length of the cochlea, being atrophic and folded upon itself. Whether these changes represented extension of the surgical trauma or were secondary to the hydrops is not known. Because the implant in this ear was inserted less deeply than on the right side, the initial damage to the spiral ligament and the basilar membrane appeared to have been less severe at the time of surgery than in the opposite ear (Fig. 2).

General Pathology. Extensive hydrops labyrinthi was present in the left ear. Reissner membrane was bulging in a highly irregular fashion and was attached to the bony wall of the scala media in the lower basal turn where hydrops was most severe. For the most part the epithelial cells were reminiscent of the regular polygonal type seen in infants. This probably indicated new growth of the membrane in response to endolymph volume increase. About 5 mm from the basal end of the cochlea a small hole or fistula was found in Reissner membrane. One marginal defect of the epithelial cell layer plus several smaller ones in the middle of the membrane were also present in the basal turn. These changes of Reissner membrane were all attributed to the hydrops.[11,13] Numerous vacuoles were also present. They have been observed before in association with both presbycusis and hydrops. Minimal pigmentation of the membrane was present on this side.

Sensorineural Degeneration. The degeneration in the left cochlea was even more severe than in the right ear, in that the organ of Corti was completely absent and no myelinated nerve fibers were seen in the osseous spiral lamina (Fig. 13A, B). Numerous

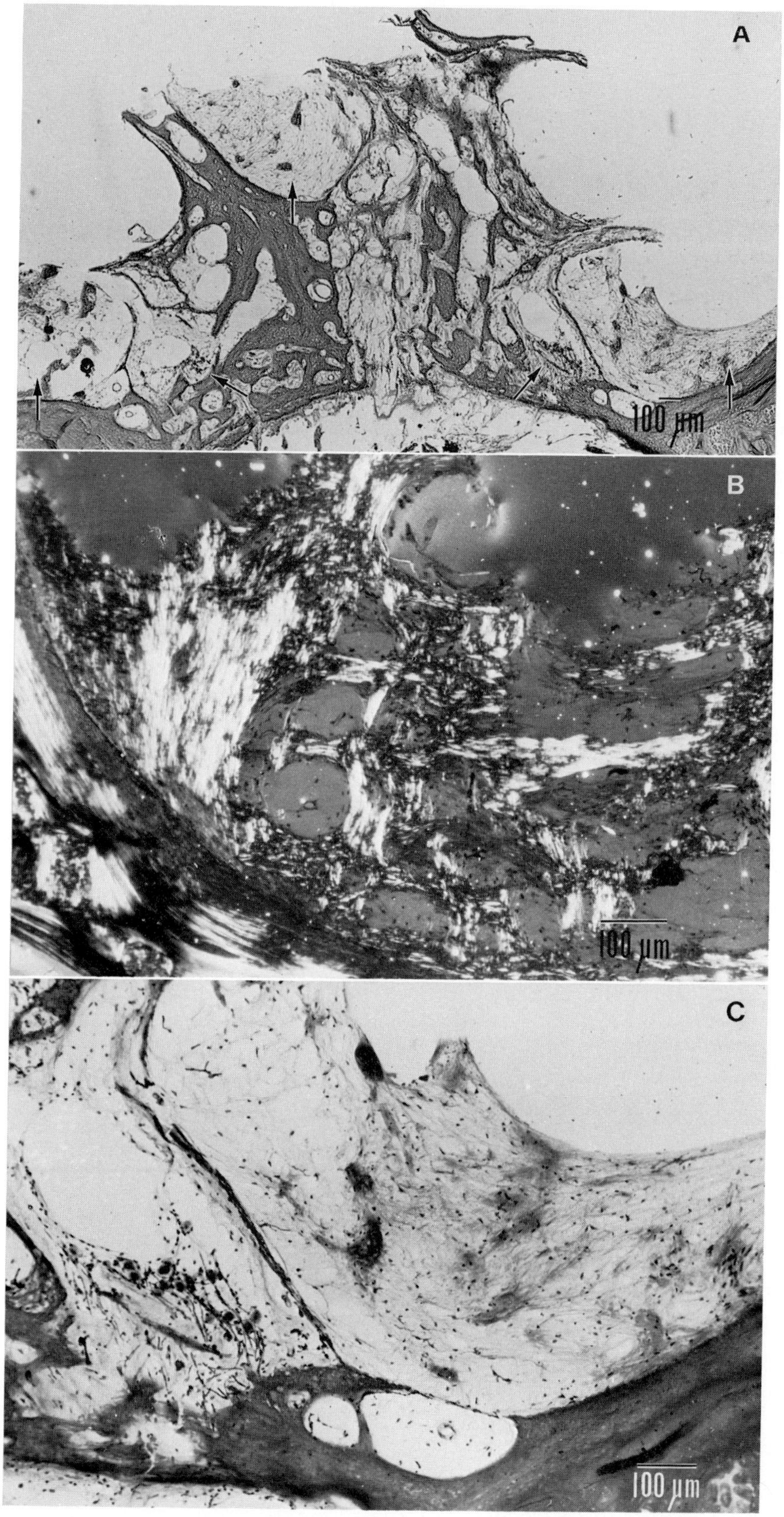

Fig. 12. Left ear, midmodiolar section, lower half of the basal turn to the left and the upper half to the right. A) A few scattered ganglion cells remain at the base of the modiolus (oblique arrows). Note the new tissue formation in scala tympani (vertical arrows) which in the middle and apical turn probably was unrelated to surgery. B) Higher magnification, in polarized light, of scala tympani in the lower half of the basal turn. Curved outline of the original wall to the left. Note formation of new, immature trabecular bone. C) Higher magnification of the upper half of the basal turn. Note the loose connective tissue, similar to that in Fig. 3B but with a few small islands of trabecular bone. (OsO_4, H & E)

spindle-shaped melanocytes arranged radially were seen in the apical turn. Cross sections of samples of the osseous spiral lamina studied in transmission electron microscopy revealed no nerve fibers. The spiral lamina was thinner than normal and contained no empty nerve channels as on the right side.

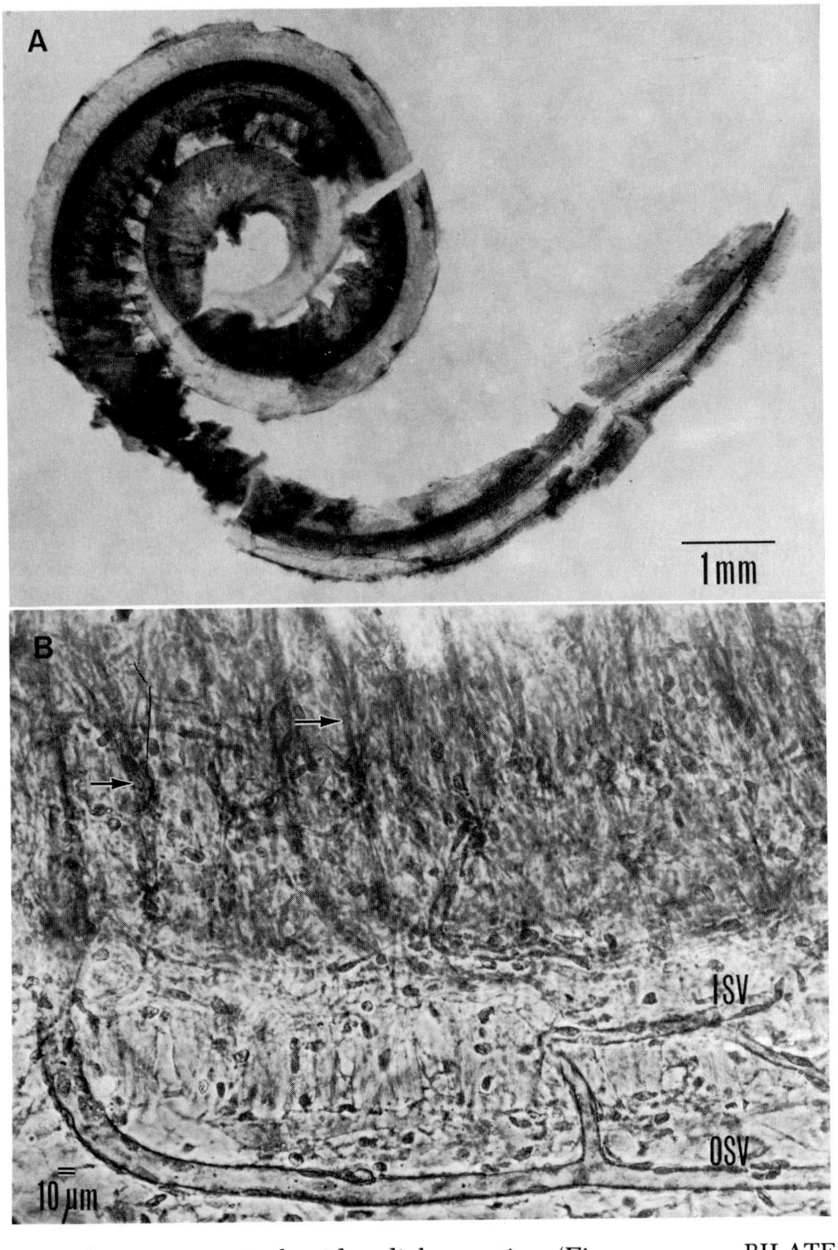

Fig. 13. Left ear. A) Basilar membrane and osseous spiral lamina dissected out (cf Fig. 4). No nerve fibers are seen. Darkly stained connective tissue from scala tympani is adherent to the undersurface of the lamina. No nerve fibers are seen. (OsO_4) B) Higher magnification of the nonosseous portion of spiral lamina in the upper basal turn in A. Radial pattern of dark, smudgy lines suggesting the presence of myelinated nerve fibers represents remnants of degenerated myelin sheaths. ISV - Inner spiral vessel; OSV - Outer spiral vessel beneath the basilar membrane. (OsO_4, phase-contrast)

In this ear a typical midmodiolar section (Fig. 12A) revealed only two single ganglion cells in the center of the modiolus plus a group of eight cells in its base. It is noteworthy that despite complete absence of myelinated distal processes in osseous spiral lamina, several proximal processes were seen taking a course toward the remaining ganglion cells. In neither ear could it be determined whether the surviving ganglion cells represented the myelinated or the unmyelinated type.

Spiral Ligament and Stria Vascularis. The strial atrophy was even more severe than in the opposite ear. Seven small, thin patches of stria remained in the middle and apical turns. The strial tissue present was clearly clustered around the branches coming from the radiating arterioles in the spiral ligament. Also in this ear there was uneven atrophy of the spiral ligament in the basal turn.

BILATERAL VESTIBULAR PATHOLOGY

The posterior membranous and bony canals in both ears were more or less completely scarred by connective tissue and occluded. They were in the process of becoming ossified. The walls of the membranous ampullae were thickened, and no hair cells were present on the crista in either ear (Fig. 14A, B).

In the left hydropic ear the thin portion of the membranous wall of the saccule was partially collapsed and adherent to the otoconia. All hair cells had degenerated. The saccular otoconia were abnormal (Fig. 15). They were analyzed using powder x-ray diffraction and scanning electron microscopy. They consisted of spheroid particles of apatite fused together into a rigid crust on the neuroepithelium. No separate otolithic membrane could be discerned.[13] We have observed identical otoconia previously in

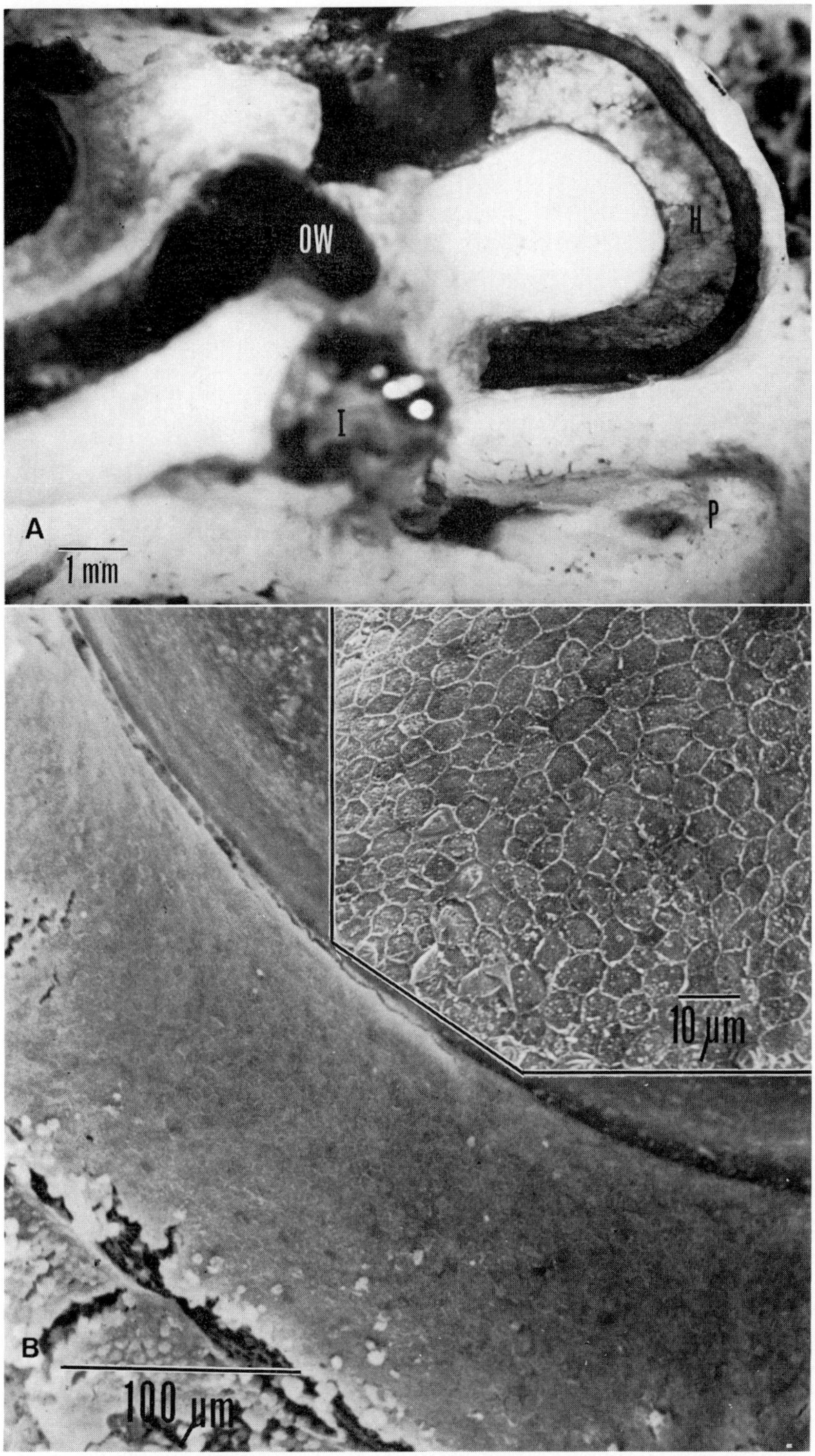

Fig. 14. Left ear. A) View of the horizontal (H) and posterior (P) ampulla and canals. Note that the posterior canal is obliterated by connective tissue and partially unstained. OW - Oval window; I - Implant. (OsO_4) B) Scanning electron micrograph of the left posterior ampullary crista showing the complete absence of hair cells. Insert) Higher magnification showing the epithelium covering the crista.

cases of hydrops or in association with ruptures or collapse of the membranous walls in the vestibular system.[14] Abnormal otoconia will be described in detail elsewhere. Saccular otoconia were absent in the right ear, and no utricular otoconia were found in either ear. Degeneration of the nerve fibers to the saccule was very severe on both sides, notably in the left ear, but degeneration of the utricular fibers was mild. In fact, on the right side an almost normal utricular network was present.

The degree of degeneration of the vestibular system in general was difficult to evaluate, due to poor preservation of the neuroepithelium. From the left ear fairly good scanning electron micrographs were obtained from the utricle and the superior and hori-

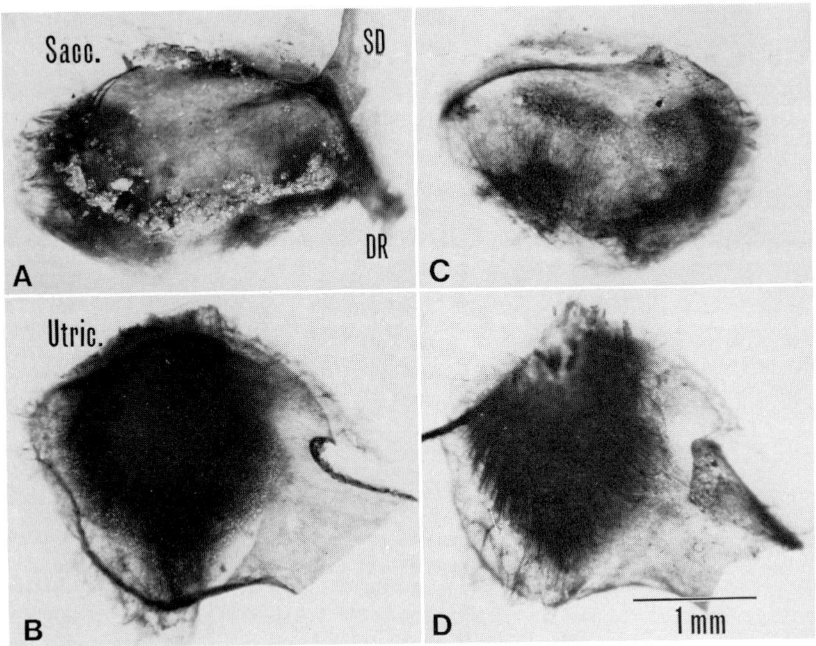

Fig. 15. Macular organs from both ears. Saccular maculae above, utricular below. A, B) Left ear. C, D) Right ear. Wall of left saccule was collapsed, and most of the otoconia removed. Abnormal otoconia consisting of apatite remain along inferior margin. Note marked degeneration of saccular nerve network on both sides. Network of right utricle, photographed from the outside, is of almost normal density. SD - Saccular duct; DR - Ductus reuniens. (OsO_4)

zontal ampullary crista. Severe hair cell degeneration was present in both cristae (Fig. 16). The utricular macula showed a lesser degree of sensory cell degeneration than the cristae.

DISCUSSION

The anatomy and degeneration behavior of the cochlear neuron is reviewed in several works.[15-27] The secondary type of nerve degeneration is effectively delayed by the presence of the supporting cells and pillar cells.[15-17,21,23,26] According to Spoendlin,[25] injury to the unmyelinated portion of the nerve fibers inside Corti organ represents the crucial factor that initiates degeneration. Therefore, all implantation surgery should aim at preserving the remaining organ of Corti in the deaf ear as nearly as possible. Any disruption of the walls of the cochlear duct, notably the basilar membrane and Reissner membrane, will, in addition to mere mechanical damage, cause contamination of endolymph with perilymph which, in turn, is likely to cause further damage to Corti organ[28-30] and accelerate the ongoing secondary nerve degeneration. In experimentally produced ruptures of Reissner membrane which, it should be noted, usually have been relatively small, damage to Corti organ is limited to the region of the rupture, and there is only limited longitudinal spread of the degeneration. One may hope that this also holds true for the human cochlea if a rupture should occur during implantation surgery.

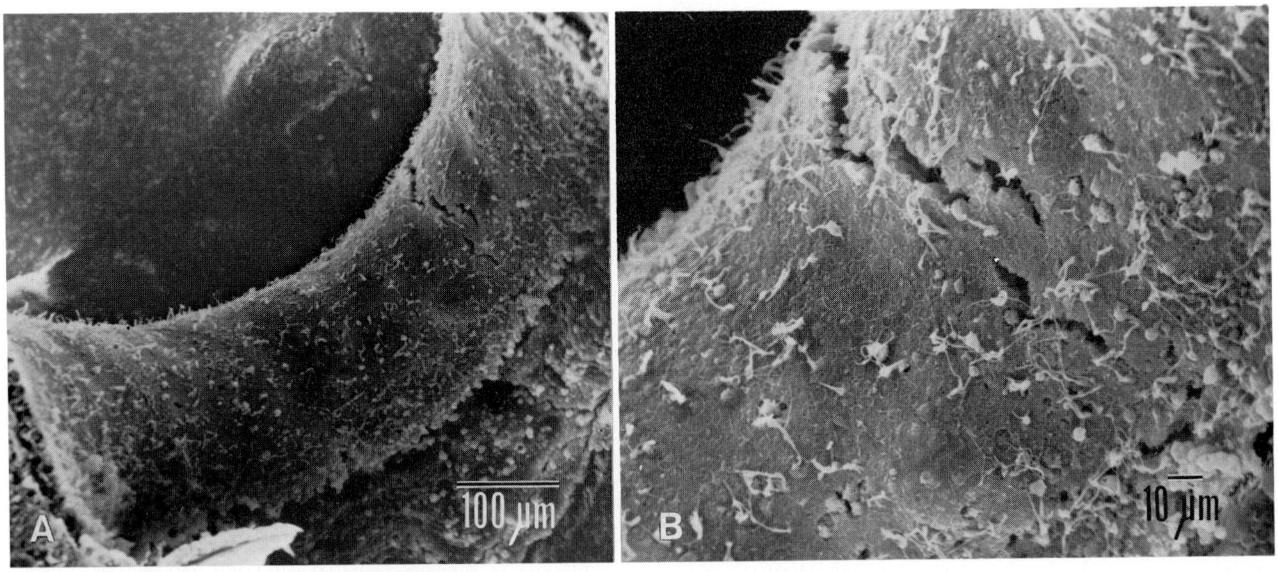

Fig. 16. A, B) Left ear. Scanning electron micrograph of the superior crista showing severe hair cell loss.

The cause of the bilateral sudden deafness in the present case remains obscure. The otic capsule appeared normal on both sides and there were no signs of luetic osteitis or fistula. The cochleosaccular hydrops found in the left ear could perhaps have been related to the patient's acquired lues but usually it is syphilis in its congenital form which causes hydrops and mimics Menière's disease.[31] Atrophy of the spiral ligament and stria was unusually severe, especially in the basal turn, but such changes are commonly associated with aging and with many other forms of deafness[10,32-34] and it is unclear to what extent implantation enhanced the pathology of these tissues. No severe regional or generalized loss of the vasculature was observed which would have indicated a blockage of a major cochlear vessel or its branches. Such occlusions would in all likelihood also have led during the patient's many years of deafness to ossification of the cochlea unless a revascularization occurred soon after the vascular accident. Our observation in this case is in agreement with the results of Schuknecht and his associates.[35] He reviewed his entire sudden deafness material and failed to find a clear-cut vascular cause for sudden auditory deficit. The severe cochlear hydrops, the fistula of Reissner membrane, and the partial collapse of the saccular wall in the left ear suggests that the hydrops, and perhaps ruptures of Reissner membrane, may have played a role in causing the deafness in this ear. The connective tissue formed in the scala tympani of the middle and apical turn in the left ear was separated from the new tissue formed around the implant by an intact stretch of bony wall (Fig. 11A) and may, therefore, have represented an incipient ossification of the apical portion of the cochlea, perhaps secondary to poor vascular supply.[31]

It may be misleading to compare the respective tissue responses to the two implants of different types because the one in the left ear was worn longer than the one in the right. Neither do we know if and how the hydrops and lues were related to the response. Nevertheless, it appears that the single induction coil on the right side was relatively well tolerated, while the multipolar device on the opposite side clearly was not. The thick, uneven multipolar electrode probably caused considerable endosteal irritation or damage on this side resulting, as one would expect, in the extensive new bone formation in the scala tympani. Furthermore, circumscribed ossification of the spiral ligament occurred at the tip of the electrode in the scala media and scala vestibuli (Figs. 2 and 11A).

It is noteworthy that on the right side, where minimal adverse reaction to the electrode was visible in the scala tympani, there was circumscribed formation of loose, darkly stained connective tissue located at the first curvature of the basal turn. The implant had probably scratched the endosteum in that region during insertion. In the future new bone might have grown at this site and invaded the weblike tissue. The tissue layer surrounding both implants was relatively thick. A thin layer of endosteal membrane has been found around intralabyrinthine tantalum wires in cats, but these prostheses were placed in the vestibule and the ears were studied 3 to 6 months after surgery so it is difficult to compare those findings with the present ones.[36]

Both implants deviated in a symmetrical fashion from their intended course c 12 mm from the round window and took an "uphill" direction along the curved bony wall of the scala tympani toward the basilar membrane, finally bending posteriorly. This result was clearly dictated by the geometry and shape of the basal turn. It is not clear whether such a deflection can be avoided with an electrode of this type and length. A continuous twist of the electrode medially during insertion could possibly prevent the implant from taking a destructive course. More likely, however, it will only shift the point of deviation slightly higher up, further increasing the risks of damage to surviving nerve fibers in the apical half of the cochlea (Figs. 1 and 2). From the otopathologist's point of view it would not have been feasible to extract either one of the electrodes, had a reimplantation been contemplated, without causing very severe damage to the cochlea and the remaining nerve fibers.

The walls of the cochlear duct apparently are capable of regrowth and repair processes, at least with time. Lawrence and Yantis[37] have described closure of ruptures of Reissner membrane in guinea pigs. A similar healing of Reissner membrane, the basilar membrane, and perhaps the spiral ligament, must have occurred in our case, where the damage to the cochlear duct at the time of surgery obviously was severe. The significance of the regular arrangement of the epithelial cells of infant type in Reissner membrane of both ears is difficult to evaluate especially in view of the cochlear hydrops on the left side. The finding could possibly imply an increased growth of cells in Reissner membrane secondary to the implantation.

Shorter electrodes of 10 mm or less would probably have created less damage and would perhaps have resulted in little or no aggravation of nerve degeneration. Another alternative would have been to stop the insertion immediately when resistance was felt. Furthermore, the ball at the tip of the electrode may have provided less protection during the insertion than a bullet-shaped tip would have done.

It is possible that the scala tympani of the lower half of the basal turn has a specific tendency to respond to endosteal damage with formation of bone, which is not matched by the more apical portions of the cochlea. In otosclerosis the formation of new lamellar bone, presumably secondary to endosteal stimulation, is usually limited to the lower half of the basal turn, even though other regions of the cochlea also are involved.[12] The same may be true concerning surgical insults of the cochlea.

The cochlear disorders in this patient probably were responsible for most of the severe sensorineural degeneration observed. This must have been the case at least in the left ear, which had no hearing for almost two decades. The specimen did, however, show more severe neural degeneration than we usually find in specimens representing long-term deafness, including those with hydrops. In view of this finding, plus the fact that the cochlear duct in all likelihood was ruptured on both sides during surgery, it is probable that the implant further aggravated the ongoing sensorineural degeneration.[28-30]

Judging from the present case and other types of deafness represented in our material, the secondary nerve degeneration began or at least initially was most severe in the distal end of the peripheral process and then proceeded centripetally in osseous spiral lamina, leaving only a few ganglion cells and their proximal processes remaining in the modiolus and the internal auditory canal. This is in agreement with our own and other investigators' observations of the degeneration pattern. Liberman and Kiang[38] have shown in experimental animals that such nerve fibers without distal processes can still be electrically excitable.

An unexpected finding in both ears, from a functional point of view, was the complete destruction of the posterior ampulla and canal. This is presumably the result of the close proximity of the implant to these structures. Similar changes have not been observed in our material before or in the large temporal bone collection of HF Schuknecht (personal communication). The shortest distance between the wall of the round window niche and the ampulla was measured in the specimens and found to be c 1 mm.

The sensorineural degeneration of the vestibular system in general was severe in both ears, especially on the left hydropic side. This is in agreement with clinical observations. Electronystagmography demonstrated decreased vestibular response in most of the implanted patients both before and after surgery.[39] It was assumed that the disorders or factors causing deafness also affected the vestibular system. Again it is impossible to say whether or to what extent the vestibular degeneration in the present case was accelerated by the implantation.

Apparently the patient had some benefit from both implants. This raises the questions of whether just a few ganglion cells and their proximal processes, or perhaps just nearby tissues and tissue fluids, could conduct stimuli to the auditory centers in the brainstem. It seems possible that this indeed is what occurred in the present case. This hypothesis would also explain the lack of deterioration of hearing thresholds in patients with long-term implants.[40]

The patient was reported to have had some degree of crude pitch discrimination for frequencies of 50 to 800 Hz when direct electrical stimulation was applied to the multipolar electrodes on the left side.[4] Considering the extreme sparsity of neural elements in this ear, this finding is difficult to understand. It is not known whether the radially running nerve canals in osseous spiral lamina can act as spatially arranged preferential current pathways to the modiolus.[41] As the nerves degenerate the canals contain remnants of myelin sheaths and in all likelihood become filled with perilymph. In any case, the osseous spiral lamina in the left ear was thin and atrophic and most of the canals had disappeared.

SUMMARY

A patient with bilateral cochlear implants died in 1976. He had carried a single-electrode induction coil system in the right ear for two years and a multiple-electrode hard-wired system in the left ear for seven years. Both implants were functional at the time of death.

Both implants were found to have deviated in a more or less symmetrical fashion away from the scala tympani and to have entered the scala media c 13 mm from the basal end of the cochlea. In the right ear, the cochlear duct in the upper half of the basal turn was displaced by the implant, but there was only minimal formation of connective tissue in the scala tympani. No osteoneogenesis was observed. Two islands of Corti organ remained in the right ear in the upper end of the basal turn and in the apical turn, respectively. Each was supplied by several bundles of nerve fibers in the osseous spiral lamina.

In contrast to the right ear with a single-electrode implant, the multiple-electrode implant in the left ear was completely buried in bone along its entire course in the scala tympani. In this ear, which had cochlear hydrops, no nerve fibers were present in the osseous spiral lamina.

There was a severe to subtotal reduction of ganglion cells in both ears, the degeneration of this distal process being more severe than that of the proximal processes. In spite of the severe degeneration present, the implants continued to function. It appears that the single-electrode induction coil implant on the right was relatively well tolerated, while the multiple-electrode on the left was not.

ACKNOWLEDGMENTS — The clinical history and audiological findings were reviewed and summarized by Karen I. Berliner, PhD.

REFERENCES

1. House WF, Berliner K, Crary W, et al. Cochlear implants. Ann Otol Rhinol Laryngol 1976; 85 Suppl 27:1-93.

2. Bilger RC, Black FO, Hopkinson NT, et al. Evaluation of subjects presently fitted with implanted auditory prostheses. Ann Otol Rhinol Laryngol 1977; 86 Suppl 38:1-176.

3. Johnsson L-G, House WF, Linthicum FH. Bilateral cochlear implants: histological findings in a pair of temporal bones. Laryngoscope 1979; 89:759-62.

4. Mladejovsky MG, Eddington DK, Dobelle WH, et al. Artificial hearing for the deaf by cochlear stimulation: pitch modulation and some parametric thresholds. Trans Am Soc Artif Int Org 1975; 21:1-5.

5. Eddington DK, Dobelle WH, Brackmann DE, et al. Auditory prostheses research with multiple channel intracochlear stimulation in man. Ann Otol Rhinol Laryngol 1978; 87 Suppl 53:1-39.

6. Bredberg G. Cellular pattern and nerve supply of the human organ of Corti. Acta Otolaryngol (Stockh) 1968; Suppl 236:1-135.

7. Hawkins JE Jr, Johnsson L-G. Microdissection and surface preparations of the inner ear. In: Smith CA, Vernon JA, eds. Handbook of auditory and vestibular research methods. Springfield, Ill: Thomas, 1976:5-52.

8. Johnsson L-G, Hawkins JE Jr. A direct approach to cochlear anatomy and pathology in man. Arch Otolaryngol 1967; 85:599-613.

9. Johnsson L-G. Cochlear blood vessel pattern in the human fetus and postnatal vascular involution. Ann Otol Rhinol Laryngol 1972; 81:22-40.

10. Johnsson L-G, Hawkins JE Jr. Vascular changes in the human inner ear associated with aging. Ann Otol Rhinol Laryngol 1972; 81:364-76.

11. Johnsson L-G. Reissner's membrane in the human cochlea. Ann Otol Rhinol Laryngol 1971; 80:425-38.

12. Johnsson L-G, Hawkins JE Jr, Linthicum FH Jr. Cochlear and vestibular lesions in capsular otosclerosis as seen in microdissection. Ann Otol Rhinol Laryngol 1978; 87 Suppl 48:1-40.

13. Johnsson L-G, Hawkins JE Jr. Otolithic membranes of the saccule and utricle in man. Science 1967; 157:1454-6.

14. Johnsson L-G, Hawkins JE Jr. Hydrops and cupulolithiasis as seen in microdissections of human temporal bones. In: Meniere's disease: Proceedings of Fourth Extraordinary Meeting of the Barany Society, Anaheim, California, 1975. Pacific Palisades, Calif: Palisades Pub Co (in press).

15. Johnsson L-G. Sequence of degeneration of Corti's organ and its first-order neurons. Ann Otol Rhinol Laryngol 1974; 83:294-303.

16. Johnsson L-G, Hawkins JE Jr. Sensory and neural degeneration with aging, as seen in microdissection of the human inner ear. Ann Otol Rhinol Laryngol 1972; 81:179-93.

17. Johnsson L-G, Hawkins JE Jr. Degeneration patterns in human ears exposed to noise. Ann Otol Rhinol Laryngol 1976; 85:725-39.

18. Lawrence M, Johnsson L-G. The role of the organ of Corti in auditory nerve stimulation. Ann Otol Rhinol Laryngol 1973; 82:464-72.

19. Lindsay JR. Profound childhood deafness: inner ear pathology. Ann Otol Rhinol Laryngol 1973; 82 Suppl 5:1-121.

20. Lindsay JR, Hinojosa R. The acoustic ganglion in profound sensorineural deafness. In: Naunton RF, Fernandez C, eds. Evoked electrical activity in the auditory nervous system. New York: Academic Press, 1978:301-21.

21. Otte J, Schuknecht HF, Kerr AG. Ganglion cell populations in normal and pathological human cochleae: implications for cochlear implantation. Laryngoscope 1978; 88:1231-46.

22. Rasmussen AT. Studies of the VIIIth cranial nerve of man. Laryngoscope 1940; 50:67-83.

23. Schuknecht HF. Lesions of the organ of Corti. Trans Am Acad Ophthalmol Otolaryngol 1953; 57:366-82.

24. Spoendlin H. Anatomisch-pathologische Aspekte der Elektrostimulation des ertaubten Innenohres. Arch Otorhinolaryngol 1979; 223:1-75.

25. Spoendlin H. The afferent innervation of the cochlea. In: Naunton RF, Fernandez C, eds. Evoked electrical activity in the auditory nervous system. New York: Academic Press, 1978:21-41.

26. Spoendlin HH, Gacek RR. Electronmicroscopic study of the efferent and afferent innervation of the organ of Corti in the cat. Ann Otol Rhinol Laryngol 1963; 72:660-86.

27. Sutton D, Miller JM, Pfingst BE. Comparison of cochlear histopathology following two implant designs for use in scala tympani. Ann Otol Rhinol Laryngol 1980; 89 Suppl 66:11-4.

28. Duvall AJ, Rhodes VT. Ultrastructure of the organ of Corti following intermixing of cochlear fluids. Ann Otol Rhinol Laryngol 1967; 76:688-708.

29. Lawrence M. Histological evidence for localized radial flow of endolymph. Arch Otolaryngol 1966; 83:406-12.

30. Schuknecht HF, El Seifi A. Experimental observations on the fluid physiology of the inner ear. Ann Otol Rhinol Laryngol 1963; 72:687-712.

31. Schuknecht HF. Pathology of the ear. Cambridge, Mass: Harvard University Press, 1974.

32. Johnsson L-G, Hawkins JE Jr. Strial atrophy in clinical and experimental deafness. Laryngoscope 1972; 82:1105-25.

33. Johnsson L-G, Hawkins JE Jr, Muraski AA, et al. Vascular anatomy and pathology of the cochlea in Dalmation dogs. In: de Lorenzo AJD, ed. Vascular disorders and hearing defects. Baltimore: University Park Press, 1973:249-95.

34. Schuknecht HF, Watanuki K, Takahashi T, et al. Atrophy of the stria vascularis, a common cause for hearing loss. Laryngoscope 1974; 84:1777-821.

35. Schuknecht HF, Kimura RS, Naufal PM. The pathology of sudden deafness. Acta Otolaryngol (Stockh) 1973; 76:75-97.

36. Schuknecht HF, Oleksiuk S. The metal prosthesis for stapes anklyosis. Arch Otolaryngol 1960; 71:287-95.

37. Lawrence M, Yantis PA. Individual differences in functional recovery and structural repair following overstimulation of the guinea pig ear. Ann Otol Rhinol Laryngol 1957; 66:595-621.

38. Liberman MC, Kiang NYS. Acoustic trauma in cats: cochlear pathology and auditory-nerve activity. Acta Otolaryngol (Stockh) 1978; Suppl 358:1-63.

39. Eisenberg LS, Nelson JR, House WF. Effects of the single-electrode cochlear implant on the vestibular system of the profoundly deafened adult. Ann Otol Rhinol Laryngol 1982; 91 Suppl 91:47-54.

40. Michelson RP. Cochlear implants. J Laryngol Otol 1976; 90:441-4.

41. Black RC, Clark GM. Differential electrical excitation of the auditory nerve. J Acoust Soc Am 1980; 67:868-74.

RISK VERSUS BENEFIT IN COCHLEAR IMPLANTATION

KAREN I. BERLINER, PhD

The impact of deafness and the potential risks and benefits of cochlear implantation are discussed, both for adults and for children. Experience with the House single-electrode cochlear implant in humans is now considerable and provides a clinical basis for evaluating risks and benefits. From the evidence to date, it is concluded that the implant does not pose a serious risk to the health, safety, or welfare of the patient and that the benefits to be gained by the patient can be considerable.

Many have asked whether the cochlear implant provides enough benefit to warrant performing a surgical procedure. To answer such a question, one must examine the impact of deafness, the potential risks associated with the implant, adverse effects to date, and the available alternatives, as well as the benefit to be expected. Experience with the House single-electrode cochlear implant in human subjects is now considerable and provides a clinical basis for evaluating risks and benefits. A large number of patients have been assessed medically, audiologically, and psychologically. Detailed discussions of these assessments can be found elsewhere in this supplement, but an attempt is made here to integrate the available information into a more global evaluation of the risks and benefits of cochlear implantation in humans.

COCHLEAR IMPLANTATION IN ADULTS

IMPACT OF DEAFNESS

To understand the need for an auditory prosthesis such as the cochlear implant, one must first consider the impact of deafness. Loss of hearing is the nation's number 1 health problem in incidence. One out of every 10 or 15 persons is affected to some degree. One out of nearly 100 has extreme difficulty understanding speech. Hundreds of thousands are deaf; each year, thousands more are born deaf or will acquire the impairment. A study in 1969[1] by the National Advisory Neurologic Diseases and Stroke Council of the National Institute of Neurological Diseases and Stroke estimated the total direct annual cost to the nation for the education, health care, and compensation of deaf or hearing-impaired people to be $410,115,000. The estimated proportion of those costs for the deaf was $100,000,000. Assuming yearly inflation of at least 6%, this amount would be more than doubled today. Indirect costs have been estimated at 2 to 3 times the direct cost. Clearly, deafness has a major financial impact on the nation.

The impact of deafness on the individual must be viewed in light of the functions that hearing normally serves. It is one of our two distance senses. The other, vision, is directional and can focus only on that area immediately in front of the individual. Audition, however, encompasses all directions simultaneously, persists even during sleep, and keeps the individual in continual contact with the environment. Sound is nature's surest sign of activity. Myklebust[2] goes so far as to state that it is difficult to conceive of an organism attaining the level of function found in humans without a sense which provides constant environmental contact. The evolutionary importance of hearing is illustrated by the fact that auditory contact with the environment begins prenatally, maybe as early as the third or fourth fetal month, and the cochlea is adult size at birth.

As hearing individuals, most of us typically have never given much thought to the functions that audition serves. Language/communication, the symbolic function of hearing, is perhaps the most recognized. Little need be said about the importance of this function to humankind as well as to the individual. Almost universally, languages have developed that depend on auditory reception. This is clearly the most effective means of communication, and only in more recent history has this auditory-based communication system been available to the visual modality through the development of writing.

In daily life, sound is the primary source of information regarding events that are occurring in the environment. We are usually first alerted to an event through hearing, and only then do we visually search to "see" what is happening. Hearing is vitally important to competent interaction with the environment. This crucial function, hearing environmental sounds which signal events, has too often been underestimated in its importance.

In addition to serving as a direct signal of events in the environment, sound also serves as a background to daily living and helps maintain a feeling of being part of a living world. Background noise provides a sense of security and reassurance. Most warning signals are auditory: for example, fire alarms, sirens, the shouted warning, the sound of a fast-approaching vehicle, and so on. In fact, the deaf individual would seem to be at some risk to safety by virtue of not being able to hear.

There are two general categories of deaf individuals, those born deaf or who have lost their hearing prior to language acquisition (prelingual), and those who became deaf after acquiring language or later in life (postlingual).

The postlingually deafened acutely feel the loss of environmental and speech sounds. They had learned, as all hearing individuals do, to depend heavily on audition for information about what was happening in the world around them. This loss often produces feelings of isolation and depression, as well as a lessening of competence in dealing with the environment. The postlingually deafened may lose their jobs when they lose their hearing, or be restricted to only certain types of employment. Inability to use the telephone is a particular vocational handicap.

Communication becomes difficult. Although a few deaf individuals can speechread (lipread) successfully, only a small portion (less than 40%) of the speech signal is visible on the lips, and most people cannot easily communicate solely by this means. It requires great concentration on the part of the deaf person and patience and repetition on the part of the speaker. A group of speakers is almost impossible to speechread adequately. Therefore, deafness often has a profound impact on the social and interpersonal aspects of life. Both quality and quantity of interactions with others are diminished.

The prelingually deaf have extreme difficulty in achieving oral language skills, and this communication deficit is probably the major consequence of their deafness. Because they may find communicating difficult, because they may not respond to safety signals, because they cannot work with equipment based on the auditory sense (eg, telephone), and because they may not speak intelligibly, the prelingually deaf have a difficult time finding employment.

Deafness from an early age is also associated with serious reading problems. The 1969 Annual Survey of Hearing Impaired Children and Youth[3] indicated that by 15½-16½ years of age the mean reading achievement grade equivalent is 3.5. Many deaf adults never achieve more than a third or fourth grade reading level. This has severe implications for academic achievement, and its effects are life-long.

In all, the impact of deafness on an individual is great, in many cases extreme, leaving that individual isolated, at risk to physical safety, less competent in interacting with the environment in daily life and vocationally, and in many ways diminished in quality of life.

RISK ANALYSIS

The risks associated with the cochlear implant device fall into three basic categories: 1) risks of mastoid surgery, 2) risks of the implantation of electrodes and induction coil, and 3) risks of stimulation of the auditory system by electric currents.

Risks of Mastoid Surgery. The surgical approach for the cochlear implant is essentially a mastoid operation and involves the same risks as that common otologic procedure: infection, facial paralysis, fluid drainage resulting in meningitis, and anesthetic risks. These are all remote risks and have not occurred to a significant degree in any of the patients implanted to date.

Risks of Implantation of Electrodes and Induction Coil. Conceivable risks associated with the implantation of electrodes and induction coil fall into two general categories: biocompatibility and surgical trauma to cochlear structures.

BIOCOMPATIBILITY. The materials currently used for the cochlear implant have a long history of biocompatibility. There have been no "rejections" of the internal coil, nor any evidence of production of toxic substances from wire electrolysis. Electron microscopic studies of electrodes implanted and used in human subjects, then removed, show no evidence of breakdown of insulation or wire.[4]

SURGICAL TRAUMA. Does insertion of the electrode into the cochlea cause damage to the cochlear structures or nerve elements? Most of the evidence on this question comes from animal studies, and these have indicated good tolerance for insertion and presence of electrodes in the cochlea.[5] Histological studies on one deceased implant patient also indicate minimal adverse reaction to the insertion and presence of the single-electrode cochlear implant.[6,7] Bilger et al[8] studied patients using a cochlear implant and from audiological assessment of each patient's implanted and unimplanted ears, concluded that the single-wire electrode has little deleterious effect on hearing in the implanted ear.

Although there is potentially a risk that insertion of the electrode might scratch the endosteum and stimulate new bone growth, electrodes have been successfully removed and replaced in eight cases. Apparently no obliterating bone growth had occurred. One subject has had removal and replacement of electrodes twice with no evidence of bone obliteration. Should bone growth in the scala occur, it would probably make replacement of a nonfunctioning implant more difficult.

Animal studies indicate that cochlear damage, should it occur, will produce degeneration of sensory and neural elements in a normal ear. This risk, however, must be viewed in light of the fact that ears suitable for cochlear implantation have already undergone severe degeneration of these elements as a consequence of the etiology of deafness. Those nerve fibers surviving are probably among the hardiest and may therefore be more resistant to further trauma.

In summary, both animal and long-term human studies (ten years in one subject) would seem to indicate that the risks due to implantation of electrodes and induction coil are minimal. This is particularly so when the status of the ear prior to implantation is considered, ie, profound deafness.

Risks of Electrical Stimulation. The long-term risks of electrical stimulation must still be classified as only partially documented. However, convincing evidence has been obtained that electrical stimulation does not pose a serious risk to the health, safety, or welfare of the patient using a cochlear implant.

When considering the safe limits of electrical stimulation at the cochlea, two major issues must be examined. First, what is an acceptable waveform? Second, what stimulus levels will effect electrode breakdown, ie, platinum dissolution, or electrolysis, which may destroy tissue at the electrode-tissue interface?

Acceptable stimulus waveforms for direct neural stimulation have been studied extensively. It is well known that direct current (DC) will destroy nerve tissue.[9] The literature reveals that stimuli such as monopolar pulses introduced directly without capacitor or transformer coupling will introduce a net DC charge which produces neural damage. Balanced bipolar pulses and sinusoids do not yield a significant net DC and, therefore, are the stimuli of choice in neurological stimulation studies. The cochlear implant stimulator operates by amplitude-modulating a 16 kHz sinusoid and then transformer (magnetic induction)-coupling the pulsed sinusoid to the implanted electrodes. This system is optimal since even in direct stimulation the pulsed sinusoid produces no net DC and, further, transformer-coupled signals do not have a DC component.

The present standard of safety for platinum (Pt) electrodes is based on the work of Brummer and Turner[10] and Brummer and McHardy.[11] Their work indicates that during biphasic pulsing, charges up to +/− 400 $\mu C/cm^2$ can be used without gas formation at the electrode tissue interface. More conservatively, Walsh et al[12,13] have shown that no measurable histological changes are seen in inner ear structures if stimulation is limited to 40 $\mu C/cm^2$/phase or less. The Pt electrodes used in the House cochlear implant system consist of a 0.5 mm diameter ball on the tip of a 0.2 mm diameter wire exposed over 15 mm in the active electrode and over 53 mm in the ground. For the active electrode, this computes to a geometric surface area of about 0.1 cm^2 or an estimated real area of 0.14 cm^2. Direct electrical measurements from a hard-wired cochlear implant patient, as well as calculated measurements from six additional implant patients, have shown that the levels at which patients report uncomfortably loud sensations are less than about 1000 μA rms. Over the range of audio frequencies of interest, this measured stimulation current equates to electrode current densities of less than 0.21 $\mu C/cm^2$/phase, roughly two orders of magnitude less than the limit based on the work of Walsh et al.

It has been shown by Leake-Jones et al[14] that using bipolar intracochlear electrodes and biphasic pulsatile stimuli (100/200 μS/phase) at current levels from 4 to 8 mA produced significant cochlear and auditory neuron degeneration in cats. It is important to note, however, that these current levels applied through the small-area bipolar electrodes resulted in charge densities much greater than those which are delivered to patients wearing the House cochlear implant system. A more representative series of experiments performed on monkeys has been reported.[15] Behaviorally verified operating ranges of intracochlear and extracochlear electrode systems for pulsatile and sinusoidal stimuli were studied with subsequent histological analysis.[16] It was found that thresholds for sinusoids were obtained at current levels approximately 0.5 dB lower than for pulses, a finding that supports the use of a sinusoidally based system. It was also noted that at low frequencies maximum acceptable stimulus currents were determined by the theoretical electrolysis limits of Brummer and Turner; at middle and high frequencies limits are psychophysical, a finding favoring a high frequency carrier system. It was also found that either widely spaced intracochlear electrodes or, optimally, an intracochlear electrode paired with an extracochlear electrode required the lowest stimulus currents to achieve threshold. Since it is clear that the extent of neural damage is directly related to the current densities required for stimulation, these data argue that an electrode configuration similar to that used in the House implant, ie, an intracochlear active electrode with a large surface area, and an extracochlear ground electrode is the safest. The findings of Clopton et al[15] have been verified in our laboratory for a human subject using a hard-wired multiple-electrode system containing both intracochlear and extracochlear electrodes.

One of the most important findings in the monkey studies was the relationship between both behavioral and objective electrical thresholds and the population of surviving neural and cochlear elements:[16]

> Animals with relatively little damage to the organ of Corti and a high percentage of surviving myelinated nerve fibers and spiral ganglion cells show low thresholds and large dynamic ranges. Animals with extensive damage to the organ of Corti and degeneration of myelinated nerve fibers and spiral ganglion cells show relatively elevated thresholds and much smaller dynamic ranges.

The relationship between the behavioral or evoked potential thresholds and the underlying physiological condition has also been reported by Walsh et al[13] and Leake-Jones et al.[14] Based on the above research, it is reasonable to evaluate the safety, with respect to long-term auditory nerve survival, of a specific cochlear implant system by monitoring thresholds over time. This is being done in all of the patients implanted with the House system, and to date there has been no significant change in thresholds over time.[17]

At this point, the House Ear Institute (HEI) has had considerable experience with human implanted subjects. As of November 1, 1981, 199 patients have received the single-electrode cochlear implant. In total, these patients have had approximately 800,000 hours of electrical stimulation. This is approximately 160 "person-years" of use of the implant for a 14-hour waking day. One patient has had electrical stimulation for ten years, with daily use for almost nine years — about 45,000 hours of electrical stimulation. Eight patients have each used the implant daily for seven or more years. More than 50 patients have used the implant for a year or more. There has been no deterioration over time in audiological performance or electrical thresholds. Psychological and neuropsychological assessments show no evidence of organic brain damage or other psychological problems. Studies at HEI have shown that the electric current does not even seem to spread to or affect the vestibular system[18] or the facial nerve.

Thus, other than animal studies specifically aimed at finding what current level will in fact produce damage, the evidence is great that for those levels being used in the cochlear implant prosthesis, the patient is at minimal risk.

Finally, the risk of producing further damage to the auditory system must be weighed against the fact that the auditory system already has a profound loss (almost 50% of House's implant patients had no response audiometrically to the limit of the audiometer for any of the speech frequencies, well beyond the definition of a profound hearing loss).

Other Risks. Other conceivable risks of cochlear implantation might be an increase in otologic symptoms such as tinnitus or dizziness. Although temporary changes in these symptoms often occur following an otologic surgery, there has been no permanent increase in such symptoms as a result of the cochlear implant. It has also been speculated that the electrode transversing the middle ear area and entering the cochlea might provide a potential pathway for the spread of otitis media to the inner ear fluids. One implanted patient did, in fact, experience an otitis media which was successfully treated with antibiotics and resolved with no measurable sequelae.

ADVERSE EFFECTS TO DATE

Sixteen patients have experienced an implanted coil device failure. Eleven of the 16 have had revision surgery under a local anesthetic and now have functioning implants. Five patients still do not have working internal devices. However, besides the fact of the device failure itself, there have been no observed adverse effects in these 16 patients.

There has been one report by an investigator of the removal of the internal device as a precautionary measure after a patient developed a cerebrospinal fluid fistula following surgery. There have been no continuing effects nor any continued fluid leakage in this patient. The investigator felt that due to the patient's history of syphilis she may have had abnormal patency of the cochlear aqueduct. Three investigators have reported one case each of an internal coil extruding through the skin at or near the incision. All cases were remedied satisfactorily.

There have been no other reports of postoperative problems, no surgical complications, no infections, no meningitis, and in general no occurrence of any of the potential risks of the surgical procedure.

There have also been no measurable adverse effects in patients after beginning use of electrical stimulation. Patients do occasionally report experiencing uncomfortably loud sounds, but even this is rare since the stimulator units are set to cut off before the patient's uncomfortable loudness level is reached. A few patients have reported episodes of slight soreness in the area around the implanted coil. This typically is a result of the fit of the patient's glasses and is easily corrected. A few patients have also reported an isolated and brief episode of increased tinnitus. However, tinnitus has not been produced in any patient who did not have it prior to implant, and occasional worsening of this symptom is not uncommon even in unimplanted deaf patients. Actually, a large number of patients report reduced tinnitus with use of the implant.

In conclusion, there have been few observed or reported adverse effects in patients using the House single-electrode cochlear implant.

AVAILABLE ALTERNATIVES

A major consideration in deciding whether a patient should undergo a surgical procedure is whether an alternative, noninvasive treatment is available. The two primary alternative prostheses for the deaf are hearing aids and vibrotactile devices.

Many patients with the level of loss that would be considered appropriate for an implant will not or cannot wear a conventional aid. They may have little or no tolerance for the vibrotactile sensations accompanying use of the aid. They may experience increases in tinnitus or vertigo. They may have a temporary threshold shift, with the aid activated, that leads to loss of any sensation after a short time period. Or they may require a greater power input than could be in their best interests. The level of amplification required is such that it may actually produce further damage to the auditory system.[19,20] Additionally, many of those who have tried amplification simply do not find it of enough subjective benefit that they are willing to wear it. Yet many of these same individuals will wear the cochlear implant in spite of its greater size.

The data at HEI have shown performance on many auditory discrimination tasks is statistically significantly better with the single-electrode cochlear implant than with a conventional hearing aid.[17,21,22] Qualitative differences in performance that indicate greater benefit from an implant have also been noted.

The other alternative, often touted as a potential prosthesis for the deaf, is a device that uses tactile stimulation to provide information about auditory events. Although research on vibrotactile devices has been in progress for decades, no sophisticated wearable prosthesis is available. Furthermore, a vibrotactile device does not produce a sensation of hearing, which is what the postlingually deafened so desperately desire. Even if a vibrotactile device could transmit as much information as the cochlear implant, it might not fully serve the needs of the profoundly deaf patient. Many patients have objected to a hearing aid because it seemed to provide only tactile, and not auditory, information. A small number of patients who were prospective candidates for the implant have tried a vibrotactile device, with training, at HEI. None of these patients chose to continue using such a prosthesis, even though they did not all receive the implant either.

In general, then, there has been no other satisfactory form of treatment for those selected profoundly deaf individuals who would be accepted for the cochlear implant investigation.

EXPECTED BENEFIT

It is not an easy task to determine how a cochlear implant affects the quality of life of a profoundly deaf individual. There is certainly no argument that the current generation of cochlear prostheses does not restore normal hearing. However, there is a wide range of levels of hearing between normal and no hearing, and a wide variety of potential benefits, from restoration of speech discrimination (which is not yet possible) to a decrease in the feelings of isolation that haunt the profoundly deaf. Detailed discussions of audiological and psychological results can be found elsewhere in this supplement, but will be reviewed briefly here.

Auditory warble tone thresholds can be obtained across the frequency range tested, 125-8000 Hz. With the stimulator unit set at the most comfortable level for speech, thresholds range approximately from 40 to 70 dB SPL at all frequencies, with means at 55 to 60 dB SPL. Thus, implant patients can hear some soft and most medium and loud sounds that occur in the environment (eg, normal conversational speech occurs at about 70 dB SPL). Patients can also score significantly above chance on a number of closed-set auditory discrimination tasks that include speech and environmental sounds stimuli.

The implant provides normal or near normal intensity and durational difference limens. That is, patients can tell differences in intensity and timing very well. Frequency discrimination is good for low frequencies, below about 500 Hz, but poor at higher frequencies. Patients cannot understand speech with the implant alone, but those aspects of speech based on intensity and timing are accessible to the implant user — stress patterns, rhythm, syllabication, and so on. These are referred to as the prosodic elements of speech.

Subjects report hearing a wide variety of sounds in their daily environment. Most subjects can distinguish between voices and other sounds and between male and female voices. They can hear their own voices and this allows better control of volume, intonation, and other aspects of voice production. Some indicate that they can recognize the voices of highly familiar persons. The hearing of voices helps them tremendously in social situations by both aiding speechreading and by eliminating embarrassment caused by interrupting another speaker. Implant users report feeling safer since they can hear warning signals such as sirens and fire alarms. They feel more secure because they are able to hear doorbells, telephones, someone's calling out to get their attention, and so on. In their homes, subjects usually learn to identify commonly occurring sounds. Many also are able to enjoy music, even though the postlingually deaf do not find it as pleasant as it was prior to their deafness.

Subject files at HEI contain many reports by the implant subjects on how their implant has helped them to deal more competently with their environment. "Anecdotal" as this information may be, subjects are amazingly consistent in their reports of what they hear, how it sounds, and how they use the auditory information.

Some subjects have experienced a "nonauditory" benefit: a reduction in the level or amount of their tinnitus. For some, these changes occur only while the implant unit is activated. For others, the effect has lasted for extended periods when the implant was not in use; up to two weeks in one case, at which time implant use was resumed.

One final comment should be made in regard to what benefit is obtained from a cochlear implant. For the postlingually deafened individual, the onset of deafness usually leads to changes in lifestyle and, nearly always, to a decrease in the quality of life. Not only the deaf person is affected. His or her family and friends are affected, too. Social interactions, in particular, often decrease in quality and quantity. We have found that, at least for some patients, the implant has had a profound positive effect in this area. The psychosocial benefits of the cochlear implant are reported in some detail in Wexler et al.[23]

The cochlear implant is a rehabilitative device. No matter what "benefit" can be shown on objective measures, no benefit will occur unless the patient uses the prosthesis. Willingness to use the implant is an important indication of its subjective value to the patient. Less than 13% of the patients implanted have chosen not to use their implants. The vast majority of patients are currently wearing their cochlear implant stimulator units on a regular basis. Most wear the device all day long, every day, in spite of its rather bulky size and the frequent expense of buying batteries. The use of the implant by profoundly deaf individuals must be regarded as the ultimate judgment that it is of significant benefit.

Summary. Many hours of cochlear implant use by numerous profoundly deaf patients have yielded no evidence that the patient is at risk. Animal studies also appear to indicate that a patient can be implanted with minimal harm to remaining auditory structure, and that for the time periods studied and the current levels considered appropriate, electrical stimulation does not cause measurable degeneration of the auditory neural elements. One study, in fact, provides evidence that electrical stimulation may reactivate "silenced" neuronal populations. Wong-Riley et al[24] found the level of cytochrome oxidase activity was significantly higher in chronically implanted and stimulated cats than in implanted but nonstimulated cats, and even approached that of the normal. The oxidase enzyme activity presumably reflects rate of energy utilization by functioning auditory neurons.

The question that remains, then, is whether the unknown long-term effects of electrical stimulation carry a significant risk to the safety or welfare of the patient. From the evidence to date it would appear not. One patient has had electrical stimulation over a period of ten years with no measurable negative effects. Even if further degeneration of the auditory system occurs, it would seem not to affect the functioning of the single-electrode cochlear implant. Histology studies on a deceased implant patient indicated almost no surviving neural elements in the auditory periphery, yet this patient experienced sound sensations to electrical stimulation through each of five electrodes in his multiple-electrode cochlear implant.

Thus the greatest risk, that of further damage to an already profoundly deaf ear, should it occur, seems not a major factor to the functioning of this prosthetic device, and most certainly does not produce a life-threatening risk or serious bodily harm.

All risks and probable benefits are discussed with prospective patients, both in written materials and in counseling sessions. Every effort is made to insure that the patient has realistic expectations for the implant and an understanding of the potential risks. Given that the patient has been as fully informed as is possible, and given the evidence to date regarding safety, it becomes appropriate to allow the patient to choose for himself or herself whether to undergo a surgical procedure.

COCHLEAR IMPLANTATION IN CHILDREN

It is clearly the hope of those working in the field of cochlear implantation that we may one day be able to provide hearing to the deaf child, to allow that child to grow up in a world of sound. The potential for benefit from an auditory prosthesis is likely to be much greater for the child than for the adult. Children are more adaptive than adults, and more readily learn to make use of new information. The impact of deafness and the risks and benefits of implantation involve some additional issues when discussing children. These are presented below.

IMPACT OF DEAFNESS

Estimates are that 1 of every 1,000 children is born deaf or deafened before age 3. The effects of early deafness are severe. A recent foreword to a book regarding hearing loss in children states:[25]

> Only recently have we fully understood the enormous negative impact of auditory deprivation in children. If unrecognized or untreated, it stunts intellectual growth, impairs emotional maturation, limits the development of creative and occupational skills, and diminishes the quality of life.

Language is learned primarily through auditory channels. A hearing child at age five is estimated to have a vocabulary of 5,000 to 26,000 words and the skills to combine them into meaningful sentences. A deaf child age five has usually acquired no more than a speaking vocabulary of 200 words with little comprehension of sentence structure.[26] As noted earlier for 16-year-old prelingually deaf individuals, the mean reading achievement grade equivalent is 3.5. That is, deaf children of about 16 years of age read at the level of a normal hearing 9-year-old. Conrad[27] has reported equivalent findings for British deaf children. Additionally, he looked separately at the deafer children, those with a greater than 85 dB loss (profoundly deaf), and found that 50% of them had no reading comprehension at all. Many deaf children will never achieve more than a third or fourth grade reading level. These language deficits have severe implications for educational achievement and the consequences are life-long, with vocational, socioeconomic, and quality of life effects.

Myklebust[2] emphasizes the fact that a sensory deprivation limits the world of experience and deprives the organism of some of the material resources from which the mind develops. Schwab[26] points out that in the early preschool years, the hearing child derives much information and education from random sources. Conversations at mealtime, conversation with peer groups, radio, television, etc, are all omitted from the deaf child's background. Even reading of nursery rhymes, fairy tales, and other such activities are not part of the deaf child's day-to-day life.

The auditory function helps us process distant stimuli. Eventually hearing children learn to auditorily recognize and label objects without any visual or tactual contact. This may be what helps the hearing child move from the realm of the concrete to the realm of the abstract. Deaf children do not get much practice in attaching labels to objects they cannot see. Conrad[27] provides a theoretical basis as well as objective evidence for believing that there are differences in cognitive functions between the hearing and the deaf.

Social, behavioral, and emotional consequences of deafness have also been documented. Most authors agree that the rate of emotional/behavioral problems is significantly higher among deaf children than among hearing children of otherwise comparable circumstances.[28,29]

In addition to the child who is born deaf or who loses hearing during the first few years of life, there are those children who become deaf following childhood disease or trauma at an age where at least some language acquisition has already occurred. Even though spoken language has been obtained, these children can become extremely isolated from their environment, family, friends, and peers. Communication is difficult and frustrating. Often such a child is transferred to a school for the deaf where the class may be well behind the level the child had already obtained in his or her hearing school. Without hearing, monitoring vocal productions is difficult, and the child's speech may become more and more difficult to understand. In fact, the effects of normal exposure to auditory language for a period of three years appears to become totally erased in many cases.[26] The cessation of auditory input has an almost immediately damaging effect. This child's vocational choices may be severely limited by educational achievement and lack of ability to communicate effectively, just as is the case for the prelingually deaf.

In summary, the impact of early deafness on the child is often extreme — limiting communication with the "hearing world," educational achievement, and quality of life.

EXPECTED BENEFIT

The benefit to be expected from the cochlear implant in children can be judged from the results obtained in adults combined with knowledge of the impact of deafness. Based on the findings in adults using the cochlear implant, and given the greater ability of children to learn to use new information, it might be expected that the potential benefit to be gained by the child is even greater than that obtained by the adult. The most devastating effect of early deafness is the impairment of language acquisition and oral/aural communication skills. There is reason to believe that the cochlear implant can lead to significant improvement in communication skills.

It is consistently found that the child with a severe hearing loss (80-95 dB) who can make some use of that residual hearing with a hearing aid is much more successful in acquiring oral skills than the profoundly deaf child. The "hearing-impaired" child (60-80 dB) does better yet and can often be successfully mainstreamed rather than educated in schools for the deaf. Even minimal auditory input can make a significant difference in language acquisition and educational success. This is why educators of the deaf feel so strongly about the necessity of fitting hearing aids on children with hearing losses at as young an age as possible, in spite of the potential risk that powerful aids may further damage residual hearing. The cochlear implant can provide auditory thresholds that would put the profoundly deaf child into the range of hearing-impaired. This does not necessarily mean that the implanted child would have discrimination as good as the child with better hearing who is using a hearing aid, but it certainly means that auditory input from speech and environmental sounds can be detected.

There is no reason to expect that children would get any less information from the cochlear implant than adults, and therefore we can assume that they will get intensity and timing information. The importance of this kind of information should not be underestimated. Even if the child can lipread a sentence, much of the meaning or connotation is carried by intensity or stress differences that cannot be lipread. Intensity information is also particularly important to speech production and intelligibility. Brooks[30] has suggested that learning to read might well depend on experience with the prosodic characteristics of speech. She discusses a model that suggests that the rhythm patterns in speech production determine the locus of important content. This aspect of linguistic structure may be very important in reading development. Scott[31] has suggested that although the traditional way to view vowels is by spectrum analysis, they can also be viewed in terms of temporal patterns, and fine temporal analysis play an important role in vowel perception.

Finally, we can expect some frequency discrimination at least at the low frequencies. Simmons[32] has reported that he knows of at least three cases of children who had no functional hearing above 750 Hz, but relatively normal hearing below that, all of whom communicated effectively. This situation is not dissimilar to that provided by the implant. He emphasized that children may be much better able to learn to use rate-pitch information than can adults.

Besides those benefits related to communication skills, there are a number of other areas for potential benefit to children from the implant. It might be expected that the experiential deficiencies produced by deafness (eg, cognitive, social, emotional, behavioral) may be partially remedied or at least that a wider range of experiences can be made available to the child. Liben[33 p 991] notes that "sound also has important implications for the quantity, quality, and effectiveness of the child's experience with objects." Further, noises made by objects and by actions upon objects excite the child toward exploration.

Early auditory experience may be important in developing basic concepts about sound and its meaningfulness. Some early opportunity to learn that objects produce sounds, that sounds signal an action in the environment, and therefore that sound contains meaningful information about events in the environment may be an important determinant in whether a child can later in life make effective use of auditory input. Thus, a potential benefit for children implanted while they are young may be a greater ability to benefit maximally from improved auditory prostheses developed later in their lives.

Lastly, there is some reason to believe that stimulation of the system as early as possible may help to prevent further degeneration or in some way have a positive physiological effect.[24] On the other hand, sensory deprivation studies do show that degeneration and/or failure to mature is likely to occur in a system that is not stimulated.

RISK VERSUS BENEFIT IN CHILDREN

To summarize, considerable clinical evidence has been gathered regarding safety and efficacy of the single-electrode cochlear implant in adults. It is clear that the impact of deafness on the child is severe and that the potential benefits to be gained from an auditory prosthesis are great.

The literature indicates that there probably is a critical age for language development as well as for general plasticity of the nervous system and that this seems to be up to about 5 years of age.

One author goes so far as to state that the ability to develop language peaks at about the age of 3 or 4, declines steadily thereafter, and that any language development program initiated after the age of 5, no matter what methods are used, is doomed to failure for the majority of deaf children.[34] Sensory deprivation studies suggest degeneration or lack of maturation is likely to occur if the system is not stimulated. Further, early auditory experience may be important to later auditory learning. And, lastly, there is evidence that it may not be possible to judge from results in adults how well children might be able to do even with the current implant devices. That is, children might do surprisingly better than adults.

CONCLUSIONS

Considerable clinical experience with cochlear implantation in selected profoundly deaf adults suggests that benefit to be expected far outweighs the potential risks involved. Adverse effects to date have been extremely minimal. In fact, the lack of surgical or postoperative complications has been quite remarkable.

When one considers the risks to children in remaining deaf, the benefits that might be gained, and the safety record obtained with adults, the balance would seem to favor use of the cochlear implant in children, too. Only from such clinical trials will we be able to evaluate the full potential of cochlear implants and accurately define the risk to benefit ratio. Meanwhile, the record to date would seem to warrant allowing the patient, or in the case of children, the legal guardian, to choose for himself or herself whether to undergo this surgical procedure.

ACKNOWLEDGMENT — All calculations regarding stimulus current levels and the discussions of the stimulus waveform, electrode breakdown and safe levels of current were prepared by Bradly J. Edgerton, PhD.

REFERENCES

1. Human communication and its disorders — an overview. Report of the National Advisory Council, National Institute of Neurological Diseases and Stroke, National Institutes of Health. Bethesda, Md: 1969.

2. Myklebust HR. The psychology of deafness: sensory deprivation, learning, and adjustment. 2d ed. New York: Grune and Stratton, 1964.

3. Gentile A, DiFrancesca S. Academic achievement test performance of hearing impaired students — United States: Spring 1969. Washington, DC: Gallaudet College, 1969.

4. Graham M. Long term intracochlear implantation in man: scanning electron microscopic observations. In: House WF, Berliner K, Crary W, et al. Cochlear implants. Ann Otol Rhinol Laryngol 1976; 85 Suppl 27:58-61.

5. Schindler RA, Merzenich MM, White MW, et al. Multielectrode intracochlear implants. Arch Otolaryngol 1977; 103:691-9.

6. Johnsson L-G, House WF, Linthicum FH. Bilateral cochlear implants: histological findings in a pair of temporal bones. Laryngoscope 1979; 89:759-62.

7. Johnsson L-G, House WF, Linthicum FH. Otopathological findings in a patient with bilateral cochlear implants. Ann Otol Rhinol Laryngol 1982; 91 Suppl 91:74-89.

8. Bilger RC, Black FO, Hopkinson NT, et al. Evaluation of subjects presently fitted with implanted auditory prostheses. Ann Otol Rhinol Laryngol 1977; 86 Suppl 38:1-176.

9. Lilly JC, Hughes JR, Galin RW, et al. Production and

avoidance of injury to brain tissues by electrical current at threshold values. Electroencephalogr Clin Neurophysiol 1955; 7:458-9.

10. Brummer SB, Turner MJ. Electrical stimulation of the nervous system: the principle of safe charge injection with nobel metal electrodes. Bioelectrochem Bioenerget 1975; 2:13-25.

11. Brummer SB, McHardy J. Current problems in electrode development. In: Hambrecht FT, Reswick JB, eds. Functional electrical stimulation: applications in neural prostheses. New York: Marcel Dekker, 1977:499-514.

12. Walsh SM, Leake-Jones PA, Vurek LS, et al. Chronic electrical stimulation with introcochlear electrodes: electrophysiological results. Ann Otol Rhinol Laryngol 1981; 90 Suppl 82:27-9.

13. Walsh SM, Leake-Jones PA, Vurek LS, et al. Effects of chronic electrical stimulation of auditory nerve in cat. Paper presented at West Coast Cochlear Prostheses Conference, Seattle, July 1980.

14. Leake-Jones PA, Walsh SM, Merzenich MM. Cochlear pathology following chronic intracochlear electrical stimulation. Ann Otol Rhinol Laryngol 1981: 90 Suppl 82:6-8.

15. Clopton BM, Miller JM, Pfingst BE, et al. Animal studies of a cochlear prosthesis. Ann Otol Rhinol Laryngol 1980; 89 Suppl 66:1-17.

16. Pfingst BE, Spelman FA, Sutton D. Operating ranges for cochlear implants. Ann Otol Rhinol Laryngol 1980; 89 Suppl 66:1-4.

17. Thielemeir MA, Brimacombe JA, Eisenberg LS. Audiological results with the cochlear implant. Ann Otol Rhinol Laryngol 1982; 91 Suppl 91:27-34.

18. Eisenberg LS, Nelson JR, House WF. Effects of the single-electrode cochlear implant on the vestibular system of the profoundly deafened adult. Ann Otol Rhinol Laryngol 1982; 91 Suppl 91:47-54.

19. Humes LE, Bess FH. Tutorial on the potential deterioration in hearing due to hearing aid usage. J Speech Hear Res 1981; 24:3-15.

20. Rintelmann WF. Effects of over-amplification on hearing of children. Paper presented at International Symposium on Childhood Deafness. Mt. Pleasant, Michigan, 1976.

21. House WF, Berliner KI, Eisenberg LS. Present status and future directions of the Ear Research Institute cochlear implant program. Acta Otolaryngol (Stockh) 1979; 87:176-84.

22. House WF, Berliner KI, Eisenberg LS, et al. The cochlear implant: 1980 update. Acta Otolaryngol (Stockh) 1981; 91:457-62.

23. Wexler M, Miller LW, Berliner KI, Crary WG. Psychological effects of the cochlear implant: patient and "index relative" perceptions. Ann Otol Rhinol Laryngol 1982; 91 Suppl 91:59-61.

24. Wong-Riley MTT, Walsh SM, Leake-Jones PA, et al. Maintenance of neuronal activity by electrical stimulation of unilaterally deafened cats demonstrable with the cytochrome oxidase technique. Ann Otol Rhinol Laryngol 1981; 90 Suppl 82:30-2.

25. Schuknecht HF: Forward. In: Jaffe BF, ed. Hearing loss in children. Baltimore: University Park Press, 1977.

26. Schwab WA. Effects of hearing loss on education. In: Jaffe BF, ed. Hearing loss in children. Baltimore: University Park Press, 1977:650-4.

27. Conrad R. The deaf school child: language and cognitive function. London: Harper & Row, 1979.

28. Emerton RG, Hurwitz TA, Bishop ME. Development of social maturity in deaf adolescents and adults. In: Bradford LJ, Hardy WG, eds. Hearing and hearing impairment. New York: Grune and Stratton, 1979:451-60.

29. Meadow KP, Trybus RJ. Behavioral and emotional problems of deaf children: an overview. In: Bradford LJ, Hardy WG, eds. Hearing and hearing impairment. New York: Grune and Stratton, 1979:395-403.

30. Brooks PH. Some speculations concerning deafness and learning to read. In: Liben LS, ed. Deaf children: developmental perspectives. New York: Academic Press, 1978:87-101.

31. Scott BL. Temporal factors in vowel perception. J Acoust Soc Am 1976; 60:1354-65.

32. Simmons FB. The electrical stimulation of the acoustic nerve. In: Merzenich MM, Schindler RA, Sooy FA, eds. Proceedings of the first international conference on electrical stimulation of the acoustic nerve as a treatment for profound sensorineural deafness in man. San Francisco: University of California; 1974: 123-5.

33. Liben LS. Developmental perspectives on the experiential deficiencies of deaf children. In: Liben LS, ed. Deaf children: developmental perspectives. New York: Academic Press, 1978:195-215.

34. Moores DF. Projected trends in language development for the deaf. Deaf American 1967; 20:5-7.

PART 2

EXPERIMENTAL SYSTEMS

COMPARISON OF PROMONTORY AND COCHLEAR IMPLANTS WITHIN A SINGLE SUBJECT

BRADLY J. EDGERTON, PhD

WILLIAM F. HOUSE, MD

KAREN JO DOYLE, MS

Audiometric pure tone, speech, and psychoacoustic data were obtained from a patient who had worn a promontory electrode for two years. Subsequently the promontory implant was replaced by a scala tympani electrode (cochlear implant) and testing was repeated. Warbled tone thresholds ranged from 52-68 dB SPL for the octave frequencies 250-8000 Hz with the cochlear implant (CI), and from 65-74 dB SPL with the promontory electrode (PE). Speech discrimination scores were better with the CI than with the PE, although performance on an environmental sounds test was slightly better with the PE. Smaller intensity difference limens (DLs) were obtained with the CI (1 dB) than with the PE (about 4 dB). Frequency discrimination was poor with both electrode systems. The CI provided better frequency DLs at 250, 500, and 1000 Hz; the PE produced better DLs at 2000 Hz. When the CI was combined with a hearing aid worn on the better implanted ear, performance improved over that with either prosthesis alone.

At least one group of researchers has contended that stimulation of the cochlea at the promontory or round window provides as much information as intracochlear implants with less risk of trauma to the cochlea, and with reduced surgical risk.[1] However, to date no data have been provided to clearly support this viewpoint. The diverse range of performance found for intracochlear implant subjects[2-4] makes the comparison of extracochlear and intracochlear implants on different subjects questionable. However, recently we have had the opportunity to compare a single subject's performance with promontory and scala tympani electrodes implanted in the same ear at different times.

PATIENT PROFILE

The subject is a 76-year-old male who was originally seen in 1962 for treatment of symptoms later diagnosed as Menière's disease. He had experienced some significant hearing loss in his right ear since 1940 and in his left ear since 1960. In 1957 he underwent stapes surgery in his right ear which resulted in a dead ear. The subject has worn a hearing aid at his left ear since 1960. By 1967, the subject was experiencing severe difficulty with dizziness, tinnitus (bilaterally), and fluctuant hearing loss in the left ear. Several endolymphatic sac shunts were done in the left ear with temporary improvements. By 1974 the subject had a profound loss in the left ear, and severe tinnitus bilaterally. Electrical stimulation (60 and 2500 Hz at 1-2 V) at the promontory was tried on both ears to reduce the tinnitus. The subject reported reduced tinnitus in both ears after stimulation. In 1975, the subject was implanted with a right hard-wire promontory electrode to facilitate the tinnitus treatments. In 1977 a new promontory electrode (PE) and induction coil system were implanted, and by 1978 the subject was using a House-Urban cochlear implant (CI) stimulator. In 1979 the subject reported deriving minimal benefit from the promontory implant and it was noted that extremely high voltages were required for stimulation. Thus, a revision surgery was done and the PE was replaced by a scala tympani CI. From 1975 to the present the subject has worn a high-gain, body-type hearing aid at the left ear in conjunction with the right-worn CI. The present experiment permits comparisons to be made among test performances with hearing aid (HA), PE, and CI.

METHODS

Instrumentation. All testing was done in a sound-treated booth (IAC-1202A). Speech and warbled tone thresholds and uncomfortable loudness level testing was done with an audiometer (Grason-Stadler 1704) calibrated to ANSI standards for audiometers.[5] Audiometer output was either to a matched pair of earphones (TDH-39) mounted in cushions (MX41/AR) or to a speaker (Maico), depending on the testing paradigm. Tape recorded speech stimuli were routed from an Ampex model ATR-700 recorder to the speech audiometer. Sound field levels were measured using a microphone (Bruel & Kjaer[B&K]4133) placed at the approximate center of the patient's head and routed to a measuring amplifier (B&K 2609). A speech spectrum noise was used for sound field calibration. Psychoacoustic tests were done using independent tone sources (Wavetek 171, 186) which were led to a logic system (Coulbourn series) for shaping and timing, and which were then routed to subject or examiner controls, or were input to a special test chamber (B&K HA test box 4212). The special test chamber was used so that HA or implant microphones alone could be placed directly into the chamber, thereby eliminating sizable sound field artifacts. Sound levels in the test chamber were monitored using a microphone (B&K 4131) and measuring amplifier (B&K 2609). A spectrum shaper (B&K 5612) was used in conjunction with the test chamber for frequency difference limen measurements.

Procedure. The subject was evaluated in five conditions: 1) unaided under earphones, 2) PE — right ear, 3) HA — left ear, 4) CI — right ear, and 5) CI — right ear and HA — left ear. Testing was performed under earphones, in the sound field, and using the test chamber. Under headphones, pure tone thresholds, speech detection thresholds (SDT), and uncomfortable loudness levels (ULL) were obtained bilaterally. In the sound field, warbled tone thresholds, SDT, and ULL were measured, and the Monosyllable-Trochee-Spondee test (MTS),[6] Environmental Sounds test (ES), and the Hearing Rehabilitation Research Center (HRRC)

TABLE 1. AVERAGE THRESHOLDS AND UNCOMFORTABLE LOUDNESS LEVELS FOR SIX TEST CONDITIONS (dB SPL)

Condition	250	500	750	1000	1500	2000	3000	4000	6000	8000	SDT	ULL
	Pure or Warbled Tone Frequency (Hz)											
Unaided R	NR	NR	NR	NR	NR	NR	NR	NR	NR	NR	NR	NR
Unaided L	NR	114	107	117	NR	NR	NR	NR	NR	NR	115	NR
PE (R)	70	67	67	66	67	67	65	67	70	74	70	95+
CI (R)	65	59	56	58	53	52	52	52	58	68	46	95+
HA (L)	66	59	55	64	66*	74*	NR	NR	NR	NR	56	84
CI/HA	67	61	56	58	57	55	56	54	60	64	53	86

*Vibratory response.

NR - No response at the output limit of the audiometer.

Rhyme test were administered. The latter three tests have been developed for use with subjects having minimal auditory capabilities. In the test chamber, intensity difference limens (△I) and scaling and frequency difference limens (△F) were measured.

Pure and warbled tone thresholds and speech detection thresholds under earphones and in the sound field were measured using an up-down adaptive procedure;[7] threshold was defined as the level where the subject responded on 3 out of 5 trials. Warbled and pure tone thresholds were measured at octaves and half octaves from 250 to 8000 Hz. For SDT and ULL a selected sample of tape recorded spondees with amplitude peaks +1 dB were used. The ULL was determined using the ascending procedure and instructions outlined by Edgerton et al.[8] During all aided or implant testing the prosthesis was set to a comfortable level with a sound field spondee level of 70 dB SPL.

The MTS, ES, and HRRC Rhyme tests are closed response format tests. The MTS consists of four common monosyllables, four trochees, and four spondees, repeated twice in a semirandom sequence. The ES is composed of 20 commonly occurring sounds, with each stimulus presented in the context of four foils. The HRRC Rhyme test consists of 50 monosyllables, each of which is grouped with three rhyming foils.

Intensity difference limens were measured using standard reference tones of 250, 500, 1000, and 2000 Hz. The stimuli were gated on for 500 ms with a 300 ms interstimulus interval. A stimulus rise-fall time of 20 ms was used to avoid transients. Tests were done with the standard at a level of 70 dB SPL with the prosthesis adjusted to a comfortable setting. To reduce the effect of subject attenuator reference bias, ascending and descending trials were alternated and the starting level of the comparison stimulus was varied by an independent experimenter-controlled attenuator. Ten ascending and descending trials were used to estimate the △I. The subject was instructed to adjust an attenuator (0.5 dB step) to the point at which both tones were equal in loudness.

Frequency difference limens were measured at 250, 500, 750, and 1000 Hz. The standard and comparison stimuli were generated from two different oscillators and monitored using two frequency counters. The tones were gated on for 1 second with a 500 ms interstimulus interval (rise/fall = 20 ms). A spectrum shaper was used to establish a rough approximation to an equal loudness contour prior to testing. Ten ascending and ten descending trials were done at each frequency to estimate the △F. The subject was instructed to adjust the comparison tone to the pitch of the standard tone. The starting point for each trial was varied by the experimenter.

RESULTS AND DISCUSSION

Sound Field Thresholds. Unaided pure tone and warbled tone thresholds obtained in each of the aided conditions are given in Table 1. Unaided thresholds range from 107 to 114 dB SPL at frequencies 500-1000 Hz in the left ear. No unaided thresholds could be measured at the limits of the audiometer (110 dB HL) above this frequency in the left ear, while no auditory responses were obtained at any frequency in the right ear. With the HA worn at the left ear, auditory responses were noted at 55-66 dB SPL from 250 to 750 Hz, vibratory responses at 66 and 74 dB SPL for 1500 and 2000 Hz, and no responses at higher frequencies. In the PE, CI, and CI/HA conditions, pure auditory thresholds could be measured at each frequency between 250 and 8000 Hz. Of these three conditions, the PE produced the poorest thresholds, in the range of 65 to 74 dB SPL. Better thresholds were measured for the CI and CI/HA conditions (ranging from 52-68 dB SPL across frequencies). Threshold levels for the CI condition are comparable to narrow-band noise thresholds obtained by Bilger et al[3] for a sample of cochlear implant wearers.

Speech detection thresholds and ULL are also given in Table 1. For each condition, SDT is within ±6 dB of the thresholds for the two best frequencies. The CI and CI/HA provide the most sensitive thresholds to speech, followed by the HA and PE conditions, respectively. ULL for speech, as shown in Table 1, could not be reached at the limits of the audiometer (95 dB SPL) for either the CI or the PE. This finding was not unexpected since the CI stimulator unit is set to peak-clip any acoustic signal that would exceed the subject's comfort level. ULLs obtained in the HA and CI/HA conditions were somewhat poorer than either the CI or PE ULLs. Because of this, the CI condition provided the largest dynamic range (49+ dB), followed by that of the CI/HA condition (33 dB), the HA condition (28 dB), and finally the PE (15+ dB).

Speech and Sound Discrimination. In Table 2, mean test scores and ranges are presented for word discrimination as measured by the MTS and the HRRC Rhyme test, and for the Environmental Sounds test. The subject scored highest on each word discrimination task in either the CI/HA or HA conditions; the CI scores were 25-45% poorer than for the HA or HA/CI conditions. PE results were the poorest, with just above chance level performance for all word discrimination tests. Stress perception scores for the MTS follow the same pattern as the discrimination scores, with the CI/HA and HA yielding higher percentages (96%) than the CI (75%) or PE (50%) scores. For the ES test, scores across conditions did not differ as much as for

TABLE 2. AVERAGED SPEECH AND SOUND DISCRIMINATION TEST SCORES AND SCORE RANGES FOR FOUR CONDITIONS

	MTS Word Discrim.		*MTS Stress*		*HRRC Rhyme Test*		*Env. Sounds*	
	Mean(%)	*Range(%)*	*Mean(%)*	*Range(%)*	*Mean(%)*	*Range(%)*	*Mean(%)*	*Range(%)*
PE	17	4-29	50	38-71	30	20-34	55	50-60
CI	30	21-46	75	63-92	46	46	45	20-70
HA	79	70-91	93	91-100	67	60-74	60	55-65
CI/HA	74	67-79	99	96-100	74	74	62	60-65

the speech tests. However, the same trends held, with the exception that PE performance exceeded that of the CI. It should be noted that under most conditions the range of the subject's performance for any given test was sufficiently great to warrant considerable caution when comparing means.

Psychoacoustics Results. The results of intensity discrimination experiments are presented in Figure 1, which shows △I expressed in decibels as a function of stimulus frequency for the CI, HA, and PE conditions. Normal △I (difference limens [DL] of about 1 dB) are obtained with the CI. DLs measured in the HA condition are larger (2 dB) while the PE condition demonstrates the largest DLs at about 4 dB. Intensity DLs, which were measured at a comfortable loudness level, remain essentially constant across stimulus frequencies for each condition. Constant intensity DLs would be expected with normal-hearing subjects at levels greater than 40 dB SL.[9] Results of △I testing with this subject compare favorably with the results of Simmons et al[10] who measured △I in two modiolar implant wearers and found DLs of about 5%. Intensity DLs with the subject of this study, by comparison, are approximately 2%.

Figure 2 provides a comparison of △F (median values and their ranges) and Weber fractions for sine wave stimuli of 250, 500, and 1000 Hz in the CI and PE conditions. Weber fractions (percentage of change in the standard stimulus required for the subject to detect a difference) obtained with the CI are approximately ten times greater than those expected from normal-hearing listeners (0.2 for CI, 0.02 for normal-hearing listeners), while Weber fractions measured with the PE are about 20 times larger (about 0.4) than normal Weber fractions. At 2000 Hz, however, the median △F with the CI (1920 Hz) is far poorer than the PE △F (573 Hz). A wide range of variability is noted for △F results in both the CI and PE conditions. The PE and CI △Fs compare favorably with those measured by Fourcin et al,[1] who measured frequency discrimination in four subjects with PEs. Only one of their subjects yielded Weber fractions better than 0.3 for the frequencies 75 to 250 Hz, and this single subject could not detect any pitch differences at higher frequencies. Results of the pitch discrimination experiment are comparable with those obtained by Bilger et al,[3] who found that some subjects implanted with the type of CI device worn by this subject had near-normal Weber fractions ($\triangle F/F = 0.02$) for frequencies below 2000 Hz, with poor △F at and above 2000 Hz. Ranges obtained for the subject of the present study indicate that △F is poor at and above 500 Hz for the CI condition, but that frequency discrimination with the CI is substantially better than that measured with the PE.

The above results may serve to further clarify two fundamental issues raised by CI researchers, namely, 1) is the intracochlear implant superior to the ex-

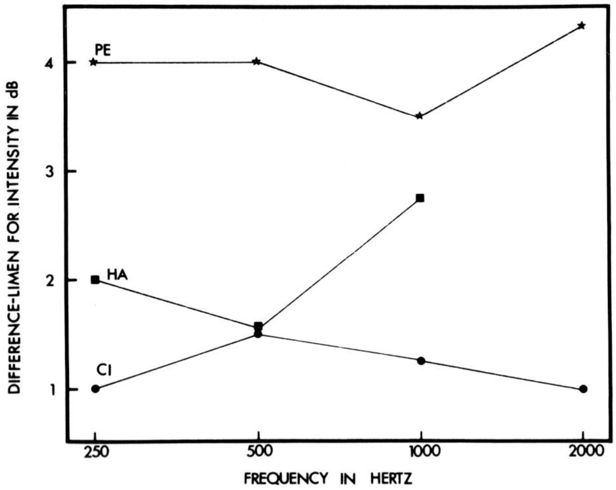

Fig. 1. Difference limens for intensity in decibels for standard tones at 250, 500, 1000, and 2000 Hz for promontory electrode (PE), hearing aid (HA), and cochlear implant (CI).

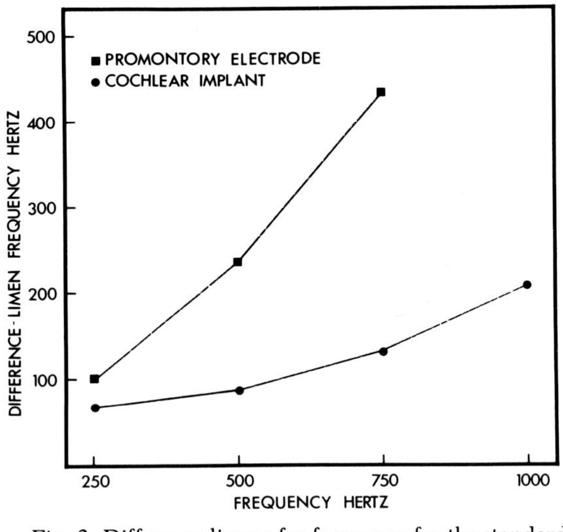

Fig. 2. Difference limens for frequency for the standard tones 250, 500, 750, and 1000 Hz for the promontory electrode and cochlear implant.

tracochlear (promontory) implant? and 2) are further advantages derived from the CI in a subject who benefits from a HA worn in the unimplanted ear? To address these questions, this study allows for direct comparison of audiometric, speech, and sound discrimination, and psychoacoustic data obtained with CI and PE, as well as comparison of audiometric and speech discrimination results obtained with CI, HA, and both CI and HA worn together.

When comparing CI and PE performances, the CI demonstrates marked superiority over the PE for every speech discrimination, threshold, and psychoacoustic test. PE performance surpassed CI performance only for the Environmental Sounds test. Though CI and PE conditions produced identical ULLs, the poor thresholds obtained with the PE resulted in the smallest dynamic range measured in any condition.

For this subject, speech and environmental sound discrimination are clearly better with an HA worn on the better ear than they are in the CI ear, despite the improved warbled tone thresholds, $\triangle$Is, and ULLs noted with the CI. On the basis of this comparison alone (CI and HA), it would be difficult to justify the wearing of the CI alone, since performance with the HA worn in the better ear is clearly superior. However, when the CI and HA are worn together and are compared to the HA alone condition, the combination of the two produces improvement in speech and sound discrimination, warbled tones, and dynamic range. The fact that our subject is able to decrease the gain of his HA in the CI/HA condition not only can account for the improvement in ULL, but may have the further advantage of preserving the residual hearing in the aided ear, which could be otherwise damaged further through continued use of his high output, powerful body-type HA. Naturally, the issue of whether this additional benefit is obtained with the CI for other subjects will depend on the level of hearing in the aided ear, as well as on the performance of the CI. Further clinical research is being carried out to address this issue.

REFERENCES

1. Fourcin AJ, Rosen SM, Moore BCJ, et al. External electrical stimulation of the cochlea: clinical, psychophysical, speech-perceptual, and histological findings. Br J Audiol 1979; 13:85-107.

2. House WF, Berliner K, Crary W, et al. Cochlear implants. Ann Otol Rhinol Laryngol 1976; 85 Suppl 27:1-93.

3. Bilger RC, Black FO, Hopkinson NT, et al. Evaluation of subjects presently fitted with implanted auditory prostheses. Ann Otol Rhinol Laryngol 1977; 86 Suppl 38:1-176.

4. Eddington DK, Dobelle WH, Brackman DE, et al. Auditory prosthesis research with multiple channel intracochlear stimulation in man. Ann Otol Rhinol Laryngol 1978; 87 Suppl 53:1-39.

5. American National Standards Institute, New York. American national standard specifications for audiometers (ANSI-S3.6-1969). New York: 1969.

6. Erber NP, Alencewicz CM. Audiologic evaluation of deaf children. J Speech Hear Dis 1976; 41:256-67.

7. Carhart R, Jerger JF. Preferred method for clinical determination of pure-tone thresholds. J Speech Hear Dis 1959; 24:330-45.

8. Edgerton BJ, Beattie RC, Wides JW. Loudness discomfort levels of hearing-impaired listeners using speech material. Ear Hear 1980 1:206-10.

9. Reisz RR. Differential intensity sensitivity of the ear for pure tones. Phys Rev 1928; 31:867-75.

10. Simmons FB, Walker MG, Mathews RG, et al. Percepts and discrimination by auditory nerve stimulation: a summary of results and some proposals for nerve viability evaluation. In: McPherson DL, Davis MS, eds. Advances in prosthetic devices for the deaf: a technical workshop. Rochester, NY: National Technical Institute for the Deaf, Rochester Institute of Technology, 1978 (NTID/CO/AU-79/0100);271-4.

A MULTIPLE-ELECTRODE COCHLEAR IMPLANT

William F. House, MD

Bradly J. Edgerton, PhD

A multiple-electrode cochlear implant comprised of three intracochlear and four extracochlear electrodes is described. A percutaneous plug allowed for direct electrical measurements and presentation of stimuli to selected electrode combinations. Electrical impedance measurements revealed functions that decreased as frequency increased to about 20 kHz. Absolute impedance magnitude varied across electrodes. Equal loudness contours were similar in shape for all three cochlear electrodes, although dynamic range was significantly reduced for the most apical electrode. Periodicity and place pitch were demonstrated; effects were most salient for low frequency stimuli. A 3-channel sound processor was built and multiple-channel stimulation was compared to single-channel stimulation. Significant performance differences were not found between single-channel and multiple-channel systems for environmental or speech sounds. However, the patient subjectively reported superior quality with the multiple-channel system.

Although the greatest amount of clinical experience with implantable auditory prostheses for the deaf has been achieved using single-electrode intracochlear implants, the potential value of multiple-channel cochlear stimulation has long been recognized. The belief is that by using multiple-channel cochlear implants, the temporal spatial characteristics inherent in the normal cochlea can be more closely approximated than is possible using a single channel of stimulation. It is hoped that by increasing the information transmission in this manner, auditory speech recognition might be restored.

Normally, acoustic activation of the hearing mechanism requires a large number of surviving hair cells and neural ganglion cells in order to achieve high levels of speech recognition. For example, Otte et al[1] suggest that speech discrimination requires at least 10,000 spiral ganglion cells with at least 3,000 located in the apical third of the cochlea. Other researchers, such as Kiang et al,[2] have hypothesized that although this large hair cell and neuron population may be necessary when stimulation is acoustic, fewer numbers may be required when electric stimulation is used. Kiang et al have demonstrated with model neurograms that a 48-channel system could transmit much of the important information necessary for speech discrimination. Even when the number of channels was reduced to six, intensity, spectral content, and on/off information still survived. Thus, even in cases of grossly damaged inner ears, if the surviving neural distribution is such that individual channels of stimulation can be obtained, the potential for achieving high levels of speech discrimination and recognition are much better than in the single-channel case.

The primary limitation of the single-electrode cochlear implant is in frequency coding. The normal cochlea codes frequencies in two ways: first, low frequencies are usually coded by a volley mechanism;[3] second, middle and high frequency components are usually considered to be coded by a place mechanism. Many of the frequency elements which are necessary for speech discrimination/understanding are present above the normal eighth nerve neural volley limit, which in humans is probably between 300 and 500 volleys per second. To improve frequency discrimination above the 300 to 500 Hz limit, it would be necessary to localize stimulation to discrete places along the cochlear gradient, evoking the place pitch mechanism.

In 1961, a 5-wire scala tympani induction coil system, with remote ground, was implanted in a patient by House.[4] Unfortunately, it was rejected due to sensitivities of the patient to the materials used in the induction coils, and was removed before much testing could be performed. In 1964, Doyle et al published a report on results with a 4-electrode intracochlear array.[5] They hoped that by sequential stimulation, the discriminable frequency range could be extended from about 600 to 2400 Hz. Although their report was brief, they did conclude that the multiple-electrode array provided speech discrimination which enabled the patient to "repeat phrases."

Subsequently, House implanted two patients in 1969 and one patient in 1970 with 5-wire scala tympani arrays.[4,6] With this 5-electrode system, the presence of place pitch and periodicity pitch could be demonstrated for all electrodes. In addition to experiments of pitch and intensity, an intensive investigation was undertaken to determine how speech signals should be processed to yield the best intelligibility. Among the experiments completed with one patient were 1) definition of the stimulus waveforms providing the largest dynamic ranges, 2) frequency transposition effects, 3) performance with a 5-channel vocoder with variable frequency bandwidth and amplitude compression characteristics, and 4) the use of delay lines in single-channel and multiple-channel stimulation to approximate the temporal patterns of the traveling wave in the cochlea. However, none of the experimental systems yielded speech discrimination that was appreciably better than when all electrodes were driven as a single-channel system.

Clark et al, using a 9-electrode intracochlear array, demonstrated both place and periodicity pitch phenomena, although high levels of speech recognition were not achieved.[7] Pialoux et al have also reported data obtained from both 8-electrode and 12-electrode systems showing frequency discrimination limited to two thirds to one octave.[8] Speech recognition was reported to be relatively poor. Results by Bosch et al, using a 4-electrode intracochlear array in one subject revealed poor periodicity pitch discrimination at any of the electrodes and an inability of the patient to discriminate between electrodes.[9] On the other hand, Eddington has reported patient performance with multiple-electrode, multiple-channel cochlear arrays which is very encouraging.[10]

The importance of the electrode itself should not be underestimated, since very high levels of speech recognition performance have been reported using multiple-electrode arrays which were activated in a single-channel mode.[11,12] However, it has been demonstrated that the speech discrimination and speech recognition abilities even of single-electrode cochlear implant patients vary considerably.[13] Thus, it is very difficult to compare the performance of patients with multiple-channel systems to patients with single-channel systems. At the present time, multiple-electrode, multiple-channel cochlear implant systems have not provided speech recognition levels which approximate normal performance.

HOUSE MULTIPLE-ELECTRODE DESIGN

Multiple electrodes used to stimulate the cochlear structures have been configured in at least four ways: 1) as a bundle of individual electrode wires of different lengths inserted through the round window into the scala tympani,[6,14] 2) as a number of electrodes arranged in opposing pairs and cast in a Silastic carrier that either fits tightly[11] or loosely[12] in the scala tympani, 3) as a tightly bound modiolar array inserted into the eighth nerve,[15] and 4) as individual electrodes introduced along the cochlea through a series of fenestra.[8]

The present House multiple-electrode system incorporates both round window/scala tympani and cochlear fenestra techniques of electrode placement. The procedures and electrode design were selected to maximize localization of electrical currents within the cochlea and to make possible the comparison of the standard House single-electrode scala tympani implant with a multiple-electrode system.

A diagram of the multiple-electrode is provided in Figure 1. The electrode array consists of 7 electrodes, 3 designed as actives and placed into the cochlea and 4 designed as grounds and placed outside of the cochlea. All of the electrodes are fabricated from 0.02 cm (0.008 in) diameter platinum wire terminated at 0.05 cm (0.02 in) fired balls. The electrode wires are insulated with silicone sleeves that allow about 0.5 mm exposure of wire on two of the active electrodes and 15 mm exposure on the third active. Approximately 32 mm of exposed wire is used on all four ground electrodes. All of the electrode wires are terminated at an ITT subminiature connector which is sealed in a silicone sleeve and insulated with bone wax. The subminiature connector was designed to allow for easy disconnect so that when an optimal signal processor was developed, an across-the-skin transmission system could be implanted. The wires are then routed to a second subminiature ITT connector mounted in a hydrolyzed carbon button. The carbon button is secured to the bone in the area of the mastoid and extends through the postauricular scalp area.

CASE HISTORY

The patient selected for the multiple-electrode device was a 54-year-old female with a long history of deafness due to otosclerosis. The patient reported some hearing loss since the age of 18 years, and in 1956 bilateral stapes mobilization surgery was done. Surgery resulted in a profound sensorineural loss in the left ear and a severe mixed loss in the right ear. An unsuccessful stapes revision was done in the right ear in 1960 which resulted in a severe to profound sensorineural loss. The patient did successfully wear a high-power body hearing aid in the right ear until 1972. In 1972, the patient experienced a sudden total hearing loss in the right ear which resulted in her deriving minimum benefit from hearing aids. At this time, she was seen at the Otologic Medical

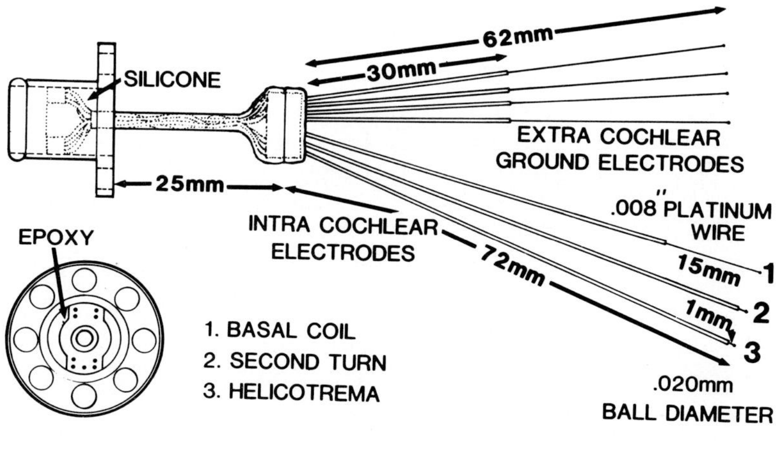

Fig. 1. Multiple-electrode cochlear implant. Percutaneous connector and electrodes, showing insulated and uninsulated dimensions.

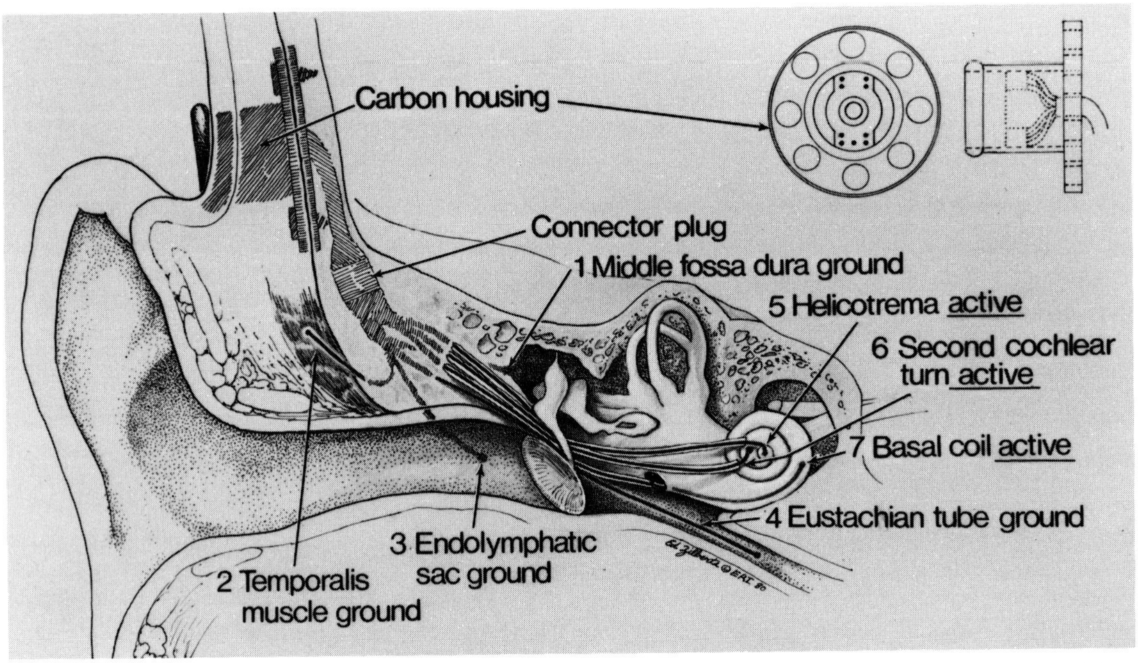

Fig. 2. Multiple-electrode system after implantation. Seven electrodes, three intracochlear and four extracochlear, terminating at a connector housed in a percutaneous carbon plug placed posterior and superior to the pinna.

Group, was later evaluated for the cochlear implant program, and in 1977 a successful single-electrode cochlear implant surgery was performed on the left ear. The patient's overall performance with the cochlear implant in the left ear was very good. In 1980, she was asked to consider a multiple-electrode cochlear implant for the right ear. The patient was informed at the time that the multiple-electrode cochlear implant was a new device requiring a more extensive surgery, and postoperative performance with the implant could not be predicted. She was cautioned that previous experimentation with multiple-electrode arrays had not in all cases provided superior performance to single-electrode systems. The risks of the surgery along with the additional risk of having a percutaneous plug behind the ear were explained to her. She made the decision to have the multiple-electrode implant.

Surgical Description. With the patient under general anesthesia, a postauricular incision was made about 2 cm posterior to the fold of the pinna, and the flap was turned forward to expose the cortex of the mastoid process and the squamous part of the temporal bone. A mastoidectomy was then done, and the facial recess was opened widely to visualize the round window niche. The round window niche was removed with a diamond stone in order to visualize the round window membrane, and an opening was made into the scala tympani just anterior to the round window membrane. The surgical approach was then changed. Through an ear speculum in the external auditory canal, a posterior canal wall flap was elevated and the eardrum was dissected off the handle of the malleus so that it could be laid forward in the external canal. Using a specially prepared tapered burr, a hole was drilled just in front of the oval window and just posterior to the malleus. This hole extended down to the second coil of the cochlea. Cadaver dissection had previously shown that this opening was usually in the scala vestibulae of the second coil. Using the same tapered burr, another hole was drilled into the promontory just anterior to the handle of the malleus and just inferior to the cochleariform process. Previous dissection had shown that this opening invariably came at the helicotrema.

At this point, the hydrolyzed carbon button which was designed to extend through the postauricular scalp area was secured to the bone with bone screws, and the electrodes were then run into the mastoid cavity. The four ground wires were placed: one in contact with the dura of the posterior fossa at about the area of the endolymphatic sac; one into the attic above the cochleariform process and down to the eustachian tube, one in contact with the dura just above the additus and the attic area by making a little opening in the bone at this point and inserting an electrode between the surface of the bone and the dura, and the fourth in contact with the temporalis muscle.

The three active electrodes were routed through the facial recess. One was inserted through the round window about 15 mm into the scala tympani, and fascia was placed around the electrode to seal it at its entrance into the scala tympani. The second active electrode was inserted approximately 1.5 mm into the opening drilled in the second cochlear coil. It is estimated that at least the 0.5 mm ball extended into the cochlea and possibly a little bit of the exposed wire. Again, fascia was placed around the electrode to help seal the opening. The third electrode was then placed into the helicotrema opening, and it was estimated that the 0.5 mm ball and a small portion of the wire extended into the fluids of the helicotrema. Fascia was placed around the electrode. The eardrum was then replaced and the external auditory canal was filled with Gelfoam. The postauricular incision was closed and sutured around the protruding connector. A head dressing was placed and the patient was transferred to the recovery room.

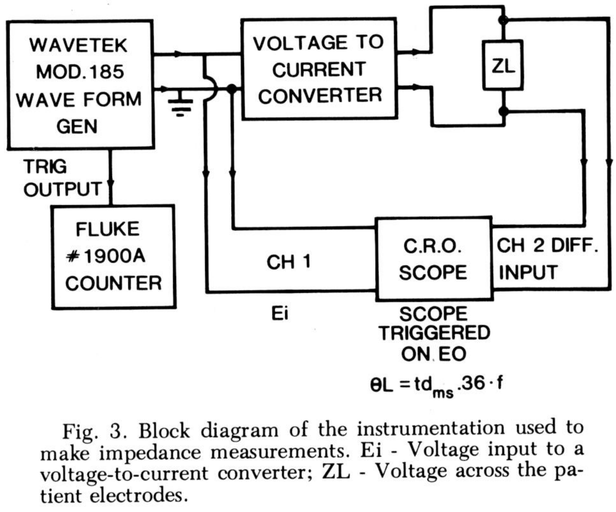

Fig. 3. Block diagram of the instrumentation used to make impedance measurements. Ei - Voltage input to a voltage-to-current converter; ZL - Voltage across the patient electrodes.

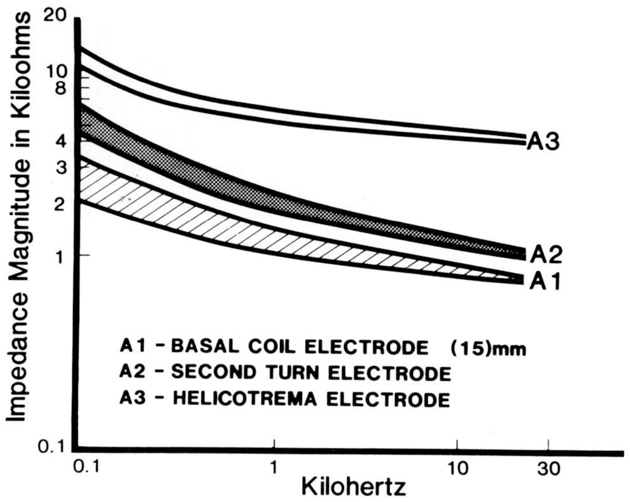

Fig. 4. Ranges of absolute impedance magnitude as a function of frequency for basal, 2nd turn, and helicotrema electrodes, paired with grounds at the temporalis muscle, eustachian tube, endolymphatic sac, and middle fossa dura.

In Figure 2, the approximate locations of the ground and active electrodes within the ear structures are shown. Four different ground wires were used because no research to date has identified, in the human ear, the natural current pathways for unipolar scalar electrodes. We felt that the location of the extracochlear ground electrodes could affect thresholds and possibly channel separation for multiple-electrode stimulation.

ELECTRICAL IMPEDANCE MEASUREMENTS

After approximately six weeks of healing, a series of impedance measurements were undertaken to define the electrical characteristics of the implanted electrode system. Figure 3 provides a block diagram of the impedance measurement apparatus.* The output of an oscillator was routed to a voltage-to-current converter. The voltage input to the voltage-to-current converter was displayed on channel 1 of a 2-channel oscilloscope. It should be noted that when converted, the applied voltage represented a specific current value at the electrodes. The output of the voltage-to-current converter was routed to the patient electrodes, and the voltage across the patient electrodes was read with a differential input on channel 2 of the oscilloscope. Using this apparatus, channel 1 served as a representation of current across the electrodes, and channel 2 represented the voltage across the electrodes. Comparison of the voltage to current levels allowed an estimation of the absolute impedance magnitude.

Figure 4 provides the impedance functions for the three intracochlear electrodes, and indicates the range of performance for each active electrode paired with each of the four grounds. The variation between grounds was not large. The variability among the grounds was greatest for the basal coil electrode and least for the helicotrema electrode. In all cases, the variability across grounds was largest at low frequencies, being on the order of 1,000 Ω or more at 100 Hz and decreasing to less than 100 Ω at 20,000 Hz for all electrodes. For all active electrodes, the highest impedance functions were obtained when paired with the middle fossa dura ground and the lowest when paired with the eustachian tube ground.

Impedance measurements were also taken by pairing the three intracochlear electrodes with each other. In Figure 5 it is seen that the general shape of the functions is very similar to the functions obtained with the extracochlear grounds. However, the overall impedance magnitudes are greater for the intracochlear pairs than when remote grounds were used. The lowest impedance function was obtained for the basal turn electrode paired with the second turn electrode. However, pairing either the basal or the second turn electrode with the helicotrema electrode yielded relatively high impedance functions. The high impedance functions obtained for the helicotrema electrode may be related to the amount of bone which is acting as an insulator in the helicotrema region in addition to the reduced electrode surface area as compared to the basal turn electrode.

ELECTRICAL THRESHOLD STUDIES

Electrical thresholds were measured using an ascending up/down adaptive technique. Measurements were made with sinusoidal stimuli ranging from 100 to 19,000 Hz. All threshold measurements began at zero stimulation level and increased in approximately 50 mV steps. Threshold was defined as the lowest stimulus level yielding a correct response about 50% of the time.

Instrumentation and Stimuli. A block diagram of the instrumentation used in the threshold and uncomfortable loudness measurements is provided in Figure 6. Sinusoidal stimuli were routed to a fre-

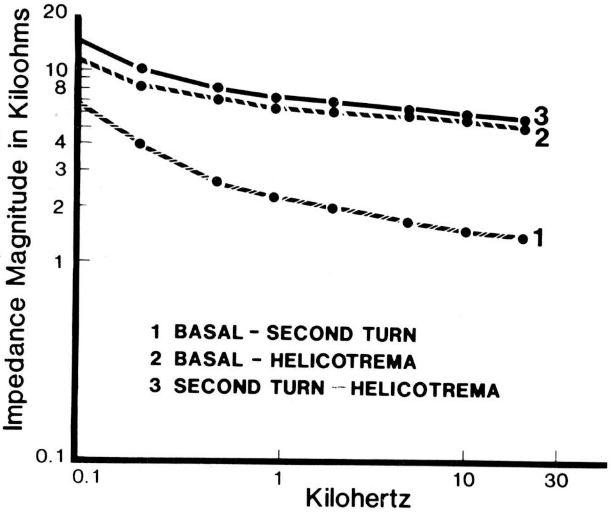

Fig. 5. Absolute impedance magnitudes as a function of frequency for the basal-2nd turn, basal-helicotrema, and second turn-helicotrema intracochlear electrode pairs.

*Francis A. Spelman, PhD, University of Washington, designed the impedance measuring apparatus and assisted in the collection of the data.

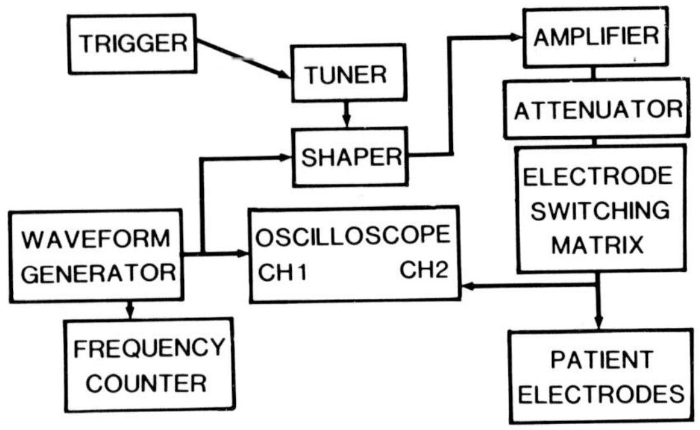

Fig. 6. Block diagram of instrumentation used for threshold and uncomfortable loudness measurements.

quency counter and one channel of an oscilloscope for monitoring, and then directed to a signal shaper and timer before terminating at the amplifier section leading to the patient electrodes. Threshold and uncomfortable levels were measured using sinusoids gated on for one second with a rise/fall time of 25 ms. The signal being delivered at the patient electrodes was monitored on a second channel of the oscilloscope.

Results. Table 1 presents the electrical thresholds obtained, expressed in peak-to-peak mV, for the intracochlear actives paired with the extracochlear grounds. From the table it can be seen that in all cases the basal turn active provided the lowest electrical thresholds, and that there was little difference in threshold among the different ground placements.

The same general results, ie, no large differences among grounds, were obtained for the second turn active electrode. For the helicotrema active, the thresholds across grounds were very similar at the low frequencies, but at the high frequencies were unobtainable when the middle fossa dura or the endolymphatic sac grounds were used.

Differences among the voltage thresholds obtained using the basal, second turn, and helicotrema actives are reflective of the differences among the electrodes in surface area, insulating properties of the tissues immediately surrounding the elec-

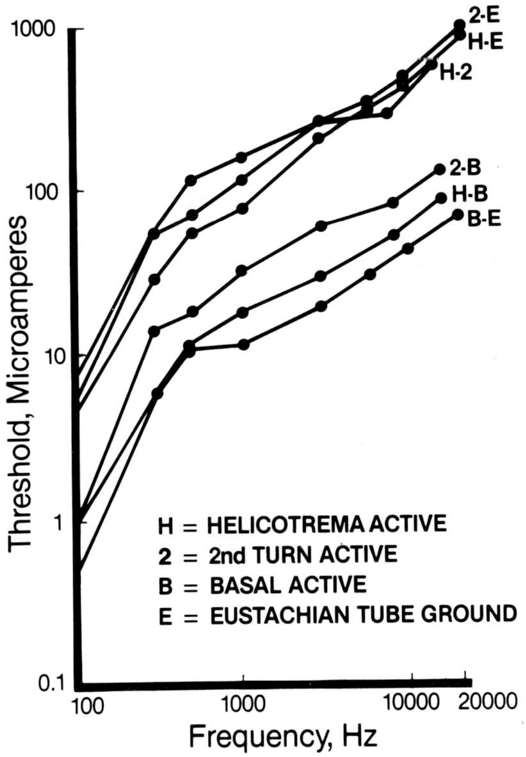

Fig. 7. Electrical thresholds in peak-to-peak microamperes for frequencies from 100 to 19,000 Hz. Helicotrema, 2nd turn, basal, and eustachian tube electrodes were paired to obtain thresholds.

trodes, and the proximity of the electrodes with respect to the stimulable neural elements. However, in all cases, thresholds increased as stimulus frequency increased.

Perhaps a more accurate picture of the differences in stimulation levels that were necessary to elicit thresholds can be obtained by measuring or estimating current rather than voltage. Therefore, in Figure 7 threshold functions are plotted in current levels. Functions are similar to those obtained using voltage threshold measurements, although the effect of high frequencies is more marked. Threshold current functions are not provided for all electrode

TABLE 1. MEDIAN THRESHOLDS IN MILLIVOLTS FOR EACH ACTIVE-GROUND ELECTRODE PAIR*

	Frequency (Hz)							
Electrode Pair	*100*	*300*	*500*	*1000*	*3000*	*6000*	*10,000*	*19,000*
AB — ET	1	11	19	16	23	32	40	59
AB — TMP	3	12	17	23	23	30	42	69
AB — ES	4	16	18	25	26	37	43	78
AB — MFD	3	15	18	25	27	38	40	64
A2nd — ET	41	196	312	366	428	483	612	993
A2nd — TMP	35	172	255	297	355	488	542	824
A2nd — ES	36	220	300	348	299	439	550	851
A2nd — MFD	90	215	266	299	452	538	636	1018
AH — ET	50	214	356	453	1070	1452	1980	3520
AH — TMP	72	286	383	450	725	1078	2050	3010
AH — ES	29	322	359	434	718	†	†	†
AH — MFD	60	240	553	465	825	†	†	†

*Basal active (AB), 2nd turn active (A2nd) and helicotrema active (AH) paired with the eustachian tube ground (ET), temporalis ground (TMP), endolymphatic sac ground (ES), and middle fossa dura ground (MFD).

†Thresholds not obtainable.

TABLE 2. ELECTRODE SAFETY LIMITS FOR CURRENT IN MICROAMPERES PEAK-TO-PEAK

Electrode	Frequency (Hz) 100	1000	10,000	16,000
Basal coil	300	27,000	274,000	437,000
Second turn	41	410	4,000	65,000
Helicotrema	41	410	4,000	65,000

pairs in Figure 7. However, those that are demonstrate that there are essentially two categories of functions: 1) those which include the basal turn active electrode, and 2) those which do not include the basal active. The lowest thresholds were obtained when the basal turn electrode was one of the pair, and the basal active with eustachian tube ground — the standard single-electrode system — required the least current to achieve threshold.

Pure platinum electrodes were selected for implantation since platinum is a chemically inert material and should be well tolerated by the tissues and fluids of the inner ear. The primary consideration, from a damage risk standpoint, was the current levels which would have the potential of causing damage directly to the neural elements being stimulated. An estimate of maximum safe stimulation levels based on histologic findings is provided by Walsh et al.[16] They report that as long as charge densities do not exceed approximately 40 $\mu C/cm^2/$phase, the risk of damage to neural elements from intracochlear electrical stimulation is very small. Using 40 $\mu C/cm^2/$phase, we have computed the maximum safe limits in peak-to-peak current at frequencies from 100 to 16,000 Hz. These are shown in Table 2. Although the helicotrema and second turn electrodes do require low overall current levels to maintain safety, comparison with Figure 7 reveals that the levels used for stimulation are substantially below the maximum safe limits.

UNCOMFORTABLE LOUDNESS LEVELS

Uncomfortable loudness levels were measured using an ascending technique and an instruction set which requested that the patient indicate when a signal was "too loud to be tolerated for at least five minutes." Sinusoidal stimuli were used ranging from 100 to 10,000 Hz. The uncomfortable loudness levels were taken as the median for 3 to 5 ascending trials. The median uncomfortable loudness levels for the three active electrodes paired with the eustachian tube ground are presented in peak-to-peak

TABLE 4. DYNAMIC RANGES IN DECIBELS FOR EACH ACTIVE ELECTRODE PAIRED WITH THE EUSTACHIAN TUBE GROUND

Electrode Pair	Frequency (Hz) 100	500	1000	3000	5000	10,000
AB — ET	39	19	24	22	20	21
A2nd — ET	19	11	15	15	14	*
AH — ET	16	12	14	9	11	*

*Not measured.

voltage and microamperes in Table 3. The uncomfortable loudness levels were lowest for the basal turn active and highest for the second turn active. The current levels tolerated by the patient increased as frequency increased. The current required to achieve uncomfortable level is generally less than the safe limits presented in Table 2. In addition, signals presented to the patient are always lower than uncomfortable level, except during the procedure to determine that level, in which case they are uncomfortably loud for only a brief presentation.

Comparison of the thresholds obtained for the three active electrodes paired with the eustachian tube ground and the uncomfortable levels for these same electrodes reveals that the dynamic ranges differed significantly for the three intracochlear electrodes. Table 4 presents the dynamic ranges, converted to decibels, at frequencies from 100 to 10,000 Hz. In general, all active electrodes yielded the largest dynamic range at 100 Hz, with a relatively constant dynamic range at higher frequencies. The basal active electrode yielded the largest or widest dynamic range (about 20 dB) followed by the second turn electrode (about 15 dB) and the helicotrema electrode (about 10 to 15 dB).

THRESHOLD AUDITORY FATIGUE

During the early stages of multiple-channel stimulation, the patient reported that a low-pass-band (250-700 Hz) stimulator system, which was routed to the apical electrode, changed its characteristics after several hours of listening. Testing of her stimulator equipment showed no abnormal functioning. Reexamination of electrical thresholds at this point found a shift upward, ie, thresholds were poorer than earlier in the session. A brief study of auditory fatigue was undertaken to determine whether the patient's perceptions could be attributed to physiological phenomena.

TABLE 3. UNCOMFORTABLE LOUDNESS LEVELS IN PEAK-TO-PEAK MILLIVOLTS AND MICROAMPERES FOR EACH ACTIVE ELECTRODE PAIRED WITH THE EUSTACHIAN TUBE GROUND

Electrode Pair	Frequency (Hz) 100	300	500	750	1000	1500	2000	3000	5000	10,000
AB — ET (mV)	84	140	167	191	250	230	256	268	300	427
(μA)	30	70	93	112	167	164	197	223	286	427
A2nd — ET (mV)	367	1105	1300	1586	1900	2145	2265	2533	2400	*
(μA)	66	345	481	659	844	1073	1224	1490	1600	
AH — ET (mV)	380	970	1435	1720	2200	2140	2550	3136	4933	*
(μA)	35	129	217	267	367	375	455	603	987	

*Not measured.

TABLE 5. AUDITORY THRESHOLD AND FATIGUE FOR EACH ACTIVE ELECTRODE PAIRED WITH THE EUSTACHIAN TUBE GROUND USING A 16,000 Hz SINUSOIDAL STIMULUS

Electrode	*Threshold*	*Fatigue*
Basal	0.1 V	0.23 V held for 60s
Second turn	1.1 V	3.00 V held for 25s 3.30 V held for 16s 3.50 V held for 26s 4.00 V held for 13s 4.50 V startle
Helicotrema	5.0 V	12.00 V could not perceive a steady tone

Thresholds were measured using a 16 kHz sinusoid, pulsed on/off for 0.5 seconds with a rise/fall time of 20 ms. An up/down adaptive threshold procedure was used. After establishing threshold, the level of the tone was increased slightly and the tone was switched on continuously. The tone was then increased in level as the patient fatigued to keep it at the *just audible* level for 60 seconds. Experiments were conducted with the basal, second turn, and helicotrema electrodes referred to the eustachian tube ground.

The results are reported in Table 5. Stimulation at the basal coil electrode yielded no appreciable fatigue. However, both the second turn and helicotrema actives showed substantial fatigue. This fatigue effect most likely relates to the limited number of neurons excited by these electrodes. Some of the tables and figures presented in subsequent sections of this paper present data only for the basal and second turn electrodes due to the severe fatigue effect at the helicotrema electrode.

EQUAL LOUDNESS CONTOURS

Equal loudness functions were derived using frequencies ranging from 25 to 5,000 Hz for the helicotrema and second turn actives paired with the eustachian tube ground and from 5 to 10,000 Hz for the basal coil active paired with the eustachian tube ground. The equal loudness contours were obtained using a 1,000 Hz sinusoidal referent adjusted to levels 1) just above threshold, 2) "medium loudness," 3) "moderate loudness," and 4) just below uncomfortable loudness.

The results of the loudness matches are presented in Figure 8A-C for the basal coil, second turn, and helicotrema active electrodes, respectively. From the figure it can be seen that the general shape of the contours is the same across all electrodes, and that the shape does not change as the intensity level is increased. It is apparent that the dynamic range differs substantially across the electrode pairs. The equal loudness experiments produced a dynamic

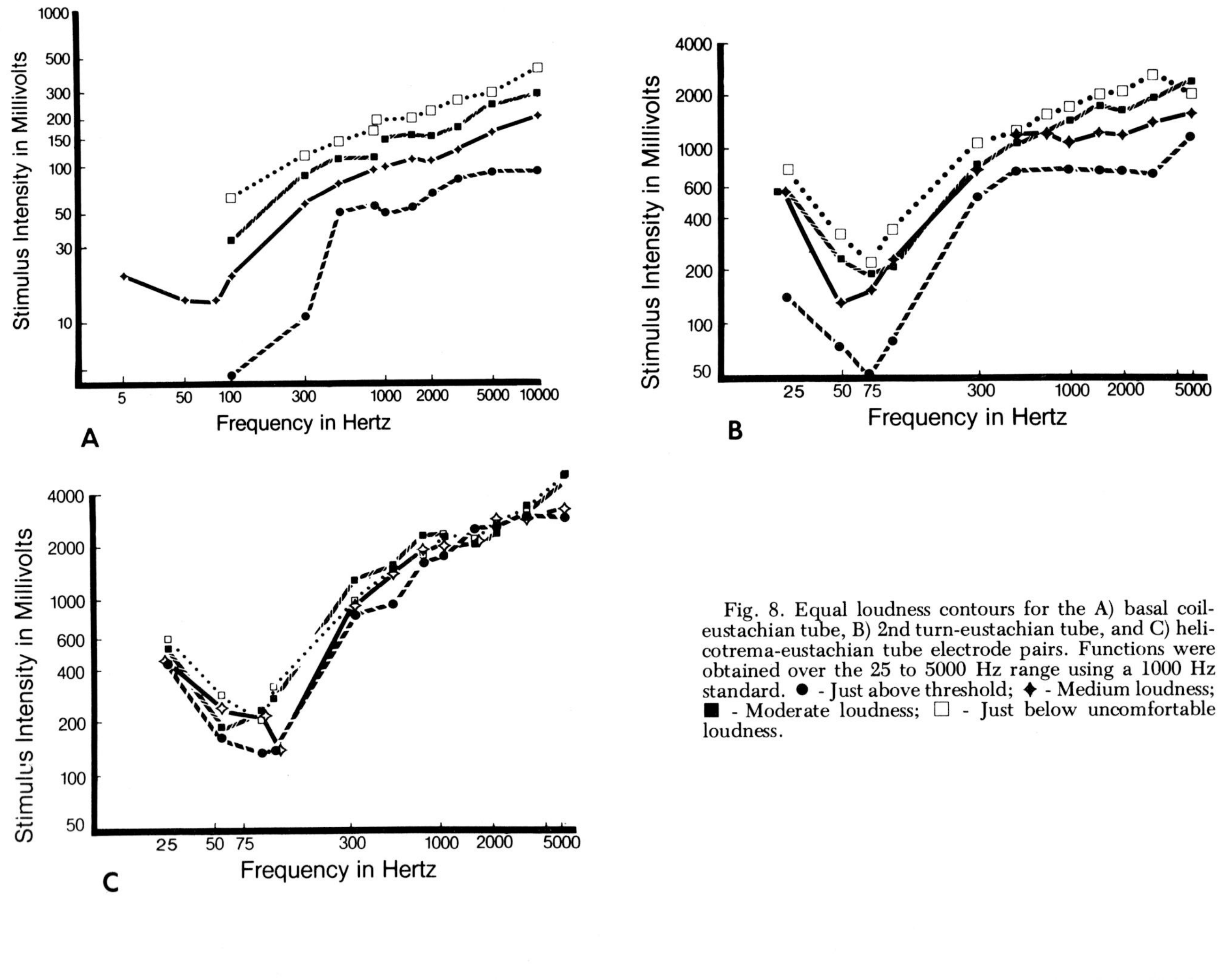

Fig. 8. Equal loudness contours for the A) basal coil-eustachian tube, B) 2nd turn-eustachian tube, and C) helicotrema-eustachian tube electrode pairs. Functions were obtained over the 25 to 5000 Hz range using a 1000 Hz standard. ● - Just above threshold; ✦ - Medium loudness; ■ - Moderate loudness; □ - Just below uncomfortable loudness.

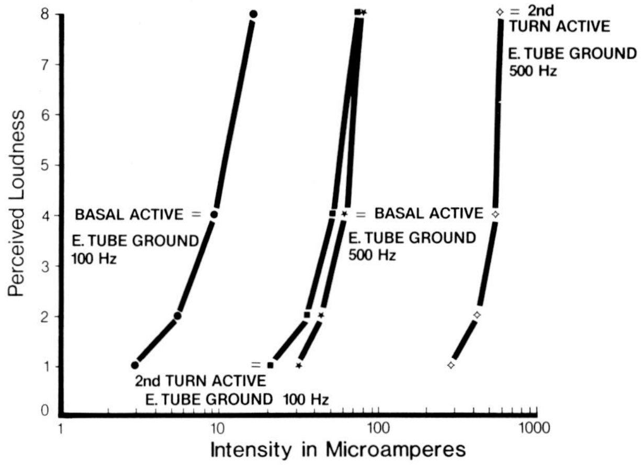

Fig. 9. Loudness growth at 100 and 500 Hz plotted as a function of current in peak-to-peak milliamperes for the basal coil-eustachian tube and 2nd turn-eustachian tube electrode pairs.

range for the helicotrema active which was even more constricted than when standard threshold and uncomfortable level measurements were taken. It is interesting to note that in the normal ear, increasing signal amplitude has the effect of flattening the equal loudness contour, but this did not appear for electrical stimulation.

LOUDNESS GROWTH FUNCTIONS

Figure 9 presents growth of loudness for 100 and 500 Hz tones over a range of stimulus intensities for the basal and second turn active electrodes paired with the eustachian tube ground. A doubling technique was used to estimate loudness growth. The obtained loudness growth functions are very similar to those reported by previous researchers.[7,17] For all the functions, there is a gradually increasing portion which extends over the first doubling of perceived loudness, and then there is a very rapid growth in loudness as signal intensity is increased. In general, the functions differ very little for the basal and second turn actives. However, as the level at which the functions were initiated was increased, the gradual tail portion of the functions decreased.

INTENSITY DIFFERENCE LIMENS

The intensity difference limens for the basal and second turn actives paired with the eustachian tube ground are presented in Table 6. The difference limens were measured at a most comfortable listening level using a method of adjustment technique.

TABLE 6. INTENSITY DIFFERENCE LIMENS IN MICROAMPERES AND WEBER FRACTIONS FOR TWO OF THE ELECTRODES PAIRED WITH THE EUSTACHIAN TUBE GROUND FOR SINUSOIDAL STIMULI

	Frequency (Hz)				
Electrode	*100*	*300*	*500*	*750*	*2000*
AB — ET △I	.33 μA	1.7 μA	1.4 μA	5.0 μA	5.2 μA
△I/I	.05	.06	.02	.06	.05
A2nd — ET △I	5.8 μA	6.6 μA	9.6 μA	40.0 μA	63.0 μA
△I/I	.15	.03	.02	.07	.08

△I - Intensity difference limens; △I/I - Weber fractions.

TABLE 7. PATIENT DESCRIPTION OF PITCH FOR TWO SINUSOIDAL STIMULI AT THREE INTRACOCHLEAR STIMULATION SITES

Electrodes	*Stimulus (Hz)*	*Patient Description*
Basal/2nd turn	100	Basal *much higher* than 2nd turn
Basal/apical	100	Basal *much higher* than apical
2nd turn/apical	100	2nd turn *higher* than apical
Basal/2nd turn	500	Basal *higher* than 2nd turn
Basal/apical	500	Basal *much higher* than apical
2nd turn/apical	500	*Same* medium pitch

From the table it can be seen that the intensity difference limen increased as frequency was increased. The just noticeable difference in current was greater for the second turn active electrode than for the basal turn active electrode. However, when the data are presented in the form of Weber fractions, it can be seen that with the exception of 100 Hz, large differences between the basal active and the second turn active are not present. It might be noted that the Weber fractions were more variable for the second turn electrode than for the basal electrode.

FREQUENCY DISCRIMINATION STUDIES

Frequency discrimination studies for the multiple-electrode cochlear implant included experiments evaluating rate or periodicity pitch, and place pitch phenomena. All frequency and pitch measurements were made along an equal loudness contour. The importance of determining frequency and pitch perceptions using the equal loudness contour was demonstrated in early pilot experiments. For example, when signal intensity was not taken into account and our patient was asked to report which of two successively stimulated electrodes yielded the highest pitch, using 100 or 500 Hz sinusoids, it was relatively easy to rank the stimuli at the basal turn electrode as highest and those at the helicotrema as lowest and the second turn electrode as intermediate (Table 7). However, when this experiment was repeated with the stimuli adjusted to equal loudness at the three electrodes, the task was very difficult, and no reliable ranking could be obtained.

Table 8 provides a summary of the frequency difference limens for the basal and second turn active electrodes paired with the eustachian tube ground. The data were collected over three test sessions. A method of limits technique was used to establish difference limens for frequency, and ascending and descending trials were averaged. From the table it can be seen that for both electrodes, frequency discrimination is near normal at 75 Hz and then gets progressively poorer as frequency increases. Overall, frequency discrimination was similar at both active electrodes. An exception was in the region of 300 Hz, where the second turn active yielded much poorer frequency difference limens than the basal turn active. The frequency difference limens obtained in this series of experiments are

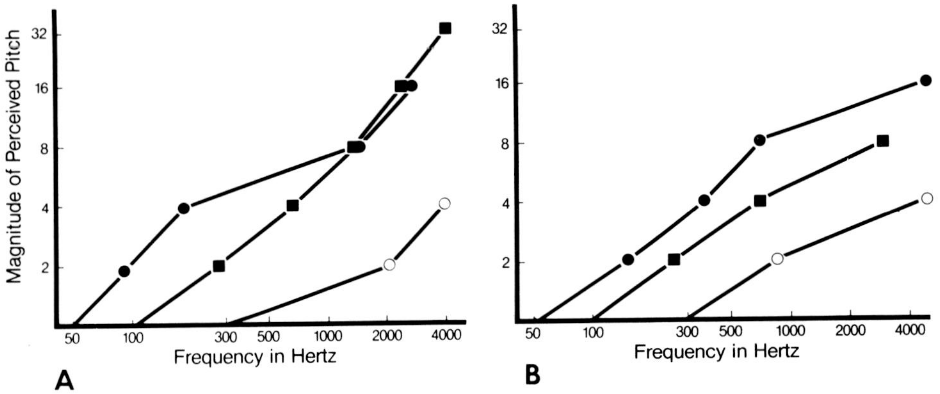

Fig. 10. Pitch ratings as a function of frequency for the A) basal-eustachian tube and B) 2nd turn-eustachian tube electrode pairs. Base frequencies: ● - 50 Hz, ■ - -100 Hz, ○ - 300 Hz.

probably larger than would have been obtained if a method of constant stimuli had been used instead of a method of limits. In addition, we recognize that while we pooled the ascending and descending trials, there are substantial differences between ascending and descending frequency difference limens, especially as the standard frequency is increased above 500 Hz.[18]

The magnitude of pitch as a function of frequency of stimulation was measured using both the doubling technique and a direct magnitude estimation technique. The results of the multiplication or doubling method of estimating pitch growth for the basal and second turn actives paired with the eustachian tube ground are presented in Figure 10A, B for standard base stimuli of 50, 100 and 300 Hz sinusoids. In general, pitch increases with frequency at about the same rate for both the basal and second tu.¬ electrodes up to about 700 Hz, above which larger frequency increments were required to achieve similar pitch doublings for the second turn electrode than for the basal electrode. This effect may be attributable to the ability of the larger basal coil electrode to maintain a more synchronous neural discharge at higher rates of stimulation than could the second turn electrode.

In the second pitch matching experiment, the effects of pulse repetition rate and place of stimulation on pitch magnitude were both evaluated. With the assistance of D. Eddington, an experiment was run whereby pitch ratings were obtained for 1 ms biphasic pulses having repetition rates of 100, 175, and 300 pulses per second (pps). The pulses were adjusted to equal loudness. Mean data for 27 trials under each frequency and electrode condition are presented in Figure 11 along with data reported by Eddington[14] for his most apical (1) and basal (6) electrodes. From the figure it can be seen that there was a consistent ranking of pitch, with the highest ranking corresponding to the most basal electrode and the lowest corresponding to the most apical electrode, at all pulse rates. In addition, for all electrodes, increases in pulse rate resulted in increase in perceived pitch. However, with the exception of the repetition rate of 100 pulses per second, the pitch ratings obtained at different electrodes by Eddington's patient were much more distinctive than those we obtained.

PERCEPTIONS OF LOW FREQUENCY STIMULI

It was demonstrated that, for any given electrode, the limiting factor in pitch perception was the maximum neural volleying rate. However, relatively little was known about the perceptions that patients would have for extremely low frequency stimuli. An experiment was undertaken to determine what our patient's perceptions were for sinusoids in the 5 to 80 Hz region. Stimuli were routed through a spectrum shaper to achieve an equal loudness condition for a 1,000 Hz stimulus at a comfortable listening level. The tones were gated on for one second and off for 500 ms. The patient was allowed to listen to as many stimulus repetitions as necessary to formulate her description. The results of the experiment are provided in Table 9. The descriptions in Table 9 suggest that major transitions were made in the regions of 10 to 12 Hz, 12 to 15 Hz, and 25 to 30 Hz. Interestingly, the transitions at which perceptual changes occurred for these electrical stimuli roughly correspond to those reported by normal-hearing listeners for low frequency tones. Wever and Bray[3] reported that at 5 Hz normal listeners perceived a high frequency pumping

TABLE 8. FREQUENCY DIFFERENCE LIMENS FOR THE BASAL AND 2ND TURN ACTIVE ELECTRODES*

	Frequency (Hz)									
	50		*75*		*100*		*300*		*500*	
Session	*(AB)*	*(A2nd)*	*(AB)*	*(A2nd)*	*(AB)*	*(A2nd)*	*(AB)*	*(A2nd)*	*(AB)*	*(A2nd)*
1	1	1	3	1	21	18	200	825	1080	750
2	1	1	4	1	14	2	95	425	300	500
3	1	1	<1	2	5	8	60	625	380	400
Mean	1	1	2	1	13	9	118	625	587	550

*All frequency difference limens rounded to the nearest 1 Hz.

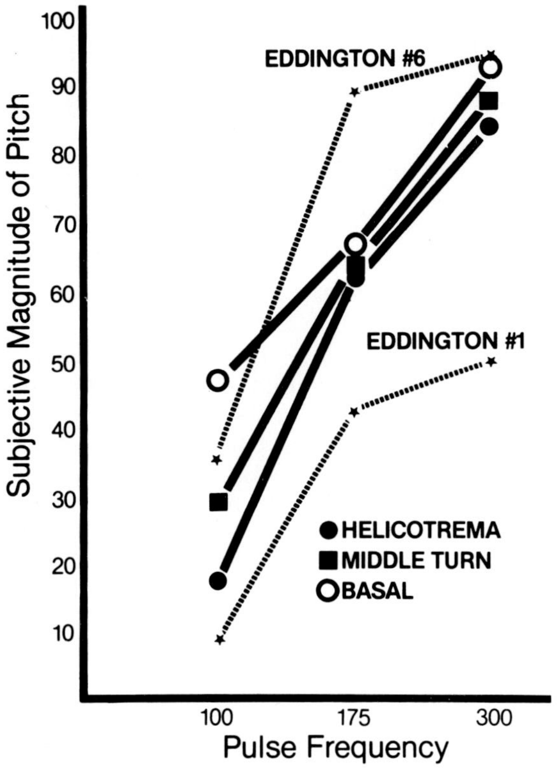

Fig. 11. Pitch magnitude estimates for the helicotrema, 2nd turn, and basal active electrodes paired with a remote ground, at pulse repetition rates of 100, 175, and 300/s. For comparison, data obtained by Eddington[14] under similar test conditions but using a different electrode array are presented for basal (No. 6) and apical (No. 1) electrodes.

noise like "choo-choo." Our patient perceived "chi-chi." At 10 Hz the pumping was louder, faster, more definite, that is, the noise outlined particular pulses or blows when at a definite point in each cycle. At 12 Hz our patient reported "put-ta" which implies a similar compaction. At 15 to 17 Hz, Wever and Bray found a sensation they called "thrusting effect" which was likened to loose bearings or pistons. This phenomenon was not reported by our patient, which seems reasonable, since Wever and Bray hypothesized that the effect was due to a middle ear artifact. At 25 Hz, Wever and Bray found a definite tonal component, as we did. Both Wever and Bray and our patient reported that as frequency increased up to 60 Hz, the pitch increased, but a rough or buzz-like quality persisted.

TABLE 9. PATIENT'S DESCRIPTIONS OF LOW FREQUENCY SINUSOIDS

Stimulus (Hz)	*Description*
5	"Chi-chi" (/tʃI/) repeated over and over like birds
7	"Chi-chi" (/tʃI/) faster and running together like a car starting
10	"Chi-chi" (/tʃI/) faster like car about to turn over
12	"Put-ta, put-ta" (/PΛtΛ, PΛtΛ/), etc
15	Medium pitch motor idling
16	Smoother motor, same pitch
20	Smoother motor, same pitch
25	Smoother motor, same pitch, faster
30	Buzz of medium pitch
35	Buzz of medium pitch
40	Buzz of medium pitch
45	Buzz getting faster, medium pitch
50	Buzz getting faster, medium pitch
55	Buzz getting faster, medium pitch
60	Smooth buzz a little above medium pitch
65	Faster and smoother, pitch not much different
70	Higher pitch but still a buzz
75	About the same pitch buzz
80	Higher pitch but still a buzz

TABLE 10. WORD AND STRESS IDENTIFICATION SCORES* FOR MULTIPLE- AND SINGLE-ELECTRODE STIMULATION USING EUSTACHIAN TUBE GROUND

Electrodes Activated	*Filter Bands†*	*Mean*		*Range*	
		Word	*Stress*	*Word*	*Stress*
Helicotrema 2nd turn Basal	Low, middle & high	10	19	8-20	18-24
2nd turn Basal	Middle & high	12	16	9-14	16-16
2nd turn	Middle	6	16	6-6	16-16
Basal	High	8	18	6-9	17-18
Basal	Broad	10	19	10-10	18-19

*Monosyllable-Trochee-Spondee Test.

†Filter bands: High = 1500-3000 Hz, Middle = 750-1500 Hz, Low = 200-750 Hz.

Probably the most significant information from the preceding comparison relates to the origin of extremely low frequency perceptions. Wever and Bray hypothesized, for example, that the perceptions in the region of 15 to 20 Hz were attributable to activities of middle ear structures. Our data lend support to this hypothesis since our patient did not experience the "thrusting effect." Bekesy reported that frequencies of 10 Hz or less were perceived as tactile stimuli, while 20 Hz or more were perceived as auditory.[9] However, since our patient was stimulated electrically, it is unlikely that external or middle ear structures played an important role in the perceptions elicited. We would also note that no vestibular responses were felt even to the very low frequency stimuli used in the present experiment. Thus, it is more likely that the auditory perceptions obtained below 20 Hz reflected the transition from neural asynchrony to synchrony. Bekesy further elaborated on the importance of low frequency stimuli for understanding the quantal character of the neural processes. He reported that this quantal property was most clearly demonstrable at 18 Hz where there was an increase in loudness and a fused tonal sensation. Our data support this conclusion

TABLE 11. SPONDEE IDENTIFICATION SCORES FOR MULTIPLE- AND SINGLE-ELECTRODE STIMULATION USING THE EUSTACHIAN TUBE GROUND

Electrodes Activated	*Filter Bands**	*Mean*	*Range*
Helicotrema 2nd turn Basal	Low, middle & high	9 (50%)	8-10
Basal	Broad	10 (56%)	9-11

*Filter bands: High = 1500-3000 Hz, Middle = 750-1500 Hz, Low = 200-750 Hz.

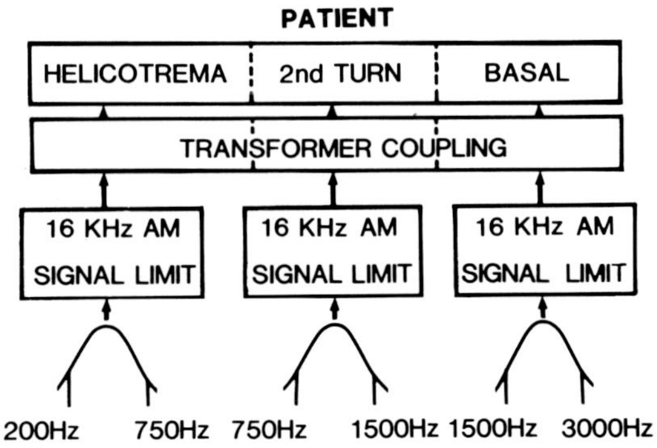

Fig. 12. Block diagram of the signal processing and coupling used in the wearable multiple-channel stimulator.

since our patient reported a medium pitch motor idling at 15 Hz but no pitch associated with the 12 Hz stimulus.

COMPLEX SOUND DISCRIMINATION

Our clinical experiences have demonstrated clearly that there is a significant learning effect with electrical stimulation that is very marked over the first several months, and then continues to occur even after years. Therefore, it was decided that a wearable multiple-channel stimulator should be constructed for this patient and that evaluations of environmental sound and speech perception should take place after some period of stimulation.

In Figure 12, a block diagram of the multiple-channel stimulator system is presented. The signal processor divides the speech spectrum into three pass-bands, 200 to 750 Hz, 750 to 1500 Hz, and 1500 to 3000 Hz, routing the output of these pass-bands to separate 16 kHz modulators and limiters, and then transformer-coupling the modulated 16 kHz to the respective helicotrema, second turn, and basal turn electrodes. Essentially the same signal processing was used as in the standard single-channel House-Urban stimulator, with the exception of some prefiltering which was designed to provide carrier modulation at rates most appropriate for the place of the various electrodes in the cochlea.

Tables 10 to 13 present the results of speech and environmental sound discrimination tests which

TABLE 12. NORTON RHYME TEST SCORES FOR MULTIPLE- AND SINGLE-ELECTRODE STIMULATION USING THE EUSTACHIAN TUBE GROUND

Electrodes Activated	*Filter Bands**	*Mean*	*Range*
Helicotrema 2nd turn Basal	Low, middle & high	24 (48%)	22-27
2nd turn Basal	Middle & high	24 (48%)	22-25
2nd turn	Middle	18 (36%)	17-19
Basal	High	19 (38%)	17-21
Basal	Broad	30 (60%)	29-31

*Filter bands: High = 1500-3000 Hz, Middle = 750-1500 Hz, Low = 200-750 Hz.

TABLE 13. HRRC ENVIRONMENTAL SOUNDS TEST SCORES FOR MULTIPLE- AND SINGLE-ELECTRODE STIMULATION USING THE EUSTACHIAN TUBE GROUND

Electrodes Activated	*Filter Bands**	*Mean*	*Range*
Helicotrema 2nd turn Basal	Low, middle & high	14 (70%)	14-16
2nd turn Basal	Middle & high	14 (70%)	14-15
Basal	Broad	14 (70%)	11-17

*Filter bands: High = 1500-3000 Hz, Middle = 750-1500 Hz, Low = 200-750 Hz.

were obtained under a variety of multiple- and single-electrode stimulation conditons. All conditions used the eustachian tube ground. In Table 10, the results of the Monosyllable-Trochee-Spondee Test[20,13] are presented. All stimuli were presented at comfortable listening levels. It should be noted that activation of the basal coil electrode was done using both high-pass-band and broad-band (200 to 3,000 Hz) filter systems. The inclusion of a broad band of stimulation on the basal coil electrode paired with the eustachian tube ground made it possible to compare the results obtained in the various multiple-channel modes directly with what could be achieved using a standard House-Urban single-electrode, single-channel system. From Table 10 it can be seen that word recognition scores were best for 2-channel stimulation (second turn, basal), with nearly equivalent performance from the 3-channel multiple-electrode scheme and the broad-band basal electrode stimulation. Word recognition scores in the vicinity of 10 to 12 out of a total of 24 possible are consistent with what are normally attained by single-channel cochlear implant patients. The best stress recognition was obtained using the 3-channel and the single-channel broad-band modes of stimulation. Stress discrimination scores of 19 out of 24 are within the range usually achieved by single-channel cochlear implant users.

In Table 11 the results of a spondee identification test are reported. The task required the patient to select the correct spondee from a closed set of six spondees, each repeated three times. Stimulation using the multiple-electrode, multiple-channel system yielded scores which were slightly poorer than those obtained using broad-band stimulation at the basal electrode only, although this is clearly not a significant difference. Similar performance was obtained with the Norton Rhyme Test, a 4-alternative choice, 50-item monosyllabic word test. From Table 12 it can be seen that broad-band stimulation on the basal coil alone yielded the highest score (60%), followed by the multiple-electrode combinations. The poorest performance was obtained from a limited band-width stimulation of either the basal or second coil electrodes.

Table 13 presents the results of the HRRC Environmental Sounds Test for the single- and multiple-channel stimulation conditions. Performance across all conditions was the same, roughly 70%, which is consistent with performance achieved using a standard House-Urban stimulator and single-electrode system.

In general, the results for speech tests and environmental sounds tests do not suggest any significant advantage was obtained from multiple-electrode, multiple-channel stimulation as compared to single-channel, single-electrode stimulation when a broad frequency band is used to active the single channel. Limiting the frequency band to any of the electrodes did reduce performance as compared to broad-band or multiple-band stimulation. This is to be expected since even though our patient did not demonstrate strong place-specific frequency perceptions, timing and intensity cues were detected over the full range from 200 to 3000 Hz. Thus, high frequency cues that are related to intensity or timing would be eliminated if only low-pass bands were used for stimulation.

Although no significant difference could be demonstrated between multiple-channel stimulation and single-channel stimulation with a broad-band signal in the laboratory, the patient subjectively felt that both speech and environmental sounds were perceived with greater clarity and were more easily recognized in daily use with the multiple-electrode, multiple-channel stimulation mode. There may be qualitative differences that are not easily measured with our standard tests.

SUMMARY

In summary, this paper has presented some of the recent electric and perceptual results obtained with a multiple-electrode cochlear implant. The multiple-electrode array consisted of three active electrodes implanted in the cochlea and four grounds implanted external to the cochlea. In general, impedance functions were similar in shape for all electrodes, although the absolute magnitude of the impedance was highest with the apical electrode and lowest with the basal coil electrode. It is also noted that impedance functions obtained using intracochlear electrode pairs were generally higher than those obtained using an intracochlear active and an extracochlear ground.

Electrical thresholds were lowest for the basal coil electrode and highest for the helicotrema electrode. Dynamic ranges were correspondingly largest for the basal coil electrode and smallest for the apical or helicotrema electrode. Equal loudness contours were found to be similar in shape for all active electrodes and did not change shape as a function of stimulus intensity. Loudness growth functions were similar to those reported by previous researchers, with a gradual loudness increase in the vicinity of threshold and rapid increases in loudness with relatively small intensity changes above threshold. Both periodicity and place pitch were demonstrated. Periodicity pitch was near normal at very low frequencies, with progressive deterioration and practically no frequency resolution beyond 500 Hz. Place pitch phenomena were present, although at stimulation rates above 100 Hz the effect was not marked.

The results of speech and environmental sounds tests did not reveal performance to be superior with the multiple-electrode, multiple-channel system as compared to a single-channel broad-band system. Overall, the results obtained to date with this multiple-channel system are similar to those reported by House et al[6] for earlier multiple-channel systems.

POSTSCRIPT

Following this series of studies, the hard-wired percutaneous plug was disconnected from the electrodes and replaced by three of our standard induction coils. That is, the patient now has totally implanted hardware. Testing is continuing to determine if a signal processing scheme can be devised which will provide better speech discrimination using the multiple-channel system.

ACKNOWLEDGMENT — The authors wish to acknowledge the assistance of Ms. Lori Eberle who was instrumental in the collection of these data.

REFERENCES

1. Otte J, Schuknecht HF, Kerr AG. Ganglion cell populations in normal and pathological human cochleae: implications for cochlear implantation. Laryngoscope 1978; 88:1231-46.

2. Kiang NY, Eddington DK, Delgutte B. Fundamental considerations in designing auditory implants. Acta Otolaryngol (Stockh) 1979; 87:204-18.

3. Wever EG, Bray CW. A perception of low tones and the resonance volley theory. J Psychol 1937; 3:101-14.

4. House WF, Urban J. Long term results of electrode implantation and electronic stimulation of the cochlea in man. Ann Otol Rhinol Laryngol 1973; 82:504-10.

5. Doyle JB, Doyle JH, Turnbull FM. Electrical stimulation of the eighth cranial nerve. Arch Otolaryngol 1964; 80:388-91.

6. House WF, Berliner K, Crary W, et al. Cochlear implants. Ann Otol Rhinol Laryngol 1976; 85 Suppl 27:1-93.

7. Clark GM, Tong WC, Bailey QR, et al. A multiple-electrode cochlear implant. J Otolaryngol Soc Austral 1978; 4:208-12.

8. Pialoux P, Chouard CH, Meyer B, Fugain C. Indications and results of the multichannel cochlear implant. Acta Otolaryngol (Stockh) 1979; 87:185-9.

9. Bosch J, Prades J, Colomina R, Monferre A. A model multichannel intracochlear implant. Ear and Hearing 1980; 1:226-8.

10. Eddington DK. Multiple channel intracochlear stimulation. Presented at Third International Workshop on Surgery of the Ear and Skull Base, Newport Beach, Calif., 1981.

11. Michelson RP, Schindler RA. Multichannel cochlear implant: preliminary results in man. Laryngoscope 1981; 91:38-42.

12. Hochmair-Desoyer IJ, Hochmair ES. An eight channel scala tympani electrode for auditory prostheses. IEEE Trans Biomed Eng 1980; BME-27:44-50.

13. Thielemeir MA, Brimacombe JA, Eisenberg LS. Audiological results with the cochlear implant. Ann Otol Rhinol Laryngol 1982; 91 Suppl 91:27-34.

14. Eddington DK, Dobelle WH, Brackmann DE, et al. Auditory prostheses research with multiple channel intracochlear stimulation in man. Ann Otol Rhinol Laryngol 1978; 87 Suppl 53:1-39.

15. Simmons FB, Walker MG, Mathews RG, White RL. Percepts and discrimination by auditory nerve stimulation: a summary of results and some proposals for nerve viability evaluation. In: McPherson DL, ed. Advances in prosthetic devices for the deaf: a technical workshop. Rochester, NY: National Technical Institute for the Deaf, 1979:271-4.

16. Walsh SM, Leake-Jones PA, Vurek LS, Merzenich MM. Chronic electrical stimulation with intracochlear electrodes: electrophysiological results. Ann Otol Rhinol Laryngol 1981; 90:27-9.

17. Shannon RV. Human psychophysical results of electrical stimulation: effects of waveform and electrical configuration. Presented at the West Coast Cochlear Prosthesis Workshop, Seattle, 1980.

18. Helmerich LH, Edgerton BJ. Psychoelectric measurements and results from cochlear implant patients. Ann Otol Rhinol Laryngol 1982; 91 Suppl 91:35-40.

19. Bekesy GV. Experiments in hearing. New York: McGraw-Hill Book Co, 1960:257-61.

20. Erber N, Alencewicz C. Audiologic evaluation of deaf children. J Speech Hear Dis 1976; 41:256-67.

HEARING BY COCHLEAR NUCLEUS STIMULATION IN HUMANS

BRADLY J. EDGERTON, PhD

WILLIAM F. HOUSE, MD

WILLIAM HITSELBERGER, MD

Many bilaterally profoundly deaf individuals cannot benefit from a cochlear implant because the eighth nerve is not intact from the cochlea to the brainstem. This paper provides the results of preliminary investigations into the effects of direct electrical stimulation of the cochlear nucleus in one patient. Results of intensity, frequency, and speech perception studies are reported. In general, performance is very similar to that obtained from single-channel cochlear implant patients.

Twenty years of effort have now made possible the reliable restoration of limited hearing in the totally deaf through the cochlear implant. This device, obviously still in the early stage of development, is designed to stimulate an anatomically intact but functionally damaged cochlea and auditory nerve. It is now established that in most cases of total deafness the problem is primarily at the hair cell level and most patients have some degree of survival of spiral ganglion nerve fibers.[1-4]

Apparently only a few fibers of cochlear nerve are necessary for stimulation to give a sensation of sound.[5] Some patients, however, have total bilateral loss of the auditory nerve due to such conditions as severe meningitis with total calcification of the inner ear, congenital inner ear agenesis (Michel deformity) and bilateral acoustic tumors.

This paper records the first attempt at chronic electrical stimulation of the *ventral* cochlear nucleus in a patient totally deafened by bilateral acoustic tumors.

PREVIOUS CENTRAL AUDITORY STIMULATION EXPERIENCE IN HUMANS

In 1964 Simmons stimulated the cochlear nerve in a patient undergoing removal of a recurrent cerebellar tumor.[6] The patient had had one cerebellar hemisphere removed and subsequently developed hydrocephalus. He had normal hearing. Before surgery he was instructed in listening to various sounds such as those produced by square waves and sawtooth waves. At surgery with use of local anesthesia a small recurrent tumor was removed. Previous removal of the cerebellar hemisphere made the floor of the fourth ventricle and the eighth nerve clearly visible. A bipolar electrode with the tips spread 4.5 mm was applied to the cochlear nerve, and 2.5 ms square wave biphasic stimuli of various frequencies were applied at a 2V level. The patient reported sound sensations similar to the square wave sounds he had heard during the auditory training on the previous day. As stimulation rates varied between 20 and 4,000 Hz, the patient reported a sensation of higher pitch with increasing stimulation rates. Stimulation of the inferior colliculus, also visible in the same surgical field, gave no auditory sensation.

Chronic stimulation of the auditory cortex to produce hearing is difficult in humans. The principal reason is anatomic. The primary auditory cortex projection areas are areas 41 and 42 on the opicular surface of the superior temporal gyrus. These areas are deep in the sylvian fissure and to visualize them the sylvian fissure must be widely spread. The middle cerebral artery courses through this fissure, and damage to the branches of this artery by surgical manipulation could cause serious neurologic deficit from brain infarction.

Direct stimulation of central nervous system structures is possible in humans. We therefore decided to try ventral cochlear nucleus (VCN) stimulation in one patient who had bilateral acoustic tumors.

AREA OF THE COCHLEAR NUCLEUS

The area of the cochlear nucleus is frequently visualized during acoustic tumor surgery through the translabyrinthine approach.[7] The acoustic recess is seen as a pocket flanked by cerebellum, pons, and medulla. The acoustic nerve enters the recess, covered dorsally by cerebellar flocculus and terminates on the lateral surface of the medulla at its junction with the pons.[8]

The cochlear nuclei are included among structures supplied by the anterior inferior cerebellar artery, or by aberrant or collateral branches of the superior or the posterior cerebellar arteries; the pattern of supply by the cerebellar arteries may vary considerably. The anterior inferior cerebellar artery, with variable tributaries, can be seen extending along the cochlear nerve into the acoustic recess. The anterior inferior cerebellar artery must be avoided during surgery since occluding it can result in tinnitus, ipsilateral total deafness, and slight impairment of hearing on the opposite side.[9,10]

Tsuchitani[11] and Kane[12] published excellent reviews of the morphologic and electrophysiologic studies of the primary afferents and the cochlear nucleus cells. These reports indicate that at the VCN the primary auditory nerve afferents and their nuclear synapses seem to be excitatory (as contrasted to inhibitory). This would favor direct electrical stimulation to activate the central auditory pathways.

The cellular architecture of the cochlear nuclei in the human has been described.[13,14] The various cell types tend to be concentrated in certain regions of the nuclei, but unlike lower animals they are intermingled considerably.[15] The major divisions of human cochlear nuclei are dorsal (DCN), inferior ventral (IVCN), and superior ventral (SVCN). The spheroid cells, of particular importance to hearing, are large, spherical to ovoid cells, and are the most numerous of the cell types. These cells receive the synaptic terminals of the majority of sensory cochlear nerve fibers. Injury of the spheroid cells is the pathologic basis of sensorineural deafness of central origin. Comparable to the situation in the cochlea, where a tonotopic frequency pattern has been demonstrated, such a gradient has been confirmed in the human superior ventral cochlear nucleus: low frequencies ventral to high frequencies dorsal.[16]

The optimal site for electrical stimulation is over the SVCN. However, direct access to the spheroid cells is limited due to overlying DCN and pontine tissue. The point at which the cochlear nerve enters the brainstem, the hilum, provides the best access and was chosen as the place of electrode implantation in this first patient.

CASE REVIEW

The patient, when first examined in 1964, was a 31-year-old employee of a grocery market. Three years previously she had noted a bilateral sudden loss of hearing accompanied by a right-sided facial weakness. She attributed these symptoms to severe emotional strain. The hearing in the left ear returned and the right facial paralysis disappeared, but total right hearing loss remained. Family history revealed that her mother had had "tumor along her spine."

Temporal bone x-ray films showed a large right canal. Pantopaque studies showed a 1-cm right acoustic tumor. A filling defect of the left internal auditory canal was not found. At this time we were using only fluoroscopic studies. It is possible, therefore, that a very small tumor in the left internal auditory canal could have been missed.

In July 1964 the tumor was totally removed through a translabyrinthine approach. A slight facial weakness cleared in about two months. The patient was seen yearly until 1973 when she moved out of town. On each visit she reported unsteadiness when tired and when in the darkness. A trial of medical management of allergy was of no help. In retrospect it is possible that an inferior vestibular tumor was developing on the left at that time.

In 1976 her local ENT specialist referred her back to us because of an episode of hearing loss in the left ear. There had been several episodes of fluctuation of hearing. Examination showed her hearing to be at a 57 dB level with 46% speech discrimination. Electronystagmography (ENG) showed total loss of vestibular function. Computerized axial tomography (CAT) scan showed a 2-cm left acoustic tumor and a 1½-cm tumor in the right cerebellopontine angle.

The diagnosis now was von Recklinghausen disease. The right tumor could have been a recurrence but more likely was a new tumor on a nerve other than the eighth. Previous experience was that partial removal of acoustic neuromas in von Recklinghausen cases has resulted in total hearing loss. Linthicum attributed this result to the multicentric origin of these tumors.[17] This causes acoustic nerve fibers to be dispersed throughout the tumor rather than to remain outside along the capsule.

The feeling was that neither tumor at this time was large enough to be life-threatening. Therefore, to preserve the residual hearing as long as possible, the top of the internal auditory canal on the left was unroofed to allow room for tumor expansion and release pressure on the acoustic nerve fibers. After this procedure in October 1976, the patient's hearing improved slightly and stabilized at 48 dB and 88% speech discrimination. In 1½ years, however, the speech discrimination began to drop. A CAT scan showed slight enlargement of the left tumor.

In May 1979, the patient's hearing was totally gone except for a response at 80 dB at 250 Hz. The CAT scan revealed considerable enlargement of the left tumor and early hydrocephalus. The right tumor had remained the same size. Total translabyrinthine removal of the left tumor was therefore recommended.

The patient accepted the recommendation and was asked if she would try an electrode placement to the left VCN. She was told that this had never been done before and therefore the risk was largely unknown. The principal risk was increased chance of postoperative infection. She was told that if it occurred, the electrode would have to be removed. She was also told that we did not know if she would gain any hearing from the electrical stimulation through the electrode and, if sound sensation occurred, what it would sound like. The implanted electrode was constructed of 7 mil platinum wire terminating at fired 0.5 mm balls. The electrodes were insulated with silicone tubing up to the ball. The ball terminals were separated by 1.5 mm.

On May 24, 1979, through a translabyrinthine approach, the left acoustic tumor was totally removed with preservation of the facial nerve. The time of surgery, from incision to total control of bleeding in the tumor bed, was three hours ten minutes. The choroid plexus, the posterior inferior cerebellar artery, and the remnant of the acoustic nerve just inferior to the pons at the opening of the foramen of Luschka were easily visualized. The surgeon inserted the terminals of the electrode into the area of the VCN by gently pushing them through the ependyma overlying the nucleus. The 15 cm of insulated wire were led out through the mastoid cavity and secured to the bone by a 4-0 silk suture placed through a hole in the bone. The ends of the wire were brought out through the incision. The entire placement took approximately ten minutes.

The total surgical time was three hours 38 minutes. Estimated blood loss was 800 cc with 0.47 l replacement. The patient responded well on the operating table and was transferred to the intensive care unit. She had a 30% facial weakness but was able to totally close her left eye. An arterial line used for blood pressure monitoring during surgery was left in place. There had been no vital sign changes during surgery.

The following day the patient was alert and stable with no increase in facial weakness. She complained of some headache. With her consent she was returned in her bed to the operating room for testing. The operating room was selected as the place of testing since it had the proper electrical isolation systems to insure patient safety.

During electrical testing the patient's blood pressure was constantly monitored through the arterial line placed the day before. Pulse and respiration were also monitored. No significant fluctuations in these measures were noted.

IMPEDANCE MEASUREMENTS

Method. Impedance magnitude of the bipolar electrode was measured using a variable resistor in series between a sine wave source and the electrode pair. At each test frequency, the series resistance R_o was adjusted so that the magnitude of the voltage

TABLE 1. IMPEDANCE DATA FOR THREE TEST SESSIONS USING STIMULI FROM 90 TO 18,500 Hz

Frequency (Hz)	*Session 1*	*Session 2*	*Session 3*
90	38	50	156
250	—	—	124
500	—	—	98
1,000	10	22	81
10,000	—	—	21
16,000	9	7	17
18,500	—	6	—

applied to the electrode pair was one half the source voltage. If Z represents electrode pair impedance, then the applicable relationship from which Z may be determined is:

$$\frac{/Z/}{/R_o + Z/} = \frac{1}{2}$$

In general, for the above procedure, impedance magnitude will be somewhat less than R_o. However, if the reactive (capacitance) component is not too large, the difference between /Z/ and R_o will not exceed a few percent. This situation prevails for electrode impedances such that the value of R_o can be interpreted as /Z/ within experimental error.

Results. Impedance data were collected one day, one week, and one month following surgery (sessions 1, 2, 3 respectively) with use of sinusoids from 90 to 18,500 Hz. As seen in Table 1, for all sessions R_o was greatest at low frequencies and decreased with increasing frequency. The general shape of the impedance function for the VCN implant was probably determined by the electrodes used. For sessions 1 and 2 the impedance of the implanted electrodes decreased at a rate of about 14 dB per octave over the most linear portion of the function (100 to 1000 Hz). The impedance function of a similar electrode derived in physiological saline decreased at a rate of about 11 dB/octave over the same frequency range. These findings are consistent with those of Spelman et al[18] and suggest that the electrode system alone contributed significantly to the observed frequency-dependent effects.

Table 1 also reveals a significant increase in impedance magnitudes over the test sessions. Although it is not clear what caused this increase in electrode impedance, some of the change could be attributed to a shift in the position of the electrodes. During the period that the impedance data were collected for session 3, significant amounts of auditory threshold fatigue were measured. Also, some sensations of feeling, ie, twitching, were reported in the leg contralateral to the implant at moderate stimulus intensity levels.

ELECTRICAL THRESHOLD AND DISCOMFORT LEVELS

Method

EQUIPMENT. Electrical thresholds (ET) and electrical discomfort (ED) levels were measured with use of sinusoidal stimuli generated by a waveform synthesizer (Wavetek model 186) and shaped and timed by a logic control system (Coulbourn series). A rise/fall time of 10 ms was used to avoid detection of on-off transients. Stimuli were gated on for 500 ms and off for 300 ms, and were presented in triads to eliminate patient confusion due to tinnitus. Frequency was monitored continuously with a digital frequency counter (Fluke 9000). Stimulus level was controlled by routing the shaped signal to a variable amplifier (Crown 075) and then to a half-decibel step attenuator (Shallco Custom) before termination at the electrode leads. An oscilloscope (Tektronix D-15; 5A-18N; 5B-12N) monitored the signal at the electrode leads; all intensity measurements were made in peak-to-peak voltage from the oscilloscope display.

The patient was instructed to raise a finger to indicate when she could "just detect" the presence of the triadic pattern of test stimuli. Initially the patient required some training for the ET measurements. Training consisted of pairing the visual representation of the test signal displayed on the oscilloscope with the auditory stimulus.

THRESHOLD MEASUREMENTS. All threshold measurements were made with use of an up-down adaptive procedure.[19] Measurements began with an ascending (half-decibel step) trial to determine the region of ET. Threshold was defined as the level at which signals were audible for 3 of 5 trials. Thresholds and EDs were obtained for 50, 90, 250, 500, 1000, 2000, 4000, 10,000, and 16,000 Hz sinusoids (not all tones were presented during every test session).

THRESHOLD OF DISCOMFORT. Thresholds of discomfort were established with use of an ascending method of adjustment technique. The signal levels were determined with use of a patient-controlled half-decibel step attenuator. The patient was instructed to adjust the attenuator setting to "a level that would not be tolerable for more than five minutes." The patient was urged to work slowly and not increase the signal to a painfully loud level. The stimulus (5000 ms on, 300 ms off) was immediately turned off when the patient indicated discomfort. The ED was taken as the median of three trials.

Results. Table 2 presents ETs and EDs in peak-to-peak voltage for the frequencies 50, 90, 250, 500, 1000, 2000, 4000, 10,000, and 16,000 Hz. The table presents data chronologically from the first to the last test sessions. It is apparent that ETs and EDs are greater at the low and high frequencies than at the middle frequencies. The frequency/sensitivity dependence is most likely the result of impedance and neuronal membrane characteristics. Table 1 showed that impedances (R_o) were highest for the low frequencies and lowest for the high frequencies. Thus, at the lowest frequencies greater input voltages were required to maintain a current capable of

TABLE 2. THRESHOLDS AND ELECTRICAL DISCOMFORT IN PEAK-TO-PEAK MILLIVOLTS FOR SINUSOIDAL STIMULI PRESENTED DIRECTLY TO THE VENTRAL COCHLEAR NUCLEUS VIA AN IMPLANTED ELECTRODE

Date* 1979	50 ET	50 ED	90 ET	90 ED	250 ET	250 ED	500 ET	500 ED	1000 ET	1000 ED	2000 ET	2000 ED	4000 ET	4000 ED	16,000 ET	16,000 ED
5/25	1300	2000	600	1200	260	400	200	400	230	550	390	580	380	580	1400	2200
5/31	—	—	650	2500	—	—	280	640	300	700	400	1100	600	1000	1100	2200
6/27	—	—	900	2900	—	—	520	—	580	1520	500	—	—	—	1740	4150
6/29	—	—	850	2200	450	1500	410	1500	450	1400	540	1750	—	—	1800	5200
7/03	—	—	880	2800	480	1500	500	1800	600	2200	680	2650	—	—	2350	6000

*Measurements span the time from the first stimulation to the point at which experimental studies were terminated.
ET - Electrical threshold; ED - Electrical discomfort.

exciting neural elements. The current level required for threshold excitation at low and middle stimulation frequencies was approximately 42 μA. Table 2 shows that, although the impedances were least at 16,000 Hz, the voltages required for threshold were higher than at any other frequency. This could be attributable to charge-dependent neural membrane properties that develop at high frequencies requiring significantly greater currents to achieve excitation.[20]

Table 2 also shows that thresholds (voltages) increased substantially over time. Table 1, however, shows that impedances also increased over time. Thus, the data in Table 2 alone do not allow us to ascertain if threshold changes were likely to have been caused by perceptual accommodation, neural degeneration, electrode migration, electrode-tissue interface breakdown, or other conditions. Table 3 provides some approximations of current levels required for stimulation at the frequencies from 50 to 16,000 Hz for sessions 1, 2, and 3. Thresholds (μA) were nearly identical for sessions 1 and 2 except at 16,000 Hz, where a higher current was required for session 2. Thus, it is not likely that voltage threshold changes were attributable to any large scale reduction in the number of stimulable neural fibers. On the other hand, session 3 required current levels 10 to 20 μA lower than either session 1 or 2 at all test frequencies. This finding supports the hypothesis that the electrode may have migrated away from its original position.

PITCH PERCEPTION

Method

EQUIPMENT. Two oscillators (Wavetek 186; Wavetek 185) were set to equivalent output voltages and routed to the Coulbourn logic system for shaping (rise/fall = 10 ms) and timing. Their frequencies were monitored independently by two frequency counters (Fluke 9000). The outputs of the two rise/fall gates (Coulbourn) were led to the input of a mixer/amplifier (Coulbourn) and then routed to a spectrum shaper (B & K 5612) and terminated at the patient's electrodes. The spectrum shaper was used to establish an approximation to an equal loudness contour. The standard (S) and comparison (C) tones were alternated with a 1-second on-time and a 500 ms interstimulus interval. The S and C were calibrated to have identical rise/fall and on-times by an oscilloscope with memory (Tektronix).

PROCEDURE. A two-step procedure was used to measure the difference limen for frequency. First, an equal loudness contour was established to reduce the confusion between loudness-induced pitch or quality changes and frequency-specific effects.[21,22] An equal loudness function was established with use of a 1000-Hz referent presented at a level judged "comfortably" loud by the patient. A spectrum shaper was then used to achieve an approximation of the loudness contour. Second, frequency discrimination testing was done with use of standard tones of 250 and 500 Hz. The patient was given the instructions: "Two tones will be alternated. Ignore differences in loudness and indicate if the tones are the same or different in pitch." A method of limits procedure was employed. Ascending and descending trials were averaged to derive frequency limens. The initial ascent or descent was begun well beyond the point at which the frequency limen was anticipated based on practice trials.

Results. Table 4 presents the ascending, descending, and grand mean difference limen along with the Weber fraction for the grand mean difference limen. Frequency discrimination was generally poor, with discrimination at 250 Hz better than

TABLE 3. PEAK-TO-PEAK CURRENT LEVELS IN MICROAMPERES REQUIRED TO OBTAIN BEHAVIORAL THRESHOLDS FOR SINUSOIDAL STIMULI

Session*	50	90	250	500	1000	2000	4000	16,000
1	33	16	13	11	23	39	42	1561
2	—	18	—	15	26	42	—	249
3	—	6	4	5	7	10	—	138

*Testing performed on 3 different days.

TABLE 4. FREQUENCY DIFFERENCE LIMENS AND WEBER FRACTIONS FOR THE STANDARD TONES OF 250 AND 500 HERTZ

Reference Frequency (Hz)	*Mean Ascending Trials (Hz)*	*Mean Descending Trials (Hz)*	*Grand Mean (Hz)*	*Grand Mean* △f/f
250	30	170	86	34%
500	263	348	261	52%

that at 500 Hz. The difference limens of 86 Hz and 261 Hz for standards at 250 and 500 Hz respectively can be contrasted to difference limens of 5 Hz for normal ears over the frequency range from 200 to 2000 Hz.[23-25] The difference limens obtained by VCN stimulation were also poorer than researchers have reported for electrical stimulation at the cochlea. Simmons et al[26] have reported difference limens on the order of 6 to 15 Hz in the region of 200 Hz. They state that the upper limit of frequency discrimination in cochlear or eighth nerve (modiolar) stimulation is about 350 to 400 Hz. Dillier et al[27] found a frequency limen of about 3 Hz for a loud 200-Hz standard and frequency limens of 50 to 75 Hz for a medium and soft 500-Hz standard. Walker reported that Weber fractions were 10 to 20% of the standard for frequencies up to 350 Hz.[28] Helmerich and Edgerton found frequency limens on the order of 5 Hz at frequencies of 100 Hz or below. As frequency increased, the frequency limen also increased, resulting in unmeasurably wide limens beyond 1000 Hz.[29]

Table 4 also reveals a methodological problem that can occur when an ascending/descending measurement procedure is used near the limits of a perceptual continuum. Note that the ascending trial frequency limen for the 250-Hz standard was about six times smaller than the descending frequency limen; the effect was present, but less pronounced, for the 500-Hz standard. Thus, to obtain a clear indication of a patient's ability to discriminate pitch, grand mean data should not be presented alone. That is, the results of ascending and descending trials should be provided in addition to the grand means.

LOUDNESS PERCEPTION

Method

EQUIPMENT. Difference limens for intensity, and loudness growth were measured. Standard (S) and comparison (C) were generated from a single audio oscillator (Wavetek 186). The oscillator output was shaped (rise/fall = 10 ms) and then split. The split signals were led to independent channels of an amplifier (Crown 075). One channel was further routed to a patient-controlled half-decibel step attenuator (Shallco) and then both channels were mixed (Coulbourn S82-24) and terminated at a pair of electrode clips. The mixed output voltage was monitored continuously on an oscilloscope (Tektronix D-15, 5A-18N, 5B-12N). Frequency was monitored continuously by a frequency counter (Fluke 1900A).

TABLE 5. VENTRAL COCHLEAR NUCLEUS INTENSITY DIFFERENCE LIMENS IN MICROAMPERES AND WEBER FRACTIONS FOR SINUSOIDAL STIMULI

Stimulus (Hz)	*VCN* △I (μA)	*VCN* △I/I(%)
90	1.8	17
500	0.3	2
1000	0.3	5
2000	0.6	2

VCN - Ventral cochlear nucleus; △I - Difference limens.

PROCEDURE. Difference limens for intensity were measured by use of standard reference tones of 90, 250, 500, 1000, and 2000 Hz. A method of adjustment procedure was used. The S and C stimuli were on for 500 ms with a 300-ms interstimulus interval. Testing was done at a level 100 mV (peak-to-peak) higher than the threshold. To reduce the effect of patient attenuator reference bias, the ascending and descending trials were alternated, and the starting levels were varied by the experimenter. The patient's attenuator box contained a switch that allowed her to initiate each stimulus pair. The patient was instructed to listen to the stimulus pairs and "adjust the attenuator dial to the point at which both stimuli are equal in loudness." The intensity limen was based on five ascending and five descending trials.

Results. Table 5 presents the intensity difference limens in μA (peak-to-peak) for the standard frequencies 90, 1000, and 2000 Hz for the VCN subject. Intensity limens ranged from 0.6 μA at 2000 Hz to 1.84 μA at 90 Hz. The larger limens for the low frequencies were verified during a later test session. Conversion of intensity limens to Weber fractions yields values as high as 0.17 at 90 Hz and as low as 0.02 at 2000 Hz. For comparison, Table 6 provides the intensity limens obtained from a direct coupled cochlear implant (CI).[22] The experiments using a similar test protocol with the direct coupled cochlear electrode system yielded intensity limens ranging from 0.6 μA at 100 Hz, to 3.5 μA at 2000 Hz; Weber fractions were approximately 0.04. Other researchers have reported that, for cochlear stimulation, intensity limens usually range between 1 and 5 μA.[21,27,30] Tables 5 and 6 reveal that the major differences between the VCN and CI were 1) cochlear stimulation required a greater range of

TABLE 6. COCHLEAR IMPLANT INTENSITY DIFFERENCE LIMENS IN MICROAMPERES AND WEBER FRACTIONS FOR SINUSOIDAL STIMULI

Stimulus (Hz)	*CI* △I (μA)	*CI* △I/I(%)
100	0.6	6
500	1.3	3
1500	2.6	4
2000	3.5	4

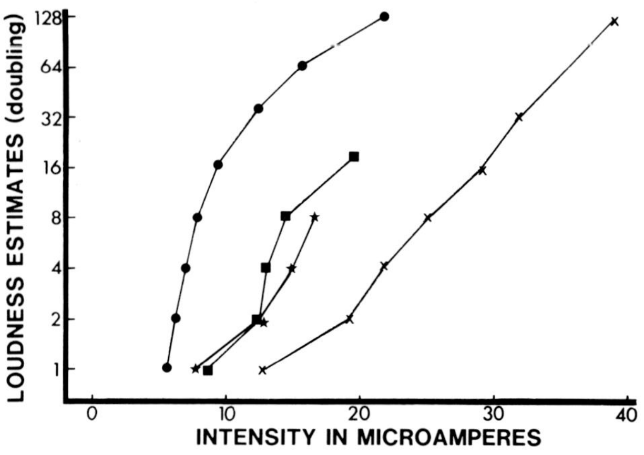

Perceived loudness as a function of intensity. ● - 90 Hz, ★ - 250 Hz, ■ - 1000 Hz, X - 2000 Hz.

signal intensity to derive intensity limens over the 500- to 2000-Hz region, and 2) at the low frequencies (VCN = 90 Hz; CI = 100 Hz) greater signal intensity was required to obtain the intensity limens for the VCN than for the CI.

LOUDNESS SCALING

Method. A loudness-scaling experiment was done with the same instrumentation previously described for intensity limen measurements. Test stimuli consisted of 90, 250, 1000, and 2000 Hz sinusoids. Stimuli were gated on for 1 second with a 500 ms interstimulus interval. The standard tone was always the first stimulus of the pair. The subject initiated each stimulus presentation and was instructed to "adjust a handheld dial (attenuator) so that the loudness level of the second tone is twice that of the first tone." Testing began with the standard and comparison tones set at equal amplitude 100 mV peak-to-peak above threshold. The patient adjusted the comparison tone to twice the standard. This level then served as the standard for the next trial. Several practice trials preceded each test session. The median of 3 to 5 trials was taken as the final loudness judgment.

Results. The results of the scaling experiments are presented in the figure. Scaling data are plotted in a log/linear fashion. Loudness growth is similar at 250, 1000, and 2000 Hz, but differs substantially at 90 Hz. For functions at 250, 1000, and 2000 Hz, doubling of perceived loudness was achieved with increases of 3 to 4 μA in stimulus intensity level. However, at 90 Hz the function may be best described as having two parts. The loudness growth near threshold was rapid, ie, approximately a doubling of perceived loudness for a 1 μA signal intensity change. At moderate and high intensity levels loudness grew more gradually, requiring a signal intensity increase of approximately 5.5 μA to achieve a doubling of loudness. The difference between the loudness growth curve at 90 Hz and the curves obtained at higher frequencies is difficult to interpret at this time.

TABLE 7. SOUNDS HEARD BY PATIENT WITH COCHLEAR NUCLEUS IMPLANT

Closing of a sliding glass door	Spoon on ice tea glass
Closing of a pill box	Door closing
Garbage disposal	Blowing of own nose
Footsteps on cement	TV channel selector switch
Golf ball being hit	Light switch
Phone being hung up	Closing of glasses case
Tearing apart of postage stamps	A knife being put onto a tray
Door knock	Telephone ring
Dog bark	Water running
Airplane	Zipper
Toilet flushing	Vacuum cleaner
	Voices (own and others')

SUBJECTIVE PATIENT EVALUATION

The preceding results represent an attempt to quantify in a controlled fashion the perceptions of a patient stimulated at the VCN with sinusoids. In addition to these data, the patient provided descriptions of sinusoidal stimuli. A 90-Hz sinusoid introduced at a level just above threshold sounded similar to the stretching of a rubber band. As intensity was increased, the sound was more like a drum but not a solid beat. As signal intensity was further increased, the patient reported that the sound was getting louder and was similar to a foghorn. When a 500-Hz signal was introduced near threshold, the subject reported a faint banging on a tin can that turned to the sound of a foghorn as intensity increased. At frequencies below 500 Hz both pitch and loudness changes were perceived. Remaining stimuli from 1000 to 18,650 Hz were heard as foghorns of varying intensity. At high signal levels the 16,000-Hz tone became noisy or sounded like static. It is notable that on the first stimulation, frequency difference limens could not be measured since changes in frequency were always perceived as changes in loudness. This effect was seen for stimuli at 50 and 1000 Hz.

A standard 16,000-Hz amplitude-modulated CI stimulator was tried on the patient for about two weeks. The patient was capable of recognizing differences in the voices of three male speakers and achieved 100% recognition of the spondees "cowboy," "sailboat," and "railroad" without seeing the speaker during the first session after the stimulator was fit. During the first session she also described a cowbell as sounding like a doorknock, a ratchet as sounding like a rattle, a knock as sounding like a knock, and a triangle as sounding like a bell. The patient was given the stimulator unit to wear at home and was asked to keep a daily diary of the sounds that she heard. Table 7 contains a listing of the sounds the patient reported hearing during the week after the stimulator was taken home.

A brief experiment was done with this patient wearing the standard CI stimulator to determine the patient's ability to discriminate between paired consonant-vowels (CV) or paired vowels. A 30-year-old male speaker (General American Dialect)

recorded a series of CV and vowel pairs that were randomized ten times and presented to the patient. For the consonant and vowel discrimination task the patient was asked to indicate if paired stimuli were the same or different. Consonants consisted of /s,p,m,l/ paired with the vowels /i, e, æ, u, ɛ, ʌ. The patient was able to consistently discriminate the /p/ from /m/, indicating that she may have perceived the features of voicing and nasality. Nasality may have been the more salient feature, since the patient also reported that /s/ and /l/ and /p/ and /l/ sounded the same. For the vowel stimuli, the patient consistently discriminated between /i/ and /a/, /i/ and /u/, and /i/ and /ʌ/. This suggests that the feature front/back may have been used to discriminate vowels. It is emphasized, however, that the data obtained are extremely limited and should be cautiously interpreted.

The patient was enthusiastic about the sound she was receiving through the stimulator unit. She reported that, although she could not understand conversational speech without visualizing the speaker's face, her ability to speechread was much improved with the stimulator on.

CONCLUSION

Results of this study suggest that cochlear nucleus stimulation may have possibilities for patients with total bilateral cochlear nerve loss. During the six weeks of stimulation, no serious side effects were noted, although at some frequencies high current levels did produce sensations in the patient's left leg. Our experience from this first VCN case encourages us to improve our electrode design for long-term stimulation, and to continue to evaluate the clinical value of VCN stimulation for rehabilitation of the deaf.

POSTSCRIPT

After the initial 6-week period of hard-wired stimulation there was a failure of the system due to electrode breakage just under the skin. A new surface electrode was designed and manufactured and in a subsequent surgery, with the patient under local anesthesia, placed on the VCN area of the brainstem. After healing, the patient was fitted with an external analog stimulator device.

The patient's progress with her present VCN implant has been very similar to that seen with the CI patients. That is, after a period of several months with daily stimulation, she moved rapidly from the perception of sound as a periodic noise to sounds that have "natural" quality, are discriminable, and in some cases recognizable. Her present performance scores on our standard test battery are 8/24 word recognition and 20/24 stress recognition for the Monosyllable-Trochee-Spondee test. These scores are within the range of our CI patients.[31]

An indication of the value of this VCN implant for everyday communication can be seen in the speechreading scores obtained with and without auditory stimulation. The Utley Sentence Test Form A was presented at a distance of 1 m with and without auditory stimulation. For both conditions stimuli were spoken aloud but in one condition the electrical stimulator was turned off. The score for the vision only condition was 37/125, for the auditory plus vision condition the score was 84/125. Thus, at the present time there is no question of the benefit this device provides to this patient. Research is continuing with this patient to define more precisely the limits of perception and to devise more efficient methods of stimulation. A major effort is also underway to optimize the design of the electrodes used to stimulate the VCN.

REFERENCES

1. Hinojosa R, Lindsay JR. Profound deafness. Associated sensory and neural degeneration. Arch Otolaryngol 1980; 106:193-209.

2. Lindsay JR, Hinojosa R. The acoustic ganglion in profound sensorineural deafness. In: Naunton RF, Fernandez C, ed. Evoked electrical activity in the auditory nervous system. New York: Academic Press, 1978:301-21.

3. Linthicum FH Jr. Cochlear otosclerosis and other treatable sensori-neural hearing loss. Audiol Hear Educ 1976; 2:20-7.

4. Otte J, Schuknecht HF, Kerr AG. Ganglion cell populations in normal and pathological human cochleae. Implications for cochlear implantation. Laryngoscope 1978; 88:1231-46.

5. Johnsson LG, House WF, Linthicum FH Jr. Bilateral cochlear implants: histological findings in a pair of temporal bones. Laryngoscope 1979; 89:759-62.

6. Simmons FB, Mongeon CJ, Lewis WR, et al. Electrical stimulation of the acoustical nerve and inferior colliculus. Arch Otolaryngol 1964; 79:559-67.

7. Bebin JB. Pathophysiology of acoustic tumors. In: House WF, Luetje C, eds. Acoustic tumors. VI. Diagnosis. Baltimore: University Park Press, 1979; 45-83.

8. Dublin WB. Fundamentals of sensorineural auditory pathology. Springfield, Ill.: Charles C Thomas, 1976.

9. Adams RD. Occlusion of the anterior inferior cerebellar artery. Arch Neurol Psychiatr 1943; 49:765.

10. Gillilan LH. The correlation of the blood supply to the human brainstem with clinical brainstem lesions. J Neuropathol Exp Neurol 1964; 23:78.

11. Tsuchitani C. Lower auditory brain stem structures of the cat. In: Naunton RF, Fernandez C, eds. Evoked electrical activity in the auditory nervous system. New York: Academic Press, 1978:373-401.

12. Kane ES. Primary afferents and the cochlear nucleus. In: Naunton RF, Fernandez C, eds. Evoked electrical activity in the auditory nervous system. New York: Academic Press, 1978: 337-51.

13. Dublin WB. The cochlear nuclei revisited. Otolaryngol Head Neck Surg (in press).

14. Moore JK, Osen KK. The cochlear nuclei in man. Am J Anat 1979; 154:393-416.

15. Lorente de No R. Anatomy of the eighth nerve. III: Gen-

eral plan of structure of the primary cochlear nuclei. Laryngoscope 1933; 43:327-50.

16. Dublin WB. Cytoarchitecture of the cochlear nuclei. Arch Otolaryngol 1974; 100:355-9.

17. Linthicum FH Jr. Unusual audiometric and histologic findings in bilateral acoustic neurinomas. Ann Otol Rhinol Laryngol 1972; 81:433-7.

18. Spelman FA, Clopton BM, Pfingst BE, et al. Design of the cochlear prosthesis: effects of the flow of current in the implanted ear. Ann Otol Rhinol Laryngol 1980; 89 Suppl 66:8-10.

19. Levitt H. Adaptive testing audiology. In: Ludvigsen C, Barfod J, eds. Sensorineural hearing impairment and hearing aids. Scand Audiol 1978; Suppl 6:241-91.

20. Spelman FA. Biophysics of the implanted ear: electrical parameters. In: McPherson DL, ed. Advances in prosthetic devices for the deaf: a technical workshop. Rochester, NY: National Technical Institute for the Deaf, 1979:312-23.

21. Eddington DK, Dobelle WH, Brackmann DE, et al. Auditory prostheses research with multiple channel intracochlear stimulation in man. Ann Otol Rhinol Laryngol 1978; 87 Suppl 53:1-39.

22. House WF, Edgerton BJ. A multiple-electrode cochlear implant: preliminary test results. Presented at the West Coast Cochlear Prosthesis Conference, Seattle, Washington, 1980.

23. Harris JD. Pitch discrimination. J Acoust Soc Am 1952; 24:750-5.

24. Nordmark JO. Mechanisms of frequency discrimination. J Acoust Soc Am 1968; 44:1533-40.

25. Weir CC, Jesteadt W, Green DM. Frequency discrimination as a function of frequency and sensation levels. J Acoust Soc Am 1977; 61:178-84.

26. Simmons FB, Mathews RG, Walker MG, et al. A functioning multichannel auditory nerve stimulator: a preliminary report on two human volunteers. Acta Otolaryngol (Stockh) 1979; 87:170-5.

27. Dillier N, Spillmann T, Fisch UP, et al. Encoding and decoding of auditory signals in relation to human speech and its application to human cochlear implants. Audiology 1980; 19:146-63.

28. Walker MG. Technical Report No. 5306-4. Palo Alto, Calif: Integrated Circuits Laboratories, Stanford University, 1978.

29. Helmerich LF, Edgerton BJ. Psychoelectric measurements and results from cochlear implant patients. Ann Otol Rhinol Laryngol 1982; 91 Suppl 91:35-40.

30. Simmons FB, Walker MG, Mathews RG, White RL. Percepts and discrimination by auditory nerve stimulation: a summary of results and some proposals for nerve viability. In: McPherson DL, ed. Advances in prosthetic devices for the deaf: a technical workshop. Rochester, NY: National Technical Institute for the Deaf, 1979:271-4.

31. Thielemeir MA, Brimacombe JA, Eisenberg LS. Audiological results with the cochlear implant. Ann Otol Rhinol Laryngol 1982; 91 Suppl 91:27-34.

FIBROUS DYSPLASIA: A REVIEW OF THE DISEASE AND ITS MANIFESTATIONS IN THE TEMPORAL BONE

George T. Nager, MD
David W. Kennedy, MD
Ernest Kopstein, MD

DEDICATION

To my former teachers, Professor F. R. Nager, Professor E. Uehlinger, Professor L. Ruedi, Sir Terrence Cawthorne and Mr. C. S. Hallpike.

G.T.N.

CONTENTS

Introduction 5
Definition 5
Historical Background 6
Overall and Age Incidence 6
Sex Distribution 7
Localization and Distribution of Bone Lesions 7
Structural Changes and Skeletal Deformities 8
Skin and Mucosal Pigmentation 9
Fibrous Dysplasia in Association with Endocrinopathies 10
Fibrous Dysplasia in Association with Other Disorders 15
Neurological Symptoms 16
Radiological Aspects 16
Biochemical Data 18
Macroscopic Appearance 18
Microscopic Appearance 19
Sarcomatous Transformation 20
Familial Monostotic and Polyostotic Fibrous Dysplasia 22
Differential Diagnosis 22
Treatment 30
Prognosis 31
Review of Literature 31
Case Reports 36
Discussion and Conclusions 42
Summary 47

ACKNOWLEDGMENTS

I am indebted to the late Professor Edwin Uehlinger, Institute of Pathology, Zürich University School of Medicine, and to Georg Thieme Verlag, Stuttgart, for allowing me to reproduce their illustrations in Figures 1 and 2. My warmest thanks are extended to my colleagues Drs. Jack W. Bowerman and John Dorst of the Russell H. Morgan Department of Radiology for their assistance and generosity in letting me reproduce a number of their excellent roentgenograms. I wish to thank my colleague Dr. Bernard R. Marsh of the USPHS, Baltimore, and the Departments of Radiology and Pathology of that hospital for their permission to use the clinical records, roentgenograms and histologic sections of their patient for Figures 4 and 5. My special thanks are due Mr. Chester Reather, RBP, FBPA, Director of Photography, for his outstanding technical skill and unfailing care in the reproduction of the numerous roentgenograms and in the preparation of photographs and photomicrographs. I am very grateful to Dr. Jerome Taxy of the Department of Pathology for reviewing the chapter on histopathology and for his advice in the selection of the photomicrographs. I also want to thank Captain Vincent Hyams, Chief of Otolaryngic Pathology at the Armed Forces Institute of Pathology in Washington for his critical review of the manuscript and for his valuable recommendations. I wish to thank especially Professor E. Steinbach and Professor D. Plester, Department of Otolaryngology of Tübingen University School of Medicine, for their generosity in sending me their outstanding clinical and pathological material for review, and for their permission to include biopsies from two of their patients in Figures 43 and 44. In conclusion, I wish to express my sincere appreciation to Mrs. Patricia Edwards for her assistance in typing the manuscript.

G.T.N.

FIBROUS DYSPLASIA: A REVIEW OF THE DISEASE AND ITS MANIFESTATIONS IN THE TEMPORAL BONE

GEORGE T. NAGER, MD

DAVID W. KENNEDY, MD

ERNEST KOPSTEIN, MD

BALTIMORE, MARYLAND

Fibrous dysplasia is a fairly common, localized misdifferentiation of the bone-forming mesenchyme affecting a single or many bones, in which skeletal aberrations represent the cardinal feature, but in which certain endocrinopathies, abnormal pigmentation of skin and mucous membrane, and occasionally other abnormalities form part of the entire disease process. The craniofacial skeleton is one of its predilective sites and therefore the temporal bone may become involved. In such instances the disease manifests itself with 1) progressive loss of hearing, 2) increasing obliteration of the external ear canal, and 3) enlargement and distortion of the temporal bone. The first part of this communication is concerned with a review of the clinical and pathological aspects of the disease in general. The second part is concerned with a discussion of the clinical manifestations in the temporal bone, based upon an analysis of the entire literature and the authors' personal experience. The indications for surgical intervention include 1) maintenance of a normal outer ear canal, 2) preservation of cochlear and vestibular function, and 3) prevention of secondary complications.

INTRODUCTION

Fibrous dysplasia of bone is a disorder of unknown etiology, in which skeletal aberrations constitute the cardinal feature, but in which certain endocrinopathies, abnormal pigmentation of skin and mucous membrane, and, at times, other abnormalities, form part of the total disease process. Fibrous dysplasia is by no means a rare disorder. Although some of the clinical manifestations had been described earlier, the condition was not recognized as an independent disease entity until about four decades ago. In fibrous dyplasia a single bone, a few, or many bones may be affected. In the monostotic form of the disease, characterized by involvement of a single bone, a rib, the femur, the tibia, or a facial bone, especially a jaw bone, may be the site of a lesion. In the polyostotic form, in which several bones are affected, one limb, more often a lower extremity, may be the site of multiple bone lesions. Involvement of an upper limb is not uncommonly associated with lesions of the skull. Since the facial and cranial bones are among the predilective sites, and since their involvement may produce symptoms of disturbance and dysfunction, fibrous dysplasia becomes of particular interest to the otolaryngologist.

Some of the more recent clinical information about the disease is unfortunately scattered throughout the literature. In the first part of this communication, therefore, an attempt has been made for the convenience of the otolaryngologist to compile all pertinent data on the pathological and clinical aspects of fibrous dysplasia. The second part discusses the clinical manifestations of fibrous dysplasia as they involve the temporal bone. This investigation is based on a scrutinous review of all available published material and the careful examination and long-term observation of our own patients. The case histories of three are reported here in detail to portray the salient clinical features. The understanding of the mechanism and behavior of fibrous dysplasia enables the otolaryngologist to adopt a more meaningful treatment and to join in the search for its etiology.

DEFINITION

Fibrous dysplasia of bone is a fairly common, well-recognized, locally circumscribed, slowly progressive, benign disorder of fibro-osseous tissue of undetermined etiology. Normal bone, undergoing physiological resorption is replaced by an abnormal proliferation of an isomorphous fibrous tissue of spindle cells and poorly formed bony trabeculae of woven bone. The trabeculae have an irregular size, form and distribution. They display no orientation or apparent relation to the function of the affected cylindrical or flat bone. The disease may be considered as an arrest of bone maturation at the immature stage of woven bone,[1] as a disturbance of postnatal cancellous bone maintenance,[2] or as a misdifferentiation of the bone-forming mesenchyme.[3] This proliferation process may sooner or later extend beyond normal boundaries and give rise to expansion, distortion and structural weakness. Since it involves primarily the cancellous and seldom the cortical bone formation, a lesion replaces normal cortex by erosion from within but in most instances it is always covered with a shell, however thin, of normal cortical bone.

From the Department of Laryngology and Otology, Johns Hopkins University School of Medicine and Hospital, Baltimore. This study was supported by Grant 5 ROI-NS-02182-22 from the National Institute of Neurological and Communicative Disorders and Stroke, USPHS.

Fibrous dysplasia may affect a single, several or many bones but never all bones. Accordingly, monostotic, oligostotic and polyostotic forms are distinguished. The preferred sites include the diaphyses and metaphyses of long bones, ribs, pelvis, shoulder and craniofacial skeleton. The lesions tend toward a unilateral distribution. The monostotic form generally comes to an arrest at puberty, whereas the polyostotic form may progress beyond the third and even later decades. The initial clinical symptoms usually appear during the first decade of life. They include pain, deformity and repeated spontaneous fractures.

The McCune-Albright syndrome represents a special category of polyostotic fibrous dysplasia. It is characterized by extensive, circumscribed, predominantly ipsilateral skin pigmentations and precocious sexual development. Females are primarily affected. Fibrous dysplasia may be associated with additional endocrine disorders, particularly with hyperthyroidism.

Fibrous dysplasia may be observed in combination with nonendocrine diseases, such as hypophosphatemic vitamin D-resistant rickets or osteomalacia,[4] adamantinoma of the long bones,[5,6] paraosseous fibromas of the soft tissue,[7,8] and intraosseous and extraosseous arteriovenous aneurysms.[9,10] Sarcomatous dedifferentiation is a rare complication. The estimated incidence is about 0.5%.[11]

HISTORICAL BACKGROUND

The first description of the bone lesions was found by von Recklinghausen in 1891.[12] Elmslie[13] in 1914 discussed a case of a 6-year-old male with disseminated skeletal lesions and skin pigmentation in the back of the neck. Weil[14] in 1922 reported on a 9-year-old female with pigmented skin patches and precocious skeletal and sexual development, calling the condition an unusual variation of osteopsathyrosis. During the following years, evidence was increasing that despite some apparently common features, essential differences existed between hyperparathyroidism, or generalized osteitis fibrosa cystica (von Recklinghausen), and localized or disseminated osteitis fibrosa, soon to be recognized as fibrous dysplasia.[15] Jaffé[16] also acknowledged that the hitherto unrecognized disease entity differed from hyperparathyroidism and osteitis deformans Paget. Furthermore, it became obvious that this bone disease could sometimes be associated with certain extraskeletal manifestations. Freund and Meffert[17] reviewed the condition in 1936, under the heading of "fibrous osteodystrophy," and the year after, McCune and Bruch[18] in confirming the separate entity, used the term "osteodystrophia fibrosa." Albright and coworkers[19] in 1937 reported five cases of bone involvement associated with endocrine disturbances and pigmented patches in the skin, using the term "osteitis fibrosa disseminata." The authors realized its similarities to hyperparathyroidism and neurofibromatosis, but regarded it as a separate entity. The condition which thereafter has been known as "Albright syndrome" or "Albright triad," ie, polyostotic, predominantly unilateral bone lesions, precocious sexual development and skin pigmentation, had already been mentioned earlier by several investigators.[20-22] The polyostotic form of the disease associated with skin pigmentation but not accompanied by precocious sexual development had already been described by Hummel in 1934.[23] In 1938 Lichtenstein[24] reported eight cases with detailed studies of bone lesions. He proposed the term "fibrous dysplasia," or "polyostotic fibrous dysplasia" in the presence of multiple bone involvement. In 1942, Lichtenstein and Jaffé[3] added 15 more cases. By 1947, Schlumberger[25] had collected 67 cases of monostotic fibrous dysplasia. Thus the study of a sufficiently large clinical material during the first half of this century led to the general recognition of fibrous dysplasia as an independent entity which, from the standpoint of the pathologist, should probably be called more correctly "fibro-osseous dysplasia"[26-28] or "fibrous-osteodysplasia."[29]

Although recognized clinically as a distinct entity only in recent decades, fibrous dysplasia has affected the human skeleton for centuries. Several reports of the disease have appeared in the literature of paleontopathology. Wells[30] in 1963 described a polyostotic form of fibrous dysplasia in the skeleton of a seventh century Anglo-Saxon. A monostotic form of fibrous dysplasia involving the right temporal bone was discovered in the skull of an approximately 39- to 44-year-old male recovered from an archaeological site in the Monroe County of East Tennessee. It dates from the Late Mississippian period with a radiocarbon-derived date of AD 1,480 ± 130 (Geochrom GX-4205) and provides documentation of the antiquity of the disease in the southeastern portion of the United States.[31]

OVERALL AND AGE INCIDENCE

The fact that by 1971 the number of reported cases exceeded 1500[32] confirms that fibrous dysplasia is not an uncommon disease. Available data seem to indicate that the monostotic form acounts for about 70%, the polyostotic form without endocrine disturbances for about 30%, and the polyostotic form with endocrine disturbances (McCune-Albright syndrome) for about 3%.[29] The actual incidence of each form, however, cannot be assessed precisely since the monostotic form may remain asymptomatic only to be detected accidentally, and thus can often escape clinical detection. Even the polyostotic form may occasionally exist unnoticed for decades and present as an incidental finding. Sante et al,[33] McIntosh et al,[9] and Harris et al[34] reported such instances. Among them are two females, aged 43 and 57, who are typical examples of late discovery rather than late manifestation of the

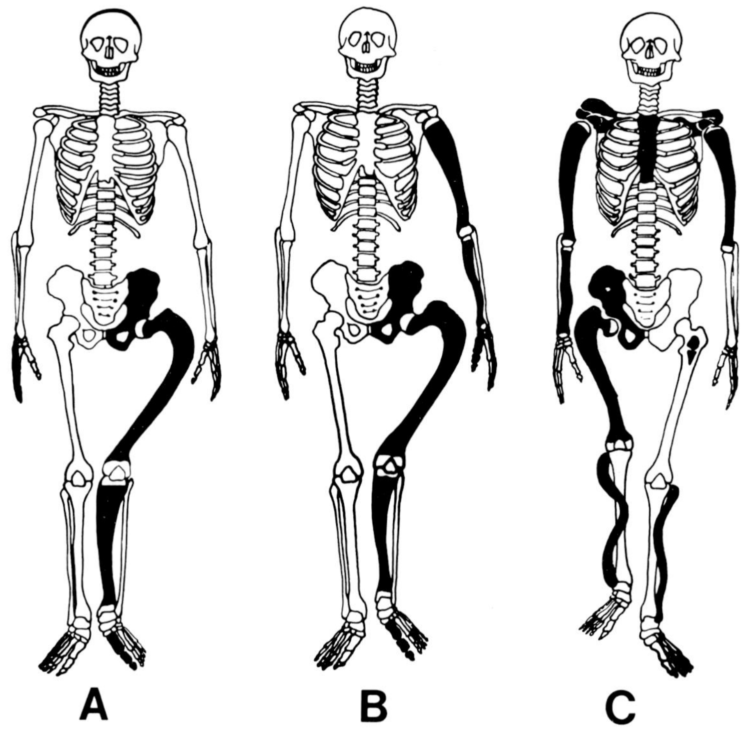

Fig. 1. Distribution patterns of polyostotic fibrous dysplasia. A) Monomelic, B) unilateral, C) bilateral distribution. (Reprinted with permission.[35])

disease.[35] Furthermore, there exists a general tendency to report primarily the more remarkable cases, namely examples of polyostotic disease.

Fibrous dysplasia generally makes its appearance in late childhood. Some severe forms, however, may manifest themselves in infancy (Fig. 16). Each form of the disease has a different average age of onset which varies slightly from clinic to clinic. One study, based upon 57 patients, showed that the monostotic form manifests itself initially around the age of 14, the polyostotic form without endocrine disorders around the age of 11, and the polyostotic form associated with endocrine disturbances around the age of 8.[36] Two other studies indicate a slightly earlier onset for the monostotic and polyostotic form of the disease.[34,37] Although it is not uncommon for certain lesions to be detected during later decades of life, there is good evidence that the majority, if not all bone lesions, develop during the period of skeletal growth.[3]

SEX DISTRIBUTION

A review of the earlier literature reveals a considerable variation in sex distribution. Lichtenstein[24] and Jaffé[26] found a higher incidence among females. Spjut et al[38] observed that among young adults more males than females were affected. According to Uehlinger,[35] monostotic and polyostotic fibrous dysplasia not accompanied by endocrine disorders reveal an even sex distribution. By contrast, polyostotic fibrous dysplasia with endocrine disorders (McCune-Albright syndrome) displays an obvious predilection for the female sex.

LOCALIZATION AND DISTRIBUTION OF BONE LESIONS

Fibrous dysplasia may present as a solitary lesion (monostotic form) or as multiple lesions in a single or in several bones (polyostotic form). The term oligostotic form is occasionally used for a very small number of lesions. Polyostotic fibrous dysplasia may be limited to a single limb (monomelic distribution), or may involve both sides of the skeleton (bilateral distribution, Fig. 1).

Monostotic Fibrous Dysplasia. A review of 269 patients with monostotic fibrous dysplasia collected from the literature[1,10,34,37,39-42] disclosed the skeletal locations shown in Figure 2A and Table 1. A survey by Eversole et al[43] of a large number of patients with monostotic fibrous dysplasia involving the jaws revealed that the maxilla was almost twice as frequently affected (64%) as the mandible (36%).

Polyostotic Fibrous Dysplasia. A review of 66 patients with polyostotic fibrous dysplasia not associated with endocrine disturbances collected from the literature[1,10,36,37,42,44-46] showed the instances of individual bone involvement as given in Figure 2B and Table 2. The polyostotic form distinguishes itself from the monostotic form by the following features: 1) in the extension of the skeletal involvement to the shoulder and pelvic girdle, and in the more frequent involvement of the craniofacial skeleton and vertebral column; 2) in the tendency to affect entire limbs; 3) in the severity of deformities which may lead to extensive crippling (ie, shepherd-crook deformity of the proximal femur); and 4) in the higher incidence of spontaneous and often recurrent fractures.[35]

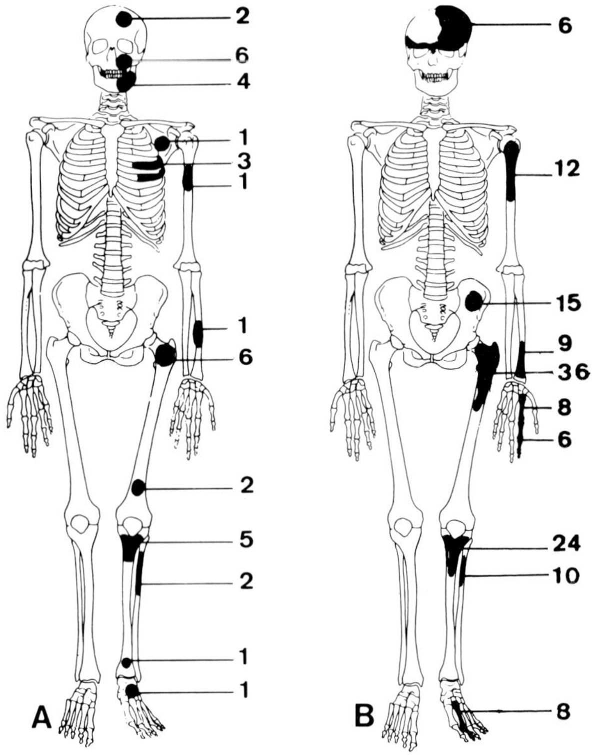

Fig. 2. Localization of A) monostotic and B) polyostotic fibrous dysplasia in 35 cases of monostotic and 36 cases of polyostotic disease from the Institute of Pathology in Zürich. (Reprinted with permission.[35])

The number of bones involved varies and may be very high. Hopf[47] describes a 43-year-old female, followed roentgenologically for more than 20 years, with 79 single lesions involving 75 bones. This represents about a 39% involvement of the entire skeleton. Occasionally, the involvement of a limb may display a certain "ray-pattern" characterized by affection of the metacarpal, proximal, middle and distal phalangeal bones, with the severity and number of lesions decreasing toward the periphery.[29] In some instances of monomelic distributions every bone of an entire extremity may be involved.

The incidence of craniofacial involvement is about 10% in monostotic disease, about 50% in polyostotic disease with moderate skeletal involvement, but reaches 100% in polyostotic disease with extensive skeletal involvement.[48] The disease seems to affect the neural and facial cranium with nearly equal frequency.[49]

TABLE 1. SKELETAL LOCATIONS OF MONOSTOTIC FIBROUS DYSPLASIA IN PATIENTS (N = 269)

Bone	*Instance (Times)*	*Bone*	*Instance (Times)*
Ribs	65	Fibula	7
Femur	45	Base of Skull	3
Tibia	36	Pelvis	3
Maxilla	33	Clavicle	3
Mandible	32	Tarsals	3
Calvaria	16	Zygoma	2
Humerus	11	Vertebrae	2
Radius and Ulna	7	Metatarsals	1

TABLE 2. INSTANCE OF INDIVIDUAL BONE INVOLVEMENT OF PATIENTS WITH POLYOSTOTIC FIBROUS DYSPLASIA (N – 66)

Bone	*Instance (Times)*	*Bone*	*Instance (Times)*
Femur	45	Calvaria	8
Skull	45	Scapula	6
Tibia	35	Sacrum	5
Humerus	22	Maxilla	4
Ribs	17	Metacarpals	4
Fibula	16	Carpals	3
Radius and ulna	15	Phalanges	2
Mandible	13	Metatarsals	2
Vertebrae	11	Tarsals	1

Van Tilburg[29] tried to determine the localization of skull lesions in monostotic and polyostotic disease by reviewing 144 patients from the literature. His observations disclosed the incidence shown in Table 3. It follows that the frontal and sphenoid bones are most often affected, frequently together, sometimes unilaterally, occasionally bilaterally, and that the temporal bones are afflicted in 18% of skull involvement. The majority of cranial lesions display an asymmetrical distribution.

The monostotic form is neither a forme fruste nor a precursor of the polyostotic form. So far there has been no report of a transition from a monostotic to a polyostotic manifestation of the disease. In spite of an identical histological appearance, the two forms distinguish themselves in their clinical course, in the tendency toward spontaneous fractures, in the frequency and severity of fracture deformities, and in the continuation of activity beyond the second decade of life.[35] It would, therefore, appear appropriate to regard the two forms as relatively independent clinical entities, a concept already suggested by Gibson and Middlemiss,[46] Hall and Warrick,[50] and Schlumberger.[25]

STRUCTURAL CHANGES AND SKELETAL DEFORMITIES

The progressive changes involving the osseous structure in fibrous dysplasia result in alteration of size, form and stability. The weight-bearing long bones tend to bend as the cortex becomes eroded from within. The ongoing replacement of cortical bone by tissue of diminished strength predisposes to recurrent spontaneous fractures (Figs. 7C and 31). The firm structure of the dense fibrous tissue on the other hand provides a certain amount of splinting

TABLE 3. INCIDENCE OF LOCALIZATION OF SKULL LESIONS IN MONOSTOTIC AND POLYOSTOTIC DISEASES[29]

Bone	*Instance (Times)*
Frontal	90
Sphenoid	72
Ethmoid	39
Parietal	32
Temporal	26
Occipital	14

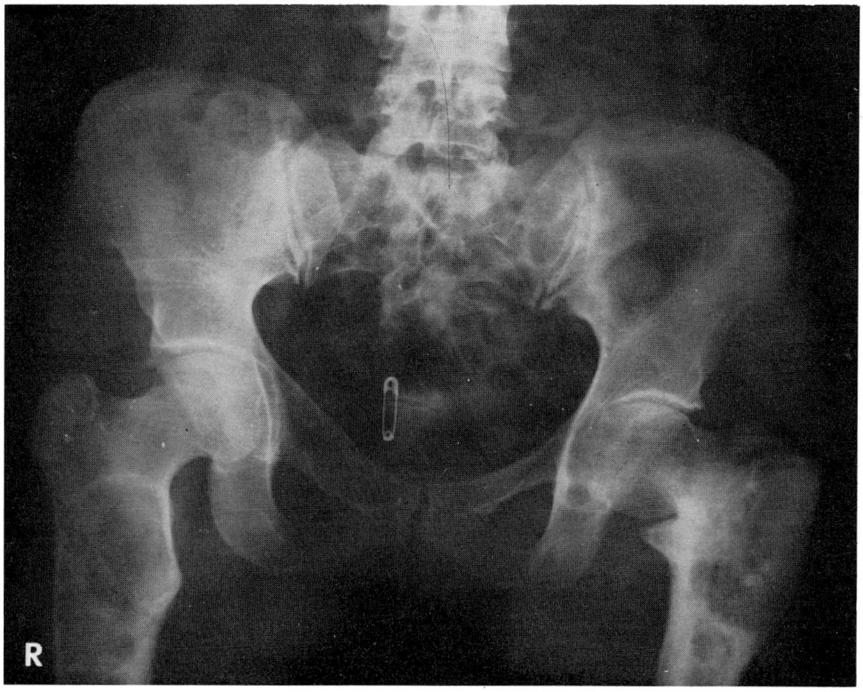

Fig. 3. Bilateral polyostotic fibrous dysplasia with involvement of the pelvis and both femora in a 45-year-old female. The extensive involvement of the femora resulted in the characteristic shepherd-crook or jug-handle deformity of their neck. (Courtesy of USPHS Hospital, Baltimore).

and, in preventing dislocation, enhances healing.[51] The proximal end of the femur is a predilective site of skeletal deformity. The outward bend of the neck, the inward protrusion of the acetabula and the association with coxa vara produce the pathognomonic shepherd-crook or jug-handle deformity (Figs. 3 and 32). A lesion invading the epiphysis, and subsequently interfering with bone growth, may result in shortening of a limb. Telescoping of a long bone is not an uncommon phenomenon. Occasionally the opposite may occur in that a lesion may actually produce lengthening of a cylindrical bone.[17,51-53] In a rare instance a lesion can reach enormous proportions to the extent that the enlargement of a single rib can obliterate half of the thoracic cavity,[49] or the involvement of the ethmoid and sphenoid bone can cause obstruction of the entire nasal cavity (Marsh B, Nager GT, personal observations) (Figs. 4A-C and 5A,B). Involvement of the occipital bone may give rise to the formation of the pathognomonic "occipital pug"[19] (Figs. 7A, 20A, and 26A). Asymmetrical enlargement and deformity of the cranial and facial bones may lead to unilateral cranial hyperostosis.[38] A symmetrical enlargement and deformity of the cranial and facial skull may lend the face a leonine appearance (Figs. 18 and 20A). Leontiasis ossea, however, occurs in a number of other skeletal disorders and is therefore not a specific feature of this disease.

SKIN AND MUCOSAL PIGMENTATION

Abnormal cutaneous pigmentation is the most common of the extraskeletal expressions of the disease. In the monostotic form, it is an occasional finding.[34,54-57] In the polyostotic form without endocrine disturbances, it is present in over 50% of patients. In the polyostotic form with endocrine disturbances, it is hardly ever absent.[29]

The pigmented areas are due to an increased amount of melanin in the basal cells of the epidermis. Their color varies from dark brown to café au lait, to yellow. They are not raised above the adjacent skin. They are generally distributed about the midline (Fig. 18). Their predilective sites are, in order of decreasing frequency, lower lumbar region, buttocks, back of the neck, shoulders, chest, face, scalp, hands, lips and oral mucosa, etc.[29] Their margins are irregular, their number is small, but their size may vary considerably. In Benedict's series[58] of 42 patients, their location generally coincided with the side of the skeletal involvement. Similarly, when the bone lesions are distributed bilaterally, so tend to be the skin pigmentations.[29] They are usually present at birth, but may develop later and precede the skeletal and endocrinological manifestations. The irregularity of their margins and the absence of the giant pigment granules in the malpighian cells or melanocytes differentiates them from very similar pigmented skin areas encountered in von Recklinghausen disease.[29]

An example of mucosal pigmentation on the undersurface of the lower lip is shown in Figure 6. It was observed in a 32-year-old female with McCune-Albright syndrome. The skeletal involvement was widespread and included the entire skull, spine, numerous ribs, pelvis, right scapula, humerus, radius and ulna, right femur, tibia and fibula, metacarpal, metatarsal, and phalangeal bones of both hands and feet. The patient had suffered numerous fractures involving ribs and limbs. Precocious sexual development was characterized by the onset of menstrual bleedings and breast

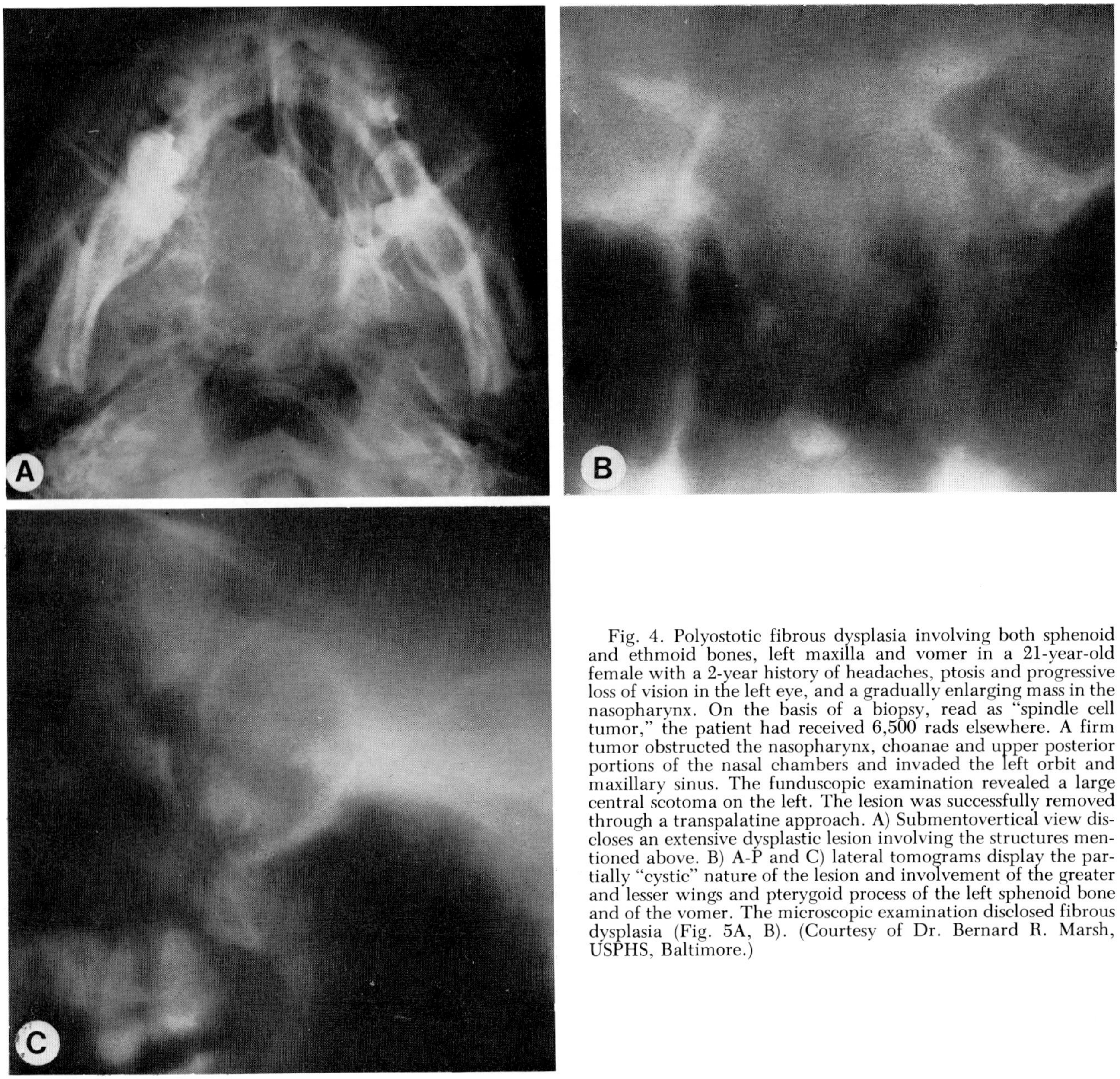

Fig. 4. Polyostotic fibrous dysplasia involving both sphenoid and ethmoid bones, left maxilla and vomer in a 21-year-old female with a 2-year history of headaches, ptosis and progressive loss of vision in the left eye, and a gradually enlarging mass in the nasopharynx. On the basis of a biopsy, read as "spindle cell tumor," the patient had received 6,500 rads elsewhere. A firm tumor obstructed the nasopharynx, choanae and upper posterior portions of the nasal chambers and invaded the left orbit and maxillary sinus. The funduscopic examination revealed a large central scotoma on the left. The lesion was successfully removed through a transpalatine approach. A) Submentovertical view discloses an extensive dysplastic lesion involving the structures mentioned above. B) A-P and C) lateral tomograms display the partially "cystic" nature of the lesion and involvement of the greater and lesser wings and pterygoid process of the left sphenoid bone and of the vomer. The microscopic examination disclosed fibrous dysplasia (Fig. 5A, B). (Courtesy of Dr. Bernard R. Marsh, USPHS, Baltimore.)

enlargement at the age of 6. Progressive obliteration of the left optic foramen by the fibrodysplastic process had resulted in total loss of vision in that eye. The serum alkaline phosphatase level was in excess of 115 units (normal: 10-32).

FIBROUS DYSPLASIA IN ASSOCIATION WITH ENDOCRINOPATHIES

McCune-Albright Syndrome. One of the earliest descriptions of polyostotic fibrous dysplasia associated with skin pigmentation and precocious sexual development was that of McCune and Bruch[18] in 1937 and McCune[20] in 1936. It concerned a 2-year-old female who displayed skin pigmentation, enlargement of the breasts and vaginal (menstrual) bleeding. Spontaneous fractures of the femur marked the appearance of skeletal manifestations at the age of 5. At 9, skeletal involvement was extensive and included the skull, vertebral column, hands and feet. Between 5 and 10, the patient had suffered 22 spontaneous fractures which had led to progressive crippling. The patient subsequently developed hyperthyroidism. A thyroidectomy induced regression of the hyperthyroidism but had no influence upon the skeletal lesions. Two years later, in 1938, Albright et al[19] described five patients with the triad of 1) polyostotic fibrous dysplasia, 2) extensive, predominantly ipsilateral, brown, nonelevated skin pigmentation, which tended to be on the side of greater skeletal involvement, and 3) precocious sexual development.

In the McCune-Albright syndrome, the skeletal involvement is characteristically polyostotic and

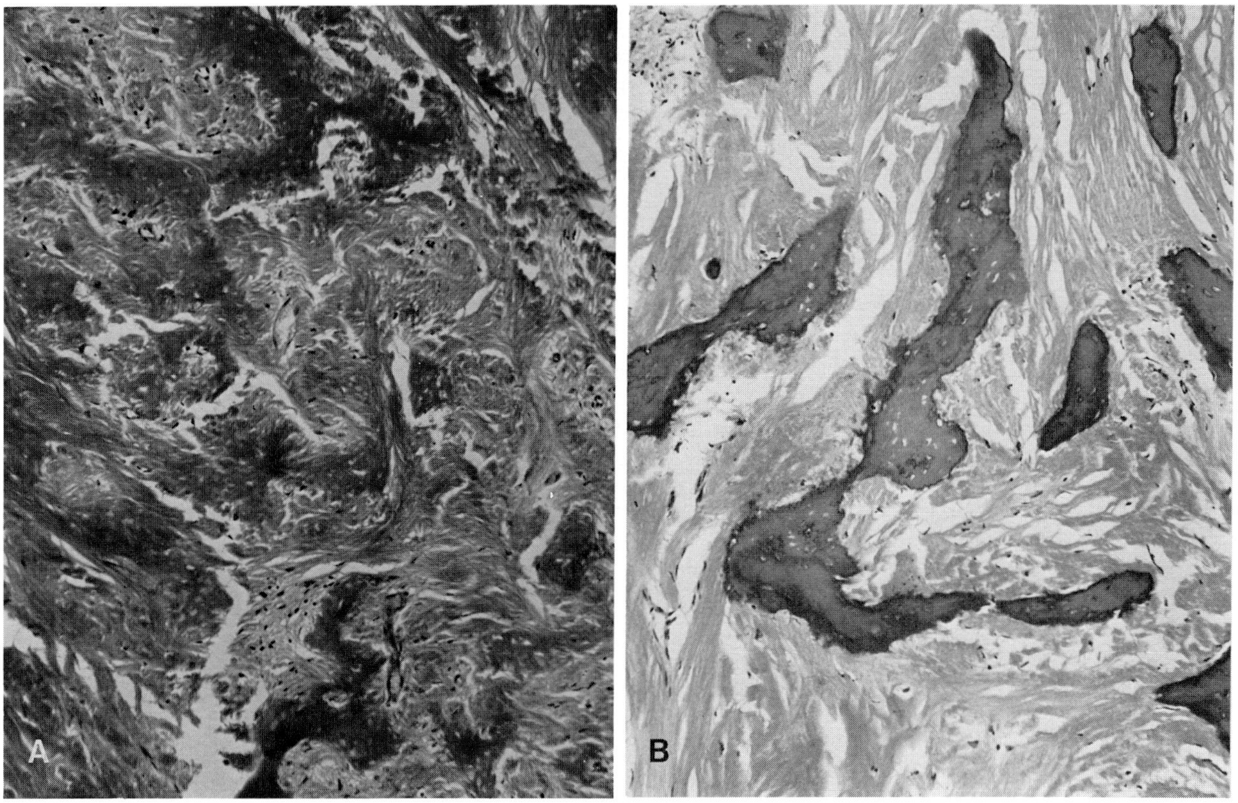

Fig. 5. A, B) Biopsy from the nasopharyngeal tumor of patient described in Fig. 4. Sections display areas of densely textured, acellular connective tissue containing tiny devitalized, in some areas (B) focally calcified, trabeculae of woven bone with irregular size and shape. Devitalization resulted from radiotherapy (6,300 rads). The morphology reflects a formerly live fibrodysplastic process. (H & E stain, x 150)

there is a tendency of the bone lesions toward unilateral distribution.[59] The area of skin pigmentation may be very large and affects primarily the neck, chest, back, shoulder and pelvic girdle.

The McCune-Albright syndrome is encountered almost exclusively in females. However, in 1966, Benedict[60] collected five cases of Albright syndrome in males and added one of her own. Figure 7 is an example of a 16-year-old male with bilateral polyostotic fibrous dysplasia, skin pigmentation, precocious sexual development, and acromegaly associated with a large pituitary adenoma and elevated growth hormone levels (male McCune-Albright syndrome).

Precocious sexual development manifests itself in females by premature occurrence of irregular menstrual bleedings at the age of 5 to 6, occasionally much earlier, and by the development of secondary sexual characteristics, with the latter usually following the former. In males the McCune-Albright syndrome is characterized by the early appearance of secondary sexual characteristics, gynecomastia, and occasionally by spermatogenesis. There is good evidence that the precocious sexual development represents true precocious puberty. Circulating levels of ovulatory luteinizing hormone (LH) have been identified in a female with McCune-Albright syndrome, and spermatogenesis with production of

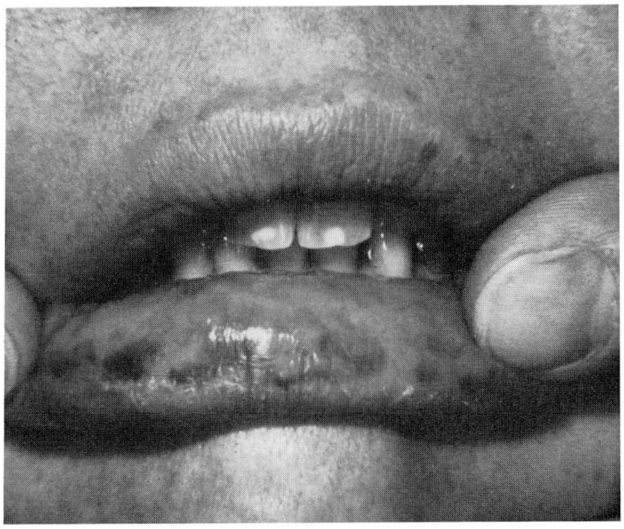

Fig. 6. Mucosal pigmentations on the undersurface of the lower lip in a 32-year-old female with McCune-Albright syndrome. Polyostotic fibrous dysplasia with widespread skeletal involvement (entire skull and spine, numerous ribs, pelvis, right scapula, humerus, radius and ulna; right femur, tibia and fibula, metacarpal-metatarsal, and phalangeal bones of both hands and feet. History of numerous fractures involving ribs and extremities. Skin and mucous membrane pigmentations (posterior neck and oral mucosa). Precocious sexual development (menarche and breast development at age 6). Alkaline phosphatase in excess of 115 I.V. (normal 10-32). Amblyopia left eye from fibrodysplastic obliteration of optic foramen. (Courtesy of Dr. L. Stefan Levin, Director Genetic Clinic, Department of Otorhinolaryngology.)

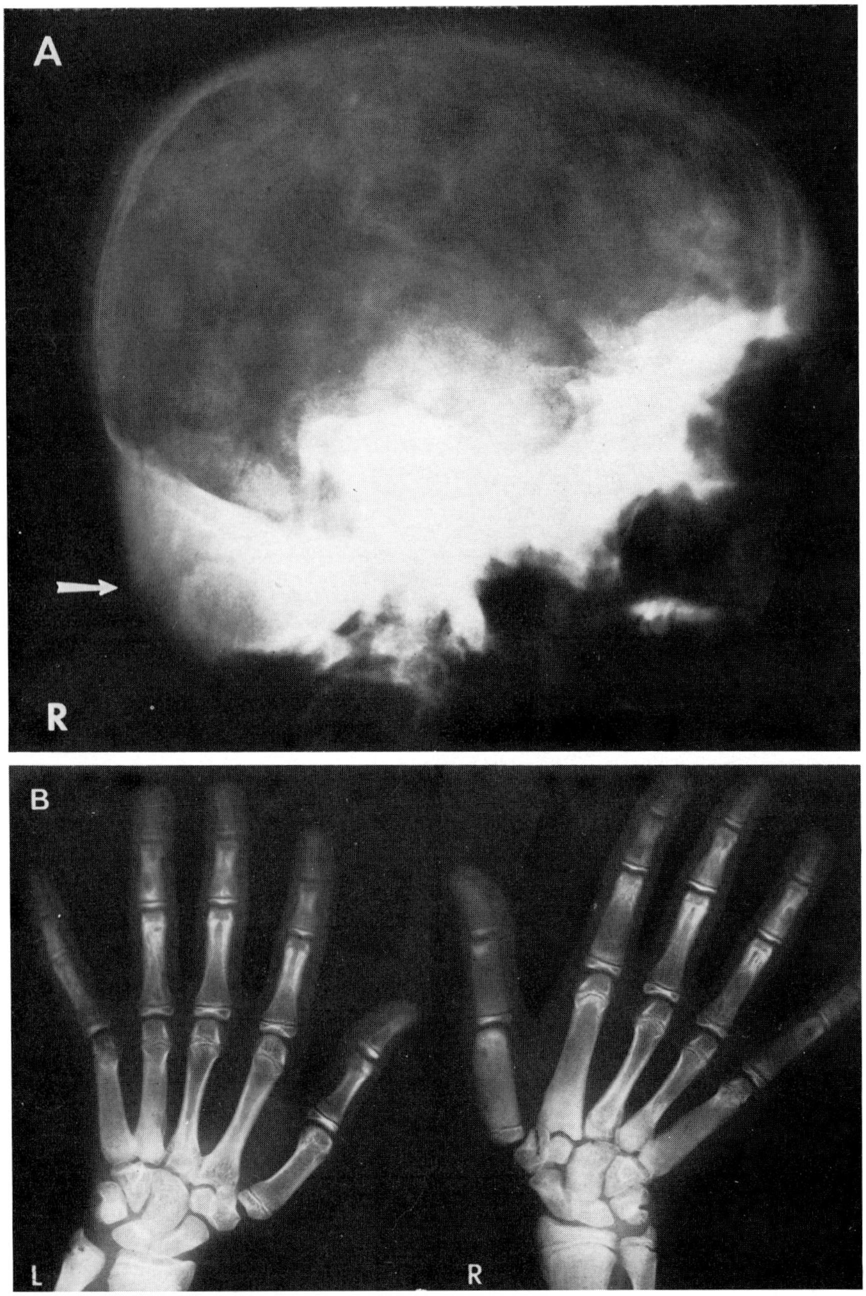

Fig. 7. Sixteen-year-old male with bilateral polyostotic fibrous dysplasia, skin pigmentation, precocious sexual development and acromegaly associated with a large pituitary adenoma and elevated growth hormone levels (male McCune-Albright syndrome). A) Massive thickening and sclerosis of the entire base of the skull, involvement of the right temporal bone, occipital pug (arrow) and enlargement of the sella are well recognized. B) Several of the metacarpal bones of both hands and the phalangeal bones of the right digits 1, 2 and 5 exhibit evidence of bone involvement.

spermatozoa, and mature Leydig cells, have been demonstrated on biopsy in a 6½-year-old male.[60]

Precocious sexual development may be accompanied by an accelerated skeletal growth, subsequently followed by premature closure of the epiphyses. In the unilateral distribution of the disease the abnormal skeletal growth is limited to the side of skeletal involvement. Adult patients with McCune-Albright syndrome, compared with healthy individuals of the same age, are therefore often of smaller stature.[35]

Association with Other Endocrinopathies. In addition to precocious sexual development, accelerated skeletal growth, and premature closure of the epiphyses, fibrous dysplasia may occasionally be associated with goiter and hyperthyroidism,[18] acromegaly,[9,61] Cushing disease,[62,63] extrainsular hypothalamic diabetes mellitus[64] and hyperparathyroidism.[10,58,60,65] The association of these endocrinopathies with fibrous dysplasia is encountered only with the polyostotic form. The incidence of hyperthyroidism and polyostotic disease is about 5%.[66] The thyroid dysfunction generally manifests itself a few years after the appearance of the skeletal lesions. One patient with polyostotic disease and hyperthyroidism also had blue sclerae.[67] The coexistence of polyostotic fibrous dysplasia and Cushing disease is rare.

The simultaneous occurrence of fibrous dysplasia and extrainsular hypothalamic diabetes mellitus is even less common.[64] The association of polyostotic

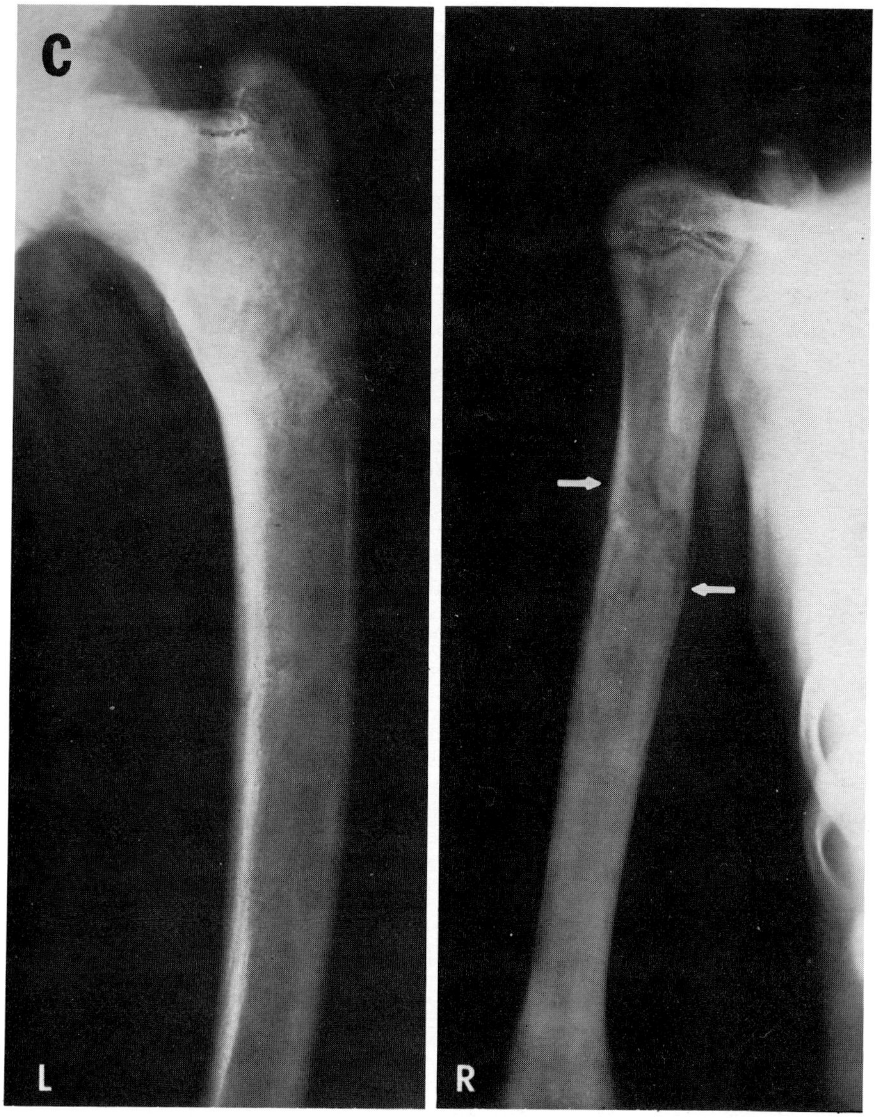

Fig. 7, cont'd. C) Extensive involvement of the left femur and right humerus resulted in a shepherd-crook deformity of the femur neck and a pathological fracture of the proximal humerus shaft (arrows). (Courtesy of Dr. Jack W. Bowerman, Russell H. Morgan Dept. of Radiology, Johns Hopkins Hospital, and the Genesee and Highland Hospitals, Rochester, NY.)

disease and acromegaly was described by Wortham and Hamblen[68] and Scurry et al.[61] Firat and Stutzman[10] observed the familial occurrence of craniofacial fibrous dysplasia and hyperparathyroidism in a mother and daughter. The mother, in whom the skeletal disease was limited to the mandible and maxilla, had two hyperplastic parathyroid glands and a chief-cell adenoma involving the third parathyroid gland. The daughter had fibrous dysplasia of the mandible and a 3-cm chief-cell adenoma of the left inferior parathyroid gland. With the exception of these two instances of familial hyperparathyroidism, all secondary endocrinopathies encountered in polyostotic disease could be traced to an anomaly or dysfunction of the hypothalamus.

It was Albright[69] who first suggested that stimuli arising in the hypothalamic-pituitary system mediate the abnormal release of pituitary hormones. Since then it has been recognized that the hypothalamus controls the function of the anterior lobe of the pituitary by the production of releasing hormones.[70] These releasing hormones are synthesized in specific areas of the hypothalamus and are stored in the median eminence. In response to appropriate stimuli they are released to reach the anterior lobe, where they initiate the synthesis and release of the organotropic hormones. A number of independent releasing hormones have so far been identified which increase release of TSH, corticotropin, LH, FSH and GH, and inhibit release of melanocyte-stimulating hormone and prolactin. Their structures as short-chain peptides have already been determined.[50]

In all of the endocrinopathies encountered in fibrous dysplasia, there is evidence of involvement of one or more anterior pituitary tropic hormones. The histologic evidence of glandular hyperplasia indicates stimulation of the pituitary from higher centers. Certain anomalies involving the hypothalamus have indeed been described in patients with fibrous dysplasia associated with endocrinopathies. Hall and Warrick's hypothesis[50] that endocrine

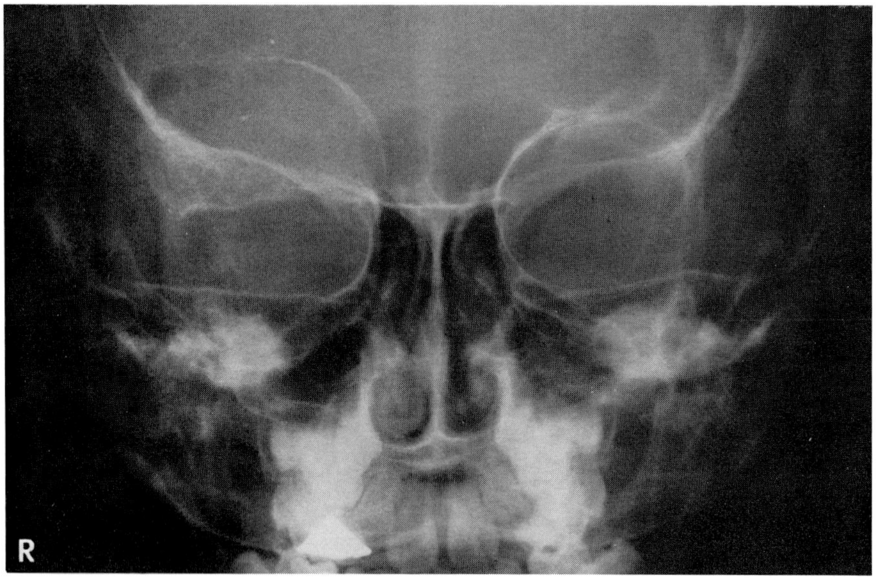

Fig. 8. Ten-year-old male with unilateral polyostotic fibrous dysplasia of the right frontal and sphenoid bones leading to secondary involvement of the right orbit. (Courtesy of Dr. John Dorst, Russell H. Morgan Dept. of Radiology, Johns Hopkins Hospital.)

manifestations in fibrous dysplasia are the result of a hitherto undetermined disorder of the hypothalamus, which leads to overproduction of certain releasing hormones, becomes very attractive. Precocious sexual development would correspond to an increased release of LRH, enlargement of the thyroid and hyperthyroidism to an overproduction of TSH, acromegaly to an overproduction of growth-hormone-releasing hormone (GRH), Cushing syndrome to an overproduction of corticotropin-releasing hormone (CRH), and acceleration of skeletal growth and maturation could possibly be associated with a minor overproduction of several releasing hormones. There is already existing clinical evidence that one form of hyperthyroidism is associated with a chronic overproduction of TSH and an enlargement of the pituitary fossa.[71,72] Similarly in some patients with acromegaly, an associated dysfunction of the hypothalamus has been identified.[73] Microscopic and histochemical investigation of that area of the hypothalamus related to the pituitary gland in patients with fibrous dys-

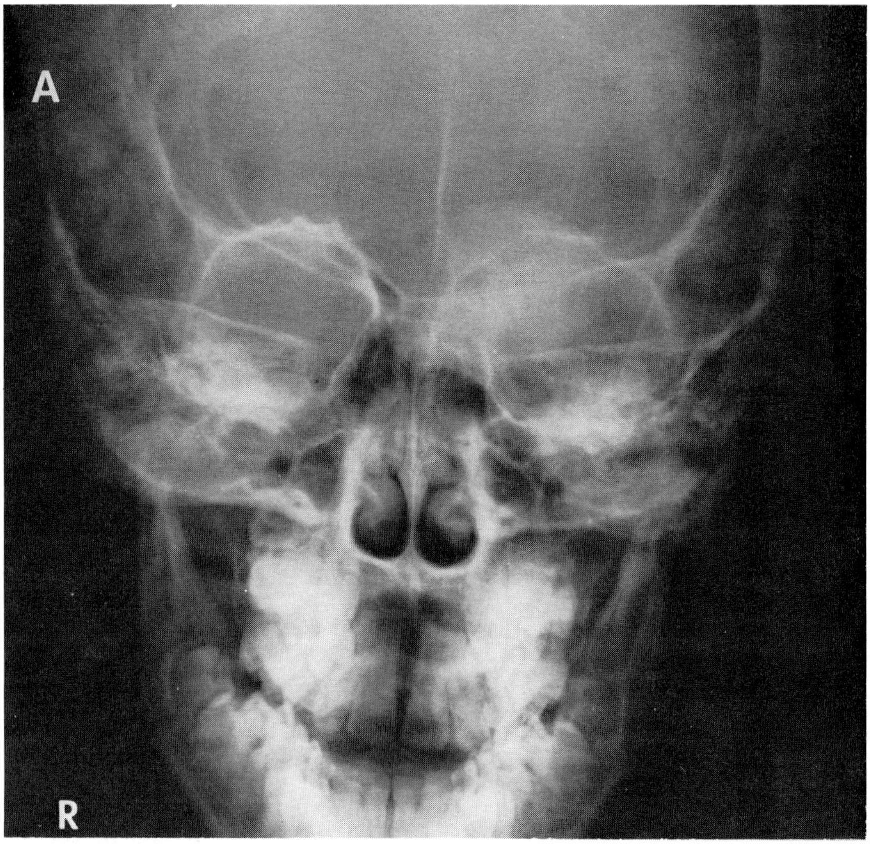

Fig. 9. Unilateral polyostotic fibrous dysplasia of the left frontal and ethmoid bone in a 9-year-old male. A) The lesion has a uniform ground-glass appearance.

plasia and endocrine disorders thus becomes of great significance.

FIBROUS DYSPLASIA IN ASSOCIATION WITH OTHER DISORDERS

A rare associated disorder is the vitamin D-resistant hypophosphatemic osteomalacia or rickets. This condition follows rather than precedes the bony lesions. It manifests itself in childhood or adolescence with skeletal pains, broadening of the epiphyses, and elevation of the renal phosphate clearance, a decrease in serum phosphate, and the presence of osteoid seams in bone biopsies. The surgical resection of the osseous lesions, which are suspected to synthesize a hormone influencing the renal phosphate clearance, induces healing of the rickets.[4]

Polyostotic fibrous dysplasia may occasionally be associated with extraskeletal tumors, such as multiple intramuscular fibromyxomas.[7,8,74] Cohen et al[5] and Johnson[6] reported on the simultaneous occurrence of adamantinoma of long bones and fibrous dysplasia. The combination of fibrous dysplasia and osteitis deformans Paget was mentioned by Daves and Yardley.[75] Gatewood and Esterly[76] reported the

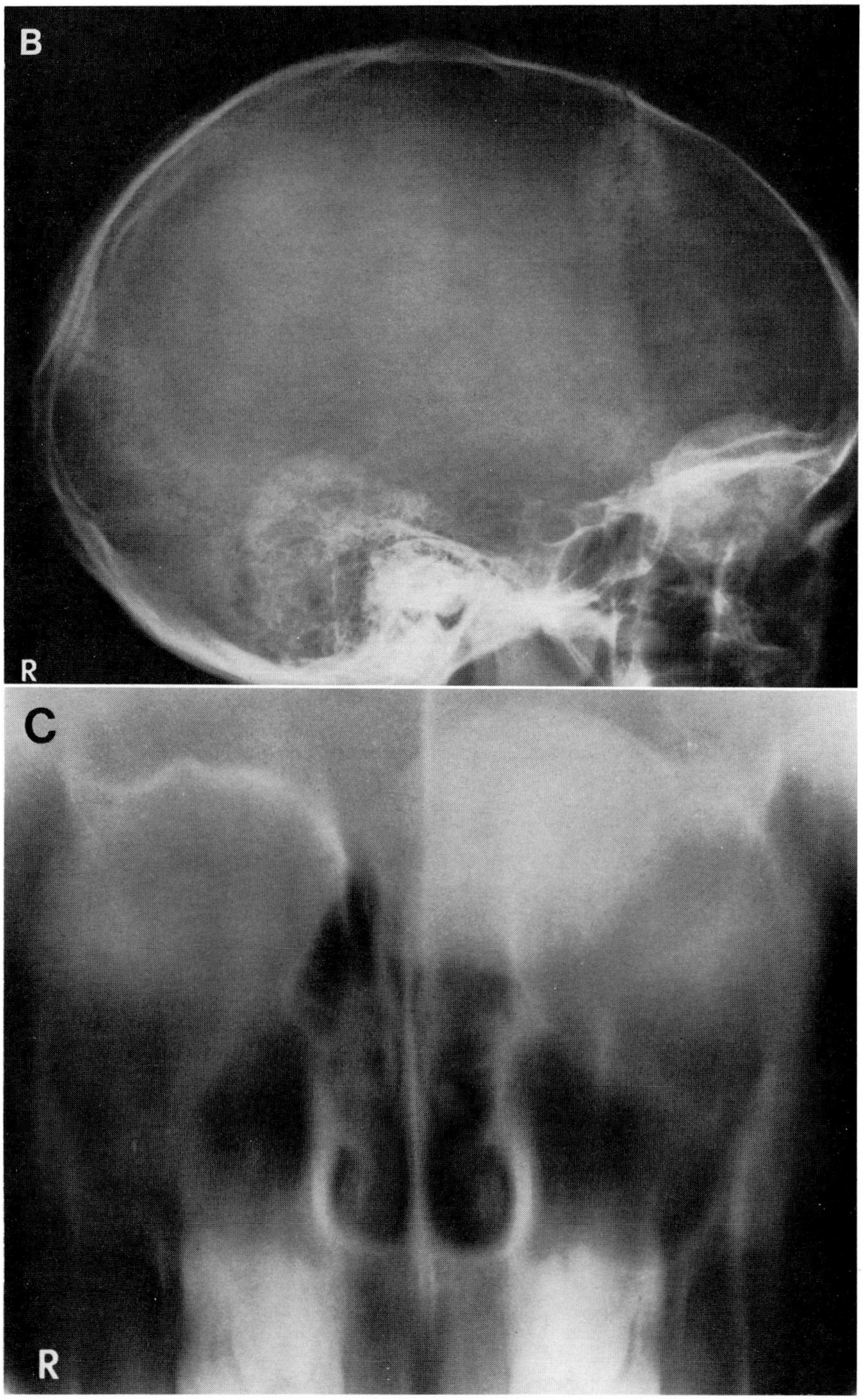

Fig. 9, cont'd. Extension into the left B) anterior cranial fossa, C) orbit and ethmoid sinus, and involvement of the cribriform plate. (Courtesy of Dr. John Dorst, Russell H. Morgan Dept. of Radiology, Johns Hopkins Hospital.)

coexistence of eosinophilic granulomas and fibrous dysplasia.

The presence of arteriovenous shunts in the osseous lesions was first recognized by Stauffer et al,[77] and subsequently confirmed by McIntosh et al,[9] and Fischer et al.[78] McIntosh et al[9] and Firat and Stutzman[10] also observed their extraosseous occurrence. Widespread shunting of that nature may in turn lead to a high output cardiac failure.

NEUROLOGICAL SYMPTOMS

The neurological symptoms in fibrous dysplasia are for the most part caused by a lesion involving an adjacent bone of the skull or spinal column. A deformity of the neural and facial cranium should raise the suspicion of an underlying neurological deficit. Involvement of the frontal, ethmoid, nasal and sphenoid bone may lead to invasion and distortion of the orbit which can result in lateral or inferior displacement of the globe, exophthalmus and hypertelorism[19,51,71,79] (Figs. 4, 8, and 9). Diplopia may be a manifestation of nerve involvement or of mechanical interference with globe mobility. Of Sassin and Rosenberg's[80] 50 patients with cranial fibrous dysplasia, 10 revealed involvement of the optic canal and in 3 of them the involvement was bilateral. All had significant visual symptoms, often severe and of long duration. Blurred and failing vision, scintillating and central scotomas, diplopia and optic nerve atrophy comprised the ophthalmological findings. The funduscopic examination may show varying abnormalities ranging from slight venous congestion to pronounced papilledema and nerve atrophy.[81,82] Pressure upon the optic chiasm may lead to a variety of bilateral impairments of the visual field. Involvement of the cribriform plate may produce hyposmia or anosmia.[48,83] Similarly involvement of the internal auditory canal and of the otic and vestibular capsule can cause tinnitus, sensorineural hypacusis and disturbance of vestibular function.[80,84,85]

Involvement of the spinal cord or nerve roots is evidence of vertebral localization of the disease. The cervical and dorsal spine are the predilective locations (Fig. 10). Varying degrees of paraplegia have been observed associated with a compression fracture or an expanding lesion in a vertebral body, vertebral arch, or an articular process.[55,86-89]

Mental retardation has been seen in association with fibrous dysplasia by several investigators. It is thought to be more than just a coincidental finding. This is exemplified for instance by the case history of a male who developed generalized seizures at 5 months, displayed evidence of severe mental deficiency at 9 months, could never stand, walk or talk, and developed skeletal deformities at the age of 3 years. At 5 he was obviously microcephalic, of short stature and exhibited extensive, disseminated bone lesions, skin pigmentation and thyromegaly. At autopsy the brain disclosed marked generalized atrophy involving particularly the frontal and parietal lobes. Disorganization of the cytoarchitecture and various cell anomalies in different regions of the cortex were the striking observations on microscopic examination. Most instances of mental retardation have been associated with the more extensive forms of the disease. Since there has been no confirmed correlation between narrowing of the intracranial space and impairment of intellectual faculties, some investigators consider mental retardation a cause of primary cerebral involvement rather than a secondary manifestation of the disease.[83] The same may apply to seizure disorders and muscular hypotonia which has been observed in association with mental retardation in fibrous dysplasia.[19,90,91]

Fries' observation[49] of schizophrenia in two patients with extensive involvement of the frontal bone, in each of whom the bone involvement preceded the abnormal behavior by many years, raises the thought of a possible correlation. Similar observations of mental disturbances suspected to have resulted from pressure by newly formed bone upon the frontal lobes leading to secondary cerebral atrophy have been made in osteitis deformans Paget. Dull and nonthrobbing headaches are frequent complaints in patients with fibrous dysplasia involving the skull.

RADIOLOGICAL ASPECTS

Monostotic fibrous dysplasia presents itself initially in a long bone generally in the proximal metaphysis where it appears as a unicameral, "cyst-like" radiolucency, demarcated from the epiphysis and diaphysis, with a slightly bulging, thinned, but usually intact wall (Fig. 11). The distention results from erosion from within. Occasionally the disease may manifest itself as a conglomerate of round or ovoid "cysts" with sclerotic margins and a tendency towards spindle-shaped expansion. In a rare instance, the lesion may appear in the diaphysis as a chestnut-like, smooth-walled radiolucency, whose margins, as it grows, display increasingly sharper demarcation. As the diaphysis becomes progressively distended, the enlarging marrow space begins to show a certain subdivision by the development of endocortical ridges. The replacement of the original cancellous bone by the fibro-osseous tissue lends the lesion characteristic "smoky," "ground-glass," or fine granular appearance (Fig. 12). The resulting structural weakness predisposes to spontaneous fractures (Fig. 13A). Eventually a certain remodeling of the original bone may take place. In this phase the remaining cortical bone displays a certain axial lamellar splintering and incorporation of rows of thread-like spongiosa along lines of pressure and traction (Fig. 14B). The disease process then be-

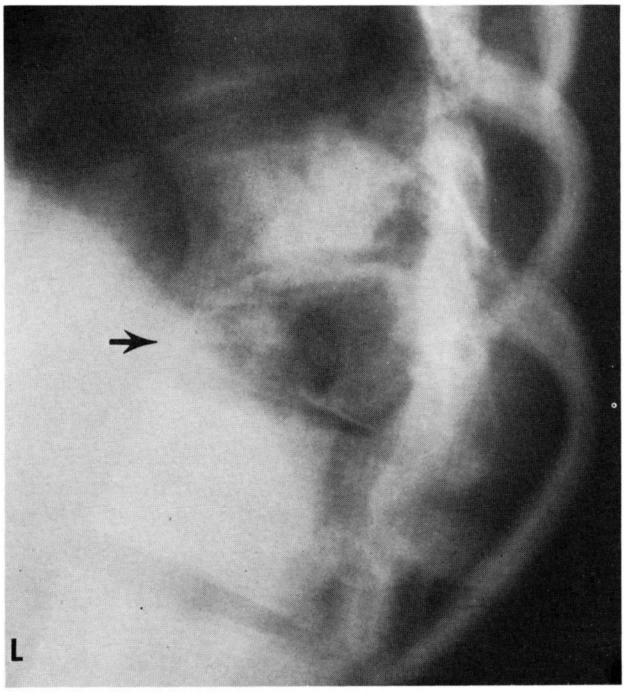

Fig. 10. (Case 2) Involvement of 12th thoracic vertebra in a 42-year-old male with bilateral polyostotic fibrous dysplasia associated with skin pigmentation and hyperthyroidism. Collapse of the vertebral body (arrow) required a spinal fusion.

comes indistinguishable from osteitis deformans Paget.[35]

Polyostotic fibrous dysplasia frequently involves the entire shaft of a cylindrical bone (Fig. 13A). Progressive erosion of cortical bone up to the outer "general lamella" with replacement of fibro-osseous tissue, persistent overload and stress upon the structurally weakened bone, and recurrent pathological fractures ultimately lead to the characteristic bony deformities. The shepherd-crook deformity of the proximal femur with the elevation of the greater trochanter, the anterior bowing of the tibia and the serpentine torsion of the fibula, and the bending and cracking of the humerus are typical examples of structural alterations encountered in polyostotic disease (Figs. 3, 7C, 31, 32 and 35). Telescoping of a cylindrical bone results in shortening of the shaft and widening of the marrow space. Severe bending of a cylindrical bone may produce incomplete and radial clefts.[35] This distortion of long bones is usually more pronounced in the lower extremities.

In polyostotic disease the ribs are less commonly involved. Often more than one rib is affected (Fig. 29). Involvement may be unilateral or bilateral, and the distribution may be asymmetrical. The lesion generally produces a spindle-shaped multicystic expansion which can reach 1-15 cm in length. It protrudes primarily into the thoracic cavity. An unusually large process can lead to compression of an entire lung. In general most rib lesions remain asymptomatic, only to be detected incidentally during a routine chest film or after a spontaneous fracture.

The pelvis, scapulae, vertebrae, flat and short bones generally exhibit a "polycystic" pattern. In the pelvis, like elsewhere in the skeleton, the disease tends toward unilateral distribution, and often one side is much more severely involved. Involvement of the whole pelvis may give rise to extreme distortion of its entire architecture with inward protrusion of the acetabula (Fig. 32). At times, however, a relatively extensive process in the ileum may remain asymptomatic.

The metacarpal, metatarsal and phalangeal bones are infrequently afflicted, but when affected, are usually involved in their entirety. In such instances they exhibit distention, cortical thinning and a uniform "ground glass-like" texture (Figs. 7B and 13B).

Based on their roentgenological appearance, three forms of craniofacial involvement may be distinguished:[10,49,92] 1) pagetoid, 2) sclerotic, 3) "cystic." The pagetoid form accounts for about 56%, the sclerotic for about 23%, and the cystic for about 21%.[49]

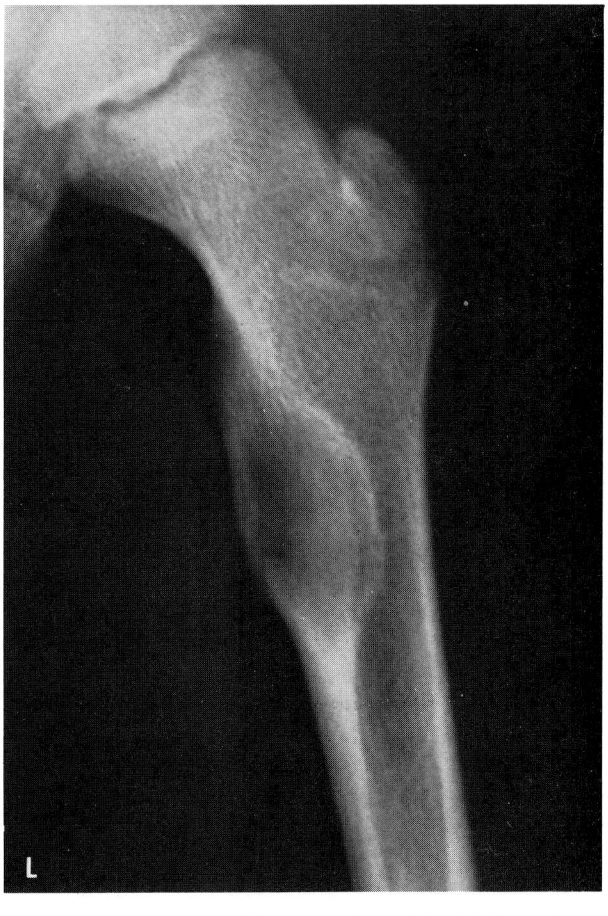

Fig. 11. Monostotic fibrous dysplasia of the left femur in a 5-year-old male. Slightly eccentric localization and cortical thinning are well recognized. (Courtesy of Dr. Jack W. Bowerman, Russell H. Morgan Dept. of Radiology, Johns Hopkins Hospital and Harford Memorial Hospital, Havre de Grace.)

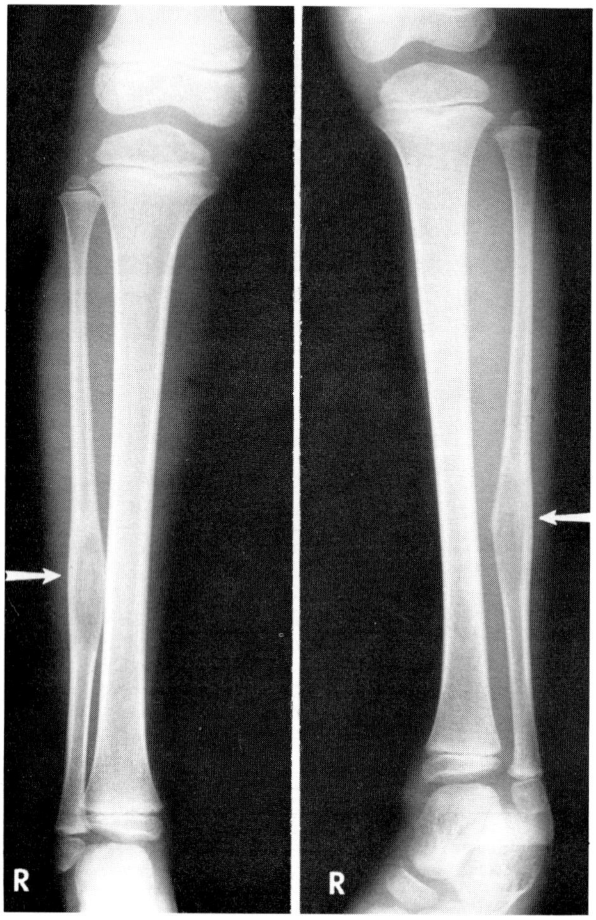

Fig. 12. Monostotic fibrous dysplasia of the right lower fibula in a 6-year-old female. Asymptomatic until kicked by brother. Subsequently developed swelling and pain. Expansile radiolucent lesion displays marked cortical thinning, a ground-glass pattern, and includes a pathological fracture (arrows). (Courtesy of Dr. John Dorst, Russell H. Morgan Dept. of Radiology, Johns Hopkins Hospital.)

The pagetoid form of fibrous dysplasia is usually an expression of polyostotic disease. The calvaria may be increased in thickness by several centimeters. The external table of the frontal and parietal bone often displays a unilateral bubble-shaped distention. The internal table is enlarged toward the diploe and the cranial cavity. The broadened calvaria displays localized and diffuse areas of radiolucency and increased density side by side. This coexistence of bone resorption and sclerosis strongly resembles the roentgenological appearance of osteitis deformans Paget (Fig. 26A). The base of the skull is usually quite enlarged and sclerotic. The sclerosis may extend from the frontal to the occipital bone. The enlargement of the external table can give rise to frontal bossing and the formation of an "occipital pug" (Figs. 7, 20A, and 26A). Remodeling of the base may in a rare instance lead to basilar impression. The sella turcica may remain unaffected. The facial bones may become involved to a varying degree. This involvement in turn may produce progressive narrowing of orbital and nasal cavities and obliteration of the paranasal sinuses (Figs. 15A, 17, 21B,D and 26A,B).

The sclerotic form of fibrous dysplasia is often accompanied by hyperostosis of the maxilla (Figs. 14A, 15A, 20, and 21), which may cause distortion of the teeth and constriction of nasal and sinus cavities. The maxilla, as mentioned earlier, is more often involved than the mandible, and its involvement usually is an expression of monostotic disease. The lesion may exhibit a "ground-glass" or dense sclerotic pattern. By contrast a mandibular lesion is more often encountered in polyostotic disease and generally appears as a solitary, smooth-walled, radiolucent defect.

The cystic form of fibrous dysplasia is characterized by solitary or multiple circular or rosette-like defects in the calvaria. Most of them are surrounded by a thin sclerotic margin. A defect may reach several centimeters in diameter. A solitary lesion may mimic an eosinophilic granuloma, and multiple defects may be mistaken for Hand-Schüller-Christian disease. As would be expected, more than one roentgenological form of craniofacial fibrous dysplasia may occasionally be encountered simultaneously in one individual.[49]

There are no radiological characteristics which would permit a differentiation between polyostotic fibrous dysplasia with or without one or several specific endocrine disorders.

BIOCHEMICAL DATA

In Pritchard's series[51] of 124 patients with predominantly polyostotic disease, serum calcium was elevated to 11-13 mg% in 25% of patients and serum phosphate to 5-6 mg% in 11% of patients. Van Horn et al[36] found an elevation of serum alkaline phosphatase in 25% of monostotic and 67% of polyostotic disease. According to Uehlinger,[35] the serum calcium may vary between 9.2-12.2 mg% and the serum phosphate may fluctuate between 2-5 mg%. During periods of exacerbation of the disease or consolidation of a spontaneous fracture, the serum alkaline phosphatase is expected to be elevated.

MACROSCOPIC APPEARANCE

Fibrous dysplasia involving the rib manifests itself as a fusiform or spherical enlargement with a surface of thin, intact, cortical bone. It may measure up to several centimeters in diameter. On a longitudinal section, the cancellous bone has been replaced by a yellowish-white, resilient tissue which occasionally includes small cysts filled with an amber fluid. The transition to normal bone is often abrupt. A cross section of a tubular bone with a fibrous dysplastic lesion generally reveals a widening of the shaft, and a thinning of the cortex (Figs. 11 and 12). The expansion resulted from eccentric erosion of the medulla and subsequent replacement by

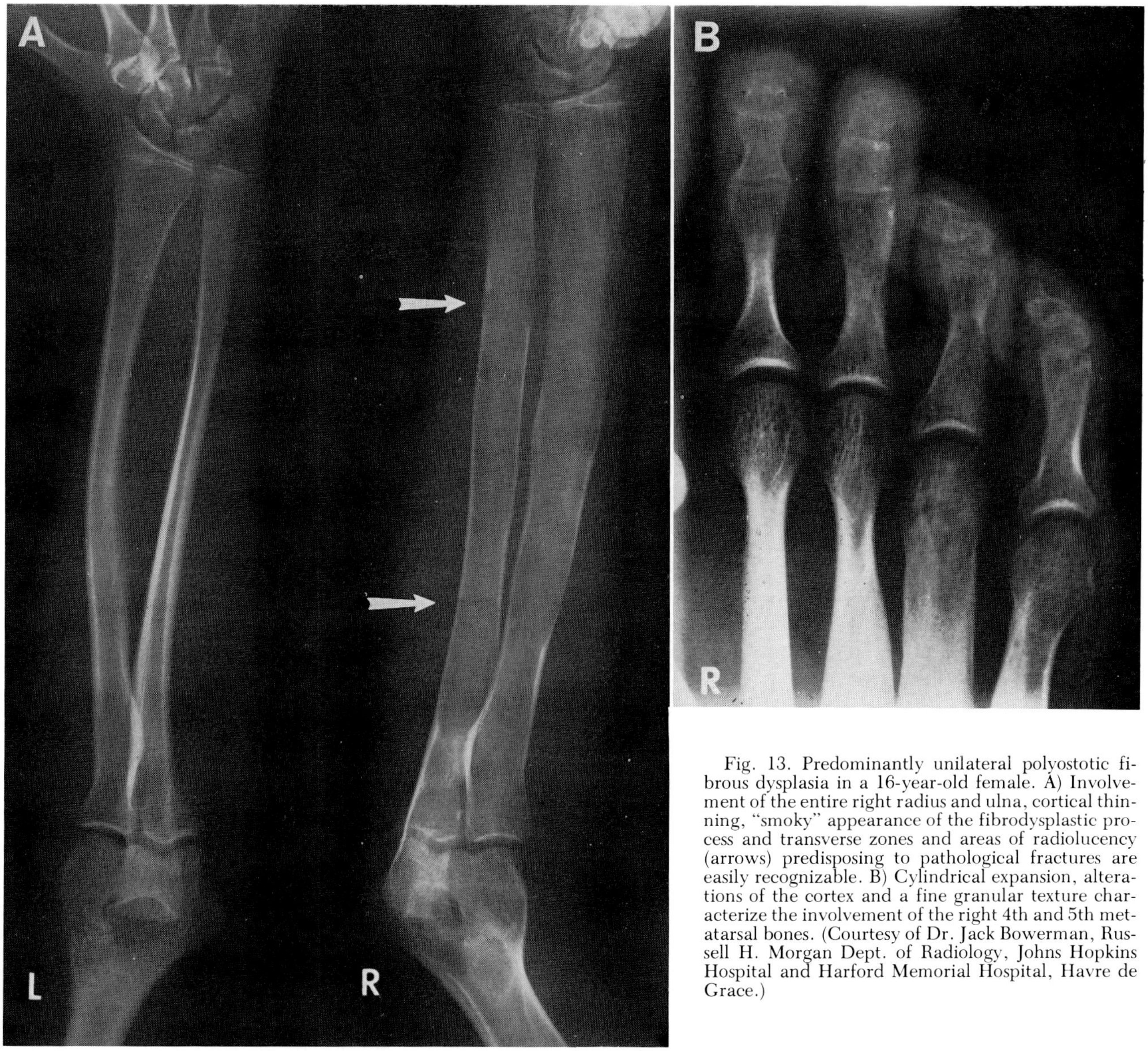

Fig. 13. Predominantly unilateral polyostotic fibrous dysplasia in a 16-year-old female. A) Involvement of the entire right radius and ulna, cortical thinning, "smoky" appearance of the fibrodysplastic process and transverse zones and areas of radiolucency (arrows) predisposing to pathological fractures are easily recognizable. B) Cylindrical expansion, alterations of the cortex and a fine granular texture characterize the involvement of the right 4th and 5th metatarsal bones. (Courtesy of Dr. Jack Bowerman, Russell H. Morgan Dept. of Radiology, Johns Hopkins Hospital and Harford Memorial Hospital, Havre de Grace.)

connective tissue. The connective tissue is firm and rubbery and includes irregularly disseminated bone spicules. Occasionally foci of myxomatous tissue, cystic spaces, small hemorrhages, and rarely islands of cartilage may be incorporated.[3] Lesions in the base of the skull or maxilla generally possess a firmer consistency than those in the ribs or long bones because they include a greater amount of bone spicules. Skull lesions, therefore, commonly produce a much greater radiodensity and display extensive sclerosis (Figs. 14A and 15B). The reduced amount of bone spicules in dysplastic lesions of ribs and cylindrical bones, on the other hand, results in an obvious radiolucency.[38] A small lesion will not affect the external appearance of a bone. A larger lesion through erosion and expansion attenuates the cortex of a tubular or flat bone, causes it to bulge (Figs. 11 and 12), and, in a rare instance, may even destroy it. As a rule, the fibrous tissue may be readily cut with a knife. Its content of poorly ossified bone spicules lends it a certain elastic gritty consistency, comparable to sand embedded in putty. The cut surface of a dysplastic lesion in general reveals a grayish or whitish color and considerable variation in vascularity.

MICROSCOPIC APPEARANCE

A representative lesion of monostotic or polyostotic fibrous dysplasia exhibits in general a fairly characteristic picture, and the identification of the disease process therefore presents no major difficulties. Irregular trabeculae of woven bone varying in size, shape and distribution, without apparent functional orientation, are embedded in a loosely or densely textured, cellular and vascular connective tissue stroma. This histologic appearance is the end result of a probable metaplasia of proliferating connective tissue.[38] The configuration of the trabeculae varies greatly. In many it is spherical. This lends them, on a cross section, a curved, C-shaped or

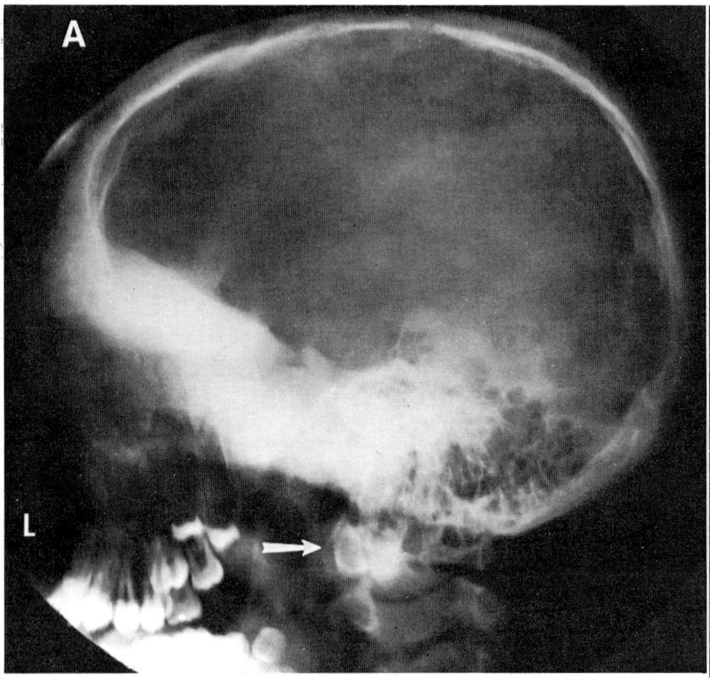

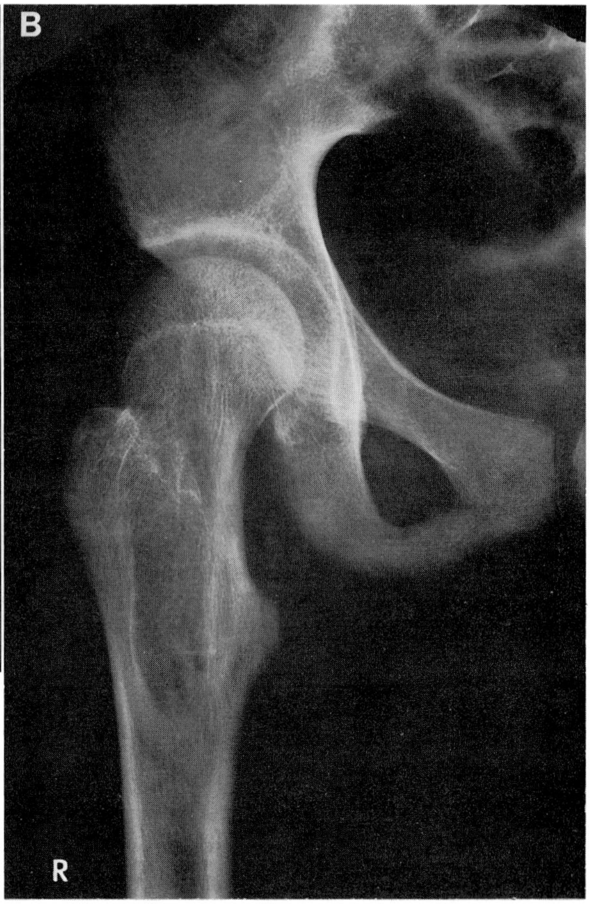

Fig. 14. Polyostotic fibrous dysplasia in a 10-year-old female with a skeletal development of a 15-16-year-old. Epiphyseal fusion has already occurred in numerous areas including the head and greater trochanter of the femur. A) The most striking features are enormous thickening and sclerosis of the anterior two thirds of the base of the skull involving the frontal and sphenoid region, distortion and constriction of the sella turcica, and sclerosis of the anterior portion of the first cervical vertebra (arrow). B) Extensive "cystic" lesions involve the upper end and neck of the right femur and right ischial-pubic junction. (Courtesy of Dr. John Dorst, Russell H. Morgan Dept. of Radiology, Johns Hopkins Hospital.)

arch-shaped appearance. Their edges are irregular, feathered, and their osteocytic lacunae are wide. At times the trabeculae close rank to form a meshwork of bone. The trabeculae are made up of coarse-fibered, primitive bone, which under polarized light, appears woven rather than lamellar (Fig. 43). Their woven structure differentiates them from similar trabeculae in other fibro-osseous disease entities. Occasionally a lamellar transformation of woven bone may be encountered. At times an arch-forming trabecula may encircle a central vessel (Fig. 44). Characteristically most trabeculae reveal a lack of osteoblastic rimming. This feature distinguishes fibrous dysplasia from ossifying fibroma. However, in some instances, one may discover trabeculae lined by osteoblasts. The matrix surrounding the bony trabeculae is made up of cellular fibrovascular connective tissue. At times it may contain islands of cartilage. The morphologic pattern of the stroma varies with the age of a lesion. In a younger lesion, the stroma displays a looser arrangement, and there is less collagen formation. In an older lesion, the stroma is usually quite dense.

SARCOMATOUS TRANSFORMATION

In rare instances fibrous dysplasia may be associated with malignant change. This phenomenon was probably first described by Coley and Stewart.[93] In 1964, Schwartz and Alpert[11] reported a series of 28 patients which included 26 cases from the literature and 2 of their own. Fourteen had monostotic and 14 polyostotic disease. The age at which fibrous dysplasia was diagnosed varied from 4 to 39, the mean age being 16. The age at which the sarcomatous transformation was recognized varied between 8 and 61, with a mean age of 32. The latency period between the diagnosis of fibrous dysplasia and subsequent sarcomatous dedifferentiation varied between 2 and 30 years. The sarcoma, on the average, developed $13\frac{1}{2}$ years later. It was somewhat more prevalent among males. The incidence was higher in the polyostotic form. Among the 28 patients 18 developed an osteogenic sarcoma, 7 a fibrosarcoma, 2 a chondrosarcoma, and 1 a giant cell sarcoma. In the monostotic form, the bones of the facial and neural cranium are most frequently affected (50%). In the polyostotic form the femur is the predilective site (62%). Only 11 of the 28 patients had previously received radiation therapy. In 1972, Huvos et al[94] reported 12 instances of sarcomatous transformation among the patient records of the Sloan-Kettering Memorial Cancer Institute. Only 1 of the 12 patients had been previously radiated. The conclusions from their statistical analysis supported the previous findings of Schwartz and Alpert,[11] who estimated the incidence of sarcomatous transformation in fibrous dysplasia at 0.5%. This percentage might be somewhat high

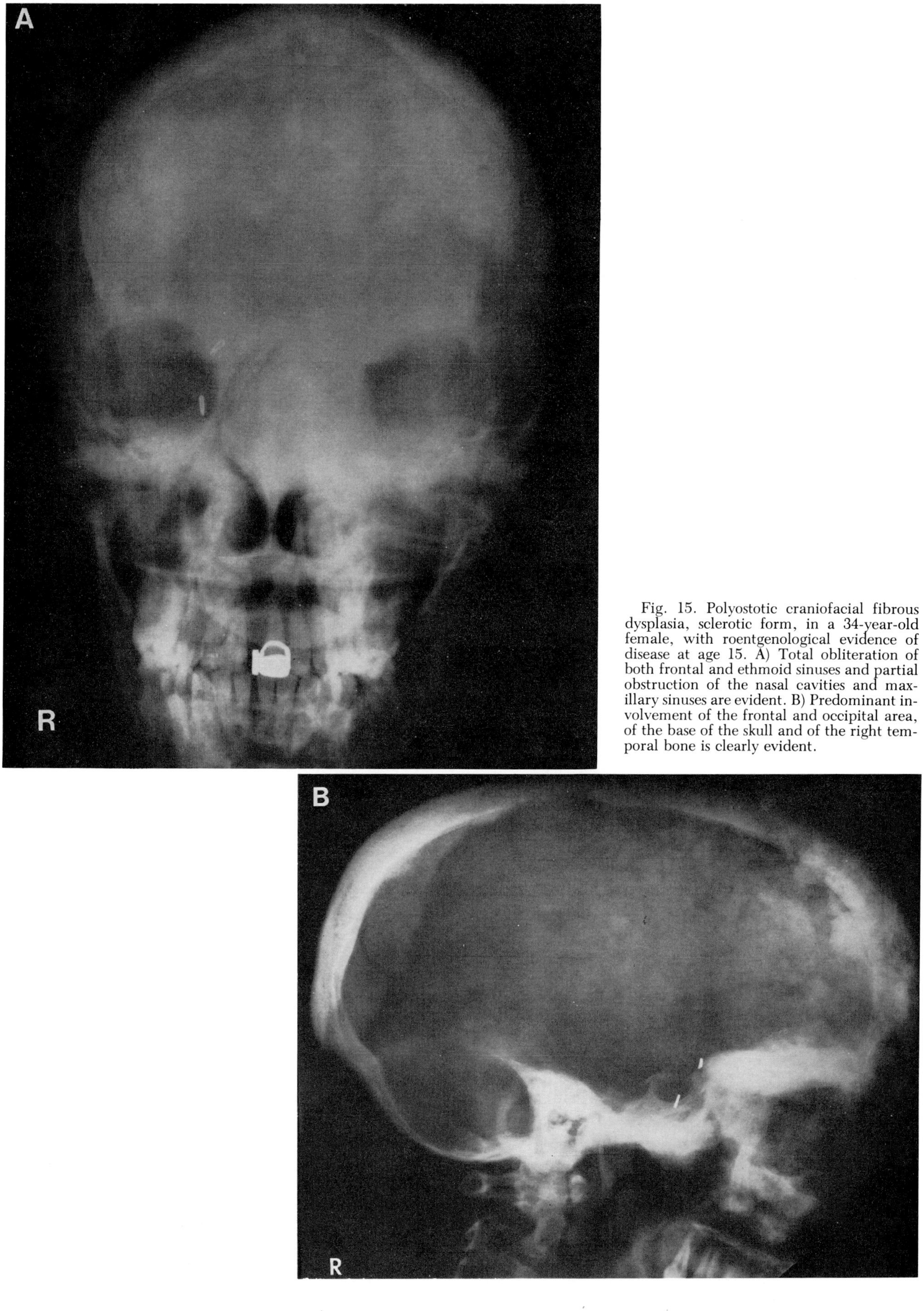

Fig. 15. Polyostotic craniofacial fibrous dysplasia, sclerotic form, in a 34-year-old female, with roentgenological evidence of disease at age 15. A) Total obliteration of both frontal and ethmoid sinuses and partial obstruction of the nasal cavities and maxillary sinuses are evident. B) Predominant involvement of the frontal and occipital area, of the base of the skull and of the right temporal bone is clearly evident.

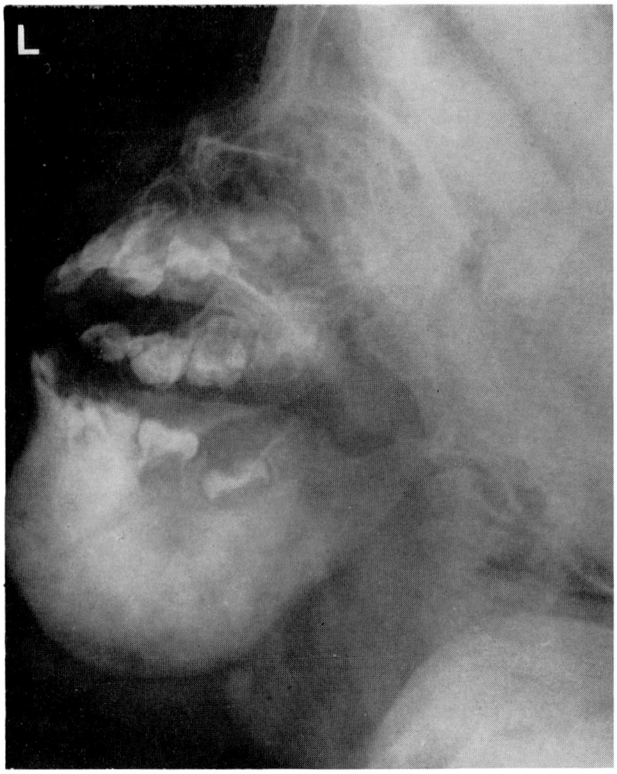

Fig. 16. Monostotic fibrous dysplasia in an 18-month-old female with a history of progressive swelling of the left mandible since 3 months of age. Lesion extends across the mental symphysis and includes numerous cystic radiolucencies in an area of increased density. (Courtesy of Dr. John Dorst, Russell H. Morgan Dept. of Radiology, Johns Hopkins Hospital.)

considering that there are presently no accurate figures available on incidence of clinically manifest and asymptomatic forms of the disease. The predilective sites for malignant degeneration are the femur, maxilla and mandible, followed by the tibia, humerus, scapula, pelvis and fibula. The clinical features include pain, local swelling and radiologically localized bone destruction and interruption of the cortical bone.[29,35] The etiology of malignant degeneration is still unknown. In a few instances radiation therapy might have been responsible. In the majority of instances, however, the same hitherto unidentified factor which induces the proliferation of the fibro-osseous tissue might also produce the sarcomatous transformation.[95]

FAMILIAL MONOSTOTIC AND POLYOSTOTIC FIBROUS DYSPLASIA

Although it would appear that there is no evidence for a genetic basis to fibrous dysplasia,[96] Rietzik and Lownie[97] reported a case of familial craniofacial polyostotic fibrous dysplasia. This 10-year-old male had noticed a hard, smooth, nontender swelling of the right side of the mandible in the premolar region for six months. The expansion of the bone extended from the mandibular right canine to the first permanent molar. Radiologically it presented as a well-defined, unilocular radiolucency measuring about 4 cm. Further examination disclosed several similar lesions in various regions of the skull 1-3 cm in diameter with either a radiolucent or radiopaque mottled pattern. Alkaline phosphatase was 28.9 King-Armstrong units (normal: 8-14 KA units). There was no evidence of café au lait pigmentation or premature sexual development. The patient's father, his paternal grandmother, and several other members of his family had similar lesions all over the skull. A biopsy of the mandibular lesion was characteristic for fibrous dysplasia. The disease was also confirmed histologically in 1 of the 12 affected relatives. Based on the observation that the disease had appeared in every generation but only in children of affected parents, the authors assumed an autosomal dominant trait.

El Deeb et al[98] reported two siblings, a 3-month-old male and a 12-day-old female infant, both presenting with an anterior mandibular lesion at birth. The clinical, radiologic, laboratory and histologic examination revealed a monostotic fibrous dysplasia. Their observation seems to be the first reported example of congenital monostotic disease in siblings. There was no consanguinity between the parents. The authors suggested the possibility of a new autosomal-recessive disorder.

Lemli in 1977[99] published a report of female monozygotic twins with and without the McCune-Albright syndrome. To his knowledge, no twins with this disease had hitherto been described. The markedly different clinical patterns of fibrous dysplasia in these two females is evidence that the phenotypic expression can vary greatly in spite of the identical genotype. Twin 1 had the classic picture of McCune-Albright syndrome, whereas her cotwin, 2, had only minor radiologic anomalies and an elevation in serum alkaline phosphatase.

DIFFERENTIAL DIAGNOSIS

MONOSTOTIC FIBROUS DYSPLASIA

This disease is not always readily identifiable roentgenographically and therefore requires histologic confirmation. It has to be differentiated from the a) solitary unicameral cyst, b) nonosteogenic fibroma, c) giant cell tumor of bone, d) aneurysmal bone cyst, e) adamantinoma of the long bones, f) eosinophilic granuloma, g) plasma cell myeloma, and h) certain fibro-osseous lesions of the jaws and a few other less common lesions.

Solitary Unicameral Cyst. The solitary unicameral cyst, the only truly cystic lesion of bone, is a disease of the growing skeleton. It is generally located in the proximal end of the humerus and femur. Its gaseous or liquid content lends the over-

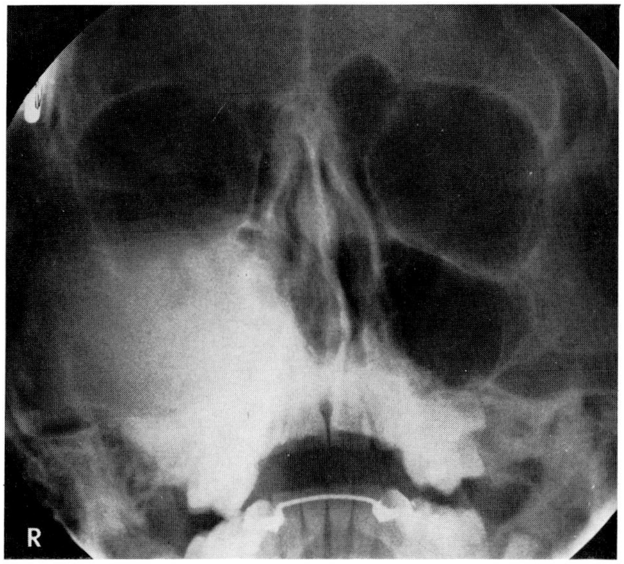

Fig. 17. Monostotic fibrous dysplasia of the right maxilla in a 16-year-old female who at the age of 8 developed a gradual, painless enlargement of the right cheek, alveolar process, epiphora and right nasal obstruction. Examination at age 9 disclosed a short stature but normal skeletal development, no skin pigmentation nor endocrinopathies, alkaline phosphatase: 106 m/ml (normal values 30-85 m/U/ml), and slight exophthalmos of the right eye. Biopsy revealed a fibrous dysplasia. Water's x-ray film of the sinuses discloses a diffuse ground-glass and sclerotic lesion involving the right maxilla extending in all directions, invading the orbit, alveolar process, turbinal bones and adjacent nasal chamber. Tomograms confirmed total obliteration of right maxillary sinus and elevation of the orbital floor. (Courtesy of Dr. Blair Webb, Washington, DC.)

lying periosteum and cortex a bluish color. It originates in the metaphysis. However, as the bone grows in length, it gives the illusory impression of drifting toward the middiaphysis. The monostotic lesion, rather than drifting toward the diaphysis may extend into it. Roentgenologically, the unicameral cyst appears as a round or oval lytic defect with the density of soft tissue and little bone reaction about it. Spontaneous fractures are common. Sarcomatous transformation has not been observed.[2]

Nonosteogenic Fibroma. The nonosteogenic fibroma is a fairly common, nonneoplastic degenerative and proliferative lesion involving the medullary and cortical bone. It is most commonly encountered near the ends of the diaphysis of the femur, tibia and fibula, and occasionally also in flat bones. It makes its appearance in late childhood, adolescence or early adult life. This frequently multiple lesion has a characteristic behavior and appearance. Its natural course is one of healing. The radiological defect usually displays a clear demarcation, often with a narrow, bosselated sclerotic margin. It too gives the illusory impression of migrating toward the middiaphysis as endochondral growth removes the epiphysis away from it.[2]

Giant Cell Tumor. The giant cell tumor or osteoclastoma generally occurs after the age of 20. Its highest incidence is in the third decade.[100-102] It affects females more frequently than males. It arises most commonly in the epiphyses of long bones. The location of the neoplasm is characteristically eccentric. This totally radiolucent lesion lacks any periosteal new bone formation and reactive bony sclerosis in its advancing margins. It may erode the overlying cortex from within. At times it may extend through the cortex into the soft tissue. Its tendency toward sarcomatous transformation is relatively high (15-30%).[2,101]

Aneurysmal Bone Cyst. The aneurysmal bone cyst is a solitary, benign and expansile lesion of bone with a predilection for the metaphysis of long bones, vertebrae and flat bones, but any bone of the skeleton may potentially become involved. It is most commonly observed in the second and third decades of life, and affects females more frequently than males. Swelling, pain and tenderness are the salient clinical features. Expansion may lead to involvement of more than one bone. Its size may vary from 2 to more than 20 cm. In a cylindrical bone, the location may be central or eccentric. Occasionally the major portion of the lesion may be located outside the bone in the soft tissue. In such instances, the shaft displays only a slight cortical erosion. Roentgenologically, the cyst presents itself as a radiolucent area with the density of soft tissue, including multiple, delicate incomplete septa. Its margins are scalloped and clearly demarcated.[2]

Adamantinoma. Adamantinoma is an uncommon, slow-growing, malignant neoplasm, observed generally in the third decade of life. It affects males more frequently than females. Its usual location is the diaphysis or occasionally the metaphysis of long bones. The tibia is by far the most frequently affected bone. The lesion generally produces a well-demarcated, occasionally multicystic-appearing defect. The cortex ordinarily remains intact but may be destroyed when the tumor extends into the soft tissue.[38]

Eosinophilic Granuloma. The eosinophilic granuloma is a benign nonneoplastic solitary, lytic lesion which probably arises from the reticuloendothelial system. It is most frequently encountered in the frontal and parietal bones, mandible, humerus, ribs and proximal metaphysis of the femur.[38] In the calvaria and mandible, the defect is generally sharply defined whereas in the long bones the lesion appears as a mottled radiolucency. Most of the cases are discovered before the age of 30. There is a slight male predominance.

Plasma Cell Myeloma. The plasma cell myeloma is a neoplastic proliferation of plasma cells of the bone marrow. It may present as a clinically localized bone lesion or as a systemic disease and occasionally as an extraosseous mass. It affects predominantly older people. The most frequently involved bones include the vertebrae, rib, skull, pelvis and

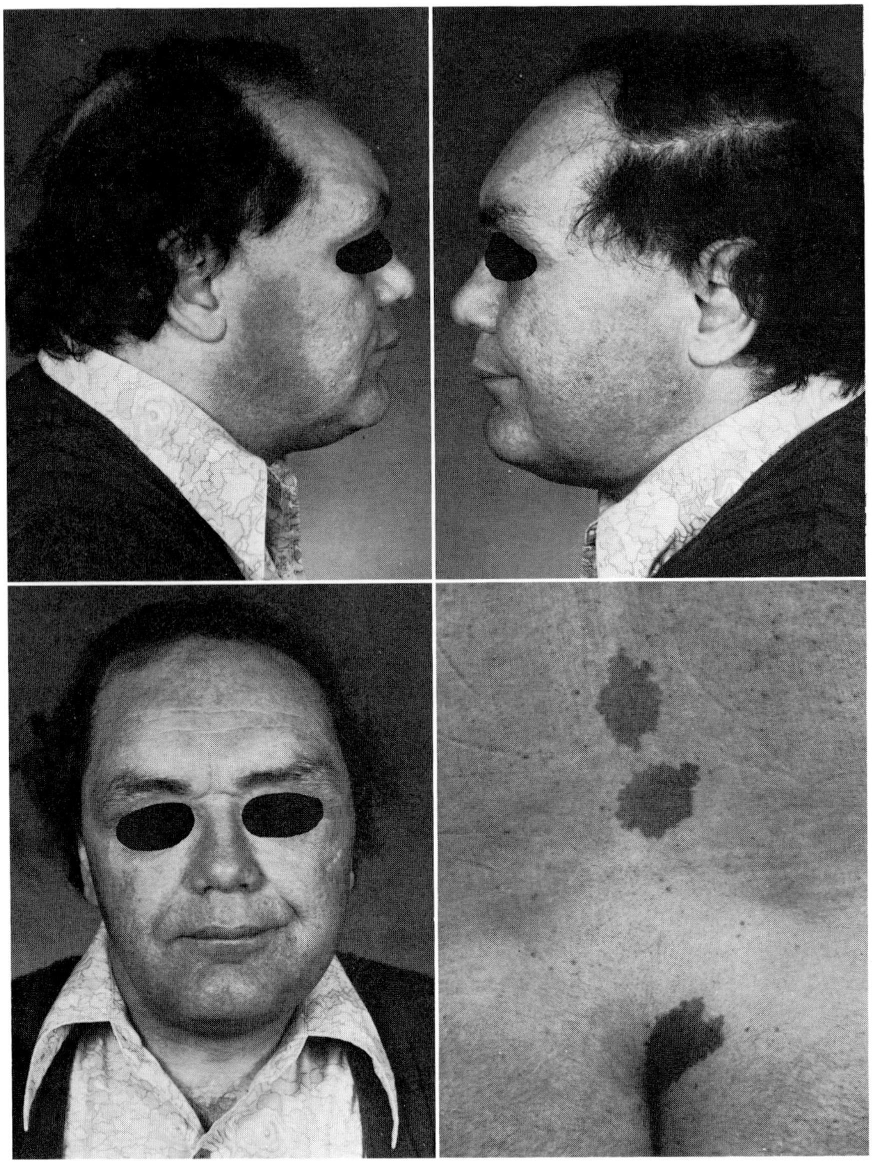

Fig. 18. (Case 1) Forty-five-year-old patient with leonine facies with frontal bossing and hypertelorism and occiptal prominence evident. The irregular, non-elevated skin pigmentations in the lumbosacral area are distributed along the midline.

femur. Radiologically, the lesion nearly always causes bone destruction, but in a rare instance, however, it may be partly or overwhelmingly sclerotic. The characteristic bone lesion appears as a punched-out, radiolucent defect.[2,38]

Fibro-osseous Lesions of the Jaws. A variety of fibro-osseous lesions in the gnathic area, whether they be dysplastic, benign-neoplastic or reactive, share overlapping clinical, radiographic and morphological features, and therefore confront the clinician and pathologist with problems in nosology and management. These lesions include in addition to fibrous dysplasia and nonosteogenic fibroma a) ossifying fibroma, b) chronic sclerosing osteomyelitis, c) Gardner syndrome, d) gigantiform cementoma, e)desmoplastic and odontogenic fibroma, f) osteoid osteoma, and g) cemental lesions.[43]

OSSIFYING FIBROMA. This is a controversial lesion, both clinically and pathologically. It was first described by Menzel,[103] but it was Montgomery[104] who introduced the term. The debate over the identity of the disease still continues. Schlumberger[105] and Zimmerman and Dahlin[106] and Zimmerman et al[107] consider monostotic fibrous dysplasia and ossifying fibroma of the jaws to be variants of the same dysplastic process. However, Sherman and Sternbergh[108] and Sherman and Glauser[109] regard them as separate diseases, making the distinction on radiographic grounds. They regard monostotic fibrous dysplasia as an expansile, dysplastic process with diffuse and blending margins, and ossifying fibroma, on the other hand, as an expansile, benign-neoplastic process with clearly delineated boundaries. Other investigators differentiate exclusively on a morphological basis, specifically on the presence or absence of woven or lamellar bone, osteoblastic rimming and spheroid calcification.

The histologic differentiation alone may cause some difficulties because some pathologists have in-

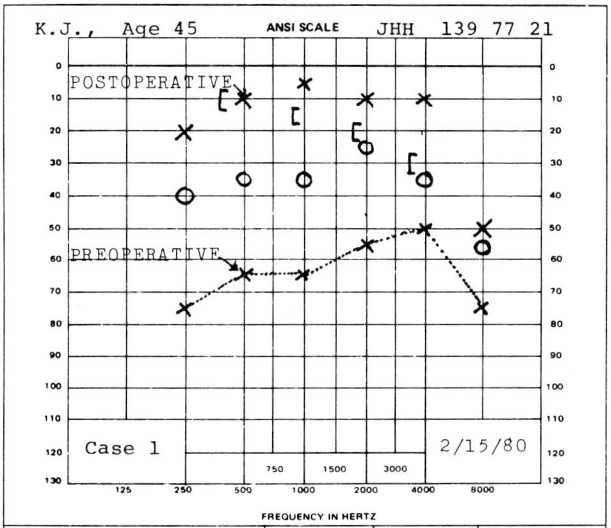

	SPEAKER	RT. EAR	LT. EAR	AID	EAR(S)
SPEECH RECEPTION THRESHOLD (SRT)	dB	30 OEM dB	10 dB		dB
DISCRIMINATION	%	100 %	100 %		%
dB ABOVE SRT		35 OEM	35		

Fig. 19. (Case 1) Audiogram reflects the postoperative thresholds for pure tones and speech in the operated left ear.

terpreted histologic features of both lesions to be present in a single specimen. In recent years, however, several comprehensive reviews of fibro-osseous lesions have appeared in the literature. They share Reed and Glagy's[110] criteria and view that fibrous dysplasia and ossifying fibroma are two different entities, and emphasize that these diseases can be differentiated on combined clinical, radiological, and morphological grounds.

Ossifying fibroma is a rare, generally slow-growing, solitary lesion, affecting primarily the jaws, occasionally the frontal and ethmoid bones, but rarely the long bones. It involves the mandible more frequently than the maxilla. Females are more often affected. It usually manifests itself clinically between the ages of 15 to 26. Whereas some ossifying fibromas reach a static phase, others tend to be more aggressive and may lead to deformities. On radiographic examination the disease presents itself as a well-delineated expansile lucency which may display a mottled center, central opacity, or pattern of opaque flecks.[43] On macroscopic examination the lesion exhibits a clean demarcation from the adjacent normal bone. On microscopic examination the fibrous component of the fibro-osseous process predominates. Irregular bony trabeculae, made up in the center of woven bone but in the periphery of lamellar bone and rimmed with osteoblasts, are distributed randomly in a fibrous stroma. The fibrous tissue consists of spindle-shaped fibroblasts arranged in whirls. The cellular density can vary considerably. "Psammona-like" islands of bone displaying a dark calcified nidus with a pale osteoid rim and occasionally lined with osteoblasts and transitional stages between such spheroidal calcifications and more fully developed bony trabecula can be observed. The variable picture of differentiation of these bony units influenced some investigators to further classify the ossifying fibroma into "juvenile, moderately mature, and mature forms."[43]

In fibrous dysplasia the maxilla is more frequently involved than the mandible. The lesion appears radiographically more homogenous. The margins are irregular, and due to their poor definition, blend into the adjacent normal bone. The expansile lesion may exhibit a ground-glass character, a mottled, or a diffuse loculated pattern. On microscopic examination the fibrous tissue is quite uniform. Nuclear atypia is infrequent and mitoses are rare. The bony trabeculae are irregular, display the same random distribution, but generally are devoid of parallel lamellae. The osteocyte lacunae are wider than in mature lamellar or haversian bone.[43] As a rule, osteoblastic rimming is absent.

Ossifying fibroma is in general adequately treated by enucleation.[111-113] When conservative management fails in preventing recurrences, partial resection becomes the treatment of choice.[114,115] An aggressive lesion, when located in the long bones, necessitates a wide excision and periosteal stripping combined with bone grafting. The possibility of sarcomatous change should preclude the use of radiation as a treatment modality.[38]

CHRONIC SCLEROSING OSTEOMYELITIS. Chronic, diffuse, sclerosing osteomyelitis, a disease entity predominantly encountered in the middle-aged female, may affect one or several jaw quadrants in dentulous or edentulous areas. It is encountered in the tooth-bearing areas, above all in the premolar regions. The lesion manifests itself radiographically as a conglomeration of radiopaque densities with a cotton-wool pattern.[43] Its localized form, the focal sclerosing osteitis, usually presents as a periapical radiodensity associated with a grossly carious molar.[116,117]

GARDNER SYNDROME. The syndrome is characterized by the association of multiple osteomas involving the mandible, maxilla, calvaria and occasionally long bones, with intestinal polyps, dermoid cysts, desmoid tumors and localized and wavy cortical thickening of long bones. The well-defined osteomas of the jaws and other features make the identification easy.[118]

GIGANTIFORM CEMENTOMA. The lesion usually involves all four quadrants of the jaw and may produce cortical expansion. Radiologically it presents as a conglomerate of dense masses. It frequently follows a genetic pattern. In general, no source of infection can be identified histologically.[43]

DESMOPLASTIC AND ODONTOGENIC FIBROMA. The desmoplastic fibroma is an uncommon lesion, considered by some a benign-neoplastic, by others a re-

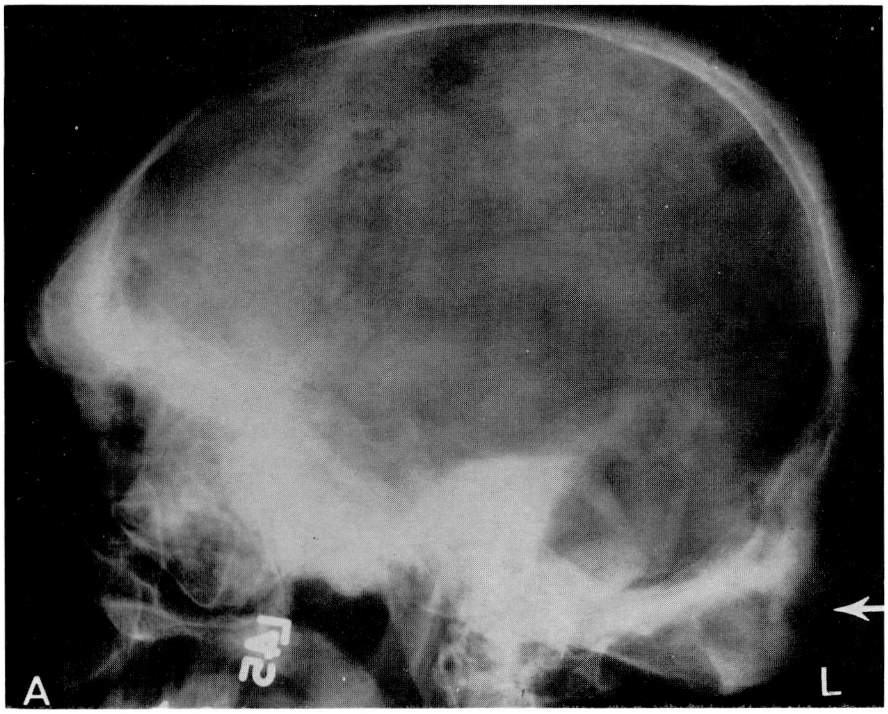

Fig. 20. (Case 1) A) Marked overgrowth and sclerosis of bone in the frontal and occipital area led to the development of the leonine facial structures and the occipital pug (arrow). Together with the thickening and sclerosis of the base of the skull, they exemplify the extensive skull involvement.

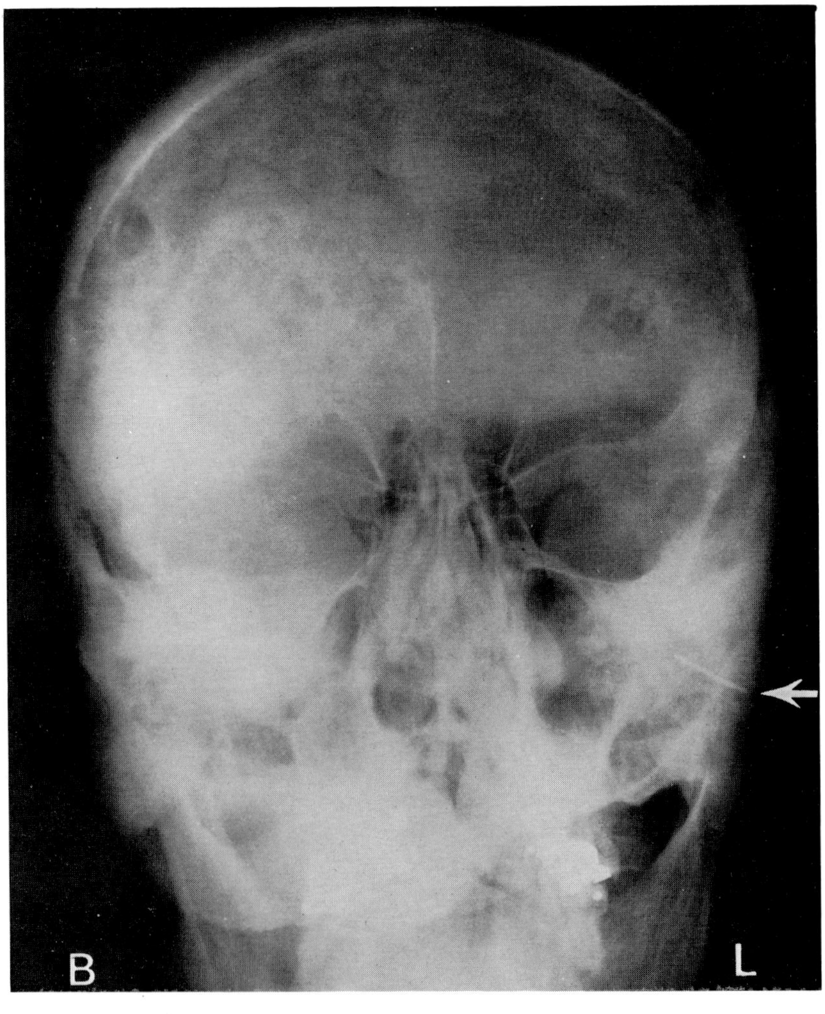

Fig. 20. B) Diffuse sclerosis characterizes the widespread involvement of the neurocranium and facial cranium. The radiopaque thread-like marker in the wall of the Silastic stent in the left external auditory canal is clearly visible (arrow).

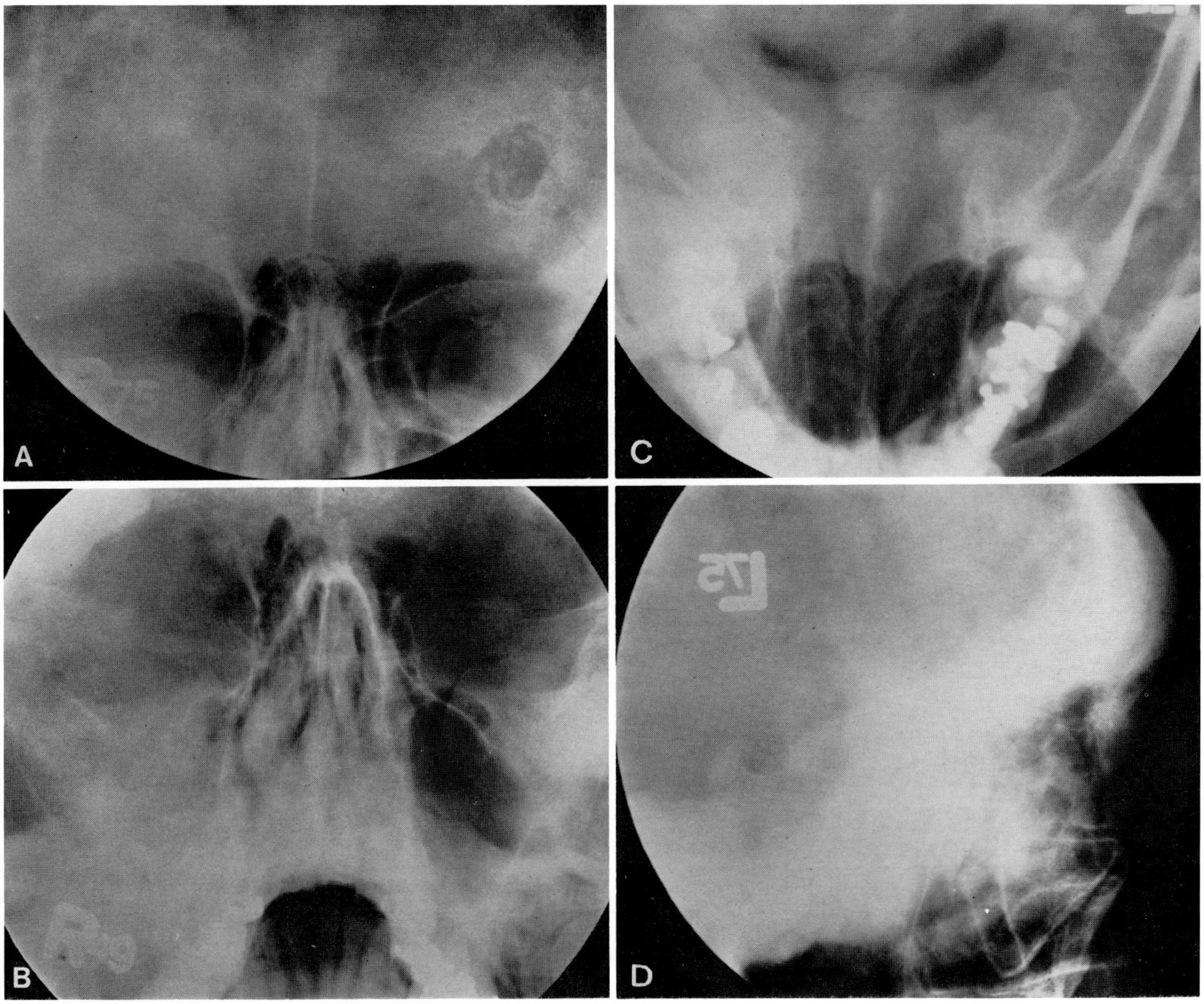

Fig. 21. (Case 1) A, C) Both frontal sphenoid sinuses and the B) right maxillary sinus are completely obliterated by the disease process, whereas the B, D) ethmoid and the left maxillary sinuses display only partial involvement.

active process. It affects primarily individuals under 30 years of age. It affects mainly the long bones, yet has also been encountered in the pelvis, mandible, scapula, vertebrae and clavicle, etc. Localized pain and occasionally a pathologic fracture may be the presenting symptom. Small, benign-appearing fibroblasts with abundant intercellular substance and numerous collagen fibers compose the lesion. It distinguishes itself from fibrous dysplasia by the absence of bone formation.[38]

OSTEOCHONDROMA, OSTEOBLASTOMA, AND OSTEOID OSTEOMA. These are additional localized lesions with a fibrous and an osseous component arising in the jaws. Another group of similar lesions are, because of their content of cementum, referred to as cemental lesions, periapical cemental dysplasia, and benign cementoblastoma. The cementifying fibroma is a designation given to localized or diffuse expansile lesions with ovoid calcifications encountered also in extragnathic fibrous processes.[119,120] Their differentiation from fibrous dysplasia, too, should be made on combined clinical, radiographic and morphologic grounds.[43]

POLYOSTOTIC FIBROUS DYSPLASIA

Unlike the monostotic form, the polyostotic form of fibrous dysplasia may be readily recognized roentgenographically. Its tendency toward unilateral distribution, propensity to involve the lower extremities, disposition toward recurrent spontaneous fractures, and pathognomonic shepherd-crook deformity of the upper end of the femur characterize the disease entity.

Polyostotic fibrous dysplasia has to be differentiated from a) hyperparathyroidism (osteitis fibrosa cystica generalista or von Recklinghausen disease of bone), b) polyostotic osteitis deformans Paget, c) predominantly unilateral enchondromatosis or Ollier disease, d) neurofibromatosis, or von Recklinghausen disease, and e) cherubism.

Hyperparathyroidism. Hyperparathyroidism (os-

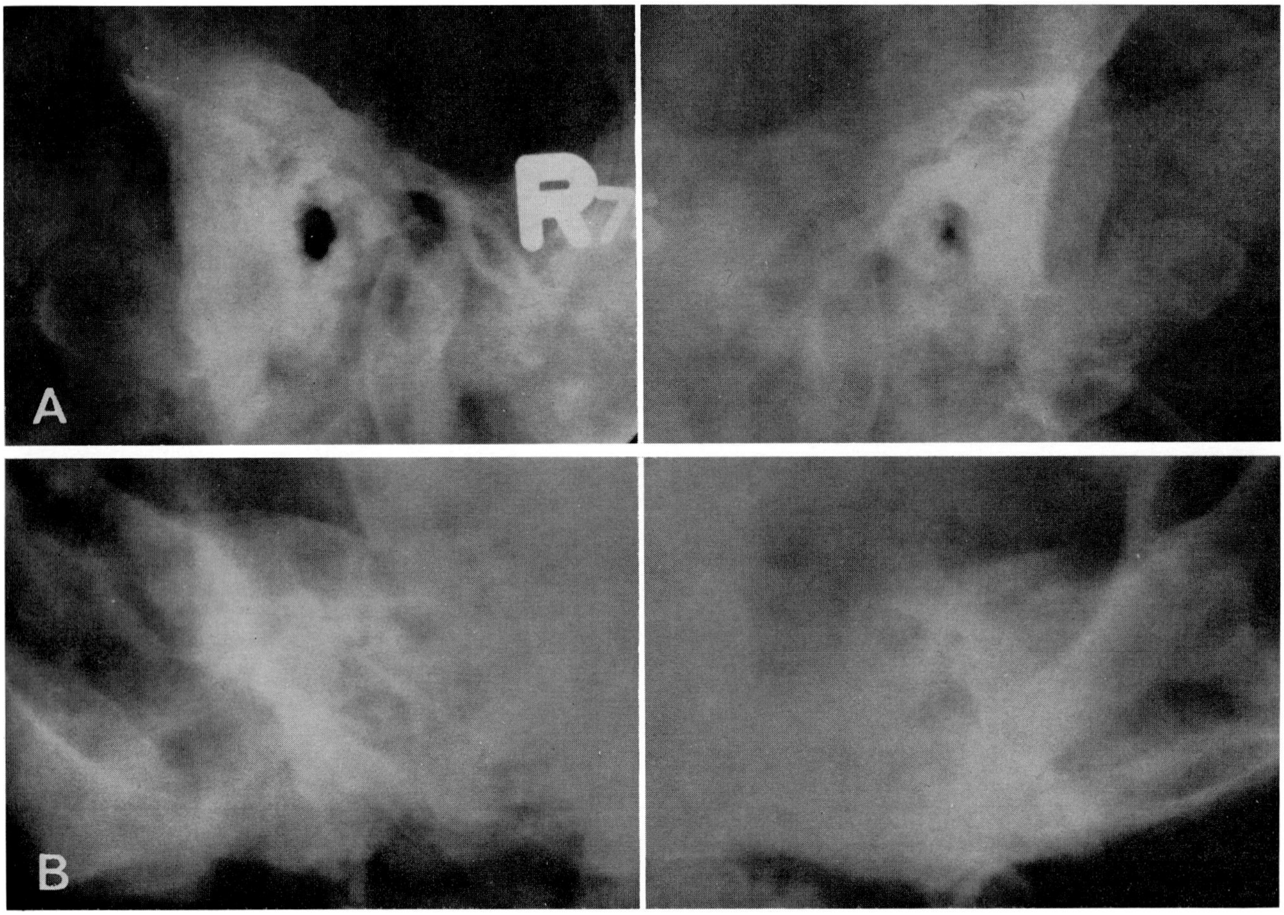

Fig. 22. (Case 1) Dense sclerosis marks the severe involvement of the temporal bone as seen in the A) Schuller and B) Stenver views. Narrowing of both, particularly the left external auditory canal, is well recognized.

teitis fibrosa cystica generalisata or von Recklinghausen disease of bone) distinguishes itself roentgenologically from polyostotic fibrous dysplasia by 1) generalized osteoporosis of the skeleton, 2) diffuse granular radiolucency of the calvaria, 3) cortical cysts, 4) subperiosteal erosion of the phalanges, 5) lack of osteosclerotic areas, 6) pronounced skeletal tenderness, 7) hypercalcemia, and 8) late onset in the middle and later decades of life. In hyperparathyroidism every single bone of the skeleton is involved, whereas in polyostotic fibrous dysplasia never are all bones affected.[35]

Osteitis Deformans Paget. Polyostotic osteitis deformans Paget distinguishes itself from polyostotic fibrous dysplasia by 1) more even, bilateral distribution of the bone lesions, 2) predominance of bending deformities over fracture deformities (ie, anterior bowing of the tibia), 3) coarse strand-like sclerosis of the spongiosa along lines of stress and strain, and 4) late onset of the disease after the age of 40. The thickening of the calvaria seldom reaches the dimensions encountered in fibrous dysplasia. The structural changes involving the external table provide a distinctive criterion. In osteitis deformans Paget the outer table is markedly thickened; in fibrous dysplasia it is thinned to a delicate cortex.[35]

Enchondromatosis (Ollier Disease). Unilateral enchondromatosis or Ollier disease is characterized by the predominant involvement of the hands and feet, combination with cartilaginous exostoses, absence of skull involvement, and presence of spotty calcification of cartilage.[35]

Neurofibromatosis. Neurofibromatosis or von Recklinghausen disease may be confused with fibrous dysplasia in that one of its skeletal features, erosion of bone caused by a neurofibroma, may display an identical cyst-like appearance. A neurofibroma may originate within a bone or in the periosteum. A neurofibroma arising in the periosteum may cause a pressure defect in the cortex and simulate an intrinsic lesion unless examined roentgenologically in more than one plane.[29] Long bones are rarely involved. In the skull the predilective sites are the orbital, sphenoid and temporal bones, calvaria, particularly in the vicinity of the lambdoid suture, zygomatic arch, and ascending ramus of the mandible. The lesions in the calvaria have an irregular sclerotic margin. The hereditary, often congenital, aspect of this hamartoblastomatosis which, in its full-blown syndrome includes neurofibromas of the skin, pigmented nevi, racemous angiomas, and a variety of intracranial tumors (schwannomas

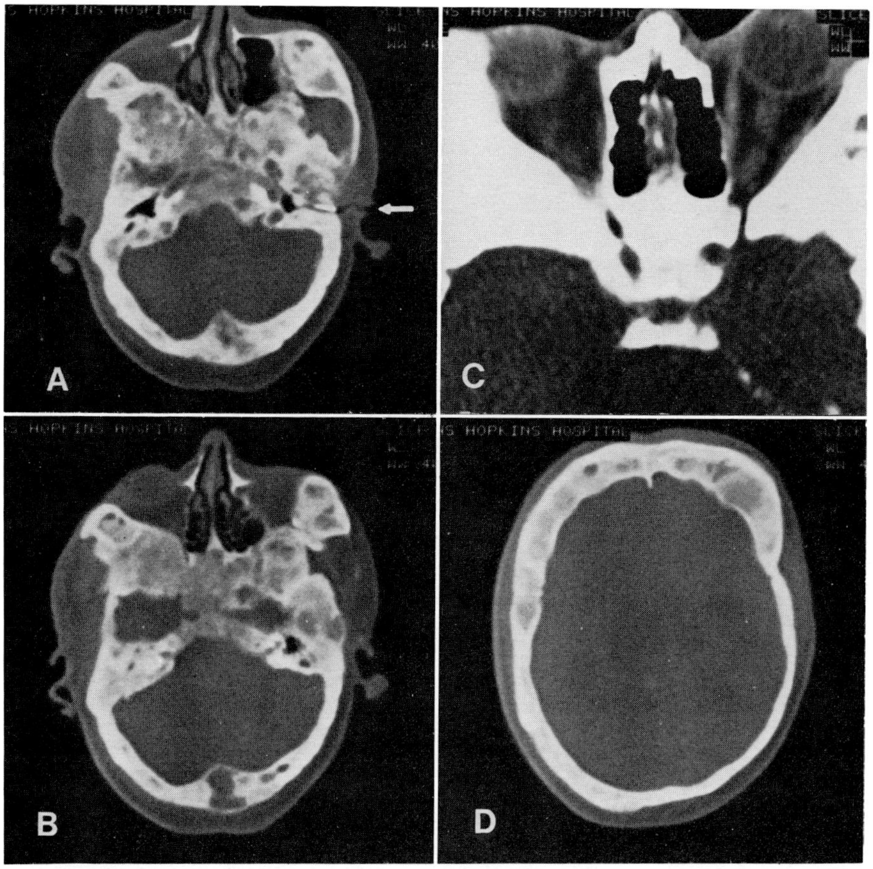

Fig. 23. (Case 1) Computerized axial tomography of the skull. A) Massive thickening of entire base of the skull, left zygoma, and midoccipital area. Arrow points to the open, cylindrical, radiopaque stent in the reconstructed left external auditory canal. B) Diffuse involvement of the sphenoid, petrous, and occipital bones. C) Exophthalmos resulted from progressive constriction of the orbital cavity caused by diffuse hyperostosis of the sphenoid bone. D) Extensive involvement of the calvaria and cystic expansion of the frontal bones.

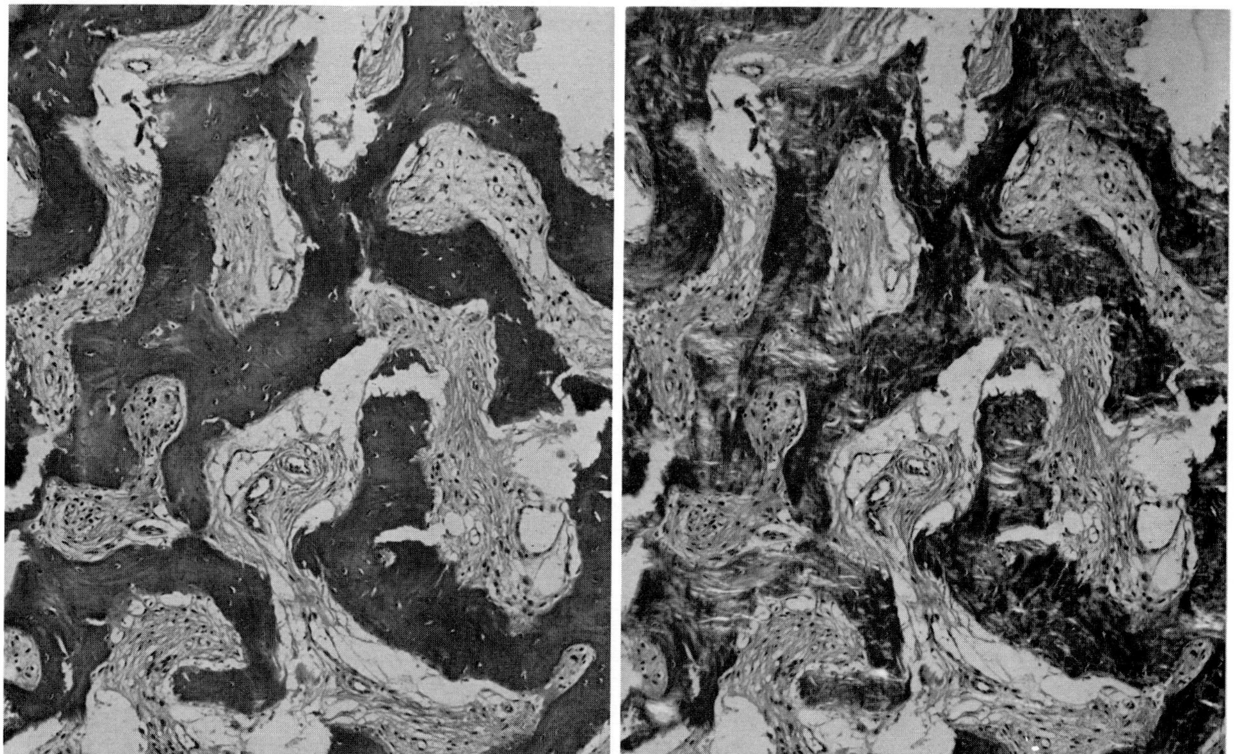

Fig. 24. (Case 1) A) Biopsy from left tympanic bone. Proliferation of vascular fibrous connective tissue and trabeculae of woven bone characterize the fibrodysplastic process. B) Same section under polarized light shows the random distribution of birefringent collagen fibers, typical for immature bone. (H & E, x 150)

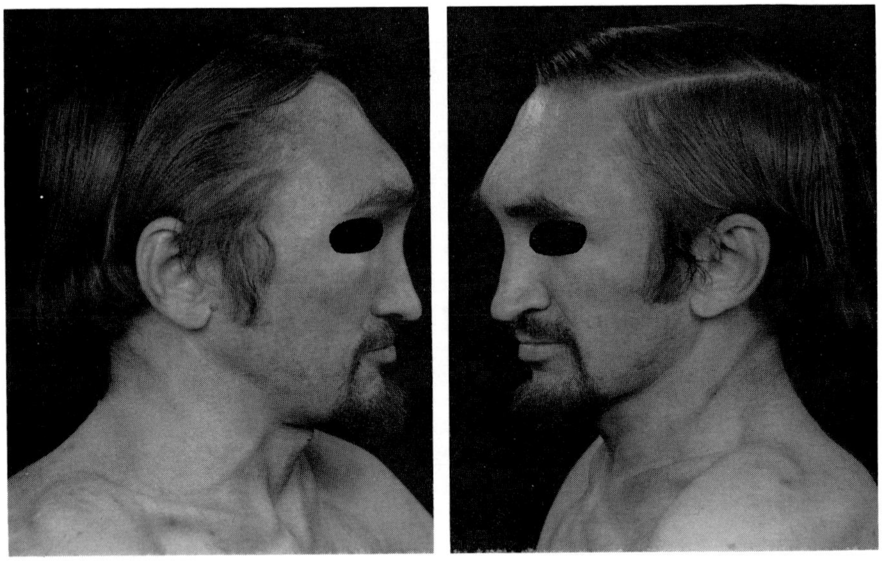

Fig. 25. (Case 2) Enlargement and deformity of the neurocranium accompanied by frontal bossing and an occipital pug reflect the massive involvement of the skull.

of the cranial nerves, multiple meningiomas, spongioblastomas of the midline, ependymomas, etc), facilitates its recognition.

Cherubism. Cherubism is a familial fibrous dysplasia of the jaws, characterized by swelling of the lower face. It is inherited as an autosomal dominant trait with an 80% penetrance and an expressivity varying in severity. It is usually recognized between the ages of 18 months and 2 years, then becomes stationary and regresses spontaneously during puberty. It affects primarily the mandible, occasionally the maxilla. Multilocular cystic lesions in a symmetrical distribution in the mandible and maxilla are responsible for the characteristic changes in facial configuration.[121,122]

TREATMENT

There is presently no conservative treatment available for the control of fibrous dysplasia. The sole presence of a lesion does not justify surgical intervention. This applies particularly to a monostotic lesion which does not impair neural or motor function and does not involve an important adjacent structure. A patient with fibrous dysplasia of the cranium and vertebral column should be followed carefully at regular intervals. Involvement of the frontal, ethmoid, and sphenoid bone demands accurate evaluation of the optic foramen. Progressive narrowing and impairment of vision call for a surgical procedure with an attempt to decompress the optic canal. Increasing constriction of the external auditory canal resulting from temporal bone involvement is an indication for reconstruction of the osseous canal followed by permanent stenting. Concentric narrowing of the internal acoustic meatus associated with progressive impairment of cranial nerve function may in selected instances justify a surgical decompression. However, such procedures on the optic foramen and internal auditory canal may result only in a temporary improvement and retardation of the disease process.

Some lesions because of their continuous, diffuse, expansile growth will require conservative osseous contouring,[123] which at times may have to be repeated until the process has reached a stable level.[124-128] Occasionally a monostotic lesion involving the maxilla may exhibit an accelerated aggressive growth tendency causing a severe facial deformity. In such situations, depending upon the natural history and local behavior of that particular disease process, a partial resection may become necessary to preserve the orbital contents.[116] It has, however, been observed that in some patients in whom a resected portion of a tubular bone or jaw had been replaced by a bone graft, the grafted bone later developed a recurrence of the dysplastic process.[43]

Recurrent spontaneous fractures require either curettage with replacement of bone chips, or local resection if the lesion involves a bone such as a rib. In spite of careful curettage, the incidence of local recurrence remains quite high. Among 37 patients of the Mayo Clinic, the recurrence rate was 21% in monostotic and 36% in polyostotic disease. An enormous spindle-shaped enlargement of a rib with compression of the lung calls for surgical resection.

Polyostotic fibrous dysplasia, particularly when complicated by progressive deformity of the femur, may demand corrective osteotomies before skeletal growth is completed. Repeated fractures of the femur neck in older individuals may require replacement of the upper end of the femur by a prosthesis. However, since the dysplastic process generally involves the neck as well as the proximal metaphysis of the femur, and thus cannot be totally removed, the possibility of a recurrence always remains.[35]

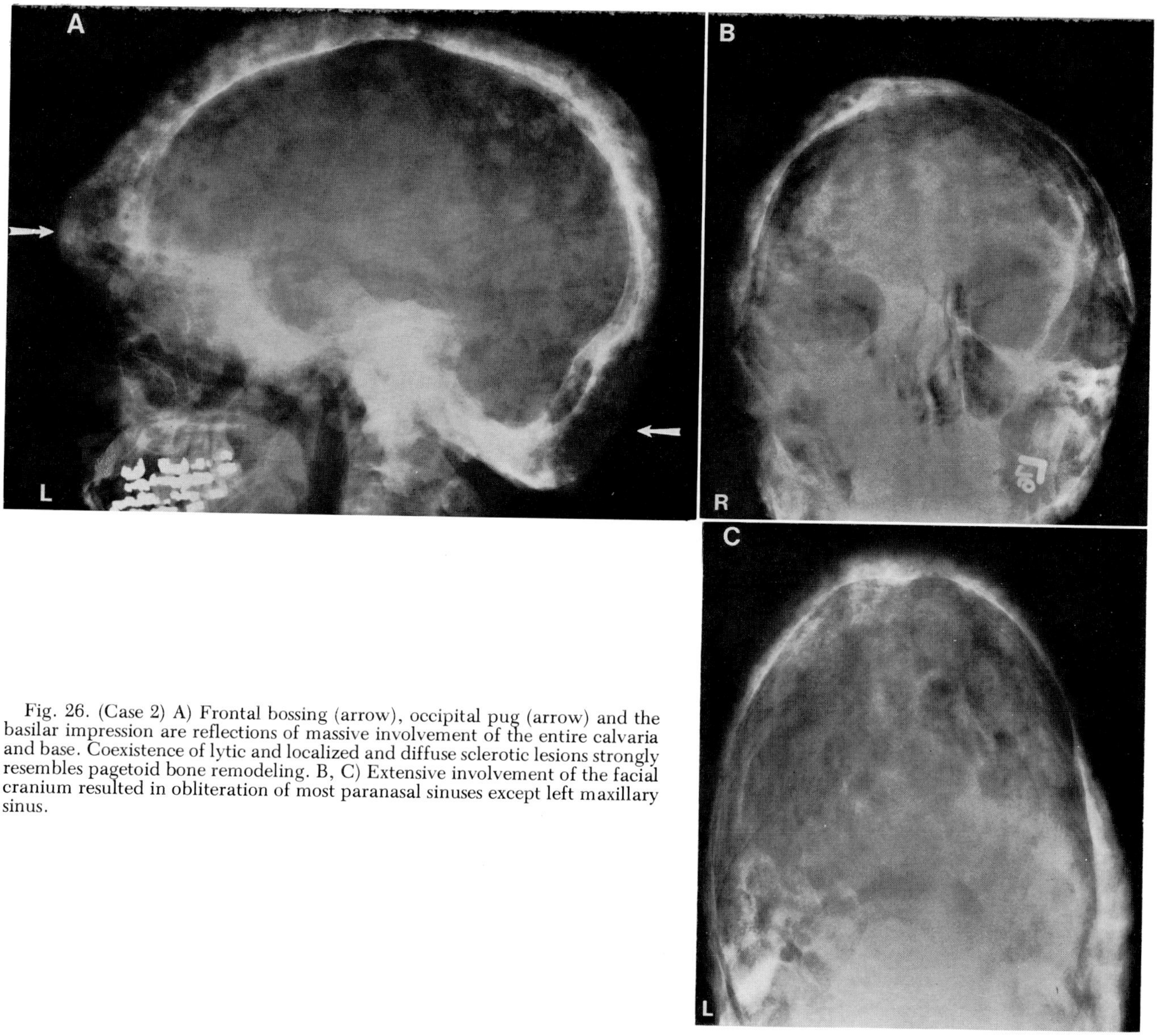

Fig. 26. (Case 2) A) Frontal bossing (arrow), occipital pug (arrow) and the basilar impression are reflections of massive involvement of the entire calvaria and base. Coexistence of lytic and localized and diffuse sclerotic lesions strongly resembles pagetoid bone remodeling. B, C) Extensive involvement of the facial cranium resulted in obliteration of most paranasal sinuses except left maxillary sinus.

Treatment by radiation therapy is absolutely contraindicated as malignant transformation is a possibility. Slow et al[32] estimated that the incidence of malignant transformation rises from 0.4 to 44% following radiation therapy.

PROGNOSIS

The prognosis of fibrous dysplasia is usually good. It depends upon the form and extent of the disease, the location of the lesions and their association with endocrine disturbances and other disorders. At puberty the monostotic form in general comes to a standstill, and the polyostotic form displays some evidence of decrease in activity. However, there are numerous exceptions.[34,129,130] Occasionally new lesions appear after puberty. These are usually encountered in the pelvis and ribs.[29] Early onset of a severe form of polyostotic disease involving one or both sides of the skeleton may lead to severe unilateral or bilateral deformity, crippling, and even complete invalidity. In polyostotic disease fresh lesions may develop and existing ones can spread. Reactivation after a prolonged period of quiesence is not uncommon. It may be observed during pregnancy.[15,131,132] In instances where fibrous dysplasia is associated with endocrine disturbances (McCune-Albright syndrome), the latter determines the outcome.[35] When sarcomatous transition takes place in a dysplastic lesion, the prognosis changes accordingly.

REVIEW OF THE LITERATURE

To estimate the incidence, and to evaluate the clinical features, regional behavior and surgical end results of fibrous dysplasia involving the temporal bone, a survey of the literature of the past four decades has been conducted.[25,28,31,41,133-174] Since 1946, 48 investigators reported 69 cases. All but six were otolaryngologists. There may have been a few more cases reported in scientific journals through-

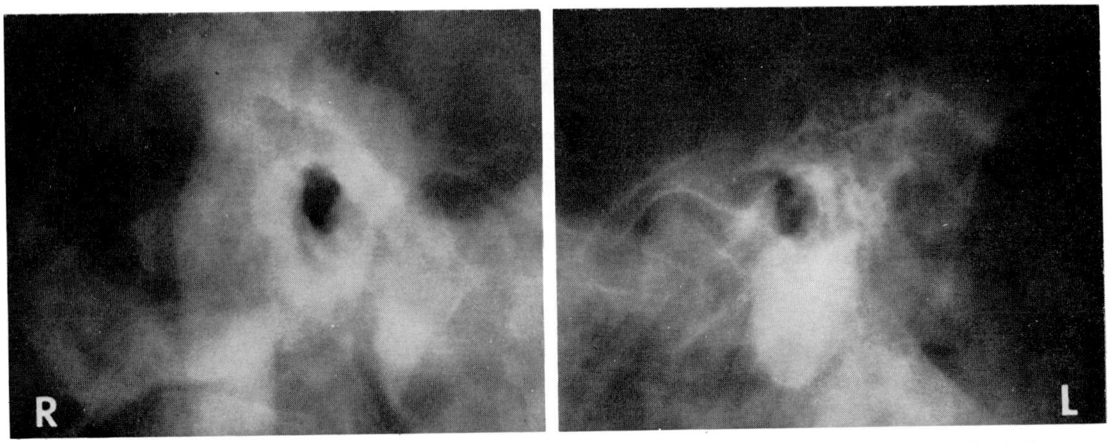

Fig. 27. (Case 2) Lateral (Schuller) view displays diffuse sclerosis of the right and left mastoid bones and a slight narrowing of the external auditory canals.

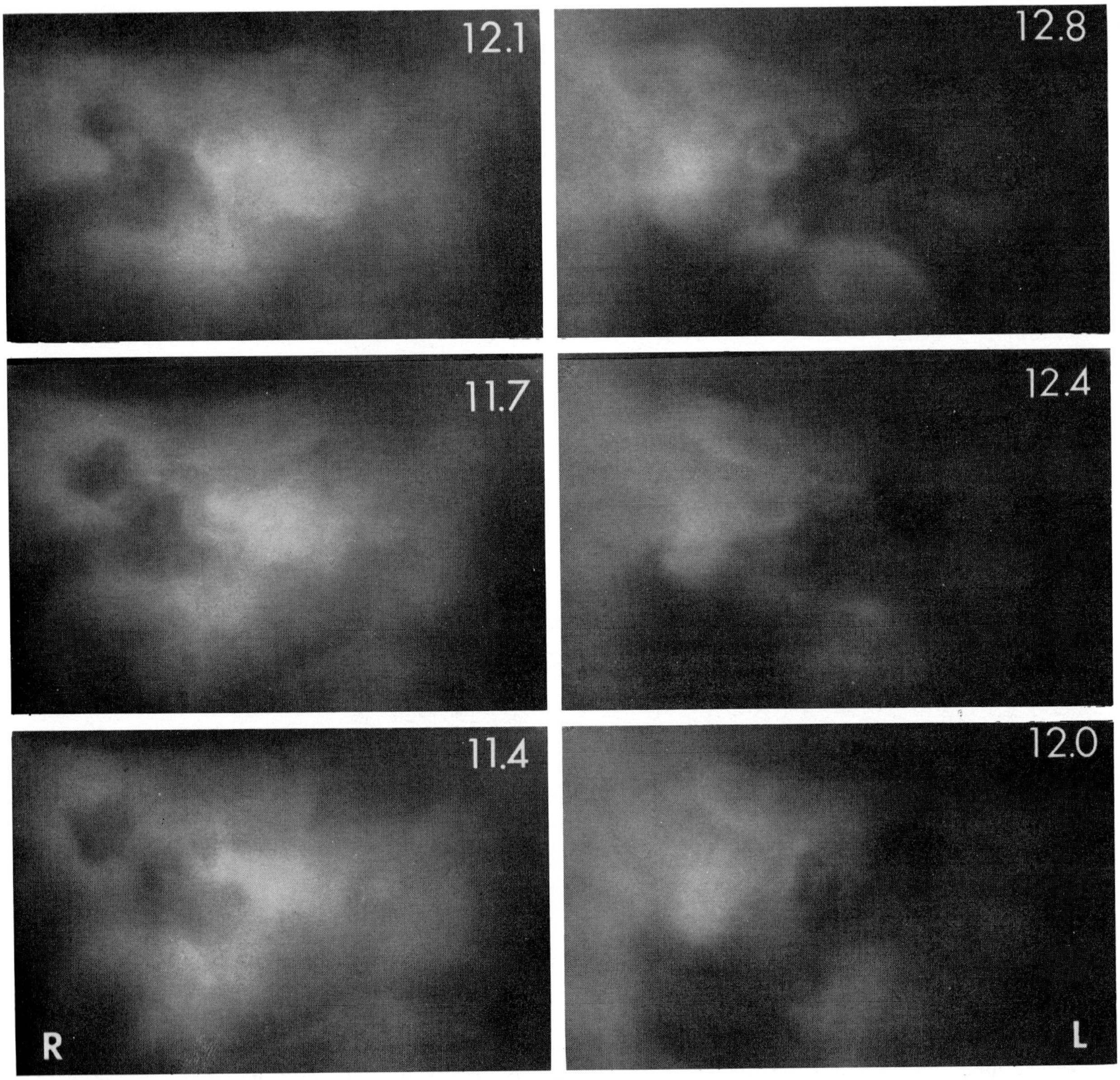

Fig. 28. (Case 2) Frontal tomograms of the right and left petrous pyramids reveal the downward bending of the external and the upward slanting of the internal auditory canals regularly encountered in basilar invagination. Diffuse sclerosis tends to obscure landmarks of the cochlear and vestibular capsule. Malleus in both ears is enlarged but there is no encroachment on the seventh and eighth cranial nerves.

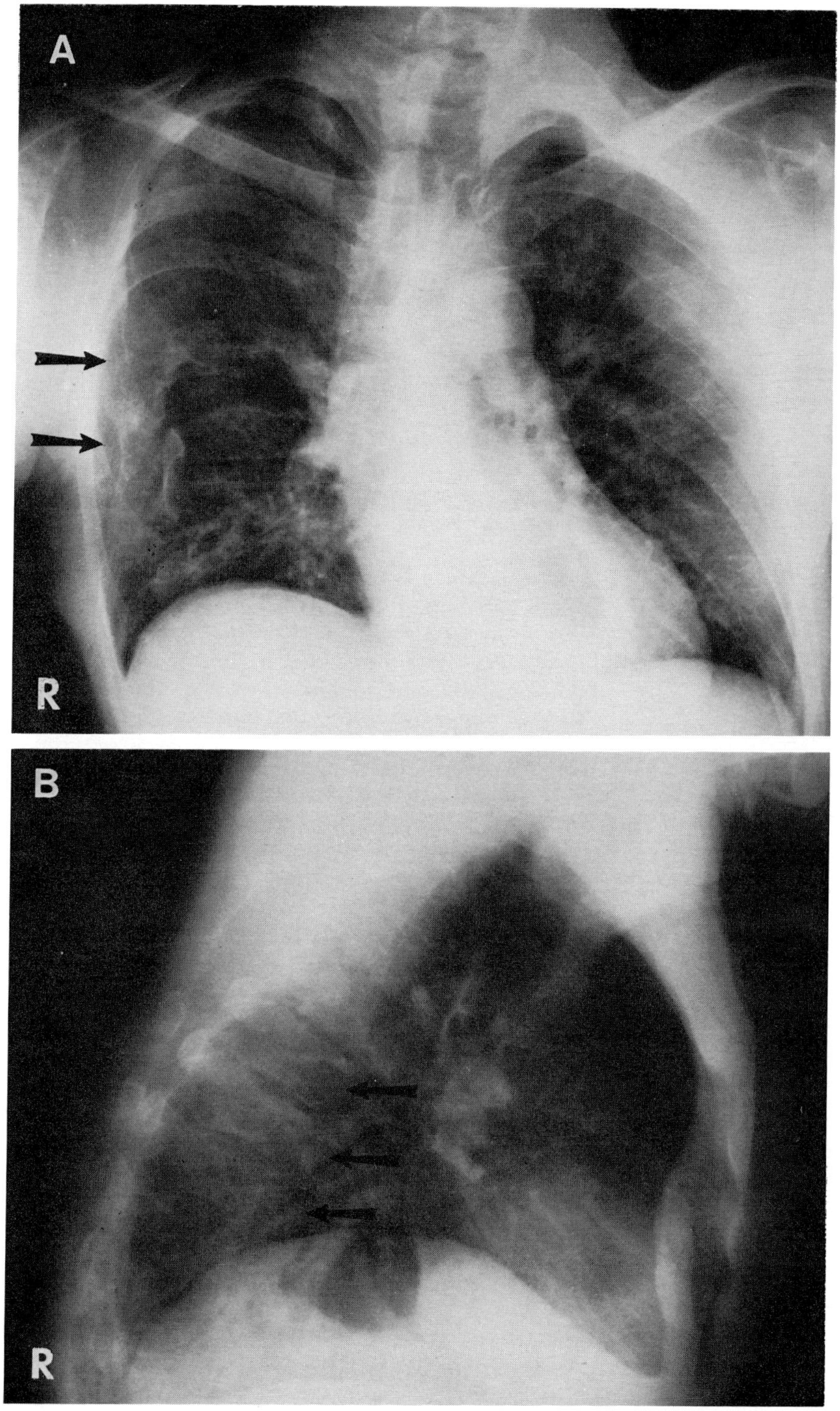

Fig. 29. (Case 2) A) A-P and B) lateral views of chest. Involvement of several right thoracic ribs is manifested by obvious spindle-shaped enlargement (arrows). On the lateral view three of the thoracic vertebrae display areas of bone resorption (arrows).

out the world which for one or another reason escaped the search. Our review, therefore, even though done with great care, does not claim to include every case reported within that particular time period. The number of 69 clinical reports, however, appears sufficient to study some of the clinical and pathological aspects of the disease entity. The available data have been tabulated with respect to 1) age incidence, sex and race distribution, 2) age at onset of clinical symptoms and sequence of clinical symptoms, 3) otological findings, 4) neurological manifestations and complications, 5) radiological appearance, 6) form of fibrous dysplasia, 7) endocrine and other associated disorders, 8) skin pigmentation, 9) serum analysis, 10) biopsies, 11) indication for surgical procedures, numbers and types of operations, 12) operative findings, and 13) complications from the disease and from opera-

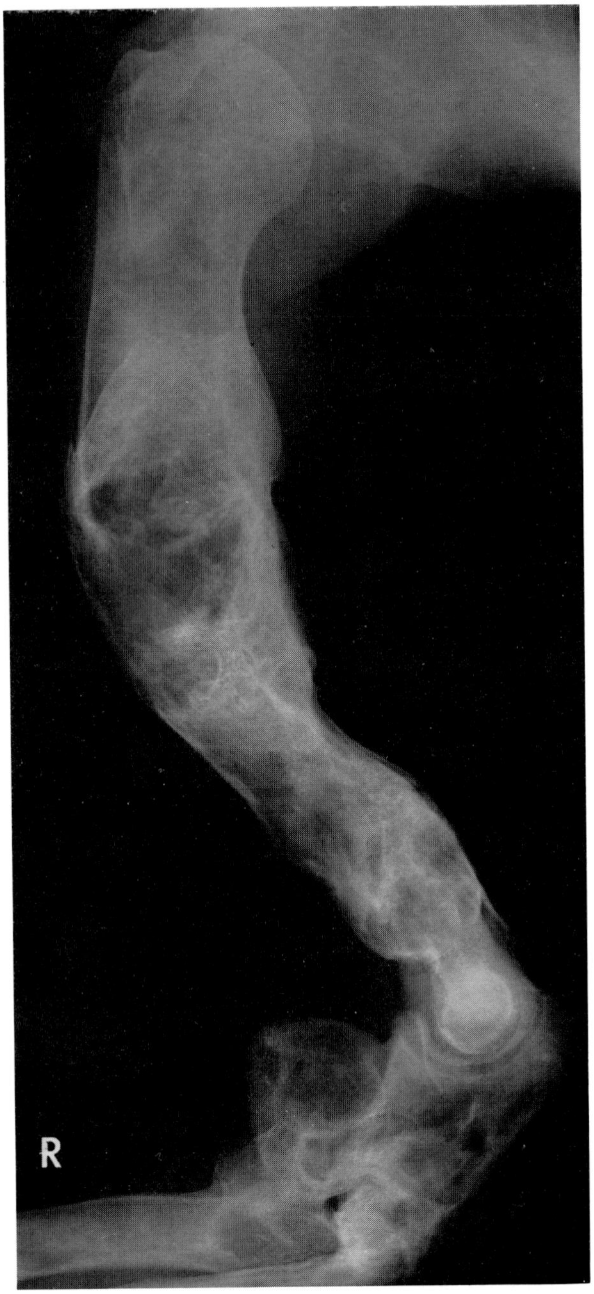

Fig. 30. (Case 2) Policyclic loosening, distension and severe deformity of the right humerus and adjacent portions of radius and ulna are obvious.

tions. The analysis of the available data reveals the following.

Of these 69 patients with fibrous dysplasia involving the temporal bone, 38 were males, 18 were females, and in 13 the sex was not stated. This would suggest a male to female relationship of about 2:1. Fifty-five were white, 2 were orientals, 3 were blacks and in 8 the race was not mentioned. Twenty-six of the 69 patients had the monostotic form, 15 had the polyostotic form, but in 28 the form of fibrous dysplasia was not specified. In 37 instances, biopsies confirming the diagnosis were made. In obviously many more patients positive biopsies were obtained but not mentioned in the paper.

The age at which the patient first consulted a physician was known in 55. It varied between 3 and 80; the mean age was 28 years. The age of onset of the initial clinical manifestation was not known in 37. It varied between birth and 59; the mean age was 15 years.

The most common presenting symptoms in order of decreasing frequency were 1) progressive loss of hearing (39), 2) increase in size of the temporal bone (35), and 3) progressive bony occlusion of the external auditory canal (29). Except for 7 with total loss of cochlear function and 1 with a profound sensorineural hearing loss, all 35 had a conductive hearing loss. In 11 patients constriction or obliteration of the external auditory meatus had given rise to an external epidermoid inclusion cyst or cholesteatoma. The cholesteatoma was associated with a labyrinthitis in 2 instances and with a semicircular canal fistula in 1, and with a postauricular abscess in another patient. Five patients had a peripheral ipsilateral facial nerve palsy. One patient presented with ipsilateral cranial nerve involvement IV to VI. In three patients fibrous dysplasia presented as an intracranial space-occupying lesion. In two of them with massive involvement of the right middle and posterior cranial fossa, the cranial nerves I to XII, and II, V to XII respectively, were affected. The increase in size of the temporal bone was manifested primarily by a postauricular, but in some instances also by a periauricular, preauricular, and supra-auricular swelling. In three patients, the marked swelling of the mastoid process produced an anterior and inferior protrusion of the auricle. Trismus was observed in three patients and reflected involvement and distortion of the temporomandibular articulation. In eight instances the disease was associated with pain. Otorrhea or symptoms of external otitis were hardly ever observed. In one instance, a secondary mastoid infection had led to a basal meningitis, in another to a facial nerve palsy.

The roentgenological examination in general revealed an enlargement of the temporal bone associated with sclerosis, or a uniform "ground-glass" appearance of the augmented bone. Occasionally areas of radiolucency and cortical thinning were observed. The constriction or obliteration of the external auditory canal was regularly confirmed by x-ray studies, but only in two instances was there evidence of narrowing of the internal auditory canal.

Among the 69 patients with temporal bone involvement, the left ear was involved in 28 and the right ear in 27 instances. In 14 the side of involvement was not known. In none of the 69 patients, however, were both temporal bones affected.

Forty-one patients underwent surgical treat-

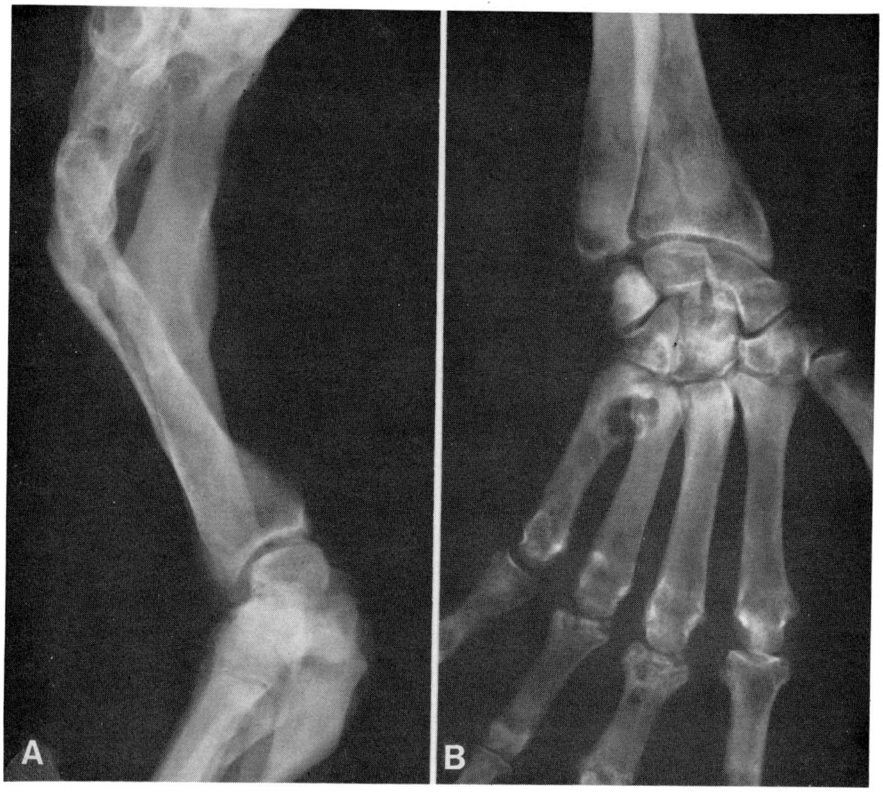

Fig. 31. (Case 2) A) Right forearm shows severe deformity and shortening as a result of diffuse bony involvement and recurrent, healed, spontaneous fractures. A recent unhealed fracture involves the radial shaft. B) Fragmentation of the bases of the proximal phalanges and cystic changes in metacarpal and phalangeal bones are all manifestations of the disease.

ment. In 14 the indication was removal of a bone growth (exostoses) obliterating the external canal, and meatal reconstruction. In 20 who had undergone a mastoid operation, an abnormal swelling of the temporal bone or a postauricular bone mass were the indications. Many of these patients also had meatal stenosis. Of these 41 patients, 20 were operated once, 11 twice, 6 three times, 3 had four operations and 1 had seven operative procedures. Thus, half of all patients (20) required two or more operative procedures, but surgery was rarely curative. In the patients who did not develop a recurrence, the impression was that it was due to a decrease in activity of the disease, rather than because of a surgical cure.

One of the 69 patients, a 9-year-old female, had McCune-Albright syndrome. A 35-year-old patient

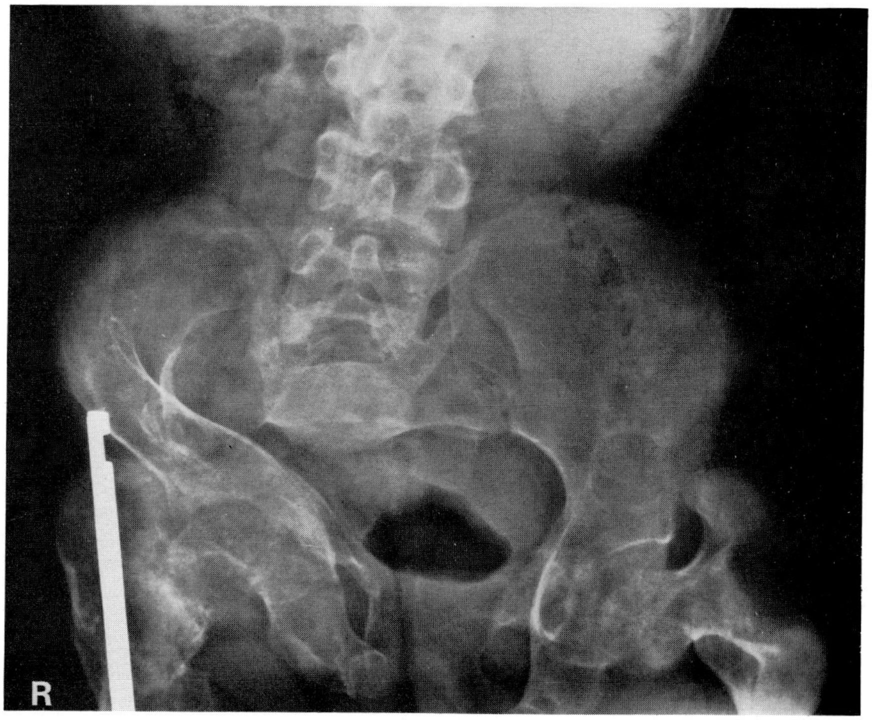

Fig. 32. (Case 2) Diffuse polycystic involvement of entire pelvis resulted in severe deformity and oblique constriction. Extreme shepherd-crook deformity of the upper portion of the femora, inward protrusion of the acetabula and scoliosis of the lumbar spine are obvious.

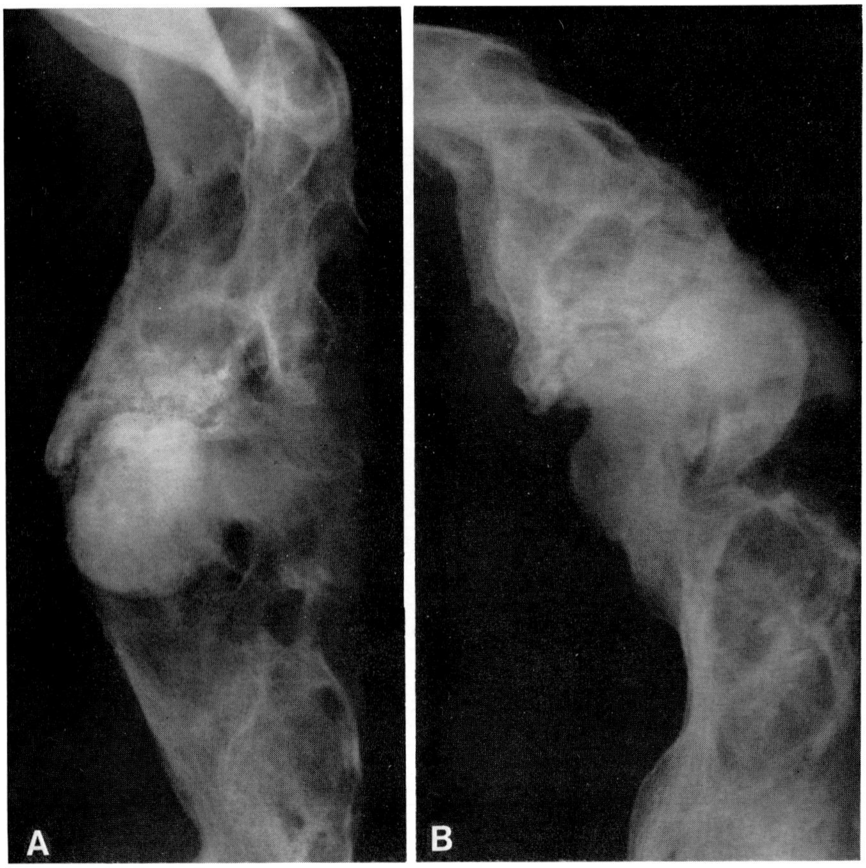

Fig. 33. (Case 2) A) A-P and B) lateral projection of right knee. Distal portion of the right femur and adjacent proximal portion of the tibia exhibit very extensive polycystic involvement which resulted in extreme distortion and deformity of the articulation.

with polyostotic disease and extensive craniofacial involvement, already manifest at birth, also showed several soft tissue tumors involving the right cheek, the right lower lip, and enlargement of the right side of his tongue, all on the side of the skeletal involvement. One 30-year-old female in whom the form of fibrous dysplasia was not stated, who displayed massive involvement of her left temporal bone, was of short stature (4 ft. 4 in.).

Three patients complained of dizziness and four of tinnitus. One patient with tinnitus[149] was a 40-year-old male with a 2½-year-history of fullness, pulse-synchronous tinnitus and hearing loss. Otoscopic examination revealed a reddish mass behind an immobile eardrum. At operation an extremely vascular, soft, pedunculated, bony mass was removed from the midhorizontal section of the fallopian canal. An almost identical case of vascular, sponge-like, gritty, osseous lesion, arising from the promontory in an 11-year-old male suspected of having a glomus tumor, diagnosed as "ossifying fibroma," was reported by Stecker.[156] His initial complaints too were pulsatile tinnitus and progressive loss of hearing.

At operation in nearly every instance all four portions of the temporal bone (mastoid, tympanic, petrous, and squamous) were found to be involved. In every case the diseased bone had a soft, spongy, crumbly and gritty consistency which could easily be scooped out with a curette and which was uniformly very vascular.

The primary complications of fibrous dysplasia were mentioned earlier and include 1) progressive loss of hearing, 2) increase in size of the temporal bone, and 3) gradual obliteration of the external auditory canal. The secondary complications of this disease comprise 1) secondary external cholesteatoma, 2) erosion of the middle ear ossicles, inner ear capsule, and fallopian canal, 3) exposure of the middle and posterior cranial fossa dura, lateral sinus, jugular bulb and carotid artery, 4) blockage of the eustachian tube leading to serous otitis media, and 5) monocranial and polycranial neuropathy.

One of the 69 patients, a 14½-year-old male with a 7 x 7 cm cystic, fibrodysplastic lesion which protruded 4 cm into the cranial cavity died in shock following severe blood loss several hours after his third operation, a neurosurgical procedure.

All patients had normal serum calcium and phosphorous levels and in all but one the serum alkaline phosphatase level was within normal limits.

CASE REPORTS

The case histories of three of our patients are presented here to illustrate the pertinent features of fibrous dysplasia involving the temporal bone. Two

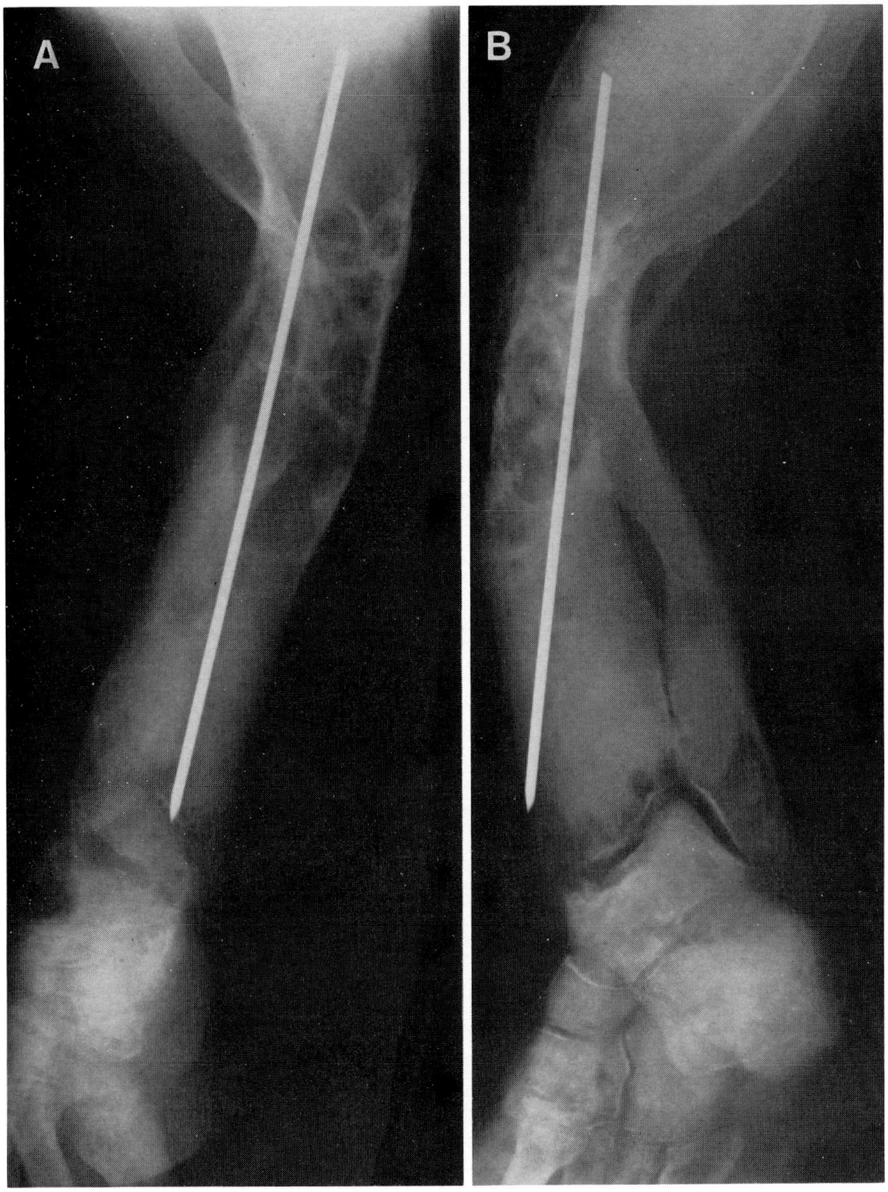

Fig. 34. (Case 2) A) A-P and B) lateral view of right lower extremity. Metal pin in the right lower tibia stabilizes the pathological fracture. Bony bridges unite the severely deformed and bent tibia and fibula which display extensive monocystic radiolucencies and a fine granular osseous pattern. Medial articular surface of the talus exhibits some fragmentation.

of them have polyostotic disease with skin pigmentation and hyperthyroidism. Their widespread skull disease led to bilateral temporal bone involvement. The third has monostotic disease without skin pigmentation but evidence of mild gynecomastia. His temporal bone involvement led to the development of an intracranial space-occupying mass. All are males and developed the initial clinical symptoms during the first decade of life.

Case 1. Polyostotic fibrous dysplasia with skin pigmentation and hyperthyroidism was diagnosed. This included massive involvement of the entire skull, several ribs and metatarsal bones; marked enlargement and deformity of facial and neural cranium; "leonine facies," hypertelorism, exophthalmus and obliteration of paranasal sinuses; and progressive stenosis of external auditory canals resulting in secondary external cholesteatoma on the left, requiring surgical removal and meatal reconstruction. There was a history of recurrent spontaneous rib fractures, pigmented skin patches in lumbar and sacral region, hyperthyroidism requiring thyroidectomies at ages 10 and 11, and subsequent thyroid-depressing medication until age 20.

Our patient was a 45-year-old attorney with a family history of hyperthyroidism. At the age of 10, after an apparently minor head injury, he developed a hard swelling involving the occipital bone, which on biopsy proved to be fibrous dysplasia, and also symptoms of hyperthyroidism. Also noticed at that time were three unelevated brownish pigmented skin patches in the lumbar and sacral area. A few months after the initial partial thyroidectomy (age 10), symptoms of hyperactive thyroid disease recurred. A subtotal thyroidectomy was performed at the age of 11, followed by radioactive and other antithyroid therapy until 20, when the condition was thought to be stabilized. His adolescence had been uneventful with puberty developing at normal age.

The family history is significant in that his mother was treated for hyperactive thyroid disease and finally underwent a total thyroidectomy.

At age 33, following a sneeze, the patient suffered a spontaneous fracture of a right thoracic rib in an area of localized fibrous dysplasia. Thereafter he suffered repeated pathological fractures in the same location. In recent years he was found to have fibrous dysplasia involving several metatarsal bones.

Already at the age of 10 he was found to have a very narrow and irregular left external auditory canal which produced in-

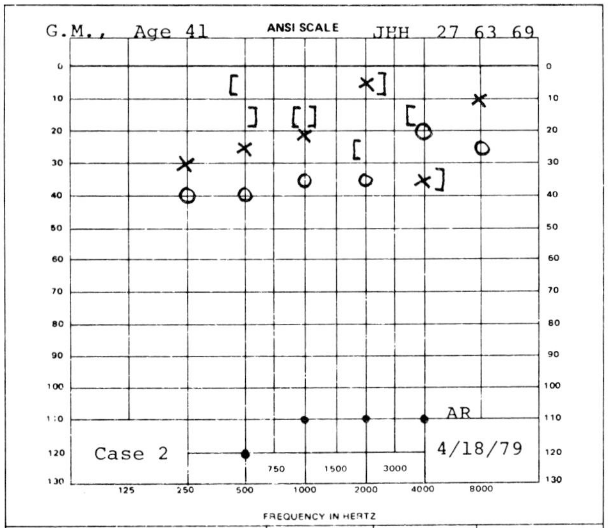

	SPEAKER	RT. EAR	LT. EAR	AID	EAR(S)
SPEECH RECEPTION THRESHOLD (SRT)	dB	35 dB	25 dB		dB
DISCRIMINATION	%	100 %	100 %		%
dB ABOVE SRT					

Fig. 35. (Case 2) Audiogram.

creasing difficulties with cleaning. At the age of 34, he was operated elsewhere for an external cholesteatoma in that ear. Shortly thereafter he was referred to us with a nearly complete closure of the canal, an underlying recurrent cholesteatoma, progressive loss of hearing and otalgia in that ear.

Examination on admission revealed considerable enlargement and deformity of the facial and neural cranium, characterized by a leonine facies, hypertelorism, bilateral exopthalmus and an occipital pug (Fig. 18). His stature was normal. Three irregular, nonelevated, dark brownish skin pigmentations, of the size of a half-dollar, were located in the lumbar and sacral area slightly to the right of the midline (Fig. 18). An enlarged right thyroid node was palpable beneath the thyroidectomy scar. The patient was found to be again hyperthyroid. There was no evidence of additional endocrine disturbances or other associated disorders.

Otoscopic examination disclosed a near complete osseous obliteration of the left external auditory canal associated with an external otitis and an underlying cholesteatoma. The right external auditory canal revealed some narrowing with irregular contours. Cochlear function studies showed a bilateral conductive hearing loss with an SRT of 65 dB on the left and 30 dB on the right and 100% discrimination bilaterally (Fig. 19).

Roentgenological examination of the skull displayed marked enlargement and deformity with diffuse sclerosis involving the neurocranium and facial cranium (Fig. 20 A, B). As a result, the frontal and maxillary sinuses were totally or incompletely obliterated by concentric new bone formation (Fig. 21 A-D). Roentgenograms of the temporal bones exhibited in addition to narrowing of the middle ear cavity, an enlargement of malleus and incus with some increase in density. They also showed a marked narrowing of the external auditory canals (Fig. 22A).

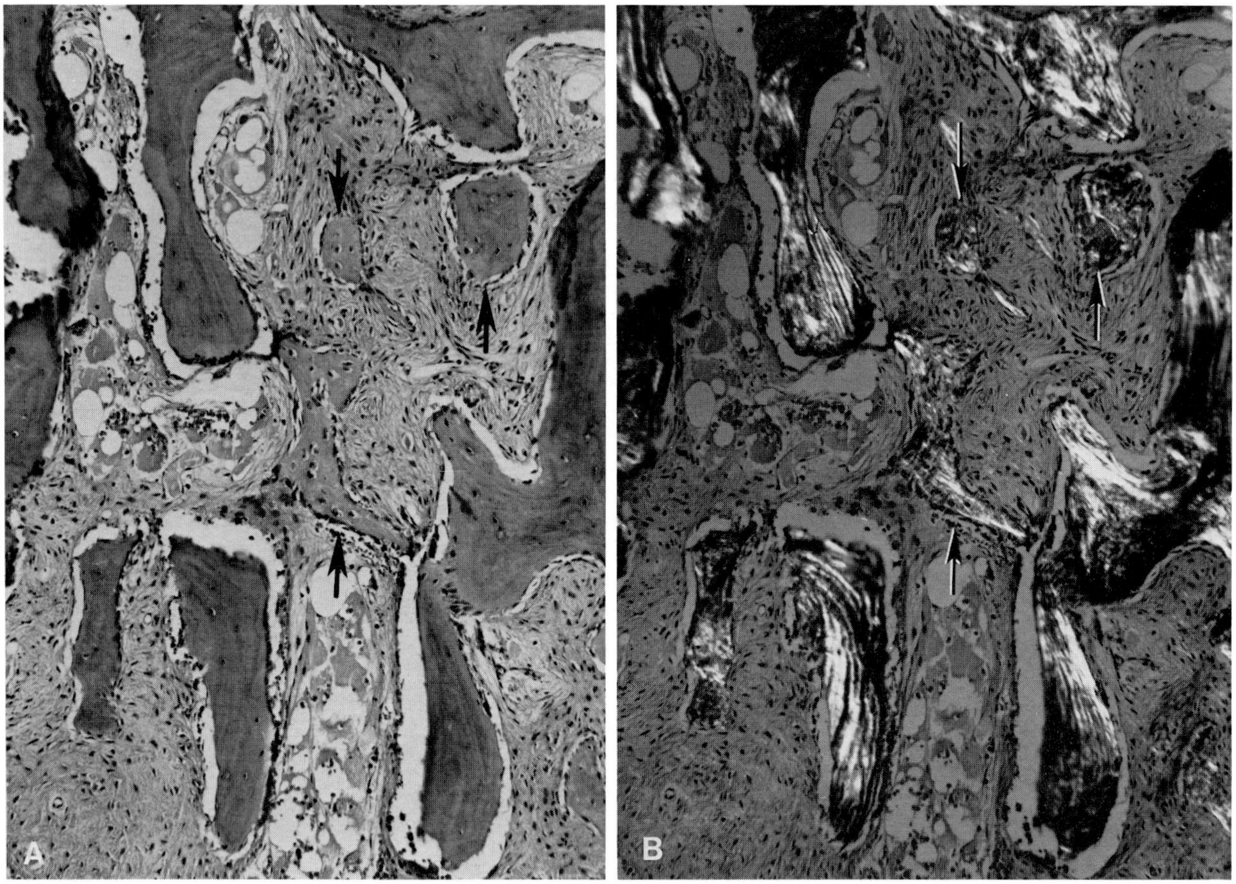

Fig. 36. (Case 2) A) Biopsy from the medullary cavity beneath the attenuated cortex of the anterior aspect of the left proximal tibia. It shows three central trabeculae of woven bone (arrows) embedded in a cellular fibrous tissue surrounded by larger trabeculae of lamellar bone. B) Same section under polarized light displays the characteristic birefringence of woven bone compared with that of the mature bone. (H & E, x 150)

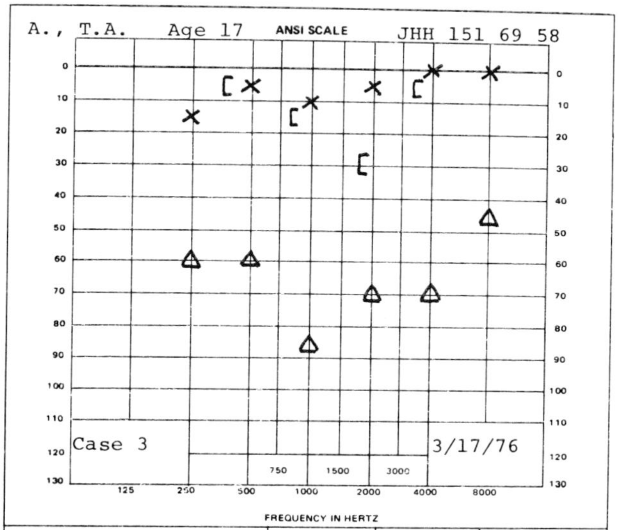

	SPEAKER	RT EAR	LT EAR	AID EAR(S)
SPEECH RECEPTION THRESHOLD (SRT)	dB	65 dB	5 dB	BC SRT (R) 15 dB
DISCRIMINATION	%	96 %	100 %	OEM 60 %
dB ABOVE SRT		40	40	

Fig. 37. (Case 3) Audiogram.

The serum alkaline phosphatase was elevated (44 IU/l); calcium (8.8 mg/d) and phosphate were decreased (3 mg/dl).

Under general anesthesia the left external auditory canal was reconstructed and a large external cholesteatoma removed. The dysplastic process involved all four portions of the temporal bone. It had the consistency of a pumice stone, felt gritty and was very vascular. The middle ear cavity was constricted. Many of the landmarks were distorted by new bone formation. The middle ear ossicles were also involved in the bony process. The biopsy revealed fibrous dysplasia (Fig. 24). The postoperative course was uneventful. The patient was started on a course of antithyroid medication. A permanent Silastic stent was placed in the external canal for prevention of restenosis, to be exchanged and cleaned at regular intervals (Figs. 20B and 23). It has been tolerated well for many years. The patient's most recent hearing test disclosed an SRT of 10 dB and a discrimination score of 100% in the operated ear. He has been treated with phosphate supplements and vitamin D by mouth. His alkaline phosphatase has been decreasing to 46 IU/l, reaching almost normal values (10-32 IU/l); serum calcium 8.8 mg/dl (normal 9-11) and phosphate levels (3 mg/dl) also have been approaching normal values (normal phosphate: 3-4.5 mg/dl).

Case 2. Bilateral polyostotic fibrous dysplasia with skin pigmentations and hyperthyroidism was diagnosed. The patient had extensive involvement of all extremities, entire skull, spine, several ribs, right scapula, both clavicles and pelvis; enlargement and deformity of facial and neural cranium; frontal bossing, occipital pug and basalar invagination; numerous spontaneous fractures of the extremities requiring multiple orthopedic procedures; premature closure of the epiphyseal centers; severe deformity of the entire skeleton resulting in crippling and short stature; gradual narrowing of external auditory canals, secondary external otitis and involvement of outer middle ear ossicles; and pigmented skin patches over the left anterior chest, back of neck and right lumbosacral area.

A 42-year-old data retrieval specialist at the age of 4 developed the first of what subsequently amounted to a total of about 50 pathological fractures resulting in the establishment of the diagnosis of bilateral polyostotic fibrous dysplasia. The skeletal lesions and injuries required numerous orthopedic procedures. The number and extent of dysplastic lesions, the spontaneous fractures, and the premature closure of the epiphyseal centers resulted in severe skeletal deformity, crippling and short stature. At the age of 30 he suffered a collapse of a thoracic vertebra, requiring a spinal fusion (Fig. 10). At the age of 32, he was found to have hyperthyroidism, clinically and biochemically, and from then on received antithyroid therapy. He developed pubic hair growth at the age of 14. He had a lifelong history of allergies.

On *physical examination*, the patient was found to be very short in stature. He displayed numerous, severe musculoskeletal deformities, but nevertheless ambulated with remarkable adroitness with the aid of a pelvic brace and crutches. The head revealed severe frontal bossing, asymmetry and deformity (Fig. 25). A large, nonelevated, irregularly contoured "coast of Maine" café au lait skin patch was noticed over the left upper anterior chest wall, in the back of the neck, and in the right lumbosacral area. The thyroid gland disclosed an obvious nodular enlargement, the right lobe being larger than the left.

During the past six years, the patient had had recurrent episodes of unsteadiness and dizziness, occasionally with a sensation of swaying, often following sudden head movements and change of position, occurring on a daily basis. On bending over they were often accompanied by a sensation of spinning. For three years he had bilateral tinnitus and periods of fullness and pressure in both, but more severely in the right ear. He had also noticed a mild loss of hearing, more marked in the right ear. Occasionally discrimination seemed to be impaired. Four years ago he was found to have a concentric narrowing of the right visual field. The serum calcium levels generally were around 9.5 mg/dl (normal 9-11) but

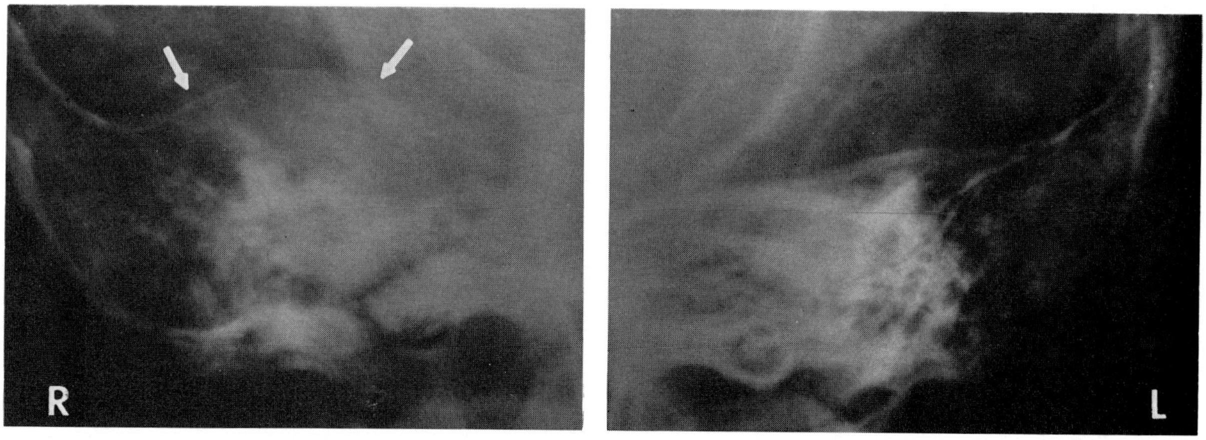

Fig. 38. (Case 3) Longitudinal (Stenver) view of right and left petrous pyramids. The fibro-osseous lesion which caused a ballooning of the right pyramid displays a uniform ground-glass structure and is covered by an extremely thin layer of cortical bone (arrows).

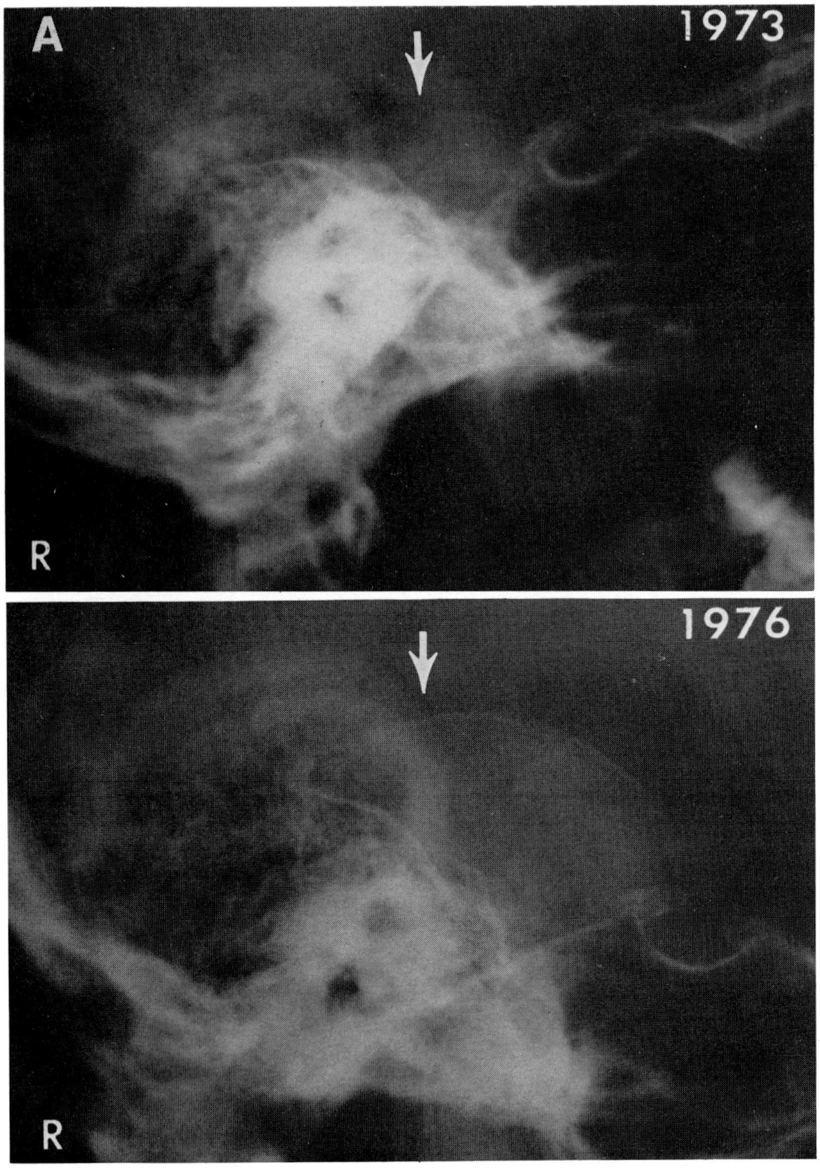

Fig. 39. (Case 3) A) Lateral projections of the right temporal bone projections of the skull in 1973 and 1976 clearly show the increase in size of the dysplastic process over the 3-year period (arrows).

occasionally had been as low as 7.9 mg/dl. Serum phosphate levels were around 2.5 mg/dl (normal 3-4.5). Alkaline phosphatase initially was much elevated, reaching levels up to 265 units but more recently dropped to 91 units (normal 10-32 μ). At one time the patient had had some polydipsia with serum glucose levels rising slightly above 120 mg/dl, but subsequent glucose tolerance tests failed to show significant abnormalities.

The *neurological examination* revealed an old Horner syndrome on the right thought to be related to an abnormality of his cervical spine. There was no evidence of central nervous system involvement or basilar artery insufficiency.

The *roentgenological examination* revealed extensive involvement of the neurocranium and facial cranium with lytic lesions, and scattered focal and diffuse sclerosis, thickening of the diploic space, inner and outer tables, enlargement of the frontal and occipital bone, and basilar invagination (Fig. 26 A, B). Both frontal, right ethmoid, right maxillary and a portion of the left maxillary sinus were opacified. The temporal bones displayed diffuse sclerosis which obscured the otic capsule, the internal auditory canal and the mastoid cell system, leaving the middle ear cavity fairly well demarcated (Figs. 27 and 28). A kyphoscoliosis involving the spine was most marked in the dorsal-lumbar junction (Fig. 29). Whereas the spinous process of cervical C-2 and the body of C-6 disclosed lytic and sclerotic lesions, involvement of lumbar L-1 through L-5 was characterized by diffuse sclerosis of the vertebral body. The right seventh and eighth and the left fifth rib displayed fusiform expansile lytic lesions (Fig. 29). The right scapula and both clavicles exhibited bone involvement. The right humerus disclosed widespread disease (Fig. 30). The right elbow was hardly recognizable. Extensive involvement of the right radius and ulna had resulted in expansion, deformity and an unhealed fracture in the distal radial shaft (Fig. 31). Cystic lesions were encountered in some of the metacarpal and phalangeal bones of the right hand (Fig. 31). Massive involvement of the pelvis and femora had led to severe oblique constriction of the pelvis with inward protrusion of the acetabula of the femur and to a shepherd-crook deformity of the latter (Fig. 32). The right knee was almost unrecognizable due to widespread involvement of predominantly cystic lesions (Fig. 33). The right tibia and fibula displayed grotesque deformities characterized by medial bowing, distention and a conglomerate of radiolucent lesions in the cental tibial shaft and spiraling of the fibula (Fig. 34). The left upper and lower extremities exhibited similar changes, and both feet showed evidence of localized disease.

On *otological examination* both external auditory canals disclosed a moderate degree of irregular, concentric narrowing, more obvious on the right, and a mild diffuse external otitis. There was a small epidermoid inclusion cyst embedded in the

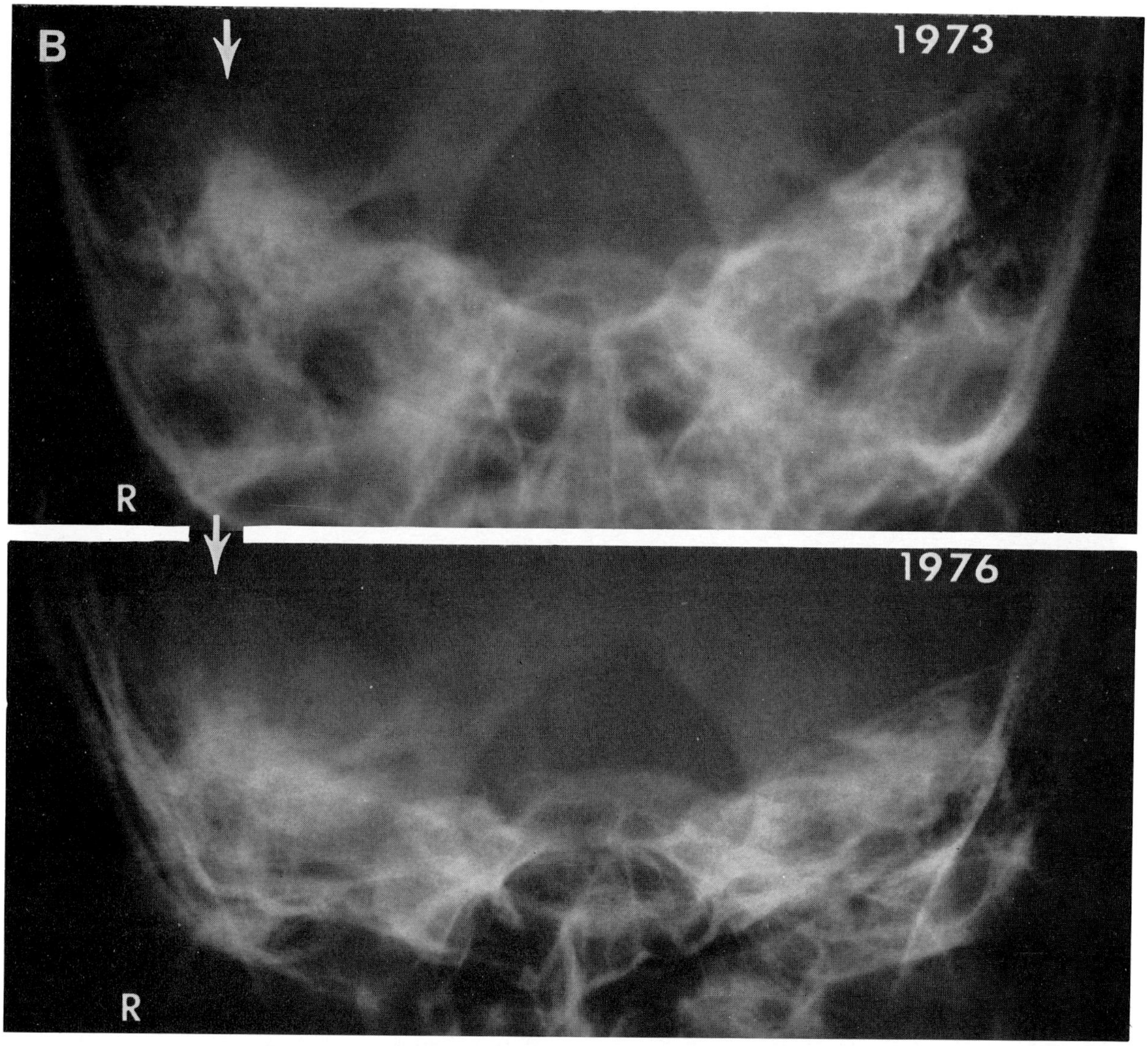

Fig. 39, cont'd. B) A-P (Town) projection showing similar findings.

right meatal skin. The right and left malleus showed a definite increase in size as a result of bone involvement (Fig. 28). Cochlear function studies revealed a mild bilateral conductive hearing loss with an SRT of 30 dB on the right and 25 dB on the left (Fig. 35). Discrimination was 100% bilaterally. Vestibular function studies revealed a poor optokinetic nystagmus, a positional nystagmus in head-hanging positions with Frenzel glasses, bidirectional gaze nystagmus and rather feeble responses to caloric stimulation bilaterally, suggesting the possibility of brainstem involvement. (Testing was done by Dr. L. Proctor.)

A biopsy from the right tibia in 1971 had identified the bone lesion as fibrous dysplasia (Fig. 36). The patient has been followed regularly for the past ten years. His gradually progressive skeletal deformity necessitated retirement at the age of 40.

Case 3. Monostotic fibrous dysplasia involving the right temporal bone associated with gynecomastia was diagnosed. Progressive tumorous enlargement of the right petrous pyramid with extension into the middle and posterior cranial fossa and increasing narrowing of the right external auditory canal were found.

A 17-year-old male at the age of 10 was referred for evaluation of a right-sided progressive conductive hearing loss. On *physical examination* no skeletal anomalies or skull deformities were noted.

The *otological examination* showed no significant narrowing of the right external auditory canal. The right tympanic membrane appeared normal. The audiometric evaluation revealed a 55 dB flat conductive hearing loss in the right but normal hearing in the left ear (Fig. 37).

The *roentgenological examination* (1973) disclosed a recognizable increase in size of the right petrous pyramid which extended laterally into the base of the squamous portion and into the anterior and superior tympanic portion of the temporal bone. The augmented petrous bone which was bounded superiorly by distended, eggshell-thin cortical bone, had a ground-glass appearance (Figs. 38-40).

On *surgical exploration* the roof and anterior wall of the right external auditory canal were replaced by an abnormally soft, vascular, gritty, yellowish, fibro-osseous tissue, which on microscopic examination proved to be fibrous dysplasia (Fig. 41).

In 1976, at the age of 13, there still was no recognizable external deformity of the right temporal bone. However, the external auditory canal had become markedly constricted. The tympanic membrane had become retracted and the middle ear filled with an amber fluid. The long process of the incus had undergone necrosis, and a natural myringostapediopexy had formed. The conductive hearing loss had increased by 10 dB to a 65 dB level. The roentgenological examination showed a considerable increase in size and additional cortical expansion of the right petrous pyra-

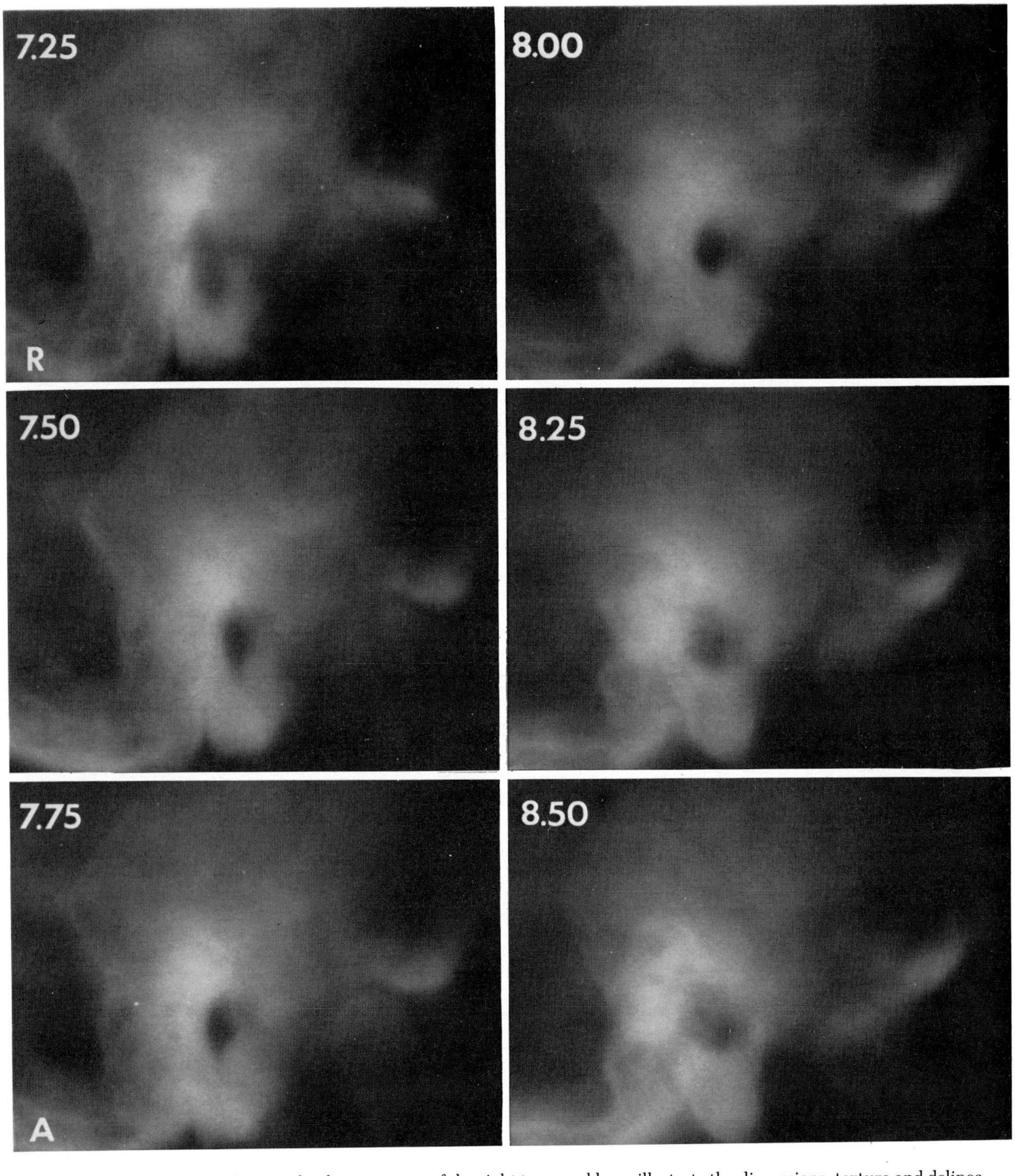

Fig. 40. A, B) (Case 3) Lateral polytomograms of the right temporal bone illustrate the dimensions, texture and delineation of the fibro-osseous lesion.

mid. The three dimensional enlargement of the petrous portion was well recognized in the CAT scan. A bone survey failed to demonstrate additional skeletal lesions. The serum levels for calcium, phosphorus and alkaline phosphatase were normal. Besides a mild form of gynecomastia, there was no evidence of other endocrinopathies. The EEG was normal. A right myringotomy was performed and a ventilation tube inserted.

In 1978, at the age of 15, a CAT scan (Fig. 42) showed little increase in size of the intracranial extension of the temporal bone lesion, and at the present time, the patient exhibits no additional changes or neurological deficits.

DISCUSSION AND CONCLUSIONS

Perusal of the literature reveals that fibrous dysplasia is no longer an uncommon skeletal disorder and that involvement of the temporal bone is not an exclusive rarity. At least 69, very likely more, patients with temporal bone involvement have been reported during the past four decades. It thus becomes a challenge for the otolaryngologist to acquaint himself with the clinical features of the dis-

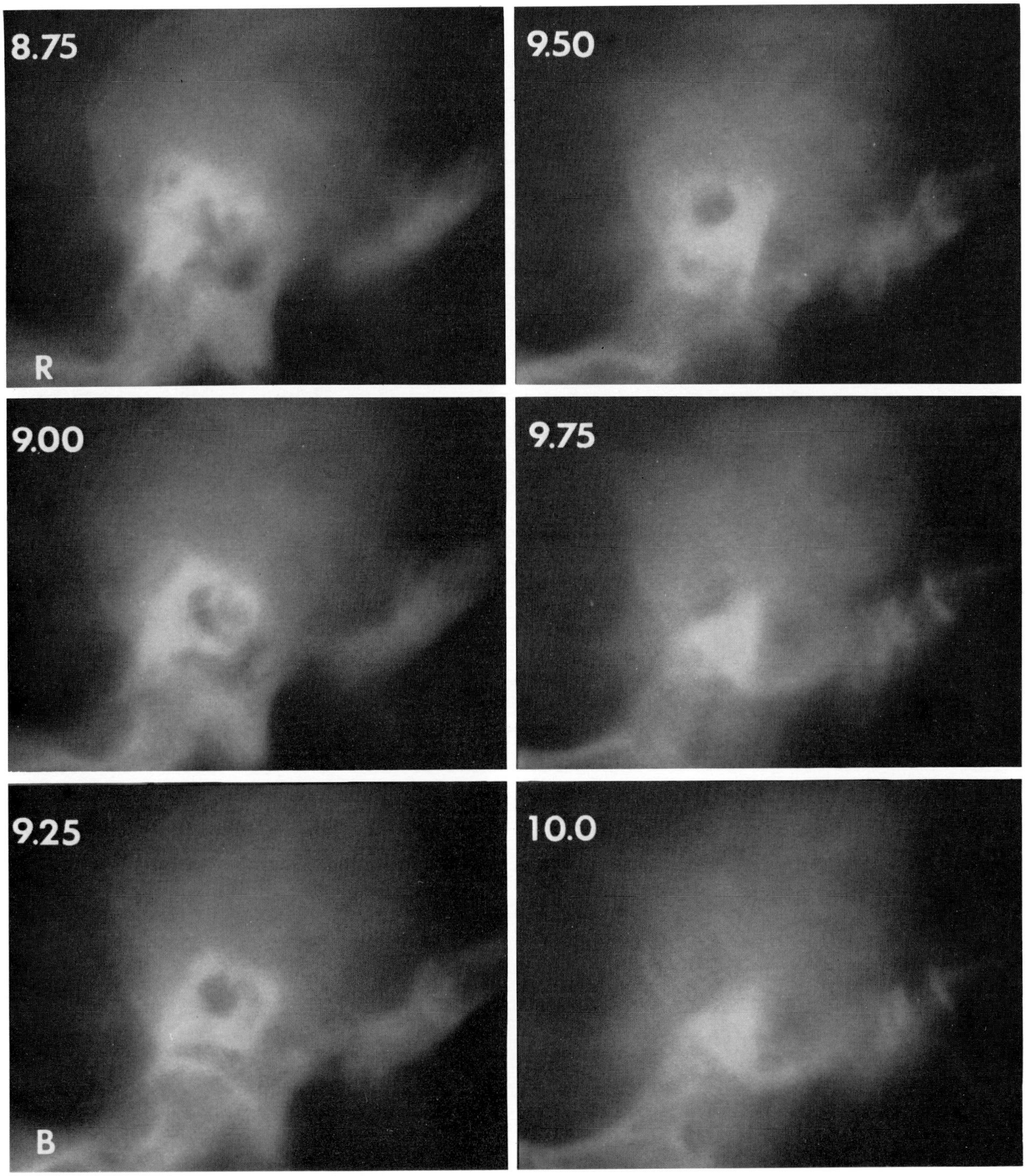

Fig. 40, cont'd.

ease. To provide him with the pertinent information, an attempt was made initially to review the clinical, radiological, and pathological aspects of the disease in general and secondarily, to study the manifestations of the condition in the temporal bone. This enables us to draw the following conclusions.

Fibrous dysplasia is a disease of younger people usually manifesting itself in childhood or early adolescence. In some instances, it has been observed at birth.[175] Most investigators therefore assume a congenital nature for this developmental anomaly of the bone-forming mesenchyme. With the rare exception of sarcomatous transformation, it generally is a benign, self-limiting disease which usually ceases to grow after having reached a certain stage. In many instances puberty does not have a stabilizing effect.

Fibrous dysplasia is the most frequent benign skeletal disease affecting the skull. The skull is one

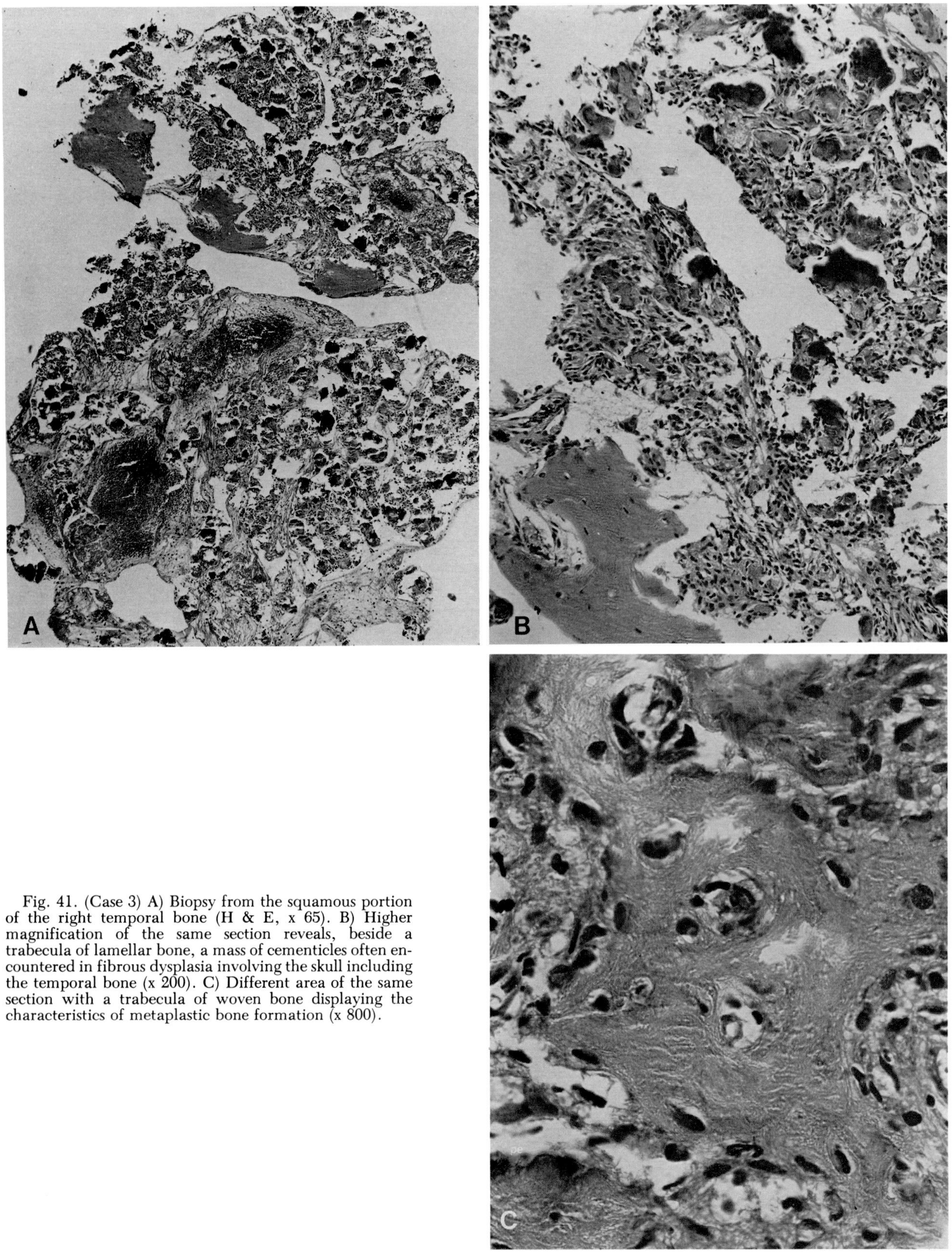

Fig. 41. (Case 3) A) Biopsy from the squamous portion of the right temporal bone (H & E, x 65). B) Higher magnification of the same section reveals, beside a trabecula of lamellar bone, a mass of cementicles often encountered in fibrous dysplasia involving the skull including the temporal bone (x 200). C) Different area of the same section with a trabecula of woven bone displaying the characteristics of metaplastic bone formation (x 800).

of the most common sites of skeletal involvement. It may be affected exclusively in the monostotic form of the disease, but on the other hand, one or several lesions can represent the initial manifestation of the polyostotic form. In monostotic disease the incidence of craniofacial involvement is about 10%. In polyostotic disease, the incidence rises to 50% in the presence of moderate skeletal involvement, but

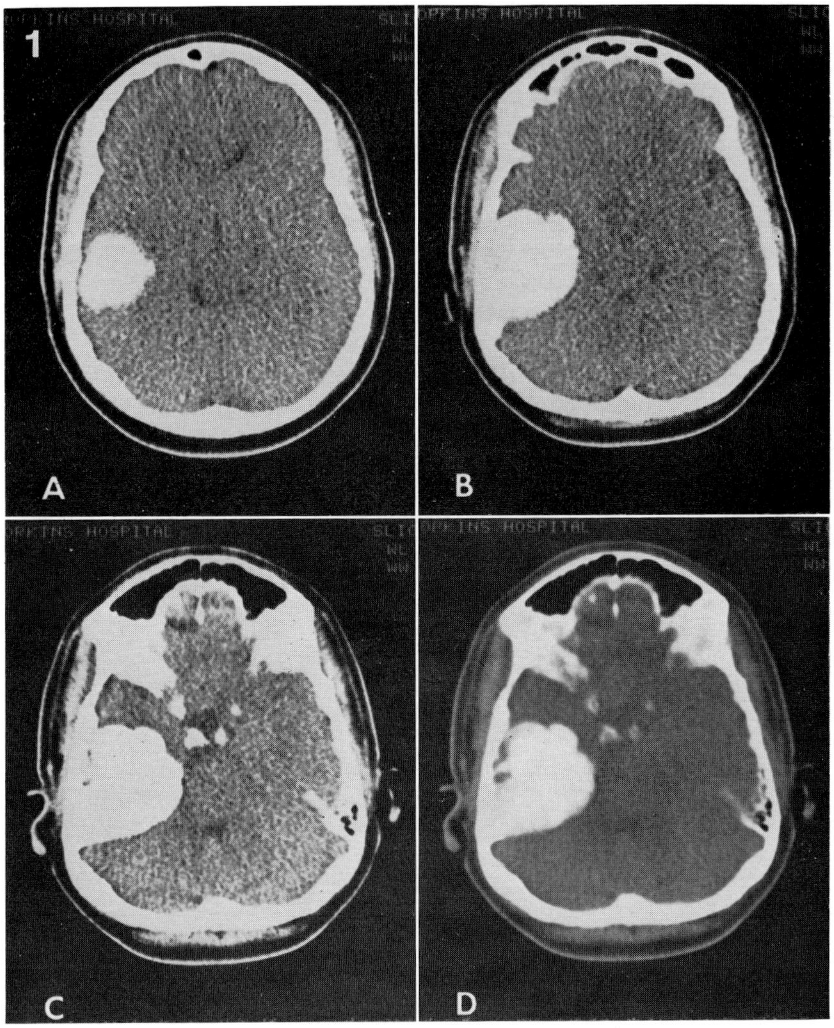

Fig. 42. (Case 3) 1 A-D) Computerized tomography of the skull in the axial projection to show the monostotic fibrodysplastic process involving the right temporal bone. Diffusely enlarged and sclerotic petrous pyramid extends considerably into the right middle and posterior cranial fossa.

reaches 100% with extensive skeletal involvement.[48] It generally begins as a hardly noticeable, gradually progressive, painless swelling in the neurocranium or facial cranium. If the lesion is small, located in the base, or covered by a thick layer of soft tissue, it remains unnoticed only to be detected incidentally. The process usually is not limited to a single bone, rather it extends across a suture line into an adjacent bone. There is a tendency toward a unilateral distribution. In some instances, vast areas of the entire skull may be affected. The skull bones most frequently involved are the frontal and the sphenoid bones, followed by the ethmoid, parietal, temporal, and occipital bones. The temporal bones are affected in about 18% of skull involvement. As a rule only one temporal bone is affected, but in widespread polyostotic disease, both temporal bones may become involved, as illustrated in two of our cases. The disease regularly affects all four portions of the temporal bone. Our survey indicates that involvement of the temporal bone is more often a manifestation of monostotic than polyostotic disease, the ratio being 2:1. However, since the majority of the 69 patients probably did not have skeletal surveys, the actual ratio could be different.

In the temporal bone, the process generally begins as a painless, slowly progressive swelling involving the mastoid process or squama, or occasionally with asymmetry of the skull, at times with a preauricular protrusion interfering with mobility in the temporomandibular joint, or with progressive obliteration of the external auditory canal. Thus the deformity of the temporal bone is a pathognomonic feature.

The radiological features of temporal bone involvement include an increase in size and bone density associated with areas of sclerosis and radiolucency. They reflect the underlying histologic architecture and vary with the amount of fibrosis and degree of calcification. Areas of prevailing fibrosis and cyst formation produce a radiolucency, whereas areas with predominating new bone formation create regions of increased bony density. The disease process may obliterate the entire cellular system and replace vast areas with a uniform, dense, ground-glasslike bony pattern. In addition to the features mentioned earlier, the hyperostotic process may give rise to a remarkable intracranial enlargement of the petrous pyramid. Our survey

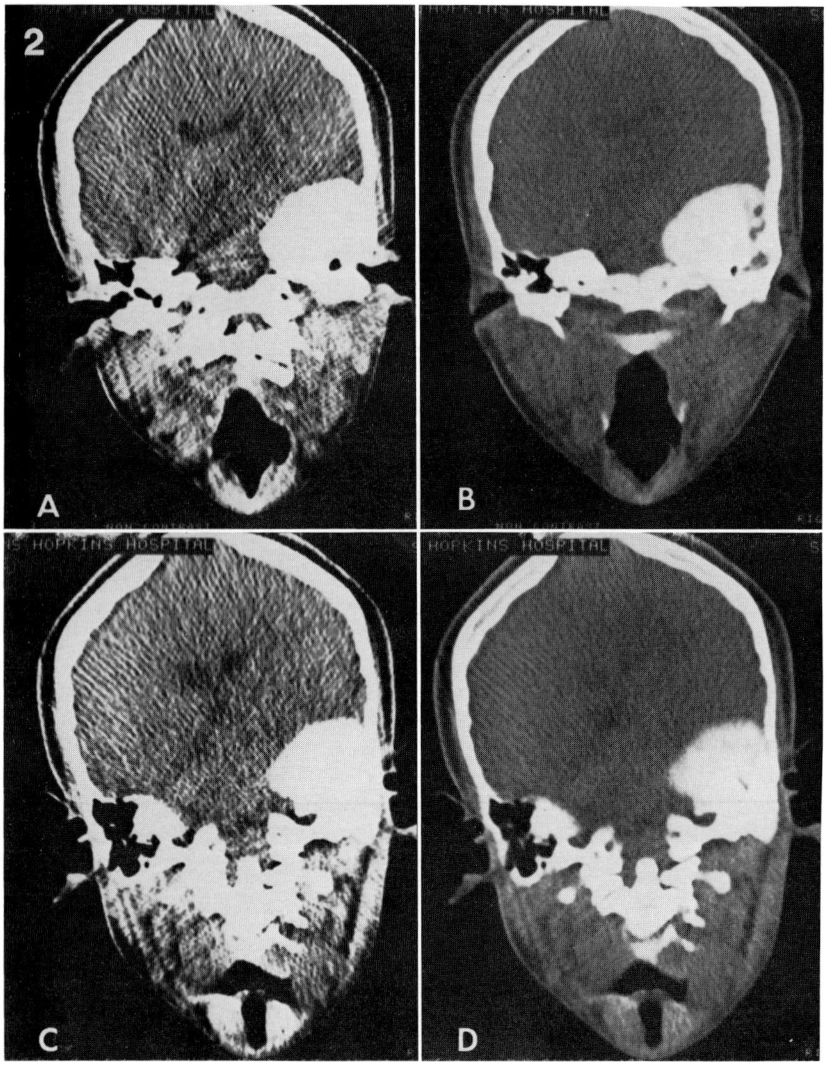

Fig. 42, cont'd. 2 A-D) Computerized tomography of the temporal bone in the coronal projection. A - Brain setting, B - Bone setting at the level of the internal auditory canal. C - Brain setting, D - Bone setting at the level of the jugular foramen. Three dimensional enlargement and sclerosis of the petrous pyramid is again demonstrated in the coronal plane.

revealed no difference between the sides involved. The serum levels for calcium, phosphorus and alkaline phosphatase are usually normal, but in widespread and bilateral involvement the alkaline phosphatase is elevated, as observed in two of our patients. Sarcomatous transformation has not yet been reported, but should it occur, an increase in growth rate, evidence of bone destruction and pain would herald such a process in the temporal bone. One patient presented the McCune-Albright syndrome. One patient with evidence of polyostotic disease at birth showed several soft tissue tumors involving the right cheek, right lower lip, an enlargement of the right side of his tongue, all on the side of the skeletal involvement.

The clinical features of temporal bone involvement are as follows. The age at which the patients first seek medical advice varied between 7 and 80; the mean age was 27 years. The age of onset of initial clinical manifestation varied between birth and 59; the mean age was 15 years. The male to female ratio was about 2:1. The most common presenting symptoms in order of decreasing frequency were 1) progressive loss of hearing, 2) increase in size of the temporal bone, and 3) progressive bony obliteration of the external auditory canal. The great majority of patients had a conductive hearing loss resulting from canal occlusion, but in several with total loss of hearing and one with a profound sensorineural loss, involvement of the otic capsule by the disease process was the cause. The secondary complications included 1) development of secondary cholesteatoma behind the canal stenosis or obliteration, in an incidence of 16%, 2) erosion of the middle ear ossicles, inner ear capsule, and fallopian canal, leading to a labyrinthitis and facial palsy, 3) exposure of the dura of the middle and posterior cranial fossa and of the greater vessels, 4) monocranial and polycranial neuropathy, and 5) blockage of the eustachian tube. Very few patients complained about otalgia, dizziness or tinnitus. In two patients with pulsatile tinnitus and a reddish mass behind the eardrum, a fibrodysplastic lesion originating from the medial wall of the tympanic cavity simulated an intratympanic paraganglioma. In a rare instance, fibrous dysplasia simulated an intracranial tumor and twice caused narrowing of

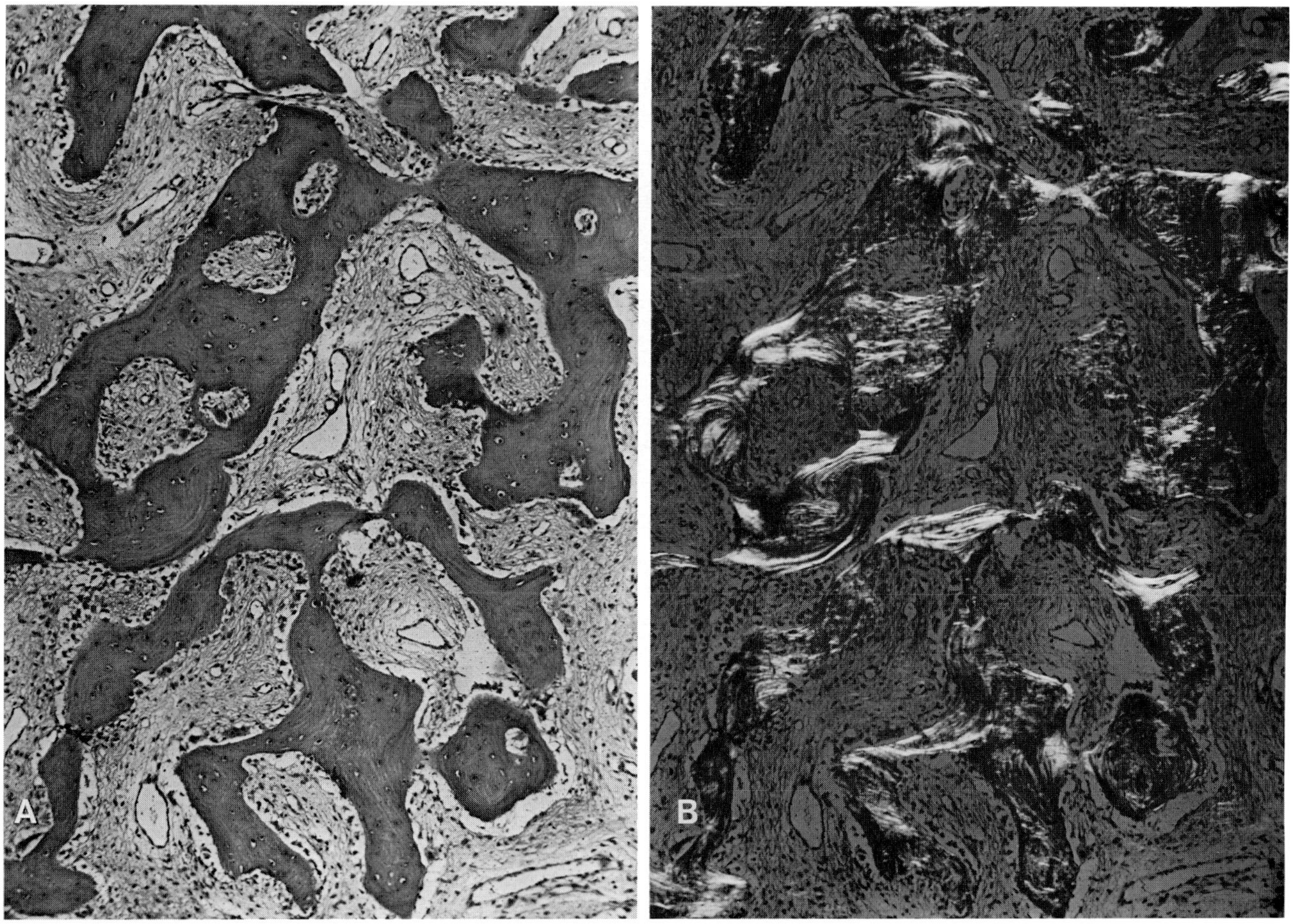

Fig. 43. Biopsy from left external auditory canal of a 12-year-old male with onset of progressive loss of hearing at the age of 10 and obliterative fibrous dysplasia of the tympanic portion of the temporal bone; a 50 dB conductive hearing loss and a secondary external cholesteatoma were present. Three operative procedures were required (1970, Katharinen Hospital, Stuttgart, Prof. Kirstein; July 12, 1971, and July 2, 1975, ORL Clinic, Tübingen, Prof. D. Plester) (H & E, x 120). A) Irregular, poorly oriented, partly calcified trabeculae of immature bone with B) irregular, randomly distributed birefringent fibers under polarized light, embedded in a fairly cellular and vascular stoma, identifies this lesion as fibrous dysplasia. (Courtesy of Prof. E. Steinbach, ORL Clinic, Tübingen).

the internal auditory canal. The majority of patients underwent an operation for exploration of an unidentified swelling involving the lateral aspect of the temporal bone, or for removal of exostoses from the outer ear canal. In every instance, the diseased bone had a soft, spongy, crumbly and gritty consistency which could be easily shelled out by curette, and which was uniformly very vascular. About half of all patients required two or more operative procedures, but surgery was rarely curative with restenosis developing. The management, therefore, should be conservative and restricted to reestablishment of function, to prevention of complications, and when indicated, to cosmetic remodeling. Restenosis of the external auditory canal can be prevented by placement of a permanent Silastic stent, as illustrated in one of our patients. In monostotic disease, the diagnosis has to be confirmed by biopsy, whereas in polyostotic disease the presence of other typical lesions elsewhere may suffice. Radiation therapy should be avoided. The differential diagnosis should include 1) osteitis deformans Paget, 2) hyperparathyroidism,3) a local reaction to a meningioma, and 4) an osteoma.

SUMMARY

Fibrous dysplasia of bone is a fairly common, possibly congenital, locally circumscribed misdifferentiation of bone-forming mesenchyme into an isomorphous fibrous tissue of spindled cells comprising poorly formed trabeculae, spicules and cementicles of metaplastic woven bone.

It may affect a single, several or many bones. Accordingly, monostotic, oligostotic and polyostotic forms are distinguished. Its predilective sites include the metaphyses and diaphyses of long bones, ribs, shoulders, pelvic region and the craniofacial skeleton. The localization of bone lesions favors a unilateral distribution. The etiology so far has remained obscure.

The initial clinical symptoms may include recurrent pains in affected bones and adjacent joints,

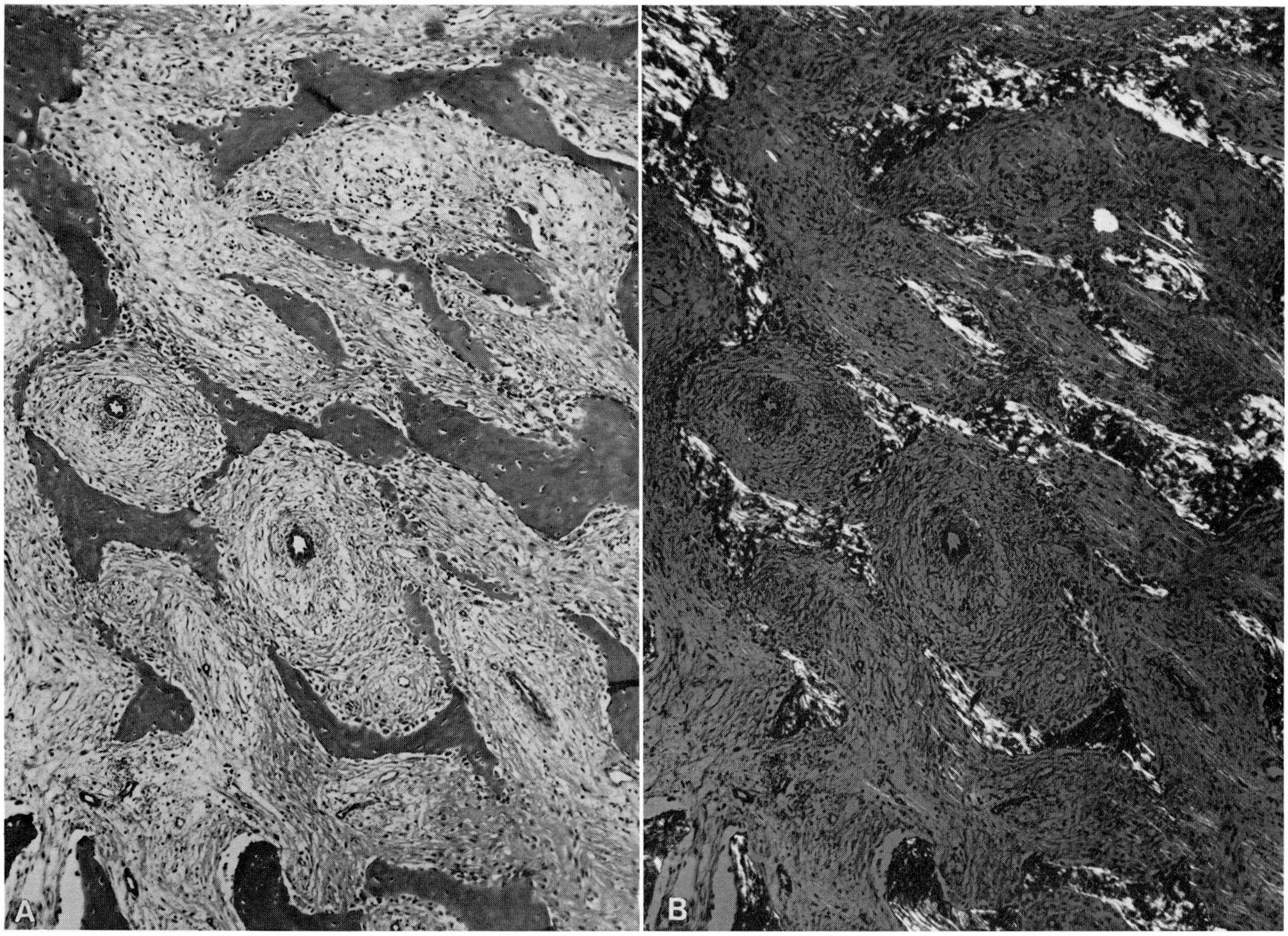

Fig. 44. Biopsy from the right ear canal of an 11-year-old female with fibrous dysplasia presenting as two spherical, pea-sized osteomas arising from the posterior bony canal wall of six month's duration with a 30 dB conductive hearing loss. (Operation by Dr. J. Helms, ORL Clinic, Tübingen, April 3, 1974). The appearance, distribution and orientation of the A) C-shaped bony trabeculae and the nature of their immature bone B) with the disorderly distribution of the birefringent fibers characterizes the lesion as fibrous dysplasia. (H & E, x 120)

swelling, and repeated spontaneous fractures. They generally appear during the first decade of life.

The McCune-Albright syndrome is a variant of the polyostotic form. It is characterized by the association of multiple bone lesions with generally ipsilateral skin pigmentation, occasionally by accelerated bone growth but early bone maturation, and by precocious sexual development. Females are almost exclusively affected.

Fibrous dysplasia may be associated with a number of other endocrine disorders, above all, with hyperthyroidism. The disease may occur in combination with other, nonendocrine disorders. Sarcomatous degeneration does occur but is very rare.

The temporal bone may occasionally become the site of monostotic, or less frequently, of polyostotic disease. In such instances, the disease manifests itself with progressive loss of hearing, increasing narrowing of the outer ear canal, and occasionally with an increase in size of the temporal bone. The hearing loss is predominantly conductive and usually related to the canal stenosis. The enlargement of the temporal bone may present itself as a painless, flat or spherical postauricular swelling which may produce a forward and downward displacement of the auricle, by an anterior, superior, or inferior auricular bulge, or by an intracranial space-occupying mass. The roentgenogram, in addition to confirming the enlargement of the temporal bone and the expansion and the thinning of the cortex, also reflects the morphology of the disease. A dense network of well-calcified bony trabeculae will produce a sclerotic pattern whereas a predominant proliferation of fibrous tissue with few and poorly calcified trabeculae or cementicles will lend a lesion a radiolucent, smoky or ground-glass appearance.

Progressive narrowing of the external meatus may be misinterpreted as diffuse or multiple exostoses. However, exostoses are hardly ever encountered during the first and second decade of life when fibrous dysplasia makes its clinical appearance. Obliteration of the external canal may give rise to an external cholesteatoma. A cholesteatoma, in turn, may lead to the development of a chronic tympanomastoiditis, facial palsy, labyrinthitis, or an endocranial complication.

The indications for surgical intervention include 1) maintenance of a normal ear canal, 2) preservation of cochlear and vestibular function, and 3) prevention of secondary complications.

The fibrodysplastic bone has a characteristic soft, gritty, and vascular texture. Restenosis of a surgically enlarged canal is a common observation. The majority of patients had several operative procedures. Since restenosis is today a rare complication, it should raise the suspicion of an underlying fibrous dysplasia. Restenosis can be prevented with a permanent Silastic tubular prosthesis.

In a rare instance fibrous dysplasia of the middle ear may mimic a vascular tumor. An expanding lesion of the petrous pyramid may produce symptoms of a middle or posterior fossa lesion. However, unless indicated, it is hazardous to attempt a total removal, since surgery is rarely curative and the vascularity of the process may lead to serious complications.

REFERENCES

1. Reed RJ. Fibrous dysplasia of bone. Arch Pathol 1963; 75: 480-95.

2. Aegerter EE, Kirkpatrick JA Jr. Orthopedic diseases. 3rd ed. Philadelphia: WB Saunders Co, 1968: 182-92.

3. Lichtenstein L, Jaffé HL. Fibrous dysplasia of bone. Arch Pathol 1942; 33:777-816.

4. Dent CE, Gertner IM. Hypophosphataemic osteomalacia in fibrous dysplasia. Q J Med 1976; 45:411-20.

5. Cohen DM, Dahlin DC, Pugh DG. Fibrous dysplasia associated with adamantinoma of the long bones. Cancer 1962; 15:515-21.

6. Johnson LC. Congenital pseudarthrosis, adamantinoma of long bones and intracortical fibrous dysplasia of the tibia. J Bone Jt Surg 1972; 54A:1355-62.

7. Uehlinger E. Osteofibrosis deformans juvenilis. (Polyostotische fibröse dysplasie (Jaffé-Lichenstein). Virchows Arch Pathol Anat Physiol 1940; 306:255-99.

8. Wirth WA, Leavitt D, Enzinger FM. Multiple intramuscular myxomas. Cancer 1971; 27:1167-73.

9. McIntosh HD, Miller DE, Goldner JL. The circulatory dynamics of polyostotic fibrous dysplasia. Am J Med 1962; 32:393-403.

10. Firat D, Stutzman L. Fibrous dysplasia of bone. Am J Med 1968; 44:421-9.

11. Schwartz DT, Alpert M. The malignant transformation of fibrous dysplasia. Am J Med Sci 1964; 247:35-54.

12. Von Recklinghausen F. Die Fibröse oder deformierende Ostitis, die Osteomalacie und die osteoplastische carcinose in ihren gegenseitigen Beziehungen. Festschrift Rudolf Virchow zum 13. Oktober, Berlin, 1891.

13. Elmslie RC. Fibrocystic disease of the bones. Br J Surg 1914; 2:17-67.

14. Weil A. Pubertas praecox und Knochenbrüchigkeit. Klin Wochenschr 1922; 1:2114-5.

15. Hunter D, Turnbull HL. Hyperparathyroidism: generalized osteitis fibrosa. Br J Surg 1931; 32:203-84.

16. Jaffé HL. Hyperparathyroidism. Arch Pathol 1933; 16: 63-7.

17. Freund E, Meffert CB. On the different forms of nongeneralized fibrous osteodystrophia. Surg Gynecol Obstet 1936; 62:451-61.

18. McCune DJ, Bruch H. Osteodystrophia fibrosa: report of a case in which the condition was combined with precocious puberty, pathologic pigmentation of the skin and hyperthyroidism, with review of the literature. Am J Dis Child 1937; 54:806-48.

19. Albright F, Butler MA, Hampton AO, Smith P. Syndrome characterized by osteitis fibrosa disseminata, areas of pigmentation and endocrine dysfunction with precocious puberty in females. N Engl J Med 1937; 216:727-46.

20. McCune DJ. Osteitis fibrosa cystica: the case of a nine year old girl who also exhibits precocious puberty, multiple pigmentation of the skin and hyperthyroidism. Am J Dis Child 1936; 52:745-8.

21. Gaupp V. Pubertas praecox bei Osteodystrophia fibrosa. Monatsschr Kinderheilkd 1932; 53:312-22.

22. Goldhammer K. Osteodystrophia fibrosa unilateralis. Fortschr Röntgenstr 1934; 49:456-81.

23. Hummel R. Zwei Fälle von Ostitis deformans Paget juvenilis. Röntgen Lab Prax (Stuttgart) 1934; 6:513-9.

24. Lichtenstein L. Polyostotic fibrous dysplasia. Arch Surg 1938; 36:874-98.

25. Schlumberger HG. Fibrous dysplasia of single bones. (Monostotic fibrous dysplasia). Mil Surg 1947; 99:504-27.

26. Jaffé HL. Tumors and tumorous conditions of the bones and joints. Philadelphia: Lea and Febiger, 1958: 117-42.

27. Panders AK. Fibro-osseuze en fibro-osseuze-cementeuze dysplasie van de kaken, thesis. Groningen, 1970.

28. Tembe D. Fibro-osseous dysplasia of temporal bone. J Laryngol Otol 1970; 84:107-14.

29. Van Tilburg W. Fibrous dysplasia. In: Vinken PJ, Bruyn GW, eds. Handbook of clinical neurology. Vol. 14. Amsterdam: North Holland Publishing Co, 1972: 163-212.

30. Wells C. Polyostotic fibrous dysplasia in a 7th century Anglo-Saxon. Br J Radiol 1963; 36:925-6.

31. Gregg JB, Reed A. Monostotic fibrous dysplasia in the temporal bone: a late prehistoric occurrence. Am J Phys Anthropol 1980; 52:587-93.

32. Slow IN, Stern D, Friedman EW. Osteogenic sarcoma arising in pre-existing fibrous dysplasia: report of case. J Oral Surg 1971; 29:126-9.

33. Sante LR, Bauer W, O'Brien RM. Polyostotic fibrous dysplasia (Albright syndrome) and its comparison with dyschondroplasia (Ollier's disease). A correlation of radiological and pathological findings. Radiology 1948; 51:676-90.

34. Harris WH, Dudley HR Jr, Barry JR. The natural history of fibrous dysplasia. J Bone Jt Surg 1962; 44A:207-33.

35. Uehlinger E. Fibröse Dysplasia (Jaffé-Lichtenstein): Osteofibrosis deformans juvenilis (Uehlinger); Albrightsches Syndrome. In: Schinz HR, Baensch WE, Frommhold W, Glauner R, Uehlinger E, Wellauer J, eds. Lehrbuch der Röntgendiagnostik. 6th ed. Band II/Teil I. Stuttgart: Georg Thieme Verlag, 1979: 947-82.

36. Van Horn PE Jr, Dahlin DC, Bickel WH. Fibrous dysplasia: a clinical pathologic study of orthopedic surgical cases. Proc Mayo Clin 1963; 38:175-89.

37. Stewart MJ, Gilmer WS, Edmonton AS. Fibrous dysplasia of bone. J Bone Jt Surg 1962; 44A:302-18.

38. Spjut HJ, Dorfman HD, Fechner RE, Ackerman LV. Fibrous dysplasia. In: Tumors of bone and cartilage. Atlas of tumor pathology. Sec series, pt 5. Armed Forces Institute of Pathology, 1970: 270-80.

39. Hadders HN. Dysplasia fibrosa monostotica. Ned Tijdschr Geneeskd 1957; 101:378-80.

40. Henry A. Monostotic fibrous dysplasia. J Bone Jt Surg 1969; 51B:300-16.

41. Talbot IC, Keith DA, Lord IJ. Fibrous dysplasia of the cranio-facial bones. A clinicopathological survey of seven cases. J Laryngol Otol 1974; 88:429-43.

42. Becker MH. Fibrous dysplasia. In: Ranniger K, ed. Encyclopedia of medical radiology. Vol 5. New York: Springer-Verlag, 1977: 488-512.

43. Eversole LR, Sabes WR, Rovin S. Fibrous dysplasia. A nosologic problem in the diagnosis of fibro-osseous lesions of the jaws. J Oral Pathol 1972; 1:189-220.

44. Furst NJ, Shapiro R. Polyostotic fibrous dysplasia: review of literature with two additional cases. Radiology 1943; 40:501-15.

45. Hoboek A. Polyostotic fibrous dysplasia of bone. Acta Radiol (Stockh) 1951; 36:145-53.

46. Gibson MJ, Middlemiss JH. Fibrous dysplasia of bone. Br J Radiol 1971; 44:1-13.

47. Hopf M. Zur Kenntnis der polyostotischen fibrösen Dysplasie. Radiol Clin (Basel) 1949; 28:129-59.

48. Windolz F. Cranial manifestations of fibrous dysplasia of bone. Am J Roentgenol 1947; 58:51-63.

49. Fries JW. The roentgen features of fibrous dysplasia of the skull and facial bones: a critical analysis of thirty-nine pathologically proven cases. Am J Roentgenol 1957; 77:71-88.

50. Hall R, Warrick CH. Hypersecretion of hypothalamic releasing hormones: a possible explanation of the endocrine manifestations of polyostotic fibrous dysplasia. (Albright syndrome). Lancet 1972; 1:1313-6.

51. Pritchard JE. Fibrous dysplasia of the bones. Am J Med Sci 1951; 22:313-32.

52. Ivimey M. Bone dystrophy with characteristics of leontiasis ossea, osteitis fibrosa cystica. Am J Dis Child 1929; 38:348-69.

53. Revers FE. Albright's disease (osteitis fibrosa cystica). Ned Tijdschr Geneeskd 1947; 91:1695-704.

54. Jaffé HL. Fibrous dysplasia of bone. Bull NY Acad Med 1946; 22:588-604.

55. Proffit JN, McSwain B, Kalmon FH. Fibrous dysplasia of bone. Ann Surg 1949; 130:881-95.

56. Russell LW, Chandler FA. Fibrous dysplasia of bone. J Bone Jt Surg 1950; 32A:323-37.

57. Fairbank HAT. An atlas of general affections of the skeleton. Edinburg: E and S Livingstone, 1951.

58. Benedict PH, Szabo G, Fitzpatrick TB, Sinesi SJ. Melanotic macules in Albright's syndrome and in neurofibromatosis. JAMA 1968; 205:618-26.

59. Dahlmann J. Zur Kenntnis des Albright's Disease. Fortschr Röntgenstr 1955; 82:723-40.

60. Benedict PH. Sexual precocity and polyostotic fibrous dysplasia. Am J Dis Child 1966; 111:426-31.

61. Scurry MT, Bichnell JM, Fajans SS. Polyostotic fibrous dysplasia and acromegaly. Arch Intern Med 1969; 114:40-5.

62. Benjamin DR, McRoberts JW. Polyostotic fibrous dysplasia associated with Cushing syndrome. Arch Pathol 1973; 96:175-8.

63. Aarskog D, Tveteraas E. McCune-Albright's syndrome following adrenalectomy for Cushing's syndrome in infancy. J Pediatr 1968; 73:89-96.

64. Peck FB, Sage CV. Diabetes mellitus associated with Albright's syndrome. Am J Med Sci 1944; 208:35-46.

65. Benedict PH. Endocrine features in Albright's syndrome (fibrous dysplasia of bone). Metabolism 1962; 11:30-45.

66. Moldawer M, Rabin ER. Polyostotic fibrous dysplasia with thyrotoxicosis. Report of a complete autopsy and skeletal reconstruction. Arch Intern Med 1966; 118:379-85.

67. Kim JP, Kbera SAK. Polyostotic fibrous dysplasia associated with hyperthyroidism. J Bone Jt Surg 1961; 43A:897-904.

68. Wortham JT, Hamblen EC. Polyostotic fibrous dysplasia with sexual precocity and pigmentation (Albright's syndrome) and associated non-neoplastic acromegaly. J Clin Endocrin 1952; 12:975-6.

69. Albright F. Polyostotic fibrous dysplasia: a defense of the entity. J Clin Endocrinol Metab 1947; 7:307-24.

70. Schally AV, Bowers CY. The nature of thyrotropin-releasing hormones [THR]. In: Kenny AD, Anderson R, eds. Proceedings of the sixth midwestern conference on the thyroid and endocrinology. Columbia: University of Missouri, 1970:25.

71. Hamilton CR, Maloaf F. Unusual types of hyperthyroidism. Medicine 1973; 52:195-215.

72. Faglia G, Ferrari C, Beck-Peroz P, Ambrosi B, Valantini F. High plasma thyrotropin levels in two patients with pituitary tumors. Acta Endocrinol (Kbh) 1972; 69:649-58.

73. Sherman L, Kolodny HD. The hypothalamus, brain catecholamines and drug therapy for gigantism and acromegaly. Lancet 1972; 1:682-5.

74. Mazabraud A, Toty L, Roze R, Semat P. Un nouveau cas d'association de dysplasie fibreuse des os avec un myxome des tissues mous. Sem Hop Paris 1969; 45:862-8.

75. Daves ML, Yardley JH. Fibrous dysplasia of bone. Am J Med Sci 1957; 234:590-606.

76. Gatewood OMB, Esterly JR. Coexistent polyostotic fibrous dysplasia and eosinophilic granuloma of bone. Am J Roentgenol 1966; 97:110-7.

77. Stauffer HM, Arbukle RK, Aegerter EE. Polyostotic fibrous dysplasia with cutaneous pigmentation and congenital arteriovenous aneurysm. J Bone Jt Surg 1941; 23:323-34.

78. Fischer JA, Bollinger A, Lichtlen P, Wellauer J. Fibrous dysplasia and high cardiac output. Am J Med 1970; 49:140-6.

79. Moore RT. Fibrous dysplasia of the orbit. Surv Ophthalmol 1969; 13:321-34.

80. Sassin JF, Rosenberg RN. Neurological complications of fibrous dysplasia of the skull. Arch Neurol (Paris) 1968; 18:363-9.

81. Feiring W, Feiring EH, Davidoff ML. Fibrous dysplasia of the skull. J Neurosurg 1951; 8:377-97.

82. Falconer MA, Cope CL, Robb-Smith, AHT. Fibrous dysplasia of bone with endocrine disorders and cutaneous pigmentation (Albright's disease). Q J Med 1942; 11:121-54.

83. Dieckmann H, Tänzer A. Zur Klinik der Fibrösen Dysplasie und des Albright Syndroms. Dtsch Z Nervenheilkd 1957; 176:615-36.

84. Kanavel AB. Surgical intervention in leontiasis ossea. Surg Gynecol Obstet 1917; 4:719-34.

85. Evans J. Leontiasis ossea. Critical review with reports of 4 original cases. J Bone Jt Surg 1953; 35B:229-34.

86. Teng P, Gross SW, Newman CM. Compression of the spinal cord by osteitis deformans (Paget's disease), giant cell tu-

mor and polyostotic fibrous dysplasia (Albright's syndrome) of vertebrae. J Neurosurg 1951; 8:482-93.

87. Jirout J, Lewit K. Cases of fibrous dysplasia with disturbances of the nervous system. Cesk Roentgenol 1957; 10:163.

88. Lecocq M. Un cas de localisation vertebral de la dysplasie fibreuse de l'os ou maladie, Jaffe-Lichtenstein. J Belge Med Phys Rhum 1956; 11:17-24.

89. Rosendahl-Jensen SV. Fibrous dysplasia of the vertebral column. Acta Chir Scand 1956; 6:490.

90. Vial A. De ziekte van Jaffé-Lichtenstein of "osteofibromatosis cystica." Ned Tijdschr Geneeskd 1948; 92:1784-7.

91. Jervis GA, Schein H. Polyostotic fibrous dysplasia (Albright's syndrome); case showing central nervous system changes. Arch Pathol 1951; 51:640-50.

92. Cahill P. Fibrous dysplasia of the skull. Med J Aust 1963; 50:843-7.

93. Coley RL, Stewart FW. Bone sarcoma in polyostotic fibrous dysplasia. Ann Surg 1945; 121:872-81.

94. Huvos AG, Higinbotham NL, Miller TR. Bone sarcomas arising in fibrous dysplasia. J Bone Jt Surg 1972; 54A:1047-56.

95. Fuchsbrunner E, Kolb E, Schoenwald A. Oberkiefersarkom bei polyostotischer fibröser Knochendysplasia (Morbus Jaffé-Lichtenstein). Zahnärzt Prax 1964; 15:105-7.

96. Standish SM, Gorlin RJ. Bone disorders affecting the jaws. In: Gorlin RJ, Goldman HM, eds. Thoma's oral pathology. 6th ed. Vol. I. St. Louis. C. V. Mosby Co, 1970:541.

97. Reitzik M, Lownie JF. Familial polyostotic fibrous dysplasia. Oral Surg 1975; 40:769-74.

98. El Deeb M, Waite ED, Gorlin RJ. Congenital monostotic fibrous dysplasia — a new, possibly autosomal-recessive disorder. J Oral Surg 1979; 37:520-5.

99. Lemli L. Fibrous dysplasia of bone. Report of female monozygotic twins with and without the McCune-Albright syndrome. J Pediatr 1977; 91:347-9.

100. Goldenberg RR, Campbell CJ, Barfiglio M. Giant-cell tumor of bone. An analysis of two hundred and eighteen cases. J Bone Jt Surg 1970; 52A:619-64.

101. Hutter RVP, Worcester JN Jr, Francis KC, Fotte FW Jr, Stewart FW. Benign and malignant giant-cell tumors of bone. A clinicopathological analysis of the natural history of the disease. Cancer 1962; 15:653-90.

102. Dahlin DC. Bone tumors. 2nd ed. Springfield, Ill: Charles C Thomas, 1967:78-89.

103. Menzel A. Ein Fall von Osteofibrom des Unterkiefers Langenbecks Arch Chir 1872; 13:212-9.

104. Montgomery AH. Ossifying fibromas of the jaws. Arch Surg 1927; 15:30-44.

105. Schlumberger HG. Fibrous dysplasia (ossifying fibroma) of the maxilla and mandible. Am J Orthod Oral Surg (Oral Surg) 1946; 32:579-87.

106. Zimmerman DC, Dahlin DC. Myxomatous tumors of the jaws. Oral Surg 1958; 11:1069-80.

107. Zimmerman DC, Dahlin DC, Stafno EC. Fibrous dysplasia of the maxilla and mandible. Oral Surg 1958; 11:55-68.

108. Sherman RS, Sternbergh WCA. The roentgen appearance of ossifying fibroma of bone. Radiology 1948; 50:595-609.

109. Sherman RS, Glauser OJ. Radiological identification of fibrous dysplasia of the jaw. Radiology 1958; 71:553-8.

110. Reed RG, Glagy DM. Benign non-odontogenic fibro-osseous lesions of the skull. Oral Surg 1965; 19:214-27.

111. Budol J. The surgical removal of large osteofibromas. Oral Surg 1970; 30:303-8.

112. Slaughter DP, Roeser EH, Smejkal WF. Excision of the mandible for neoplastic disease. Indications and techniques. Surgery 1949; 26:507-22.

113. Thoma KH, Holland DJ, Rounds CE. Miscellaneous case reports: ossifying fibroma of mandible treated by excision. Am J Orthod Oral Surg (Oral Surg) 1947; 33:351-7.

114. Kemper JW. Hemi-resection of the mandible for ossifying fibroma. Report of case. J Oral Surg 1946; 4:340-2.

115. Ramsey HE, Strong EW, Frazell EW. Fibrous dysplasia of craniofacial bones. Am J Surg 1968; 116:542-7.

116. Schoff J. A new technique for the surgical removal of osteoma of the jaw. Oral Surg 1949; 2:1422-7.

117. Shafer WG, Hine MK, Levy BM. A textbook of oral pathology. 2nd ed. Philadelphia: WB Saunders, 1963.

118. Gorlin RJ, Pindborg JJ. Syndromes of the head and neck. New York: McGraw-Hill, 1964.

119. Cohn LR. The jaws in generalized skeletal disease. Ann R Coll Surg Engl 1951; 8:115-40.

120. Hamner JE, Scofield HH, Cornyn J. Benign fibro-osseous jaw lesions of periodontal membrane origin: an analysis of 249 cases. Cancer 1968; 22:861-78.

121. Anderson DA, McClenden JL, Cornelius EA. Cherubism — hereditary fibrous dysplasia of the jaw. Oral Surg 1962; 15 Suppl 2:5-16, 17-42.

122. Cornelius EA, McClenden JL. Cherubism — hereditary fibrous dysplasia of the jaws. Am J Roentgenol 1969; 104:136-43.

123. Gutman D, Gellei B, Laufer D, Tomaskewski A. Fibrous dysplasia of maxilla and zygoma treated by intra-oral approach: report of case. J Oral Surg 1967; 25:367-70.

124. Carson IH. Polyostotic fibrous dysplasia: report of a case. Oral Surg 1954; 7:524-33.

125. Levin ML. Fibrous dysplasia of the mandible. Am J Surg 1955; 90:951-61.

126. Levin ML. Fibrous dysplasia of the mandible in children. Plast Reconstr Surg 1960; 25:161-73.

127. Levin ML. Non-malignant maxillofacial tumors in children. Plast Reconstr Surg 1966; 38:186-96.

128. Rushton MA. Fibrous dysplasia of bone: arrested jaw lesions. Br Dent J 1950; 89:185-9.

129. Harris HW, Dudley R Jr, Barry RJ. The natural history of fibrous dysplasia. An orthopedic, pathological and roentgenographic study. J Bone Jt Surg 1962; 44A:207-33.

130. Ramsey HE, Strong EW, Frazell EL. Progressive fibrous dysplasia of the maxilla. J Am Dent Assn 1970; 81:1388-91.

131. Dockerty MD, Ghormley BK, Kennedy RLJ, Pugh DG. Albright's syndrome. Arch Intern Med 1945; 75:357-75.

132. Bonduelle M, Claisse R. Dysplasie fibreuse des os et syndrome d'Albright. Leur place nosologique. Sem Hop Paris 1948; 24:514-21.

133. Cohen A, Rosenwasser H. Fibrous dysplasia of the temporal bone. Arch Otolaryngol 1969; 89:31-43.

134. Berger R. Fibrome envahissant de la mastoide. Presse Medicale 1947; 55:202.

135. Cooke SL, Powers WH. Monostotic fibrous dysplasia. Report of two cases. Arch Otolaryngol 1949; 50:319-29.

136. Towson CE. Monostotic fibrous dysplasia of the mastoid and the temporal bone. Arch Otolaryngol 1950; 52:709-24.

137. Jezek K. Pripad Fibrosni Dysplasie Kostni Výenelku Soscovitehó. Cas Lék Ces 1951; 90:1386-8.

138. Brunner H. Fibrous dysplasia of facial bones and paranasal sinuses. Arch Otolaryngol 1952; 55:43-54.

139. Skolnik EM, Perrelli SL, Pornoy RA. Fibrous dysplasia of the skull and temporal bone. ENT Month 1958; 57:755-72.

140. Deuber JW. Dissertation. University of Zürich, 1958.

141. Kearney HL. Fibrous dysplasia of the temporal bone. Laryngoscope 1959; 69:571-4.

142. Kleinsasser O, Friedmann G. Die fibröse Knochendysplasie des Gesichts und Hirnschädels. Laryngol Rhinol Otol Ihre Granzgeb 1960; 39:201-20.

143. Sussman HB. Monostotic fibrous dysplasia of the temporal bone. Report of a case. Laryngoscope 1961; 71:68-77.

144. Clay A, Deguine C. Un cas de dysplasie fibreuse a localisation occipitomastoidienne. J Fr Oto-Rhino-Laryngol Chir Maxillo-Fac 1962; 11:393-400.

145. Leeds N, Seaman WB. Fibrous dysplasia of the skull and its differential diagnosis. Radiology 1962; 78:570-82.

146. Wong A, Vaughan CW, Strong StM. Fibrous dysplasia of temporal bone. Arch Otolaryngol 1965; 81:131-3.

147. Flurr E, Soderberg G. Monostotic fibrous dysplasia (ossifying fibroma) of the mastoid. J Laryngol Otol 1966; 80:678-85.

148. Shiffman F, Aengst FE. Fibrous dysplasia of temporal bone. Arch Otolaryngol 1967; 86:528-34.

149. Basek M. Fibrous dysplasia of the middle ear. Arch Otolaryngol 1967; 85:26-9.

150. Deshmukh SS, Gandhi RK, Mody SN, Deshmukh SM. Fibrous dysplasia of temporal bone. J Postgrad Med 1967; 13: 198-200.

151. Samy LL, Girgis IH, Wasef SA. Fibrous dysplasia in relation to the paranasal sinuses and the ear. J Laryngol Otol 1967; 81:1357-71.

152. Privara M, Cerny E. Osteodysplasia fibrosa kosti spankove. Cesk Otolaryngol 1968; 17:141-4.

153. Antonova NA, Kosakova EI, Fostovsky JA. Fibrous dysplasia of the temporal bone. Vestnik ORL 1968; 30:101-2.

154. Kinnman JEG, Hong CE, Lee EB, Shin HS. Fibrous dysplasia of the face and skull. Pract Oto-Rhino-Laryngol 1969; 31:11-21.

155. Brusis T. Extensive deformation of the skull in fibrous dysplasia (Jaffé-Lichtenstein). J Laryngol Otol 1970; 49:643-53.

156. Stecker RH. Ossifying fibroma of the middle ear. Arch Otolaryngol 1971; 94:80-2.

157. Sharp M. Monostotic fibrous dysplasia of the temporal bone. J Laryngol Otol 1970; 84:697-708.

158. Venker DH. Monostotische fibreuze dysplasie uitgaande van het mastoid. Ned Tijdsch Geneeskd 1971; 115:327-9.

159. Bouche J, Freck C, Chaix G. Fibrous dysplasia in otorhinolaryngology. Apropos of 17 personal cases. Ann Otolaryngol Chir Cervicafaciale 1971: 88:421-3.

160. Steinbach E. Die Gehörgangsstenose als Folge der fibrösen Dysplasie. Arch Klin Exp Ohren Nasen Kehlkopfheilkunde 1972; 202:623-7.

161. Mündnich K. In discussion, Steinbach E. Die Gehörgangstenose als Folge der fibrösen Dysplasie. Arch Klin Exp Ohren Nasen Kehlkopfheilkunde 1972; 202:627.

162. Mathieu L, Martin C. Essential fibrous dysplasia: several uniosseous forms of the temporal bone and superior maxillary bone. Ann Odontostomatol (Lyon) 1972; 29:87-105.

163. Deringuia BA. Fibrous dysplasia of the temporal bone. Vestn Otorinolaryngol 1973; 35:88-9.

164. Pokrajcic M. Ostitis fibrosa localisata of the temporal bone. Srp Arh Celok Lek 1972; 10:419-21.

165. Sienkiewicz M. A case of fibrotic degeneration of the temporal bone. Otolaryngol Pol 1971; 25:241-3.

166. Mizuno M. Monostotic fibrous dysplasia. Otolaryngology (Tokyo) 1972; 44:15-20.

167. Scott MJ. Nonprogressive calcified mass of the skull involving unilateral cranial nerves. J Neurosurg 1974; 40:779-82.

168. Canigiani G, Ferreira CS, Czech W, Wilhenhauser J. Beitrag zur fibrösen dysplasie des os temporale. Monatsschr Ohrenheilkd Laryngo-Rhinol 1974; 108:285-93.

169. Ward PH, Foster CH. Monostotic fibrous dysplasia of the temporal bone. Trans Pac Coast Otoophthalmol Soc 1975; 56:147-57.

170. Williams DML, Thomas RSA. Fibrous dysplasia. J Laryngol Otol 1975; 88:359-74.

171. Ukleja J, Domawiewski J. Case of fibrous osteodysplasia of the temporal bone complicated by cholesteatoma. Otolaryngol Pol 1975; 29:605-8.

172. Chatterji P. Massive fibrous dysplasia of the temporal bone. J Laryngol Otol 1974; 88:179-83.

173. Fernandez E, Calavita U. Fibrous dysplasia of the skull with complete unilateral cranial nerve involvement. Case report. J Neurosurgery 1980; 52:404-6.

174. Barrinuevo CE, Marcallo FA, Coelho A, Cruz AG, Mocellin M, Patrocinio JA. Fibrous dysplasia and the temporal bone. Arch Otolaryngol 1980; 106:298-301.

175. Jacobson HH, Vraa-Hansen G. Fibrous dysplasia of bone. Acta Radiol (Stockh) 1949; 31:1-16.

EXPERIMENTAL OTITIS MEDIA IN CHINCHILLAS

I. BASELINE IMMUNOLOGICAL INVESTIGATION

Noritake Watanabe, MD

Bruce R. Briggs, BS

David J. Lim, MD

II. COMPARISON OF THE MIDDLE EAR IMMUNE RESPONSES TO *S PNEUMONIAE* TYPES 3 AND 23

Noritake Watanabe, MD

Thomas F. DeMaria, MD

Daniel M. Lewis, PhD

Goro Mogi, MD

David J. Lim, MD

This publication was supported in part by Parke-Davis Division of Warner-Lambert Company.

EXPERIMENTAL OTITIS MEDIA IN CHINCHILLAS
I. BASELINE IMMUNOLOGICAL INVESTIGATION

NORITAKE WATANABE, MD
BRUCE R. BRIGGS, BS
DAVID J. LIM, MD
COLUMBUS, OHIO

Baseline immunological data on the chinchilla were obtained, and a detailed method for purification of each immunoglobulin is described. Antiserum to each chinchilla immunoglobulin was made by immunizing rabbits with immunoglobulins purified from serum and colostrum. The main classes of serum immunoglobulins in the chinchilla are G, A and M, similar to those in other rodents and humans. The immunohistochemical study showed that the distribution of immunocytes in lymphoid organs is similar to that of other rodents and humans. In the eustachian tube the glandular acinar cells were distinctly positive for IgA staining. A few IgA-forming cells and very rare IgG- and IgM-forming cells were found in the eustachian tube mucosa, but all were very rare in the middle ear mucosa. These findings suggest that the secretory immune system of the chinchilla eustachian tube may be active in the normal state and that the local immune system of the normal middle ear mucosa may be latent but could become active following antigenic stimulation.

INTRODUCTION

The chinchilla *(Chinchilla laniger)* has been widely used in recent years as a laboratory animal for experimental otitis media because of: 1) its large and easily accessible bulla, which allows the collection of large quantitites of effusion; 2) its thin bullar bone, which allows the injection of inoculum directly into the bulla without puncturing the tympanic membrane; 3) the resistance of its middle ear to natural infection; and 4) the susceptibility of its middle ear to pathogenic organisms causing otitis media in humans.[1-4]

Hook[5] investigated the humoral immune response of the adult chinchilla against several antigens and suggested that there might be two classes (19S and 7S) of immunoglobulin in chinchilla serum. Visco and Kinkler[6] studied the cellular immune system in chinchillas by investigating in vitro lymphocyte transformation using specific and nonspecific mitogens and suggested that there might be two subpopulations of chinchilla lymphocytes, T-cells and B-cells. According to these studies the chinchilla seems to have humoral and cellular immune systems like those of humans. However, the basic immunological and immunochemical characteristics of the chinchilla eustachian tube and middle ear have not been adequately established. In an effort to clarify the normal immune mechanism of the middle ear of the chinchilla, purification of immunoglobulins (G, M and A) from serum and colostrum was attempted. Antisera to the major immunoglobulins were produced in rabbits and used to assess the distribution of immunoglobulin-forming cells in the middle ear and eustachian tube of normal chinchillas using immunofluorescence.

MATERIALS AND METHODS

Materials. Chinchilla blood for sera was obtained from 41 animals by cardiac puncture under methoxyflurane inhalation anesthesia. Following centrifugation (at 1500 rpm for 15 minutes) to remove clots and red blood cells, the sera were pooled and stored at -20°C until use. Chinchilla colostrum was collected manually for up to one week postparturition from about 20 animals, and about 0.5 ml/animal/day of colostrum could be collected after an 8-hour separation from its litter. A total of 200 ml of colostrum was used for this study.

Purification of Chinchilla Serum Immunoglobulins. Chinchilla IgG and IgM were purified by gel filtration on Sephadex G-200 (Pharmacia, Piscataway, NJ) and DEAE-cellulose (Whatman, Maidstone, Kent) ion exchange column chromatography according to the procedure of Vaerman and Heremans.[7] Crude gamma globulins were prepared by two successive precipitations of sera with saturated ammonium sulfate (SAS) at 45% final saturation. This precipitate was then resuspended in 1/20 of the original volume of sera, dialyzed against distilled water for three 1 L changes, then dialyzed against borate buffered saline (BBS) at 0.01M, pH 8.3, for three additional 1 L changes. The crude gamma globulins were applied to the Sephadex G-200 column, which was equilibrated with BBS. The column was run at a rate of 1 ml every 4 minutes and fractions collected by a fraction collector in 5-ml aliquots. Fractions were assayed at 280 nm, and the first protein peak was used as a source of IgM and the second protein peak as a source of IgG.

The IgM peak was concentrated by lyophilization and rechromatographed twice as above through a Sephadex G-200-BBS column equilibrated with BBS. The first protein peak was saved each time. The resulting IgM-rich fraction was applied to a Sepharose 6B column equilibrated with BBS. Again the first protein peak was concentrated and dialyzed against veronal buffer at pH 8.6 for preparative block electrophoresis on Pevikon C-870 (Calbiochem-Behring, La Jolla, Calif), as outlined by Müller-Eberhard and Osterland.[8] Pevikon block electrophoresis (1.5 x 15 x 60 cm) was performed on this fraction at 3 V/cm for 24 hours. Upon completion 1.5-cm segments were cut from the block. The proteins contained in the segment were eluted with 10 ml BBS on a sintered glass filter, and the protein concentration was determined by the Folin-Lowry method.[9] The protein peak closest to the point of introduction of the sample (origin) was collected and concentrated as chinchilla IgM.

From the Otological Research Laboratories, Department of Otolaryngology, Ohio State University College of Medicine, Columbus. This study was supported in part by grants from the NIH-NINCDS (R 501 NS08854), Deafness Research Foundation and E.A.R. Foundation.

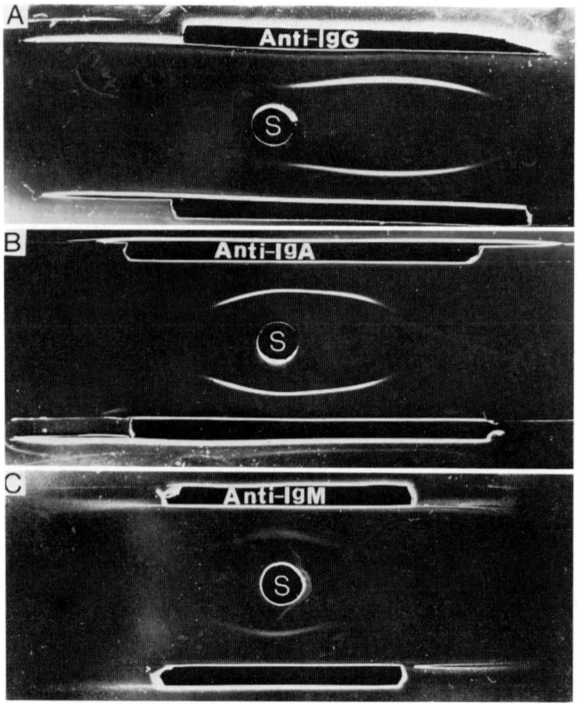

Fig. 1. A-C) Immunoelectrophoretic patterns of chinchilla sera (S), which develops a single precipitation arc to each antisera, demonstrating monospecificity.

The IgG peak from Sephadex G-200 was concentrated, dialyzed against 0.005M phosphate buffer at pH 7.6 and was then applied to a DEAE-cellulose ion exchange column equilibrated with 0.005M phosphate buffer. The proteins were eluted by a stepwise gradient of 0.005M, 0.01M, 0.02M, and 0.1M phosphate buffer, all pH 7.6. The eluate of 0.005M phosphate buffer, pH 7.6, was used as chinchilla IgG.

Purification of Chinchilla Milk IgA. IgA from the chinchilla milk was purified as described previously.[7,10,11] The colostrum was centrifuged at 16,100g for one hour, and the intermediate layer between the top fatty layer and the bottom casein precipitate was collected and salted out with 50% SAS. The precipitate was redissolved, dialyzed against 0.01M phosphate buffer at pH 7.6, and was applied to a DEAE-cellulose ion exchange column. Similarly, elution was performed by a stepwise gradient procedure. The first elution was conducted using a 0.01M phosphate buffer at pH 7.6, followed by 0.02M, 0.1M and 0.2M phosphate buffers at pH 7.6. Eluates of 0.1M and 0.2M buffers at pH 7.6 were concentrated and applied to a Sephadex G-200 column. The first protein peak was further purified by Sepharose 6B gel filtration. The second peak from Sepharose 6B gel filtration served as a source of IgA.

Preparation of Antisera. Antisera were prepared in rabbits by immunization, with each antigen mixed 1:1 with complete Freund's adjuvant. Rabbits were immunized with 1 mg of the antigen subcutaneously once a week for four weeks. The monospecificity of each antiserum was analyzed by immunodiffusion and immunoelectrophoresis (Fig. 1). Antisera were adsorbed with appropriate serum components by affinity chromatography in order to render them monospecific.

Fluoresceinated Antisera. Each antiserum against chinchilla IgG, IgA and IgM was conjugated with fluoresceinated isothiocyanate (FITC) by the method of Kawamura.[12] The FITC-conjugated antisera were absorbed with chinchilla liver powder in order to remove nonspecific background staining.[10]

Immunofluorescent Studies. Specimens of the fresh tissues were fixed in cold 95% ethanol and prepared according to the method of Hamashima and Kyogoku.[13] Immunoglobulin-positive cells were counted and averaged from 3-5 microscopic fields at 160x. The cell counts are expressed in this paper as "very rare" (fewer than 1/field), "rare" (1-2/field), "few" (3-5/field), "moderate" (6-10/field), or "many" (over 11/field).

Measurement of IgG, IgA and IgM. Levels of IgG, IgA and IgM in serum samples from 41 healthy chinchillas were determined by single radial immunodiffusion according to the method of Mancini et al.[14] IgG (IgG_2) and IgM purified from chinchilla serum and IgA purified from chinchilla colostrum were used as standards.

RESULTS

CHARACTERISTICS OF CHINCHILLA SECRETORY IgA AND SECRETORY COMPONENT

The antisera against chinchilla milk IgA developed a spur between precipitation lines of chinchilla milk and serum. The antiserum also developed a precipitation line against the third peak of Sephadex G-200 gel filtration of protein fractions that were obtained by 0.01M and 0.02M buffers on DEAE-cellulose chromatography of the colostrum (Fig. 2). This suggests the existence of an extra antigenic determinant in chinchilla milk IgA (secretory IgA) as compared with serum IgA, and the extra antigenic determinant is assumed to be the secretory component.

LEVELS OF IgG, IgA and IgM IN SERA

Mean levels of each immunoglobulin in sera from 41 normal adult chinchilla are shown in Figure 3. The mean level of IgG was 1016 mg/100 ml (mean ± 2SE: 889-1148). The mean value of IgA was 98

Fig. 2. Ouchterlony gel diffusion experiment. A) A major precipitation line between anti-SIgA and milk (M) is interpreted to be secretory IgA. The minor precipitation line formed between anti-SIgA and serum (S) is partially fused with that of milk, demonstrating immunological partial identity. This minor line is interpreted to be serum IgA. B) Anti-SIgA against SIgA and peaks I, II, and III from Sephadex G-200 gel filtration to which 0.01M and 0.02M eluates of DEAE-cellulose chromatography of chinchilla colostrum were applied. A single precipitation line between anti-SIgA and peak III is interpreted to be secretory component.

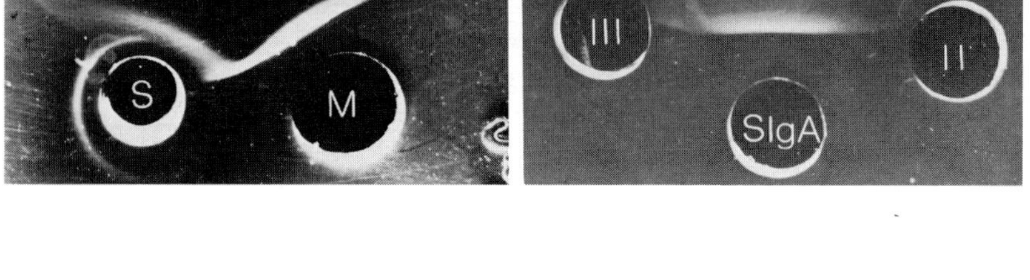

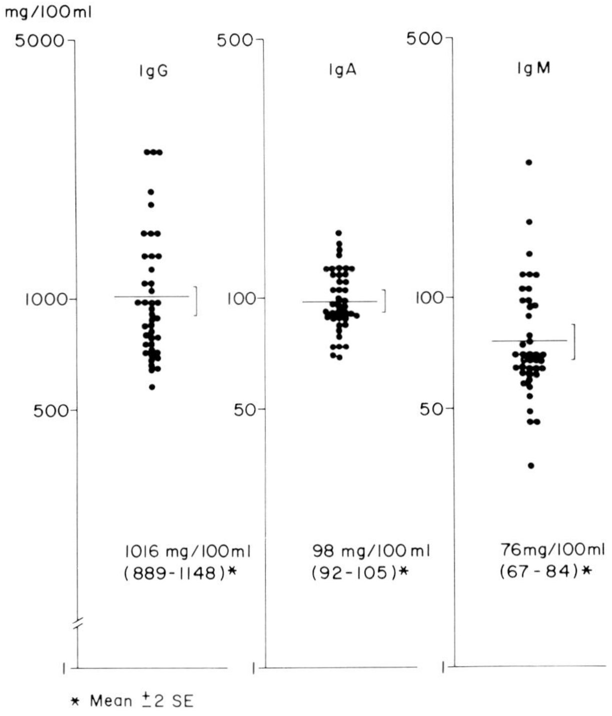

Fig. 3. Concentrations of different classes of immunoglobulins in normal chinchilla sera.

mg/100 ml (92-105) and of IgM 76 mg/100 ml (67-84).

IMMUNOFLUORESCENT STUDIES

Immunoglobulin-Forming Cells in Mucous Membranes of the Eustachian Tube and Middle Ear Cavity. In the mucous membrane of eustachian tubes a few IgA-forming cells were found in the subepithelial connective tissue and between the glands, whereas the presence of both IgG- and IgM-forming cells was very rare. A few IgA-forming cells were found in the cartilaginous portion and pharyngeal orifice of the tubes, but the number of IgA-forming cells became rare in the bony portion (Fig. 4).

Epithelial cells of the eustachian tube mucosa were not stained with FITC-conjugated antisera to IgA, whereas acinar cells of tubal glands were positive for IgA staining. These IgA-positive glands were of mixed type (seromucous) and distributed mainly in the cartilaginous portion and pharyngeal orifice. In the bony portion of the eustachian tubes the lamina propria was thin and tubal glands were not found.

Any type of immunoglobulin-forming cells was very rare in the middle ear mucosa of normal adult chinchillas as compared with the eustachian tube,

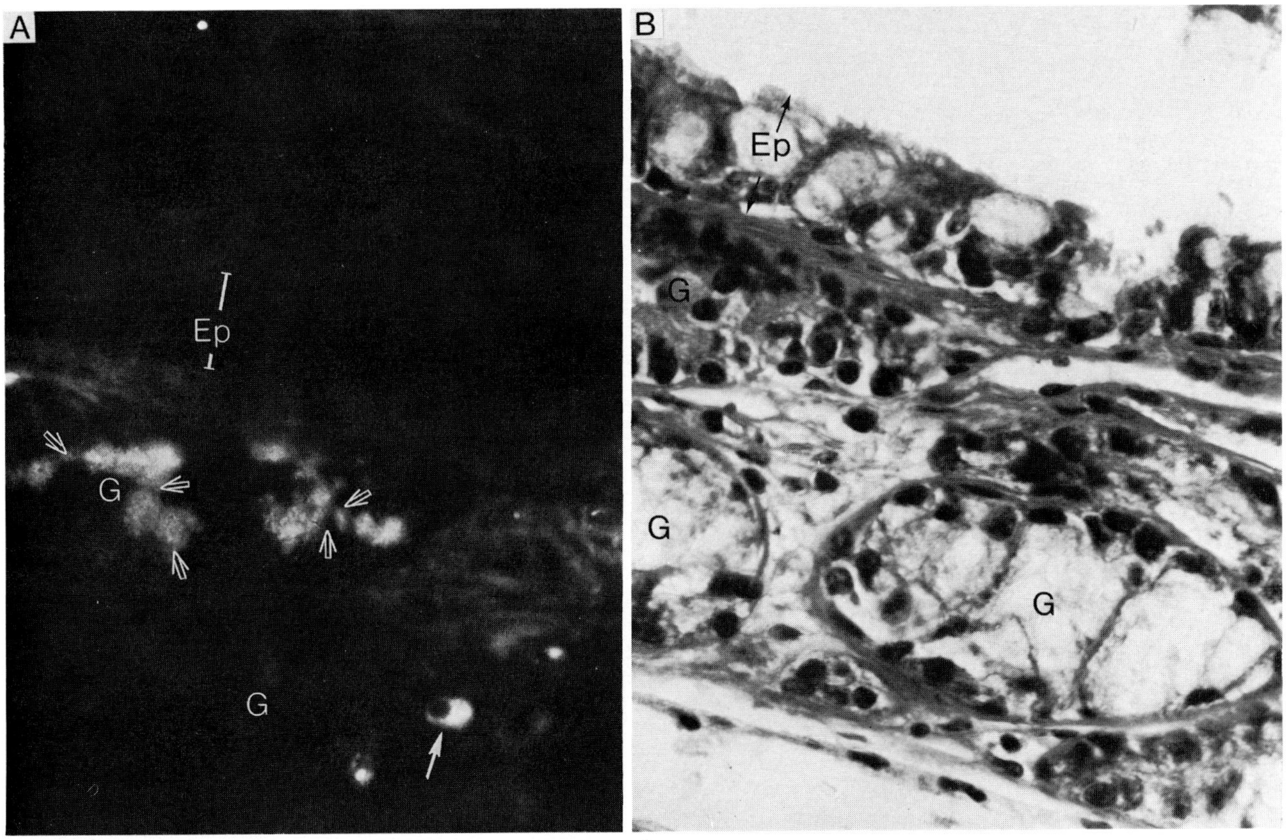

Fig. 4. A) IgA-forming cells (single arrow) and glandular acinar cells (double arrows) were found in the eustachian tube in this immunofluorescent stained section. B) Adjacent section to A, stained by H & E. Ep - Epithelium; G - Glands. (x160 original magnification)

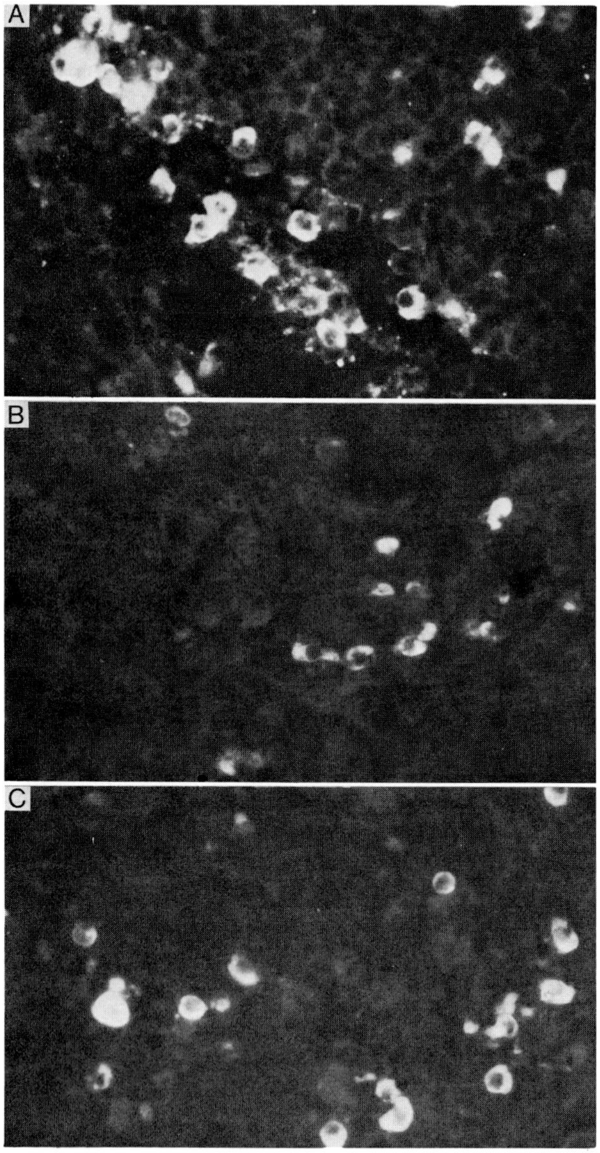

Fig. 5. Immunoglobulin-forming cells in chinchilla spleen stained with FITC-conjugated A) anti-IgA, B) anti-IgM, and C) anti-IgG. (x160 original magnification)

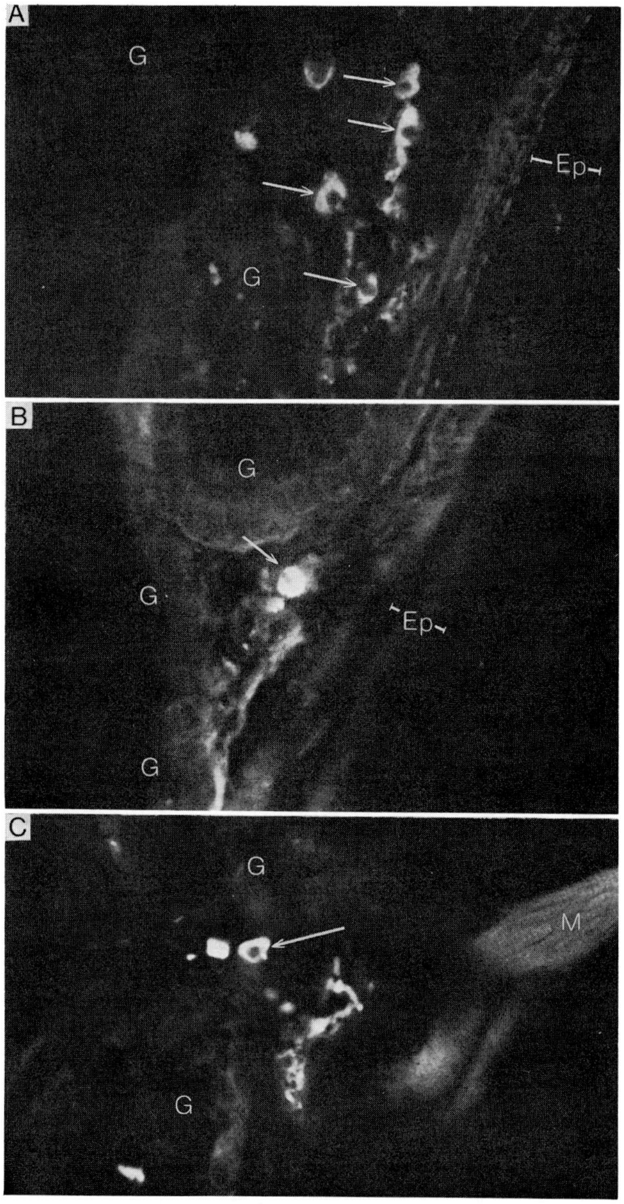

Fig. 6. Immunoglobulin-forming cells in chinchilla trachea stained with A) FITC-conjugated anti-IgA, B) anti-IgM, and C) anti-IgG. M - Muscle. (x160 original magnification)

although there were some IgA-forming cells. The epithelial cells were cuboidal or flat in the middle ear mucosa, and they were not stained with FITC-conjugated antisera to each immunoglobulin. Glands could not be found in the normal middle ear mucosa.

Immunoglobulin-Forming Cells in Lymphoid Organs and Respiratory and Alimentary Tracts. The spleen, mesenteric lymph nodes, and peripheral lymphoid organs were examined as controls for the middle ear tissue. There were many immunoglobulin-forming cells present in the interfollicular area of the lymph nodes and red pulp of the spleen. The most common immunoglobulin-forming cells were IgG-forming cells, which accounted for 70% of the immunoglobulin-forming cells. The percentage of IgM-forming cells was 20% and of IgA-forming cells only 10% (Fig. 5).

In the trachea a few IgA-forming cells were scattered in the subepithelial connective tissue and between glands, whereas IgG- and IgM-forming cells were very rare. This finding is similar to those of the eustachian tube and middle ear mucosa (Fig. 6).

Many IgA-forming cells were found in the subepithelial connective tissue of the small and large intestines, and the luminar contents and acinar cells of intestinal glands were also brilliantly stained with FITC-conjugated anti-IgA. The IgA-forming cells accounted for 80% of the immunoglobulin-forming cells present in the alimentary tract. In contrast, IgM-forming cells were few in number (20%), and IgG-forming cells were very rare (Fig. 7).

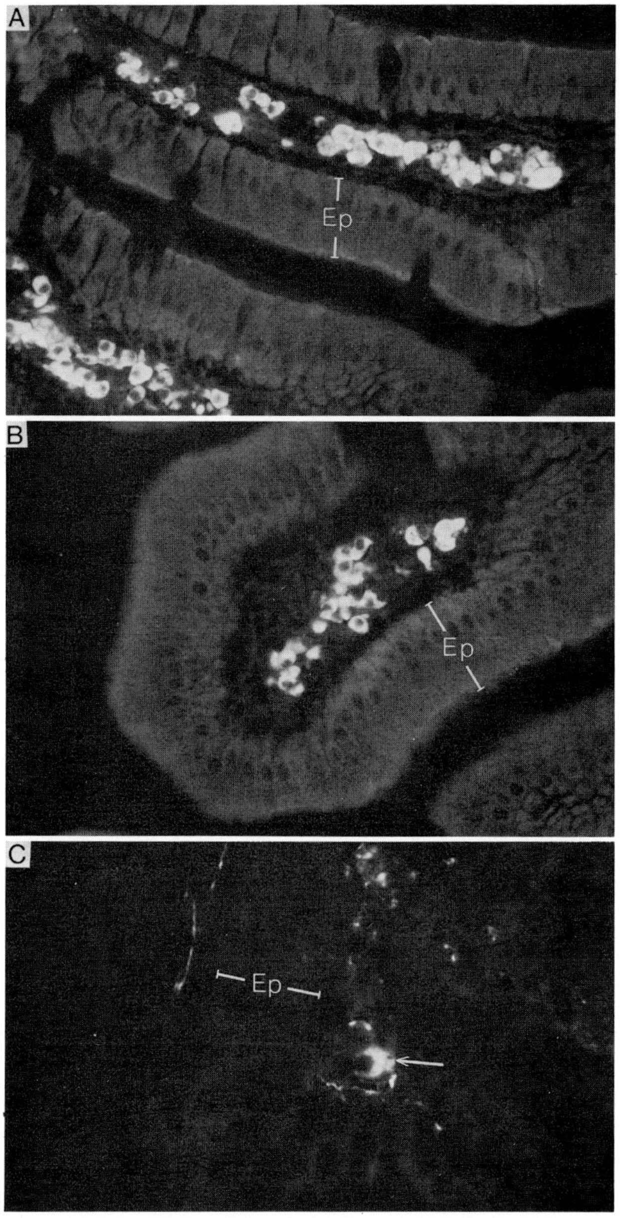

Fig. 7. Immunoglobulin-forming cells in chinchilla intestine stained with FITC-conjugated A) anti-IgA, B) anti-IgM, and C) anti-IgG (arrow). (x160 original magnification)

DISCUSSION

The present study identified at least three main classes of immunoglobulin (IgG, IgA and IgM) in chinchilla serum, which correspond to those in humans in their chromatographic and electrophoretic characteristics. Results of this study showed that the predominant immunoglobulin in chinchilla serum is IgG, followed by IgA and IgM. This finding is in accordance with that from other laboratory animals, such as the guinea pig,[7,15] mouse,[16] rat,[17] and hamster,[18] and humans.[10,19,20]

Rodents have two subclasses of IgG, IgG_1 and IgG_2, as determined by electrophoretic and chromatographic properties.[7] Electrophoretically IgG_2 moves to the anode faster than IgG_1 and also can be eluted by 0.005M Tris HCl buffer at pH 8 from the DEAE-cellulose column, while IgG_1 is eluted by higher than 0.005M buffer, as shown in guinea pigs.[7] Our study suggests that subclasses of IgG in the chinchilla are similar, if not identical, to those in guinea pigs.[21]

The immunofluorescent investigation of this study demonstrated that IgG-positive cells were the predominant type of immunoglobulin-forming cells in the peripheral lymphoid organs, whereas IgA-positive cells were the main immunoglobulin-forming cells in the respiratory and alimentary tracts and middle ear mucosa. This finding suggests that the chinchilla possesses both systemic and local immune systems, as demonstrated in other rodents (guinea pig,[7] mouse,[16] rat,[17] hamster[18]) and humans.[11,19,20]

Hussl and Lim[22] studied immunoglobulin-forming cells in the mucosa of middle ears and eustachian tubes of squirrel monkeys and reported that immunoglobulin-forming cells were occasionally encountered in normal middle ear mucosa and that their number increased following inflammatory changes in the middle ear. Mogi et al[15] investigated immunoglobulin-forming cells in the middle ear mucosa of developing and mature guinea pigs and suggested that the local synthesis of IgA is latent in the middle ear mucosa of normal guinea pigs because the middle ear cavity has less opportunity to receive antigenic stimulation than other areas of the respiratory and alimentary tracts because of its anatomic arrangement. The present study confirms these previous observations in which IgA-forming cells were predominant in the cartilaginous portion and pharyngeal orifice of the tube and less prominent in the tympanic cavity.

Recent studies[23,24] have suggested that the human and laboratory animal middle ear mucosa maintains a local mucosal immune system.[25-28] Bernstein et al[23] demonstrated the local synthesis of SC in the middle ear epithelium, and Mogi et al[24] identified free SC and bound SC in the middle ear effusions. More recently it has been demonstrated that secretory IgA possesses antibody activity in the middle ear effusions from patients with otitis media with effusion.[29] These findings indicate that there is active function of the local immune system in the human middle ear mucosa. It is known that secretory IgA plays an important role in the first-line defense system of the mucous membranes that face the external environment.[25] The demonstration of secretory IgA in chinchilla colostrum in this study supports the notion that the chinchilla possesses a mucosal immune system like that in humans, making the chinchilla an immunologically appropriate animal model for experimental otitis media.

At the time of this study, Dr. Watanabe was a Research Fellow in the Department of Otolaryngology, Ohio State University, Columbus, on leave of absence from the Department of Otolaryngology, Yamaguchi University School of Medicine, Ube, Japan. His present address (1982) is Oita Prefecture Hospital, Oita, Japan.

ACKNOWLEDGMENTS — The authors wish to express thanks for their invaluable assistance to Karen Targgart, Thomas Lee, Ilija Karanfilov, Linda Cox, Steven Lee McBride, Nancy Sally, Scott Gordon, Laurence Owens, and Katherine Adamson. The experimental animals were donated mainly by members of the Columbus, Dayton, Cincinnati, and Lima Units of the Ohio Empress Chinchilla Breeders Cooperative. We are particularly grateful for the critical review of the manuscript by Dr. Thomas F. DeMaria.

REFERENCES

1. Giebink GS, Payne EE, Mills EL, Juhn SK, Quie PG. Experimental otitis media due to *Streptococcus pneumoniae:* immunopathogenic response in the chinchilla. J Infect Dis 1976; 134:595-604.

2. Giebink GS, Quie PG. Comparision of otitis media due to types 3 and 23 *Streptococcus pneumoniae* in chinchilla model. J Infect Dis 1977; 136:S191-5.

3. Juhn SK, Giebink GS, Hanson DG, Paparella MM. Experimentally induced acute otitis media — an animal model. Arch Otolaryngol 1977; 215:95-6.

4. Lewis DM, Schram JL, Meadema SJ, Lim DJ. Experimental otitis media in chinchillas. Ann Otol Rhinol Laryngol 1980; 89 Suppl 68:344-50.

5. Hook RR Jr. Humoral immune response of the adult chinchilla. Lab Anim Sci 1973; 23:837-42.

6. Visco RJ, Kinkler RJ. Cell mediated immunity in the chinchilla *(Chinchilla laniger)*: in vitro lymphocyte transformation. Lab Anim Sci 1976; 26:751-7.

7. Vaerman JP, Heremans JF. The IgA system of the guinea pig. J Immunol 1972; 108:637-48.

8. Müller-Eberhard HJ, Osterland CK. Zone electrophoresis on powder block. In: Williams CA, Chase MW, eds. Methods in immunology and immunochemistry. Vol. II. New York: Academic Press, 1968:57-67.

9. Lowry OH, Rosebough NJ, Farr AL, Randall RJ. Protein measurement with Folin phenol reagent. J Biol Chem 1951; 193: 265-75.

10. Mogi G. Secretory immunoglobulin A in oral and respiratory passage in man. Ann Otol Rhinol Laryngol 1975; 83 Suppl 20:1-20.

11. Watanabe N. Immunochemical and immunohistochemical studies on chronic paranasal sinus infection. Bull Yamaguchi Med Sch (Japan) 1977; 24:25-48.

12. Kawamura A. Fluorescent antibody techniques and their applications. 2nd ed. Tokyo: University of Tokyo Press, 1977: 45-65.

13. Hamashima Y, Kyogoku K. Immunofluorescent technique, immunoelectron microscopic technique, radioisotopic labeled antibody technique. 2nd ed. Tokyo: Igaku Shoin Ltd, 1968.

14. Mancini G, Carbonara AO, Heremans JF. Immunological quantitation of antigens by single radial immunodiffusion. Immunochem 1965; 2:235-54.

15. Mogi G, Maeda S, Watanabe N. The development of mucosal immunity in guinea pig middle ear. Int J Pediatr Otorhinolaryngol 1980; 1:331-49.

16. Nash DR, Vaerman JP, Bazin H, Heremans JF. Comparative molecular size of mouse IgA in different body fluid. Int Arch Allergy Appl Immunol 1970; 37:167-74.

17. Stechschulte DJ, Austen KF. Immunoglobulins of rat colostrum. J Immunol 1970; 104:1052-62.

18. Bienenstock J. Immunoglobulins of the hamster. II. Characterization of the γA and other immunoglobulins in serum and secretions. J Immunol 1970; 104:1228-35.

19. Tomasi TB Jr, Zeigelbaum S. The selective occurrence of γ_1A globulins in certain body fluids. J Clin Invest 1963; 42:1552-60.

20. Tomasi TB Jr. The immune system of secretions. Englewood Cliffs: Prentice-Hall, 1976.

21. Mogi G, Lim DJ, Watanabe N. Immunologic study on the inner ear: immunoglobulins in perilymph. Arch Otolaryngol 1982; 108:270-5.

22. Hussl B, Lim DJ. Experimental middle ear effusions: an immunofluorescent study. Ann Otol Rhinol Laryngol 1974; 83: 332-42.

23. Bernstein JM, Hayes ER, Ishikawa T, Herd JK. Secretory otitis media: a histopathologic and immunochemical report. Trans Am Acad Ophthalmol Otolaryngol 1972; 76:1305-17.

24. Mogi G, Honjo S, Maeda S, Yoshida T, Watanabe N. Secretory immunoglobulin A (SIgA) in middle ear effusions: a further report. Ann Otol Rhinol Laryngol 1974; 83:92-101.

25. Liu YS, Lang R, Lim DJ. Microorganisms in chronic otitis media with effusion. Ann Otol Rhinol Laryngol 1976; 85 Suppl 25:245-9.

26. Lim DJ, Shimada T. Secretory activity of normal middle ear epithelium. Scanning and transmission electron microscopic observation. Ann Otol Rhinol Laryngol 1971; 80:319-29.

27. Lim DJ. Functional morphology of the lining membrane of the middle ear and eustachian tube. Ann Otol Rhinol Laryngol 1974; 83 Suppl 11:5-26.

28. Mogi G, Maeda S, Yoshida T, Watanabe N. Immunochemistry of otitis meda with effusion. J Infect Dis 1976; 133: 126-36.

29. Mogi G, Maeda S, Yoshida T, Watanabe N. Otitis media with effusion: specific antibody activities against exotoxins in middle ear effusions. Laryngoscope 1976; 86:1042-55.

EXPERIMENTAL OTITIS MEDIA IN CHINCHILLAS
II. COMPARISON OF THE MIDDLE EAR IMMUNE RESPONSES TO *S PNEUMONIAE* TYPES 3 AND 23

NORITAKE WATANABE, MD

THOMAS F. DEMARIA, PHD
DANIEL M. LEWIS, PHD
GORO MOGI, MD
DAVID J. LIM, MD

COLUMBUS, OHIO

The present study shows that two different serotypes of *Streptococcus pneumoniae* (types 3 and 23) when inoculated through the bulla elicit distinctly different immune responses in chinchillas. The passive hemagglutination assay shows that type 3 is a better immunogen than type 23 and that type 3 primarily elicits immune responses in the middle ear. When class-specific antibody activity was measured with the red cell linked antigen-antibody reaction test, antibody activities of serum IgG to type 3 slightly declined and of effusion IgM and IgA to type 3 increased following type 3 infection, whereas following type 23 infection antibody activities of serum IgG to type 23 increased and no antibody activities of IgA and IgM to type 23 were present in the effusions.

INTRODUCTION

Streptococcus pneumoniae is reported to be one of the most common bacteria involved in acute otitis media[1,2] and otitis media with effusion (OME),[3,4] and it can elicit immune response in middle ear effusions (MEEs).[1,5] In pneumococcal otitis media it has been suggested that the clinical course may depend to a certain extent on the serotype.[6] In a recent animal experiment on otitis media using the chinchilla and type 23 pneumococcus,[7,8] the animals were capable of clearing the infection over a 6-week period without treatment, whereas otitis media caused by type 3 persisted throughout the 6-week study. The resolution of type 23 pneumococcal otitis media paralleled the development of type-specific serum antibody, and the prolonged course of type 3 pneumococcal infection was associated with a fall in the levels of type-specific antibody in serum.[7] This observation suggests that serum antibodies may play an important role in dictating the clinical course. On the other hand, Lewis et al[9] observed that prior infection of *S pneumoniae* type 3 in the middle ear made that middle ear resistant to a second challenge, even though the systemic antibody specific to type 3 fell following infection.

Secretory IgA, the predominant immunoglobulin in external secretions, plays an important role in local immunity, which is independent from systemic immunity.[10,11] Several investigators[1,12-15] have demonstrated that MEEs have specific antibody activity against bacterial and viral antigens and that secretory IgA in MEE possesses specific antibody activity.[13,14] These results suggest that the middle ear is an organ capable of responding immunologically to antigenic stimulation independently from the systemic immune system. The preceding study from this laboratory demonstrated the presence of the IgA system in chinchillas, suggesting a similarity in the human and chinchilla middle ear immune systems.[16]

The serotype specificity of the immune response, the directional preference as to whether a local or systemic response is induced by pneumococcal otitis media, and the relative value of serum antibodies versus locally produced effusion antibodies are important research questions. This information is useful not only for understanding the clinical course of pneumococcal otitis media but also for evaluating the potential use of a pneumococcal vaccine for otitis media.

MATERIALS AND METHODS

Animals. Sera and effusions from 124 healthy chinchillas (*Chinchilla laniger*, 1-2 years; 200-500 g) were used in this experiment. Forty-one of these chinchillas served as controls; 55 chinchillas that had been used in an earlier study had been inoculated with live *S pneumoniae* type 3; and the remaining 28 were infected with *S pneumoniae* type 23.

Antisera. Antisera against chinchilla IgG, IgA and IgM were prepared in rabbits, as previously described.[16]

Bacterial Inoculum. S pneumoniae type 3 was obtained from the Center for Disease Control (Atlanta) and *S pneumoniae* type 23 from the American Type Culture Collection (Rockville, Md). The virulence of these organisms was maintained by intraperitoneal passage in mice. The bacteria were cultured overnight in brain-heart infusion broth supplemented with 10% horse serum. After being washed twice with sterile 0.1M phosphate buffered saline (PBS) at pH 7.4, the bacteria were suspended in saline and the concentration adjusted to 10^6 organisms/ml spectrophotometrically by reference to a standard curve. Standard plate counts on blood agar were used to confirm the concentration in the original inoculum. The chinchillas were aseptically inoculated directly into the superior bulla with 0.3 ml of the bacterial suspen-

From the Otological Research Laboratories, Department of Otolaryngology, Ohio State University College of Medicine, Columbus. This study was supported in parts by grants from the NIH-NINCDS (R 501 NS08854) and Deafness Research Foundation.

TABLE 1. TOTAL CONCENTRATION OF EACH IMMUNOGLOBULIN CLASS IN MEEs AND SERA AS MEASURED BY SINGLE RADIAL IMMUNODIFFUSION

		Normal Sera (n=41)		Otitis Media due to S pneumoniae			
				Type 3	(n=16)	Type 23	(n=10)
IgG	Sera	1016*	(1148-900)**	1058	(1342-832)	1026	(1531-687)
	MEEs			695	(1198-403)	481	(697-332)
	MEE/Serum			0.66		0.47	
IgA	Sera	98	(105-92)	103	(130-81)	94	(106-83)
	MEEs			51	(81-32)	42	(54-33)
	MEE/Serum			0.50		0.45	
IgM	Sera	76	(84-67)	88	(110-70)	93	(96-91)
	MEEs			49	(70-34)	58	(81-33)
	MEE/Serum			0.56		0.62	

* mg/100ml
**Mean ± 2 SE

sion. The number of organisms in the inoculum is the optimal quantity that effectively induces otitis media in chinchillas without killing the animals.[9] The volume of the inoculum was appropriate for inoculation into the chinchilla bulla without rupturing the tympanic membrane.

Fluoresceinated Antisera. Each antiserum against chinchilla IgG, IgA and IgM was conjugated with fluoresceinated isothiocyanate (FITC) by the method of Kawamura[17] and absorbed with chinchilla liver powder in order to remove nonspecific staining for connective tissue.

Preparation of Tissues and Immunofluorescent Study. The immunofluorescent study of the middle ear mucosa and eustachian tube and the blocking test were carried out as previously reported.[18] Immunoglobulin-positive cells were counted in a 160x-power field in five different areas and averaged.

Indirect Fluorescent Antibody Technique. In order to detect the specific antibody activity of each immunoglobulin class in MEEs and sera, the indirect fluorescent antibody technique was employed as reported by Sloyer et al.[1]

Collection of MEEs and Sera. Sixteen of 55 chinchillas (29%) developed MEEs within two weeks after the inoculation of *S pneumoniae* type 3, and 10 of 28 chinchillas (36%) inoculated with *S pneumoniae* type 23 had MEEs. MEEs were collected by puncturing the inferior bulla using 21-gauge needles fitted to a tuberculin syringe between 10 and 14 days after inoculation. Blood samples were obtained by cardiac puncture before sacrifice.

Quantitative Analysis of IgG, IgA and IgM in MEEs and Sera. Levels of total IgG, IgA and IgM in MEEs and sera were determined by single radial immunodiffusion according to the method of Mancini et al.[19] Milk IgA was used as the standard for IgA, and IgG and IgM purified from sera as standards for IgG and IgM, respectively.

The use of a serum IgA (7S) for IgA measurements underestimates levels of secretory IgA (11S) by approximately three times.[13] Conversely, when secretory IgA is used for the standard, the levels of 7S IgA overestimate by three times. Although we have not determined whether IgA in MEEs in this study is of the secretory type (11S) or serum type (7S), we divided the values of IgA by three in this study in order to estimate the secretory IgA value since Mogi et al[14] reported that 89% of total IgA in MEE was of the serum type.

Passive Hemagglutination (PHA) Titers and Specific Antibody Titers of Each Immunoglobulin Class. The PHA test was done to detect antibody titers, regardless of their immunoglobulin classes, according to the method of Baker et al.[20] For the PHA test rabbit red blood cells (RRBC) were sensitized with pneumococcal capsular polysaccharides (provided by the Eli Lilly Research Laboratory, Indianapolis, Ind) using chromic chloride. Ten milligrams per milliliter pneumococcal capsular polysaccharide were mixed with an equal volume of 0.1% $CrCl^3$ in saline. The mixture was added to a half volume of washed packed RRBC and incubated for 4 minutes at room temperature. The sensitized RRBC were immediately washed four times with 0.1M PBS at pH 7.4 and adjusted to 2% with 0.1M PBS at pH 7.4. The titration was performed by the microtiter method, and the reagents used were dispensed or diluted in 25 μl volumes in the titration. Serial twofold dilutions of the samples were made in 0.2% bovine serum albumin in 0.1M PBS at pH 7.4. After two hours of incubation at room temperature the titers of the PHA test were determined.

The red cell linked antigen-antibody reaction (RCLA-AR) test was carried out to detect specific antibody titers of each immunoglobulin class in MEEs and sera by the method of Toyoshima and Tamaki.[21] The negative wells of the microtiter plate in the PHA test were used. Supernatants of all wells were removed by centrifugation, and the precipitated RRBC were washed four times with 100 μl of PBS. The RRBC of each well were resuspended in 25 μl of PBC, after which 25 μl of a 1/100 dilution of the appropriate anti-immunoglobulin solution against each immunoglobulin was added. The mixture was incubated overnight at 4°C. The titers were determined as in the PHA test. In the RCLA-AR test if the antibody activity in one of the immunoglobulin classes was lower than the titer determined by the PHA test, the antibody activity was unmeasurable and the result of the RCLA-AR test was judged to be negative. The specificity of this test was examined by the absorption of specific antibody in samples with pneumococcal polysaccharides and by the inhibition of antiserum with each chinchilla immunoglobulin.

The mean titers of specific antibody in the PHA and RCLA-AR tests were calculated logarithmically in log 2, and in this calculation the negative titers were calculated as zero (= $\log_2 2^0$).

Statistics. The χ^2 test was employed to estimate the incidence (of detectable antibodies) differences between the control and experimental sera and between the experimental sera and MEEs. Due to the nonparametric distribution of antibody titers, we used the Wilcoxon rank-sum test, which is equivalent to the nonparametric Mann-Whitney U-test, for analysis of these titers.

RESULTS

Total Immunoglobulin Levels in Sera and MEEs. In order to see whether the value of each immunoglobulin class reflected a possible increase in specific antibody following infection with type 3 or 23, mean values of total IgG, IgA and IgM in MEEs and sera were measured (Table 1). There were no significant differences in the mean values of IgG, IgA and IgM in sera between normal and infected

TABLE 2. SPECIFIC ANTIBODY TITERS TO TYPE 3 OF EACH IMMUNOGLOBULIN CLASS IN MEEs AND SERA AS MEASURED BY RCLA-AR

	Normal Sera (n = 20)		Otitis Media due to Type 3 S. pneumoniae			
			Sera (n = 16)		MEEs (n = 14)	
	Titer	Incidence (%)	Titer	Incidence (%)	Titer	Incidence (%)
PHA*	A_1 —	a_1 0 **	B_1 1.1 (1.5 - 0.9)	b_1 6.3	C_1 1.3 (1.7 - 1.1)	c_1 35.7
IgG	A_2 3.0 (4.1 - 2.1)***	a_2 70	B_2 2.8 (4.9 - 1.6)	b_2 50	C_2 2.2 (3.6 - 1.5)	c_2 57
IgA	A_3 1.3 (1.7 - 1.0)	a_3 20	B_3 1.4 (2.1 - 1.0)	b_3 19	C_3 1.9 (2.9 - 1.2)	c_3 43
IgM	A_4 1.1 (1.2 - 0.9)	a_4 5	B_4 1.2 (1.7 - 0.9)	b_4 13	C_4 1.5 (1.8 - 1.2)	c_4 50

— Undetectable
* Total antibody to Type 3
** Percent of positive cases
*** Mean ± 2 SE

$b_1 < C_1$ ($p = 0.0441$)
$b_3 < c_3$ ($p = 0.1506$)
$b_4 < c_4$ ($p = 0.0253$)

groups and between the groups infected with the two serotypes, with the exception of serum IgM in type 23-infected animals. The serum IgM level was higher in type 23-infected animals than in controls ($p < 0.06$). The mean value of each immunoglobulin in MEEs from infected animals was significantly lower than that in sera from infected animals ($p < 0.10$). There were no significant differences between mean immunoglobulin values of MEEs from animals infected with the two serotypes. The data from the measurement of total immunoglobulins following infection failed to reflect the increase in class-specific antibody, except in the case of IgM after type 23 infection (see following section on specific antibody activities).

In order to determine the source of immunoglobulins in the MEEs, the E/S ratio of each immunoglobulin class was determined (Table 1). The E/S ratios of IgG, IgA and IgM from animals infected with the two serotypes were smaller than one (0.45-0.66). The IgA/IgG ratio in MEEs from the type 3-infected group was 0.07 and from the type 23-infected group 0.08. The IgA/IgG ratios of MEEs were smaller than those of sera (0.09) from animals infected with each serotype. This finding suggests that the total IgG level is proportionally greater than the IgA level in both MEEs and sera. Based solely on the total immunoglobulin measurement, this could be interpreted to mean that IgG is the main immunoglobulin class in the MEEs and that the effusion immunoglobulins are derived from serum transudation.

Specific Antibody Activities against Different Serotypes in MEEs and Sera from Infected Chinchillas. The specific antibody activities against type 3 in normal sera and MEEs from infected animals are shown in Table 2. Anti-type 3 antibody activity could not be detected in normal sera by the PHA test but was demonstrable in the MEEs and sera after infection with type 3. The incidence of anti-type 3 antibody was significantly higher in MEEs than in sera of infected animals ($p < 0.05$).

When the second antibody was added to the test system for the RCLA-AR test, specific anti-type 3 IgG antibody was detected in 70% of the normal sera. The mean titer and incidence of anti-type 3 IgG were significantly higher than those of IgA ($p < 0.005$) and IgM ($p < 0.004$) in normal sera. These data suggest that the antibody activity against type 3 in normal sera primarily resides in the IgG class.

Although the mean titers and incidence of anti-type 3 IgG are slightly reduced following infection with type 3, the differences are not significant. In contrast to IgG antibody, the mean titer and incidence of anti-type 3 IgA antibody in MEEs in type 3-infected animals were higher than those in sera from normal and type 3-infected animals. This increase was not significantly different, possibly due in part to the small sample size and large variance between samples.

The levels and incidence of IgM in the serum and MEE after type 3 infection also increased over the normal serum values, and the incidence of IgM in the MEEs was significantly higher ($p < 0.02$) than the corresponding level in the sera of type 3-infected animals.

The distribution of specific antibody titers in the MEEs and sera from animals infected with type 23

TABLE 3. SPECIFIC ANTIBODY TITERS TO TYPE 23 OF EACH IMMUNOGLOBULIN CLASS IN MEEs AND SERA AS MEASURED BY RCLA-AR

	Normal Sera (n=20)		Otitis Media due to Type 23 S. pneumoniae			
			Sera (n=10)		MEEs (n=10)	
	Titer	Incidence (%)	Titer	Incidence (%)	Titer	Incidence (%)
PHA*	A_1 —	a_1 0 **	B_1 —	b_1 0	C_1 —	c_1 0
IgG	A_2 1.2 (1.5 - 1.0)***	a_2 15	B_2 2.5 (3.9 - 1.6)	b_2 70	C_2 1.6 (2.3 - 1.2)	c_2 50
IgA	A_3 1.1 (1.2 - 0.9)	a_3 10	B_3 1.4 (1.9 - 1.0)	b_3 30	C_3 —	c_3 0
IgM	A_4 1.2 (1.5 - 0.9)	a_4 10	B_4 1.5 (2.2 - 1.1)	b_4 40	C_4 —	c_4 0

— Undetectable
* Total antibody to Type 23
** Percent of positive cases
*** Mean ± 2 SE

$A_2 < B_2$ ($p = 0.0175$)
$a_2 < b_2$ ($p = 0.0026$)
$a_4 < b_4$ ($p = 0.0528$)
$b_3 < c_3$ ($p = 0.0603$)
$b_4 < c_4$ ($p = 0.0253$)

pneumococci was substantially different from that of type 3. Although the PHA test failed to show antibody activity in normal sera or in sera and MEEs from infected animals, when class-specific antibody titers were examined the antibody activity against type 23 in normal sera was equally distributed among the three immunoglobulin classes (Table 3).

The specific antibody titers as measured by RCLA-AR showed that the titer of serum IgG antibodies to type 23 was twice as high in the infected animals as in the controls, and this difference was statistically significant ($p < 0.02$). The level of specific IgG in the MEEs reflected the levels of IgG present in the sera of infected animals, and the difference between the two values is not statistically significant (Table 3).

The titer and incidence of IgA against type 23 in infected sera was higher than that in normal sera, but the difference was not statistically significant. Anti-type 23 IgA could not be detected in the MEEs of type 23-infected animals, which is in striking contrast to the increased levels of specific IgA in the MEEs of type 3-infected animals mentioned previously.

There was a slight but not significant increase in the mean titer of anti-type 23 IgM in the sera of infected animals, but the incidence of IgM increased significantly in the type 23-infected animals ($p < 0.06$). This finding is consistent with the increased total serum IgM levels (Table 1). The IgM response following infection was similar to the IgA response in that no anti-type 23 IgM was demonstrable in the MEEs following type 23 infection.

Comparison of Specific Antibody Titers between Paired MEEs and Sera. In order to demonstrate variation in immune response, we compared speci-

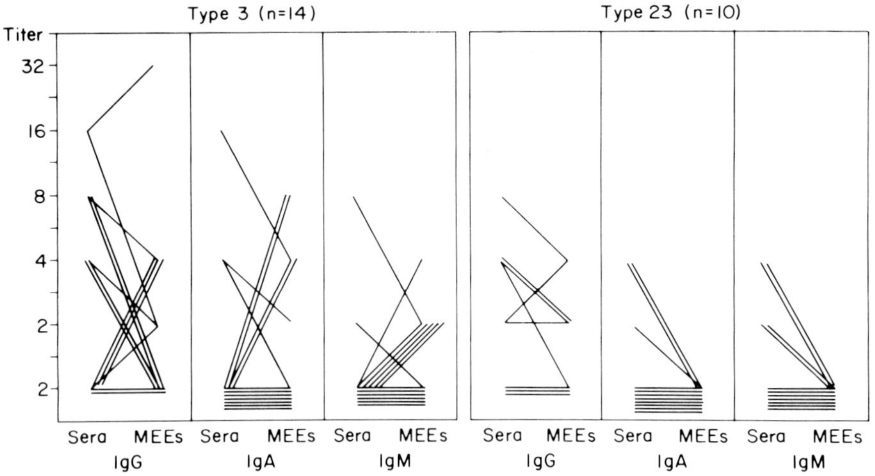

Fig. 1. Comparison of specific antibody titers to *S pneumoniae* type 3 and type 23 of each immunoglobulin class in paired samples.

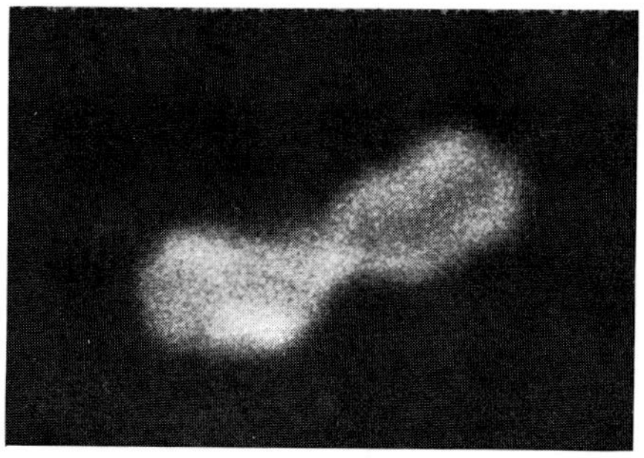

Fig. 2. Immunofluorescent demonstration of specific antibody against *S pneumoniae* type 3. The capsule of *S pneumoniae* type 3 is stained with FITC-conjugated antichinchilla IgA antiserum. (x640 magnification)

fic antibody titers between paired MEEs and sera for each serotype. The results of such a comparison for type 3 are shown in Figure 1. IgG in 36% of the samples, IgA in 29%, and IgM in 32% were greater in the MEEs than in the paired sera, but in the remainder the immunoglobulin values in MEEs were either equal to or less than those of sera. On the other hand, a comparison of paired samples from type 23-infected animals revealed that all the immunoglobulin values (IgG, IgM, IgA), with one exception, were less than those of sera (Fig. 1).

Immunofluorescent Demonstration of Specific Antibody to Bacterial Antigens in Each Immunoglobulin Class. Antibody activity of all three immunoglobulin classes in both MEEs and sera against *S pneumoniae* types 3 and 23 was demonstrated using the indirect immunofluorescence technique of Sloyer et al.[1] A bacterial smear was incubated with a sample of MEE or serum from each infected animal. After the slides were washed with PBS the bacteria were stained by FITC-conjugated antisera against each chinchilla immunoglobulin (Fig. 2). Antibody activity of all three classes against type 3 was detected in sera and MEEs from type 3-infected animals. On the other hand, only IgG antibody to type 23 was found in MEEs from type 23-infected animals although antibodies of all classes were detectable in sera from the infected animals. This finding is consistent with the specific antibody levels measured by the RCLA-AR test (Tables 2 and 3).

Immunohistochemistry. Immunoglobulin-forming cells in the middle ear mucosa were investigated. There were abundant immunoglobulin-forming cells in the middle ear mucosa of the infected animals. The IgG-forming cells were greatest in number (15-20 cells/field), followed by IgM-forming cells (8-10 cells/field), and IgA-forming cells (4-6 cells/field) (Fig. 3). These indicate a five- to tenfold increase in immunocytes in the infected animals as compared with the control ears. In the immunofluorescent study, no differences were found between the two groups infected with the two types of *S pneumoniae.* This finding is consistent with the presence of all three classes of immunoglobulins in the MEEs following experimental infection regardless of serotype (Table 1). Since we have not stained immunocytes with specific antipneumococcal antibody FITC conjugates we cannot correlate the immunochemistry with the RCLA-AR data.

DISCUSSION

The striking differences in the clinical courses of pneumococcal otitis media induced in laboratory animals by two different serotypes (types 3 and 23)

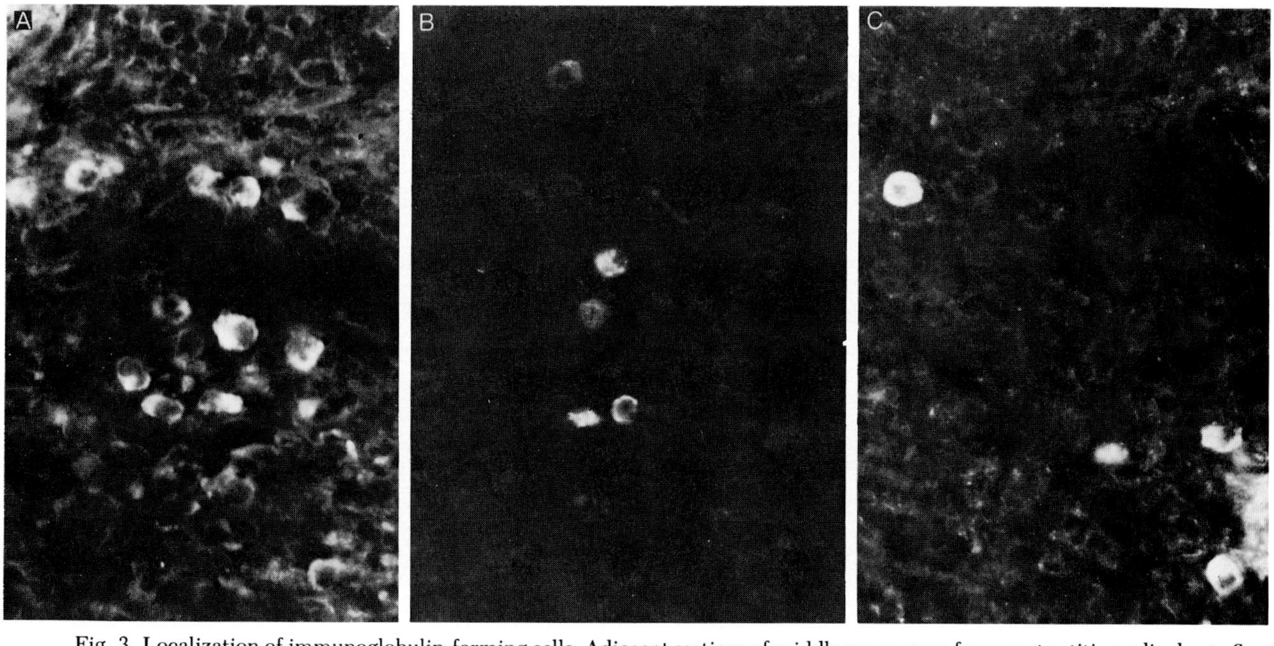

Fig. 3. Localization of immunoglobulin-forming cells. Adjacent sections of middle ear mucosa from acute otitis media due to *S pneumoniae* type 3 treated with A) anti-IgG, B) anti-IgM, and C) anti-IgA, showing that the number of IgG-forming cells was greatest and that IgM-forming cells outnumbered IgA-forming cells. (x160 magnification)

have been suggested to be related to the differences in the immune responses elicited by each pneumococcal serotype.[7,9] The present data are essentially in agreement with previous observations in that type 3 elicited antibody response predominantly in the effusion and type 23 elicited antibody response primarily in the serum, at least in terms of the incidence of measurable antibody detected. This finding is also consistent with the middle ear response in human pneumococcal otitis media as reported by Sloyer et al.[1] Therefore, type 3 may be a much better immunogen than type 23, as suggested by these authors.

Serum antibody decline following type 3 infection has been observed by radioimmunoassay.[7,9] However, this decline was not evident in our data obtained by the PHA technique, which may be attributable to the poor sensitivity of the method. Giebink and Quie[7] suggested several possibilities to explain the underlying mechanism for this peculiar response: 1) immune paralysis; 2) neutralization either by newly formed type-specific antibodies[22] or by a cross-reactive antibody such as enterobacterial antigens, which are known to occur in *S pneumoniae* type 3.[23] The RCLA-AR, which measures serotype-specific antibodies of different immunoglobulin classes, revealed a trend of decline in serum IgG in the titer and incidence of measurable IgG antibody to type 3 following infection, but because of the sample size the difference is not statistically significant. This decline of IgG is nevertheless consistent with an earlier report.[7] However, the incidences of measurable specific antibody (particularly IgM and, to a lesser extent, IgA) to type 3 in the effusions of infected animals were significantly greater than those in sera, supporting earlier reports regarding the measurement of total antibody activity in the effusions.[7,9,24]

In contrast with type 3, the RCLA-AR titers showed a twofold increase in IgG ($p<0.02$) and a significant increase in the incidence ($p<0.003$) of measurable IgG antibody to type 23 in sera following infection. This finding is consistent with earlier reports that serum antibody to type 23 increased following infection as measured by radioimmunoassay.[7,24] The slight increases in IgA and IgM in both titers and incidence of measurable antibody in sera following infection were not statistically significant. It is important to note that there were no detectable IgA and IgM antibodies in the effusions, although effusion IgG to type 23 was detected. This finding could be interpreted to mean that the systemic immune system is stimulated more than the local immune system as a result of *S pneumoniae* type 23. This interpretation also is consistent with the suggestion that the spontaneous clearance of middle ear infection from type 23 is parallel to the rise of serum antibodies.[7] Another piece of supporting evidence for this notion is that the 14 valent pneumococcal vaccines (which include types 3 and 23) seemed to reduce the rate of recurrence of otitis media.[25] Giebink et al[24] tested the efficacy of pneumococcal vaccine using the capsular polysaccharide from *S pneumoniae* type 7 and reported a twofold rise in serum antibody. Only 7% of the seroconverted animals developed otitis media, but 62% of the unvaccinated group developed otitis media following challenge. On this basis they suggested that high serum antibody levels are associated with the protection of the ear against pneumococcal infection.

The abovementioned concept may hold true for *S pneumoniae* type 23 but not for type 3. Even with slightly depressed IgG antibody to type 3 following infection, the chinchilla has a considerable amount of antibody in both serum and effusion, and yet infection lingers in the middle ear.[7,9] Obviously the antibody to type 3 that is present in serum does not afford complete protection. As mentioned above, *S pneumoniae* type 3 is known to cross-react with various other bacterial antigens such as enteric bacteria,[23] and perhaps this naturally occurring cross-reactive antibody may not be protective against *S pneumoniae* type 3.

A mucosal membrane facing the external environment is known to possess its own immune system that is largely independent from the systemic immune system.[11] Secretory IgA (SIgA) is considered to be the major immunoglobulin in the external secretion, although IgM and, to a lesser extent, IgG also can be produced locally.[11] The role of the secretory immune system in providing protection against viral and bacterial infection on a mucosal surface has been studied by numerous investigators in recent years.[26,27] Recent evidence suggests that the local immune system comprises not only mucosal immunoglobulins but also the cell-mediated immune system via lymphocytes.[28] The mechanism by which this local immune system affords protection has not been fully determined. One possibility is that the SIgA provides the protection by preventing, delaying, or reducing the intensity of bacterial colonization on the mucosal surface; another is agglutination.[27] There is ample evidence to suggest that SIgA does not function as an opsonin for phagocytes[29,30] and does not fix complement unless aggregated.[31,32] The secretory piece may provide protection against proteolytic enzyme, as shown in the intestinal tract[27] and may be involved in facilitating IgA and IgM transport across the mucosal membrane.[11] In the latter regard, it is interesting to note that IgA and IgM antibodies are absent in the effusion following *S pneumoniae* type 23 but that the serum IgA and IgM increase after type 3 infection. It is not clear whether the IgA and IgM antibodies to type 3 found in MEEs following type 3 infection are transported across the membrane with the help of the secretory piece.

MEE is considered to be a mixture of serum transudates and secreta, based on its biochemical and immunochemical composition.[28,32-34] There appears to be a drastic increase in immunoglobulin-producing cells of all classes in the connective tissue following middle ear infection, suggesting that all classes of antibody are locally produced and transported across the mucosal membrane and/or transudated through injured (inflamed) epithelium. The total immunoglobulin levels in the MEEs are roughly parallel with the immunohistochemical data of immunoglobulin-producing cells in the middle ear mucosa following *S pneumoniae* type 3 and 23 infections (Table 1). Although our present immunohistochemical data tend to suggest that there is no difference in the numbers of immunocytes between the two experimental groups, because we have not completed a histochemical study using serotype-specific antiserum we cannot fully explain the lack of IgM and IgA antipneumococcal antibody in the effusions following type 23 infection.

Lewis et al[9] compared the efficacy of different immunization methods using *S pneumoniae* type 3 for preventing middle ear infection and found that direct inoculation of bacteria into the middle ear cavity was far superior to inoculation via the intranasal or intramuscular route. The present data are in line with this observation if increased titer and incidence of IgA and IgM antibodies in the effusion have any bearing on local immunological defense. As discussed above, there is ample evidence that it does. However, the fact that *S pneumoniae* type 3 is known to cause a lingering infection[7,9] raises a rather perplexing question regarding the efficacy of mucosal immunity against *S pneumoniae* type 3. Further study is needed to clarify the mechanisms by which the middle ear provides protection against various serotypes of *S pneumoniae* as well as other pathogenic organisms.

At the time of this study Drs. Watanabe and Mogi were on leave of absence from the Department of Otolaryngology, Yamaguchi University School of Medicine, Ube, Japan. Dr. Watanabe's present address (1982) is Oita Prefecture Hospital, Oita, Japan.

ACKNOWLEDGMENT — The animals were donated mainly by members of the Columbus, Dayton, Cincinnati, and Lima Units of the Ohio Empress Chinchilla Breeders Cooperative. The authors wish to express thanks for their invaluable assistance to Bruce R. Briggs, Karen Targgart, Thomas Lee, Kay Herouvis, Ilija Karanfilov, Steven Lee McBride, Nancy Sally, and Katherine Adamson.

REFERENCES

1. Sloyer JL Jr, Howie VM, Ploussard JH, Amman AJ, Austrian R, Johnston RM Jr. Immune response to acute otitis media in children. I. Serotype isolated and serum and middle ear fluid antibody in pneumococcal otitis media. Infect Immunol 1974; 9:1028-32.

2. Klein JO. Microbiology of otitis media. Ann Otol Rhinol Laryngol 1980; 89 Suppl 68:98-101.

3. Liu YS, Lim DJ, Lang RW, Birck HG. Chronic middle ear effusions. Immunological and bacteriological investigations. Arch Otolaryngol 1975; 101:278-86.

4. Riding KH, Bluestone CD, Michaels RH, Cantekin EI, Doyle WJ, Poziviak CS. Microbiology of recurrent and chronic otitis media with effusion. J Pediatr 1978; 93:739-43.

5. Austrian R, Howie VM, Ploussard JH. The bacteriology of pneumococcal otitis media. Johns Hopkins Med J 1977; 141: 104-11.

6. Howie VM, Ploussard JH, Sloyer J. The "otitis-prone" condition. Am J Dis Child 1975; 129:676-8.

7. Giebink GS, Quie PG. Comparison of otitis media due to type 3 and 23 *Streptococcus pneumoniae* in the chinchilla model. J Infect Dis 1977; 136:S191-5.

8. Giebink GS, Payne EE, Mills EL, Juhn SK, Quie PG. Experimental otitis media due to *Streptococcus pneumoniae:* immunopathogenic response in the chinchilla. J Infect Dis 1976; 164:595-604.

9. Lewis DM, Schram JL, Meadema SJ, Lim DJ. Experimental otitis media in chinchillas. Ann Otol Rhinol Laryngol 1980; 89 Suppl 68:344-50.

10. Tomasi TB Jr, Grey HM. Structure and function of immunoglobulin A. Prog Allergy 1972; 16:81-213.

11. Tomasi TB Jr. The immune system of secretions. Englewood Cliffs: Prentice-Hall, 1976.

12. Bernstein JM, Tomasi TB Jr, Ogra P. The immunochemistry of middle ear effusions. Arch Otolaryngol 1974; 99:320-6.

13. Bienenstock J, Tourville D, Tomasi TB Jr. The secretion of immunoglobulins by the human salivary gland. In: Botelho SY, Brools FP, Shelly WB, eds. The exocrine glands. Philadelphia: University of Pennsylvania Press, 1969:187-98.

14. Mogi G, Maeda S, Yoshida T, Watanabe N. Otitis media with effusion: specific antibody activities against exotoxins in middle ear effusions. Laryngoscope 1976; 86:1042-55.

15. Lewis DM, Schram JL, Birck HG, Lim DJ. Antibody activity in otitis media with effusion. Ann Otol Rhinol Laryngol 1979; 88:392-6.

16. Watanabe N, Briggs BR, Lim DJ. Experimental otitis media in chinchillas. I. Baseline immunological investigation. Ann Otol Rhinol Laryngol 1982; 91 Suppl 93:3-8.

17. Kawamura A Jr. Fluorescent antibody techniques and their applications. Tokyo: University of Tokyo Press, 1977.

18. Watanabe N. Immunochemical and immunohistochemical studies on chronic paranasal sinus infection. Bul Yamaguchi Med Sch 1977; 24:25-48.

19. Mancini G, Carbonara AO, Heremans JF. Immunological quantitation of antigens by single radial immunodiffusion. Immunochem 1965; 2:235-54.

20. Baker PJ, Stashaka PW, Prescott B. Use of erythrocytes sensitized with purified pneumococcal polysaccharides for the assay of antibody and antibody-producing cells. Appl Microbiol 1969; 17:422-6.

21. Toyoshima K, Tamaki H. Simple method for the measurement of antibody activity of each immunoglobulin class: red cell linked antigen-antibody reaction. In: Migita S, ed. Methods of immunology. Vol. VIII. Kanazawa, Japan: Jap Soc Immunol 1979:2369-73 (in Japanese).

22. Jones JM, Amsbough DF, Prescott B. Kinetics of the antibody response to type III pneumococcal polysaccharide. II. Factors influencing the serum antibody levels after immunization with an optimally immunogenic dose of antigen. J Immunol 1975; 116—52-64.

23. Robbins JB, Myerowitz RL, Whisnant JK, et al. Enteric bacteria crossreactive with *Neisseria meningitidis* groups A and C and *Diplococcus pneumoniae* types I and III. Infect Immunol 1972; 6:651-6.

24. Giebink GS, Berzins IK, Quie PG. Animal models for

studying pneumococcal otitis media and pneumococcal vaccine efficacy. Ann Otol Rhinol Laryngol 1980; 89 Suppl 68:339-43.

25. Karma P, Luotonen J, Timonen M, et al. Efficacy of pneumococcal vaccination against recurrent otitis media. Preliminary results of a field trial in Finland. Ann Otol Rhinol Laryngol 1980; 89 Suppl 68:357-62.

26. Waldman RH, Ganguly R. The role of the secretory immune system in protection against agents which infect the respiratory tract. In: Mestecky J, Lawton AR, eds. The immunoglobulin A system. New York: Plenum Press, 1974:283-94.

27. Cantey JR. Prevention of bacterial infections of mucosal surfaces by immune secretory IgA. In: McGhee JR, Mestecky J, Babb JL, eds. Secretory immunity and infection. New York: Plenum Press, 1977:461-70.

28. Drucker M, Drucker I, Neter E, Bernstein J, Ogra PL. Cell mediated immune responses to bacterial antigens on human mucosal surfaces. In: McGhee JR, Mestecky J, Babb JL, eds. Secretory immunity and infection. New York: Plenum Press, 1977: 479-88.

29. Eddie DS, Schulkind ML, Robbins JB. The isolation and biologic activities of purified secretory IgA and IgG anti-*Salmonella typhinurium* "O" antibodies from rabbit intestinal fluid and colostrum. J Immunol 1971; 106:181-90.

30. Steele EJ, Chacumpa W, Rowley D. Isolation and biological properties of three classes of rabbit antibody to *Vibrio cholerae.* J Infect Dis 1974; 130:93-103.

31. Fubara ES, Freter R. Protection against enteric bacterial infection by secretory IgA antibodies. J Immunol 1973; 111:395-403.

32. Lim DJ. Microbiology and cytology of otitis media with effusion: a review. In: Sadé J, ed. Secretory otitis media and its sequelae. New York: Churchill Livingstone, 1979:125-43.

33. Bernstein, JM, Ogra PL. Mucosal immune system: implications in otitis media with effusion. Ann Otol Rhinol Laryngol 1980; 89 Suppl 68: 326-32.

34. Juhn SK, Giebink GS, Huff JS, Mills EL. Biochemical and immunochemical characteristics of middle ear effusions in relation to bacteriological findings. Ann Otol Rhinol Laryngol 1980; 89 Suppl 68: 161-7.

MICROCRYPT EXTENSIONS OF TONSILLAR CRYPTS

SHOICHI MAEDA, MD
OITA, JAPAN

GORO MOGI, MD
OITA, JAPAN

MOTOW OH, MD
UBE, JAPAN

The crypts of human palatine tonsils were examined electron microscopically. The cryptal epithelia contained three types of micropores (termed microcrypt). Type I microcrypts opened between intercellular spaces of the epithelial cells. Free cells were observed in the micropores. Type II microcrypts opened near the center of a cryptal epithelial cell. Type III microcrypts appeared after "specialized epithelial cells" degenerated and fell off. Many mature plasma cells are attached to the walls of the sinusoidal vessels in the lower boundary zone of the epithelium and subepithelial layer. Lymphocytes were observed migrating from the postcapillary venules of the subepithelial zone. The findings indicate that the microcrypts are probably orifices for tunnel-like passages of free cells and that they are located in the walls of the tonsillar crypts. The lymphocytes in the passages perhaps come from lymphoid tissues in the subepithelial layer and postcapillary venules, and the antibodies produced in the cryptal epithelia of the palatine tonsils may contribute to humoral immunity.

INTRODUCTION

The human palatine tonsil has 10 to 20 board-like or tubular crypts that penetrate deeply into the parenchyma. The organ has a widespread surface and receives antigenic stimulation from the external environment.

Recent studies have demonstrated that the palatine tonsil has the function of both antibody production and cell-mediated immunity.[1-4] Although it produces all five immunoglobulin classes, Schmedtje and Batts[5] and Mogi[3,6] reported that the cryptal epithelium did not produce secretory IgA. Secretory IgA blocks the adherence of certain bacteria to the mucosal surface.[7] It is a well accepted finding that bacilli, as well as cell debris and food particles, are present in the cryptal lumens of normal and inflamed tonsils. The cryptal epithelium may not be similar to the defense wall of the oral cavity and pharyngeal space, and it may also differ in function from the upper respiratory tract mucosa.

Recent SEM studies[8-11] have demonstrated the presence of micropores on the cryptal epithelia of palatine tonsils. However, the exact function of the micropores is obscure, and the present study was designed to clarify the functional morphology of tonsillar crypts.

MATERIALS AND METHODS

Forty-two palatine tonsils were obtained from 21 patients, 5 to 15 years of age, who underwent tonsillectomy because of recurrent tonsillitis or hypertrophy. The samples were immediately rinsed with cold saline and placed in buffered 2.5% glutaraldehyde. They were trimmed under a dissecting microscope, and split through the crypts for scanning electron microscopy. The adjacent areas were trimmed to small blocks for transmission electron microscopy. The specimens were fixed in cold fresh buffered 2.5% glutaraldehyde for 2 to 3 hours, thoroughly rinsed in cold 0.1 M cacodylate buffer at pH 7.4, and then fixed with cold 1% osmium tetroxide for 1 to 2 hours. The specimens were dehydrated in graded ethanol to 100%, and then dried by the critical point method using liquid carbon dioxide as transitional fluid. Some dehydrated specimens were embedded and stored in Epon 812 (Shell Chemical Co, New York), and cryofractured in liquid nitrogen. After four washings with propylene oxide in one hour, the specimens were placed in acetone and dried by the critical point method. Then they were sputter-coated with gold and examined under SEM (Model JSM-F7 [SEM] JEOL Ltd, Tokyo). Transmission electron microscopic specimens embedded in Epon 812 were cut with a microtome (Model MT-1, Nissei Industrial Co, Tokyo). The ultrathin sections were stained with uranyl acetate and lead citrate, and examined (Model JEM 100B, JEOL Ltd). Immunofluorescent studies were carried out as prevously reported.[6]

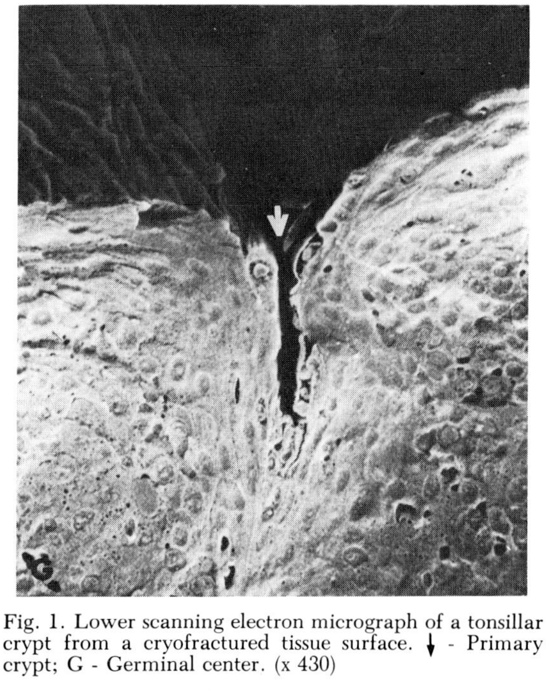

Fig. 1. Lower scanning electron micrograph of a tonsillar crypt from a cryofractured tissue surface. ↓ - Primary crypt; G - Germinal center. (x 430)

From the Department of Otolaryngology, Medical College of Oita; and the Department of Anatomy, Yamaguchi University School of Medicine, Ube, Japan.

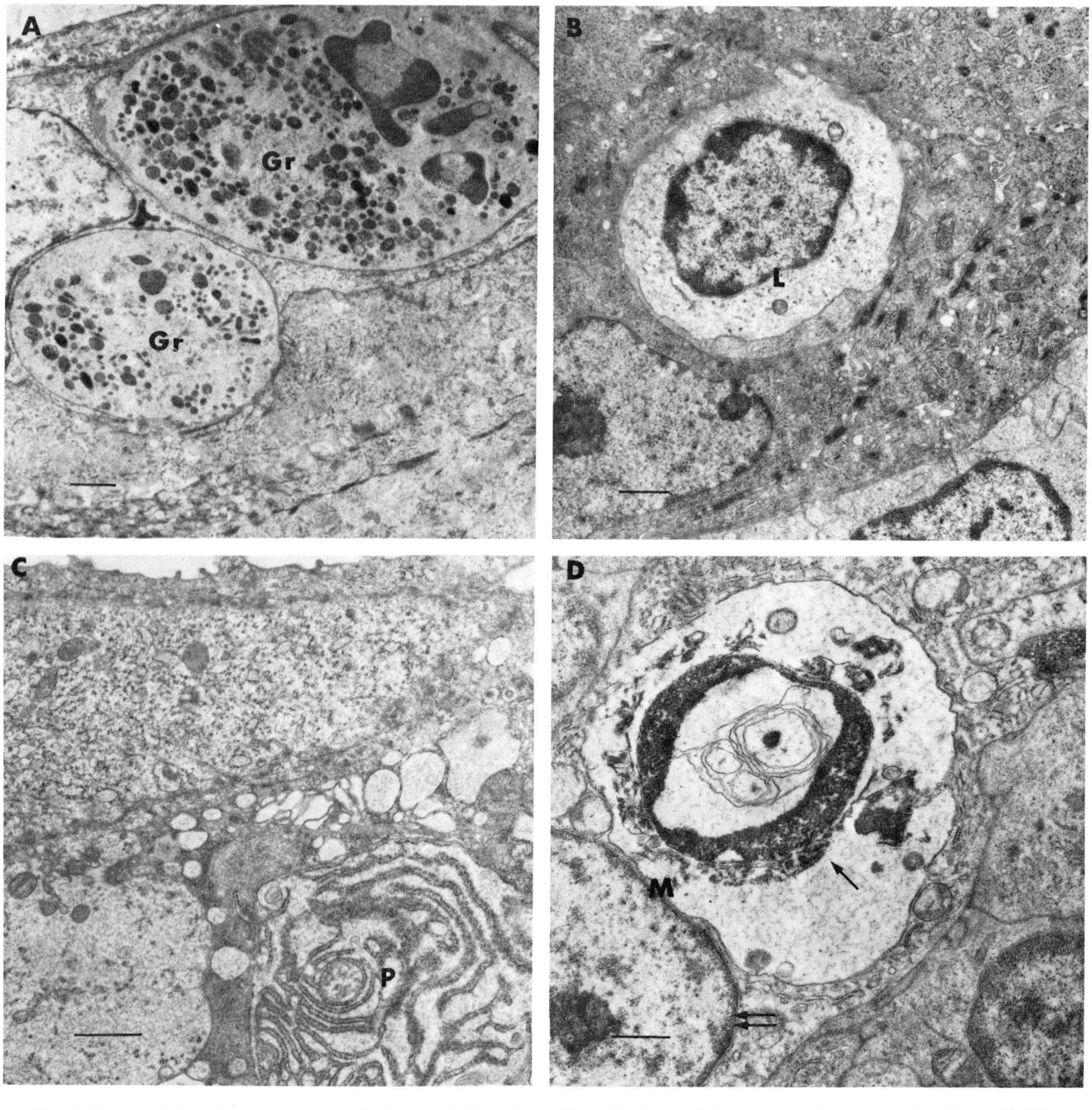

Fig. 2. Transmission electron micrograph showing infiltrating cells in the intercellular space of the crypt epithelium. A) GR - Granulocyte. (x 6,150) B) L - Lymphocyte. (x 6,890) C) P - Plasma cell. (x 9,600) D) Macrophage contains undigestible residues of phagocytized material. Single arrow - Phagocytized material. Double arrow - Nucleus of the macrophage. (x 8,270)

RESULTS

Cryptal Lumen and Epithelium of the Palatine Tonsil. The external surface facing the oropharynx was covered by stratified squamous epithelium with numerous microridges. Crypts penetrated and branched deeply into the lymphoid tissue of the tonsils, widening the surface to the external environment. Figure 1 shows a scanning electron micrograph of the cryptal entrance exposed in cryofracture. The free surface formed furrows running along the edge of the cryptal entrance.

The cryptal epithelium consisted of flat and polygonal cells with many microridges on the surface, arranged in a cobblestone pattern. There were many infiltrating cells in the cryptal epithelial layer, but cell identification was difficult under SEM. Under transmission electron micrograph

Fig. 3. Scanning electron micrographs of the cryptal epithelial surface showing the three types of microcrypts. A) Type I at a cellular junction of the cryptal epithelium and a round cell with microvilli in the microcrypt. (x 8,330) B) Type II is a micropore opening near the center of a squamous epithelial cell and a round cell with microvilli in the microcrypt. (x 7,500) C) A smooth round cell in type II microcrypt. (x 8,300) D) Type II microcrypt opening near the center of a squamous epithelial cell. (x 10,000) E) Low power view of a type III opening in the crypt. (x 700) F) High power view of picture E (rectangle), showing a ciliated cell and nonciliated cells with microvilli. (x 4,800)

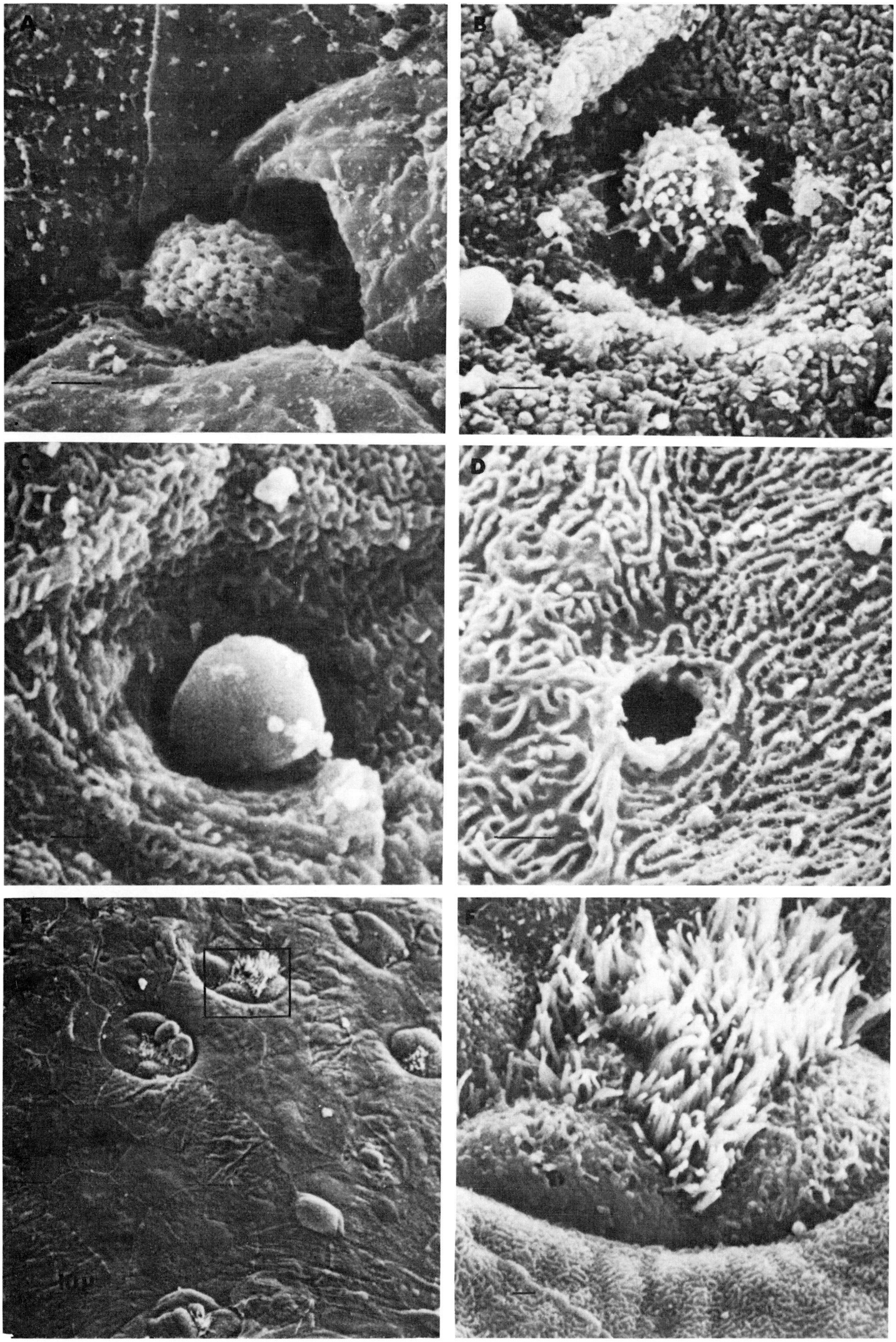
A
B
C
D
E
F
10 µ

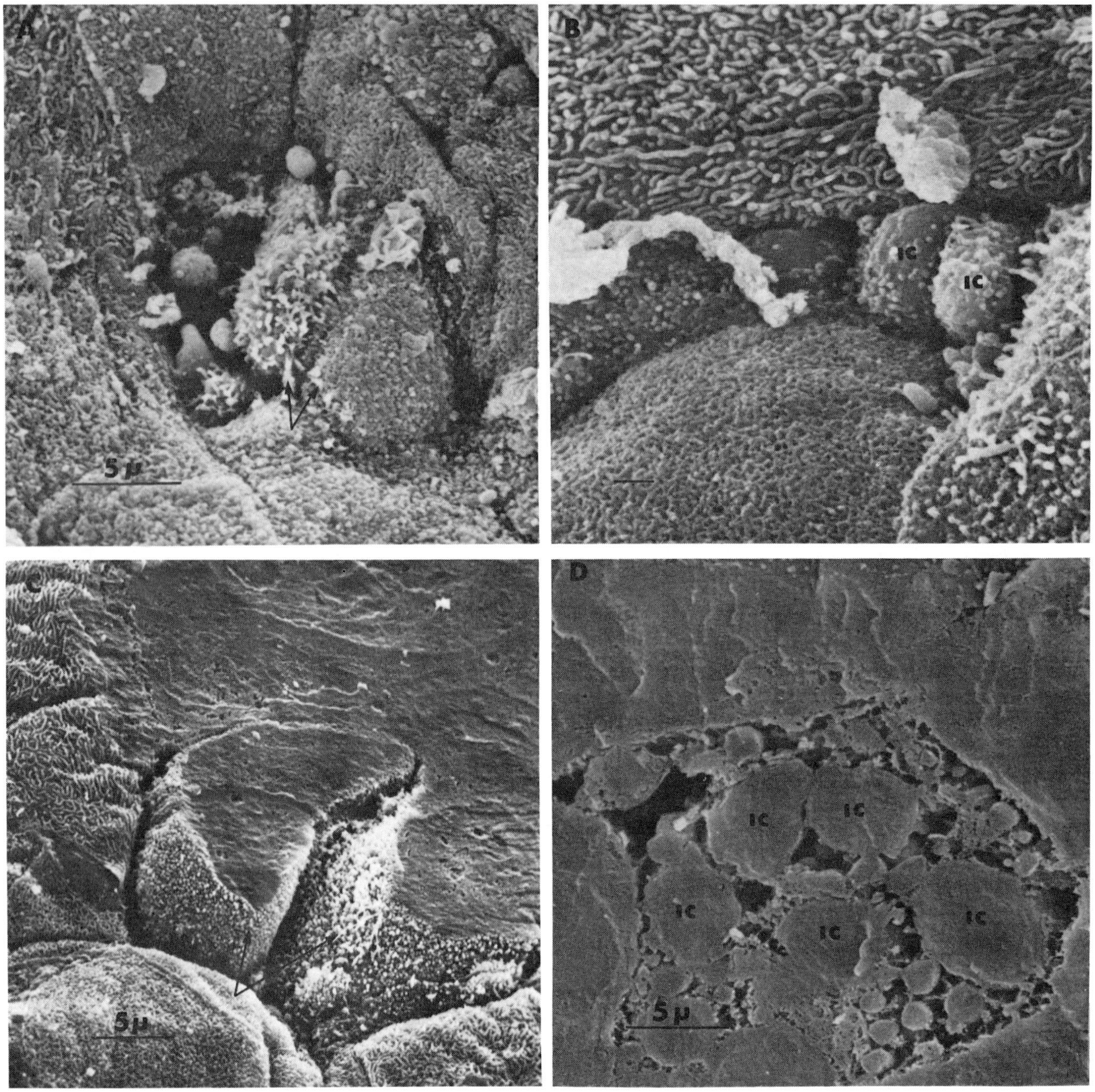

Fig. 4. Scanning electron micrographs showing the varying functional stages of type III microcrypt. A) Type III microcrypt appears after degeneration of a specialized epithelial cell (arrow). (x 3,200) B) Some infiltrating cells (IC) projecting through the space between a specialized epithelial cell and adjacent cryptal epithelial cell. (x 5,630) C) Fractured surface of specialized epithelial cells with microvilli (arrow) and adjacent cryptal epithelial cells. Note the loose intercellular junction. (x 2,500) D) Clusters of infiltrating cells (IC) just beneath the specialized epithelial cells. (x 3,000)

(TEM), these cells are granulocytes, lymphocytes, plasma cells and macrophages (Fig. 2).

On the surfaces of the cryptal epithelia, small pores 1-50 μm in diameter were observed. The shape and size of the micropores varied. The reason for using the term microcrypts will be stated in the Discussion. These microcrypts were classified into three types. Type I microcrypt is usually 5-15 μm in diameter, and opens tunnel-like passages between epithelial cell junctions (Fig. 3A). Round cells with microvilli, perhaps wandering cells, are often seen in the microcrypt. Type I microcrypt is the most common type of microcrypt. Type II microcrypt is 1-6 μm in diameter and opens near the center of a cryptal epithelial cell (Fig. 3B-D). In the microcrypt, two kinds of round cells were often seen. One is a round cell with villous surface (Fig. 3B), and the other with smooth surface (Fig. 3C). Figure 3D shows a micropore of type II opening near the center of a squamous epithelial cell. Type III microcrypt is between ordinary epithelial cells with microridges and "plugging" epithelial cells which are usually respiratory type cells (Fig. 3E, F). When a plugging cell falls off, a pore appears (Fig. 4A). The plugging cells were termed "specialized" epithelial cells, since they are interspersed as different type epithelial cells among the ordinary epithelial cells of

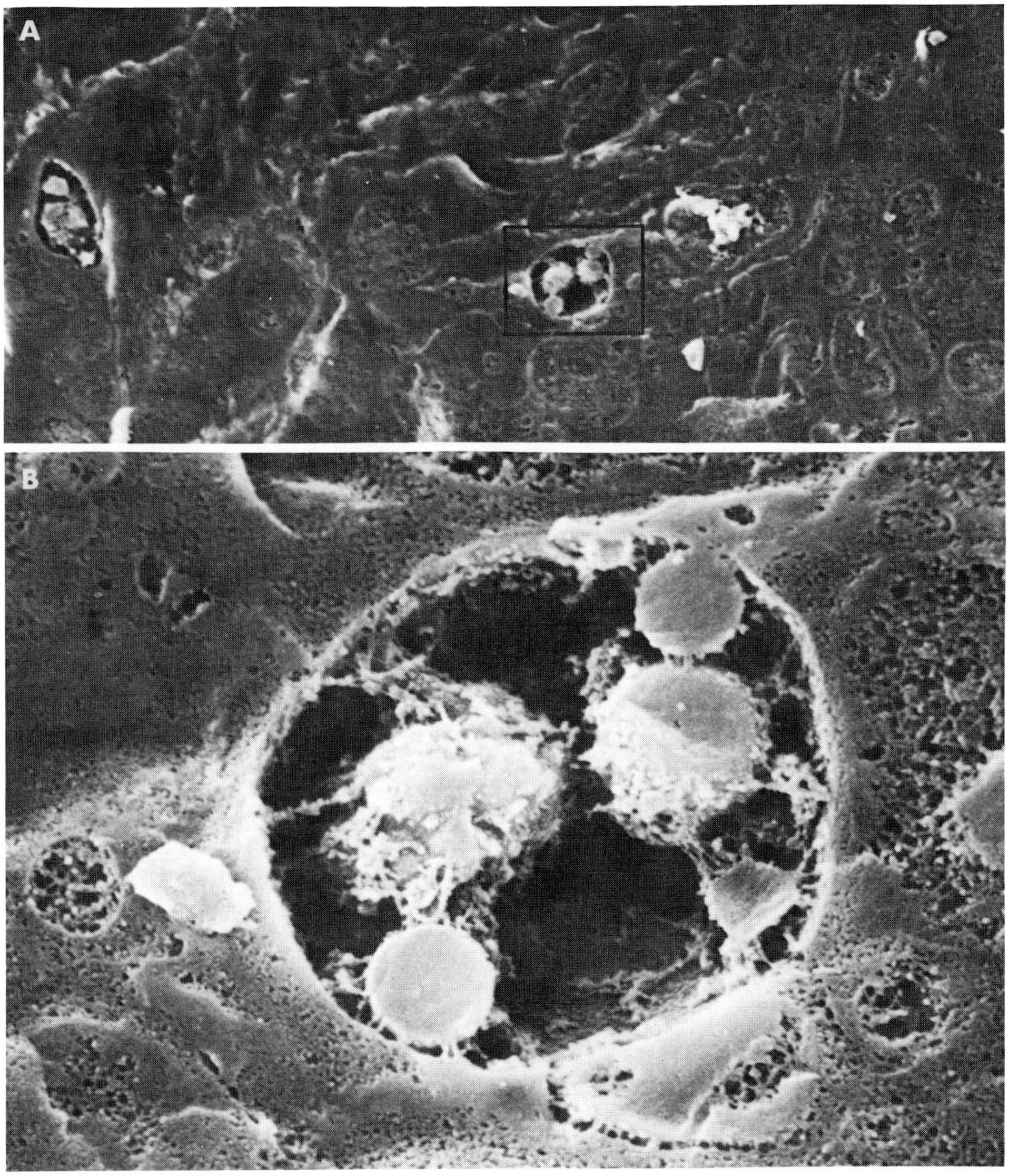

Fig. 5. SEM view of a vertically fractured face of the cryptal epithelium showing a mode of epithelial passage of lymphoid cells in the lower boundary zone. A) Low power view. (x 2,100) B) High power view of box in A. (x 14,000)

palatine tonsils. The size of the type III microcrypts was larger than that of the other two. Figure 4B shows some round cells with smooth or villous surface protruding to the cryptal lumen from the epithelial tunnel-like passage between the specialized epithelial cells and squamous epithelial cells surrounding the microcrypt. Figure 4C shows a cryofractured surface of the specialized epithelial cells with microvilli. A cluster of lymphoid cells is seen under the specialized cells (Fig. 4D). In the lower zone of the crypt epithelial layer, the epithelial tunnel-like passages are present with infiltrating lymphoid cells (Fig. 5). The wall of these tunnel-like passages consisted of squamous type epithelial cells.

Blood Vessels of the Cryptal Epithelium of Palatine Tonsil. Two kinds of blood vessel were seen under TEM. One was a sinusoidal blood vessel. Figure 6 shows a cluster of plasma cells in contact with the wall of a sinusoidal vessel in the cryptal epithelial, subepithelial and interfollicular areas. Many plasma cells close to the vessel wall contained dilated cisternae of rough endoplasmic reticulum with much homogenous substance. An electron-dense substance was seen in the intercellular spaces between the endothelial cells and basal lamina. Immunofluorescent technique reveals many immunoglobulin (usually IgG and IgA)-containing cells in the crypt epithelium, accumulating around sinusoidal vessels (Fig. 7).

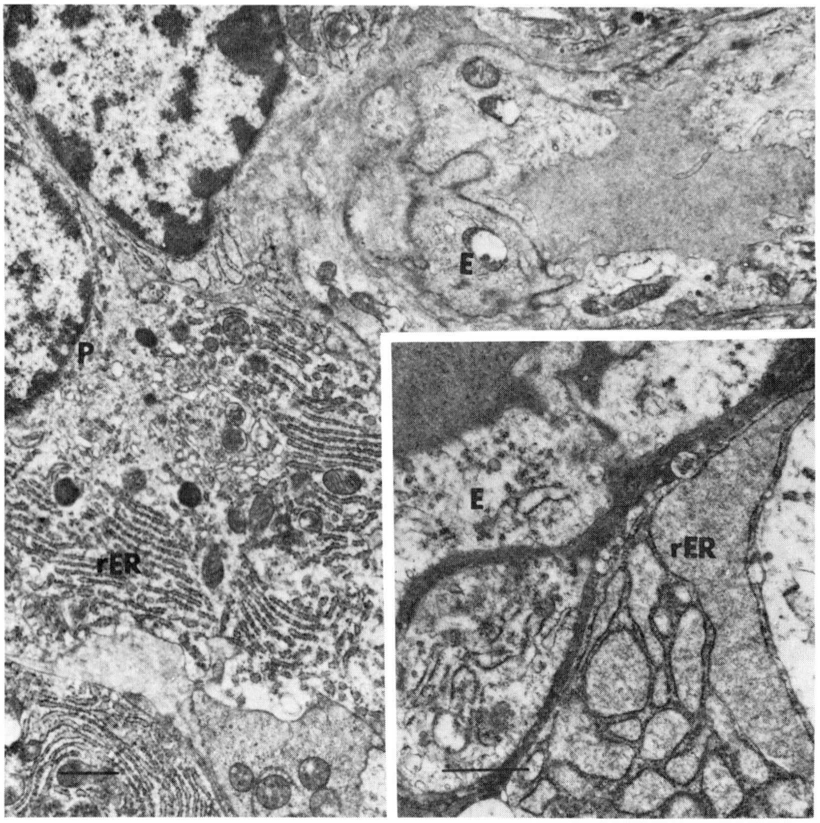

Fig. 6. TEM photograph showing plasma cells in contact with a small venule wall in the lower boundary zone of the cryptal epithelium. (x 8,600) Insert) A plasma cell in contact with basal lamina. (x 13,200) P - Plasma cell; E - Endothelium; rER -Rough endoplasmic reticulum.

The other type of vessel was the postcapillary venule which was often located in the lower boundary zone of the epithelium and interfollicular zone. This venule was characterized by high endothelial cells and migrating small lymphocytes. Figure 8 shows a migrating hourglass-shaped lymphocyte between endothelial cells of the postcapillary venule.

DISCUSSION

Lenz[11] in 1971 first reported the existence of micropores on the cryptal epithelium of human palatine tonsils and used the term "ultrakrypte." Kodama and Hoshino,[8] Mogi and Maeda[9,12] and Kawabata[10] then demonstrated micropores on human tonsillar crypts. Kawabata used the term "crypt epithelial micropore" and a 2-type classification. His type I pore was deep on the enlarged intercellular area in the cryptal epithelium. Kawabata suggested that his type I pore served as an entrance for passage of wandering cells. His type II pore was round, 10-20 μm in diameter and relatively shallow. The function of the type II pore was unclear.

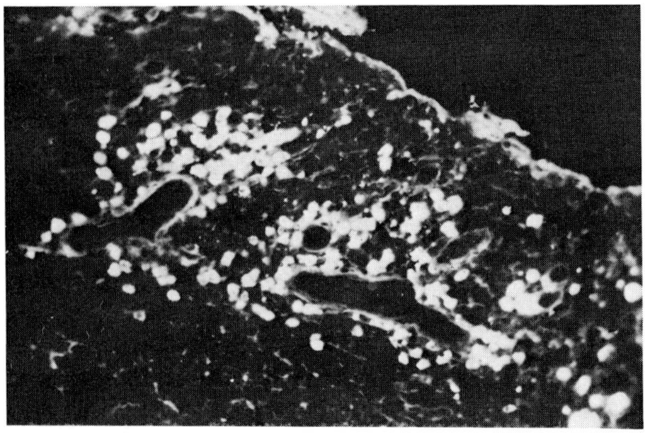

Fig. 7. IgA-containing cells in the lower boundary zone of cryptal epithelium, aggregated near the small venules. (x 260)

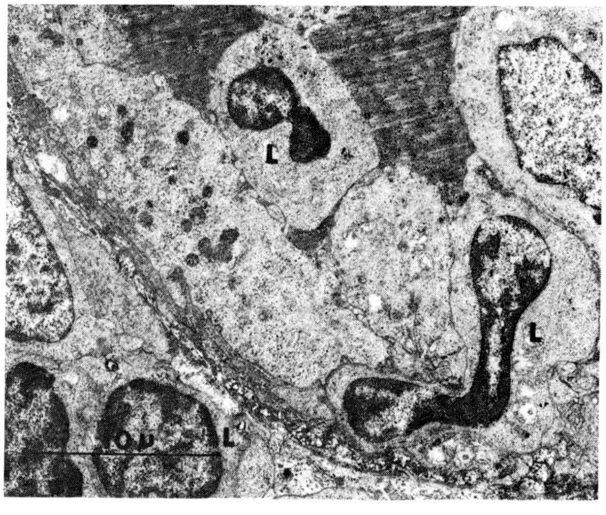

Fig. 8. TEM view of postcapillary venule immediately beneath the cryptal epithelium. Lymphocyte (L), shaped as an hourglass in the intercellular space of the endothelia, is migrating through the postcapillary venule wall to the parenchyma. (x 2,670)

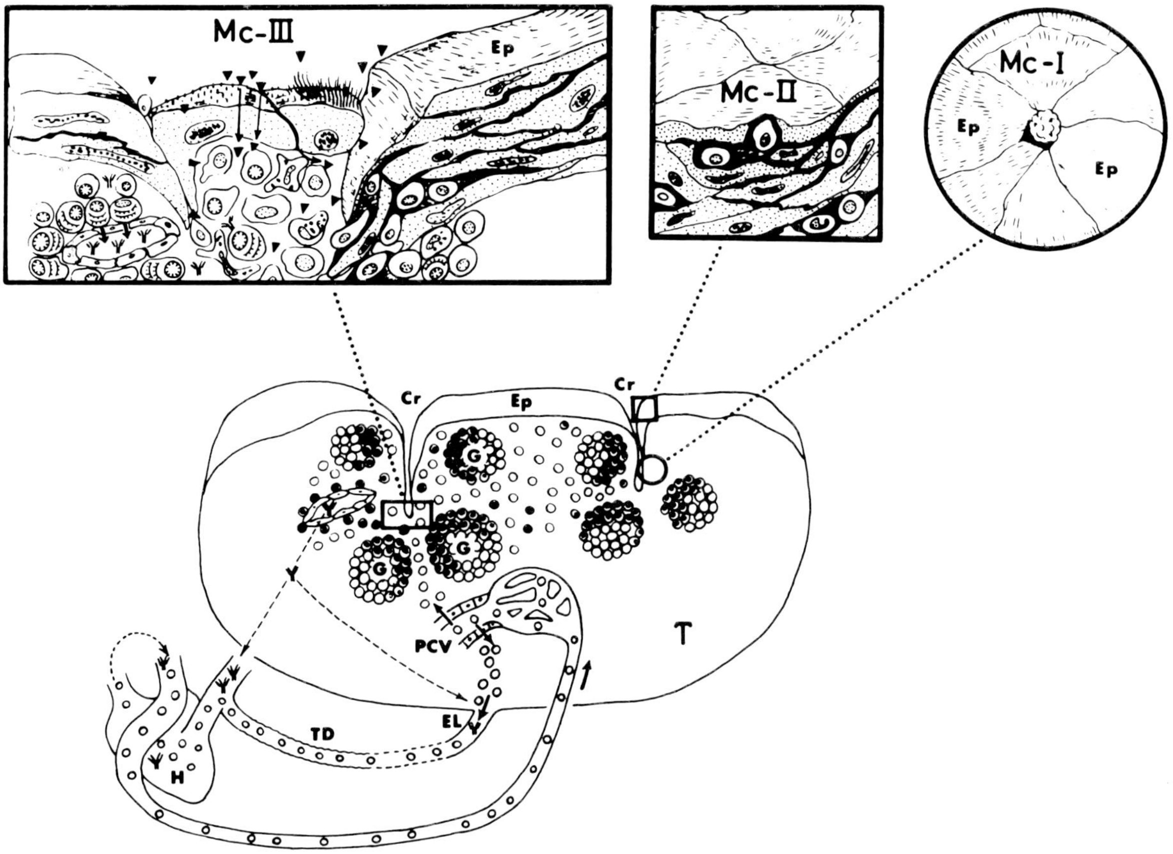

Fig. 9. Immune response of tonsil. Schematic illustrations of the microcrypts of the palatine tonsil. Type I microcrypt (Mc-I) opens at a junction of epithelial cells. Type II microcrypt (Mc-II) opens near the center of a flat epithelial cell. Type III microcrypt (Mc-III) usually opens between specialized epithelial cells and the adjacent ordinary cryptal epithelial cells of the tonsil. When these plugging cells fall off, a pore appears. Microcrypts are orifices of tunnel-like passages for wandering cells. Lower diagram shows circulating lymphoid cells from postcapillary venules and germinal centers. T - Tonsil; H - Heart; Cr - Crypt; Mc - Microcrypt; Ep - Epithelium; G - Germinal center; PCV - Postcapillary venule; EL - Efferent lymphatic; TD - Thoracic duct; ▼ - Antigen; Y - Antibody.

Our results indicate that microcrypts can be divided into three types. Figure 9 illustrates the three types of microcrypts. Type I microcrypt is a widened intercellular space between epithelial cells, continuing to a tunnel-like passage which penetrated deeply to the subepithelial area. The diameter of this type microcrypt was between 5-15 μm. The wall of the tunnel-like passage was composed of epithelial cells, and wandering cells were often found in the passages. Under TEM these wandering cells were seen to be lymphocytes, macrophages, granulocytes and plasma cells. Sometimes infiltrating cells protruded to the cryptal lumen from the microcrypt. Our type I microcrypt is probably the same as Kawabata's type I crypt epithelial micropore. Our findings support his suggestion that the pore is an orifice for intraepithelial passages of wandering cells. Our type II microcrypts, 1-6 μm in diameter, were found near the center of flat epithelial cells. These microcrypts are different from Kawabata's type II in their size and localization in the epithelia. Moreover, our study here revealed a few free cells with a villous surface and a smooth surface in type II microcrypts, although their incidence was rare. Type II microcrypts are probably also passages for free cells. Type III microcrypts were larger, and in the normal state plugged by a specialized epithelial cell with microvilli and cilia which differed from the ordinary squamous epithelial cells of the tonsil. Type III microcrypts appeared after the epithelial cells fell off. In inflamed tonsils the falling off was remarkable. These epithelial cells seemed to be ciliated or nonciliated cells with microvilli on the surface (Fig. 3 E, F). Our specialized epithelial cells are similar to the "crypt epithelial plug" of Kawabata,[13] "M-cell" of Owen and Jones[14] and Owen and Nemanic[15] and the "special epithel-cell" of Törö and Oláh.[16] Owen and Nemanic[15] reported that M-cells were commonly present in lymphoepithelial organs, such as Peyer patch, appendix and tonsil, and suggested that M-cells enhanced the trapping and uptake of antigenic and particular substances. Oláh et al[17] and Williams and Rowland,[18] using horseradish peroxidase or India ink as a tracer, demonstrated that M-cells transport antigens to lymphocytes through the tubulovesicular system. Our study did not investigate these aspects of specialized epithelial cells; however, as wandering cells were occasionally seen between the specialized cells and squamous epithelial cells surrounding the type III microcrypt, this microcrypt probably is an opening for a passage that induces wandering cells.

Although there are various types of microcrypts, we would consider all of them orifices with tunnel-like passages for wandering cells. As the walls of the passages are made of squamous epithelial cells, the passages are the terminal portions of the tonsillar crypt. Therefore, we called these micropores microcrypts. Microcrypts are usually found on the cryptal epithelium, which forms a network of intercellular spaces called the reticular area. This area is accorded to the epithelium covering the cap zone of the lymph follicles. Lymph follicles appear upon exogenous antigenic stimulation. Such secondary follicles are formed after antigenic stimulation. Microcrypts have not been observed in fetal tonsils. Kodama and Hoshino[8] suggested that lymphoid cells approach the cryptal lumens from the lymphoid tissue directly through these microcryptal tunnels. Although we did not observe direct connections between microcrypts and lymphoid tissues, particularly in the cap zone, it appears reasonable to assume that lymphoid cells, as well as other wandering cells in the microcrypts, are from the subepithelial lymphoid tissue.

The present investigation found postcapillary venules in the interfollicular zone and lower boundary zone of the cryptal epithelium. The postcapillary venules are characterized by high endothelial cells, and occasionally small lymphocytes migrated between the endothelial cells (Fig. 8). Since the postcapillary venule is a route for lymphoid cells to move from general circulation to the lymphoid organs,[19] our finding suggests that some lymphocytes in microcrypts are derived from the general circulation.

It was also noted that many mature plasma cells with dilated cisternae of rough endoplasmic reticulum with homogenous substance were attached to the walls of the sinusoidal vessels in the lower boundary region of the cryptal epithelia (Fig. 6). This suggests that plasma cells secreted substances into the sinusoidal lumen. Our fluorescent investigation showed accumulations of IgG-containing and IgA-containing cells around sinusoidal vessels. The antibodies produced in the cryptal epithelia of the palatine tonsils may contribute to systemic humoral immunity.

The exact role of the microcrypts is still not determined. Moreover, the difference in function between these three microcrypts remains unclear, even though morphologically they differ from each other. However, since the present study showed that all of the microcrypts are orifices, which open to cryptal lumens, with tunnel-like passages for wandering cells, it would be assumed that lymphocytes (or macrophages), which come from the subepithelial lymphoid tissue or general circulation via postcapillary venules, contact exogenous antigens in the crypt and that after the antigen-trapping the lymphocytes go back to the subepithelial tissue or general circulation or lodge in the intraepithelial layer. However, the going back of the lymphocytes is yet to be proven. The palatine tonsil positively receives exogenous antigens and contributes to the development of systemic immunity rather than protects the host mechanically against foreign invasions.[9] The microcrypts are beneficial to this function of the tonsil.

REFERENCES

1. Surján L, Surján L Jr, Surján M. Further investigations into the immunological role of tonsils. Acta Otolaryngol (Stockh) 1972; 73: 222-6.

2. Ishikawa T, Wicher K, Arbesman CE. Distribution of immunoglobulins in palatine and pharyngeal tonsils. Int Arch Allergy 1972; 43:801-12.

3. Mogi G. Secretory immunoglobulin A in oral and respiratory passages in man. Ann Otol Rhinol Laryngol 1975; 84 Suppl 20:1-23.

4. Morag A, Morag B, Bernstein JM, et al. In vitro correlates of cell-mediated immunity in human tonsils after natural or induced rubella virus infection. J Infect Dis 1975; 131:409-16.

5. Schmedtje JF, Batts AF. Immunoglobulins and blood vessels in the tonsillar crypt epithelium. Ann Otol Rhinol Laryngol 1973; 82:359-69.

6. Mogi G. IgA immunocytes in tonsils. Acta Otolaryngol (Stockh) 1977; 83:505-13.

7. Williams RL, Gibbons RJ. Inhibition of bacterial adherence by secretory immunoglobulin A. A mechanism of antigen disposal. Science 1972; 177:697-9.

8. Kodama A, Hoshino T. Scanning electron microscopic study of human tonsillar crypt. Practica Otologica (Kyoto) 1977; 70:479-86.

9. Mogi G, Maeda S. The function of tonsillar crypts. J Tonsil Jpn 1978; 17:221-311.

10. Kawabata I. Scanning electron microscopic observations of the crypt epithelium of the human tonsil. J Tonsil Jpn 1979; 18:17-8.

11. Lenz H. Rater-elektronenmikroskopische Beobachtungen an den menschlichen Tonsillen. Arch Klin Exp Ohren-Nasen Kehlkopfheilkd 1971; 199:599-604.

12. Maeda S, Mogi G. Ultrastructure of human tonsillar crypts. II. Chronic tonsillitis. J Tonsil Jpn 1979; 18:28-36.

13. Kawabata I. The surface structure of human tonsillar crypt. Scanning electron microscopic observation. J Tonsil Jpn 1978; 17:204-10.

14. Owen LR, Jones AL. Epithelial cell specialization within human Peyer's patches: An ultrastructural study of intestinal lymphoid follicles. Gastroenterology 1974; 66:189-203.

15. Owen LR, Nemanic P. Antigen processing structures of the mammalian intestinal tract: an SEM study of lymphoepithelial organs. IITRI/SEM/1978, Chicago, 367-78.

16. Törö I, Oláh I. Elekronenmikroskopische Structur und Antigenrezeption in der Garmenmandel des Kaninchens. Verh Anat Ges 1971; 66:109-19.

17. Oláh I, Surján L Jr, Törö I. Electronmicroscopic observations on the antigen reception in the tonsillar tissue. Acta Biol Acad Sci Hung 1972; 23:61-73.

18. Williams DM, Rowland AC. The palatine tonsils of the pig — an afferent route to lymphoid tissue. J Anat 1972; 113:131-7.

19. Gowans JL, Knight EJ. The route of recirculation of lymphocytes in the rat. Proc R Soc Biol (London) 1964; 159:257-82.

ENDOTRACHEAL ARTIFICIAL LARYNX

Vijay S. Dayal, MB, FRCS(C)

Michael L. G. Joy, PhD, PEng

Richard E. Moon, MD, FRCP(C)

Alex Lo, BASc

Anthony Jares

From the Departments of Otolaryngology, University of Toronto and Toronto General Hospital, and the Institute of Biomedical Engineering, University of Toronto. Supported by Grants PR 386 from the Ontario Ministry of Health, Charlie Conacher Research Fund, Ontario Cancer Treatment and Research Foundation Grant 451, MRC Operating Grant and NSERC Operating Grant A8006.

ENDOTRACHEAL ARTIFICIAL LARYNX

An endotracheal artificial larynx, capable of performing basic laryngeal functions, has been developed. Placed in laryngectomized dogs, in whom a large tracheopharyngeal fistula has been created, it is effective in acting as a laryngeal sphincter, thereby preventing aspiration. It provides an adequate and satisfactory normal airway. In laboratory bench studies it is shown to be capable of producing sound. Tissue studies show no untoward reaction from its long-term use in dogs.

CONTENTS

Rationale and Surgical Technique for the Endotracheal Artificial Larynx. V. S. Dayal, MB, FRCS(C); M. L. G. Joy, PhD, PEng 7

Design of the Endotracheal Artificial Larynx. M. L. G. Joy, PhD, PEng; R. E. Moon, MD, FRCP(C); V. S. Dayal, MB, FRCS(C) 11

Actuation of the Endotracheal Artificial Larynx. M. L. G. Joy, PhD, PEng; A. Lo, BASc; V. S. Dayal, MB, FRCS(C); A. Jares 18

Evaluation of the Endotracheal Artificial Larynx. R. E. Moon, MD, FRCP(C); V. S. Dayal, MB, FRCS(C); M. L. G. Joy, PhD, PEng 21

Considerations in the Design of an Airflow-Activated Sound Source for an Endotracheal Artificial Larynx. R. E. Moon, MD, FRCP(C); V. S. Dayal, MB, FRCS(C); M. L. G. Joy, PhD, PEng 26

RATIONALE AND SURGICAL TECHNIQUE FOR THE ENDOTRACHEAL ARTIFICIAL LARYNX

VIJAY S. DAYAL, MB, FRCS(C)

MICHAEL L. G. JOY, PhD, PEng

The incidence of laryngeal cancer has been estimated at 1 per 100,000 population.[1] Laryngeal cancer is treated by surgery, radiation or a combination of both. Many of those undergoing laryngectomy will have satisfactory vocal rehabilitation.

Esophageal speech is poor at best in comparison to natural human speech. Vocal rhythm is inferior because of the necessarily small air reservoir. Consonants cannot be enunciated well because an unvocalized airstream cannot be produced. The technique, furthermore, is often difficult or impossible to learn for a given patient. Approximately one third of patients in all cannot learn the technique.[2,3] Fistula speech has superior vocal rhythm, but voice quality is generally poor as in esophageal speech.[4] This is a result of the unphysiologic nature of the vibrator, which may be the cricopharyngeal muscle, the base of the tongue, or the hypopharyngeal soft tissue. Many patients suffer from salivary leakage, and the necessary surgery often cannot be performed because of prior irradiation.[5] External electrolarynxes may be used with little training; however, they require the use of one hand, are cosmetically poor, and the resulting speech they produce is inferior to other modes of artificial voice production.[2,6,7]

Our aim is to replace the surgically removed larynx with a device to be situated in the position of the original larynx and that can reproduce most of the functions of the original organ: low resistance to airflow, voice, cough, and the prevention of aspiration. Figures 1 and 2 show the intended position of the device in humans. The surgery includes the creation of a large diameter fistula between the trachea and the pharynx using the rigidity of the upper tracheal rings to maintain patency. The device will be easily inserted and removed through a conventional tracheostomy situated below the level of the anastomosis. This article describes the surgical results obtained from experimental canine preparations. The design, evaluation, and power pack for the artificial larynx will be discussed in the following article.

PRINCIPLES

The present approach is based on the fistula method; ie, a large tracheoesophageal fistula following removal of the larynx. An electromechanically activated laryngeal device (US Patent 4274162) has been developed (described in detail in this supplement; a brief preliminary report has been published[8]) which in dogs effectively prevents aspiration into the trachea.

Our approach is based on simple and well-known physiological facts. It is known that during the second phase of swallowing the tongue moves up and the laryngeal glottis closes to prevent aspiration of food in the tracheobronchial tree. Other activities such as the elevation of the larynx and movements of the epiglottis and the aryepiglottic fold also help in preventing aspiration, but the critical and essential movements are the movement of the vocal cords and the closure of the glottis.

Our device performs this function by actively blocking the passage to the trachea when it detects that a swallow has occurred. A number of events occur during this second phase of swallowing, eg, muscle movement in the tongue, movement of the hyoid bone, and increase in pharyngeal pressure. Any of these can be detected and used to trigger closure of a laryngeal device (sitting on top of a tracheopharyngeal fistula) and thereby prevent aspiration. We have considered several detection techniques. Muscle contraction in the tongue during the second phase of swallowing generates motor unit potentials that can be detected and used to trigger closure of the laryngeal device.

Likewise, movement of the hyoid bone (as it rises during swallowing) can be detected by an electromagnet attached to it, and this displacement can also be used to trigger closure of a laryngeal device. We have experimented with both of these methods of detection but have chosen the following, more direct, method instead. We use a pressure transducer as the trigger for closure. It is placed so the leading edge of the food bolus hits it and enables the closure of the device. Details are described in the following article.

Different theories ascribe to the vocal cords both an active and a passive role in voice production. It is clinically known that in patients with paralyzed vocal cords (positioned in the midline) the voice is

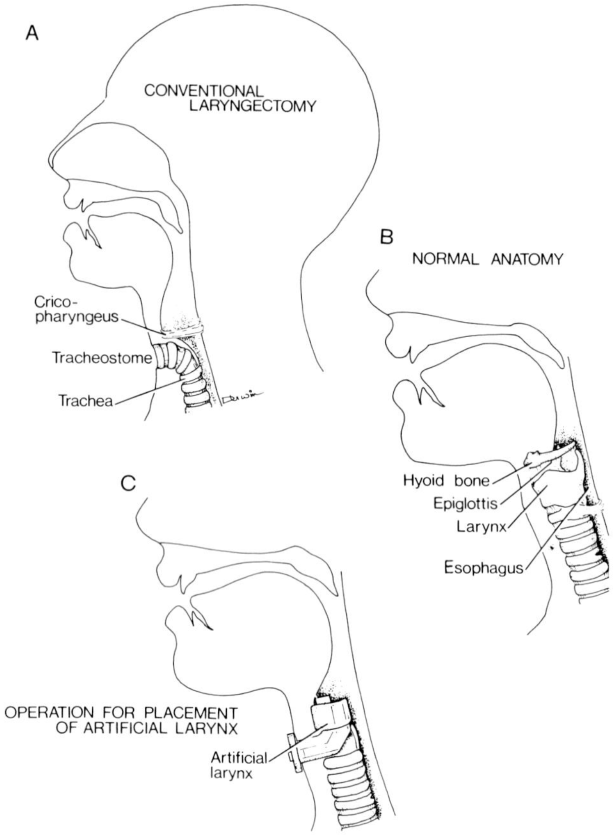

Fig. 1. A-C) Intended position of artificial larynx.

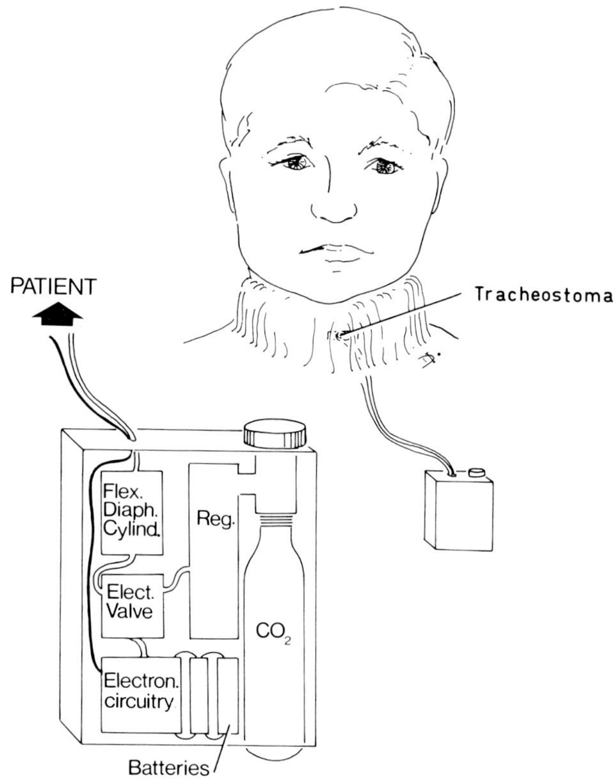

Fig. 2. Artificial larynx with power pack as planned for patient use.

almost unaffected. Based on this, passive vibrators have been used in this device for voice production (described in detail in the final article in this supplement.

Another important consideration in the development of this device has been that it should not be permanently in the tissues because of the rejection which commonly occurs with implants in this area. Therefore, a device that is removable, much like a tracheotomy tube, has been developed. In experimental animals the surgical procedure was designed with these facts in mind.

Because the device is active, close attention must be paid to the design of a portable power source for its activation. These matters are discussed in this supplement in the paper on actuation of the endotracheal artificial larynx. The article on evaluation of the endotracheal artificial larynx deals with the evaluation of the sphincter and respiratory functions of a prototype system, without the power of vocalization, in dogs. The final article in the series deals with the sound source. This article describes in detail the surgical results obtained from experimental canine preparations.

SURGICAL PROCEDURE

The experimental animals chosen were 20-kg mongrel dogs. These animals have similar anatomy to the human in the region of the larynx and pharynx; the tracheal size is similar to human size; furthermore, timing of swallowing motions is similar to that of the human.[9] Experimentation on acute preparations established the surgical anatomy and feasibility of the operation. The trachea was found to be mobile to the same degree as the human trachea and could be pulled cephalad 4 to 5 cm without undue tension.

Initially the surgical plan was to perform the procedure in two stages: the first stage to remove the larynx, repair the pharynx, and create a tracheostomy, with the opening in the anterior wall of the trachea three or four cartilaginous rings below the upper edge; the second stage to anastomose the upper end of the trachea to the anterior pharyngeal wall. Three dogs were operated on in this way. One died postoperatively after the first stage. In the other two dogs at the time of the second stage, performed two weeks after the initial operation, there was considerable fibrosis; some difficulty in mobilizing the trachea and moving it upward was encountered. To prevent aspiration after the second stage, a dummy larynx was inserted through the tracheostomy at the time of surgery. This device had the same shape as the artificial larynx, with the vertical lumen obliterated to prevent the passage of food, water, and saliva.

Breathing occurred via the horizontal limb of the device (see following article). Radiographic examination of the surgical area was performed eight

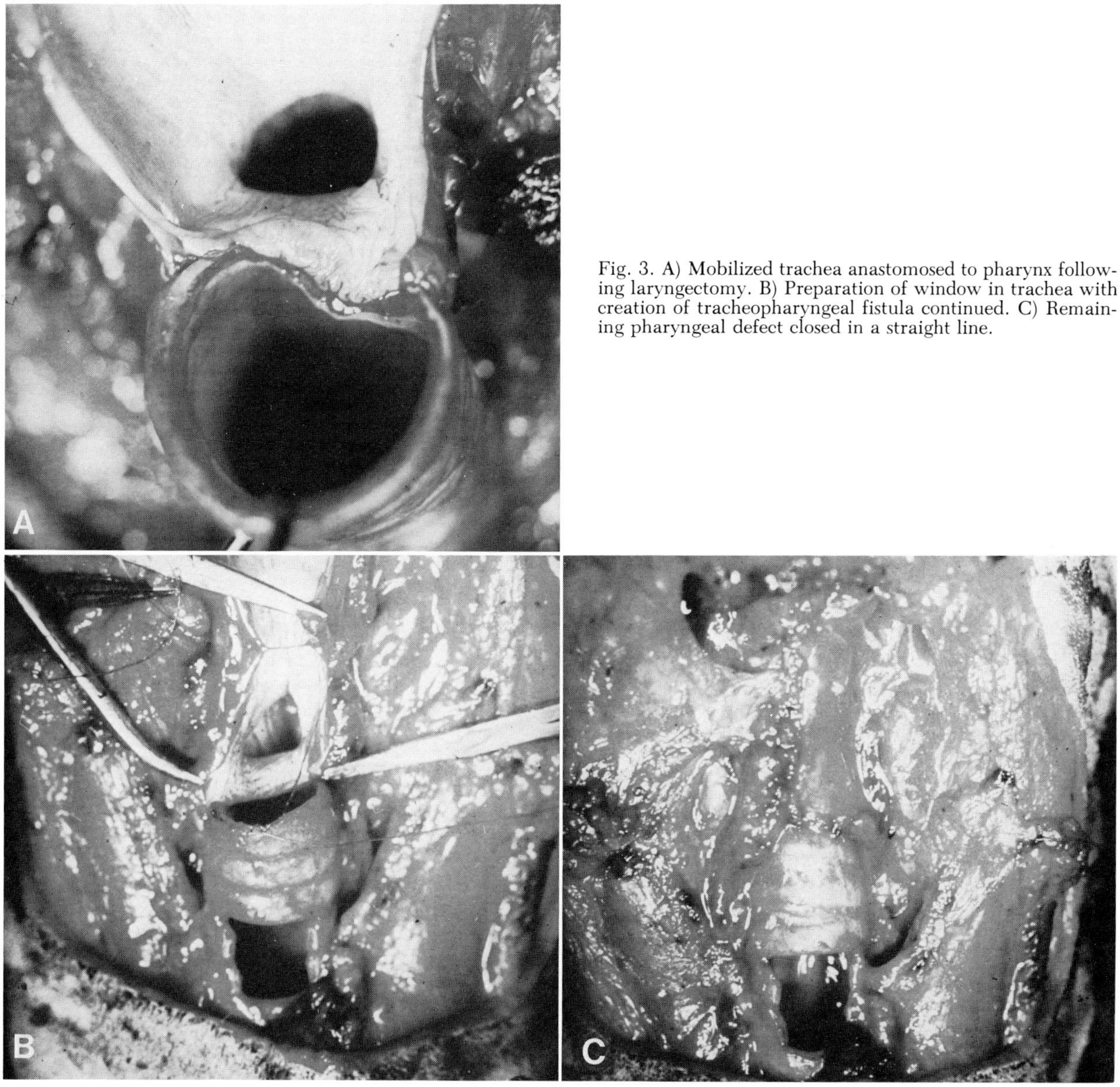

Fig. 3. A) Mobilized trachea anastomosed to pharynx following laryngectomy. B) Preparation of window in trachea with creation of tracheopharyngeal fistula continued. C) Remaining pharyngeal defect closed in a straight line.

and nine days after the second operation in the two animals. Healing appeared to be adequate, although the area of the anastomosis was somewhat narrowed. One dog died 22 days postoperatively of asphyxia caused by a mucus plug in its dummy larynx. At postmortem examination there was marked narrowing of the anastomosis. The surgical area of the remaining dog was examined with a rigid bronchoscope 21 days postoperatively. The fistula between the trachea and pharynx was 2 to 3 mm in diameter. By 61 days postoperatively the fistula had narrowed to such an extent that the dog could not breathe through it when its tracheostomy was plugged. The fistula could not be demonstrated radiographically with contrast material, and on day 72 the dog was sacrificed. Narrow probe patency was demonstrated.

Because of this experience a decision was made to attempt the entire procedure in one operation. After performing a conventional laryngectomy the trachea was mobilized and anastomosed to the pharynx using chromic gut suture, taking particular care that the sutures did not penetrate the mucosa (Fig. 3A).

A window was then cut into the anterior portion of the trachea for the tracheostomy (Fig. 3B). Three tracheal rings were left intact between the window and the anastomosis; the window was two tracheal rings long. The remaining line pharyngeal defect was closed in a line anterior to the anastomosis (Fig. 3C). A Penrose drain was left in for four days. Procaine penicillin was administered intramuscularly for seven days postoperatively. To allow eating without aspiration, dummy valves that had been gas-autoclaved were inserted after the operation. Seven dogs were operated on in this way. Of the first four, one survived for 112 days and was used for multiple evaluations. The fistula remained widely patent until the dog died of asphyxia secondary to mucus plugging. Autopsy showed a perfectly satisfactory anastomosis with only mild narrowing, which was acceptable for the purpose of inserting the artificial larynx. Three of the first four died within a week of surgery. All had breakdown of suture lines in the pharynx and two had associated purulent infection of their wounds. Once these complications had occurred in the dogs, it was difficult to maintain hydration and nutrition, and the dogs had to be sacrificed.

With this in mind, a nasogastric tube was inserted into the fifth animal at the time of surgery and sutured in place at the nose. This allowed food and water to be given without the dog having to swallow. This dog died 11 days postoperatively of mucus plugging of its dummy. Autopsy showed dehiscence of the anterior half of the pharyngeal anastomosis, as well as of the pharyngeal closure.

As a result of this early experience, it was felt that the immediate placement of a dummy larynx into the trachea, with its cuff pressing on the suture line, may have impeded healing and caused early dehiscence of the anastomosis. The next two dogs operated on had Portex tracheostomy tubes inserted downward into their tracheas at the time of surgery. The placement of dummy larynges was delayed until 14 days postoperatively. Each dog turned out to be a long-term survivor, one dying 79 days postoperatively, the other at 386 days, both dogs dying of asphyxia secondary to mucus plugging. Autopsy performed on these animals revealed an intact anastomosis with minimal inflammation of the tracheal mucosa adjacent to the pneumatic cuff of the artificial larynx.

The majority of the problems we encountered in the experimental preparations were related to the difficulty of nursing uncooperative dogs. Maintenance of hydration with intravenous fluid was virtually impossible during the early postoperative period, and it was necessary to feed these dogs with both food and liquid through nasogastric tubes. On occasion these tubes were pulled out by the dogs, and it was difficult to reinsert them without some degree of trauma to the surgical area. To reduce drying of mucus a humidifier was kept running in the rooms housing the dogs. All but one of our long-term survivors died of mucus plugging of their tracheostomies; the last one was sacrificed one year and ten months postoperatively for tissue studies. That animal cages are not continuously supervised for the 24 hours in the day, we believe, was the main reason for accumulation of dry mucus and mucus plugging. In humans this would not be a problem; early mucus plugging could be relieved by the patients after temporarily removing the device.

CONCLUSION

A satisfactory surgical technique has been devised to create the necessary anatomic relationships for the insertion of an engineered endotracheal artificial larynx. We have gained experience with postoperative care. Satisfactory healing occurred in three out of four dogs fed via nasogastric tube for 14 days postoperatively, with conventional cuffed tracheostomy tube for airway protection. We anticipate using a similar regimen when similar surgery is performed on humans.

Autopsies performed on four dogs revealed that the tracheopharyngeal fistula remained wide open for prolonged periods after surgery. A fifth dog was sacrificed 22 months postoperatively for studies. It had a wide open fistula with no evidence of stenosis. Clearly the goal of maintaining a patent anastomosis has been achieved. Barium swallows, chest x-ray studies, and tissue examinations are discussed under the paper on evaluation of the endotracheal artificial larynx.

This surgical technique and device will be applied in a few carefully selected human subjects to determine its more general applicability. Interested and motivated patients will be selected from the following two groups: 1) patients who have had conventional laryngectomy but who have experienced unsatisfactory vocal rehabilitation, and 2) patients who require laryngectomy, either primarily or postirradiation, who would prefer to try the new operation. In either case, in the event of an unsatisfactory result, it would be relatively easy to close the tracheopharyngeal anastomosis. If, in the first group of patients undergoing the new procedure, the vocal result is superior to that generally achieved with esophageal voice, the indications for the new technique might be extemely wide.

DESIGN OF THE ENDOTRACHEAL ARTIFICIAL LARYNX

MICHAEL L. G. JOY, PhD, PEng
RICHARD E. MOON, MD, FRCP(C) VIJAY S. DAYAL, MB, FRCS(C)

INTRODUCTION

The previous article has discussed the fundamental design decisions for the electromechanical larynx. It is a removable active valve that can be inserted through a tracheostoma. It allows normal respiration but prevents aspiration by closing during a swallow. In this article we discuss design alternatives in greater detail. We then describe the devices we have evaluated in dogs. The next article discusses the power source used to close the valve.

The artificial larynx is shown in Figure 4. The device is L-shaped, consisting of a vertical limb containing the swallow detector, valve and cuff, and a horizontal limb to anchor the device and provide conduits for the tubing and wires. The horizontal limb also holds the reed mechanism and provides an emergency breathing route in case of blockage of the vertical section. Breathing normally occurs through the lumen of the vertical limb.

DESIGN ALTERNATIVES AND DECISIONS

VALVE MECHANISM

The valve itself may either close passively when food touches it (for example, a trapdoor design) or actively, when triggered by some event occurring near the beginning of swallowing. A passive valve has the advantage of simplicity, whereas an active valve may resist pressure from either direction and, therefore, enable cough and Valsalva maneuver. The latter is not essential, although certainly helpful during urination, defecation, and lifting extremely heavy weights. It has been reported, for example, that bladder pressure may drop by 20% if the larynx is rendered incompetent.[10] Both types of valve were considered and experimented with. Our final choice was to construct an active device. We felt its positive closure and the other benefits just mentioned justified the additional complexity of the device.

Constraints While Closing and Closed. First, the valve must be able to close quickly to prevent any aspiration of food or liquid into the trachea. From the onset of the involuntary stage of swallowing, when the hyoid bone and larynx elevate, until the food reaches the cricopharyngeal sphincter, about 1 to 2 seconds elapses.[11] The total time from triggering the valve to closing must certainly be less than this, although the exact constraint will depend on the means of detecting swallowing.

Second, the device should tend to expel, during closure, any material that may have begun to enter the valve. Sometimes closure may be slightly delayed for a number of reasons and a part of the bolus may enter the artificial larynx. Mucus and small amounts of food left behind after the swallow may also enter the device. One method of clearing these bits of debris is to provide a milking action when the valve closes.

Third, the valve must be able to withstand momentary increases in pressure up to 100 mmHg at the superior end and 120 mmHg from below. These are the peak pressures that have been measured in normal adults respectively in the pharynx[12] during swallowing and in the esophagus (approximately equal to subglottic pressure) during cough.[13]

Fourth, the valve should function so that closure would not be prevented by mucus buildup or small particles of food.

Fifth, the valve must be reliable. Adults swallow an average of 550 times per 24 hours, with a 95% confidence range of 491 to 680.[14] An average of 45 of these swallows occurred while asleep. If an artificial larynx is expected to last two months the valve might have to close and open 40,000 times. It must not miss more than one in several hundred swallows, otherwise the unfortunate patient will spend most of his day trying to remove aspirated material from his trachea.

Constraints While Opening and Open. First, the valve must offer low resistance to airflow. Measurements on the human larynx in vivo show that the pressure drop across it at a flow of 2000 ml/s is approximately 1 cm H_2O.[15] If a person breathes sinusoidally with a tidal volume of 500 ml at a rate of 12 breaths/min, his peak flow rate will be 314 ml/s; therefore, the valve must have a small pressure drop across it at that order of magnitude of airflow, otherwise the patient will find it uncomfortable to breathe. During cough the airflow may reach 5000 to 6000 ml/s with a pressure drop across the larynx of 80 to 100 mmHg.[15] These figures give approximate values to aim for in design.

Second, by the nature of its shape, the section of valve sticking above the pharyngeal junction must divert small amounts of saliva away from the opening. In normal humans the epiglottis does this by forcing liquids to dribble out each side into the

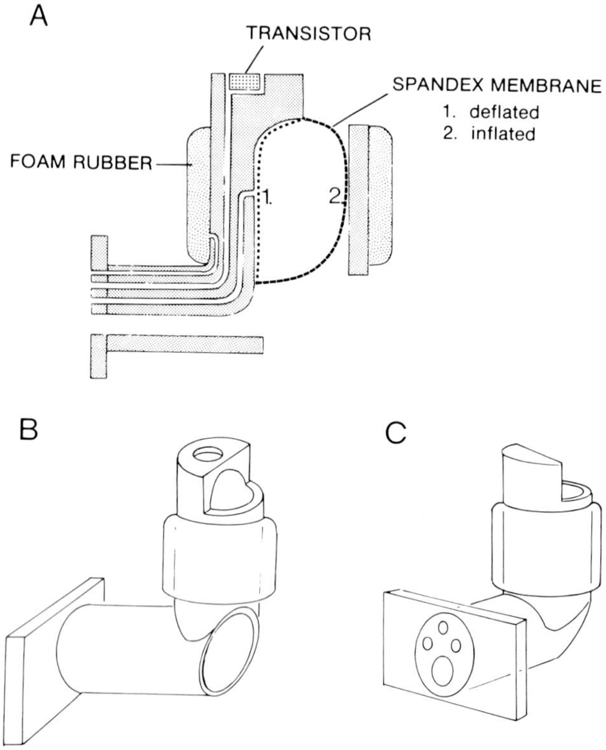

Fig. 4. Prototype endotracheal artificial larynx with valve mechanism. A) Central section. B, C) Views from back and front of device. (Reed used for voice production not shown.)

pyriform fossae. Following laryngectomy there is no epiglottis, and the shape of the pharyngeal floor is likely to be smooth, allowing saliva to roll down the posterior surface of the tongue directly into the valve. These small amounts of liquid might not be detected by any swallow detection system.

Third, the valve should be able to open quickly to allow a large airflow during cough. It is difficult to predict exactly what "quickly" means in this context. However, qualitatively it means that when the valve opens to permit cough it must do so to allow a sufficiently high linear velocity of air to develop to clear the trachea and artificial larynx of debris before the volume of air in the lungs is depleted.

SWALLOW DETECTION

Detection of swallowing other than by the direct physical force of flow is necessary only for an active valve. Many events occur during swallowing that might be transduced, and a discussion of some feasible methods is given below. The possibility of using some voluntary manipulation by the patient, such as a particular movement of the tongue, is not ruled out. For safety and for the convenience of being able to test the device on animals we chose an involuntary method for the initial implementation.

Myoelectric Potentials. These are the electrical potentials developed during the contraction of muscle motor units. They may be transduced either from electrodes in the muscle or from surface electrodes. A wealth of literature exists on the electrical activity of various muscles during swallowing in experimental animals.[9] It appears that electrical activity in the mylohyoid muscle just before elevation of the hyoid is the first electrical event in swallowing. This event occurs about one second before the food reaches the level of the larynx; thus it would be a useful signal to trigger the valve. However, there are considerable disadvantages to this method. Electrode implantation usually leads to infection, and surface electrodes inject considerable noise and unreliability. Implanted transmitters can circumvent both of these problems, but implants may become infected shortly after surgery, surrounding tissue reaction may eventually change the electrical contact resistance, and, of course, power supplies must periodically be replenished.

Mechanical Force Developed by Muscle Contraction. An implantable pressure transducer could be placed inside a suitable muscle (for example, digastric or geniohyoid) which is of sufficient size for implantation of a probe and contract early in swallowing. All of the disadvantages of implants listed in the previous section apply. A pressure transducer might also be placed in the pharynx and positioned so it can be caused to impinge on surrounding tissue when a swallow occurs. This motion might be voluntary or possibly caused by secondary motion of the walls of the pharynx caused by the act of swallowing; ie, the approach of the food bolus or contraction of the tongue muscles. The disadvantage of this approach is there is no way to predict what the appropriate position might be for the transducer in each individual. Also, if this positioning is critical it is not clear how it could be reliably achieved. These problems might be overcome with the aid of a cooperative patient but are insurmountable with dogs. Our final design does not rule out this triggering technique.

Motion of Surrounding Structures. The hyoid bone moves vertically upward at the onset of the second stage of swallowing. This motion can be detected by attaching a passive device such as a magnet to the bone during surgery and transducing its motion by means of an external detector. The first objection to this method is that removal of the hyoid bone is a standard feature of laryngectomy; surgeons feel its removal is necessary to facilitate evacuation of the pre-epiglottic space. Dayal et al[16] have shown, however, that the contents of the pre-epiglottic space may be satisfactorily separated from the hyoid with preservation of the latter. Other disadvantages include the conspicuousness and discomfort of the external detector; that the hyoid and detector may move relative to each other during head turning, stretching, and tongue movements; and all the disadvantages of implantation.

Intrapharyngeal Pressures. The increase in intrapharyngeal pressure that occurs during swallowing has been well documented.[12] However, after the proposed tracheopharyngostomy leaving the trachea open, it is difficult to predict what the increase in pressure might be, if any, because is would appear intuitively that any increase would be dissipated through the low impedance trachea into the lungs. This method, therefore, does not seem promising. It is not precluded in our final design, however.

Acoustic Signals. Inexpensive miniature microphones for hearing aids are available. It might be possible to transduce the intensity of sound at a particular frequency that might be characteristic of food moving through the upper pharynx. No data to our knowledge have been published on such a phenomenon. It would be difficult, however, to keep extraneous noise, such as laryngeal or other speech, from triggering such a sensor.

Impulse of Food. Our final choice was to place a pressure transducer at the pharyngeal entrance to the artificial larynx.[17] We anticipated that when the leading edge of a food bolus hits the transducer, the resulting pressure change could be detected and used as a trigger for closure. A lower estimate of the magnitude of this pressure change can be derived from the known velocity and density of the food bolus in the pharyngeal region. The velocity of the food bolus in humans can be estimated from the cineradiographic data of Ingervall and Lantz.[18] In the standing position the mean velocity of watery barium in the first 50 mm of travel beyond the mandibular contour was 416 mm/s, with a range of 278 to 833 mm/s.

Viscous barium was slower, with a mean velocity of 294 mm/s and a range of 227 to 500 mm/s. The predicted pressure range exerted on a transducer placed in the path of the food is 0.53 to 7.1 g/cm^2. This prediction assumes an inelastic collision. In practice with dogs we found that the signals we obtained were about 45 g/cm^2, considerably larger than those predicted here. This point is discussed in the fourth article in this supplement.

This pressure may be conveniently transduced by a number of simple devices. The ones considered were a compliant spring surrounding but not touching a center post (the pair acting as a sensitive contact switch); a pneumatic diaphragm comparator (for example, Johnson FON-201, 3-way valve, Wainbee Ltd, Rexdale, Ont) or moving iron miniature microphones (Knowles BI—1585 subminiature transducer, Knowles Electronics Inc, Franklin Park, Ill); a commercial microswitch; or a pressure-sensitive transistor (Pitran, Stow Laboratories Inc, Hudson, Mass).

Preliminary testing was done on all of these. The spring-center post contact switch is feasible but difficult to manufacture reproducibly with a continously adjustable threshold level. The pneumatic diaphragms commercially available were not reliable at low pressure. The miniature microphone was also feasible but not particularly sensitive to low frequencies; therefore, extremely high gain was required to detect the signals. Available microswitches were found to be too bulky and not sufficiently sensitive. Pressure-sensitive Pitran devices were our final choice for the transducer. Although quite temperature-sensitive, they can be compensated. They are very pressure-sensitive, small, and light. They are, however, also expensive, fragile, and without a "second source." Our next model will probably use a sensor based on a strain gauge transducer.

TRACHEAL SEAL

One obvious way to construct a seal is to surround the device with a pressurized cuff. The first constraint to consider is the pressure at which it is to be maintained. Endotracheal intubation with cuffed tubes has been followed by mucosal inflammation, ulceration, stenosis of the trachea and tracheoesophageal fistula.[19]

The major etiologic factor appears to be excessive pressure, and it has been suggested that occlusion of mucosal capillaries and the resulting ischemia initiates the process. Grillo et al[20] showed that tracheal damage could be minimized by keeping the intracuff pressure below 60 mmHg. This has been confirmed by the clinical experience of others (A. Scott, MD, personal communication). Tracheal capillary occlusion pressures have been measured in dogs by Galoob et al.[21] These investigators found that occlusion pressure depended on the size and position of the blood vessel in the trachea. The mean occlusion pressure for mucosal capillaries over the tip of a cartilaginous ring was 23 mmHg; over the lateral wall if a cartilaginous ring it was 38 mmHg. It would be reasonable, therefore, to attempt to keep the tracheal contact pressure below 23 mmHg.

It has been shown analytically that tracheal contact pressure is in fact less than cuff inflation pressure because of the stiffness of the inflated cuff.[22] The proportion of the cuff pressure transmitted to the trachea is a function of the fractional length of the cuff in contact with the wall. If this fractional length = 0.7, only about 30% of the cuff inflation pressure acts on the tracheal mucosa. Therefore, the allowable inflation pressure should be about 75 mmHg, depending on the fractional contact length. Maintaining the inflation pressure at a constant level may be accomplished by using a supply of compressed gas and a regulator. This would, of course, add weight and bulk. Furthermore, currently available miniature regulators are not stable enough for this purpose. Another solution is to fill the cuff with an isotropic springy material such as polyurethane foam. Such a technique has already been successfully implemented for endotracheal tube cuffs.[23]

The type of material is also critical. Tracheal damage produced by toxic materials has been reported.[24] A material must be chosen for the ease with which it can be shaped, and also for its biocompatibility. Criteria for choosing a material for vascular grafting were listed by Wilkes and Samuels.[25] Some of these apply to material used for the manufacture of tracheal cuffs. The material must not be physically modified by tissue fluids; must be chemically inert; must not excite inflammatory or foreign body response; must not be carcinogenic; must not produce allergy or hypersensitivity; must be capable of being sterilized; must be capable of withstanding the mechanical strains imposed on it inside the body; and must not lose its strength. Several materials fulfill these criteria. One other practical criterion is important: the elastomer must bond readily to the base material used for the structural components.

Segmented polyurethane (Spandex, Lycra T-126, DuPont Co, Montreal) in particular, is well suited. Tests for physical strength, flexion fatigue, abrasion resistance, and resistance to change when exposed to high temperatures have been reported.[26] Acute toxicity studies, 18-month implantation studies in dogs,[26] and 36-month implantation studies in dogs[27] have also been reported. The material does not elicit skin sensitivity when worn by people hypersensitive to other materials.

All results have shown so far that Spandex is a material of superior physical strength when compared with other elastomers. It fulfills all of the criteria for biocompatibility mentioned above. Furthermore, it bonds readily to polyvinyl chloride (PVC), a suitable material for making the structural components. It is quite easy to coat all exposed PVC surfaces of a prosthetic device with Spandex or silicone.

CONSTRUCTION

STRUCTURAL ELEMENTS

The structural elements, the horizontal and vertical limbs, and the faceplate are constructed with PVC. In the earlier models each piece was individually machined. Injection molding techniques have now been implemented to facilitate rapid manufacture. The horizontal limb and faceplate (Figs. 1 and 4) are molded in one piece. One large central hole is used to house the reed mechanism and provide an emergency breathing and suction port. Two smaller holes allow flow of gas to the valve and cuff balloons. A third hole contains wires that connect the transistor food-sensing unit with its circuitry.

The vertical limb holds the valve and cuff. At its lower end the vertical limb widens to form a shoulder to which the cuff is bonded during manufacture of the latter. At the upper end is a 50% overhang that houses the pressure-sensitive transistor (Pitran).[17] This overhang helps deflect food around the device away from its lumen. Dummy devices, used for the majority of feedings of experimental animals and to be used during sleep in human trials, contain a permanently plugged vertical limb. When a dummy is worn, breathing occurs via the horizontal limb. Airtight bonding is obtained by using Spandex as the glue. All conduits within the device are pneumatically isolated from each other.

CUFF

The cuff is manufactured from Spandex membrane. This is made by dipping a mold of appropriate shape into a solution (of syrup-like consistency) of Spandex in N, N-di-methylacetamide. The mold with a thin coating of the solution is then placed in an oven at about 50°C, allowing the solvent to evaporate. Additional coats may be added to produce a membrane of the desired thickness. The mold was designed so the PVC portion of the vertical could be inserted axially, allowing the Spandex to bond simultaneously to the shoulder.

The foam cuff fillers are made in toroidal shape from high quality polyurethane foam. Each piece is machined on a lathe after impregnation with hard wax. The wax is removed with heated halocarbon solvent such as tetrachloroethylene. The dimensions of the foam filler were found not to be critical. Reasonable cuff pressure and deformity characteristics were obtained when filler was approximately 30% larger in diameter and length than the outer margin of the membrane.

VALVE

The valve is a balloon made from Spandex. It has the form, when inflated, of a cylinder capped by a hemisphere at its upper end. When inflated it fills the lumen in the vertical limb, closing the valve. When deflated the balloon collapses against the wall of the lumen and the overhang at its upper end. An alternative type of valve was considered in which an electromagnetic actuator would be placed inside the larynx. This approach was abandoned when we were unable to develop a device that could provide the forces required without excessive heating.

To close the valve (unfold the balloon) the balloon is filled rapidly with gas from an external source. The unfolding action of the balloon during this phase helps eject any material that may stray into the device from above. The gas is removed to open the valve and a small negative pressure difference maintained to keep the balloon pressed tightly to the walls of its housing. Two potential sources of gas for inflating the balloon have been considered. In all devices built to date we have used compressed carbon dioxide as a source of power to drive a spring-loaded piston that caused air to inflate the balloon. We are currently considering replacing this with an external electrically driven piston. Such a design would be simpler and more efficient than our current power source.

SWALLOW DETECTOR ELECTRONICS

Pitran devices are available with linear ranges of ±3.5 g/cm², ±8.8 g/cm², ±17.6 g/cm² and higher. The overload pressure that might permanently change the device characteristics is five to seven times the linear pressure range. In the human pharynx with valve closed, the pressure may be expected to be as high as 140 g/cm².[12] Therefore, the ±17.6 g/cm² (PT-H2) devices were used. (Note: 1 psi = 70.3 g/cm² = 51.7 mmHg [Torr]). Manufacturer's specifications indicate that one may expect a 20% change in βDC over the entire linear range of this device (2 x 17.6 g/cm² in our case). The rise time of the device is specified as 10 μs, much faster than we will require. Temperature variation of the transducer is probably reduced by the thermal buffering of the structural components and surrounding tissues; however, upper and lower bounds of the temperature range are the temperatures of the hottest (say 45 to 50°C) and coldest (0°C) liquid that can comfortably be swallowed.

The uncompensated thermal stability of a Pitran is very poor. The manufacturer's specifications suggest 7% of linear range per degree Centigrade. We designed two detector circuits, described in the following sections. Simple circuits have been designed by the manufacturer to compensate for temperature effects by removing the dc component of the signal. Compensation is based on the assumption that pressure changes of interest are fast while temperature changes are slow. This method of compensation leads to three difficulties. First, calibration of the device is made quite difficult. Second, drop in the output pulse might lead to errors during a prolonged swallow. Finally, it is possible that temperature changes within the pharynx are indeed rapid.

SWALLOW DETECTOR MARK I

The swallow detector circuit used in our initial work was designed to detect changes in the small signal current gain (βAC) of the Pitran. We later found that this parameter depends more strongly on temperature than on pressure. This circuit, with which most of our experimental results were obtained, is described here.

A model PT-H2 Pitran with a nominal linear range of ±17.6 g/cm² was biased at a base current of 1 mA in a conventional emitter-follower configuration. A high-pass filtered square wave was applied to the base. The resulting signal at the collector (AC load resister 1.5 k Ω) was AC coupled to an active peak detector. The DC output of this circuit was linearly related to the negative excursion of the collector voltage from its quiescent value of about 2.3 V. This output was therefore linearly dependent on βAC. It was used to trigger valve closure. With this device we were able to obtain a sensitivity of 1.5 mV cm²/g (range 1 to 1.6). The temperature sensitivity was −6.8 g/cm²/°C. For some values of square wave amplitude this sensitivity could double. The minus sign indicates that an increase in temperature appeared to be a drop in pressure.

SWALLOW DETECTOR MARK II

The detector circuit just described was unsatisfactory because of its temperature sensitivity. For this reason it was redesigned to take advantage of the strong dependence of βAC on temperature. The new circuit develops a signal proportional to βAC and therefore (principally) to temperature. This signal is used to adjust the biasing base current of the Pitran so its collector current becomes independent of temperature (at constant pressure). A pressure change (at constant temperature) causes a larger change in the DC current gain (βDC) than in βAC. Thus the collector current can be made to depend on pressure and not temperature over a certain range of temperatures and pressures.

Figure 5 is a block diagram of the Mark II circuit. The timing circuit provides three logic pulses T_A, T_B, and P, which are of equal length. The two T pulses define the temperature phase during which the analog signal TEMP is determined. The P pulse defines the pressure phase during which the signal PRES is determined. These pulses control the various voltage sources and switches as indicated.

The Pitran and the amplifier which control its emitter voltage (amplifier 1) constitute the gain stage of two separate negative feedback loops. During the temperature phase the collector current is proportional to value of V_T. During the pressure phase the base current is proportional to the value of TEMP. This proportionality follows from the very small differential voltage maintained at the input to amplifier 1 by negative feedback. The double pole double throw switch determines whether it is i_B or i_C that is controlled by the negative feedback.

We next consider the derivation of the signal TEMP. The valve of V_T is proportional to the logic signal not T_A. Thus the collector and base currents are lower during T_A than during T_B. Because the collector current, i_C, is fixed by V_T, the difference in the base current, i_B, is inversely proportional to the current gain βAC. The triple pole single throw switch samples this difference and stores it on the two capacitors at the input to amplifier 2. The voltage V_1 is also proportional to the logic signal not T_A. Because i_B is lower during T_A than T_B the voltage V_1 can be adjusted to make the output of amplifier 2 equal to zero for any choice of V_T. This output voltage is added to the voltage V_2 (for

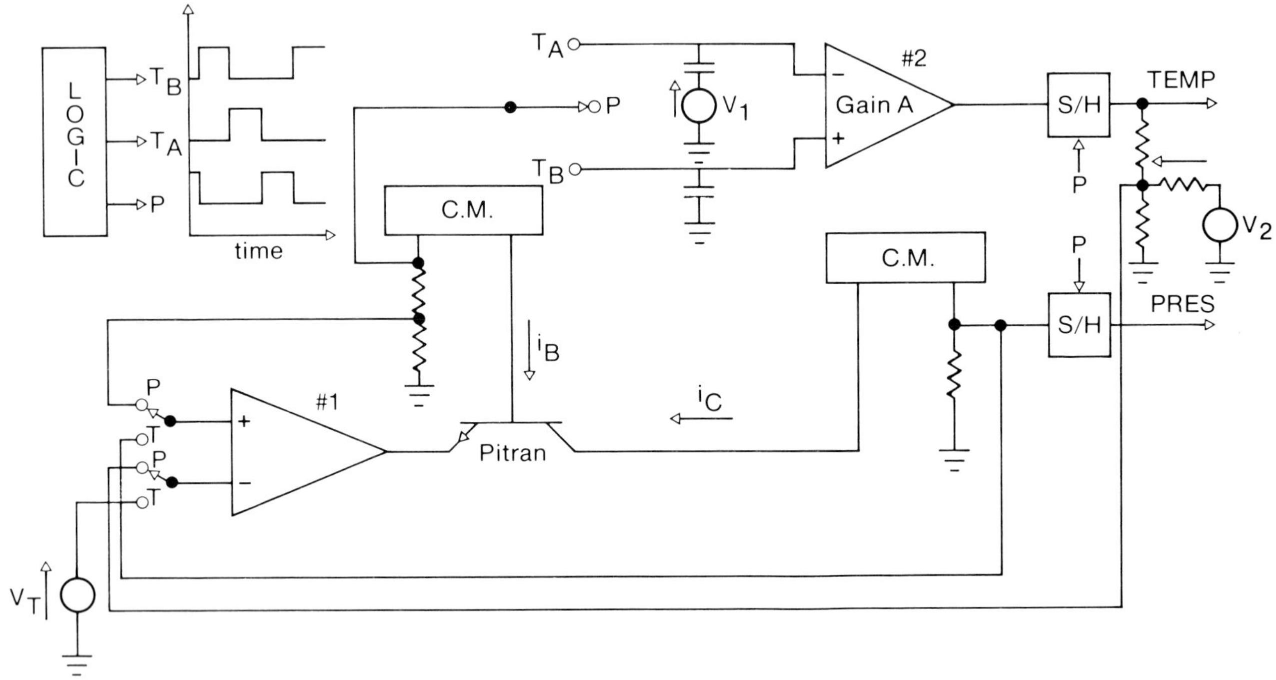

Fig. 5. Mark II swallow detector circuit. C.M. - Current mirror; S/H - Sample and hold. (See text for additional abbreviations.)

reasons to be discussed shortly) and sampled at the start of the pressure phase to form the signal TEMP.

We now show that TEMP varies inversely with temperature. As the temperature goes up the value of β_{AC} rises. Thus the differential signal derived from the base current drops. The actual relationship between temperature change and TEMP is found to be roughly linear. If V_1 is used to set the output of amplifier 2 to zero for some temperature then V_2 and the amplifier gain A determine the intercept and slope of the TEMP versus temperature relation.

It can be seen now how the temperature compensation is achieved. First, suppose the signal TEMP was independent of temperature. Then as temperature increased so would β_{DC} and thus so would i_C (because TEMP did not change). However, TEMP actually drops as the temperature rises, as we have just shown. Now, because of the negative feedback during the pressure phase, i_C is proportional to TEMP. Thus the rising value of i_C resulting from the change in β_{DC} is offset by a falling value of TEMP. With proper adjustment of V_1, V_2, and A, compensation for temperature change can thus be achieved. Two offset voltages (V_1 and V_2) are used to simplify the calibration procedure.

A potential problem with this compensation method is that reduces the pressure sensitivity. This reduction is a consequence of the fact that both β_{AC} and β_{DC} drop as the pressure rises. As we have noted, however, β_{AC} is quite insensitive to pressure and, therefore, the loss in sensitivity is slight in our circuit.

Calibration of the circuit is performed by first placing the Pitran in a water bath at about 0°C. (The Pitran is mounted in an aluminum container of mass 24.9 g to keep it dry and to allow it to be subjected to various pressures.) The voltage V_1 is adjusted so the output of amplifier 2 is 0 V. The voltage V_2 is then adjusted to make the signal PRES so i_C is about 3 mA during the pressure phase. The temperature of the water bath is then raised to about 45°C. Any drift in the voltage PRES is removed by changing the Gain A of amplifier 2. These steps are repeated once again and the calibration is complete.

The pressure sensitivity we achieve is from 1.5 to 2.5 mV cm²/g. The temperature sensitivity is very low. If we plunge the Pitran from one water bath to the other we find a transient variation in PRES occurs, equivalent to ±12 g/cm² of pressure. We attribute this to strain caused by nonuniform heating of the case and the aluminum container. The steady state sensitivity of PRES to temperature is typically less than the equivalent of 0.3 g/cm² °C.

The stability of the PRES signal was monitored by exposing the Pitran to air at room temperature and monitoring both PRES and the output of amplifier 2. We found that although the latter signal indicated short term fluctuations of ±1°C there were no corresponding fluctuations in the PRES signal. This signal did, however, drift by the equivalent of 2 g/cm² over the test period of 7½ hours. The circuit is powered by six AA cells, which can be carbon-zinc, alkaline-manganese dioxide, or rechargeable nickel-cadmium. It is designed to operate for cell voltages down to 0.95 V and will fail totally below this voltage. A flashing light is provided that stops when the batteries have failed. The quiescent current drain is 50 mA. The current drain caused by the solenoid valve (discussed in the next article), which actuates the larynx, is 250 mA while the valve is active. A further two silver-oxide cells provide reference voltages for a voltage regulator and for the detection of battery failure.

A bench test of the circuit indicates that if Duracell MN1500 alkaline cells are used with a 10 h/day — 500 swallows/day schedule we may expect the batteries to last for about three days. About 90% of the power is used up in the swallow detector circuit and the rest in the solenoid valve, which activates the pneumatic CO_2 circuit. When Eveready CH15 rechargeable nickel-cadmium batteries are used with the same schedule, we find that two sets of cells will be required to operate the device. Each set will last for 10 hours but then must be charged for 14 hours before reuse.

CONCLUSION

We have presented the specifications for an endotracheal artificial larynx and discussed the design alternatives we considered to meet these specifications. We have described the basic construction of our larynx and discussed the electronic design in detail. A discussion of the actuation of the valve, the pneumatic and acoustic aspects of the larynx, and its evaluation in dogs will be found in other articles in this supplement.

The electronic swallow detector described in this article (MK II) is capable of reliably detecting swallows, which give rise to pressure signals greater than 5 g/cm^2. Its reliability is a result of the temperature compensation of its sensor. This compensation is effective in the range 0 to 45°C. The power requirement of the electronic components is such that frequent charging or replacement of its batteries will be required. This is partially a result of over design of the complex temperature compensation circuit. Future versions of this circuit will focus on the reduction of the power drain by simplifying this circuit. The more radical approach of using a strain gauge sensor will also be attempted.

ACTUATION OF THE ENDOTRACHEAL ARTIFICIAL LARYNX

MICHAEL L. G. JOY, PhD, PEng
VIJAY S. DAYAL, MB, FRCS(C)
ALEX LO, BASc
ANTHONY JARES

The basic design of the endotracheal artificial larynx has been discussed in the previous articles in this supplement. Details of the surgical technique are given in the first article[28] and of the electronic swallow detector in the second article.[29] In this article we discuss the design of the system that inflates the balloon valve in the artificial larynx.

The volume of the balloon is from 2 to 3 ml when inflated. The inflation pressure is 140 to 200 g/cm.^{2} This is sufficient to seal the valve against any anticipated pharyngeal pressure. (Note: 1 psi = 70.3 g/cm^2 = 51.7 mmHg [Torr]). The balloon must be inflated when a swallow occurs and must have done so before food has passed into the tracheal limb of the artificial larynx. In our current design the distance from the Pitran sensor and the uppermost portion of the seat of the balloon is 1.3 cm. The velocity of a bolus of barium during a swallow can be estimated from the cineradiographic data from Ingervall and Lantz.[18] In the standing position the mean velocity of watery barium so estimated was 41.6 cm/s and of viscous barium was 29.4 cm/s. The highest velocity for watery barium was 83.3 cm/s. Thus if the latency of closure was less than 16 ms one could be certain of meeting the above goal. The average transit times, however, would be from 30 to 40 ms. Further objectives of the actuator design are ease and economy of use and maintenance. Finally, the actuator should be reliable and pose no direct threat to its user's safety.

POWER SOURCE

The two potential sources of power for the actuator are compressed gas and electrical batteries. Although the latter are more efficient in their storage of energy, we initially chose compressed gas because of the availability of components for the actuator's construction. There are also two choices of compressed gas, liquid carbon dioxide (CO_2) or liquid freon. The significant difference between these is their vapor pressure. At room temperature this is 56 atm for CO_2 and about 7 atm for freon. A second difference concerns the useful volume of gas that can be obtained from a given volume of its liquified form. This useful volume is greater for CO_2 than for freon by as much as 50%.

The basic pneumatic circuit used to actuate the larynx is shown in Figure 6. Gas is delivered to an electromechanical solenoid valve at a pressure of about 7 atm. The crosshatched area of this valve represents a moving member that connects the linear actuator either to the source of compressed gas or to the atmosphere. When the solenoid valve is activated this gas pushes a piston in the linear actuator forward against a spring. This motion forces air into the balloon, which inflates it, closing the valve in the larynx.

When the solenoid valve is deactivated the gas that forced the piston forward is vented to the atmosphere by the return of the piston because of the force of the spring. This return of the piston also evacuates the balloon, causing it to lie flat against the inside wall of the tracheal limb of the larynx. The patient is thus isolated from the high pressure gas. Because the vapor pressure of the liquid CO_2 is much too high to be controlled by reasonably small electromagnetic valves, a regulator is required. This regulator has proven to be the weak link in this design. One problem is that it limits the flow of CO_2 from the liquid gas bottle. This resistance can be alleviated by increasing the volume between the regulator and the solenoid valve using an accumulator as shown in Figure 6. This step reduces the drop in pressure at this point when the solenoid valve is opened.

A second consequence of the high vapor pressure of CO_2 is the heavy weight of its container. When charged the gas may account for only 30% of the gross weight. When the bulk of the regulator (about 350 g), accumulator, and container are considered, the advantage of CO_2 over freon in useful volume is lost.

Despite these negative aspects of CO_2 we chose it for our initial work because of the ready availability of components. We are now in the process of evaluating the use of freon for our pneumatic device. We are also constructing an electrical solenoid pump with a very short stroke as an alternative motive force. This pump would provide the convenience of a single power source for the whole system, a rechargable battery pack.

The amount of gas required to operate the larynx depends on the design of the linear actuator and the pressure of the gas that enters it. For example, if we use the simple actuator suggested in Figure 6, we will use a volume of gas equal to the stroke volume of the piston for each swallow. This gas will be at the regulated pressure. If, for example, this pressure is 4 atm and we start with 25 g of CO_2, we will be

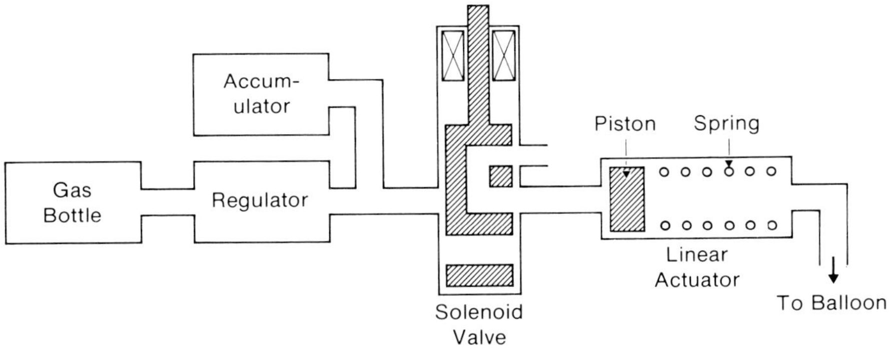

Fig. 6. Pneumatic circuit used to actuate larynx.

able to expend about 3,200 ml of gas. If the stroke volume is 2.2 ml this will allow 1,454 swallows. The average number of swallows per day is 550 with a range of about 500 to 700.[14] Thus the gas bottle would last from two to three days in this case. If the pressure were halved the number of swallows would double but the speed of response would drop. These considerations are discussed in greater detail in the following sections.

LINEAR ACTUATOR

In the experiments described in the next article in this supplement,[30] we used the simple actuator shown in Figure 6. The piston diameter of this actuator was 1.5 cm and it delivered a stroke volume of 2.2 ml. This volume of CO_2, at the regulated pressure (usually 4 atm), is consumed for each swallow. The measured number of swallows per 25 g of CO_2 was 1,010 for this actuator. This is less than predicted in the previous simple calculation (1,454) because of the nonisothermal expansion of the gas and losses during the actuation of the solenoid valve.

An improved version of the linear actuator has been built and tested. It has a 1.9-cm piston and delivers a stroke volume of 2.84 ml. This allows us to fill a slightly larger balloon if required. It also incorporates a second seal that prevents any communication between the high and low pressure circuits when the piston has reached the end of its stroke. Because of the larger stroke volume this actuator delivers only 860 swallows at 4 atm for 25 g CO_2. Two modifications to the design were tested, each of which resulted in a large improvement in this figure. In the first modification a second valve was added on the high pressure side of the actuator, which cut off the inlet when the piston reaches the end of its stroke. This valve prevents the gas pressure in the actuator from climbing any higher than is required to finish its stroke. The second modification achieved the same end by reducing the time for which the solenoid valve was open and adding a second valve to control the venting of the gas at the end of the swallow.

The first modification resulted in 1,680 swallows per 25 g CO_2 and the second in 1,960 swallows per 25 g CO_2. The first modification has been adopted because it is simpler, lighter, and less expensive. The actuator is constructed from aluminum and uses a rolling diaphragm (Bellofram Corp) to ease tolerances. This diaphragm can withstand 34 atm pressure and a million cycles.

CONTROL VALVE

The control valve is a Clippard model EV3. It requires about 250 mA to actuate. The opening time depends on the applied voltage and source resistance. Measured values ranged from 8 to 15 ms. We found the resistance to gas flow through the valve was an important factor in determining the time required to inflate the balloon. For this reason we modified the EV3 valve by enlarging the orifice in the poppet seat from 0.63 mm to 0.91 mm. We also increased the stroke by 0.12 mm. The resulting improvement is discussed in the next section.

RESPONSE TIME

We have measured the time required to fill the balloon by placing electrical contacts on its seat in such a way that contact is made when the balloon is fully inflated. We define the transfer time as the interval between the receipt of the logic signal and the full inflation of the balloon.

The transfer time is the sum of the delay in opening the solenoid valve, the piston travel time, and the delay caused by the distributed volume of the tube connecting the actuator and the balloon and the volume of the balloon itself. The solenoid delay is affected by the battery voltage and the length of the stroke of the poppet. It is typically 7 ms (range 6 to 13 ms). The delay in the tubing and balloon is affected by tubing length and inner diameter and the volume of the balloon. The tubing we use has an inner diameter of 1.6 mm. In the dog experiments it was 90 cm long. For the bench tests recorded in Figure 7 it was 50 cm long. This reduction in length reduces the delay from about 8 ms to 5 ms at 4 atm pressure.

The piston travel time is strongly affected by the properties of the solenoid valve. The actuator's piston is light enough to have a negligible effect on this time. Also, the spring has little effect on the

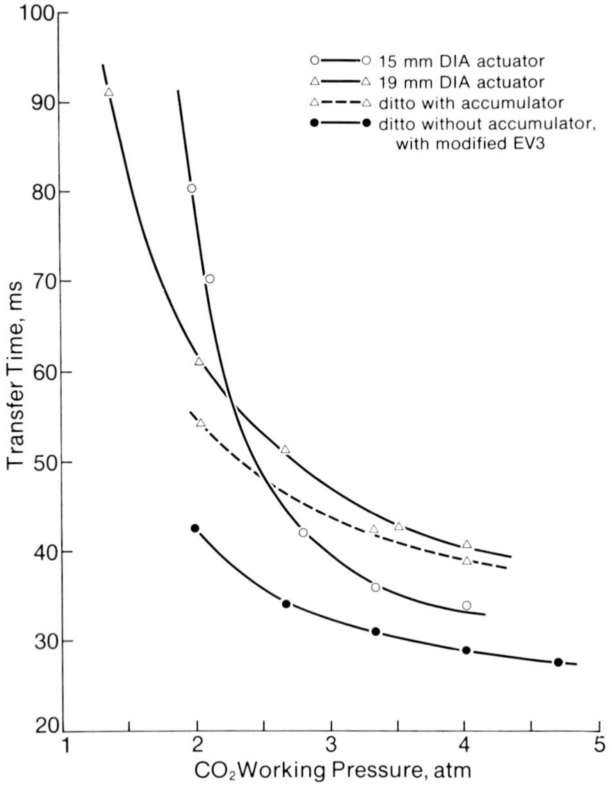

Fig. 7. Transfer time of various pneumatic systems as function of gas pressure at solenoid valve. Transfer time is interval between receipt of logic signal and full inflation of balloon.

travel time when inflating the balloon. Figure 7 shows transfer time as a function of nominal regulated pressure for various combinations of actuator and solenoid. Note that the 15 mm actuator has a smaller stroke volume than the newer 19 mm actuator (2.2 ml versus 3 ml). It also has a longer stroke. Numerical comparison of its transfer time with those of the other actuator are therefore not simple.

The relatively longer times at low pressures probably arise because the resistive force caused by the diaphragm increases linearly with its diameter, while the force on the piston increases as the square of the diameter. Thus the smaller diameter piston is more sensitive to the resistance of the diaphragm than is the larger piston. A very simple model of this system would neglect all effects resulting from the piston or the diaphragm and would also assume laminar flow. For such a model we would expect an inverse proportionality between pressure and the difference between transfer time and solenoid delay time. In fact, Figure 7 shows that for pressures over 2.5 atm the transfer time does not drop quite as rapidly as would be predicted by this model. We hypothesize that the efforts of turbulent flow in the valve and actuator account for this observation.

The most satisfying result of this work is the marked reduction in transfer time that resulted from the modification of the solenoid valve. This modification reduced the transfer time at 4 atm pressure from about 40 ms to about 30 ms. It also resulted in uniformly low transfer times than we obtained from the 15 mm actuator used in our experiments with dogs.[30] Finally, we note that the pressure drop caused by poor regulation increases the transfer time by several milliseconds. This increase is not as large as that caused by the constricted orifice of the solenoid valve.

CONCLUSION

The smallest transfer time we have achieved is about 30 ms. This would be adequate for viscous barium swallows and the average watery barium swallow. It would, however, let the fastest watery barium swallows enter the valve. In the next article in this supplement[30] we describe experiments with dogs in which we found the 30 ms transfer time was adequate for watery as well as viscous meals. Thus it appears that, in dogs, our specification of the minimum closure time was overly stringent. Our next in vivo experiment with a dog will attempt to obtain more exact information concerning the relative positions of food and larynx when the valve is activated. This will allow us better to predict the triggering mechanism in humans. Initial work with an electric pump indicates the 15 ms limit can be achieved. We therefore are still attempting to reach this goal.

Carbon dioxide is one choice for powering the linear actuator. At present freon is being evaluated as a substitute. We have demonstrated closure times with freon of 32 ms at 4.5 atm by simply substituting a bottle of freon for one of CO_2. Our goal is to develop the electric pump to a point where 15 ms transfer times can be achieved. We will also develop the freon-activated system as a backup but expect that 30 ms transfer times will be the best that can be obtained.

EVALUATION OF THE ENDOTRACHEAL ARTIFICIAL LARYNX

RICHARD E. MOON, MD, FRCP(C)
VIJAY S. DAYAL, MB, FRCS(C)
MICHAEL L. G. JOY, PhD, PEng

This article deals with the evaluation of the effectiveness of the artificial larynx in preventing aspiration, and the assessment of tissue reaction caused by it.

CUFF

Evaluation of the cuff consisted of a) a pressure-volume measurement of the sponge-filled cuff; b) gross and histologic examination of the tracheas of experimental animals that died spontaneously or were sacrificed; c) cineradiographic data showing that the cuff with sponge filler can prevent aspiration in the short term; d) periodic radiographic examination of the lungs of experimental dogs dependent on cuff integrity to prevent aspiration; and e) examination of the cuff each day to look for loss of strength, tears, etc.

A typical pressure-volume plot of a cuff with foam filler of the proportions described earlier is shown in Figure 8. The plot was made by measuring the pressure change within the cuff induced by evacuation of small amounts of air. Cuffs with any desired characteristics can be manufactured by changing the size of the foam filler. The mean intracavitary pressure exerted by the foam inside a dog or simulated trachea can be estimated by first inserting the cuff to allow equilibirum to be established, then attaching the tubing from the cuff port to a manometer and removing the cuff from the trachea. The manometer reading gives the intracavitary pressure.

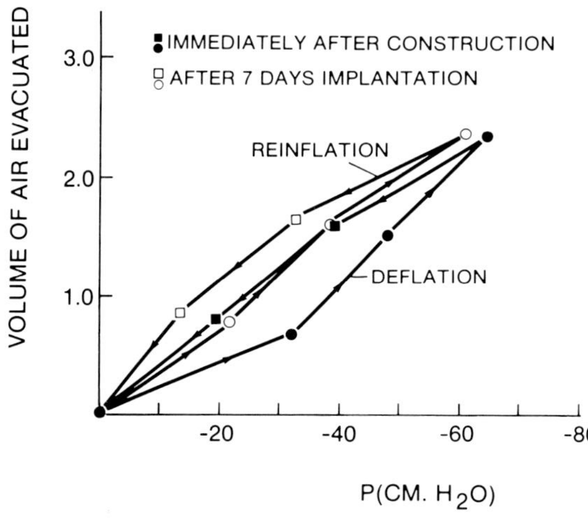

Fig. 8. Typical pressure-volume relationships of cuff with foam filler immediately after construction and seven days after implantation.

All autopsied dogs had their tracheas examined grossly; the mucosa was graded according to the following scale: grade 1 — normal in appearance; grade 2 — injected in appearance, no ulceration; grade 3 — superficial ulceration; grade 4 — gross ulceration exposing cartilaginous rings.

Histologic sections were made of the 79- and 386-day survivors from the following areas: the tracheopharyngeal anastomosis, trachea adjacent to the cuff, and control trachea caudad to the tracheostomy. The gross examination results are shown in Table 1. All of the fistulas after the one-stage operation were widely patent and the anastomoses were healed satisfactorily. Figure 9 shows the anastomosis at autopsy in a dog dead 386 days postoperatively. Microscopic examination of the tissue sections were performed by a pathologist. Control trachea showed patchy squamous metaplasia and minimal to moderate chronic inflammation (Fig. 10A).

Trachea in contact with the cuff showed submucosal fibrosis with both acute and chronic inflammation in the 79-day survivor (Fig. 10B). The

TABLE 1. OPERATION, IMMEDIATE POSTOPERATIVE MANAGEMENT, SURVIVAL TIME, AND GROSS TRACHEAL APPEARANCE AT AUTOPSY

Dog No.		*NG Tube Insertion*	*Dummy Insertion*	*Death*	*Trachea Grade*
21	2-stage	Yes	Not inserted	Day 3 Mucus	2
34	2-stage	No	Immediate	Day 72 Sacrificed*	2
36	2-stage	No	Immediate	Day 22 Mucus	2
38	1-stage	No	Immediate	Day 4 Sacrificed†	4
39	1-stage	No	Immediate	Day 112 Mucus	2
40	1-stage	No	Immediate	Day 7 Sacrificed†	4
41	1-stage	No	Immediate	Day 7 Sacrificed†	4
42	1-stage	Yes	Immediate	Day 11 Mucus	2
44	1-stage	Yes	Day 14	Day 386 Mucus§	2
45	1-stage	Yes	Day 14	Day 79 Mucus§	2
46	1-stage	Yes	Day 14	1 yr, 2 mo Sacrificed for study	2

*Dog sacrificed because fistula was no longer patent.

†Dog sacrificed because of overwhelming infections in region of surgery.

§Histologic sections made.

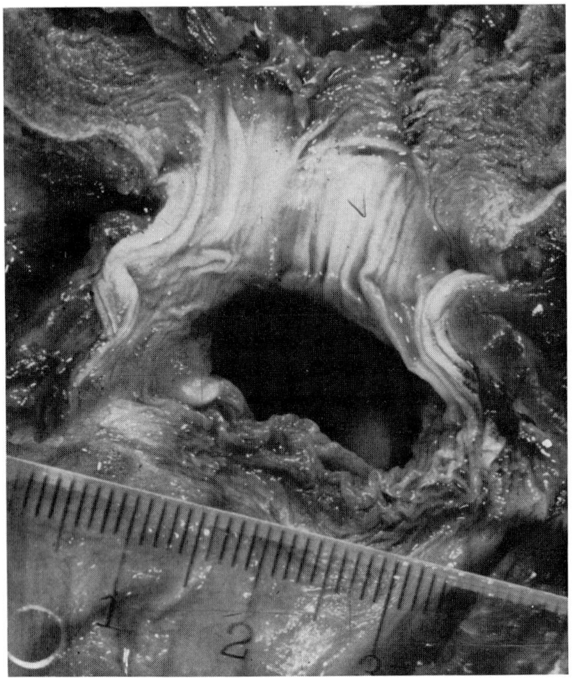

Fig. 9. Patent tracheopharyngeal anastomosis at autopsy in dog who died 386 days postoperatively.

386-day survivor had less inflammation but marked vascular congestion. This was compatible either with resolving inflammation or obstruction to venous drainage. Figure 10C shows a section of the tracheopharyngeal anastomosis from the 79-day survivor. This shows satisfactory healing. There were no malignant changes. The inflammatory changes seen were much less than the ones seen in patients who have been intubated for periods as short as 24 hours.

Cineradiographic studies were performed with the dog held in a stand. A mixture of food and barium sulfate was eaten by the dog as cineradiographs were taken at a rate of 100 frames per second. Figure 11 shows a sequence of enlargements of individual frames with one line drawing (E) delineating the structures more clearly. It can be seen that the barium-food mixture does not spill into the trachea.

Chest x-ray films were taken at times shown in Table 2. All radiographs were examined for the presence of chronic aspiration pneumonia. All of the films were normal. A sample chest radiograph is shown in Figure 12. The cuff material remained intact throughout all studies. The only change in cuff membrane characteristics appeared to be a yellowish discoloration. The factor that limited the operating lifetime of a cuff was gradual loss of resiliency of the foam filler.

VALVE

Evaluation of the valve and closure mechanisms consisted of a) measurement of the pressure at which the valve leaks; b) measurement of elapsed time for Pitran triggering until valve closure, ie, transfer time (detailed in preceding article); c) cineradiographic studies of the pharyngeal area during swallow of contrast material to prove the valve is necessary to prevent aspiration and can perform the task; d) polygraph recordings of the pressure signal output during a meal to establish consistency of operation; e) fatigue-testing of a valve.

TABLE 2. CHEST X-RAY FILMS ON LARYNGECTOMIZED DOGS

Dog No.	*Postoperative Days on Which Studies were Performed*
34	8
36	10
39	21
44	85, 127
45	40
46	386

To measure leakage pressure of the valve, an artificial larynx was inserted into a 20-mm inside diameter transparent cylinder that was closed at one end except for a pressure port. The larynx was attached to its power pack and then triggered to produce valve closure. Unless specified otherwise the Mark I version of the swallow detection electronics was used.[29]

Water was introduced through the pressure port and then pressure applied until leakage occurred. The valve was capable of withstanding 50 g/cm^2 steady state pressure and 140 g/cm^2 when pulsed at 50% duty cycle with pulse length of one second. Transfer time depends on the pressure at which the pneumatic cylinder (which derives air pulses to the valve balloon) is activated. As activation pressure is increased, transfer time decreases (see preceding article for details).

Cineradiograph studies were performed as in the cuff evaluation. Valve closure was indeed necessary for the prevention of aspiration. During a swallow with the valve power pack turned off, part of the food bolus entered the artificial larynx. When the valve was activated it effectively prevented aspiration. This result was obtained reproducibly throughout a meal. During six meals using two different dogs polygraph recordings were made. Each dog was observed carefully during each meal and every swallow seen was recorded on the chart by manually pressing an event marker.

Also recorded were the pressure signal from the Pitran and the final output pulse used to trigger valve closure. During these meals a total of 223 swallows were successfully detected; valve closure occurred each time. No swallows were missed by the detection circuit. A total of 42 valve closures occurred in the absence of swallows. Of these false triggers, 31 occurred while the dog was panting rapidly and, therefore, creating significant pressure changes within the pharynx.

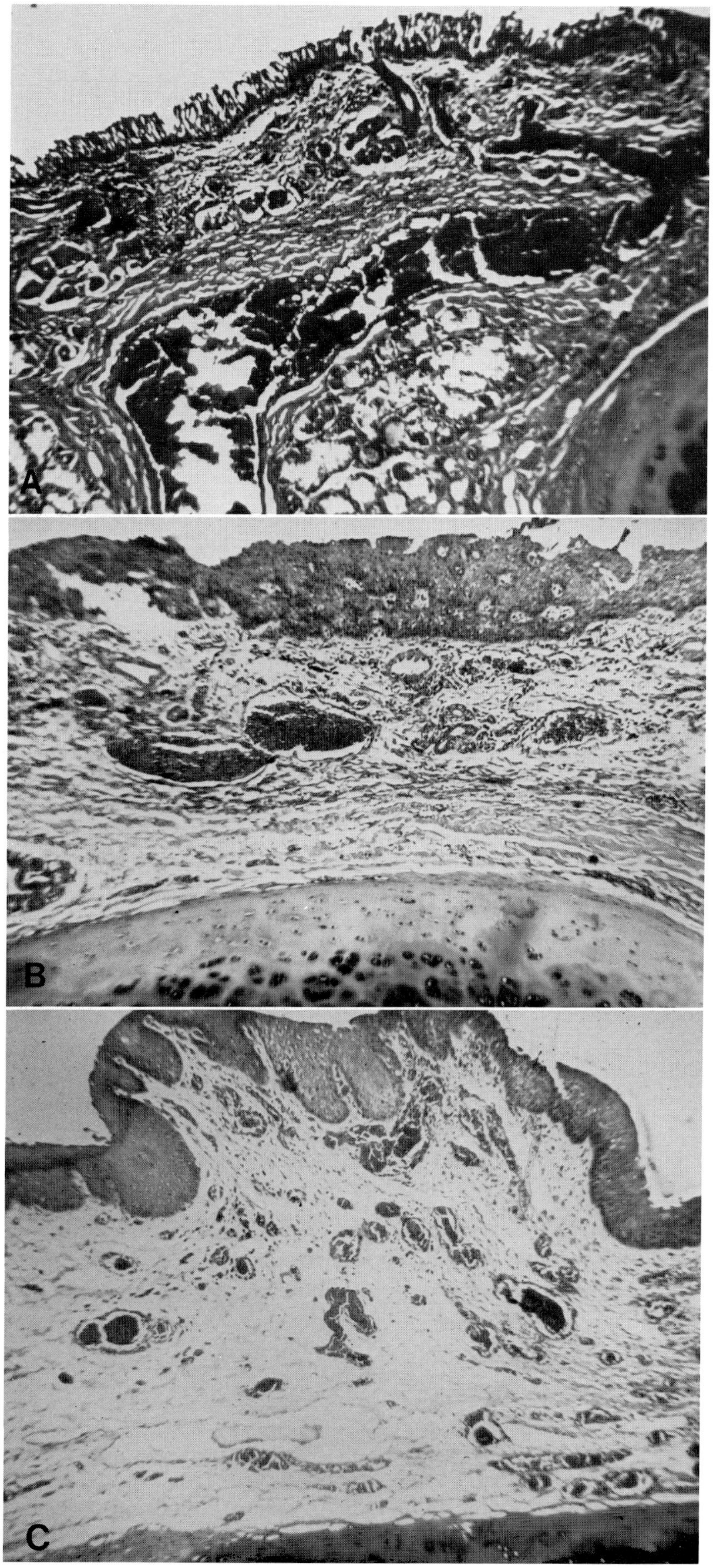

Fig. 10. A) Patchy squamous metaplasia and minimal to moderate chronic inflammation in control trachea. B) Submucosal fibrosis with acute and chronic inflammation in trachea at cuff site in 79-day survival. C) Satisfactory healing at tracheopharyngeal anastomosis site in 79-day survival.

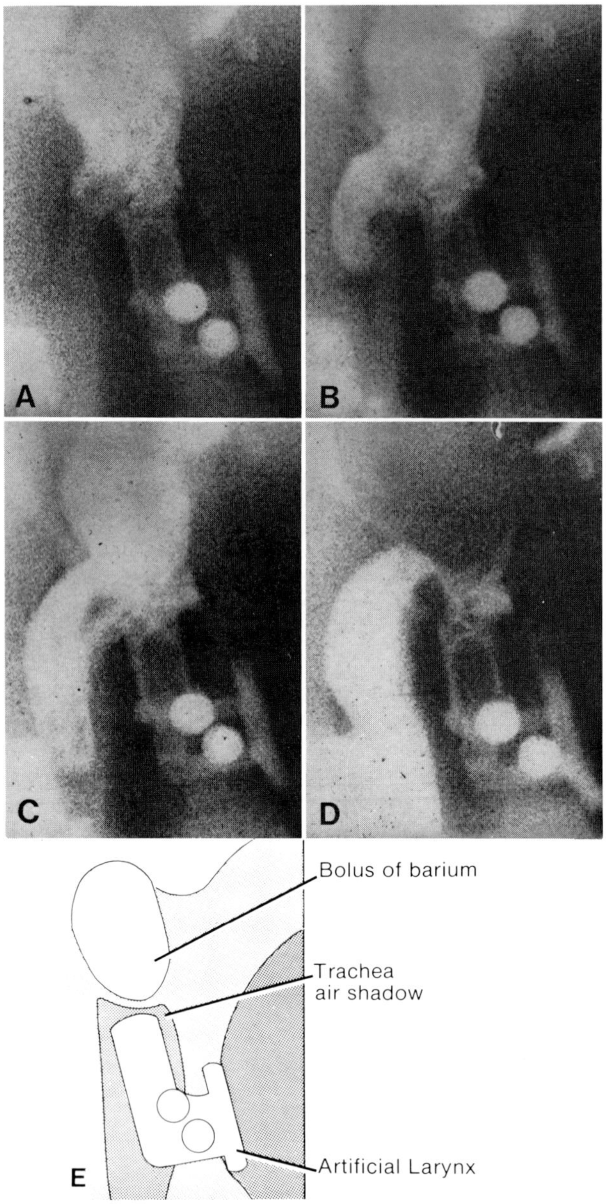

Fig. 11. A-E) Barium swallow with artificial larynx in place. Line drawing (E) delineates structures and applies specifically to A. Barium food mixture does not spill into trachea.

To test the physical integrity of the valve balloon after multiple closures the following test was performed. A balloon installed in an artificial larynx was tested for leaks by inflating it under water. During the next 24 hours it was subjected to 29,000 cycles of inflation and deflation. It was again tested for leaks. The balloon remained intact and no leaks developed.

The artificial larynx can be activated to close either automatically during swallowing (by food contact) or manually by pushbutton. This latter maneuver will allow the patient to cough: valve closure followed by Valsava maneuver then valve opening.

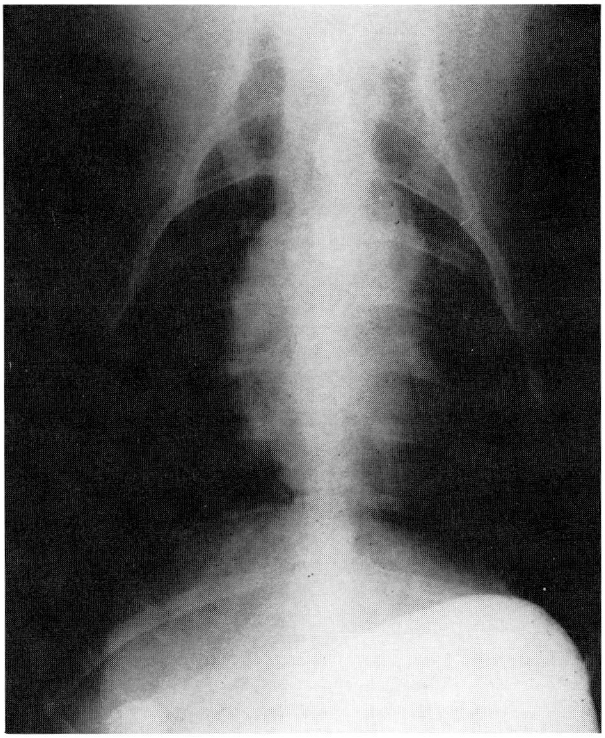

Fig. 12. Long-term follow-up chest radiograph showing normal examination with no evidence of aspiration pneumonitis.

SWALLOW DETECTION

The newer version of the swallow detection electronics is discussed in the second article in this supplement. It is capable of monitoring the temperature as well as the pressure of the Pitran sensor. This circuit has been tested on a single dog during four meals. The valve functioned well. Food entered the trachea only once, when it was discovered we had torn the balloon during a bench test before inserting the larynx. During these trials we noted the effects of cold food (ice cream) on the temperature of the device. We also determined (for this animal) the appropriate threshold levels for the triggering circuit.

It was found that a typical swallow's pressure signal had two phases. The first phase lasted about 50 ms and consisted of a rapid increase equivalent to about 50 g/cm^2 pressure. This increase was often followed by a number of rapid fluctuations of smaller or larger amplitude. The second phase lasted about 1000 ms and consisted of a single peak of high pressure that reached a maximum at about 600 ms. This maximum varied from the equivalent of 50 g/cm^2 to 100 g/cm^2 pressure.

To detect swallows we set a threshold at the equivalent of 35 g/cm^2 pressure. This was sufficient to detect all of the several hundred swallows observed. About 3% of valve closures were not caused by swallows but by other activities such as licking and looking backwards. When the dog was fed ice cream or drank ice water (0°C) the temperature of the Pitran dropped by as much as 14°C. This temperature change did not cause any noticeable change in the pressure signal.

CONCLUSION

A device has been designed that can replace those functions of the normal human larynx related to preventing aspiration. The device is suitable for use in patients in whom, following laryngectomy, a tracheopharyngeal fistula is created, as described in the first article of this supplement. The apparatus has been tested in experimental dogs for which the surgical approach has been designed. Four long-term survivors were studied. Three of these have died so far, all from mucus plugging. These deaths resulted because the animals could not be observed for more than a short time each day. Mucus plugging would not be a problem in humans because each patient could easily remove the device and clean it as often as desired. The last dog in this group was sacrificed after one year, ten months for study. In dogs the device has been proven to be capable to preventing aspiration of food during meals.

CONSIDERATIONS IN THE DESIGN OF AN AIRFLOW-ACTIVATED SOUND SOURCE FOR AN ENDOTRACHEAL ARTIFICIAL LARYNX

RICHARD E. MOON, MD, FRCP(C)
VIJAY S. DAYAL, MB, FRCS(C)
MICHAEL L. G. JOY, PhD, PEng

INTRODUCTION

A successful design for a voice source powered by pulmonary air must incorporate two main features: a) ease and efficiency of excitation by expired air, and b) appropriate loudness and timbre such that the normal human voice may be approximated. In addition, the sound source should ideally be amenable to modulation to allow vocal inflexion.

Considerable information on the first of these features exists in the literature. Parameters relevant to ease of speaking include glottic airflow, subglottic pressure, and efficiency of the sound generator. This last parameter may be defined as the proportion of power dissipated (by airflow through the larynx) that is converted into sound. Subglottic pressure during speech varies between 5 and 50 cmH_2O.[31,32] Kitzing and Lofquist have measured transglottic pressure and have reported values between 1 and 10 cmH_2O.[33] Airflow during speech has been measured in normal subjects and patients with bilateral vocal cord paralysis.

Isshiki and von Leden[34] reported that phonation in their normal subjects required 100 to 182 ml/s in males and 76 to 172 ml/s in females. Patients with bilateral vocal cord paralysis with fixation in the median or paramedian position required a range of 200 to 760 ml/s for normal phonation. For artificial larynx design, this latter range should be considered the upper limit of acceptability; patients with this disability generally have acceptable speaking voices.[35,36] Plots of sound pressure level versus the logarithm of the power dissipated by airflow through the glottis have been constructed by van den Berg.[31] The relative efficiencies of different sound generators, or the same sound generator under different conditions, may be compared using this method provided the necessary sound pressure level measurements are made in exactly the same way. Absolute measures of efficiency cannot easily be obtained because of the difficulty of measuring total sound energy produced by the larynx.

The timbre of the human larynx is more difficult to measure. Most of the information contained in the terms "timbre" or "quality" of voice may be depicted in spectral analysis of the emitted sound. Such an analysis consists of a plot of sound pressure level versus frequency. It contains peaks at the fundamental frequency of vibration (or first partial) and at multiples of this frequency (overtones or higher partials). It does not contain phase information, which most physiologists consider to be of minor importance in determining sound quality. Any such analysis of human voice represents sound from the glottis considerably filtered by the supraglottic vocal tract. Therefore, sound spectra of the in situ human larynx can only be constructed indirectly. This has been done in several ways. Van den Berg[37] inserted a loudspeaker with known spectrum through the tracheostomy of a hemilaryngectomized patient and observed the quality of vowel sounds. Flanagan[38] obtained volume velocity spectra from photoglottograms, which are plots of glottal area versus time. He used a function derived by van den Berg[39] relating volume velocity of air passing through the glottis to subglottic pressure and glottic area. Volume velocity functions of time were transformed into frequency spectra. Stevens et al[40] constructed an electrical analog of the supraglottic vocal tract and varied the spectrum of the source of excitation until optimal vowel quality was obtained. Spectra obtained by these methods show decay of harmonics at a rate of 6 to 12 dB per octave.[41]

The mean fundamental frequency of the larynx in normal males is about 130 Hz. In females it is about one octave higher.[42] The fundamental frequency may be raised voluntarily over a range of 2 to $2\frac{1}{2}$ octaves. This is partially accomplished by adjusting the intrinsic laryngeal musculature under neural control. However, some variation in pitch may occur without changing the laryngeal "setting." This may be demonstrated by voicing constant pitch for a few seconds then pressing suddenly on the abdomen. A rise in pitch will occur simultaneously with the increase in glottic airflow. Patients with paralyzed vocal cords may also produce a range of fundamental frequencies as great as two octaves by expiring at different flow rates.[35] Van den Berg demonstrated the same phenomenon in his experiments on isolated human larynges.[43] It is possible, therefore, that some degree of pitch control may be obtained from other types of passive voice sources.

A reed assembly has been designed to provide voice for the artificial larynx described in a previous article in this supplement. The reeds used are made

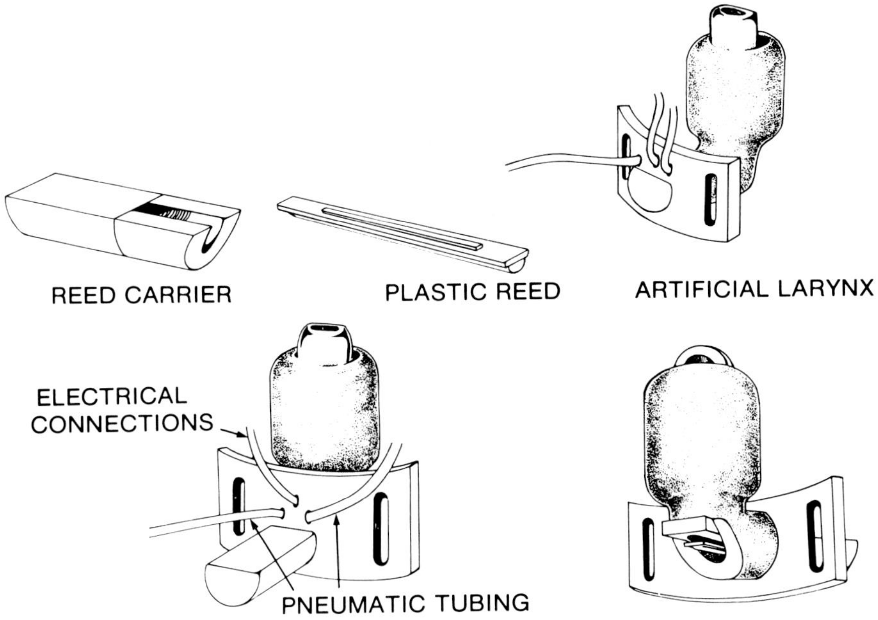

Fig. 13. Endotracheal artificial larynx showing position of reed and carrier.

of plastic and are available in a range of frequencies from about 130 Hz upward (Proll reeds, Bloomfield, NJ). An aluminum carrier holds the reed; the reed and carrier can easily be inserted into the horizontal limb of the artificial larynx as shown in Figure 13. This article describes the evaluation of the reed system in the artificial larynx.

METHODS

To measure the parameters just described an apparatus similar to the one used by van den Berg[43,44] was constructed. It is illustrated in Figure 14. Compressed air from a cylinder passed through a regulator, an airflow meter, then a heater. The warmed air was then humidified in the chamber filled with polyurethane foam into which warm water was continuously dripped. The second chamber, containing loosely packed gauze, served to remove water droplets. The warmed, humidified air then passed into the aluminum subglottic tube and through the larynx attached to the top. The subglottic tube was adapted so that either human cadaver larynges or artificial larynges could easily be connected. The system was allowed to run for about 30 minutes before any experiments were performed to allow the subglottic tube and larynx to warm sufficiently so condensation did not occur. The air heater was provided with a thermistor at the efferent end to sense air temperature, and a control box with feedback circuit to maintain a constant temperature. Naturally there was some cooling of air between the heater and the larynx; therefore, the setting on the air heater control box was adjusted until the steady state air temperature at the larynx was 37°C as measured with a mercury thermometer.

A U-tube manometer as shown was initially used to measure subglottic pressure. This was replaced by a precision manometer (Wilhelm Lambrecht), which could measure low pressure with much greater accuracy. A sound level meter (Bruel & Kjaer 2203) fitted with a 2.5-cm [1-in] condenser microphone (Bruel & Kjaer 4145) was used to measure the sound pressure level and provide the input signal to the spectrum analyzer (Hewlett-Packard 3580A). The sound level meter was suspended vertically, with the microphone 80 mm from the sound source. A permanent record of each spectral analysis was obtained with an X-Y plotter (Hewlett-Packard Moseley 7005A). The subglottic tube was 283 mm long and 12 mm in diameter. These dimensions approximate those of the human subglottic system.

Seven fresh cadaver larynges were obtained from the autopsy service of one of the local teaching hospitals. None of the patients had had any history of laryngeal pathology. Five of the larynges were grossly normal. Two had vocal fold trauma from prolonged intubation and were not used for study. All larynges were dissected down to the level of the vocal cords. Connective tissue and fat were removed to expose the arytenoid cartilages posteriorly and a separate nylon thread was passed through each one. A third thread was affixed to the connective tissue of the anterior surface of the thyroid cartilage in the midline at the level of intersection of the vocal ligaments. Inferior to the larynx the trachea was removed below the third tracheal cartilage. The internal diameter of the tracheal stub that remained attached was measured by carefully inserting a series of plastic cylinders of graduated size. The internal diameter was taken as the diameter of the largest cylinder that could be inserted without stretching the tissues.

For analysis each larynx was placed over the top of the subglottic tube and tied in place to prevent leaks. Each arytenoid thread was passed over a pulley and attached to an aluminum weight pan. The larynx was anchored by attaching the anterior thread to the support pole. Recordings were made only with larynges set in chest voice mode.[44,45] This setting produces the quality of sound present in conversational speech. To produce this in the isolated larynx preparations the arytenoids were forced together by crossing and aligning the attached threads in a transverse plane. There was no stretching of the vocal cords. Sufficient weight was added to each pan to force the arytenoids together (0 to 20 g was sufficient). Recordings were made of four larynges.

After analyzing the spectra of several human larynges, the artificial larynx was installed. It would not utter a sound when placed on the experimental apparatus although it vibrated with ease when it was inserted upside down and air drawn backwards through the apparatus. One possible explanation was acoustic coupling. Many physiologists believe that coupling between the vocal cords and subglottic air changes the glottic sound spectrum very little in humans.[38,46,47] This cannot be assumed for an artificial sound source, however. It is possible that if at certain frequencies the driving point impedance of the subglottic system viewed from the glottis is of the same order of magnitude as the sound source impedance, then pressure fluctuations in the vicinity of the source may be so large that vibration is severely disturbed or inhibited.

To test this hypothesis a glass reservoir with a volume of 3.5 l

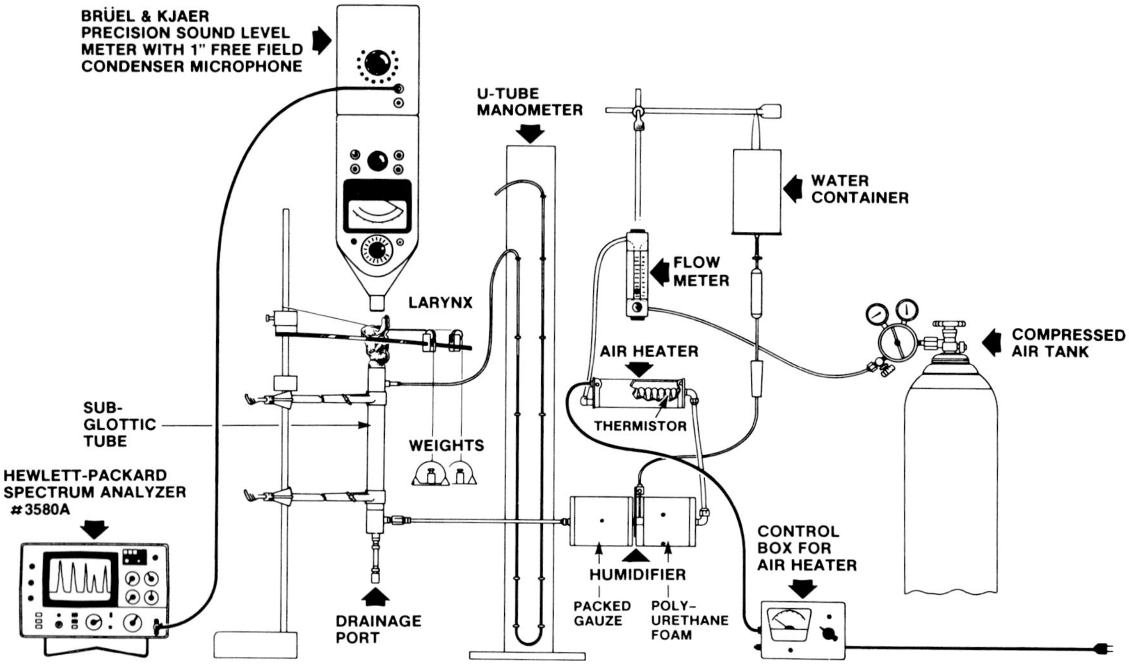

Fig. 14. Instrument for measuring sound spectra from isolated human larynges.

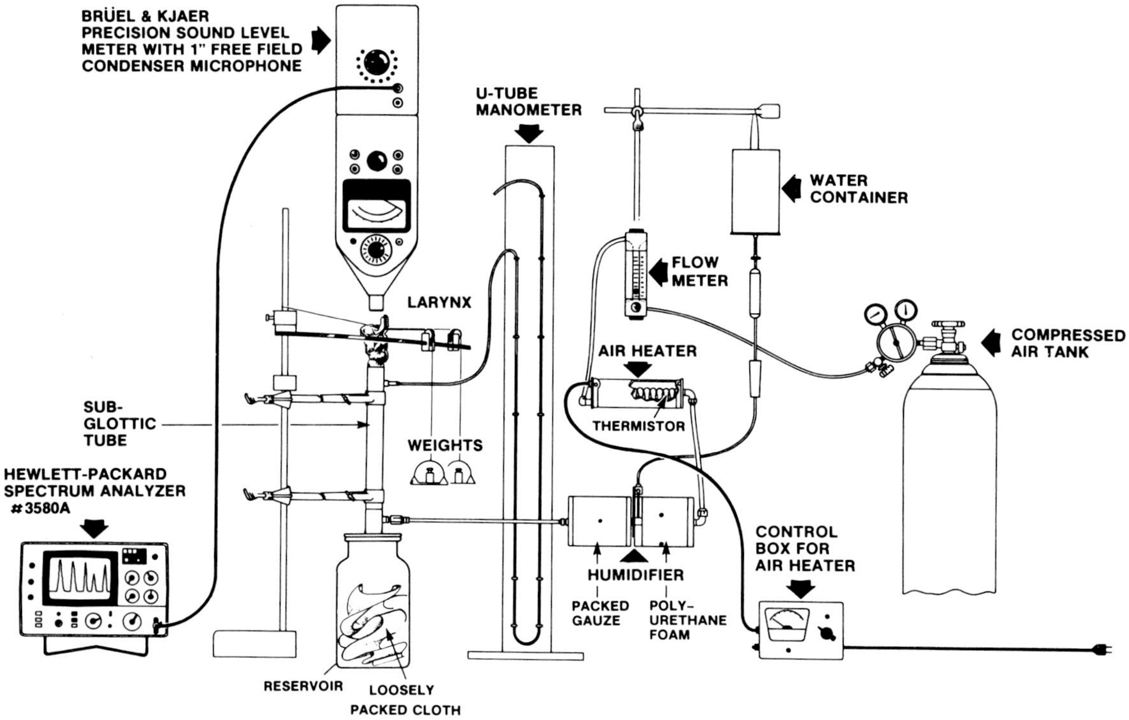

Fig. 15. Instrument shown in Fig. 14 with addition of reservoir.

was attached to the bottom of the subglottic tube (Fig. 15). Cloth rays were loosely packed into the reservoir to dampen reverberation. This modified system more closely models the human subglottic system, which to a first approximation behaves like a pipe open at one end.[46,48] The reed system vibrated satisfactorily with reservoir attached. Acoustic impedances were calculated for both configurations.

After discovering the necessity for the reservoir when testing the plastic reeds, a further larynx was tested both with and without the reservoir. A rubber cork was allowed to hang from a thin wire in the reservoir. The wire was passed up the lumen of the subglottic tube and out through a tiny hole in the tube wall. The cork could then be pulled up by the wire to block the bottom of the tube to allow the reservoir to be removed acoustically from the apparatus while the larynx was vibrating. Recordings were made at airflow rates from 83 to 412 ml/s. In exactly the same way recordings were made of sound from the artificial larynx.

To estimate the resistance of airflow in patients with bilateral vocal cord paralysis after surgical laterofixation, three larynges were prepared in the following way. A straight surgical needle

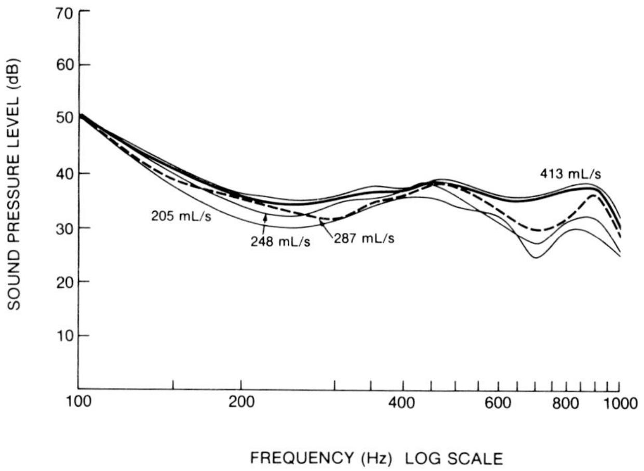

Fig. 16. Noise spectra in room where vocal spectra of larynx at different airflow rates were obtained.

was used to transfix both arytenoids, allowing them to be held any desired distance apart. Transglottic pressure was then measured at various airflow rates with the posterior edges of the vocal cords separated by a distance of 2 to 5 mm.

RESULTS

The height of each peak of a spectral analysis was measured in decibels and plotted against frequency with a correction factor according to the following formula: dB corrected + dB measured = 20 $\log_{10} f$ + 60, where f = frequency. In effect a boost in sound pressure level was given to the low frequency harmonics to offest the 6 dB per octave increase in measured sound pressure level that occurs because of the radiation characteristics at the mouth.[41] The resulting spectra could then be compared directly with the volume velocity spectra published in the literature. Spectra of room noise recorded under the same conditions as the vocal spectra, with various airflow rates, are shown in Figure 16. Noise sound pressure level was always at least 10 dB below the measured signal from the vocal cords or artificial larynx reed; over most of the spectrum it was 20 dB or more below. The possible effects of noise on the

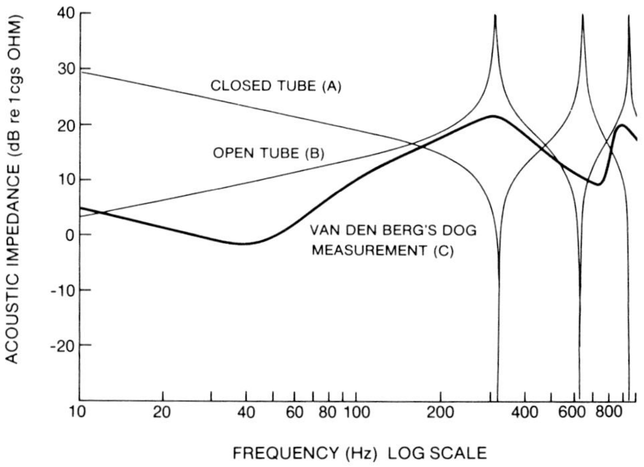

Fig. 17. Acoustic impedances of experimental subglottic tube and canine subglottic system.

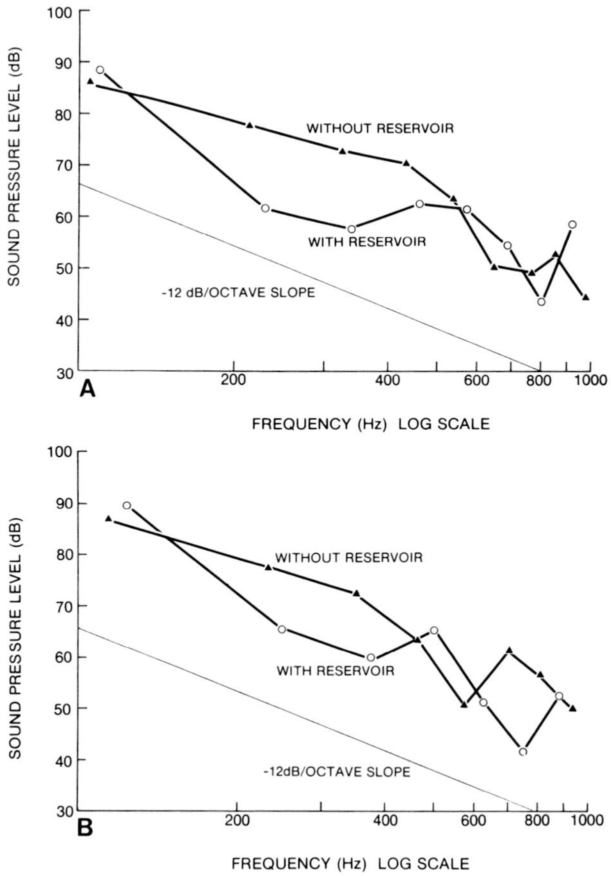

Fig. 18. Frequency spectra of isolated larynx at two different flow rates. A) 288 mL/s; B) 412 mL/s.

resulting spectra was therefore considered insignificant.

Values of acoustic input impedance were calculated[49] for the subglottic tube, assuming that the bottom end was either closed or open. The two curves are plotted in Figure 17 along with the subglottic impedance of a dog measured and reported by van den Berg.[46] Impedances are expressed as dB re 1 cgs acoustic ohm. The glass reservoir, because of its capacitance, acts almost as an open space. The impedance of the subglottic system with reservoir can therefore be approximated closely by curve B. The actual impedance curves will not have such sharp peaks and valleys as the theoretical ones shown because of damping. It can be seen that the tube with reservoir approximates the human subglottic system more closely than the tube alone.

There was no difficulty forcing the isolated larynges to make sound. Once the arytenoids were brought together by lateral tension on the threads, reproducible spectra could be obtained. There was a definite difference between the isolated human larynx spectra obtained with and without the reservoir.

Figure 18 shows spectra from a larynx excited at two different airflow rates under both conditions. It is apparent that significant acoustic coupling occurs

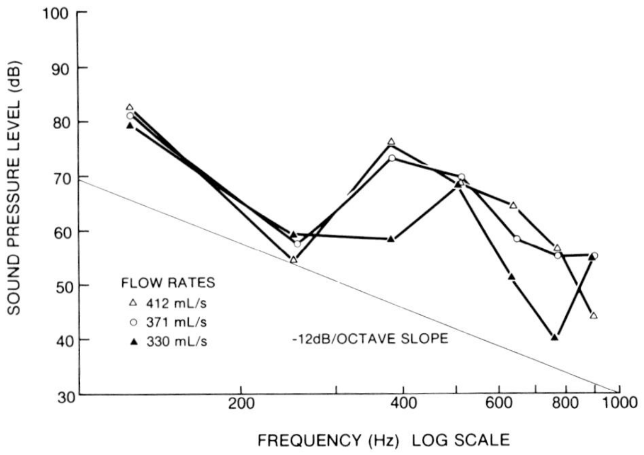

Fig. 19. Frequency spectra of artificial larynx at various flow rates.

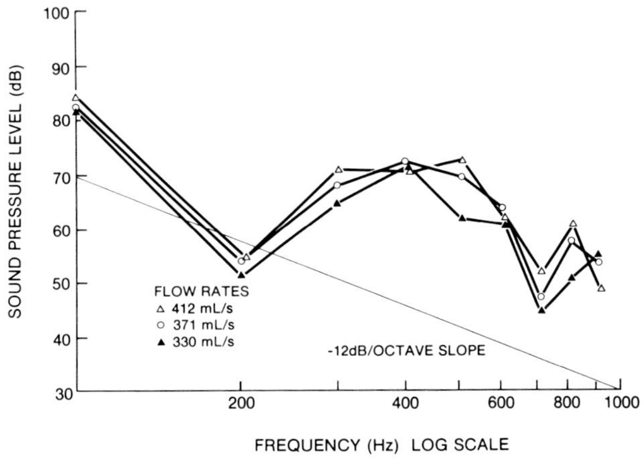

Fig. 20. Frequency spectra of artificial larynx with reed shown in Fig. 19 with a 27-mg weight attached to tip.

between the vocal folds and the subglottic air column at least in one of the two configurations. Also shown is a line with negative slope of 12 dB per octave. The laryngeal spectra generally conforms to this slope. Considering the curves generated with the reservoir present (the more relevant ones), the general pattern consists of a rapid fall-off of sound pressure level with frequency, a nadir at 250 to 450 Hz, a peak at 450 to 550 Hz, a second nadir at 750 to 825 Hz, and then a final upturn.

Spectra of the reeds in the artificial larynx showed a somewhat similar pattern (Fig. 19). The major difference is that the third, fourth, and fifth harmonics are relatively accentuated compared to the human laryngeal spectra. There was no variation of fundamental frequency with airflow rate. Furthermore, the frequency of vibration of the system was different from the resonant frequency of the reed. This indicates significant coupling between the reed and the subglottic air. Of interest is that the fundamental frequency of vibration does not at all correspond to the resonant frequency of the reed. Figure 19 shows the spectra of the C#3 reed at three rates of airflow. The fundamental frequency of vibration is approximately 14 Hz lower than its resonant frequency (138.6 Hz).

Subglottic coupling with the plastic reeds is therefore significant. Figure 20 shows the spectrum of the same reed with a 27-mg weight attached to the tip. The fundamental frequency is lower, as would be expected; however, the overall spectrum is very similar to that of the unweighted reed.

When the artificial larynx with plastic reed is put in the apparatus and air is passed through at low flow there is no vibration. As airflow rate is gradually increased the threshold flow for vibration is eventually reached (cut in) and the reed vibrates. If the airflow rate is then slowly decreased a second flow rate will be reached at which vibration ceases (cut out). For all three reed configurations tested the cut-out flow rate was lower than the cut-in rate. Table 3 shows cut-in and cut-out airflow rates for the plastic reeds. Transglottic pressure in the artificial larynx during unvoiced expiration with the reeds in place is higher than in human cadaver larynges. Figure 21 shows the transglottic pressure measured in the artificial larynx with and without reeds and in cadaver larynges.

The relative vocal efficiency of several configurations of the artificial larynx and an isolated human larynx are shown in Figure 22. Total sound pressure level is plotted against power dissipated by the air passing through the glottis. All of the reed configurations are more efficient than the human larynx. It is also evident that the D3 reed (resonant frequency 146.8 Hz) was more efficient than the C#3 reed (resonant frequency 138.6 Hz). The efficiency of the C#3 reed could be increased by gluing the small lead weight to the reed tip.

DISCUSSION

It appears that coupling between the vibrating source and the adjacent air cavities may influence the behavior of the source, particularly the plastic reeds. It is interesting that the fundamental frequency of vibration of the plastic reed system is not the same as the resonant frequency of the reed. This suggests that the system might be modeled as a pair of coupled oscillators. The current belief that coupling between the vocal cords and subglottic air changes the glottic sound spectrum very little obviously cannot be assumed for an artificial sound source.

Coupling between the vocal cords and the unconstricted supraglottic vocal tract is considered insig-

TABLE 3. CUT-IN AND CUT-OUT AIRFLOW RATES FOR DIFFERENT REEDS

	Flow Rate (ml/s)	
Reed	*Cut-In*	*Cut-Out*
C#3	370	285
C#3 (loaded)	330	205
D3	330	205

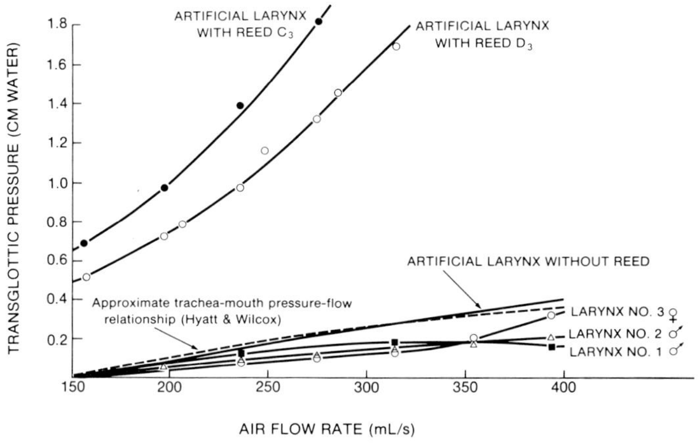

Fig. 21. Transglottic pressure of artificial and cadaver larynges as function of airflow rate.

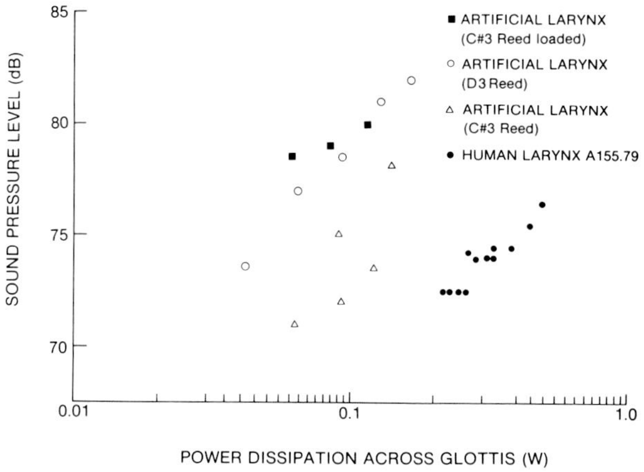

Fig. 22. Relative vocal efficiency of several configurations of artificial larynx and isolated human larynx.

nificant except at the frequencies near about 500 Hz.[38,44] When the tract is constricted, however, coupling may be enhanced and the glottic spectrum may be affected considerably.[50] No attempt was made to reproduce supraglottic coupling. Many configurations of the pharynx, palate, tongue, and lips may be produced at will by the patient and continuously adjusted according to the sound output fed back through the ear. This acoustic filter system is inside the feedback loop. Therefore, the overall effect of supraglottic coupling is extremely difficult to simulate.

With the plastic reeds in the artificial larynx it appears that the fundamental frequency of vibration cannot be varied by changing the airflow rate; however, the frequency spectrum can be varied in this manner. The corresponding change in vocal timbre might convey some degree of vocal intonation. Free breathing is possible with the artificial larynx with all expired air passing through the reed. Laryngeal resistance to airflow is higher in artificial larynges than in human cadaver larynges.

Whether this degree of resistance would be objectionable to a patient is presently unknown. It is possible, however, by moving the reed anteriorly, to create a space for air to bypass the reed within the larynx. This would lower expiratory resistance that would at the same time increase the cut in airflow rate for vocalization. Each patient would, therefore, be able to adjust the reed for his own compromise between ease of speaking and of breathing. For strenuous exercise the reed assembly may be removed entirely to provide airflow resistance of an order of magnitude similar to the resistance during unvoiced breathing in intact human larynges. The voice hysteresis demonstrated in the reed assemblies is an obvious advantage in that airflow rate during vocalization is less than would be required if there were no hysteresis.

CONCLUSIONS

A bench test apparatus has been described that can measure the frequency spectra of isolated human larynges and reed sound sources within an artificial larynx. Objective criteria have been stated, whenever possible, by which artificial sound sources may be judged. An assembly has been designed to allow the use of plastic reeds in an artificial larynx. The reed mechanism can easily be removed and cleaned. A means of increasing the efficiency of sound production has been described.

ACKNOWLEDGMENTS — The authors thank Mr. Abul Quashem for invaluable technical assistance with all aspects of this research, and Mrs. Elizabeth Wood for typing the manuscript.

REFERENCES

1. Batsakis JG. Tumors of the head and neck. Baltimore: Williams and Wilkins, 1979.

2. Martin H. Rehabilitation of the laryngectomee. Cancer 1963; 16:823-41.

3. Snidecor JC. Some scientific foundations for voice restoration. Laryngoscope 1975; 85:640-8.

4. Shedd DP, Bakamjian VY, Sako K, Schaff NG, Mann MB. Post-laryngectomy speech rehabilitation by a simplified, single-stage surgical method. Am J Surg 1974; 128:505-11.

5. Sisson GA, McConnel FMS, Logemann JA, Yeh S. Vocal rehabilitation after laryngectomy. Arch Otolaryngol 1975; 101:178-81.

6. Arnold GE. Alleviation of a laryngeal aphonia with the modern artificial larynx. Logos 1960; 3:55-67.

7. Goode RL. Artificial laryngeal devices in post-laryngectomy rehabilitation. Laryngoscope 1975; 85:677-89.

8. Dayal VS, Joy MLG, Moon RE, Lo A. Endotracheal artificial larynx — preliminary report. J Otolaryngol 1981; 10:41-4.

9. Doty RW. Neural organization of deglutition. In: Handbook of physiology IV: 1861-1902. Baltimore: Williams & Wilkins, 1968.

10. Pressman JJ, Keleman G. Physiology of the larynx. Physiol Rev 1955; 35:506-54.

11. Saunders JB deC M, Davis C, Miller ER. The mechanism of deglutition (second stage) as revealed by cine-radiography. Ann Otol Rhinol Laryngol 1951; 60:897-919.

12. Fyke FE Jr, Code CF. Resting and deglutition pressures in the pharyngo-esophageal region. Gastroenterology 1955; 29:24-34.

13. Ross BB, Gramiak R, Rahn H. Physical dynamics of the cough mechanism. J Appl Physiol 1955; 8:264-8.

14. Lear CSC, Flanagan JB Jr, Moorrees CFA. The frequency of deglutition in man. Arch Oral Biol 1965; 10:83-100.

15. Ferns BG Jr, Mead J, Opie LH. Partitioning of respiratory flow resistance in man. J Appl Physiol 1964; 19:653-8.

16. Dayal VS, Bahri H, Stone PC. Pre-epiglottic space: an anatomic study. Arch Otolaryngol 1972; 95:132-3.

17. Moon RE. The design and evaluation of an endotracheal artificial larynx. MSc thesis, University of Toronto, 1979.

18. Ingervall B, Lantz B. Significance of gravity on the passage of bolus through the human pharynx. Arch Oral Biol 1973; 18:351-6.

19. Andrews MJ, Pearson FG. Incidence and pathogenesis of tracheal injury following cuffed tube tracheostomy with assisted ventilation: analysis of a two-year prospective study. Ann Surg 1971; 173:249-63.

20. Grillo HC, Cooper JD, Geffin B, et al. A low-pressure cuff for tracheotomy tubes to minimize tracheal injury. J Thorac Cardiovasc Surg 1971; 62:898-907.

21. Galoob HD, Norris CW, Toledo PS. *In vivo* observation of tracheal microcirculation in dogs. Ann Otol Rhinol Laryngol 1977; 86:204-8.

22. Doyle JM, Dobrin PB. Transtracheal pressure exerted by endotracheal cuffs. J Biomech 1977; 8:247-52.

23. Kamen JM, Wilkinson CJ. A new low-pressure cuff for endotracheal tubes. Anesthesiology 1971; 34:482-5.

24. Stetson JB, Guess WL. Causes of damage to tissues by polymers and elastomers used in the fabrication of tracheal devices. Anesthesiology 1970; 33:635-52.

25. Wilkes GL, Samuels SL. Porous segmented polyurethanes — possible candidates as biomaterials. J Biomed Mater Res 1973; 7:541-54.

26. Boretos JW, Detmer DE, Donachy JH. Segmented polyurethane: a polyether polymer. II. Two years experience. J Biomed Mater Res 1971; 5:373-87.

27. Boretos JW. Tissue pathology and physical stability of a polyether elastomer on a three year implantation. J Biomed Mater Res 1972; 6:473-6.

28. Dayal VS, Joy MLG. Rationale and surgical technique for the endotracheal artificial larynx. Ann Otol Rhinol Laryngol 1982; 91 Suppl 95:7-10.

29. Joy MLG, Moon R, Dayal VS. Design of the endotracheal artificial larynx. Ann Otol Rhinol Laryngol 1982; 91 Suppl 95:11-7.

30. Moon R, Dayal VS, Joy MLG. Evaluation of the endotracheal artificial larynx. Ann Otol Rhinol Laryngol 1982; 91 Suppl 95:21-5.

31. Van den Berg J. Physiology and physics of voice production. Acta Physiol Pharmacol Neerl 1956; 5:40-55.

32. Van den Berg J. Direct and indirect measurement of the mean subglottic pressure. Folia Phoniatr (Basel) 1956; 8:1-24.

33. Kitzing P, Lofquist A. Subglottal and oral air pressures during phonation — preliminary investigation using a miniature transducer system. Med Bio Eng 1975; 13:644-8.

34. Isshiki N, von Leden H. Hoarseness: aerodynamic studies. Arch Otolaryngol 1964; 80:206-13.

35. Woodman de G. Rehabilitation of the larynx in cases of bilateral abductor paralysis. Arch Otolaryngol 1949; 50:91-6.

36. Arnold GE. Vocal rehabilitation of paralytic dysphonia. Arch Otolaryngol 1959; 70:444-53.

37. Van den Berg J. Imitation of Dutch vowels and words by a hemilaryngectomized subject using a throat loudspeaker as a pseudolarynx. J Acoust Soc Am 1955: 27:169-72.

38. Flanagan JL. Some properties of the glottal sound source. J Speech Hear Res 1958; 1:99-116.

39. Van den Berg J, Zantema JT, Doornenbal P Jr. On the air resistance and Bernonilli effect of the human larynx. J Acoust Soc Am 1957; 29:626-31.

40. Stevens KN, Kasowski S, Fant CGM. An electrical analog of the vocal tract. J Acoust Soc Am 1953; 25:734-42.

41. Stevens KN, House AS. An acoustical theory of vowel production and some of its implications. J Speech Hear Res 1961; 4:303-20.

42. Murry T. Biophysical requirements for new and projected procedures and devices for vocal rehabilitation after total laryngectomy. Can J Otolaryngol 1975; 4:571-8.

43. Van den Berg J, Tan TS. Results of experiments with human larynxes. Pract Otorhinolaryngol 1959; 21:425-50.

44. Van den Berg J. Sound production in isolated human larynges. Ann NY Acad Sci 1968; 155:19-27.

45. Van den Berg J. Register problems. Ann NY Acad Sci 1968; 155:129-35.

46. Van den Berg J. Modern research in experimental phoniatrics. Folia Phoniatr (Basel) 1962; 14:81-149.

47. Van den Berg J. Myoelastic-aerodynamic theory of voice production. J Speech Hear Res 1958; 1:227-44.

48. Van den Berg J. An electrical analogue of the trachea, lungs and tissues. Acta Physiol Pharmacol Neerl 1960; 9:361-85.

49. Morse PM. Vibration and sound. New York: McGraw-Hill, 1948.

50. Flanagan JL. Speech analysis synthesis and perception. New York: Springer-Verlag, 1972.

POSTNATAL DEVELOPMENT OF THE VESTIBULAR AQUEDUCT AND ENDOLYMPHATIC SAC

DIMENSIONAL ANATOMY OF THE VESTIBULAR AQUEDUCT AND THE ENDOLYMPHATIC SAC (RUGOSE PORTION) IN HUMAN TEMPORAL BONES

STATISTICAL ANALYSIS OF 79 BONES

Akira Kodama, MD

Isamu Sando, MD, DMS

This publication was supported in part by
Parke-Davis Division of Warner-Lambert
Company.

POSTNATAL DEVELOPMENT OF THE VESTIBULAR AQUEDUCT AND ENDOLYMPHATIC SAC

AKIRA KODAMA, MD ISAMU SANDO, MD, DMS

PITTSBURGH, PENNSYLVANIA

The purpose of this study was to gain basic information about the postnatal development of the vestibular aqueduct (VA) and the endolymphatic sac (ES). For this study, serial horizontal sections of 31 normal temporal bones of individuals whose ages ranged from 0 to 13 years were used. Medial view graphic reconstruction of the VA and rugose portion (RP) of the ES was performed in every case for analysis of the VA and RP. The findings of this study revealed the following new information about the postnatal development of the VA and ES. 1) The VA and RP undergo significant growth postnatally up to age 3 years. 2) In the newborn, individual variations in the VA and RP already exist and at age 3 years significantly wide individual variations which can be classified into three groups (hypoplastic, normoplastic, hyperplastic) may be recognized. 3) Hypoplastic VAs are of two types: one is fairly elongated and tubelike while the other is short and funnel-shaped. The tubelike VA seems to be the prenatal form. 4) The changes that occur with development postnatally in the area of the VA are more closely related to the changes that occur in the length of the external aperture of the VA than they are to the changes that occur in the length of the VA. 5) Development of the area of the VA is closely correlated with development of the area of the RP.

INTRODUCTION

While the rest of the labyrinth attains its adult size by the middle of fetal life, the vestibular aqueduct (VA) and the endolymphatic sac (ES) undergo great changes in late fetal and postnatal life.[1] However, to our knowledge, no thorough investigation has so far been performed into the postnatal development of the VA and ES in the human ear. Clinically, however, hypoplasia of the VA and ES has recently become of interest to otologists, who feel that pathology of these structures may possibly be associated with endolymphatic hydrops[2] or Menière's disease.[3] The purpose of this study is to report new anatomical findings on the postnatal development of the VA and ES in children.

MATERIALS AND METHODS

From the collection of 1,342 temporal bones in our Otopathology Laboratory, 31 bones from 31 different children were carefully chosen to meet the following three conditions: 1) no congenital middle ear or inner ear anomaly was present; 2) the entire VA was included in the specimen; 3) the rugose portion (RP) of the ES was included.

Temporal bones from individuals whose ages ranged from 0 to 13 years were classified into seven groups according to age. Classification and age distribution of the temporal bones are shown in Table 1. In addition, as control cases, three temporal bones from adults with no history of ear disease were selected from 157 bones to show normoplasia, hypoplasia, and hyperplasia of the VA. The variations in form of the VA and RP noted in the adult bones were compared to those observed in the bones from children.

The temporal bones were removed at autopsy and immediately fixed in formalin. After decalcification and dehydration, they were embedded in celloidin and sectioned horizontally at 20-μ. Every tenth section was stained with hematoxylin and eosin (H & E), and mounted on a glass slide for light microscopic study.

The VA is a complicated 3-dimensional structure that shows wide individual variations in form.[4,5] In studying the normal development of such an organ it is necessary to analyze an adequate number of cases, and to choose the method of analysis carefully. Recently, Egami et al[2] and Sando et al[6] reported on a new method of cochlear graphic reconstruction to study the VA and the paravestibular canaliculus (PVC); their modification of Schuknecht's graphic reconstruction techniques was used to study the morphology of these structures in the medial view. This method is relatively simple in comparison to other methods[5] used previously and enables an easier reconstruction of 3-dimensional structures graphically as 2-dimensional structures. In addition, this method allows for qualitative and quantitative analysis of these complicated structures. This graphic reconstruction method was used for all cases in the present study. The method was also used to reconstruct and draw the RP on the same medial view graph as that used to represent the VA. In each horizontal section the limit of the RP was measured from the anterior end to the posterior end of the lumen.

Because it was difficult to establish the location of the RP, particularly in specimens in which the VA was hypoplastic, we used three criteria to decide where this structure lay. Under the microscope we looked for the following three histological features to define the RP:[7] 1) rugosity; 2) loose, vascular, subepithelial connective tissue; and 3) cuboidal to columnar form of the epithelial cells.

After graphically reconstructing the VA and RP, we made several measurements (Fig. 1): 1. The areas of the VA and the RP were measured by compensating polar planimeter. 2. The length of the external aperture (EA) was taken as the distance between points a and b on Figure 1. The length of the VA was determined by drawing a line from the midportion of the internal aperture (i) to that of the external aperture (e) of the VA such that the line (ie) passed as closely as possible through the middle of the VA. This was accomplished by drawing lines parallel to line ab at 2-mm intervals and then connecting the midpoints of these lines. This resulted in line ie. The length of the line ie was then equal to the length of the VA.

For statistical analysis of the present study, the *f* test and Student's *t* test were used. In addition, for studying the relationship of the development of the VA to that of the RP and the mastoid, we also noted the rugosity of the RP and the degree of pneumatization of the temporal bone.

From the Department of Otolaryngology and Pathology, University of Pittsburgh School of Medicine, Eye and Ear Hospital of Pittsburgh. This study was supported by Research Grant NS 13787 from the National Institute of Neurological and Communicative Disorders and Stroke.

TABLE 1. MEAN VALUES (M ± SD) AND RANGES OBTAINED IN MEASUREMENTS FOR AREAS OF VA AND RP AND LENGTHS OF EA AND VA IN EACH AGE GROUP

Age Group	No. Cases	Area (mm^2) VA	Area (mm^2) RP	Length (mm) EA	Length (mm) VA
0-1 mo	4	3.3 ± 0.7 (2.5 – 4.3)	2.4 ± 1.4 (1.2 – 4.4)	1.7 ± 0.4 (1.3 – 2.2)	4.4 ± 0.2 (4.1 – 4.4)
2-12 mo	6	4.1 ± 0.8 (3.0 – 5.3)	3.2 ± 1.6 (0.8 – 5.7)	2.0 ± 0.4 (1.4 – 2.5)	5.1 ± 0.8 (4.4 – 6.2)
1-2 yr	2	3.8 ± 1.5 (2.7 – 4.8)	2.2 ± 0.8 (1.6 – 2.7)	2.1 ± 0.9 (1.4 – 2.7)	4.7 ± 0.3 (4.5 – 4.9)
3-4 yr	6	9.7 ± 5.4 (3.7 – 18.4)	5.8 ± 3.0 (2.7 – 11.2)	3.5 ± 1.1 (2.2 – 5.5)	6.1 ± 1.2 (4.4 – 7.5)
5-7 yr	4	10.4 ± 5.0 (3.7 – 14.7)	5.7 ± 3.5 (2.5 – 10.0)	3.4 ± 1.7 (1.4 – 5.4)	7.3 ± 0.9 (6.2 – 8.3)
8-10 yr	6	9.8 ± 5.7 (2.8 – 20.1)	4.6 ± 2.4 (0.9 – 7.9)	3.9 ± 1.4 (1.8 – 6.0)	6.6 ± 1.1 (5.0 – 8.3)
11-13 yr	3	16.6 ± 11.8 (5.3 – 28.8)	8.7 ± 5.9 (2.1 – 13.5)	4.6 ± 2.2 (2.4 – 6.8)	8.7 ± 1.3 (7.6 – 10.2)

VA - Vestibular aqueduct; RP - Rugose portion; EA - External aperture.

RESULTS

DEVELOPMENT OF THE VA AND RP IN CHILDREN

Figure 2 shows the areas of the VA and RP measured for each case as a function of the age of the child. Table 1 summarizes the mean values (M ± SD) and the ranges obtained for areas of the VA and RP and for lengths of the EA and VA, in each age group.

Newborns (4 Cases). In this group the areas of the VA and RP were small and the EA and VA were short; there was some individual variation except in the area of the RP. When the VA and RP were represented graphically, the EA was located inside the inner arch of the posterior semicircular canal (PSC) and the RP extended to the posterior cranial fossa in all cases. In three cases, the ES and the sigmoid sinus overlapped slightly. Figure 3 shows a medial view reconstruction of the area of the ES outside the VA for two representative cases (one with the largest VA and the other with the smallest VA) in this group. Histologically, the specimen with the

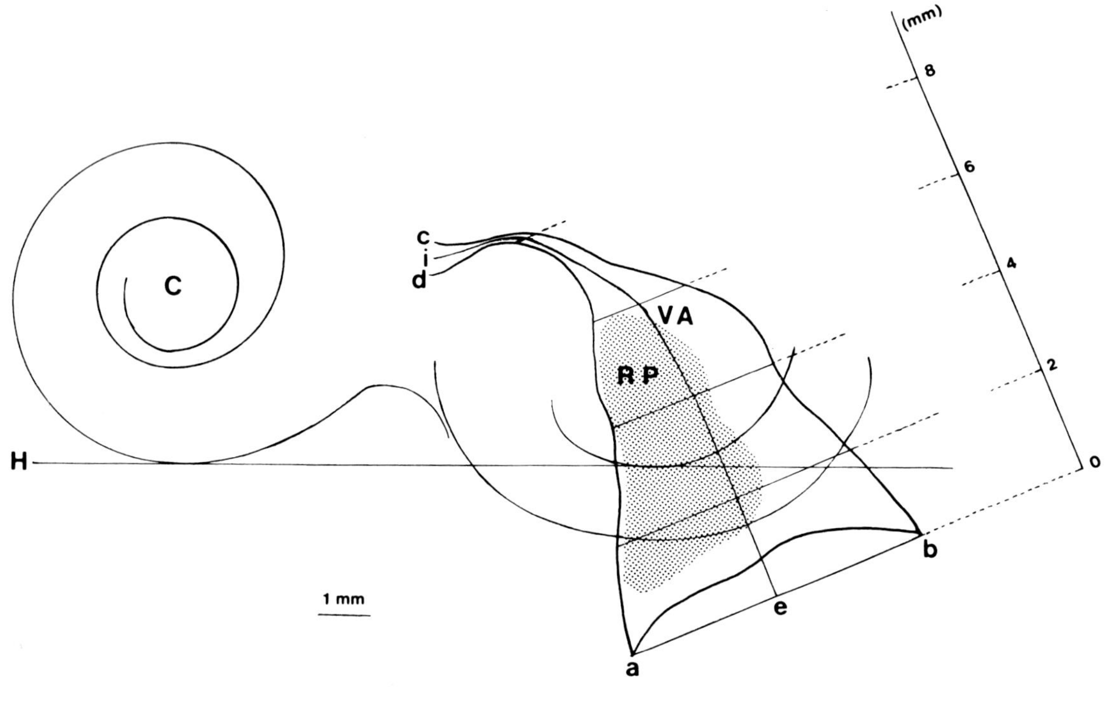

Fig. 1. Medial view reconstruction graph of VA and RP used to make measurements. Area of VA is indicated by thick lines (a-b-c-d) and area of RP is indicated by shading. Length of EA is indicated by straight line (ab) and length of VA is line (ie) made by connecting midpoint of internal aperture (i) to that of external aperture (e) of VA along middle of course of VA as marked at 2-mm intervals parallel to line ab. C - Cochlea; H - Horizontal line tangential to arches of lower basal turn of cochlea and lower inner circle of posterior canal.

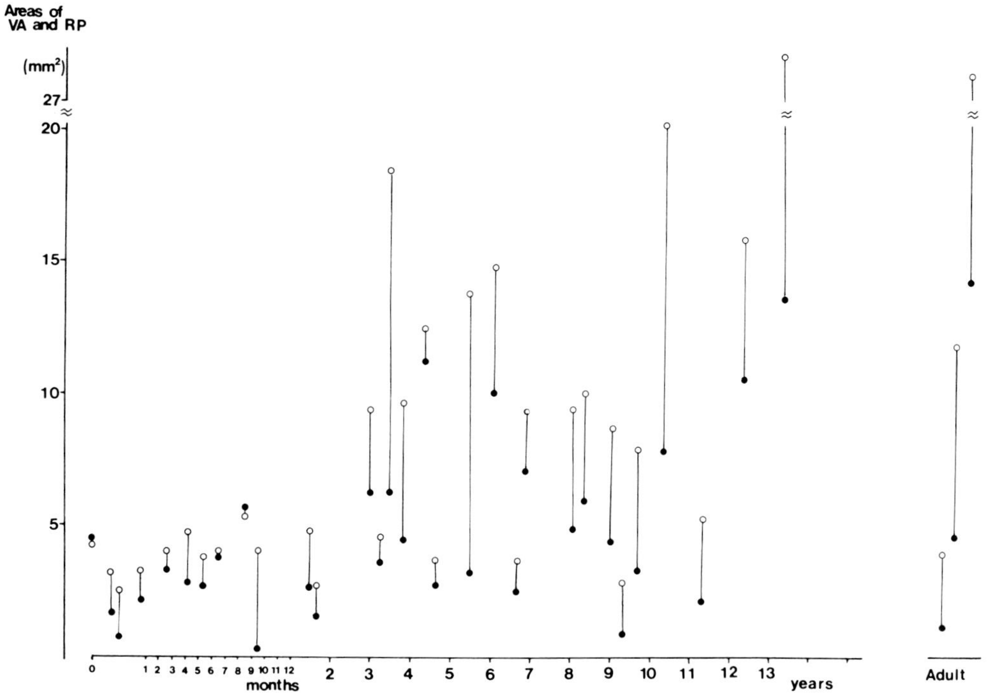

Fig. 2. Results of measuring areas of VA and RP of 31 cases shown as function of specimen age. Areas of three different types of adult VA (hypoplastic, normoplastic, and hyperplastic) are also shown. ○ - VA area; ● - RP area. Areas of VA and ES for each case are connected by line.

largest VA was highly rugose, whereas in the case with the smallest VA the rugose portion had few folds (rugosities). In every case in this group the periantral air cells were extremely poorly developed and the periaqueductal air cells could not be seen.

Two to Twelve Months (6 Cases). In this group the areas of the VA and RP and the lengths of the EA and VA were slightly greater than those in the newborn group, but the ratios of the areas of the largest VA to that of the smallest VA and of the areas of the largest RP to the smallest RP were similar to those calculated in newborn specimens. In 4 of the 6 cases, the EA was still located inside the inner arch of the PSC. The RP extended into the posterior cranial fossa to a varying distance in four

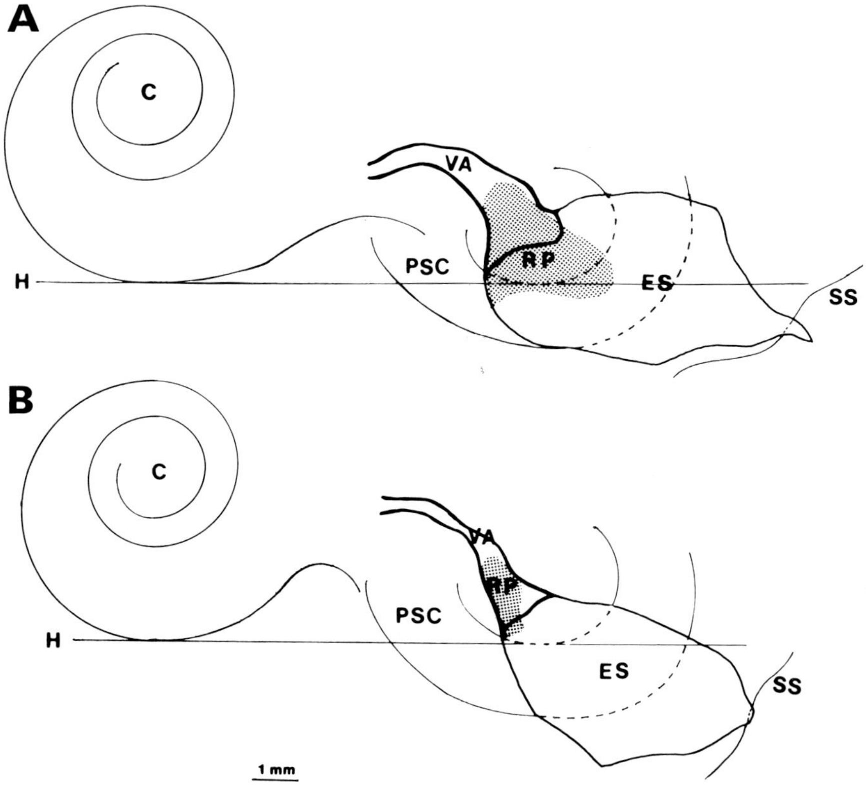

Fig. 3. Reconstruction graphs showing largest and smallest VAs observed in newborn group. A) Largest VA, from 2-day-old infant. Medial view reconstruction shows VA to be relatively small and short with somewhat funnel-shaped dilatation. ES is located inside inner arch of PSC. ES outside VA is shown by thin line extending from external aperture of VA; distal portion overlaps sigmoid sinus slightly. Area of RP is also the largest in this group, extending from VA to intraduralis of posterior cranial fossa. Ratio of segment of RP in intraduralis to entire RP is 55%. B) Smallest VA, from 12-day-old infant. Medial view reconstruction shows VA to be small, short, and tubelike. EA is located inside inner arch of PSC. Area of RP is also smallest in this group, with most of RP being contained in VA. Distal portion of ES overlaps sigmoid sinus very slightly. SS - Sigmoid sinus.

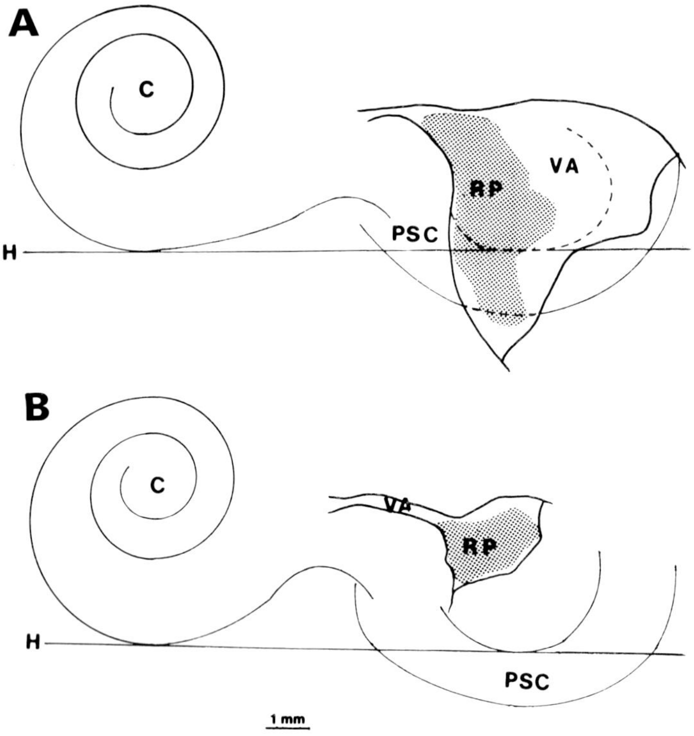

Fig. 4. Reconstruction graphs showing largest and smallest VAs observed in group aged 3 to 4 years. A) Largest VA, from 3-year-old male. Medial view reconstruction shows VA to be large, elongated, and to have marked funnel-shaped dilatations. VA extends to arch of PSC. RP is located within VA. B) Smallest VA, from 4-year-old female. Medial view reconstruction of VA shows it to be small and short with funnel-shaped dilatation. EA is located inside inner arch of PSC. Small RP is located in VA.

cases. The degree of folding evident in the RP showed about as much variation between specimens as was evident among specimens in the newborn group. The periantral air cells were poorly developed in the greater part of the mastoid region and the periaqueductal air cells were undeveloped in the specimens.

One to Two Years (2 Cases). The specimens in this group were from two children, aged 13 and 14 months. There was no evident increase in the areas of the VA and RP or in the lengths of the EA and VA from those measured in the group of specimens from children aged 2 to 12 months. In both cases, the EA was located inside the inner arch of the PSC. In one case the RP extended to the posterior cranial fossa, while in the other case the VA and RP were smaller and the RP was located within the VA. The folds of the RP were distinct in one case and relatively distinct in the other case. The periantral air cells were more developed in the specimens of this group than in those from the children aged 2 to 12 months, particularly in the upper part of the mastoid. The periaqueductal air cells were still undeveloped.

Three to Four Years (6 Cases). In this group the degree of development and the evidence of wide individual variations in the shapes of the VA and RP became marked (Figs. 2 and 4, Table 1). The mean area of the VA was 2.9 times that in the newborn group, while the mean area of the RP was 2.4 times that in the newborn group. The mean length of the EA was 2.1 times that in the newborn group, and the mean length of the VA was 1.4 times that in the newborn group. In the medial view reconstructions of the specimens in this group, all VAs showed funnel-shaped dilatations, but there was wide variation in size. The VA extended to or through the arch of the PSC in 4 of the 6 cases; in the other 2 cases it remained inside the inner arch of the PSC. In five cases, almost the entire RP was located within the VA, while in the remaining case the RP extended to the posterior cranial fossa. The largest and the smallest VAs in this group are presented in Figures 4 and 5. The folds of the RP were distinct in every case, including the smallest, funnel-shaped VA. The periantral air cells were hollowed out and moderately or well developed in every case, but no periaqueductal air cells could be seen in any specimen.

Five to Seven Years (4 Cases). In this group the areas and lengths of both the VA and RP and their wide individual variations were very similar to those of the specimens from children aged 3 to 4. In three cases, medial view reconstruction showed a funnel-shaped VA of varying size, while in the remaining case the VA was small and tubelike. In every case, the VA extended to or through the arch of the PSC and the RP was located within the VA. The folds of the RP were distinct in the three cases in which the VA was funnel-shaped, but indistinct in the other case in which the VA was tubelike (Fig. 6). The periantral air cells were moderately or well developed in each case, but the periaqueductal air cells were observed only in one case, that with the largest VA.

Eight to Ten Years (6 Cases). The areas of both the VA and the RP and the degree of individual variation in this group were similar to those seen in the

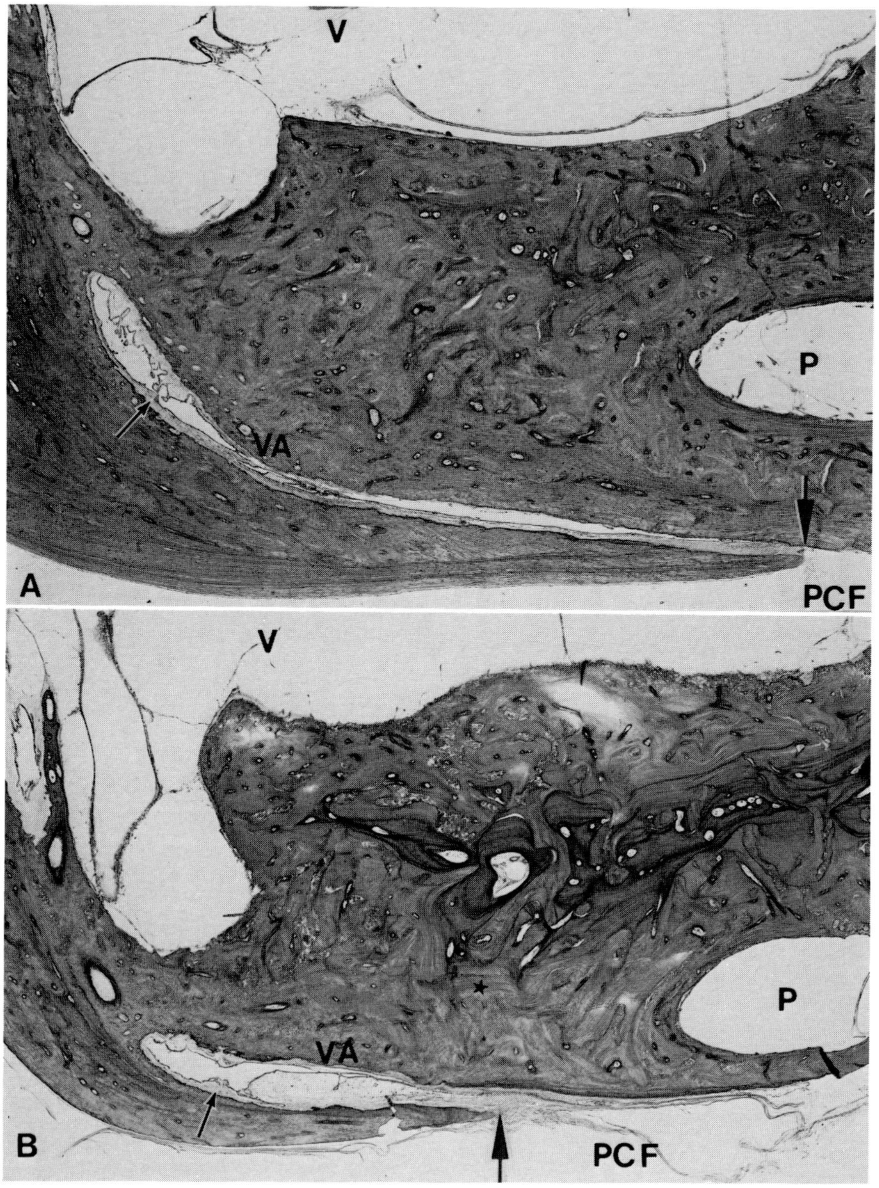

Fig. 5. Horizontal sections showing largest and smallest VAs observed in group aged 3 to 4 years. A) VA is elongated and extends to area (large arrow) near most posterior portion of PSC (P). RP is located in VA and folds are distinct (small arrow). B) VA has funnel-shaped dilatation and is short; external aperture (large arrow) of VA leading to posterior cranial fossa (PCF) is close to midportion (★) of plane of PSC (P). RP is located in VA and folds are moderately well developed (small arrow). V - Vestibule. (H & E stain, x 20)

specimens from children aged 3 to 4 years. The degree of variation in the appearance and the location of both the VA and the RP in medial view reconstructions were also similar to that seen among specimens in the 3 to 4-year-old and the 5 to 7-year-old groups. The folds of the RP were distinct in every case except one, in which the VA was tubelike. The periantral air cells were underdeveloped in two cases and moderately developed in the other four cases. The periaqueductal air cells could be seen only in the specimen with the largest VA.

Eleven to Thirteen Years (3 Cases). The degree of variation in development of the VA and ES among the cases in this group was similar to that seen in the other three groups of cases older than three years. The folds of the RP were distinct in two cases in which the VA was funnel-shaped, but the RP was extremely poorly developed in the third case, in which the VA was tubelike. The periantral air cells were moderately to well developed in each case. The periaqueductal air cells were observed only in the specimen which had the largest VA.

FORMS OF THE VA AND RP IN ADULT SPECIMENS

In addition to measuring the areas of the VA and RP and the lengths of the EA and VA in children's bones, we measured these structures in three different types of adult temporal bones. These measurements are shown in Figure 2 and Table 2 and were used as controls in our study. These three cases are described below.

Hypoplastic VA (38-year-old male). The RP was indistinct. Its folds were extremely poorly developed and there was very little subepithelial connective tissue in this portion. Medial view reconstruction showed the VA to be small and short and somewhat funnel-shaped. The EA remained inside the

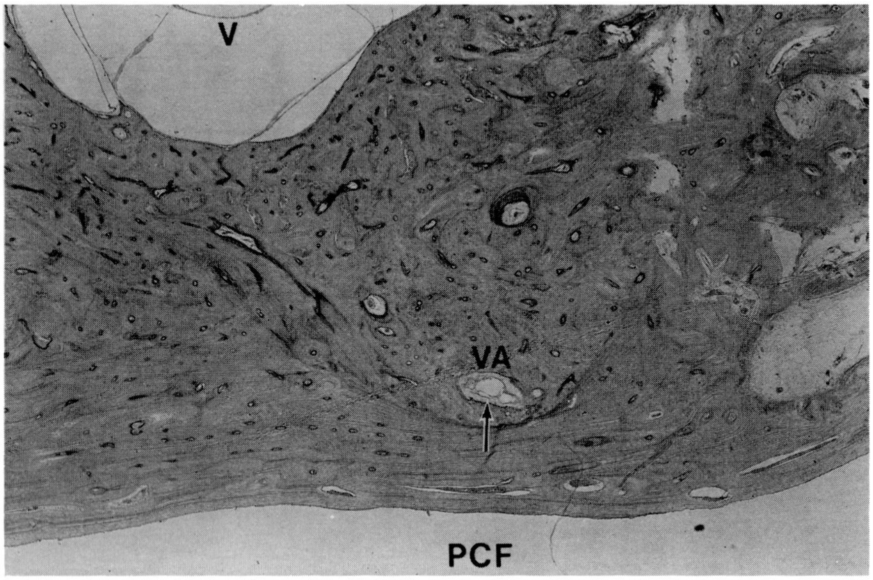

Fig. 6. Horizontal section showing tubelike VA observed in specimen in group aged 5 to 7 years. VA has no funnel-shaped dilatation and its distal portion is dislocated anteriorly. RP is extremely small and folds are extremely poorly developed (arrow). (H & E stain, x 20).

inner arch of the PSC. The extremely small RP was located in the VA. The periantral air cells were underdeveloped and the periaqueductal cells could not be seen.

Normoplastic VA (65-year-old female). The folds of the RP and the subepithelial loose connective tissue were distinct. Medial view reconstruction showed that there was a well-developed, funnel-shaped dilatation of the VA. The EA extended to the area posteromedial to the outer arch of the PSC. The RP was located in the VA. The periantral air cells were moderately developed, but the periaqueductal air cells could not be observed.

Hyperplastic VA (69-year-old female). The RP was distinctly rugose and contained subepithelial connective tissue. Medial view reconstruction showed that an extremely well-developed, funnel-shaped dilatation of the VA was present. The VA extended to the area posteromedial to the PSC and the EA was far removed from the outer arch of the PSC. The large RP was located in the VA. The periantral air cells were well developed but the periaqueductal air cells could not be observed.

STATISTICAL ANALYSIS

The mean values (M ± SD) and ranges for the areas of VA and RP and the lengths of the EA and VA obtained in each age group are presented in Table 1. A statistically significant difference ($p<0.05$) existed between the areas of the VA and RP in the specimens from children aged less than 12 months and those from children aged 3 to 4 years (Fig. 2 and Table 1). However, we could not find any significant difference ($p<0.2$) between the areas of the VA and RP in bones from children aged 3 to 4 years and these areas in bones from older children. Wide variations and a marked increase in the area of both the VA and RP were noted in the 19 cases from children aged 3 years or older in comparison with these measurements in the 12 cases from children aged younger than 3 years.

DISCUSSION

Some interesting aspects of the developmental anatomy of the ES and VA are presented by previous reports. In the human fetus, the endolymphatic sac undergoes great changes throughout fetal life and even into early postnatal life,[1,7] whereas the labyrinth reaches its maximum size and fully differentiates by the middle of fetal life. By midterm, the endolymphatic sac (in which the low rugae had developed by eight weeks of gestation) is small and fairly straight, lying almost parallel to the common crus. During the latter half of fetal life and in early postnatal life[1] as the posterior cranial fossa enlarges three significant gross changes in the endolymphatic duct and sac occur: 1) bending of the duct, 2) enlargement of the sac, and 3) tendency of the sac to separate from the sigmoid sinus. During the same period remodeling of the otic capsule in the region of the vestibular aqueduct takes place[8] and the shape of the external aperture of the VA alters to accommodate changes in position of the ES.[9]

Observations on the postnatal development of the VA and ES made in the course of this study are as follows.

TABLE 2. MEASUREMENTS OF THREE TYPES OF VA OBSERVED IN ADULT TEMPORAL BONES

Type of VA	*Area of VA* (mm^2)	*Area of RP* (mm^2)	*Length of EA* (*mm*)	*Length of VA* (*mm*)
Hypoplastic	4.0	1.2	3.1	5.2
Normoplastic	11.8	4.6	3.8	7.8
Hyperplastic	28.3	14.3	5.9	11.1

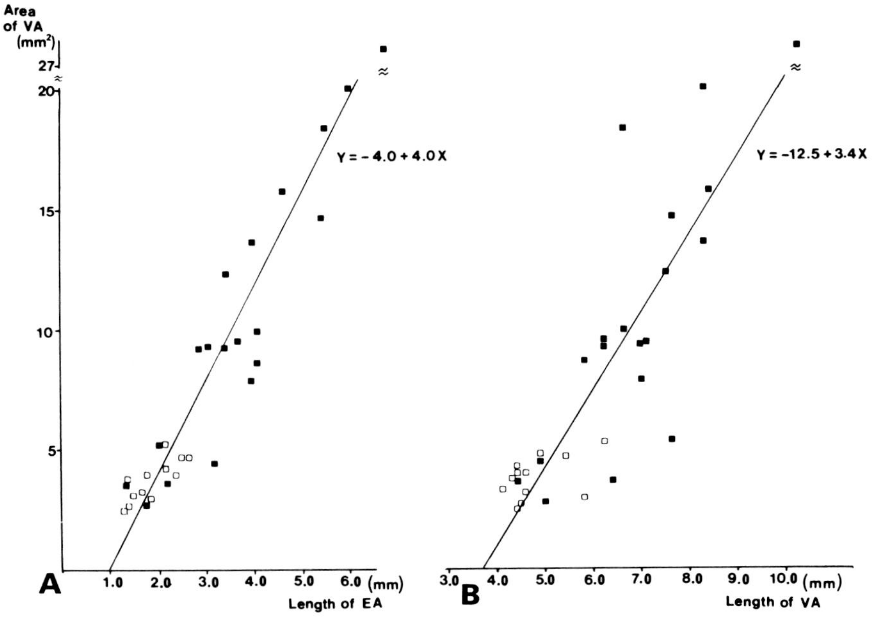

Fig. 7. Relationships of A) area of VA to length of EA and B) area of VA to length of VA. Area of VA is more closely correlated to length of EA than it is to length of VA. □ - Under age 3; ■ - Age 3 or older.

DEVELOPMENT OF THE VA AND RP

For the first year after birth the VA is small and shows some individual variations in form. The RP is also small but shows wide individual variation in form. By ages 3 to 4 years marked development of the VA and RP may be noted. Wide individual variations, similar to those seen in the VA and ES of adults[4,5] may be observed. The VAs and RPs of children aged 5 to 7 years, 8 to 10 years, and 11 to 13 years were not statistically different from those of children aged 3 to 4 years. Our findings may be summarized as follows: for the first year after birth, growth of the VA and RP is fairly gradual. By age 3 years, the VA and RP have reached nearly adult size. However, there is wide variation in the sizes of the VA and RP among individuals. By age 3 to 4 years the average length of the EA is close to that of adults as measured by Anson et al.[4]

Significant increase in head circumference continues until age 3 years,[10] and although pneumatization of the mastoid usually begins in late fetal life, significant mastoid cell formation takes place postnatally. Mastoid air cells form as the mastoid process grows, a process that becomes marked by age 2 years, and by age 3 years the mastoid is fairly well developed.[11,12] The development of the VA and ES appears to be closely associated with the development of the posterior cranial fossa and of the mastoid region of the temporal bone, and to be mostly completed by age 3 years.

ANATOMICAL CORRELATION

Both the relationships of the area of VA to the length of the EA and of the area of the VA to the length of the VA during development showed statistically significant correlations. However, the former relationship (correlation coefficient = 0.94) was more closely correlated than the latter (correlation coefficient = 0.85) (Fig. 7). It appears that during postnatal development of the VA the lengths of the EA in particular and of the VA in general increase as the area of the VA increases. Statistically significant correlations ($p<0.01$) exist between the area of the VA and that of the RP at all developmental stages. However, the correlation for the group of specimens from children younger than age 3 years is somewhat different from that for the children aged 3 years or older. The correlation coefficient and regression line for the former group were r

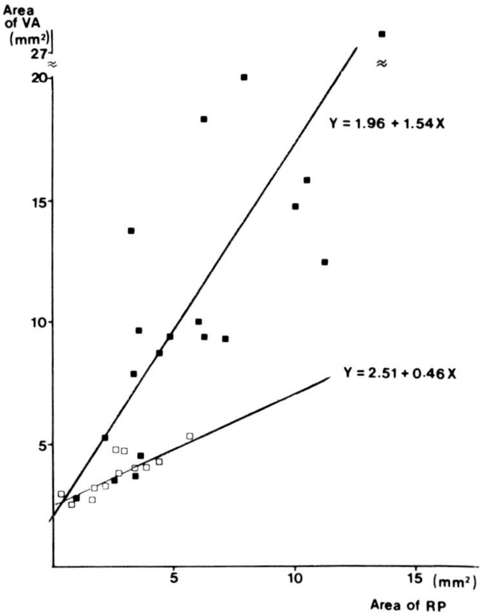

Fig. 8. Relationship between area of VA and area of RP. □ - Under age 3; ■ - Age 3 or older.

TABLE 3. MEAN AREAS (M ± SD) OF EACH TYPE OF VA IN SPECIMENS AGED 3 YEARS OR OLDER (19 CASES)

Type of VA	No.	Area of VA (mm^2)	Area of RP (mm^2)	Length of EA (mm)	Length of VA (mm)
Hypoplastic	5	4.0 ± 0.9	3.4 ± 1.2	2.2 ± 0.7	5.8 ± 1.4
Normoplastic	11	11.0 ± 2.7	6.5 ± 2.9	3.9 ± 0.7	7.1 ± 0.8
Hyperplastic	3	22.4 ± 5.6	9.2 ± 3.8	6.1 ± 0.7	8.4 ± 1.8

= 0.9, Y = 2.51 + 0.46X, and those for the latter group were r = 0.81, Y = 1.96 + 1.54 X (Fig. 8).

In regard to the relationship between position of the VA and RP and age, Zechner and Altman[13] reported that the RP in the newborn lies outside of the VA and gradually becomes incorporated into the bony capsule. In our study, medial view reconstruction of the specimens demonstrated that the RP extends from the VA to the posterior cranial fossa in newborns. In children aged 2 to 12 months the relationship between these structures was similar to that seen in newborns. By age 3 to 4 years, however, almost the entire RP was located within the VA in all of our specimens but one. In the specimens from children older than age 4 years most of the RP was located within the VA in every case. The statistical and positional alterations in the relationship between the VA and RP during development that we have reported appear to be the result of differences in rate of development of these structures. Although both the VA and RP grow postnatally and both appear to achieve almost their adult sizes by age 3 years, and although their growth is correlated, in actuality the VA grows more than does the RP (Fig. 8). Thus, most of the RP appears to become incorporated into the VA by the time a child is aged 3 years.

CLASSIFICATION OF VA

Assuming that the VA is mostly developed by age 3 years, the 19 specimens in our study group of 31 specimens that were from individuals older than age 3 years may be classified into three groups on the basis of size of the VA — hypoplastic, normoplastic, and hyperplastic (Fig. 7 and Table 3). According to the classification system established by studying 79 adult normal temporal bones,[14] the VAs with areas measuring 8 to 18 mm^2 are classified as normoplastic, those with areas under 8 mm^2 are classified as hypoplastic, and those with areas over 18 mm^2 are classified as hyperplastic. Of the 19 specimens, 5 (26%) in our study group that were older than age 3 years were classified as hypoplastic, 11 (58%) as normoplastic, and 3 (16%) as hyperplastic.

As shown in Table 3, VAs of each type are markedly different in area, and the area of the RP and the lengths of the EA and VA also differ among specimens of the three groups. The mean areas of the hypoplastic VA and RP are approximately one third and one half of those of the VA and RP of the normoplastic group, respectively, and the areas of the hyperplastic VA and RP are approximately 2 times and 1.5 times larger, respectively, than those of the normoplastic VA and RP. The average length of the EA varied more from group to group than did the average length of the VA (Table 3 and Fig. 9).

Hypoplastic VA. When the lengths and areas of both the VA and the RP in specimens with hypoplastic VAs are compared to those in newborns, it may be seen that the EA and VA in the former group are slightly larger: the area of the VA is 1.2 times that of the newborns, the area of the RP is 1.4 times that of newborns, and the lengths of the EA and of the VA are both 1.3 times those of newborns (Fig. 9 and Tables 1 and 3). The hypoplastic VAs in this group may be subclassified into two different types as follows: in 3 of the 5 hypoplastic VA cases the VA was small, fairly elongated, and tubelike as seen in Figure 6, while in the remaining two cases the VA was small and short with a funnel-shaped dilatation such as seen in Figures 4B and 5B.

In the specimens that had tubelike VAs, the EA extended to the arch of the PSC in two cases and the EA was located inside the inner arch of the PSC in another case. The RP was located within the VA in every case. In all three cases the areas of the RP were extremely small, the folds were poorly developed, and the loose subepithelial connective tissue was hypoplastic. The VA and RP were only slightly larger than those of the newborns, but the VA was fairly elongated. The features, size, and location of the tubelike hypoplastic VA and RP were similar to those of the tubelike hypoplastic VA and RP in the newborn group and the adult control case. The periantral air cells were moderately developed and pneumatized in every case, but no periaqueductal air cells were found (Table 4).

In both specimens that had funnel-shaped VAs, the EA was located inside the inner arch of the PSC. The RP was incorporated in the VA in one case, but extended to the posterior cranial fossa in the other case. The areas of the RPs were small in these two cases, the folds were moderately well developed, and the loose subepithelial connective tissue was fairly thick. The features, size, and location of the VA and ES in these two cases were similar to those in three cases (excluding the specimen with the smallest VA) in the newborn group. In these two cases, the periantral air cells were underdeveloped and the periaqueductal air cells were not developed.

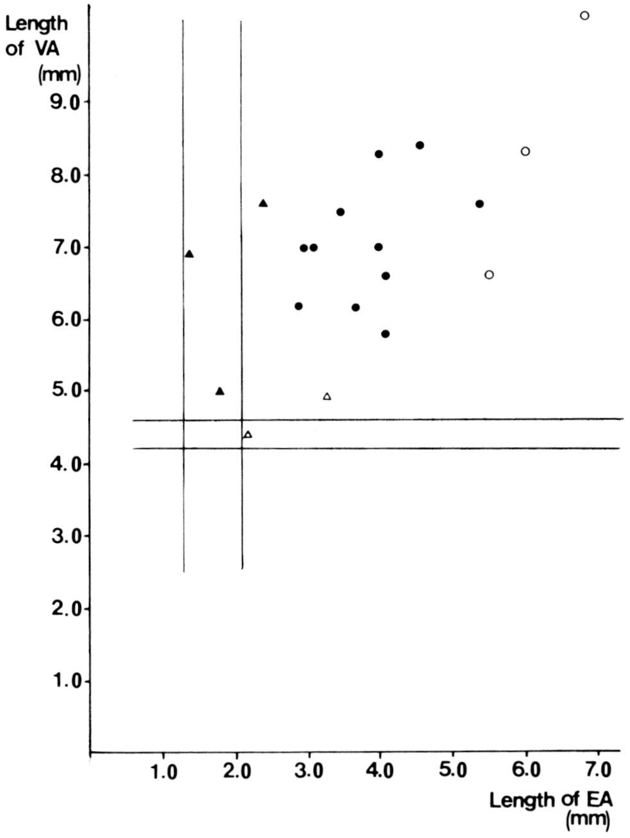

Fig. 9. Lengths of EA and VA for each of four different types of VA: ▲ - Tubelike hypoplasia; △ - Funnel-shaped hypoplasia; ● - Normoplasia; ○ - Hyperplasia. Parallel vertical lines indicate limits of 1 SD of mean of length of EA; parallel horizontal lines indicate limits of 1 SD of mean of length of VA in newborn group.

In specimens in which the VA was tubelike, pneumatization of the temporal bone had apparently proceeded as it had in the majority of specimens with normoplastic VAs, whereas extremely poor pneumatization was observed in the specimens from newborns. In spite of the postnatal growth of the temporal bone evident in those cases, the VA was still hypoplastic and the folds of the RP were poorly developed, just as they were in the specimens with tubelike VA in the newborn group. Thus, we feel that tubelike VAs are likely to be the result of prenatal hypoplasia of this structure; to contain hypoplastic ES; and to persist even after maximum postnatal growth of the posterior cranial fossa has been obtained.

Normoplastic VA. In the specimens with normoplastic VAs, the VA and RP were on the average 3.3 and 2.7 times, and the lengths of EA and VA were 2.3 and 1.6 times those of the newborn group, respectively. All VAs of this group showed funnel-shaped dilatations and extended to or through the arch of the PSC. Almost the entire RP was located within the VA in every case. The area of the RP was moderate in size in all the cases. The features, size, and location of the normoplastic VAs and RPs were similar to those of the normoplastic VAs and RPs in the adult control cases. The folds of the RPs were distinct and the loose subepithelial connective tissue was thick. Development of periantral air cells varied from underdeveloped to well developed in this group, but in the majority of cases (6 cases) the mastoid was moderately well pneumatized. Periaqueductal air cells were poorly developed in most of the cases in this group.

TABLE 4. RELATIONSHIP BETWEEN THREE TYPES OF VA AND DEVELOPMENT OF MASTOID AIR CELLS

Type of VA	No.	*Periantral Air Cells* Under-developed	Moderately Developed	Well Developed	*Periaqueductal Air Cells* (−)	(+)
Hypoplastic	5	2F	3T		3T,2F	
Normoplastic	11	2	6	3	10	1
Hyperplastic	3		2	1	1	2

T - Tubelike VA; F - Funnel-shaped VA.

Hyperplastic VA. The areas of the VAs and RPs in these specimens were approximately 6.8 and 3.8 times those of the VA and RP in the newborn specimens, and the lengths of the EA and VA were 3.6 and 1.9 times those of newborns. Medial view reconstruction of the VAs in this group showed that all specimens had funnel-shaped VAs with wide dilatations and that all the VAs extended to or through the arch of the PSC (Fig. 4A). Almost the entire RP was located within the VA. In every case the areas of the RP were large. The features, size, and location of the hyperplastic VAs and RPs in these specimens were quite similar to those in the adult specimens with hyperplastic VAs and RPs. The folds of the RP were distinct and the loose subepithelial connective tissue layer was thick. The periantral air cells were moderately to well pneumatized, and periaqueductal air cells were observed in 2 of the 3 cases.

CONCLUSION

In conclusion, summarizing the findings of this study, the following observations may be made regarding the postnatal development of the VA and ES.

1. In newborns the VA and RP are small, but already show individual variations.
2. The VA and RP grow postnatally. They increase in area until age 3 years, by which time they have attained almost their adult sizes. They show wide individual variations in form.
3. Statistically significant correlations exist between the area of the VA and the length of the EA, and between the area of the VA and the length of the VA. However, the former shows a higher correlation.
4. The development of the area of the VA is correlated with that of the area of the RP.
5. Postnatally developed VAs can be classified into three groups (hypoplastic, normoplastic, and hyperplastic) based on the size of the VA.

6. There are two types of hypoplastic VA: a fairly elongated, tubelike VA with poorly developed RP, and a short, funnel-shaped VA with fairly distinct rugosities. The tubelike VA appears to represent prenatal hypoplasia.

Using the findings obtained in this study as normal controls, further statistical investigations to find a correlation between hypoplastic VA and ES and endolymphatic hydrops or Menière's disease would be extremely worthwhile.

Dr. Kodama is presently Assistant Professor at the Department of Otolaryngology, University of Teikyo School of Medicine, Toyko.

ACKNOWLEDGMENTS — The authors wish to express their gratitude to Eugene N. Myers, MD, Professor and Chairman, and to Franklin Owen Black, MD, Department of Otolaryngology, University of Pittsburgh School of Medicine, for encouraging them to study this subject and for giving helpful criticism during the preparation of this paper. Appreciation is also expressed to Mrs. Ruth Anderson for her assistance in preparing this paper.

REFERENCES

1. Watzke D, Bast TH. The development and structure of the otic (endolymphatic) sac. Anat Rec 1950; 106:361-79.

2. Egami T, Sando I, Black FO. Hypoplasia of the vestibular aqueduct and endolymphatic sac in endolymphatic hydrops. Trans Am Acad Ophthalmol Otolaryngol ORL 1978; 86:327-39.

3. Stahle T, Wilbrand H. The vestibular aqueduct in patients with Meniere's disease: a tomographic and clinical investigation. Acta Otolaryngol (Stockh) 1974; 78:36-48.

4. Anson BJ, Donaldson JA, Warpela RL, Winch TR. A critical appraisal of the anatomy of the perilymphatic system in man. Laryngoscope 1964; 74:945-66.

5. Ogura Y, Clemis JD. A study of the gross anatomy of the human vestibular aqueduct. Ann Otol Rhinol Laryngol 1971; 80: 813-25.

6. Sando I, Egami T, Harada T. Course and contents of the paravestibular canaliculus. Ann Otol Rhinol Laryngol 1980; 89: 147-56.

7. Bast TH, Anson BJ. The temporal bone and the ear. Springfield: Charles C Thomas, 1949; chap 2.

8. Anson BJ, Bast TH. The development of the otic capsule in the region of the vestibular aqueduct. Quart Bull Northw U Med Sch 1951; 25:96-104.

9. Anson BJ, Donaldson JA. Surgical anatomy of the temporal bone. Part II. 3rd ed. Philadelphia: W B Saunders, 1981.

10. Westropp CK, Barber CR. Growth of the skull in young children. Part 1. Standards of head circumference. J Neurosurg Psychiatr 1956; 19:52-4.

11. Anson BJ. The sense organ. Part 2. Organ of hearing and equilibrium. In: Anson BJ, ed. Morris' human anatomy. New York: McGraw-Hill Company, 1966; 1171-227.

12. Pearson AA. Developmental anatomy of the ear. In: English GM, ed. Otolaryngology. Hagerstown: Harper & Row, 1979: 15-40.

13. Zechner G, Altman F. Histological studies on the human endolymphatic duct and sac. Pract Otorhinolaryngol 1969; 31: 65-83.

14. Kodama A, Sando I. Dimensional anatomy of the vestibular aqueduct and the endolymphatic sac (rugose portion) in human temporal bones. Statistical analysis of 79 bones. Ann Otol Rhinol Laryngol 1982; 91 Suppl 96:13-20.

DIMENSIONAL ANATOMY OF THE VESTIBULAR AQUEDUCT AND THE ENDOLYMPHATIC SAC (RUGOSE PORTION) IN HUMAN TEMPORAL BONES

STATISTICAL ANALYSIS OF 79 BONES

AKIRA KODAMA, MD

ISAMU SANDO, MD, DMS

PITTSBURGH, PENNSYLVANIA

The purpose of this study was to investigate the anatomy of the vestibular aqueduct (VA) and rugose portion (RP) of the endolymphatic sac. Serial horizontal sections of 79 normal temporal bones of individuals aged 20 to 102 years were used. Medial view graphic reconstruction of the VA was performed for each specimen to determine the area, length, angle and position of the VA. The relationship between the width of the VA and the area of the VA, and the relationship between the degree of development of the VA and the degree of development of the temporal bone (periaqueductal pneumatization and the otic capsule in the periaqueductal region) were also investigated. Measurements of the RP were also made and further histological study of the RP was performed on 30 selected specimens. We found that 1) the VA in adult temporal bones varies in size and can be classified as hypoplastic, normoplastic, or hyperplastic; 2) many of the VAs in each group have similar sizes, although they vary in length, angle, or position; 3) all or most of the RP was located within the VA in all but one specimen, which had a hypoplastic VA (in this specimen more than half of the entire RP extended into the posterior cranial fossa); 4) the histology of the RP was characteristic in each type of VA; and 5) the degree of development of the VA seems to correlate with the degree of development of the otic capsule in the periaqueductal region.

INTRODUCTION

The vestibular aqueduct (VA), which is the bony canal containing the endolymphatic duct and endolymphatic sac (ES), and the rugose portion (RP) of the ES have recently become of particular interest to otologists because apparent hypoplasia of these structures in some cases has been observed in the temporal bones from patients with endolymphatic hydrops or Menière's disease. Several articles[1-7] have discussed whether this hypoplasia of the VA and ES was abnormal (anomalous) or whether hypoplasia was simply a normal variation. To answer this question, we examined in great detail the anatomical variations of the VA and ES, especially the RP of the ES, which occur in normal adult temporal bones.

MATERIALS AND METHODS

Seventy-nine normal temporal bones from 79 human adults, aged 20 to 102 years, were used for this study. The temporal bones were removed at autopsy and immediately fixed in 10% formalin. After decalcification and dehydration they were embedded in celloidin and sectioned horizontally at 20-μ intervals. Every tenth section was stained with H & E for light microscopic study.

The anatomy of the VA, RP, and their related structures was studied by making the following quantitative and qualitative analyses.

GRAPHIC RECONSTRUCTION (79 SPECIMENS)

Graphic reconstruction was used to determine the area, length, angle, and position of the VA in all 79 specimens. The medial view graphic reconstruction method developed by Egami et al,[8] which enables an easier reconstruction of 3-dimensional structures graphically as 2-dimensional structures, was used.

Area of VA. The area of the VA in each specimen was measured by compensatory polar planimetry. The VAs were classified as described previously[9] into three groups on the basis of size of the VA: hypoplastic, normoplastic, and hyperplastic. These terms were also used to describe degree of development of the VA. In addition, we developed the LAP system to analyze and classify the individual VAs statistically. By this system, the length (L) of the VA, the angle (A) of the VA, and the position (P) of the VA with respect to that of the posterior semicircular canal (PSC) were used to categorize each VA studied. The parameters of these three components were defined as follows (Fig. 1).

Length of VA (L). The length of the VA was taken to be the distance along the middle of the VA (i to e in Fig. 1) from the internal to the external aperture of the VA. Short VAs located in the area superomedial to the inner arch of the bony PSC were categorized as belonging to group L_1. Intermediate VAs extended to or through the area medial to the PSC, but not far (within 1 mm) from the outer arch of the PSC (L_2). Long VAs (L_3) extended inferomedially beyond the outer arch of the PSC.

Angle of VA (A). The angle of the VA was defined as the angle obtained by extending two lines drawn tangential to the anterior and posterior margins of the distal portion of the VA to their point of intersection. In narrow VAs this angle was less than 20° (A_1). Some VAs had moderately wide angles (20 to 40°)(A_2). Other VAs had even wider angles, over 40° (A_3).

Position of VA (P). The position of the VA was determined according to which portion of the PSC the midportion of the distal part of the VA lay against: P_1, anterior portion of the PSC; P_2, inferior portion of the PSC; P_3, posterior portion of the PSC.

Width of VA (79 Specimens). The width of the VA was measured at the proximal rugose portion of the ES. It was equal to the length of the line cd in Figure 2.

DETAILED ANALYSIS OF THE RP AND ES IN THE VA (30 REPRESENTATIVE SPECIMENS)

The following analyses were performed on 30 specimens, 10 carefully selected from each of the three categories of VA, because the ES were sufficiently well preserved for detailed study.

From the Departments of Otolaryngology and Pathology, University of Pittsburgh School of Medicine, Eye and Ear Hospital of Pittsburgh. This study was supported by Research Grant NS 13787 from the National Institute of Neurological and Communicative Disorders and Stroke.

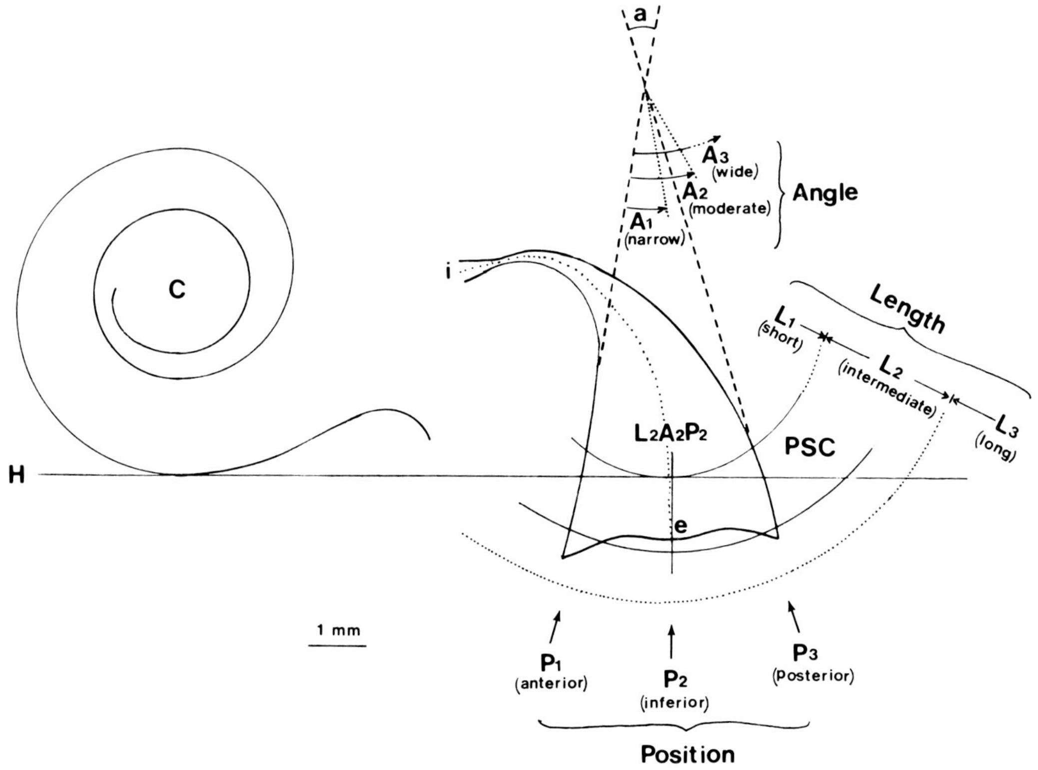

Fig. 1. Schematic drawing of VA showing how each of the following three components was measured: length (L) of VA, angle (A) of VA, and position (P) of VA with relation to posterior semicircular canal (PSC) (see Methods). In VA graphically reconstructed, midportion of external aperture (e) extends to area medial to PSC (L2), angle of VA (a) is 26° (A2), and external aperture (e) of VA is located in vicinity of inferior part (P2) of PSC. Thus, this VA is symbolically represented as L2A2P2. Line H (tangential to arches of lower basal turn of cochlea and lower inner circle of PSC) is determined as constant horizontal line for comparison in each case. This comparison is essential to correct any erroneous impressions of location and configuration of VA created by various horizontal sectioning angles. C - Cochlea.

Certain areas of the ES in the VA and RP were graphically drawn on the same medial view graph as that used to represent the VA and were measured carefully. For this measurement the most anterior and posterior ends of the ES in the VA and RP in each horizontal section were defined as their respective borders. The ES in the cranial fossa was not drawn because conventional serial horizontal sections of temporal bones do not contain the distal part of the ES in the cranial fossa.

The morphological condition of the epithelial cells, folds, loose subepithelial connective tissue, and vascularity in the RP were noted. The vascularity in the RP was measured by projecting the slides of the temporal bone section that contained the RP with a microprojector so an area of 1.3 mm on the microscope slide filled a circular area of diameter 18.2 cm on the paper. This magnification by 140 times allowed us to count every vessel in this area. Vessels were counted in the same way in another area of the RP about 400 μ distant. The average number of vessels in the two areas of the RP was then defined as the vascularity of the RP.

DEGREE OF PNEUMATIZATION AND THICKNESS OF THE OTIC CAPSULE (79 SPECIMENS).

We investigated the mastoid pneumatization in the periaqueductal region and development of the otic capsule in the periaqueductal region.

The degree of periaqueductal pneumatization was classified according to Stahle and Wilbrand,[1] and Plantenga and Browning,[5] as group I (large air cells), group II (varying types of pneumatization, mostly small air cells, or small bone marrow spaces), and group III (no pneumatization).

A quantitative assessment of the degree of development of the otic capsule in the periaqueductal region was performed as follows (Fig. 2). A horizontal temporal bone section at the lowest level of the inner arch of the PSC was selected in each specimen. Using the microprojector, the periaqueductal region of the temporal bone section was projected and drawn. A line (S) on the posterior cranial fossa surface close to the PSC and a line tangential to the medial PSC perimeter (ab) were drawn; then line mn was drawn at right angles to line S, connecting it to the midpoint of line ab. The length of line mn then represents the thickness of the bone between the PSC and posterior cranial fossa, and was used as an indication of the degree of development of the otic capsule in the periaqueductal region.

RESULTS

CLASSIFICATION OF SIZE OF THE VA

The results obtained from measuring the areas of the VA in each specimen are shown in Figure 3. In 17 of the 79 specimens the VA was classified as hypoplastic (under 8 mm^2), in 38 as normoplastic (8 to 18 mm^2), and in 24 as hyperplastic (over 18 mm^2). In 14 of the 24 specimens with hyperplastic VAs the entire area of the VA could not be measured because a part of the VA extended below the level of the lowest section available for study.

The difference in size between the VAs in the three different groups was marked: the mean values (M $\pm$ SD) for the area of the VA were 5.5 $\pm$ 1.1 mm^2 in the hypoplastic VA group, 12.7 $\pm$ 5.3 mm^2 in the normoplastic VA group, and more than 24.2

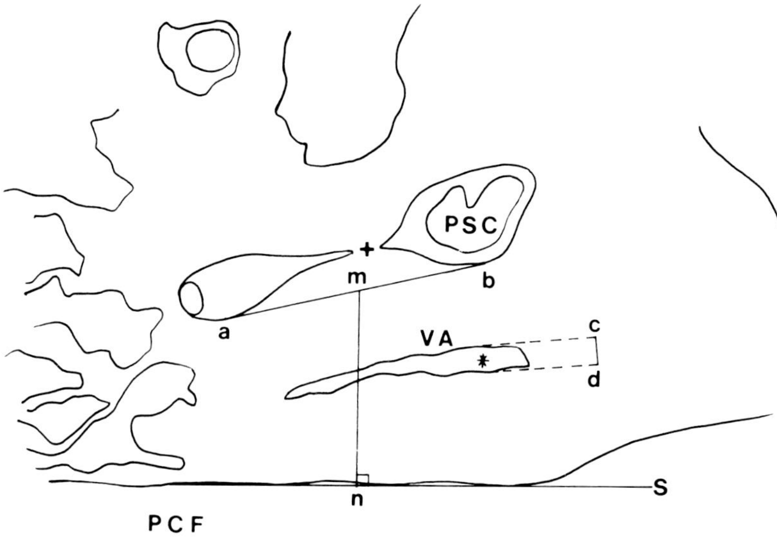

Fig. 2. Methods for measuring width of VA on horizontal sections and thickness of otic capsule in periaqueductal region. Width (cd) is measured in area (*) where proximal rugose portion of ES is located. Line (mn) is thickness of otic capsule in periaqueductal region, and is at right angles to surface (S) of posterior cranial fossa (PCF) and connects S to midpoint (m) of line (ab) which is tangential to medial PSC perimeter at lowest level (+) of inner arch of PSC.

± 5.3 mm^2 in the hyperplastic VA group.

ANALYTIC REPRESENTATION OF LENGTH, ANGLE, AND POSITION OF THE VA

Hypoplastic VA (17 Cases). According to the LAP system (Fig. 4), common types of the VA in this group were $L_1A_2P_1$ (3 cases, 18%), $L_1A_2P_2$ (3 cases, 18%), and $L_2A_1P_1$ (3 cases, 18%). The results of analyzing these three parameters (L,A,P) in bones in this group are presented in Figure 5. In many specimens (10 cases, 59%) the VA was located in the area superomedial to the inner arch of the PSC (L_1) and was tubelike, with the angle being under 20° (A_1). The position of the VA with respect to the PSC was anterior (P_1; 6 cases, 35%) or inferior (P_2; 8 cases, 47%) in most specimens.

Normoplastic VA (38 Cases). Common types of the VA in this group (Fig. 4) were $L_2A_2P_3$ (16 cases, 42%) and $L_2A_3P_3$ (6 cases, 16%). Analysis of these three parameters (L,A,P) is seen in Figure 5. In most of the specimens the VA extended to or through the area medial to the arch of the PSC (L_2; 29 cases, 76%), was funnel-shaped with an angle of between 20 and 40° (A_2; 27 cases, 71%), and overlapped or crossed medially over the posterior portion of the PSC (P_3; 31 cases, 82%).

Hyperplastic VA (24 Cases). Common types of the VA in this group (Fig. 4) were $L_3A_2P_3$ (10 cases, 42%) and $L_2A_2P_3$ (5 cases, 21%). Analysis of each parameter in this group is shown in Figure 5. In most of these specimens the VA extended inferomedially beyond the outer arch of the PSC (L_3; 14 cases, 58%), was funnel-shaped with an angle of between 20 and 40° (A_2; 16 cases, 67%), and was positioned posteriorly (P_3; 23 cases, 96%).

RELATIONSHIP BETWEEN AREA OF VA AND WIDTH OF VA

The relationship between the area of the VA and the width of the VA as measured on horizontal sections in the three groups is shown in Figure 6. Mean (M ± SD) of the width of the VA in the specimens with hypoplastic VAs was 0.4 ± 0.13 mm, while in specimens with normoplastic or hyperplastic VAs it was 0.54 ± 0.13 and 0.63 ± 0.17 mm, respectively. There was a statistically significant difference ($p<0.05$) between the widths of the VAs in the specimens with hypoplastic VAs and those with normoplastic VAs, and also between those in the normoplastic VA group compared to those in the hyperplastic VA group.

DETAILED STUDY OF THE ES IN THE VA AND RP IN 30 REPRESENTATIVE SPECIMENS

Hypoplastic VA (10 Specimens). Mean values for the areas of the ES in the VA and the RP in this group were 4.3 ± 1 mm^2 and 2.7 ± 1 mm,², respectively; these values were the smallest of the three groups. The area of the ES in the VA averaged 79.3% of the area of the VA, and the area of the RP averaged 50.8% of that of the VA. In two of the specimens the entire RP was located within the VA. In seven specimens, however, although most of the RP was located within the VA, a small area of the distal RP extended into the posterior cranial fossa. In the remaining specimen with a tubelike VA, more than half of the entire RP extended to the posterior cranial fossa.

The epithelial lining of the RP was cuboidal or mostly cuboidal in many specimens (8 cases), but was cuboidal in some parts and squamous in others in the remaining two specimens. The folds of the RP were minimal or absent in most specimens (8 cases), while folding was moderate in the remaining two specimens. Loose subepithelial connective tissue was almost absent, or was poorly developed in most of the specimens (8 cases); it was moderately well developed in the other two specimens. The vascularity of the RP in these specimens was very poor

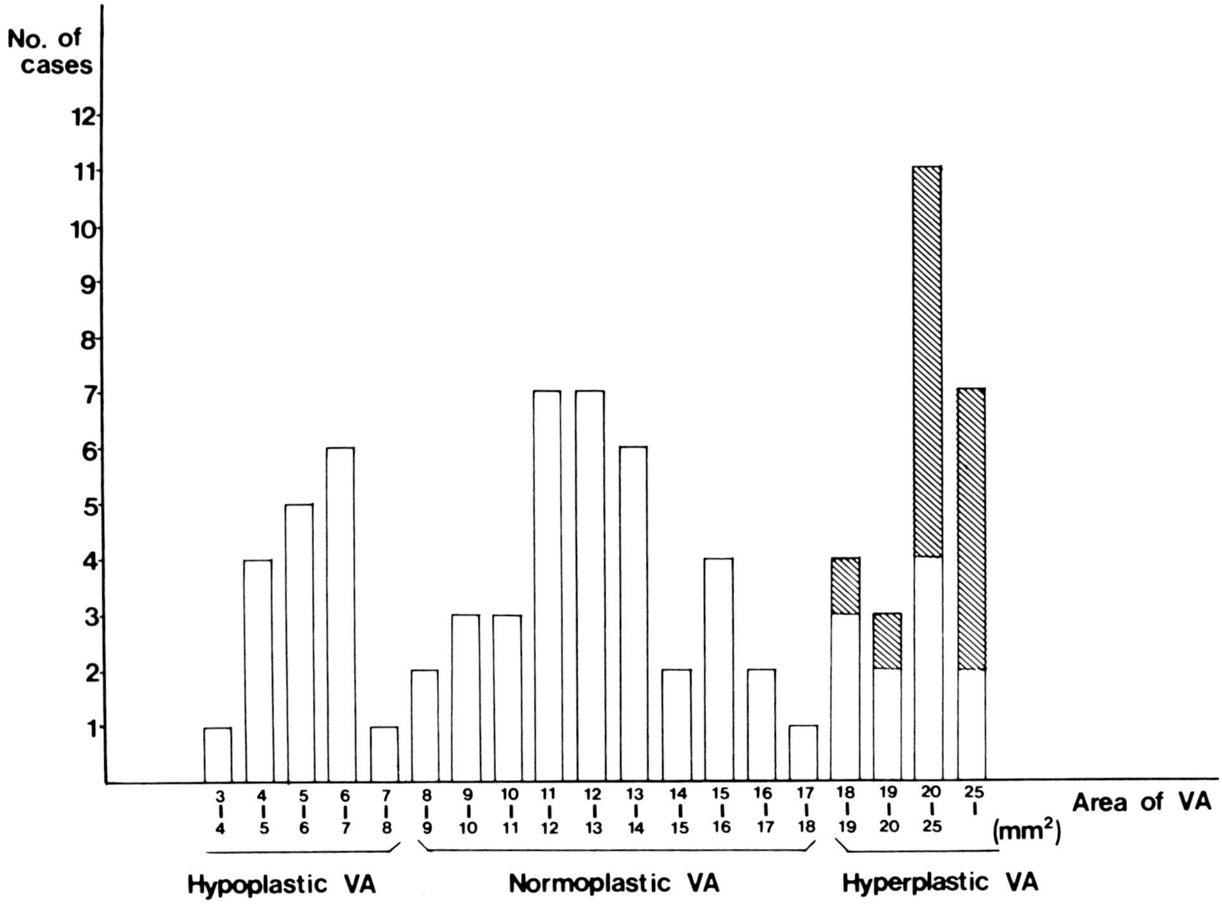

Fig. 3. Histograms indicating numbers of temporal bone specimens having VAs with areas indicated on abscissa. Seventy-nine temporal bones were measured. Hatched areas indicate specimens in which total area of VA could not be measured because lower part of VA was not included in specimen.

(15.7 ± 5.3 vessels in 1.3 mm^2), being two thirds of that noted in the specimens of the normoplastic VA group. Polyplike eosinophilic tissue with calcified deposit was observed in part of the subepithelial layer in two specimens.

Normoplastic VA (10 Specimens). The mean values of the area of the ES in the VA and the area of the RP in specimens of this group were 11.6 ± 1.8 mm^2 and 6.5 ± 2 $mm,^2$ respectively. These areas are larger than those in hypoplastic VAs but smaller than those in hyperplastic VAs. The area of the ES in the VA averaged 85.9% of the area of the VA, and the area of the RP was 47.5%, on average, of the area of the VA. In six of the ten specimens, the entire RP was located within the VA. In four specimens a small area of the distal RP extended into the posterior cranial fossa.

The epithelial cells of the RP were cuboidal in every specimen. The folds of the RP were moderate in many specimens (6 cases), while folding was poorly (3 cases) or well developed (1 case) in the remaining specimens. The loose subepithelial connective tissue was moderately developed in most specimens (7 cases), and in the remaining specimens it was poorly (2 cases) or well developed (1 case). The vascularity of the RP averaged 24.3 ± 4.4 vessels in 1.3 $mm.^2$ Broadbased apposition of a lamellar bone to the wall of the VA was seen in a part of the subepithelial layer in one specimen.

Hyperplastic VA (10 Specimens). The mean values for the areas of the ES in the VA and the area of RP were the largest (20.1 ± 2.9 mm^2 and 12 ± 3.5 $mm,^2$ respectively) of the three VA groups. The ratios of the area of the ES in the VA to the area of the VA, and of the area of the RP to the area of the VA averaged 84.5% and 48.9%, respectively. In seven specimens the entire VA and RP could be reconstructed. In four of these the entire RP was located within the VA. In three specimens, a small area of the distal RP extended into the posterior cranial fossa.

In most specimens (9 cases), the epithelial cells of the RP were cuboidal or mostly cuboidal; in the tenth specimen the epithelial cells were mostly squamous. The folds of the RP were well developed in most specimens (8 cases), moderately developed in one specimen, and poorly developed in one specimen. The loose subepithelial connective tissue was moderately or well developed in every specimen except one in which the loose subepithelial connective

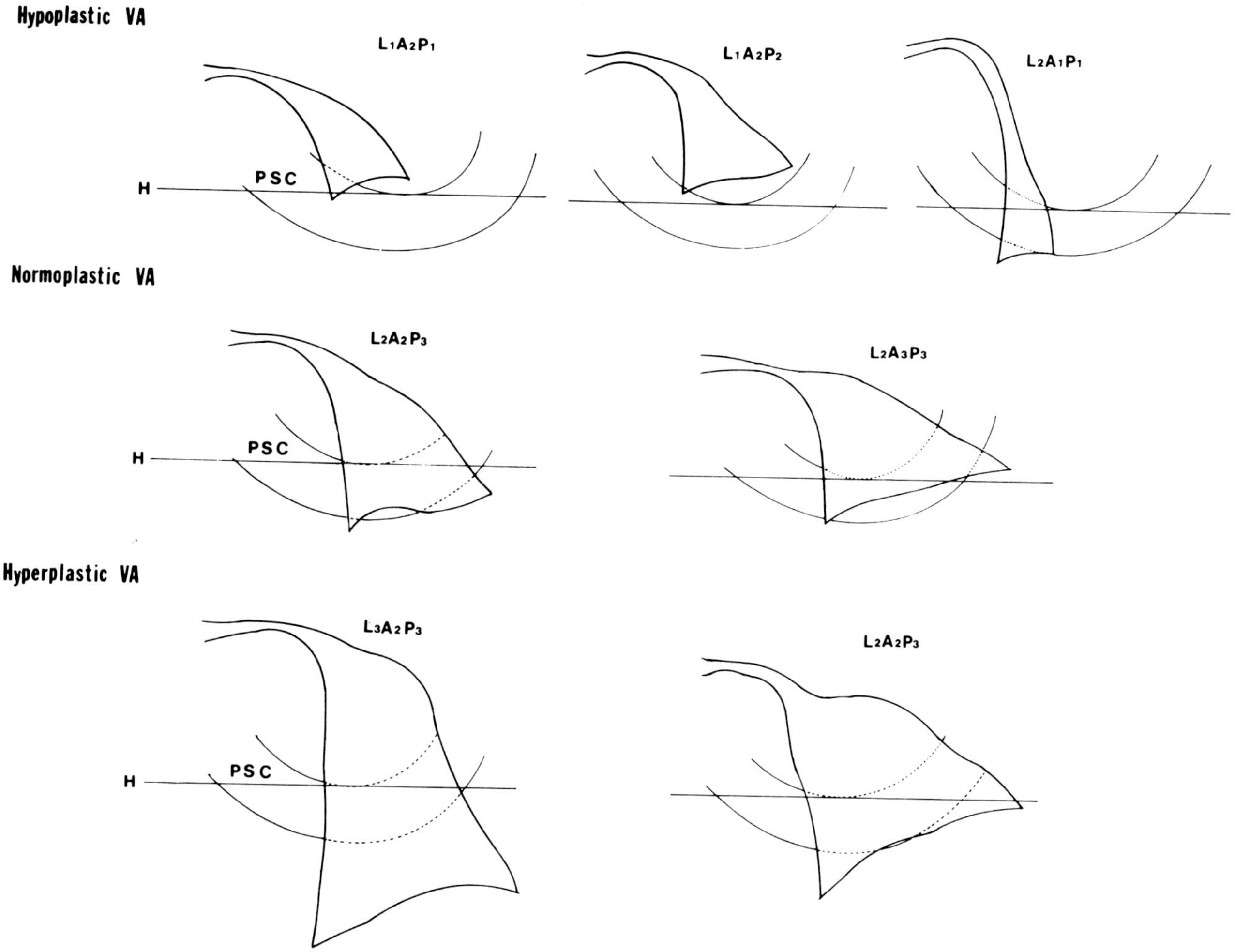

Fig. 4. Medial view graphic reconstructions of representative cases from each of three groups of temporal bones: those with hypoplastic, normoplastic, and hyperplastic VAs. There were evident differences between VAs characteristic of each group.

tissue was poorly developed. The vascularity was the richest (28.4 ± 7.4 vessels in 1.3 mm^2) of the three VA groups, and was 1.2 times that of specimens with normoplastic VAs. We noted new bone formation with dense fibrotic connective tissue in a part of the subepithelial layer in one specimen.

RELATIONSHIP OF DEGREE OF DEVELOPMENT OF VA TO DEGREE OF DEVELOPMENT OF THE TEMPORAL BONE (PERIAQUEDUCTAL PNEUMATIZATION AND OTIC CAPSULE IN THE PERIAQUEDUCTAL REGION)

Analytic data obtained regarding the degree of development of the VA and degree of periaqueductal pneumatization are presented in the table. Large periaqueductal air cells (group I) were often associated with hyperplastic VAs (9 cases, 60%; Fig. 7A), while small periaqueductal air cells or small bone marrow spaces (group II) were associated with normoplastic VAs in many of the specimens (11 cases, 55%). However, lack of periaqueductal pneumatization (group III) was more often associated with normoplastic VAs (22 cases, 50%) than with hypoplastic VAs (14 cases, 32%).

The mean value for the thickness of the otic capsule in the periaqueductal region was 2.5 ± 1.2 mm in the group with hypoplastic VAs (Fig. 7B), 3.5 ± 1.1 mm in the group with normoplastic VAs, and 4.5 ± 1.1 mm in the group with hyperplastic VAs (Fig. 7A). There was a statistically significant difference ($p < 0.05$) between the thickness of the otic capsule in the specimens with hypoplastic VAs and the thickness in specimens with normoplastic VAs. The difference in thickness of the otic capsule was also statistically significant ($p < 0.05$) between specimens with normoplastic VAs and those with hyperplastic VAs.

An additional interesting finding is that in specimens with tubelike hypoplastic VAs the thickness of the otic capsule was 3.3 ± 1.3 mm, whereas it was 1.7 ± 0.5 mm in specimens with funnel-shaped hypoplastic VAs. We found that the difference between these two types of specimens in thickness of the otic capsule was statistically significant ($p < 0.05$).

DISCUSSION

The ES, as well as the VA, is a 3-dimensional

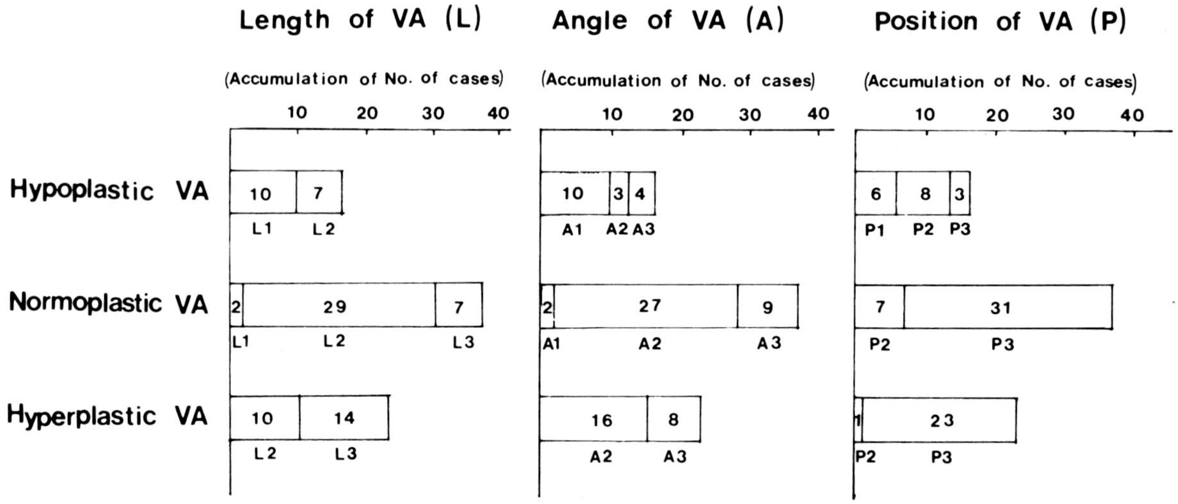

Fig. 5. Statistical analysis of each parameter (L, A, P) for three different groups of VA. Numbers indicate number of cases in each different category. Differences are notable between groups in length, angle, and position of VA.

structure that shows wide individual variations.[10,11] However, to our knowledge, no systematic (qualitative and quantitative) investigation into the dimensional anatomy of the VA and the ES using the graphic reconstruction method has been performed on a large number of temporal bones.

After careful examination of normal temporal bone specimens, we can now classify the VA into

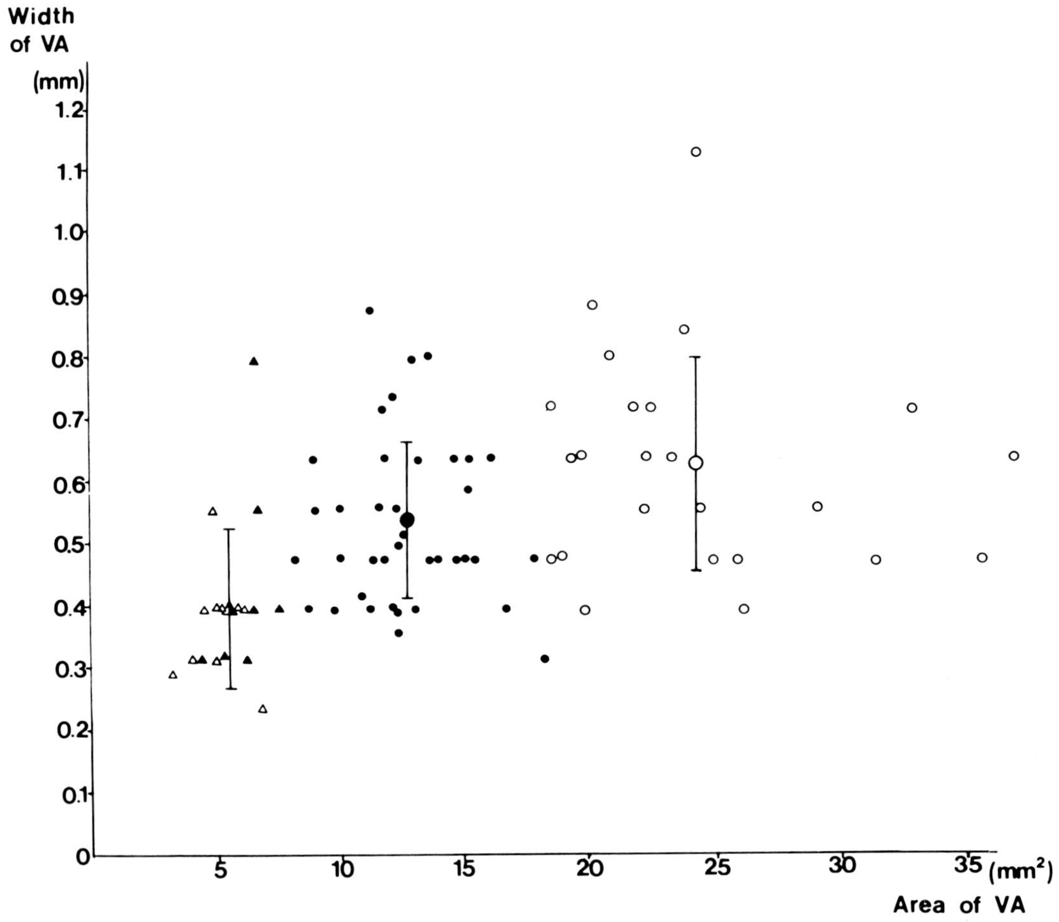

Fig. 6. Relationship between width and area of VA. Abscissa indicates VA area and ordinate indicates VA width. There is a significant difference between widths of VAs in specimens with hypoplastic VAs (△ - Tubelike hypoplasia; ▲ - Funnel-shaped hypoplasia) and those with normoplastic VAs (●), and also between those with normoplastic VAs compared to those with hyperplastic VAs (○). ▲, ● and ○ indicate mean value (M ± SD) of width of VA in specimens with hypoplastic, normoplastic, and hyperplastic VAs, respectively.

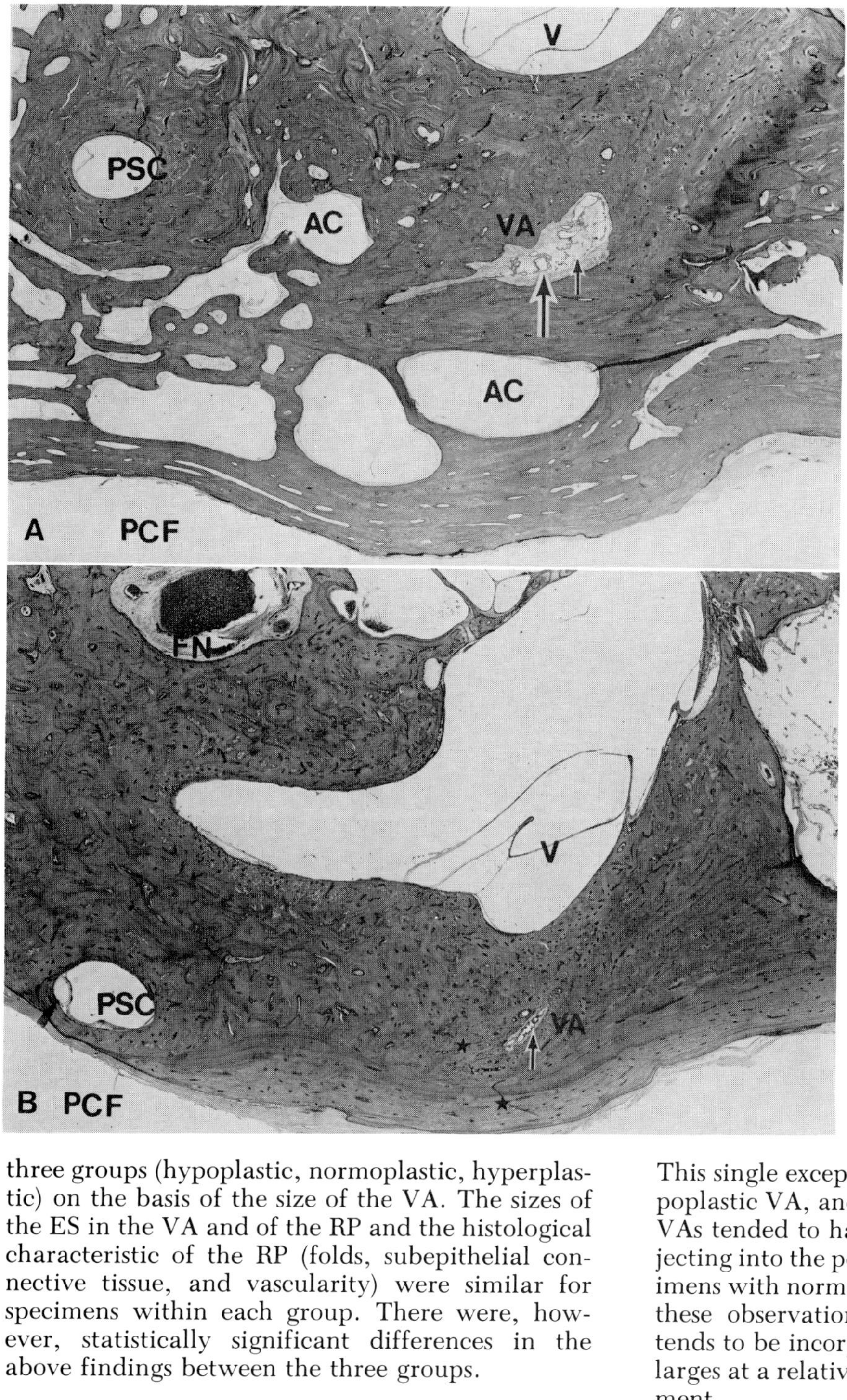

Fig. 7. A) Horizontal section of left temporal bone showing large air cells (AC) in periaqueductal region (group I). VA is hyperplastic. Epithelial folds (large arrow) and loose subepithelial connective tissue (small arrow) of RP are also well developed. V - Vestibule; PCF - Posterior cranial fossa. B) Horizontal section of left temporal bone showing absence (*) of periaqueductal air cells (group III). VA is hypoplastic (tubelike). RP (arrow) shows almost absent folds and loose subepithelial connective tissue. FN - Facial nerve. (H & E, x 20)

three groups (hypoplastic, normoplastic, hyperplastic) on the basis of the size of the VA. The sizes of the ES in the VA and of the RP and the histological characteristic of the RP (folds, subepithelial connective tissue, and vascularity) were similar for specimens within each group. There were, however, statistically significant differences in the above findings between the three groups.

An increase in VA width correlated with an increase in VA area. Therefore VA volume would also be expected to increase proportionately with increase in VA width. These histological measurements theoretically could be compared with roentgenographic measurements of the VA.

Whereas it has been found that the RP in newborns extends from the VA to the posterior cranial fossa, most of the RP comes to be located within the VA by 3 to 4 years of age,[9] and was so located in all but one of the adult temporal bones in this study. This single exception was a temporal bone with hypoplastic VA, and more specimens with hypoplastic VAs tended to have a distal portion of the RP projecting into the posterior cranial fossa than did specimens with normoplastic or hyperplastic VAs. From these observations it would appear that the RP tends to be incorporated into the VA as the VA enlarges at a relatively greater rate during its development.

RELATIONSHIP OF DEGREE OF DEVELOPMENT OF VA TO DEGREE OF PERIAQUEDUCTAL PNEUMATIZATION

Development of VA	*Periaqueductal Pneumatization* I	*II*	*III*	*Total*
Hyperplastic VA	9	7	8	24
Normoplastic VA	5	11	22	38
Hypoplastic VA	1	2	14	17
Total	15	20	44	79

Numbers indicate number of temporal bones observed in each of specific entities.

After reviewing the data we obtained from studying the relationships between development of the VA and the temporal bone as a whole, we have the following comments. The development of the otic capsule seems to be correlated with the development of the VA. However, although funnel-shaped hypoplastic VAs were associated with poorly developed, thin otic capsules in all of the specimens we examined (7 cases, 100%), the tubelike hypoplastic VAs were associated in many specimens (7 cases, 70%) with moderately developed, thick otic capsules. This finding may indicate that the tubelike VAs are of prenatal origin[9] because they persist even after development of the otic capsule in the periaqueductal region is completed postnatally.

Clinically, a controversy[1-4,6,12] exists concerning whether or not roentgenographic narrowing or nonvisualization of the VA and histologically confirmed hypoplasia of the VA are associated with Menière's disease. In the present histopathological study, hypoplastic VAs (which are difficult to visualize roentgenographically) were noted in normal temporal bones. Thus, our findings support the hypotheses of other investigators[3,4] who felt that a narrow or nonvisualizable aqueduct (ie, a tubelike VA) may also be present in temporal bones with diseases other than Menière's disease, as well as in normal ears.

Histologically, Hallpike and Cairns[13] observed that absence of the loose subepithelial connective tissue (perisaccular fibrosis) of the RP was present in the temporal bones of individuals with Menière's disease. Altmann and Zechner[14] also observed perisaccular fibrosis and decreased folding of the RP on the diseased side and felt that these conditions might predispose to the development of endolymphatic hydrops. In the present series, however, absence or poor development of the loose subepithelial connective tissue and the folds of the RP were common histological features in the normal temporal bones with hypoplastic VAs and were observed even in a few bones with normoplastic or hyperplastic VAs. Accordingly, we feel that these conditions of the RP are not necessarily related to hydrops.

In conclusion, we feel that the findings obtained in this study reflect the range of normal variations that can occur in the VA and ES of adult human temporal bones. We recommend that further investigations be undertaken to discover any relationships that may exist between the normal but hypoplastic VA and the RP which would have any bearing on the development of endolymphatic hydrops.

Dr. Kodama is presently Assistant Professor at the Department of Otolaryngology, University of Teikyo School of Medicine, Tokyo.

ACKNOWLEDGMENTS — The authors wish to express their deep gratitude to Eugene N. Myers, MD, Professor and Chairman, and Franklin Owen Black, MD, Department of Otolaryngology, University of Pittsburgh School of Medicine, for encouraging them to study this subject and for giving helpful criticism during the preparation of this paper. Appreciation is also expressed to Mrs. Ruth Anderson for her kind assistance in this study.

REFERENCES

1. Stahle J, Wilbrand H. The vestibular aqueduct in patients with Meniere's disease. Acta Otolaryngol (Stockh) 1974; 78: 36-48.

2. Arenberg IK, Rask-Anderson H, Wilbrand H, Stahle J. The surgical anatomy of the endolymphatic sac. Arch Otolaryngol 1977; 103:1-11.

3. Øigaard A, Thomsen J, Jensen J, Dorph S. The narrow vestibular aqueduct. An unspecific radiological sign? Arch Otorhinolaryngol 1975; 211:1-4.

4. Kraus EM, Dubois PJ. Tomography of the vestibular aqueduct in ear disease. Arch Otolaryngol 1979; 105:91-8.

5. Plantenga KF, Browning GG. The vestibular aqueduct and endolymphatic sac and duct in endolymphatic hydrops. Arch Otolaryngol 1979; 105:546-52.

6. Antunez JM, Galey FR, Linthicum FH, McCann GD. Computer-aided and graphic reconstruction of the human endolymphatic duct and sac. A method for comparing Meniere's disease cases. Ann Otol Rhinol Laryngol 1980; Suppl 76:23-32.

7. Rizvi SS, Smith LE. Idiopathic endolymphatic hydrops and the vestibular aqueduct. Ann Otol Rhinol Laryngol 1981; 90:77-9.

8. Egami T, Sando I, Black FO. Hypoplasia of the vestibular aqueduct and endolymphatic sac in endolymphatic hydrops. Trans Am Acad Ophthalmol Otolaryngol ORL 1978; 86:327-39.

9. Kodama A, Sando I. Postnatal development of the vestibular aqueduct and endolymphatic sac. Ann Otol Rhinol Laryngol 1982; 91 Suppl 96:3-12.

10. Anson BJ, Donaldson JA, Warpeha RL, Winch TR. A critical appraisal of the anatomy of the perilymphatic system in man. Laryngoscope 1964; 74:945-66.

11. Ogura Y, Clemis JD. A study of the gross anatomy of the human vestibular aqueduct. Ann Otol Rhinol Laryngol 1971; 80: 813-25.

12. Black FO, Sando I, Hildyard VH, Hemenway WG. Bilateral multiple otosclerotic foci and endolymphatic hydrops. Ann Otol Rhinol Laryngol 1969; 78:1062-74.

13. Hallpike CS, Cairns H. Observation on the pathology of Meniere's syndrome. J Laryngol Otol 1938; 53:625-55.

14. Altmann F, Zechner G. The pathology and pathogenesis of endolymphatic hydrops. New investigations. Arch Klin Exp Ohren Nasen Kehlkopfheilkd 1968; 192:1-19.

PAPERS PRESENTED AT THE MEETING OF THE AMERICAN OTOLOGICAL SOCIETY, INC.

PART 2

CONTENTS

Cochlear and Otoconial Abnormalities in Capsular Otosclerosis with Hydrops.
L-G. Johnsson, MD; J. E. Hawkins, Jr, DSc; R. C. Rouse, PhD; F. H. Linthicum, Jr, MD 3

Behavior of the Vestibular Nerve Following Labyrinthectomy.
H. F. Schuknecht, MD 16

The Facial Canal: Normal Anatomy, Variations and Anomalies.
B. Proctor, MD; G. T. Nager, MD 33

Speech and Language Development in a Parent-Infant Total Communication Program.
A. Dee, MA; I. Rapin, MD; R. J. Ruben, MD 62

COCHLEAR AND OTOCONIAL ABNORMALITIES IN CAPSULAR OTOSCLEROSIS WITH HYDROPS

LARS-GÖRAN JOHNSSON, MD
HELSINKI, FINLAND

JOSEPH E. HAWKINS, JR, DSc
ANN ARBOR, MICHIGAN

ROLAND C. ROUSE, PHD
ANN ARBOR, MICHIGAN

FRED H. LINTHICUM, JR, MD
LOS ANGELES, CALIFORNIA

Temporal bones from four patients with capsular otosclerosis were examined by microdissection. Otoconia and abnormal crystalline deposits were studied by scanning electron microscopy and x-ray analytical methods. One patient showed more or less symmetrical invasion of the basilar membrane and osseous lamina by connective tissue from thickened endosteum adjacent to the larger anterior foci. In one ear sensorineural degeneration was circumscribed; in the other it was extensive and associated with cochleosaccular hydrops. Two other patients were deaf, with severe sensorineural degeneration; one had multiple active foci and evidence of cochleosaccular hydrops. In the fourth patient, who had small anterior foci, no specific inner ear pathology was found related to otosclerosis. In the hydropic labyrinths, apatite was present as abnormal deposits in the cochlear duct and as rigid crusts replacing the otoconia. Apparently these changes had been associated with abnormal labyrinthine fluid dynamics rather than with the otospongiotic process per se.

INTRODUCTION

This paper presents further observations on the effect of capsular otosclerosis on the inner ear as seen by microdissection complemented by celloidin sectioning of the remaining bone, including the modiolus and the floor of scala tympani. The term capsular otosclerosis is used to denote the condition involving extensive spread of the otosclerotic process from the margin of the oval window to invade other portions of the otic capsule. It is thus distinguished from histological otosclerosis, which denotes the presence of an otosclerotic lesion not affecting either the conductive or the sensory component of hearing, and cochlear otosclerosis, which has been postulated to affect the sensory component only, without fixation of the stapes.

Microdissection is not, as indicated in an earlier publication, an ideal method for histological observation of the changes in bone.[1] On the other hand, it does show the histological changes in the membranous labyrinth and its vasculature in relation to the otosclerotic process better than other techniques. Furthermore, microdissection leaves pathological crystalline deposits and otoconia unaffected by decalcifying agents used in conventional histology. As a result, we have been able to employ the techniques of x-ray diffraction and x-ray energy dispersive analysis to reveal new features of otoconial pathology and to identify abnormal crystalline deposits in the labyrinth.[2-6]

In our previous report we concluded that there is a common, characteristic pattern of expansion of an anterior focus from the margin of the oval window toward the apex of the cochlea. Therefore, the upper half of the basal turn located just anterior to the oval window becomes a target for possible toxic substances released by the focus and a site of predilection for sensorineural degeneration, which occurs especially when an active process invades or involves the endosteum of the scalae.[1]

Causse and Chevance[7] identified proteolytic enzymes in perilymph samples from patients with otosclerosis and showed a correlation between abnormal enzyme activity in the perilymph and the degree of sensorineural hearing loss. Such enzymes could act directly upon Corti's organ and could thus be responsible for the types of circumscribed degeneration we have described.[1] They could also diffuse into perilymph and cause sensorineural degeneration in the lower half of the basal turn close to the focus, or more extensive cochlear injury depending on the size and activity of the otosclerotic process.[1]

In cases where the endosteum of the cochlea has been invaded by otosclerosis, we have observed a loss of overlying blood vessels which presumably affected the microcirculation of the cochlea. Forms of vestibular pathology which had not been documented before were also found.[1] In the present paper evidence is presented that supports the findings of our previous investigation, and a new form of pathology is described in the specific region of the cochlea which we proposed as a predilectional site of damage in otosclerosis.

From the Department of Otorhinolaryngology, University of Helsinki Central Hospital, Finland (Johnsson); the Department of Otorhinolaryngology, Kresge Hearing Research Institute, University of Michigan Medical School, Ann Arbor (Hawkins, Rouse); and the House Ear Research Institute, Los Angeles (Linthicum). This investigation was supported by a grant from the Research Fund of the American Otological Society, Inc., by USPHS Program Project Grant NS 05785, and Research Grants NS 05065 and NS 12706 from the National Institute of Neurological and Communicative Disorders and Stroke, and by Paulo Sääpiö, Helsinki, Finland.

Presented in part at the meeting of the American Otological Society, Inc., Palm Beach, Florida, May 2-3, 1982.

REPRINTS — Joseph E. Hawkins, Jr., DSc, Kresge Hearing Research Institute, University of Michigan, Medical School, Ann Arbor, MI 48109.

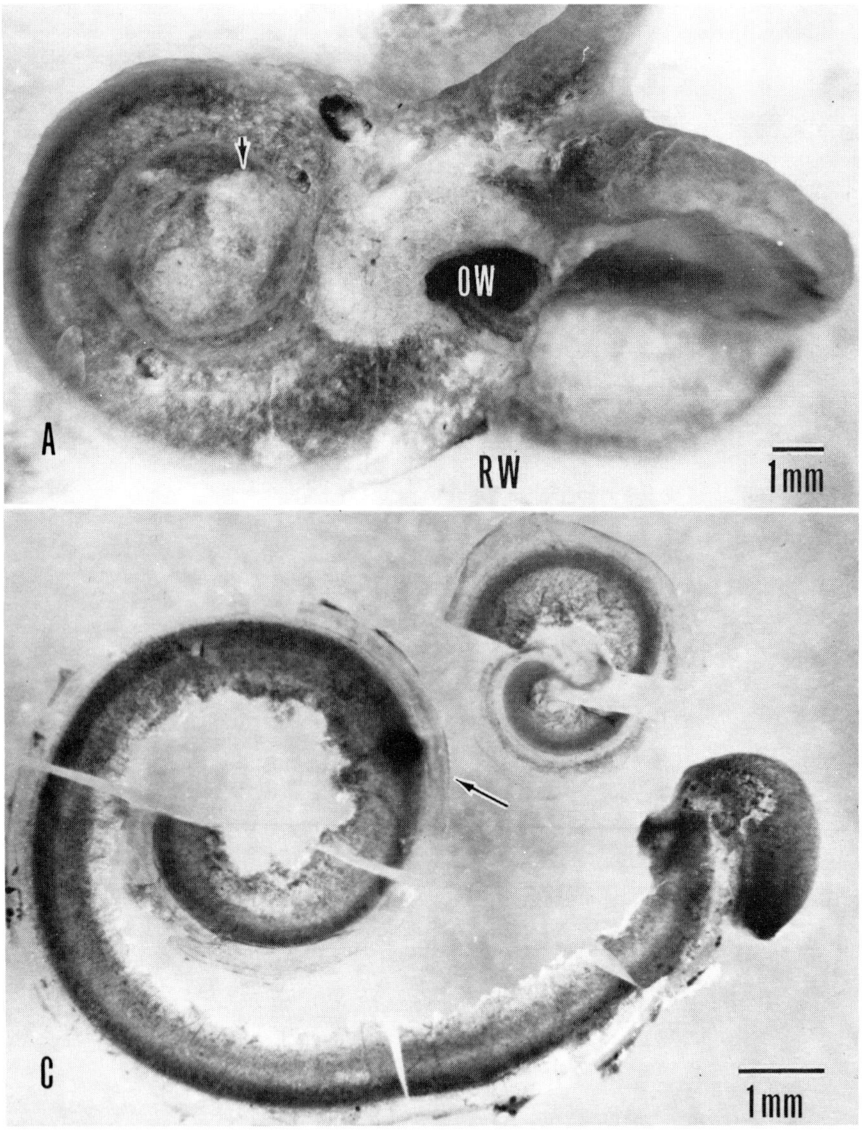

Fig. 1. (Case 1) Left (A, C) and right (B, D) ears. A and B show respective otic capsules; C and D, osseous spiral laminae and basilar membranes. OW - Oval window, RW - Round window. A) In addition to anterior focus, note separate apical focus (arrow). B) Expansion of anterior focus to involve apical turn. C) Complete degeneration of Corti's organ

MATERIALS AND METHODS

The temporal bones were processed using the technique of microdissection and surface preparations described in two of our previous papers.[1,8] The inner ears were fixed and stained with repeated perilymphatic perfusion of 1% osmium tetroxide injected through the round window. Otosclerotic foci are distinguished from normal capsular bone by their different texture and color. Foci which are active or in a spongiotic state are soft, vascular, and darkly-stained. Inactive foci are hard, white, dense, and poorly vascularized. An estimate of the state of activity of each focus was made during removal of the otic capsule with a dental drill and during the microdissection.[1]

CASE REPORTS

Case 1

HISTORY

The most interesting findings were made in this case, which showed unique cochlear pathology. The patient was a 73-year-old woman with severe arteriosclerosis, who had undergone abdominal aneurysmectomy and bilateral amputation below the knee. She never recovered from surgery and died five months later in the intensive care unit, after several attempts to treat a postoperative intermittent sepsis with antibiotic had failed. In addition to the sepsis, renal insufficiency was considered to be an underlying cause of death. The BUN was approximately 50-60 mg% and the creatinine clearance was approximately 15-20 ml/min during the last month of her life.

The patient had been hard of hearing for several years, the right being the better ear. Because of the sepsis, she was given tobramycin 20 mg every eight hours for about a month. Before that she underwent a month of treatment with tobramycin at another hospital. After her last tobramycin treatment she was given a combination of amikacin 150 mg and vancomycin 200 mg every 12 hours for about a week. Her hearing gradually worsened during this treatment. The physicians and nurses in the inten-

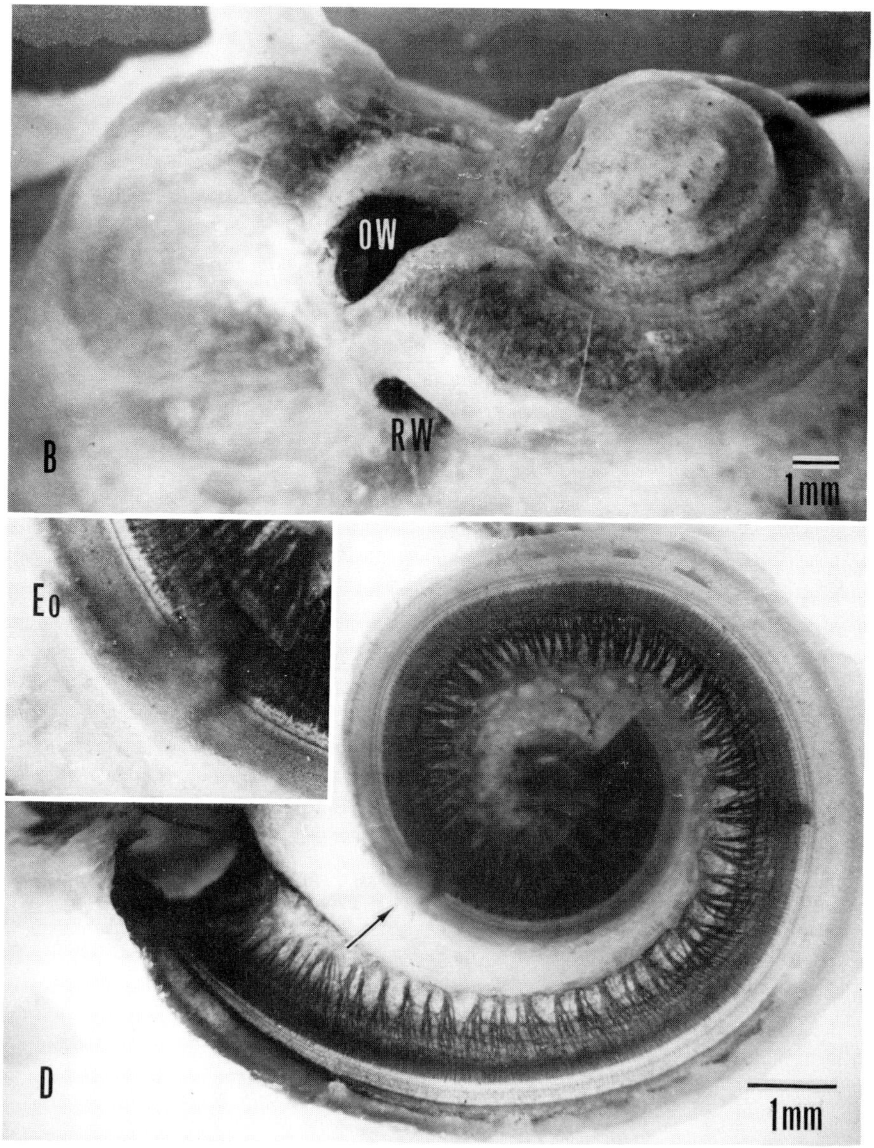

and nerve fibers. Arrow points to growth of connective tissue, located 19.7 mm from basal end. D) Cochlea, showing thickening of endosteum (Eo) next to otosclerotic focus and growth of connective tissue (arrow) onto basilar membrane in region located 22.4 mm from basal end. Inset) Close-up of area of basilar membrane pathology. (OsO_4)

sive care unit thought her to be completely deaf, but in the absence of audiometric studies one cannot be certain that she had no residual hearing at the time of death. In view of the labyrinthine hydrops found in both ears, it is important to note that according to her next of kin she never complained of dizziness, tinnitus, or feelings of aural fullness.

HISTOPATHOLOGY

Extent and Nature of the Foci. Both temporal bones were obtained at autopsy 24 hours postmortem. The stapes were completely ankylotic. The extent and nature of the otosclerotic process was similar in both ears (Fig. 1). The pathological bone surrounded the oval window and extended anteriorly in the characteristic fashion described earlier[1] to involve the upper end of the basal turn and the apical turn. The left ear actually had a separate apical process set apart from the main focus by a narrow bridge of normal-appearing bone; in addition there was a small focus in the wall of the scala tympani just anterior to the round window. There was a clearly visible border between the normal and the otosclerotic bone, which was white, hard, and sclerotic in both ears. The process was therefore considered to be inactive at the time of death.

In the right ear the otosclerotic process reached the endosteum in all three scalae in the upper half of the basal turn. In the apical turn only the walls of the scala media and scala vestibuli were involved. In the left ear the process reached the endosteum only in the scala media and the scala tympani of the upper basal turn. In neither ear was there any visible thickening of the endosteum directly underlying otosclerotic bone. The main otosclerotic process in this ear also extended into the lateral third of the spheroid recess where the pathological bone impinged upon the saccular nerve.

Cochlear Pathology Adjacent to the Foci. Two forms of pathology were observed involving the

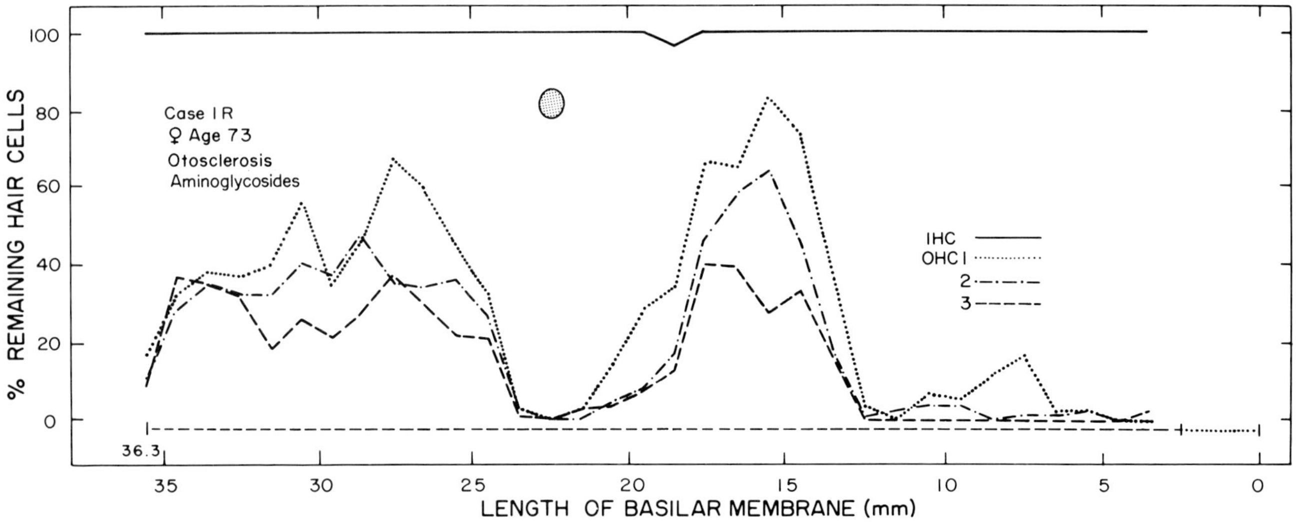

Fig. 2 (Case 1) Cytocochleogram for right ear, showing loss of hair cells at basilar membrane lesion in Fig. 1D. Note maximal degeneration at 18 to 25 mm (upper basal turn), site of predilection. Oval spot indicates location of connective tissue growth shown in Fig. 1D. Dashed horizontal bar below curves represents condition of peripheral processes of cochlear neurons in osseous spiral lamina. They were severely degenerated at extreme basal end (dotted line, 0 to 3 mm), and partly degenerated throughout rest of cochlea. Total length of basilar membrane, 36.3 mm.

basilar membrane and the spiral ligament, respectively; both appeared to be directly related to the otosclerotic process.

In both ears connective tissue was present on a small portion of the basilar membrane or the osseous spiral lamina in the upper half of the basal turn. On the right side there was a localized thickening of the endosteum just apical to the upper margin of otosclerotic bone, 22.42 mm from the basal end. The total length of the cochlea was 36.3 mm. From this area connective tissue extended to cover both sides of the basilar membrane and the margin of the osseous spiral lamina (Fig. 1D). The maximum width of clumps of tissue was 0.48 mm. It was highly cellular and dense, but no fibrillar structures could be discerned. Vascularization was poor, but two capillaries were seen to enter the growth, one from each side. The capillaries came from the inner and outer spiral vessels, respectively. There was complete hair cell loss at the site of the lesion and hair cell degeneration on both sides of it (Fig. 2). The distal ends of the nerve fibers covered by the tissue had degenerated, much as they do after ototoxic injury.[9]

The changes in the left ear were different, in that there was no visible thickening of the endosteum, and the tissue formation was not clearly in continuity with the bony wall of the cochlea, although it was located adjacent to otosclerotic bone just anterior to the oval window. The growth, which was similar in appearance to that in the right ear but avascular, covered both sides of the osseous spiral lamina and the inner margin of the basilar membrane but was not in contact with the endosteum covering the otosclerotic bone (Fig. 1C). The growth was 0.46 mm wide and located 19.74 mm from the basal end of the cochlea (total length 36.3 mm).

In the left ear the spiral ligament was partially calcified and atrophic in an area which precisely corresponded to the location and extent of otosclerotic bone reaching the upper half of the basal turn (Fig. 3).

Left Cochlea. The most severe changes were found on this side (Fig. 1C). No hair cells were present and the tectorial membrane was rolled in a narrow, distorted ribbon which was partly pulled away from the limbus. No nerve fibers were seen in the osseous spiral lamina except in the apical turn. There a faint network of nerve fibers was present in a narrow segment where some supporting elements remained on the basilar membrane. The width of this area measured at the habenula perforata was 1 mm.

It was obvious that severe cochleosaccular hydrops had been present at some time in life and that Reissner's membrane had subsequently collapsed, presumably after overexpansion and rupture. No separate endolymphatic space was found. Reissner's membrane was adherent to large areas of the spiral ligament and to the bony wall of the modiolus in the scala vestibuli. In the upper half of the basal turn next to the otosclerotic focus, Reissner's membrane formed a cyst-like space above the basilar membrane. In the apical turn the membrane had herniated through the helicotrema into the scala tympani. There were also two small oblong holes in the outermost third of the basilar membrane in the apical turn. The size of the holes was approximately

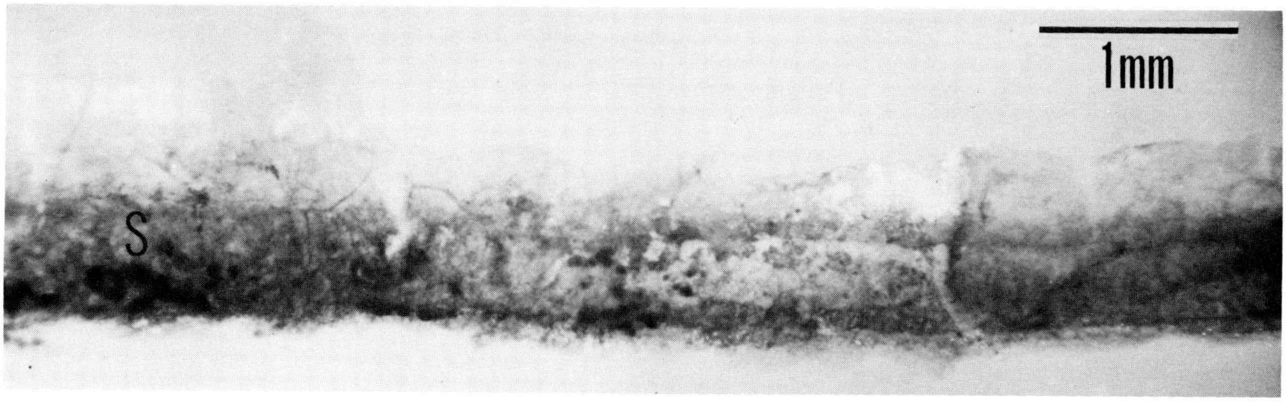

Fig. 3. (Case 1) Spiral ligament from upper half of basal turn of left ear. S - Area normally covered by stria, which has atrophied. Note calcification (white area) of spiral ligament adjacent to focus. (OsO_4)

35 by 15 μm. We have observed similar defects in the basilar membrane previously in a case of labyrinthine hydrops and otosclerosis.[1]

The cells in Reissner's membrane were not larger than in nonhydropic specimens. On the contrary, in some areas the cells were smaller, indicating an increase in the number of cells per unit area in response to the increase in the volume of endolymph. A few individual epithelial cells had very light cytoplasm and appeared abnormal. In the middle turn epithelial cells were missing in small areas at the margin of the membrane. This is in agreement with our previous observations in hydropic ears.[2,10,11]

There was complete strial atrophy in the basal and middle turns. Small clumps of osmiophilic tissue were seen in the area normally covered by the stria; this gave the lateral cochlear wall an appearance reminiscent of that seen in deaf Dalmatian dogs.[12] In the apical turn a thin stripe of stria remained. In the lower half of the basal turn portions of the spiral ligament ordinarily covered by the stria were also atrophic, with numerous small roundish spaces within the tissue. This gave the spiral ligament a spongy appearance similar to what we have observed in Alport's syndrome.[13] In the upper half of the basal turn there was a focal calcification of the spiral ligament, as previously mentioned (Fig. 3).

Numerous crystalline deposits were found on the basilar membrane and on the bare surface of the spiral ligament once covered by the stria. The largest deposits were seen on the basilar membrane in the "hook" and in the upper half of the basal turn. Two samples of the latter material proved to be spherulitic apatite similar to that described previously.[2,3] The distribution of the deposits appeared random except in the basal turn, where small deposits were seen along the distorted tectorial membrane and the limbus.

Right Cochlea. Reissner's membrane was in normal position in this ear. There was almost complete loss of sensory cells in the first 12 mm of the basal turn and a mild nerve degeneration in the first half of this turn. These changes were probably age-related.[14] The extent and degree of sensorineural degeneration are shown in Figure 1D and in the cytocochleogram in Figure 2. Considering the patient's age and the extent of outer hair cell loss, there was remarkably little nerve fiber degeneration in the osseous spiral lamina. The inner hair cells were almost intact. The most striking finding was the circumscribed hair cell degeneration associated with the tissue growth already described, shown as a dip in the cytocochleogram.

There was a diffuse atrophy of the stria vascularis throughout the basal and middle turns. In the apical turn, the stria was narrowed by atrophy at both margins, and a large, dilated capillary ran longitudinally through the remaining strip.

Vestibular Pathology. In the left (hydropic) ear the wall of the saccule was collapsed. Only a small, isolated, tent-like space remained along the striola line. This space was occupied by the displaced remnant of the otoconial membrane, ie, only the gelatinous layer;[15] no saccular otoconia were present in either ear. The saccular maculae in both ears showed severe nerve degeneration, which was almost complete on the left side. The utricular maculae showed only a mild nerve degeneration, and most of the otoconia were present (Fig. 4). In the right utricle these otoconia were of normal calcite, but the left utricle contained some apatite mixed with the calcite.

The vestibular neuroepithelia were studied with the scanning electron microscope. They were poorly preserved and only a crude picture of the condition of the neuroepithelia was obtained, but both ears showed a severe loss of vestibular sensory cells. The degeneration was somewhat more severe on the cristae than on the maculae. In the right utricle the loss of hair cells was most pronounced along the striola line.

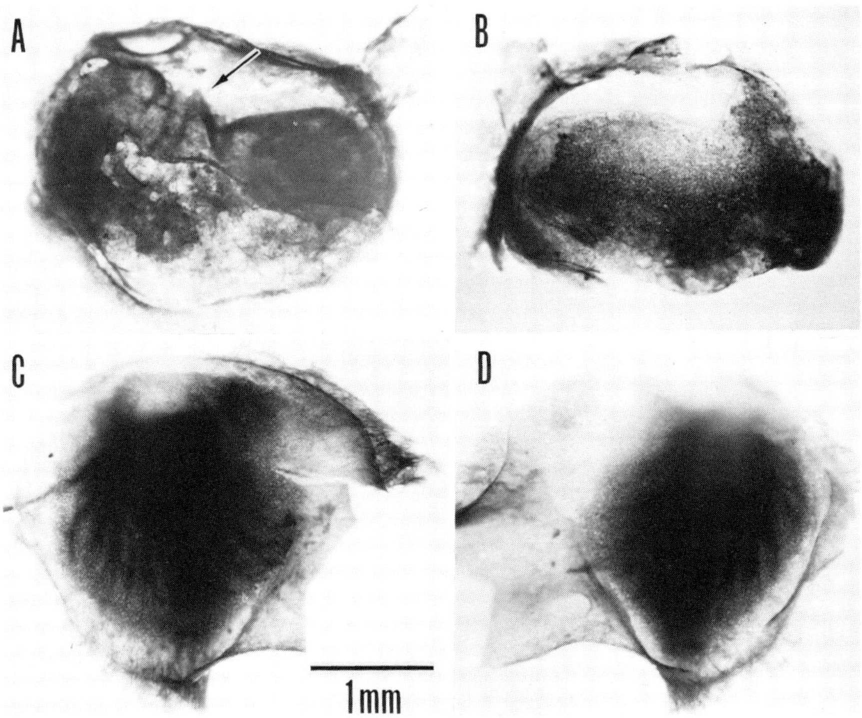

Fig. 4. (Case 1) A) Left and B) right saccular maculae; C) left and D) right utricular maculae. Note in A collapsed saccular wall (arrow) forming pocket enclosing folded otoconial membrane. Compare marked neural degeneration beneath saccular maculae with milder utricular neural degeneration. (OsO_4)

Case 2

HISTORY

The patient was a 78-year-old man. At the age of 14 he noticed a hearing loss, which he believed had begun when he was hit in the left ear by a baseball. The hearing loss progressed and by the time the patient was 19 years old, he was quite hard of hearing but able to use a hearing aid. Apparently, he wore a bone-conduction aid until he was about 40 years old. In his 60s he visited an otologist and was found to be completely deaf. There was no history of ear infections or bone fractures and no visible anomalies except that the patient had blue sclerae.

Judging from a questionnaire the patient answered at the age of 64, he suffered almost constantly from tinnitus which sounded like escaping steam. He had no dizzy spells, but reported that his sense of balance was poor. His father had become hard of hearing in later life, and 5 of 7 members of the father's family had blue sclerae. Two of them were hard of hearing. The patient had one daughter who was also hard of hearing.

HISTOPATHOLOGY

Extent and Nature of the Foci. Both temporal bones were obtained 15 hours postmortem. The stapes were ankylotic and their footplates thickened, but otherwise they were of normal shape. The otic capsule in both ears was almost completely invaded by multiple foci in an irregular and diffuse fashion so that the precise spread of the pathological process was difficult to determine. In addition, well-defined, soft or spongiotic foci were seen adjacent to the upper half of the basal turn anterior to the oval window and in the middle of the basal turn adjacent to the scala tympani.

Right Cochlea. No hair cells were present, and there was complete loss of nerve fibers in the osseous spiral lamina. The tectorial membrane was rolled up, distorted, and partly displaced peripherally on the basilar membrane, presumably as a result of hydrops. In the middle turn a portion of the tectorial membrane had become attached to that part of the spiral ligament normally covered by the stria. A narrow strip of supporting elements remained on the basilar membrane. This is an unusual occurrence in association with complete nerve degeneration. It may have been the result of an independent neural degeneration preceding or simultaneous with the sensory cell degeneration. There were faint traces of radial nerve fibers in the osseous spiral lamina. They probably represented remnants of myelin sheaths in the empty bone channels which once had contained nerve fibers passing to the modiolus.[16]

Severe hydrops was present; Reissner's membrane bulged outward and adhered to the spiral ligament and to the bony wall of the modiolus in the scala vestibuli. In the apical turn the membrane had herniated through the helicotrema into the scala tympani and extended in the basal direction well into the middle turn.

The changes in Reissner's membrane were similar to those seen in the left ear of the patient in case 1. There was marked hyperplasia of epithelial cells, especially in the basal turn, where the cells were small and greatly increased in number per unit

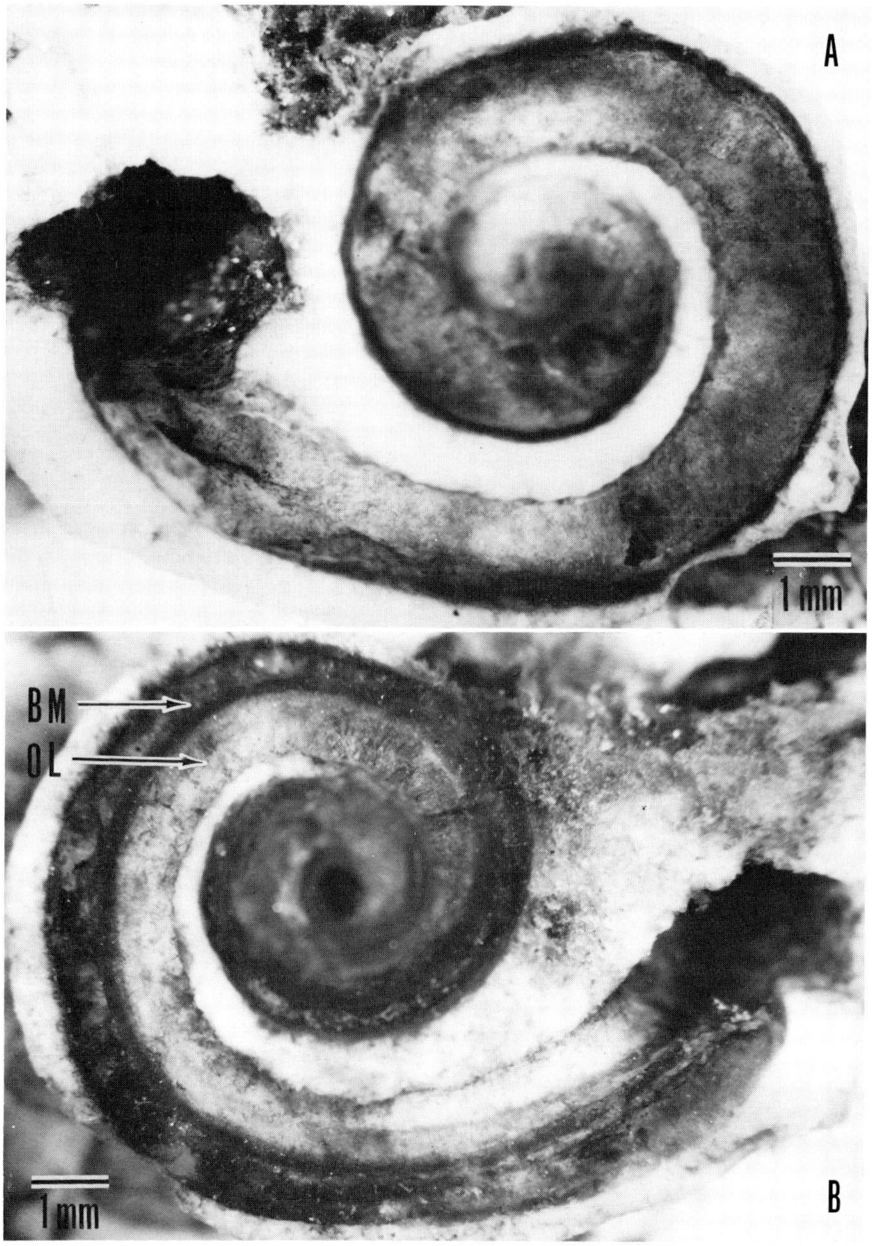

Fig. 5. (Case 2) A) View of floor of scala tympani in right ear, showing thin layer of diffuse bone growth. Note loss of venules and capillaries normally seen as distinct network (see Fig. 6D) (OsO_4). B) Complete sensorineural degeneration in left ear in presence of extensive, multiple foci. BM - Basilar membrane; OL - Osseous spiral lamina, devoid of nerve fibers, opaque, and attached to new bone occluding scala tympani.

area. A few minute perforations were seen in the membrane in the middle turn.

There was complete strial atrophy in the apical turn and in the upper half of the middle turn. The stria in the rest of the cochlea was atrophic and poorly vascularized. Some of the remaining capillaries were dilated. Several glassy-appearing roundish crystals were seen on the surface once covered by stria. Most frequently there was a clump of crystals surrounded by scattered smaller crystals. In the basal turn beads of crystalline material were arranged along atrophied strial capillaries. Similar calcification has been seen in the stria of old dogs and in an aged chimpanzee.[17]

The spiral ligament was atrophic, but its outer surface adjacent to the endosteum was dense and fibrotic. There was a severe loss of capillaries and of some arterioles, much more so than one would expect in an ear from this age group.[18] Some of the remaining arterioles were markedly dilated.

The scala tympani was slightly narrowed by some new bone formation in the first 7 mm of the cochlea, and the osseous spiral lamina, which is usually somewhat flexible in this area, was rigid and opaque. The endosteum in the scala tympani was thickened in all three turns and darkly stained. There was a severe loss of the capillary network on the wall of the scala tympani, and most of the venules normally taking a radial course toward the modiolus were missing (Fig. 5A). The remaining vessels were severely dilated.

Left Cochlea. The pathological changes were

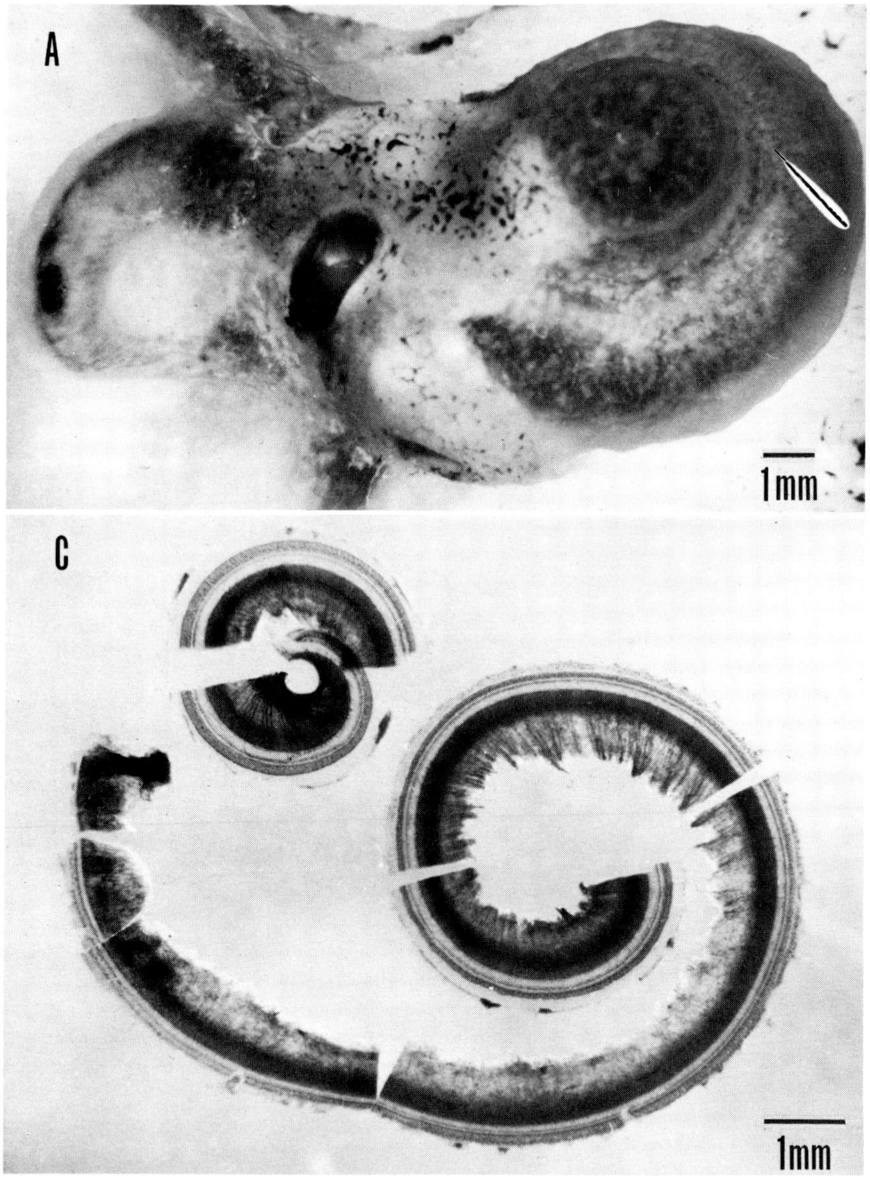

Fig. 6. (Case 3) A) Right ear showing commonly occurring extension of white, sclerotic anterior focus. Superficial layer of focus extends more anteriorly than in B) deeper layer. C) Entire osseous spiral lamina with Corti's organ dissected out; note nerve degeneration in all turns.

similar to those in the right ear but more severe. No hair cells or even supporting cells were present, and no nerve fibers were seen in the osseous spiral lamina (Fig. 5B). The tectorial membrane was distorted and rolled up. In the apical turn it was covered by a thin layer of colorless, glassy spherulites composed of apatite. In the hook area a thick layer of apatite spherulites covered the entire spiral limbus and the basilar membrane.

Severe hydrops apparently had been present at some time in life, but Reissner's membrane was now collapsed and adhered to the walls of the scala vestibuli. In the apical turn the membrane had herniated through the helicotrema into the scala tympani and now extended to the upper end of the basal turn. Only small samples of the membrane could be removed for study. The results were similar to those in the opposite ear.

The stria vascularis was more or less completely atrophied, and only a thin, uneven avascular layer of osmiophilic tissue remained. Crystals similar in appearance and distribution to those in the right ear adhered to the atrophic stria. Most of the spiral ligament had been replaced by a dense and fibrotic tissue representing endosteal proliferation. There was an almost complete loss of blood vessels from the spiral ligament. Only a few radiating arterioles were left, and these were extremely dilated. The basilar membrane in the middle and apical turns was in a markedly abnormal position, being pulled downward because its outer attachment to the spiral ligament was shifted toward the scala tympani.

In the scala tympani there was profuse new bone formation, which completely occluded the first 9 mm of the scala, including the round window and the opening of the cochlear aqueduct. Apical to this portion, the new bone under the basilar membrane

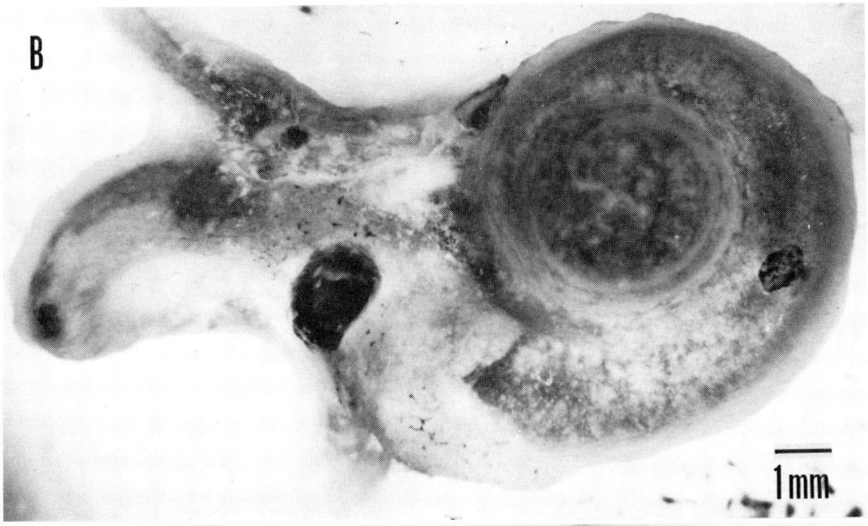

D) Scala tympani showing extension of focus (arrows) to round window (RW), which is narrowed. Note normal pattern of collecting venules and capillaries, and lack of involvement of endosteum at site of predilection. (OsO_4)

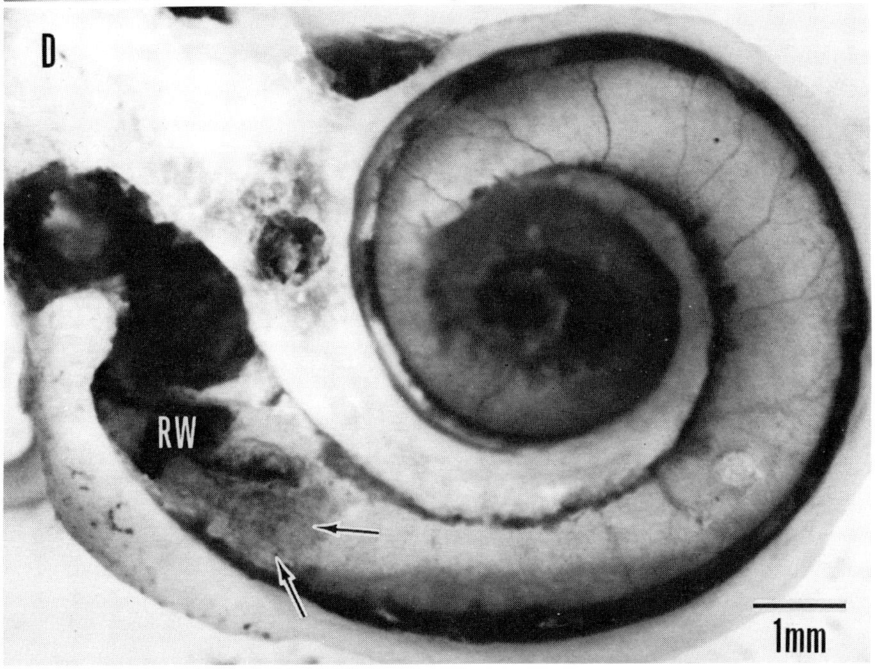

showed a shallow, uneven groove, which extended to the upper end of the basal turn, where the scala tympani gradually expanded and became normal in shape. The new bone, as well as the unoccluded portions of the scala tympani in the middle and apical turns, was covered by a thickened endosteum and a loose, uneven meshwork of connective tissue. The latter had the appearance of an accumulation of cotton or of cobwebs under the osseous spiral lamina, which was completely rigid and opaque throughout the cochlea. In the scala tympani of the middle turn there were several large irregularly shaped masses of apatite surrounded by loose connective tissue.

Vestibular Pathology. In both ears the otosclerosis extended to the vestibular portion of the labyrinth, and the endosteum of the entire horizontal canal and ampulla was markedly thickened. In the left ear the endosteum of the superior bony ampulla and of the canal adjacent to the ampulla was involved as well. Both saccules had collapsed, and the maculae were covered with a thick crust of white apatite spherulites. The same was true for the utricular macula in the right ear.

The neuroepithelia in both ears (with the exception of the saccular macula and utricular macula in the left ear) were studied by scanning electron microscopy. In the right ear there was a marked loss of sensory cells in all organs. The loss was complete on the superior and posterior cristae, but a few scattered hair cells remained on the horizontal crista. The saccular macula exhibited an almost complete loss of nerve fibers. Nerve degeneration in the utricular macula was less severe, and numerous hair cells were still present there.

In the left ear there was an almost complete loss of sensory cells, the degeneration being most severe in the crista of the horizontal canal. The changes in

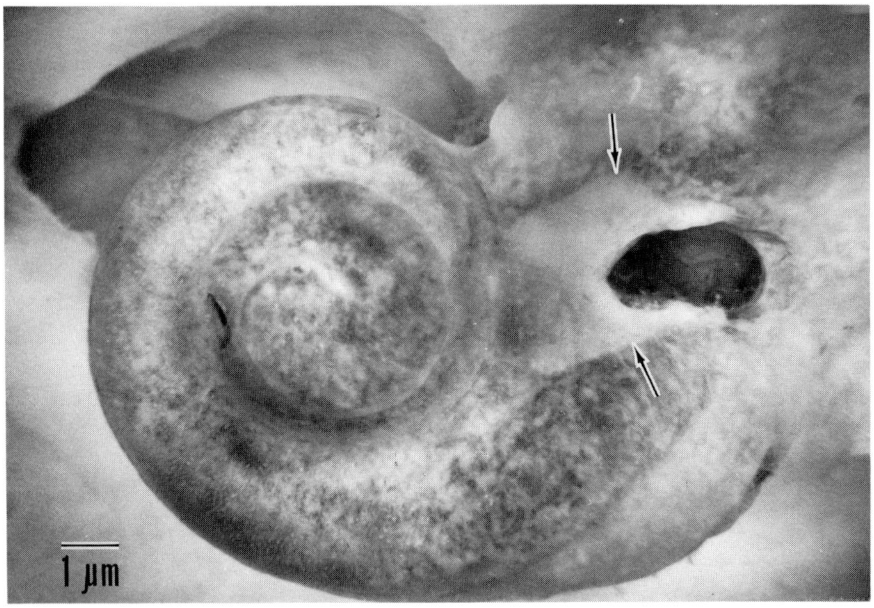

Fig. 7. (Case 4) Otic capsule of left cochlea showing sclerotic anterior focus (arrows) extending toward but not invading middle turn. Right ear had similar focus.

the utricle were unusual. It appeared that the patient had had an extensive utricular hydrops at some time, followed by marked atrophy or thinning of the wall and its subsequent collapse. The walls around the macula were folded over the neuroepithelium and adhered to it. No normal otoconia were seen. A crystalline covering in the form of apatite spherulites was found only along the posterior tip of the macula. Thin membranes extended in folds into the membranous ampullae.

The ampullae were partly collapsed. The cupulae were missing, as were the plana semilunata. Scattered, irregular layers of concretions were found on the inside of the ampullae and the ampullary ends of the canals; they were particularly numerous in the posterior ampulla and canal.

There was a complete loss of nerve fibers in the saccular macula, whereas some nerve fibers remained in the utricular macula. A few nerve fibers had grown into the collapsed membranous wall. Apparently these represented an abnormal regeneration of vital nerve fibers. This phenomenon is most unusual, although we have made a few similar observations in the cochleas of experimental animals.[17]

The vasculature of the membranous walls of the labyrinthine organs in both ears was reduced, and some of the remaining vessels were dilated. There appeared to be a marked loss of dark cells in the wall of the utricle.

Case 3

HISTORY

The right temporal bone of an 87-year-old woman was obtained from the House Ear Research Institute. The patient had suffered from hearing loss in both ears for many years, but the history of her auditory deficit was not well known. She underwent audiometric testing a few years before her death and was found to be completely deaf in her right ear. Tests indicated that the hearing on her left side was at the 80-dB level for all frequencies. No bone conduction responses were obtained.

HISTOPATHOLOGY

Extent and Nature of the Focus. Only the right ear was examined. The stapes was ankylotic and there was a large, white, sclerotic anterior focus which was considered inactive (Fig. 6). The superficial layer of the otosclerotic bone was slightly vascularized and extended to the apical turn. The deeper layer was also sclerotic and reached close to the upper end of the basal turn but did not impinge upon the scalae to involve their endosteum. The focus extended around the round window, which was narrowed. The endosteum overlying the otosclerotic bone anterior to the round window was slightly thickened.

Right Cochlea. A severe sensorineural degeneration was present in all turns. In the first half of the basal turn the degeneration of nerve fibers was considerably more severe than that in Corti's organ, suggesting that an independent neural degeneration had preceded or dominated the process which led to the severe loss of sensory cells and nerve fibers (Fig. 6C). Although supporting cells and some hair cells remained even in the hook region, most of the nerve fibers in the osseous spiral lamina in the first half of the basal turn had degenerated. A sparse, uneven network of single nerve fibers remained, discernible only in high-power microscopy by bright-field illumination. A thin network of radial nerve fibers in the osseous spiral lamina was visible in the upper half of the basal turn and in the middle and apical turns. An exception was an area about 5 mm long in the middle turn, where the nerve fibers were particularly sparse.

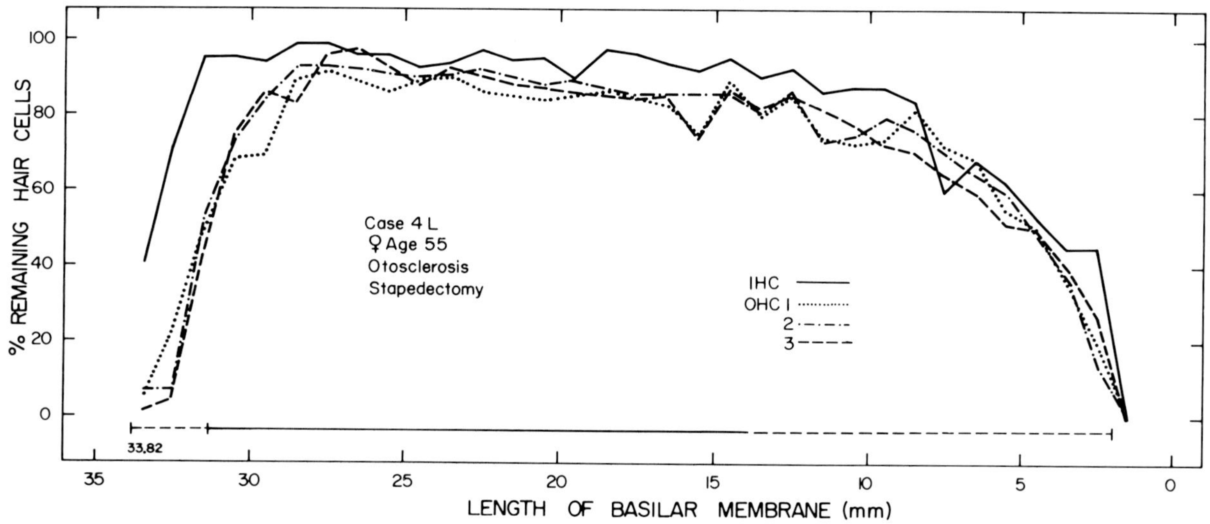

Fig. 8. (Case 4) Cytocochleogram for left ear showing hair cell loss restricted to basal and apical ends of Corti's organ. Horizontal bar below curves represents condition of peripheral processes of cochlear neurons in osseous spiral lamina. They were completely degenerated in most basal 2 mm, partly degenerated from 2 to 14 mm (broken line), normal in appearance from 14 to 32 mm (solid line), and partly degenerated at extreme apex. Total length of basilar membrane, 33.82 mm. Similar changes were present in right cochlea.

There was atrophy of the stria vascularis and of the spiral ligament including its capillaries, which is invariably seen in our specimens from this age group.[18] A narrow strip of partially atrophic stria extended as far as the upper half of the middle turn, above which there was complete atrophy.

Case 4

HISTORY

The patient was a 55-year-old woman who had suffered from hearing loss for about 25 years, and who died of bronchogenic carcinoma. At the age of 43 she had had a stapedectomy in her left ear, and two years later a similar operation in the right ear. There was no history of dizziness.

HISTOPATHOLOGY

Extent and Nature of the Focus. A fat-wire prosthesis was found in the oval window of the right ear and a Teflon piston in the left ear. There were sclerotic anterior foci in both ears, which did not reach the upper end of the basal turn and were thus classified as "small" or "moderate" in Guild's[19] and our classification.[1] The left cochlea, with the sclerotic focus extending to but not encroaching upon the middle turn, is illustrated in Figure 7.

Right and Left Cochlea. No labyrinthine pathology that could be specifically related to otosclerosis or to its surgical treatment was found in this pair of temporal bones. The cytocochleogram for the left ear (Fig. 8) shows a relatively mild sensorineural degeneration in the first 14 mm of the cochlea, and a limited sensorineural degeneration in the apical turn. These changes, which were more or less symmetrical in the two ears, are characteristic of the age-related pathology underlying presbyacusis, and it is impossible to say to what extent, if any, otosclerosis and its surgical treatment may have been responsible for them.

DISCUSSION

The most striking findings in the present study were those in case 1, which showed ingrowth of connective tissue on the basilar membrane and osseous spiral lamina (Fig. 1). In the right ear there was a thickening of the endosteum just at the apical margin of the anterior focus, and it was obvious that endosteal proliferation had led to a circumscribed invasion of the basilar membrane by connective tissue. In comparing the cytocochleograms for this case (Fig. 2) and for case 1 in our previous publication (Fig. 6 in Johnsson et al[1]), where there was a localized sensorineural degeneration adjacent to the active focus, it is obvious that the two curves are similar. The center for maximal hair cell loss in both ears is in the area located approximately between 18 and 25 mm from the basal end of the cochlea. This region represents the specific site of predilection for cochlear lesions induced by the anterior focus.

The causation of the comparable lesion in the left ear is more difficult to understand. The tissue formation occurred on the osseous spiral lamina adjacent to otosclerotic bone, but there was no thickening of the endosteum and the lesion was separated from otosclerotic bone by an intact basilar membrane. Therefore, it is not clear how the otosclerotic process could have induced the growth of the neoplasm on this side. However, the location of the lesion 19.74 mm from the basal end adjacent to otosclerotic bone in the area of predilection, and its identical appearance with the formation in the opposite ear, make it all but certain that this neoplasm was caused by otosclerosis. Because of the extensive sensorineural degeneration in this ear, one could not estimate the possible damage the otosclerotic process had caused to hair cells and nerve fibers. It should also be noted that the spiral ligament next to the abnormal bone was impregnated with some refractile material, probably apatite. This finding may explain the focal hyalinization of the spiral ligament seen in conventional serial sections by Lindsay and Beal.[20] Removal of the impregnating apatite by decalcifying agents had presumably left the hyalinized tissue they observed.

Considering the common occurrence of the otosclerotic foci extending anteriorly toward the upper half of the basal turn, surprisingly few temporal bones have been reported with cochlear lesions in this area. Besides our three specimens, only four other similar temporal bones have been described.[21,22] We can only assume that this form of cochlear pathology must be less rare than an examination of the current literature would suggest.

The reduction in the vasculature of the spiral ligament in cases 1 and 2 and the marked loss of venules and capillaries in the scala tympani in case 2 are similar to conditions in the mucosa overlying otosclerotic bone in the middle ear.[23] Such devascularization is bound to alter the microcirculation of the cochlea, and it appears to be a far more important defect than the vascular shunts which have been held to induce sensorineural degeneration in otosclerosis through venous stasis.[24] An extensive otosclerotic process is required for substantial loss of blood vessels to occur. It is likely that such a change occurs relatively late in the disease when sensorineural degeneration has already begun, so that vascular pathology may not play an important role in the causation of the sensorineural hearing loss, at least in its earlier stages.

Both our previous study[1] and the present one show that multiple foci can cause severe sensorineural degeneration. This fact is also well documented in the literature.[20,25] The question of whether otosclerosis can cause labyrinthine hydrops is, however, unresolved. It has generally been considered that the association of otosclerosis and hydrops is coincidental. Nevertheless, Wittmaack depicted a case of extensive otosclerosis and severe hydrops in his 1919 monograph[26] and later stated that "chronischer Reizhydrops" is common in extensive capsular otosclerosis.[27] Both cases 1 and 2 showed evidence of cochleosaccular hydrops, and in our previous report[1] we described a case of hydrops associated with extensive otosclerosis. Black et al[28] have also published a case with bilateral multiple foci and hydrops. These observations lead us to believe that extensive capsular otosclerosis can cause labyrinthine hydrops. The dizziness associated with clinical otosclerosis is, however, probably related to an altered composition and density of the labyrinthine fluids rather than to hydrops.[1]

It is of interest to note that Reissner's membrane in the three specimens with hydrops apparently responded to the increase in endolymph volume with hyperplasia, ie, increase in the number of cells per unit area. Aspects of the relationship between hydrops and Reissner's membrane have been discussed in earlier papers.[10,11]

The precise nature of the disease in case 2, which involved blue sclerae and total deafness, remains unclear. Our histological findings indicate that the patient had otosclerosis. He had no history of fractures and apparently did not have osteogenesis imperfecta in a clinically manifest form. The disease is known, however, to show great variations in its genetic expressitivity.

While the severe sensorineural degeneration in cases 1 and 2 in all likelihood was caused by otosclerosis, the cause for the severe sensorineural degeneration in case 3 is unclear. It appeared that an independent neural degeneration had at some time dominated the disease process. Considering the long history of hearing loss as well as the patient's advanced age, otosclerosis, and hereditary factors could all have contributed to the cochlear pathology. The otosclerotic focus had a characteristic pattern of expansion which was almost identical with that observed in case 7 in our previous report.[1] The process was considered inactive at the time of death, but it could have caused cochlear injury during an earlier, active phase.

The labyrinthine endosteal thickening in response to active otosclerosis has been well documented in conventional sections as well as in our microdissections. There appeared to be no relation between the amount of endosteum involved and the degree of sensorineural degeneration. The corresponding reaction in the vestibular labyrinth is seen less often. Case 2 showed considerable thickening of the endosteum in the semicircular canals; in particular, the endosteum of the ampulla of the horizontal canal was markedly thickened. It is conceivable that the horizontal canal and ampulla are more likely to become damaged than the others because of their proximity to the oval window.

Numerous abnormal crystalline deposits were found in the cochlear duct in case 2 on the atrophied stria vascularis, on the basilar membrane, and on the tectorial membrane. We have described similar deposits both in man[2,3] and in experimental animals.[12] Crystalline deposits are not uncommon in association with strial atrophy.[17,18] Concretions having a similar mineralogical composition occur elsewhere in the human body in association with atrophy, eg, in the pineal gland and in the choroid plexuses. The original source for the deposits on the basilar membrane may have been the tectorial membrane, which, like other gelatinous membranes in the inner ear, represents a site of predilection for abnormal calcification.[3] The large crystalline masses found in the loose connective tissue in the scala tympani are probably closely associated with the process of ongoing calcification in the scala.

Both the saccular and utricular mineralization in case 2 were in the form of a thick crust of spherulites instead of the thin, flexible layer of discrete crystals found on the macula in normal ears. All abnormal crystalline deposits found in this case, including the abnormal otoconia, consisted of apatite. New mineralization in the inner ear tends to be in the form of phosphate salts rather than calcite, which is the normal constituent of otoconia. We believe that the abnormal crystalline deposits are not a direct consequence of otosclerosis, but are associated with abnormalities of the labyrinthine fluid dynamics brought about by otosclerosis and labyrinthine hydrops. The cochlear deposits were certainly formed de novo, while the apatite layers on the maculae were probably due to "phosphatization" of pre-existing normal calcite otoconia. The phosphatization process and other features of abnormal mineralization in the inner ear have been discussed in detail by Johnsson et al.[3]

ACKNOWLEDGMENT — Case 1 was obtained from the University of Michigan Hospital, cases 2 and 4 from the National Temporal Bone Banks Program, and case 3 was supplied by the House Ear Research Institute.

REFERENCES

1. Johnsson L-G, Hawkins JE Jr, Linthicum FH Jr. Cochlear and vestibular lesions in capsular otosclerosis as seen in microdissection. Ann Otol Rhinol Laryngol 1978; 87 Suppl 48.

2. Johnsson L-G, Rouse RC, Hawkins JE Jr. Kingsley TC, Wright CG. Hereditary deafness with hydrops and anomalous calcium phosphate deposits. Am J Otolaryngol 1981; 2:284-98.

3. Johnsson L-G, Rouse RC, Wright CG, Henry PJ. Hawkins JE Jr. Pathology of neuroepithelial suprastructures of the human inner ear. Am J Otolaryngol 1982; 3:77-90.

4. Wright CG, Weinberg AG, Hubbard DG, et al. Ear anomalies in an infant with Potter's syndrome. Am J Otol 1981; 3:134-8.

5. Wright CG, Rouse RC, Johnsson L-G, Weinberg AG, Hubbard DG. Vaterite otoconia in two cases of otoconial membrane dysplasia. Ann Otol Rhinol Laryngol 1982; 91:193-9.

6. Wright CG, Rouse RC, Zajic GH, et al. A calcareous concretion in the posterior semicircular duct of a human labyrinth. Am J Otolaryngol 1982; 3:196-201.

7. Causse JR, Chevance L-G. Sensorineural hearing loss due to cochlear otospongiosis: etiology. Otolaryngol Clin North Am 1978; 11:125-34.

8. Hawkins JE Jr, Johnsson L-G. Microdissection and surface preparations of the inner ear. In: Smith CA, Vernon JA, eds. Handbook of auditory and vestibular research methods. Springfield, Ill: Charles C Thomas, 1976:5-52.

9. Johnsson L-G, Hawkins JE Jr, Kingsley TC, et al. Aminoglycoside-induced cochlear pathology in man. Acta Otolaryngol (Stockh) 1981; Suppl 383.

10. Johnsson L-G, Hawkins JE Jr. Hydrops and cupulolithiasis as seen in microdissections of human temporal bones. In: Pulec JL, ed. Menière's disease. Proceedings of the Fourth Extraordinary Meeting of the Barany Society, Anaheim, Calif, 1975: Palisades Publishing Company (in press).

11. Johnsson L-G. Hydrops of the membranous labyrinth as seen by microdissection. In: Shambaugh GE Jr, Shea JJ, eds. Proceedings of the Shambaugh Fifth International Workshop on Middle Ear Microsurgery and Fluctuant Hearing Loss. Huntsville, Ala: The Strade Publisher, 1981:219-27.

12. Johnsson L-G, Hawkins JE Jr, Muraski AA, et al. Vascular anatomy and pathology of the cochlea in Dalmatian dogs. In: de Lorenzo AJ, ed. Vascular disorders and hearing defects. Baltimore: University Park Press, 1973:249-95.

13. Johnsson L-G, Arenberg IK. Cochlear abnormalities in Alport's syndrome. Arch Otolaryngol 1981; 107:340-9.

14. Johnsson L-G, Hawkins JE Jr. Sensory and neural degeneration with aging as seen in microdissections of the human inner ear. Ann Otol Rhinol Laryngol 1972; 81:179-93.

15. Johnsson L-G, Hawkins JE Jr. Otolithic membranes of the saccule and utricle in man. Science 1967; 157:1454-6.

16. Johnsson L-G, House HF. Linthicum FH. Otopathological findings in a patient with bilateral cochlear implants. Ann Otol Rhinol Laryngol 1981; 91 Suppl 91:74-89.

17. Johnsson L-G, Hawkins JE Jr. Strial atrophy in clinical and experimental deafness. Laryngoscope 1972; 82:1105-25.

18. Johnsson L-G, Hawkins JE Jr. Vascular changes in the human inner ear associated with aging. Ann Otol Rhinol Laryngol 1972; 81:364-76.

19. Guild SR. Histologic otosclerosis. Ann Otol Rhinol Laryngol 1944; 53:246-66.

20. Lindsay JR, Beal DD. Sensorineural deafness in otosclerosis. Ann Otol Rhinol Laryngol 1966; 75:436-57.

21. Sando I, Hemenway WG, Hildyard VH, English GM. Cochlear otosclerosis: a human temporal bone report. Ann Otol Rhinol Laryngol 1968; 77:23-36.

22. Dietzel K. Kausal-analytischer Beitrag zur cochleären Otosclerose. Presented at V. Symposion über Cochleaforschung, Halle (Saale), 1977.

23. Arnold W, Plester D. Gefässveränderungen bei der Otosklerose und ihre Auswirkungen auf die mesenchymale Reaktion des Mucoperiostes. Arch Otorhinolaryngol 1975; 209:127-43.

24. Ruëdi L, Spoendlin H. Pathogenesis of sensorineural deafness in otosclerosis. Ann Otol Rhinol Laryngol 1966; 75:525-52.

25. Lindsay JR. Histopathology of otosclerosis. Arch Otolaryngol 1973; 97:24-9.

26. Wittmaack K. Die Otosklerose auf Grund eigener Forschungen. Jena: Fischer, 1919:171.

27. Wittmaack K. Die Ortho- und Pathobiologie des Labyrinthes. Stuttgart: Georg Thieme Verlag, 1956.

28. Black FO, Sando I, Hildyard VH. Hemenway WG. Bilateral multiple otosclerotic foci and endolymphatic hydrops. Ann Otol Rhinol Laryngol 1969; 78:1062-73.

BEHAVIOR OF THE VESTIBULAR NERVE FOLLOWING LABYRINTHECTOMY

HAROLD F. SCHUKNECHT, MD

BOSTON, MASSACHUSETTS

Transtympanic labyrinthectomy was performed on 24 cats, and after survival times of one month to three years, the temporal bones were prepared for light microscopic study. The operated ears showed mean neuronal losses of 12% in six months, 24% in 1 year, 35% in 2 years, and 53% in 3 years. There was no evidence of regeneration of vestibular nerve fibers nor of formation of traumatic neuromata. The temporal bones of two human subjects who had undergone transtympanic labyrinthectomy are also presented; one shows atrophy of the vestibular nerves while the other exhibits proliferation of nerve fibers not resembling a neuroma. It is concluded that the afferent vestibular nerves undergo slow but progressive atrophy following labyrinthectomy and that they have no potential for the creation of amputation neuromata. The evidence suggests that excision of the vestibular nerves may have no therapeutic advantage over labyrinthectomy in the treatment of intractable vertigo.

Ablation of vestibular function is a method of treatment sometimes used to alleviate the intractable vertigo associated with diseases of the labyrinth. Among these disorders are Menière's disease, severe positional vertigo, dysequilibrium complicating unsuccessful reconstructive ear surgery, and the delayed hydrops syndrome.[1] Ablation can be accomplished at three anatomical levels in the vestibular system: 1) the vestibular sensory cells (hair cells), 2) the sense organs (including the afferent nerve endings), and 3) the vestibular nerve trunks. The vestibular sensory cells can be decimated by the administration of ototoxic doses of streptomycin.[2] The sense organs can be obliterated by surgical invasion of the labyrinth (labyrinthectomy) by approaches through the mastoid[3] or the external auditory canal.[4] Vestibular nerve section or excision can be done by approaches through the posterior cranial fossa,[5] the middle cranial fossa,[6] or the middle ear (translabyrinthine).[7]

There is ample clinical evidence to show that when the technical objectives of these various procedures are fully achieved, each can be successful in alleviating the disabling dysequilibrium caused by peripheral vestibular disease. Once it has been decided that ablation may be of therapeutic value, the conditions which determine the method to be employed for any given patient are 1) unilateralism or bilaterialism of disease, 2) the auditory function of each ear, 3) the age and health of the patient, and 4) the clinical experience, surgical skill and biases of the clinician.

Some surgeons[8,9] believe that any procedure accomplishing less than total excision of the vestibular nerves may fail to relieve the symptoms of dysequilibrium. They believe that persisting vestibular neurons can be responsible for dysequilibrium, even though the sense organs have been obliterated. Additionally, it is suggested that amputation neuromata of the vestibular nerves can develop after labyrinthectomy and act as a nidus for continuing dysequilibrum.[10]

Other surgeons[1,11,12] point out that labyrinthectomy, particularly via the transtympanic route, is a direct, safe and effective method for accomplishing vestibular ablation. They believe that the reported failures of labyrinthectomy are due to incomplete removal of vestibular sense organs and therefore may be attributed to poor surgical technique. A further argument given in favor of labyrinthectomy is the lesser morbidity and the fewer postoperative complications than are seen with nerve section. The stated risks of nerve section are facial palsy, postoperative intracranial hemorrhage, edema of adjacent brain structures, cerebrospinal fluid leak and meningitis. While the incidence of these complications is small, it is very real and abundantly documented in the literature.[5,13,14]

There can be no question that the transtympanic labyrinthectomy is simpler and safer than vestibular nerve excision. The argument regarding continuing or recurring vertigo after labyrinthectomy is greatly disaffirmed by the observation that labyrinthectomies are sometimes performed in a haphazard manner with incomplete destruction of the vestibular sense organs. In such cases a caloric response can be elicited postoperatively, attesting to the incompleteness of the labyrinthectomy. Moreover, when revision labyrinthectomy is performed in such cases, the utricular maculae are usually still

---

From the Department of Otolaryngology, Massachusetts Eye and Ear Infirmary, and the Department of Otolaryngology, Harvard Medical School, Boston. Supported by NINCDS Grant No. 5ROL NS13425.

Presented in part at the meeting of the American Otological Society, Inc., Palm Beach, Florida, May 2-3, 1982.

REPRINTS — Harold F. Schuknecht, MD, 243 Charles Street, Boston, MA 02114.

present and their removal under local anesthesia precipitates severe vertigo, further indicating the inadequacy of the initial labyrinthectomy.[1]

A matter of some importance in comparing the relative merits of nerve excision versus labyrinthectomy is the behavior of the vestibular nerves following labyrinthectomy. If the nerves atrophy after labyrinthectomy, there is no advantage to nerve excision. If amputation neuromata are a common occurrence after labyrinthectomy, that fact might weigh against the use of this procedure.

The vestibular ganglion (Scarpa's ganglion) consists of bipolar neurons lying in two linearly arranged cell masses extending in a rostral-caudal direction in the internal auditory canal. It consists of superior and inferior cell groups related to the superior and inferior divisions of the vestibular nerve trunk. The superior division supplies the cristae of the lateral and superior canals, the macula of the utricle, and the anterosuperior part of the macula of the saccule. The inferior division supplies the crista of the posterior canal and the main portion of the macula of the saccule. Central to the vestibular ganglion, the nerve fibers of both divisions merge into a single trunk which enters the brainstem. Richter and Spoendlin[15] describe two types of vestibular neurons: large neurons with central spherical nuclei, and small neurons with eccentric indented nuclei. All neurons contain single nucleoli having diameters of about 3 μm.

The purpose of this report is to provide further information on the behavior of the vestibular nerves following labyrinthectomy. The observations derive from two sources: 1) a controlled experimental study in which labyrinthectomy was performed on cats, and 2) a histological study of the temporal bones of two human subjects who had had labyrinthectomy for presumed Menière's disease.

EXPERIMENTAL STUDY

Labyrinthectomy was performed on the right ear of each of 24 adult cats with the left ear serving as a normal control. (Animals used in this study were maintained in accordance with the guidelines of the Committee on Animals of the Harvard Medical School and those prepared by the Committee on Care and Use of Laboratory Animals of the Institute of Laboratory Animal Resources, National Research Council [DHEW publication No. (NIH) 78-23, revised 1978].) The surgical technique was identical to that used by the author for human patients except that the cat's ear canal was entered via a postauricular approach.

A tympanomeatal flap was elevated and a small section of the posterosuperior margin of the bony tympanic annulus was removed to expose the posterior part of the mesotympanum. The incus and stapes were removed. The saccule was removed by aspiration with a 24-gauge suction tube. The utricular macula, which is hidden from view in the superior part of the vestibule, was engaged by a right-angled hook and removed through the oval window. A longer right-angled hook was then used to probe blindly the ampullae of the semicircular canals. Small pledgets of Gelfoam were placed in the vestibule. The tympanomeatal flap was returned to its normal anatomical position, and the postauricular incision was closed with a row of absorbable sutures.

The cats were divided into six groups of four animals each, distinguished by postoperative survival periods of 1 month, 3 months, 6 months, 1 year, 2 years and 3 years. They were sacrificed by intraarterial perfusion with Heidenhain-Susa fixative solution. The temporal bones were removed and processed for light microscopic study. The standardized method included fixation, decalcification, embedding in celloidin, serial sectioning at a thickness of 20 μm, staining every tenth section with hematoxylin and eosin, and mounting on glass slides.

The total number of neurons for the superior and inferior divisions of the ganglion was determined by counting the nucleoli of the stained sections (every tenth serial section) with the aid of an ocular grid and multiplying the resultant number by 10. A factor of 0.87 was used to correct for double counting of split nucleoli. The formula of Abercrombie (cited by Konigsmark[16]) was used:

$$N_1 = n_1 \frac{t}{t+d}$$

where N_1 = the estimated number of neurons, n_1 = the counted number, t = the thickness of the sections, and d = the diameter of the nucleoli. No attempt was made to differentiate between large and small neurons.

RESULTS

Histological study showed all 24 control ears to be normal.

The tympanic membranes of the operated ears showed fibrous thickening but all were intact. The middle ear spaces and mucosal surfaces of 15 operated ears were normal, while 9 showed moderate fibrous tissue proliferation, and 2 had mild otitis media. The incudes and stapedes were missing. Each oval window was sealed by fibrous tissue continuous with fibrous tissue in the vestibule. Twelve of the vestibules were partly obliterated and 12 were totally obliterated by fibrous tissue and bone. The bony labyrinths appeared normal in 23 ears. The ear of one animal, sacrificed 12 months after labyrinthectomy, showed chronic labyrinthitis characterized by destruction of both the bony and membranous labyrinths, obliteration with fibrous tissue and bone, and abscess formation in the cochlea. This ear showed no evidence of infection in

TABLE 1. VESTIBULAR SENSE ORGANS

Cat No.	Survival Time (months)	Maculae Utricle	Maculae Saccule	Cristae Lat.	Cristae Sup.	Cristae Post.
1	1	A	D	A	A	A
2	1	A	D	D	D	N
3	1	A	S	A	A	D
4	1	A	D	D	D	S
5	3	A	A	A	A	A
6	3	A	D	D	D	S
7	3	A	S	D	D	N
8	3	A	D	D	D	N
9	6	A	A	A	A	A
10	6	A	D	A	A	D
11	6	A	A	A	A	A
12	6	A	D	S	S	N
13	12	A	A	A	A	A
14	12	A	D	D	D	A
15	12	A	A	A	A	A
16	12	A	D	D	D	S
17	24	A	A	D	D	N
18	24	A	A	A	A	A
19	24	A	A	D	D	D
20	24	A	A	A	A	A
21	36	A	A	D	D	A
22	36	A	A	D	D	S
23	36	A	A	A	A	A
24	36	A	A	A	A	A

A - Absent; D - Degenerated epithelium; S - Some sensory cells; N - Normal sensory cells; Lat. - Lateral semicircular canal; Sup. - Superior semicircular canal; Post. - Posterior semicircular canal.

the middle ear or subarachnoid space of the internal auditory canal.

The cochleas of 20 ears manifested endolymphatic hydrops. It is reasonable to assume that the cochlear hydrops is the result of blockage of the ductus reuniens causing interruption of the longitudinal flow of endolymph. The three cochleas without hydrops each appeared to have a surgically-induced fistula of the cochlear duct permitting the escape of endolymph into perilymphatic spaces. The cochlear hair cell populations were normal in 2 ears, partially missing in 12 and totally missing in 10. The cochlear neuronal populations showed losses proportional to the severity of atrophy of the supporting cells of the organ of Corti.

There was partial resorption of the bone of the cribrose area for the superior division of the vestibular nerve in five ears, including the one with chronic labyrinthitis. The bony configuration and fluid spaces of the internal auditory canals were normal in all ears.

The utricular maculae were absent and replaced by fibrous tissue and bone in all 24 operated ears. The saccular maculae were absent and replaced by fibrous tissue and bone in 13 ears, degenerated and without hair cells in 9, and partially degenerated but with some hair cells remaining in 2. The ampullae of the lateral and superior semicircular canals showed similar changes consisting of absence of the cristae and replacement by fibrous tissue and bone

TABLE 2. SUMMARY OF PATHOLOGICAL CHANGES IN VESTIBULAR SENSE ORGANS

	Absent	Severe Degeneration	Partial Degeneration
Maculae			
Utricle	24		
Saccule	13	9	2
Cristae*			
Lateral	12	11	1
Superior	12	11	1
Posterior	12	3	4

*Normal in 5 ears.

in 12, degeneration of the cristae with total loss of hair cells in 11, and partial degeneration of the cristae with loss of some hair cells in 1 ear. The cristae of the posterior semicircular canals were absent and replaced by fibrous tissue and bone in 12, degenerated and without hair cells in 3, partly degenerated but with some hair cells remaining in 4, and normal in 5 ears. A summary of the pathological changes in the vestibular sense organs appears in Tables 1 and 2. The neuronal populations for both operated and control ears are shown in Table 3 as well as in Figures 1 and 2.

Figures 3 to 9 are representative photomicrographs of the superior divisions of the vestibular nerves and their ganglia. These photographs also show the cribrose areas and the region of the labyrinth normally occupied by the utricular macula, as well as the cristae of the lateral and superior semicircular canals. In each case the operated ear shows fibrous tissue and bone occupying the intralabyrinthine space. In each case the terminal ends of the peripheral fibers of the vestibular neurons have been amputated and the compartment filled with fibrous tissue and bone. These peripheral fibers show retrograde degeneration which begins in the cribrose area and progresses in the direction of the vestibular ganglia. A loss of neuronal population is first seen at six months and is progressive for the three-year duration of this study. At three years it appears that most of the peripheral nerve fibers have undergone retrograde degeneration to the cell bodies of the Scarpa's ganglia. The mean total neuronal populations show mean losses of 12% at six months, 24% at 1 year, 35% at 2 years and 53% at 3 years. At 3 years the losses are 58% for the superior division and 40% for the inferior division.

There was no evidence of nerve fiber regeneration or neuroma formation.

HUMAN TEMPORAL BONE STUDY

In the collection of temporal bones at the Massachusetts Eye and Ear Infirmary there are two specimens from subjects who underwent labyrinthectomies for presumed Menière's disease.

Case 1. In 1953, at the age of 50, this patient began having acute vertiginous episodes characterized by a sensation of rotation associated with right-

TABLE 3. VESTIBULAR NEURONAL POPULATIONS

Cat No.	Experimental Survival Time (months)	Superior Division Operated	Superior Division Control	Inferior Division Operated	Inferior Division Control	Total Operated	Total Control
1	1	6,953	6,128	2,813	3,476	9,766	9,604
2	1	3,204	4,301	6,604	6,587	9,808	10,888
3	1	8,024	7,548	3,187	2,890	11,211	10,438
4	1	8,576	8,627	3,102	2,881	11,678	11,508
	Mean	6,689	6,651	3,926	3,958	10,615	10,609
5	3	6,579	6,553	3,111	2,796	9,690	9,349
6	3	7,539	7,828	3,000	2,915	10,539	10,743
7	3	7,930	7,590	4,012	4,131	11,942	11,721
8	3	8,389	8,831	2,924	3,298	11,313	12,129
	Mean	7,609	7,700	3,261	3,285	10,871	10,985
9	6	6,273	7,335	3,298	3,408	9,751	10,743
10	6	7,284	7,446	3,187	3,459	10,471	10,905
11	6	6,706	7,573	3,340	4,292	10,046	11,865
12	6	7,743	9,163	3,119	3,689	10,862	12,852
	Mean	7,001	7,879	3,236	3,712	10,237	11,591
13	12	5,508	6,179	1,470	2,252	6,978	8,431
14	12	6,230	8,500	2,201	2,473	8,431	10,973
15	12	5,950	8,704	2,694	3,910	8,644	12,614
16	12	5,822	7,310	3,332	4,216	9,154	11,526
	Mean	5,877	7,673	2,424	3,212	8,301	10,886
17	24	4,190	6,519	2,091	3,697	6,281	10,216
18	24	4,760	7,871	2,822	2,949	7,582	10,820
19	24	4,267	7,497	3,374	4,326	7,641	11,823
20	24	4,785	7,905	2,907	3,561	7,692	11,466
	Mean	4,501	7,448	2,799	3,633	7,299	11,081
21	36	2,150	7,590	722	2,737	2,872	10,327
22	36	2,610	7,777	2,048	3,009	4,658	10,786
23	36	3,434	6,519	1,921	3,043	5,355	9,562
24	36	4,173	7,369	2,116	2,533	4,793	9,902
	Mean	3,091	7,313	1,701	2,830	4,793	10,144
	Mean Total	5,915	7,445	2,945	3,439	8,807	10,884

sided tinnitus and vomiting. At the age of 55 she complained of a feeling of constant light-headedness but no longer had severe attacks with vomiting. Audiometric study at that time showed a mild right sensorineural hearing loss with 58% speech discrimination score. Ice water caloric testing elicited brisk, symmetrical responses. She noted a tendency to veer to the right. She was suspected of having a posterior fossa tumor, possibly a vestibular schwannoma. Numerous tests, including pneumoencephalogram, were negative. In 1960, at the age of 57, she complained of recurrent syncopal attacks, as well as vertiginous episodes. Audiometry showed mild progression of the right sensorineural hearing loss with speech discrimination of 62% (Fig. 10). There was no response to ice water caloric testing in the right ear. A right transtympanic labyrinthectomy was performed (not by the author) by removing the stapes, followed by introducing the aspiration tip into the vestibule and aspirating its contents. Postoperatively she was nauseated and had a spontaneous nystagmus to the left; this gradually subsided, and she had no further complaints of vertigo. She died of unrelated causes in 1974 at the age of 71, 14 years following labyrinthectomy.

Histological study of the right ear shows the stapes to be absent and an open oval window (Fig. 11). The vestibule and semicircular canals obviously contain air in continuity with the middle ear. The endosteum of the vestibule shows slight thickening; however, there is neither bone nor fibrous tissue proliferation in the inner ear. Reissner's membrane is displaced into the scala vestibuli in all three turns (Fig. 12). The organ of Corti is missing in some areas, and consists of a mound of undifferentiated tissue in other areas. The tectorial membrane is either missing or spherically deformed and encapsulated. About 50% of the stria vascularis and roughly 70% of cochlear neurons are missing. The utricle and ampullae are widely dilated. The saccular wall appears to be collapsed on the macula (Fig. 13). The stroma of the maculae of the utricle and saccule are thickened by fibrous tissue proliferation (Fig. 14). There is partial preservation of supporting cells of the maculae and cristae, but all sensory cells are missing (Figs. 14 and 15). The vestibular nerves are severely atrophied. Only a few scattered nerve fibers are seen in the cribrose areas and only a few neurons (possibly 5%) remain in Scarpa's ganglia.

The left ear shows slight atrophy of the organ of Corti and neurons at the extreme basal end of the cochlea, which appears to be normal for age. The sensory and neural structures of the vestibular sys-

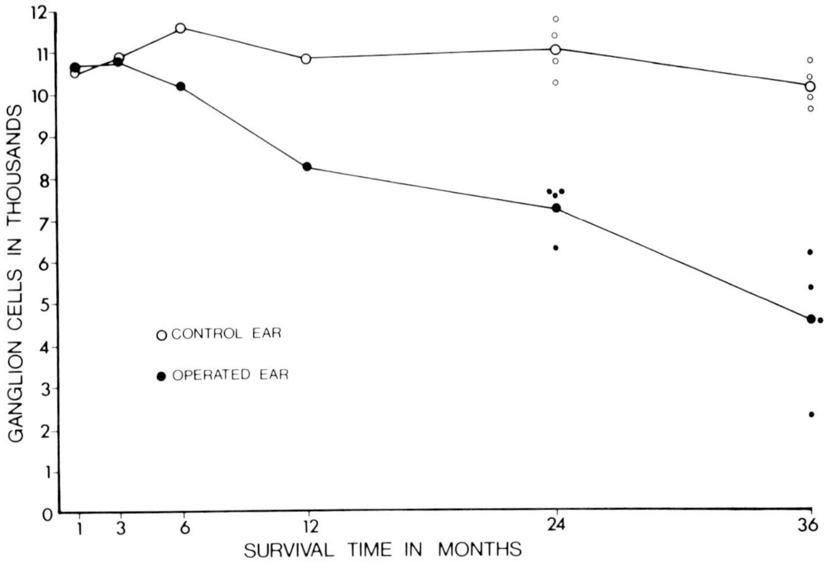

Fig. 1. Vestibular neuron populations in 1000s plotted against survival time in months following labyrinthectomy. Each entry represents mean for four cats. Small circles show populations for each of four cats at 24 and 36 months survival times.

tem are normal.

COMMENT. The diagnosis of Menière's disease seems to be substantiated by endolymphatic hydrops of both the cochlear and vestibular parts of the labyrinth. Histological study shows that labyrinthectomy failed to accomplish removal or maceration of the vestibular sense organs; nonetheless all sensory cells of the vestibular sense organs have degenerated. The severe loss of vestibular neurons is most logically attributed to trauma to the peripheral nerve ending associated with atrophy of the hair cells and supporting cells of the sensory epithelium.

Case 2. In 1964, at the age of 63, this retired merchant sought treatment at the Ambulatory Services Clinic of the Massachusetts Eye and Ear Infirmary for bilateral progressive hearing loss of 13 years' duration. He also stated that he had experienced two episodes of vertigo; the first, which lasted four days, occurring one year prior to evaluation, and the second, lasting for one week, 11 months later. There was no hearing change associated with these attacks. Audiometry showed a severe hearing loss in the right ear with 68% speech discrimination score, and a profound hearing loss in the left ear with zero discrimination. Bithermal caloric tests showed hypoactive response bilaterally with right directional preponderance. Tests for positional nystagmus were unremarkable. Plain radiographic films of the temporal bones were normal. Neurological evaluation was negative. He had no further vertigo until the age of 65, at which time he complained of progressive hearing loss, episodes of vertigo with vomiting, and headache. Audiometry documented progression of the hearing loss (Fig. 16). Cold caloric responses were reduced in both ears, more so on the left. There was a right-beating nystagmus in the left-ear-down position which had no onset latency and lasted 11 seconds. Again, neurological evaluation was negative.

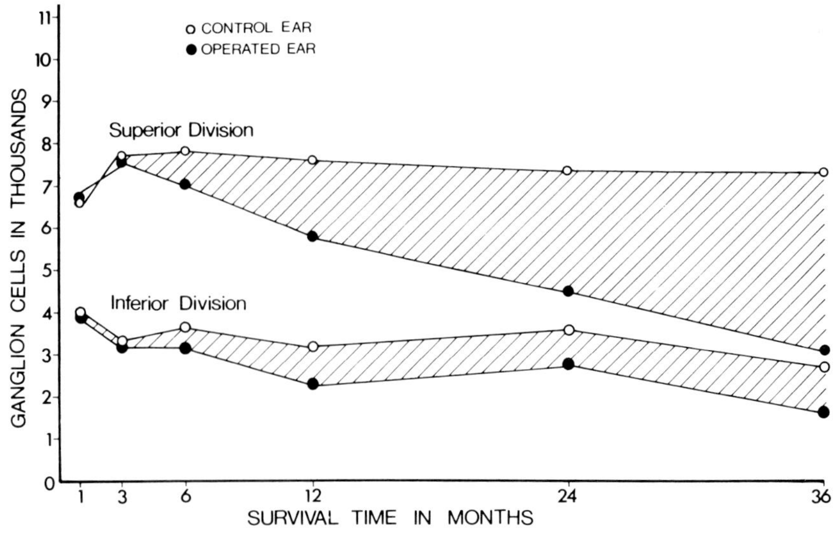

Fig. 2. Vestibular neuron populations of superior and inferior divisions in 1000s plotted against survival time in months following labyrinthectomy. Each entry represents mean for four cats.

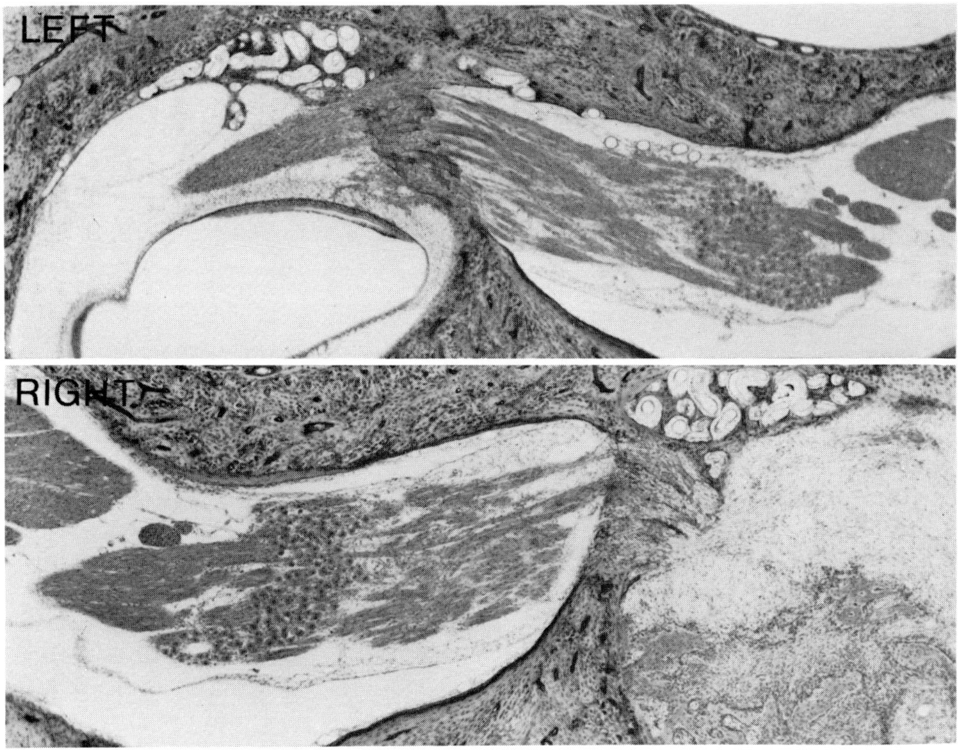

Fig. 3. (Cat 1) Vestibular sensorineural structures one month following labyrinthectomy. Control (left) ear - 9,604 neurons; operated (right) ear - 9,766 neurons. In operated ear there is bone and fibrous tissue in vestibule and peripheral nerve fibers are degenerated in cribrose area.

The patient was presented at the weekly clinical conference at the Massachusetts Eye and Ear Infirmary and the consensus of those present held that a left labyrinthectomy should be performed in an attempt to alleviate the vertiginous symptoms, even though no specific etiology had been determined. The labyrinthectomy was performed via a transtympanic approach (not by the author). The footplate of the stapes was perforated and fluid was aspirated from the vestibule for chemical analysis. The operative report states "the saccule and utricle were grasped with a cupped forceps and removed from the vestibule. The walls of the vestibule were scraped and the round and oval windows were con-

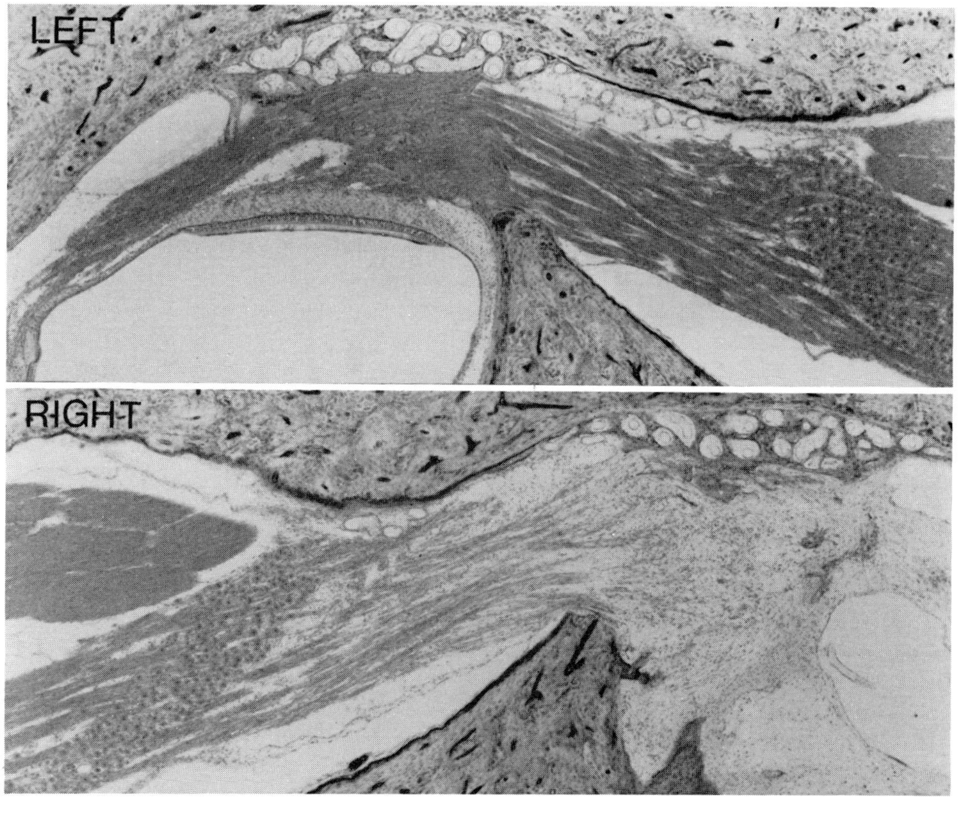

Fig. 4. (Cat 6) Vestibular sensorineural structures three months following labyrinthectomy. Control ear - 10,743 neurons; operated ear - 10,539 neurons. In operated ear there is fibrous tissue and small amount of bone in vestibule. Cribrose area shows partial resorption of bone. Degeneration of peripheral nerve fibers has advanced toward Scarpa's ganglion.

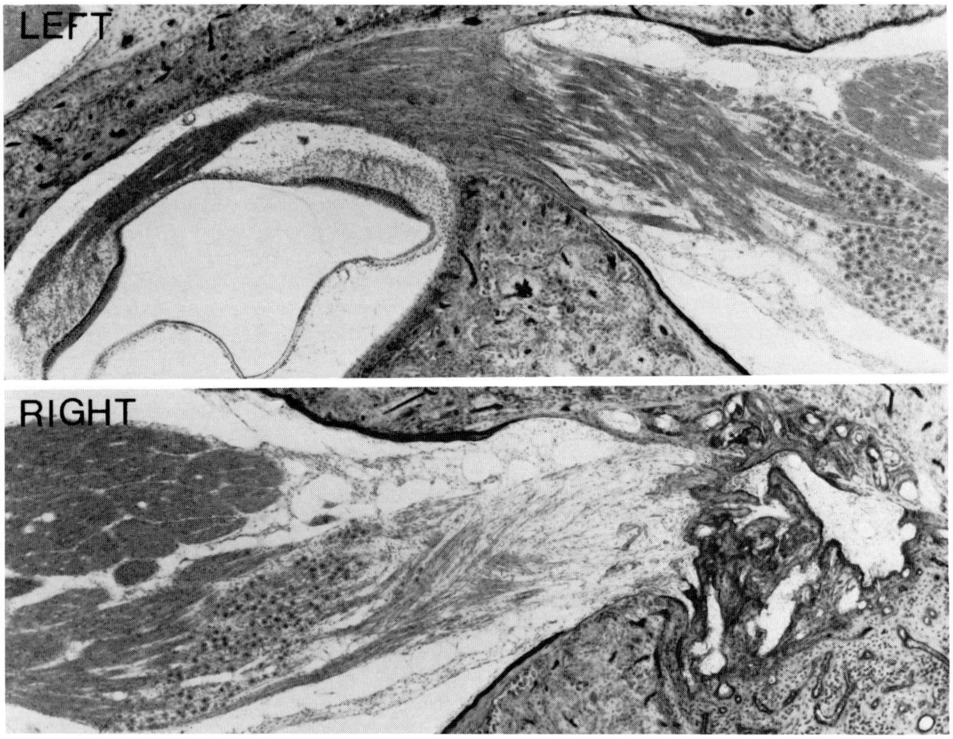

Fig. 5. (Cat 10) Vestibular sensorineural structures six months following labyrinthectomy. Control ear - 10,905 neurons; operated ear - 10,471 neurons. Vestibule of operated ear is filled with bone and small amount of fibrous tissue. There is severe degeneration of peripheral nerve fibers, but as yet no significant loss of neurons. Also see Fig. 9.

nected with the aid of a drill."

The fluid from the vestibule contained 15 mEq/L of potassium, 120 mEq/L of sodium, and 127 mg% of protein, all of which were considered to be normal for perilymph. Therefore, the fluid analysis did not support the diagnosis of Menière's disease (in which case the potassium value should have been elevated), or vestibular schwannoma (in which case the protein should have been elevated).[17]

Postoperatively the patient exhibited a right-beating nystagmus and ataxia, both of which subsided during the following month. He had no further episodes of severe vertigo, but he continued to be unsteady. Three months after labyrinthectomy

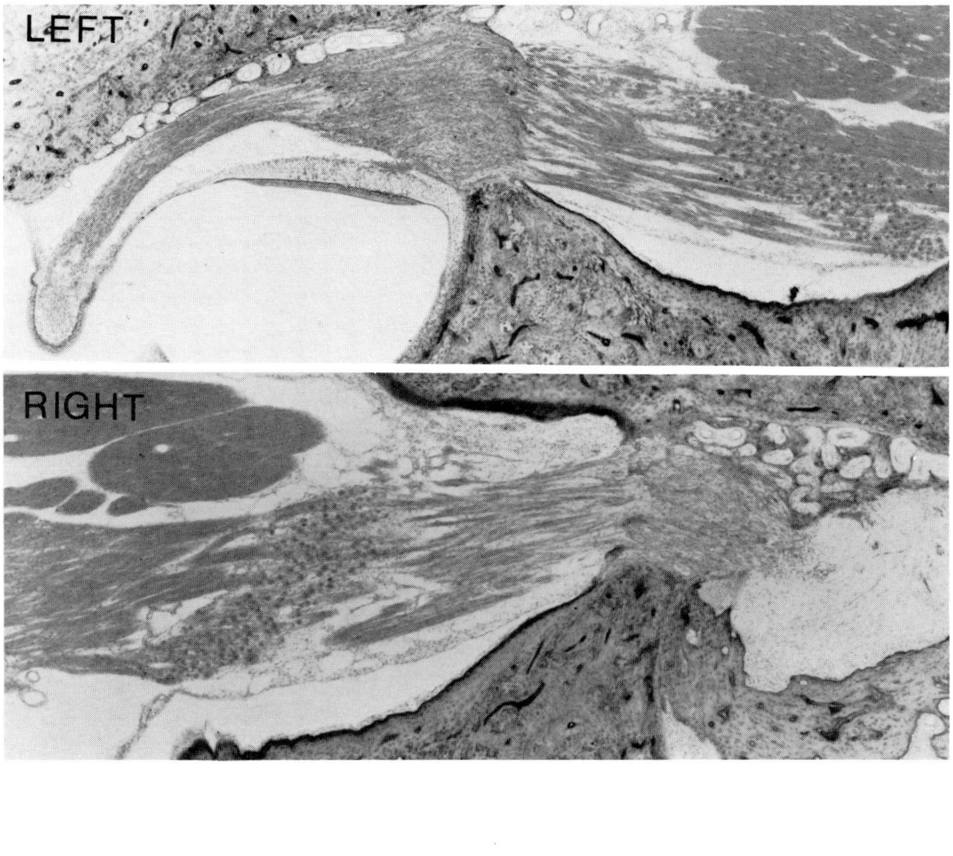

Fig. 6. (Cat 13) Vestibular sensorineural structures 12 months following labyrinthectomy. Control ear - 8,431 neurons; operated ear - 6,978 neurons. Operated ear shows bone and fibrous tissue in vestibule, severe degeneration of peripheral nerve fibers, and slight loss of neurons.

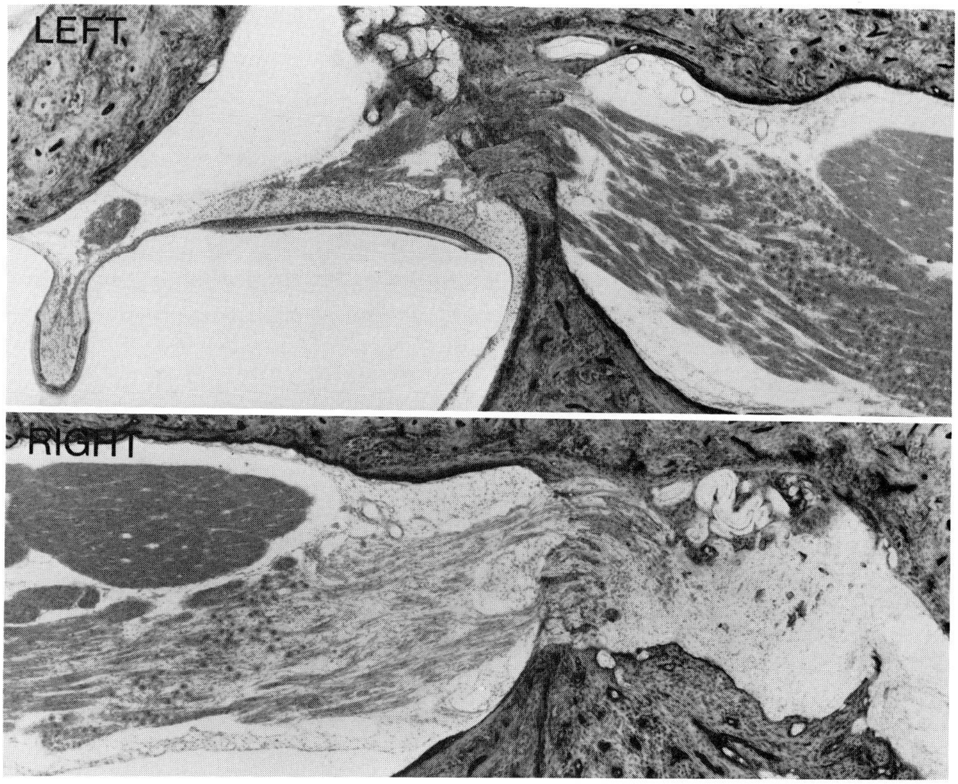

Fig. 7. (Cat 17) Vestibular sensorineural structures 24 months following labyrinthectomy. Control ear - 10,216 neurons; operated ear - 6,281 neurons. Control ear shows bone and fibrous tissue in vestibule, severely degenerated peripheral nerve fibers, and moderate loss of neurons.

he was admitted to the hospital because of right-sided headaches, vomiting, left hemiparesis, left facial weakness, and papilledema. Craniotomy revealed a large neoplasm of the right temporal lobe which was removed and subsequently identified as an astrocytoma. He died of cerebral edema the day following surgery. Histological study of the temporal bones showed the membranous structures of both labyrinths to have moderately severe postmortem autolytic changes.

The right cochlea has a nearly total loss of neurons in the basal and middle turns with 50% remaining in the apical turn. The vestibular sensory

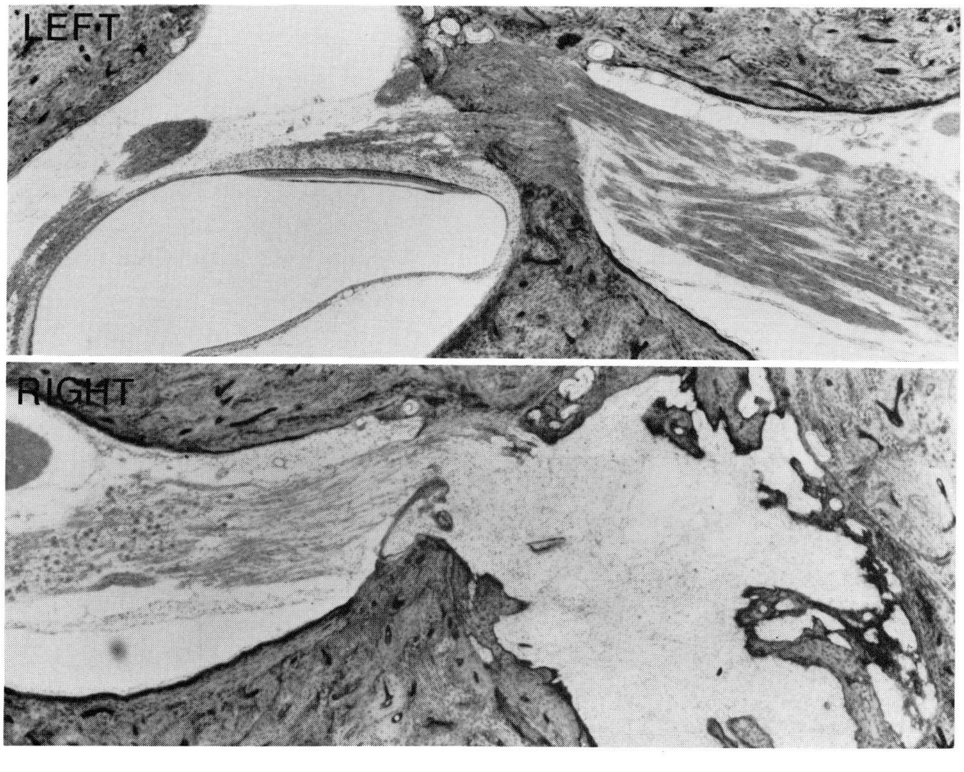

Fig. 8. (Cat 23) Vestibular sensorineural structures 36 months following labyrinthectomy. Control ear - 9,562 neurons; operated ear - 5,355 neurons. Control ear shows bone and fibrous tissue in vestibule, partial resorption of bone in cribrose area, severe degeneration of peripheral nerve fibers, and loss of nearly half of neurons.

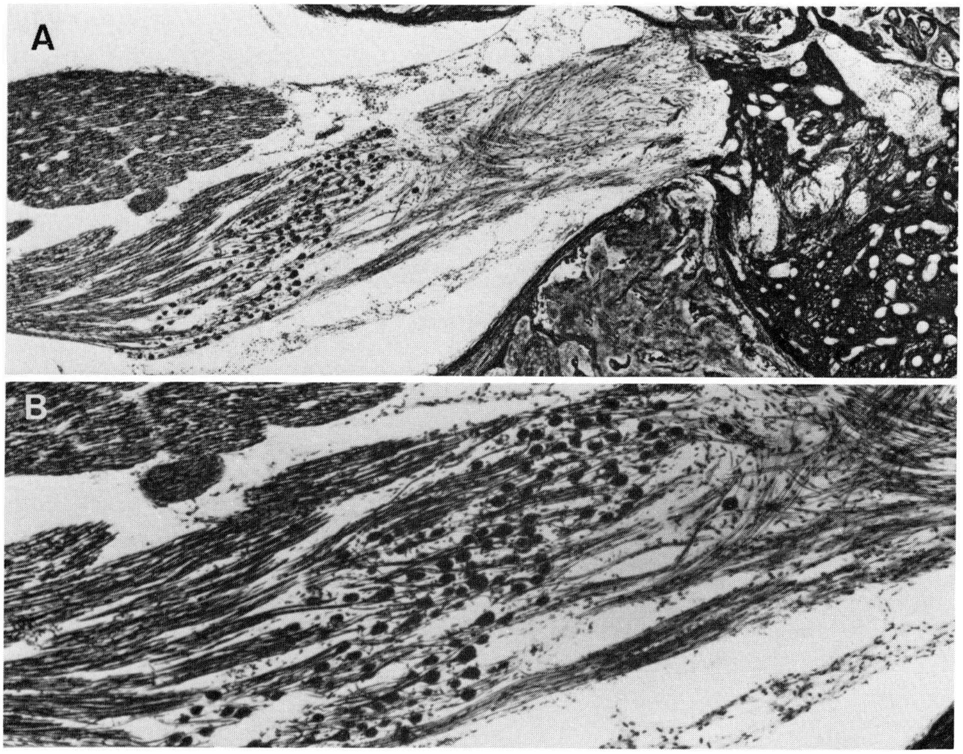

Fig. 9. (Cat 10) Vestibular sensorineural structures six months following labyrinthectomy. A) Same operated ear as in Fig. 5, showing partly degenerated peripheral nerve fibers six months following labyrinthectomy (protargol stain). B) Enlargement of Scarpa's ganglion from A view.

and neural structures show moderate postmortem autolysis but otherwise appear normal.

The left ear, in which the labyrinthectomy was performed, is lacking the incus and stapes; in addition, the bony wall between the oval and round windows is absent. The vestibule and semicircular canals are partly filled with fibrous tissue and bone (Fig. 17A). The organ of Corti, stria vascularis, tectorial membrane, and cochlear neurons are severely degenerated. Reissner's membrane is displaced into the scala vestibuli in all turns (Fig. 18). There is atrophy of the spiral ligament and a rupture of the basilar membrane in the basal turn. The utricular macula and cristae are present; however, their sensory epithelia are totally degenerated.

The saccular macula is missing and the spherical recess contains bundles of nerve fibers interspersed with fibrous tissue (Fig. 17B). There is a remarkable proliferation of nerve fibers within the supporting stromata of the utricular macula and cristae (Figs. 19-21). The nerve fibers are arranged in orderly interlacing bundles of 10 to 30 fibers each. The identification of these bundles as nerve fibers was confirmed by protargol staining. The nerve bundles cannot be traced centrally beyond the cribrose areas because the vestibular nerves were avulsed from the internal auditory canals at the time of autopsy.

COMMENT. It is not clear whether this patient's symptoms should be attributed solely to the brain tumor or whether Menière's disease was coexistent. The cochlear endolymphatic hydrops could have followed the labyrinthectomy as the result of blocking the ductus reuniens and saccule. The stimulus for the proliferation of nerve fibers in the subepithelial stroma of the vestibular sense organs is not evident. The sensory epithelium is atrophied but, in the case of the utricular macula and cristae, the nerve fibers were not surgically traumatized by the labyrinthectomy. The histological pattern of interlacing bundles of fibers is somewhat different from the more disorderly, tightly intertwining pattern characteristic of traumatic neuromata and schwannomata.

DISCUSSION

Gacek and Rasmussen[18] found cats to have an average of 2,652 nerve fibers to each crista, 1,821 to the macula of the saccule, and 2,693 to the macula

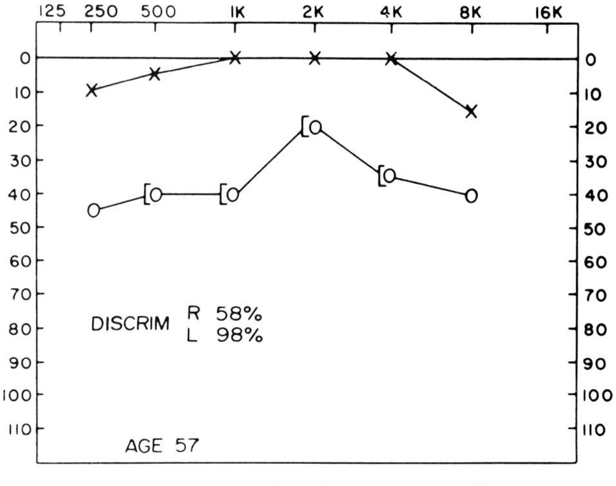

Fig. 10. (Case 1) Audiogram at age 57.

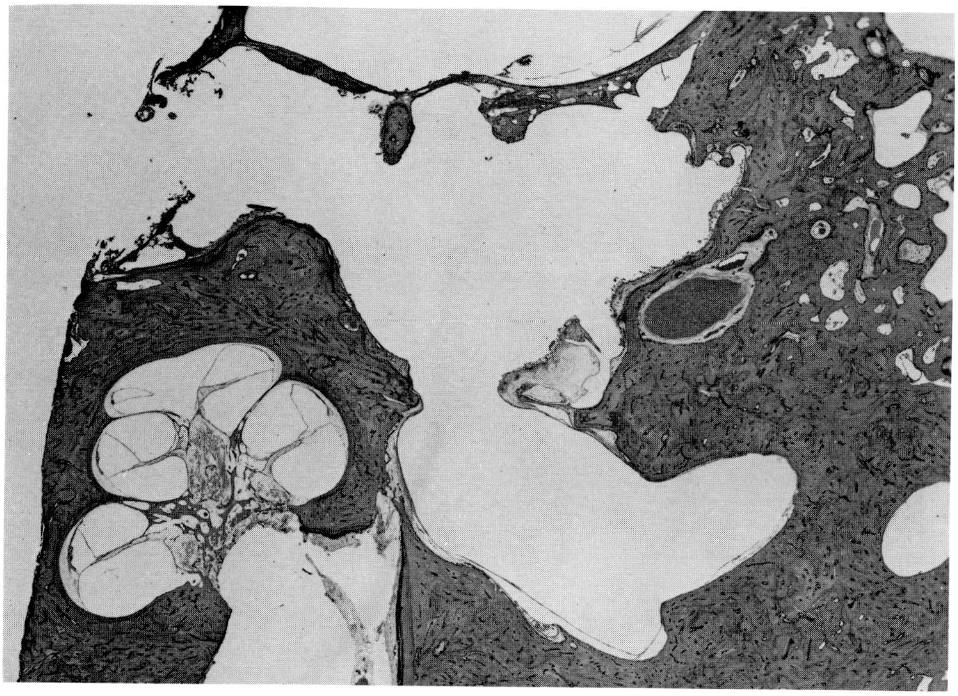

Fig. 11. (Case 1) Right ear showing vestibule and semicircular canals in communication with middle ear 14 years following transtympanic labyrinthectomy.

of the utricle. The total of 12,470 includes Voit's anastomosis and the efferent fibers. In the present experiment, neuronal cell bodies were counted, and all, of course, are of the afferent type. This method has been used previously for both cochlear ganglia[19-21] and vestibular ganglia.[22] Using this method on eight normal cat ears, Richter and Spoendlin[15] found a mean of 11,809 neurons in the vestibular nerve trunk, of which 8,015 were in the superior division and 3,794 in the inferior division. In the present study the mean total population for the normal ears of the 24 cats was 10,884, of which 7,445 were in the superior division and 3,439 in the inferior division. Working in our laboratory, Richter[23] reported a 30% reduction in vestibular neurons in three cats one year after labyrinthectomy. Transmission electron microscopy showed the neurons to be less densely packed in the ganglia, and there was more fibrous tissue between the cells and nerve processes in the operated ears than in the opposite control ears.

By comparison, Richter[24] found the mean human vestibular neuronal population to be about 18,000

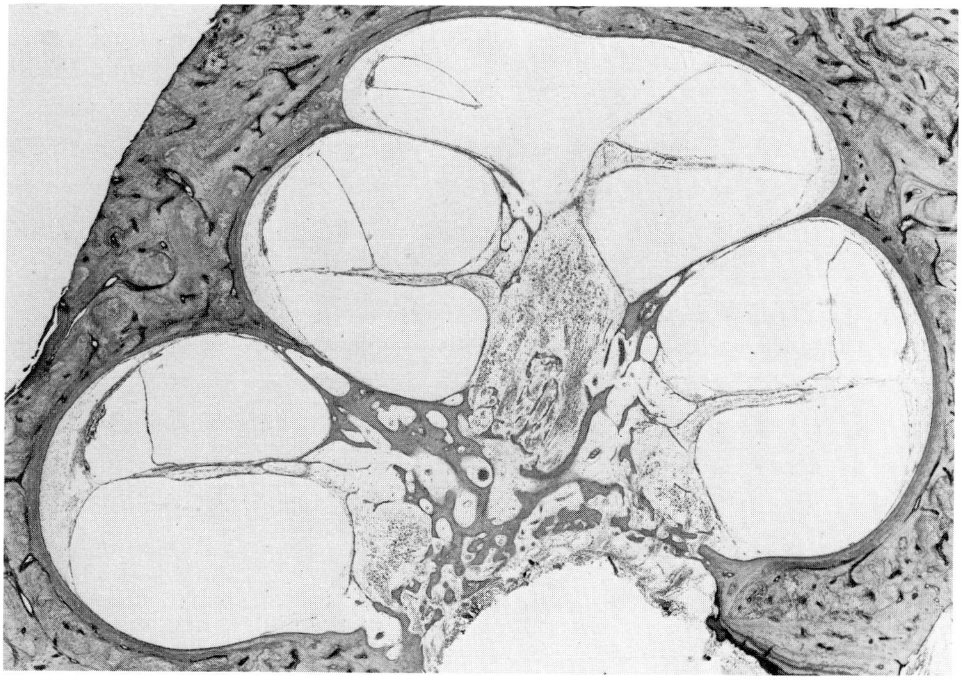

Fig. 12. (Case 1) Right ear showing cochlear hydrops, severe atrophy of organ of Corti, partial atrophy of stria vascularis, and partial loss of cochlear neurons.

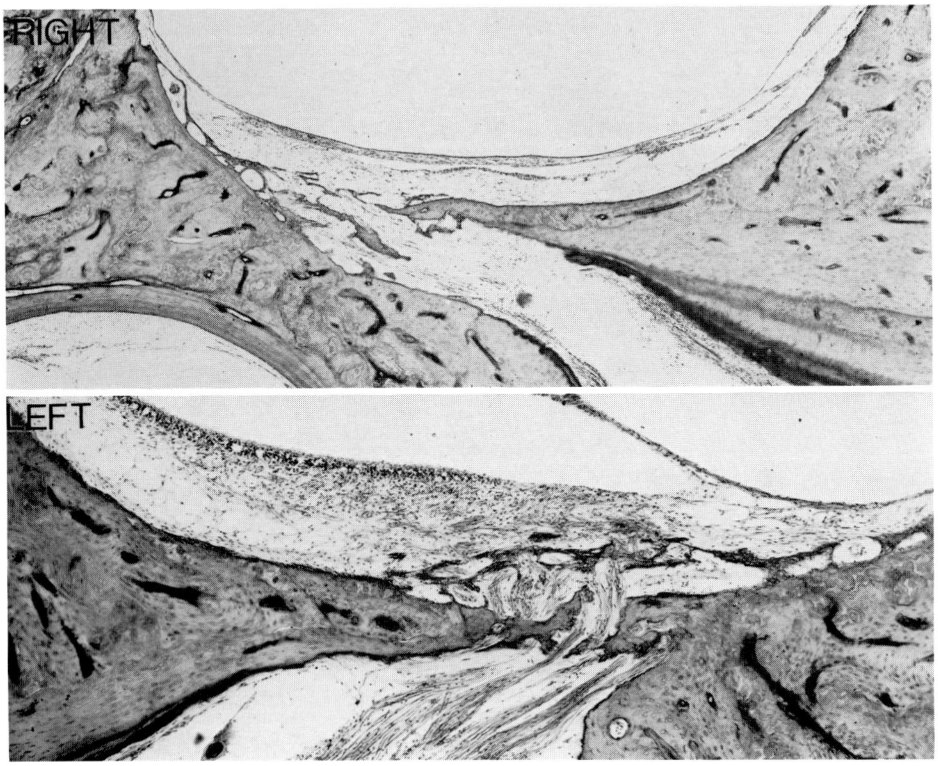

Fig. 13. (Case 1) Saccules. Atrophy of the right macula and nerve; left macula is normal.

with about two thirds in the superior division and one third in the inferior division. This compares closely with a mean of 18,439 in 15 normal ears studied by Naufal and Schuknecht.[22]

Following labyrinthectomy, the first change, observed as early as one month postoperatively, was degeneration of the peripheral nerve fibers in the cribrose areas. With time the degeneration extended progressively toward the ganglion. A loss of cell bodies of the ganglion was first noted at six months postoperatively and continued at a steady rate, so that about 53% were missing at three years.

Histological studies show that labyrinthectomy failed to achieve total destruction of sensory cells of

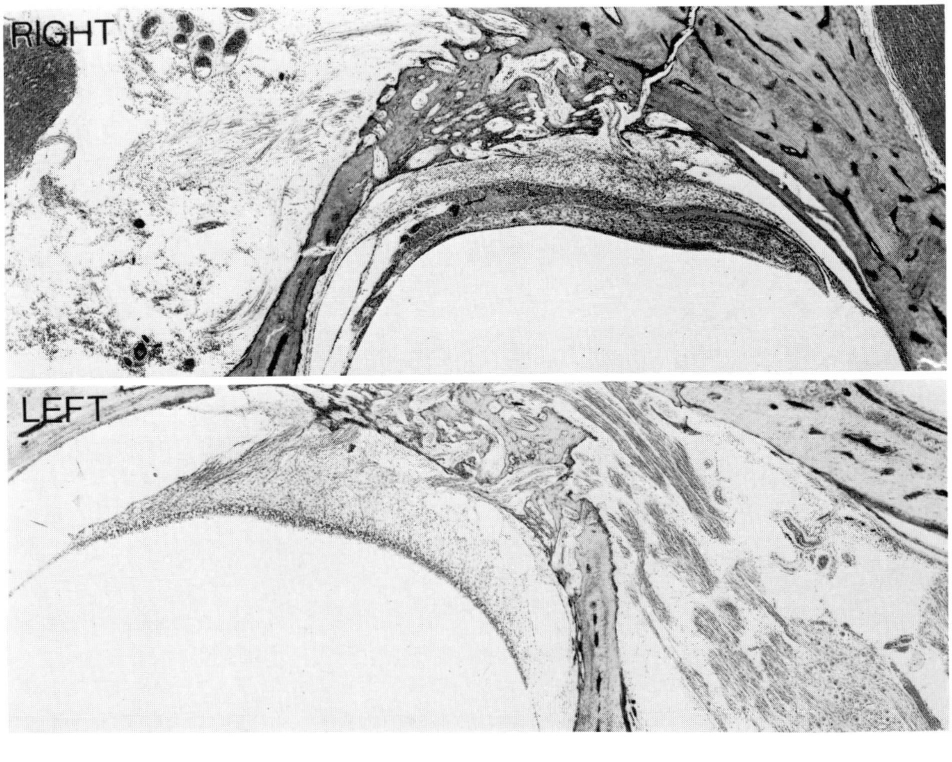

Fig. 14. (Case 1) Utricles. Atrophy and fibrosis of right macula and atrophy of nerve; left macula is normal.

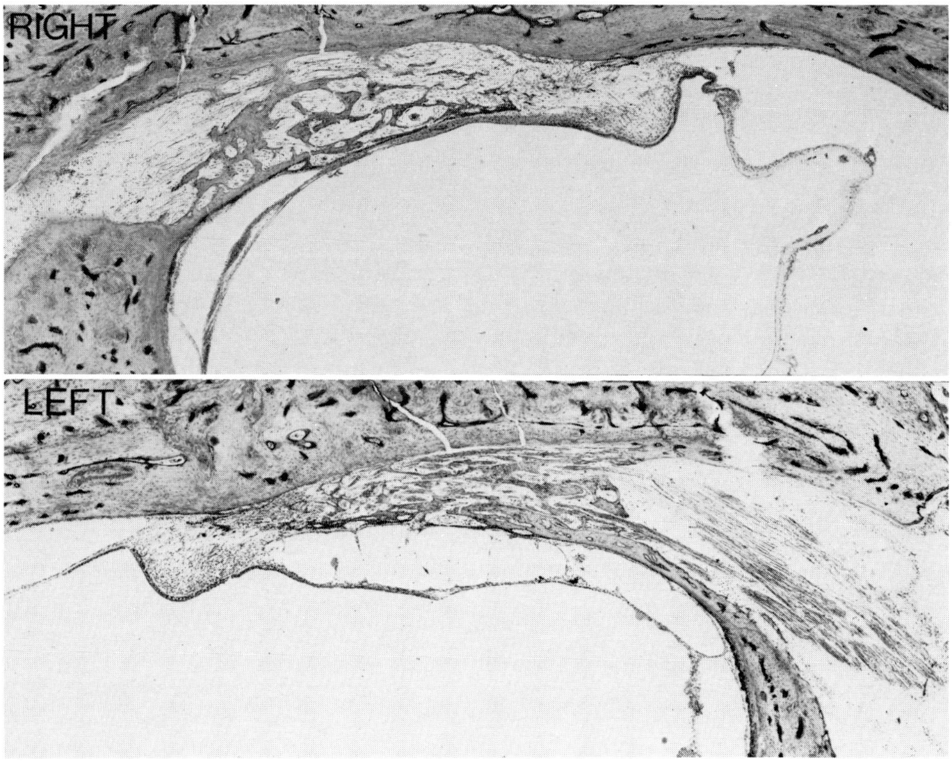

Fig. 15. (Case 1) Cristae of lateral canals. Atrophy of sensory epithelium and nerve on right side; left crista is normal.

the vestibular system in 10 of the 24 operated ears. Most of these failures were due to inadequate probing of the posterior canal ampulla which, because of its more remote location from the oval window, is more difficult to reach. This observation suggests that a more aggressive approach may be needed to reach and destroy the posterior canal crista in human labyrinthectomy also.

A question of some importance is whether any vestibular symptoms arise from the slowly progressive atrophy of the vestibular nerves following destruction of their sense organs. Certainly if the sensory ablation is complete, the nerves cannot be stimulated physiologically; therefore episodic dysequilibrium could not be attributed to the remaining nerve elements. The experiment provides no information as to whether nerves deprived of their sense organs have the potential for creating vestibular sensations or symptoms.

In none of the animal ears was there evidence of vestibular nerve regeneration. It seems quite improbable, therefore, that neuromata will occur at the site of amputation of the peripheral nerve fibers. Moreover, a neuroma must be clearly differentiated from a schwannoma. A neuroma is a mass of intertwining, regenerating nerve fibers proliferating in response to nerve injury. A schwannoma, often mistakenly referred to as an acoustic neuroma, is a neoplasm arising from the Schwann cells. A neuroma may be difficult to differentiate histologically from a schwannoma, particularly on biopsy or small excisional specimens. Temporal bone studies show that occult schwannomata are not rare, occurring in 0.17% of the population, and they may be entirely intralabyrinthine (author, unpublished data).

The literature contains four case reports of traumatic neuromata following labyrinthectomy. The first case, reported by Hilding and House in 1965,[25] had unsuccessful stapes surgery (not by the authors) in 1959, complicated by intractable vertigo; a transtympanic labyrinthectomy was performed in 1961 (not by the authors), but dizziness continued. A repeat transtympanic labyrinthectomy was performed in 1963 by W. House and the contents of the vestibule were removed for histological examination. Electron microscopic study showed myelin-

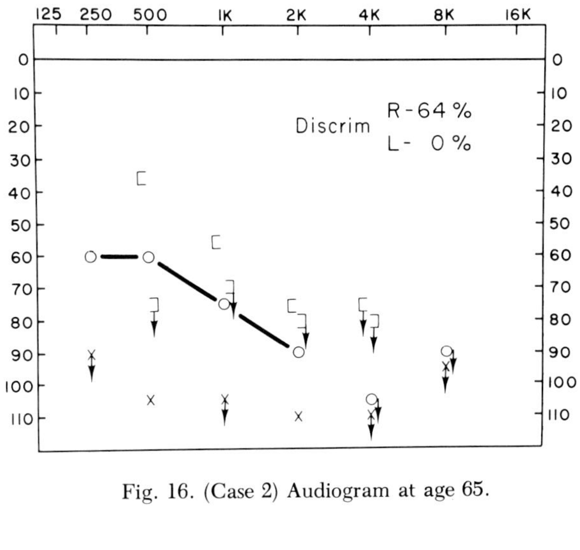

Fig. 16. (Case 2) Audiogram at age 65.

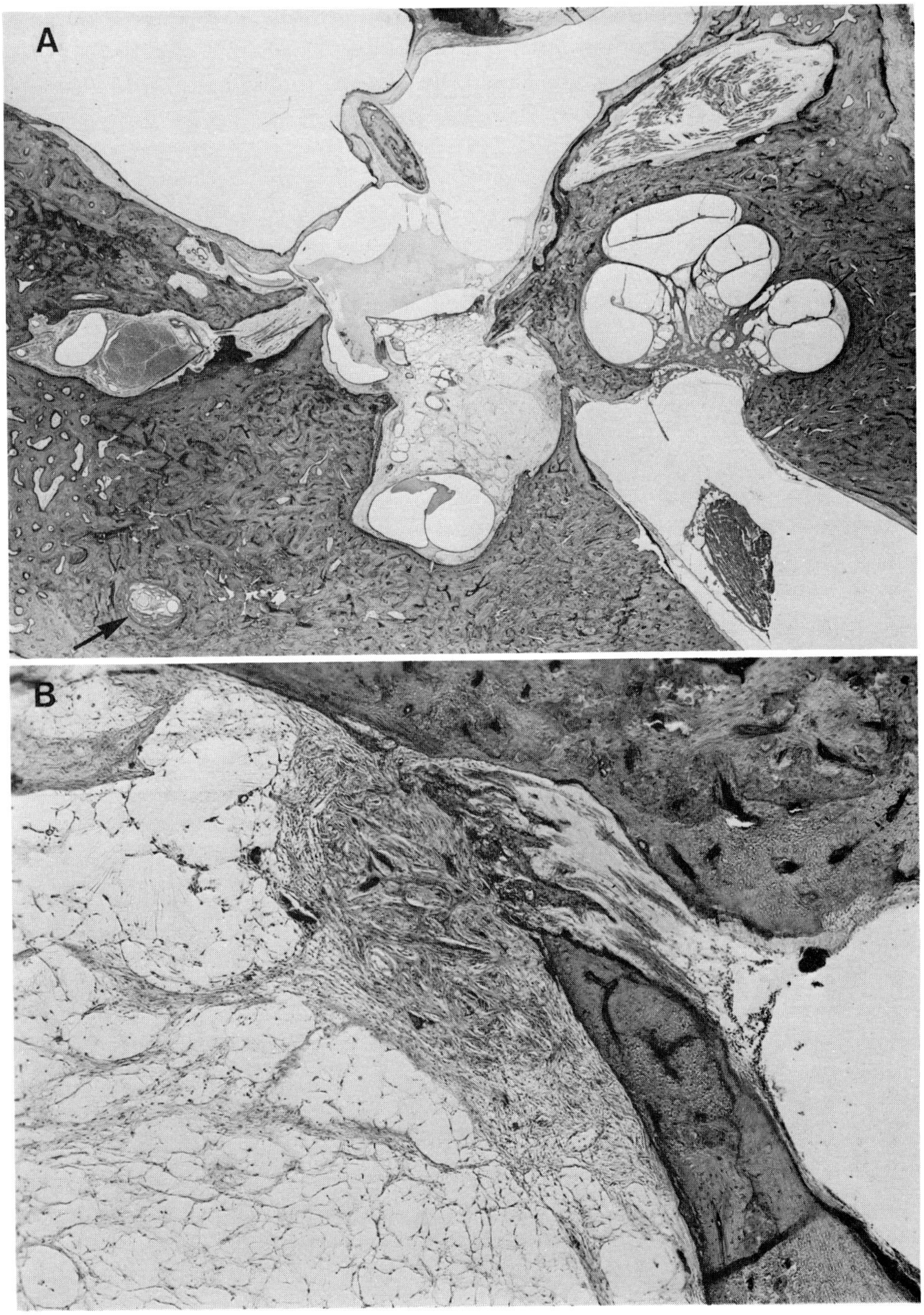

Fig. 17. (Case 2) Left ear three months following labyrinthectomy. A) Fibrous tissue in vestibule, bone in posterior semicircular canal (arrow), cochlear endolymphatic hydrops, and severe atrophy of structures of cochlear duct and cochlear nerve. B) High-power view of spherical recess area showing saccular macula containing fibrous tissue mixed with nerve fibers.

ated and unmyelinated nerve fibers twisted together among a few strands of connective tissue, a situation which Hilding and House interpreted to be consistent with traumatic neuroma. No clinical follow-up report was given. The second case, reported by Pulec in 1974,[9] had a transtympanic labyrinthectomy by Linthicum in 1960. The stapes was removed, the contents of the vestibule were aspirated and the stapes was replaced. Following the labyrinthectomy the patient "had constant poor balance and was severely disabled." Four years later she exhibited no response to bithermal caloric testing in that ear. The patient continued to complain of vertigo until the time of her death in 1970 at age 78, ten years following labyrinthectomy. Histological study of the temporal bone revealed vestibular contents consisting of fibrous tissue, bone, and a mass interpreted to represent a traumatic neuroma (Fig. 22). There was cochlear endolymphatic hydrops, and the ampulla of the posterior semicircular canal was intact. The third and fourth cases were reported by Linthicum et al in 1979.[10] In both cases the patients had undergone transtympanic labyrinthectomy (not by the authors), but had persistent vertigo. Repeat transtympanic labyrinthectomy revealed tissue masses in the vestibules which on histological study were believed to be traumatic neuromata. The patients were reported

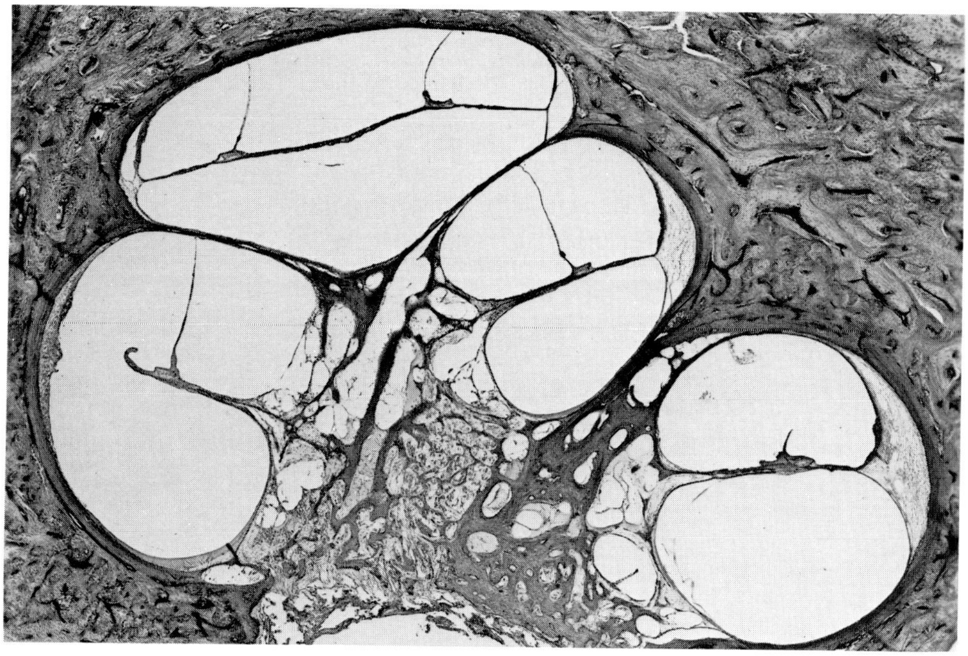

Fig. 18. (Case 2) Left ear showing cochlear endolymphatic hydrops, atrophy of organ of Corti and cochlear neurons, and atrophy of spiral ligament with rupture of basilar membrane in basal turn.

to be free of vertigo following the repeat labyrinthectomies.

The histological appearance of these traumatic neuromata is somewhat different from the nerve fiber proliferation seen in case 2. The histological features in the former resemble more the Antoni type A schwannomata consisting of merging and diverging streams of elongated spindle cells, with a tendency for the nuclei to be aligned in straight or curved rows, their long axes parallel to one another. The pathognomonic feature of neuromata is the proliferation of axons; this condition can be demonstrated with silver stains as was done in case 2. The histological appearance of the proliferating axons in case 2 is characterized by interlacing bundles of 10 to 30 fibers each, with growth restricted to the subepithelial stromata of the sense organs. It is possible that the nerve fiber proliferation in this case is unrelated to the labyrinthectomy and may represent some other disease entity.

SUMMARY AND CONCLUSIONS

Experimental transtympanic labyrinthectomies

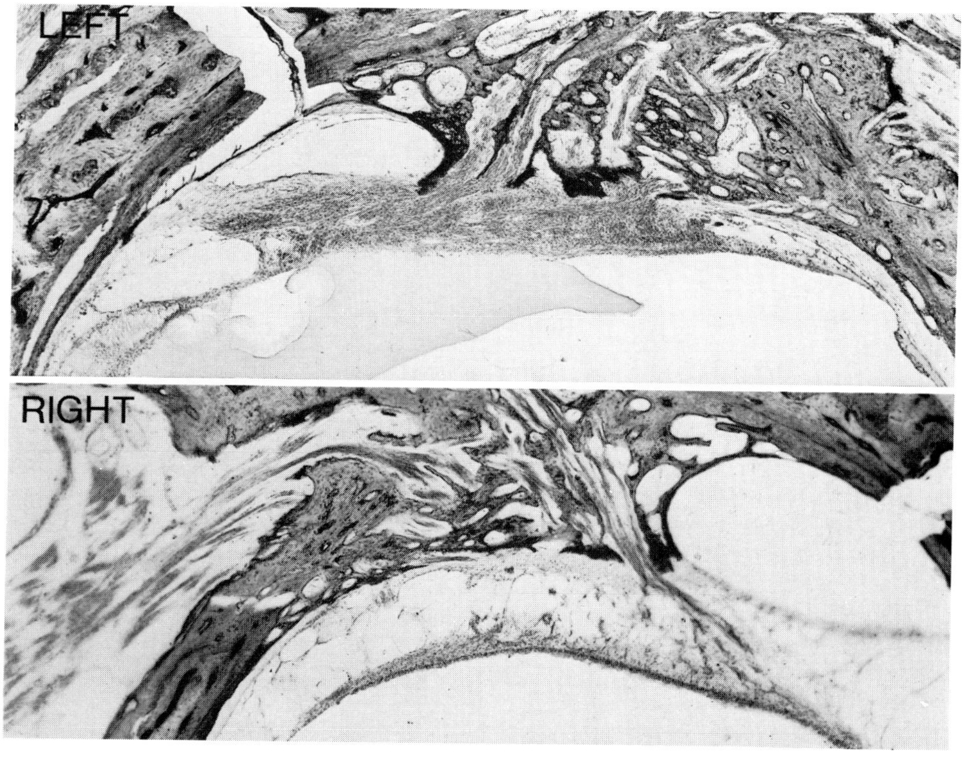

Fig. 19. (Case 2) Utricles. Atrophy of sensory epithelium and proliferation of nerve fibers in stroma of macula on left side; right macula is normal.

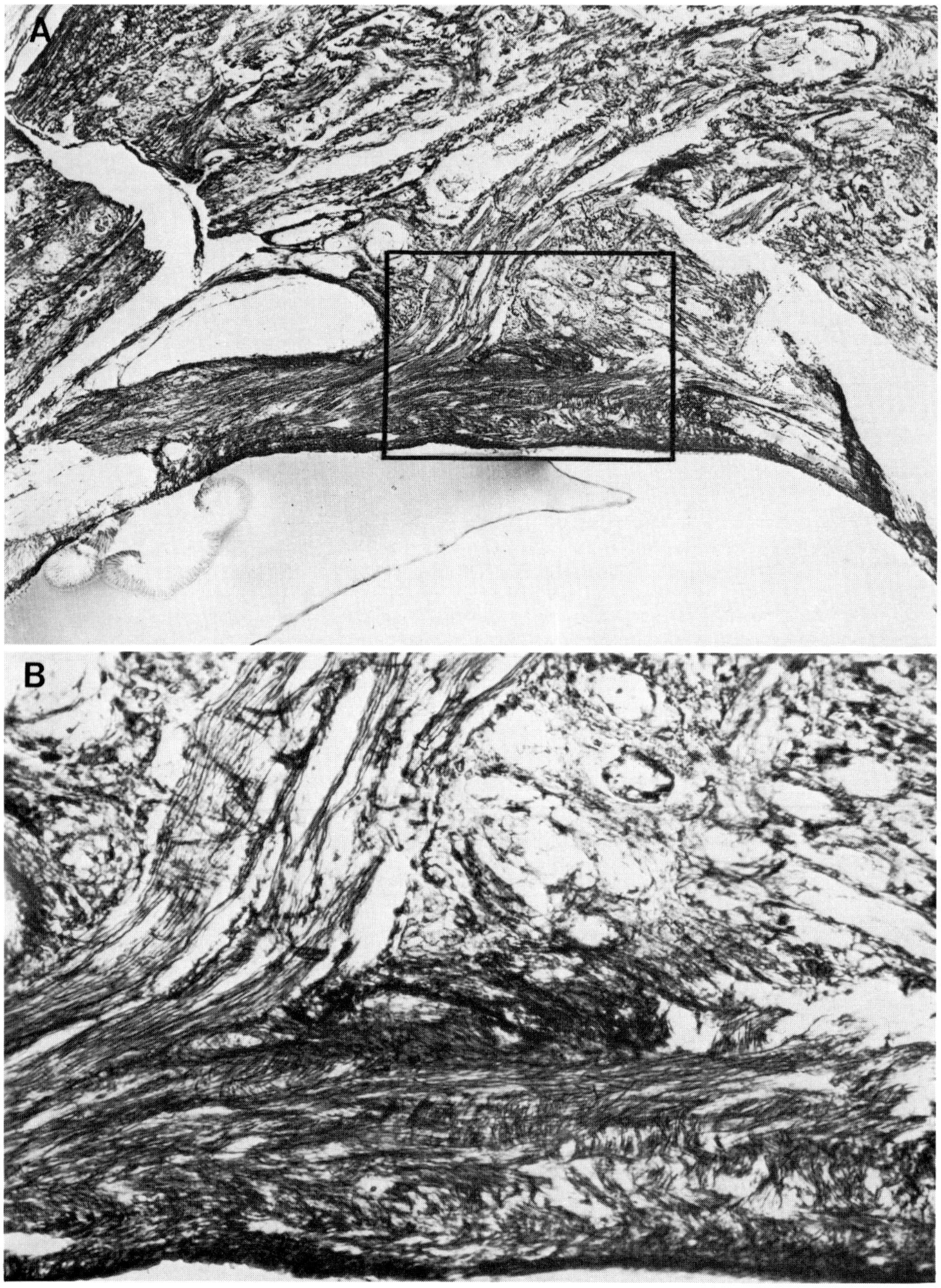

Fig. 20. (Case 2) A) Left utricle, protargol stain showing proliferation of nerve fibers in stroma of macula. B) High-power view of macula (rectangle in A) showing nerve fibers in stroma of macula and degenerated sensory epithelium.

on 24 cats showed that destruction of the vestibular sense organs incited a slowly progressive degenerative change in the vestibular nerves. Atrophy began at the peripheral ends of the fibers at the sites of trauma and progressed centrally to include the cell bodies of Scarpa's ganglia. Three years following labyrinthectomy the peripheral nerve fibers appeared totally degenerated and about half of the cell bodies had disappeared. There was no evidence of regeneration of the vestibular nerve fibers.

The temporal bones of two human subjects who had had transtympanic labyrinthectomy for presumed Menière's disease showed disparate neural changes. In both cases the sensory epithelia had degenerated, but the supporting stromata of the maculae and cristae were preserved. In one case, 14 years following surgery, there was nearly total loss of vestibular nerve fibers and cell bodies. In the other case, three months following surgery there was a proliferation of nerve fibers in the supporting stromata of the maculae and cristae. The growth pattern was characterized by interlacing bundles of fibers rather than intertwining single fibers in a fibrous tissue matrix as would be expected in a traumatic neuroma. It is assumed that these fibers originated from Scarpa's ganglia; however, positive identification could not be made because the vestibular nerve trunks, including Scarpa's ganglia, had been avulsed from the internal auditory canal at the time of autopsy.

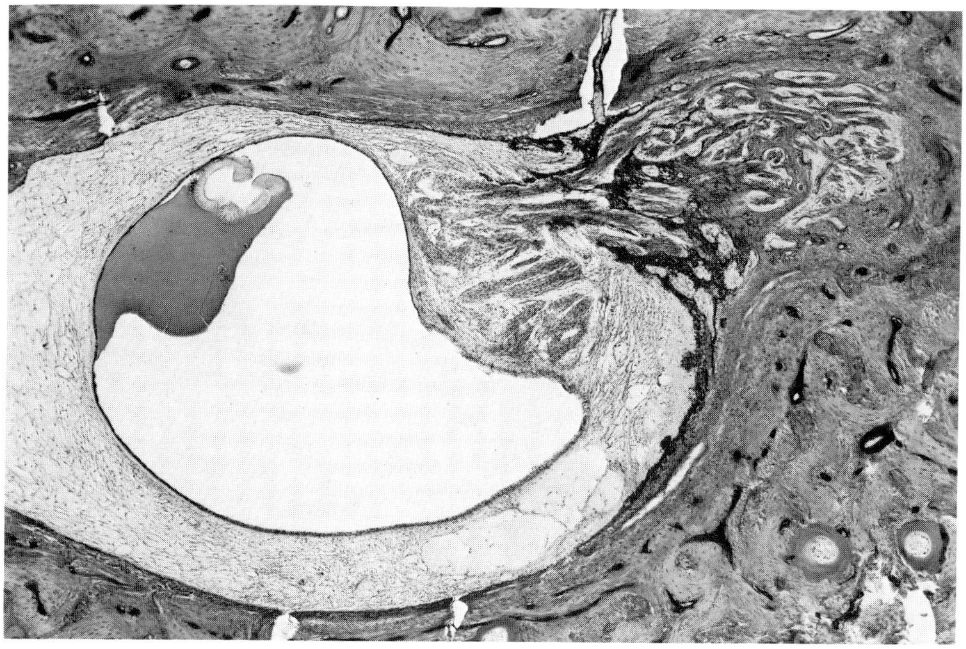

Fig. 21. (Case 2) Ampulla of left posterior semicircular canal showing proliferation of nerve fibers in stroma of crista. Sensory epithelium is degenerated and perilymphatic space contains fibrous tissue.

The principal objective of these studies was to determine the morphological behavior of the vestibular nerve following surgical ablation of the vestibular sense organs. It was anticipated that this knowledge would provide a more rational basis for determining the relative merits of labyrinthectomy versus vestibular nerve excision for the ablation of vestibular function in the treatment of intractable vertigo. Should the vestibular nerve promptly degenerate following labyrinthectomy, there would be no need to subject the patient to the risks involved in vestibular nerve excision. The question is noteworthy only if it is assumed that the vestibular nerve can cause vertigo after being deprived of its sensory stimulus, which is by no means certain. Be that as it may, the studies show that following labyrinthectomy the vestibular nerves undergo progressive atrophy, but only very slowly. Moreover, the condition of total atrophy would not be attained for many years. The question not yet answered is

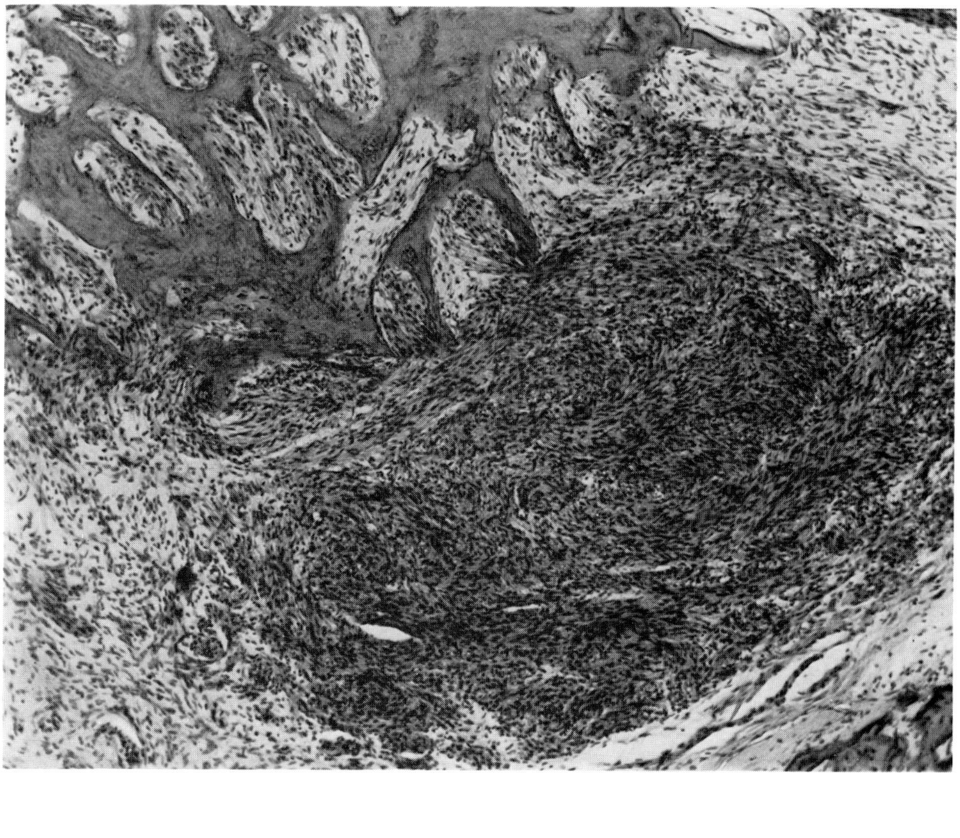

Fig. 22. Tissue in vestibule ten years following labyrinthectomy; question of traumatic neuroma or proliferation of Schwann cells. (Photomicrograph courtesy of Fred Linthicum, Jr, MD.)

whether a vestibular nerve devoid of sensory stimulation can cause vertigo. The very high therapeutic success rate achieved with a well-performed labyrinthectomy,[1] however, augurs well for the proposition that a barren vestibular nerve is sensorially impotent.

A closely related question is whether the afferent fibers of the vestibular nerve are capable of regeneration to the extent that labyrinthectomy could cause formation of traumatic neuromata. The experimental studies show quite clearly that the afferent vestibular nerves of the cat do not have regenerative capability.

Linthicum has kindly provided us with unstained sections of one of his cases of postlabyrinthectomy neuroma. We have performed protargol stains on this tissue and, indeed, it is composed of intertwining bundles of nerve fibers consistent with the diagnosis of traumatic neuroma. The origin of the nerve fibers cannot be determined because the vestibular nerves have been avulsed from the internal auditory canal.

Thus, we face an enigma. The afferent vestibular nerves of the cat show no inclination for regeneration, yet temporal bone studies of postlabyrinthectomy ears of human patients show neuromata. Are these fibers of efferent origin or of some other source, or alternatively do the human afferent vestibular nerves behave differently from those of the cat? But here again the question is noteworthy only if it is assumed that traumatic neuromata would be sensorially potent, a fact which is unknown.

In summary, an experimental study showed that traumatized afferent vestibular nerve fibers of the cat show no inclination for regeneration. Human temporal bone studies, however, have shown regeneration of nerve fibers within the labyrinth following labyrinthectomy. It has not been shown that these fibers are from afferent vestibular neurons, nor has it been shown that regenerating afferent vestibular neurons, devoid of sensory epithelium, can cause dysequilibrium. The total evidence favors the proposition that vestibular nerve excision has no advantage over a well-performed labyrinthectomy in the treatment of intractable vertigo.

ACKNOWLEDGMENTS — The author gratefully acknowledges the assistance of the following persons: Richard Cortese for help with the animal surgery and determination of neuronal populations; Edward Lenard for care of the animals; Diane Jones for the preparation of histological materials; Carla Wittig, Alan Lucas, Arthur Bowden and Laurel Cook for the microphotographs and graphs; and Eileen Nims, Carol Ota, Anne Schuknecht and Julie Gulya for assistance in preparing and editing the manuscript.

REFERENCES

1. Hammerschlag PE, Schuknecht HF. Transcanal labyrinthectomy for intractable vertigo. Arch Otolaryngol 1981; 107: 152-6.

2. Wilson WR, Schuknecht HF. Update on the use of streptomycin therapy for Meniere's disease. Am J Otol 1980; 2:108-11.

3. Cawthorne T. The treatment of Meniere's disease. J Laryngol Otol 1943; 58:563-71.

4. Schuknecht H. Ablation therapy in the management of Meniere's disease. Acta Otolaryngol (Stockh) 1957; Suppl 132: 14-42.

5. Dandy WE. Effects on hearing after subtotal section of the cochlear branch of the auditory nerve. Bull Johns Hopkins Hosp 1934; 55:240-3.

6. House W. Surgical exposure of the internal auditory canal and its contents through the middle cranial fossa. Laryngoscope 1961; 71:1363-85.

7. Antoli-Candela F Jr, Lavarez de Cozar F, Antoli-Candela F Sr. Transvestibular approach to the internal auditory canal. Ann Otol Rhinol Laryngol 1975; 84:145-51.

8. Fisch UP. Excision of Scarpa's ganglion. Arch Otolaryngol 1973; 97:147-9.

9. Pulec JL. Labyrinthectomy: indications, technique and results. Laryngoscope 1974; 84:1552-73.

10. Linthicum F Jr, Alonso A, Denia A. Traumatic neuroma. A complication of transcanal labyrinthectomy. Arch Otolaryngol 1979; 105:654-5.

11. Lempert J. Lempert decompression operation for hydrops of the endolymphatic labyrinth in Meniere's disease. Arch Otolaryngol 1948; 47:551-70.

12. Ariagno R. Transtympanic labyrinthectomy. Arch Otolaryngol 1964; 80:282-6.

13. Fluur E, Tovi D. Microscopic intracranial section of the vestibular nerve in Meniere's disease. Acta Otolaryngol (Stockh) 1965; 59:604-6.

14. Bryan V, Bucy P. Vestibular nerve section for Meniere's disease. Arch Otolaryngol 1973; 97:115-7.

15. Richter E, Spoendlin H. Scarpa's ganglion in the cat. Acta Otolaryngol (Stockh) 1981; 92:423-31.

16. Konigsmark B. Methods for the counting of neurons. In: Nauta W, Ebbeson S, eds. International conference on contemporary research methods in neuroanatomy. Berlin: Springer-Verlag, 1970:316.

17. Silverstein H, Schuknecht H. Biochemical studies of inner ear fluid in man. Arch Otolaryngol 1966; 84:395-402.

18. Gacek RR, Rasmussen GL. Fiber analysis of the statoacoustic nerve of the guinea pig, cat and monkey. Anat Rec 1961; 139:445-63.

19. Schuknecht H, Woellner R. Hearing losses following partial section of the cochlear nerve. Laryngoscope 1953; 63:441-65.

20. Kerr A, Schuknecht HF. The spiral ganglion in profound deafness. Acta Otolaryngol (Stockh) 1968: 65:586-98.

21. Otte J, Schuknecht HF, Kerr A. Ganglion cell populations in normal and pathological human cochleae. Implications for cochlear implantation. Laryngoscope 1978; 88:1231-46.

22. Naufal P, Schuknecht H. Vestibular, facial and oculomotor neuropathology in diabetes mellitus. Arch Otolaryngol 1972; 96:468-74.

23. Richter E. Scarpa's ganglion in the cat one year after labyrinthectomy. Arch Otorhinolaryngol 1981; 230;251-5.

24. Richter E. Quantitative study of human Scarpa's ganglion and vestibular sensory epithelia. Acta Otolaryngol (Stockh) 1980; 90:199-208.

25. Hilding DA, House WF. Acoustic neuroma: complications of traumatic and neoplastic. J Ultrastruct Res 1965; 12:611-23.

THE FACIAL CANAL: NORMAL ANATOMY, VARIATIONS AND ANOMALIES

BRUCE PROCTOR, MD
DETROIT, MICHIGAN

GEORGE T. NAGER, MD
BALTIMORE, MARYLAND

Modern otologic surgery revolves around the use of the operating microscope. The surgeon must have a thorough knowledge of all structures in the temporal bone, particularly since surgery may now be directed to areas in its deeper portions. Of concern here is the whereabouts of the facial canal in its complex course through the temporal bone. A detailed descriptive anatomy with emphasis on the relations of the facial canal to adjacent structures is presented. The variations in the course of the facial canal are discussed. The location of dehiscences in the bony canal wall are described. Finally, great stress is laid upon presentation of these anomalies known to us which can occur in the course of the facial nerve through the temporal bone. These anomalies have clinical and surgical significance.

I. NORMAL ANATOMY OF THE FACIAL CANAL

BRUCE PROCTOR, MD

Surgery directed to the skull base has become more frequent due to new diagnostic techniques and the development of microsurgical procedures. The intricate course of the facial nerve through the temporal bone becomes of vital concern to all otological surgeons since it often traverses the operative field. Therefore, we will review the course of the facial canal through the petrosal portion of the temporal bone from the internal auditory meatus to the stylomastoid foramen, paying particular attention to its relations to adjacent structures.

The facial nerve, along with the intermediate nerve of Wrisberg and the auditory nerve, passes through the internal auditory canal (5 to 12 mm) (Figs. 1-3). The facial nerve occupies the anterosuperior segment of the meatus and lies in a shallow gutter (Fig. 1) which is limited above by the superior wall of the internal auditory canal and below by a barely perceptible crest which becomes progressively accentuated until it forms a sharp horizontal projection at the bottom (fundus) of the internal auditory meatus, dividing it horizontally into two levels (falciform crest, transverse crest) (Figs. 2, 4-6).

The superior level contains (from front to back) the facial nerve, the intermediate nerve of Wrisberg, the utricular nerve and the horizontal and superior ampullary nerves (Figs. 1-3). The inferior level contains the cochlear, saccular and inferior ampullary nerves. The latter exits through the singular foramen. These nerves all reach the lateral wall or terminus of the internal auditory meatus. The facial nerve and the intermediate nerve of Wrisberg pass obliquely into the facial canal (fallopian aqueduct), whereas the remaining nerves (auditory and vestibular) penetrate into the labyrinth.

The facial canal runs a very tortuous course across the petrosa (Figs. 7 and 8). This course may be divided as follows:

1. A first horizontal course which goes from the internal auditory canal to the site of the geniculate ganglion (Figs. 5-11).
2. A first turn with an acute angle (Figs. 8, 10-13).
3. A second straight course which runs along near the top of the tympanum (Figs. 8, 11-16).
4. A second turn which is a curvature with a large radius and which is directed vertically downward (Figs. 8, 15 and 16).
5. A third and last straight portion directed inferiorly and a little posteriorly to end at the stylomastoid foramen (Figs. 8, 15 and 16).

FIRST PART OF THE FACIAL CANAL (LABYRINTHINE SEGMENT)

The orifice of the facial canal in the internal auditory meatus measures 0.68 mm in diameter.[1] It opens on the anterosuperior wall of the meatus very near the fundus of the meatus. Above the facial canal we have the ceiling of the internal auditory meatus; below, the falciform crest (transverse crest); and externally, a vertical crest (Bill's bar) which separates it from the superior vestibular area. The latter contains several small openings of

From Wayne State University, School of Medicine, Detroit (Proctor), and the Department of Laryngology and Otology, Johns Hopkins University School of Medicine and Hospital, Baltimore (Nager).

Presented in part at the meeting of the American Otological Society, Inc., Palm Beach, Florida, May 2-3, 1982.

REPRINTS — Bruce Proctor, MD, 3535 West 13 Mile Road, Royal Oak, MI 48072, or George T. Nager, MD, Dept. of Laryngology and Otology, Johns Hopkins Hospital, 601 North Broadway, Baltimore, MD 21205.

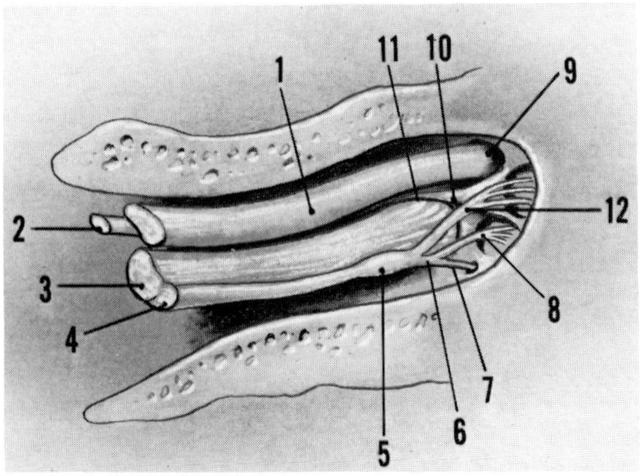

Fig. 1. Schema of internal auditory meatus and contents viewed anteriorly on right. 1 - Facial nerve, 2 - Intermediate nerve of Wrisberg, 3 - Cochlear nerve, 4 - Vestibular nerve, 5 - Scarpa's ganglion, 6 - Inferior branch of vestibular nerve, 7 - Posterior ampullary nerve exiting through singular foramen, 8 - Saccular nerve in saccular fossa, 9 - Facial nerve in facial fovea at origin of facial canal, 10 - Falciform or transverse crest, 11 - Cochlear nerve in cochlear fossa, 12 - Superior branch of vestibular nerve in vestibular fossa.

canals that conduct branches of the upper terminal ramus of the vestibular nerve through the lamina cribrosa to the superior cribrosa macula to the utricle and to the ampullae of the lateral and superior semicircular canals. The facial canal crosses the petrosa in an anterior direction and almost perpendicular to the petrosal axis to empty into the geniculate fossa.

This first horizontal part (portion) of the facial canal contains the facial nerve and the intermediate nerve of Wrisberg. Its length varies from 3 to 5 mm. It is slightly inclined from above, below, and from behind forward, paralleling the zygomatic line. It describes a curve with internal concavity to arrive at the geniculate fossa with a direction, if prolonged following its curvilinear movement, that would go toward the facial hiatus (ie, anteriorly). It passes in the intervestibulocochlear groove.

At the very beginning of the first portion of the facial canal (Fig. 7) there is a slight constriction from the vertical crest. The periosteum of the internal meatus is thicker than that in the facial canal so that the facial nerve is more constricted at this point than in the remainder of the canal. If decompression of the facial nerve is carried out in the labyrinthine segment of the nerve for Bell's palsy, this constricting ring of periosteum should be cut.

As the facial nerve enters the facial canal three morphological peculiarities are to be noted:[2]

1. Whereas the nerves have an individual sheath of pia mater in the internal auditory meatus, this sheath curves up as the nerve enters the facial canal and continues with the arachnoid. This arachnoid-pia mater-dura mater junction generally lies in the fundus of the meatus but it can occur in the neighborhood of the foramen or even far into the facial canal.

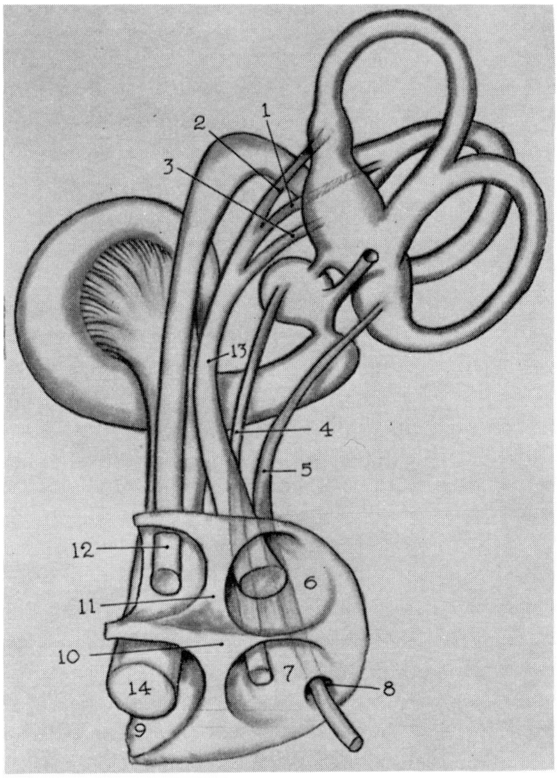

Fig. 2. Fundus of internal auditory canal and distribution of eighth nerve to membranous labyrinth. 1 - External ampullary nerve, 2 - Superior ampullary nerve, 3 - Utricular nerve, 4 - Saccular nerve, 5 - Posterior ampullary nerve, 6 - Superior vestibular fossa, 7 - Inferior vestibular fossa, 8 - Singular foramen of Morgagni, 9 - Cochlear fossa, 10 - Falciform crest, 11 - Vertical crest, 12 - Facial nerve, 13 - Superior vestibular nerve, 14 - Cochlear nerve.

2. There is a slight constriction (0.68 mm) of the nerve. This normal stricture must not be confused with a pathological stricture.

3. There is a change in the direction of the nerve which produces a 132° angle, open anteriorly and medially (Fig. 8).

RELATIONS

As it leaves the internal auditory canal, the facial canal is in relation with the canaliculi of the utricular and the superior and lateral ampullary nerves as well as with the vestibule in its anterior, medial and superior region — immediately adjacent to the elliptical or utricular fossa.

When surgery is carried out in the vestibule, gentle manipulations are necessary to avoid penetration into the internal auditory meatus and facial canal. The party wall between vestibule and internal auditory meatus is very thin (Figs. 6, 10 and 11). It is further weakened by passage of the numerous nerves into the vestibule.

The facial canal (only 3 to 5 mm long in this first portion) quickly leaves the region of the vestibule and approaches the geniculate fossa. The first portion of the facial canal constitutes the internal arm

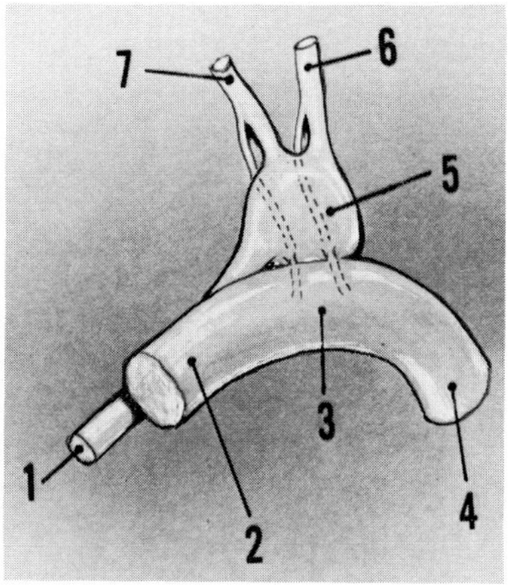

Fig. 3. Schema of right geniculate ganglion and its connections. 1 - Intermediate nerve of Wrisberg, 2 - First part of facial nerve, 3 - Genu or first turn of facial nerve, 4 - Second part of facial nerve, 5 - Geniculate ganglion, 6 - Lesser superficial petrosal nerve, 7 - Greater superficial petrosal nerve.

of the first turn whose external arm becomes the tympanic portion of the facial canal. The two arms of the turn form an acute angle between them of 74° on a nearly horizontal plane[2] and are separated from each other by a small triangular space filled with compact bone whose base rests against the vestibule and whose summit projects like a wedge into the acute turn in the facial canal (Figs. 7, 12 and 14).

Medially, the first portion of the facial canal includes in its curvature with internal concavity the top of the first cochlear turn (Figs. 7, 10 and 11).

Inferiorly, near the internal auditory canal, the facial canal rests on the superior external flank of this first spiral in the intervestibulocochlear groove. Near the geniculate fossa it rests on the second spiral and on the cupula (Figs. 10 and 16).

Superiorly, it is in relation to the petrosal space covered by the petrosal cortex stretched from the top of the arch of the superior semicircular canal to the cupula of the cochlea (Fig. 10). This space is frequently pneumatized by cells belonging to the superior prelabyrinthine tract.

FIRST TURN OF THE FACIAL CANAL AND THE GENICULATE FOSSA

The geniculate fossa is the crossroad of four nerve canals: the central and peripheral extremities of the facial canal, the conduit for the greater superficial petrosal nerve, and the conduit for the lesser superficial petrosal nerve. The geniculate fossa is usually quadrilateral in shape with sides of 2 or 3 mm when both petrosal nerves are large. However, the canaliculus for the lesser superficial petrosal nerve is often minute and in this case the crossroads take a triangular form whose base faces the anterior wall of the vestibule and whose apex corresponds medially to the facial hiatus (Figs. 3 and 7). The latter

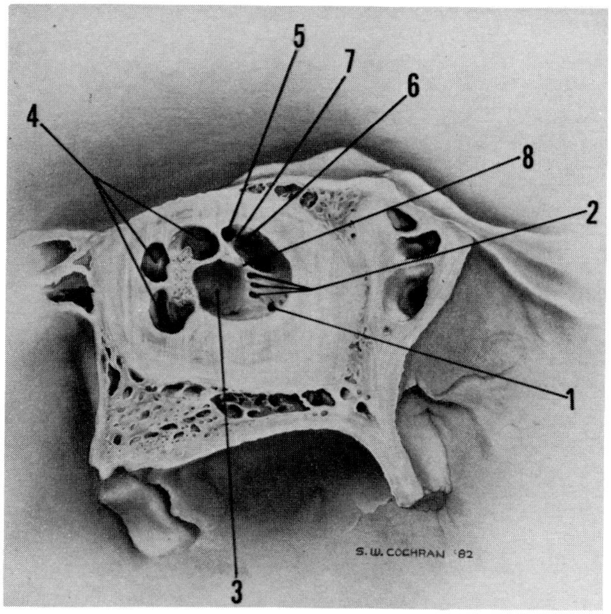

Fig. 4. Vertical cut through temporal bone showing details of fundus of internal auditory meatus. 1 - Singular foramen, 2 - Saccular fossa, 3 - Cochlear fossa, 4 - Cochlea, 5 - Facial canal, 6 - Superior vestibular fossa, 7 - Vertical crest, 8 - Transverse crest.

opens on the anterior surface of the petrosa for passage of the superficial petrosal nerves. These run from the surface of the petrosa in two small grooves which are directed toward the anterior lacerated foramen. More often, the geniculate fossa is completely encased in bone, but sometimes the canaliculus for the greater superficial petrosal nerve does not form, and then the facial hiatus is carried back to the geniculate fossa itself, so that it is covered directly by the dura mater (Fig. 7).

If such a situation is encountered in doing a middle fossa approach to the internal meatus, there is danger of injury to the exposed facial nerve. Care must be taken in elevating the dura from the petrosa whenever the dura penetrates through the petrosal cortex to contact venous lacunae, as shown by Walker.[3]

RELATIONS

Externally, the geniculate fossa contacts the anterior and superior angle(s) of the tympanum in front of the cochleariform process. A bed of small cells conceals it from view (Figs. 7, 13 and 14).

Inferiorly, the geniculate fossa rests on the cupula of the cochlea, which it overhangs to a considerable degree on the medial wall of the tympanum (Figs. 11 and 16).

Internally, it is in relation with the compact tissue which unites the cupula of the cochlea to the cortex of the anterior petrosal wall (Fig. 11).

Superiorly, the geniculate fossa is in contact with the cortex of the anterior wall of the petrosa; but in

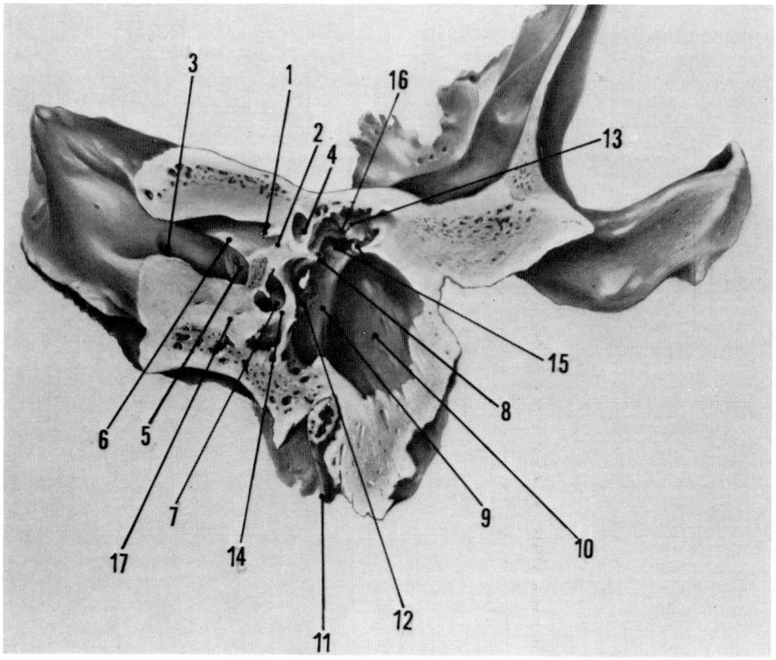

Fig. 5. Vertical cut through internal and external auditory meatuses showing anterior wall of internal auditory meatus and anterior tympanum. 1 - Vertical crest with facial fovea immediately in front, 2 - Utricular fossa above dot, 3 - Internal auditory meatus, 4 - Facial canal at geniculum, 5 - Cochlear fossa (spiral cribriform plate of cochlea), 6 - Transverse crest, 7 - Cochlea, 8 - Cochleariform process, 9 - Tympanic sulcus, 10 - External auditory canal, 11 - Styloid process, 12 - Protympanum, 13 - Pretympanic sinus, 14 - Promontory, 15 - Glaserian fissure, 16 - Canal of Huguier, 17 - Cochlear aqueduct.

some cases, there is a space of as much as 3 mm, containing air cells of the superior labyrinthine tract (Figs. 5, 9, 14 and 15).

Posteriorly, the geniculate fossa is in relation to the anterior wall of the vestibule, from which it is separated by 2 to 3 mm of compact bone (Figs. 7, 9 and 11).

The geniculate fossa contains the geniculate ganglion. It is a bulbous enlargement of the facial canal. The intermediate nerve of Wrisberg terminates in the ganglion but emerges from the ganglion as the greater superficial petrosal nerve, passing through the facial hiatus (Fig. 3). A portion continues on for 1 mm or so and emerges as the lesser superficial petrosal nerve. Running parallel to the greater superficial petrosal nerve, it passes through the accessory facial hiatus.

The first portion of the facial canal is directed anteriorly; but at the geniculate fossa, its course is abruptly changed, and it courses posteriorly and slightly laterally, thus forming an acute angle of variable degree but usually at an angle of 75° (Figs. 7, 11-13).

Anterior to the turn, the facial canal is anterior to the vestibule, but once it turns, its course is along the side of the vestibule. Thus, the two arms of the facial canal embrace the anterior portion of the vestibule (Figs. 7, 11 and 12). It is at this point where the facial canal passes the labyrinthine barrier after leaving the cranial cavity.

The external relations of the geniculate fossa have been studied in some detail in recent years. The anterior epitympanic sinus was studied by Wigand and Trillsch.[4] This sinus lies between the bony compartment of the tensor tympani muscle and the floor of the middle cranial fossa which slopes down to meet it anteriorly. The length, height, and width of this space vary from 1.8 to 5 mm. Its medial wall is in contact with the geniculate ganglion and may be dehiscent. A preferred nomenclature for this sinus, when present, is geniculate sinus to indicate its position. This same area was studied by Hawke et al[5] who reported frequent nonlamellar new bone

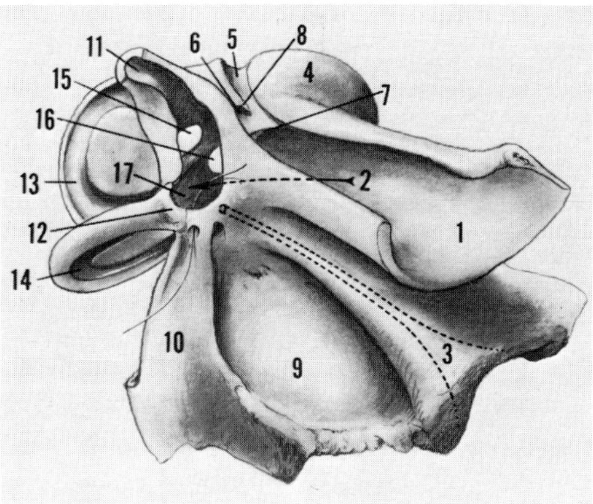

Fig. 6. Posterosuperior view of skeletonized otic capsule of adult showing cochlear and vestibular aqueducts, their relations, and first part of facial canal in intercochleovestibular course. 1 - Internal auditory meatus, 2 - Singular foramen (arrow), 3 - Cochlear aqueduct, 4 - Top coil of cochlea, 5 - Geniculate fossa, 6 - Superior vestibular foramen, 7 - Transverse crest, 8 - Vertical crest, 9 - Jugular dome, 10 - Opened vestibular aqueduct, 11 - Superior semicircular canal, 12 - Ampullary end of superior semicircular canal, 13 - Lateral semicircular canal, 14 - Posterior semicircular canal, 15 - Oval window, 16 - Round window, 17 - Vestibule.

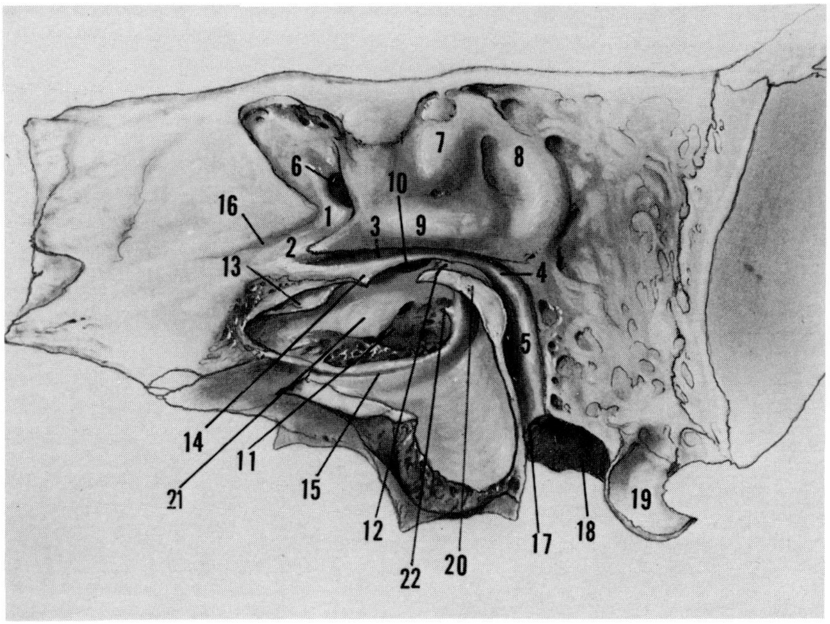

Fig. 7. Facial canal in its entire length. 1 - First part of facial canal (intercochleovestibular), 2 - Geniculate fossa with first turn of facial canal, 3 - Transverse or second part of facial canal, 4 - Second turn of facial canal, 5 - Vertical or third part of facial canal, 6 - Internal auditory meatus, 7 - Superior semicircular canal, 8 - Posterior semicircular canal, 9 - Lateral semicircular canal, 10 - Oval window, 11 - Round window niche, 12 - Pyramidal eminence, 13 - Tensor tympani canal, 14 - Cochleariform process, 15 - Tympanic sulcus, 16 - Facial hiatus, 17 - Stylomastoid foramen, 18 - Digastric groove, 19 - Mastoid tip cell, 20 - Posterior wall of external auditory canal, 21 - Promontory, 22 - Chorda tympani nerve.

formation in the sinus in the absence of ear or systemic disease. This appeared to be a normal anatomic feature for this sinus.

A tiny bony plate extending down (1.5 to 3 mm) from the epitympanum in front of the malleus head and extending from the facial canal to the scutum was described by Hoshino and Suzuki.[6] This structure is not uncommon. It represents the anterior bony wall of the attic. The space anteriorly (supratubal recess) is in communication with the protympanum.[7] This same structure was reported by Gacek[8] who uses it as a surgical landmark when seeking the facial nerve at the geniculate ganglion level. He shows the temporal bone of a 4-month-old fetus wherein this structure forms the outer wall of the facial canal in its tympanic or second part.

SECOND PART OR TYMPANIC PORTION OF THE FACIAL CANAL

The tympanic portion of the facial canal is straight and measures 10 to 12 mm in length. It extends from the geniculate fossa to the posterior wall

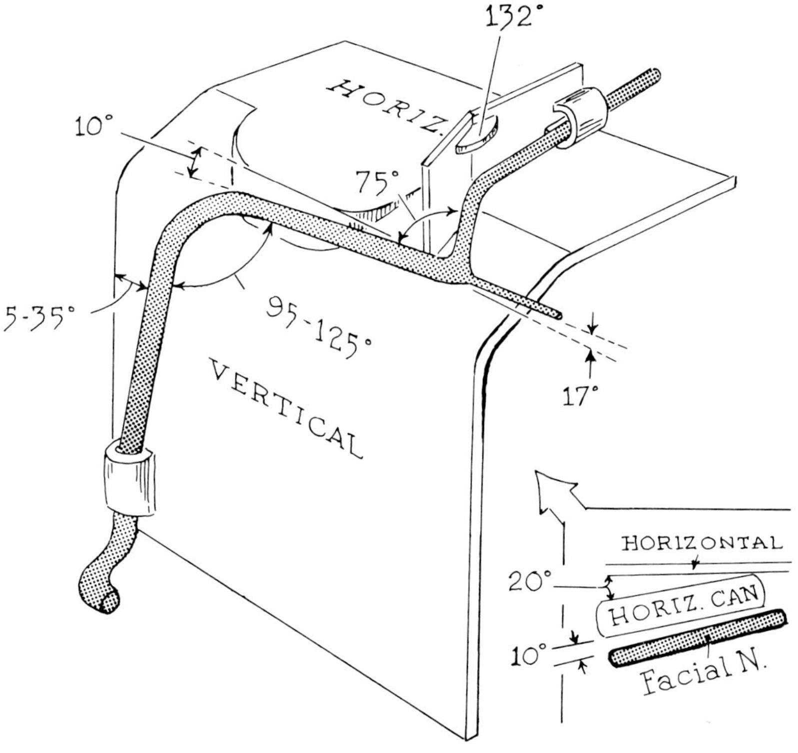

Fig. 8. Schematic course of facial canal. Length of facial nerve in internal auditory meatus varies from 5-12 mm. Upon entering facial canal there is immediately angulation forward of 132° as well as downward inclination for 3-5 mm to reach geniculate fossa. Canal then turns 75° to continue posteriorly for 10-12 mm. At the same time it is directed outward 17° and inclined inferiorly 7-10° from plane of lateral semicircular canal which in turn is inclined 20-25° below true horizontal plane. At second turn curve formed between second and third parts of facial canal varies from 95-125°. Third part of facial canal (13 mm) deviates posteriorly as well as laterally from vertical plane by 5-35°. (After Guerrier[2] in part.)

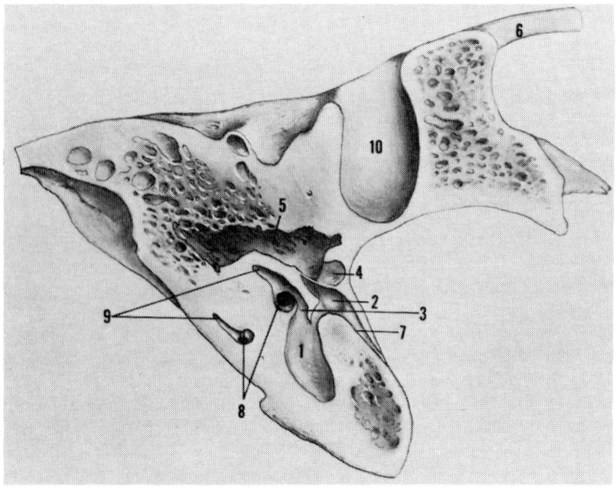

Fig. 9. Upper half of horizontal cut through internal auditory meatus and geniculate fossa. 1 - Roof of internal auditory meatus, 2 - Geniculate fossa, 3 - Canal for superior vestibular nerve, 4 - Geniculate sinus, 5 - Tympanum, 6 - Zygoma, 7 - Canal and hiatus for greater superficial petrosal nerve, 8 - Superior semicircular canal, 9 - Lateral semicircular canal, 10 - Temporomandibular joint. Note thin bony wall separating geniculate sinus from facial nerve in geniculate fossa.

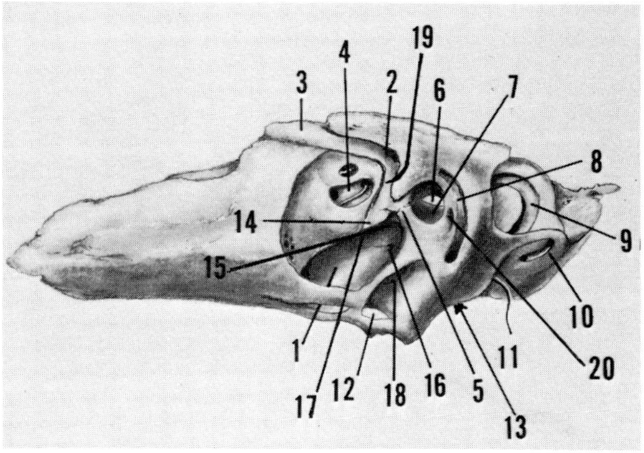

Fig. 10. Dissection of bony labyrinth from posterior fossa showing relations of facial nerve canal. Note proximity of first part of facial canal to basal turn of cochlea and to anterior wall of vestibule. 1 - Internal auditory meatus, 2 - Geniculate fossa, 3 - Canal for greater superficial petrosal nerve, 4 - Cochlea, 5 - Canal for superior vestibular nerve, 6 - Oval window, 7 - Vestibule, 8 - Superior semicircular canal, 9 - Horizontal semicircular canal, 10 - Posterior semicircular canal, 11 - Vestibular aqueduct, 12 - Termination of cochlear aqueduct at the pyramidal fossa, 13 - Jugular dome (arrow), 14 - Transverse crest (falciform crest), 15 - Saccular fossa (inferior vestibular area), 16 - Singular foramen, 17 - Cochlear fossa, 18 - Tympanic canaliculus opened (Jacobson's nerve), 19 - First part of facial canal, 20 - Petromastoid canal.

of the tympanum, running the length of the superior edge of the internal wall of the tympanum. Sometimes its course is parallel to the plane of the horizontal semicircular canal, but more often it is slightly inclined inferiorly and forms an angle of less than 10° with the plane of the horizontal canal (Fig. 8).

The longitudinal axis of the petrous pyramid forms an angle of 50 to 53° with the sagittal plane, whereas the tympanic course of the facial canal forms an angle of 35 to 40° with the same sagittal plane. If one were to extend the plane of the tympanic portion of the facial canal anterior to the geniculate fossa, the line would follow the gutter for the superficial petrosal nerves into the facial hiatus. Passing through the facial hiatus we find the greater superficial petrosal nerve, the artery of the geniculate ganglion and especially the homonymous veins, whose diameter is five times that of the nerve, all passing in a common fibrous sheath.[2]

The tympanic (second) part of the facial canal forms an angle of 37° with the horizontal plane opening posteriorly with the anteroposterior axis

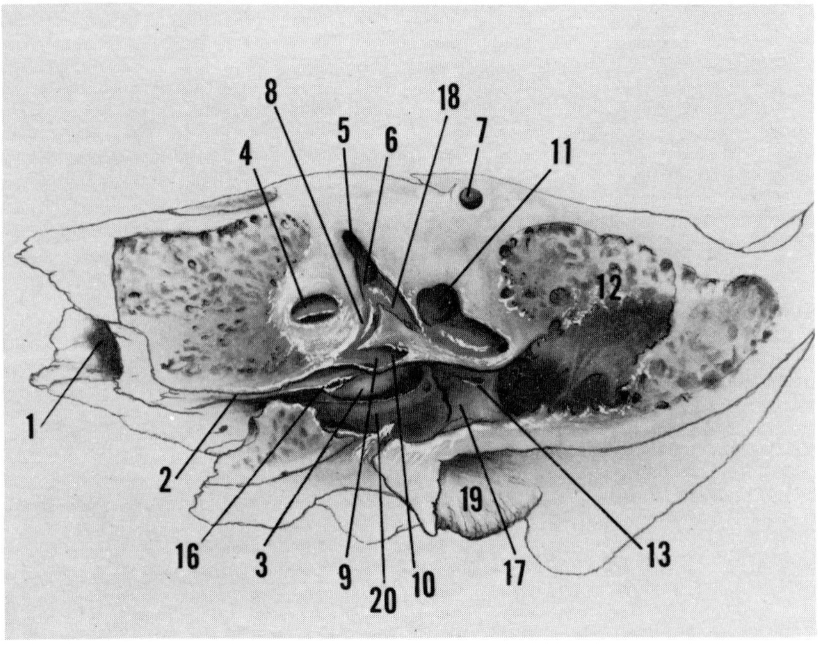

Fig. 11. Horizontal cut with anterior inclination at upper level of internal auditory meatus showing first part of facial canal and its relations to cochlea, vestibule and middle ear. 1 - Carotid canal, 2 - Tensor tympani canal, 3 - Promontory, 4 - Cochlea, 5 - Internal auditory meatus, 6 - Transverse crest, 7 - Superior semicircular canal, 8 - First part of facial canal, 9 - Geniculate fossa, 10 - Beginning of second part of facial canal, 11 - Vestibule at ampullary end of lateral semicircular canal, 12 - Mastoid antrum, 13 - Facial sinus, 16 - Cochleariform process, 17 - Incudal fossa, 18 - Utricular canal, 19 - External auditory meatus, 20 - Tympanic sulcus. Second part of facial canal and lateral semicircular canal overhang oval window and posterior tympanic sinus to remarkable degree.

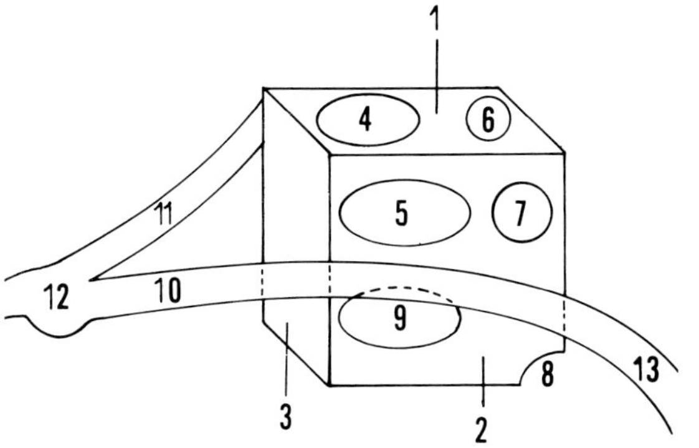

Fig. 12. Schema showing relations of vestibule with facial canal (left side). Corners of vestibule are all rounded and walls are convex externally except superior wall. 1 - Superior wall of vestibule, 2 - External wall of vestibule, 3 - Anterior wall of vestibule, 4 - Ampullary orifice of superior semicircular canal, 5 - Ampullary orifice of lateral semicircular canal, 6 - Nonampullary orifice of superior semicircular canal, 7 - Nonampullary orifice of lateral semicircular canal, 8 - Ampullary orifice of posterior semicircular canal, 9 - Oval window, 10 - Tympanic or second part of facial canal, 11 - First part of facial canal, 12 - Geniculate fossa, and 13 - Second turn of facial canal.

but this time laterally so that its anterior part is deep and its posterior part superficial.

Relative positions of the tympanic facial canal are indicated below.

1. Anteriorly it lies above and medial to the cochleariform process.
2. In its middle portion it runs over the oval window forming the roof of the posterior tympanic sinus.[2,9]
3. It then runs under the lateral semicircular canal.
4. The lateral semicircular canal forms an angle of 30° with the horizontal plane. Therefore, the second part of the facial canal forms a backward and downward opening angle of 7°.
5. The facial nerve forms a backward and outward opening angle of 17° with the labyrinthine wall of the tympanic cavity.

RELATIONS

The principal relations are established externally with the tympanum and internally with the vestibule.

External Surface. This faces the tympanum. It is free, except at its two extremities: 1) at its exit from the geniculate fossa, where it is concealed by small air cells (Figs. 14 and 15); and 2) at the level of the pyramid, where it enters the bony mass of the styloid complex (Reichert's cartilage) (Fig. 17).

Between these two extremities the external wall of the facial canal is made up of a very thin bony lamella which is easily fractured at surgery if delicate techniques are not used. In such instances, the facial nerve may be seriously damaged even by a tiny bone spicule.

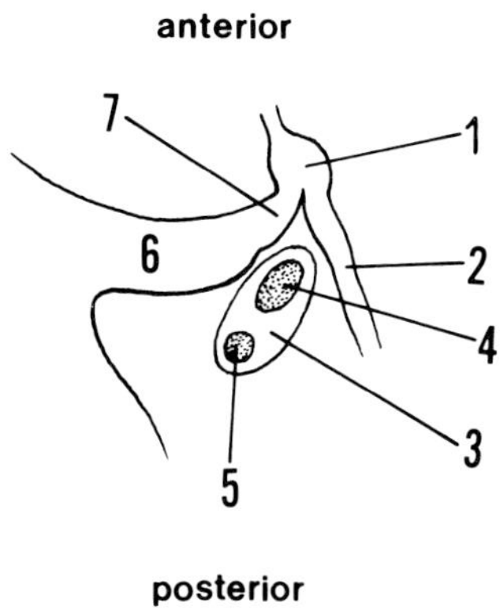

Fig. 13. Schema showing divergence of tympanic part of facial canal with external wall of vestibule. 1 - Geniculate fossa, 2 - Tympanic (second) part of facial canal, 3 - Superior wall of vestibule and its external border, 4 - Ampulla of superior semicircular canal, 5 - Nonampullary orifice of superior semicircular canal, 6 - Internal auditory meatus, 7 - First part of facial canal.

At the level of the aditus, the facial canal forms a semicylindrical projection, running from front to back on the floor of the aditus passage, thus constituting its threshold; below, it is the tympanum; above, it is the aditus ad antrum, or passage into the antrum (Fig. 11). This portion of the canal, which is 3 mm long, is usually seen clearly at surgery. If not, its position may be indicated by its relation to the anterior extremity of the projection of the lateral semicircular canal, below which it can be localized, or by finding it directly across the oval window niche from the projecting cochleariform process.

The tympanic portion of the facial canal lies medial to the attic and its contents from front to back are the malleus head, the incudomallear joint, the incus body and its horizontal or short process.

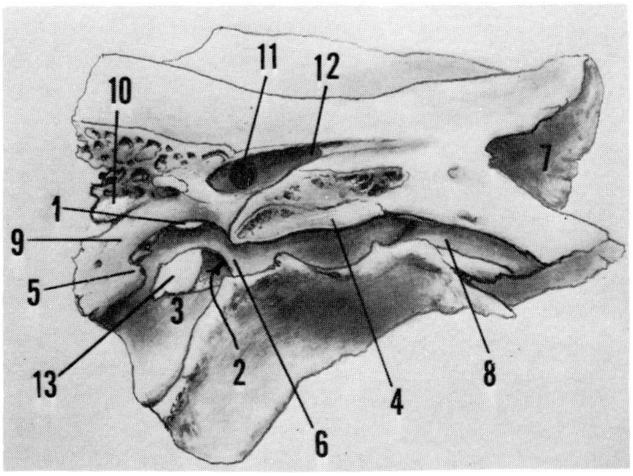

Fig. 14. Medial wall of tympanum showing large dehiscence over geniculate fossa extending to facial hiatus as well as one over jugular dome. 1 - Oval window, 2 - Round window niche (arrow), 3 - External auditory meatus, 4 - Groove for tensor tympani muscle, 5 - Pyramidal orifice, 6 - Promontory, 7 - Carotid canal, 8 - Protympanum, 9 - Facial canal, 10 - Lateral semicircular canal, 11 - Dehiscence over geniculate fossa, 12 - Facial hiatus, 13 - Dehiscence over jugular dome.

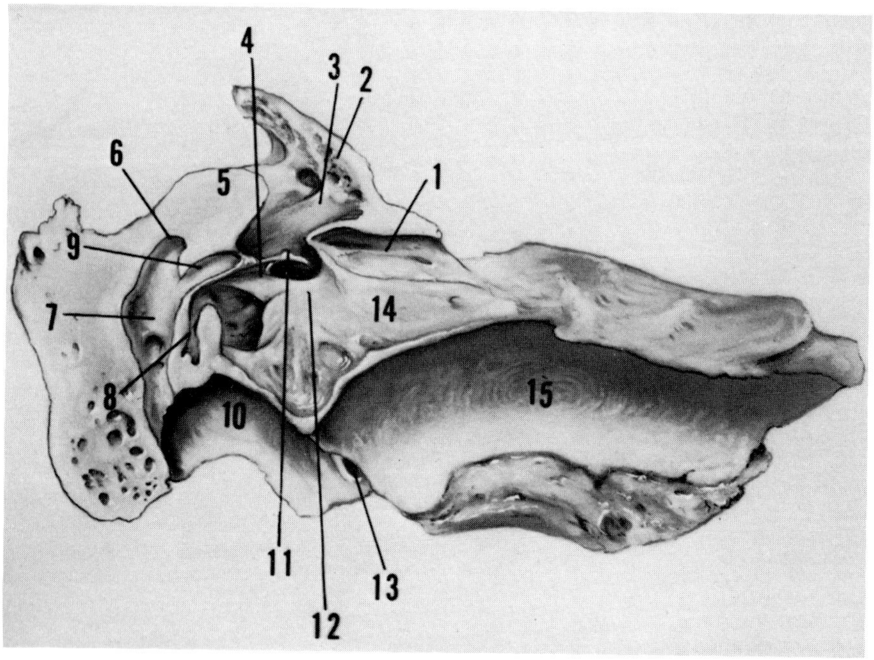

Fig. 15. View of medial tympanic wall with high jugular dome and high stylomastoid foramen. Pyramidal eminence is a shell. Note small geniculate cells in anterior tympanum. 1 - Tensor tympani canal, 2 - Geniculate cells, 3 - Facial canal (second part), 4 - Large ponticulus, 5 - Lateral semicircular canal, 6 - Second turn of facial canal, 7 - Third part of facial canal, 8 - Lateral tympanic sinus, 9 - Pyramidal muscle canal, 10 - Jugular dome, 11 - Stapes, 12 - Promontory, 13 - Opening of cochlear aqueduct, 14 - Protympanum, 15 - Carotid canal.

The posterior extremity of the short process of the incus marks the point where the facial canal begins its second turn.

Inferior Surface. The inferior surface of the tympanic portion of the facial canal can be divided into three parts: anterior, middle and posterior.

The anterior part goes from the geniculate fossa to the extremity of the cochleariform process which advances up over the anterior border of the oval window niche. It has a length of 3 to 4 mm (Figs. 7, 11, 14 and 15). Its internal border rests on the superior and external side of the cochlear cone, and its external border overhangs the promontory and adheres to the superior lip of the cochleariform process (Fig. 7).

The middle part of the inferior surface of the facial canal goes from the cochleariform process to the pyramidal apex and measures 3 to 4 mm. It is made up of a very thin bony lamella and is often dehiscent. Thus, the facial canal in the middle part of its tympanic course is covered by very thin and fragile bone which overhangs the oval window. It may conceal the top of the oval window so that in order to see the top of the oval window, one must look at it from below (Figs. 7, 11, 14 and 16).

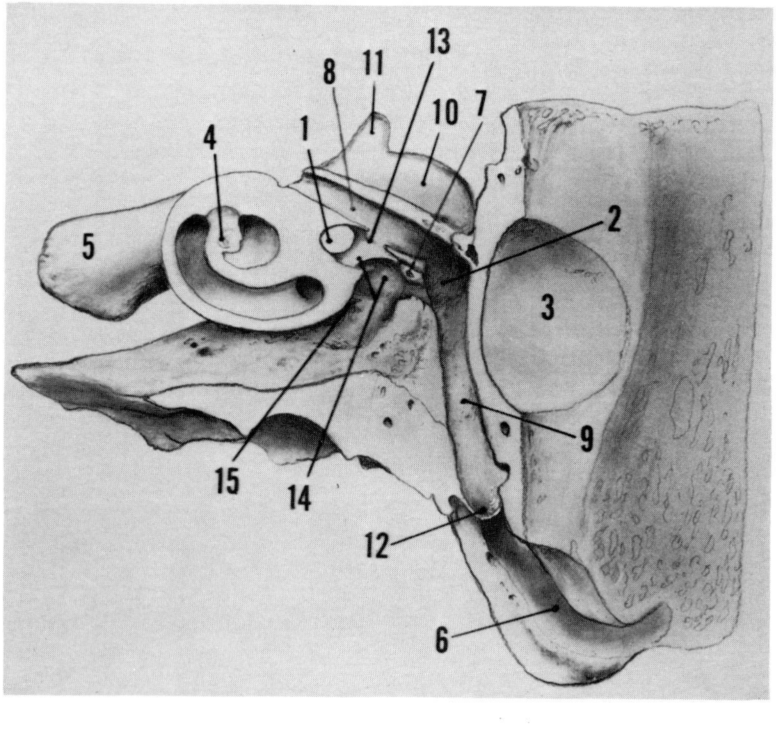

Fig. 16. Medial wall of tympanum showing details at second turn of facial canal. 1 - Oval window, 2 - Facial canal at second turn, 3 - External auditory canal, 4 - Helicotrema of cochlea, 5 - Skeletonized wall of internal auditory meatus, 6 - Digastric groove, 7 - Pyramidal eminence, 8 - Second part of facial canal, 9 - Third part of facial canal, 10 - Lateral semicircular canal, 11 - Vertical semicircular canal, 12 - Stylomastoid foramen, 13 - Dehiscence in facial canal, 14 - Tympani sinus ponticulus, and 15 - Subiculum.

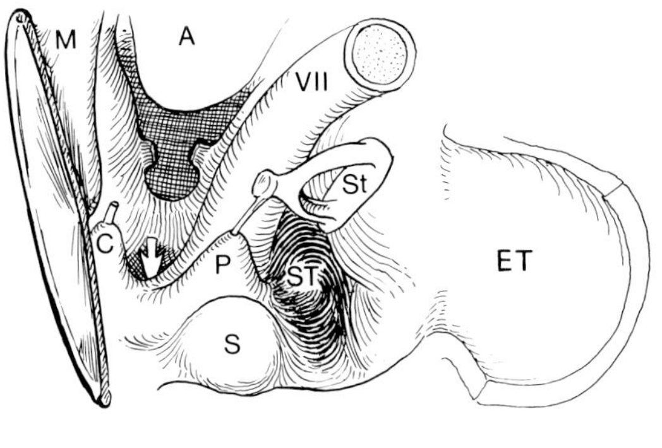

Fig. 17. Schema of posterior tympanum showing position of facial sinus (arrow) lying on posterior aspect of styloid complex (C, P and S) between chorda tympani nerve (C) and descending facial canal. Posteriorly it is limited by incudal fossa and pars squamosa of mastoid. A - Mastoid antrum, ET - Eustachian tube, St - Stapes, ST - Tympanic sinus, P - Pyramidal eminence, S - Styloid protuberance of Politzer, C - Chordal eminence (iter chordae posticus), and M - Malleus handle.

The posterior part of the inferior surface of the facial canal is about 2 mm long. It adheres closely to the pyramid and overhangs the posterior tympanic sinus or the upper portion of the tympanic sinus (Figs. 7, 11, 14-16).

Superior Surface. The superior surface of the tympanic portion of the facial canal is at first in relation with the small prelabyrinthine air cells in front of the projection of the semicircular canal (Figs. 9, 14 and 15); then, exactly at the point where it passes above the anterior commissure of the oval window, the facial canal engages under the ampulla of the horizontal semicircular canal. Its superior surface enters in very intimate contact with the inferior surface of the ampulla for a length of about 2 mm (Figs. 7 and 14). The bony plate separating the cavity of the horizontal ampulla and the facial canal is often less than 1 mm thick (Fig. 16). More posterior, the facial canal passes under the horizontal canal until it reaches the middle of the arch of the canal. It then begins its second turn in order to assume a vertical direction downward (Figs. 7 and 16). The facial canal slopes slightly downward in relation to the plane of the horizontal canal. If only 1 mm separates it from the anterior edge of the ampulla, there are often 2 mm at the level of the arch of the canal.

The horizontal canal covers the superior surface of the facial canal to a variable degree. If the facial canal takes a more transverse direction in its relation to the petrosa, it engages deeply under the semicircular canal (Fig. 11). On the other hand, if it tends to become parallel to the longitudinal axis of the petrosa, the facial canal is only slightly engaged under the anterior arm of the horizontal canal.

Internal Surface. On leaving the geniculate fossa for 2 to 3 mm, the internal surface of the facial canal corresponds to the triangular space which separates the two arms of its first turn in front of the vestibule (Fig. 7). It then arrives at the anteroexternal angle of the vestibule just above the anterior commissure of the oval window and just below the anterior edge of the ampulla of the external canal (Fig. 7). This is the point where the facial canal and the vestibule are the closest to each other. Only the labyrinthine capsule separates their cavities by 1 mm of bone or less (Figs. 12-14 and 16).

At this level, the facial canal passes in a sort of groove formed above by the ampulla of the horizontal canal and, medially, by the portion of the vestibular wall which extends from the ampulla to the superior edge of the oval window. This section of the wall rarely has more than 1 mm of height in the middle of the window. It is a little wider at the level of the commissure because of the rounded shapes of the ampulla and of the lintel of the window which it faces on their convexity. That is why the facial canal, which often has nearly a 2-mm diameter, cavity and walls included, cannot lodge completely

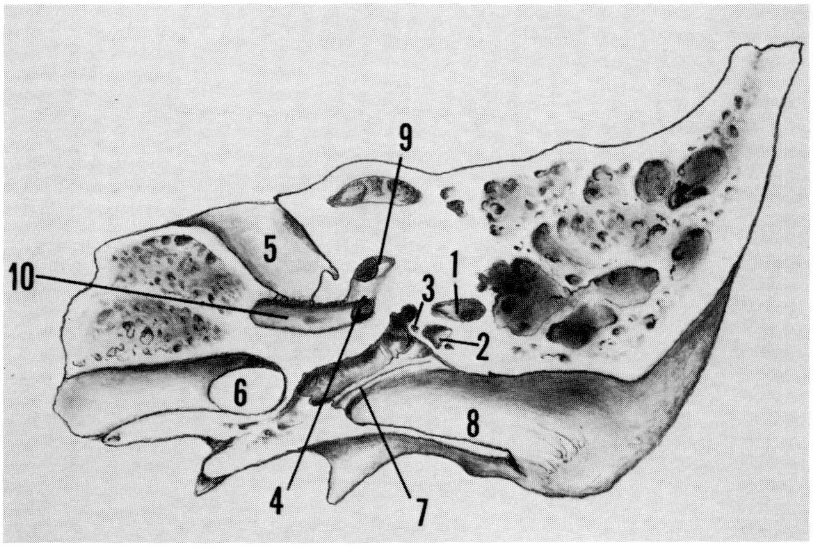

Fig. 18. Horizontal cut near floor of internal auditory meatus. 1 - Descending facial canal, 2 - Facial sinus, 3 - Pyramidal foramen, 4 - Round window, 5 - Internal auditory meatus, 6 - Carotid canal, 7 - Tympanic sulcus, 8 - External auditory meatus, 9 - Vestibule, 10 - Basal turn cochlea.

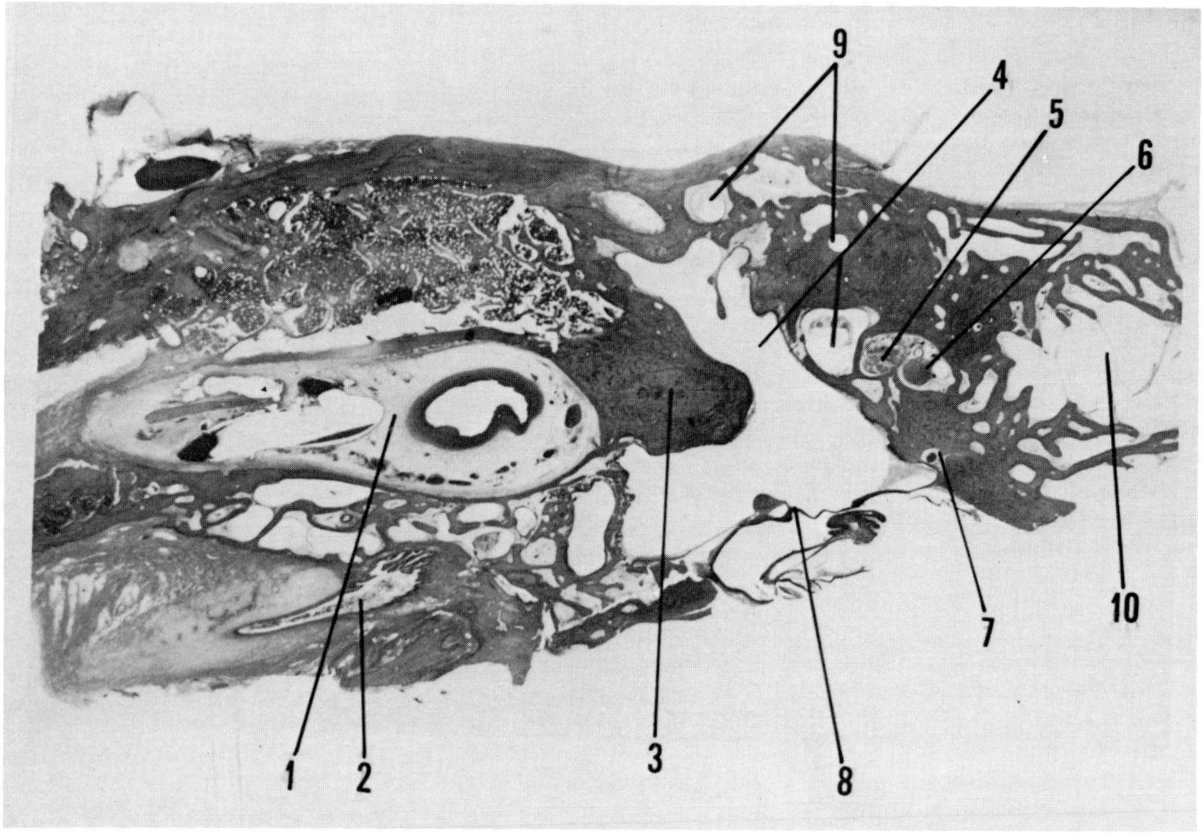

Fig. 19. Horizontal section of temporal bone showing relation of third part of facial canal just below its second turn. 1 - Carotid canal, 2 - Eustachian tube, 3 - Base of cochlea, 4 - Tympanic sinus, 5 - Stapedius muscle, 6 - Facial nerve, 7 - Chorda tympani nerve, 8 - Umbo, 9 - Posterior semicircular canal, and 10 - Mastoid antrum. Note dense bone of styloid complex lateral to facial nerve and dense bony labyrinth medial to it.

in the groove and instead hangs over the lintel of the oval window below. That is why the top of the oval window is often found concealed by the facial canal (Figs. 7, 11, 12 and 14).

The facial canal is closest to the ampulla of the horizontal canal, to the external wall of the vestibule and to the oval window at the level of the anterior commissure of the oval window. At that point, the facial canal is equidistant from the ampulla above, from the vestibule medially and from the oval window below. This distance is usually less than 1 mm.

Posterior to this point, the facial canal tends to swerve externally, while the external wall of the vestibule is inclined toward the interior (Fig. 13). That is why the relations of these structures at the level of the posterior commissure of the oval window are no longer the same as before. Here the facial canal can be 2 mm from the window and a lesser distance from the vestibule. The facial canal would be even more separated if the external wall of the vestibule did not present an external convexity.

On leaving the posterior commissure of the oval window, the external wall of the vestibule turns medially, while the facial canal goes externally, so that at the level of the posterior edge of the vestibule the two structures can be found separated from each other by 3 or 4 mm (Figs. 7 and 13).

It is possible for the facial canal to lose contact with the bony labyrinth because an accessory cavity of the tympanum, the tympanic sinus or the posterior tympanic sinus is insinuated between them while occupying the angle formed by the posterior half of the external wall of the vestibule medially, the posterior semicircular canal posteriorly and the horizontal semicircular canal above.

SECOND TURN OF THE FACIAL CANAL

The second turn of the facial canal is a curvature with a wide, graceful radius which starts in the horizontal plane and then becomes almost vertical. Sometimes this curvature is double, not only bending inferiorly, but also a bit posteriorly and medially to approach the posterior semicircular canal and the vestibule.

The angle formed by the second and third portion(s) of the facial canal is never a right angle, but varies from 95 to 125°. The curvature presents various forms; sometimes it is short and at other times very large, with the inflexion beginning at the level of the posterior commissure of the oval window and

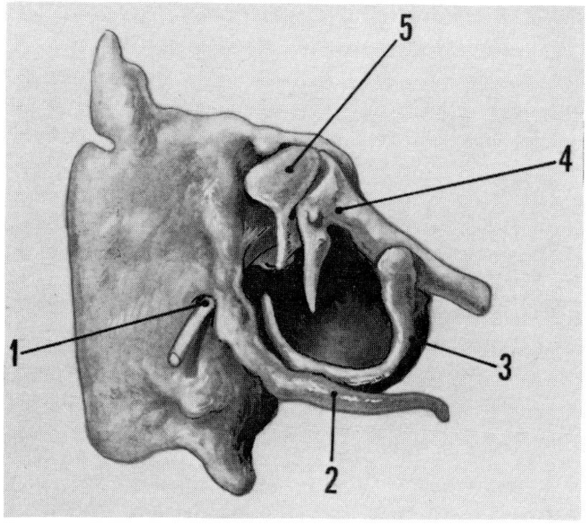

Fig. 20. Temporal bone of premature infant showing high level at which stylomastoid foramen located. 1 - Facial nerve at stylomastoid foramen, 2 - Styloid process (Reichert's cartilage), 3 - Tympanic ring, 4 - Malleus with large anterior mallear process (Meckel's cartilage) and 5 - Incus.

ending at the inferior third of the vertical portion of the facial canal.

In the newborn and young child the second turn appears to stretch backward like a loop. This disposition can also be found in the adult and then represents an anomaly in its course.

The tympanomastoid course of the facial canal is extremely variable; hence, descriptions vary considerably.

RELATIONS

The concavity of the second turn corresponds to the posterosuperior region of the tympanum. It is divided by the pyramidal eminence for the stapedius muscle which is seen at the bottom of the bend (Fig. 18). The concavity faces the rounded eminence of the promontory separating the oval and round windows. The bend of the facial canal is 3 to 4 mm from the posterior commissure of the oval window and 3 mm from the tympanic sulcus. The latter distance is fairly constant and represents the thickness of the styloid complex, which is derived from Reichert's cartilage.

The convexity of the second turn of the facial canal has relations posteriorly with the posterior semicircular canal and the posterior cranial fossa. In large pneumatized petrosas, 10 to 12 mm separate the turn from the posterior fossa (Fig. 7); and in small, narrow petrosas, the distance may be only 4 mm. In the first case the ampullary arm of the posterior canal is 3 to 4 mm from the turn, but in the second, the facial canal and posterior canal contact each other, and their cavities are separated only by the thickness of the labyrinthine capsule and the facial canal wall — a distance of 1.5 mm.

The distance separating the turn of the facial from the summit of the angle formed by the horizontal semicircular canal and the posterior vertical canal is at most 3 to 4 mm (Fig. 7).

Above the second turn of the facial canal lies the arch of the horizontal semicircular canal, but the turn in the facial canal quickly separates from it as it proceeds posteriorly and inferiorly (Fig. 7).

Medially, the second turn of the facial canal is separated from the ampulla of the posterior semicircular canal by 4 to 5 mm of compact bone or cells in large petrosas (Fig. 7) and by only 2 mm of compact bone in contracted petrosas. In the first case, the tympanic sinus often separates it from the posterior ampulla (Fig. 19). This does not occur in the second case.

Externally, on leaving the posterior third of its tympanic portion, the facial canal immediately encounters progressively thickening bone on its external and superior surface. This heavy bone separates the posterior tympanum from the mastoid cells up to the level of the fossa incudis, which is the floor of the mastoid antrum. It is referred to as the posterior buttress and as the "massif du facial" by the French otologists. It is of second branchial arch origin (Reichert's cartilage). The facial nerve is the nerve of the second branchial arch. It takes a position on the posterior and medial portion of this extension up into the complex posterior tympanum of the styloid complex. The term "styloid complex" is applied to the styloid process, posterior wall of the tympanum up to the fossa incudis, the pyramidal process, ponticulus, and subiculum and chordal eminence.[9] The facial canal keeps this relationship until it emerges at the stylomastoid foramen.

From the surgeon's view, the facial canal and the posterior limb of the horizontal canal are suddenly covered by this styloid complex. If one dissects carefully through this mass of bone, one can uncover the facial sinus (Fig. 17), which is a recess descending along the external surface of the facial canal as far down as the level of the canal for the chorda tympani nerve.[9] Once this sinus is uncovered laterally, it is usually possible to see the descending facial canal beneath its thin, smooth medial wall. Laterally, the styloid complex fuses with the tympanic bone.

THIRD PART OR VERTICAL PORTION OF THE FACIAL CANAL

The vertical portion of the facial canal extends from the second turn to the stylomastoid foramen (13 mm). It is nearly rectilinear. It forms an angle of 95 to 125° with the tympanic portion of the facial canal (Figs. 7, 8, 15 and 16). It deviates from the vertical posteriorly. It runs through the mastoid process and thus merits the name "mastoid portion."

The vertical portion of the facial canal tends to swing laterally, and at the level of the stylomastoid foramen the nerve is found more external than at the level of the last turn. This lateral deviation may reach 2 or 3 mm. In some individuals, however, the canal may be found to have deviated medially instead of laterally.

The superior half of the third portion of the facial canal rarely deviates from its vertical course except for a minimal external shift. The second turn lies beneath the posterior portion of the horizontal canal. Therefore, the facial canal is very rarely external to the projection of the horizontal canal. If the surgeon remains 1 or 2 mm external to the horizontal canal, there is no risk of injury to the facial nerve.

Posteriorly, the vertical portion of the facial canal is separated from the posterior fossa by a distance of 4 to 12 mm. This retrofacial space is usually occupied by the retrofacial air cells. The inferior third of the descending mastoid portion of the lateral sinus lies directly behind the facial canal at a distance varying from 3 to 10 mm. The mastoid portion of the facial canal deviates posteriorly from the vertical by 5 to 35°, a point to always remember when operating in the mastoid (Fig. 8).

Medially, the vertical portion of the facial canal enters in relation to the jugular bulb (Fig. 15). These relations are very variable. When the jugular fossa is high, the facial canal is accessible from the posterior via the retrofacial space or anteriorly via the tympanum. The facial canal can be found 8 mm external to the jugular dome, and at other times (rarely) its thin bony shell can adhere to the dome along its entire vertical length. The facial canal may even be dehiscent in the jugular fossa (Fig. 15). If the jugular fossa is nonexistent, the facial canal is not in relation with the jugular bulb, which remains below the level of the stylomastoid foramen.

When the facial canal is not in contact with the jugular dome (this is the usual case), the space which separates them is filled with compact bone separating the tympanum from the occipitojugular region. However, this endofacial region can be filled by air cells, the jugular fossa may be absent, and the sublabyrinthine space is found pneumatized. In such a case tympanum, occipitojugular cells, and sublabyrinthine spaces can form a very large pneumatic area, which could be difficult to eradicate in cases of infection. The tympanic sinus often passes medial to the facial canal as far up as the inferior arm of the posterior canal.

The third portion of the facial canal is in relation anteriorly with the tympanum and the external auditory canal. In its superior region, it is in relation to the posterior wall of the tympanum, which is made up by the styloid complex (Fig. 17) and which varies from 2 to 4 mm in thickness. At the level of the round window, it crosses the tympanic bone in an "X" and is found hereafter behind the external auditory canal (Fig. 15). This crossing results from the fact that the tympanic membrane is more or less strongly inclined from above below and from externally internally, while the facial canal is nearly vertical.[10] The tympanic ring is thus a good landmark for the facial canal, 3 mm separating it constantly. Further down, the posterior wall of the external auditory canal and the facial canal deviate a little more from each other. The external auditory canal being horizontal and the facial canal vertical, their relationships are measured by the height of the external canal and cease completely at the level of its floor, which corresponds to the junction of the middle and inferior thirds of the facial canal.

STYLOMASTOID FORAMEN

The stylomastoid foramen opens at the base of the petrosa between the mastoid process and the styloid. It is always very close to the styloid process, and often it is contiguous to its base and lies on its posteroexternal surface. Viewed from the profile of the head, it is projected on the suture of the tympanic bone and the mastoid (tympanopetrosal suture). At the time of mastoid surgery, the stylomastoid foramen can be localized by following the middle of the digastric groove forward to the base of the styloid process. The foramen lies immediately posterior to the styloid process (Figs. 7, 15 and 16). To avoid injury to the facial nerve at the stylomastoid foramen, the surgeon should limit the surgery to the anterior extremity of the diagastric groove or to the anterior edge of the base of the mastoid process.

In the newborn the stylomastoid foramen (Fig. 20) is at a very high level with the facial nerve emerging at the level of the floor of the mastoid antrum. With the growth of the squamosal portion of the mastoid the facial canal is displaced downward while adhering to the styloid process. The position of the facial nerve in the newborn must be kept in mind whenever surgery is done in this area.

Extensive studies of the anatomy of the facial canal have been made by Bellocq,[11] Girard,[12] and Paturet.[13] Further information may be obtained from these sources.

II. ANATOMICAL VARIATIONS AND ANOMALIES INVOLVING THE FACIAL CANAL

George T. Nager, MD

Bruce Proctor, MD

All portions of the temporal bone are subject to variations and anomalies. They concern the formation of the components that constitute the temporal bone, the extent of pneumatization, the configuration of the middle ear cavity, the differentiation of the middle ear structures, and the development of the otic and vestibular capsule. They also involve the anatomy of the facial canal, the architecture of the internal and external auditory meatuses, the position of the endolymphatic sac, the location of the major blood vessels, and the persistence of certain embryonic vascular structures.

The facial canal, as it traverses the temporal bone, may display congenital bony dehiscences, variations and anomalies of its natural course, and in a rare instance, include a large persisting embryonic artery or vein. Each of these features may have clinical and surgical significance.

The otologic surgeon must be familiar with these variations and anomalies, suspect them and identify them preoperatively whenever indicated, so that he can adjust his surgical approach or leave them undisturbed, in order to avoid an injury to the facial nerve.

CONGENITAL BONY DEHISCENCES IN THE FACIAL CANAL

It is not surprising that the facial canal can be defective since it is made from two separate embryologic structures, the primordial otic capsule and Reichert's cartilage from the second branchial arch.[14] In the 10-week-old fetus, the facial "canal" is a deep sulcus in the canalicular portion of the primordial otic capsule. The otic capsule is at that time entirely cartilaginous. Reichert's cartilage becomes attached to the otic capsule and provides the remaining cartilaginous circumference to the labyrinthine and tympanic segments of the facial canal. Its ossification begins at that time. This contribution from Reichert's cartilage persists as a readily identifiable histologic structure through the first postnatal year. By the end of the year ossification is generally completed. In some instances closure of the facial canal is never fully accomplished, and in localized areas or dehiscences the canal remains open to mucoperiosteum of the middle ear, just as the tissue of the facial sulcus in fetal life was continuous with the mesenchyme beneath the epithelium of the expanding tympanic cavity.[14]

A gap in the continuity of the osseous wall may be observed in any portion of the facial canal; the majority, however, is observed along the tympanic segment (Fig. 21). Such dehiscences may involve the inferior, lateral and medial wall. They are most frequently located above and posterior to the oval window, and occasionally at the cochleariform process over the lateral aspect of the geniculate ganglion. The remaining gaps are found along the mastoid segment, and very rarely over the superior aspect and medial to the geniculate ganglion. Their greatest width varies from 0.5 to 3 mm. As a rule they are less numerous and smaller in a well-pneumatized temporal bone, and they are regularly observed bilaterally and symmetrically in location and extent. The presence of more than one gap is not unusual.

The most accurate information concerning their incidence, size and location has been derived from histologic examination of serially sectioned temporal bones. Baxter[15] examined 535 temporal bones from 332 individuals from the collection of the Massachusetts Eye and Ear Infirmary. His observation revealed an incidence of 55%. Ninety-one percent of dehiscences were located in the tympanic segment and 9% in the mastoid segment. Of all dehiscences in the tympanic segment, 83% were located adjacent to the oval window involving the lateral, inferior and medial portion of the canal, with the facial nerve protruding from its canal in 26%. Their greatest diameter ranged from 0.5 to 3.1 mm. In less than 1% (0.8%) did a dehiscence involve the entire length of the tympanic segment. Of all the dehiscences in the mastoid segment 79% opened into the facial recess and 21% into the tympanic sinus or into the retrofacial cells, with the nerve protruding from its canal in 12%. Their greatest diameter ranged from 0.4 to 2 mm. Baxter's findings are very similar to those of Dietzel's[16] who had examined 211 temporal bones and found an incidence of 57%, identical predilective sites and comparable dimensions. The frequency of dehiscences in the facial canal is therefore sufficient to regard them as a variation rather than an anomaly. Guild[17] emphasized the clinical and surgical significance. Since Politzer[18] wrote about them in his textbook in 1894, numerous aural surgeons reported their observations.

Dehiscences in the tympanic segment of the facial canal may lead to an inferior protrusion of the nerve from its canal (Figs. 21-24). This protrusion

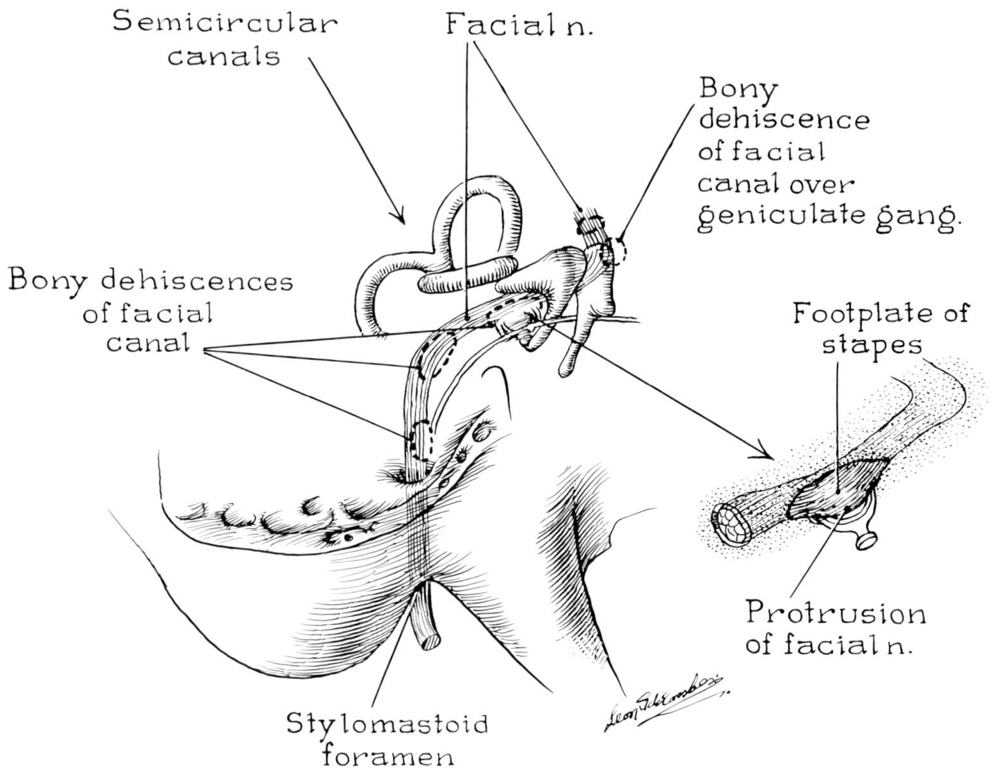

Fig. 21. Locations of bony dehiscences in facial canal.

may vary from a slight bulge of the nerve through a small opening to a situation in which the greater portion of the nerve has emerged from the facial canal and has come to lie upon the superior aspect of the crural arch and upon a portion of the footplate of the stapes (Figs. 23 and 24). Occasionally the entire lateral and inferior circumference of the facial canal may be missing around the posterior crus of the stapes leaving the facial nerve widely exposed (Fig. 25). That such an exposed nerve has a higher risk to become involved in an inflammatory process (Fig. 26) or any other form of injury is readily understandable. Similarly, a facial nerve injury may result, for instance, from elevation of the middle cranial fossa dura during an approach to the trigeminal nerve in a patient with a bony dehi-

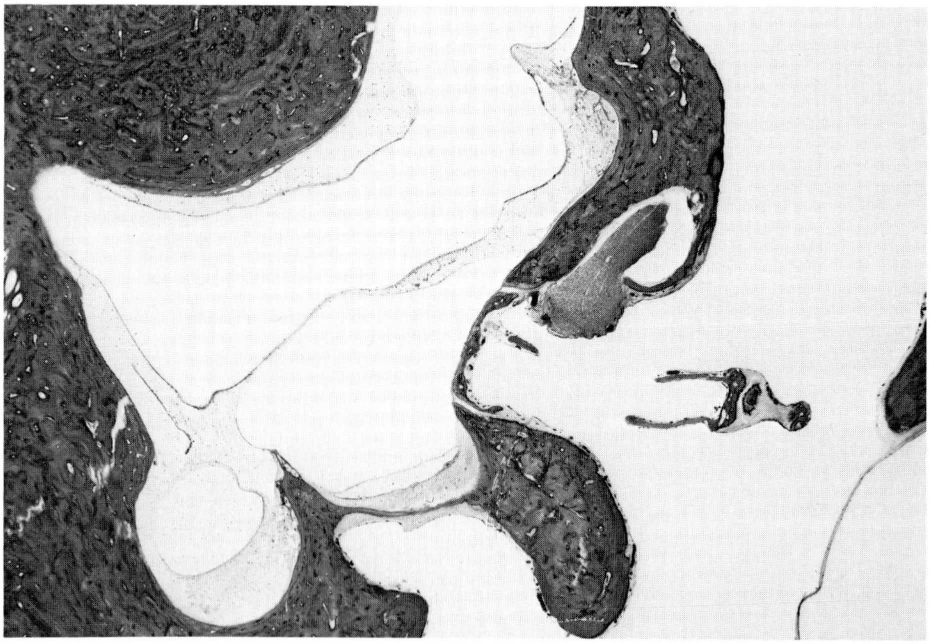

Fig. 22. Vertical section through left temporal bone at level of vestibular and cochlear fenestra in adult. Facial nerve partially protrudes through congenital dehiscence in inferior wall of tympanic segment of facial canal. (H & E, x 16)

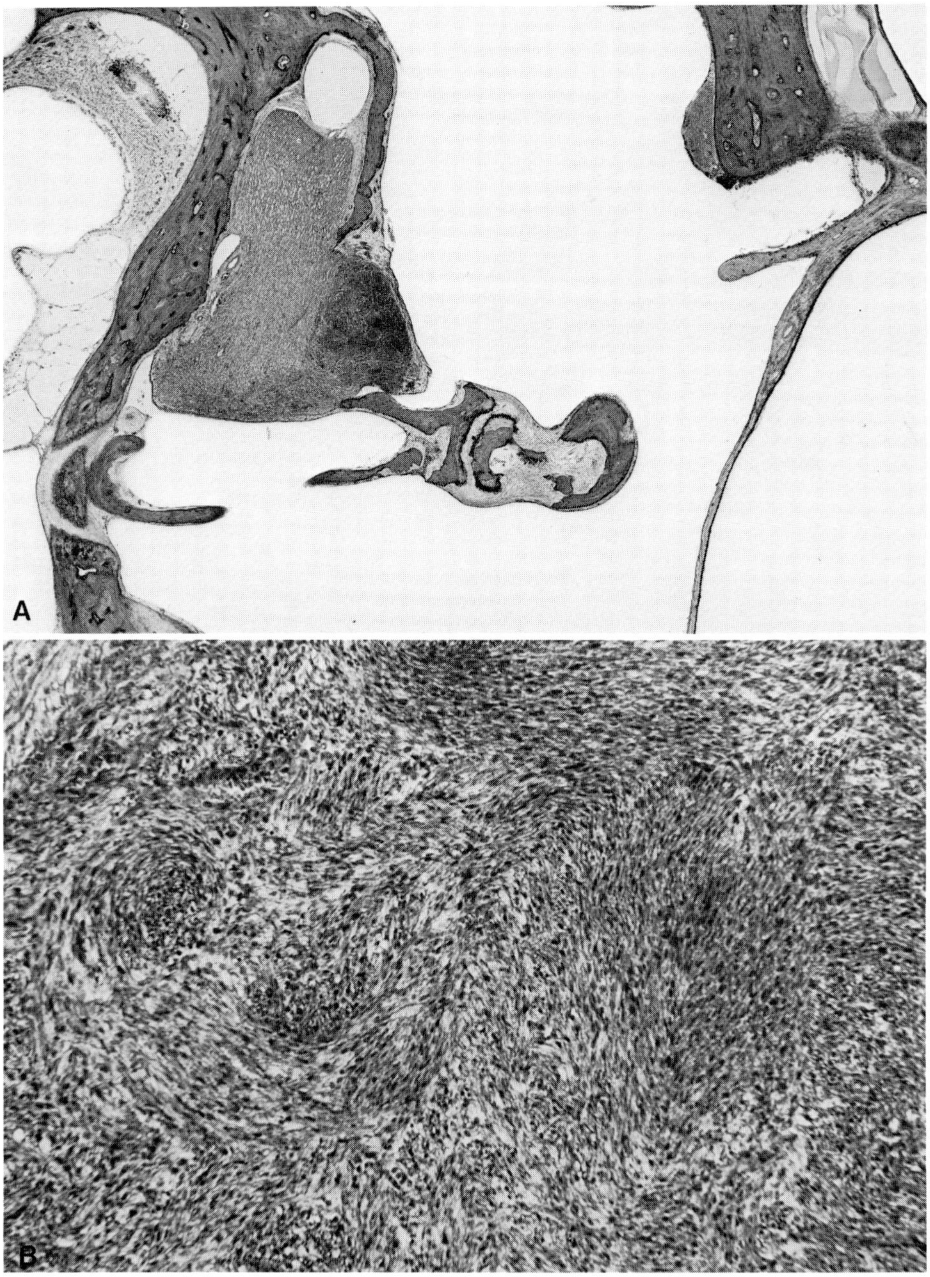

Fig. 23. Vertical section through left temporal bone at posterior end of stapes footplate in adult. A) Abnormal vein (persistent lateral capital vein) occupies one third of facial canal. Major portion of facial nerve lies outside canal on posterior crus of stapes. Its lateral portion reveals early asymptomatic schwannoma (H & E, x 12). B) Tumor is composed of interwoven bundles of long bipolar spindle cells with ovoid or rod-shaped central nuclei containing variable amounts of chromatin and inconspicuous nucleoli (type A tissue of Antoni) (H & E, x 250).

scence in the labyrinthine segment of the facial canal, above or just medial to the geniculate ganglion (Fig. 27). The observation that in a dehiscence the mucoperiosteum of the middle ear is in direct apposition with the epineurium may explain the potential effect of a local anesthetic in the middle ear upon the facial nerve. The inferior sagging of the seventh nerve through a bony defect above the oval window (Fig. 21) should not be confused with an aberrant course of the facial canal in that particular area.

A dehiscence in the lateral wall of the facial canal at the geniculate ganglion exposes the nerve to the anterior epitympanic recess. Care, therefore, must be exercised when eradicating disease from that area.[19] Similarly the aural surgeon must be aware of the frequent occurrence of dehiscences in the lateral, inferior and medial wall of the facial canal above and posterior to the oval window.[17,20] A dehiscence over the vestibular fenestra may be so large as to permit the facial nerve to slide out of its bony canal and rest on the stapedial arch where it may produce a conductive hearing loss. Marked protrusions of an exposed facial nerve have been observed by many surgeons and reported in the literature.[21] Their occasional presence in middle ear dysplasias is well recognized.[22] Many years ago one of the authors (GTN) discovered a small asymptomatic schwannoma in a herniated facial nerve in this location in the left temporal bone of one of our patients (Fig. 23). A subsequent report of a tumor-like her-

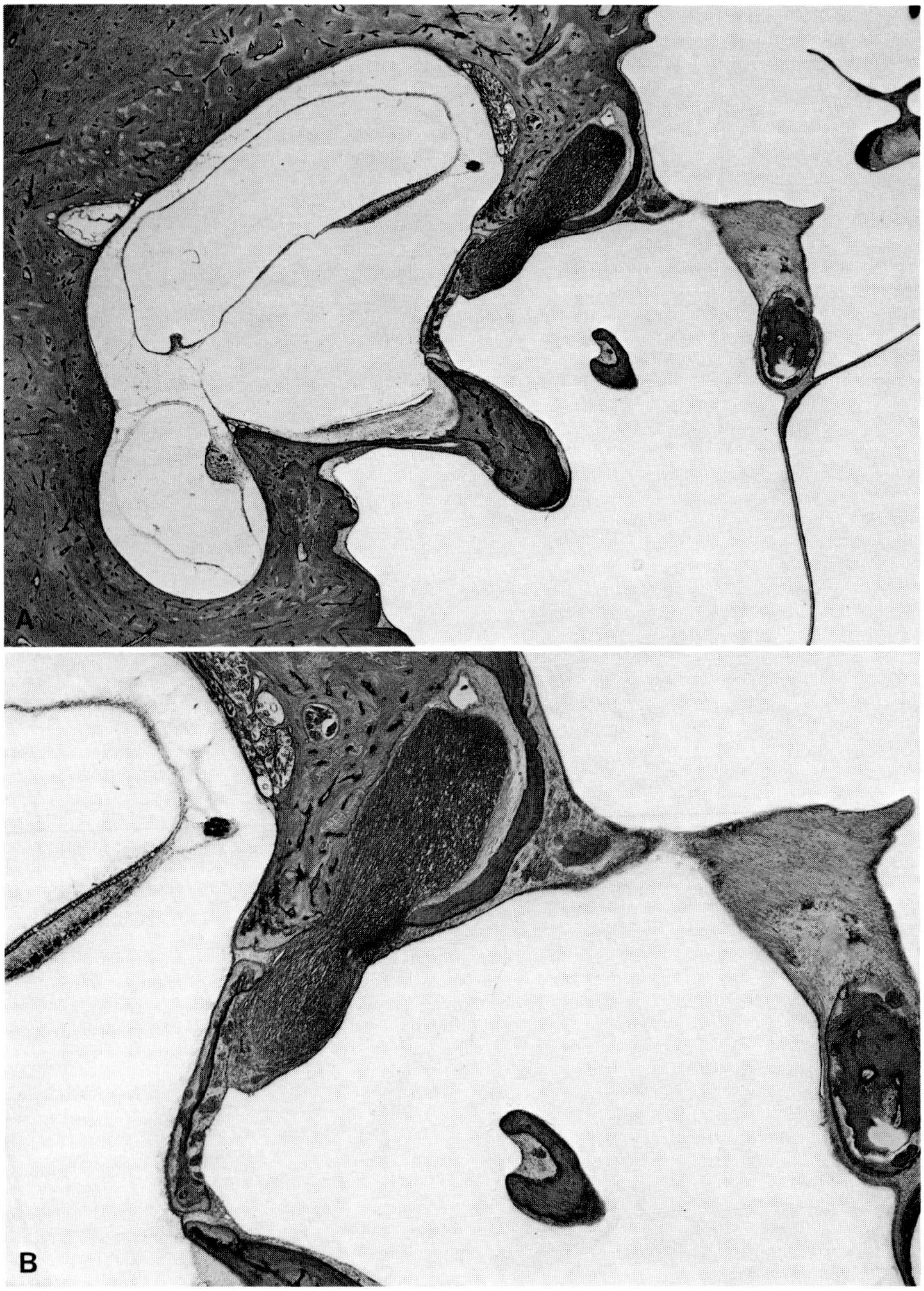

Fig. 24. Vertical section through left temporal bone at center of stapes footplate of adult. A) Almost half of facial nerve protrudes into oval window niche through congenital dehiscence in floor of facial canal (H & E, x 15). B) Extracanalicular portion of facial nerve covers cranial half of stapes footplate in its entire length. There is no separation between epineurium of nerve and mucoperiosteum of footplate (H & E, x 30).

niation of the tympanic portion of the right facial nerve in a 17-year-old girl[23] raises the question of a possible causal relationship. Of interest in this respect are the observations by Babin et al[24] of a "traumatic" neurinoma of the facial nerve in such a herniation in two patients with a history of long-standing chronic otitis media.

ANATOMICAL VARIATIONS IN THE COURSE OF THE FACIAL CANAL

The labyrinthine segment of the facial canal extends from the fundus of the internal acoustic meatus to the geniculate ganglion across the axis of the petrous pyramid. It varies in length between 2.5 and 6 mm.[25] The tympanic segment runs from the geniculate ganglion posteriorly to the lateral semicircular canal in a more or less inclined plane parallel to the axis of the pyramid. As it courses along the medial wall of the tympanic cavity above the oval window it follows an oblique direction from inside out. It varies in length from 7 to 11 mm.[25] The mastoid segment generally runs straight downward from the posterior margin of the oval window to the stylomastoid foramen. Its length varies between 9 and 16 mm.[26] It may form a slight anterior, posterior or medial curve when viewed laterally (Fig. 28 C-E). In most instances its course is straight downward. In some patients, however, the stylomastoid foramen is located more laterally

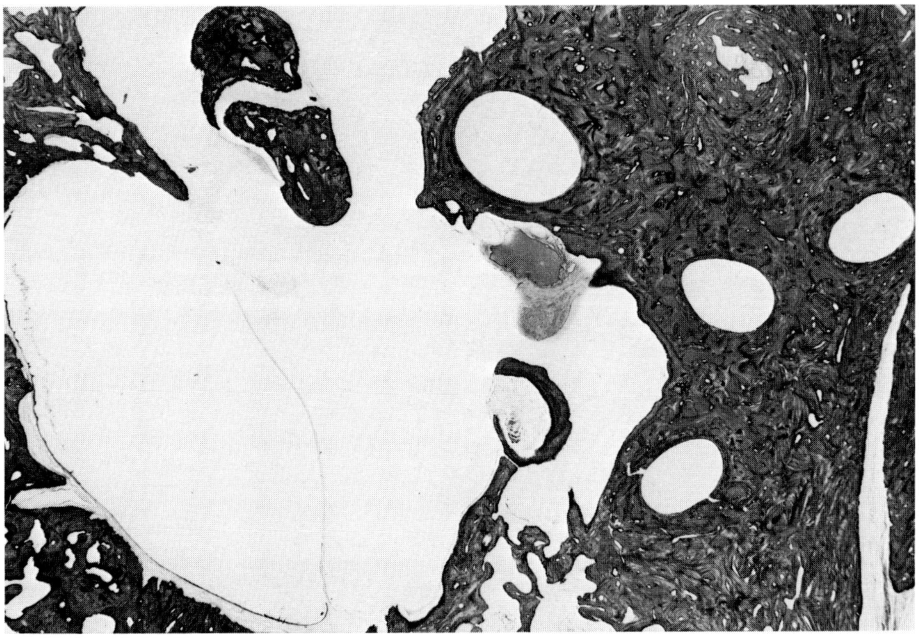

Fig. 25. Vertical section through right temporal bone at junction of tympanic with mastoid segment of facial canal in adult. Congenital absence of lateral, inferior and part of medial portion of bony canal wall resulted in almost total exposure of facial nerve in that location. (H & E, x 12)

when viewed from behind, and in such instances the mastoid segment of the facial canal follows, instead of a vertical, an outward oblique direction (Fig. 28 F). Rarely does the mastoid segment follow an inward oblique course.

ANATOMICAL ANOMALIES OF THE COURSE OF THE FACIAL CANAL

In addition to the variations, there are a number of recognized anomalies involving the course of the facial canal. These anomalies are seldom encountered in the normally developed temporal bone, but frequently are observed in its malformations. Fowler[27] collected the most pertinent forms from the literature and depicted them in a diagrammatic manner. Whereas the observations involving the mastoid segment may be found in a normally developed temporal bone, the ones involving the tympanic segment are frequently associated with a dysplasia of the stapes, lack of differentiation, or agenesis of the oval window. Severe dysplasias of the middle and inner ear are, with few exceptions, regularly accompanied by an aberrant course of the facial canal.

The anomalies of the course of the facial canal may be conveniently classified according to the level at which they involve the facial nerve or the segment of the facial canal in which they are encountered.

Canalicular Segment of the Facial Canal. In an exceptional instance the facial nerve may enter the petrous pyramid instead of via the internal acoustic meatus through the subarcuate fossa and run through the center of the superior semicircular canal to the stylomastoid foramen, bypassing the middle ear cavity[28] (Fig. 29 A). In a rare situation a bifurcation of the nerve may be encountered within the internal auditory canal.

Labyrinthine Segment of the Facial Canal. Rare cases of a bifurcation of the facial nerve within the labyrinthine segment of the facial canal were described by Altmann[29] and Miehlke and Partsch.[30]

Tympanic Segment of the Facial Canal. Aberrations in the course of the facial nerve in this segment of the facial canal can be subdivided into the following categories:

1. Facial nerve coursing along the superior aspect of the lateral semicircular canal (Fig. 29 B).
2. Bifurcation of the facial nerve anterior or proximal to the oval window (Fig. 29 C-F).
3. Facial nerve coursing horizontally over the oval window (Fig. 29 G).
4. Facial nerve coursing through the stapedial arch (Fig. 29 H, I).
5. Facial nerve coursing posteriorly between the oval and round window (Fig. 29 J).
6. Facial nerve coursing posteriorly inferior to the round window (Fig. 29 K).
7. Facial nerve coursing from the geniculate ganglion straight downward over the promontory (Fig. 29 L).
8. Hypoplasia of the facial nerve (Fig. 29 N, X, Y).

H. House (personal communication) has seen the facial nerve coursing along the superior aspect of the lateral semicircular canal in two instances (Fig. 29 B). One observation was in a cadaver, the other in a patient scheduled for a fenestration operation.

Bifurcations of the facial nerve anterior to the oval window are commonly associated with developmental anomalies of the vestibular fenestra and stapes whereby the greater or lesser portion of the nerve may run above or below the totally or partial-

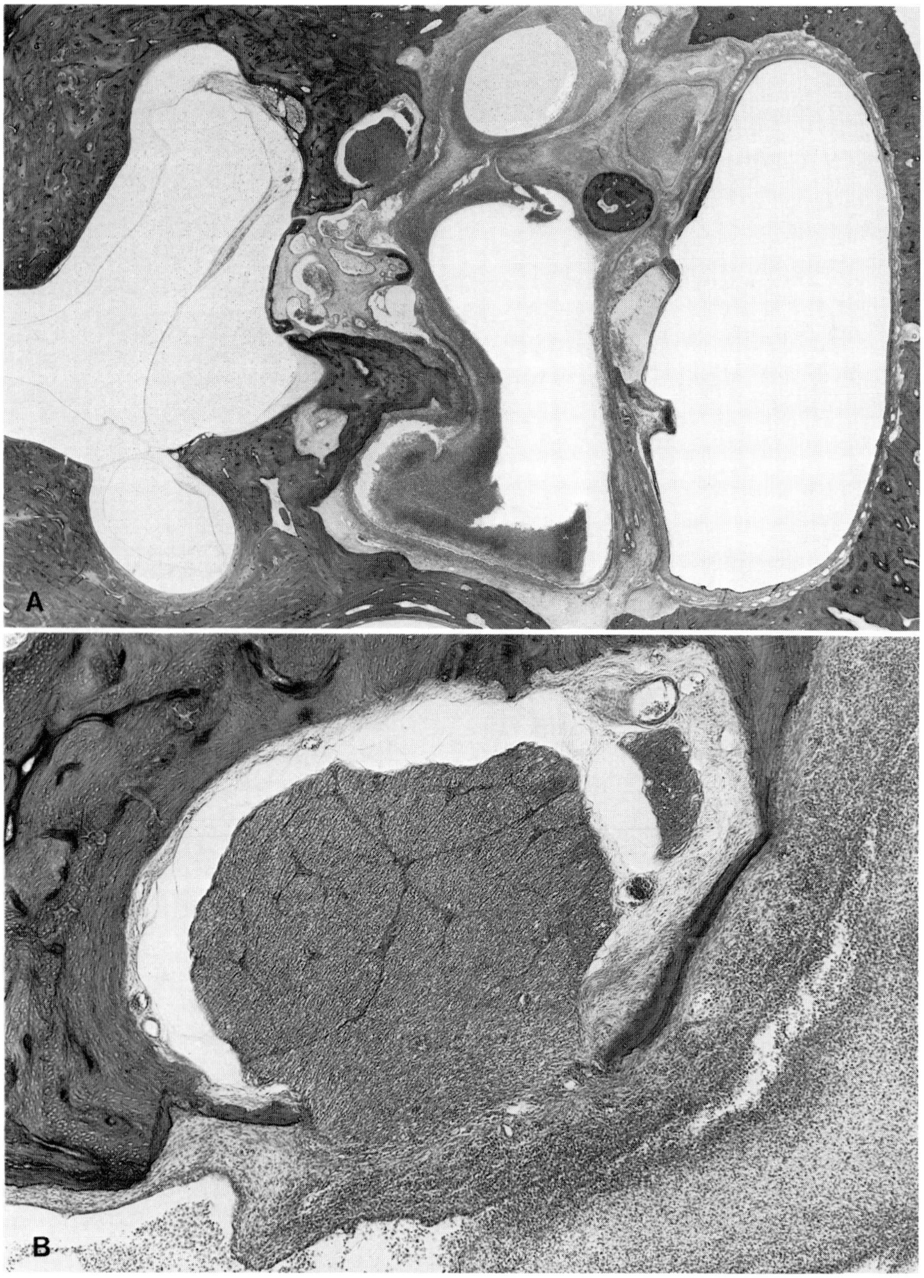

Fig. 26. Vertical section through left temporal bone at level of oval window in child with congenital dehiscence in tympanic segment of facial canal and acute bacterial otitis media. A) Purulent exudate occupies most of middle ear cavity and drains through central perforation in inferior tympanic membrane into external auditory canal (H & E, x 12). B) Acute cellulitis involves mucoperiosteum covering facial canal and extends through dehiscence in bony canal into exposed underlying facial nerve (x 75).

ly undifferentiated oval window. This form of bifurcation has been observed by the authors and others on many occasions[21,27,31] (Fig. 29 C-F).

A transcrural course of a facial nerve has been observed on several occasions[29,32,33] (Fig. 29 H, I). Marquet[34] reported a patient in whom one portion of a bifid facial nerve passed through the center of the stapedial arch (Fig. 29 I). Butler,[32] during the removal of a cholesteatoma, found an exposed facial nerve passing through the stapedial arch almost totally occupying its lumen. The facial nerve reentered a bony facial canal which continued its course downward posterior to the round window (Fig. 29 H).

Fowler[27] observed a facial nerve crossing the promontory in a patient with congenital fixation of the footplate and a persistent stapedial artery. Martin and Martin[35] reported a bilateral course of the facial nerve below the oval window in association with bilateral congenital fixation of the footplate and ossification of the stapedius tendon. Mayer and Crabtree[36] added three additional patients and reviewed nine previous cases from the literature. All 12 patients had a congenital conductive hearing loss and the facial canal was dehiscent in that segment. The exposed nerve appeared normal in nine, but as a "boggy mass" in three patients. In ten instances the stapedial arch was markedly anomalous and the stapedial footplate lacked differentiation. In one of these author's three patients the lateral semicircular canal and vestibule were abnormally large.

Durcan et al[21] discussed three patients in which

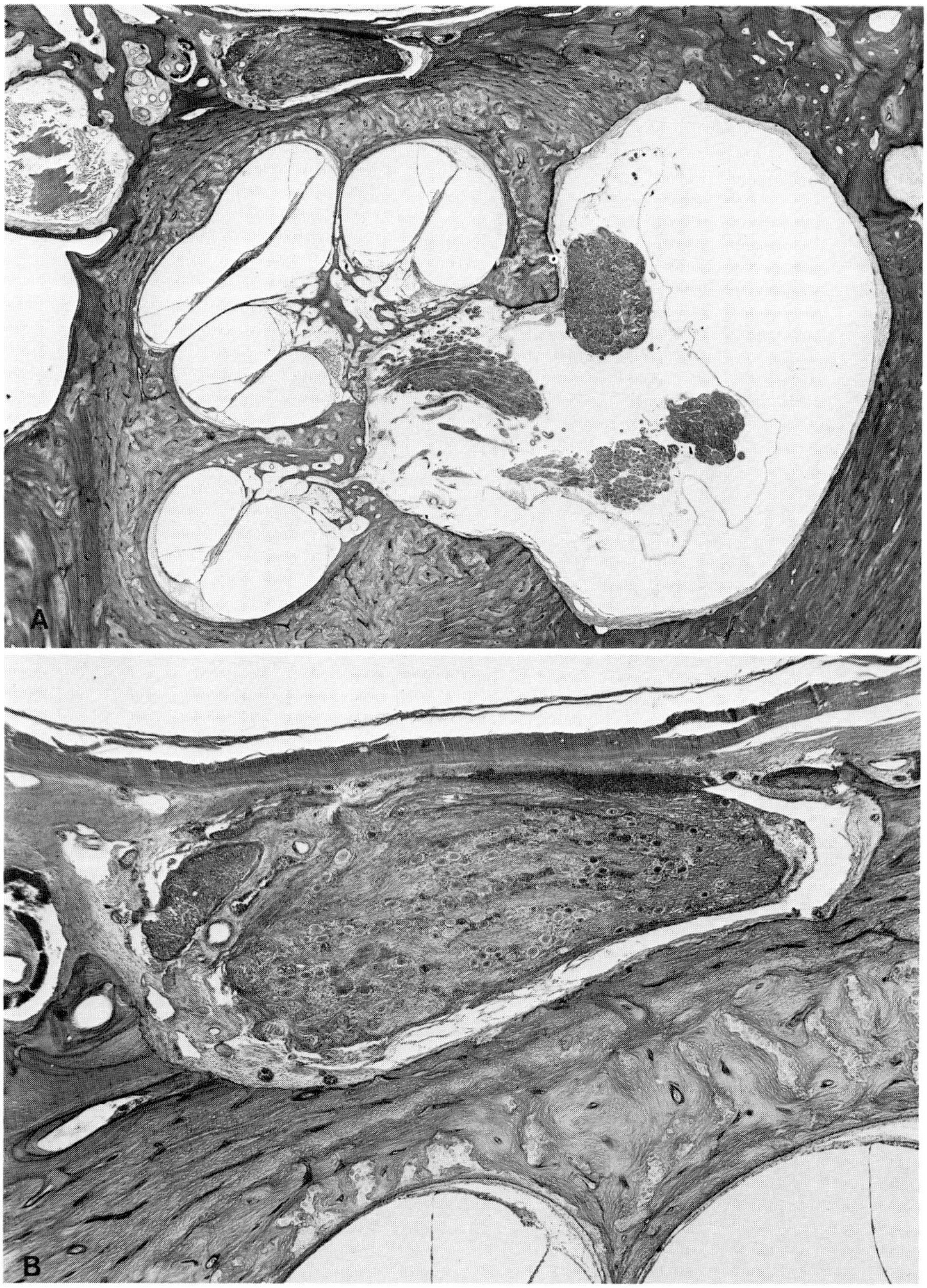

Fig. 27. A) Paramodiolar section through right temporal bone at level of geniculate ganglion and origin of greater superficial petrosal nerve in adult (H & E, x 14). B) Same section. Due to complete absence of superior bony wall of labyrinthine segment of facial canal, geniculate ganglion is exposed and has become firmly attached to overlying dura of middle cranial fossa (x 50).

the facial nerve ran over the promontory between the oval and round window. The nerve appeared slightly larger than normal and overlaid the oval window from below. Leek[37] and Henner[38] made a similar observation in one patient with an otosclerotic process, and another with a dysplasia of the stapedial arch and oval window. Jahrsdoerfer[22] observed anomalies of the facial nerve in 13 of 54 ears (24%) operated for minor malformations of the ear (patent outer ear canal and identifiable tympanic membrane). The most frequent abnormalities were an exposed facial nerve devoid of any bony cover (10/13 patients), and an abnormal position of the facial nerve. The position of the tympanic segment of the facial nerve was normal, above the oval window, in two patients. In two it was impinging the stapedial arch from above. In 4 patients it was covering the oval window, in 4 it was below the oval window, and in 1 the exposed nerve segment was suspended in midair. In these 13 patients the anomaly of the facial nerve was associated with a normal stapes in 3, with a malformed stapes in 8, and with an absent stapes in 2 patients. The oval window was present in four but absent in nine patients. The round window was present in 7 patients, absent in 2 and not visualized in 3 patients.

A facial nerve, descending over the promontory anterior to both windows and leaving the temporal bone through the hypotympanum, associated with an empty facial canal in a normal position was reported by Dickinson et al[39] (Fig. 29 L). Angell-

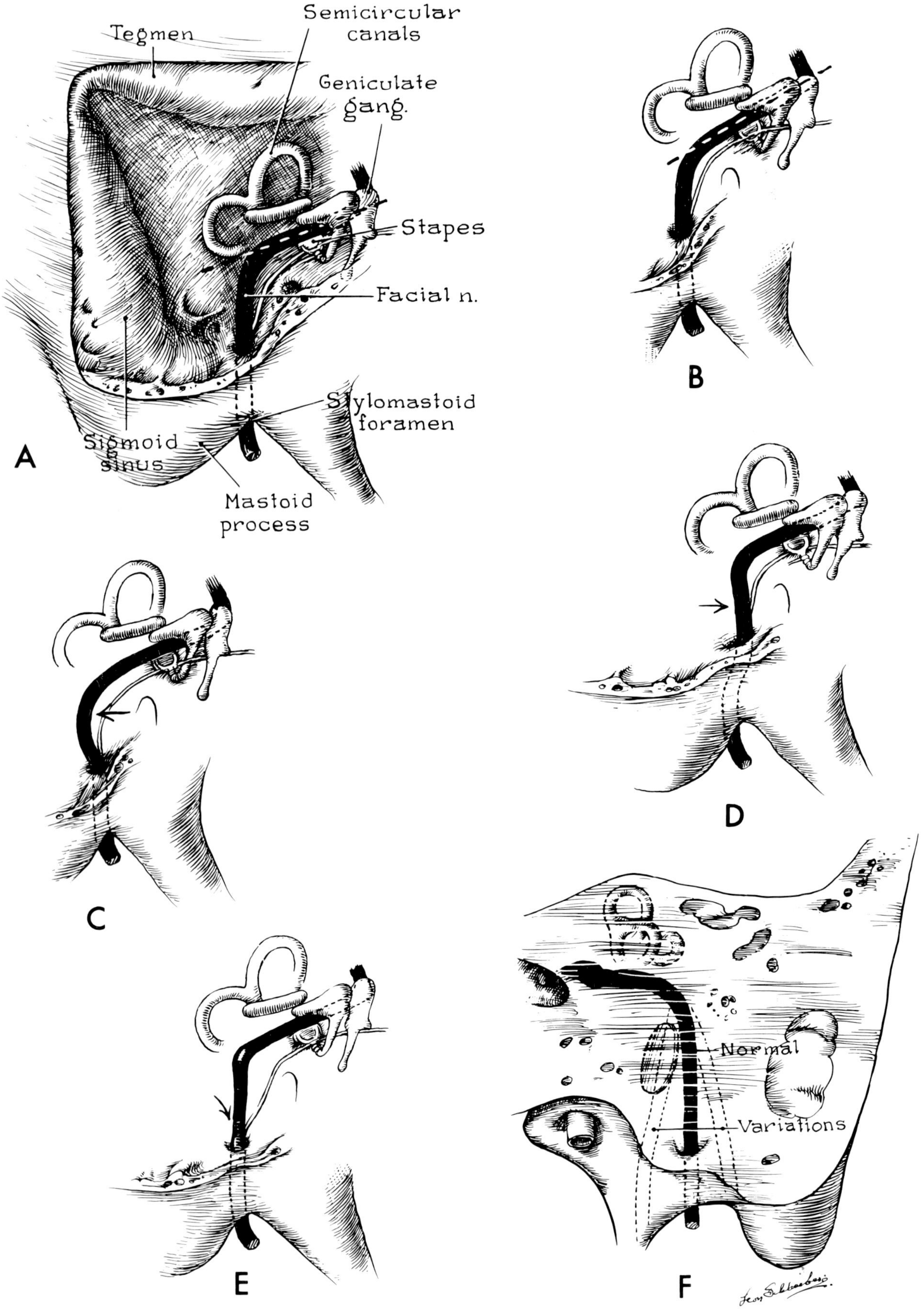

Fig. 28. Variations in course of facial nerve.

James (personal communication to Fowler[27]) describes a patient in whom the facial nerve ran through the anterior wall of the external auditory canal wall (Fig. 29 M).

Kodama et al[40] discussed the histologic findings in the left temporal bone of a 9-year-old girl, born with a deformed left auricle and left facial nerve paralysis. The extremely hypoplastic left facial nerve ran together with a large persisting stapedial artery within a bony canal downward over the promontory anterior to the oval and round window (Fig. 29 N). The stapedial artery entered the middle cranial fossa at the facial hiatus. Failure of certain portions of the branchial arch cartilages to develop, and nonunion or a delayed union between these branchial arch elements and the primordial otic capsule, may permit the developing facial nerve to assume the abnormal forward position in these malformations. Similarly a delay in the fusion of the stapedial crura with the lamina stapedialis of the primordial otic capsule may be responsible for a partial or total transcrural course of the facial nerve.[41,42]

Mastoid Segment of the Facial Canal. Aberrations in the course of the facial canal in this segment can be subdivided into the following three categories:

1. Facial nerve following an abnormal posterior, lateral or anterior course (Fig. 29 O-T).
2. Bifurcation and trifurcation of the facial nerve posterior or distal to the oval window (Fig. 29 U-W).
3. Hypoplasia of the facial nerve (Fig. 29 X, Y).

The most frequent anomaly so far observed is the one characterized by a distinct posterior and lateral bulge ("dorsal hump") of the canal just beneath the prominence of the lateral semicircular canal[27,43] (Fig. 29 O). In that instance the nerve is in a more lateral position than usual and closer to the operator. Fowler[27] and Angell-James (personal communication to Fowler[27]) together had observed seven patients with that anomaly. Wright[44] reported seeing vascular prominences in that location. They represent anastomoses between the descending superficial petrosal vessels and the ascending pharyngeal vessels. Their usual location is just above the level of the pyramidal process of the facial canal.

Fowler[27] and Kettel[43] described an abnormal posterior position of the mastoid segment, with the nerve overlying the anterior wall of the lateral sinus. This situation may be associated with an unusual lateral displacement of the nerve[27,45] (Fig. 29 P).

The entire mastoid segment of the facial nerve may be in an abnormal posterior location[46] (Fig. 29 Q). In such a situation it may course 2 to 4 mm posterior to its usual location which is posterior to the posterior wall of the tympanic cavity. The mastoid segment is therefore located between the external meatus and the sigmoid sinus.

Glasscock[47] reported an S-shaped anomaly of the right mastoid segment of the facial canal in a 5-year-old female with a history of two episodes of right facial palsy preceded in each instance by acute otitis media. An abnormally large chorda tympani nerve joined the facial nerve at the level of the pyramidal process (Fig. 29 R).

Pou[48] reported an infant with agenesis of the mastoid segment of the facial canal. In its absence the facial nerve made an anterior turn somewhat anterior and lateral to the level where normally the second turn of the facial canal would be encountered, to follow the chorda tympani nerve (Fig. 29 S).

Bellucci[49] noted that in 9 of 71 patients with congenital aural dysplasia, the facial nerve followed an abnormal course in the hypotympanum, turning anteriorly at the level of the round window instead of continuing downward toward the stylomastoid foramen (Fig. 29 T). During the removal of the atresia plate in congenital aural dysplasia, on two occasions, Pracy[50] observed the facial nerve taking a lateral turn below the short process of the incus, passing forward at this level to leave the temporal bone at the height of the temporomandibular articulation.

The tympanic segment of the facial nerve is formed by the 35th week of fetal life. The posterior opening of the canal is located at the end of the second turn. This aperture is referred to as the primitive mastoid foramen. The formation of the mastoid portion of the facial canal occurs during the subsequent development of the mastoid process. Any disturbance in the development of that segment of the canal may result in an abnormal location or division of the nerve. Harpman[51] presented a radiograph of the mastoid process of a patient in whom the facial nerve emerged from the lateral surface of the mastoid, about 1.27 cm (0.5 in) above the tip.

A bifurcation of the facial nerve posterior or distal to the oval window, with the two branches continuing in separate canals and leaving the mastoid process through individual foramina, was mentioned by several otologists[25,45,52] (Fig. 29 U,V). The separate branches may cross on their way to individual stylomastoid foramina, or reunite either at or just outside the stylomastoid foramen into a single trunk again.[25,44] The lateral of the two trunks is usually the larger and the one which received the chorda tympani nerve[44] (Fig. 29 U, V). Basek[53] found bifurcations in 3 of 500 individuals, or in 0.6%. A trifurcation of the facial nerve in the same location and with identical characteristics (separate canals and separate stylomastoid foramina), was reported by Botmann and Jongkees,[54] and also by Heermann[55] (Fig. 29 W).

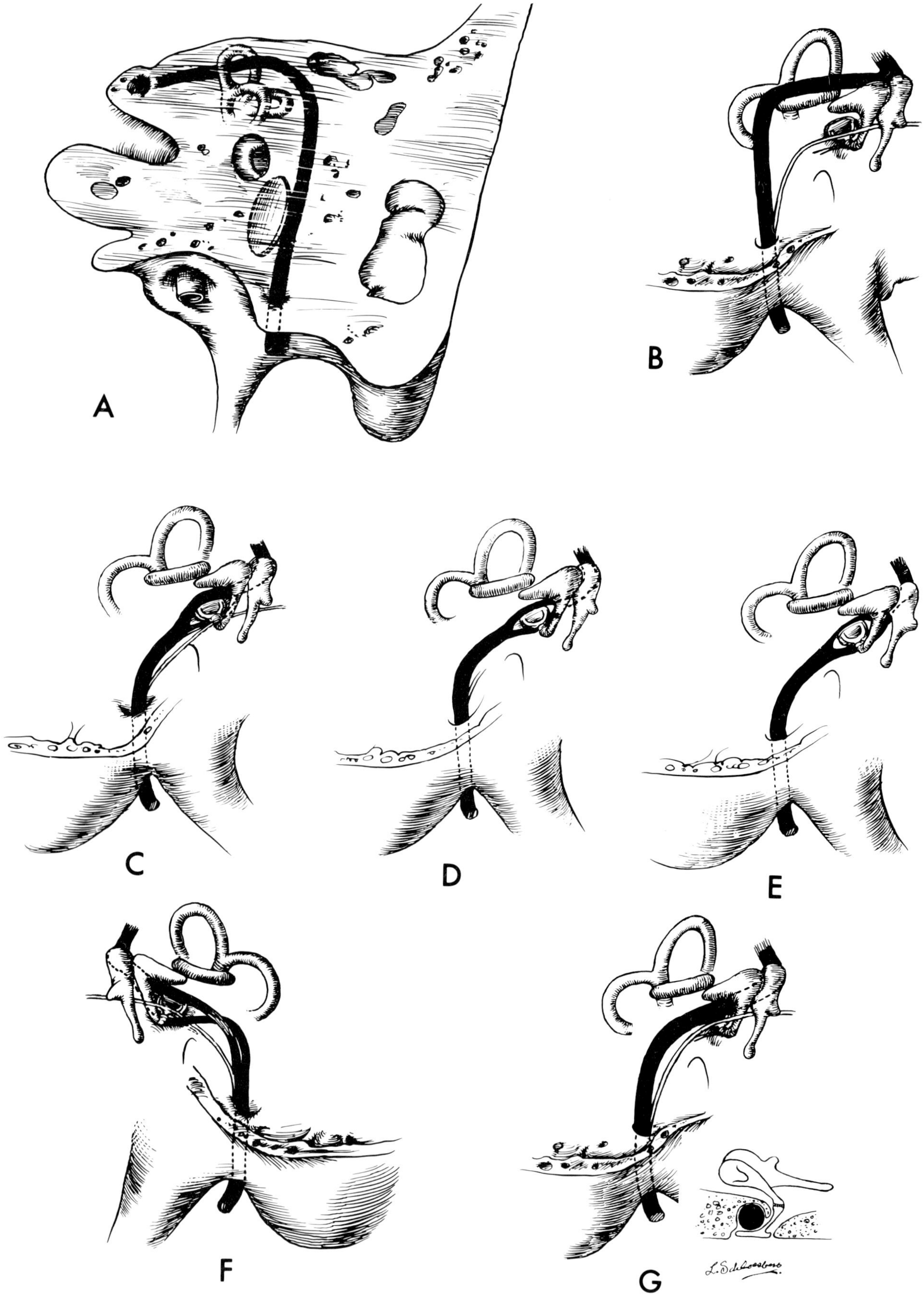

Fig. 29. Anatomical abnormalities in course of facial nerve.

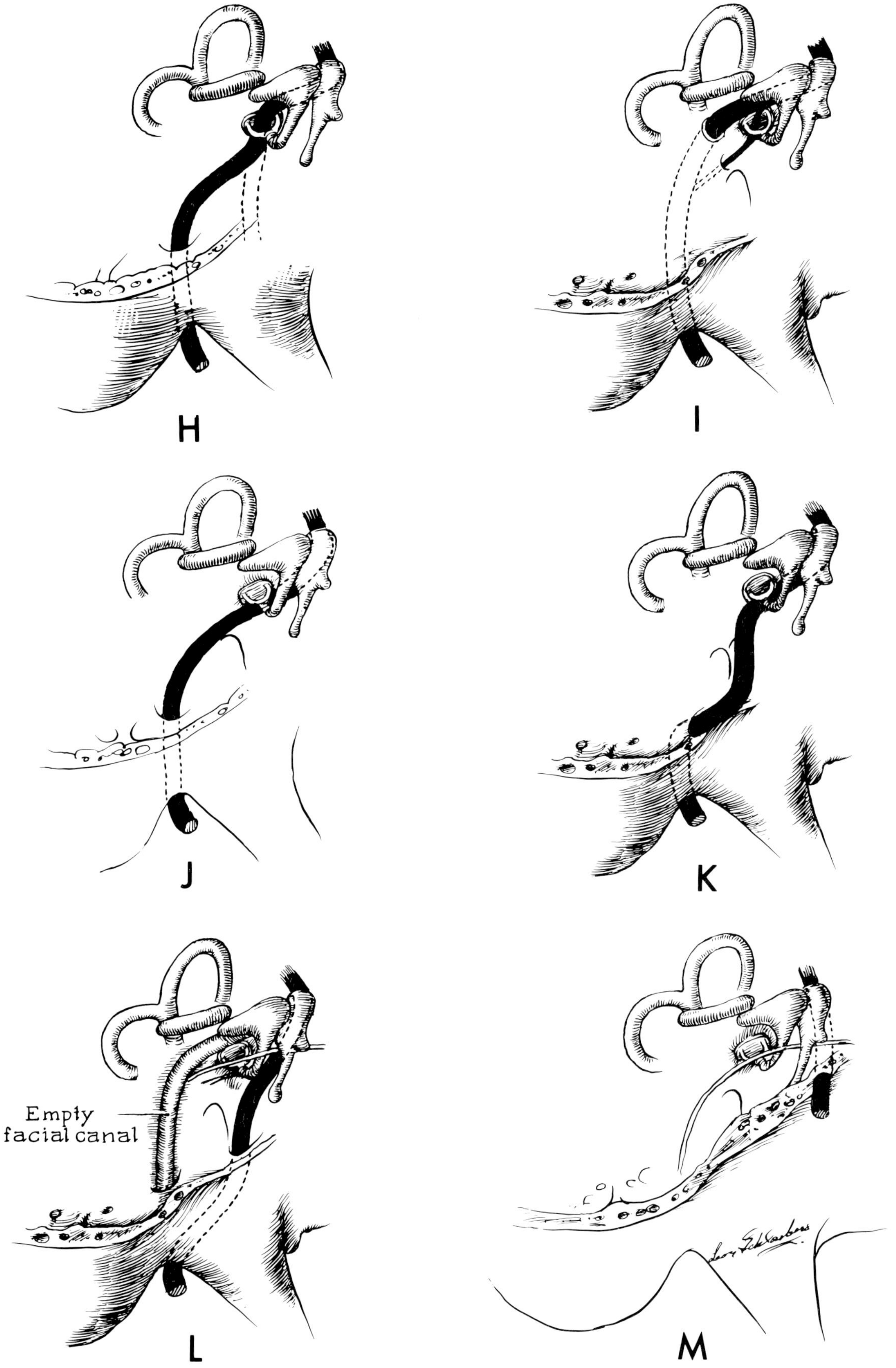

Fig. 29, cont'd.

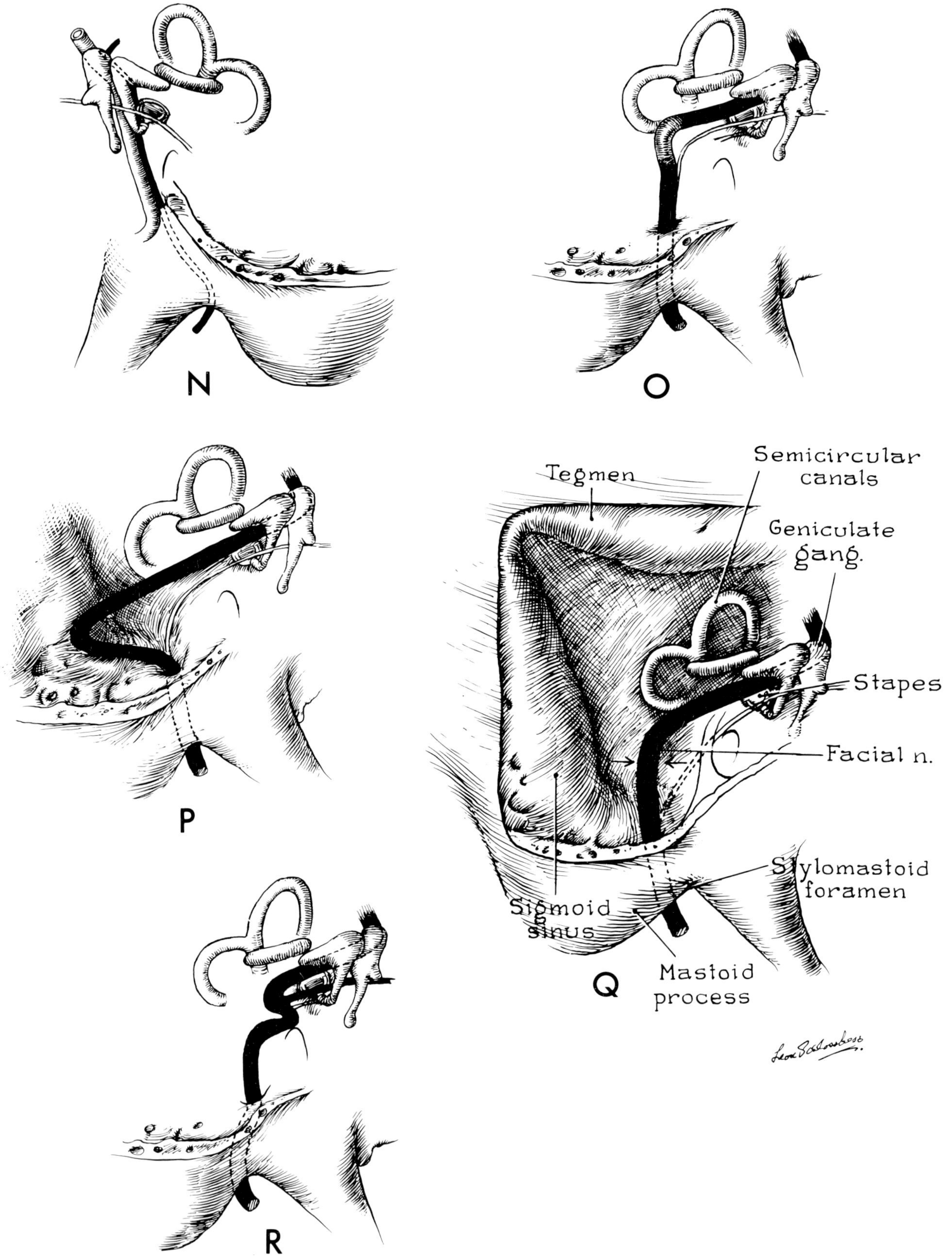
N
O
P
Tegmen
Semicircular canals
Geniculate gang.
Stapes
Facial n.
Stylomastoid foramen
Sigmoid sinus
Mastoid process
Q
R

Fig. 29, cont'd.

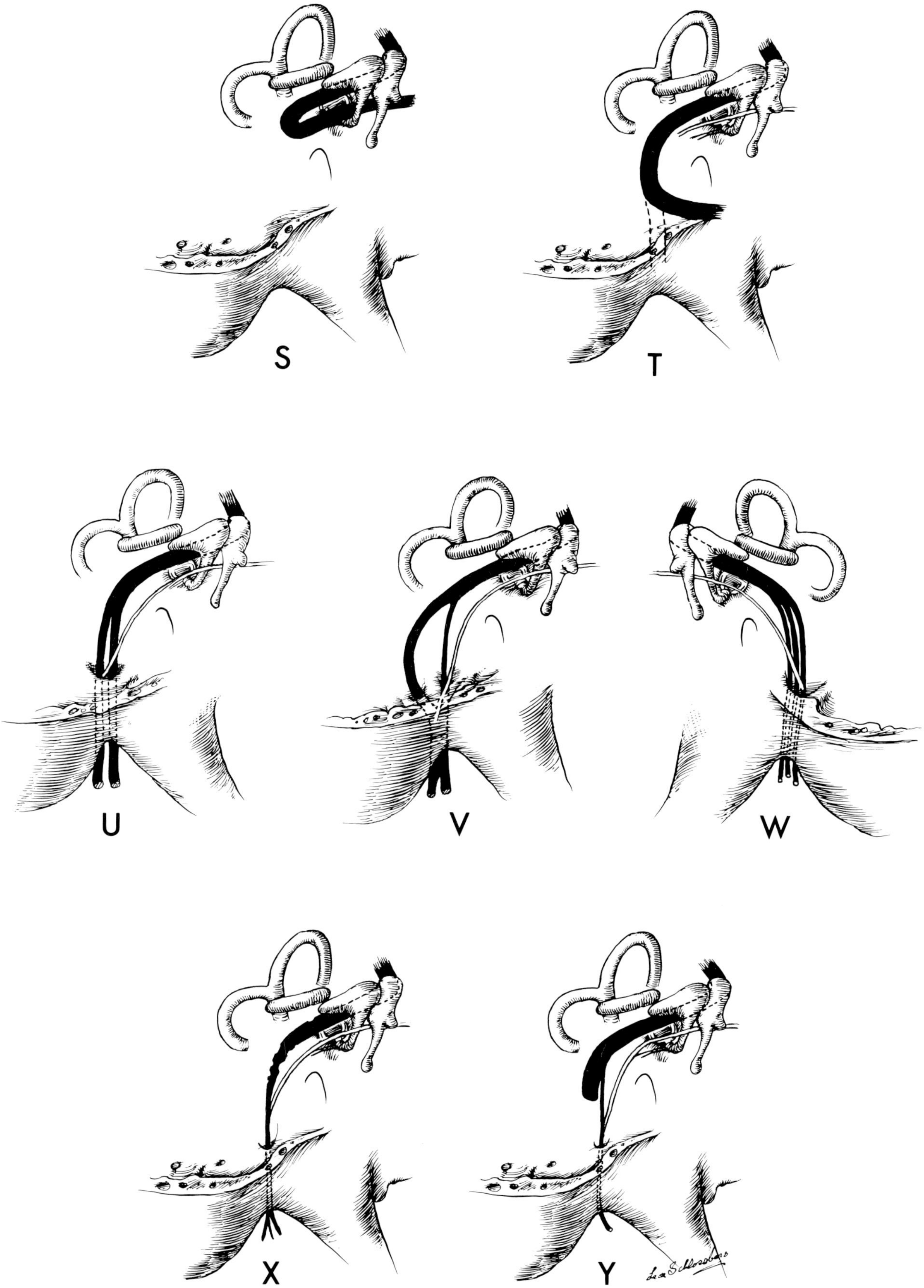

Fig. 29, cont'd.

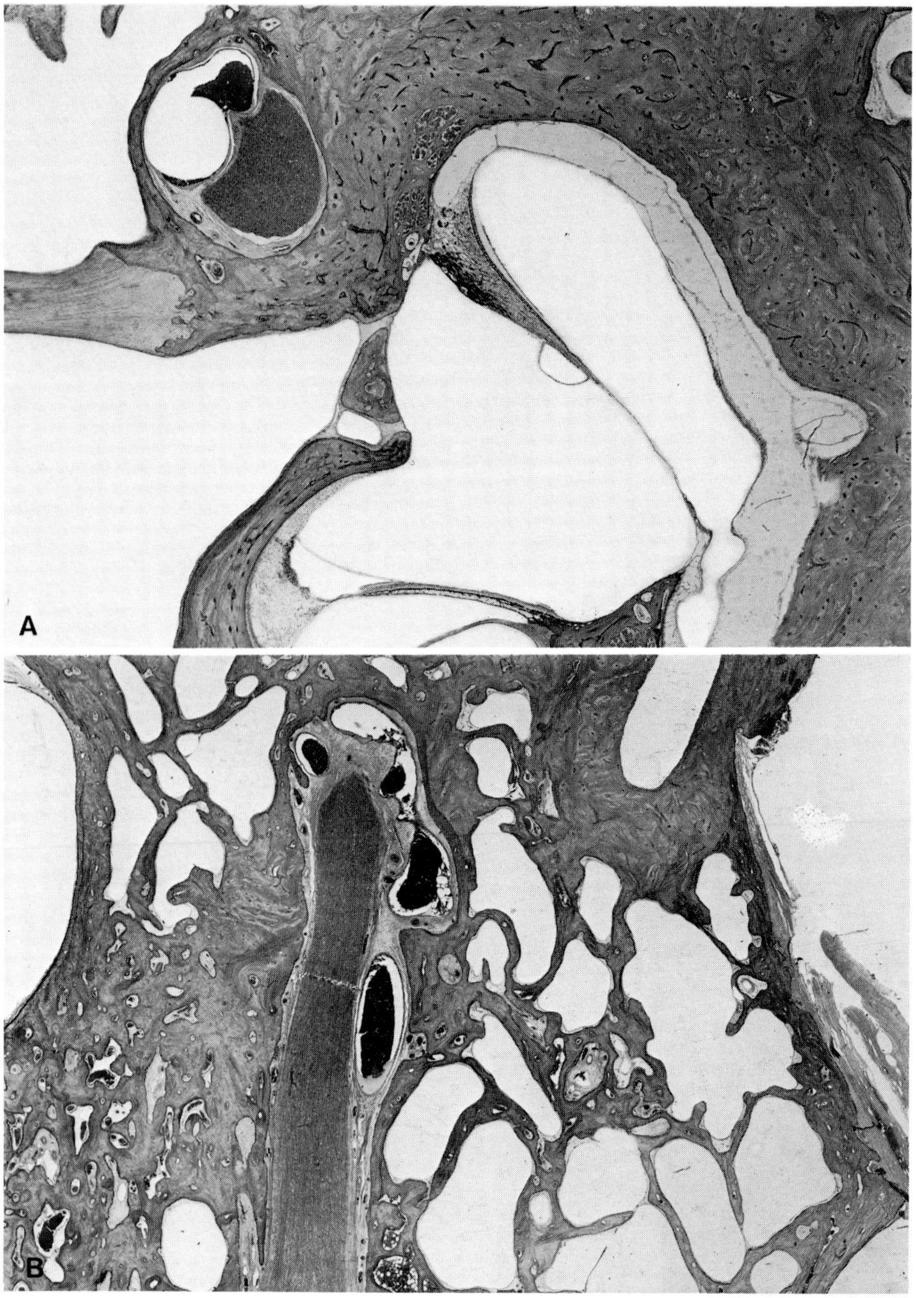

Fig. 30. Vertical section through right temporal bone at level of cochleariform process in adult. A) Abnormally large vein (persistent lateral capital vein) occupies half of lumen of tympanic segment of facial canal (H & E, x 10). B) Same abnormal vein is seen accompanying right facial nerve in mastoid segment of facial canal (H & E, x 10).

Hawley,[56] Tobeck[57] and Miehlke[45] found the main trunk of the facial nerve to end in a blind pocket of the mastoid process while only a very small branch continued the normal course of the nerve (Fig. 29 Y). Marquet[34] reported a similar dysplasia of the facial canal and nerve (Fig. 29 X).

The most severe malformations of the facial canal and nerve, including their total agenesis, have been observed in the thalidomide embryopathy.[45]

ANATOMICAL VARIATIONS OF THE CHORDA TYMPANI NERVE

The chorda tympani nerve may exhibit variations and aberrations in relation to its origin from the facial nerve as well as its course through the mastoid process.[29] Its origin may vary from 1 mm distal to 11 mm proximal to the stylomastoid foramen. On the average the chorda arises 5 mm above the stylomastoid foramen. In the rare situation of an extratemporal origin (2%) the chorda travels in its own separate bony canaliculus parallel to the facial canal. In an exceptional middle ear malformation, the chorda may join the facial nerve in its tympanic segment at the cochleariform process.[27] Three instances of a bifurcation of the chorda tympani nerve have been described by Durcan et al.[21]

Abnormal Artery and Vein. Occasionally a persisting stapedial artery may be encountered entering the tympanic segment of the facial canal through the stapedial arch. It is a remnant of the

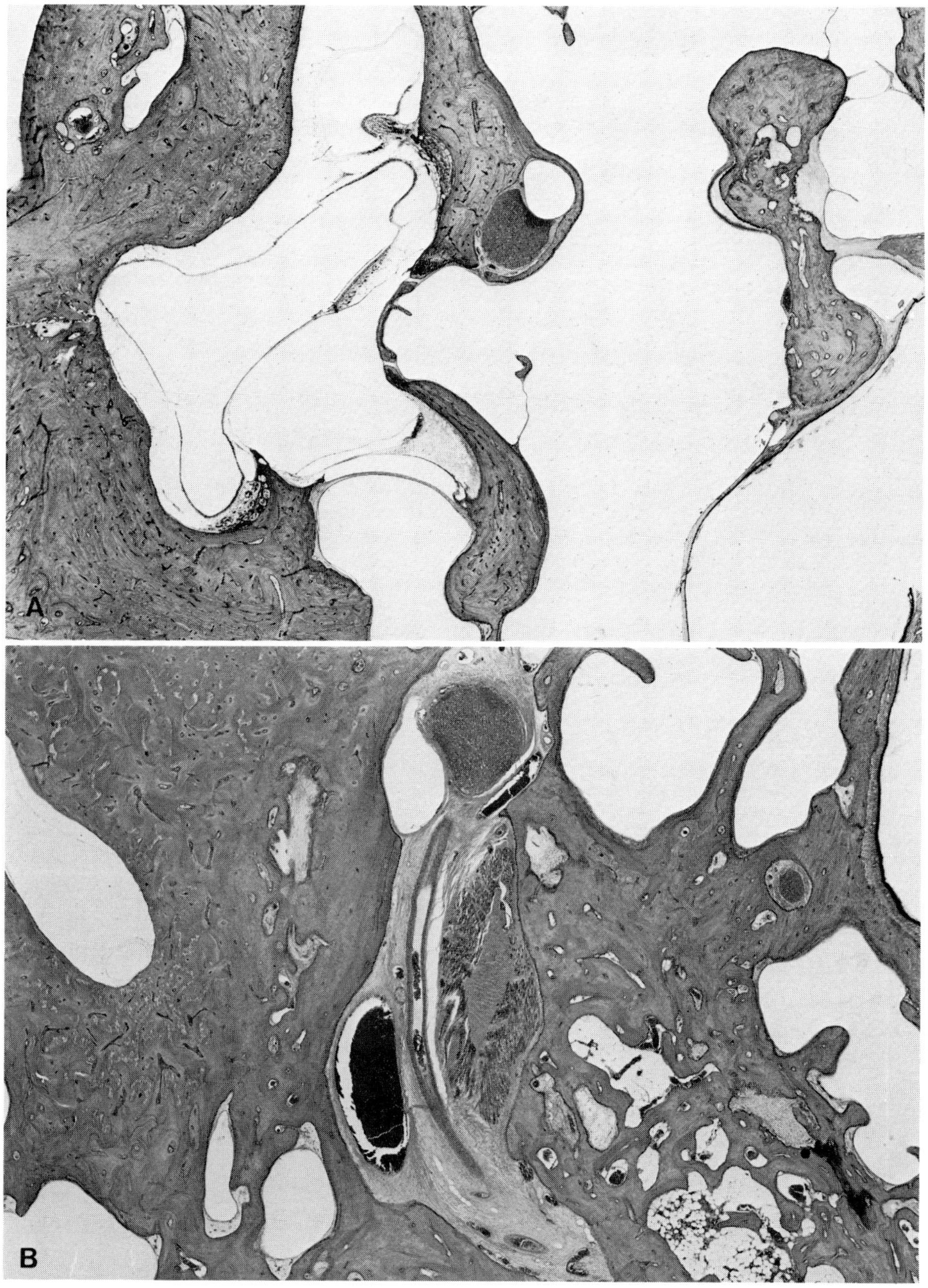

Fig. 31. Vertical section through left temporal bone of same patient in Fig. 30 at level of oval and round window. A) Abnormal vein, accompanying facial nerve, is well recognized (H & E, x 12). B) Same abnormal vein accompanies left facial nerve and stylomastoid artery in mastoid segment of facial canal (H & E, x 16).

dorsal end of the second aortic arch which usually disappears early in fetal life. The persisting stapedial artery arises from the internal carotid artery, traverses the floor of the hypotympanum, ascends along the promontory within its own bony canal, passes through the stapedial arch, and enters the facial canal above the oval window. It accompanies the facial nerve upward and supplies the outer surface of the dura in a similar fashion as the middle meningeal artery does.[58]

In a rare instance a large vein, of equal size or larger than the facial nerve, may be observed joining the nerve in the facial canal near the geniculate ganglion and accompanying it to the stylomastoid foramen. This vessel represents a persisting lateral capital vein (Figs. 30 and 31). During early embryonic life it provides the main venous drainage from the anterior and middle portions of the brain. It normally undergoes involution in later fetal life when the anterior and middle cerebral veins begin to drain into the posterior cerebral vein.

SUMMARY

The regional and surgical anatomy of the facial canal as it traverses the temporal bone and relates to important adjacent structures is reviewed in detail.

Congenital bony dehiscences in the facial canal are encountered in about 55% of temporal bones. They result from incomplete closure of the canal wall during its development. Dehiscences may be observed in any portion of the facial canal. The majority, about 90%, are located in the tympanic segment, and about 10% are situated in the mastoid segment. In the tympanic segment, about 80% are located adjacent to the oval window, involving the lateral, inferior and medial portion of the canal, with the facial nerve protruding in about 25%. In the mastoid segment about 80% of the dehiscences open into the facial recess and about 20% communicate with the tympanic sulcus or with the retrofacial cells, with the nerve protruding in about 12%.

The variations of the facial canal may involve the length and direction of each segment, the angular relation between the tympanic and the mastoid segment, and the downward course of the mastoid segment.

Anomalies of the facial canal are seldom encountered in the normally developed temporal bone, but frequently are observed in its malformations. They include aberrations of the course of a single or of all segments of the canal, an abnormal relation to the oval and round window, bifurcations and trifurcations of the nerve, and associations with dysplasias of the stapes, oval window, external ear canal and auricle. In a rare instance the facial nerve may be severely hypoplastic or totally absent.

Two abnormal vessels may occasionally accompany the facial nerve in the facial canal: a persistent stapedial artery and a persistent lateral capital vein.

AXIOMS AND CONCLUSIONS

1. Always be on the lookout for the facial nerve.
2. Know exactly where you are at all times. Being careful is not enough.
3. If the surgical procedure involving the facial nerve makes corrective surgery difficult, then the operation should not be pursued to the point that makes facial paralysis a possibility.
4. Anticipate dehiscences all along the course of the facial canal.
5. If the facial canal is opened without injury to the nerve, there is no need to do a decompression.
6. If a soft tissue mass involves the promontory and hypotympanum, check the facial nerve at the geniculate and follow it peripherally before curetting soft tissue. A boggy mass on the promontory can be the facial nerve.[38]
7. When cholesteatoma obscures the course of the facial nerve, identify the nerve in an uninvolved area, and using important landmarks (promontory, lateral semicircular canal, cochleariform process), follow the nerve into and through the diseased tissue.
8. Remove matrix if it is present on the facial nerve — even if there is a dehiscence.
9. If in doubt, probe the facial nerve gently with a blunt probe.
10. Never avulse the stapedial muscle or tendon but rather cut it with a sharp scissors or knife — it may be firmly attached to the facial nerve.
11. Polytomography is essential when anomalies are suspected.
12. Look for minor anomalies (preauricular cysts, etc) which may indicate other anomalies.
13. A bifurcated facial nerve can easily be cut accidentally — the two parts are usually unequal and the smaller overlooked.
14. Beware of any soft tubular structure in the middle ear regardless of its location.
15. If an anomaly is evident, do not cut a large chorda tympani nerve — it may have facial nerve fibers.
16. Never ligate the stapedial artery — it may compromise cerebral circulation.
17. Abnormalities should be carefully documented and reported.

ACKNOWLEDGMENTS — We are indebted to Leon Schlossberg, Assistant Professor, Department of Art as Applied to Medicine, Johns Hopkins University, and to William Loechelle for the superb quality of their illustrations. We wish to thank Chester Reather, RBP, FBPA, Director of Photography, Johns Hopkins University, for his exceptional technical skill in the preparation of the photomicrographs. We wish to express our sincere appreciation to Ms Kathy King and Mrs Patricia Edwards for their assistance in typing the manuscript.

REFERENCES

1. Fisch U. Surgery for Bell's palsy. Arch Otolaryngol 1981; 107:1-11.

2. Guerrier Y. Surgical anatomy, particularly vascular supply of the facial nerve. In: Fisch U, ed. Facial nerve surgery. Birmingham: Aesculapius, 1977.

3. Walker AE. Attachment of dura mater over base of skull. Anat Rec 1933; 55:291-5.

4. Wigand ME, Trillsch K. Surgical anatomy of the sinus epitympani. Ann Otol Rhinol Laryngol 1973; 82:378-84.

5. Hawke M, Farkashidy J, Jahn AJ. Non-lamellar new bone formation in the anterior attic recess. Arch Otolaryngol 1975; 101: 117-9.

6. Hoshino T, Suzuki J. Anterior attic wall anatomy. Arch Otolaryngol 1978; 104:588-90.

7. Proctor B. The development of the middle ear spaces and their surgical significance. J Laryngol Otol 1964; 78:631-48.

8. Gacek RR. Surgical landmark for the facial nerve in the epitympanum. Ann Otol Rhinol Laryngol 1980; 89:249-50.

9. Proctor B. Surgical anatomy of the posterior tympanum. Ann Otol Rhinol Laryngol 1969; 78:1026-41.

10. Litton W, Krause C, Anson B, Cohen W. Relationship of facial canal to the annular sulcus. Laryngoscope 1969; 79: 1584-1604.

11. Bellocq P. L'os temporal. Paris: Masson et Cie, 1924.

12. Girard L. Atlas d'anatomie et de médecine opératoire du labyrinthe osseux. Paris: Libraire Maloine, 1939.

13. Paturet G. Traité d'anatomie Humaine. Vols 1 & 4. Paris: Masson et Cie, 1951.

14. Anson BJ, Harper DG, Warphea RL. Surgical anatomy of the facial nerve. Ann Otol Rhinol Laryngol 1963; 72:713-34.

15. Baxter A. Dehiscence of the fallopian canal. J Laryngol Otol 1971; 85:587-94.

16. Dietzel K. Ueber die Dehiszenzen des Facialiskanals. Z Laryngol Rhinol Otol 1961; 40:366-76.

17. Guild SR. Natural absence of part of the bony wall of the facial canal. Laryngoscope 1949; 59:668-73.

18. Politzer A. A textbook of the diseases of the ear and adjacent organs. Dalby W, ed; Dodd O, trans. Philadelphia: Lea Brothers & Co, 1894.

19. Schuknecht H. Anatomical variants and anomalies of surgical significance. J Laryngol Otol 1971; 85:1238-41.

20. Donaldson JA, Anson BJ. Surgical anatomy of the facial nerve. Symposium on disease and injury of the facial nerve. Otolaryngol Clin North Am June 1974.

21. Durcan DJ, Shea JJ, Sleeckx JP. Bifurcation of the facial nerve. Arch Otolaryngol 1967; 86:619-31.

22. Jahrsdoerfer RA. The facial nerve in congenital middle ear malformations. Laryngoscope 1981; 91:1217-25.

23. Johnsson LG, Kingsley TC. Herniation of the facial nerve in middle ear. Arch Otolaryngol 1970; 91:598-602.

24. Babin RW, Fratkin J, Harker LA. Traumatic neuromas of the facial nerve. Arch Otolaryngol 1981; 107:55-8.

25. Arndt HJ. Zweiteilung des Nervus facialis zwischen Ganglion geniculi und Foramen stylomastoideum. HNO (Berlin) 1967; 15:116-8.

26. Kullman GL, Dyck PJ, Cody TR. Anatomy of the mastoid portion of the facial nerve. Arch Otolaryngol 1971; 93:29-33.

27. Fowler EP Jr. Variations in the temporal bone course of the facial nerve. Laryngoscope 1961; 71:937-44.

28. Dworacek H. Die anatomischen Verhältnisse des Mittelohres unter operationsmicroscopischer Betrachtung. Acta Otolaryngol (Stockh) 1960; 51:31-45.

29. Altmann F. Zur Anatomie und formalen Genese der Atresia auris congenita. Monatsschr Ohrenheilkd Laryngo-Rhinol 1933; 67:765-71.

30. Miehlke A, Partsch CJ. Ohrmissbildung, Facialis und Abducenslähmung als Syndrom der Thalidomidschädigung. Arch Ohren Heilk Z Hals Heilk 1963; 181:154-74.

31. Caparosa RJ, Klassen D. Congenital anomalies of the stapes and facial nerve. Arch Otolaryngol 1966; 83:420-1.

32. Butler GE. Transstapedial congenital malposition of the facial nerve. Arch Otolaryngol 1968; 88:268.

33. Ombrédanne M. Chirurgie des surdités congénitales par malformation ossiculaire. Ann Otolaryngol (Paris) 1960; 77:423.

34. Marquet J. Congenital malformations and middle ear surgery. J R Soc Med 1981; 74:119-28.

35. Martin H, Martin C. Anomaly of the facial nerve pathway and congenital ankylosis of the footplate. J Fr Oto-Rhino-Laryngol Chir Maxill-Fac 1977; 26:543-5.

36. Mayer TG, Crabtree JA. The facial nerve coursing inferior to the oval window. Arch Otolaryngol 1976; 102:744-6.

37. Leek JF. An anomalous facial nerve; the otologist's albatross. Laryngoscope 1974; 84:1535-44.

38. Henner R. Congenital middle ear malformations. Arch Otolaryngol 1960; 71:454-8.

39. Dickinson JT, Srisomboon P, Kamerer DB. Congenital anomaly of the facial nerve. Arch Otolaryngol 1968; 88:357-9.

40. Kodama A, Sando I, Meyers EN, Hashida Y. Severe middle ear anomaly with underdeveloped facial nerve. Arch Otolaryngol 1982; 108:93-8.

41. Hanson JE, Anson BJ, Strickland EM. Branchial sources of the auditory ossicles in man. Arch Otolaryngol 1962; 76: 200-15.

42. Bast JH, Anson BJ, Richany SF. The development of the second branchial arch (Reichert's cartilage), facial canal and associated structures in man. Q Bull Northwest Univ Med School 1956; 30:235-49.

43. Kettel K. Abnormal course of the facial nerve in the fallopian canal. Arch Otolaryngol 1946; 44:406-8.

44. Wright JW. Polytomography and congenital external and middle ear anomalies. Laryngoscope 1981; 91:1806-11.

45. Miehlke A. Surgery of the facial nerve. München: Urban and Schwarzenberg Verlag, 1973. Philadelphia: W. B. Saunders, 1973.

46. Kettel K. Surgery of the facial nerve. Arch Otolaryngol 1963; 77:327-41.

47. Glasscock M. Unusual facial nerve problems. Laryngoscope 1971; 81:669-83.

48. Pou JW. Congenital anomalies of the middle ear: presentation of two cases. Laryngoscope 1971; 81:831-9.

49. Bellucci RJ. Congenital aural malformations, diagnoses and treatment. Otolaryngol Clin North Am 1981; 95-124.

50. Pracy R. Surgery for congenital conductive deafness. Proc R Soc Med 1977; 70:823-6.

51. Harpman JA. A congenital aural deformity and its correction. Eye Ear Nose Throat Month 1971; 50:10-3.

52. Hahlbrock KH. Zweiteilung des N facialis im Warzenfortsatz. Arch Ohren Nasen Kehlkopfheilkd 1960; 174:465-9.

53. Basek M. Anomalies of the facial nerve in normal temporal bones. Ann Otol Rhinol Laryngol 1962; 71:382-90.

54. Botman J Wm, Jongkees LBW. Endotemporal branching of the facial nerve. Acta Otolaryngol (Stockh) 1955; 45:111-4.

55. Heermann J Jr. Zwei und dreigeteilter Facialis in der Pauke mit Aplasie des ovalen Fensters. Facialis neurinom unter dem Ambosschenkel. Z Laryngol Rhinol 1967; 46:451-7.

56. Hawley CW. Abnormalities of the mastoid with special reference to the facial nerve. Illinois Med J 1922; 41:116-20.

57. Tobeck A. Ueber den Verlauf des Facialiskanals im Roentgenbild. Arch Ohren Nasen Kehlkopfheilkd 1938; 144: 276.

58. Altmann F. Missbildungen des Ohres. In: von Berendes J, Link R, Zöllner F, eds. Hals Nasen Ohrenheilkunde. Vol III. Stuttgart: Thieme, 1965:653-4.

SPEECH AND LANGUAGE DEVELOPMENT IN A PARENT-INFANT TOTAL COMMUNICATION PROGRAM

A. Dee, MA

I. Rapin, MD

R. J. Ruben, MD

Bronx, New York

In the program described, the use of total communication (TC) did not impede speech development in preschool deaf children. Evidence indicates that sign language facilitated the young hearing-impaired child's acquisition of communicative oral speech. Exposure to sign language combined with speech enhanced the meaningfulness of residual hearing and lipreading. Milestones in sign language acquisition paralleled the milestones of spoken language. Young hearing-impaired TC children appeared to learn and express more language at an earlier age than is typical of orally trained hearing-impaired children. This implies that their cognition may not be as severely inhibited because their language acquisition is less severely delayed. This should have favorable consequences for later educational and social development. The families in the TC program were able to normalize their child-rearing activities and relationships.

INTRODUCTION

A long-term controversy exists between educators advocating a strictly oral and those a total communication (TC) approach to the habilitation of deaf children. A TC program mandates early exposure to manual signs and finger-spelling, always combined with speech and with speechreading training.

Advocates of TC point to research findings that indicate the failure of oral educational environments to foster adequate language development among most deaf children and adults.[1-4] These reports conclude that a deaf child who cannot hear or understand connected speech has minimal opportunity to learn language if his/her exposure is limited to oral communication. When manual signs are incorporated into the habilitation approach, more normal language acquisition can occur during the critical early years.[5-7] Language, once learned, can then be expressed verbally as speech skills develop.[8] One need not stress the importance of language for the optimum social, psychological, and educational development of the hearing-impaired child.[3,9-17]

Advocates of oralism contend that the ability of young deaf children to develop speech is inhibited if they are permitted to communicate in sign language.[18] The null hypothesis of our investigation is that the use of sign language in the early habilitation of the significantly hearing-impaired child will inhibit the development of speech.

This null hypothesis was examined in the total population of deaf infants, ages 14 to 42 months, enrolled in an early intervention parent-infant program which used TC. This longitudinal study documents the acquisition of speech and language in these infants. The data were collected by means of diaries maintained at least weekly on each of the children. A description of the audiometric and medical information on each of the children is provided.

METHOD

Population. The subjects of this study were all of the hearing-impaired children enrolled in a regional TC parent-infant program from September 1977 to September 1980. The children were entered in the program on the basis of age, geographic location, and handicap. Selection of the program by the parents was not based on its educational method as the parents were not aware, at intake, of the characteristics of TC.

Subjects. The 11 subjects ranged in age from 14 to 30 months at entry into the TC program. They left the program at ages 31 to 42 months (Table 1). There were no uniform intake or exit dates for the subjects, and the total number of months spent in the program varied from 6 to 21 months. None of the subjects had known intellectual deficits. One, subject 4, was multiply handicapped, with a cleft palate and a tracheotomy because of subglottic stenosis that impaired his ability to produce speech (Table 2). Subject 9 had Goldenhar's syndrome with velopharyngeal insufficiency which decreased the intelligibility of her speech. Subject 1 had a progressive neurological illness with ataxia, myoclonus, and retinitis pigmentosa.

All children had hearing parents who agreed to be trained in TC. Six of the children had normal-hearing siblings who were also involved in sign language training. The families' social background was predominantly middle income (Table 3).

The children were all thought to have severe to profound sensorineural hearing losses on the basis of brainstem auditory evoked potentials and/or behavioral audiometry when they entered the program. Subject 11 was found to have a severe loss with a pure-tone average of 83 dB in the left ear and 75 dB in the right ear. The audiometric data on 7 of the 11 children in which audiograms are available are given in Table 4. Subjects 3, 6, and 7 had soundfield responses of greater than 90 dB. Subject 1 had soundfield responses at 75-80 dB. Information was available concerning responsiveness to hearing aids in all 11 children (Table 5).

From the Departments of Otolaryngology and Neurology, and the Rose F. Kennedy Center for Research in Mental Retardation and Human Development of The Albert Einstein College of Medicine, and Montefiore Hospital and Medical Center, Bronx, New York.

Presented in part at the meeting of the American Otological Society, Inc., Palm Beach, Florida, May 2-3, 1982.

REPRINTS — Robert J. Ruben, MD, Department of Otolaryngology, Albert Einstein College of Medicine, 1300 Morris Park Avenue, Bronx, NY 10461.

TABLE 1. AGE AT DIAGNOSIS AND TIME IN PROGRAM (MONTHS)

Subject No.	*Age at Intake*	*Age at Exit*	*Time in Program*	*Age Aided*
1	23	41	18	18
2	30	36	6	30
3	16	37	21	19
4	28	41	13	27
5	16	37	21	19
6	20	35	15	20
7	14	34	20	13
8	20	37	17	22
9	20	33	13	24
10	18	31	13	14
11	22	42	20	22
Average	20.6	36.7	16.1	20.7

Teaching Method. The TC method integrated speech, sign language, finger-spelling, aural/oral training, and amplification. Total communication was used to stimulate the language and cognitive development of the infants and to allow communication between infant and parents.

Speech and auditory training were coordinated into the normal day-to-day living activities appropriate for each infant's developmental level. Supplementary formal speech and auditory training outside of the program was recommended as soon as the infant appeared to be able to respond to such training; it was instituted in subjects 4, 8, 10 and 11 (Table 6).

Family Instruction Sessions. Each family met weekly for two-hour sessions with the parent-infant teacher in the infant room of the local public school in which the program was located. Fathers participated as often as their work schedules permitted. All of the fathers were able to attend sporadically throughout the year and received training in TC. Siblings and other family members were encouraged to attend these sessions. Occasional home visits were made on an "as needed" basis. This enabled the teacher to monitor compliance with the program in the home environment. Two of the 11 infants (subjects 4 and 5) received almost all of their instruction in the home setting.

These family instruction sessions were structured to give the family members skills for the habilitation of their hearing-impaired child. This was done by demonstration-teaching of the child with the parent observing, and then by having the parent interact with the child under the guidance of the parent-infant teacher. Routine age-appropriate activities such as eating, playing, toilet training, storytelling, bathing, etc, were used as a basis for this instruction, in addition to educational games and tasks.

The parents were trained in TC techniques designed to develop the infant's awareness of voice, to foster maximum use of residual hearing and lipreading skills, to develop language input strategies and concept formation, and to promote age-appropriate sensorimotor and cognitive skills. In addition, the parents were made aware of the implications of their child's hearing impairment in terms of his/her emotional, social, and educational development.[19] At the end of each session, the teacher gave specific assignments for home reinforcement to be carried out during the next week. The family sessions helped the family group cope with the initially overwhelming problem of having a hearing-impaired child.

TABLE 2. ETIOLOGIES OF DEAFNESS

Uncomplicated, idiopathic	7
Meningitis	1
Malformation syndromes	2
Vater syndrome with absent labyrinth and no vestibular function (subject 4)	
Goldenhar's syndrome (subject 9)	
Progressive ataxia, myoclonus and retinitis pigmentosa (subject 1)	1

Weekly parent education sessions supplemented the weekly instructional sessions.

Data Collection. The data for this study were derived from weekly diary entries for each child collected in a systematic manner. The information came from three sets of observations and was entered after each of the family sessions: 1) each family kept a diary of the day-to-day development of its child; 2) the parent-infant teacher kept a diary of the progress of each child and family while in the instructional environment; and 3) information obtained at the weekly parent instructional session was recorded by the teacher.

Diary information used for this report concerned the expressive and receptive speech and language development of each of the children (Tables 8-11), together with an assessment of the families' communicative competence at the time the child left the program (Tables 12 and 13).

RESULTS

Findings at Intake. The communicative characteristics of the subjects at intake are summarized in Table 7. All of the subjects attempted to communicate with their parents by means of various combinations of voice, gesture, body language, and facial expression. The children would get attention by tugging at their parents' clothing, arms or legs, or by the use of some form of vocalization, eg, whining or crying. Vocal output, at intake, varied from minimal (subjects 4, 5, 9 and 11) to occasional (subjects 1, 3 and 6), to frequent (subjects 2, 7, 8 and 10). There were significant differences between subjects in the character of this vocal behavior, which ranged from minimal, nondifferentiated sounds, through more varied and consistent vocal play, to actual and deliberate first speech attempts by subjects 2 and 8. Some families used their own system of basic gesture language. The overall communication competence of each of the families was inadequate and inappropriate. Each experienced a high degree of frustration because of their inability to communicate with their hearing-impaired child.

Sign Language Development — Receptive and Expressive. The development of receptive and ex-

TABLE 3. SOCIOECONOMIC STATUS OF FAMILIES

Level of education	Mother		
		High school	3
		College	7
		Unknown	1
Level of education	Father		
		High school	2
		College	7
		Unknown	2
Marital status			
		First marriage	8
		Second marriage	2
		Single parent	1
Occupation	Mother		
		Homemaker	11
Occupation	Father		
		Blue collar	1
		Skilled trades	4
		Executive/professional	5
		Unknown	1

TABLE 4. HEARING STATUS OF SUBJECTS

Ear	*Subject*	*Age (months)*	*Frequency (Hz)*					
			250	*500*	*1000*	*2000*	*4000*	*8000*
Right	1*							
	2	36	85	100	105	105	NR	NR
	3†							
	4	51	85	90	NR	NR	NR	NR
	5	58	85	NR	NR	NR	NR	NR
	6†							
	7†							
	8	52	85	90	100	105	NR	NR
	9	56	NR	NR	NR	NR	NR	NR
	10	36		95	105	95	80	
	11	52	60	75	95	75	50	80
Left	1*							
	2	36		100	110	110		
	3†							
	4	51	85	105	NR	NR	NR	NR
	5	58	90	NR	NR	NR	NR	NR
	6†							
	7†							
	8	52	90	90	95	105	100	NR
	9	56	NR	NR	NR	NR	NR	NR
	10	36		100	110	NR	NR	
	11	52	75	85	100	75	65	55

NR - No response.
*Pure tone audiogram not available. Behavioral response in free field at >90 dB.
†Pure tone audiogram not available. Behavioral response in free field at 75-80 dB.

pressive sign language is detailed in Tables 8 and 9. There was significant and orderly development of expressive and receptive sign language, closely paralleling the stages of spoken language development of normal-hearing children.

Comprehension of a number of basic first signs, eg, eat, drink, bed, etc, was almost immediate. Acquisition of these signs resulted in prompt subsidence of what, in some families, was a destructive feeling of impotence and frustration brought about by the parents' feeling of hopelessness in their inability to communicate with their hearing-impaired child. Within a few months, all subjects were understanding simple directions and could respond to "yes/no," "either/or," and "where" questions, eg, "Do you want milk or juice?" and "Where are your shoes?" "Where" was the first wh- question word of the English language learned. "What," "who," "when," "why" and also "how" were acquired later. There was a minimum lag of 1 to 30 days between the understanding of a first sign and its production. Thereafter, the children all moved rapidly from understanding to the expressive use of signs. All of the 11 infants started using signs in a communicative mode within a month of entering the program (Table 10).

TABLE 5. AWARENESS OF SOUND WITH HEARING AID

Subject No.	*Awareness Level (dB)*
1	55
2	45
3	90
4	85
5	NR
6	85
7	80
8	30
9	75
10	40
11	35

NR - No response.

Subjects 6, 8 and 9 produced their first sign as a meaningful communication within one week of exposure. The oldest, subject 4, who was 28 months at intake, mastered several signs receptively and expressively during his first day of instruction. The youngest, subject 7, who was 14 months at intake, used his first sign at 15 months of age, only slightly later than the age a normal-hearing child produces a first word.

The first communicative signs resembled the first words used by hearing children. These identified people, objects, and events important to the child's life, such as favorite food and toys, highlights of the daily routine, and words to influence parents, peers, and siblings. The earliest signs produced by the

TABLE 6. SUPPLEMENTAL INTERVENTION (SI)

Subject	*Age SI Instituted (mo)*	*Months of SI Before Exit from Program*	*Type of Intervention*
4	39	2	Oral, motion and swallowing therapy
8	31	6	Speech therapy
10	29	2	Speech therapy
11	36	6	Speech therapy

TABLE 7. COMMUNICATIVE CHARACTERISTICS OF SUBJECTS AT ENTRANCE

	Subjects 1	2	3	4	5	6	7	8	9	10	11
Communicates with body language, gesture and/or facial expression	+ + + +	+ + + +	+ + + +	+ + + +	+ + + +	+ + + +	+ + + +	+ + + +	+ + + +	+ + + +	+ + + +
Gains attention by using voice or crying	+ +	+ +	+ +	+ +	+ +	+ +	+ + +	+ + +	+ +	+ + +	+ +
Gains attention by tugging	+ + +	+ + +	+ +	+ +	+ + +	+ + +	+ + +	+	+ + +	+ + +	+
Vocalizes when playing	+ +	+ + +	+ +	+	+	+ +	+ + +	+ + +	+	+ + +	+
Makes speech attempts	+	+ +	+	+	+	+	+	+ +	+	+	+
Frustrated at needs not being met by parents	+ + +	+ + +	+ + + +	+ + + +	+ + +	+ + +	+ + +	+ +	+ + +	+ + + +	+ + + +

+ - Almost never; + + - Occasionally; + + + - Frequently; + + + + - Almost always.

youngest signers (subject 7, 15 months; subject 5, 17 months; and subject 10, 19 months) were infantile approximations of adult signs, just as the first words of hearing infants are approximations of adult speech.

After learning their initial signs the subjects displayed a number of behaviors commonly seen in normally hearing children who are first beginning to communicate in recognizable speech. These included visual-attending behavior, experimental finger and hand play, and both imitative echoic type signing and spontaneous jargon signing. These visual and signing behaviors of the hearing-impaired children correspond qualitatively to the auditory and oral behaviors of hearing children.

Like hearing children, the hearing-impaired children's first (signed) utterances were single signs that stood for an entire sentence. Depending upon the context in which it was used, a single sign would communicate a number of diverse meanings. The sign for "shoe" could mean "My shoe lace is untied again", "My milk spilled on Daddy's shoe", or "Put on my shoes so I can go outside."

The sign "hurt" was a particularly functional sign for these children who had a limited signing vocabulary. Even the youngest signer quickly learned to position the "hurt" sign over the injured area to show which specific area needed parental attention: eg, "I hurt my knee." This communicative behavior parallels the "one-word sentence" holophrastic stage that marks the beginning of expressive language in hearing children.

The sequential development of signs paralleled that of speech (Tables 8-10). Both the signers and hearing children progressed from one-word sentences to the "telegraphic speech" stage of two- and three-word sentences.[20-22] Only subject 9 progressed beyond this stage and was signing age-appropriate standard English phrases and sentences when he finished the program at 37 months.

"Shortcut" questions and negative forms often preceded the appearance of more standard two-sign phrases expressing question and negation. "Who" and "what" questions were first expressed by pointing, accompanied by a questioning facial and body expression. "Where" was almost immediately used as a formal sign when it was introduced into the child's lexicon. Negative statements were observed very early. For example, one child made the sign for medicine and shook his head vehemently in the negative fashion, conveying emphatically that he did not want his medicine.

The two-sign phrases used by the subjects expressed the same relationships recorded in the speech of hearing children, eg, "More milk" (recurrence); "Daddy shoe" (possessive); "baby cry" (agent action).[21] Negative constructions were also identical to the first negative phrases of hearing children, eg, "no eat," "no bed," etc.

Assessment of finger-spelled items included in Table 9 show that 8 of the 11 subjects were able to finger-spell the entire alphabet imitatively or from a wall chart before they were 3 years old. Three of the subjects were beginning to finger-spell simple words or familiar names. They could also produce the hand formation corresponding to four or more printed letters of the alphabet.

The comparison of the growth of vocabulary in speech and sign is found in Tables 10 and 11. All of the subjects except subject 8 learned more signs faster than spoken words.

Speech Development and Verbal Behavior. Seven of the 11 children had a hearing aid at the time of intake. The remaining four acquired them within three months of entering the program (Table 1).

At intake seven of the subjects used their voice minimally, while the other four produced frequent vocalizations (Table 7). Most of the vocalizations were in the category of nondifferentiated sounds. Subject 2 and subject 8, who was unaided, produced several differentiated sounds in apparent speech attempts before entering the program.

All of the children (Tables 12 and 13) learned to understand and respond to the signed directions

TABLE 8. DEVELOPMENT OF SIGNING SKILLS — RECEPTIVE

Skill	*Subject by Age in Months* 1	2	3	4	5	6	7	8	9	10	11	*Average*
Understands and responds to yes/no questions	23	31	17	29	17	25	18	20	21	20	23	22.2
Understands 10 everyday basic signs	24	31	17	29	17	25	18	20	22	21	24	22.5
Understands (and follows) simple requests	24	32	18	30	18	25	22	20	22	23	24	23.5
Understands "where?"	25	31	21	30	20	26	22	20	21	24	25	24.1
Can "give me," "show me" on request	25	32	28	38	24	28	24	21	22	26	29	27.0
Understands "help me," "do you need help?"	30	34	28	38	24	28	24	23	24	26	34	28.5
Will point to familiar objects when signed	35	32	28	30	24	28	34	21	24	23	28	27.9
Will point to 3-5 pictures in a book when signed	27	32	28	30	24	28	34	20	26	24	28	27.4
Understands "same"	35	32	32	30	24	28	28	20	24	26	26	27.7
Understands "open," "close"	31	32	21	30	18	27	22	20	24	27	29	25.5
Understands "in," "out"	25	32	21	30	18	27	24	20	24	24	25	24.5
Understands "on," "off"	26	34	21	30	20	28	34	23	24	24	25	26.3
Understands "put it back"	27	34	36	38	36	28	30	23	24	23	23	29.3
Understands "clean-up time"	25	34	22	38	18	29	30	23	24	24	30	27.0
Understands "under"	25		(48)	40	(40)			30			42	37.5*
Understands "over"	35		(48)	40	(40)			30			42	39.2†
Understands several animal signs	27	32	20	28	20	27	30	21	23	23	28	25.4
Recognizes name signs of family members	26	32	18	36	18	27	26	21	24	23	30	25.5
Recognizes own name sign	31	32	35	40	35	30	34	24	26	31	36	32.2
Understands "your turn — my turn"	31	32	28	36	28	30	30	24	26	27	36	28.8
Understands "finished! — next!"	31	33	28	36	20	30	26	24	26	26	36	28.7
Understands "where does this belong?"	40		(48)	38	(40)			28	27			36.8**
Understands "not now . . . later"	45	33	30	40	24	31	34	24	24	26	36	31.5
Understands toilet sign for bathroom needs	31	31	24	39	24	31	30	24	24	26	28	28.4
Understands at least two color signs	30	33	34	36	33	33	33	24	28	(33)	30	31.5***
Appears to understand "who"	40		36	40	35			21	(38)	31	(43)	35.5††
Understands and responds to "what's this?" "what's that?"	35	35	(41)	39	(41)		(41)	22	33	31	34	35.2†††
Appears to understand "what happened?"	41		36		33			27		38	35	
Understands and follows series of two related commands	31	34	32	40	32	34	34	21	24	26	36	31.3
Appears to understand simple signed stories	36		(49)	36	(39)			21	(36)			36.2
Can "read and understand" finger-spelling of simple words or familiar names	40	(53)	41	(53)				28	32		40	41
Understands "which one do you want?"	36	36	(48)	34			34	28	30	31	31	34.2
Understands "why" questions	(48)		(57)		(56)		37					49.5

( )Information obtained after the subject left the program.
*Average = 34.3 without subjects 3 & 5.
**Average = 33.3 without subjects 3 & 5.
***Average = 31.4 without subject 10.
†Average = 36.8 without subjects 3 & 5.
††Average = 33.8 without subjects 9 & 11.
†††Average = 32.7 without subjects 3, 5, 7.

given for speech training and speech stimulation. The child (subject 4) with the tracheotomy and cleft palate mouthed visible lip movements and would produce an occasional "ah" vowel and an "m" consonant when his airway permitted vocalization. The other ten children imitated an increasing number of speech sounds and single words. They learned how to combine sounds with signs in response to the frequently signed direction, "Use your voice — I want to hear you when you sign to me." There was considerable variation in the difficulty each child experienced in producing audible words. Four of the 11 children did so with less effort than the other 7.

Subjects 4, 8, 10, and 11, whose development suggested they would be able to utilize this additional help, were given speech and auditory training by speech and hearing clinicians outside of the program (Table 6). These four children responded favorably to the additional intervention when they worked with signing speech clinicians.

Ten of the 11 subjects used spontaneous verbalizations on occasion when signing, and 3 could verbalize two- or three-word utterances, in combination with sign, when they left the program (Tables 12 and 13). The only child who could not do this was subject 4, with the tracheotomy and cleft

TABLE 9. DEVELOPMENT OF SIGNING SKILLS — EXPRESSIVE

Skill	*Subjects by Age in Months* 1	2	3	4	5	6	7	8	9	10	11	*Average*
First sign used	24	31	19	28	17	20	15	20	20	19	23	21.5
Used 10-20 signs	27	32	24	29	19	26	23	22	22	22	25	24.6
Signs "where?"	25	31	28	30	34	30	26	20	22	30	29	27.7
Signs "no"	25		24	29	23	30	16	23	23	19	29	24.1
Signs "yes"	25			41	41	35	28	23	23	27	29	30.2
Signs "up," "down"	25	32	24	34	18	28	27	20	23	22	25	25.3
Signs "in," "out"	29	33	31	34	30	32	31	21	26	24	26	28.8
Signs "open," "close"	25	33	35	34	24	31	22	20	26	26	27	27.5
Signs "on," "off"	29	34	35	34	27	31	34	23	26	(34)	26	30.3*
Can sign toilet needs	25	32	30	38	31	31	34	23	26	24	26	29.1
Uses 50 + signs	29	36	29	34	21	30	27	22	26	24	29	27.9
Uses "mine" (possession)	29	34	30	41	20	32	32	22	27	23	41	30.1
Uses "same" appropriately	31	32	35	38	32	29	29	23	26	31	30	30.5
Uses name signs of family members	29	32	28	36	34	31	28	22	28	27	27	29.3
Uses 75 + signs	29		30	35	24	31	32	22	28	29	30	29.0
First 2 sign phrases	28	34	29	36	31	34	28	21	24	31	28	29.5
"I want" phrases	36			38	(46)			23	28	31	35	33.9**
Names at least two colors	35	33	35	36	33	35	33	23	29		30	32.2
"Reads" books by signing picture contents	31	34	36	34	36	32		21	24	27	30	30.5
Signs to self and toys in make-believe play activities	29	34	30		24	31	28	21	24	27	36	28.4
Uses 100 + signs	32		32	39	28	34	34	23	28	31	33	31.4
First 3 sign phrases	28		30	36	32	35	(34)	22	28	(34)	35	31.4†
Uses "what?," "what's this"	(48)							30			33	37.0††
Uses "who," "who's that?"	(48)							30			(45)	41.0
Begins to communicate about past experiences	41				(51)			30				40.7
Begins to describe feelings, eg, "scared," "tired," "angry"	36		36	41	36			24	28		42	34.7
Uses 200-300 signs	36		37	41	36	35		27	33		42	35.9
300 + signs								36				
Uses signs continuously to express wants and needs	29		29	34	24	31	30	22	24	27		27.8
Uses signs conversationally, to share experiences with others	36		36	41	32	34	30	22	30	30	29	32.0
Can sign 6 letters of manual alphabet	36	34		38	34		(36)	23	30		36	33.4***
Can sign entire manual alphabet from wall chart	38	36		40	36		(38)	24	32		42	35.8****
Can sign 4 or more letters of alphabet in correct correspondence with printed symbol	(48)			41	(40)			24			40	38.6†††
Can finger-spell simple words or names	40			41	(50)			29	(36)		42	39.7††††

( )Information obtained after the subject left program.
*Average = 29.0 without subject 10.
**Average = 31.8 without subject 5.
***Average = 33.0 without subject 7.
****Average = 35.4 without subject 7.
†Average = 30.8 without subjects 7, 10.
††Average = 31.5 without subject 1.
†††Average = 35 without subjects 1, 5.
††††Average = 38 without subjects 5, 8.

palate. Two of the children (subjects 2 and 8) made occasional speech attempts without sign. Follow-up studies on these children at 5 years of age show that they use speech alone when attempting to communicate with individuals who do not sign.

All except subject 8 acquired new sign words more quickly than new speech words. Except for subject 8, all children had larger active signing vocabularies than speech vocabularies at exit (Tables 10 and 11).

The intelligibility of the children's speech generally was poor. The most intelligible words were the simplest, such as "mama," "bye-bye," etc. Signs were necessary with almost all speech efforts to clarify the meaning of the speech utterance. The variability of children's acquisition of speech is noted in Table 11. All of the subjects showed an increase in oral behavior and speech attempts as their signing proficiency increased.

Follow-up information was obtained for 9 of the 11 children. Of those nine, eight were using speech, while speech development was slow in one. Eight of the nine were attending preschool for hearing-impaired children, and one attended a regular kindergarten with a resource program.

DISCUSSION

This study provides information about the speech development, auditory training, language acquisition, and communication competence of young deaf

TABLE 10. DEVELOPMENT OF EXPRESSIVE SIGN LANGUAGE

Subject	*First Sign*		*10-20 Signs*		*50 + Signs*		*75 + Signs*		*100 + Signs*		*200 + Signs*		*300 + Signs*		*Signs At Exit*	*Age Began Program (Months)*	*Age Left Program (Months)*
	A	*No.*	*A*	*No.*	*A*	*No.*	*A*	*No.*	*A*	*No.*	*A*	*No.*	*A*	*No.*			
1	24	(1)	27	(4)	28	(5)	29	(6)	30	(7)	36	(13)			200 +	23	41
2	31	(1)	32	(2)	36	(6)									65 +	30	36
3	17	(1)	24	(8)	29	(13)	30	(14)	32	(16)	37	(21)			200 +	16	37
4	28	(0)	29	(1)	34	(6)	35	(7)	36	(8)	40	(12)			200	28	41
5	17	(1)	19	(3)	21	(5)	24	(8)	28	(12)	36	(20)			200 +	16	37
6	20	(0)	24	(4)	28	(8)	30	(10)	32	(12)	35	(15)			200	20	35
7	15	(1)	23	(9)	27	(13)	32	(18)	34	(20)					100 +	14	34
8	20	(0)	21	(1)	22	(2)	22	(2)	23	(3)	27	(7)	33	(13)	300 +	20	37
9	20	(0)	22	(2)	26	(6)	28	(8)	28	(8)	33	(13)			200 +	20	33
10	19	(1)	22	(4)	26	(8)	29	(11)	31	(13)					100	18	31
11	23	(1)	25	(3)	29	(7)	30	(8)	33	(11)	42	(20)			200 +	22	42
Average		(0.6)		(3.7)		(7.2)		(9.2)		(11)		(15)		(13)			

A - Age in months; No. - Number of months in program.

children in a total communication environment. It also highlights psychological, social, and educational consequences of this approach.

Acquisition of Speech with Sign. The data do not support the null hypothesis that the use of sign language inhibits the development of speech. The data clearly show that all of the children with an intact speech tract acquired speech vocabularies and made oral attempts while signing. The findings in this study are consistent with those of Meadow and Schlesinger,[8,13] who recorded similar findings in four children. The children in the present study all increased their verbal behavior as their signing skills increased. More speech attempts were made in conjunction with signs than without signs, suggesting that sign language makes speech production more relevant.

Intelligibility. The lack of the intelligibility of the speech of significantly hearing-impaired children and adults, especially the congenitally deaf, is well documented.[1,18,23,24] Conrad[1] reports that in England only 10% of profoundly deaf 15- to 16-year-old teenagers who had received at least ten years of strictly oral training spoke well enough to be understood by strangers. This communication barrier did not exist for the children in this study since all their speech efforts, no matter how imperfect or distorted, acquired immediate meaning because they were associated with the corresponding sign.

Intelligibility, the ability to associate a verbalization with its sign so as to communicate unambiguously, begins with the earliest attempts at language. The first word of the oral deaf toddler, "buh," will have a variety of meanings which are important to the child. Thus "buh" could mean, in different contexts, "bottle," "ball," "balloon," "boat," "bubble," etc. The parent will have difficulty determining which of these words the child is conveying when he says "buh." The TC family escapes the frustration of degraded intelligibility and its barrier to understanding since the child will also produce a sign which clarifies the meaning of the speech word. There will be no ambiguity about the meaning of "buh" with the sign for "bath" as opposed to the combination of "buh" with the sign for "bottle."

Comparison of Rate, Complexity and Extent of Acquisition of Verbal and Sign Language. All of the children, except subject 8, acquired new signs faster and with greater ease than new verbal words. This was an expected finding in view of the known difficulties hearing-impaired children experience in acquiring speech.[25] The complexity and extent of the children's active sign vocabulary was greater than that of their oral vocabulary, with the one exception. Ten of the 11 children would be considered substantially delayed in language development if only their oral language was measured. However, when their total language skills, including sign, are measured, they are all found to approach age level for expressive and receptive language. This information supports the concept that language is not dependent upon the mode of reception or expression. Furthermore, there may be a "critical" period for the establishment of language.[26-28] The children in this study acquired language during this critical period and should be able to build upon this language base as they grow. Children who are deprived of a language base during the critical period may be significantly impaired in their ability to acquire normal linguistic skills and thus become functionally retarded.

The manual signs provided the children with an adequate channel for communication without having to wait for speech to have developed to the point of giving them a functional verbal vocabulary. These early manual signs laid the foundation of language and enabled the children to acquire more extensive, complex, and varied lexicons than that of deaf oral-

TABLE 11. DEVELOPMENT OF EXPRESSIVE SPEECH

Subject	First Word A	First Word No.	1-5 Words A	1-5 Words No.	5-10 Words A	5-10 Words No.	10-20 Words A	10-20 Words No.	20-25 Words A	20-25 Words No.	No. of Words At Exit	Age Began Program (Months)	Age Left Program (Months)
1	25	(2)	26	(3)	27	(4)	36	(13)	41	(18)	23	23	41
2*	25		30	(0)	32		36				16	30	36
3	30	(14)	33	(17)	35	(19)					7	16	37
4†											0	28	41
5	17	(1)	18	(2)	20	(4)	33	(17)	37	(21)	25	16	37
6	31	(11)	32	(12)	35	(15)					6	20	35
7	23	(9)	33	(19)							5	14	34
8*	17		18		19		20		21	(1)	300 +	20	37
9	28	(18)	33	(13)							4	20	33
10	25	(7)	26	(8)	28	(10)	31	(13)			13	18	31
11	25	(3)	28	(6)	29	(7)	30	(8)	32	(10)	66	22	42

A - Age in months; No. - Number of months in program.

*Had first words before entering program.

†Had cleft palate and tracheotomy; could not produce speech.

ly trained children of a comparable age.[25,29,30]

Subject 8 developed differently from the rest of the group: he had the more extensive sign and speech vocabulary of all of the children and his speech and sign developed at the same rate. Yet his speech was often unintelligible, requiring him to use sign to convey his meaning clearly. He also used his knowledge of sign to understand and respond to his communicative environment. This child's hearing loss was no less than that of many of the other children in the group. The biological or psychological reasons for his rapid linguistic development is not known, except that his parents, both hearing, became very good signers and provided an enriched linguistic environment. This boy has progressed to the point where he is now partially mainstreamed in an oral classroom with a sign language interpreter.

Distinction Between Speech and Language Development. A clear distinction must be made between speech and language acquisition when one considers the communication handicap of deafness. When a deaf child is taught how to speak or lipread a particular word, this does not guarantee that the child knows language or the meaning of the word. Language ability is the child's ability to understand and communicate ideas, needs, and feelings. Children learn language by using it freely, first with parents, then with peers, and with other adults. A deaf child who cannot hear or understand connected speech has a minimal opportunity to learn language if his/her exposure to language is limited to oral communication.

A young TC child can develop and expand both language competence and communication skills through constant and meaningful usage of the language of signs, thereby reaching closer to normal levels of linguistic and communicative functioning.

Language Acquisition and Communication Competence: Comparison of Young TC and Young Oral Child. There is no substantive data base concerning the language acquisition and communication competence of young deaf children who have been exposed to an exclusively oral program. The only available information is its outcome in older schoolchildren. These data uniformly demonstrate that almost all orally trained children have substantial language and communication retardation in receptive and expressive abilities for both speech and reading.[5]

One area in which the TC children in our study had a clear advantage over orally trained children was in their knowledge and use of question and an-

TABLE 12. COMMUNICATION COMPETENCE OF SUBJECTS AT EXIT

	Yes	No
Two-word sentence	11	0
Three-word sentence	7	4
Mostly holophrastic	9	2
Mostly phrases and sentences	2	9
Imitates oral speech with signs spontaneously	7	4
Initiates oral speech on commands	9	2
Initiates oral speech spontaneously without sign	6	5
Communicative competence in family sufficient for normal activities	11	0
Conversational language	7	4
Conversational language age - appropriate for hearing child	1	10
Concept of "where" receptive	11	0
Spontaneous and appropriate use of "where"	10	1
Can finger-spell manual alphabet from wall chart	8	3
Can finger-spell more than 4 letters in correct correspondence to 2 printed symbols	3	8
Beginning to finger-spell single words and familiar names	4	7
Using "my," "mine" appropriately	10	1
Has concept of "same/different" and uses "same" sign appropriately	11	0
Answers "what's this?", "who's this?" question	9	2

TABLE 13. COMMUNICATION CHARACTERISTICS OF SUBJECTS AT EXIT

	Never	*Almost Never*	*Occasionally*	*Frequently*	*Almost Always*
Verbal response or verbalization for speech tasks at imitation or on command	0	1	2	4	4
Single words elicited	0	1	5	2	3
Two-word utterance elicited	0	7	2	0	2
Three or more words and/or phrases elicited	0	9	0	1	1
Spontaneous vocalization while signing	0	1	3	2	5
Initiates deliberate speech attempts while signing single words	0	1	6	2	2
Initiates while signing two-word utterances	0	8	1	1	1
Initiates while signing three words or more and/or phrases	0	9	1	0	1
Deliberate speech attempts without sign	0	8	3	0	0
Intelligible without sign	1	8	2	0	0
Intelligible with sign	0	0	0	0	11
Signs without vocalizing	0	5	2	3	1
Vocalizes while signing	0	2	2	2	5
Signs with meaningful speech or speech attempts	0	1	6	2	2
Uses spontaneous speech or speech attempts without signing	0	8	3	0	0
Frustration at needs not being met by parents	0	1	10	0	0

swer forms. Quigley et al[31] showed that this was an area of serious linguistic deficit in older deaf children in that many of them were neither able to ask nor to answer questions appropriately.

All of the children in this study were able to process and respond to a variety of question and answer forms. This suggests that TC may make a significant difference in early language and communication competence. The TC children in this study were able to communicate at an age-appropriate level in the sense that their parents could fulfill their normal child-rearing roles. There was social communication and communication concerning environmental events and the daily routine of family life. The children were able to make themselves understood and to understand language close to their age level. This is not the case of older orally trained children or those exposed to TC only by school age. One would expect that children exposed to TC from infancy or toddler age will continue to develop language at a more nearly normal rate and that the final outcome will be a person with more functionally appropriate communication skills to interact in society.

The enjoyment and relative ease with which the children in this study acquired receptive and expressive language stands in stark contrast to the frustrations and difficulties of young children attempting to communicate in the oral mode.[32] Total communication families used a wide range of channels for satisfactory interpersonal communications which, in our experience, few strictly oral families achieve. Effective communication with teachers and peers was also facilitated.

In the oral deaf child, communication is limited to the child's ability to understand and produce intelligible speech. His communicative capacity is much more restricted than that of the TC child whose skills approach those of the hearing child both quantitatively and qualitatively. The TC child's ability to use both speech and sign greatly enhances his/her intelligibility. Previous data[25] show that the orally trained deaf child has little or no verbal capacity at age 5 or 6. The children in this study, at 3 years of age, were communicating with greater ease, flexibility, and diversity than many older oral deaf children. Language development appears to depend on the acquisition of certain basic communicative skills in early life. The TC children's acquisition of this basic substrate affords them the opportunity for language growth. The oral children's markedly retarded language may be attributed to the lack of this basic language substrate. Quigley et al[31] predicted that the use of TC during the early stages of language development would foster better language skills in deaf children. Our observations support this prediction.

Implications of Parent-Infant TC for Speech Development, Speechreading Skills and Utilization of Residual Hearing. Signs ensured that each newly developed speech sound would be incorporated into a meaningful communicative act. For example, "m" used with the sign for "milk," "mom," etc, was reinforced in a meaningful manner, rather than being taught through meaningless repetition of a speech drill. Sign language enabled the speech therapist, the teacher, and the parent to give clearly understood directions for speech training tasks, speech games, and speech situation activities. It also enabled the instructor to develop more effective speech skills, using signs to tell the child to use his/her voice, make a loud sound, make two short sounds, etc. The child was not dependent on his/her mastery of the meaning of oral words to acquire specific speech skills since the meaning of the word

TABLE 14. TOTAL COMMUNICATION COMPETENCE OF PARENTS AT EXIT FROM PROGRAM

	Beginner	*Fair*	*Good*	*Excellent*
Mothers	1	2	6	2
Fathers	5	1	3	1
Total	6	3	9	3

could be conveyed through its sign. The use of sign also improved the efficacy of lipreading. Signs fostered the use of residual hearing by giving meaning to the auditory component of the spoken communication. Both parent and teacher were more effective in reinforcing the traditional auditory training procedures by bringing environmental sounds to the child's attention, helping him/her to localize them and explaining their source, their significance, and other attributes. Signs were an efficient means of informing the child of the auditory environment; in fact they were the tools with which the child could come to understand his/her world.

Effect on Parents. Early intervention programs for deaf infants place special demands on parents. Parents are expected to participate in many aspects of their infant's remediation and to become knowledgeable about deafness and its implications.[19] They are also expected to support and enhance the optimum development of their child by becoming skilled in home reinforcement of therapies and in training procedures. A TC program commits the parents to learn sign language and to create an effective home environment for total communication. Parents need ongoing counseling and sustained educational services to allow them to become effective in the program. Experience from this study indicates that the sign language program for the parent should emphasize the signs needed for day-to-day living.

There needs to be an appreciation of the parents' overwhelming feeling of loss when they first realize that their child is deaf. Continued involvement of the parents, from the start of habilitation, allows them to begin to function in such a way as to help their child to overcome his/her handicap. Their ability to communicate with their child enables them to fulfill their natural need to parent. When parents are limited to the oral mode of communication there will be much that they cannot convey to their child; this results in deep feelings of frustration, anger, and despair within the family. How can a parent communicate the concepts of good and bad, religious beliefs and cultural values, or even tell a story or make a joke with the extremely limited avenue of oral communication? Signs allow the parents to communicate all of the above and more to the child and ensure a much more normal child-parent relationship.

Table 14 shows the parents' variable fluency in use of sign. All of the parents did advance to at least the level of an advanced beginner. Mothers were usually more proficient than fathers; this was probably due to mothers' more consistent use of signs. Even in those families in which TC skills were minimal, signs provided a pleasurable mode of communication between child and parent. Most importantly, all of the families established communicative competence. It was our feeling that their level of competence was greater than that of families limited to oral communication alone.

Despite the difference in communication competence among families, all had, at the time of exit from the program, adequate and appropriate basic communication skills for their day-to-day needs.

CRITIQUE

The original purpose of the diaries used in this report was to provide the parent-infant teacher with ongoing information so that she could assess progress in parent-infant communication and so that she could set new goals and/or make changes in the individual educational plan. All the diaries represent a sample in time of the progress of each child; they document the child's and the parents' progress over time.

Quantification of the growth in the vocabulary for the first 100 signs and the first 100 verbal utterances was precise. Once the child had more than 100 items in his vocabulary, counts became less accurate. The parents found it difficult to keep track of new signs. Data on all lexical items above 100 are only approximations and probably represent minimal estimates. It would have been ideal to have audiovisual documentation of each child's progress. This avenue of data collection should be explored in the future.

The number of subjects is small but they do represent the total population of this program. This sample appears to be representative of the total population of congenitally hearing-impaired children in terms of etiology and the extent of their hearing loss. Therefore, the observations made from these children can probably be generalized to other hearing-impaired infants without significant mental retardation or other neurological deficits. Multiply handicapped deaf children may even benefit more from a TC program than "normal" deaf children because of their curtailed ability to process information.

CONCLUSIONS

Total communication (the use of manual signs with oral/aural language) does not inhibit the development of speech. There is evidence suggesting that it facilitates the development of speech. Total communication provides a channel for early communication between the hearing-impaired child and his/her family. In addition, total communication fosters the development of linguistic skills that begin to approach those of hearing children.

REFERENCES

1. Conrad R. Facts and fantasies about the verbal abilities of deaf school leavers. Br Deaf News 1977; Oct: 145-7.

2. Conrad R. Profound deafness as a psycholinguistic problem. In: Fant G, ed. International symposium on speech communication ability and profound deafness. Washington, DC: Alexander Graham Bell Association for the Deaf, Inc., 1972.

3. Furth HG. Thinking about language: psychological implications of deafness. New York: Free Press, 1966.

4. Moores DF. Psycholinguistics and deafness. Am Ann Deaf 1970; 15:37-48.

5. Quigley SP. Environment and communication in the language development of deaf children. In: Bradford LJ, Hardy WC, eds. Hearing and hearing impairment. New York: Grune & Stratton, 1979.

6. Stuckless ER, Birch JW. The influence of early manual communication on the linguistic development of deaf children. Am Ann Deaf 1966; 111:452-60; 499-504.

7. Vernon M, Koh SD. Early manual communication and deaf children's achievement. Am Ann Deaf 1970; 115:527-36.

8. Schlesinger HS, Meadow KP. Sound and sign: childhood deafness and mental health. Berkeley: University of California Press, 1972.

9. Brill RG. A study in adjustment of three groups of deaf children. Except Child 1960; 26:464-6.

10. Brill RG. The superior I.Q.'s of deaf children of deaf parents. California Palms 1969; 1-4.

11. Freeman RD. Psychosocial problems associated with childhood hearing impairment. In: Bradford LJ, Hardy WG, eds. Hearing and hearing impairment. New York: Grune & Stratton, 1979:405-15.

12. Harris RI. Mental health needs and priorities in deaf children and adults: a deaf professional's perspective for the 1980's. In: Stein LK, Mindel ED, Jabaley T, eds. Deafness and mental health. New York: Grune & Stratton, 1981:219-50.

13. Meadow KP. Early manual communication in relation to the deaf child's intellectual, social, and communicative functioning. Am Ann Deaf 1968; 113:29-41.

14. Meadows KP, Trybus RJ. Behavioral and emotional problems of deaf children: an overview. In: Bradford LJ, Hardy WG, eds. Hearing and hearing impairment. New York: Grune & Stratton; 1979:395-403.

15. Moores DF. Educating the deaf: psychology, principles and practices. Boston: Houghton Mifflin, 1977.

16. Stevenson EA. A study of the educational achievement of deaf children of deaf parents. California News 1964; 80:1-3.

17. Stokoe WC, Buttison, RM. Sign language, mental health and satisfactory interaction. In: Stein LK, Mindel ED, Jabaley T, eds. Deafness and mental health. New York: Grune & Stratton, 1981:179-94.

18. Ling D. Speech and the hearing impaired child: theory and practice. Washington, DC. The Alexander Graham Bell Association for the Deaf, Inc., 1976.

19. Dee AD. Meeting the needs of the hearing parents of deaf infants: a comprehensive parent-education program. Language Speech and Hearing Services for Schools. Rockville, MD: ASHA Publications, 1981; 12:13-9.

20. Bloom L. Language development: form and function in emerging grammars. Cambridge, Massachusetts: M.I.T. Press, 1970.

21. Brown R. Psycholinguistics. New York: Free Press, 1970; 220.

22. Dale PS. Language development: structure and function. Hinsdale, Illinois: Dryden Press, 1972.

23. Markides A. The speech of deaf and partially hearing children with special reference to factors affecting intelligibility. Br J Disord Commun 1970; 5:126-40.

24. Nober EH. Articulation of the deaf. Except Child 1967; 33:611-21.

25. Mindel E, Vernon M. They grow in silence. Silver Spring, Maryland: National Association for the Deaf, 1971.

26. Lenneberg EH. Biological functions of language. New York: Wiley Press, 1967.

27. McNeill D. Developmental psycholinguistics. In: Smith F, Miller GA, eds. The genesis of language: a psycholinguistic approach. Cambridge, Massachusetts: M.I.T. Press, 1966.

28. Mussen PH, Conger JJ, Kagan J. Child development and personality. New York: Harper & Row, 1969.

29. Curtis S, Prutting CA, Lowell EL. Pragmatic and semantic development in young children with impaired hearing. JSHR 1979; 22:534-52.

30. McNeill D. The acquisition of language: the study of developmental psycholinguistics. New York: Harper & Row, 1970.

31. Quigley S, Wilbur R, Montanelli D. Question formation in the language of deaf students. JSHR 1974; 17:699-713.

32. Stark RE. Speech of the hearing impaired child. In: Bradford LJ, Hardy WG, eds. Hearing and hearing impairment. New York: Grune & Stratton, 1979:229-48.

TISSUE IMPEDANCE AND CURRENT FLOW IN THE IMPLANTED EAR

IMPLICATIONS FOR THE COCHLEAR PROSTHESIS

Francis A. Spelman, PhD
Ben M. Clopton, PhD
Bryan E. Pfingst, PhD

NEURAL MECHANISMS RELEVANT TO THE DESIGN OF AN AUDITORY PROSTHESIS

LOCATION AND ELECTRICAL CHARACTERISTICS

Ben M. Clopton, PhD
Francis A. Spelman, PhD

This publication was supported in part by Parke-Davis
Division of Warner-Lambert Company.

TISSUE IMPEDANCE AND CURRENT FLOW IN THE IMPLANTED EAR

IMPLICATIONS FOR THE COCHLEAR PROSTHESIS

FRANCIS A. SPELMAN, PHD

BEN M. CLOPTON, PHD BRYAN E. PFINGST, PHD

SEATTLE, WASHINGTON

Tissue impedance was measured in the cochleas of monkeys and guinea pigs implanted with electrode arrays. The impedances were measured within the scala tympani and between the scala tympani and the internal auditory meatus of the modiolus. The measurements revealed several impedance properties. 1) The impedances inside and outside of the scala tympani are resistive for frequencies between 8 Hz and 12.5 kHz. 2) The impedances measured between the scala tympani and the internal auditory meatus were larger in magnitude than the impedances measured in the scala tympani. 3) Impedance was not affected significantly by changing stimulus current flow from 0.45 to 45 μA rms. 4) Impedance magnitude increased rapidly by different factors inside and outside the scala tympani after sacrifice of the subject animals. Measurements of the tissue impedance made in conjunction with measurements of threshold of response to electrical stimulation revealed that the threshold of response to electrical stimuli was lowest when the stimulating currents were highest outside the scala tympani. We conclude that the excitable elements of the auditory nerve are being stimulated within the modiolus rather than within the scala tympani.

INTRODUCTION

An optimal cochlear implant would provide the maximum transfer of information to the patient for the minimum expenditure of energy. The former criterion requires that suprathreshold electrical stimuli be delivered to the appropriate nerve cells for a given effect; stimulation of too many, or too few, or inappropriate cells may distort the auditory information underlying the process and make interpretation difficult for the patient. The latter criterion allows a maximum dynamic range within the limits imposed by considerations of safety and prolongs the life of both the electrodes and the energy source that powers the implant. To meet these criteria, one must know the locations of the surviving neural elements within the patient's ear, and understand the best way to apply suprathreshold stimuli to those elements.

The interaction of electrical energy with implanted tissues has been under investigation for decades. In large peripheral nerves, stimuli can be minimized when electric currents parallel the axes of nerves, when electrodes are separated by at least 1-2 mm, and when electrical currents are applied at frequencies below 100-200 Hz.[1] Similar effects have been demonstrated with respect to the relation between electrodes and nerve fibers in tissues of the central nervous system.[2-4] The frequency dependence of thresholds of stimulation in the nervous system also has been studied over the last several decades.[5,6]

The behavioral thresholds of electrical stimulation in the inner ear are less at low frequencies than at higher frequencies, and dynamic ranges are greater at lower than at higher frequencies.[7,8] It is necessary to know whether the similarities between the excitable tissues of the inner ear and other excitable tissues are due to properties of the cells or to redirection of stimulating currents through the tissues surrounding them. This understanding is particularly important if stimulus frequency is to be used as part of the code delivered to patients via cochlear implants.

The vocoder model of the cochlear prosthesis assumes it is possible to convey frequency information to patients by stimulating particular electrodes within an array, and thus exciting nerves that are associated with particular regions of the basilar membrane.[9-13] It is not yet clear whether a cochlear prosthesis can be built successfully on this vocoder model. A basic concern is whether the patient retains sufficient fibers to allow multichannel stimulation and whether stimulus current can be directed to independent sets of cells within a given ear.

To help determine the basis of stimulation of cells of the inner ear, we embarked on a series of studies in two directions. The first was to determine the threshold of stimulation of evoked responses as a function of stimulus frequency and electrode position;[14] the second was to determine the paths taken by stimulus currents applied to the prosthesis, as functions of the stimulus frequency and electrode placement. The investigation reported here is an extension of previous studies of the latter kind.[15,16] In those studies, we investigated current flow with the existing electrodes of the implanted array and included the electrode impedance in the measure of current flow. In the present study we used a 4-ter-

---

From the Regional Primate Research Center, Center for Bioengineering, and Department of Otolaryngology, University of Washington, Seattle. This work was supported by NIH grants RR00166, NS13056, and NS13052.

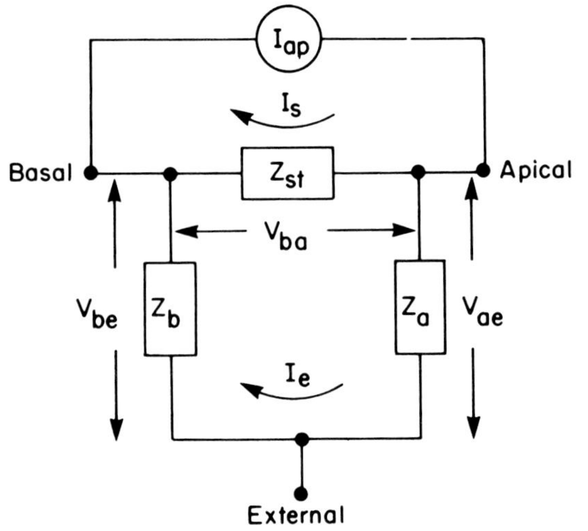

Fig. 1. Schematic diagram of implanted ear. Six electrodes are shown as filled circles. For one of the three stimulus arrangements, stimulus is applied between basal and apical electrodes in scala tympani. Voltages are measured between two additional electrodes in scala tympani (V_{ba}), as well as from basal sensing electrode to external sensing electrode (V_{be}) and from apical to external sensing electrodes (V_{ae}). External stimulating electrode is not used in this measurement. Applied current (I_{ap}) is split into scalar (I_s) and external (I_e) components. These currents are determined by scalar (Z_{st}), apical-external (Z_a) and basal-external (Z_b) impedances.

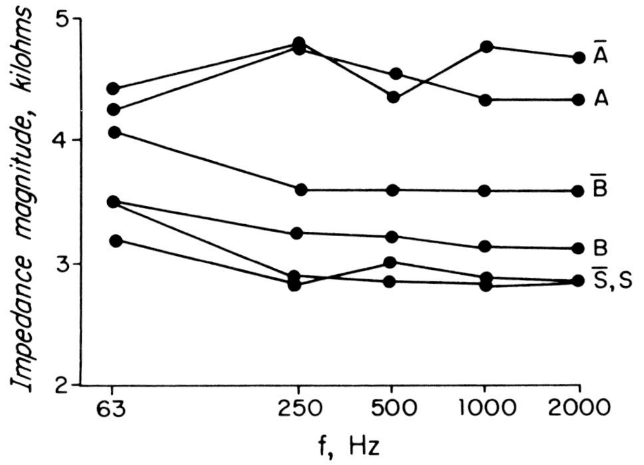

Fig. 2. Magnitudes of average impedances of apical (Ā), basal (B̄), and scala tympani (S̄) paths of four guinea pigs for frequencies of 63-2,000 Hz. Apical path is path taken by current that flows between most apical electrode and internal auditory meatus; basal path is path taken by current that flows between most basal electrode and internal auditory meatus; scala tympani current is sum of basal and apical currents. Same impedances are shown for a single animal (A,B,S).

minal technique with independent stimulation and voltage measurement electrodes to estimate tissue impedance, thus eliminating the electrode impedance from the measurements.

METHODS

Measurements were made on 12 healthy guinea pigs and one healthy rhesus macaque *(Macaca mulatta)*. The guinea pigs were selected specifically for this study. The monkey was also used in a series of psychophysical experiments, the results of which are reported elsewhere.[17]

The guinea pigs were anesthetized with ketamine hydrochloride (100 mg/kg, supplemented as necessary during the experiment). The implant was placed in the scala tympani[14] and held in place with dental acrylic. The animals' heads were stabilized with stainless steel screws fixed to their skulls and with dental acrylic and small screws threaded into the bones. Surgical procedures for the monkey are described elsewhere.[8]

The implants were modified slightly from our previous design.[8] They originally had two pairs of closely spaced electrodes (0.2-0.5 mm) that were separated by 1.5-2 mm on a substrate of Silastic rubber (Dow Corning, Midland, Mich). The electrodes were made of platinum-iridium (90-10%) 25-μm-diameter wire flamed to a 200-μm-diameter ball. The electrode carrier was curved to fit within the scala tympani, but was not molded to fit snugly in the scala.[18] In addition to the scalar electrodes, external electrodes were placed in the internal auditory meatus in the guinea pig and in the mastoid cortex in the monkey. Both external electrodes had the same dimensions as the scalar electrodes. The external electrodes were placed near each other (within 0.2-0.5 mm).

Measurements were made of the magnitude and phase angle of the voltage elicited within the tissues of the inner ear when a constant current stimulus was applied via the implant electrodes. Currents were applied at three pairs of electrodes: the two most widely spaced electrodes in the scala tympani array, the most basal electrode in the array paired with the external stimulating electrode, and the most apical electrode in the array paired with the external stimulating electrode. Voltage measurements were made between each pair of the three monitoring electrodes that were placed in the inner ear (Fig. 1). Two of those electrodes were in the scala tympani array and one was implanted within 0.5 mm of the external electrode. For each applied stimulus current, three voltage measurements were made. The magnitude of the applied current varied from 1 to 32 μA rms, while frequency varied from 63 to 2,000 Hz. Current was taken as the reference for the phase shift measurements. The voltage measurements were made with a differential amplifier (AD 521, Analog Devices, Norwood, Mass) and averaged with a minicomputer (MED-80, Nicolet Instrument Corp, Madison, Wisc). Twenty-five cycles were averaged in each case. The reference current signal and the measured voltage signal were analyzed for magnitude and phase on the minicomputer and saved for later analysis.

The resulting data formed three-by-three complex voltage matrices, which were analyzed as previously described.[15] Briefly, it is necessary to solve the complex matrix equation $[I] = [V \times Y]$, where [I] is the vector of applied current, [V] is the complex voltage matrix, and [Y] is the complex admittance vector. In a totally deterministic system, three applications of current and three measurements of voltage would be sufficient to determine the admittances and thus to determine the current flow within the ear for a given stimulus pair. As this system is noisy, more measures and analyses are necessary. The system is reciprocal, ie, independent of the direction of current flow (the cofactors of the matrix are symmetrical with respect to the principal diagonal) but it contains noise. The data were reduced by averaging the reciprocal terms and requiring that each equation fit Kirchoff's Voltage Law. The modified voltage matrix was inverted, the equation solved for admittances, and the currents were calculated. The admittance magnitudes were inverted and phases negated to obtain complex impedance values.

For 6 of the 12 guinea pigs, the stimuli were broadband (8-12,500 Hz) white noise waveforms generated by the computer as signals for the current generator. The voltage responses were averaged, and complex spectra were obtained for the stimulus current and the response voltage. Impedances were calculated over the full frequency range.

In two guinea pigs, impedance was measured with a white noise current just before sacrifice, for two hours immediately following sacrifice (in five-minute intervals) and at 16 hours after sacrifice. The purpose of these measurements was to determine whether cochlear current paths are changed postmortem and thus

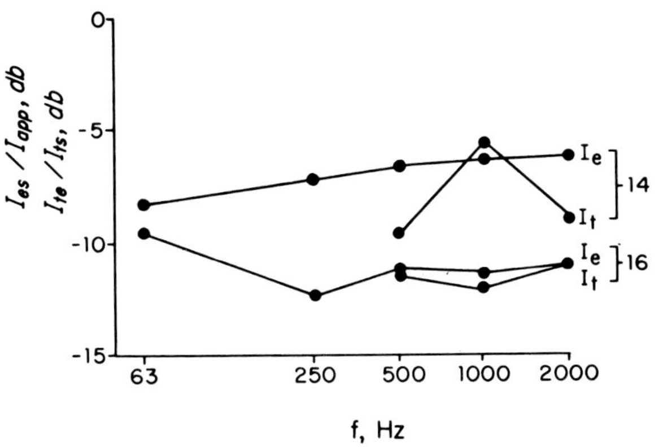

Fig. 3. Ratio of external current (I_{es}) to applied current (I_{app}) when current is applied to two scalar electrodes (I_e), and ratio of thresholds (I_{te}/I_{ts}) to elicit brachial evoked response when current is applied scalarly or between scalar electrode and external electrode (I_t). Ratios are plotted as function of frequency (63-2,000 Hz) for guinea pigs 14 and 16.

whether these measurements could be made in the temporal bones of human or nonhuman primate cadavers.

RESULTS

Measurements made within the basal turn of the cochleas of four of the guinea pigs are shown in Figure 2, along with measurements made in a single animal for comparison. The impedance is larger in magnitude for the paths from both the basal and apical electrodes to the internal auditory meatus than it is within the scala tympani. The impedance had a negative phase angle, which indicates a capacitive component in the tissues. The phase angle never exceeded 20°. The magnitude of the impedance remained within 3 dB of its low-frequency value throughout the range for frequencies measured (63-2,000 Hz). The impedances in the ear of the monkey were similar to those in the guinea pigs, except that the measured magnitudes were less by 20%.

The measurements of current flow within the implanted ear show that the shunting effect of the fluid in the scala tympani has marked influence. When a constant current is applied to the electrodes of the scala tympani, approximately 75% flows through the scala and 25% flows outside of it. The relation is not changed significantly as frequency is varied from 63 to 2,000 Hz. If, on the other hand, current is applied to one of the scalar electrodes and to the external electrode, all of the applied current must flow through external pathways. The circuit model in Figure 1 shows that when stimulus current is applied to either the basal or the apical electrode and the external electrode, all of the applied current flows externally. The amount of current flow through the scala tympani and the unstimulated path is 25% when current is applied to the basal and external electrodes, while 40% of the current flows through the scala tympani when current is applied to the apical and external electrodes. The amount of current flowing through the scalar path is not significantly affected by changing frequency.

When the data acquired by measuring current flow in the ear are compared with those acquired by measuring the neural evoked responses to electrical stimulation (Fig. 3),[14] the crucial parameter for threshold neural stimulation was the current that flowed outside the scala tympani. When the animals were stimulated with currents applied basal-externally or apical-externally, the thresholds were similar (usually within 1 dB in both cases). When current was applied scalarly, the thresholds measured were 9 dB greater than in either of the other two cases. The difference in threshold does not change markedly over a frequency ranging from 500 to 16,000 Hz.[14]

In the monkey, the electrodes were arrayed so there were two pairs spaced 4 mm apart in the scala. The electrode pairs were two platinum-iridium electrodes, each 4 mm apart. The behavioral detection threshold at 1 kHz was 10-15 dB greater for stimulation of either closely spaced pair of electrodes than it was for the widely spaced pairs (either the inner pair or the outer pair). The mea-

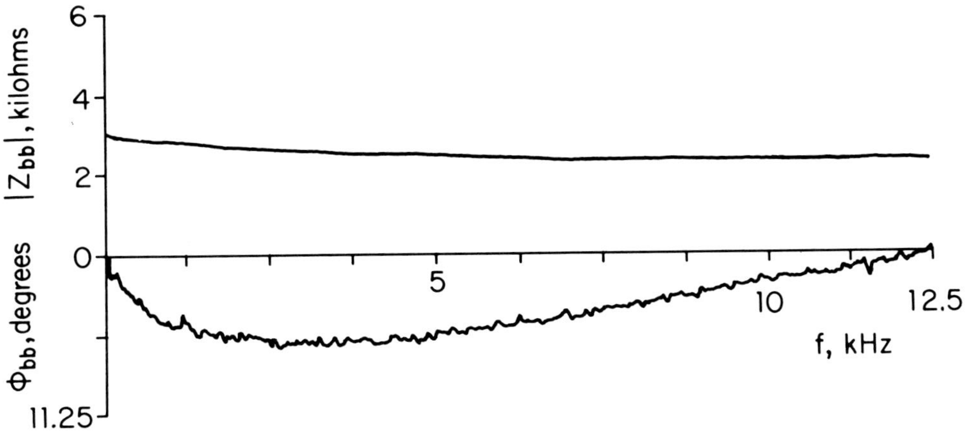

Fig. 4. Magnitude, $|Z_{bb}|$, and phase Φ_{bb}, of basal impedance as function of frequency from 8-12,500 Hz for a white noise stimulus.

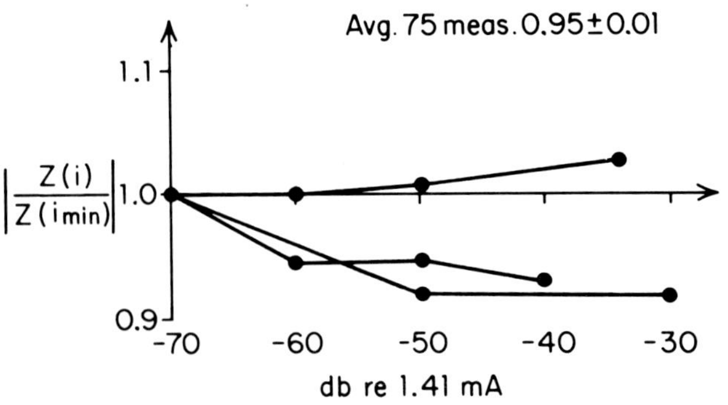

Fig. 5. Ratio of magnitude of impedance measured at various applied currents to magnitude measured at minimum current (−70 dB re 1.41 mA rms). Stimulus was broadband white noise from 8-12,500 Hz.

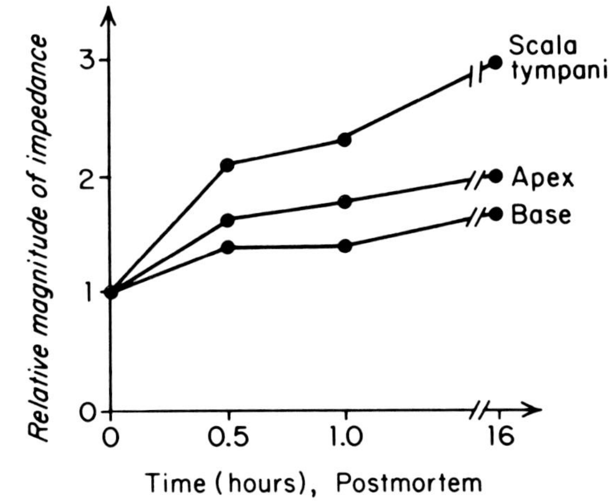

Fig. 6. Ratio of impedance measured postmortem to that measured just before sacrifice. Impedance ratio is shown as function of time postmortem.

sured magnitude of the tissue impedance of the path terminated by two electrodes 4 mm apart in the scala tympani was 2,170 Ω, while the paths from the scala to the external electrode have magnitudes of 2,540 and 2,990 Ω for the basal and scalar electrodes.

A typical set of impedances obtained in the noise studies is shown in Figure 4. The magnitude of the impedance varies less than 10% over the entire frequency range and the phase lag has a maximum value of 6°. The results obtained with sinusoids at discrete frequencies agree with those shown for the white noise current, indicating that the system is, to a first approximation, resistive in nature. It is therefore reasonable to employ the magnitude of the impedance, independent of its phase, for the other measures shown here.

In three guinea pigs, we measured the variation in the magnitude of the tissue impedance as a function of applied current. The results are summarized in Figure 5. Current was varied from 0.45 to 45 μA rms. In no case did the magnitude of impedance vary more than 10% as current was varied, and impedance varied by less than 2% over all 75 measurements. The ratio of impedance at test currents to that measured at 0.45 μA is shown in Figure 5.

The results of the tests made just before and after sacrifice are shown in Figure 6. The magnitude of impedance is expressed as a ratio of the magnitude measured postmortem to that measured immediately before sacrifice. The impedances increased with the most rapid rate of change occurring during the 30 minutes following sacrifice. The increase was most pronounced in the tissue of the scala tympani and least pronounced in the tissue between the apical electrode and the external electrode in the internal auditory meatus.

CONCLUSIONS

In previous studies of the electrical properties of the inner ear, we measured impedance with a two-electrode technique. That technique is misleading, since it requires one to measure the sum of the electrode impedance and the tissue impedance. The electrode impedance contributed significantly to the magnitude of the impedance and to the frequency-dependent effects that were measured, and it led to erroneous conclusions with respect to the current paths in which the greatest current flowed (we concluded previously that the primary paths of current were outside of the scala tympani). However, the present results and the companion neural observations[14] support the previous conclusion that the location at which cells are excited is outside the scala tympani, despite the shunting effects of the scala tympani.

Our current results are consistent with earlier results in other laboratories. Like Ranck,[2] we obtained, in a volume of neurons, tissue impedances with magnitudes between 1 and 10 kΩ and negative phase angles of less than 20°. Like Strelioff[19] and Black and Clark,[20] we found that the impedance measured more apically is greater than that measured basally. The technique described here is useful in investigations of the characteristics of the implanted ear because it not only leads us to descriptions of the location of excitable elements, but it also has shown us anomalies in the implant. In the case of one animal (guinea pig 15), we found that the voltage matrix was not reciprocal. That result suggests either that there were sources of voltage in the implanted ear that led to voltage levels on the order of 30 mV, or that there was something wrong with the electrode array. Calculation showed that a nonreciprocal result could be measured if one of the sensing electrodes had an extremely high impedance or was not in contact with the solution. Histological study revealed a folded electrode array, with the suspect electrode hidden in the innermost fold.

Two observations support our conclusion that the excitable cells lay outside the scala tympani. First, the threshold current to elicit an evoked potential decreased by nearly the same value that external current increased when stimulus was applied between electrodes within the basal turn of the scala tympani. Second, the threshold remained essentially the same when current was applied with a basal-external electrode or with an apical-external electrode. The current changed substantially in the two external paths, but the total external current remained unchanged. The elements excited by stimulation in the basal turn of the implanted cochlea were not markedly different in location whether the stimulating electrode was located basally or 2 to 4 mm apically. It remains to be seen what the effect of stimulation from other turns will be. We cannot state on the basis of these data what the site of excitation is: whether it is in the habenula perforata where the dendrites of the cells of the eighth nerve develop their myelin sheaths, at the cell bodies, or along the axons.

The fluids of the scala tympani shunt current from excitable cells. That conclusion is drawn from the currents measured in the cochleas of guinea pigs and from the data collected in the single monkey measured in this study. It is possible to calculate a difference in current flow for stimuli applied between either widely spaced or closely spaced pairs of electrodes. If it is assumed that the impedance per unit distance of the scala tympani is constant over the length occupied by the implant,[21] the scalar impedance for closely spaced electrodes in this implant would be 216 Ω. The change in external current flow for closely spaced electrode pairs would be 17 dB less than it would be for the widely spaced pair. This calculated effect is slightly larger than the measured threshold effect (10-15 dB).

Measurements made here in the guinea pig and preliminary measurements in the monkey (Spelman, unpublished results) indicate that tissue impedance is invariant with current up to 45 μA rms. The linearity of the tissue impedance means that two currents directed to the same location within the inner ear will operate additively on the cells in that location. The cells will respond nonlinearly to summed currents because of their imposition of a threshold, but electrode arrays can be designed to increase or decrease local currents by algebraic summation.

These results indicate that current paths within the inner ear can be resolved with spatial and spectral detail. However, significant questions remain. The longitudinal and transverse impedances within the modiolus must be measured. Current flows must be measured concurrently with evoked behavioral or electrophysiological responses. These studies should be conducted in damaged cochleas to provide a useful model of patient implant candidates. It is essential to understand the change in the paths of current flow that result as 1) electrode positions are varied, 2) extraneous tissues grow in the implanted cochlea, and 3) current drive is varied between electrode pairs (in the hope of focusing currents in the regions that contain excitable cells). The values of tissue impedance obtained in guinea pigs premortem and postmortem show it is unwise to infer particular values in vivo that are based on postmortem studies. To understand how to direct stimulus currents to particular tissues in the inner ear, we will have to make acute or chronic measurements in live animals. A more complete understanding of the electrical properties of the implanted ear should result in the design of an electrode array that will minimize drive currents, maximize dynamic range, and maximize the useful life of implants for human patients.

REFERENCES

1. Rushton WAH. The effect upon the threshold for nervous excitation of the length of nerve exposed, and the angle between current and nerve. J Physiol 1927; 63:357-77.

2. Ranck JB. Analysis of specific impedance of rabbit cerebral cortex. Exp Neurol 1963; 7:153-74.

3. Ranck JB Jr. Which elements are excited in electrical stimulation of the mammalian central nervous system: a review. Brain Res 1975; 98:417.

4. MacNeal DR, Teicher DA. Effect of electrode placement on threshold and initial site of excitation of a myelinated nerve fiber. In: Hambrecht FT, Reswick JB, eds. Functional electrical stimulation. New York: Marcel Dekker, 1977.

5. Hill AV, Katz B, Solandt DY. Nerve excitation by alternating current. Proc R Soc 1936; B121:74-133.

6. Guttmann R, Hachmeister R. Effect of calcium, temperature, and polarizing currents upon alternating-current excitation of space-clamped squid axons. J Gen Physiol 1971; 58: 304-21.

7. Simmons FB. Electrical stimulation of the auditory nerve in man. Arch Otolaryngol 1966; 84:24-76.

8. Pfingst BE, Donaldson JA, Miller JM, Spelman FA. Psychophysical evaluation of cochlear prostheses in a monkey model. Ann Otol Rhinol Laryngol 1979; 88:613-25.

9. Merzenich MM, Michelson RP, Pettit CR, Schindler RA, Reid M. Neural encoding of sound sensation evoked by electrical stimulation of the acoustic nerve. Ann Otol Rhinol Laryngol 1973; 82:486-503.

10. Eddington DR, Dobelle WH, Mladejovsky MB, Parkin JL. Auditory prostheses: research with multiple channel intracochlear stimulation in man. Ann Otol Rhinol Laryngol 1978; 87 Suppl 53:1-39.

11. Mercer HD, White RL. Photo lithographic fabrication and physiological performance of microelectrode arrays for neural stimulation. IEEE Trans Biomed Eng 1978; BME 25:494-500.

12. Hochmair E, Hochmair-Desoyer I, Burian K. Investigations towards an artificial cochlea. Int J Art Org 1979; 2:255-61.

13. Hochmair E, Hochmair-Desoyer I, Burian K. Un implant cochleaire a 8 canaux. Cah Otol Rhinol Laryngol 1979; 14:691-5.

14. Clopton BM, Spelman FA. Neural mechanisms relevant to the design of an auditory prosthesis: location and electrical characteristics. This supplement.

15. Spelman FA, Clopton BM, Pfingst BE, Miller JM. Design of the cochlear prosthesis: effects of the flow of current in the implanted ear. Ann Otol Rhinol Laryngol 1980; 89 Suppl 66:5-7.

16. Spelman FA, Pfingst BE, Miller JM, Hassul M, Powers

WE, Clopton BM. Biophysical measurements in the implanted cochlea. Otolaryngol Head Neck Surg 1980; 88:183-7.

17. Pfingst BE, Spelman FA, Sutton D. Operating ranges for cochlear implants. Ann Otol Rhinol Laryngol 1980; 89 Suppl 66:1-4.

18. Sutton D, Miller JM, Pfingst BE. Comparison of cochlear histopathology following two implant designs for use in scala tympani. Ann Otol Rhinol Laryngol 1980; 89 Suppl 66:15-7.

19. Strelioff D. A computer simulation of the generation and distribution of cochlear potentials. J Acoust Soc Am 1973; 54: 620-9.

20. Black RC, Clark GM. Differential electrical excitation of the auditory nerve. J Acoust Soc Am 1980; 67:868-74.

21. Honrubia V, Strelioff D, Sitko S. Electroanatomy of the cochlea: its role in cochlear potential measurements. In: Ruben RJ, Elberling C, Salomon G, eds. Electrocochleography. Baltimore: University Park Press, 1976; 23-39.

NEURAL MECHANISMS RELEVANT TO THE DESIGN OF AN AUDITORY PROSTHESIS

LOCATION AND ELECTRICAL CHARACTERISTICS

BEN M. CLOPTON, PHD FRANCIS A. SPELMAN, PHD

SEATTLE, WASHINGTON

A cochlear prosthesis designed to electrically stimulate eighth nerve fibers in deaf subjects was studied in acute guinea pig preparations. The prosthesis, which consisted of two pairs of platinum-iridium electrodes, was inserted into the scala tympani through the round window. The electrical impedances of different current paths and their effectiveness in evoking neural responses in the central auditory system are compared. Assuming lumped neural elements, the results indicate that the sites of neural excitation lie outside the scala tympani. Frequency-response characteristics of neural excitation are in agreement with resistive spread of current through tissue to the site of stimulation. Neural membrane characteristics similar to those previously studied in nonmammalian nerves seem to account for the response initiation.

INTRODUCTION

In the normal ear, the mechanical fluid motion of the cochlea is changed into neural firing through the mediation of hair cells. In damaged ears, these hair cells are often missing, and cochlear prostheses have been developed to alleviate profound hearing loss by direct electrical activation of whatever neural elements remain in the region of the cochlea. Quantitative criteria for a successful cochlear prosthesis have not yet been established because its limits and variations are still unclear. Qualitative criteria may be specified as a maximum transfer of information with the minimum possibility for damage or postoperative complications. Based on our knowledge of cochlear function, a multichannel implant that selectively stimulates spatially discrete portions of the afferent auditory array would seem to have advantages for the transfer of sound information. Attempts have been made to provide multichannel stimulation through electrodes introduced through the scala tympani,[1,2] the modiolus,[3,4] and the lateral wall of the cochlea.[5] While most implants are still used as single-channel devices, there is continuing support for multichannel stimulation.[6,7]

Introduction of speech signals through a multichannel implant poses problems. We need to devise an encoding strategy for separating and introducing signal features through independent transmission channels, and we have to find the most effective arrangements for electrodes and optimal stimulating waveforms for the discrete activation of these channels. At the center of these problems is a lack of knowledge about which neural elements are likely to remain in profoundly deaf individuals, and the ways in which cochlear implants stimulate these elements. While there are currently no suitable diagnostic techniques for electrically determining which excitable neural elements remain in damaged cochleas, many patients probably have few spiral ganglion cells remaining in the basal turns of the cochlea, which are most accessible to the scalar implants currently in use.[8-10] Given an unpredictable population of surviving neural elements, which must be stimulated more or less discretely, it is of paramount importance that we clarify the electrical properties and neurophysiological mechanisms relevant to the operation of cochlear implants.

Cochlear prostheses evidently effect stimulation through mechanisms associated with neural membranes. Neural and behavioral thresholds to electrical stimulation[11-13] through these implants show a frequency dependence that agrees with known properties of nerve membranes.[14,15] Manipulation of the biochemical environment in the cochlea affects neural responsiveness to prosthetic stimulation[13] in a manner predictable from the behavior of squid axons.[15] These observations aid in the search for the location and function of the neural elements that mediate electrical stimulation in the cochlea.

In this paper is described a series of neurophysiological observations made in conjunction with studies of the pathways of electrical current for electrical signals introduced through scalar and extrascalar electrodes. These measurements were designed to locate the neural elements responsible for central activation under these conditions. Electrical observations, described in a companion paper,[16] consisted of voltage measurements at selected sites in and around the cochlea during stimulation with sinusoidal and white noise waveforms through scalar and extrascalar electrodes. The neurophysiological observations included threshold estimates of responses evoked at the inferior colliculus by transient signals.

From the Department of Otolaryngology, Regional Primate Research Center, and Center for Bioengineering, University of Washington, Seattle. This work was supported by NIH grants RR00166, NS13056, and NS13052.

METHODS

Subjects and Procedures. Six pigmented guinea pigs weighing 200-350 g were anesthetized with ketamine hydrochloride (100 mg/kg) and xylazine (20 mg/kg) supplemented as necessary. Respiratory problems were minimized with a presurgical dose of atropine sulfate (0.8 mg/kg) and a tracheotomy. The head was stabilized by a small bolt, attached to the rostral skull with dental acrylic, and stainless steel screws threaded into the bone.

The middle ear was widely exposed by removal of overlying tissues, the tympanic membrane, and the cochlear bulla caudal to the tympanic membrane. A free-fit cochlear prosthesis containing at least two pairs of bipolar electrodes within a Silastic mold[17] was inserted through the round window and fixed in place with Durelon. The electrodes in a pair were separated by 0.2-0.5 mm, and the pairs were 1.5-2 mm apart along the axis of the scala next to the basilar membrane. An electrical connector to the implanted prosthesis was attached to the skull near the defect in the bulla. Pairs of stimulating and measuring electrodes were also implanted external to the cochlea at one or more of the following sites: the internal meatus near the modiolus as approached through the vestibule, the internal auditory meatus as exposed through a posterior fossa approach, the junction of the eighth nerve and cochlear nucleus as exposed by aspiration of the overlying cerebellum, and the neck muscles. All animals used for impedance measurements had external electrodes in the internal auditory meatus and some had electrodes at the cochlear nucleus and neck muscles. Electrodes for recording evoked potentials in the rostral auditory pathways consisted of a silver wire insulated except for its terminal 1.5 mm. This exposed portion was bent 90° to form a boot, which was placed on the brachium of the inferior colliculus opposite the implanted ear. A reference electrode was placed near the sagittal sinus.

Stimulation and Voltage Measurement Procedures. One aspect of these experiments was the introduction of constant currents either between pairs of electrodes in the scala tympani or between an electrode in the scala tympani and an external electrode. Voltage differences were measured between all nonstimulated electrodes in the system, and a later analysis provided estimates of tissue impedance for characterization of the electrical properties of the cochlea and the surrounding tissues. The techniques for these measurements and calculations used for data analysis are described in a companion paper.[16]

Recording of Evoked Responses. Electrical artifact from stimulation through a cochlear prosthesis interferes significantly with any electrophysiological recording in the area of the brainstem. While the components of the stimulus resulting from capacitance coupling and electromagnetic radiation can be minimized, a significant component resulting from current spread remains. To minimize this interference and yet obtain frequency-specific information about the electrophysiological response, we presented single cycles of sinusoids to electrode pairs through a constant-current stimulator.[18] The frequency of the sinusoids was varied in 1-octave steps from 500 Hz to 16 kHz. These electrode pairs were separated by 1.5-2 mm along the scala tympani, or one was in the scala and the other outside the cochlea. To reduce the duration of the electrical artifact, we set all filters in the recording circuit at their widest point to achieve an impulse response of minimal duration. The brachial potential resulting from these transient stimuli was sampled at 25 kHz for 10.24 ms and averaged 50 times with a Nicolet MED-80 computer. The averaging was repeated while the intensity of the stimulating current was adjusted to estimate the threshold for an evoked response. The threshold was established as a minimally detectable evoked waveform on the cathrode-ray computer display. Suprathreshold observations were made with 1-dB increases in stimulus intensities so we could follow the growth of the evoked response from threshold to a maximum value, determined by either 1) interference from electrical artifact or limitations dictated by current spread to nonauditory nerve or muscle or 2) gassing limits of the platinum-iridium electrodes.[19] Threshold estimates could be made rapidly and safely in conjunction with impedance observations throughout an acute experiment (8-18 hours).

TABLE 1. MEAN DIFFERENCE IN THRESHOLDS (dB) BETWEEN THREE ELECTRODE COMBINATIONS ACROSS FREQUENCIES (N = 5)

	Electrode Pairs Compared		
kHz	*S-A*	*S-B*	*B-A*
0.5	11.49	9.89	1.60
1	8.21	6.91	1.30
2	8.56	7.23	1.33
4	8.37	6.13	2.24
8	7.65	6.21	1.44
16	8.06	5.69	2.27
Overall mean	8.72	7.01	1.70
95% confidence intervals	7.18-10.26	8.69-5.33	1.20-2.19

Confirmation of Electrode Location. The placements of stimulating and recording electrodes both on the prosthesis and external to the cochlea were confirmed after the experiment by dissection of the cochlea and surrounding tissue under an operating microscope. Twisting, folding, and other displacements of the prosthesis were noted, along with any other unanticipated electrode placements. Some preparations were unsuitable because of poor electrode placement, or because of defective implants or other technical or physiological considerations.

RESULTS

Relatively stable thresholds were obtained for all electrode combinations and frequencies in acceptable preparations. Independent replications were always possible to within ± 2 dB and commonly within ± 1 dB. Thresholds for detectable evoked potentials at the brachium of the colliculus were below 10 μA rms for optimal electrode placements and stimulating frequencies in every animal except guinea pig (GP) 15. In this animal, the implant was folded within the scala tympani so that the platinum electrodes were isolated from scalar fluids by the Silastic carrier. For GP 15, therefore, measurements of both impedance[16] and neurophysiological thresholds deviated from those obtained for the other preparations. Thus the following results do not apply to GP 15 except where indicated.

At every frequency in every preparation except GP 15 (n = 5), current passing from a scalar electrode to an external one evoked a neural response more effectively than did current passing between electrodes within the scala. The apical-to-external (A) and basal-to-external (B) electrode pairs had thresholds that were significantly lower than the base-to-apex or scalar (S) pair (Table 1). While the A electrode configuration yielded consistently lower thresholds than the B configuration, the difference was less than 2 dB. In contrast, the S configuration was 7-9 dB less effective than either the A or B configuration. Clearly, directing current across the scalar-external boundary increases its effectiveness by 2 to 3 times.

The relation between log threshold and log frequency of stimulation was an increasing, curvilinear one (Fig. 1). This form of relationship has been reported previously for middle ear stimulation,[13] is qualitatively predictable from experimental observations on squid giant axon,[15] and agrees

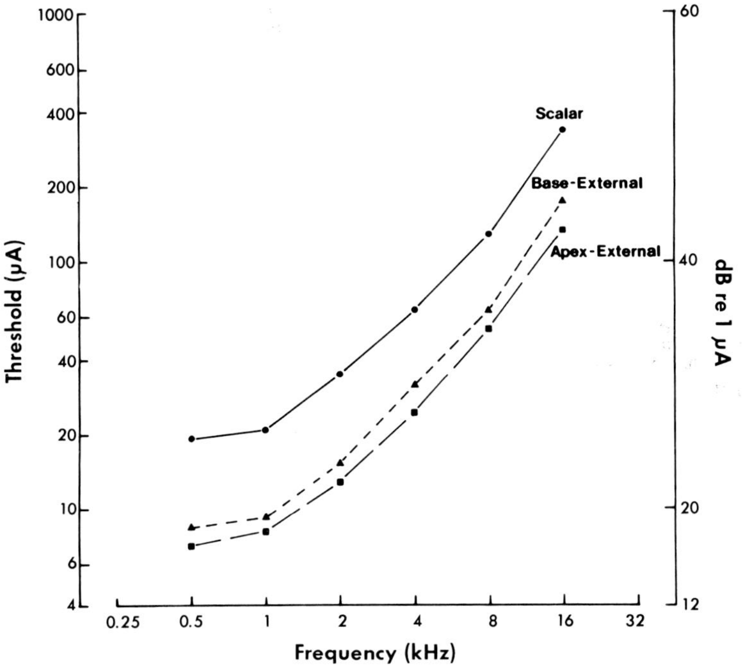

Fig. 1. Threshold for evoked response versus frequency of stimulation for three electrode pairs. Both extrascalar current paths were associated with thresholds 7-9 dB less than those for scalar pathway throughout frequency range (Table 1). Shapes of functions are very similar, with increasing slopes at higher frequencies (Table 2).

qualitatively with behavioral measures.[17] Threshold-frequency functions can be compared by noting their slopes. These slopes in decibels per octave changed in an orderly manner, ranging from less than 1 dB/octave at 0.5-1 kHz to 8.46 dB/octave at 8-16 kHz (Table 2). The S, A, and B electrode pairs were not different with respect to these slopes, only in absolute thresholds.

Electrical analysis of the cochlea revealed that the current paths were primarily resistive, ie, little phase shift was seen between the applied voltage and measured current flow.[16] For comparison of measured electrical and neurophysiological characteristics, the following results and analyses are given for three animals. These animals had complete impedance and threshold observations, confirmed placements of prostheses, stable physiological signs throughout all procedures, and appropriate replications. The following analysis is for data at 1 kHz, but entirely comparable results would hold at 500 and 2,000 Hz; the other frequencies overlap for the neural and electrical data.

It was assumed that a discrete site of neural excitation existed regardless of the site of stimulation, and that these neural elements could be exclusively associated with one of the three current paths. The electrical characteristics for each pathway were also assumed to be lumped and resistive. Because no current-voltage phase shifts exceeded 6° for these preparations, the assumption of resistive characteristics appeared valid. Absolute threshold for excitation at the site of neural activation could not be determined from the overall current threshold because of the possibility of an undetermined portion of the threshold current being shunted through an alternate, ineffective pathway. However, changes in thresholds for changes in pairs of stimulating electrodes can be predicted from measured impedances for the three possible sites of neural activation. The site associated with the most accurate prediction of the observed threshold changes is thus supported.

TABLE 2. MEAN SLOPES OF THRESHOLD-FREQUENCY RELATIONS (dB/OCTAVE) ACROSS FREQUENCY

	Electrode Pair				95%
Frequency	S	A	B	*Mean*	*Confidence Interval*
0.5-1	0.67	1.04	0.74	0.816	0.59-1.04
1-2	4.48	4.13	4.16	4.26	3.80-4.71
2-4	5.28	5.47	6.38	5.71	4.33-7.09
4-8	6.00	6.72	5.92	6.21	5.18-7.25
3-16	8.43	8.00	8.95	8.46	7.34-9.58

The first step is to determine the relative current magnitudes in the direct and indirect current pathways. A single impedance characterizes the direct current path, while the indirect pathway has two serial impedances. As shown in Table 3, the direct pathway for the S path has 2,574 Ω impedance, and the indirect (extrascalar) pathway has 8,520 Ω impedance (5,119 + 3,401). For a constant current injected through the scalar pair of electrodes, the decibel ratio of indirect to direct current is 20 log (2,754/8,520) = −9.81 dB.

Also shown in Table 3 are the mean neural threshold current values for the S, A, and B pairs of

TABLE 3. ELECTRICAL PARAMETERS AND OBSERVED NEURAL THRESHOLDS AT 1 kHz FOR S, A, AND B PATHWAYS IN THREE GUINEA PIGS

Pathway	*Mean Impedance*	*Current Out of Pathway (dB re Current in Pathway)*	*Threshold (μA, rms)*
S	2,754	−9.81	25.88
A	5,119	−1.60	8.46
B	3,401	−7.29	9.59

TABLE 4. CHANGE IN THRESHOLD (dB) FOR CHANGE IN STIMULATION ELECTRODES FOR OBSERVED THRESHOLD VALUES IN TABLE 3

Electrode Change	*Threshold Change*
S to A	−9.71
S to B	−8.62
A to B	+1.09

TABLE 5. DISCREPANCIES (dB) BETWEEN PREDICTED AND OBSERVED CHANGES IN THRESHOLDS FOR THREE POSTULATED LUMPED LOCI OF STIMULATED NEURAL ELEMENTS

Postulated Site	*Change in Stimulation Locus*				*95% Confidence Interval*
	S to A	*S to B*	*A to B*	*Mean*	
S	11.31	15.91	4.60	10.61	4.97-16.24
A	0.1	6.1	6.2	4.13	0.67-7.59
B	1.5	1.19	2.69	1.79	1.01

stimulation electrodes. Table 4 gives the relative change in threshold for changes in stimulation configuration from the data of Table 3. For example, changing from the S to the A stimulating electrode pair yielded a change of −9.71 dB = 20 log (25.88/8.46). These data allow a comparison of the evidence for assumed loci of excitable neural elements (Table 5).

DISCUSSION

Describing pathways of current flow in the inner ear is particularly difficult because of the complex, three-dimensional structure of soft tissues, bone, and cochlear fluids. These tissues and their interfaces are characterized by specific electrical properties. We must know the current densities that a cochlear prosthesis induces in these tissues if we are to approximate the sites of neural excitation. In the present case, we made simplifying assumptions to estimate these current pathways. At the center of these assumptions is a linear, lumped-constant, resistive model of the inner ear during stimulation with a scalar prosthesis. Our data support the assumption of a relatively pure resistance, and checks on the assumption of a linearity across different intensities indicate that it holds within the range where the electrode-fluid interface is stable.[16] The assumption of lumped-constant elements is not directly supportable by observation; it is, of course, an assumption of necessity and not conviction. In the absence of an adequate field model and greatly improved resolution of voltage samples in the spatial domain, some variation on the lumped-constant assumption is indicated.

Neurons are distributed elements in terms of electrical stimulation.[20] Obtaining relative thresholds for spike initiation with, for example, an exploring stimulation electrode is not an adequate characterization of the mechanisms of a cochlear prosthesis placed in the scala tympani. A low threshold at one stimulating electrode position does not ensure that the site is a successful competitor with other sites for spike initiation, given that current injected through a prosthesis will affect many possible loci of spike initiation simultaneously. Current injected into the cochlea spreads through an apparently resistive medium that, in turn, determines local increases and decreases in transmembrane potentials. Different sites of current injection may thus induce membrane depolarization and hyperpolarization at the same place on a neuron. The resulting activation process is likely to reflect integrative processes of neurons that are unique to an individual arrangement for stimulation through a prosthesis. The only method of completely describing this current activation process involves simultaneous measurements of current flow patterns and neural thresholds across different conditions of current injection. The overall strategy is to establish variations in neural thresholds that correlate positively with variations in current densities specific to anatomical loci. The data presented here represent an attempt to implement this strategy using three stimulation and measuring sites and their three associated interelectrode pathways. Table 5 contains the results of this implementation.

The prediction of changes in neural thresholds from measured electrical characteristics of the cochlea most closely agrees with the excited neural elements lying in the scalar-external current pathway. The basal-external pathway is most congruent with the observed results, although both external pathway assumptions are more consonant with the data by a factor of more than 2 to 1 over the scalar assumption.

These results agree with other estimates of the location of excited neural elements. Using middle ear stimulation, Clopton and Bosma[13] found that a modiolar locus was probably based on the manipulation of cochlear biochemistry and the survival of structures on the basilar membrane. Clopton et al[11] also found support for a similar locus on the basis of relative thresholds with different electrode positions, although an analysis lacking an incorporation of electrical impedance data compromised this conclusion. The somas of spiral ganglion neurons are the probable foci of excitation. Previous investigations have indicated restricted spatial activation of elements conforming to tonotopic organization for closely spaced scalar electrodes.[21,22] The most parsimonious basis for this observation is that electrical stimulation of ganglion cells occurs immediately adjacent to the electrodes, where a restricted segment of the tonotopic map would be influenced. Current invasion of the nerve would be expected to yield much less spatially discrete excitation patterns as, in fact, occurs with higher stimulation levels.

The membrane mechanisms involved in spike generation seem to have properties similar to those observed in squid giant axon[15] and frog axon[14] over the frequency range observed. The mechanism is

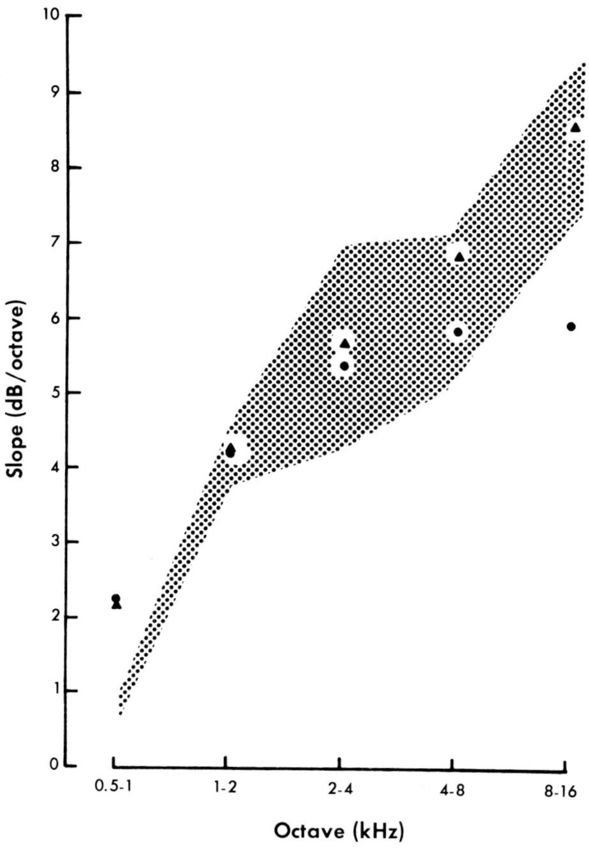

Fig. 2. Ninety-five percent confidence intervals for slopes of threshold vs frequency functions (shaded area) compared with those predicted from first-order (circles) and second-order (triangles) systems. Physiological data agree more with characteristics of second-order system than with those of first-order system, although both are inaccurate at lowest octave.

similar to the operation of a threshold device preceded by a low-pass filter. Figure 2 shows the 95% confidence intervals for the slopes of the threshold-versus-frequency relation in Table 2. Any effort to fit absolute threshold values with parameters would involve assumptions about the values of membrane electrical characteristics, but the shape of threshold-versus-frequency relations as reflected by their slopes can be compared with simple models. The circles of Figure 2 represent a first-order system response (eg, a resistance-capacitance circuit) with a break frequency of 894 Hz. The high-frequency slopes of first-order systems asymptote at 6 dB/octave. The triangles represent a second-order, parallel-resonance system (eg, resistance-capacitance-inductor circuit) with a break frequency of 3,450 Hz and a damping factor of two. Such systems asymptote at 12 dB/octave. Both approximations are fit by trial and error. The second-order system better describes the data at 8-16 kHz, although both systems diverge from the observed slopes at 0.5-1 kHz.

A simple charge integration mechanism such as a resistance-capacitance low-pass filter followed by a threshold device seems inadequate to describe the data at higher frequencies. This is not surprising in light of knowledge about the dynamics of membrane mechanisms.[23] One could extrapolate nonlinear differential equations derived for the squid axon[24] to the mammalian nerve to approximate the observed data, but the usefulness of such an exercise is doubtful for this data base. The distortion of membrane response characteristics within this experimental paradigm must be considered. The thresholds observed were for a population of neurons, and the measurement used is open to possible frequency selectivity resulting from central processing, although we do not believe this is a factor. We did not observe changes in current paths with frequency,[16] so it is unlikely that the slopes of the threshold-versus-frequency relations were distorted by nonmembrane mechanisms.

In summary, threshold variations correlate with changes in current densities in extrascalar pathways. The basal-external pathway is especially in agreement with the observations as a site of excitable neural elements. These conclusions are based on the assumption of a linear, resistive current-spread model supported by physical measurement. The observed threshold-versus-frequency relations may reflect membrane mechanisms, but we need to obtain further observations on single neurons.

REFERENCES

1. House WF, Urban J. Long term results of electrode implantation and electronic stimulation of the cochlea in man. Ann Otol Rhinol Laryngol 1973; 82:504-17.

2. Michelson RP. Electrical stimulation of the human cochlea: a preliminary report. Arch Otolaryngol 1971; 93:317-23.

3. Simmons FB, Epley JM, Lummis RC, et al. Auditory nerve: electrical stimulation in man. Science 1965; 148:104-6.

4. Simmons FB. Electrical stimulation of the auditory nerve in man. Arch Otolaryngol 1966; 84:2-54.

5. Chouard CH, MacLeod P. Implantation of multiple intracochlear electrodes for rehabilitation of total deafness: preliminary report. Laryngoscope 1976; 86:1743-51.

6. Eddington DK. Speech discrimination in deaf subjects with cochlear implants. J Acoust Soc Am 1980; 68:885-91.

7. Simmons FB, Mathews RG, Walker MG, White RL. A functioning multichannel auditory nerve stimulator. Acta Otolaryngol Scand 1979; 87:170-5.

8. Bredberg G. Cellular pattern and nerve supply of the human organ of Corti. Acta Otolaryngol Scand 1968; Suppl 236: 1-325.

9. Johnsson LG. Sequence of degeneration of Corti's organ and its first order neurons. Ann Otol Rhinol Laryngol 1974; 83: 294-303.

10. Otte J, Schuknect HF, Kerr AG. Ganglion cell populations in normal and pathological human cochleae. Implications for cochlear implantation. Laryngoscope 1978; 88:1231-46.

11. Clopton BM, Spelman FA, Miller JM. Estimates of essential neural elements for stimulation through a cochlear prosthesis. Ann Otol Rhinol Laryngol 1980; 89 Suppl 66:5-7.

12. Pfingst BE, Spelman FA, Sutton D. Operating ranges for cochlear implants. Ann Otol Rhinol Laryngol 1980; 89 Suppl 66: 1-4.

13. Clopton BM, Bosma MA. Effectiveness of middle ear electrical stimulation for activating central auditory pathways. Ann Otol Rhinol Laryngol 1982; 91:285-91.

14. Hill AV, Katz B, Solandt DY. Nerve excitation by alternating current. Proc R Soc 1936; B121:74-133.

15. Guttman R, Hachmeister L. Effect of calcium, temperature, and polarizing currents upon alternating current excitation of space-clamped squid axons. J Gen Physiol 1971; 58:304-21.

16. Spelman FA, Clopton BM, Pfingst BE. Tissue impedance and current flow in the implanted ear: implications for the cochlear prosthesis. Ann Otol Rhinol Laryngol 91 Suppl 98.

17. Pfingst BE, Donaldson JA, Miller JM, Spelman FA. Psychophysical evaluation of cochlear prostheses in a monkey model. Ann Otol Rhinol Laryngol 1979; 68:613-25.

18. Spelman FA, Pfingst BE, Miller J. A constant current stimulator for use with chronic cochlear implants. Proc San Diego Biomed Symp 1978; 1-3.

19. Brummer SB, Turner MJ. Electrical stimulation with Pt electrodes: II. Estimation of maximum surface redox (theoretical non-gassing) limits. IEEE Trans Biomed Eng 1977; BME 24: 440-3.

20. Ranck JB Jr. Which elements are excited in electrical stimulation of the mammalian central nervous system: a review. Brain Res 1975; 98:417-40.

21. Merzenich MM, Michelson RP, Pettit CR, Schindler RA, Reid M. Neural encoding of sound sensation evoked by electrical stimulation of the acoustic nerve. Ann Otol Rhinol Laryngol 1973; 82:486-503.

22. Clopton BM, Silverman MS. Central correlates of intracochlear electrical stimulation determined by single-unit recording. First Annual Meeting of the Association for Research in Otolaryngology, Jan 23, 1978.

23. Hodgkin AL, Huxley AF. A quantitative description of membrane current and its application to conduction and excitation in nerve. J Physiol 1952; 117:500-44.

24. Huxley AF. Ion movements during nerve activity. Ann NY Acad Sci 1959; 81:221-46.

THE ANNALS PUBLISHING COMPANY
4949 FOREST PARK BLVD.
ST. LOUIS, MISSOURI 63108

COMPUTED TOMOGRAPHY OF THE NECK

Carlos R. Martinez, MD
Bob W. Gayler, MD
Haskins Kashima, MD
Stanley S. Siegelman, MD
Baltimore, Maryland

Thorough familiarity with the anatomy of the neck depicted in axial sections is fundamental to the interpretation of computed tomography (CT) scans. Fifteen consecutive sections are selected at 1 cm-intervals beginning at the level of the nasopharynx and extending down to the level of the thoracic inlet. Each scan is referenced to a profile drawing of the neck. Each CT scan is reproduced in line drawing, which is labeled for major organs and discrete structures appearing in that section. Twelve representative cases illustrate the usefulness of CT in the evaluation of neck masses by documenting tumor size, location and relationship to adjacent structures. Intravenous contrast improves recognition of vascular structures and distinguishes lymph nodes from blood vessels. The location and relative density of lesions facilitate their specific identification. Demineralization of bone and cartilage is accurately documented in the illustrative cases. Symmetry is the key to the interpretation of subtle pathologies.

INTRODUCTION

Computed tomography (CT), with its unique capacity for displaying bone, soft tissue and airway detail in a single image, has become the imaging modality of choice in the evaluation of patients with neck masses. Thorough knowledge of cross-sectional anatomy is essential for full appreciation of the CT image. This communication reviews the cross-sectional anatomy using 15 reference levels extending from the mastoid tip to the thoracic inlet. The capabilities and limitations of this technique are presented with particular attention to the infratemporal fossa, the parapharyngeal space, salivary glands, larynx, and thyroid gland.

MATERIAL AND METHODS

This report is derived from the study of 140 patients evaluated for lesions of the head and neck. Scans were obtained with an AS&E/Pfizer 500 CT unit.

Normal Anatomy (Figs. 1-16). To represent the normal anatomy 15 scans were selected, beginning at the level of the nasopharynx and extending to the thoracic inlet. The composite reference diagram (Fig. 1) depicts some of the structures occurring at each scan level. For clarity, line drawings are derived from each scan; a few anatomical structures not visualized on the reference scans were included in the line drawings because of their clinical importance and constant relationship to demonstrable anatomical landmarks.

Illustrative Cases (Figs. 17-28). Twelve representative cases, each with CT scan, line drawing and relevant additional documentation, are presented.

TECHNICAL ASPECTS

The reference sections of 1-cm thickness are obtained at 1-cm intervals. The examination is performed with the patient supine, the neck slightly hyperextended, and during quiet breathing. Ten-millimeter sections are obtained with a 10-second exposure, at 20 mA and 120 kilovolt peak (kVp). The scanning time can be reduced to 5 seconds and 50 mA tube current is used. For examination of the larynx, 5-mm sections are obtained at 5-mm intervals. Patients for evaluation of neck masses are preferably studied with intravenous contrast enhancement. Variation of window widths and level settings is helpful for optimal imaging of structures.

NORMAL ANATOMY

Analysis of the image is based on the identification of normal structures as visualized by CT and the relatively constant symmetry of paired structures, ie, major vessels, salivary glands, major muscle groups, etc. The symmetry of deep fat planes which separate the different compartments of the neck is particularly helpful in the assessment of palpable masses.

Identification of the carotid arteries and internal jugular veins is necessary to predict the location of cranial nerves IX through XII and for detection of enlarged lymph nodes. Normal lymph nodes, usually less than 5 mm in size, have a CT density similar to muscle and blood prior to contrast administration. Normal lymph nodes do not enhance with intravenous (IV) contrast. Consequently, opacification of blood vessels after contrast permits improved identification of normal and abnormal lymph nodes, particularly those in the internal jugular chain. The carotid arteries are of nearly identical size; the size of the jugular veins is frequently asymmetrical. The infratemporal fossa is pyramidal in shape and is limited anteriorly by the maxillary antrum; laterally by the zygomatic arch and the mandible; medially by the styloid process, the pterygoid plates, and the medial pterygoid muscle; and superiorly by the greater wing of the sphenoid bone. The infratemporal fossa contains pterygoid muscles, temporalis muscle, internal maxillary artery, pterygoid venous plexus, lingual nerve, and branches of

From the Russell H. Morgan Department of Radiology and Radiological Services (Martinez, Gayler, Siegelman), and the Department of Laryngology and Otology (Kashima), The Johns Hopkins Medical Institutions, Baltimore.

the mandibular nerve. The parapharyngeal space is located between the pharyngeal musculature medially and the pterygoid muscles laterally, and is continuous with the retropharyngeal space. The internal carotid artery, internal jugular vein, cranial nerves IX to XII and the sympathetic trunk lie within this space. Normal lymph nodes are usually very small in this space.

High resolution CT scanning permits identification of parotid and submandibular glands due to their relatively low CT density. This is particularly true in older patients and reflects increasing amounts of fat in the gland parenchyma, an accompaniment of aging. In children, the density of the gland is similar to that of muscle and, due to the small amount of fat in the deep soft tissue planes, identification of the precise boundaries of the parotid may be difficult. The appearance and size of the pharyngeal airway is variable depending on the phase of respiration, fat content, the thickness of the parapharyngeal musculature, the position of the carotid arteries, and the volume of pharyngeal lymphoid tissue. Appearance of the parapharyngeal space, however, should be symmetrical.

The pattern and extent of the ossification of laryngeal cartilages is variable, but usually symmetrical. The hyoid bone is readily identified; its greater horns are at the same level as the carotid bifurcation. The thyroid gland is at the level of the upper trachea, about 2 cm inferior to the cricoid arch. The density of the normal thyroid gland is high (80-100 Hounsfield units) due to the high iodine content. Following contrast administration the CT number increases due to glandular vascularity and iodine content. The esophagus is visualized as a rounded mass of muscle density, posterior to the trachea. Occasionally, a small amount of air is seen in its lumen; this is a normal finding. The esophagus may bulge into the lumen of the trachea, due to the thinness and elasticity of the posterior tracheal membrane. At the level of the thoracic inlet the esophagus is to the left of the midline. Displacement of the esophagus to the right of the midline should be viewed with suspicion.

DISCUSSION

Infratemporal Fossa — Parapharyngeal Space. The exact location and extent of tumors of the infratemporal fossa and parapharyngeal space is best evaluated by CT. Tumors in these compartments are frequently the result of direct extension from maxillary sinus, pharyngeal or deep lobe parotid tumors. Primary sarcomas from the mandible or skull base may also invade this space. Metastatic nodes are a frequent cause of subclinical and symptomatic parapharyngeal masses. Benign tumors of neurogenic origin are common in the parapharyngeal space. Neurofibromas in this location usually arise from the vagus nerve, but may originate from other major nerves within this area. Glomus tumors (inferior extension of glomus jugulare, glomus vagale and carotid body tumors) also occur here. Examination with contrast media is helpful in their delineation.

The detection of parapharyngeal tumors depends more on asymmetry of the tissue compartments, less on asymmetry of the pharynx airway. Inflammatory processes in the parapharyngeal space may mimic tumor infiltration and the differentiation of benign or malignant tumors is not possible on CT findings alone.

Parotid Gland. Computerized tomography is valuable for evaluation of tumefactions and swellings of the parotid gland. Previous reports have stressed the advantages of opacifying the gland parenchyma and ductal system during the CT examination, the so-called CT sialogram. We have studied 24 patients with parotid swelling or localized parotid mass using a high-resolution scanner, intravenous contrast, and 8-mm sections. By this technique, we delineated 12 of 14 (85%) benign tumors and 5 of 5 (100%) malignant tumors. Computerized tomography does not distinguish the benign from the malignant lesion, but it defines the location, number and extent of the lesion(s).

Five patients who had a documented diagnosis of sialodenitis or autoimmune sialectasis were studied. Computerized tomography detected enlargement and increased density of the gland in all cases and the absence of a discrete mass. High resolution CT scanning obviates the need for parotid gland opacification for these cases. We presently recommend combined CT sialography for patients with a palpable mass and a negative CT examination. Conventional sialography remains the imaging modality of choice for the evaluation of patients with diffuse parotid swelling and a history of clinical features suggestive of inflammatory disease or autoimmune disorders.

Larynx. Previous reports have demonstrated the value of CT in the evaluation and staging of laryngeal carcinoma. Our experience with 40 patients supports this view. Computed tomography of the larynx is the best imaging modality for evaluation of cartilage involvement and tumor extension into the preepiglottic, paraglottic and subglottic spaces. Sequential images in the axial plane are helpful in accurate staging based on these factors. Current limitations of CT of the larynx are a) motion artifacts, b) lack of dynamic information, c) failure to differentiate edema from tumor infiltration, and d) lack of adequate characterization of mucosal surfaces. Contrast enhancement is used to improve detection of lymph node metastases. The clinical examination, operative endoscopic examination, and CT are complementary and should be carefully correlated. Contrast laryngography continues to be helpful when dynamic information is important or when there is discrepancy between the CT and clinical findings.

Thyroid. The role of CT in the evaluation of thyroid nodules has been limited by the diagnostic accuracy achieved by isotopic and ultrasound evaluations. However, CT is helpful in defining the extent of tumors, evaluating mediastinal extension or nodal metastases from thyroid carcinoma, and in differentiating tracheal compression or transmural invasion by thyroid tumors.

CONCLUSIONS

Computed tomography is helpful in the evaluation of neck masses by documentation of tumor size, location and relationship to contiguous structures. It demonstrates routes of tumor-spread and provides clues supporting a specific diagnosis. Thorough knowledge of the normal cross-sectional anatomy and meticulous technique are mandatory. The examination should be customed according to the clinical presentation and specific questions. Intravenous contrast medium delineates vascular anatomy and should be given as a continuous infusion to maintain higher iodine levels in plasma. Evaluation of adenopathy is improved by IV contrast enhancement.

Computed tomography is a versatile and highly informative imaging procedure for the evaluation and staging of laryngeal, pharyngeal, parapharyngeal, parotid and infratemporal fossa lesions. It is a helpful adjunct in the management of thyroid and paratracheal tumors.

ACKNOWLEDGMENTS — We gratefully acknowledge the cooperation of our colleagues in the Departments of Otolaryngology and Radiology and the expert assistance of the technical staff. We appreciate the typing of Mrs. Liz Novak and Mrs. Rose Walker. The photography of Mr. Henri Hessels is much appreciated. The illustrations were done by Marjorie Gregerman and Molly Dunker, Department of Art as Applied to Medicine.

BIBLIOGRAPHY

Carter BL, Karmody CS, Blickman JR, Panders AK. Computed tomography and sialography. 1. Normal anatomy; 2. Pathology. J Comput Assist Tomogr 1981; 5:42-53.

Doubleday LC, Jing BS, Wallace S. Computed tomography of the infratemporal fossa. Radiology 1981; 138: 619-24.

Larsson S, Mancuso AA, Hoover L, et al. Differentiation of pyriform sinus cancer from supraglottic laryngeal cancer by CT. Radiology 1981; 141:427-32.

Mancuso AA, Calcaterra TC, Hanafee WN. Computed tomography of the larynx. Radiol Clin North Am 1978; 16:195-208.

Mancuso AA, Bohman L, Hanafee W, et al. Computed tomography of the nasopharynx: normal and variants of normal. Radiology 1980; 137:113-21.

Mancuso AA, Hanafee WN. Computed tomography of the head and neck. Baltimore/London: Williams & Wilkins, 1982.

Mancuso AA, Maceri D, Rice D, et al. CT of cervical lymph node cancer. AJR 1981; 136:381-5.

Martinez CR, Kashima HK, Gayler BW, et al. Computed tomography of the neck. Presented at the Scientific Exhibit - 65th Scientific Assembly, The Radiology Society of North America, Nov 1981.

Miller EM, Normal D. The role of computed tomography in the evaluation of neck masses. Radiology 1979; 133:145-9.

Som PM, Shugar JMA. Combined CT sialogram. Radiology 1980; 135:387-90.

Som PM, Shugar JMA, Train JS, et al. Manifestation of parotid gland enlargement: radiographic, pathologic and clinical correlations. Part I. The autoimmune pseudosialectasis. Part II. The diseases of Mikulicz syndrome. Radiology 1981; 141:415-26.

Stove DN, Mancuso AA, Rice D, et al. Parotid CT sialography. Radiology 1981; 138:393-7.

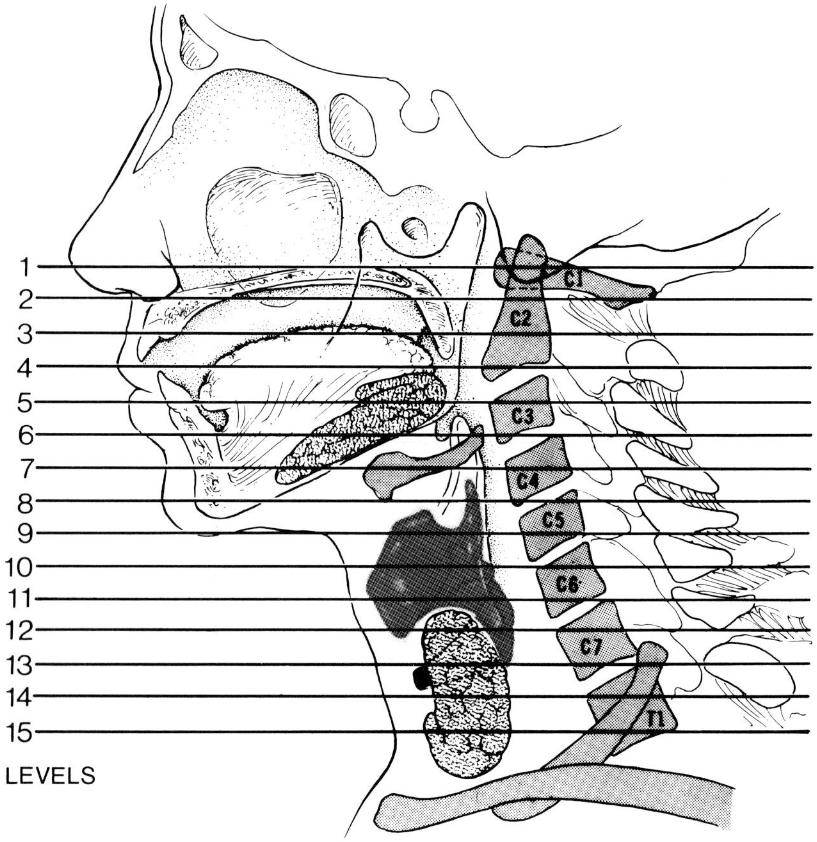

Fig. 1. Diagram of reference levels.

Fig. 2. A,B) (Level 1) Upper nasopharynx. Section demonstrates relationship of nasopharynx, prevertebral and pharyngeal musculature and anterior arch of C-1, and torus tubarius at opening of eustachian tube. Appearance of airway may be asymmetrical due to variable amounts of lymphoid tissue. Deep soft tissue planes in parapharyngeal space should be symmetrical. Close relationship of lateral wall of nasopharynx to pterygomaxillary space and its neural and muscular elements clarifies basis for complex syndromes which arise from disease in this region.

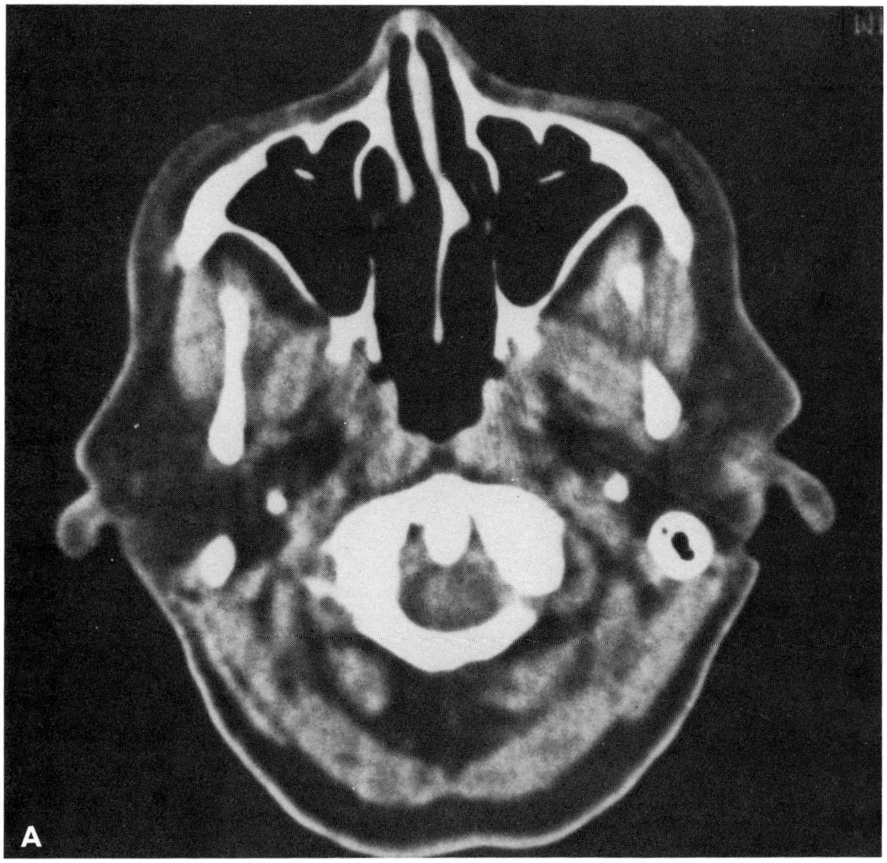

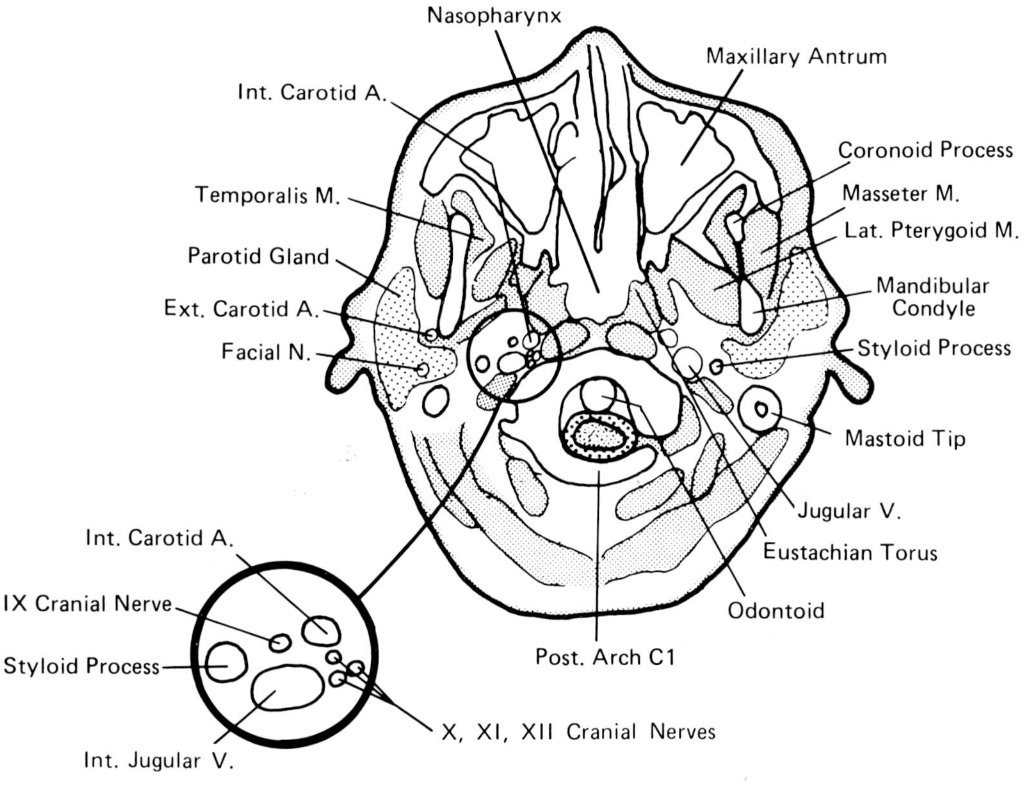

B

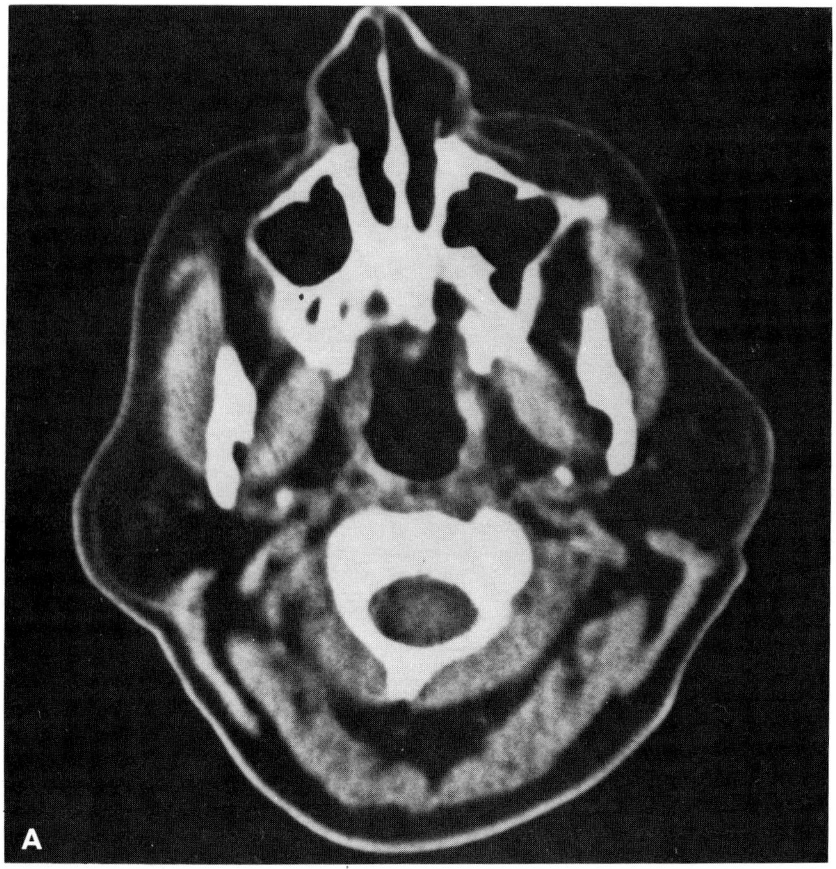

Fig. 3. A,B) (Level 2) Lower nasopharynx. Infratemporal fossa is well seen, limited laterally by mandibular ramus and parotid gland and anteriorly by posterolateral walls of maxillary antrum. Notice medial extension of deep lobe of parotid and its relationship with medial pterygoid muscle and carotid sheath contents. External carotid artery is usually embedded in parotid gland at this level, just proximal to origin of internal maxillary artery. Low density (fatty) tissue is normally present between pharyngeal musculature and pterygoid muscles.

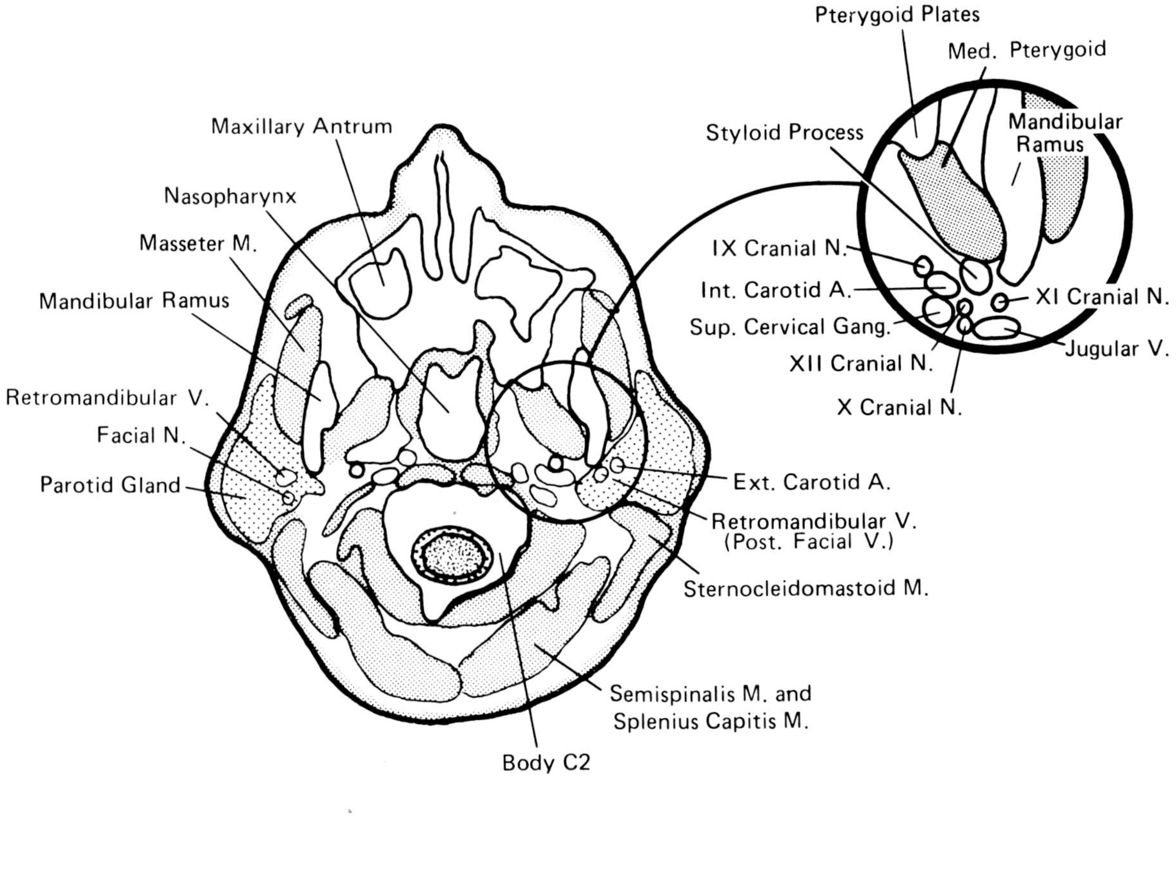

Fig. 4. A,B) (Level 3) Upper alveolar ridge — soft palate. Oral cavity and isthmus of pharynx are seen. Midportion of parotid gland is usually of relatively low density (less than surrounding muscles and vascular structures) due to variable amounts of fatty infiltration of parenchyma. Posterior facial vein is commonly visualized just posterior to mandibular ramus. Main trunk of facial nerve, although not visualized on CT images, is posterior to posterior facial vein.

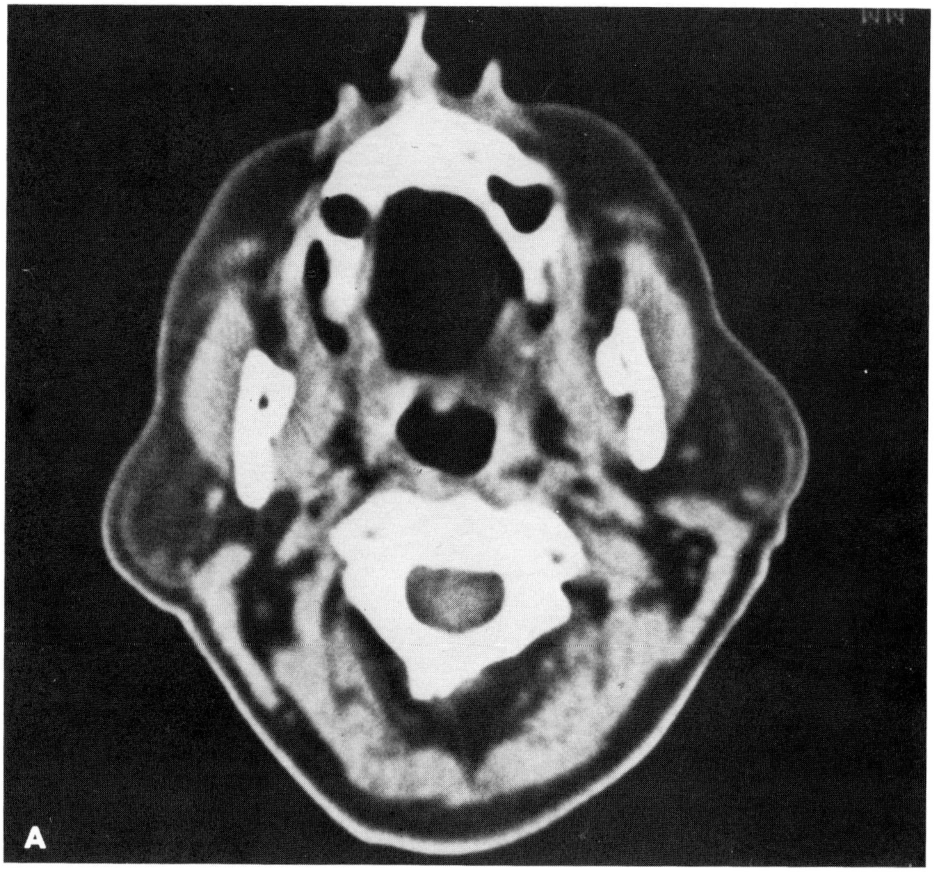

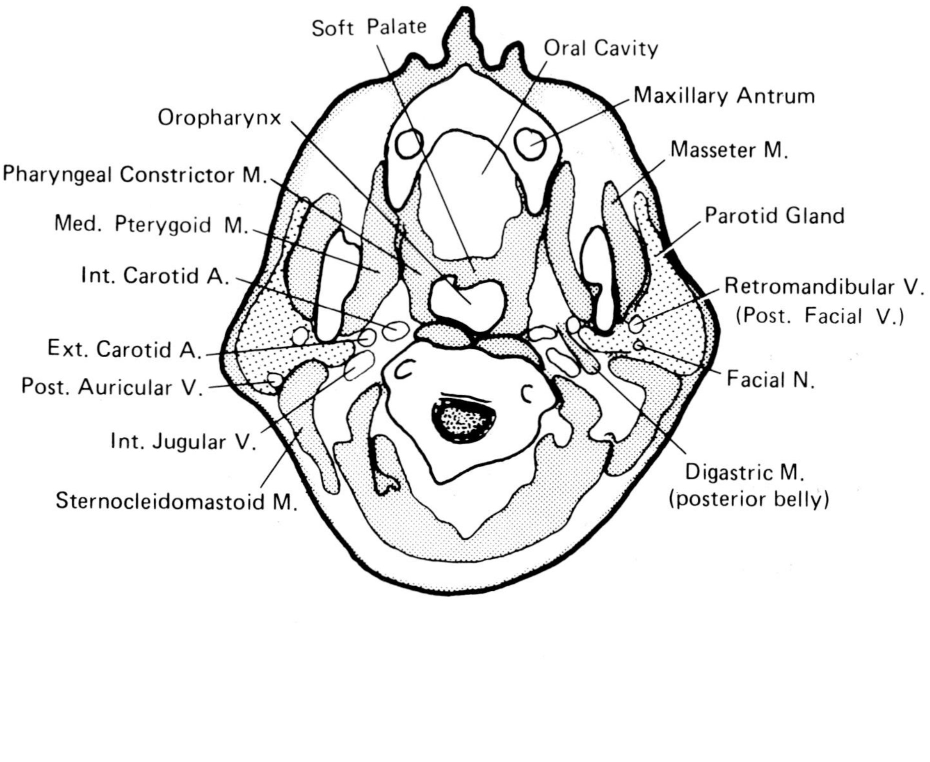

B

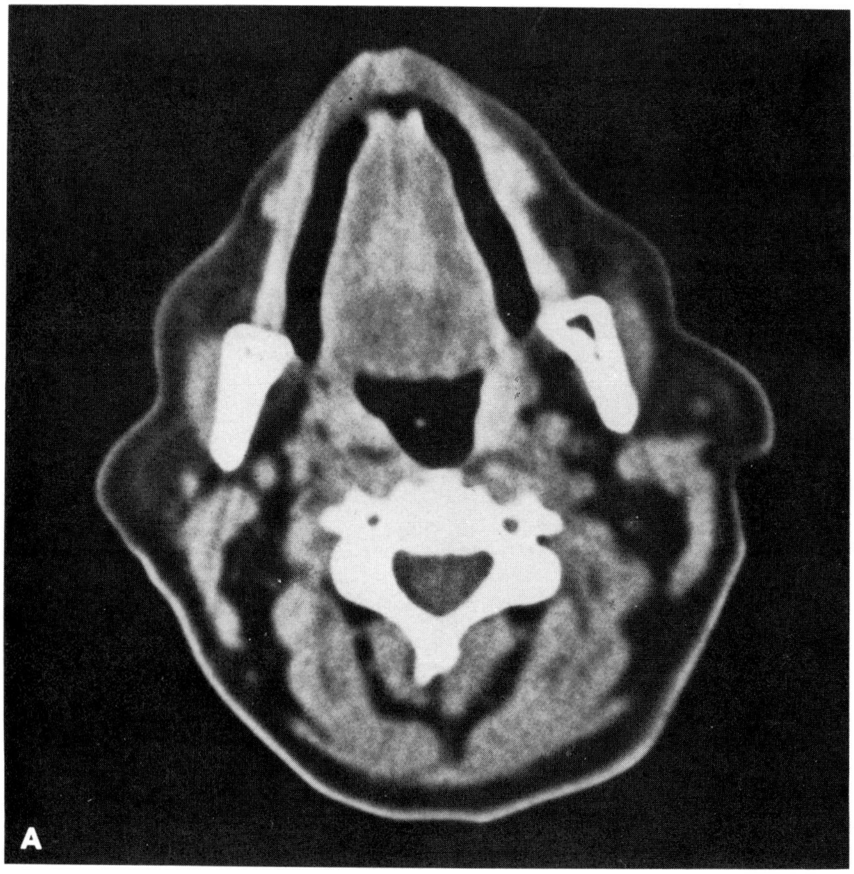

Fig. 5. A,B) (Level 4) Oral cavity — uvula. Uvula appears in cross section as round structure in middle of oropharynx, surrounded by palatine tonsils and oropharyngeal musculature (pharyngeal constrictor, palatoglossus and palatopharyngeus). Posterior belly of digastric muscle, an important anatomical landmark, is lateral to carotid sheath and external carotid artery. Posterior facial vein becomes external jugular vein after exiting parotid gland.

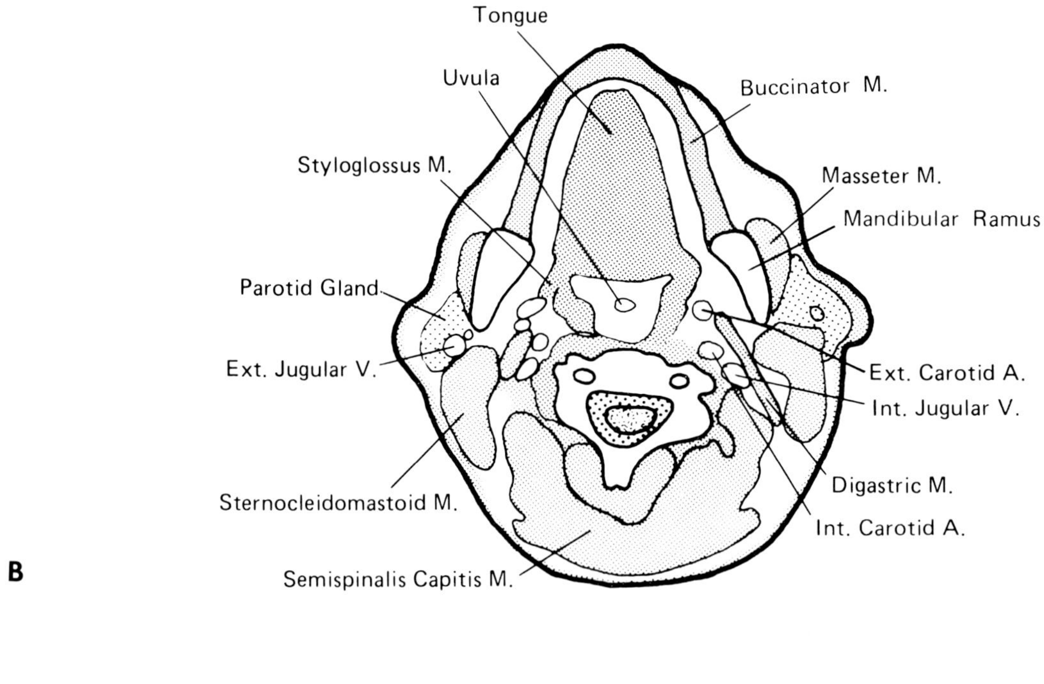

Fig. 6. A,B) (Level 5) Mandibular angle — submandibular gland. Oropharynx, base of tongue, and upper portion of submandibular gland are well visualized at this level. Internal and external carotid arteries and jugular veins are in close proximity to oropharynx. Inferior-most portion of parotid gland is separated from submandibular gland by stylomandibular ligament. Stylohyoid and digastric muscles separate carotid sheath structures from submandibular gland. Note that submandibular gland is usually denser than parotid gland.

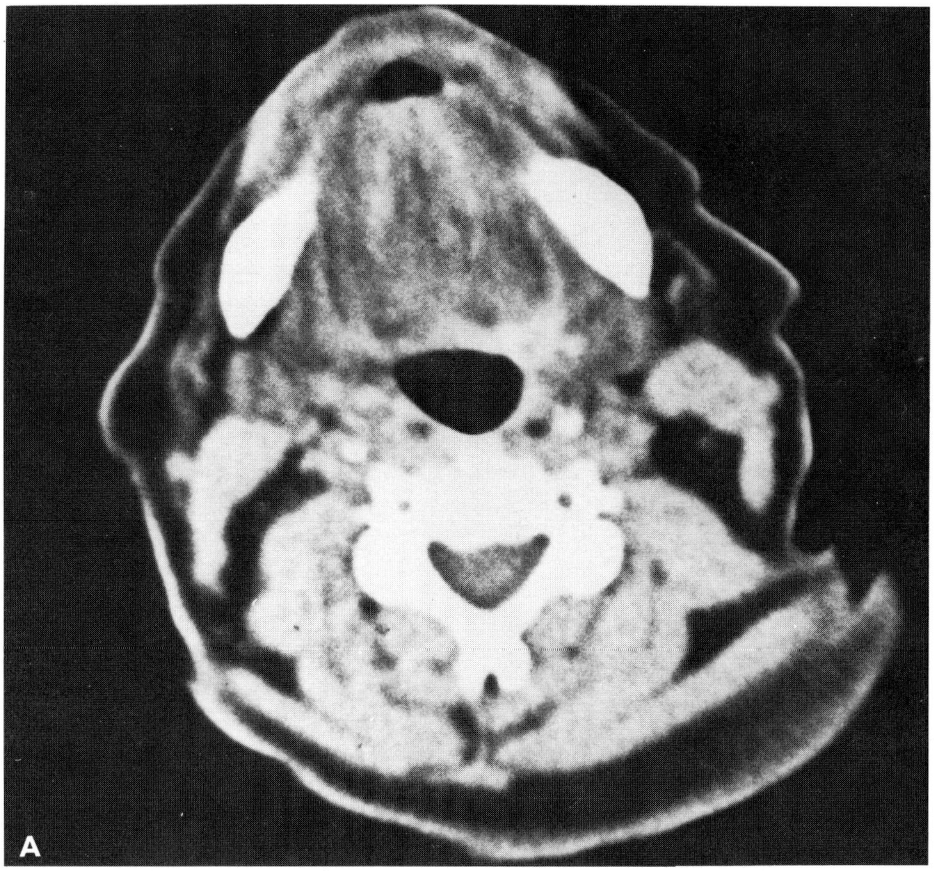

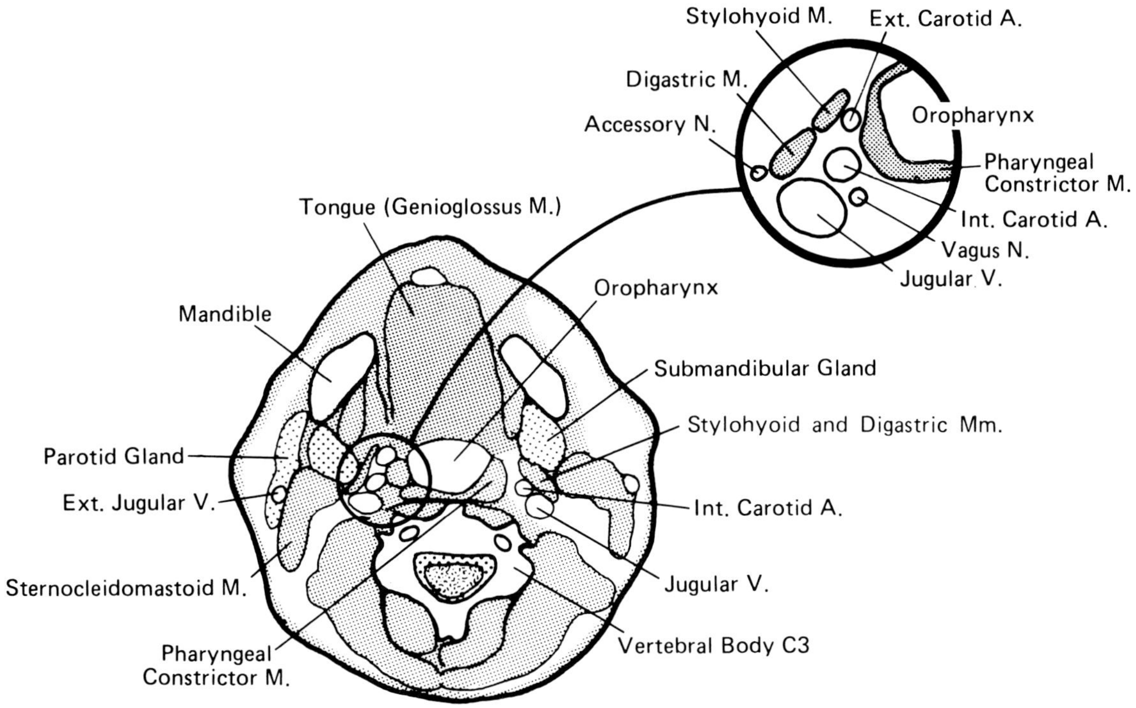

B

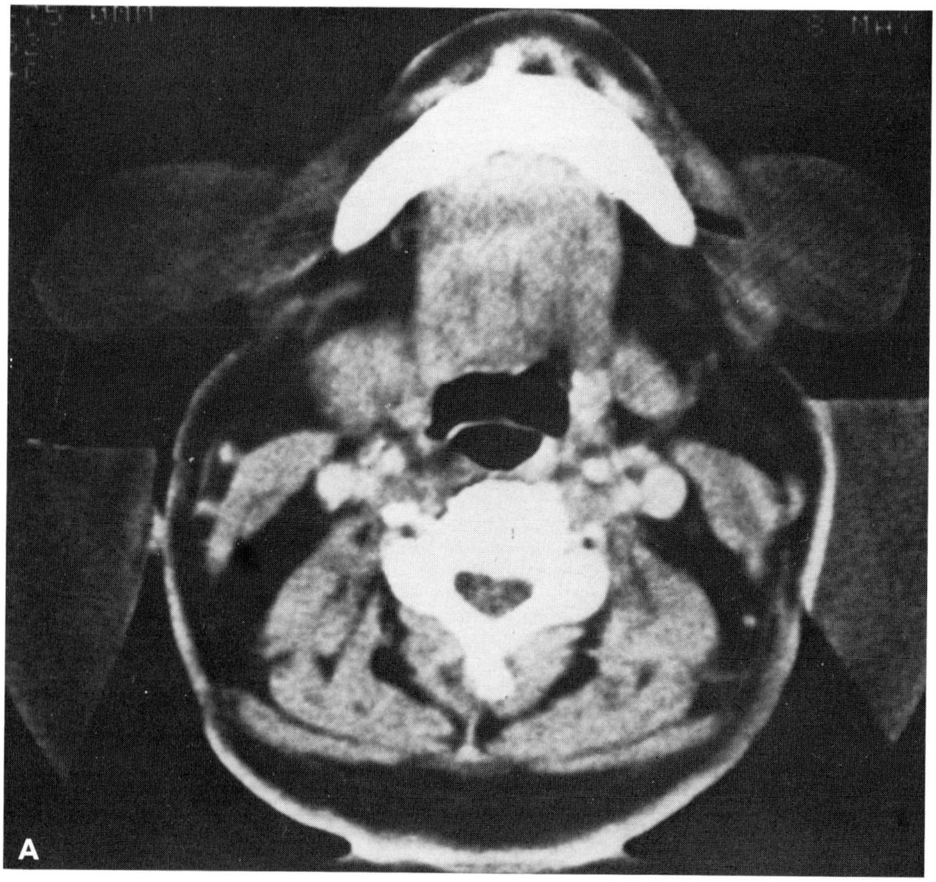

A

Fig. 7. A,B) (Level 6) Free border of epiglottis — superior horn of hyoid. Section demonstrates relationship of submandibular gland to base of tongue and free border of epiglottis. Superior horn of hyoid is adjacent to internal and external carotid arteries. Suprahyoid group of muscles (stylohyoid, mylohyoid, and geniohyoid) is visualized as group.

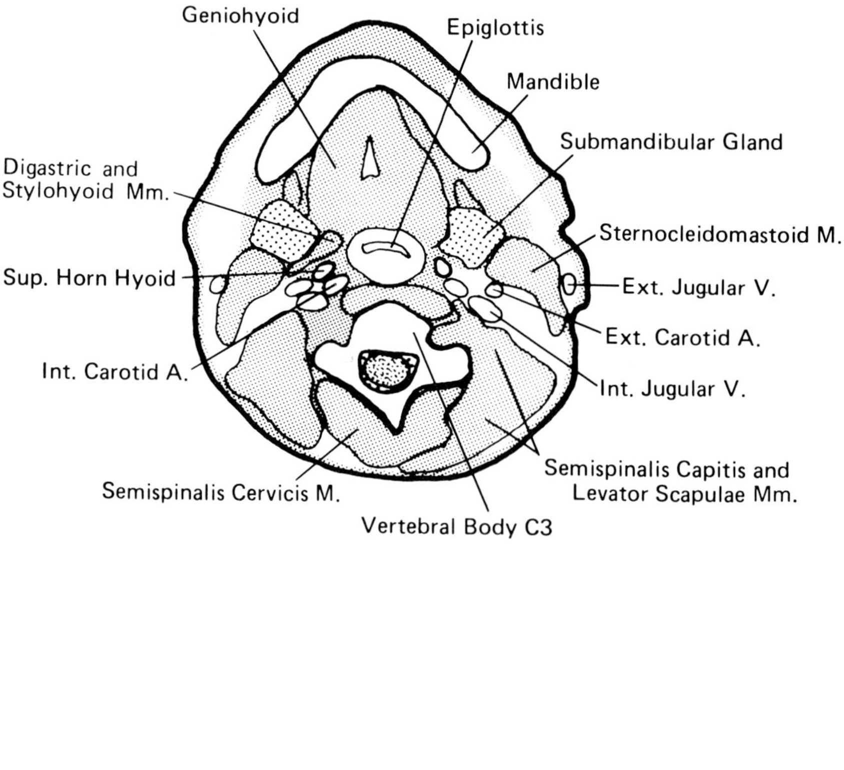

B

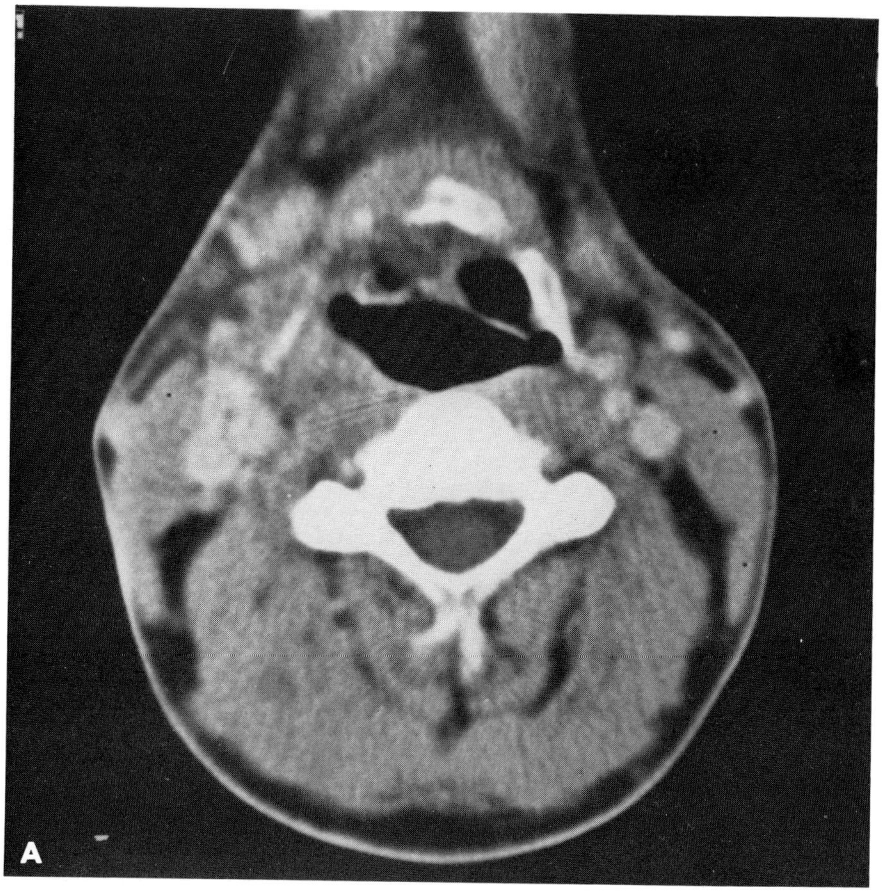

Fig. 8. A,B) (Level 7) Valleculae — hypopharynx. Valleculae, epiglottis and median glossoepiglottic fold are seen. Vallecular asymmetry is accounted for by secretions on right side. Vallecular spaces are best seen if scans are obtained while tongue is protruding. Fat layer deep to sternocleidomastoid is regularly seen irrespective of body habitus. Muscle definition is dependent on intermuscular fat rather than on muscle size. Hyoid body is a useful reference structure.

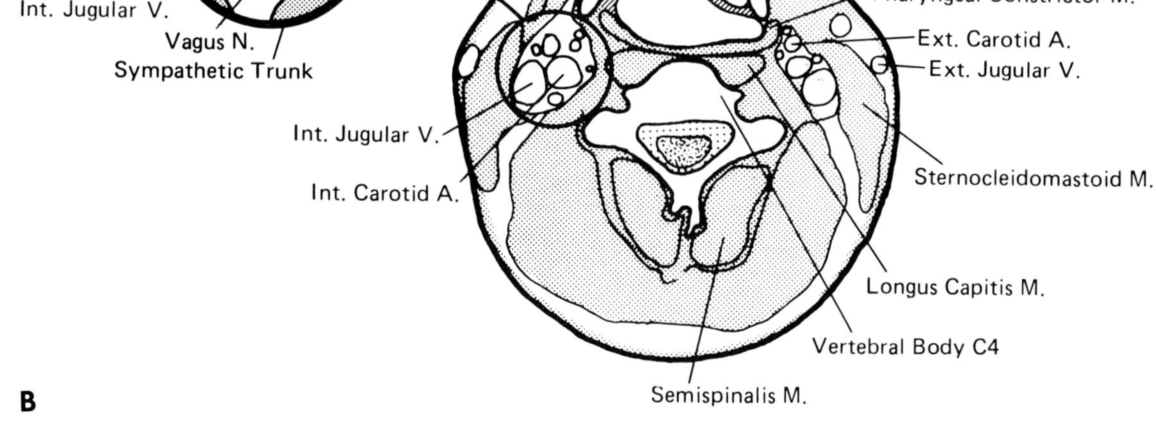

B

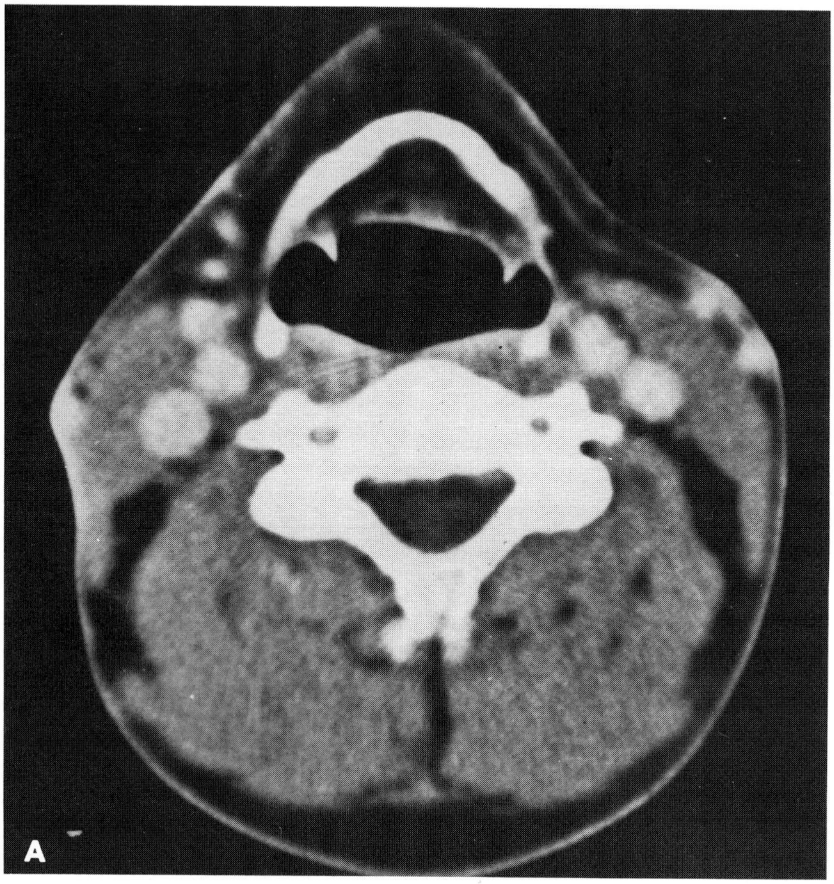

Fig. 9. A,B) (Level 8) Hyoid body — carotid bifurcation. Preepiglottic space is well demonstrated due to low density (fat). Portion of aryepiglottic fold is seen laterally. Carotid bifurcates at this level in most individuals. This section is at level of fourth or fifth cervical vertebral body. Note posterolateral portion of jugular vein in relation to carotid bifurcation. Foramina for vertebral arteries can be visualized in favorable sections.

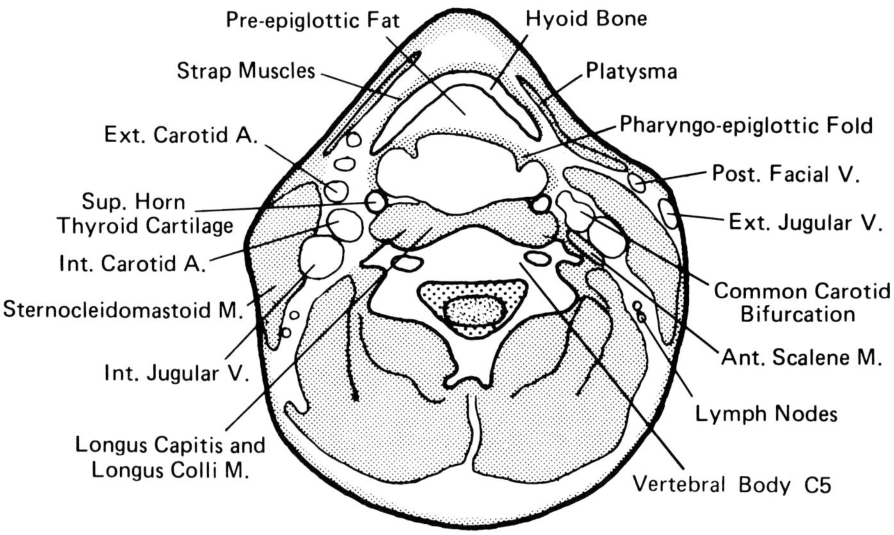

Fig. 10. A,B) (Level 9) Thyroid notch — aryepiglottic folds. Thyroid alae are seen at level of thyroid notch. Pattern and extent of ossification of thyroid cartilage is variable but usually symmetrical. Aryepiglottic folds separate laryngeal vestibule from piriform sinuses. Common carotid artery and jugular vein lie under sternocleidomastoid posterolateral to thyroid lamina.

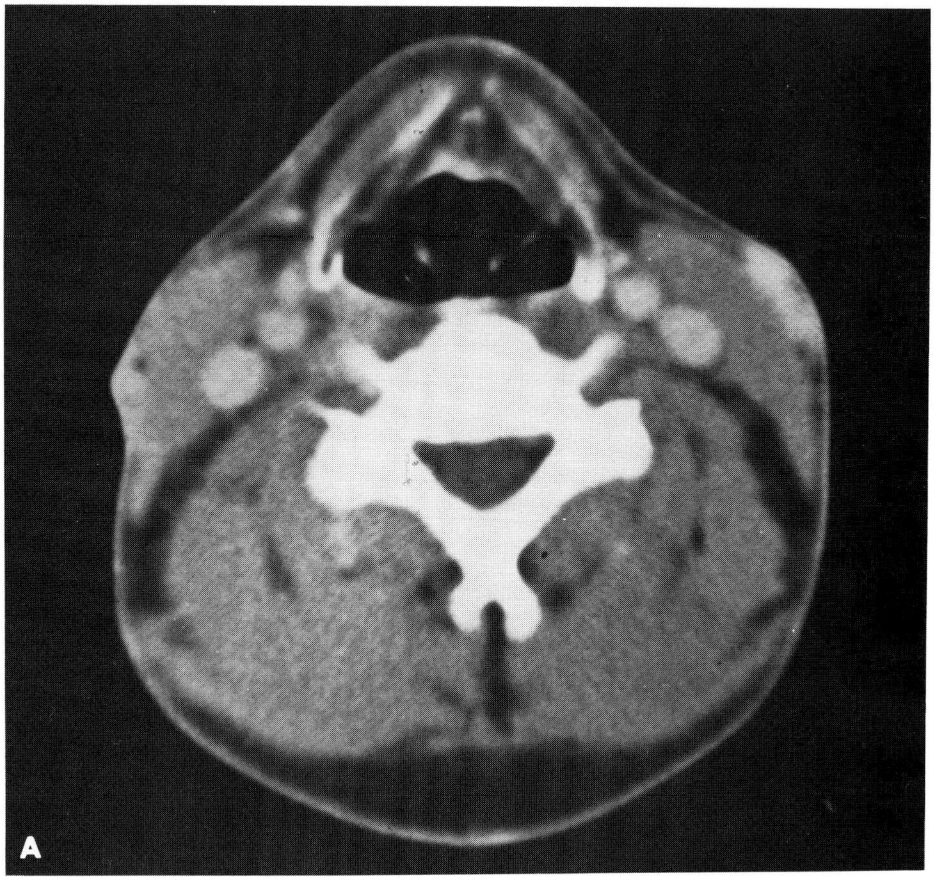

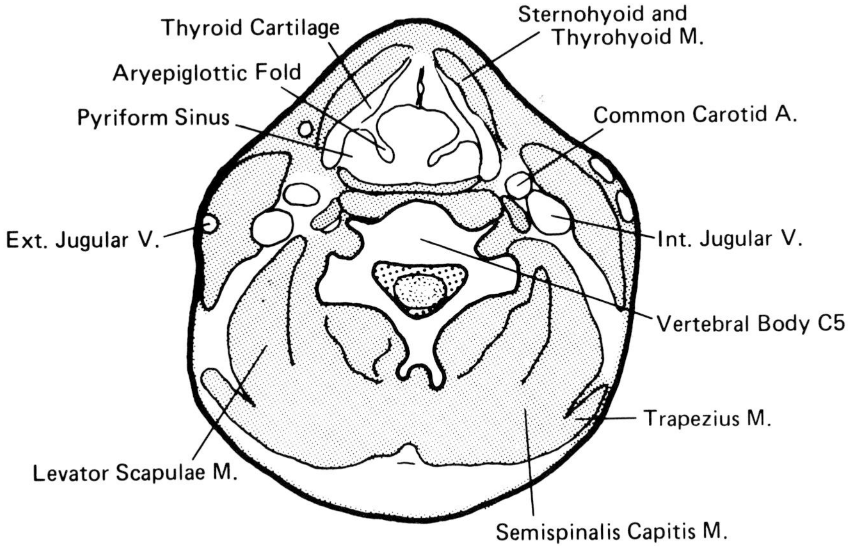

B

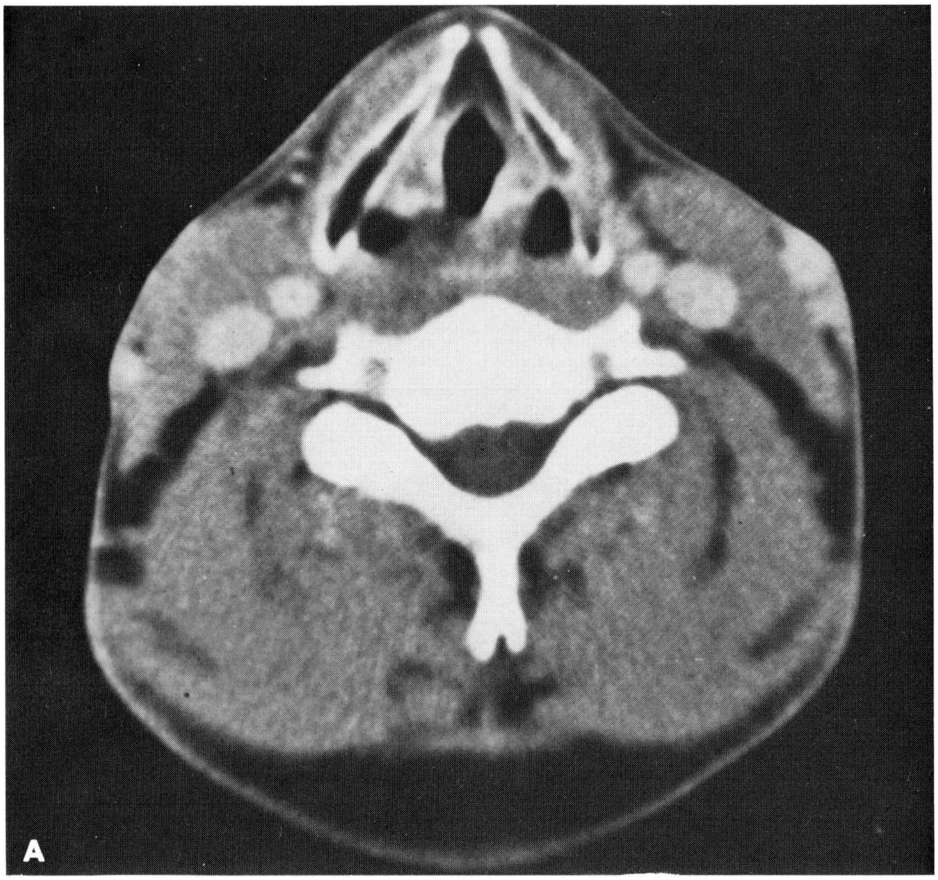

Fig. 11. A,B) (Level 10) Arytenoid cartilages — laryngeal vestibule. Upper portion of arytenoid cartilages is present at posteroinferior aspect of aryepiglottic folds. Corniculate cartilages are very seldom calcified and cannot be identified within aryepiglottic fold.

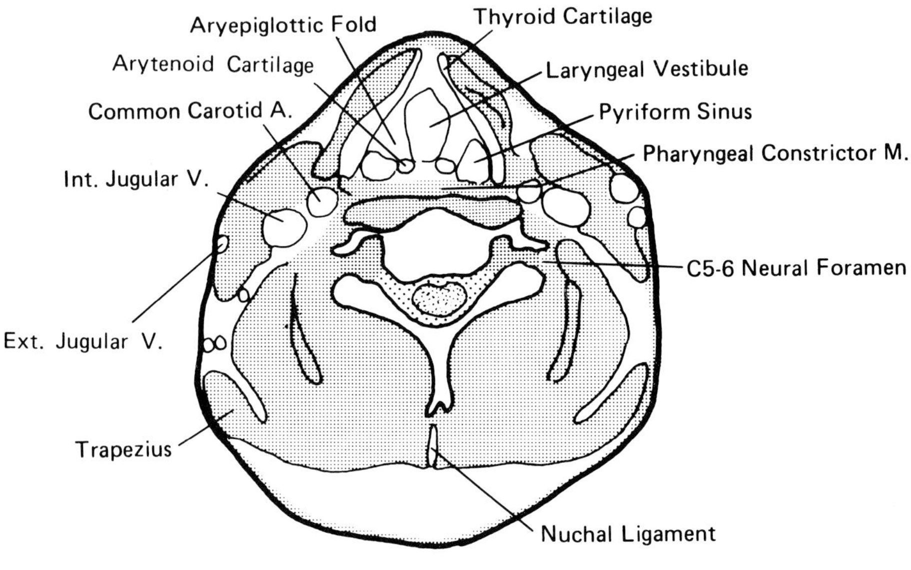

B

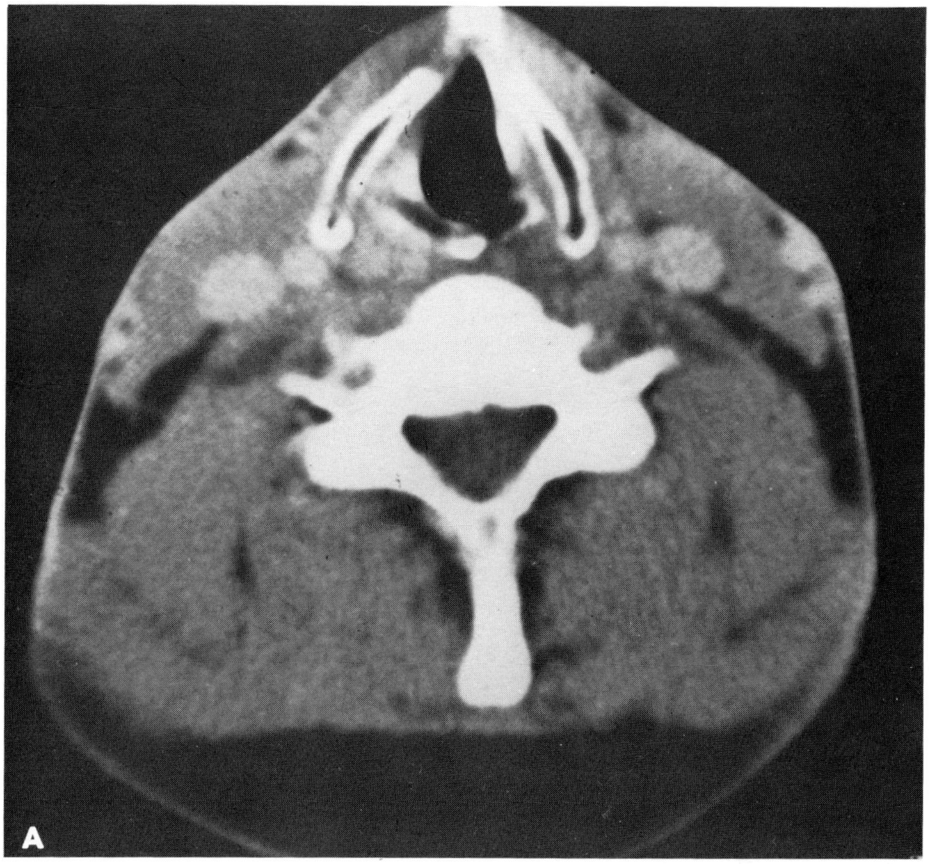

Fig. 12. A,B) (Level 11) Vocal cords. True vocal cords are identified by close apposition of anterior commissure to inner surface of thyroid cartilage. Uppermost portion of cricoid may be noted at this level.

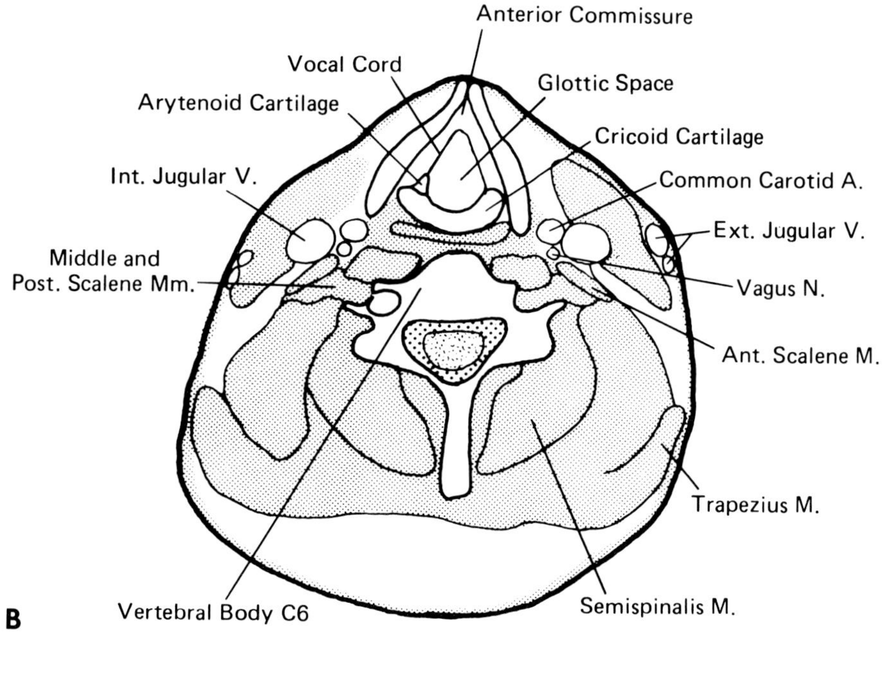

B

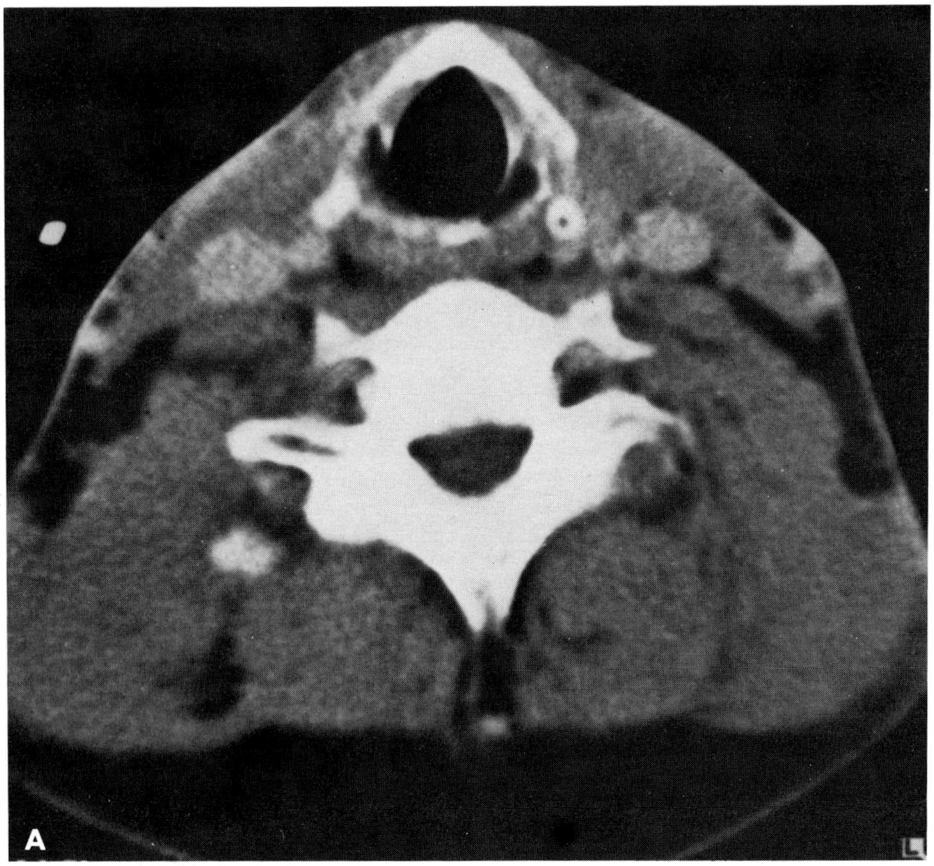

Fig. 13. A,B) (Level 12) Subglottis. Mucosa of subglottis is closely applied to cricoid ring and thyroid cartilage. Cervical esophagus is posterior to posterior lamina of cricoid. Note relationship of cricoid lamina, especially on left, to inferior cornu of thyroid cartilage. In children and young adults carotid arteries and jugular veins may be difficult to separate from adjacent muscles unless rapid infusion of contrast material is employed during examination. Normal lymph nodes usually measure less than 1 cm in diameter.

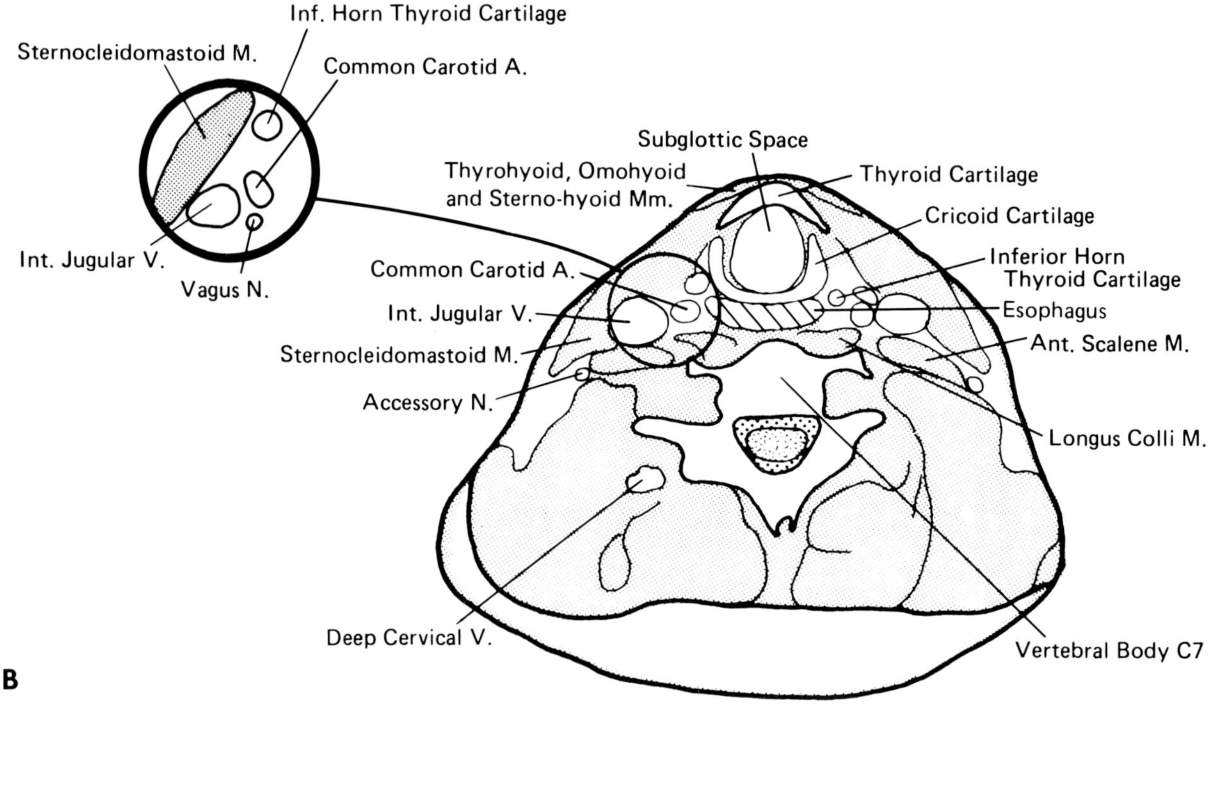

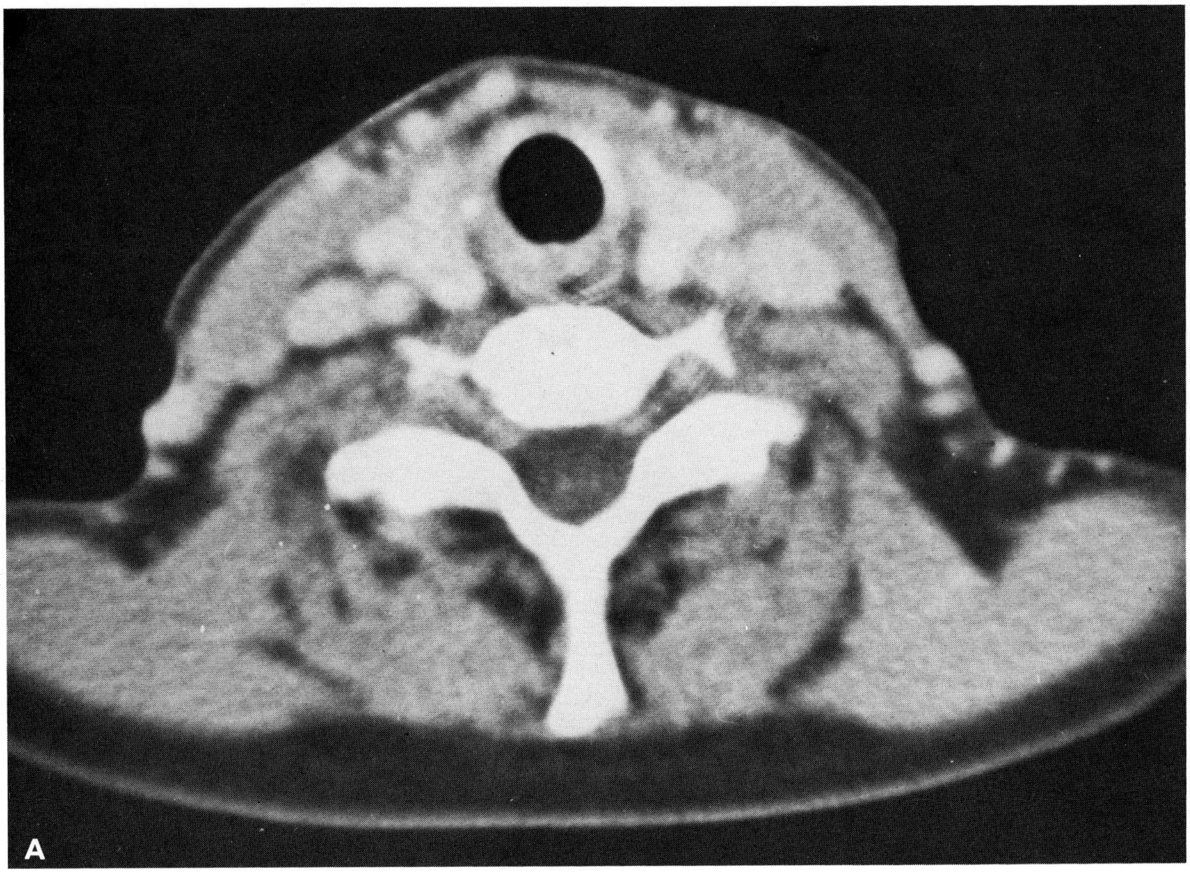

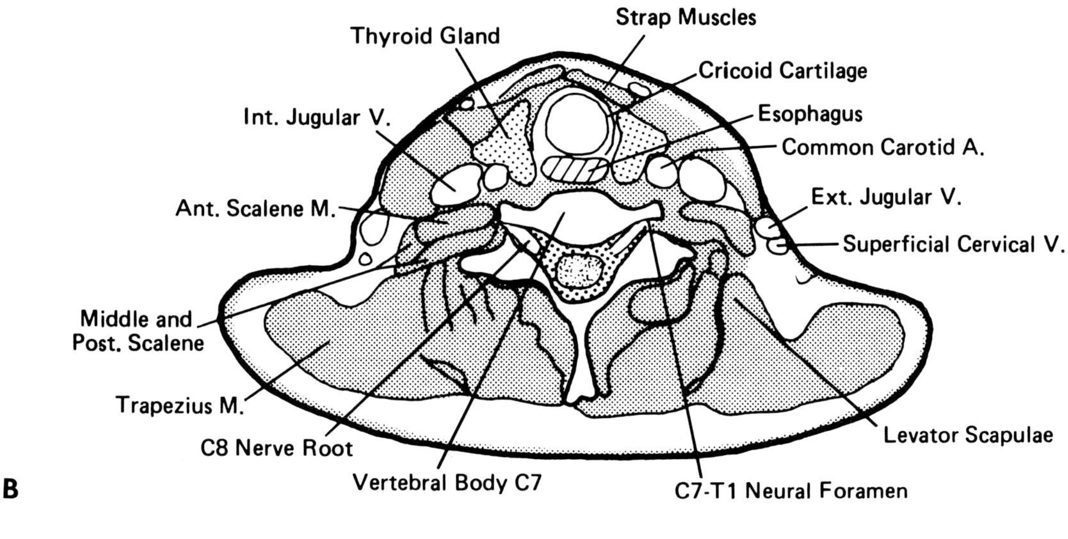

Fig. 14. A,B) (Level 13) Cricoid ring — laryngotrachea. Cricoid ring surrounds airway. Upper poles of thyroid gland are readily identified due to their high density which is result of high vascularity of thyroid gland and its high iodine content.

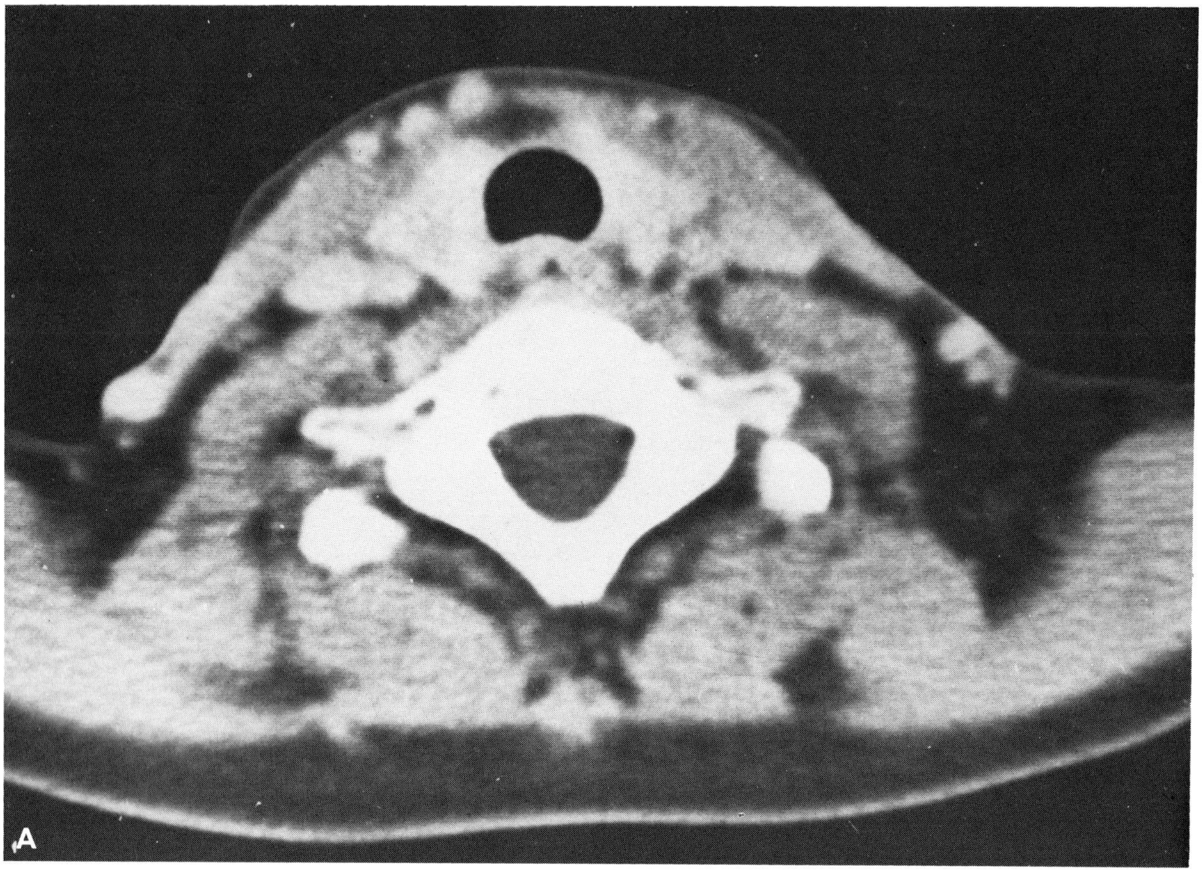

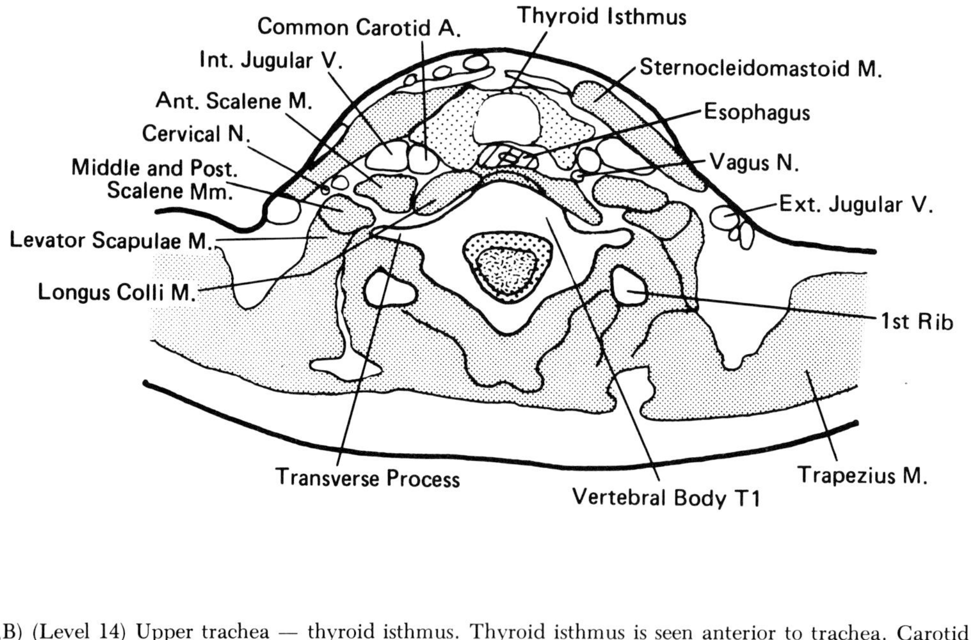

B

Fig. 15. A,B) (Level 14) Upper trachea — thyroid isthmus. Thyroid isthmus is seen anterior to trachea. Carotid arteries lie posterior to thyroid gland while jugular veins are more laterally placed between anterior scalene muscles and sternocleidomastoid. Jugular veins are usually asymmetrical, right being larger in most subjects.

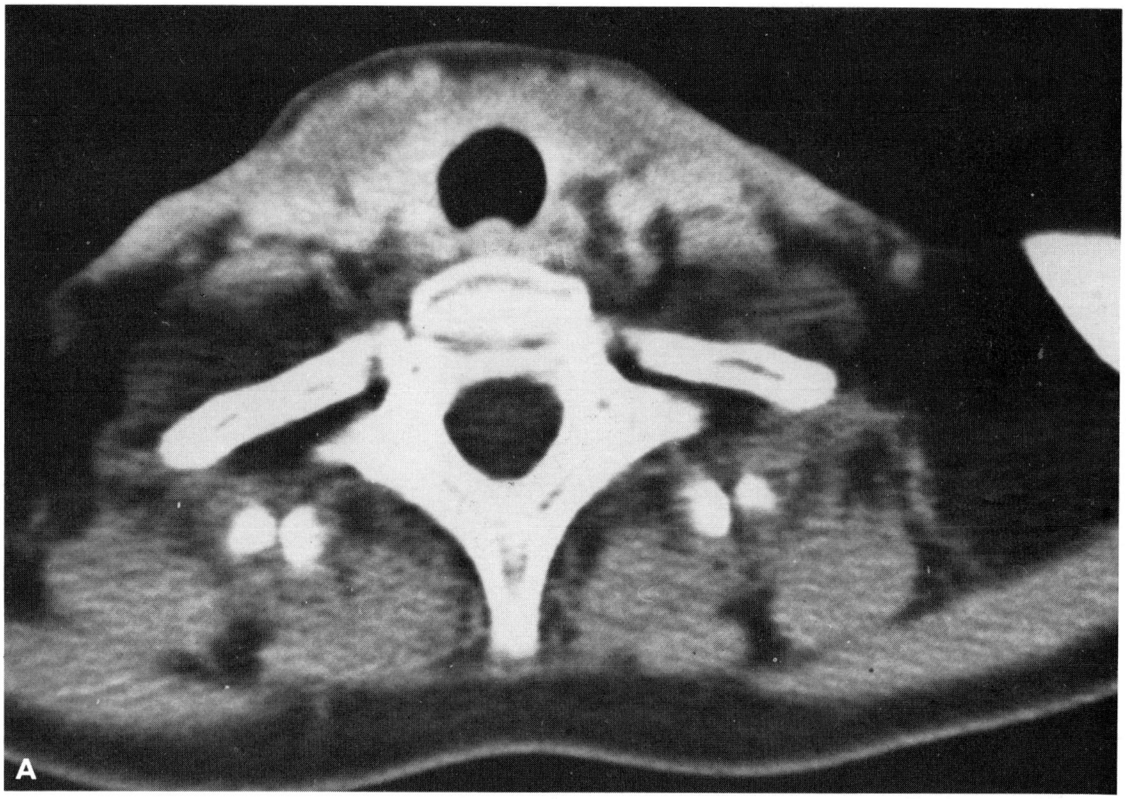

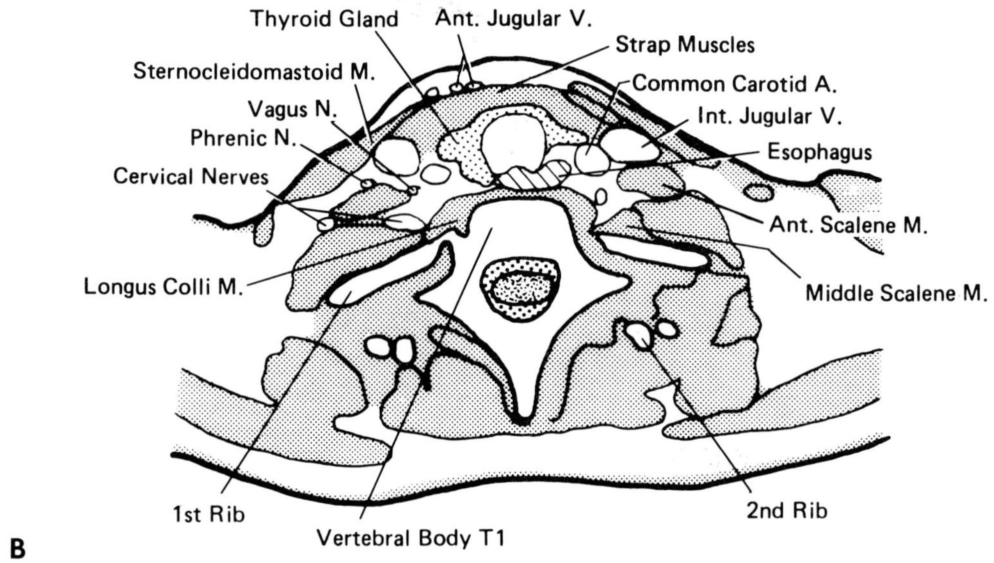

Fig. 16. A,B) (Level 15) First rib — lower thyroid gland. This section, just above thoracic inlet, is at level of first rib. Individual tracheal rings are visible in older individuals only as they become calcified. Esophagus is commonly just to left of midline at this level. Lower cervical nerves may be seen directed inferolaterally between anterior scalene and middle and posterior scalenes group. Anterior scalenes may be prominent in patients with chronic obstructive pulmonary disease and should not be mistaken for masses or adenopathy.

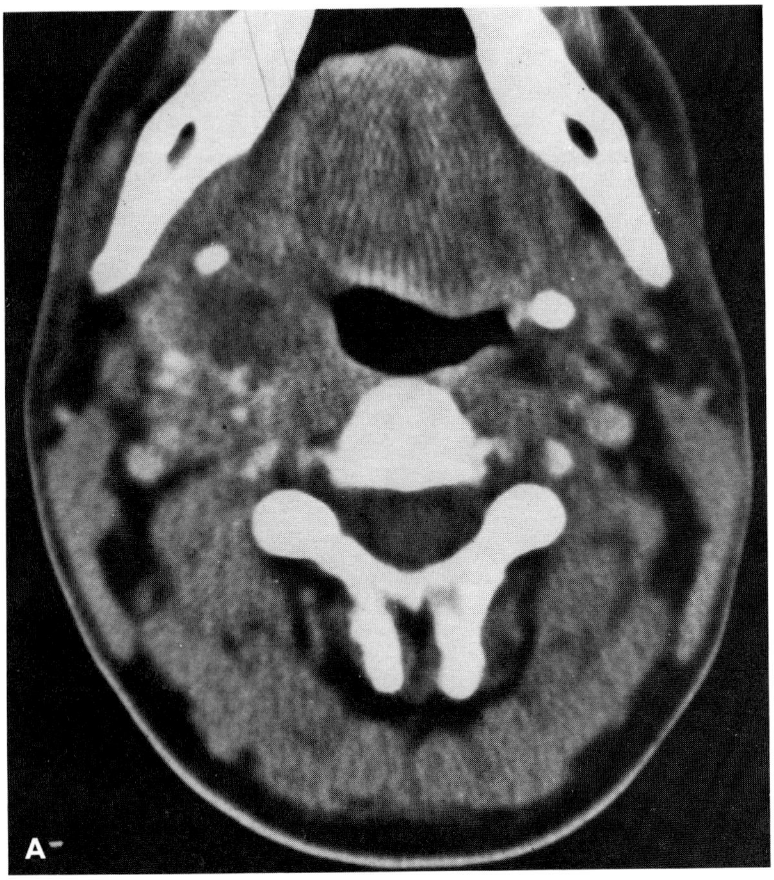

Code for diagrams in Figures 17-28.

Pathology

Major salivary gland or thyroid

Muscle and soft tissue

Fig. 17. (Case 1) Metastatic papillary carcinoma of thyroid gland. Patient was 35-year-old man with past history of papillary carcinoma of thyroid presenting with right parapharyngeal mass. A) Level 3. Cystic mass, 2.5-cm, in right parapharyngeal space displaces styloid process anteriorly and laterally. B) Level 6. Lateral pharyngeal wall is distorted and right submandibular gland is displaced anteriorly. Relationship of cystic mass to carotid artery and jugular vein is demonstrated. Note tip of epiglottis. C) Drawing from level 6. Box - Density scanner.

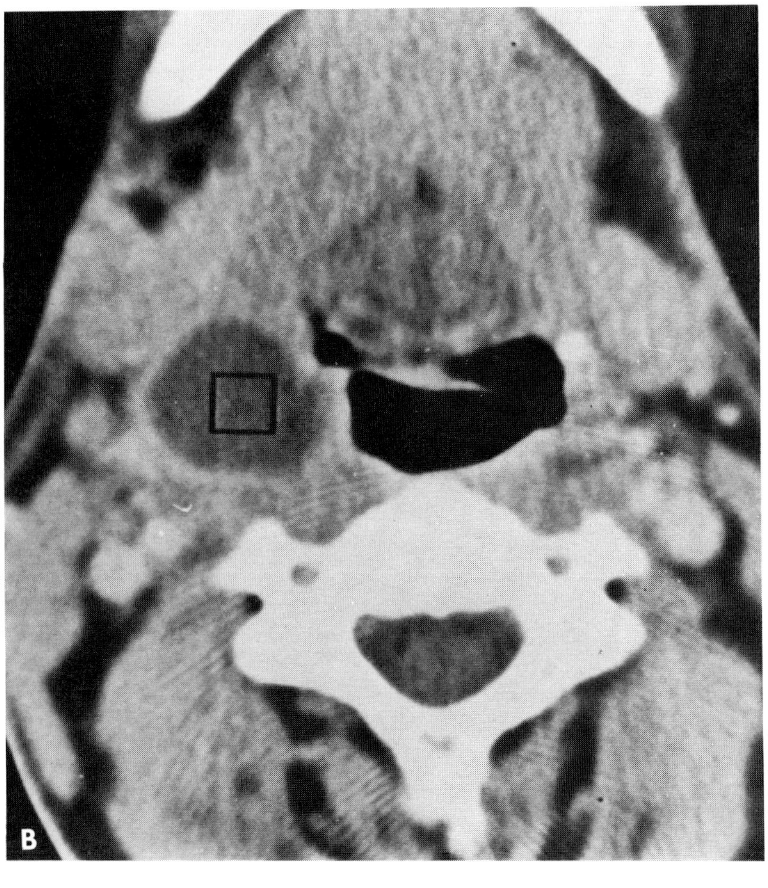

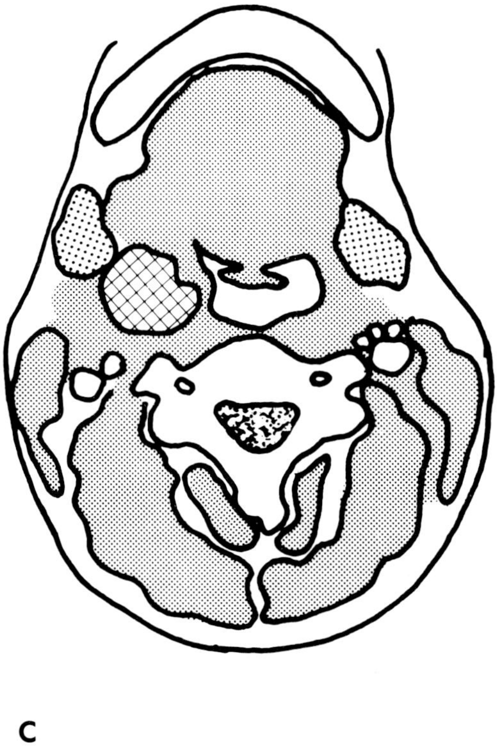

C

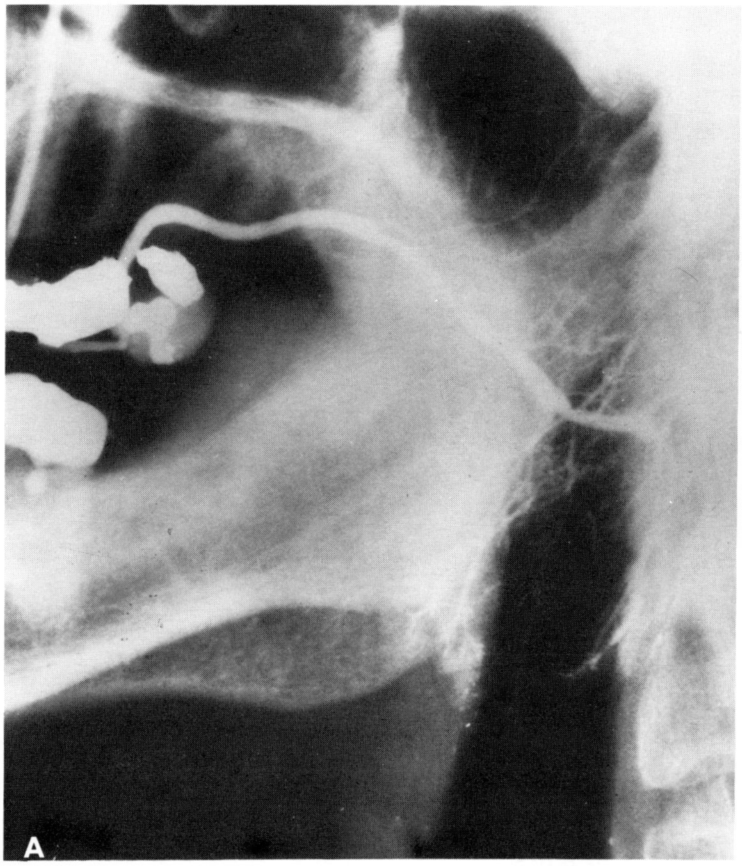

Fig. 18. (Case 2) Adenopathy, Hodgkin's disease. Patient was 68-year-old man with two palpable masses in right parotid region. A) Dialogram. Displacement and distention of ducts suggests single intraparotid mass lesion. B,C) Level 3. Two sharply defined masses are present in right parotid. Note clear visualization of posterior facial vein within normal left parotid gland between two masses. Vein is clearly seen because study was done during contrast media infusion.

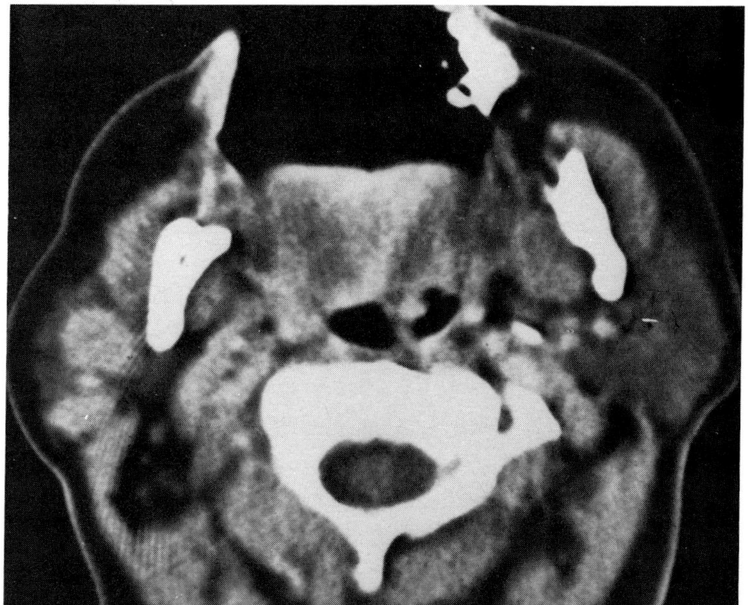

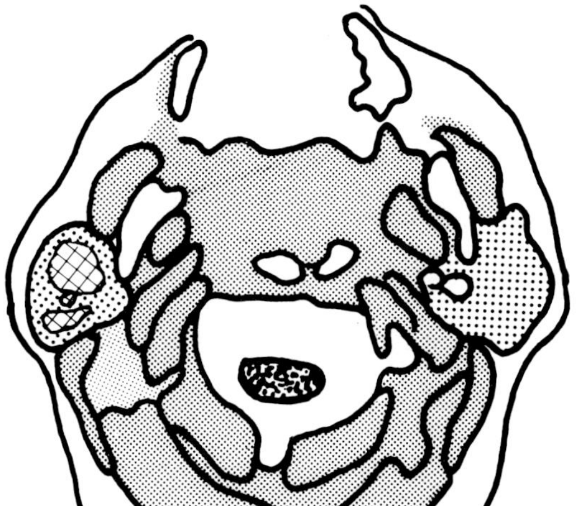

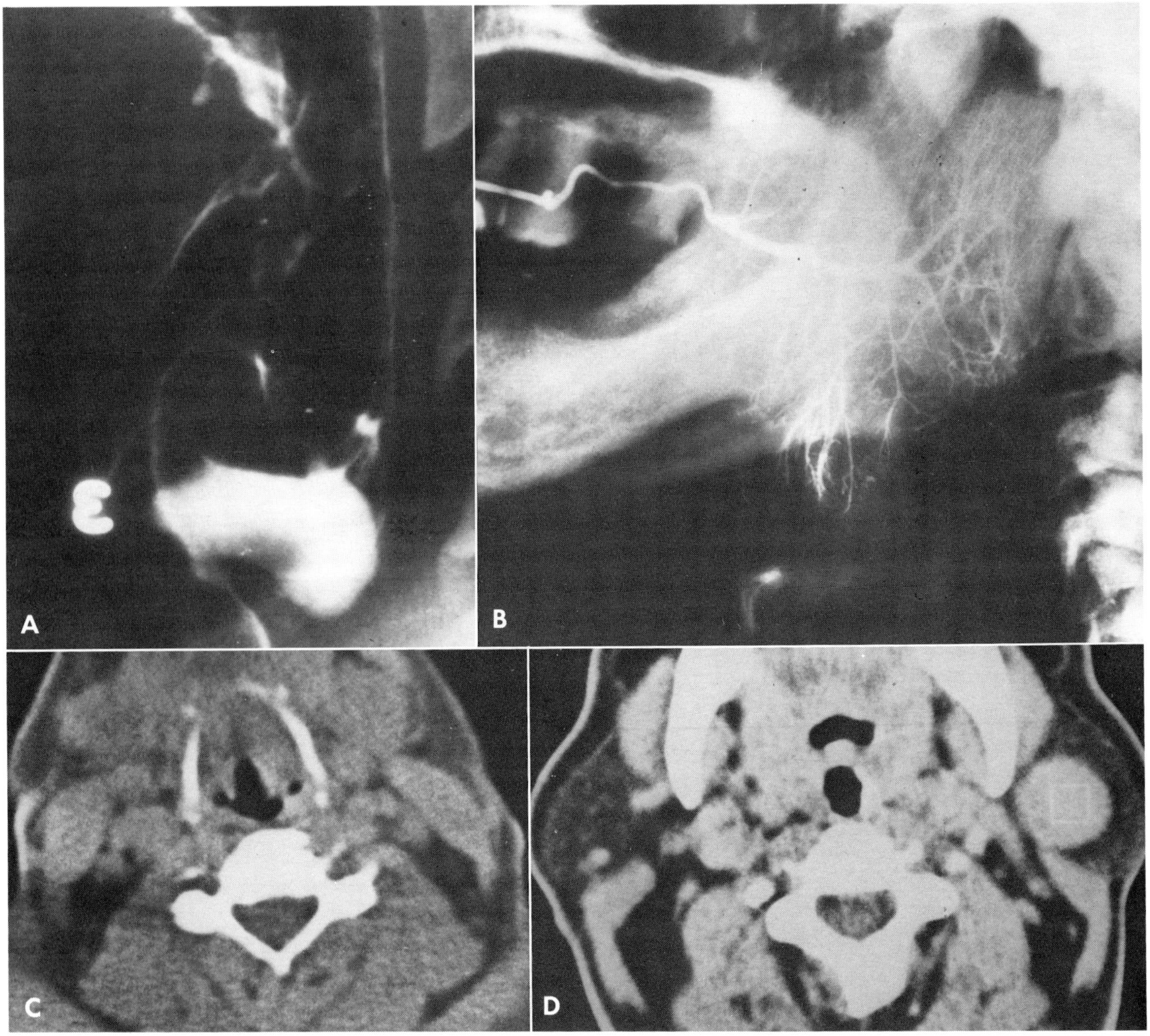

Fig. 19. (Case 3) Carcinoma of epiglottis and left parotid Warthin's tumor. Patient was 53-year-old man admitted for evaluation of supraglottic lesion. He had asymptomatic left parotid mass noted on physical examination. A) Laryngogram. Thickened epiglottis and distortion of valleculae. B) Sialogram. Ductal displacement in lower portion of superficial lobe suggests intraparotid mass. C) Level 7. Thickened epiglottis, obliteration of valleculae and infiltration of preepiglottic space. D) Level 4. Sharply defined mass within left parotid gland. Moderate fatty infiltration of parenchyma accounts for low density of both parotid glands. Uvula and portion of soft palate separate oral cavity from oropharynx. E) Line drawing from level 4.

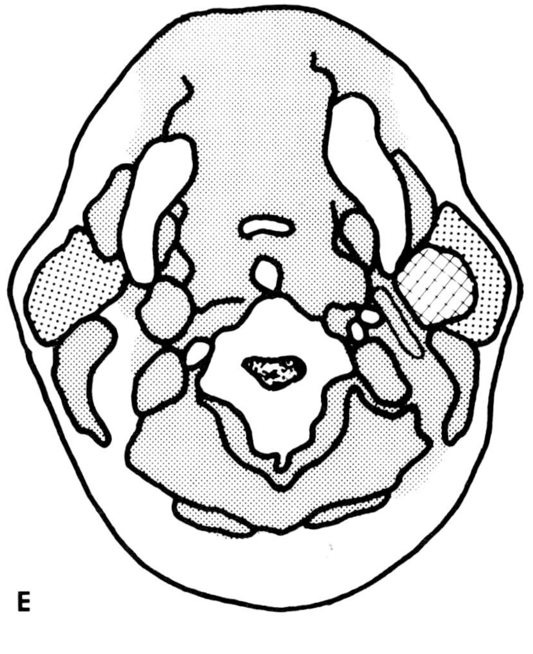

E

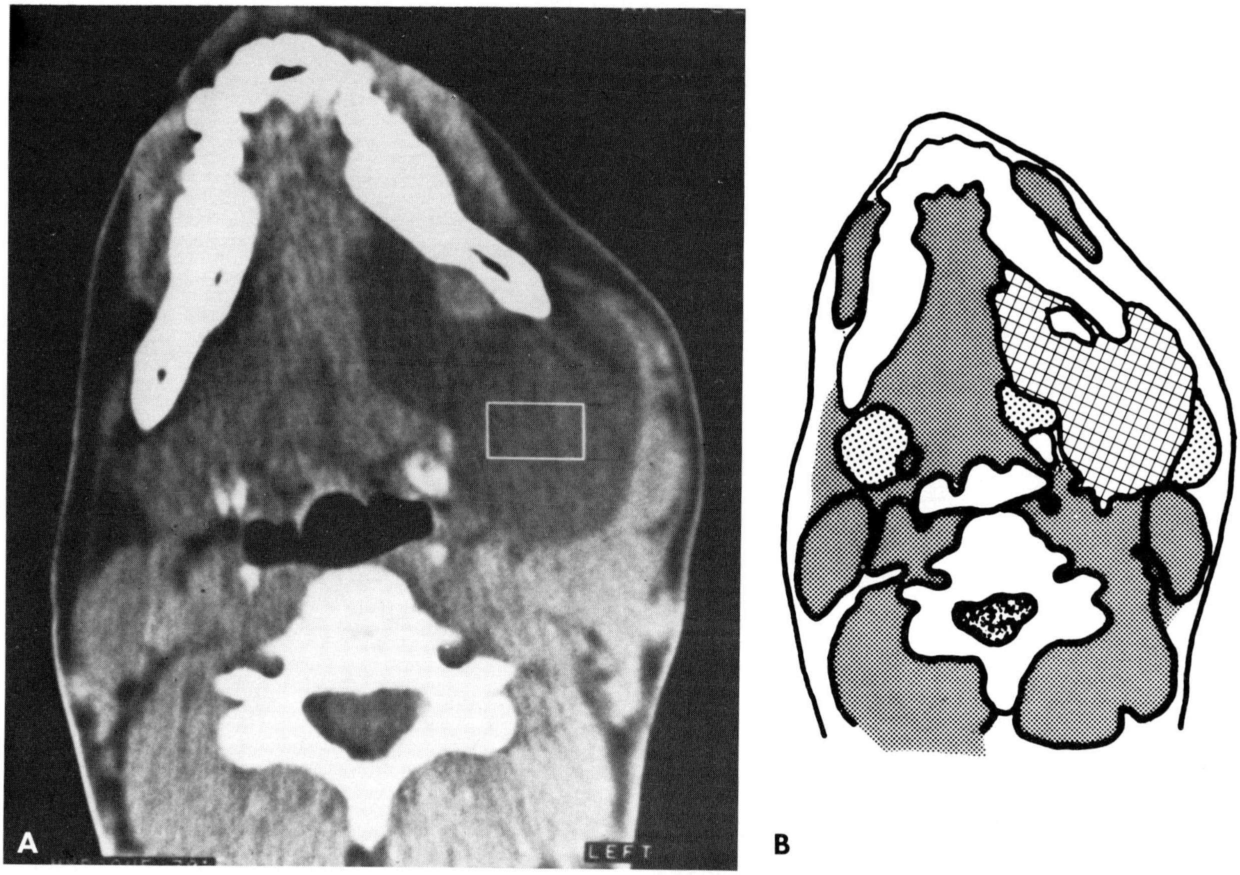

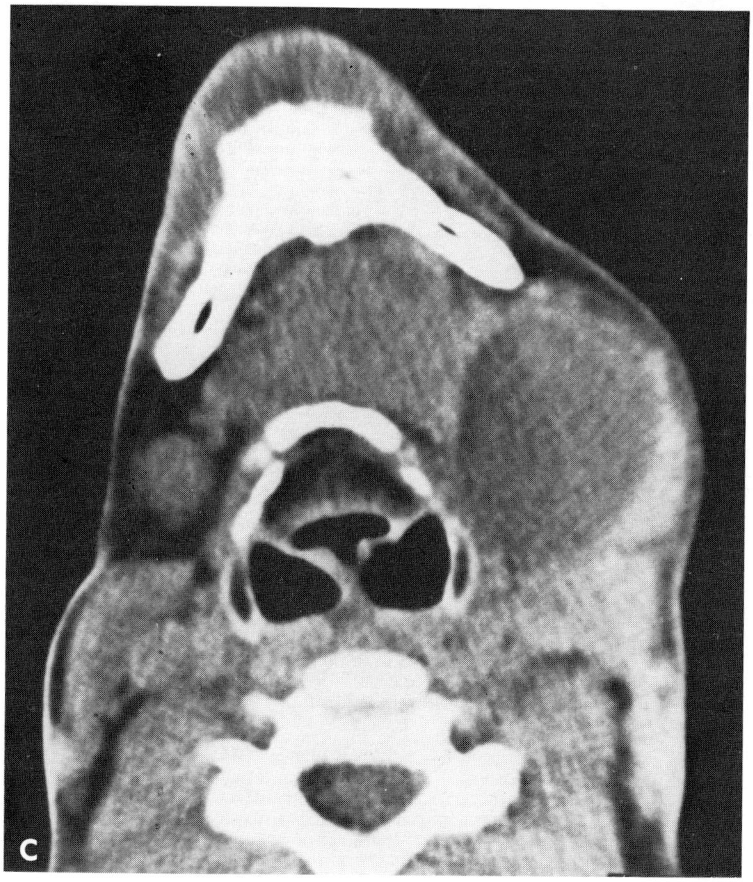

Fig. 20. (Case 4) Left sublingual gland cyst, ranula. Patient was 26-year-old man with slowly enlarging left neck mass. A,B) Level 6. Cystic mass located between mylohyoid muscle and deformed left submandibular gland. Anterior portion of mass extends to floor of mouth. C) Level 8. Hyoid is displaced to right by lower portion of mass.

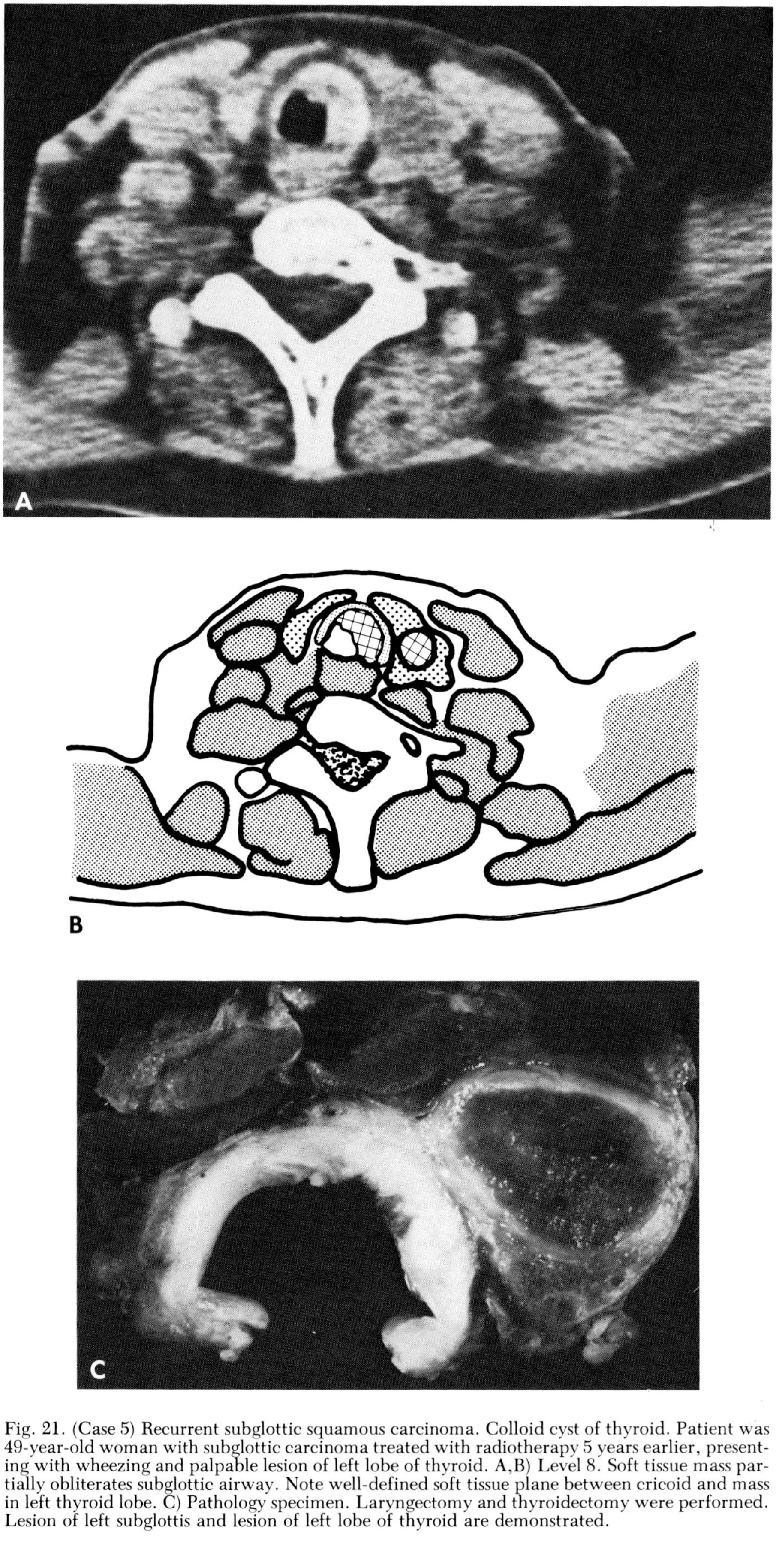

Fig. 21. (Case 5) Recurrent subglottic squamous carcinoma. Colloid cyst of thyroid. Patient was 49-year-old woman with subglottic carcinoma treated with radiotherapy 5 years earlier, presenting with wheezing and palpable lesion of left lobe of thyroid. A,B) Level 8. Soft tissue mass partially obliterates subglottic airway. Note well-defined soft tissue plane between cricoid and mass in left thyroid lobe. C) Pathology specimen. Laryngectomy and thyroidectomy were performed. Lesion of left subglottis and lesion of left lobe of thyroid are demonstrated.

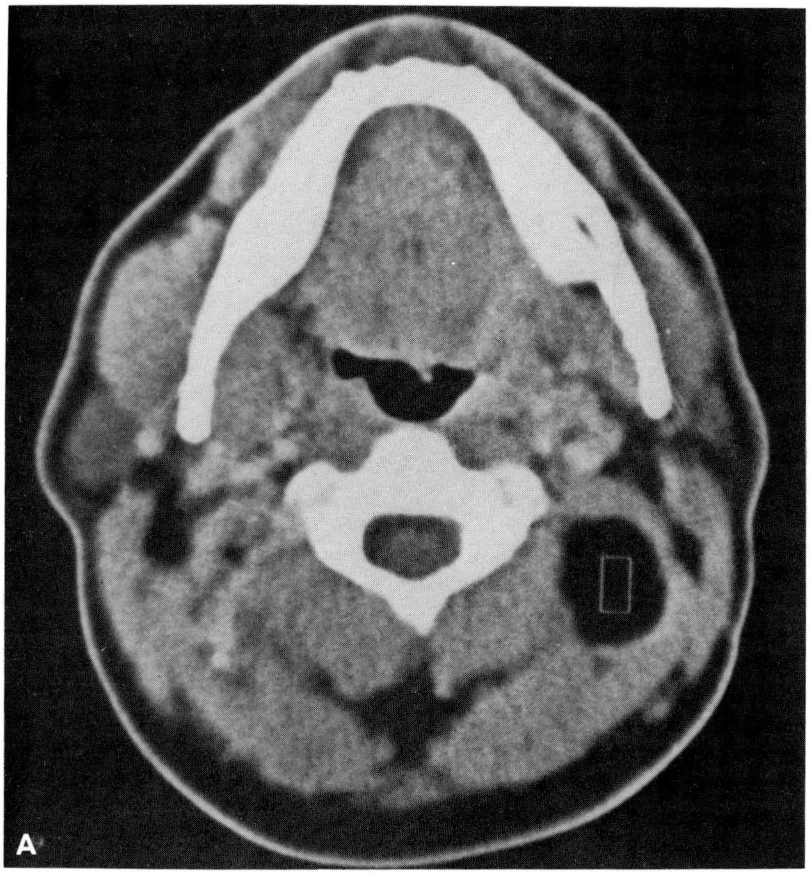

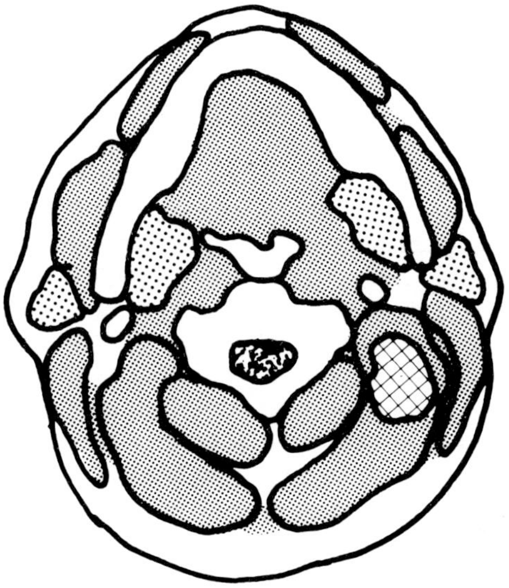

B

Fig. 22. (Case 6) Lipoma. Patient was 50-year-old man with mass in posterior neck. A,B) Level 4. Sharply defined mass with very low density (fat), located between semispinalis muscle and spenius capitis muscle is visualized.

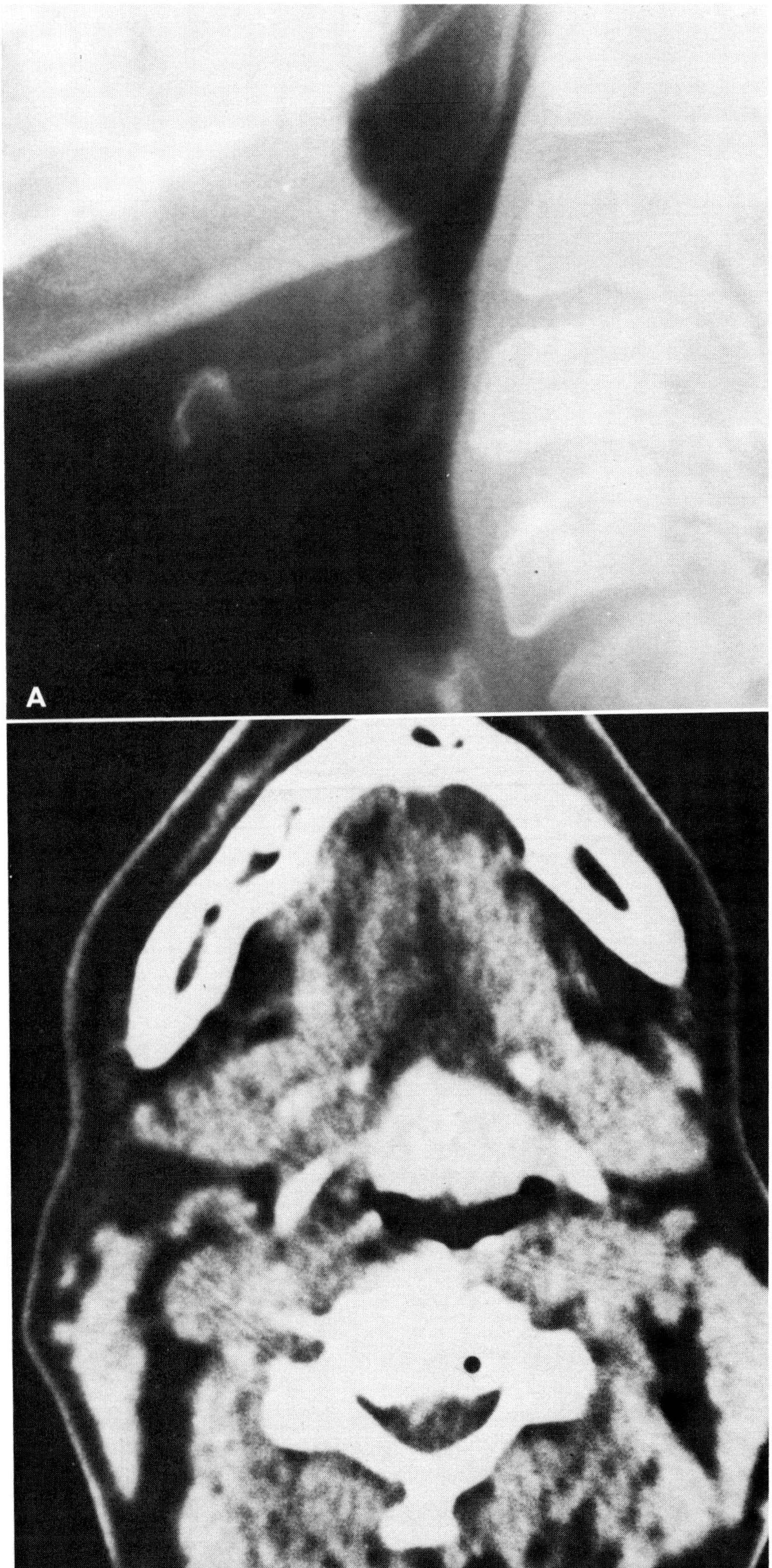

Fig. 23. (Case 7) Lingual thyroid. Patient was 39-year-old woman with lump in throat. A) Radiograph. Smooth mass in base of tongue displacing epiglottis posteriorly. B,C) Level 6. CT done without contrast. High density "mass" in base of tongue. Density of this lesion is same as that of normal thyroid tissue, result of high iodine content. Superior horns of hyoid are seen in either side of mass.

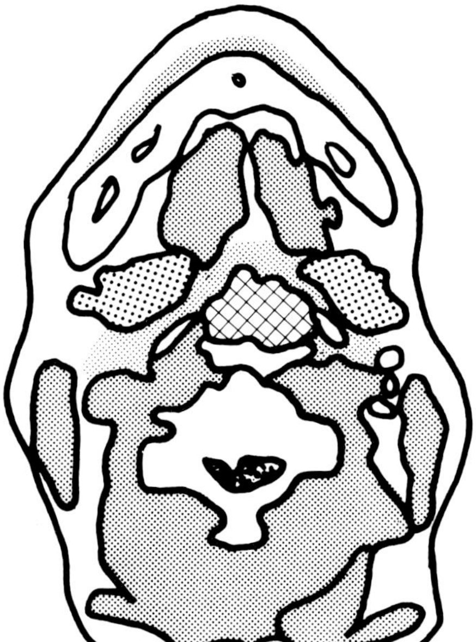

C

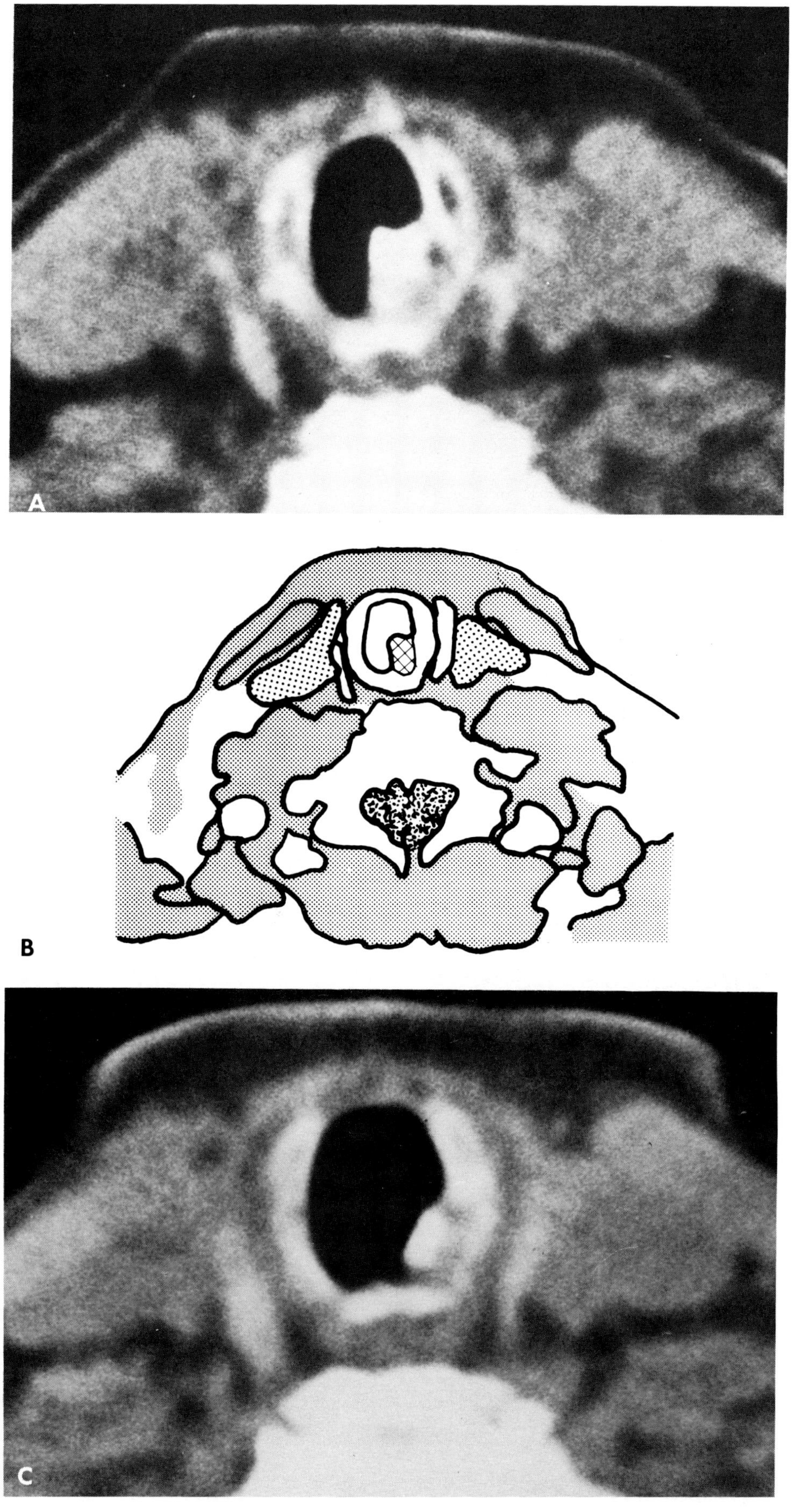

Fig. 24. (Case 8) Chondrosarcoma of larynx. Patient was 76-year-old woman with 2-year history of progressive airway obstruction. A,B) Level 13: July 25, 1980. Partially calcified subglottic mass arising from inner lamina of cricoid. Outer lamina of cricoid cartilage appears intact. C) Level 13; Nov 18, 1980. Follow-up after partial laser excision of tumor. Clinical improvement was corroborated by CT appearance.

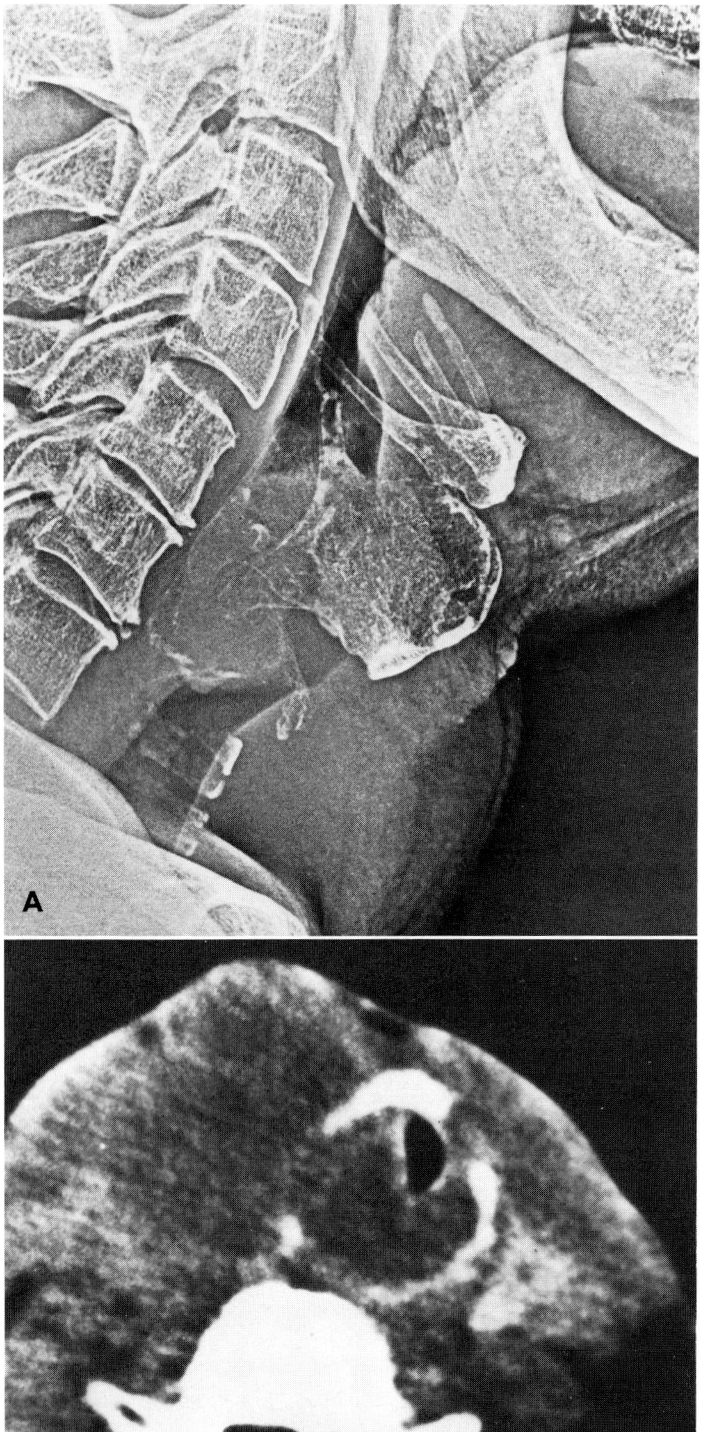

Fig. 25. (Case 9) Carcinoma of thyroid with transmural extension. Patient was 48-year-old man with enlarging goiter and stridor. A) Xeroradiograph. Large neck mass with erosion of cricoid ring and narrowing of subglottic airway. B,C) Level 11. Large mass arising from right lobe of thyroid. Erosion of cricoid ring posteriorly and transmural extension.

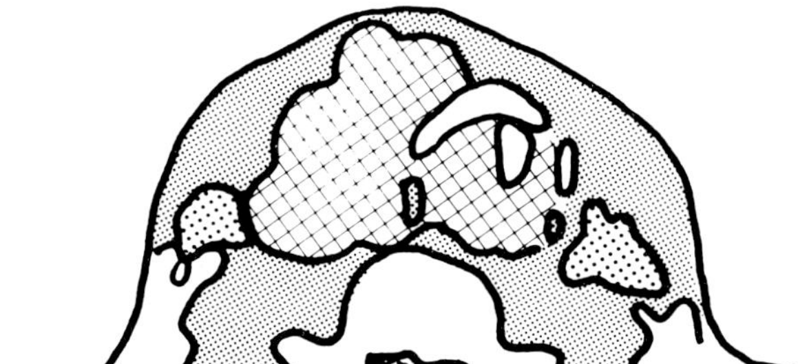

C

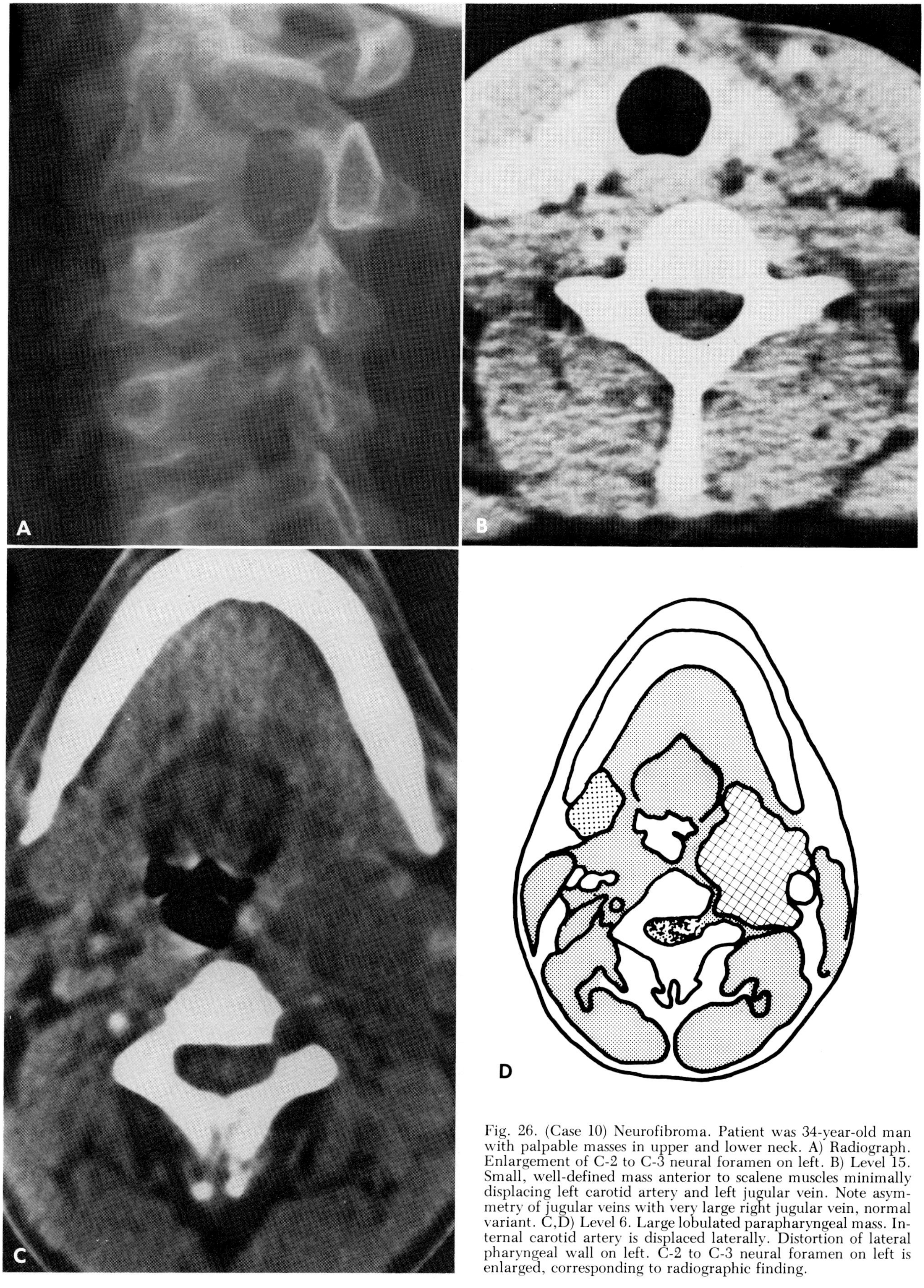

Fig. 26. (Case 10) Neurofibroma. Patient was 34-year-old man with palpable masses in upper and lower neck. A) Radiograph. Enlargement of C-2 to C-3 neural foramen on left. B) Level 15. Small, well-defined mass anterior to scalene muscles minimally displacing left carotid artery and left jugular vein. Note asymmetry of jugular veins with very large right jugular vein, normal variant. C,D) Level 6. Large lobulated parapharyngeal mass. Internal carotid artery is displaced laterally. Distortion of lateral pharyngeal wall on left. C-2 to C-3 neural foramen on left is enlarged, corresponding to radiographic finding.

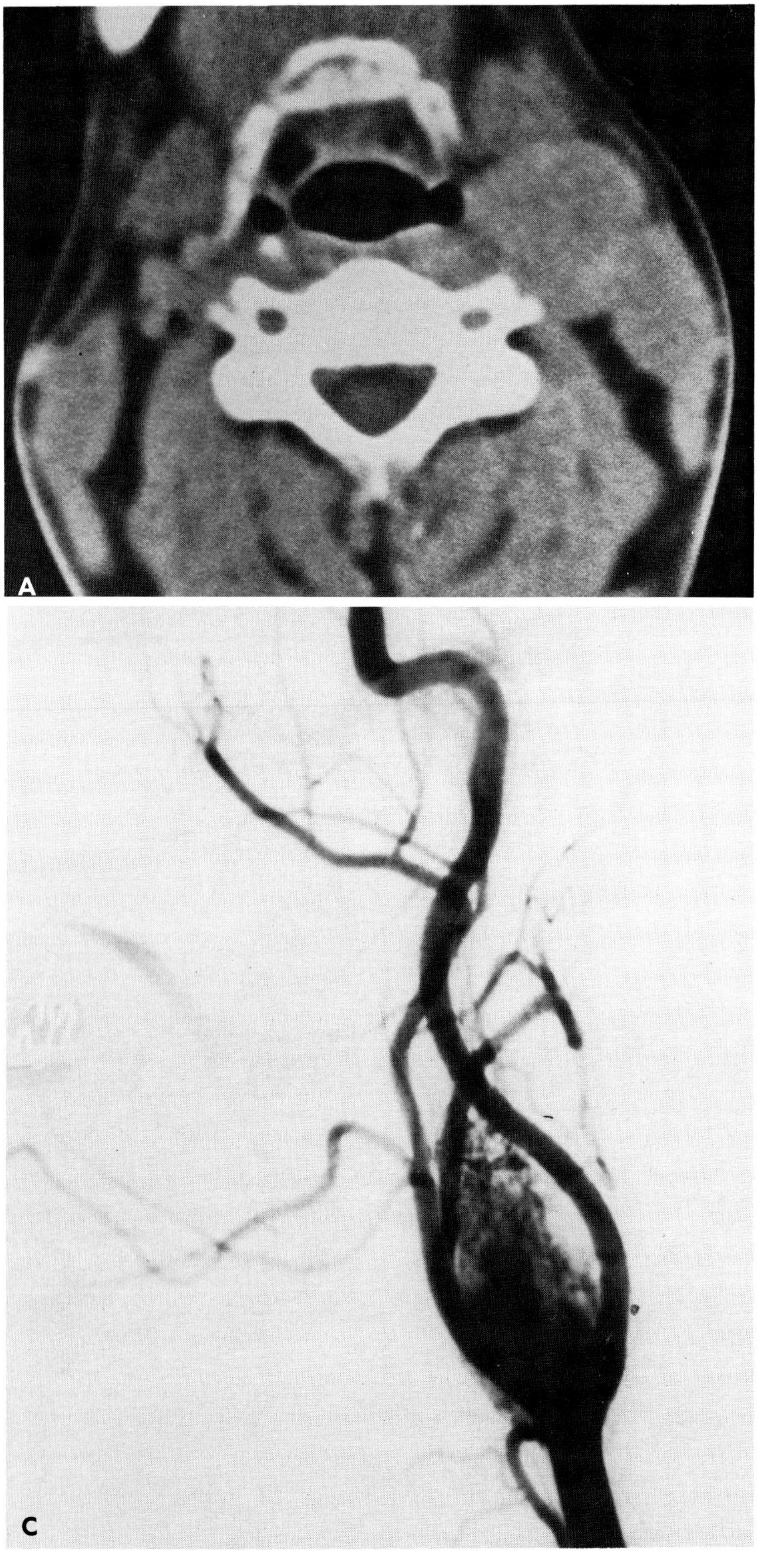

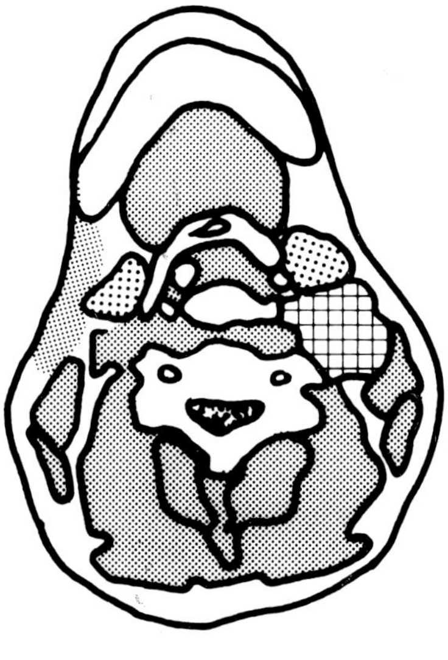

B

Fig. 27. (Case 11) Carotid body tumor (glomus caroticum). Patient was 29-year-old man with slowly enlarging left neck mass who had history of previous operation for glomus tympanicum. A,B) Level 7. Sharply defined enhancing mass under sternocleidomastoid muscle displacing left submandibular gland anteriorly. Carotid bifurcation is usually located at level of hyoid cornu. C) Angiogram. Highly vascular mass is seen at carotid bifurcation. Multiple small feeders arising from proximal internal and external carotid arteries are demonstrated.

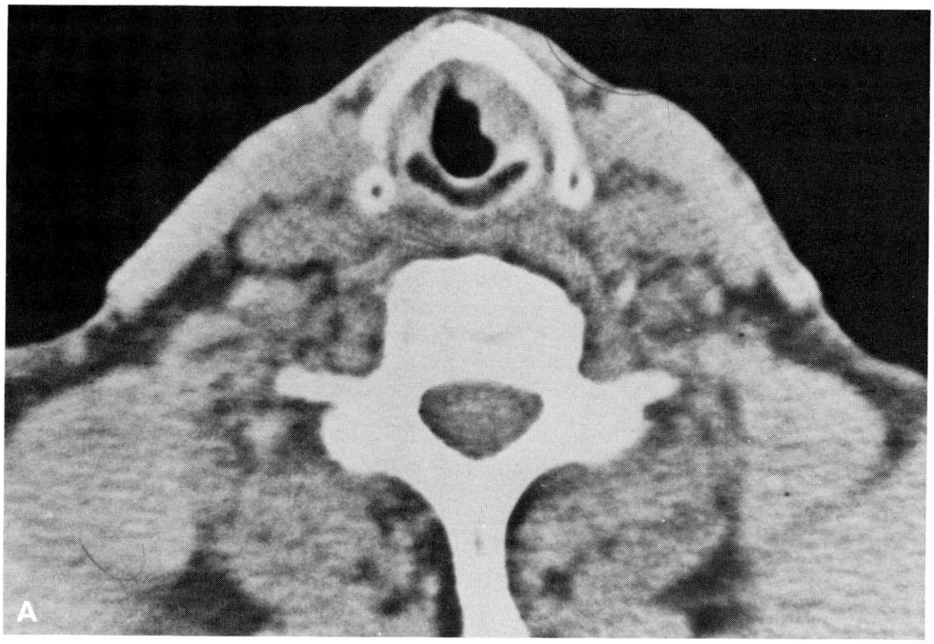

Fig. 28. (Case 12) Squamous carcinoma of left vocal cord. Patient was 62-year-old man with hoarseness. A,B) Level 11. Sections at level of vocal cords demonstrate irregular margin of enlarged left vocal cord. Note excellent definition of laryngeal cartilages. C) Level 12. Normal subglottic region 5 mm below vocal cords.

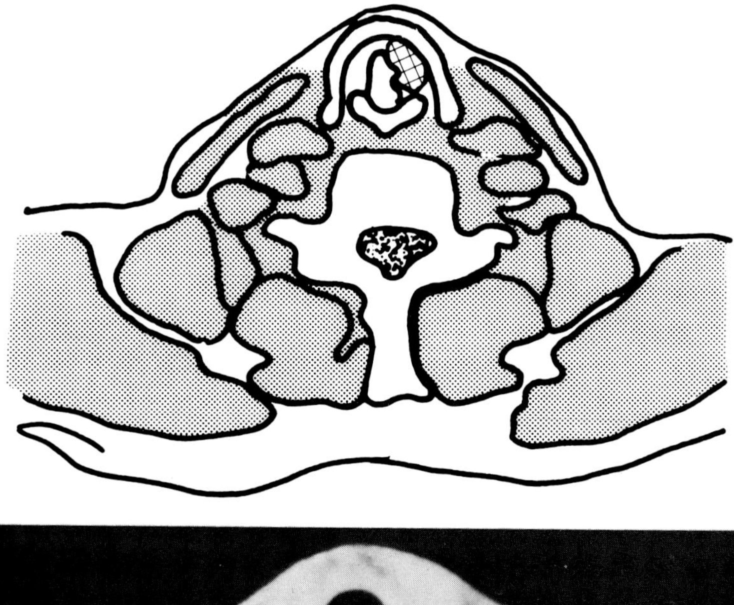

B

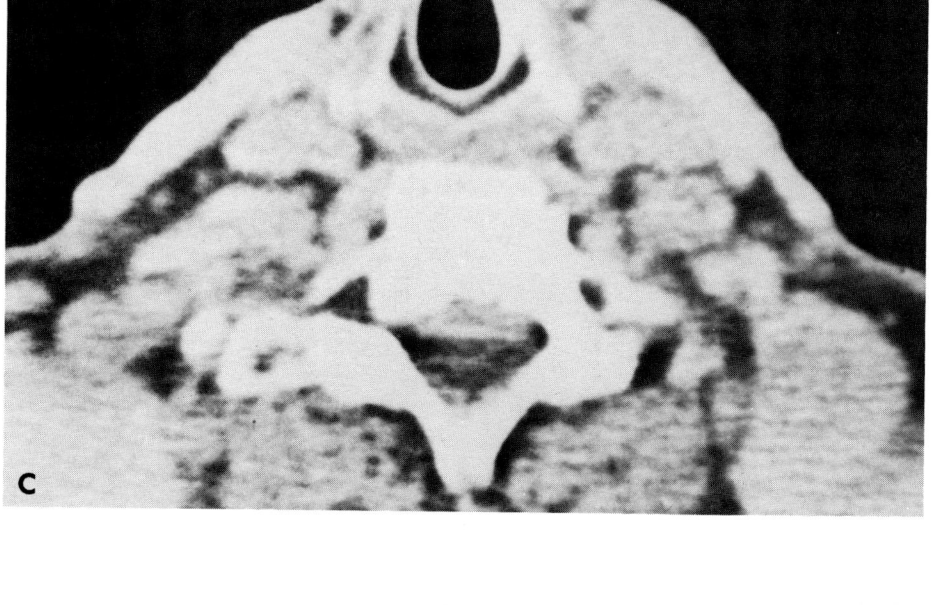

This publication was supported in part by Parke-Davis
Division of Warner-Lambert Company

FIRST NATIONAL CONFERENCE ON RESEARCH GOALS AND METHODS IN OTOLARYNGOLOGY

RECOMMENDATIONS OF THE WRITING GROUPS

George A. Gates, MD
Conference Chairman

This publication is supported in part
by Burroughs Wellcome Company.

CONTENTS

Conference Participants 4

Introduction. G. A. Gates, MD 7

Recommendations of the Writing Groups 7

1. Research Training for Residents. C. W. Cummings, MD; B. Jafek, MD; L. Proctor, MD; W. R. Panje, MD; M. L. Wiederhold, PhD 7

2. Development of Research Careers for Young Faculty. R. I. Kohut, MD; D. J. Anderson, PhD; M. E. Johns, MD; J. T. Johnson, MD; J. G. Neely, MD; D. E. Schuller, MD 9

3. Research Funding. C. D. Bluestone, MD; J. W. Bordley, MD; H. P. House, MD; M. S. Karlan, MD; M. M. Paparella, MD; F. B. Simmons, MD 10

4. Important Unanswered Research Questions. P. H. Ward, MD; D. E. Mattox, MD; J. E. Hawkins, Jr, DSc; C. J. Krause, MD; D. J. Lim, MD 11

5. Postdoctoral Research Training. R. R. Gacek, MD; L. T. Malmgren, PhD; J. H. Abbs, PhD; C. I. Berlin, PhD; R. A. Dobie, MD; J. M. Fredrickson, MD; G. Wolf, MD; E. J. Moore, PhD . 15

6. Research Facilitation. F. O. Black, MD; E. Elkins, PhD; W. E. Fee, Jr, MD; M. Igarashi, MD; J. M. Miller, PhD; E. W. Rubel, PhD 17

7. Current Research Resources. R. A. Mathog, MD; P. E. Brookhouser, MD; R. F. Naunton, MD; W. C. Stebbins, PhD; G. A. Gates, MD 19

8. Responsibilities of Otorhinolaryngology-Head and Neck Surgery to the National Institutes of Health. B. J. Bailey, MD; J. B. Snow, Jr, MD; R. J. Ruben, MD 21

Summary. G. A. Gates, MD 23

CONFERENCE PARTICIPANTS

James H. Abbs, PhD
Professor, Communicative Disorders
University of Wisconsin
Madison

Bobby R. Alford, MD
Professor and Chairman, Otorhinolaryngology & Communicative Sciences
Baylor College of Medicine
Houston

David J. Anderson, PhD
Chairman, Bioengineering
University of Michigan
Ann Arbor

Byron J. Bailey, MD
Weiss Professor & Chairman, Otolaryngology
University of Texas Medical Branch
Galveston

Charles I. Berlin, PhD
Professor, Otolaryngology
Louisiana State University Medical Center
New Orleans

F. Owen Black, MD*
Good Samaritan Hospital
Portland, Oregon

Charles D. Bluestone, MD
Director & Professor, Otolaryngology
Childrens Hospital of Pittsburgh

John E. Bordley, MD
Emeritus Professor, Otolaryngology
Johns Hopkins University
Baltimore

Patrick E. Brookhouser, MD
Professor and Chairman, Otolaryngology
Creighton University
Omaha

Erdem I. Cantekin, PhD
Director of Research, Otolaryngology
Childrens Hospital of Pittsburgh

Thomas E. Carey, PhD
Assistant Research Scientist, Otolaryngology
University of Michigan Medical School
Ann Arbor

Charles W. Cummings, MD*
Chairman, Otolaryngology
Unversity of Washington School of Medicine
Seattle

John C. Dalton, PhD
Director, Extramural Activities Program NIH-NINCDS
Bethesda, Maryland

Hallowell Davis, MD
Emeritus Director of Research
Central Institute for the Deaf
St. Louis

Robert A. Dobie, MD
Associate Professor, Otorhinolaryngology
University of Washington
Seattle

Dennis G. Drescher, PhD
Associate Professor, Otolaryngology
Wayne State University School of Medicine
Detroit

Avrim R. Eden, MD, PhD
Associate Professor, Otolaryngology
Mt. Sinai School of Medicine
New York

Earleen Elkins, PhD
Program Administrator, Communicative Disorders Program, NIH-NINCDS
Bethesda, Maryland

Willard E. Fee, Jr, MD
Head, Otolaryngology
Stanford University Medical Center
Stanford, California

John M. Fredrickson, MD
Chairman, Otolaryngology
Washington University School of Medicine
St. Louis

Richard R. Gacek, MD*
Professor & Chairman, Otorhinolaryngology
SUNY Upstate Medical Center
Syracuse

George A. Gates, MD*
Professor and Head, Otorhinolaryngology
The University of Texas Health Science Center
San Antonio

Joseph E. Hawkins, Jr, DSc
Professor, Otorhinolaryngology
University of Michigan Medical School
Ann Arbor

Jules Hirsch, MD
Professor and Senior Physician
Rockefeller University
New York

Howard P. House, MD
Otologic Medical Group
Los Angeles

Makoto Igarashi, MD
Professor, Otorhinolaryngology
Baylor College of Medicine
Houston

Bruce W. Jafek, MD
Professor and Chairman, Otolaryngology
University of Colorado Health Sciences Center
Denver

Michael E. Johns, MD
Professor, Otolaryngology
University of Virginia Medical Center
Charlottesville

Jonas T. Johnson, MD
Assistant Professor, Otolaryngology
Eye and Ear Hospital
Pittsburgh

Gerald S. Johnston, MD
Chief, Nuclear Medicine
National Institutes of Health
Bethesda, Maryland

Marc S. Karlan, MD
Associate Professor, Otolaryngology
Northwestern University
Chicago

Robert I. Kohut, MD
Professor and Head, Otolaryngology
Wake Forest University
Winston-Salem, North Carolina

Charles J. Krause, MD
Professor and Chairman, Otolaryngology
University of Michigan Medical Center
Ann Arbor

David J. Lim, MD
Professor and Director
Otological Research Laboratories
Ohio State University Hospitals
Columbus

Leslie T. Malmgren, PhD
Associate Professor, Otolaryngology
SUNY Upstate Medical Center
Syracuse

Robert H. Mathog, MD*
Professor and Chairman, Otolaryngology
Wayne State University School of Medicine
Detroit

Douglas E. Mattox, MD
Associate Professor, Otorhinolaryngology
The University of Texas Health Science Center
San Antonio

Josef M. Miller, PhD*
Professor, Otolaryngology
University of Washington School of Medicine
Seattle

Ernest J. Moore, PhD
Program Administrator, Communicative Disorders Program, NIH-NINCDS
Bethesda, Maryland

Ralph F. Naunton, MD
Director, Communicative Disorders Program, NIH-NINCDS
Bethesda, Maryland

J. Gail Neely, MD
Professor and Chairman, Otolaryngology
University of Oklahoma Health Science Center
Oklahoma City

William R. Panje, MD
Director, Head and Neck Oncology
University of Iowa Hospitals
Iowa City

Michael M. Paparella, MD
Professor and Chairman, Otolaryngology
University of Minnesota Medical School
Minneapolis

Sidney J. Peerless, MD
ENT Associates of Cincinnati, Inc
Cincinnati

Leonard R. Proctor, MD
Professor, Laryngology and Otology
Johns Hopkins University
Baltimore

Kenneth D. Rogers, MD
Professor and Chairman, Community Medicine
University of Pittsburgh School of Medicine

Edwin W. Rubel, PhD
Associate Professor, Otolaryngology
University of Virginia Medical Center
Charlottesville

Robert J. Ruben, MD
Professor and Chairman, Otorhinolaryngology
Albert Einstein College of Medicine
Bronx, New York

David E. Schuller, MD*
Assistant Professor, Otolaryngology
Ohio State University
Columbus

F. Blair Simmons, MD
Professor of Surgery, Otolaryngology
Stanford University Medical Center
Stanford, California

James B. Snow, Jr, MD
Professor and Chairman
Otorhinolaryngology & Human Communication
University of Pennsylvania School of Medicine
Philadelphia

William C. Stebbins, PhD*
Professor, Kresge Hearing Research Institute
University of Michigan Medical Center
Ann Arbor

Thomas R. Van De Water, PhD
Director, Laboratory of Developmental Otobiology
Albert Einstein College of Medicine
Bronx, New York

Paul H. Ward, MD
Professor and Head, Head & Neck Surgery
UCLA School of Medicine
Los Angeles

Michael L. Wiederhold, PhD
Associate Professor, Otorhinolaryngology
The University of Texas Health Science Center
San Antonio

George W. Williams, PhD
Chairman, Bio-Statistics
Cleveland Clinic

Gregory Wolf, MD
Associate Professor, Otorhinolaryngology
University of Michigan Medical Center
Ann Arbor

*Members of the Planning Committee.

INTRODUCTION

George A. Gates, MD, Conference Chairman

The following report comprises the recommendations of the eight writing groups which met immediately following the First National Conference on Research Goals and Methods in Otolaryngology held in Bethesda, Maryland, April 15-17, 1982. The writing groups consisted of speakers and other participants in the conference who were selected by the Planning Committee because of their active involvement in research and their commitment toward insuring that the future of research in otolaryngology will be bright.

Because the conference was held for the purpose of reversing the decline in numbers of physician-investigators and clinically oriented research projects in otolaryngology-head and neck surgery (OHNS), the Planning Committee felt strongly that positive steps should be taken without delay. The first step was obvious — to quickly distill the conference recommendations into a concise document suitable for wide dissemination.

To facilitate the report, the subject matter of the conference was divided into eight areas: 1) Research Training for Residents; 2) Development of Research Careers for Young Faculty; 3) Research Funding; 4) Research Priority Areas; 5) Postdoctoral Research Training; 6) Research Facilitation; 7) Current Research Resources; and 8) What is the Responsibility of Otolaryngology to the National Institutes of Health? Although the reports overlap to a certain extent, each provides a unique perspective on the subject as a whole as well as specific recommendations for improvement.

It is hoped that this report will be of value to program directors in OHNS, deans of medical schools, research directors, legislators and their staffs and the National Institutes of Health (NIH) in helping to develop further the research efforts aimed at meeting the unsolved needs of patients with communicative disorders and other diseases of the head and neck regions.

The conference was made possible because of the broad-based support of OHNS departments across the country, and grants from the American Academy of Otolaryngology-Head and Neck Surgery, the American Council of Otolaryngology-Head and Neck Surgery, the American Laryngological Association, the American Rhinologic Society, the American Society for Head and Neck Surgery, the Association for Research in Otolaryngology, the Association of Academic Departments of Otolaryngology, Beecham Laboratories, Burroughs Wellcome Company, Eli Lilly and Company, the Society of University Otolaryngologists and the National Institutes of Health.

RECOMMENDATIONS OF THE WRITING GROUPS

1. RESEARCH TRAINING FOR RESIDENTS

Charles W. Cummings, MD, Chairman
Bruce Jafek, MD
Leonard Proctor, MD
William R. Panje, MD
Michael L. Wiederhold, PhD

INTRODUCTION

The amount of research training for residents in otolaryngology-head and neck surgery (OHNS) varies widely from program to program, with extremes from no research training to PhD-level programs. This paper reports a survey made by the Research Committee of the Society of University Otolaryngologists for this conference. Sixteen percent of the responding programs had no research experience and 35% had a formal research rotation; but the majority had some type of informal research activity. The structure and content of the resident research experience varied considerably. In general, sources of support were tied to existing projects, but in a few instances, departmental or private funds were available for the initiation of independent new projects. It may be concluded from this brief overview that, at present, the status of resident research training and experience is inadequate to meet the needs of the profession.

RATIONALE

There is a general consensus among members of this writing group and program directors that research training for residents is desirable. The rationale for such training is based upon the following assumptions: 1) it awakens the potential for substantive academic growth by the development and use of critical reasoning and objective judgment; 2) it directly augments the resident's knowledge and provides exposure to techniques of study, review, and knowledge-generation that will be valuable for a lifetime of continued study; 3) it fosters an appreciation for the effort required and the criteria for the pursuit of an academic investigative career; 4) it provides experience in the use of the experimental method that will be valuable in the clinical as well as the laboratory setting; 5) it provides insight into the intellectual environment necessary to foster an investigative group; and 6) it provides an introductory experience so that the resident may be able to critically evaluate research papers in the literature and to learn to use constructive skepticism in evaluation of results.

In the AMA Chicago Directory of Residency Training Programs for 1981/1982, the special requirements for residency training in otolaryngology state:

> Research offers an important opportunity for the application of the basic sciences in clinical problems, and is an essential part of the preparation of the resident for a lifetime of self-education after the completion of formal training. It is essential that the training program provide a meaningful research experience for the residents, sufficient to result in an awareness of the basic principles of study design, performance, analysis and reporting. The research experience may be clinical or basic in nature and should reflect careful advice and planning with the faculty.

Thus, the Accreditation Council for Graduate Medical Education has mandated a substantial commitment to research in otolaryngology residency training.

STRUCTURE OF THE RESEARCH ROTATION

One goal is that all training programs have a well-formulated resident research rotation. The resident should receive a short-course introduction to research methods early in the training program followed by a period of independent study and review. Subsequently, time should be set aside for the completion of a supervised project in the latter part of the training period with adequate time for data analysis and report writing.

The steps that the resident should take in the development of a project are the traditional ones. Preliminary ideas and problems should be identified and studied by the resident. In concert with a research advisor, the problem is then presented to a research committee within the department, comprised of both basic science and clinical researchers. At this time, methods of research and funding are approached with respect to feasibility. A dedicated aliquot of time is spent by the resident on research, with guidance from his or her senior advisor. At the termination of this block of time the research data is collected and a report prepared. A manuscript should evolve of a high enough quality to pass the peer review process in a refereed journal. The program must be designed so that the residents' efforts will be stimulated by peer group pressure for excellence.

There should be an identified faculty member who is the director of research. There is no question that there needs to be a formalized mechanism of guidance on the part of the clinical and research faculty to introduce topics of research to the residents. The mystique of research must be eliminated so that the performance of research is brought to a realistic level and a full appreciation of the rewards and frustrations of research may be gained by the residents at an early stage. We should introduce interdisciplinary collaboration to expand the potential significance and attractiveness of research to our residents.

IMPLEMENTATION

Inasmuch as many programs have no apparent research experience the implementation of this goal may be difficult. In some programs there may be a negative attitude about resident research because it takes time away from clinical training, because of difficulties in funding, or because of the absence of qualified investigators to teach research methods. Undoubtedly there are programs with inadequate numbers of research personnel where an obligatory research rotation would impose an added burden on already compromised work loads. Appropriate steps should be taken to remove these deficiencies in such programs.

Currently the absolute requisites for a successful residency research rotation are talented aggressive residents, willing experienced faculty, space, time, necessary research funding, and avoidance of unachievable goals. The resident research experience must be kept realistic and not unduly taxing on either the resident or department.

There are unanswered questions at this time with regard to research in otolaryngology-head and neck residencies. How much time is enough? Three months? Four months? Six months? Acknowledging that any practical amount of time is inadequate, how much is satisfactory to achieve the goal of exciting those intracranial centers assigned to the quest for knowledge? How do resident research efforts compare to those undertaken by committed researchers? They will usually come up far short, but with the guidance and overview of experts, the quality of resident research need not be second-rate. At what level should the resident be immersed in research? Should it be at a clinical level? Should it be at a basic science level? The overview is that this should be inclusive of both and not selective.

CONCLUSION

Research in the residency training process is not presumably to train the resident as a skilled researcher. Rather, it enhances the potential for seeking future research opportunities and growth. Solutions to funding, expansion of research horizons beyond topics predominantly otologic, and orchestration of a uniform research experience during the residency are most achievable goals for the future.

2. DEVELOPMENT OF RESEARCH CAREERS FOR YOUNG FACULTY

ROBERT I. KOHUT, MD, CHAIRMAN — DAVID J. ANDERSON, PHD — MICHAEL E. JOHNS, MD
JONAS T. JOHNSON, MD — J. GAIL NEELY, MD — DAVID E. SCHULLER, MD

This committee agreed that a totality of combined elements was necessary for the proper development of young faculty research careers. These elements come both from the faculty member and the department/institution. The department/institution provides a milieu, time, funding, and encouragement. What must be provided by the young faculty member, if his or her research career is to thrive, are motivation, a special sense of values, and preparation.

Motivation is the key element in the personal qualities of young faculty members. They must have an indefatigable enthusiasm, being motivated and excited by new findings. To have this requires a special sense of values that is inherent, not acquired. The satisfaction of new findings through research must surpass the desire for monetary rewards.

Preferably, they will have had previous research experience and will understand the principles of question identification, protocol development, statistical analysis, and hypothesis testing, and will be skilled in writing. However, such experience is not gained sufficiently in a residency program and few current faculty applicants have had the opportunity to have postdoctoral research training. Therefore, the first few years of a young faculty member's career must be structured to incorporate research training commensurate with prior experience. Such training should be considered a strong investment in the future of the faculty members, the program and the specialty. Of course, as a clinician investigator, fully developed clinical abilities are assumed.

The department/institution must provide other necessary elements. First, within the department there must be an environment of intellectual curiosity where research is a regular, ongoing activity in which faculty and students are intensely engaged. It must never be an isolated or token activity. The excitement of sharing research-related findings is contagious, and stimulates similar activity.

Just as faculty members and departmental resources are regularly available for clinical activities, so time and resources must be provided, with equal priority, for research activities. The time must be guarded by insuring adequate, not token, clinical coverage. It is often easy and psychologically rewarding to let clinical demands interrupt research activity. In these instances, the long-term goals of research are delayed and the satisfaction of an immediate clinical result substituted. Although young faculty must be gradually prepared for future administrative tasks, the responsibilities of committee work and other administrative activities should never be so burdensome as to distract from the heavy investment of time needed for research.

There is a negative attitude that may inhibit even well-designed institutional plans for research career development for the faculty. Ingrained in some physicians' minds is the feeling that time for research may be construed as a form of shirking of clinical responsibilities. If the role model of the young faculty, usually the departmental chairperson, endorses the importance of research, this negative attitude would fade, to the benefit of all. The mature mind readily accepts a balance of activity. Being too active clinically may be an excuse to avoid more taxing research activity. One must realize that the potential clinical impact of the research effort may be far greater than the sum of the individual clinical abilities.

Lack of time becomes an increasingly compelling consideration for the young faculty member. Competing priorities leave little allowance for immediately nonproductive activities such as following up on a research idea in the face of more concrete departmental activities such as surgery, consultations, lecturing, and staffing the clinic.

Funding difficulties frustrate the beginning researcher at every step along the way. It is difficult to find start-up funds to develop, among other important elements, support personnel to perform adjunctive tasks which facilitate the development of research projects. Multispecialty interaction may be facilitated by adequate funding. Dwindling federal support for research compounds the problem so that it is increasingly necessary to look to departmental funds to support research activities. The "catch 22" of this situation is that departmental funds are not generated by young faculty members when in the laboratory. This is the department's problem, not the faculty members'.

Departmental contributions to research are expensive. Generation of funding, in particular, is costly both in terms of actual resources and the time devoted to securing them. Should faculty members invest more of their clinical earnings resulting in still lower salaries (an identified disincentive)? What is our individual obligation (ie, tax-deductible contributions)? What proportion of departmental resources should be devoted to research activities?

Considering that the 6% growth of medical faculty in the 1970s may decrease to zero-growth and that only 20% of new faculty have any research experience, a graying population of research faculty might result. Therefore, to maintain an appropriate research milieu, additional faculty will be necessary. Recruitment of young faculty with talent and vision is an important long-range goal.

3. RESEARCH FUNDING

CHARLES D. BLUESTONE, MD, CHAIRMAN JOHN W. BORDLEY, MD HOWARD P. HOUSE, MD
MARC S. KARLAN, MD MICHAEL M. PAPARELLA, MD F. BLAIR SIMMONS, MD

INTRODUCTION

In spite of the significant increase in the number of otolaryngologists who have chosen an academic career during the past decade, there has been a dramatic decline in the number of research grants submitted, approved and funded by the primary source of federal funding for diseases and disorders of the ear, nose and throat — head and neck, the Communicative Disorders Program (CDP) of the National Institute of Neurological and Communicative Disorders and Stroke (NINCDS).

The explanation for this enigma is not clear at present, but is most likely due to several factors: 1) a steady decline in available funds (real dollars) due to inflation and budget constraints; 2) apathy resulting from the feeling among otolaryngologists that the competition for funding is so great and the chances of success are slight; 3) lack of academic role models in otolaryngology to stimulate and assist young investigators to secure funding; and 4) lack of a research environment in most departments of otolaryngology.

The following recommendations made this writing group of interested otolaryngologists address the need to stimulate more otolaryngologists to become involved in research, improve the quality of research in otolaryngology, and provide funds for training in research. In order of priority they are as follows:

FORMATION OF A NATIONAL FOUNDATION FOR RESEARCH IN OTOLARYNGOLOGY

Since funding for research from both governmental and private sources remains limited and not directed to the broad needs or research questions posed by modern OHNS physicians and surgeons, a national foundation for research in otolaryngology must be established. This foundation should have an endowment from which the interest can be used to train new investigators, provide start-up or seed-money for promising new research projects, and aid departments of otolaryngology in providing a research environment.

The endowment should be generated from the following sources: 1) gifts from otolaryngologists and other interested health care professionals; 2) "planned giving" (bequests) by otolaryngologists and their patients who want to provide research support after their death to answer the important questions that faced them during their lifetimes; 3) independent, company and community foundations; 4) companies involved in health care (eg, drug and instrument companies); 5) major corporations; 6) service organizations (eg, Lions International); and 7) gifts and planned giving by other interested citizens.

The foundation should provide funding for all aspects of diseases and disorders that are the responsibility of the modern OHNS physician and surgeon.

The foundation should be under the umbrella of an existing organization that represents otolaryngology, but should have a separate board of directors and management to maintain autonomy from the parent organization.

SEPARATE IDENTIFICATION AND FUNDING FROM THE NIH FOR OTOLARYNGOLOGY

Since there are research questions and needs for funding that are unique to otolaryngology as compared to other diseases, disorders of the body and research/health care professionals, separate funding and identification should be established by the NIH to meet these specific needs.

PROMOTION OF MORE SUCCESSFUL APPLICATIONS TO NINCDS

This goal can be accomplished by encouraging senior investigators and departmental chairpersons to take active roles in stimulating and assisting young investigators to develop high quality research projects and to give the NINCDS the opportunity to support these and other projects by submitting applications for review and funding. Senior investigators and/or department chairpersons must take active roles in stimulating and assisting young investigators to apply for Teacher-Investigator Development Awards (TIDAs) and actively solicit institutional fellowship awards for their departments.

OTHER GOVERNMENTAL SOURCES OF FUNDING

Otolaryngologists should contact and inform other agencies of federal, state and local governments of their needs to secure funds for research. These include (among others) other institutes of the NIH (eg, National Cancer Institute), Biomedical Research Support Grants, National Aeronautics and Space Administration, National Science Foundation, Environmental Protection Agency, and Veterans Administration.

PRIVATE SOURCES

Otolaryngologists should seek research funding from companies involved in health care (eg, drug and instrument), major corporations and company-sponsored foundations, commercial/financial institutions in their communities, national health foundations (eg, American Cancer Society, March of Dimes), special interest groups (eg, Deafness Research Foundation, American Otological Society, Inc), and others such as the Robert Wood Johnson Foundation.

OTHER PRIVATE SOURCES

Funding should be sought by applying to local or service (hospital or institution) organizations, sponsoring special events and programs, or through private practice and patient care.

CONCLUSION

It is the consensus of this committee that we, as otolaryngologists, are facing a crisis that may potentially affect the health care of our patients. It is only through research that we can solve the unanswered problems that will allow us to manage our patients' health and prevent and/or treat the diseases and disorders that affect their well-being. Otolaryngologists, the time to act is now.

4. IMPORTANT UNANSWERED RESEARCH QUESTIONS

PAUL H. WARD, MD, CHAIRMAN

DOUGLAS E. MATTOX, MD
JOSEPH E. HAWKINS, JR, DSc
CHARLES J. KRAUSE, MD
DAVID J. LIM, MD

The report of this group lists important areas for future research in otolaryngology. Their importance derives from the frequency of occurrence, the extent of disability, the cost to society for treatment or lost productivity, and impact on quality of life. The list of research areas is not in any order of priority. All of them are important in the judgment of this group. To attempt to rank them on a meaningful priority scale is outside the scope of this review. Nonetheless, inclusion here indicates their importance in the minds of this group.

Where appropriate, likely avenues of investigation are suggested. Many of these problems will require multidisciplinary, interinstitutional collaborative efforts to solve. We place high priority on the formation of a National Advisory Panel for Research in Otolaryngology to study research needs, to develop a national policy for research in otolaryngology and to make specific recommendations for the conduct of the investigations needed. In particular, long-term studies to determine effective means of prevention, treatment, and rehabilitation of the most common and serious disorders of human communication and of the head and neck should be developed and carried out. Emphasis also must be placed on more efficient/less costly techniques for diagnosis and treatment.

INFECTIOUS DISEASE

Infectious diseases of the ear, nose, paranasal sinuses, throat, tonsils and adenoids continue to be frequent causes of morbidity in spite of advances in treatment. Assessment of the potential role of subtle immune deficiencies in recurrent infections may provide an important clue to prevention.

Otitis media with effusion is still a major cause of infant and child morbidity and concerns remain unanswered about the unproven possibility of language and intellectual retardation from conductive hearing loss in childhood. Investigation into prevention, identification and intensive treatment of high-risk cases is a pressing public health need.

HEARING

Approximately 13 million adults are hearing-impaired. Advances in the field of hearing will be dependent upon a constellation of scientific efforts in otolaryngology, anatomy, otopathology, biochemistry, engineering, psychology, audiology, physiology, embryology and molecular biology. Much of the research must of necessity be interdisciplinary.

Probably the greatest void in research on acquired sensorineural deafness is the precise definition of its cause and pathogenesis. The effects and interactions of otosclerosis, middle ear infections, noise, ototoxic drugs, diabetes, hypertension and hyperlipidemia need to be determined. We are still not certain of the individual factors and are even more uncertain about the interaction of the different genetic, environmental and disease factors that may accelerate and exacerbate susceptibility to presbycusis. This disorder, which is the most common cause of chronic disability in the adult, is becoming more common as the average age of our population increases.

The ability to detect vertebrobasilar insufficiency by hearing tests (decreased ability to detect short-tone bursts in noise) offers a new clue for noninvasive diagnosis and the potential for remediation of one form of acquired central hearing impairment.

GENETIC HEARING LOSS

Epidemiological studies and genetic analysis indicate that approximately 50% of all congenital hearing loss may be genetic. Counseling remains the only feasible prevention of genetic hearing loss. It is hoped that biochemical advances will eventually result in control. There are deaf mutant animal models available for study of the molecular, biochemical and abnormal cellular development in these genetic defects. Correlation of electrocochleography and cochlear histopathology will aid in understanding the progressive nature of genetic cochlear disorders seen in adults.

HEARING AIDS

Hearing aids are the most frequently used prosthetic device, yet many patients are unable to use them satisfactorily. Research opportunities include the use of microprocessors to adjust frequency and gain characteristics, improvements of signal-to-noise ratio (through signal extraction), and multiband compression to suit individual patient needs. Studies have indicated improved hearing can result from adjustment of frequency-gain characteristics.

Despite these achievements many sensorineurally deaf patients with poor speech discrimination are unable to function adequately with the best available conventional hearing aids. Theoretically, if feedback and distortion can be eliminated with an implantable middle ear transducer having no speaker, ear mold, or tubing, then the resulting high-fidelity signal should produce better speech comprehension. Transducers of this sort have provided "perfect fidelity" in normal human volunteers. Further bioengineering development and testing will be necessary before proceeding to a clinical trial.

COCHLEAR PROSTHESIS

This has been a much-publicized and controversial topic. There are approximately 200,000 profoundly deaf people in the United States who potentially could benefit from such a device. Several research teams worldwide are now conducting clinical trials with a variety of electrode designs and stimulus parameters.

Patients with a monopolar cochlear electrode implanted through the round window appear to tolerate the prosthesis very well over several years. Speech is not comprehensible, but environmental sounds are better recognized, lipreading scores are frequently improved and some low-frequency discrimination is possible.

Otopathological evaluation of the long-term effects of prostheses in human ears is also an essential feature of this work. Widespread use of this device should be discouraged until these long-term effects have been clarified.

TINNITUS

Tinnitus is one of the most common sequelae of sensorineural hearing loss. It is reported that in the United States there are over 7 million persons who suffer from tinnitus, 32% of all adults have tinnitus at some time, and in 6.4% the tinnitus is reported to be debilitating. Studies of clinical characterization and pathogenesis as well as the development of a scientific rationale for treatment are urgently needed. The neurophysiological and biochemical basis of tinnitus must be elucidated.

OTOSCLEROSIS

It is estimated that there are 14-15 million otosclerotic patients in this country. It is also well known that it is a genetically linked disorder with distinct family-linked traits. However, the pathogenesis of this disorder is not yet known. It is generally believed that some biochemical malfunction of the ground substance may be involved. Recently, autoimmunity to type II collagen has been proposed as a mechanism for otosclerotic bone lesions. Considerable basic work in the biochemistry, cell biology, and immunology of the otic capsule is needed. Although surgical treatment of conductive hearing loss due to otosclerosis is highly developed, there is no effective prevention or correction of the sensorineural hearing loss that also occurs in many patients.

VESTIBULAR SYSTEM

Approximately 100,000 cases of Menière's disorder are diagnosed annually in the United States, and approximately 40% of the population complains of spontaneous vertigo. Fundamental knowledge concerning the pathogenesis of Menière's disease is lacking. Before specific therapeutic trials can be developed, the disorder must be characterized on a firm scientific basis. Clearly there is much more to learn of the basic physiology and function of the vestibular system and its interaction with the visual and proprioceptive systems before we will be able to improve current methods of treating a variety of poorly understood vestibular disorders.

Many investigators are pursuing diagnostic tests designed to evaluate semicircular canal and otolith organ functions through their interaction with the visual and proprioceptive systems in the control of posture. A team approach, with basic scientists, otolaryngologists and bioengineers working together, is essential to construct diagnostic and therapeutic trials most efficiently.

RHINOLOGY

Disorders of the nose and paranasal sinuses — the common cold, allergic rhinitis, vasomotor rhinitis, and polyps — are among man's most common and least understood afflictions. Among the major research voids in this area are the prevention and treatment of upper respiratory infections, the pathogenesis and treatment of vasomotor rhinitis, and the efficient pharmacologic and immunologic prevention/treatment of nasal allergy.

TASTE AND SMELL

There is a significant deficit in our understanding of the fundamental mechanisms of taste and smell and their disorders. There is an urgent need for developing diagnostic and management programs for dealing with these disorders and dysfunctions, which detract so much from the quality of life.

LARYNX

The principal unsolved clinical laryngeal problems, other than cancer, are papillomatosis, stenosis, and paralysis. The presumed viral etiology of papillomatosis is unproven, and no method of therapy is curative. Immunologic control through interferon or other as yet unknown agents should receive close scrutiny, because no other therapeutic approach offers promise for control of this crippling childhood disorder.

Methods to prevent and treat subglottic stenosis should continue to be investigated. Restoration of laryngeal function following paralysis continues to be a goal that promises achievement through continued study.

Vocal restoration following laryngectomy should continue to receive much attention. Research is proceeding to develop a safe, long-term, tissue-compatible, retropharyngeal voice box which will produce a human speech sound.

Computer analysis of speech output to identify laryngeal pathology should continue to be pursued. A prospective clinical trial should study the variables of vocal fold activity for normals and for the entire range of voice disorders, employing such methods in parallel with aerodynamic and electromyographic techniques.

IMMUNOLOGY

Adenoids and tonsils are well-recognized lymphatic organs, but their role in the immune system is poorly understood. Systematic investigation of the function of these organs and the consequences, if any, of their removal is needed.

It has also been established that the mucosa of the middle ear and eustachian tube can mount its own immune response to antigens such as viruses and bacteria. It is postulated that some form of immune injury is responsible for otitis media with effusion. Further fundamental study of the immune mechanism is needed, not only for the understanding of the pathogenesis, but also for prevention and treatment of otitis media and its sequelae.

The immune system of the inner ear is not well explored. Available information suggests that it is independent of the CSF immune system, and the existence of autoimmune inner ear disorders has been suggested recently. Progress has been impeded in the past because of the difficulty of access to the small volume of tissue available for study. New technological developments, such as the monoclonal antibody and microchemical quantitative techniques, promise an exciting and potentially productive research future in this area.

HEAD AND NECK CANCER

Since President Nixon's "war on cancer" was announced nearly a decade ago, there has been a great deal of money and effort expended on research to determine the cause, prevention, and treatment of this dreaded disease. Thus far, this effort has not achieved the hoped-for level of clinical advances. In all but a few types of cancer, discoveries have been few in number and have not significantly changed the occurrence and success of treatment. Considering that head and neck cancer strikes 16 per 100,000 persons, resulting in death in 50% of these people, research in this area is vital.

Cancer of the head and neck lends itself to many types of analysis since specimens are easily obtained for evaluation, and the treatment site can be readily observed. Recently it has also become possible to establish cell lines in tissue culture, offering an opportunity for long-term study of a specific tumor's biological properties.

Cancer research must proceed along several key avenues. It is important that we determine the crucial biologic factors which cause the cancer cell to act so differently from normal cells, and factors which control the tumor-host interaction. Continued study of etiologic factors such as viruses, smoking, and alcohol use is critical, and this knowledge must be applied to prevention programs. Development of effective measures to assist smokers to quit their habit and establishment of patient education programs about the health consequences of smoking would substantially reduce the incidence of head and neck cancer.

We must continue to evaluate the effects of various treatment modalities (ie, heat, cold, chemotherapeutic drugs, irradiation, and surgery) used individually or in combination. The small number of patients with head and neck cancer available for study requires better classification systems to evaluate the effectiveness of the various therapeutic modalities. Multi-institutional cooperative studies appear to offer the greatest hope for accumulating a sufficient number of patients to answer these important questions.

WOUND HEALING

Because wound healing is such a basic ingredient of surgery, a clearer understanding of those biochemical and physical factors which influence the rate and amount of collagen production, epithelialization, capillary induction, and inflammatory processes are very important. Understanding these processes should lead to methods of controlling collagen production and promote more rapid healing, yet prevent hypertrophic scar formation.

RECONSTRUCTIVE SURGERY

There continues to be a need for better undertanding of flap physiology and the effects of physical and chemical factors upon flap perfusion and survival. Methods should be developed to improve patency rates in free flap while decreasing the amount of time and training required to perform the anastomoses. Methods of stretching skin to increase the area available for transfer may offer a significant advantage in planning reconstruction.

Though most of the investigation of nerve regeneration has in the past been directed toward the facial nerve, improved understanding and control of spatial distribution of axons and neurophysiology may result in improved restoration of other nerve functions, including cranial nerves X, XI, and XII. One of the most exciting areas of rehabilitation research lies in muscle regeneration and neurotization of denervated muscle. Restoration of effective muscle function of the face, palate, tongue, and larynx will provide a major advance in rehabilitation.

Vascularized bone as part of a composite flap or free flap appears to show promise of improved survival and healing. Other investigators are studying methods of procuring autogenous or homogenous mandible to provide ideal contour. New forms of prosthetic material may provide even simpler means of restoring mandibular function. New synthetic materials are constantly being developed, but the indications for their use and their long-term sequelae must be carefully evaluated.

Although recent years have brought rapid growth in knowledge about gene aberration and regulation, much remains to be learned about preventing and correcting congenital anomalies. Facial growth is a complex process under normal circumstances, and the superimposition of congenital anomalies and the surgical treatment of these anomalies creates an even more confusing picture. As surgeons, we must better understand how to correct such anomalies while avoiding those techniques which impair subsequent growth. The development of improved alternative methods for those with significant communication impairment remains a very important area for investigation.

AGING

Much remains to be learned about the biologic mechanisms which regulate the aging process, and about how these might be controlled. Development of better agents to protect the skin from the harmful effects of sun exposure and safer methods of ameliorating these effects are long-range goals.

5. POSTDOCTORAL RESEARCH TRAINING

Richard R. Gacek, MD, Chairman
James H. Abbs, PhD
Robert A. Dobie, MD
Gregory Wolf, MD

Leslie T. Malmgren, PhD, Cochairman
Charles I. Berlin, PhD
John M. Fredrickson, MD
Ernest J. Moore, PhD

The majority of information generated by basic science researchers is not being applied clinically. This may indicate an inadequacy in several areas: insufficient research manpower, inadequate research training, outdated research facilities in OHNS departments, as well as inadequate transfer of basic science findings to clinical practice.

The term "training" (Figure) is used in a general sense to include methods of information transfer that contribute to the competency of researchers. In this scheme, postdoctoral "training" events can be divided into 1) intradisciplinary training interactions which involve information transfer within an individual discipline, and 2) interdisciplinary training interactions which include information transfer between various disciplines involved in OHNS research.

A major goal of basic science research is clinical application, and therefore, the effective transfer of information from basic to applied science is important. For this reason, the various postdoctoral training interactions and the types of research expertise required in such information pathways determine success.

A directory of OHNS departments (research programs, postdoctoral training) should be developed to stimulate interest from other departments and other disciplines. Such a directory (by providing specific information on laboratory equipment, space, faculty, research interests, training, projects, etc) would provide a method for attracting research-oriented medical students and basic science fellows. In this way, the quality of postdoctoral research training in otorhinolaryngology may be improved by appropriate attention to training environment, personnel and financial support. The directory should be circulated nationally.

ENVIRONMENT

The research environment is the responsibility of the department chairperson, with the support of the institution. The chairperson and the director of research should be effective role models for the clinician-investigator and the clinically oriented basic scientist (Figure). The commitment of the chairperson to establish and maintain space, equipment, support, etc, will attract both basic and clinical (doctoral level) investigators. The chairperson and director of research will, by their examples, recruit other clinicians (residents, faculty) and basic scientists into research in otolaryngology. The commitment to research often includes the use of funds generated by clinical practice so as to provide or supplement outside support for renovations of space and special laboratory equipment.

The research environment will be enhanced not only by quality faculty research but, also, by research programs for all residents, and those medical students who have made a decision to prepare for academic careers. Such research programs will succeed, or fail, in recruiting researchers into OHNS by motivational efforts and research activities of the research faculty. Resident research training is now mandated by the Accrediting Council on Graduate Medical Education. This requirement should provide a stimulus to resident research programs due to possible loss of accreditation if not followed. Furthermore, this requirement provides justification to acquire research faculty positions and postdoctoral fellowship support. An important side effect of an expansion in resident research programs will be that the PhD research faculty responsible for directing resident research projects will probably become more knowledgeable in clinical areas as a result of interactions with residents.

The awarding of intrainstitutional research awards for superior research are desirable motivational factors. Recognition of research faculty, space and trainees by administrative titles, office and lab space designation will also be beneficial.

INTERDISCIPLINARY TRAINING

It is essential to increase the interdisciplinary training between the clinician-investigator and the clinically oriented basic scientist (area B in the Figure). As more basic scientist researchers are attracted to OHNS departments, they will add to the pool of clinically oriented basic scientists. Their productivity will encourage the association of other basic scientists. It is recommended (if institutional faculty attitudes permit) that OHNS and basic science departments jointly administer a research program, eg, a graduate student in anatomy conducting auditory, vestibular or other head and neck sys-

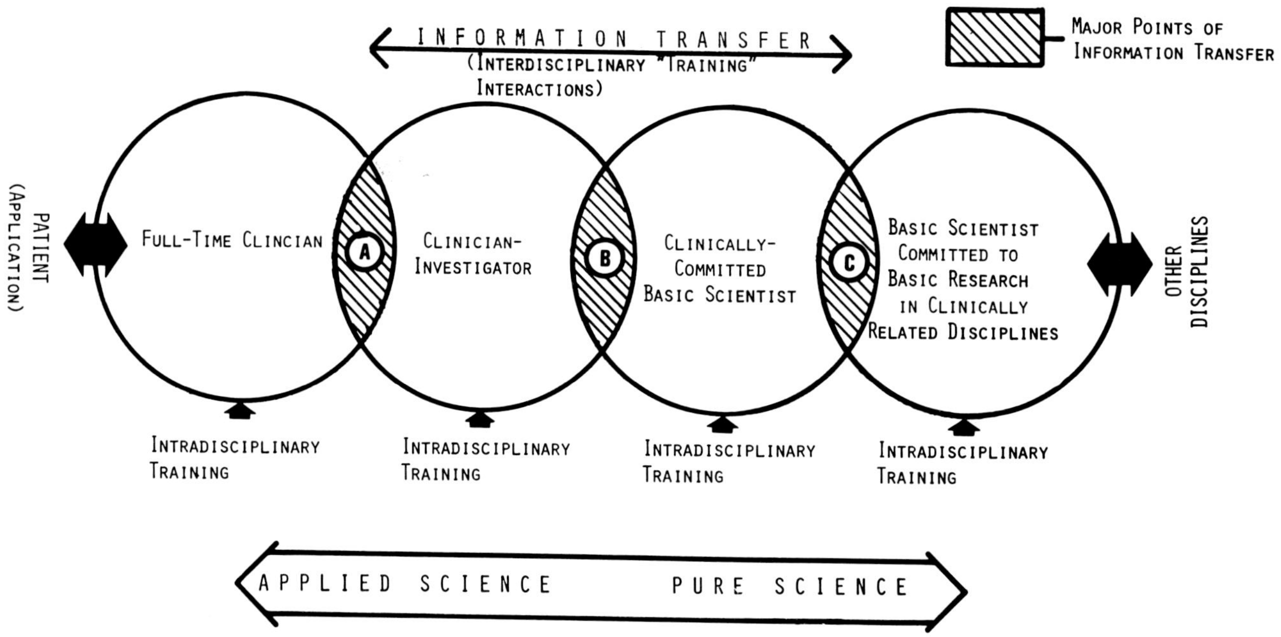

Common pathway for information transfer in otolaryngology-head and neck surgery research.

tem anatomical research/teaching in an OHNS department. The fostering of institutional interdisciplinary conferences would also promote cross-interaction of research, and attract more clinically oriented basic scientists. It is also recommended that basic scientists in an OHNS department avail themselves of clinical training (conferences, rounds, ward rotations) so as to enhance awareness of clinical problems that may relate to ongoing research. Short-term (4-8 weeks), intensive training for clinical scientists in areas of basic research, with documented clinical relevance, would also provide the clinical investigator with insight, as well as training in basic science methodology.

PERSONNEL

Resident research training and research opportunities for motivated medical students should provide future generations of OHNS researchers. Following the residency training, opportunities should be provided for in-depth research training. The location and form of this research experience will vary according to the goals of the individual, but ideally it should consist of one to two years of fellowship so as to acquire sufficient research expertise, and to initiate independent research. The financial support for postdoctoral training should be sufficient to attract, rather than discourage, individuals at this level. Since the resident graduate may not have sufficient research credentials to receive Teacher-Investigator Development Award (TIDA) support, postdoctoral fellowship support (stipend) is required. This support should, at the least, exceed the senior resident salary level.

Following a fellowship and appointment to the faculty, opportunities to acquire additional research laboratory experience should be provided by release time from clinical and administrative obligations. It is the department chairperson's responsibility to encourage clinical faculty research by providing adequate research time. For faculty with demonstrated research potential (eg, several publications), a TIDA award is useful to compensate for salary lost while conducting research.

DEVELOPMENT OF A RESEARCH TRAINING PROGRAM

One of the major causes of the currently low level of research expertise on the part of clinician-investigators is the lack of strong research training programs for residents, postresident fellows and for periodic retraining of established clinician-investigators. The future strength of such training programs depends largely upon the available technical expertise, new ideas, and information transmitted to the clinician-investigator (resident, postresident fellow, established investigator) by career investigators within OHNS departments. Although some career investigators will be trained as MD-PhDs, the majority of the scientists filling these positions will probably be recruited from the basic sciences. Individuals recruited to fill these positions should be competent and well-qualified in their respective basic science discipline. A number of difficulties, however, presently interfere with the achievement of this goal:

1. Positions in clinical departments are often considered by basic scientists to be of lower prestige than those in basic science departments.

2. There is a perception by basic scientists that possibilities for career development are more limited within clinical departments (eg, no possibility of becoming chairperson).

3. Clinician-investigators often have difficulties in accepting the independent, professional role of the clinically oriented basic scientist. It is very common for the clinician-investigator to feel that basic scientists within their departments should be satisfied to serve as highly skilled technicians. This attitude has probably been a major factor responsible for the departure of highly skilled basic scientists from clinical departments.

4. Presently there are few basic scientists within OHNS departments. Future PhD faculty will probably be initially attracted to a postdoctoral fellowship by the possibility of learning a new technique or area of expertise from a creative, established basic science investigator who is part of an OHNS department. The recruitment of the basic scientist into the pool of clinically oriented basic scientists (Figure) would then potentially take place during this postdoctoral fellowship in a clinical department. There a need would be established for clinically oriented OHNS research. The support for this experience could be competitively sought from an individual fellowship, eg, a postdoctoral fellowship, a Research Career Development Award (RCDA) or a TIDA.

SUPPORT FOR RESEARCH TRAINING

Although the institutional training grants program of the 1960s has expired, federal funding is still available, including:

1. Individual Postdoctoral Fellowships (PD): these awards have stipends that are generally too low to attract the MD investigator who has completed a residency.
2. Research Career Development Award (RCDA): these awards are aimed at the investigator with an accomplished research career two to three years after residency with credentials.
3. Teacher-Investigator Development Award (TIDA): these awards are made available to residents who have demonstrated research ability in residency programs and who are associated with programs where good research opportunities are present, and release time is provided from clinical duties.
4. Minority Access to Research Careers (MARC): these awards represent support available to investigators at minority institutions who wish additional research training otorhinolaryngology. This work can be in any research area appropriate to communicative disorders. Administered by the National Institute of General Medical Sciences (NIGMS), the program is intended to strengthen research capabilities of institutions where there is significant enrollment from minority groups.

Institutional support for salaries of clinical and basic science faculty is an absolute necessity to subsidize research time, and lessen the need to produce income from clinical practice.

OTOLARYNGOLOGY SOCIETIES

Support should be requested from otolaryngology societies (American Otological Society, Inc, American Laryngological Association, American Society for Head and Neck Surgery, American Academy of Facial Plastic and Reconstructive Surgery) to fund research fellowships. Such support should be substantial enough to be competitive; several societies may choose to contribute to a single postdoctoral research fellowship. The area of research could be rotated every year so that all special interests would be satisfied. It is recommended that fellowship stipends be approximately $25,000 to $30,000, with applicants carefully screened by a committee with representatives from all contributing societies. Laboratory qualification of the research and mentor for research experiences would also be reviewed by this committee.

Support from private foundations and industry to fund postdoctoral training opportunities should be developed.

6. RESEARCH FACILITATION

F. Owen Black, MD, Chairman
Earleen Elkins, PhD
Willard E. Fee, Jr, MD
Makoto Igarashi, MD
Josef M. Miller, PhD
Edwin W. Rubel, PhD

The development of a research group and significant research activity requires institutional resources (salary, space, funding), departmental commitment (protected time, interactive research environment), and the recruitment and support of research-oriented faculty. Given that these essentials for development have been met, what are the steps that an otolaryngology department can take to facilitate and enhance the productivity of its research group and sustain the quality of its work? While the members of this writing group had many divergent opinions regarding the priority of facilitatory efforts, there was, nonetheless, general agreement about their substance.

PRIORITY

Above all, there has to be a sufficient institutional and faculty commitment to research to grant it high priority in the utilization of resources. Unless there is protected time for scholarly and research activity, the demands of clinical, teaching, and administrative responsibilities may seriously erode the research effort. Not only should the department's priority for research be sufficiently strong to eliminate competition for time allotments, it must also eliminate competition for operational funds and other departmental resources. It was suggested that a tangible system of rewards and incentives for research productivity be developed within each department. These should include, but not necessarily be limited to honors, awards that are based on the same principles as for rewarding clinical activity, and consideration for promotion and tenure.

STRATEGY AND PLANNING

Where possible, the research-oriented members of the department should form a cohesive group or groups in which the roles, backgrounds, and experiences of the individual members are not only supportive and complementary but can be integrated. This fosters building of strength and avoids fragmentation and dilution of effort, especially in small groups.

Ideally, the group should have a common research theme, a strong leader, and a clear-cut sense of direction. It is far better to collaborate on a single important problem than to divide the group's efforts into multiple directions. Particularly important is the maintenance of state-of-the-art technical methodology in the conduct of the research activity.

Additions to the research faculty should be made with the program theme in mind. Care should be given to selection of individuals with experience and proven productivity over junior faculty who may be least costly in terms of salary and support, but very expensive in terms of lost opportunities and prolonged commitment for support. Therefore, the otolaryngology research team must be constituted by careful selection of high quality faculty, including those recruited from other disciplines. For groups whose research leader is not the departmental chairman, a director of research must be identified who has the administrative authority and qualities of leadership necessary to maintain a cohesive group.

INTERACTIVE ENVIRONMENT

Carefully developed and well-utilized mechanisms for communication among the research-oriented faculty should be a regular part of the intellectual activity of the department. The exchange of ideas, critical review of hypotheses and proposed methodology, and discussion of problems from different vantage points all contribute to the academic growth of a department. The clinical and basic scientists should meet regularly, both formally and informally to enhance the intellectual development of all members of the group and to provide a milieu in which the training of residents and young faculty in problem-solving and critical analysis skills can be fostered.

Such a mechanism is conference rounds which focus on a particular clinical research problem. Exchanges of knowledge, opinions, and philosophies will occur that may contribute to the intellectual growth, problem-solving ability, and research activities of the group.

NATIONAL INTERACTION

It is clear that the otolaryngic research community must develop a stronger sense of national identity in order to foster the most efficient utilization of limited resources. National interaction can take the form of a visiting scientist program, opportunities for specialized training, external consultants, pilot studies, and the support of professional societies and organizations. A visiting scientist program can help overcome intellectual isolationism in both individuals and programs. Whether the visitor be a young academician who comes to learn or a mature scientist who comes to teach, benefits accrue to both the visitor and the visitee through the exchange of information and attitudes. It behooves the developing research program to send its faculty to more advanced, mature programs for both short and extended periods of study. Whether these study periods should be formalized into a fellowship or serve an ad hoc purpose for the acquisition of a specific skill depends on the needs of the individual and the institution and the goals and objectives of the exchange program.

Programs should avail themselves of the opportunity to invite external consultants to review their research activities on a regular basis. This is an important form of interinstitutional cross-fertilization that usually benefits both the consultant and the program. Not only are specific questions addressed, but through the development of personal relationships, future dialogue is enhanced. By maintaining a high level of awareness of the otolaryngology research activities around the country, the visiting scientists and external consultants can be called upon to provide specific information as well as overall perspectives about the state of research efforts in the field. Thus, specific questions about training opportunities, problem-solving advice, and technical skill acquisitions may be addressed readily.

More formalized reviews of the state-of-the-art in a given field may be obtained by national research conferences in which the experts in the field are convened to address the status of knowledge in a given area. Such media of exchange provide important forums for reporting of results, both preliminary and defined, as well as discussion of controversial topics. These conferences are invaluable for the generation of new research hypotheses and the outlining of new and continuing investigations. From such conferences should come pilot studies, funded and implemented nationally, to develop concepts, test feasibility of proposed projects, and determine in advance the ability of investigators to perform a proposed project. Such pilot studies are indispensable for the formulation and conduct of studies to answer questions of national importance that cannot be addressed by a single institution. National otolaryngic organizations should collaborate with the academic institutions, industry, and the National Institutes of Health in supporting national interchange in the areas outlined above.

PEER REVIEW

Although implied in a general way in the preceding section, review of specific research projects plays an important role in the facilitation of research ideas and activities. While the peer review process maintained by each funding agency is the final arbiter of review for scientific merit and appropriateness for funding, considerable prereview should occur prior to the submission of a project. Informal reviews by colleagues and senior scientists in the department and institution should occur regularly during the development of a project. Two other types of informal review are most helpful. First is the review by a respected colleague in another institution who is working in the same general area of research. The second concerns staff review within the prospective funding agency. The review of the external consultant should address a limited number of questions raised by the applicant. These should be at an overview level. The staff of the funding agency often proves valuable on issues of appropriateness, format and technical aspects of the proposals. Staff preview is mandated by some agencies; its importance cannot be overemphasized.

In some institutions, there are inadequate numbers of trained scientists within otolaryngology available for review of fledgling projects. It would greatly facilitate the development of such projects if a national organization in otolaryngology were to develop a mechanism for peer review of such proposals where local help is not available.

It behooves the investigator to accept the criticisms of colleagues in a constructive and grateful manner. Such reviews require considerable time and effort. They are essential to identify deficiencies in a proposed investigation. Few are those who cannot benefit from the assistance of colleagues.

7. CURRENT RESEARCH RESOURCES

ROBERT A. MATHOG, MD, CHAIRMAN
PATRICK E. BROOKHOUSER, MD
RALPH F. NAUNTON, MD
WILLIAM C. STEBBINS, PHD
GEORGE A. GATES, MD

Activities that require ongoing and new investigations benefit from a knowledge of current available resources. In OHNS there is a great concern that research activity is waning, and that knowledge of available resources would facilitate and stimulate maximum utilization. To be of any major contribution, information on resources should include but not be limited to: 1) current investigators and their professional backgrounds and research interests, 2) research projects and methodology in otolaryngology, 3) available equipment and techniques, 4) training programs, and 5) institutions actively participating in research.

The rationale for a listing of currently available resources would primarily be related to its usefulness and its potential to fulfill the needs of the otolaryngologic community. Young and established researchers would be interested in information on the activity of various research projects so that they may plan their research and career objectives. There would also be an interest in the same individuals to determine with whom and where to collaborate, and where one might obtain assistance in methodology. One would also want to know where to share experiences and obtain use of certain pieces of equipment. Obviously with such a listing, duplication of effort can be avoided and areas in which collaborative research is needed might be stimulated.

Other important advantages are apparent. For the basic scientist, there would be an opportunity to evaluate the applications of basic science methods to the etiology, prevention and treatment of diseases. For the clinician-investigator, information would be available on what basic methods might be available for working out clinical problems. Others including granting agencies might seek "contracts" from one laboratory or another and consultation would be indirectly available for carrying out research, for assistance in grant writing and for suggestions in funding.

Knowledge of resources would be also useful for evaluating training opportunities with particular individuals on selected projects and in certain institutions. Since it is essential to answer requests of lay people regarding research activities, the listings would be desirable. Moreover, public relation programs dealing with particular projects or with the scope of otolaryngologic research could be facilitated.

A common knowledge of current research resources is probably best obtained through a comprehensive directory/data base. All investigators, new and established, should be listed alphabetically, as in a "Who's Who," noting their educational and professional activities. These lists should be referenced to research interests and institutions, and should not be limited to investigators in otolaryngology but to all basic and clinical scientists with relevant activity to otolaryngology.

A directory or data base should also include and categorize research projects and interests. This listing should represent the most comprehensive scope of the specialty. Areas of research should be divided according to organ system (ie, ear, nose, larynx, etc), discipline (ie, anatomy, physiology, etc), methodology (ie, electron microscopy, histology, etc), and by diseases. Since categorization of research activity is so important for obtaining information, this part of a directory/data base should have cross-references to individuals and institutions.

As a separate resource, there should also be a listing of special places of equipment, ie, computers, PET scanners, electron microscopes, etc. These items should be cross-referenced to research activities, individuals, and institutions.

Regarding training opportunities, separate categories should be provided for medical students, residents, and new and established faculty. There should also be a listing for PhD candidates, postdoctoral investigators, established investigators and clinicians. Information should be available on sabbatical appointments.

When considering a comprehensive directory on research resources, one should also include a listing of institutions carrying on research with appropriate cross-references to research projects, equipment and individuals. These institutions should include but not be limited to universities and colleges (departments and divisions), hospitals, industry, private laboratories, and federal institutions.

Finally, one should also consider a listing of funding agencies, especially those agencies that have funded projects in the past and those that will possibly fund projects in the future. This listing should include and note the interest of the funding groups as well as limitations for grant support.

In order to achieve the goal of a directory/data base in research, the specialty of otolaryngology turns to its major organizations. For example, the American Academy of Otolaryngology-Head and Neck Surgery should be considered as a sponsor and a caretaker of such a project. This organization has had interest and now has the requirement for fostering research in a specialty where research activity has been waning. Research is necessary for advancement in medicine, and otolaryngology looks to the Academy for providing this leadership. Also, the Academy is a logical choice when one considers the financial and administrative support to carry out and maintain such a project.

From a practical standpoint the methods for obtaining current research resources should be turned over to individuals with experience and training in reaching these goals. Considering the scope of the project, the data would be best stored and updated in a computer registry with printouts available to interested users. Data and management system specialists could advise on the lists, the methods of accruing data and the categorization of the data. Undoubtedly, a questionnaire would serve as one of the main mechanisms of obtaining information.

This project on resources should not only require the support of organized otolaryngology but also the cooperation of closely allied specialists in audiology, speech and language pathology, neuroscience and cleft palate research, so that the information can be comprehensive and all-inclusive. Ideally, these groups would benefit as much as otolaryngology from the information sources.

The concept of a research directory/data base is not new, but it has come of age. It will be invaluable to otolaryngology and the many other professional groups that need this information, It would improve efficiency of operations in research, the thrust of otolaryngologic research, and the recruitment of potential investigators.

8. RESPONSIBILITIES OF OTORHINOLARYNGOLOGY-HEAD AND NECK SURGERY TO THE NATIONAL INSTITUTES OF HEALTH

BYRON J. BAILEY, MD

JAMES B. SNOW, JR, MD

ROBERT J. RUBEN, MD

The purpose of this paper is to provide a descriptive listing of the responsibilities which our specialty has in regard to maintaining its relationship with the NIH. While we are more accustomed to thinking and acting in terms of the responsibilities which we feel the NIH has to us, this task gives us the opportunity to "turn the tables" and to review some very significant obligations which we have in this partnership.

The specialty of OHNS has a clear obligation to provide volunteer otolaryngologist peer reviewers who are able to meet the stringent demands of service on an NIH Study Section. Some of those who have been asked to serve have refused to do so on the basis of the volume of effort required for this service and the time that it requires, which is taken away from other pursuits. Others have preferred not to serve in this capacity because of the criticism to which they would be exposed in the course of their duties. It is clear that currently there is a limited pool of willing and qualified clinician-investigators who can serve in this capacity. We believe that OHNS and the NIH should formalize and expand the search and nomination process for candidates who are qualified to serve as members of Study Sections. The specialty should view these appointments as positions of significant stature and should reward the individuals who serve by moving them to leadership positions whenever appropriate. Both the specialty and the NIH should work more diligently to assure that this appointment is turned into a positive professional experience.

We have the responsibility to provide volunteer otolaryngologists for service on the National Advisory Council of the NINCDS. For these positions, we must identify our strongest, most experienced medical scientists for service in this distinguished capacity. We have the obligation to recommend individuals who are in close touch with the research priorities of the nation at the particular time. These otolaryngologists should be conversant with research training and manpower issues and in touch with the trends and the problems of university research centers. Again, we feel that OHNS might benefit from a closer relationship in the search, nomination, and appointment process.

As a specialty, we have the responsibility to provide accurate and detailed input into the preparation of an annual or biennial nonelaborate publication which provides a clear, concise statement of the research goals, objectives, and needs that exist jointly for the NIH and OHNS. In order to achieve success in this activity, we will have to work together more closely within our specialty and make an effort to speak with one voice. The Association for Research in Otolaryngology, the American Academy of Otolaryngology-Head and Neck Surgery, the Association of Academic Departments of Otolaryngology, and the Society of University Otolaryngologists should collaborate with all other interested parties to provide a balanced input to the NINCDS in order that the NIH priorities reflect, in major part, the needs of our patients for new scientific information. We must assume the responsibility for speaking to the NIH in an unfragmented manner and for validating our conclusions in this important area.

As a specialty, we have the responsibility to provide the NIH with supportive testimony before the Congress and before other federal agencies and to provide the informational foundation which is required if we are to be successful in the pursuit of funds and policies that will strengthen the research effort in OHNS. Our professional organizations can provide much of the support for these efforts in terms of data collection and organization and the selection of our most effective spokespersons. This may require a major effort on the part of the American Academy of Otolaryngology-Head and Neck Surgery by virtue of its 501 (c) 6 tax status which makes it the appropriate vehicle for any major lobbying effort. Coordination of these efforts with the activities of other organizations such as the National Committee for Research in Neurological and Communicative Disorders will be essential.

Otorhinolaryngology-head and neck surgery has the responsibility to participate in the on-going dialogue between our specialty and the director of the NIH and the associate director of the NINCDs on matters of importance to otorhinolaryngic research. The Association of Academic Departments of Otolaryngology has done this periodically by means of the liaison committee within NINCDS, but we have the opportunity to expand the effort and to improve upon our past successes. Appropriate topics for discussion include matters such as the funding of research in our specialty, and review of current research resources and needs.

We have the responsibility to provide the NIH with a steady flow of significant, carefully prepared, competitive, fundable research grant applications from individuals who are qualified by their training to conduct valid research investigations. In these activities, we must identify and support certain key groups and programs including investigators and potential future investigators working in resident research programs, masters of medical science programs, MD-PhD programs, postdoctoral fellowships, and young otolaryngologist faculty members with strong research commitments.

Otorhinolaryngology-head and neck surgery has the responsibility to remedy some of its internal problems which impact on its relationship with the NIH. We are currently being victimized by our defeatist attitudes with regard to research by physician-investigators. This conference will serve to initiate new research efforts based upon the developing technologies and human resources which are now available and must be recruited into the field of otorhinolaryngology-head and neck surgery. This will be built upon the substantive advances which have been made during the past two decades.

We must undertake an adjustment in our academic priorities in favor of research and researchers in the milieu of residency and the early years of faculty service where the emphasis is currently heavily focused on expanding clinical skills, delivering patient care, and generating patient-care income. We must be successful in our efforts to expand the reward system for faculty engaged in successful careers in terms of providing them with adequate salaries, regular promotion, and sufficient time away from other responsibilities to engage in research activities.

The specialty has the responsibility to assist departments which are in transition toward a position of importance as mature research resources for the specialty. We must develop an effective consultation program which is available to advise younger departments on matters relating to the development of research programs. We should develop a network of volunteers who are available for the review of research grant proposals prior to their submission to the NIH. This set of activities is within the capability of a consortium of interest which could be developed among the Association for Research in Otolaryngology, the American Academy of Otolaryngology-Head and Neck Surgery, the Association of Academic Departments of Otolaryngology and the Society of University Otolaryngologists.

We have the responsibility to provide the NIH with our views and suggestions concerning important administrative issues. We must express our opinions concerning such matters as the effect of the NIH administrative organization on the validity of such basic concepts as peer review and parity among various research disciplines, the effect of policies and procedures of the NIH on the OHNS research community, and the appointment of key staff at the NIH who will have significant interaction with researchers in our specialty.

We have the responsibility to be fair, but candid, critics of the NIH from time to time. We should express our concerns with regard to the nomination and appointment system for study sections and for the National Advisory Council when it seems to be suboptimal. We should provide input with regard to our observations of the performance or lack of effectiveness of the staff with whom we work at the NIH. We must express our concerns with regard to such matters as the NIH conferences, which seem at times to deserve our criticism and to require our input. These have been criticized in terms of appearing to be arbitrarily and narrowly organized, often leading to major funding in a minor area, and occasionally generating documents that define what is "in" and what is "out" for several years. Any group-exercise this potent deserves a great deal of attention.

We have the responsibility to generate public support for the financing of a major portion of the research in OHNS consistent with our financial partnership with the NIH and our mutual concerns for the health of the research community. We can improve our communication in this regard with foundations and with private industry. We can generate more seed money for the collection of pilot data which is so necessary in the preparation of a successful research grant application. We can participate more effectively in the publicizing of the activities and the successes of the NIH.

We have a responsibility to promote the general research interest and research priorities at the time of our major scientific meetings. Presently, research presentations are actively discouraged at some meetings, and at others they are segregated from the major sessions or scheduled at odd times. It is time for us to honor research and to recognize the support provided by the NIH, and especially to move away from the currently popular antigovernment posture.

We have the responsibility to provide medical resources for the dissemination of important new scientific information in the form of a healthy family of professional publications. We should encourage research publications in all of our specialty journals. The education of all residents and practicing otolaryngologists concerning the fundamental and essential nature of research should be an objective of our journals and could be strengthened by more timely releases of developments related to research in our specialty by the staff at the NIH. The

NIH could also support this effort significantly by the preparation of an annual report on the national state of research in OHNS.

A final item of responsibility is in the area of greater effort with regard to a strengthening of our capability to organize and execute multi-institutional research projects. We must pool our resources and develop a better mechanism for the conduct of important clinical trials designed to assess the safety and effectiveness of new diagnostic methods, drug therapy, and surgical procedures with a high degree of accuracy, in a timely manner, and in an environment free from investigator bias.

Greater attention to the responsibilities which have been elaborated will result in a system of research for otolaryngology that will generate important new scientific information needed urgently for the benefit of our present and future patients.

SUMMARY

George A. Gates, MD, Conference Chairman

The reports of the writing groups are best summarized by placing them at the three levels of organizational activity which have the capability and the responsibility for implementation. These levels are local, interinstitutional and national. Undoubtedly, these recommendations will be modified according to local conditions as they are adopted and put into effect because these are consensus recommendations and are to be used as guidelines; they are not hard and fast rules.

LOCAL INSTITUTIONAL LEVEL

The primary burden of research in otolaryngology falls upon the OHNS group within each institution wherein lies the responsibility for initiating, developing, and supporting the programs for research training, faculty development, establishment of facilities, recruitment of research faculty, and creation of the proper research environment. The extensiveness of these programs is proportional to the interest and effort of the group's leader. Unless the departmental chairperson is committed to development and support of research programs, little can be accomplished.

Research environment is predicated on the assumption that research is a high-priority activity, fostered by the intellectual curiosity of the participants, and nourished by opportunities for regular exchange of ideas through continuing dialogue between clinical and basic scientists and brought to fruition through cooperation and mutual effort.

The departmental chairperson must work with the administration of the institution in obtaining local support for research activity. Such support includes, but is not limited to, space, start-up funds and seed money, and assistance in long-term fund raising. It is clear that in this regard institutional resources are often underutilized.

INTERINSTITUTIONAL LEVEL

Once the local research environment is established, continued growth is predicated on interaction with colleagues at other institutions. This interaction can take several forms and may include a visiting scientist program, liberal use of consultants, and the establishment of collaborative projects.

Visiting Scientist Program. A visiting scientist program should be developed in which the local institution invites noted authorities to visit and exchange ideas through lectures, seminars and informal review. Such a program benefits both the institution and the visiting scientist through sharing of knowledge, intellectual stimulation, and exchange of ideas.

Consultants. Much can be gained by requesting a formal consultation from authorities in the field. This consultation can help in the development of a grant request, for the review of a research program or project already in process, and for expert opinion in interpretation of data. This activity should be arranged on a highly structured and formal basis with clear delineation of the program's expectations and the consultant's responsibilities and compensation.

Collaborative Research. This may take two forms. A visiting scientist may conduct a specific project in the laboratories of a host institution where the particular skills of the scientist are combined with the unique facilities of the institution. This type of collaboration is used widely, especially in Europe. The second area of collaborative research involves the development of interinstitutional projects. This is especially effective in conducting clinical trials where accrual of large numbers of patients at any given institution is difficult and can best be achieved by a multi-institutional study. These projects require substantial advanced planning, extensive training of the investigators in the standardization of observations and data collection, and close cooperation in the conduct of the study.

NATIONAL ORGANIZATIONAL LEVEL

Consistently mentioned throughout the Conference and the writing group recommendations was the lack of a national organized structure to support the research effort in otolaryngology. Indeed, it was a commonly held perception that this has been a lamentable void in the specialty. It is clear that a national effort is needed to make research a high-priority subject on the program of meetings, for fund raising, for leadership, and perspective. The importance of national attention to this subject cannot be overemphasized. The establishment of a separate NIH for communicative disorders and other disorders of the head and neck is a long-range goal. In addition to general support to increase the level of awareness of the importance of research by otolaryngology societies, it was felt that four specific functions need to be subserved by organizations at the national level. These functions include the establishment of a research directory, a project peer review mechanism, a foundation for fund raising and a national advisory panel.

Research Directory. Currently, there is no central source listing all of the personnel, facilities, areas of expertise, training opportunities, and fellowship opportunities in otolaryngologic research. Establishment of such a data base is a high-priority need that could be fulfilled by a national organization such as the American Academy of Otolaryngology-Head and Neck Surgery. Appointment of a coordinator for research in a national organization would greatly facilitate the development of such a directory.

Project Peer Review. An important mechanism to upgrade the level of sophistication of research projects in otolaryngology would be the establishment of an informal project review by a national organization such as the American Academy of Otolaryngology-Head and Neck Surgery. This is conceived of as a pressing but temporary need until the development of similar capabilities within or among institutions is achieved. Peer review is an essential mechanism in the facilitation of research projects. Currently, no mechanism exists for assisting otolaryngologists at institutions where local resources are incompletely developed.

National Foundation for Research in Otolaryngology. There is a pressing need to develop an autonomous foundation that would have the capability of attracting gifts, bequests, and other financial support for research in the entire field of otolaryngology. The foundation could assume the responsibilities of awarding grants for research projects as well as fellowship stipends for research training.

National Advisory Panel. A national advisory panel for research in otolaryngology should be appointed that would periodically review the status of research efforts in otolaryngology in meeting the needs of the nation. Such a panel would establish research priorities consistent with the current state of knowledge and availability of facilities and resources to conduct projects to answer the national research questions. Such a panel should be established independently of organizations or federal agencies, but should be in a position to communicate freely with them. Such a blue ribbon panel could greatly facilitate the development of important research projects in this field.